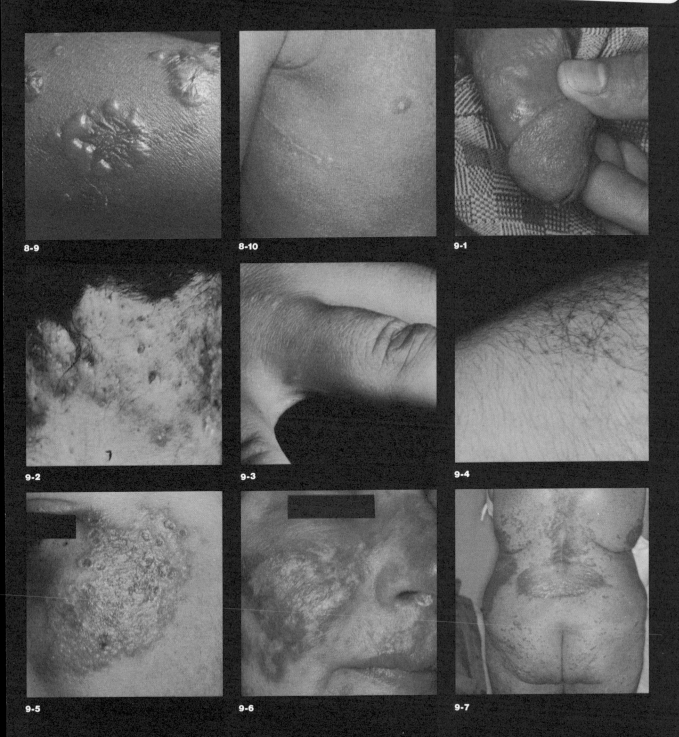

**8-9** Vesicles and bullae (umbilicated, necrotic center) in black

**9-4** Pediculus corporis. *(Courtesy of the Department of*

Dermatology The University of Michigan Medical Center.)*

# MEDICAL-SURGICAL NURSING: A CONCEPTUAL APPROACH

# MEDICAL-SURGICAL NURSING

## A CONCEPTUAL
## APPROACH

**DOROTHY A. JONES, R.N., M.S.**
Assistant Professor
Boston University School of Nursing
Nurse Clinician
Harvard Community Health Plan

**CLAIRE FORD DUNBAR, R.N., M.S.**
Formerly Assistant Professor
Boston University School of Nursing

**MARY MARMOLL JIROVEC, R.N., M.S.**
Clinical Assistant
University of Wyoming School of Nursing
Formerly Instructor
Boston University School of Nursing

McGRAW-HILL BOOK COMPANY

New York   St. Louis   San Francisco   Auckland   Bogotá   Düsseldorf
Johannesburg   London   Madrid   Mexico   Montreal   New Delhi
Panama   Paris   São Paulo   Singapore   Sydney   Tokyo   Toronto

## NOTICE

Medicine is an ever-changing science. As new research and clinical experience broaden our knowledge, changes in treatment and drug therapy are required. The editors and the publisher of this work have made every effort to ensure that the drug dosage schedules herein are accurate and in accord with the standards accepted at the time of publication. Readers are advised, however, to check the product information sheet included in the package of each drug they plan to administer to be certain that changes have not been made in the recommended dose or in the contraindications for administration. This recommendation is of particular importance in regard to new or infrequently used drugs.

This book was set in Helvetica by Monotype Composition Company, Inc. The editors were Orville W. Haberman, Jr., Michael LaBarbera, Douglas J. Marshall, and Irene Curran; the designer was Nicholas Krenitsky; the production supervisor was Robert C. Pedersen.
R. R. Donnelley & Sons Company was printer and binder.


Illustration Credits:

Charles Boyter, M.S., Medical Illustrator
Virginia W. Hughes, Jr., B.F.A., Graphic Illustrator
D. Patrick Russell, Instructional Illustrator
Alice Vickery, Graphic Illustrator
Marcia Williams, M.S., Medical Illustrator

Educational Media Support Center
Boston University Medical Center


**Library of Congress Cataloging in Publication Data**
Main entry under title:

Medical-surgical nursing.

    Bibliography: p.
    Includes index.
    1.  Nursing.  2.  Surgical nursing.  I.  Jones,
Dorothy A.  II.  Dunbar, Claire Ford.  III.  Jirovec,
Mary Marmoll.  [DNLM:  1.  Medical—Nursing texts.
2.  Nursing care.  WY156 J76m]
RT41.M48     610.73     77-13981
ISBN 0-07-032785-8

**To**
our families and friends
who have endured

# CONTENTS

# LIST OF CONTRIBUTORS

CHERYL K. AHERN, R.N., M.S.
Adult Nurse Practitioner, Hill/West Rock Community
Health Center and Instructor, Family Nurse
Practitioner Program, Community Health Nursing,
Yale University School of Nursing,
New Haven, Connecticut

IRENE B. ALYN, R.N., Ph.D.
Professor of Nursing, University of Illinois
at the Medical Center, College of Nursing,
Chicago, Illinois

BARBARA BRADEN, R.N., B.S.N., M.S.
Assistant Professor, Medical-Surgical Nursing,
Creighton University, College of Nursing,
Omaha, Nebraska

ANNE FERO CHESTNUT, R.N., M.S.
Lecturer, University of California, School of
Nursing, San Francisco; Formerly Lecturer,
Extended Bachelor of Science Degree Program,
University of California-San Francisco, School of
Nursing, San Francisco, California

ELAINE SZTYNDOR CLANCY, R.N., B.S.N.
The Johns Hopkins Hospital, Baltimore, Maryland

NANCY FAIRCHILD CLARK, R.N., M.S.
Instructor of Medical-Surgical Nursing, Boston
College School of Nursing,
Boston, Massachusetts

THOMAS H. COOK, R.N., M.S.N.
Instructor and Nurse Clinician, State University of
New York at Binghamton, New York

IRENE C. CULLIN, R.N., B.S.
Coordinator Nursing Education, Massachusetts Eye
and Ear Infirmary, Boston, Massachusetts

NANCY DIEKELMANN, R.N., M.S.
Assistant Professor, University of Wisconsin,
School of Nursing, Madison, Wisconsin

CLAIRE FORD DUNBAR, R.N., M.S.
Formerly Assistant Professor, Boston University
School of Nursing, Boston, Massachusetts

VICKIE EDWARDS, R.N., M.S.N.
Resource Person, Division of Staff Development,
University of Washington Hospital,
Seattle, Washington

SUE B. FOSTER, R.N., M.S.N.
Cardiovascular Clinical Specialist and
Nurse Clinician, Ambulatory Services,
Peter Bent Brigham Hospital,
Boston, Massachusetts

JOAN GALLAGHER, R.N., M.S.
Instructor, Boston University
School of Nursing, Boston, Massachusetts

ROSELLEN MEIGHAN GARRETT, R.N., M.S.
Family Nurse Practitioner,
School of Nursing, State University of New York at
Binghamton, New York

MARCIA MOELLER GRANT, R.N., M.S.N.
Clinical Research Nurse, Department of
Nursing Research, City of Hope National
Medical Center, Duarte, California;
Formerly Assistant Professor, University of
Hawaii, School of Nursing, Honolulu, Hawaii

DIANE CHAPELL HAGEN, R.N., M.A.
Clinical Specialist, Emergency Service,
University Hospital, Boston, Massachusetts

ANN ZIEBOL HAMORY, R.N., B.S.N., M.S.N.
Formerly Clinical Nurse Specialist in Medicine,
University of Virginia, Medical Center,
Charlottesville, Virginia; Currently in
Addis Ababa, Ethiopia

CAROL E. HARTMAN, R.N., M.S.
Assistant Professor, Medical-Surgical Nursing,
Francis Payne Bolton School of Nursing,
Case Western Reserve University; and
Associate in Nursing, University Hospital of
Cleveland, Cleveland, Ohio

ANN HALL HARVEY, R.N., M.S.
Assistant Professor of Medical-Surgical Nursing,
Graduate Program, University of Maryland
School of Nursing, Baltimore, Maryland;
Formerly Assistant Professor, Nursing Education
Program, Johns Hopkins University School of
Health Services, Baltimore, Maryland

ANN E. HINKHOUSE, R.N., B.A.
Staff Nurse-Intensive Care Unit,
Mercy Hospital, Iowa City, Iowa

NANCY L. HOLLAND, R.N., M.A.
Instructor, School of Nursing,
Jewish Hospital and Medical Center of
Brooklyn, New York

DEENA B. HOLLINGSWORTH, R.N., M.S.
Instructor, University of Wyoming School of
Nursing, Laramie, Wyoming

KARYN McGAGHIE HOLM, R.N., M.S.
Assistant Professor, Rush University; and
Clinical Specialist, Rush-Presbyterian St.
Luke's Hospital, Chicago, Illinois

SUSAN MOLLOY HUBBARD, R.N., B.S.
Clinical Specialist, Medicine Branch of the
National Cancer Institute, and Cancer Nursing
Service—Nursing Department, Clinical Center,
National Institutes of Health, Bethesda, Maryland

MARY MARMOLL JIROVEC, R.N., M.S.
Clinical Assistant, University of Wyoming
School of Nursing; Formerly Instructor, Boston
University School of Nursing,
Boston, Massachusetts

BONNY LIBBEY JOHNSON, R.N., B.S.
Formerly Clinical Specialist, Medicine Branch of the
National Cancer Institute and Cancer Nursing
Service—Nursing Department, Clinical Center,
National Institutes of Health, Bethesda, Maryland

DOROTHY A. JONES, R.N., M.S.N.
Assistant Professor, Boston University School of
Nursing, Nurse Clinician, Harvard Community
Health Plan, Boston, Massachusetts

MI JA KIM, R.N., Ph.D.
Assistant Professor, College of Nursing,
Department of Medical-Surgical Nursing,
University of Illinois at the Medical Center,
Chicago, Illinois

NELL ANN KIRBY, R.N., M.S.
Instructor, Division of Rehabilitation Medicine,
The Johns Hopkins University School of Medicine;
and Instructor, Nursing Education Programs,
The Johns Hopkins University School of Health
Services, Baltimore, Maryland

RITA L. KRAUT, R.N., B.S.
Head Nurse—Neurology/Neurosurgery,
New York Hospital, Cornell Medical Center,
New York

PATRICIA E. MAHONEY, R.N., M.A.
Clinical Nursing Specialist and Nursing
Care Coordinator, Neurological-Neurosurgical
Service, New York Hospital-Cornell Medical
Center, New York

MARGARET MANGAN, R.N., M.S.N.
Formerly Instructor, Boston University
School of Nursing, Boston, Massachusetts

JOYCE S. MARTIN, R.N., M.S.
Associate Professor, Indiana University
School of Nursing, Indianapolis, Indiana

MARY BRAMBILLA McFARLAND, R.N., M.S.N.
Associate Professor, University of Oregon,
Health Science Center—School of Nursing,
Portland, Oregon

JUDITH M. McFARLANE, R.N., M.N.
Pediatric Nurse Clinician, Hematology/
Oncology, Medical College of Georgia,
Augusta, Georgia

MARGARET A. MURPHY, R.N., M.S.
Lecturer, Boston College School of Nursing,
Boston, Massachusetts

JoELLEN WILBUR NOLAN, R.N., M.S.N.
Instructor and Nurse Practitioner, State University of
New York at Binghamton, School of Nursing, Family
Nurse Practitioner Program, New York

LYNNE A. OLAND, R.N., M.S.N.
Instructor, Catholic University
School of Nursing, Washington, D.C.

CAROL L. PANICUCCI, R.N., Ph.D.
Coordinator of Family Nurse
Practitioners and Assistant
Professor, University of Missouri,
School of Nursing, School of Medicine,
Columbia, Missouri

SARAH B. PASTERNACK, R.N., M.A.
Assistant Professor, Boston University School of
Nursing, Boston, Massachusetts

LINDA HANNAWALT RICKEL, R.N., C.F.N.P.
Oncology Nurse Practitioner, Little Rock
Veterans Administration Hospital, Little
Rock, Arkansas

LORA B. ROACH, R.N., M.S.
Assistant Professor, The University of Texas
at Arlington School of Nursing

NANCY GUARDINO SAFER, R.N., B.S., M.S.
Instructor, Boston University School
of Nursing, Boston, Massachusetts

DELORES SCHUMANN, R.N., B.S., M.S.
Lecturer, University of Wisconsin, School of
Nursing, Madison, Wisconsin

GLADYS MARY SCIPIEN, R.N., M.S.N.
Associate Professor, Boston University
School of Nursing, Boston, Massachusetts

DOROTHY L. SEXTON, R.N., Ed.D.
Associate Professor and Chairperson,
Medical-Surgical Nursing Program, Yale University
School of Nursing, New Haven, Connecticut

BARBARA SIGLER, R.N., M.N.Ed.
Oncology Nurse Clinician, Department of
Otolaryngology, Eye and Ear Hospital of Pittsburgh,
Pittsburgh, Pennsylvania

VALERIE C. STILLYARDS, R.N.
Assistant Director of Nursing, Tulane Medical
Center Hospital and Clinic, New Orleans, Louisiana

FRANCES J. STORLIE, R.N., Ph.D.
Associate Professor, Medical-Surgical Nursing,
Pacific Lutheran University, Tacoma Washington

ANN GILL TAYLOR, R.N., B.S.N., M.S.N., Ed.D.
Associate Professor of Nursing, Graduate Program
in Medical-Surgical Nursing, University of Virginia,
School of Nursing, Charlottesville, Virginia

ANDREA THOMSON, R.N., M.S.N.
In-Service and Patient Education Coordinator,
Luther Hospital, Eau Claire, Wisconsin;
Formerly Instructor, University of Wisconsin,
School of Nursing, Madison, Wisconsin

PAMELA GAHERIN WATSON, R.N., M.S.
Assistant Professor and Project Director,
N.I.H.-N.C.I., Enterostomal Therapy
Education Program, Boston University
School of Nursing, Boston, Massachusetts

NINA H. WILLIAMS, R.N., M.S.N.
Instructor of Medical-Surgical Nursing,
The University of Michigan, Ann Arbor, Michigan

ZANE ROBINSON WOLF, R.N., M.S.
Part-Time Instructor, Medical-Surgical Nursing,
Villanova University College of Nursing,
Villanova, Pennsylvania

# PREFACE

In recent years significant advances in the health-related fields have had a direct influence on nursing education and practice. The nursing knowledge drawn from these advances has expanded at an ever increasing rate. The emergence of nursing research has also contributed to this body of knowledge much information which is unique to nursing. At the same time, changing nursing roles have seen the nurse practitioner evolve into a primary health facilitators, functioning both in independent practice and in community health settings. Nurses are assuming greater responsibility for their actions and are becoming increasingly involved in the decision-making process.

The changing scope of the nurse's role in all health settings has necessitated a new approach to nursing education. To meet these challenges, nurses must develop the skills needed to establish a data base from which sound judgments can be made. Therefore, *nursing assessment,* which includes utilization of the health history, physical assessment, and diagnostic examinations, is emphasized throughout this book. In keeping with nursing's expanding role in all health environments, this textbook will focus upon nursing practice in the nonacute as well as acute settings. Throughout this text nursing is explored according to levels of nursing care. *First-level* nursing care focuses on identification of a population susceptible to a specific health problem and the ultimate prevention of health disruptions. *Second-level* nursing care discusses the care and maintenance of community-based persons with specific alterations in health. *Third-level* care is oriented toward the acute care of the hospitalized patient, and *fourth-level* care examines the rehabilitative process which begins in the hospital and continues in the community. The levels of nursing care are presented and discussed in depth in Chapter 1.

A textbook which reflects current nursing knowledge must be founded on a sound theoretical base, and the authors believe a *conceptual framework* provides such a base. "The conceptual approach is the uniting, combining, modifying and utilizing of many theories or ideas from various disciplines into a new form . . . holistic and dynamic in its approach (Murray and Zenter, 1974)." The use of concepts provides readily available vehicles with which to transmit new learnings in a holistic and more comprehensive way.

The unifying concept for this text, the *man-environment interaction,* is introduced in Part 1. Humans are seen in a constant state of interaction with physical, psychological, social, and cultural factors in both the external and internal environments. Stress and coping are viewed as integral components of this interactive process. Within this conceptual framework nursing is defined as an intrinsic part of this interaction and a nursing model is developed to examine closely the nurse-health interaction.

In the remaining parts of the text, disruptions in health are explored through the biophysical concepts of cellular growth and proliferation, inflammation and immunity, fluid and electrolyte dynamics, metabolism, oxygenation, and perception and coordination. These are broad concepts which can be applied to patients at various stages of development in all clinical settings. The initial chapters for each concept area depict normal biophysical dynamics and physical assessment techniques to be utilized in relation to these concepts. Subsequent chapters within each part delve into the pathophysiological changes that alter the healthy state. Throughout the text, *psychosocial* and *cultural factors* that affect the human-environment interaction in the presence of biophysical pathologies are examined. *Current research,* an essential component of nursing knowledge, is incorporated into the discussions as well.

*Health teaching* as well as *nursing assessment* strategies are vital to *health promotion.* These components are introduced early in each chapter and are subsequently integrated throughout the text. Because the adult in all stages of development comprises a major portion of health clients for this book, *adult development* is also viewed as essential and is explored in depth in Chapter 3.

It is the authors' intent to develop and present medical-surgical nursing practice in both acute and nonacute care settings. They believe the conceptual framework permits the greatest freedom in helping the student transfer concept commonalities to various settings. In addition the book aids the student in acquiring a basic, comprehensive indepth knowledge, data base, and the application of information to adult patients in any setting. From this application, a plan of care can be developed which reflects analysis and problem-solving components representative of individual patient needs.

## ACKNOWLEDGMENTS

An endeavor of this magnitude always requires the time, support and encouragement of families, friends, and colleagues. To this end, the editors would like to give special thanks to the following people.

Dorothy and Thomas Jones . . . for their love and the freedom to be myself

Billy and Tom Jones . . . for being there and caring

Maureen, Mary Ellen, Sippy, Sally, and Eleanore . . . for sharing . . . each in their special way

Gary Dunbar . . . for perspective, humor, and love

Judith, Sarah, and McBrien Dunbar . . . for the joy that gives life meaning

Ronald Jirovec . . . for himself and his love

Lisa Jirovec . . . for doing without

Special recognition is given to the Educational Media Support Center at Boston University, School of Medicine, especially Jerome Glickman, D. Patrick Russell, Marcia Williams, and Charles Boyter for their outstanding illustration program. Special thanks to Peter Donnovan for his friendship, legal guidance, and patience. We would like to acknowledge the assistance of the staff at McGraw-Hill Book Company. Special appreciation is given to Cathy Dilworth Somer for initiating the project. We would also like to recognize the editorial assistance of Michael LaBarbera and Doug Marshall and the administrative assistance provided by Orville W. Haberman, Jr.

Dorothy A. Jones
Claire Ford Dunbar
Mary Marmoll Jirovec

# MEDICAL-SURGICAL NURSING: A CONCEPTUAL APPROACH

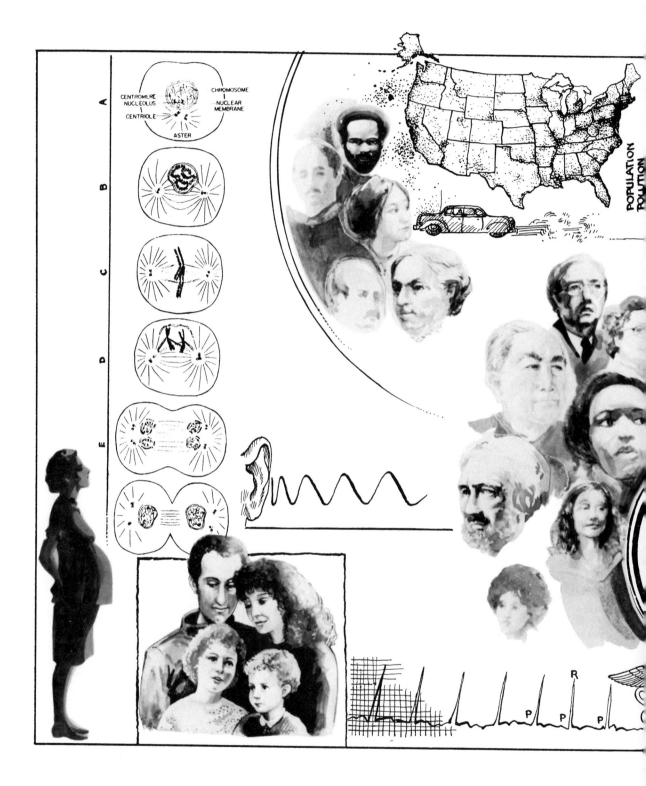

CENTROMERE
NUCLEOLUS
CENTRIOLE
ASTER

CHROMOSOME
NUCLEAR
MEMBRANE

A
B
C
D
E

POPULATION
POLLUTION

R
P P P

# PART 1

## INTERACTION

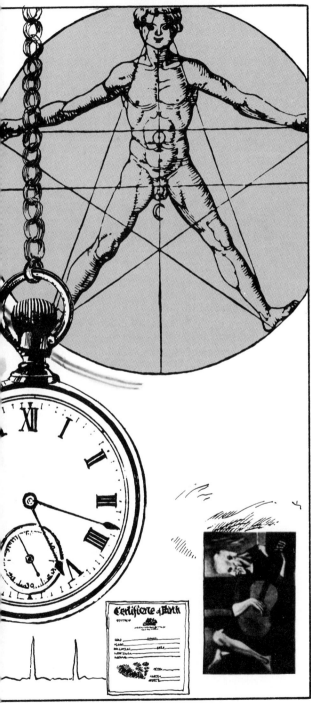

# 1

# MAN-ENVIRONMENT INTERACTION†

Sarah B. Pasternack
Mary Marmoll Jirovec

## HUMAN BEINGS: THE SYNERGISTIC LIFE PROCESS

The science of nursing is the study of the life process in people, as they interact with their environment, for the purpose of assisting individuals, families, and groups to maintain, improve, or regain their optimum levels of wellness.[1-3] In all the known universe, there is no living species comparable with human beings or *man,** a term which is commonly applied to all humanity. Not only do human beings have an intricate physiology, they also think, perceive, and interpret stimuli, formulate diverse languages, experience emotion, and respond to, as well as influence, their surroundings.

The life process in people is *synergistic:* it is a unified "whole" which emerges from the dynamic interaction among the multiple dimensions of human beings, and between human beings and their environment. There is multifaceted integration among the many dimensions which compose man's structure, function, and behavior. In addition, man's complex existence is inextricably bound to the surrounding environment. Man should, in fact, be viewed as continuous with the environment.[4,5] The term *synergistic,* then, denotes the expression of human existence as a unified phenomenon which cannot be predicted from any of its components alone.[6] Even brief reflection on man's behavior and accomplishments illustrates the elusive, and sometimes paradoxical, complexity of human existence. Both students of nursing science and experienced practitioners are likely to encounter awe and fascination as they seek an answer to the questions: Who and what is man?

It is believed that the species *Homo sapiens* has existed on the earth for approximately thirty-five thousand years.[7] During this time, not only have men been able to respond to and affect their constantly changing environment, they have also been able to unravel many mysteries about life in this vast universe. Human capacity for invention and creativity reached an unparalleled pinnacle during the present century. The resourcefulness of human beings has enabled them to devise various means

* The terms *human, humanity, man, people, persons,* and *individuals* will be used interchangeably throughout this chapter. When the term *man* is used, its purpose will be to denote individuals of both sexes. The reader should not infer that the writer views one sex as superior to the other.
† The section on biological rhythms was written by Mary Marmoll Jirovec. The section on nursing intervention during the life process was contributed by Dorothy A. Jones.

of increasing the momentum with which they travel through space and time. Every 4 years, when skilled athletes of many nations engage in the Olympic games, they invariably exceed the performance records set during previous competitions. The last century saw men forsake their own feet and beasts of burden as the primary means of travel, in favor of the automobile and the airplane. Only 100 years ago, travel between the Eastern seaboard of the United States and Western Europe was possible solely via an ocean vessel which took weeks to complete its journey. Today the supersonic Concorde jet aircraft can traverse the Atlantic Ocean in scarcely more than 3 hours.

Human beings conceived of, designed, and built a device known as the *computer,* which, on command, will gather, store, synthesize, and instantly retrieve an almost infinite amount of information. Man gave computers information-processing abilities which far exceed that of the human brain. Paradoxically, the computer is utterly useless unless it is properly programmed by a human being.

During the twentieth century, man invented instruments which capture electromagnetic waves and convert them into visual images. Not only can men transmit these television images over several thousand miles, they can also beam images to distant continents via communications satellites in outer space. The sophisticated telecommunication now possible between virtually every corner of the globe is already taken for granted.

During the last decade, man's sophisticated scientific exploration brought into reality discoveries and achievements which were not long ago regarded as science fiction. Man is now able to create a gene, the basic unit of heredity, which can perform normally inside a living bacterial cell.[8] Man has walked on the moon, not once, but several times. Human beings have built and launched unmanned spacecraft and, through remote control by earthbound electronic computers, landed them on other planets, such as Mars, in order to photograph the terrain and analyze samples of the soil and rock via computer and beam the results back to earth.

However, despite their superior intelligence and seemingly endless creativity, human beings have also pursued directions which have resulted in undesirable consequences. Man has constructed skyscrapers and sprawling superstructures to such an extent that maintaining them has seriously depleted the quantity of energy available for consumption by this and future generations. Under the guise of "progress," people have dismantled precious historical structures, destroyed forests, polluted lakes, rivers, streams, and the air, congested highways, and overcrowded cities, only to abandon them later for a "utopian" suburbia. In the fast-paced industrialized societies which have been created, man is driven to engage in fierce competition with peers in order to achieve status, success, and power. Frequently the benefits of society are won by some individuals at the expense of others.

A small minority of the world's population possesses and controls wealth of such incredible magnitude that it eludes estimation. Yet, the majority of people who inhabit this earth are suffering the ravages of hunger and malnutrition. The fact that the same species which can create the computer, formulate space technology, and give evidence of extrasensory perception is also frequently unable to communicate adequately with family, friends, and neighbors defies explanation.

It has been said that the study of human aggression is "more than any other aspect of human behavior . . . studded with dilemma, anomaly, myth and just plain irony."[9] Issues of race, religion, poverty, power, and territoriality among others have aroused human emotions, which prompt man to display violent aggression against fellow men. In the same society where pet animals are highly valued, meticulously groomed, and catered to by their owners, abuse of children reached epidemic proportions in 1976, when it was estimated that one in every seven children was abused or neglected.[10] Of the funds bequeathed to the American Humane Association, 70 percent have been donated for the protection of animals and only 30 percent have been available for the protection of children.[11] During the twentieth century, man's bellicose capacity led him to wage two world wars and several other wars of major proportion in different parts of the world. The crime rate in the United States and other countries soared dramatically in recent years; between the late 1940s and the late 1960s the murder rate in the United States doubled.[12] These dynamic interactions (achievement, aggression, etc.) all contribute to the life process.

## Characteristics of the Life Process

The theoretical framework of nursing science elaborated by Rogers[13] provides a foundation for the discussion of the life process in people. While it is not the only theoretical framework advanced for nursing, Rogers' theory has been widely accepted because of its emphasis on man as a "holistic" being who is in constant interaction with the environment. In addition, Rogers' theoretical framework has been complemented and amplified by the work of nurse researchers and those in other scientific disciplines. Rogers' theoretical framework is presented here and includes assumptions about the complexities, commonalities, and subtleties of the life process in people. It provides a framework for a holistic nursing assessment of individuals and their interaction with the environment.

**Wholeness**    It is essential that the nurse perceive human beings in terms of their wholeness. People are not an aggregate of "parts"; rather, each individual is unique and accurately discernible only as a unified whole. Scholars in a variety of disciplines dealing with people—nursing, psychology, medicine, science, philosophy, and theology among them—have, for several years, established that "man is more than and different from the sum of his parts."[14-20] In recent years, general system theory has been widely utilized as a conceptual framework for the understanding of people. This approach further supports the belief that any individual must be viewed in his or her entirety, as a "unified whole."[21,22]

The importance of a holistic approach cannot be overemphasized in nursing practice. Although the collection of information about an individual is an essential step in the nursing process, none of the facts identified, alone or in summation, can truly be representative of the unique, "whole person." Even the most intricate analyses of the multiplicity of human cells, tissues, fluids, and organs are inadequate descriptions of human beings because these analyses reflect only *parts* of the individual. A nursing assessment which focuses on only selected parts of an individual without consideration of the total person is likely to result in a nursing diagnosis which is incomplete, inaccurate, or both. An incomplete assessment is likely to result in the setting of goals which are inappropriate. For example, teaching and treatment measures directed toward an individual's attainment of optimum health following an illness may prove unsuccessful if the individual is not emotionally ready to comply. Likewise, nursing measures directed toward the relief of an individual's anxiety will not be effective when the person is also suffering physical discomfort.

**Mind-body interaction**    The wholeness of human beings is further exemplified by an elusive and only superficially understood interaction which is believed to exist between the body and mind. Prominent theorists in different fields have cited mind-body interaction as an important facet in man's wholeness.[23-28] Belief in an interaction between body and mind has been acknowledged since ancient times. Hippocrates was known to espouse the belief that the composition of certain body "humors" (fluids) could affect the "temperament" of man and that a person's emotions had bearing on his or her physical well-being.[29]

Recent acceptance of the mind-body interaction phenomenon has increased understanding of health problems such as peptic ulcer, rheumatoid arthritis, and bronchial asthma. These problems are frequently associated with psychophysiologic factors, but the precise interaction of variables which contributes to the development of these and other psychophysiologic illnesses still remains a mystery. There exists a minority of individuals who would doubt the mind-body relationship because precise information about it is lacking. However, the vast majority of experts who deal with human beings affirm their belief in mind-body interaction even though their knowledge remains, for the most part, quite nebulous.

Research into mind-body relationships has revealed new findings which have import both for the further description of the life process in man and for nursing practice. Until recently, it was believed that mind-body interaction was only involuntary, being due to the effects of the autonomic system which was assumed to be linked with the "lower" brain centers below the neocortex.[30] However, recent research in the field would indicate that "elaborate avenues of communication exist between the somatic network and the autonomic one."[31] Such findings, Miller contended, reject formerly held beliefs that "reason" and voluntary nervous system activity are "superior functioning" in contrast to the "inferior functioning" characterized by emotions and involuntary glandular responses.[32] Investigations conducted during the 1960s and 1970s have revealed that people are, to some extent, able to control involuntary functions in the body.

Methods such as biofeedback, transcendental meditation, yoga, zen meditation, and hypnosis have been employed in order to effect a desired interaction between the body and mind. The first efforts directed toward the use of biofeedback as a means of teaching humans how to modify functioning of the autonomic nervous system were largely controversial and inconclusive. However, more recent studies suggest promising clinical applications. Reports indicate that biofeedback has been successfully employed in the control of cardiac arrhythmias, hypertension, low-back pain, tension and migraine headaches, and peripheral vascular disorders.[33,34] Biofeedback may also prove to be the most significant breakthrough in the control of epileptic seizures since the discovery of anticonvulsants. Two different studies, although limited in scope and still preliminary, have reported significant reduction of seizure activity in epileptics who previously were inadequately controlled by medication.[35,36]

Investigations of correlations between electrical potentials of brain waves, behavior, and feeling states are beginning to identify other clues to the nature of the relationship between the body and mind. One investigator proposed that if the physical state of a person's brain (as recorded by an electroencephalogram) during a given interval can be determined, and this pattern correlated with the individual's actions and experiences during the same time interval, the information gleaned might further understanding of the role of the brain in producing psychological differences among people.[37]

Although gross electroencephalogram (EEG) waves have limited value, investigators have found that when electrical potentials are averaged after an individual is exposed to an auditory or visual stimulus, the response pattern can provide information about some mental processes.[38] Investigators have noted that the pattern of brain wave recovery after a strong stimulus differs between persons diagnosed as mentally ill and those deemed mentally healthy. Rapid recovery and habituation (decrement in the magnitude of evoked response) have been correlated with mental health, whereas persons with diagnosed pathology demonstrated wave patterns which were significantly slower in habituation and recovery. It has been hypothesized that these findings may reflect an individual's characteristic mode of responding to the environment and perhaps be indicative of a mental health–mental illness continuum.[39] One must remember, however, that correlations between brain electrical potentials can never precisely reflect the processes within an individual's mind, and even these correlations can be viewed only as isolated pieces of information about complex human beings.

**Human diversity** The incredible and unequivocal differences which exist between each and every human being constantly pose a challenge for the nurse. No matter how extensive a professional practice is, the nurse will never encounter two individuals who are identical in every way. Diversity characterizes all dimensions of man's existence for it transcends anatomy, physiology, perceptions, thoughts, emotions, fears, and aspirations. For example, one individual endeavors to climb Mt. Washington simply because "it is there," while another person's fear of water compels him to

avoid water sports at all costs. One man's hypertension is related to dietary factors and sodium intake, while another's is believed to be due to hereditary influences, and still another's to stressful periods associated with work. Long-time inhabitants of a high-altitude environment find no difficulty in carrying out daily activities of living without restrictions; the newcomer experiences fatigue for several days as a result of the low environmental oxygen concentration. A woman who possesses outstanding athletic ability might have one brother who excels in music and a sister who is an expert in linguistics.

Human diversity has been attributed to the interaction of two factors: the individual's genetic endowment and the influence of the environment.[40,41] Genetic variation among members of a species may result from mutation, natural selection, or recombination, but most of the observed differences in man are the result of new combinations passed on to the offspring by each parent.[42] The potential for such difference among people has long been recognized as so inexhaustible that it exceeds the number of people born in all generations combined.[43] Study of genetic inheritance has taken on added import in recent years because scientists now believe that individuals inherit behavioral traits as well as physical characteristics from their parents.[44] Although the tools to measure inheritance of these behavioral traits are imperfect, there is strong evidence to support the contention that special talents, skills, and mental ability are transmitted via genes.[45]

Attributing human diversity to the interaction of genetic inheritance and environmental influences is a deceptively simple explanation for a complex phenomenon. Scholars in several fields cite strong evidence which suggests that diversity among human beings is the result of a dynamic process which is evolutionary in nature.[46–49] They contend that this is not a discrete step-by-step process but rather the result of an interaction among a multiplicity of factors engaged in a simultaneous feedback system. Thus, man's evolutionary development includes not only physical development but also the sociocultural development resulting from differing opportunities afforded man by his environments.[50] Such dynamic changes occur continuously, as man is always in a state of "becoming."[51,52]

Rogers uses the concepts of *pattern* and *organization* to explain the evolutionary process which leads to growing complexity and diversity among humans.[53] According to Rogers' conceptual framework, *pattern* includes man's structure and function as he interacts with his environment.[54] A few visible examples of "pattern" in man include *genotype* (the particular arrangement of genes on the chromosomes), *phenotype* (individual physical traits), anatomical structures, physiological processes, and metabolism. Although they are less tangible, an individual's biological rhythms, state of consciousness, and behavior at any given point in time are also manifestations of "pattern." Pattern is not a static quality. Instead, it is a dynamic process which evolves continuously as man and environment interact. For example, one's genotype may be fixed at birth, but its expression in one's phenotype may change as environmental conditions change.[55]

In Rogers' theoretical framework, *organization* denotes the increased order and complexity toward which man's evolution is directed. Organization is closely bound to the repatterning which constantly takes place during man-environment interactions. It is postulated that the continuous flow of matter, energy, and information between man and environment creates fluctuations within the man-environment system. These fluctuations constitute *repatterning* between man and environment which allows the system to achieve a more highly organized and complex dynamic state.

Evidence for man's development in the direction of increasing complexity and order has been cited by several who have studied man's development.[56–60] While increasing complexity in pattern and organization evidenced by individuals (and the species *Homo sapiens*) is demonstrated in several aspects of man's existence, the most striking examples are provided by man's brain and nervous system. The rate of evolution of complex mental operations which man is capable of performing has exceeded the rate of human anatomical changes.[61] It is believed that the acquisition of language skills was closely related to man's ability to invent hand tools and improve manual skills. It is postulated that the emergence of manual dexterity and dominant handedness, accompanied by an increase in size of the related hemisphere of the brain, triggered similar development of the *opposite* hemisphere which is responsible for language skills.[62] Study of endocranial casts from various eras of man's development reveals steady and substantive increases in areas of the neocortex which are devoted to speech and manual skills.[63]

It is important to remember that the increasing complexity of human beings is an expression of their holistic nature. The fluctuations which occur with each repatterning between man and environment affect the individual as an organized whole.

Both body and mind interact as man progresses in complexity. It is believed by some that interrelationships between man's increasing physical and chemical complexity are correlated to abstract abilities such as memory, thinking, dreams, emotions, and other attributes.[64] The genetic changes which contribute to man's increasing complexity and diversity are never "simple." Even a very small alteration in genetic material will inevitably affect other structures and lead to numerous changes.[65] Also, influences from culture and society are as significant in man's evolutionary emergence as are changes in structure and function. It has been noted that human culture is changing the environment more rapidly than cultural evolution can respond.[66]

Man's evolutionary development holds import for all nurses. Not only is it inevitable that man will continue to progress in complexity and diversity, the *rate* of such changes will become more rapid. In addition, new technologies will enable men to significantly influence and, to a certain degree, control their evolutionary emergence.

The power to control the nature and quality of human life is compounded with numerous legal, moral, professional, and religious issues as well as with unknown factors. Scientists question whether men should endeavor to control their own biological evolution by producing a *Homo superior,* when the rate of cultural evolution may well override man's biological potential. The benefits and risks of experimentation with recombinant deoxyribonucleic acid (DNA) have been disputed at length in both scientific and nonscientific circles.[67–69] Experiments with recombinant DNA involve adding minute amounts of DNA called "plasmids" to bacterial host cells. Once the DNA is added to this host cell, it becomes part of the cell's permanent genetic complement. Some feel that the danger of leaking bacterial contamination during experiments on bacterial cells, primarily *Escherichia coli,* beyond the laboratory is the most compelling reason to exercise caution in conducting these experiments. Others believe that the overriding issue is that recombinant DNA experiments are essentially the forerunners of "genetic engineering." Not only does recombinant DNA experimentation constitute an unknown area of biological research, it may represent embarkation on research which will have a long-range and potentially dangerous impact on society and the environment.

Certainly the decisions which confront scientists, health professionals, and society in general are ominous. Promoting the health and optimum human potential of each individual is perhaps the most important role of the professional nurse. Not only does this responsibility require the nurse to *recognize* the vast differences among individuals, it also requires that the nurse utilize measures to *enhance* those factors which contribute to each person's uniqueness. It is incumbent, therefore, that the nurse, as both a professional and a citizen, assume an active role in making the crucial decisions which will have an impact on all humanity.

**Sentience and thought** Sentience and thought are vital elements of holistic human existence. Not only is an individual able to produce, communicate, and interpret information, he or she is also a sentient being who experiences and expresses feeling and emotion while maintaining awareness of self, others, and environment.[70] This quality clearly establishes man's superiority over other forms of life. Of all living creatures, only a human is able to analyze his or her own existence. Human beings' capacity for thought, perception, and feeling should be viewed as a continuously evolving correlate of their increasing complexity and diversity. The review of man's accomplishments cited at the beginning of this chapter attests to the seemingly endless capacity for creativity and invention.

Experts in various disciplines contend that man's future development is likely to proceed in the direction of heightened sensory awareness and cognitive functions. Exploration into differences

**TABLE 1-1**
COGNITIVE MODES OF THE TWO CEREBRAL HEMISPHERES

| Left Hemisphere: "Analytical" | Right Hemisphere: "Holistic, creative" |
|---|---|
| Language and verbal skills (speech, writing) | Nonverbal skills |
| Logic, order | Intuition |
| Processing information sequentially | Integration of simultaneous inputs<br>Perceiving spatial relationships and patterns |
| Mathematics and science skills | Musical and artistic ability |
| Motor skills | Proprioception |
| Temporal ordering of events: past, future | Perception of time as "present moment" |

SOURCES: Ronald H. Bailey, *The Role of the Brain,* Time-Life Books, New York, 1975, pp. 87 and 90; Enoch Calloway, *Brain Electrical Potentials and Individual Psychological Differences,* Grune & Stratton, New York, 1975, p. 96; David Galin, "The Two Modes of Consciousness and the Two Halves of the Brain," in Philip R. Lee et al. (eds.), *Symposium on Consciousness,* Viking, New York, 1976, pp. 28–30.

between hemispheres of the brain and extrasensory perception provides two fascinating examples of man's evolving sentience and thought. Until recently, it was believed that each hemisphere of man's brain possessed identical functions although one hemisphere functioned in a "dominant" manner. Thus, it was assumed that the cerebral hemisphere which controlled an individual's language and handedness was the "dominant" hemisphere. Since a person's handedness is usually controlled by the contralateral hemisphere, the left hemisphere was assumed "dominant" in a right-handed person while the right hemisphere was assumed "dominant" in a left-handed individual. The opposite ("nondominant") hemisphere was largely ignored.

We now know that neither of man's cerebral hemispheres is truly "dominant." Rather, each cerebral hemisphere controls distinctly different and specialized cognitive abilities.[71-73] (See Table 1-1.) It is estimated that the left hemisphere controls language skills in 97 percent of the world's population.[74] This estimated figure includes approximately half of the people who are left-handed and the 92 percent who are right-handed. In right-handed people, the left hemisphere is also the origin of motor skills. In left-handed people, motor skills are usually controlled by the right hemisphere.

Regardless of an individual's handedness, it is important to remember that one of the hemispheres typically functions in the "analytical" or "logical" mode, whereas the other is able to process complex patterns and relationships in an integrated, "holistic" manner.[75] For centuries, man has emphasized the development of analytical ability rather than creative cognitive traits. However, the traits which belong to man's "holistic" hemisphere more accurately reflect evolving complexity and diversity. Certainly, cultivation of the more "holistic" cognitive abilities will be essential if man is to achieve true creativity through the use of both intellect and intuition.

*Extrasensory perception* (ESP) is an important aspect of man's continuously evolving capacity for sentience and thought. Extrasensory perception, or *psi,* is the ability to perceive events and objects through means other than the five senses. Although research into ESP is still in its early stages, numerous well-documented accounts of man's "super-sensory" abilities provide compelling evidence to support its existence.[76] Some of the more commonly observed forms of ESP are listed in Table 1-2.

Because ESP is a faculty of the mind which is clearly superior to that afforded by the five senses, many believe that its emergence should be viewed as a sign of man's evolutionary progression toward greater complexity. It is believed that many people actually possess a latent form of ESP which, when given the proper conditions for development, will fully emerge.[77-79]

### The Four-Dimensional Human Field

The nurse should bear in mind the important, but seldom recognized, fact that man's existence includes *more* than the physical manifestations of the human body. Actually, man's body is only the *visible* portion of the "human field" which comprises each and every individual. Rogers pointed out that *man is actually an energy field* consisting of constantly fluctuating electrical charges.[80] The assertion that man is an energy field may strike some as rather strange, but the reader should remember that man is composed of matter and all matter, in turn, is composed of atoms. All atoms, of course, carry positive, negative, and neutral electrical charges. Furthermore, modern physics reveals that matter, energy, and space are actually the *same.* Therefore, an energy field may organize molecules in such a manner that an object, or person, is generated as a *partial manifestation* of the field, but the field actually has invisible boundaries which extend into space.

With these fundamental laws in mind, the nurse can more readily understand Rogers' contention that although they are not visible to the naked eye, boundaries of the human field expand and contract as man exchanges energy with the environment.[81] Pattern and organization, properties of the visible portion of the human field, are likewise properties which are possessed by the entire human field.[82,83]

Neither human sensory apparatus nor sophisticated instrumentation and technology adequately permit perception of the dimensions of the human field. Rogers explains that the human field is closely bound to both space and time in a four-dimensional matrix.[84] Although the concept of a four-dimensional human field is new to nursing science, its existence has been cited by scholars in physics, mathematics, philosophy, and social sciences for several years.[85]

A satisfactory definition eludes even experts who attest to the existence of the fourth dimension. Essentially, the *fourth dimension* is the term used to denote a complex relationship between time and space which cannot ordinarily be perceived or measured by man's senses or the instruments cur-

rently available to him.[86] Belief in the existence of a higher dimension in the universe has grown as a result of numerous documented events which can neither be explained by scientific laws nor disregarded.

In order to understand the nature of man's four-dimensional life field, one must conceptualize *space* and, especially, *time* in a manner very different from the usual. Space, in the fourth dimension, should not be thought of as another geometrical dimension, but rather, as a facet of man's existence in the universe which is closely interrelated to time. In the fourth dimension, time remains immutable and stationary; there is *no* past, present, or future. This goes counter to the commonly held belief that time "flows" or "passes." While one might, at first, find this concept difficult to accept, one must remember that clocks and calendars are actually *artificial* constructs which man invented in order to "measure" time. It is believed that the corporeal world known to man is actually just a facet of the higher four-dimensional world and that man and the corporeal world are actually passing *through* higher, four-dimensional space although such motion is imperceptible to the human senses[87] (see Fig. 1-1).

Perhaps, the fourth dimension may be better understood if the reader recalls that man is actually an energy field. If only a portion of the field is visible, then it follows that the remaining portion must extend into the fourth dimension. The constant expansion and contraction of this energy field results in a "present moment" which is experienced differently by each individual. This elusive interrelationship between time, space, and human existence is evidenced by numerous well-documented precognition and retrocognition experiences.[88,89] Other manifestations of the fourth dimension include documented instances where a dead person *appeared* and *spoke* to one or more indi-

**TABLE 1-2**
SOME FORMS OF EXTRASENSORY PERCEPTION
OBSERVED IN MAN

| | |
|---|---|
| Clairvoyance | Ability of the mind to acquire information about or from an inanimate object without employing the senses of sight or hearing. |
| Precognition | Ability of the mind to know or perceive an event before it actually occurs. |
| Retrocognition | Ability of the mind to see or perceive an event which occurred in the past. Frequently the event occurred before the birth of the percipient. |
| Telepathy | Direct communication of information between two minds without use of the spoken word. |

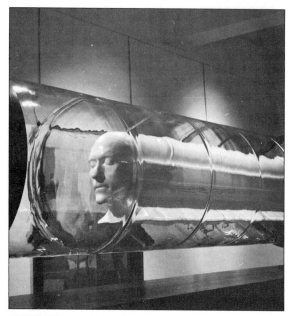

**FIGURE 1-1**
*The Accelerator* by Harold Tovish. This sculpture provides a unique visual representation of the multidimensionality of human beings and their emergent evolution. (*Courtesy of Harold Tovish,* Boston University School for the Arts, Boston, Massachusetts.)

viduals. Such apparitions have taken place in the ordinary course of events and without provocation by occult means. In many cases, the individuals who experienced apparitions were not aware that the person was actually dead. They did not realize that these manifestations were actually apparitions of the dead until some time after the event.[90] *Astral projection* may be cited as another example of man's four-dimensional life field. Astral projection is a phenomenon whereby an individual is able to project a replica of his or her body, known as an *astral body,* to almost any distance in time and space in such a manner that the astral body which is visible to other persons is mistaken for the real person.[91] Numerous examples of fourth-dimension experiences during sleep and dreaming states have been reported. It is theorized that because sleep and dreams free the individual from the ordinary limits of time and space, the individual is "free" to experience the higher four-dimensional world. Shared dreams (the identical dream experienced by more than one person simultaneously), precognitive dreams, and dreams of events actually happening, but at a distance from the dreamer, are striking examples of man's four-dimensional life field. These various manifestations of man's four-

dimensional existence involve an interrelationship between man, space, and time. In each instance, it is evident that man does, at times, possess the ability to traverse distances of space and the traditional barriers of time.

The concept of the four-dimensional life field has important implications for contemporary and future nursing practice. The most obvious, and perhaps the most important, of these implications stem from the fact that every encounter between the nurse and client involves interaction between their energy fields. If an individual's energy field is in constant flux in relationship to his or her psychophysical state and interaction with the environment, then it follows that all exchanges between the nurse and client are unique and entail much more than visible physical contact and interpersonal behavior.

For centuries, people have experienced beneficial effects from the comforting touch of a "significant other." Although touch is an integral and essential component of nursing practice, many nurses underestimate its significance. Research studies reveal that "therapeutic touch," especially when applied with the intent to heal or help, is associated with a resulting benefit to the client.[92] The precise mechanism underlying therapeutic touch is unclear at this time, but some form of energy is believed to flow from the healing or helping person to the client during the process.[93]

The nurse should be aware that experiences in the higher four-dimensional world may not be uncommon among patients during sleep and during altered states of consciousness. Because man's subconscious mind is not bound to an artificial past-present-future temporal orientation, the subconscious is actually capable of drifting into the fourth dimension.[94,95] Reports of unusual experiences involving time and space during sleep and dreaming states are quite numerous.[96,97]

More striking, however, are the growing number of *out-of-body experiences* (OOBEs) reported by individuals following periods of unconsciousness, cardiac arrest, severe injury or illness.[98] During an OOBE, individuals are able to watch all transactions which take place between themselves and others in their environment as if they were a nearby observer. Accounts of these OOBEs are quite similar. Individuals who have reported OOBEs can accurately describe their own appearance while lying in bed, the people caring for them, and even the events of their own resuscitation. Since there is reason to believe that the actual incidence of OOBEs exceeds the number of reported episodes, it is quite possible that many patients, especially those in critical-care units, experience this phenomenon unbeknown to the nurse.

## SIMULTANEOUS INTERACTION BETWEEN MAN AND ENVIRONMENT

A human is a sentient, holistic being who is inextricably bound to the environment which he or she inhabits. The interaction between man and environment can best be understood if man is viewed as a *living, open system.* A *system* is an assemblage of component parts which are organized in a unique way in order to form a unified whole. There are both *open* and *closed* systems. An *open system* constantly exchanges matter, energy, or information with the environment, whereas a *closed system* does not engage in an exchange of matter, energy, or information with the environment. The *environment* of a given system consists of all that is external to it. For man, the environment consists of the entire universe (Fig. 1-2).

Therefore, man, as a living, open system, is engaged in a mutual simultaneous interaction with the environment. This interaction is a highly dynamic, continuous process which transcends the complex, multiple dimensions of both man and environment. Although each of the components is unique, there is complementarity in all interactions between man and environment. *Complementarity* denotes the unity which is characteristic of all reciprocal interactions between man and environment. Since both man and environment are active participants, the nurse should remember that mutual simultaneous interaction is more than and different from mere passive adaptation to impinging forces.

The term homeodynamics denotes the dynamic, interacting, and reciprocal processes which continually occur in the living system and between the living system and the total environment.[99,100] There is constant flux in all exchanges which occur within man as an open system and between man and environment. This process differs significantly from the state of equilibrium. The formerly revered theories of "equilibrium" and "homeostasis" do not adequately describe the multiplicity of changes inherent in man's unique self-regulatory capacity. In an open system equilibrium is attained only in the static condition of death.

The life process of man is *unidirectional* in nature.[101] Because man is a living, open system, all interactions between man and environment are irreversible and directed toward the achievement of

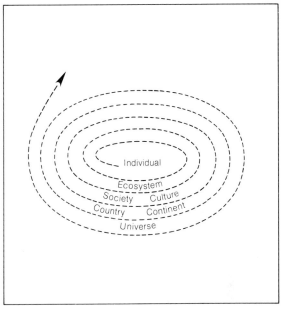

**FIGURE 1-2**
Interaction between the individual and environment. Individuals should be viewed as coextensive with the environment and the universe. The individual constantly engages in mutual simultaneous interaction with the environment and constantly responds to forces arising from the environment.

greater order and organization. Multiple changes which result from mutual simultaneous interaction between man and environment promote man's development in the direction of increasing complexity and diversity. No life stage or life situation can be repeated because each new interchange between an individual and the environment is influenced by the nature of all previous interactions. It is for this reason that Rogers states: "At each point in space-time, man is what he has been becoming but he is not what he has been."[102]

### Environmental Influences

Man is influenced by forces within the immediate environment and forces which arise from the larger environment, such as society and the total universe (Fig. 1-2). Man's immediate physical and social surroundings are frequently referred to as the *ecosystem.* Included in man's ecosystem are other human beings, such as the family and significant others, as well as the life-supporting elements of food, air, and water.

Each of the elements in an individual's ecosystem as well as his or her *pattern of interaction* with these elements will inevitably affect the individual. It is important that the nurse assess individuals in relation to their ecosystems. Analysis of the individual's interaction with impacting forces such as family relationships, ethnic background, social roles, and value systems as well as socioeconomic factors is critical to accurate assessment and formulation of the nursing diagnosis. In assessing individuals' interactions within their ecosystem, the nurse should not overlook the influence of the immediate environment. Such factors as immobility, prolonged bed rest, sensory stimuli, time of day or night, or an unfamiliar environment are likely to affect the individual's physical condition and behavior. The nurse should also be aware that architectural features, such as corridors, tunnels, reflective glass, furniture, and placement of windows, frequently serve as disorienting factors in health care facilities and hospitals.[103,104]

Since man is coextensive with the universe (Fig. 1-2), the nurse should be aware that human beings are constantly responding to forces which arise from the larger, less immediate environment. Factors such as the quality of the earth's atmosphere, water, and food supply are well-recognized forces in man's environment. However, man's simultaneous interaction with the environment also includes forces which are not readily perceptible. For example, one researcher reported that behavior among groups of the mentally ill was related to geophysical manifestations of naturally occurring variations in the earth's magnetic field.[105] It is most likely that there are numerous influential unidentified forces arising from man's environment.

## Rhythmic Phenomena

The simultaneous interaction between man and the environment is marked by continuous change. As this change occurs, its rhythmic nature emerges. Rhythms are the cyclic repetition of events. They are a universal phenomenon evidenced in the sun rotating on its axis, the moon revolving around the earth, the seasons changing, the tides coming and going, and flowers opening and closing.

A *cycle* may be defined as a coming around to the place of beginning. A cycle becomes a *rhythm* when a fairly regular period of time passes whenever the cycle returns to its beginning. A rhythm, then, is dependent on time. A *period* is the time a cycle takes to occur. All rhythms are characterized by highs and lows—the high tide and low tide, the opened and closed flower. The high point in a rhythm is called the *peak,* while the low point is the *trough.*

Rhythms are categorized according to their period. The most common rhythms found in man

are *circadian.* These rhythms fluctuate "around a day" and are 24-hour rhythms. Rhythms that occur more frequently than once in 24 hours are *ultradian* rhythms. *Infradian* rhythms are longer than 24 hours. There are also 12-month *circaannular* rhythms, *seasonal* rhythms, and *lunar* rhythms.

Because of the variability in the types of rhythms, their cause remains unclear. An *exogenous* rhythm is thought to be dependent on external environmental stimuli. Without the stimuli, the rhythm would not occur. The opening and closing of flowers were thought to be dependent on light changes. Flowers kept in complete darkness or constant light, however, continue to open and close rhythmically. The possibility of an *endogenous* rhythm, one that originates independently as an inherent property of life, has been explored.

Rhythms are influenced by both exogenous and endogenous factors. Living matter has an inherent rhythmic blueprint which can be conditioned by the environment. As the rhythm is exposed to certain environmental stimuli that reoccur regularly, it will adjust to the environmental rhythms. The day/night rhythm in nature accounts for the large number of circadian rhythms. If a person is isolated from all environmental stimuli in relation to the day/night rhythm, it has been found that his or her circadian rhythms become "free flowing." That is, they continue to demonstrate a rhythmic pattern but tend to run slightly longer than 24 hours.[106]

A rhythm that undergoes a change in timing becomes *dysrhythmic.* Jet travel causes dysrhythmia. People usually adjust to a new time zone at a rate of 1 hour per day. As environmental cues fluctuate rhythmically, they synchronize the internal rhythms. All the body's rhythmic changes occur in relation to each other. If the environmental cues are disrupted, the rhythms become dysrhythmic and *desynchronized.* For example, the body temperature curve peaks at a different time, energy peaks become troughs, and the activity/rest cycles become disturbed. This happens to nurses when they rotate shifts and adjust to a completely different circadian rhythm in a short period of time. Nurses who rotated from day work to night work were found to have difficulty sleeping, trouble staying awake, fatigue, and a disruption in bowel habits. It usually took a week before bowel movements returned to their rhythmic pattern.[107]

**Psychosocial rhythms** Rhythms occur not only in a biological sense, but in a psychological, social, and cultural context. The human mind responds to rhythms expressed in music, dance, and poetry.

would manifest the same set of GAS *symptoms,* but the initial stressors might be different for each person. Furthermore, the fact that an agent produces stress in one person does not mean that the same agent is a stressor for all persons. The GAS, Selye explains, is not synonymous with stress. Rather, it is a series of "nonspecific changes which develop throughout time during continued exposure to a stressor."[116] There are three sequential stages in the GAS: alarm, resistance, and exhaustion (see Fig. 1-3).

The complex nature of man dictates that one must continually raise questions about the nature of stress and its role in the mutual simultaneous interaction between man and environment. Is stress *always* harmful? Does stress exist only when an individual is *aware* of it? Is stress usually regarded as an undesirable factor because it is *only* when the stress becomes pronounced, harmful, or uncomfortable that it comes into conscious awareness?

Recent investigations seeking answers to these and other questions about stress suggest that the set of "predictable" responses which constitutes the GAS does not universally occur. Instead, researchers are reporting that the key factor in the stress phenomenon seems to be the individual's *perception* of the potentially stressful event or stressor.[117–121] Such variables as one's innate characteristics, past experiences, and future goals play a significant role in either mitigating the stress or facilitating its impact on the individual. Researchers have also noted a relationship between the individual's perceived control over a potentially stressful situation and lessened response to the stress.[122,123] These findings may be understood if one recalls that there is an interaction between most body organs and the impulses which travel along the autonomic and endocrine pathways. This highly complex response occurs as a result of interaction between the highest integrative levels of the nervous system and the interpretive areas of the brain.[124] Figure 1-4 depicts the physiological mechanism which underlies an individual's response to internal or external inputs. The individual's perception will largely determine whether stress will occur.

## NURSING INTERVENTION DURING THE LIFE PROCESS

A theoretical framework of nursing science becomes relevant as the professional practitioner translates nursing science theory, derived through research, into modes of practice which promote,

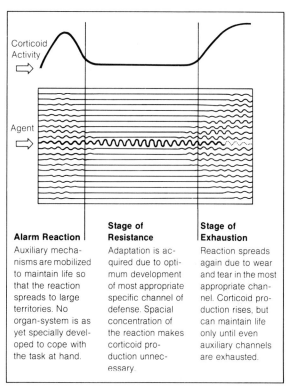

**FIGURE 1-3**
The general adaptation syndrome. (*Reprinted by permission of Hans Selye, M.D.,* The Stress of Life, *McGraw-Hill, New York, p. 121.*)

**Alarm Reaction**
Auxiliary mechanisms are mobilized to maintain life so that the reaction spreads to large territories. No organ-system is as yet specially developed to cope with the task at hand.

**Stage of Resistance**
Adaptation is acquired due to optimum development of most appropriate specific channel of defense. Spacial concentration of the reaction makes corticoid production unnecessary.

**Stage of Exhaustion**
Reaction spreads again due to wear and tear in the most appropriate channel. Corticoid production rises, but can maintain life only until even auxiliary channels are exhausted.

maintain, and improve the quality of human existence for individuals, families, and groups of people. Nursing is unique among the health professions in that its practice is directed toward the "whole person" and the person's interaction with the environment in health and during illness.

An individual's interaction with the environment can be described as simultaneous, continuous, and dynamic. A person's health status is a reflection of interacting psychological, physiological, and sociocultural variables at any given point in time. The impact of these variables on an individual changes from day to day, hour to hour, and minute to minute. Therefore, the health of an individual is continuosuly changing in quality.

At any given point in time, an individual's response to these interacting variables will be a function of the individual's status as well as the status of the environment. For example, an individual who is exposed to a virus one week may successfully resist its invasion. However, during another week, when the same individual receives inadequate sleep and inadequate nutrition, the same virus may invade the system and alter the individual's health status.

The practicing nurse must be able to apply principles of nursing science in providing health care to people of all ages in a variety of settings. In order to be successful in this endeavor, the nurse must be able to intervene appropriately during the continuous man-environment interaction process. In this text, nursing intervention will be discussed with respect to four phases, or levels, of care. These phases will be referred to as *first-level, second-level, third-level,* and *fourth-level* nursing care.

*First-level nursing care* focuses on the "healthy" individual in a "disease-free" state. The objectives of nursing care at this level are to identify those persons at risk of developing disturbances or disruptions in health and to prevent disruptions in health from actually taking place. In order to identify a "high-risk" population, the nurse must carefully analyze the physiological, psychosocial, and environmental variables which are interacting within the individual's field. In analyzing the effect of significant variables on an individual's health status, the nurse may predict situations which have the potential to disrupt the person's health and interfere with achievement of his or her maximum potential.

Nurses may identify persons at risk either through large-group screening programs or by careful assessment of individuals. Use of a careful screening program to identify factors which predispose people to a particular health problem may ultimately result in avoidance of that problem in the population at hand. Prevention of a particular health problem begins as soon as risk factors are identified. The objective is to eliminate the risk factors completely or to reduce their threatening effect on the human condition. When preventive measures are instituted early, they can significantly alter the course of a potential health problem.

Nursing intervention may include a reorganization in the "pattern" of an individual's life in order to change the person's current health trajectory. Suppose, for example, John Smith, age 40, has a significant family history of heart disease, smokes heavily, manifests a compulsive, tense personality, works in a stressful occupation and ingests a diet which is high in cholesterol. These interacting variables have a potentiating effect on each other and, thus, interfere with Mr. Smith's optimum potential for health. By changing his dietary intake and smoking habits, utilizing strategies to modify

**FIGURE 1-4**

Relationship between sensory input and stress response. (*From John Mason, "Emotions as Reflected in Patterns of Endocrine Integration," in L. Levi (ed.), Emotions— Their Parameters and Measurements, Raven Press, New York, 1975, p. 143–181.*)

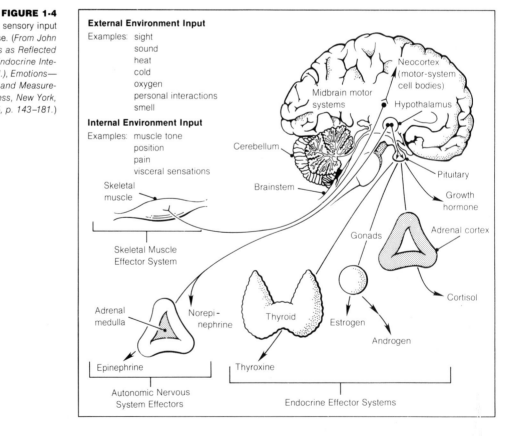

his personality, and identifying ways of coping with a stress-producing occupation, Mr. Smith is likely to reduce the risk of developing life-threatening disruptions in health.

*Second-level nursing care* focuses on the individual presenting early changes in health status. At this point, physiological and psychosocial alterations have already begun, and the individual is attempting to cope with these changes while retaining a "normal" life-style within the community. The objectives of nursing care are to help identify the extent of the problem, isolate the major problems the patient is experiencing, select appropriate interventions, and help prevent further disruptions and alteration in the individual's health.

For example, the nurse may participate in the assessment of an individual who has developed a minor upper respiratory infection. The assessment may include observations of the individual, a careful interview, and, perhaps, diagnostic tests. The individual may remain at home while being treated. The nurse's role will include conducting follow-up visits to evaluate the individual's compliance with the prescribed regime and responses to the regime. Health teaching may be employed in order to promote the changes within the individual's internal and external environment which will optimize the person's health potential and prevent further disruptions. There are times when an emergency will arise and an individual will require immediate intervention (i.e., cardiopulmonary resuscitation) lest death occur. In such situations, the nurse deals with the life-threatening situation, and the patient is transferred to an acute-care facility.

*Third-level nursing care* deals with acute health problems which require complex nursing intervention. The nurse focuses upon problems which threaten the patient's immediate health status and promptly implements interventions which are likely to reduce disruption in a component of the total system.

At this point, nursing assessment becomes complex, and it is directed toward the identification of problems involving the multiple dimensions of the individual's existence. The health history and physical examination often reveal several health problems which vary in their degrees of complexity. Rigorous diagnostic testing is a vital component in analyzing and evaluating the degree of disruption in human functions. Concomitant medical and surgical interventions may produce additional problems for the patient and require additional nursing interventions.

Extension of the physiological and psychologi-cal disruptions continually poses a threat to the patient. Continuous reassessment and goal-directed nursing intervention are imperative in halting or reducing this detrimental progression. As the patient begins to gain momentum in proceeding toward a more optimal level, activities which allow for increasing self-awareness as well as physical and emotional growth may be incorporated into the nursing care plan. Nursing interventions should support this "recovery" period and help move the patient toward independence once again.

*Fourth-level nursing care* focuses on rehabilitation. The nurse assesses the client's current health status and plans interventions which will ensure health promotion and realization of optimal human potential for the client. Health teaching of both patient and family members becomes most important in facilitating this process.

As a result of alterations in the "whole being," the patient may be faced with multiple changes in life-style. A detailed teaching plan which reflects individual human needs and limitations must be developed. The plan should be realistic and incorporate the interdisciplinary health care services which will be needed to accomplish the goals. Psychological and physiological, as well as sociocultural, variables influencing the rehabilitative period must be considered when the nurse develops the teaching plan.

Nursing intervention must also focus on patient compliance. The patient's ability to return to a state of optimum health will be influenced by individual motivation, the impact of the health teaching, and the personal significance of health.

## INTERDEPENDENCY OF NURSING PRACTICE, NURSING EDUCATION, AND NURSING RESEARCH

Nursing can be conceptualized as an "open system" which responds to the society of which it is a part. As an open system, nursing is engaged in a simultaneous interaction with the surrounding social system. Technology and research findings produced by society provide nursing with sophisticated technical and interpersonal tools which can be utilized in carrying out the nursing process. Utilization of society's inventions by nurses changes society at the same time that society responds to nursing's interventions. This process is continual, with the resulting changes in society giving rise to new needs and new inventions. These, in turn, call forth innovative nursing approaches to meet emerging human needs.

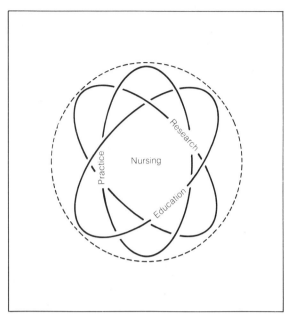

**FIGURE 1-5**
Nursing's interdependent energy sources. Nursing may be conceptualized as an "open system" which responds to society. The three interacting components, (1) nursing practice. (2) nursing education, and (3) nursing research, serve as continual energy sources for the profession.

The conceptualization of nursing as an open system includes three interacting components: (1) nursing practice, (2) nursing education, and (3) nursing research. Each of the three serves as a continual energy source for the profession, and, as such, each is essential to its existence and development (Fig. 1-5).

*Nursing practice,* perhaps the most visible of the three components, is of fundamental importance to the profession because it epitomizes the very purpose of nursing, which is service to people. When people cease to need nursing services, the profession will no longer have a reason for existence.

The effective practice of nursing requires much more from the nurse than intellectual processes and application of skills. Unless there is substantial involvement of "self" by the practitioner in each encounter with a client, the nurse's practice is no more than "educated caretaking." The truly professional practice of nursing should be typified by a therapeutic use of self which finds expression in all activities the nurse performs with and for a client. *Therapeutic use of self* within the nursing process is not merely a rote skill; rather, it is a creative undertaking, and it should be uniquely different in every nurse-client encounter. Therapeutic use of self will assume even greater significance in the future, because innovative nursing practice will be imperative in order to meet increasingly divergent needs of complex human beings.

The second component of the system, *nursing education,* is essential to the profession because its primary function is to prepare the practitioners who will be able to translate nursing science theory into relevant professional nursing practice. In addition, nursing education is responsible for preparing nurse researchers, who are charged with the task of further defining the body of nursing science knowledge and preparing future educators of nurses. The system of nursing education serves as a vital force in the continual upgrading of the nursing profession and its practitioners.

The third component, *nursing research,* is the means by which the theoretical body of nursing science is obtained. Today, the practice of professional nursing flows directly from this body of knowledge. As with other professions, the practice of nursing preceded the elaboration of its underlying theoretical basis and research component. And, just as other professions have enlarged upon original modes of practice as they developed scientific rationale, the clinical practice of nursing will continue to expand in breadth and depth as a reflection of evolving nursing science theory. Without a continually evolving knowledge base about the life process, nursing practice and nursing education would fade into obsolescence.

The process of scientific inquiry must be integrated with all aspects of professional nursing practice. Continual exploration of relationships among the variables influencing the life process in man is essential if nursing is to fulfill its purpose in society.

## REFERENCES

1    Martha E. Rogers, *An Introduction to the Theoretical Basis of Nursing,* Davis, Philadelphia, 1970.
2    Imogene M. King, *Toward a Theory of Nursing,* Wiley, New York, 1971.
3    Rozella M. Schlotfeldt, "This I Believe . . . Nursing Is Health Care," *Nurs Outlook,* **20:**245–246, April 1972.
4    Myra E. Levine, "Holistic Nursing," *Nurs Clin North Am,* **6:**255, June 1971, citing Alfred N. Whitehead, *Adventure of Ideas,* Mentor Books, New American Library, New York, 1964, p. 236.
5    Rogers, *op. cit.,* p. 53.

6   *Ibid.,* p. 93.

7   Bernard O. Davis, and Patricia Flaherty (eds.), *Human Diversity: Its Causes and Social Significance,* Ballinger, Cambridge, Mass., 1976, p. 23.

8   Robert Cooke, "First Working Artificial Gene Built at MIT," *Boston Globe,* Aug. 28, 1976, p. 1.

9   Ronald H. Bailey, *Violence and Aggression,* Time-Life, New York, 1976, p. 7.

10   Barbara Campbell, "Children's Abuse Target of Drive," *The New York Times,* Aug. 15, 1976.

11   Mark A. Stuart and George James, "Our Children: Sometimes We Kill Them," Part I of "the Unprotected," a series on child abuse, *Hackensack* (N.J.) *Record,* Nov. 22, 1970.

12   Bailey, *op. cit.,* p. 8.

13   Rogers, *op. cit.*

14   Teilhard de Chardin, *The Phenomenon of Man,* trans. by Sir Julian Huxley, Harper & Row, New York, 1959, p. 178.

15   Theodosius Dobzhansky, *Mankind Evolving,* Bantam, New York, 1962, p. 24.

16   René Dubos, *So Human an Animal,* Scribner, New York, 1968, p. 27.

17   ———, *Man Adapting,* Yale, New Haven, Conn. 1965, p. 1.

18   Rogers, *op. cit.,* pp. 44–47.

19   Kurt Goldstein, *The Organism,* Beacon Press, Boston, 1963, pp. 213–290.

20   Charles Hampden-Turner, *Radical Man,* Schenkman, Cambridge, Mass., 1970, pp. 24, 25, 32, and 33.

21   Ludwig von Bertalanffy, *General System Theory,* George Braziller, New York, 1968, pp. 186–194.

22   Ervin Laszlo, *The Systems View of the World,* George Braziller, New York, 1973, pp. 8, 29, 30, and 79–120.

23   George H. Estabrooks and Nancy E. Gross, *The Future of the Human Mind,* Dutton, New York, 1961, pp. 119–120.

24   Dubos, *Man Adapting,* p. 7.

25   Erwin W. Strauss, *Phenomenological Psychology,* Basic Books, New York, 1966, p. 164.

26   Rogers, *op. cit.,* p. 46.

27   Keith Campbell, *Body and Mind,* Anchor Books, Doubleday & Company, Garden City, N.Y., 1970, pp. 34–35.

28   Levine, *op. cit.,* pp. 255–256.

29   Alfred M. Freedman, et al.: *Modern Synopsis of Comprehensive Textbook of Psychiatry,* Williams & Wilkins, Baltimore, 1972, pp. 431–432.

30   Gerald Jonas, *Visceral Learning,* Viking, New York, 1973, p. 35.

31   *Ibid.*

32   *Ibid.,* pp. 46–47.

33   *Ibid.,* pp. 114–124.

34   Lorraine Taylor Sterman, "Clinical Biofeedback," *Am J Nurs,* **75:**2006–2007, November 1975.

35   Maurice B. Sterman, et al.: "Biofeedback Training of the Sensorimotor Electroencephalogram Rhythm in Man: Effects on Epilepsy," *Epilepsia,* **15:**395–416, September 1974.

36   W. W. Findley, et al.: "Reduction of Seizures and Normalization of the EEG in a Severe Epileptic Following Sensorimotor Biofeedback Training: Preliminary Study," *Biol Psychol,* **2:**189–203, 1975, cited by Lorraine Taylor Sterman in "Clinical Biofeedback," *Am J Nurs,* **75:**2009, November 1975.

37   Enoch Calloway, *Brain Electrical Potentials and Individual Psychological Differences,* Grune & Stratton, New York, 1975, p. ix.

38   *Ibid.,* pp. 6–7.

39   *Ibid.,* pp. 80–95.

40   Max K. Hecht, and Williams C. Steere (eds.), *Essays in Evolution and Genetics in Honor of Theodosius Dobzhansky,* Appleton-Century-Crofts, New York, 1970, pp. 4 and 576.

41   Rogers, *op. cit.,* p. 55.

42   Davis and Flaherty, *op. cit.,* p. 5.

43   Dobzhansky, *op. cit.,* p. 32.

44   Davis and Flaherty, *op. cit.,* pp. 4 and 51.

45   *Ibid.,* p. 51.

46   Rogers, *op. cit.,* pp. 23–27 and 55.

47   Davis and Flaherty, *op. cit.,* p. 51.

48   Erich Jantsch, *Design for Evolution,* George Braziller, New York, 1975, pp. 37–38 and 62–64.

49   Hecht and Steere, *op. cit.,* pp. 101–102.

50   Davis and Flaherty, *op. cit.,* p. 51.

51   *Ibid.,* p. 4.

52   Rogers, *op. cit.,* pp. 55 and 98.

53   *Ibid.,* pp. 61–66.

54   *Ibid.,* p. 62.

55   I. Michael Lerner and William J. Libby, *Heredity, Evolution and Society,* Freeman, San Francisco, 1976, p. 315.

56   *Ibid.,* pp. 37–38 and 63–64.

57   Hecht and Steere, *op. cit.,* pp. 101, 102, 105, and 109.

58   Lerner and Libby, *op. cit.,* p. 83.

59   Sylvan J. Kaplan and Evelyn Kivy-Rosenberg (eds.), *Ecology and the Quality of Life,* Charles C Thomas, Springfield, Ill., 1973, p. 11.

60   G. V. Anfang, *Man: Attempts at a Complete Description,* Exposition Press, New York, 1975, p. 4.

61   Davis and Flaherty, *op. cit.,* p. 51.

62   *Ibid.,* p. 24.

63   *Ibid.,* p. 25.

64   Anfang, *op. cit.,* p. 4.

65   Hecht and Steere, *op. cit.,* p. 101.

66   Lerner and Libby, *op. cit.,* p. 89.

67 Liebe F. Cavalieri, "New Stains of Life—or Death," *The New York Times Magazine,* Aug. 22, 1976, p. 8.

68 Harold M. Schmeck, Jr., "Keeping Watch on Deoxyribonucleic Acid," *The New York Times,* Feb. 20, 1977, p. E16.

69 Cheryl M. Fields, "Who Should Control Recombinant DNA?" *Chronicle Higher Education,* March 21, 1977, p. 1.

70 Rogers, *op. cit.,* p. 68.

71 Robert E. Ornstein, *The Psychology of Consciousness,* Freeman, San Francisco, 1972.

72 ———— (ed.), *The Nature of Human Consciousness,* Freeman, San Francisco, 1973.

73 Philip R. Lee, et al., *Symposium on Consciousness,* Viking, New York, 1976.

74 Ronald H. Bailey, *The Role of the Brain,* Time-Life Books, New York, 1975, p. 80.

75 David Galin, "The Two Modes of Consciousness and Two Halves of the Brain," in Philip R. Lee et al. (eds.), *Symposium on Consciousness,* Viking, New York, 1976, pp. 28–30.

76 Literature on extrasensory perception and paranormal phenomena is proliferating at such a rapid rate that only a few references will be suggested here. Each of the following will provide the reader with an overview of ESP and paranormal phenomena: Edgar D. Mitchell, *Psychic Exploration: A Challenge for Science,* Putnam, New York, 1974; Charles Panati, *Supersenses,* Quadrangle/The New York Times Book Company, New York, 1974; John L. Randall, *Parapsychology and the Nature of Life,* Souvenir Press, London, 1975; and Leo Talamonti, *Forbidden Universe,* Stein and Day, New York, 1975. Journals which contain reports of current research in this area include: *Fields within Fields, International Journal of Parapsychology, Journal for Study of Consciousness, Journal of Altered States of Awareness, Journal of Parapsychology,* and *Journal of the Society for Psychical Research.*

77 Edgar D. Mitchell, *Psychic Exploration: A Challenge for Science,* Putnam, New York, 1974, p. 38.

78 Rogers, *op. cit.,* p. 72.

79 Ian Stevenson, *Telepathic Impressions,* University Press of Virginia, Charlottesville, 1970, pp. 186–187.

80 Rogers, *op. cit.,* p. 90.

81 *Ibid.*

82 *Ibid.,* p. 91.

83 Bob Toben, *Space-Time and Beyond,* Dutton, New York, 1975, pp. 129–131.

84 Rogers, *op. cit.,* p. 91.

85 In the late nineteenth century (circa 1880) Edwin Abbott presented the concept of a fourth dimension in a clever combination of satire and science fiction entitled *Flatland.* Currently in its seventh edition (Dover, New York, 1952), this work is viewed by many as a classic on the subject. Other early, but noteworthy works on the fourth dimension include: C. Howard Hinton, *The Fourth Dimension,* G. Allen, London, 1921; Claude Bragdon, *Fourth Dimensional Vistas,* Knopf, New York, 1930; and P. D. Ouspensky, *A New Model of the Universe,* Knopf, New York, 1934.

86 Ramon Valdes, *The Fourth Dimension,* Exposition Press, New York, 1971, p. 85.

87 *Ibid.,* pp. 102–114.

88 *Ibid.,* p. 114.

89 Leo Talamonti, *Forbidden Universe,* Stein and Day, New York, 1975, pp. 57–62.

90 Valdes, *op. cit.,* p. 128.

91 *Ibid.,* p. 59.

92 The foremost nurse-researcher in the area of Therapeutic Touch is Dr. Dolores Krieger, R.N., who has presented the results of her research to nurses as well as other professional and lay audiences throughout the United States and abroad. Two of Dr. Krieger's works are suggested for the student who desires further study in this area. The first, "Therapeutic Touch: The Imprimatur of Nursing," *Am J Nurs,* **75:**784–787, May 1975, gives a good basic overview of this phenomenon and its use in nursing. The second, "The Relationship of Touch with Intent To Help or To Heal, to Subjects In-Vivo Hemoglobin Valves: A Study in Personalized Interaction," in *American Nurses' Association Ninth Nursing Research Conferences,* San Antonio, Tex. March 21–23, 1973, American Nurses' Association, Kansas City, Mo., 1974, pp. 39–58, provides more depth on the research methodology Dr. Krieger utilized in her earlier studies.

93 Charles Panati, *Supersenses,* Quadrangle/The New York Times Book Company, New York, 1974, pp. 82 and 91–95.

94 Valdes, *op. cit.,* pp. 135–138.

95 Talamonti, *op. cit.,* pp. 63 and 76.

96 *Ibid.,* pp. 19–20, 26, and 58.

97 Valdes, *op. cit.,* p. 167.

98 Raymond Moody, *Life after Life,* Bantam, New York, 1975.

99 Rogers, *op. cit.,* pp. 26 and 63.

100 Gean M. Mathwig, "Set II: Nursing Science Concepts," New York University Division of Nursing, 1972 (mimeograph).

101 Rogers, *op. cit.,* pp. 55–60.

102 *Ibid.,* p. 98.

103 Mayer Spivack, "Archetypal Place," *Forum,* pp. 44–49, October 1973.

104 ———, "Psychological Implications of Mental Health Center Architecture," *Hospitals,* **43:**39–44, Jan. 1, 1969.

105 Robert O. Becker, "The Effect of Magnetic Fields upon the Central Nervous System," in Madeline F. Barnothy (ed.), *Biological Effects of Magnetic Fields,* vol. 2, Plenum, New York, 1969, p. 208.

106 A. Reinberg and J. Ghata, *Biological Rhythms,* Walker, New York, 1964.

107 Geraldene Felton, "Body Rhythm Effects on Rotating Work Shifts," *J Nurs Admin,* **5:**16–19, March-April 1975.

108 W. Ya Brodsky, "Protein Synthesis Rhythm," *J Theor Biol,* **55:**167–200, November 1975.

109 Reinberg and Ghata, *op. cit.,*

110 Gay Luce, *Biological Rhythms in Psychiatry and Medicine,* NJMH, Washington, 1966, p. 147.

111 Hans Selye, *The Stress of Life,* McGraw-Hill, New York, 1956, p. 54.

112 John S. Schweppe, *Man: A Remarkable Animal,* Research and Education Fund, Chicago, 1970, p. 83.

113 J. F. Brock, "Nature and Stress in Health and Disease," *Lancet,* 702, April 1, 1972.

114 Dubos, *Man Adapting,* p. 27.

115 Selye, *op. cit.*

116 *Ibid.,* p. 64.

117 Steward Wolf and Helen Goodell (eds.), Harold G. Wolff's *Stress and Disease,* 2d. ed., Charles C Thomas, Springfield, Ill., 1968, pp. 3, 136, and 144.

118 Richard S. Lazarus, "The Self-Regulation of Emotion," in Lennart Levi (ed.), *Emotions: Their Parameters and Measurement,* Raven Press, Publishers, New York, 1975, pp. 55–57.

119 John Mason, "Emotions as Reflected in Patterns of Endocrine Integration," in Lennart Levi (ed.), *Emotions: Their Parameters and Measurement,* Raven Press, Publishers, New York, 1975, p. 171.

120 A. T. Welford, "Stress and Performance," in A. T. Welford (ed.), *Man under Stress,* Halsted Press, New York, 1974, pp. 1–2.

121 I. Pilowsky, "Psychiatric Aspects of Stress," in A. D. Welford (ed.), *Man under Stress,* Halsted Press, New York, 1974, pp. 125–131.

122 Lazarus, *op. cit.,* p. 55.

123 Marianne Frankenhaeuser, "Experimental Approaches to the Study of Catecholamines and Emotions," in Lennart Levi (ed.), *Emotions: Their Parameters and Measurement,* Raven Press, Publishers, New York, 1975, pp. 214–216.

124 Wolf and Goodell, *op. cit.,* p. 9.

## BIBLIOGRAPHY

Asimov, Isaac: *Of Time, Space and Other Things,* Lancer Books, Inc., 1968.

Baker, Marjorie G.: "The Relationship between a Change in Social Routine and Fluctuations in Blood Pressure and Temperature," unpublished doctoral dissertation, New York University, 1975.

Brodt, Dagmar: "A Synergistic Theory of Nursing," *Am J Nurs,* **69:**1674–1676, August 1969.

Calder, Nigel: *The Mind of Man,* British Broadcasting Corporation, London, 1970.

Capobianco, Anna T.: "An Investigation of Changes in Pulse Rate under Differing Auditory Environments among Bed-Confined Young Adults," unpublished doctoral dissertation, New York University, 1975.

Cassidy, Catherine A.: "The Relationship between Appraisal of Adjustment Required by Reported Daily Life Events, Physical Symptoms and Temperature Range," unpublished doctoral dissertatipn, New York University, 1975.

———: "The Relationship between Daily Life Changes, Physical Symptoms and Body Temperature Range," *Image,* **8:**30–35, June 1976.

Deely, John N., and Raymond J. Nogar: *The Problem of Evolution: A Study of the Philosophical Repercussions of Evolution,* Appleton-Century-Crofts, New York, 1973.

deEstron, Veronica Rapp: "Radiation as Agents of Somatic and Genetic Alterations," *J Am Medical Women's Assoc,* **30:**445–449, November 1975.

Dobzhansky, Theodosius: *Genetics of the Evolutionary Process,* Columbia University Press, New York, 1970.

Eccles, John C.: *The Understanding of the Brain,* McGraw-Hill, New York, 1973.

Ehrlich, Paul R., Anne H. Ehrlich, and John P. Holdren: *Human Ecology,* Freeman, San Francisco, 1973.

Gotesky, Rubin, and Erwin Laszlo (eds.): *Evolution—Revolution,* Gordon and Breach, New York, 1971.

Grovitz, Samuel, et al.: *Moral Problems in Medicine,* Prentice-Hall, Englewood Cliffs, N.J., 1976.

Jirovec, M. M., and D. Jones: *Rhythms of Life,* videotape produced at Boston University School of Nursing Audiovisual Department, 1975.

Koestler, Arthur: *The Roots of Coincidence,* Vintage Books, Random House, New York, 1973.

Leddy, Marion Susan: "Sleep and Phase Shifting of Biological Rhythms," unpublished doctoral dissertation, New York University, 1973.

Levi, Lennart (ed.): *Emotions: Their Parameters and*

*Measurement,* Raven Press Publishers, New York, 1975.

Lewin, Kurt: *Field Theory in Social Science,* Harper & Row, New York, 1951.

Mitchell, Pamela H.: *Concepts Basic to Nursing,* 2d ed., McGraw-Hill, New York, 1977.

Murray, Ruth, and Judith Zentner: *Nursing Concepts for Health Promotion,* Prentice-Hall, Englewood Cliffs, N.J., 1975.

Ouspensky, P. D.: *A New Model of The Universe,* Vintage Books, Random House, New York, 1971.

Peusner, Leonardo: *Concepts in Bioenergetics,* Prentice-Hall, Englewood Cliffs, N.J., 1974.

Rockstein, Morris (ed.): *Theoretical Aspects of Aging,* Academic, New York, 1974.

Schweppe, John S.: *Man: A Remarkable Animal,* Research and Education Fund, Chicago, 1970.

Selye, Hans: *Stress without Distress,* Signet Books, New American Library, New York, 1975.

Smith, Mary Jane: "An Investigation of Changes in Judgment of Duration with Different Patterns of Auditory Information for Individuals Confined to Bed," unpublished doctoral dissertation, New York University, 1974.

Spuhler, J. N. (ed.): *Genetic Diversity and Human Behavior,* Aldine, Chicago, 1967.

Volicer, Beverly J., and Mary W. Burns: "Pre-Existing Correlates of Hospital Stress," paper delivered at University of Pennsylvania, Philadelphia, April 27–29, 1976.

# 2

# HEALTH PROMOTION*

Dorothy A. Jones
Rosellen Meighan Garrett

**H**uman beings continuously interact with a myriad of forces in the internal and external environment. These forces create a dynamic effect upon an individual at any point in time and can lead to alterations in the health state. As these changes occur, the client and the nurse become partners in preventing, assessing, solving, and evaluating disruptions in health. The purpose of this chapter is to focus upon *health promotion* through the constructs of *health assessment* and *health education*.

## HEALTH PROMOTION

The significance of *health promotion* is based upon a definition of health. Numerous definitions are available, but for purposes of this chapter *health* will be defined as an individual's dynamic and interactive response to multiple internal and external variables, at any given point in time, in any setting.

Health is therefore a process whose ultimate goal is to optimize each individual's realization of their human potential. Contingent upon the implementation of this definition is the individual's perception of health potential. *Health potential* is described as a human being's interpretation of a personalized ideal healthy state, which includes recognition of individual potentials, choices available to achieve goals, and awareness of the influence of values, culture, education, and past experiences on one's interpretation of health. *Health promotion,* then, comprises all planned means designed to optimize those human potentials chosen by the consumer of health care.

Through effective communication, recognition of individual uniqueness, establishment of a trust relationship, and effective health teaching, the nurse can respond to the consumer as a health facilitator and counselor. In this way nursing can offer guidance to individuals in all health settings, while encouraging the consumer to make independent decisions about health care needs.

### Nursing Responsibility

Nursing practice has traditionally obtained much data from patients, family, and friends, either solicited or nonsolicited, to aid in rendering care. Until recently, however, nurses' participation in assessment was relegated to observation and identification of changing signs and symptoms. Now,

---

* Section on Nursing Assessment and Physical Assessment written by Rosellen Meighan Garrett. Section on Health Teaching written by Dorothy A. Jones.

with the role of nurses expanding, responsibility for health promotion exists in both acute care and community health settings. Today, nurses are expected to clarify and document current health status, identify major and minor health problems, and plan care as well as refer patients to appropriate resources in order to meet health care needs.

To successfully achieve these expectations, the nurse's approach to data collection is critical. The practitioner must establish a sound rapport with individuals based on trust and mutual respect. The nurse must be attuned to both nonverbal and verbal cues communicated by the patient and respond accordingly. Decisions about health care must be based on sound judgment, careful assessment, and a solid theoretical framework. Responses to health problems should not be immediate or intuitive. Instead, interventions must be selected after careful analysis of all the facts. Nursing care should be developed within the parameters of standards set for nursing practice.

A nurse who utilizes appropriate resources as necessary can provide the client with comprehensive health care. Accountable, successful health care delivery by the nurse will be manifested by improved health status of the individual.

## Nursing Assessment

Nursing assessment aims at discovering where clients are in terms of their current health status. Determination of health potential can also be evaluated at this time. Three principal tools are included in assessment proceedings, and these are the *health history,* the *physical assessment,* and *diagnostic testing.* The health history and physical assessment are integral parts of the nursing process and are used at each level of nursing care. In each situation the emphasis and setting may vary, but the components remain the same. For example, first-level nursing care is most often conducted in community settings and focuses on prevention through health education, while third-level care is delivered in a hospital setting with the patient involved in an acute health crisis.

The sequencing of data collection and physical assessment may also vary with the setting. Usually the health history should precede the physical examination and be followed by appropriate diagnostic tests; however, during an acute illness (third-level nursing care), the health history may follow the physical assessment and the diagnostic tests. In such a situation the nurse may have to rely upon obtaining much of the health history from relatives or friends.

**Health history** Despite the development of sophisticated equipment for the physical examination and a multitude of diagnostic tests, the *health history* still remains the most valuable tool in assessing the client's health status. The health history enables the nurse to obtain crucial information which cannot be detected by even the most sensitive technical tools. The personality profile, which includes feelings, life-style, relationships, exercise patterns, eating habits, housing, and environmental factors, have as much to do with health as the quality of the heartbeat, blood pressure, and blood counts. Indeed, the factors unearthed in the interview and history taking are often related to the symptoms and the disruptions in health detected by other medical procedures. Excessive smoking, for example, may be the cause of shortness of breath or a productive cough, or it may aggravate a sinus condition. Similarly, the physiological and psychosocial components identified as precipitating factors in overeating need to be uncovered in order to treat the cardiovascular problems associated with obesity.

Proper health care involves recognition of the dynamic interaction between an individual and those potential stressors within the environment that can interfere with the healthy state. Therefore, it is incumbent upon the nurse to establish a mechanism for collecting data and identifying existing or potential stressors. History taking provides an opportunity for the nurse to interview, record, and synthesize data accurately, and thus offers a more personalized approach to health care delivery.

Collection and storage of information obtained during a health history and physical assessment are essential components of patient care. Inherent in any method of data collection is the development of a mechanism to record and retain all inputed information. With the large number of patient contacts encountered daily, it is difficult to remember all the facts of a particular patient problem, much less analyze current health disruptions. A dictaphone, magnetic memory storage, punch tape, written annotations, and computerized records are but a few methods available to receive, record, and retain patient data. Careful recording of information obtained during both an initial health assessment (IHA) and follow-up visits can give a comprehensive and continuous profile of the patient and the current health status.

**Interviewing** The art of eliciting and verifying information through *interviewing* is the chief tool in taking the health history. While there is a tendency to substitute a checklist or a printed form for a personalized interview, direct contact with the client is more effective. An interviewer with the proper attitude and effective technique can obtain all the information needed. Only a personal interview can establish the *trust* necessary to obtain much of the information. It can *clarify* the questions and answers and allow the nurse to identify clues for follow-up care. The information gained from questioning should be coordinated with observations. Notes taken by the nurse during an interview should always be reviewed with the client to ensure the accuracy of the information.

*Trust*   A feeling of *trust* results from repeated successful encounters that cumulatively have a significant impact. To establish a trusting relationship, the nurse must be glad to see the client and be genuinely interested in offering comprehensive nursing care, whatever the problem. A smile, a courteous introduction of oneself, an effort to make the client feel at ease, even a little casual conversation, go a long way toward *establishing rapport.* The starched face and the haughty bearing are out of place. The interview is a human encounter between equals who should be partners in health care. Anything that makes the client feel less human or less than an equal will distort the entire process.

Trust and rapport are not only conditions for eliciting information, they are essential to the relationship which is at the core of quality health care. Proper rapport will help allay the client's anxieties and gain the cooperation needed to plan health maintenance, implement treatment, and optimize all health potentials. While the nurse is appraising the client's health status, the client is appraising the personality, competence, and trustworthiness of the nurse.

The interview can also be the occasion to assess the client's health needs and indicate areas for health teaching. The questions may focus the client's attention on items that are often overlooked, such as diet activity and rest. As the interviewer explains the purpose of certain questions, the client can become more familiar with the intricate workings of the physical as well as behavioral body components. The interview can then become a two-way flow of information and a sharing of ideas.

*Setting*   While the manner and attitude of the interviewer are the crucial items in establishing rapport, the setting for the interview can add or detract from the results. *Physical privacy* helps to assure the client of professional secrecy and thus encourages discussion of matters which are sensitive. Comfortable chairs and the absence of a barrier, such as

a desk, between the interviewer and the client also help to create an ambience which encourages human interaction. Many professionals find that they get the best results when the setting does not look like an office at all. In practice, there is often little choice about the setting, so that manner and attitude of the nurse become even more important. Creating a private space will increase patient comfort and enhance the interviewing process.

*Listening*   Because the interview is a human event aimed at obtaining information needed to optimize human potentials, *a good interviewer must be a good listener.* Listening is a total activity, a reaching out to grasp the ideas, the feelings, and the person of the speaker. Listening requires the suppression of distractions, both internal and external. The interviewer who is rehearsing the next question is not listening. Fumbling with papers and losing eye contact also detract from listening.

Good listening involves more than having open ears. Posture, body language, and the tone of voice should be observed, as they frequently say more than the words themselves. When a seemingly neutral question, for example, causes the client to tense up or avoid eye contact, the good listener will know that he or she is close to something important and will pursue the matter. The poor listener is liable to go rushing on to another area.

The good listener is particularly alert for new and unexpected leads and follows these. The client's casual mention of a trip to Mexico, of a relative who has recently moved in with the family, or of a similar incident at age 15, may be a valuable clue that contributes greatly to the health history.

*Questioning*   If listening is the prime skill required in the interview, the *art of questioning* is second. It is important to remember that an interview can be *controlled* by the proper questioning. The good listener spots the vague or the evasive answer, asks that vague statements be clarified, and pursues areas where the client is evasive. Since people often avoid crucial points precisely because they are painful or embarrassing, structuring of questions to elicit more data is critical. If the interviewer is not sure that he or she has heard the information correctly, it is well to repeat what was heard and to ask for comments. This not only clarifies issues but assures the client that the nurse is listening and is interested. The right questions asked in the right order will keep the interview on the track, help rapport, and make sure that everything is covered in a reasonable time. Before discussing the various types of questions and their use, it is first necessary to stress the need for clarity.

A good question must be *clear to the client.* Unfortunately, medical personnel often forget this and lapse into terminology which is either vague or unknown to the layman. The simple question "How often do you void?" may be heard as "How often do you avoid?" Furthermore, most people do not think of themselves as "voiding." Better to ask, "How often do you pass water or urinate?" than to risk ambiguity. It is important not to talk down to the patient, but rather to evaluate each situation individually. A simple and clear question is the most efficient way to obtain information.

To ensure clarity, practicing with children will give the nurse the opportunity to find clear language for everyday medical terms, such as rales, epistaxis, lesion, dyspnea, and vertigo. Finally, the nurse should practice until every word used can be explained with a concrete example. If the nurse cannot give a clear, specific example of what is meant, the nurse's knowledge is of no practical use to the client.

*Types of questions* The nurse must decide on what type of questions to use. In general, each section should begin with a broad open-ended question, such as "Tell me about your vision" or "Describe a typical day's menu." These questions offer the client an opportunity to discuss issues of concern and offer the nurse a chance to pinpoint questions and clarify issues. From here you can elicit information using the so-called "leading" question, such as "Do you feel your problem with chest pain increases when you are under stress?" This offers direction and focus to the questioning and forces the patient to respond with specific data about a particular subject.

The so-called loaded question confronts the patient with information that often elicits an emotional response. Asking patients a question such as whether they feel they are going to die forces them to consider a highly emotional issue, whether or not they choose to respond.

Some discussions are embarrassing to either the nurse, the client, or both. People usually do not ask even friends if they have ever had a venereal disease or how much they earn. Yet such questions have to be asked in the course of health assessment. Fortunately, a potentially embarrassing question need not be so if the client knows why the information is needed. An explanation of the reason for the question is an important part of health education. The simple question, "Can you tell me about

anything that is upsetting you emotionally?" may have very different meanings to nurse and client. The nurse sees the question as a simple harmless request for information. The client may see it as requiring the revelation of personal secrets.

At times the client's individual thought processes reflect inner confusion, paranoia, or inability to cope with situations. These fears are intensified by the thought of exposure of such information to the practitioner. It is helpful if the practitioner prefaces questions by stating that "Many illnesses are caused by, or made worse by, our feelings or emotions. Can you tell me about anything that is upsetting you?"

Perceptions of the nurse and client are influenced by background, experience, and expectations. These factors affect the way each individual processes the raw data as presented and interpreted. While this processing cannot be avoided, it is necessary to be aware of the many variables that influence our data processing.

*Anxiety* When an individual seeks medical attention, be it for prevention of a health problem or intervention for an acute or chronic problem, there are varying degrees of anxiety present. The cause can be tension created by unusual presenting symptoms, past health history, previous experiences with the health care system, or fear of death, immobility, and pain. Fears can be manifested by uncooperative behavior, agitation, anger (nonverbal), loss of eye contact, or impatience. It is important that the nurse attempt to resolve some of this hostility as it could interfere with an accurate health history. Creating a private environment, being supportive while identifying the observed behavior, and establishing a sense of confidence will help create an atmosphere for discussion. Allowing the client to express stresses and concerns early in the interaction will help reduce anxiety. By providing the patient an opportunity to share any fears, the nurse may be able to clarify terms and issues and identify specific problems that may be creating unnecessary stress.

Helping the patient see the need for prevention, talking about current health problems, and clarifying potential health issues are all necessary components of health promotion. Reducing anxiety can relieve the patient of additional stresses and create an atmosphere in which the facilitation of health care can be enhanced by careful evaluation of reliable data.

*Misinformation* Certain causes of *misinformation,*

*misinterpretation,* and *omission* are so common that they deserve special emphasis. Clients will often give misinformation because they are eager to offer the answer they think is expected. The client may assure the interviewer that he or she eats a balanced diet because everyone is expected to do so. To avoid this sort of misinformation, it is necessary to ask the client for specific details which may reveal a typical breakfast, lunch, or dinner menu. Clients may give misinformation because they are ashamed of some of their habits. People do not like to admit that they smoke three packs of cigarettes a day, drink a pint of whiskey a day, or never exercise. If the interviewer is to get a true assessment of the situation, it is necessary to maintain a *nonjudgmental attitude* and to assure the client that all these items have meaning only when looked at as a total health picture.

In addition to misinformation, many *omissions* result from the client's failure to appreciate the significance of transient symptoms and episodes. The client may not mention pains after eating fried foods 6 months ago because there has been no reoccurrence. Because such an episode may be important, the nurse must use specific questions about food intolerances and make sure that the client does not focus only on the present or immediate past.

A hurried manner on the part of the interviewer, often caused by the pressure of work, can also lead to serious omissions. The client can be made to feel uneasy about taking up valuable time and in an effort to limit excess work may omit all but the most serious complaints. Often, minor—but potentially serious—health problems go unnoticed or untreated.

The nurse also has a responsibility to avoid misinterpreting or omitting data. Not only should verbal imput be noted, but *nonverbal* mannerisms as well. Increased restlessness, distraction, disinterest, and fatigue may be subtle manifestations of personal responses to a question. Gestures which indicate stress, such as facial movements, coughing, or drying of the mouth should all be noted, since they offer clues for further development of questions.

In addition, *agreement* between what an individual says and really means is essential if one is to assess a situation accurately. Diminishing distortion between the nurse and the client will improve health care delivery and the client's health status. The productivity of health care is not measured by how many clients are seen, but rather by the number of people helped. Careful collection of, and

reflection upon, all data elicited will help in making in-depth health assessments based on accurate perceptions.

Interviewing is an art which can aid the practitioner in this process. In order to learn the technique of interviewing, the nurse needs feedback from clients, supervisors, and observers. Through repetition, the art becomes part of the interviewer and the related skills are used with ease and accuracy.

**O**bservation   As soon as the nurse and client meet, observation of the client begins. Viewing the appearance, behavior, emotional state, perception, and outward expressions of the thought process of an individual is particularly important and may suggest specific questions to be asked about the client's physical, emotional, or psychological state. When the nurse detects a short attention span or lapses in memory, it will be necessary to supplement the client's information by consulting the family. In any event, significant material gathered from general observation throughout the health assessment process should be included in the Observational Summary Client Profile. This profile (see Table 2-1) may contain content which can serve as a basis for an observational assessment.

Patient motivation may also provide a reliable source for accuracy. Health intervention is usually

**TABLE 2-1**
OBSERVATIONAL SUMMARY CLIENT PROFILE

---

1   Appearance and behavior
   *a*   Body language, including posture, gesture, movement, facial expression, nonverbal responses, personal appearance
   *b*   Dress, grooming, and personal hygiene
   *c*   Speech: the quality, quantity, coherence, and relevance, as well as pattern
   *d*   Response to persons and things around the client
   *e*   Body build, distribution of weight, and distribution of body hair
2   Emotional state
   *a*   Dominant mood and emotional response
   *b*   Reaction to stressful situations—presence or absence of anxiety and patterns of coping with anxiety
   *c*   Level of dependence or independence prior to and during current health problem
3   Thought process
   *a*   Level of consciousness, response to stimuli (verbal, noise, light, touch, pain)
   *b*   Attention, concentration, and memory
   *c*   Comprehension—intellectual development relative to age
   *d*   Orientation to time, place, and persons
   *e*   Content, coherence, and relevance of information elicited by nurse
   *f*   Perception and understanding of health problem and goals of health plan
   *g*   Soundness of judgment and ability to make decisions in collaboration with the nurse

---

sought for relief of problems. Hence, one can assume that the symptoms and related health problems are valid.

**F**ormat of the Health History  While the format of the health history can vary with the nurse's personal preferences or conceptual scheme, certain key elements must be included and should be organized for the sake of both ease and completeness. The health history consists generally of the following components: (1) An initial client profile, (2) current health status, (3) past health history, (4) review of systems, (5) family health history, (6) personal and social history, and (7) summary client profile. (Table 2-2 develops in detail each component of the health history.)

The sequencing of these steps will vary with the client and the initial contact with the nurse. If the current health problem suggests a familial disease, the nurse may wish to move directly to the family health history. On the other hand, if the client exhibits an emotional problem, it is often well to examine the personal and social history before going any further. So long as the nurse has the total format clearly in mind and covers all points, the order may be adapted to the situation at hand. In recording the health history, care should be taken to be specific about dates and length of time of foreign travel, smoking habits, illnesses, etc. It is also important to record all data clearly and accurately, communicating all information in an easily interpreted manner. If, for some reason, the nurse does not make an inquiry into an item or examine a body part, it should be recorded as "not explored at this time" or "examination deferred" and not left to speculation. The information contained within the patient's record is a legal document, and, as nurses, we are accountable for its accurate input.

*Initial client profile*  The initial client profile identifies the client and the informant, if other than the client. It is a brief, general description of the client. In certain situations it may be important to note who referred the client and the reason for the contact. Table 2-2 reflects data which aids in giving a psychosocial as well as physiological background on each individual.

*Current health status*  If the client has come for a checkup and has no current health problems, proceed to the past health history. If the client has a current health problem, the nurse should record the information about the factors listed in Table 2-2. The information should be recorded in the client's own words. No attempt should be made to translate the client's words into a diagnosis.

The data should be recorded in a logical, chronological sequence that is complete, concise, and readable. *Pertinent negatives,* that is, problems that are suggested by the clinical picture but which are not currently present, should be noted. For example, when a 16-year-old client complains of increased thirst and frequent urination, the nurse may suspect insulin deficiency. If, after inquiry, it is clear that the client lacks other signs, such as excessive eating, weight loss, or blurring of vision, the absence of these signs should be noted.

Information about the client's response to a problem(s) and its effect on individual life-style and the family should be obtained. The client who denies current health problems while seeking treatment will often resist using even simple means of intervention like bed rest. These clients require special handling to assist them in recognizing problems and accepting appropriate interventions. Sound health care demands that these issues of both a physical as well as a psychosocial nature be identified and resolved as they can seriously affect the course of a health problem.

*Health history*  The health history is recorded in chronological order for each of the headings in Table 2-2. Here the nurse is attempting to discover the client's pattern of health care, as well as strengths and weaknesses which may influence present and future health potentials.

Data collected at this point will enhance the health history by providing information of events that occurred earlier but which may have direct bearing on the present problem. Having traveled to another country 2 months prior to the onset of symptoms may significantly influence the patient's treatment.

*Review of systems*  The review of systems is intended to unearth previously noted health problems and to get detailed information about the duration, severity, and precipitants of all disruptions in the health state. Frequently this review will detect problems and related physical and/or psychosocial changes which belong in the current health section but which the client overlooked.

In line with the principles of interviewing previously presented, simple, ordinary language should be used to elicit data. Table 2-2 focuses upon specific areas which should be developed during the health history and physical examination. Asking additional questions as to location, character, type,

**TABLE 2-2**
HEALTH HISTORY FORMAT

1   Initial client profile
Identification of informant
Age and stage of development of client
Sex
Ethnic background
Marital status
Occupation
General physical description (size, condition of skin, hair, nails)
Reason for seeking health care
Source of referral

2   Current health status
Date of onset of problem(s)
Health prior to onset of problem(s)
Mode of onset of problem(s)
Duration and course (chronological progress or change in problem)
Current status of problem
Characteristics: Location, intensity, constancy, radiation, frequency
Influencing factors: Precipitating, relieving, time of day, season, position, relation to other symptoms, relation to body function, recent infection
Pertinent negative data
Previous personal or family history of current problem
Previous treatment of problem and client's response
Effect of problem on client and family
Review of information received with the client

3   Health history
General health and strength
Growth and development as a child
Previous pattern of and response to health care
Childhood diseases
Infectious diseases
Medical illnesses and/or problems
Surgical procedures
Injuries
Allergies
Immunizations
Blood transfusions
Foreign travel
Past and present use of medication and reactions
Hospitalizations

4   Review of systems
*General state of health:* Loss or gain of weight, weakness, fatigue, fever, other general symptoms
*Skin:* Texture, temperature changes, remarkable pigmentation, sun sensitivity, undue dryness or perspiration, pruritus, rashes, growths, breaks in skin, acne, bruising, dermatitis, hair texture and distribution, minute hemorrhage of skin, urticaria
*Head:* Headaches, trauma, vertigo, syncope, unsteadiness
*Eyes:* Visual acuity, redness, pruritus, pain, blurred vision, diplopia, lacrimation, edema, spots, light sensitivity, hemorrhage, scotomas, strabismus, discharges, inflammation, date of last eye examination
*Ears:* Hearing acuity, earaches, discharge, tinnitus, infection, vertigo
*Nose and sinuses:* Altered sense of smell, pain, tenderness, discharge, sneezing, obstruction, epistaxis, colds, polyps
*Mouth:* Altered sense of taste, mouth breathing, sore tongue, bleeding gums or mucous membrane, lesions, abscesses, saliva, mechanism, difficulty in chewing, caries, date of last dental examination
*Throat:* Sore throat, tonsils, hoarseness, altered voice, dysphagia, upper respiratory infections
*Neck:* Pain, stiffness, swelling, masses, injury, enlargement of the thyroid
*Breasts:* Alteration in size and shape, pain, tenderness, lumps, nipple discharge, edema, dimpling, nipple changes
*Respiratory system:* Frequency and nature of infections, pain, dyspnea, wheezing, foreign bodies, cough, amount and nature of sputum, hemaptysis, number of pillows used at night, stridor

*Cardiovascular system:* Pain, edema, palpitations, difficulty in breathing, leg cramps, hypertension, lips, fingers, or toes turning blue, syncope, orthopnea
*Gastrointestinal system:* Altered appetite, food intolerances, dysphagia, dyspepsia, pyrosis, nausea, vomiting, flatulence, diarrhea, jaundice, constipation, altered bowel habits, hematemesis, melena, rectal polyps, hemorrhoids, rectal bleeding, cramping, encopresis
*Urinary system:* Dysuria, burning, urgency, frequency, hesitancy, incontinence, dribbling, altered character or odor of urine, retention, decreased urination, polyuria, hematuria, pyuria, urethral discharge, enuresis
*Reproductive system:* Pain, burning, itching, discharge, edema, secondary sex characteristics, sexual activity and satisfaction, dyspareunia, birth control methods and side effects, venereal disease
*Gynecologic system:* Onset of menses, duration and amount of flow, interval between periods, date of last period, vaginal infections, menstrual tension, metrorrhagia, amenorrhea, menorrhagia or hypermenorrhea, polymenorrhea, leukorrhea, dysmenorrhea, cessation of menses, date of last Pap test.
*Obstetric system:* Number of pregnancies, number and types of deliveries, abortions, stillbirths, miscarriages, premature births, number of living children with their birth weights, length of labor, complications of pregnancy, delivery and postpartum period
*Musculoskeletal system:* Pain, weakness, cramps, edema, altered range of motion, deformities, ataxia, altered temperature and color of extremities, altered gait
*Neuropsychiatric system:* Altered consciousness, vertigo, seizures, weakness, somnolence, insomnia, amnesia, altered disposition, altered emotional stability, level of anxiety, altered coordination, tics, tremors, paresis, paralysis, paresthesia, twitching, altered attention span
*Hematopoietic system:* Bleeding tendencies, bruising, anemia, dyscrasias, blood type
*Endocrine system:* Temperature intolerances, abnormal growth and development, alteration in weight, remarkable pigmentation, undue dryness or perspiration, hirsutism, altered secondary sex characteristics, altered disposition, palpitations, drowsiness, polyuria, polydypsia, polyphagia, anorexia
*Lymphatic system:* Tender or enlarged area in the cervical, axillary inguinal region

5   Family health history
Current state of health and ages of living spouse, parents, siblings, children
Cause of and age at death of spouse, parents, siblings, children, grandparents, aunts, and uncles
Familial diseases: Diabetes mellitus, cancer, arthritis, heart disease, allergies, epilepsy, hypertension, mental problems, migraine headache, tuberculosis, other

6   Personal and social history
Daily living patterns: Diet, exercise, sleep, elimination, hygiene, lifestyle, stress, hobbies
Habits: Use of alcohol, cigarettes, coffee, drugs, vitamins
Relationships: Family, friends, significant others
Occupation: Current and past, position, length of time, physical conditions, attitude toward work, satisfactions, pressures, hazards
Environment: Living conditions, number in family, pets
Educational background
Community activities
Prior armed forces affiliation
Religion
Level of income and health insurance

7   Summary client profile
Summary and/or evaluation of health status
Health needs/problems
Origin and precipitating factors
Client's reactions to needs/problems
Client's strengths and assets
Client's support system

severity, and duration of problems, as well as current treatment, is appropriate.

*Family health history* The family health history is useful in detecting the presence or probability of genetic or familial diseases. The information obtained here can also be invaluable in planning preventive regimens during first-level nursing practice (see Table 2-2). If problems are suspected or the family history is positive, diagnostic testing can be done to support findings or rule out the presence of health problems. Accumulation of data related to the family health history can be incorporated into the overall assessment and provide additional data when analyzing patient information.

*Personal and social history* The personal and social history supplies information about the client as a person, as a member of a family, and as a member of society. Here, too, is an opportunity to educate the client with regard to those aspects of daily life which may be causing less than optimal functioning. A life-style characterized by hectic activity, that allows no time for exercise and too little time for sleep, reduces health potential and sets up conditions which can theoretically alter one's health state, even when it does not breed illness. Many clients, moreover, have poor nutritional habits which they mistakenly believe can be offset by vitamin supplements and over-the-counter pills. Particular attention should be paid to stress-producing situations at home and at work which can predispose, if not actually cause, many altered health states.

Inquiries about religion are relevant to the extent that a person's beliefs may prescribe or proscribe some dietary or medical regime. Religion may also become an identified source of support as serious health problems are uncovered.

*Summary client profile* The summary client profile is a brief summation of the total collection and evaluation of all data relevant to an individual's health status. It identifies health needs and problems, elicits the origin of problems and precipitating stress factors, assesses a client's reactions to health problems, determines an individual's perception of health, and recognizes personal strengths, assets, and support systems. This summary client profile indicates specific direction for the physical examination and future diagnostic tools.

**Diagnostic tests** Diagnostic testing is decided upon usually after a careful physical assessment and health history are completed. The nurse may or may not be involved in prescribing testing. Generally with a routine health assessment, specific tests may be decided upon as a matter of protocol. These tests provide baseline information for future health assessments. Additional tests needed for a more comprehensive patient profile can be determined by the nurse and/or physician on the basis of ascribed proceedings.

However, when the patient must be hospitalized or a more complicated listing is determined, this decision is usually made by the physician. In all situations it is the nurse who must prepare the patient for all components of the diagnostic procedure.

**Physical assessment** The nurse begins the *physical assessment* on the initial contact with the client. Indeed, a systematic, unobtrusive observation is perhaps the single most important technique to learn in the process. The actual physical examination becomes an extension and completion of those observations already made.

Establishment of a good rapport with the client during the taking of the health history will help make the physical assessment both a pleasant and educational experience. To ensure this, the nurse should continue to show consideration and respect for the client. Being attentive to individual client concerns may help reduce anxiety and improve the patient's cooperation. The setting should be conducive to this process. A private, warm, well-lighted room and adequate draping will provide the patient with personal dignity and security. The part(s) of the body to be examined should be accessible to the nurse. Therefore, no clothing should interfere with the examination. Care should be taken to ensure that both the nurse and the client are in comfortable and appropriate positions. Hands and instruments should be clean and warm, as cold instruments can be startling and cause tenseness. In order to provide a relaxed environment for the patient, the room should be free of interfering noises and extraneous environmental sound.

Clients often experience some anxiety during an examination. The nurse should allay anxiety by explaining each step of the procedure and eliciting an informed cooperation. A systematic and structured approach based upon in-depth knowledge of the normal range of responses helps to establish the client's and the nurse's personal confidence in the process.

Height, weight, temperature, pulse, respiration rate, and blood pressure should be recorded at the beginning of the examination. When there is any suspicion that anxiety about the examination has led to distorted readings, a second reading should be taken when the client is more at ease.

**M**ethods of Examination   The methods of examination include *visual inspection, percussion, auscultation,* and *palpation.* These should be utilized in an orderly and systematic manner so that important areas are not overlooked. The sequence of methods, while always beginning with visual inspection, will vary according to the body part being examined. For example, examination of the heart and lungs proceeds from visual inspection to palpation, percussion, and auscultation. In contrast, the abdominal examination proceeds to auscultation, percussion, and palpation. General principles of inspection, percussion, auscultation, and palpation will be discussed here. Specific physical assessment techniques and findings are discussed in detail in relation to cellular growth (Chap. 4), immune system response (Chap. 8), metabolism (Chap. 15), fluids and electrolytes (Chap. 11), oxygenation (Chap. 22), and perception and coordination (Chap. 31).

None of these methods yields any significant results unless the examiner is familiar with the normal variations. Without that yardstick, abnormalities in color, location, position, contour, movement, symmetry, and comparison will be overlooked, and normal conditions taken as abnormal. While textbooks can provide checklists and some hints, only experience and constant practice will teach the norms themselves.

*Inspection*   Four of the senses, namely, sight, hearing, smell, and touch, are involved in visual inspection. They should be used to determine not only those items mentioned in taking the *health history,* but also such specifics as body posture and general stature, gait as well as range of joint movement, skin color, symmetry and pigmentation, breath odor, discharge from lesions, edema, and cyanosis. Emotional reaction and disposition should also be evaluated at this time. The purpose is not merely to verify information given by the client, but to detect what the client cannot see or may have overlooked.

*Percussion*   The striking or thumping of the body surface, primarily the chest and abdomen, to produce sound and touch vibration is termed *percussion.* The objective of percussion is to determine the density, location, boundary, size, and shape of the underlying structures and organs. This is

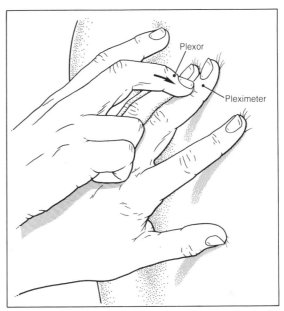

**FIGURE 2-1**
Percussion.

achieved by comparing the vibrations produced with those in the surrounding tissues. Abnormal findings will be due to fluid, air, or a solid mass present in an organ.

To percuss, the middle fingers are usually used. Place one finger, the *pleximeter,* on the body surface with the other fingers and the palm of the hand relaxed and off the skin. Press firmly while using the other middle finger, the *plexor* (the finger striking the blow) slightly bent to strike a sharp quick blow on the distal phalanx of the pleximeter between the cuticle and the first joint. Be sure the fingernail of the plexor is short to prevent injuring the pleximeter. The action must be in the flexed wrist, and the striking finger must be withdrawn after each strike. (See Fig. 2-1.)

*Percussion sounds,* or notes, have qualities of tones which reveal specific density of the body part being examined. The percussion sounds that are produced are called resonance, tympany, hyperresonance, dullness, and flatness. A *resonant* sound is heard over body parts that have both air and mass, such as the lungs. It has a low pitch that is easily heard. *Tympany* is a higher-pitched, hollow sound that is sustained as in a kettledrum. It is heard on body parts that have air in them, such as the stomach and bowel. *Hyperresonance* is an intense "booming" sound resulting from increased air, decreased tissue, or both and is of a lower pitch than normal resonance. It can be heard in patients with emphysema. *Dullness* results from increased density and solidity and is a high-pitched "thud" sound. A *flat* sound is heard in the absence of resonance. It is heard over parts of the body that have mostly solid mass, such as muscle. *Dullness* is a "thudlike" high-pitched sound that does not resonate. It can be heard when listening to the chest of a patient with obstructive lung disease.

The characteristics of sounds that are applicable to auscultation, as well as to percussion, are frequency or pitch, intensity, loudness, quality, and duration. *Frequency* or *pitch* refers to the rapidity with which vibrations occur. The faster the vibration, the higher the pitch. The reverse is also true. *Intensity* refers to the tone produced by sound, while *loudness* refers to the amplification of that sound. *Quality* of a sound refers to that intensity or pitch that allows us to distinguish tones. *Duration* of a sound helps differentiate between those that are dull and those that are sustained over a period of time. When fluid is present in the lungs, the duration of a vibration produced upon percussion, and the resonance of a sound is decreased, and the duration shortened.

*Auscultation*   Listening to sounds produced by the function of body organs, such as the heart, lungs, and stomach is termed *auscultation*. This method of examination can be performed by placing the ear against a body surface (immediate auscultation), but a *stethoscope* (mediated auscultation) is usually employed. The *bell* of the stethoscope picks up low-pitched sounds, while the *diaphram* picks up high-pitched sounds. It is advisable to use a stethoscope equipped with both. (See Chap. 22 for a complete discussion of lung auscultation.)

Auscultation is considered the most intricate and demanding method of examination. It requires concentration on one sound at a time, identifying it accurately and interpreting it as normal or abnormal. By placing the stethoscope firmly against the organ being examined, extraneous sound can be avoided. As with all methods of physical assessment, auscultation can be learned only through experience with normal variations of sounds in order to distinguish the pertinent characteristics. Care should be taken to limit movement of the stethoscope to avoid the interference of external noise.

*Palpation*   The use of the sense of touch in examining the accessible parts of the body is termed *palpation.* By feeling or pressing on the body, it is possible to examine organs, glands, skin texture, temperature, vessels, muscles, and bones in order to learn about their structure and function. During palpation, organ size, symmetry, and additional masses as well as organ location should be checked. The part of the body being examined dictates the type of palpation used, whether light or deep. All palpation should be slow and deliberate, progressing from gentle to stronger pressure in order to detect the presence or absence of organ enlargement, tenderness, pulsations, pain, swelling, masses, muscle spasms or rigidity, crepitus, fluid, sound vibrations, and abnormal texture. A light touch, using the tips of the fingers, is best to examine organs near the surface of the body, such as lymph nodes. The palm of the hand serves best for determining sound vibrations, while the back of the hand is most sensitive to temperature (Fig. 2-2a).

Both hands are needed to palpate deeper structures. In Fig. 2-2b you will note that one hand is placed on top of the other, palms down. The lower hand is placed lightly and loosely on the abdomen, and the other hand is used to apply the pressure. A technique called *ballottement* is used to examine for fluid in a body cavity and for rebound tenderness. In this technique, pressure is applied to the area and then rapidly released. If fluid is present, a wavelike effect will be observed, and tenderness will be experienced as pain on release.

If the client is experiencing tenderness or pain during the examination, the affected area should be examined last. The client who has difficulty relaxing during the examination should be asked to take deep breaths. Bending the knees will help muscle relaxation during examination of the abdomen.

It is important that bilateral assessments be made, especially when there are suspected neurological disruptions. In addition, organs such as the lungs and kidneys should be compared with one another so that a more discriminating examination can be given and more accurate results posited.

**E**quipment   The nurse should initially rely upon the hands, the senses, knowledge, and experience in order to conduct an accurate physical assessment. Necessary equipment includes flashlight, otoscope with ear and nose specula, ophthalmoscope, stethoscope, sphygmomanometer or blood pressure cuff, tuning fork for testing hearing, percussion or reflex hammer, tongue blade or depressor, safety pin and cotton, vaginal speculum plus gloves and a lubricant for the pelvic and rectal examination, tape measure, thermometer, and paper and pen or pencil. All these items will provide additional information for the examiner but cannot replace the personal skill, expertise, and experience of the nurse.

**Formulation of the problem list** When the health assessment is completed and specific diagnostic tests ordered, the nurse can develop a list of the client's nursing problems. *Pertinent data,* in this context, means any physical, psychological, socioeconomic, and demographic findings that, in the nurse's judgment, are deviations from normal. These changes, in turn, constitute a problem for the client as they interfere with optimum use of the human potential. Each problem should be stated accurately on the basis of current conclusive evidence from the health history, physical assessment, and laboratory studies. This evidence is both subjective and objective and is synthesized by the nurse according to his or her understanding and interpretation of the problems. The problem list is the basis for the health plan aimed at optimizing an individual's potential as well as preventing illness and, where necessary, solving current health problems. The assessment of each problem is then followed by a plan of care incorporating the nursing process into each level of patient care. Physical problems, such as pain and dyspnea, and psychological problems including anxiety and alteration in behavior, along with sociocultural, environmental, and occupational constraints, all need to be clearly identified and interventions planned in order to optimize the healthy state.

## HEALTH TEACHING

In order to facilitate health promotion, nurses have a responsibility to actively participate in health teaching. Nursing plays a critical role in helping members of our society sustain, retain, and regain their optimum health status.

### Nursing Role

According to a recent statement by the American Nurses' Association, "The nursing care delivery system is a distinct subtype within the health care delivery system . . . providing health teaching to selected clients in the achievement or maintenance of health. . . ."[1] Nurses must make patient teaching a priority which is assigned, documented, and evaluated; the nurse must be held accountable for patient teaching just as he or she is for taking vital signs.[2]

In a study conducted by Pohl, the majority of nurses questioned believed that patient teaching was a responsibility of nursing and an important

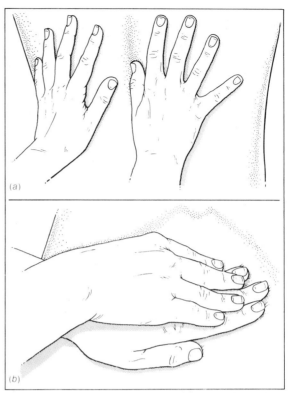

**FIGURE 2-2**
Palpation.

component of their work.[3] Powell's study of teaching with patients who sustained a myocardial infarction revealed that the majority of nurses felt that patient teaching was a priority, even though they were not teaching.[4]

Much of the discrepancy over the role of the nurse as a teacher has been long-standing. Lack of knowledge on the part of the nurse, insufficient time to teach, poor preparation for teaching, and physician dominance have all contributed to the confusion. Although patients often want to be taught new information, they do not view the nurse as the prime dispenser of this information. In a study done by Pender on patient reception of health education, physicians and nurses were both viewed as giving related health information if so asked. However, 105 patients said they received the most helpful information from the physician, while only 24 received such information from the nurse.[5] Other studies, however, argue this point, stating that nurses have given the most helpful information on preoperative teaching[6] and suggesting that teaching is a clearly identifiable area for nurses.

It is time to state unequivocally that patient teaching *is* a responsibility of the nurse in all settings. Nurses should be held accountable for delivery of this professional service. They must provide time for teaching and possess necessary knowledge to educate the public. To clearly establish the teaching role for the professional nurse, nurses must document and evaluate the effects of these teaching activities on the maintenance, retention, and attainment of maximum health.

Patient teaching facilitates the process of improving health by clarifying existing alternatives, setting limits, relieving patients' doubts, and redirecting patients in their life goals.[7] Nursing must assume this role as health educator and improve patient care delivery by actively becoming involved in the health teaching-learning process.

**Teaching within the levels of nursing care**

Opportunities for health teaching exist everywhere. The potential for enacting a teaching-learning encounter is readily available in the community or acute-care setting, with children or adults, and in both formal and informal ways.

Within the various levels of nursing practice the nursing role as a health educator can be identified. The goal of teaching in *first-level* nursing practice is prevention. Therefore, identification of high-risk populations through successful screening programs, research, interviewing, and careful history taking is critical. The learner can be found in multiple situations, and the determination of the teaching-learning encounter can be planned on an individual or group basis.

During a routine health examination, for example, the patient may be found to be overweight. Given a particular current health status, the patient is encouraged to lose weight. This involves nutritional teaching as well as identification of other variables that may aid in weight reduction. A selected plan is developed specifically for the patient with the ultimate goal of health promotion through intensive weight loss.

On the other hand, atherosclerosis and elevated cholesterol levels have been identified as potential risk factors in the development of cardiac ischemic changes. Small and large group teaching-learning seminars can be planned in local communities and industrial settings to help reduce this risk. Preventive measures such as diet and exercise can be taught. Screening programs can be developed to further identify a population at risk. The objective of the teaching-learning transaction can be to decrease ischemic changes within these high-risk groups through various interventions.

Early detection of disruptions in the healthy state are noted during *second-level* nursing care. Here, specific nursing problems can be identified in relation to a particular health problem. Nursing interventions include many teaching components such as nutrition and drug therapy. The goal of these teaching encounters is to provide the learner with knowledge about therapeutic measures that can help restore the healthy state. Teaching-learning transactions may also include instruction related to diagnostic tests, as well as elements of preventing reoccurrence complications.

During the *third level* of nursing practice, teaching occurs in response to acute health needs, with an awareness of the implications a particular health problem can have on the patient's future. Initial teaching is directed toward informing the patient about immediate life changes and implications of specific changes on life-style. Therefore, teaching-learning transactions will be geared toward preparing patients for immediate diagnostic procedures, current therapies, and pre- and postoperative interventions. Since the stress of hospitalization often interferes with learning, especially when patients are in intensive-care settings where anxiety is high, long-range teaching is minimal.[8] While teaching most often occurs on an individual basis, small groups and discussions may be feasible at this time.

As the more acute health problems subside, long-term teaching plans are developed. This phase of instruction begins to prepare the patient for discharge and rehabilitation. *Fourth-level* nursing care focuses on rehabilitation and the return of the patient to a maximum state of health. Follow-up of teaching plans begun in the acute-care setting should continue. These plans may include referral to other community health agencies as well as follow-up by the acute care facility. Prevention of further health problems or the recurrence of chronic problems is an important component of this level of care. Evaluation and reassessment of the achievement of objectives are of critical importance. If compliance to ascribed teaching strategies fails, a reassessment of the patient's needs and teaching-learning transactions is in order.

**Teaching-Learning Process**

The *teaching-learning process* is a transaction between the teacher and the learner, in which a specific learning objective(s) is met through a planned sequence of activities. These activities include selection of learning objectives, definition of content, identification of a teaching strategy, and evaluation of the encounter.

Education by another must always be a process that is planned and executed according to preconceived ideas. According to Tift, "the process of health education . . . facilitates each learner's discovery about the body and mind and feelings in order to maximize a particular potential."[9] By engaging in the teaching-learning process, the *learner* interacts with multiple internal and external experiences which lead to an eventual change in attitude and behavior. The *teacher* becomes the facilitator of this interactive process by helping the learner achieve goals through a mutually agreed-upon plan.

**Philosophy of adult education**  A *philosophy* in education is the attempt to help students develop insight into the comprehensiveness, penetration, and flexibility displayed by an individual as he or she attacks problems.[10] The philosophical approach to adult learning makes the basic assumption that learning is a lifelong process which begins at birth and lasts until death. A philosophy is usually derived after a careful assessment of the beliefs of a given group. For purposes of this chapter, the philosophy of the adult educational approach to learning will be used.

The philosophy of *adult education* evolves from a comprehension of two terms, andragogy and pedagogy. *Andragogy* is the art and science of *helping* adults learn, as distinguished from *pedagogy,* which is the art of teaching children. Adult education focuses upon the learner as a whole unit, indicating the need for harmony among all parts. The learning experience is viewed as being holistic rather than segmented.

According to Knowles the androgogical approach to learning is based upon four characteristics. These are the following:[11]

As individuals grow, the emerging adult's self-concept shifts gradually from that of a dependent personality toward becoming more of a self-directed individual. As this process continues, the adult begins to assume increased responsibility for personal learning experiences.

As individuals begin to accumulate a growing body of personal experiences, they begin to value their own learning. This suggests that learning will be better in situations which utilize the learner's previous learning experiences.

One's readiness to learn appears to be contingent more upon developmental tasks and emerging social roles than merely biological and academic development. Therefore, learning seems to improve when associated with a need.

Learners appear better able to retain knowledge or skills that will help them cope with a specific problem presently facing them than knowledge or skills acquired for their own sake.

These characteristics help formulate a basic framework within which the teaching of adults can be planned and developed. This basic philosophical approach allows for the individuality of the learner and offers the teacher some guidelines for development of an effective teaching plan.

**Types of learning**  The way an individual learns is often determined by a person's *cognitive style.* This refers to the way (or style) in which a person plans or controls the direction of a learning experience. Many events determine how, over the course of time, one acquires a learning style.

As a person interacts with the environment, inherited traits and past experiences are brought to the learning situation and contribute to the ability to learn. An individual's predisposition interacts with the learning environment itself to affect growth, behavior, and human development. According to Gagne,[12] there are eight types or sets of learning that the learner engages in throughout life. These include signal learning, stimulus-response learning, chaining, verbal association, multiple discrimination, inferencing, concept learning, and problem solving. As these learning types are briefly discussed below, note the hierarchy of learning that begins to evolve, indicating a growth from a more simple to a more complex learning style.

*Signal learning* refers to a generalized and somewhat diffuse response to an established signal. It is an involuntary response similar to the Pavlovian conditioned response. For example, the fear response, which may cause stimulation of the generalized flight-fright syndrome, can be initiated, but is not voluntarily controlled.[13] *Stimulus response learning,* on the other hand, involves more precise musculoskeletal voluntary movements. It reflects deliberation and decision as to when and where an action will be evoked. Generally, a reward is generated for a correct response to a signal which contributes to the reinforcement of the action.

The critical difference between signal learning and stimulus response learning is the process of discrimination afforded by the latter. Skinner referred to this type of learning as *discriminated operant.* The child quickly learns this process early in life when words are first uttered and then praised by the parent. The child begins to discriminate between those vocalizations which bring this reward and those which do not. With the initial reinforcement comes a continuation and development of the response.

A *chain* is a connection or sequencing of events, words, or symbols. An individual will learn a certain word, which will have a particular meaning for that person. This is then followed by *verbal association.* The learning of a chain that is verbal represents the beginning of language formation. Therefore, if a *chaining* of cues leads the child to believe "X" equals a doll, then at some point the verbal association leads to the sudden utterance of the word *doll,* and the beginning of a language link is made in the learning process.

*Multiple discrimination* requires further isolation of thought. A child chains together a series of stimuli to equal the word *car.* However, although cars may look alike, each may be different in terms of color, size, and shape. In order to achieve multiple discrimination a degree of *inferencing* (deducting) occurs. This phenomenon is a prominent characteristic of multiple discrimination.[14] It is a type of learning that allows the individual to distinguish cars from trucks and animals from plants. Some suggest it is a form of "rote" learning, inferring memorization of facts on the part of the learner.

*Concept learning* means learning which responds to stimuli in terms of abstract properties like color, shape, and position as opposed to concrete physical properties.[15] In this type of learning the learner is offered a variety of stimuli which incorporate the distinguishing properties of a concept so as to differentiate it from other forms. Concept learning is often a cumulative process occurring over time.

The activity that ensues can lead to a lengthy connection and gradual building of events until a specific activity with meaning is reached. The individual will then know that if certain sets of cues are present that which is being discussed must be a clearly defined object such as an animal or plant. Concept learning allows the learner to make assumptions about a subconcept based on identification of specific characteristics of a broader concept. In a formal sense, a principle is a chain of two or more concepts.[16] *Principle learning* allows for inductive and deductive reasoning based on knowledge of facts. Inherent in this type of learning is an element of *discovery.* The learner puts together or observes the presence of a specific set of certain concepts and "discovers," as it were, what results when ideas combine under a certain set of circumstances, and why.

The final type of learning involves the ability to problem solve a new situation by relying upon learned principles and concepts. This type of learning involves looking at a new situation, thinking it through, and "discovering" a new way of handling a problem. *Problem solving* allows for creativity and generation of new ideas which incorporate "higher order principles"[17] in order to reach a successful solution.

Many other learning theorists have suggested learning patterns which are similar to those of Gagne but differ in terminology. Thorndike's so-called "trial and error" type of learning closely resembles early signal learning, while Skinner's behavioristic model of *classical conditioning* is more aligned to stimulus response learning. In addition, the *phenomenological* school of thought views human beings as basically good with a potential to be better.[18] Carl Rogers has identified five essential components of this type of learning which are: (1) personal involvement, (2) self-initiation, (3) pervasiveness, (4) evaluation by the learner, (5) and comprehension of the meaning.[19]

Dewey, on the other hand, believes the educational experience should allow for *freedom* of choice within an environment that provides the learner with choices. An educational aim must be founded upon the intrinsic activities and needs of a given individual to be educated.[20] After identification of needs, the educator must select a learning climate that will liberate the intellectual potential in order to prepare the learner for future life experiences.

A final theory that should be mentioned in terms of health teaching is Lewin's *cognitive field theory.* It suggests that a field is considered to be the totality of coexisting facts, external and internal, which are conceived as mutually interdependent.[21] Learning is viewed as a whole, and each problem is solved by looking at all the components and making decisions as new perceptions are gained.

There are many other theoretical frameworks upon which a teaching-learning transaction can be based. All are interrelated and present specific patterns for learning which the teacher and learner will use in evolving the teaching-learning process.

**Factors influencing health teaching and learning** There are many factors which influence health teaching and learning. Of prime importance is the value an individual places on health. This is a personal decision and has significant influence on overall health perception. Many additional physical, psychological, sociocultural, and environmental factors interact with one's health perception and enhance or detract from the teaching-learning transaction. Since each person or groups of individuals will respond differently to each teaching-learning encounter, careful assessment must be made of influencing variables prior to implementing the teaching plan.

**P**hysical Variables  Many physical changes occur during one's life that influence the ability to learn. Age can affect memory retention, speed of response and reaction to a procedure, and comprehension. *Loss of body function* can diminish perception, decrease physical skills, and alter manual dexterity. Changes in *visual* and *auditory* acuity can alter the teaching-learning process and cause distortion of information. *Immobility* and decreased or diminished perception due to *sensory loss* can prolong teaching-learning and interfere with one's ability to perform normal activities.

Changes in perception caused by cerebrovascular trauma or cellular growth can influence the rate of learning and alter an individual's cognitive abilities. Loss of the sense of *touch* can interrupt normal proprioceptors and disrupt performance of manual skills. *Communication disturbances* caused by alteration in the speech center, oral surgery, or changes in verbal expression can limit interpretation of new information and frustrate the learner.

Diminished cerebral circulation can cause mental cloudiness and confusion and affect retention of data. *Fatigue,* precipitated by anemia, inflammation, or changes in oxygenation, decreases the learner's attention span and tolerance for new information. Accumulation of *toxic* substances in the body due to disruption in metabolism or fluids and electrolytes can precipitate physical changes that will interfere with retention and absorption of information.

*Pain* will distract the learner's attention and decrease attention span. It can also distort perception and interpretation of sensory input. *Anesthesia* and medication, on the other hand, can dull perceptions and decrease the intake of new data.

**P**sychological Variables  An individual's personality as well as emotional response to potential or actual disruptions in health can interfere with learning. *Anxiety* in moderation serves as a learning stimulus. However, when an individual is confronted with the *stress* of hospitalization, *fear* of surgery, or sudden illness, anxiety can interfere with the teaching-learning process. *Depression* associated with loss of a bodily function along with *grieving* about

real or anticipated fears can distract the learner and interfere with retention of knowledge.

In early grief responses the patient may be *angry* and *deny* the need for any medical assistance. For these individuals a particular health problem does not exist, and therefore teaching is viewed as unnecessary. Other *coping mechanisms,* including *rationalization,* may be used by the patient in response to a particular crisis. Until the patient can accept a particular health problem, teaching becomes almost impossible. It should be pointed out that for some individuals this process may take months. When a particular health problem threatens an individual's future, life-style, occupation, or body competence, health teaching may be most difficult to institute.

Changes in *bodily appearance* often present the patient with much conflict. These alterations can serve to threaten an already unstable *ego* and affect one's *self-esteem.* Therefore the individual may be unwilling to learn or be depressed and unable to hear what is being taught.

As some health problems may be terminal, *developmental* growth and maturity may be interrupted before *self-actualization* is reached. This may create an added stress because the patient may focus on goals that cannot be achieved. This problem must be resolved before effective teaching can begin.

Patients must first cope with any specific emotional problems they have before they can engage in active learning. At times, counseling may be required prior to enacting an effective teaching plan. Unless the learner is ready to participate in a teaching-learning transaction and accept needed change, patient teaching should be avoided. Patients will determine when they are *ready* to learn and often indicate what they want to know. They can be *motivated* by the intrinsic reward of improving their health status or preventing a particular health problem for which they are at risk.

**S**ociocultural Variables  Many sociocultural variables exist which influence a patient's response to health teaching. Among these are *regional culture,* that is, the locale in which a person lives; *social class,* which includes life-style, economy, occupation, education, language, use of leisure time, and values as well as attitudes; *religion,* which constitutes a way of living and thinking and contributes to a value system; and *family culture,* including attitudes toward the roles of men, women, and children, sexual behavior, and customs or rituals.[22] These factors contribute to an individual's health perception and influence personal receptiveness to a teaching-learning transaction. Prior to initiation of a teaching plan, changes which modify a patient's beliefs may be required before effective teaching can begin.

*Change* is often a slow process requiring much patience on the part of the nurse. The process of change involves the breaking down of old ideas, the introduction of new ways of dealing with an issue (change), and reintegration of these changes into a person's life. The longer a pattern has been followed, the harder it will be to change. *Resistance* to change may persist and present additional problems for the nurse. Often this will be manifested by verbal unwillingness to change, lack of attention and interest, lack of maturation or giving priority to other less important activities in order to avoid dealing with the problem.

Some patients may be unwilling to give up traditions, change occupations, move to a different locale, or eliminate specific rituals. These decisions must be respected by the nurse. However, when unwillingness to change seriously interferes with the patient's health potential, the nurse must utilize those resources at his or her disposal to plan changes that will be more acceptable. By offering the learner an opportunity to participate in the planning of a learning activity, personal control of the learning experience may be felt. Avoiding abrupt change will be less disruptive for the patient and diminish resistance. Use of *linkage ideas,* that is, ideas consistent with both public health and cultural beliefs, should aid in health promotion.[23]

Problems in communication and *language* can create barriers to learning and must be considered by the nurse. Much information can obviously be lost when the patient speaks a language foreign to the nurse. Efforts to know the language of a particular cultural group are important. When this is not possible, a knowledgeable translator should be obtained.

Use of sophisticated medical terminology should be avoided. Unfamiliar words confuse the patient and interfere with interpretation of specific information.

A final point to consider is the significance of the *sick role* within a particular culture. If the secondary gains of being in an unhealthy state exceed the perceived benefits of the healthy state, a patient may not *hear* specific instructions. This factor must be carefully evaluated along with other data collected in the teaching-learning assessment. Utilization of counseling by psychiatry or social service may be employed when suggested changes in life-style present multiple problems for the patient and interfere with effective coping.

**E**nvironmental Variables   The physical location of the teaching-learning transaction is of critical importance. *Noise* control is essential as it decreases distraction. The room or locale should be *comfortable, well lit,* acoustically *soundproof,* and *free of odor.* The environment should have adequate seating with provision for visual and audio teaching equipment when possible. Demonstration areas should be well equipped and have space for return demonstrations.

Care should be taken to select an area in the hospital where teaching can be effective. Crowded space, noise of visitors, machinery in a room, or the stress of the moment would distract from any teaching-learning interaction.

In the community, space should be selected for convenience to either the patient or general public. When possible, socialization periods may help attract community members and stimulate continued participation. When teaching occurs in the home, it should be done in a quiet area. If possible, family members should participate. Actual materials to be utilized by the patient can be selected, and practice sessions can be carried out with active participation by the learner(s).

Whatever the setting, the teaching transaction should not be rushed, and the patient's normal biological rhythm should not be altered or interrupted. Care can be taken to avoid teaching at such times when the patient is tired by procedures or distracted by other environmental constraints.

**Interactional instructional model**   Various models or planned strategies can be used to design a teaching-learning transaction. A systems model helps conceptualize all the components of the interaction and serves as a guide for planning learning experiences. Each model has as its goal the achievement of specific learning objectives.

The *instructional model* proposed in Fig. 2-3 is an example of an interactive educational design through which a systematic approach is used to identify a learner, select specific learning objectives, plan content and strategies, and evaluate the overall success of the transaction.

**P**reentry Behavior   In order to determine the *preentry behavior* of a learner, careful assessment must be completed at the start of each teaching-learning encounter. This assessment includes an educational history which addresses academic experience, occupation, social and cultural background, and psychological and physiological variables that can influence the learning experience. In addition, it helps to identify the learner's present knowledge of the material being presented. Pretesting offers the teacher an opportunity to assess knowledge of data to be taught and retention of factual information already presented. Following this, an overall decision can be made as to the individual's strengths and weaknesses. Information about patients can be obtained through the use of written examinations, verbal quizzes, asking for a return demonstration and observation of performance.

*Constraints* to the teaching-learning transaction should also be identified early in the encounter. Those physical, psychological, environmental, and sociocultural factors discussed earlier should be carefully evaluated. When possible, attempts to correct these constraints should be made so that the teaching-learning process will not be hampered.

It is important to note that the teacher may be a constraint to the transaction by being unprepared

or unfamiliar with the content being taught or by presenting dull, unmediated, rushed classes, thus thwarting the entire transaction. In addition, unskillful use of language, inappropriate level of content, poor use of visual or audio aids, overly large class size, and the teacher's overall style and personality can decrease teaching effectiveness.

**P**rofile of the Learner   After the learner has been pretested and any constraints to the interaction identified, a learning profile can be developed. In an assessment of a learner or groups of learners, a careful descriptive profile will be needed to enhance the teaching plan. This assessment should include the client's level of education, previous hospitalizations, previous contact with the subject being taught, any physical handicaps or language disability, sensory disturbance, physiological problems, and sociocultural limitations. The assessment is an opportunity to pretest and assess the entry level behavior of a client. Therefore, any other data that aids the teacher in knowing more about the learner will be included in this component.

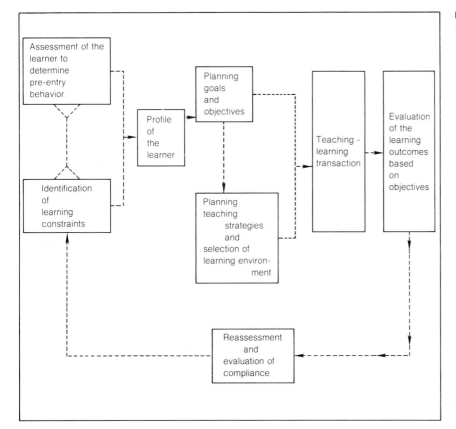

**FIGURE 2-3**
Interactional instructional model.

**P**lanning Learning Objectives and Goals Planning learning goals or the overall purpose of a transaction can be a challenging experience. Selection of specific measurable objectives to achieve goals affords the learner an opportunity to know the exact direction of the learning experience and establishes parameters for evaluation. By a plan of specific goals that are mutually agreed upon, the content can be selected and a teaching-learning transaction developed.

*Behavioral objectives* To date, there remains much controversy about the use of behavioral performance objectives (BPO). Some criticize them as self-limiting, confining, and restrictive of creativity, while proponents of BPO contend that they guide student learning, set up clear criteria for learning, and provide a way to evaluate the results of the teaching-learning encounter. Whatever the controversy, it can be said that in order for learning to occur, a goal or direction must be involved in the teaching-learning process. The learner should have some way of knowing an intended learning outcome, and the teacher must realize what the goals of the transaction are. Strict adherence to one style of objective writing to the exclusion of all other directions is to the learner's disadvantage. A balance must be reached whereby the student's goals can be easily identified and evaluated.

Behavioral objectives should describe the learner, the intended behavioral outcome, the conditions under which the learner will demonstrate competence, and identification of a standard of performance.[24] Several components compose an objective. According to Cyrs, there should be: (1) a *doer* of the action, (2) a *behavioral task,* (3) a *product* of the behavior, (4) a *stimulus condition,* and (5) a *standard of performance.*[25]

The following example will demonstrate these components. A patient (the *doer*) while working alone (*stimulus condition*) will list from memory and in writing (*behavioral task*) five out of six side effects (*standard of performance*) of decreased blood sugar. (The *product* will be the list.) Objectives and intended goals should be stated in a clear, efficient manner. They should be mutually developed and selected by the patient and the nurse, allowing the learner some control over the learning experience.

The purpose of formulating objectives is to make learning outcomes visible, to facilitate evaluation, to enhance communication between the teacher and learner, and to serve as a means of determining content and related teaching strategies. With specific criteria established, the overall teacher-learning transaction can become more effective.

*Classification of objectives* Learning behaviors are manifested in three ways: (1) cognitive, the intellectual ability, (2) affective, the status of feeling and valuing, and (3) psychomotor, the manipulative and motor skills.[26] Accordingly, a taxonomy or classification system was developed by Bloom et al.[27] in order to provide language for describing and ordering educational outcomes. By the selection of specific terminologies, rendering of a definition, and placing of these words in a hierarchical order, learning becomes more visible.

The affective and cognitive domains have been classified into learning behaviors by Bloom. The psychomotor levels used here have been developed by Dave. Table 2-3 lists the appropriate classifications for each domain and clarifying definitions. These classifications will help the teacher when planning specific transactions with the learner. It should be remembered that when writing objectives, nothing is purely cognitive, affective, or psychomotor. Rather, it should be noted that objectives overlap and when a psychomotor task is performed, cognitive and affective learning may also be present.

**S**election of Content Content selection, or that material so defined in the behavioral objectives, is usually specific and mutually planned by the patient and nurse where possible. It may be identified in response to a community need, or as a response to an individual health problem of a chronic or acute nature.

Careful delineation of content and accurate assessment of time allotment for each defined content area are important to incorporate in the teaching plan. This will help the patient and the nurse recognize the amount of time needed to present selected content. Time often is a major constraint to the teaching-learning transaction. The effect of this constraint can be limited by a careful, well-planned teaching strategy.

**T**eaching Strategy A teaching strategy is that methodology used by a teacher to transmit identified content to the learner. Multiple teaching strategies including the use of film, transparencies, lecturing, audio and/or visual taping, and discussion groups are available to the teacher to communicate data to the learner. Selection of a particular strategy is dependent upon the behavioral objective, the material being taught, the individual or group being taught, the level of the learner, the appropriateness of the medium being used, and the educational needs of the learner(s).

Since patients in a hospital setting may already feel the impact of increased sensory stimulation, it may be more appropriate to limit a teaching encounter to one or two strategies. However, if the nurse is involved in a public education program, a variety of teaching strategies may help to heighten the senses and increase awareness of the learning situation. Table 2-4 identifies a variety of teaching methods available, defines them, and indicates their use in educating a learner or groups of learners. Selection will depend upon the teacher, the learner, the content, and learning objectives.

**E**valuation  Evaluation of the teaching-learning process can occur at intervals throughout the learning experience. It should be an organized process which evolves directly from the objectives developed.

The purpose of an evaluation is generally to

decide whether the student learned all that was intended and how well. Evaluation helps the teacher and learner isolate those variables within the process that enhanced or detracted from the teaching-learning transaction.

Evaluation can measure the learner's progress over time and identify personal strengths and weaknesses. After obtaining this information, new learning experiences can be planned; when needed, remediation and reinforcement can be provided. Alternate learning experiences can be included to help the student acquire information.

Determination of what is to be evaluated is often contingent upon the appropriateness of the initial objectives. If these are vague and unclear, they can interfere with the evaluation process. Cognitive and psychomotor objectives are easier to evaluate because they are tangible and concrete. Affective learning is often value oriented, requiring changes in attitude. This is difficult to evaluate since subjectivity adds another constraint to the teaching-learning process. Following the evalua-

## TABLE 2-3

| 1 COGNITIVE DOMAIN | |
|---|---|
| Knowledge | Recall of factual information |
| Comprehension | Ability to translate or interpret information and summarize events |
| Application | Translation of concepts learned in the classroom to the real situation |
| Analysis | Investigation of the relationship of ideas, elements, principles; ability to distinguish fact from hypothesis; comparison between facts |
| Synthesis | Putting ideas together to form a whole<br>Designing an experiment<br>Formulating a hypothesis |
| Evaluation | Ability to problem solve, analyze, synthesize, make judgments based on the facts, and arrive at a solution |

| 2 AFFECTIVE DOMAIN | |
|---|---|
| Receiving (attending) | Awareness of color arrangement and design<br>Willingness to receive information when others speak<br>Tolerance for others<br>Alertness to human values and judgment<br>Some discrimination of music |
| Responding | Willingness to respond by acquainting oneself with specific rules and regulations<br>Assuming responsibility for self and others<br>Enjoying self-expression in art, music |
| Valuing | Accepting values of others; speaking, writing effectively<br>Identifying with all human beings in their struggle for survival<br>Being committed<br>Willing to hear all sides of an argument |

| Organization | Conceptualizing values<br>Making judgments regarding social issues<br>Weighing alternatives |
|---|---|
| Characterization (value or value complex) | Willing to change opinion in light of new data<br><br>Tending to be less rigid, making decisions after all the facts are in<br><br>Developing a personal philosophy of life based on individual ideals and goals . |

| 3 PSYCHOMOTOR LEVELS | |
|---|---|
| Imitation | The learner is exposed to an observable action and then imitates that action, covertly at first, then overtly by repeating the activity. The performance often reflects limited coordination of musculoskeletal system. |
| Manipulation | Involves developing skill in following directions, performing selected activities, then fixing the performance by practice. The learner can then carry out a specific activity according to a set of instructions and not merely by imitation. |
| Precision | More independent activity involved; improved coordination, refined performance. The learner can now carry out an action without a model or set of directions. |
| Articulation | Coordination of multiple activities through establishment of an appropriate sequence, achieving harmony and consistency among different acts. Well-coordinated actions. |
| Naturalization | Proficiency at performing a single act skillfully in an almost routine, automatic, spontaneous way. |

SOURCES: (1 & 2) B. Bloom: *Taxonomy of Educational Objectives*, Handbooks I & II, *Cognitive and Affective Domains*, McKay, New York, 1968. (3) Dr. R. H. Dave, Head of Curriculum and Evaluation, N.I.E., Nehravl Road, New Delhi, India.

**TABLE 2-4**
TEACHING-LEARNING STRATEGIES

| Strategy | Definition | Utilization |
|---|---|---|
| Lecture | Content is delivered orally to an audience by a qualified person in an organized way with or without the integrated use of visual material. Length of time varies. | Large-group teaching |
|  |  | Presenting didactic material, e.g., any pathophysiology of altered health states |
|  |  | Encourages further study, analysis, and inquiry |
|  |  | Limits discussion of issues, although possible |
|  |  | A medium to present controversial issues |
|  |  | Lack of stimuli or poor lecturer can lessen attention |
| Interviewing | Short presentation of material in response to a series of questions. | Informal presentation of facts |
|  | Usually conducted before an audience. Two people are usually involved in the presentation which usually lasts for no more than 30 minutes. | Allows for exploration of issues in a relaxed, clarifying manner |
|  |  | To obtain impressions on a subject from an authority in the field |
|  |  | Allows for interaction by the audience |
|  |  | To present several interventions to a specific health problem, such as open-heart surgery |
| Panel | Small group of people (two to six usually) selected to present information on a particular topic. Persons chosen should have knowledge of the subject being discussed and the ability to present the facts in an organized and clarifying way. The panel is usually presided over by a moderator. | To present varying sides of an issue |
|  |  | To clarify the pros and cons of a topic, e.g., the use of various forms of contraception |
|  |  | Allows for a number of informed persons to present a range of ideas |
|  |  | Provides the learner with an opportunity to select a side on the basis of informed opinion |
| Demonstration | A skill is taught by the acting out of a particular procedure; material being taught must be carefully prepared. | Instructing individuals in the performance of a procedure |
|  | The teacher completes all the steps of the procedure. Usually, this strategy is accompanied by actual materials, both visual and audio, as well as oral presentation. At times a *return* demonstration is used in which the learner presents material to the teacher as taught. When possible, videotaping of this encounter enhances the learning experiences and clearly identifies areas for improvement. | Providing "hands on" approach to learning |
|  |  | Promoting confidence in one's ability to successfully complete a procedure |
|  |  | Allows the teacher to observe the learner's ability to follow through with material taught |
|  |  | Particularly important when assessing how well the learner will be able to complete a procedure in the community or following discharge from the hospital, e.g., administration of insulin, colostomy irrigation, testing of urine |
| Colloquium (colloquy) | Similar to a panel but uses six to eight persons. These include resource people and individuals from the learning audience to critique or raise questions about issues presented. This format is generally presided over by a moderator. | Offers expert opinion on a topic |
|  |  | Allows for audience participation and interaction |
|  |  | Provides an opportunity for clarification of factual information by qualified resource personnel, e.g., an interdisciplinary presentation on specific health problem such as obesity, atherosclerosis, nutrition, or problems associated with aging |
| Discussion | A strategy usually carried out in small groups, with or without an identified leader. A discussion can be one of four types. (1) *Book-based: Socratic,* structured to express a particular point or present an argument. (2) *Problem solving,* dealing directly with an attempt to solve a problem. (3) *Case oriented,* focusing on a particular problem, discussing issues in a private way, usually related to a patient issue or problem. All facts presented, analyzed, and resolved. (4) Group centered inter- | Allows for personal expression for small group and seminar learning when the intent is to increase individualized and personalized learning. |
|  |  | Provides an opportunity to share personal experiences with one another and to benefit from others' successes and failures. |
|  |  | Allows for learning in a more informal, relaxed environment. |
|  |  | Helps increase personal growth and self- |

| | | |
|---|---|---|
| | action offers the most opportunity for individuals to share personal ideas and experiences with one another and to gain information from the interaction with other group members. | awareness; e.g., this can be used as a component of a preoperative teaching session to encourage expression of fears and clarification of ideas<br><br>Allows for visualization and recreation of "the real thing" |
| Role playing | This strategy offers an opportunity for realistic enactment of a particular situation or group experience before a selected audience in an impromptu or preplanned manner. It is unstructured, spontaneous, and informal and offers the learner an opportunity to experiment. | Can be taped and replayed for in-depth analysis and discussion, thereby allowing for feedback from the participants and the audience to solve complex situations often involving behavior of an individual or group, e.g., can be used to help patients express concerns, especially if there is a conflict about impending surgery, changes in body image, and fear of loss |
| Visual materials:<br>Video tape recording (VTR)<br><br>Television<br><br>Film<br><br>Slides<br><br>Film strips<br><br>Closed-circuit television<br><br>Computer | The use of visual materials combines auditory and visual senses to present a multiplicity of learning materials in a creative, stimulating manner. Visual resources are able to overcome the limitations of a teaching-learning situation by recreating actual material and making it available for continuous review. Visual media assist with learning transfer as they make steps to be enacted more tangible. | Increases the impact upon the senses<br><br>Enhances learning and retention of information<br><br>Increases its potential impact when it accompanies audio presentation.<br><br>Brings the "real world" into the learning situation<br><br>Generates thoughts and helps stimulate creativity and discovery<br><br>Can be combined with field trips<br><br>Makes words visible<br><br>Stimulates discussion to evaluate learning<br><br>Can enhance all learning situations, such as demonstration of a procedure, administration of an injection, or menu planning |
| Audio material (tapes) | Material considered important to the learner is recorded on tape by the teacher to be listened to at a later time.<br><br>Visual material may or may not accompany the presentation.<br><br>Listening to material presented can facilitate summarization of data, facilitate discussion, capture key points for review, and stimulate auditory perception. | Attention span limited to 15–30 min; without added stimuli effect of audio material diminishes<br><br>To provide learning experiences when a particular sequence cannot be attended by a learner<br><br>To reinforce learning when studying a content learned during a particular class<br><br>Tapes should never be retaped directly from presentation "in class," as they become contaminated by interruptions, questioning, etc.; teachers should retape classes, identifying key points and adding additional information as needed<br><br>Can reinforce preoperative teaching or review pathophysiology prior to a discussion with the nurse<br><br>Can be reused and duplicated without loss of effectiveness |
| Structured or interactive notes | This is a way for the teacher to identify for the learner key words, terms, or phrases that are considered important. This format usually accompanies the lecture or audio tapes and helps the learner focus on the material. | To accompany lecture or audio tapes<br><br>Effective way to store information for study or recall at a later time.<br><br>To teach a patient specific content in any area such as nutrition, insulin coverage, or stoma care; by taking notes during a particular interaction, the patient will have a ready reference following the listening period |
| Instructional learning packages | An instructional learning package (ILP) is a unit which can be completed independently by the learner outside the formal classroom setting. It contains a listing of final objectives as well as intermediate objectives and then | To facilitate independence<br><br>When selected, activities can be performed prior to actual class session<br><br>Practice demonstration |

**TABLE 2-4 (Continued)**
TEACHING-LEARNING STRATEGIES

| Strategy | Definition | Utilization |
|---|---|---|
| | requires, recommends, and suggests a series of activities which can lead to completion of the packet. It includes tests for before and after the instruction and a variety of printed and nonprinted materials, discussions, lecture, and bibliography. | Increase freedom of learner |
| | | Allow for increased choice on the part of the learner |
| | | Total self-contained learning system |
| | | Specifies all activities so that the learner knows the exact direction in which to move |
| | | To teach any learning area; by having an available guide, the patient can use this resource in the home in any subject area |

tion, careful analysis of data is critical to the evaluation process. These data can provide feedback essential for reevaluation of the learner and serve as a basis for planning new learning experiences. Many methods of evaluation are available to the teacher and learner and should be written into the objective(s). Written examinations, role playing, return demonstrations, discussions, films, etc., can provide a basis for an evaluation. These tools can include components of creativity, discovery, application, analysis, synthesis, and problem solving as determined at the outset of the transaction.

**C**ompliance  The patient's ability to follow teaching instruction, according to directions given, and for as long as needed is termed *compliance.* In order to ensure compliance, the teaching plan must be realistic and adaptable to the home setting. If the strategies to be used are confusing and require a large investment of time and money, the patient may become discouraged and disinterested.

If a procedure needs to be continually performed at home, directions should be clear, simple, and carefully written out. The equipment to be used must be easy to purchase, cost effective, easy to handle, refillable without difficulty (if appropriate), and easily adaptable to the home setting. When changes in the home are needed they should be made with minimal disruption. Return demonstration should be performed by the patient; when possible, family members should participate. The patient should be provided with a phone number so that the nurse can be consulted whenever questions arise. Often patients become frightened when they are performing a task alone and think of issues not presented earlier. Having an immediate resource will be comforting to the patient and family, and facilitate compliance.

Patient compliance is often contingent upon intrinsic reward of good health, personal motivation, personality, willingness to change, and the impact of the teaching-learning transaction. In order to facilitate compliance, teaching will often need to be reinforced and reevaluated during *follow-up* health visits.

*Missed appointments* or failure to contact the health provider might be a clue to *noncompliant behavior.* Careful follow-up by telephone is important. When possible a home visit should be made. The importance of return visits to health providers must be stressed to the patient. If necessary, reminders may have to be devised using calendars, phone calls, and letters to facilitate this objective.

The final measure of patient compliance is the actual changes that have occurred following the teaching-learning period. Did the patient's blood pressure go down? Is there still excess sugar in the urine? Is the cholesterol level lowered? Have the irrigations been successful? Is the colostomy working efficiently?

The success of the teaching-learning transaction and related patient compliance can be most accurately evaluated by the improvement noted in the patient's overall health status. Lack of patient compliance will require a reevaluation of patient needs and associated variables influencing the transaction.

**Teaching-learning transaction**  A *teaching-learning transaction* is a comprehensive example of an instructional teaching mode used by the nurse to instruct patients in any setting. It is a systematic plan which defines a learning population, lists constraints to the teaching-learning process, selects learning objectives, identifies content, plans selected teaching strategies, and provides an evaluation of learning experience and analysis of the results. It is a planned interaction by the nurse and patient to present information according to a systematic approach. Table 2-5 is an example of the

**TABLE 2-5**
TEACHING-LEARNING TRANSACTION

1 Profile of the learner
    *a* Description of the population: Factory blue collar workers, average intelligence, high school graduates
    *b* Learning environment: Local school auditorium, limited resources
    *c* Content: Normal nutrition and a well-balanced diet
2 Goal(s) of the transaction
    *a* Improve good nutrition through a well-balanced diet
    *b* Change attitudes in eating habits and food selection
3 Constraints to the interaction
    *a* Psychological: Personal problems, attention, anxiety
    *b* Physical: Current health problem, pain
    *c* Environment: Uncomfortable seats, poor acoustics, poor equipment
    *d* Sociocultural: Limited income; content presented in conflict with cultural eating pattern
    *e* Other: Disinterest in attending the workshop

| Student/Teacher Objective | Content to Be Taught | Strategy to Be Used | Evaluation of the Performance | Assessment of Achievement |
|---|---|---|---|---|
| Following a workshop on the daily components of a balanced diet the learner will: | Purpose of a balanced diet | Film on a balanced diet | | Evaluation based on achievement of the objectives |
| | Health problems that can occur when an unbalanced diet is followed | Slide tape on food selection | | Follow-up test to evaluate compliance |
| (a) List in writing all the basic foods included in a balanced diet and comprehend the value of good nutrition on one's health | Basic components of normal nutrition | Lecture | List of the basic foods with 100% accuracy | |
| | | Small group discussions on menu planning, and health maintenance | Food selection with 90% accuracy | |
| (b) Pick out the basic foods from a menu given in class with 90% accuracy | Foods that should be used to achieve a balanced diet | Food budgets | Plan menu containing all the basic foods according to the class lecture | |
| | Nutritional value of each food discussed | Nutritional laboratory sessions | | |
| (c) Plan a balanced diet according to guidelines presented in class | Discussion of a well-balanced menu and food selection | | An interview which reflects personal views | |

instructional model which can be used by the nurse when teaching patients in any setting.

## SUMMARY

Learning is a lifelong process. It begins at birth and terminates with death. Teaching is a responsibility the professional nurse assumes. In health teaching many learning opportunities exist in a variety of settings. Although the focus may differ, each teaching-learning transaction offers the learner an opportunity to gain knowledge and incorporate that information into handling the activities of daily life. The nurse must make health-related learning experiences meaningful to patients and create and sustain a curiosity about their health promotion.

Since each learner is unique and individual, so too must each learning experience be molded to the learner or groups of learners. The nurse must recognize these differences and develop a teaching plan that identifies the patient's strengths and limitations while meeting individual learning needs.

**TABLE 2-6**
GUIDELINES FOR TEACHING-LEARNING PLAN

Teaching-learning transactions should be individualized to each learner or group of learners.

Assessment of each learner, including limitations as well as strengths, prior to the learning experience facilitates the teaching-learning process.

Readiness to learn is critical to the teaching transaction and is often determined by the patient.

Teaching plans should begin at the proper level for the patient.

Mutual goals for the teaching-learning plan should be developed by the patient and nurse, when possible.

Learning should be goal directed with measurable outcomes established, where possible (cognitive, psychomotor, affective).

Intermittent evaluation is important to the teaching-learning process; therefore, a feedback mechanism should be established.

Teaching strategies should be varied and complement an individual's learning style and meet the learner's readiness.

Patient motivation to learn increases when information imparted will have a significant impact on an individual's life.

Where possible, patients should be allowed a choice in acquiring new information.

Current life-style and cultural practice as well as family participation should all be incorpated into the teaching transaction.

The learning environment should be conducive to the learning process, and, where possible, distractions should be eliminated.

The teaching plan should build in reinforcements, such as written directions for follow-up in the home and home visit, when possible.

The teacher should operate as a facilitator of the teaching-learning transaction, enhancing the learning experience whenever possible.

The teacher must be adept in the subject taught, able to adjust levels of the learner, and establish rapport early.

The learning situation must be realistic and meaningful to the learner. It should present information clearly and in a way that will complement individual learning styles. The teacher should select teaching strategies that will attract the learner's attention and enhance future retention. Each teaching-learning transaction must provide an opportunity for freedom of choice in selection of learning objectives, materials, and activities. The teacher-nurse must show trust and respect for each individual, always recognizing those physical, psychological, and sociocultural variables that are continuously interacting.

Those learning experiences prompted by need and purpose tend to be more meaningful to the learner. Hence, the motivation to retain this information increases. Involving the learner in the planning of individual learning activities can offer a sense of control over the learning situation and provide a feeling of participation in the planning of learning objectives. Table 2-6 summarizes those guidelines that can be used by the nurse to enhance the teaching-learning transaction.

As nursing becomes increasingly independent and interdependent, it must seek out new opportunities to educate. In so doing, nurses will clearly establish their role as health educators, and be viewed by the public as such.

## REFERENCES

1    American Nurses' Association, Position paper, "The Scope of Nursing Practice: Description of Practice of Nurse Practitioner/Clinician," *Clinic Nurse Specialist,* May 1976, p. 6.
2    Winslow, Elizabeth H., "The Role of the Nurse in Patient Education," *Nurs Clin North Am,* **11:**2, June 1976.
3    Pohl, Margaret L., "Teaching Activities of the Nursing Practitioner," *Nurs Res,* **14:**4–11, Winter 1966.
4    Powell, Ann H., "The Nurse's Role in Teaching Acute Myocardial Infarction Patients," unpublished master's thesis, University of Kansas, Lawrence, 1972.
5    Pender, Nola J., "Patient Identification of Health Information Received during Hospitalization," *Nurs Res,* **23:**262–267, May-June 1974.
6    Weiler, Sister M. Casbel, "Postoperative Patients Evaluate Preoperative Instruction," *Am J Nurs,* **68:** 1465–1467, July 1968.
7    Storli, Frances, *Patient Teaching in Critical Care,* Appleton-Century-Crofts, New York, 1975, p. 6.
8    Cassem, N. H., et al., "Reactions of Coronary Patients to the C.C.U. Nurse," *Am J Nurs,* **70:**319, 1970.

9  Tift, K., "Individualizing Health Instruction," *School Health Rev,* **1:**4, 2, November 1970.
10  Smith, Philip, *Philosophy of Education,* Harper & Row, New York, 1965.
11  Knowles, M., *The Modern Practice of Adult Education: Andragogy vs. Pedagogy,* Association Press, New York, 1970.
12  Gagne, P., *The Conditions of Learning,* Holt, New York, 1965, p. 33.
13  *Ibid.,* p. 35.
14  *Ibid.,* p. 46.
15  *Ibid.,* p. 47.
16  *Ibid.,* p. 52.
17  *Ibid.,* p. 57.
18  Reilly, Dorothy, *Behavioral Objectives in Nursing: Evaulation of Learner Attainment,* Appleton-Century-Crofts, New York, 1975, p. 21.
19  *Ibid.,* p. 22.
20  Rich, John M., *Readings in the Philosophy of Education,* Wadsworth, Belmont, Calif., 1968, p. 39.
21  Reilly, *op. cit.,* p. 39.
22  Murry, Ruth, and Judith Zenter, *Nursing Concepts for Health Promotion,* Prentice-Hall, Englewood Cliffs, N.J., 1975, p. 274.
23  *Ibid.,* p. 124.
24  Reilly, *op. cit.,* p. 30.
25  Cyrs, Thomas, *Working with Behavioral Objectives,* Northeastern University Press, Boston, 1971, p. 5.
26  Reilly, *op. cit.,* p. 49.
27  Bloom, B., *Taxonomy of Educational Objectives, Handbook I and II: Cognitive and Affective Domain,* McKay, New York, 1968.

## BIBLIOGRAPHY

### Physical Assessment

Bates, Barbara: *A Guide to Physical Examination,* Lippincott, Philadelphia, 1974.
Berni, Rosemarian, and Helen Readey: *Problem Oriented Medical Record Implementation,* Mosby, St. Louis, 1974.
Bernstein, Lewis, Rosalyn Bernstein, and Richard Dana: *Interviewing: A Guide for Health Professionals,* 2d ed., Appleton-Century-Crofts, New York, 1974.
Bird, Brian: *Talking with Patients,* 2d ed., Lippincott, Philadelphia, 1973.
Capell, Peter T., and David B. Cuse: *Ambulatory Care Manual for Nurse Practitioners,* Lippincott, Philadelphia, 1976.
Epstein, Charlotte: *Effective Interaction in Contemporary Nursing,* Prentice-Hall, Englewood Cliffs, N.J., 1974.
Fowkes, William C., and Virginia K. Hunn: *Clinical Assessment and the Nurse Practitioner,* Mosby, St. Louis, 1973.
Francis, Gloria, M., and Barbara A. Munjas: *Manual of Sociopsychologic Assessment,* Appleton-Century-Crofts, New York, 1976.
Gillies, Dee Ann, and Irene B. Alyn: *Patient Assessment and Management by the Nurse Practitioner,* Saunders, Philadelphia, 1976.
Hobson, Lawrence (ed.): *Examination of the Patient,* McGraw-Hill, New York, 1975.
Judge, Richard D., and George D. Zuidema: *Methods of Clinical Examination: A Physiologic Approach,* 3d ed., Little, Brown, Boston, 1973.
Lipkin, Mack: *The Care of Patients: Concepts and Trends,* New York, Oxford, 1974.
Maloney, Elizabeth Ann, Laurie Verdisco, and Lillie Shortridge: *How to Collect and Record a Health History,* Lippincott, Philadelphia, 1976.
Murray, Ruth, and Judith Zentner: *Nursing Assessment and Health Promotion through the Life Span,* Prentice-Hall, Englewood Cliffs, N.J., 1975.
——— and ———: *Nursing Concepts for Health Promotion,* Prentice-Hall, Englewood Cliffs, N.J., 1975.
Neelon, Francis A., and George J. Ellis: *A Syllabus of Problem-Oriented Patient Care,* Little, Brown, Boston, 1974.
O'Brien, Maureen: *Communications and Relationships in Nursing,* Mosby, St. Louis, 1974.
Prior, John A., and Jack S. Silberstein: *Physical Diagnosis: The History and Examination of the Patient,* Mosby, St. Louis, 1973.
Sana, Josephine M., and Richard D. Judge: *Physical Appraisal Methods in Nursing Practice,* Little, Brown, Boston, 1975.
Samuels, Mike, and Hal Bennett: *The Well Body Book,* Random House, New York, 1973.
Sherman, Jacques L., and Sylvia Kleiman Fields: *Guide to Patient Evaluation,* Medical Examination Publishing Co., New York, 1974.
Weed, L. L.: *Medical Records, Medical Education, and Patient Care,* Case Western Reserve University Press, Cleveland, 1969.

### Health Teaching

Aiken, L.: "Patient Problems Are Problems in Learning," *Am J Nurs,* **70:**1816–1818, September 1970.
Berlowitz, Marfred: "Thermal Environment and Learning," *Audio-Visual Instructor,* **15:**77, October 1970.
Bolvin, J. O.: "Materials for Individualizing Instructions: An Interpretation of Goals," *Educ Technol,* **12:**23–27, September 1972.

Bruner, J.: *Toward a Theory of Instruction,* Harvard, Cambridge, Mass., 1966.

Canfield, A.: "A Rationale for Performance Objectives," *Audio-Visual Instruction,* **13:**127–129, February 1968.

Culbert, P., and B. Kos: "Aging: Considerations for Health Teaching," *Nurs Clin North Am,* **6:**605, December 1971.

Dickinson, Gary, and Dale Russell: "A Content Analysis of Adult Education," *Adult Education,* **XXI:** 177, September 1971.

Fox, R., and K. Owen: "New Directions for Health Education through Instructional Television," *J Sch Health,* **XLI:**188, April 1971.

Hays, J., and J. Disanto: "The Implementation of Behavioral Objectives in Curriculum Development," *Education,* **90:**44, September-October 1969.

Hyman, Ronald: *Ways of Teaching,* Lippincott, Philadelphia, 1974.

Lauson, Millie: "Progressive Coronary Care," *Heart Lung,* **1:**240–253, March-April 1972.

Lindeman, C., and M. Airman: "Nursing Intervention with Pre-Surgical Patient, Effectiveness and Efficiency of Group and Individual Pre-operative Teaching," *Nurs Res,* **21:**196–209, May-June 1972.

Mager, R.: *Preparing Instructional Objectives,* Fearon, Palo Alto, Calif., 1962.

Millen, H.: *Teaching and Learning in Adult Education,* Macmillan, New York, 1969.

Palardy, J. M.: "Some Revised Learning Principles," *Education,* **91:**22–157, November-December 1970.

Palm, Mary L.: "Recognizing Opportunities for Formal Patient Teaching," *Nurs Clin North Am,* **6:**4,669, December 1971.

Pohl, M.: *Teaching Function of the Nursing Practitioner,* Wm. B. Brown Company Publishers, Dubuque, Iowa, 1968.

Redman, B.: *The Process of Patient Teaching,* Mobsy, St. Louis, 1972.

Schweer, J.: *Creative Teaching in Clinical Nursing,* Mosby, St. Louis, 1968.

Shetland, M.: "Teaching and Learning," *Am J Nurs,* **65:**9, 113, September 1965.

Smith, D.: "Writing Objectives as a Nursing Practice Skill," *Am J Nurs,* **71:**2–329, February 1971.

Smyth, Kathleen: "Symposium on Teaching Patients," *Nurs Clin North Am,* **6:**571–679, December 1971.

Solomon, G., and R. MacDonald: "Pre-Test and Post-Test Reactions to Self Viewing One's Teaching Performance on Video Tape," *J Educ Psychol,* **61:**4, Pt. I, August 1970.

# 3

# DEVELOPMENTAL PATTERNS OF INTERACTION*

Cheryl K. Ahern
Nancy Diekelmann
Carol L. Panicucci

## THE YOUNG ADULT

Late adolescence, ages 16 to 20, marks the transition from childhood to adulthood in the human life cycle. Early or young adulthood, ages 19 to 30, overlaps late adolescence and completes the transition from juvenile to adult status. At this stage, physical attributes are usually at optimal levels, and intellectual capacities are reaching their full potential, only to be enhanced by the wisdom of experiential learning. Psychologically, young adults struggle to (1) free themselves from economic, physical, and emotional dependence on their family, (2) establish intimate relationships, (3) elaborate a personal set of life values, and (4) develop a sense of personal identity and a life-style which supports that identity. Socially, they focus on career- and family-building, trying to establish themselves as accountable adults. Despite career-building efforts, young adults often experience an extended socialization process through which they are kept out of the competitive labor market and in schools. Many protest the depersonalization of the modern superindustrial technocracies and choose to explore nontraditional lifestyles, family patterns, and religious and political ideologies. Often their personal relationships reflect freer moral and sexual value systems than those of young adults in the past. They experience "future shock" in a modern world where the pace of life and rate of change are accelerated.

### Physical Changes

Physical development reaches its peak during the young adult years. Anatomically and physiologically, the human body completes its genetically determined growth pattern between the ages of 16 and 20, at which point human adult aging begins. Full stature and *skeletal development* is reached by the late teenage years and early twenties, after which there is no significant change in the length of individual bones. Maximum *muscular power* and coordination is reached at ages 25 to 30. Thereafter, the strength, speed, and endurance of muscular contractions diminish.

Development of the *human brain* in early life brings about an increase in the size of nerve cells, in supporting tissues, and in the cerebrovascular system. This growth continues until ages 20 to 30, when the maximal weight of the brain, reflecting its total cell content potential, is reached.

---

* The Young Adult section was written by Cheryl K. Ahern, the Middle Adult by Nancy Diekelmann, and the Older Adult by Carol L. Panicucci.

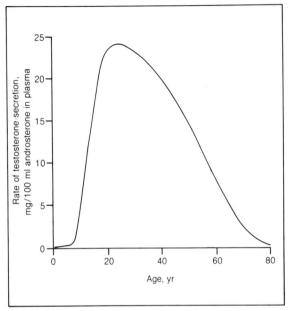

**FIGURE 3-1**
Rate of testosterone secretion at different ages based on the concentration of androsterone in the plasma. (*From Arthur C. Guyton, Textbook of Medical Physiology, Saunders, Philadelphia, 1961, p. 1074, by permission.*)

Measurements of *visual and auditory* acuity are said to reach their maximum at 10 years of age. After 10 the best viewing distance lengthens gradually until, by the age of 50, many people need to wear glasses to correct long-sightedness. The lens of the eye begins aging in infancy and becomes more opaque and less elastic in adult life.

Between 19 and 30 years of age, *bodily processes* related to cellular proliferation, fluid and electrolyte dynamics, metabolism, and oxygenation function at maximum efficiency. The *cardiac output* and *respiratory vital capacities* are high; vascular structures are elastic and readily responsive to changes in environment and body needs. It is important to note, however, that arteriosclerosis, with its potential for degenerative changes in the cardiovascular system, may well have begun earlier in life and may continue its development during the young adult years.

The *endocrine glands*—the pituitary, thyroid, parathyroids, adrenals, and gonads—function at full potential during early adulthood. The pituitary and the adrenals appear to maintain their functions well over the entire life span. Hormone secretion from the gonads rises sharply at puberty in both males and females. It peaks in the early young adult years and then gradually falls off in the middle years

of life. Testosterone secretion across the life span is summarized in Fig. 3-1. Testosterone production at puberty causes the penis, scrotum, and testes to enlarge until the male sexual organs are fully developed by age 20. It also triggers the development of the secondary sexual characteristics in the male which reach maturity at about the same age.

Like the male, the female reaches sexual maturity in transition from puberty to young adulthood, with the peak estrogen production occurring in the young adult years. Estrogens are responsible for the development of the sexual organs and the secondary sexual characteristics in the female. Figure 3-2 illustrates estrogen secretion across the life span.

**Health**

During young adulthood it is important that individuals establish a life-style that takes into account the body's needs for (1) a balanced diet, (2) a regular regimen of exercise, and (3) a pattern of work and rest that assures adequate sleep to ease strain and restore psychic energy.

**Nutritional needs**  Developing a diet pattern that establishes a functional balance between individual physical requirements and food intake is important during these years, as it sets a precedent for diet patterns later in life. In general, a balanced diet should include a wide variety of foods, a caloric intake consistent with the energy needs of the individual, and limited intake of sugar, cholesterol, and food additives. Young adult males need increased consumption of foods high in vitamins C, E, $B_6$, and riboflavin in their diets. Young adult females need high intakes of protein, vitamins C, A, E, $B_6$, $B_{12}$, and riboflavin.[2] Anemia is a common problem in young menstruating women, so an increased number of foods that are high in iron should also be a regular part of their diet.

Obesity is a significant problem among young adults. Surplus subcutaneous fat deposition may have begun in adolescence or before and may continue into the young adult years. Counseling in weight reduction and diet regulation are important aspects of the care of obese young adults.

**Exercise**  Physical activity that increases the heart rate and requires deep breathing, such as jogging, swimming, rope jumping, or hiking, should become an important part of the life-style of young adults. Regular physical exercise has been demonstrated to have a significant effect in reducing some of the physiological changes of aging, even late in life.[3] Exercise also helps to regulate appetite and is helpful in relieving tension from worries about work, school, money, and family problems which are common during young adult years.

**Sleep**  Getting adequate amounts of sleep is frequently a problem for young adults, particularly for those with a newborn baby or with financial, work, or personal difficulties. Insomnia is common during these years, as is the temptation to reduce necessary hours of sleep in order to study longer or complete unfinished work projects. Sleep is not expendable, however, as it is important in (1) restoration after new learning situations, (2) easing psychic strain, (3) repairing, reorganizing, and forming new connections in the neuronal system required for focused attention and learning, and (4) repairing synaptic endings of neurons.[4]

### Common Health Problems

The health problems of the young adult are by and large transient, nondegenerative, nondebilitating ones. They most commonly include (1) traumatic injuries, primarily resulting from athletic or automobile accidents, (2) infectious diseases such as mononucleosis, hepatitis, viral and influenza illnesses, and venereal diseases, (3) allergic and dermatologic syndromes, (4) cystitis and vaginitis in females and nonspecific urethritis in males, and (5) stress-related conditions such as back pain, headaches, and epigastric distress. Most of these problems require only short-term episodic care. Health education covering accident prevention, basic first-aid concepts, communicable diseases and their prevention, and environmental factors that influence health is a significant and necessary part of health care. Sex, birth control, pregnancy, abortion, and genetic counseling are common concerns for the 19-to-30-year old. All of these areas require thoughtful, nonjudgmental teaching and counseling from health professionals.

**Psychological issues**  The psychological adjustment from adolescent to adult status is often a traumatic and painful one. Rapid emotional and social changes occur as new roles of parent, spouse, or worker are begun. The young adult's efforts to achieve independence from parental control and develop a value system, personal identity, and life-style which is uniquely self-defined are often fraught with emotional turmoil. As a result, suicide is statistically high among causes of death in this age group (Table 3-1), and many young people seek counseling assistance for support through

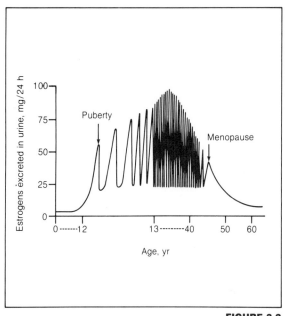

**FIGURE 3-2**
Oscillation of estrogen production throughout female sexual life. (*From Arthur C. Guyton, Textbook of Medical Physiology, Saunders, Philadelphia, 1961, p. 1090, by permission.*)

this transition. Open-minded, sensitive health professionals can play important roles in providing the needed support during this time.

**Chronic or catastrophic illness**  Serious chronic or catastrophic illness does occur in young adults, but less frequently than the more common problems discussed earlier. Table 3-2 summarizes the leading causes of cancer in young adults. Cancer of the breast occurs in young women more frequently from age 20 to menopause and is largely accountable for the statistics that show cancer as the second leading cause of death in women aged 15 to 24. Leukemia, in its acute myeloblastic or chronic myelocytic forms, is found most commonly in young adults, although it may occur at any age. Systemic lupus erythematosus is often diagnosed during this time period; it occurs most frequently in females in their second to fifth decade. Diabetes mellitus is found most frequently in older people, but does occur in the young adult. There are 10 diabetics per 1000 people between the ages 25 to 44. Duodenal ulcer is most common in men between the ages 20 to 50.[5]

Young adults experience major life adjustment crises when faced with chronic or catastrophic illness. It is difficult for them to comprehend and accept serious, limiting illness and/or possible

**TABLE 3-1**
FIVE LEADING CAUSES OF DEATH, BY AGE GROUP AND SEX: UNITED STATES, 1970

| | All ages Male | All ages Female | 1–4 Male | 1–4 Female | 5–14 Male | 5–14 Female | 15–24 Male | 15–24 Female | 25–44 Male | 25–44 Female | 45–64 Male | 45–64 Female | 65+ Male | 65+ Female |
|---|---|---|---|---|---|---|---|---|---|---|---|---|---|---|
| 1 | Heart diseases 417,918 | Heart diseases 317,624 | Accidents 2,564 | Accidents 1,736 | Accidents 5,695 | Accidents 2,508 | Accidents 19,396 | Accidents 4,940 | Accidents 18,865 | Cancer 9,902 | Heart diseases 128,955 | Cancer 55,444 | Heart diseases 274,181 | Heart diseases 264,236 |
| 2 | Cancer 180,157 | Cancer 150,573 | Congenital malformations 694 | Congenital malformations 637 | Cancer 1,389 | Cancer 1,040 | Homicide 3,333 | Cancer 1,114 | Heart diseases 13,445 | Accidents 5,114 | Cancer 66,556 | Heart diseases 47,663 | Cancer 102,769 | Cerebrovascular disease 96,738 |
| 3 | Cerebrovascular disease 93,456 | Cerebrovascular disease 113,710 | Pneumonia, influenza 601 | Cancer 449 | Congenital malformations 481 | Congenital malformations 420 | Suicide 2,378 | Homicide 824 | Cancer 7,939 | Heart diseases 4,793 | Accidents 17,528 | Cerebrovascular disease 14,028 | Cerebrovascular disease 73,313 | Cancer 82,511 |
| 4 | Accidents 79,756 | Accidents 34,882 | Cancer 578 | Pneumonia, influenza 442 | Pneumonia, influenza 327 | Pneumonia, influenza 324 | Cancer 1,817 | Suicide 750 | Suicide 5,866 | Suicide 2,506 | Cerebrovascular disease 17,165 | Accidents 6,636 | Pneumonia, influenza 21,434 | Pneumonia, influenza 18,778 |
| 5 | Pneumonia, influenza 35,148 | Pneumonia, influenza 27,591 | Meningitis 141 | Homicide 128 | Homicide 215 | Heart diseases 162 | Heart diseases 642 | Heart diseases 412 | Homicide 4,907 | Cerebrovascular diseases 2,446 | Cirrhosis 11,908 | Cirrhosis 6,158 | Bronchitis, emphysema, and asthma 16,756 | Arteriosclerosis 17,336 |

SOURCE: *Vital Statistics of the U.S. National Center for Health Statistics, Washington, D.C.*

death when they "should be at their prime." They require sensitive, high-quality long-term medical care and psychological support skills on the part of health professionals involved in their care.

## Death

The major cause of death among young adults is accidents, predominantly automobile accidents. Teaching about prevention of accidents—the importance of routinely wearing seat belts and the dangers of drinking and driving—is, therefore, an important aspect of health care to young adults.

Cancer is the second leading cause of death in females and the fourth in males between 15 and 24 years of age. Counseling about the need for routine health examination and assessment is important. Regular health care can be lifesaving. This need is accented by the fact that young adults often feel "too healthy" to need periodic health assessments or "too young" to consider the possibility of serious illness. Young women need to be taught the importance of routine Pap smears and breast examinations. Young adults should be aware of the relationship of smoking to lung cancer and of the warning signs of cancer and their significance.

## Personality Dynamics

The young adult is reaching full physical potential and this developmental process puts demands on the individual that help to shape personality development.

**Cognitive intelligence**  Authorities disagree as to when intellectual capacity "peaks." The young adult years, however, are a time when the human intellect is *biologically* maximized.[6] Biological intellectual capacity, however, is only one factor in the definition of an individual's overall intellectual performance during the life span. The two basic types of intelligence, fluid intelligence and crystallized intelligence, intertwine throughout the life process to determine an individual's intellectual performance level. Social wisdom and scientific or creative productivity grow out of this intertwining process.

*Fluid intelligence* is defined as basic intellectual endowment, derived from physiology and heredity and independent of education and experience. *Crystallized intelligence* grows out of life experience. It is based on potentials or capacities within the fluid intelligence but expands those in interaction with cultural, social, and environmental influences and experiences. Environmental influences on learning and formal educational processes play an important role in determining the development of crystallized intelligence. Both fluid and crystallized intelligence develop with age, but fluid intelligence reaches its peak and begins to decline in the early twenties. Crystallized intelligence, on the other hand, continues to develop throughout the adult life span.

Intellectual performance or achievement is a product of both natural potential and experience. In a study of intellectual productivity and achievement that is still considered one of the best on the subject, H. C. Lehman tabulated the ages at which people had made significant contributions to art, science, music, literature, technology, medicine,

**TABLE 3-2**
INCIDENCE OF CANCERS IN YOUNG ADULTS AGED 20 to 35

| Site | Rate per 100,000 Population | |
| --- | --- | --- |
| | Male | Female |
| ALL SITES | 107.98 | 161.48 |
| BUCCAL CAVITY | 3.89 | 2.88 |
| DIGESTIVE SYSTEM | 11.40 | 9.06 |
| Esophagus | 0.09 | 0.09 |
| Stomach | 1.78 | 1.05 |
| Colon | 4.97 | 4.44 |
| Rectum | 1.31 | 1.05 |
| Liver | 0.94 | 0.09 |
| Pancreas | 0.70 | 0.35 |
| RESPIRATORY SYSTEM | 5.72 | 3.49 |
| Lung | 4.08 | 2.57 |
| BONE | 2.72 | 1.13 |
| TISSUE | 4.03 | 3.22 |
| SKIN (MELANOMA) | 9.24 | 10.20 |
| URINARY SYSTEM | 5.35 | 2.48 |
| Kidney | 1.45 | 1.09 |
| Bladder | 3.52 | 1.39 |
| EYE | 0.52 | 0.57 |
| BRAIN AND CENTRAL NERVOUS SYSTEM | 7.60 | 5.45 |
| ENDOCRINE SYSTEM | 6.00 | 21.48 |
| Thyroid | 5.44 | 21.31 |
| LYMPHOMAS | 21.86 | 13.68 |
| Hodgkin's disease | 15.06 | 10.24 |
| LEUKEMIA | 7.79 | 4.66 |
| MALE GENITAL ORGANS | 19.47 | — |
| Testis | 19.04 | — |
| BREAST | — | 28.84 |
| FEMALE GENITAL SYSTEM | — | 52.55 |
| Uterus (cervix, corpus, not otherwise specified) | — | 39.74 |
| Ovary | — | 9.80 |
| Other female | — | 1.44 |

SOURCE: American Cancer Society based on *The Third National Cancer Survey: Incidence Data*, Monograph 41, National Cancer Institute, March 1975.

athletics, and other fields. He concluded from his extensive statistical data that, in general: (1) between the ages of 15 and 19, the rate of intellectual achievement in the fields of art and science is low; (2) the rate rises steeply and steadily until it reaches a peak between 30 and 34 years; and (3) after the age of 34, the rate of output falls steadily to nearly zero after age 70. In contrast to these figures, however, he found that the peak years for established leadership status and social accomplishment occurred between the ages of 50 and 70, emphasizing the effect of experience and social wisdom on social leadership ability.[7]

**Emotional development** The psychological concepts handed down by Freud made a basic assumption that the human personality is more or less determined by the time a child reaches the age of 5. As a result, much research was done on the psychological development of children. It has only been in recent years that psychiatrists and social scientists have addressed themselves to defining predictable psychological changes or stages within adulthood. It is necessary to analyze some of these developmental theories in order to discuss the emotional or psychosocial personality dynamics of young adulthood.

Charlotte Bühler was one of the first to study developmental psychology. Her focus was on the concept of developing self-determination within the personality. She defined five periods of development within the human life span, periods which she saw as "decisive" for developing self-determination including the critical tasks of occupational development and the founding of a family. During the second of these five periods, adolescence, self-determination becomes concrete in relation to life but still has a temporary or tentative character. The tasks in this stage include preparation for an occupation, the beginnings of a career, and relations with the opposite sex before marriage. During the third period, ages 25 to 45, the individual becomes established in life with a definite self-determination. The focus is on occupational activity, marriage, and the founding of a family.

One of the most important psychosocial developmental theories of the human life cycle was outlined by Erik Erikson. He described a psychosocial developmental process in which "eight ages of man" develop in predictable sequence. Each "age" represents a critical step or *crisis* point in human development; in each *crisis* there is heightened vulnerability and potential, and the need to decide between developmental progress or regression. His eight stages represent certain ego qualities that emerge from each crisis. If adjustment is successful, the emerging quality will allow the person to interact successfully within the structure of social institutions.

Erikson's last three stages represent the psychosocial crises of adulthood: intimacy vs. isolation, generativity vs. stagnation, and ego integrity vs. despair. It is the first of these, intimacy vs. isolation, that is critical to the young adult's psychological development. Erikson says: "The young adult, emerging from the search for and insistence on identity, is eager and willing to fuse his identity with that of others. He is ready for intimacy, that is, the capacity to commit himself to concrete affiliations and partnerships and to develop the ethical strength to abide by such commitments, even though they may call for significant sacrifices and compromises. Body and ego must now be masters of the organ modes and of the nuclear conflicts, in order to be able to face the fear of ego loss in situations which call for self-abandon: in the solidarity of close affiliations, in orgasms and sexual unions, in close friendships and physical combat, in experiences of inspiration by teachers and of intuition from the recesses of the self."[8]

Theodore Lidz expands Erikson's statement somewhat in describing the young adult as a person who is able to go beyond a focus on individual growth and development. Being independent of the natal family, the young adult must find a place in society. This is accomplished through vocation, marriage, and personal "involvements" in people and tasks. Various social roles are assumed and the person becomes less self-centered.

In addition to those of Bühler and Erikson, there are other "phase" theories of human psychological development that describe emotional "tasks" of early adulthood. Robert Havighurst defines six life stages, based on specific developmental tasks. The developmental task of the young adult in this schemata is to find a mate, marry, start a family, and assume a sexual and social role in society. Havighurst defines the young-adult period as one that is characterized by disorganization as the transition from an age-graded to a social-status-graded society is made.

Psychiatrist Roger Gould of the University of California, Los Angeles, has developed his own concept of the phases of adult life and presents them in more carefully defined age groupings. He delineates several major developmental issues that occur during the period of young adulthood. In phase 1, *Ages 16 to 18,* the main issue is a break from parents. At this age one's sense of autonomy is precarious and easily eroded. Negativism is common. The deep close relationships with peers that are longed for are often unstable, resulting in a temporary rebound to parents. Phase 2, *ages 18 to 22,* is a continuation of the "we have to get away from our parents" theme, but from a different standpoint. Young adults at this stage feel themselves halfway out of the family, since they are living away at school, working, and paying rent, but they are worried that they will be reclaimed by the family pull and not make it out completely. The peer group becomes an important support system, and group belief becomes a strong governing force for behavior. In phase 3, *Ages 22 to 28,* young adults feel independence has been achieved. They are adults on their "true course in life," seldom stopping to consider whether their commitments are appropriate or right for them. Feeling like adults, they are trying to act like adults. During phase 4, *ages 29 to 34,* questioning about life goals begins. They begin to wonder about the meaning of life and consider alternate life courses or paths they could take.

Building on the work of Gould and the other developmental theorists, Gail Sheehy has created her own description of the human adult life cycle which even more specifically delineates psychological and emotional tasks of young adulthood. Synthesizing her own extensive research of other developmental theories and 115 "life story" interviews with middle-class American adults, aged 18 to 55, she has formulated a more detailed conceptual framework in which to analyze adult developmental crises. Her theory describes "the strategic interplay of stable periods and critical turning points" as *passages,* rather than *crises.* During the young adult years, these passages encompass: (1) ages 16 to 22, *pulling up roots,* during which concern is focused on developing independence from the natal family; (2) ages 22 to 29, *provisional adulthood,* when attempts are made to lay the foundation for a life pattern through work, life-style, and personal relationships; and (3) ages 29 to 32, *age 30 transition,* in which restlessness with earlier decisions begins and often leads to changes in career patterns and personal relationships.

Sheehy expands other theorists' work by including a comparison between the developmental rhythms of men and women, and a description of what she sees as predictable *passages* for couples. Her work points out that men and women rarely struggle with developmental passages at the same age, although, over time, development is the same for both sexes. She finds that men become increas-

ingly confident during the twenties, while women are beginning to lose the assurance of adolescence. As a man passes 30 he begins to settle down, while the woman becomes restless. About 40 a man begins to feel like strength, power, dreams, and illusions are slipping away. Meanwhile, his wife is beginning to realize her full potential, and ambition becomes a part of her life.

**Personality-trait development** Norma Haan studied personality development from adolescence to adulthood by analyzing changes in personality traits demonstrated by different age groups on the Oakland Growth and Guidance Studies.[9] Figure 3-3 summarizes her findings. She found significant differences in personality traits between adolescence and young or early adulthood. Late adolescence was characterized by a temporary "regression" in socialization. Decreases in personality traits such as dependability, productivity, giving, or sympathetic tendencies, and a "temporary drop in guilt feelings" occurred during this period.

Young adults, on the other hand, according to Haan's research, reversed several of the trends of adolescence. Dependability and productivity became salient personality traits. They demonstrated value independence, and, as a result, socially inefficient actions such as rebellious, undercontrolled behavior, or withdrawal when frustrated became less characteristic. The young adult tended to be more internalized, guilty, repressive, accountable, and sensitive than the adolescent.

**Nursing implications** The young adult years are years of transition and emotional turmoil. The critical emotional issues involve achieving emancipation from family controls, developing the capacity for intimacy, establishing a personal set of life values, and developing a personal identity and a life-style which supports that identity. Men and women may differ in the timing and resolution of their developmental crises during these years, but the issues are the same. The nurse should be cognizant of the problems with which the young adult is struggling. Often support can be found within peer groups. Patients should be aware of local community mental health resources where both individual and group therapy can ease the transition into adulthood. High school and college nurses, health services, and academic advisors can often help give the young adult needed support and assistance with critical life and career decisions. Ministers, social workers, family-planning services, and neighbor-

| JUNIOR HIGH SCHOOL | SENIOR HIGH SCHOOL | EARLY ADULTHOOD | MIDDLE ADULTHOOD |
|---|---|---|---|
| **SEVEN** | | | 7.3 dependable |
| | | | 7.0 productive |
| **SIX** | | | |
| 6.6 gregarious | | 6.8 dependable | |
| 6.5 sex-typed behavior | | 6.7 productive | |
| 6.5 dependable | | | 6.4 sex-typed behavior |
| 6.4 repressive | | | 6.4 straightforward |
| 6.2 compares self to others | | 6.2 repressive | 6.2 giving |
| 6.2 uncomfortable with uncertainty | 6.1 repressive | 6.2 values independence | 6.2 sympathetic |
| 6.2 fantasizing | | | 6.1 arouses liking |
| 6.0 arouses liking | | 6.0 feels guilty | |
| 6.0 productive | | 6.0 sex-typed behavior | |
| **FIVE** | 5.9 sex-typed behavior | | |
| | 5.8 gregarious | 5.8 sympathetic | 5.8 values independence |
| | 5.7 uncomfortable with uncertainty | 5.8 straightforward | |
| | | 5.8 giving | |
| | 5.7 compares self to others | 5.8 arouses liking | |
| | 5.7 dependable | | |
| 5.6 feels guilty | | 5.6 compares self to others | |
| 5.5 values independence | 5.5 fantasizing | 5.5 uncomfortable with uncertainty | |
| 5.4 straightforward | 5.4 values independence | 5.4 gregarious | 5.4 compares self to others |
| 5.3 sympathetic | 5.3 arouses liking | | 5.3 gregarious |
| | 5.2 productive | | 5.1 repressive |
| 5.1 giving | | | 5.1 insightful |
| | 5.0 sympathetic | | 5.0 philosophical concern |
| **FOUR** | 4.9 feels guilty | | 4.9 uncomfortable with uncertainty |
| | 4.9 straightforward | | 4.8 feels guilty |
| 4.8 brittle | 4.7 giving | | |
| 4.6 emotionally bland | | 4.6 brittle | |
| 4.6 withdraws on frustration | 4.5 brittle | 4.5 fantasizing | 4.5 fantasizing |
| | 4.5 withdraws on frustration | 4.5 insightful | |
| 4.4 undercontrolled | | 4.3 philosophical concern | |
| | 4.2 emotionally bland | 4.1 emotionally bland | 4.1 complicates simple situations |
| | 4.1 undercontrolled | | |
| 4.1 rebellious | 4.1 rebellious | | |
| **THREE** | | 3.9 complicates simple situations | 3.9 undercontrolled |
| 3.7 complicates simple situations | | | 3.8 brittle |
| | | 3.6 withdraws on frustration | |
| | | 3.6 undercontrolled | |
| 3.4 insightful | 3.4 insightful | 3.5 rebellious | 3.4 withdraws on frustration |
| | 3.3 complicates simple situations | | 3.3 emotionally bland |
| | 3.2 philosophical concern | | 3.3 rebellious |
| **TWO** | | | |
| 2.8 philosophical concern | | | |

hood health centers may all serve as valuable needed resources to the young adult.

## Sexuality

The development of human sexual behavior is a complex issue. Biological, social, and experiential factors all interact to influence the development of sexuality. Sex may be viewed from both a physical and a psychosocial perspective. Ontologically, chromosomal sex comes first. The gonads and endocrine glands, including the thyroid, play a major role in physiological development. Child-rearing patterns, societal value systems, and life experiences, on the other hand, are major determinants of an individual's psychological and behavioral sex. Learning influences the acquisition of sexual behaviors.

During young adulthood, both men and women are sexually mature, physiologically. The gonads are fully developed and the estrogens and androgens are at peak levels of secretion. The capacity to respond quickly and repeatedly to sexual stimuli and have multiorgasmic sexual encounters is common to both sexes.

Although their physiologic potentials are similar, the sexual activity or experience of males and females may differ significantly. "According to the Kinsey studies of the early 1950s, the heterosexual patterns of males tend to cover a wider range than those of the females, the former liking variety in their sexual activities and the latter being content with less range of sexual pleasures. Furthermore, it seems to be the case that the human male is more prone than the female to acquire unusual and surrogate modes of sexual expression, as in fetishes, voyeurisms and exhibitionism, and in the variety of homosexual patterns."[10]

Societal value systems have had significant influence on the development of male and female sexual behaviors. Religious prohibitions and the "double standard" have been important factors in controlling or suppressing sexual behavior in women. This so-called double standard tends to foster the belief that men and women are different sexually. Men are expected to be aggressors and women submissive. Feelings contrary to this are denied or falsified.

"Once males and females are in their twenties, the social sorting system begins segregating them by domestic duties and career opportunities, and the massive distinction in sexual roles takes effect. They begin moving apart in every way, including sexually."[11] An overwhelming proportion of the babies are born to women in their twenties; only after completing these child-bearing years, at about 30 or 31, do women begin to lose their sexual inhibitions and reach their full sexual availability and freedom. Males, on the other hand, reach their peak level of sexual performance in their early to mid-twenties.

In recent years, however, young adults have been exploring variations in traditional sexual roles. The "era of the pill," with its development of readily available and more effective birth control measures, legalization of abortion, and feminist movements working to foster more independent feminine role models, has led to more exploration and experimentation in female sexual behaviors.

Social and moral value systems related to sexual activity, at least among young adults, have changed significantly over the past several decades. Daniel Yankelovich has documented these changes in his research on American youth, aged 16 to 25. His research in the late 1960s showed that acceptance of casual premarital sex, abortions, homosexuality, and extramarital relations was confined to a minority of college students. In 1973, however, the evidence indicated that this "new sexual morality" was much more widely prevalent, occurring both in college and working-class youths.[12]

Young people who attended the White House Conference on Youth in 1971 adopted resolutions which further delineate the contemporary sexual value system among young adults. (1) "Relationships: Human beings are sexual persons. Ideal sexual relationships are sensitive, concerned and responsible expressions of human feelings. Every person has the right to fully express his or her individual sexuality. Furthermore, any sexual behavior, when occurring between consenting, responsible individuals, must be recognized and tolerated by society as an acceptable life style." (2) "Legal restrictions: Social repression and sex role channel-

**FIGURE 3-3**
Hierarchies of trait organization for four time periods (sample averages precede trait names). Results are for 144 subjects, men and women combined, who had Q sorts for all four time periods. Solid connecting lines indicate difference is significant, that is, less than 0.05; broken lines, not significant. (*From Norma Haan, Personality Development from Adolescence to Adulthood in the Oakland Growth and Guidance Studies, Seminars in Psychiatry,* **4**:412–413, 1972, *by permission.*)

ing are manifested in our legal statutes. Laws, as those forbidding fornication, adultery, homosexuality, lesbianism, and so-called 'unnatural-acts', restrict the right of individual expression. Laws restricting or prohibiting abortion or distribution of contraceptives inhibit individual expression and attempt to legislate sexual morality. Sexual morality cannot and must not be legislated.''[13].

## Life-styles

Traditionally, young adults in modern urban industrial societies have worked hard to establish themselves socially. They acquire legal maturity and voting rights as a function of their chronological age. They usually complete their education and struggle to become economically independent and responsible, putting a significant amount of energy into developing a lucrative and/or satisfying trade or career. They often marry and begin to raise a family, taking on the socioeconomic responsibilities that family life requires.

Contemporary young adults experiment more broadly with life-style. They resist automatic acceptance of the marriage, child-rearing, career-building social role that has been traditional for those in their age group. Their search for a higher ''quality of life'' than they perceive in modern technological society leads them to test new diet and health practices, encourages ''back-to-nature'' experiments, and results in their examining the political, religious, and philosophical ideologies of other cultures. Their restlessness with the results of their own educational processes leads them to develop experimental ''free'' educational systems. Their inability to break into the labor market forces them to imagine and develop new employment modalities. Their search for closer personal relationships and their dissatisfaction with the family structures in which they grew up leads them to develop alternate family styles. The nuclear family of mother, father, and children predominates in United States society. It is, however, not the only option available. Alternatives such as childless marriages, communal families, and remaining single are recognized as legitimate and fulfilling choices.

**Societal influences** Many of the personal and social value systems and life-styles of twentieth century young adults reflect or are reactions to the social environment and changes which confront their generation. The youth of the twentieth century are ''technocracy's children.''[14] They grew up in an era in which efficiency, rational control, technical competence, and scientific knowledge were the valued ''modus operandi.'' A person's productivity in the technological environment is often the criteria used for evaluation of ''success'' or contribution to the society. The economic aspects of the social structure, productivity, the free enterprise system, and private consumption, are prominent features in the disposal of the products of industry and technology.

Young adults perceive uncontrolled technology and materialism as dehumanizing. They express their concern about this dehumanization process: ''Man's role in the process of technology lies in his ability to integrate the human factor within the materialization of an end product. The consequences of marketing must be considered before marketing is permitted. There must be checks and balances with research and development procedures, for we cannot always legislate technology into a prescribed channel.''[15]

Unlike youth of pretechnocracy times, young people today experience an extended socialization process wherein they are transformed from an asset to the family as labor to a liability as student-consumer. This occurred earlier in the United States, where prolonged education for everyone became the rule. The public willingly invested in its youth as the society was able to employ only a fraction of its untrained youngsters after high school. The longer educational process extended the economic dependency and ''freedom'' of exploration for young adults, allowing them to take economic security for granted much longer than their parents had been allowed to.

Other influential social factors contributed to the ''milieu'' in which contemporary young adults have been reared. These include wars, lost liberties, growing feelings of powerlessness, ecological concerns, and the loss of a sense of community. In total, the impact of these social influences has often bred a sense of ''alienation'' within the young. Enthusiasm and ardor are fading. The young adult especially feels the growing distance between human beings. Social commentaries are dominated by terms like alienation, estrangement, disaffection, anomie, withdrawal, disengagement, separation, noninvolvement, apathy, indifference, and neutralism.[16] Young adults sense a loss as the gap between humanity and the social environment seems to them to be increasing.

**Economic influences** Young adulthood is usually a time of struggling to become economically independent. A significant amount of energy is invested in developing a lucrative and/or satisfying trade or career. Middle-upper class and upper class youths often take economic security for granted. They are often still dependent on their parents long after their peers are financially capable. This dependence, enhanced by the willingness of their parents to accept it, is also often expected or taken for granted. When economic independence finally comes, the young adult will often experiment with alternate money styles. These may include day-to-day existence, ventures in free enterprise, communal financial arrangements, or even "panhandling." By the end of the young adult years, however, most young adults have achieved a fiscal responsibility compatible with their life-style.

**Cultural influences** Western culture today is "youth-oriented." Many of the tangible artifacts of Western culture are focused on youth. Television, radio, advertisements, magazines, clothes, automobiles, etc., all emphasize a youthful existence. Being a young adult is considered the prime of life. Entrance into young adulthood is marked by certain rituals which reconfirm passage into this select group, and becoming a young adult is considered a milestone. In many states persons are first allowed to buy alcoholic beverages. The young adult is considered "legally of age." Voting privileges are extended. Other rituals marking entrance into young adulthood often include entering the military, getting married, graduating from college, getting an apartment, and beginning a career. While Western culture tells the young adult that life is at its best, societal, economic, and family pressures prove to be very demanding.

**Family influences** Twentieth century young adults have also experienced significant changes in family structure. They have grown up in an era of broken homes. Marriage commitments are less permanent than in the past and serial marriages—successive temporary marriages—are common. Family "roots" or attachments to the surrounding social environment and extended family ties have been diminished by the transiency and mobility of the modern family. The involvement of individual family members in "outside" organizations or peer groups has splintered the family, pulling individuals away from the central family core.

Parenting of contemporary young adults has largely been "mothering," since in many cases, the father has often been absent from the home, either because of a terminated relationship or because his work commitments have dominated his time. The mode or style of parenting has been predominantly "permissive," with the intent of fostering independence and self-expression within the child.

The trend among young adult parents themselves appears to be toward fostering even greater independence in their children. The young adult parent often tolerates more freedom and demands a higher level of performance and responsibility than an older parent. This trend is partly influenced by the fact that young adult parents today are often involved in trying to develop a balance between family responsibilities and career or work roles.

## THE MIDDLE ADULT*

The middle adult years from 40 to 60 are a time of major changes emotionally, socially, and physically. The children leave home, individuals begin to feel their age, and chronic illness becomes a real threat. These are the "change of life" years, when women experience menopause, the cessation of the menstrual period. Decreasing levels of hormones from the ovaries produce hot flashes, dizzy spells, headaches, cramps and breast tenderness; all signs of change. While men do not go through the physical changes of menopause, they do experience periods of anxiety, irritability, confusion, depression, and hypochondria.

It is also a time of joy, with new opportunities to learn and time for sensing one's accomplishments and feeling secure and independent. Middle adulthood offers new opportunities to grow. The role of the nurse in supporting this growth will be emphasized throughout this section.

Just as we prepare the parents of the toddler for what they can expect in the preschool child, so we should prepare the middle adult for what life still holds. Changes that are not anticipated may be very disturbing, and they may be regarded as "abnormal" or "bad." When an individual is prepared to realize that a change is normal at a certain age, it is more easily accepted and more competently dealt with. *Anticipatory guidance* is the teaching and counseling of individuals to prevent a potential crisis. Everyday aspects of normal growth and development may evoke a crisis in the family or the individual if those involved are not aware of the usual, normal behaviors or changes to be anticipated. Anticipatory guidance, then, involves helping an individual to know what to expect before an event occurs.

There are endless opportunities for the nurse

---

\* Adapted from Nancy Diekelmann (ed.), *Primary Health Care of the Well Adult,* McGraw-Hill, New York, 1977.

to apply the concept of anticipatory guidance in professional practice. Each stage of normal growth and development carries with it a number of potential "crisis" areas. Helping the young adult to prepare for the cellular changes of the middle years can do a great deal to minimize the trauma associated with this stage of growth. Thus, the middle adult prepared for the vision changes of the middle years may seek out an eye examination every year and not "panic" the first time difficulty reading the phone book is experienced.

### Physical Dynamics

Physical changes occur throughout the life span. At various points, however, these changes may be more or less evident. The middle adult years are often the time when one's aging first begins to manifest itself. It is reflected in cellular changes, perception, coordination, metabolism, oxygenation, as well as health problems.

**Cellular changes**  The classic signs of aging that make their appearance in middle age are anticipated by the young and recognized by the old with much fear and repulsion. While some cells begin to proliferate, others atrophy. This is especially evident in the skin where decreases in cutaneous fat and shrinkage of collagen and elastic fibers first become evident with the appearance of sagging and wrinkles. There is also a loss of pigment in hair and the first strands of gray appear. Loss of hair leads to thinning in women and receding hairlines or baldness in men. These changes cause the overall balance of facial features to change and the face appears coarser or bony with a more prominent nose. Due to a more sedentary life-style and a decreased metabolic rate with no accompanying decrease in caloric consumption, weight gain is common. We are all familiar with the term "middle-aged spread."

American men and women spend billions of dollars each year on cosmetics, hoping to reverse these changes. Ignorant of the philosophy involved in aging, they purchase hormone creams, cucumber juice, or queen bee extract "guaranteed" to preserve youthful appearance, because coping with these changes in *physical appearance* in our youth-oriented society can be difficult. However, those adults who enjoy being adult will value other qualities more than they did as young adults. They may appreciate, for instance, that all of these changes taken in concert may create an elegance of appearance. While the pigment in the hair-producing cells disappears and the skin's pink tint begins to yellow, the eyes keep their color and become the dominant, exquisite features of the aging portrait.[17] The nurse should support this attitude and encourage the middle adult to experience the harmony of these changes in physical appearance.

Besides the changes in physical appearance, *musculoskeletal integrity* generally begins to decline. There is a decrease in bone density and mass, and vertebral compression may occur with resultant backache. The middle adult starts to "shrink." Arthritic complaints commonly begin in middle age, and middle adults may often complain of "feeling the weather in their bones" and talk of the soreness they feel in their joints. This is due in part to accumulated wear and tear on the joints and is aggravated by the presence of obesity.[18]

*Muscle tone* also gradually decreases, and muscle cells are replaced by adipose and connective tissue, resulting in a flabbier appearance and decreased strength. This decrease in muscle tone and muscle cells, however, only influences the strength and speed of the muscle reaction.

*Endurance* does not necessarily decrease with age so long as the middle adult participates in a routine exercise program that involves strenuous exercise. A father may no longer be able to overpower his son at tennis, but the father who routinely jogs may have more endurance than his son who only jogs on the weekend. Bicycling may have more appeal than basketball, and swimming more than volleyball. Without proper exercise, endurance may suffer during the middle years, and couples may not be able to keep up with their social activities as they once did. Comments like, "I can tell we're getting old because my husband and I can't stay out late like we used to," are common. Middle adults may need more sleep and may find themselves taking naps or scheduling events far apart to allow themselves time to "recuperate."

**Changes in perception and coordination**  The physical changes of middle age associated with the sense organs may well be the first noticeable hallmarks of aging. *Presbyopia* or "farsightedness" is extremely common even in adults who have had no previous vision problems, and glasses are typically needed for reading or for close work. The middle adult may feel embarrassed at having to admit to changing eyesight; hence the standard quip, "I had to get glasses because my arms have gotten shorter."

Other vision changes that begin in middle age are decreases in *acuity, sensitivity in the dark,* and *peripheral vision,* all due to the cornea becoming less transparent and so admitting less light. These changes have more dangerous implications than presbyopia, since acuity, peripheral vision, and dark adaptation are all important in driving a car at night. It may not be possible to correct the latter two with eyeglasses. Decreased peripheral vision could perhaps be compensated for by shifting the eyes more often, and in that way maintaining a wide field of vision, but if decreased dark adaptation becomes significant, it might be necessary to limit driving to daylight hours. In any case, these problems cannot be treated medically or behaviorally until they are recognized. This is a real problem, as their onset may be so slow that subtle changes are not detected.

*Presbycusis* or impaired auditory acuity is another common sensory change of aging and is due to sensorineuron damage. The ability to hear the higher frequencies, women's voices or bird songs, for example, is usually the first to be lost. This may well be an extremely difficult change with which the middle adult and the family have to cope. The hard of hearing are often treated with an impatience and discourtesy that is not shown the visually impaired. Hearing loss serves as an isolating factor in a way that nearsightedness or farsightedness does not; the person with impaired hearing may have difficulty taking part in conversations, especially in crowds. A hearing aid is less common and therefore more of a stigma than eyeglasses. It is also a more blatant sign of aging, for people of all ages wear glasses, while hearing aids are typically worn only by the old. All this points to the increased need for dignity and self-acceptance of the hard-of-hearing person.

**Metabolic changes** In middle age the basal, or resting, energy expenditure of the body begins to decrease, and less oxygen is utilized. Given the analogy of the body to a car, the engine idles at a slower rate. As a result, the amount of blood pumped by the heart and the volume of air expired by the lungs under resting conditions decrease.

There is a consequent decline in *physical work capacity*. Quick mobilization of energy suffers, and the middle adult may no longer be able to participate in sports as before. This has important implications in terms of the psychological adjustment which must be made in accepting a changing body and in finding new interests and activities that do not require quick mobilization.

Metabolism is especially affected by the *endocrine system* which becomes less efficient with age. In general, less hormones are secreted. The development of adult onset diabetes is thought to be due in part to the pancreas "wearing out" and thereby secreting too little insulin. Decreases in the adrenal hormones lessen the ability to cope with stress, and one finds a decreased tolerance of extremes like very high or low temperatures or going without liquid for a long period of time. Repair after trauma or illness is slower, as the body does not "bounce back" as quickly as before. This is of special concern during times of inordinate stress such as hospitalization or surgery. Common illnesses like colds and flu can require longer periods of recuperation. Finally, symptoms related to stress and illness are less conspicuous than in younger people, and the magnitude of the problem may not be realized until the condition is serious.[19] The nurse should provide anticipatory guidance to middle adults to alert them to this possibility, so that they can become more aware of their reaction to stress and illness.

**Changes in oxygenation** As a person ages there is a reduction in the number of normally functioning cells. These cells are replaced by relatively inelastic connective tissue. Every physiological system becomes less efficient due to this degeneration, and perhaps the most dramatic and far-reaching changes occur in the cardiovascular system.

Blood vessels become increasingly inelastic as a result of connective tissue replacement and calcium salt deposits. The walls become thicker and the lumen smaller leading to a variety of cardiovascular diseases. Valves in the veins of the legs may not function as well as before causing varicosities to occur, particularly in women. Capillaries become more fragile, and bruising in response to trauma is common.

**Common health problems** Middle adults have a higher incidence of disease, especially chronic problems, than young adults. These include cardiovascular diseases, obesity, arthritis, deafness, eye diseases, and diabetes. Alcoholism and its complications are more common, as are gall-bladder disease, anemia, prostate gland problems, diseases of the female reproductive system, and depression. Cancer in the female and heart disease in the male are the leading causes of death in the middle adult.[20]

**Personality Dynamics**

As the middle adult's body changes to reflect a different stage in life, so does the personality. As a result of the physical changes, as well as the societal influences that vary with age, the middle adult's personality develops to reflect a new maturity. The middle years have a minimal effect on cognition, while the effects on emotional development are profound.

**Cognitive development** There is no mental decline in middle age. Indeed for some, especially those of higher intellectual abilities, there may even be an increase in cognitive development.[21] Crystallized intelligence, which grows out of life experiences, continues to expand, and the curve of cerebral function can continue to rise throughout the middle adult years. It is true, however, that the middle adult may less readily memorize material that is not well-organized. Retention from oral presentation of information may also be less than in younger adults. Activity has been shown to be a factor under the middle adult's control that influences cognitive development. One study indicated that physically fit and active middle-aged men score higher on intelligence tests than men who engage in little physical activity.[22]

For many people the experience of middle age brings enhanced flexibility, a sense of humor, confidence, and maturity gained through experience. Motivation to improve oneself intellectually may increase. Knowledge can be applied to past life experiences, and learning becomes more meaningful. It is no longer learning for learning's sake alone.

**Emotional development** Until recently, the stages of growth and development in the adult, particularly the middle adult, have been relatively neglected by investigators. Perhaps we have always felt that once an individual reaches young adulthood and begins functioning as an adult, he or she is emotionally set for life. However, with the growing awareness of the emotional problems experienced by middle and older adults, there is now a very genuine concern among researchers for generating a theory of adult development.

*Erik Erikson* has suggested that the middle years be characterized as a period of conflict between stagnation and generativity; that is, these years are a time of tension between retaining the perspectives of the young adult and establishing a new perspective, in which the concern for others equals the concern for the self. In a broad sense, this encompasses the areas of productivity and creativity. It suggests that we focus on the potentially unique social responsibilities of middle adults as well as their sense of being able to contribute something to the future. In this context, the middle adult either becomes more and more successful or stands still and accomplishes nothing.

*Neugarten's* research on personality changes in the second half of life support Erikson's focus on generativity.[23] Forty-year-olds perceive the external environment as one that rewards boldness and risk-taking and feel they possess energy consistent to meet the demands. The decade of the fifties represents an important turning point. Introspection increases and new perceptions of self, time, and death are formulated. This time of contemplation and reflection is often marked by psychological crisis for the middle adult.

*Robert Peck* has expanded this concept of crisis in the middle adult to cover four specific stages of emotional development in which the middle adult must learn to value wisdom over physical powers, socializing over sexualizing, emotional flexibility over emotional impoverishment, and mental flexibility over mental rigidity. Individuals in their middle years face these stages in their own time sequence. What is important to remember is that as the adult ages, change is inevitable. Each of these emotional milestones must be confronted, and these changes must be acknowledged for the middle adult to profit from them; otherwise stagnation will result.

**W**isdom vs. Physical Powers As we have seen, middle adults must anticipate changes in both strength and appearance. Perhaps a man can no longer play as vigorous a game of touch football or baseball as he used to, or a woman may tire before a younger partner in a game of tennis. While physical strength and appearance can be dominant features of life for young adults, this can no longer be true for middle adults.

Adults in their middle years have, however, gained wisdom through experience and can realize this as a resource rather than physical powers. Many middle adults feel as though they are bridges between younger and older generations, both in terms of family and the community. They can begin to think seriously about helping the younger generation benefit from their greater knowledge and experience. They can justifiably begin talking about being good role models and making the world a better place to live. While they may find themselves treated as ancient adults by their children, they are in a better position to achieve important goals, to pass along knowledge and wisdom, and to be supportive of younger and older generations.

Not all middle adults make this shift in perspective successfully. With our exaggerated emphasis on youth, the challenge to make the change has become significantly more difficult. It is a temptation to cling to illusions of youthfulness and to reinforce them by buying inappropriately youthful clothes. Unfortunately, such behavior only accentuates the fact of aging, and those individuals who attempt it may be setting themselves up for an emotional crisis. Running across old yearbooks or having to drop out of a volleyball game at a family reunion come as a heavy blow to the middle adult who cannot accept the aging process. Those who can adjust and who can avail themselves of the compensations that accompany being more experienced will handle the middle years more successfully.

**S**ocializing vs. Sexualizing  During adolescence and young adulthood, the emphasis on sexuality in human relationships may be very pronounced. However, the middle adult who persists in focusing on sexuality in social relationships very likely may experience peer group alienation. Because the middle adult has begun the process of discovering other qualities, personally and in others, this carryover from earlier years becomes less and less appropriate as a social behavior.

Middle adults can discover fuller and freer relationships when they are no longer distracted by viewing themselves and others as sexual objects. While two young couples traveling together may be too conscious of their sexuality to be willing to share a motel room with two double beds, middle adults who are more secure in their sexuality may be able to save money and enjoy increased companionship by taking advantage of their increased awareness.

Some adults have difficulty making the transition from their young adult orientation to this new, middle adult perspective. They may persist in their earlier patterns of socializing by flirting with members of their own circles. Frequently, these individuals find that they have only superficial acquaintances and that attempts to develop deeper relationships are thwarted because of the discomfort others feel with the sexual overtones that are involved. Middle adults who can face these changes will find that they can find greater satisfaction by developing human contacts based on individuality, interests, and merit.

**E**motional Flexibility vs. Emotional Impoverishment Loss begins to be the rule rather than the exception during the middle years. Parents die, children grow up and leave home, retirement and death begin to make inroads into circles of relatives and friends. Consequently, transferring one's emotional investments to new outlets is both desirable and neces-

sary if the middle adult is to continue to cope with life.

The individual who has suffered a significant human loss may be able to give some of the feeling, as well as some of the time that was invested, to others. An elderly or confined neighbor would gladly accept offers of friendship or assistance. Organizations like churches, day care centers, hospitals, and nursing homes are always in need of volunteer workers. By directing emotions into these other channels, the middle adult can maintain essential emotional ties that might otherwise be lost during these years.

However, this transfer of emotions may be infinitely complicated by circumstances for which the adult is not prepared. It is relatively easy to accept the death of elderly parents as inevitable events of aging, but it is frequently very difficult to accept the loss of a son or daughter, whether it is through death or marriage. The mother who "denies" her daughter's marriage and continues to act as though her child were still single and dependent will not only be trying to destroy the marriage unconsciously, but will herself be bitterly unhappy. The reinvestment of emotional "capital," preferably in a variety of places, will open avenues for the middle adult to rewarding, productive, and perpetuating experiences.

**M**ental Flexibility vs. Mental Rigidity  It is commonly believed that change is the only constant in our world. This applies as much or more to fields of knowledge and skills as it does to any other area of our lives. In education as in business, communications, industry, agriculture, and health care, changes are so rapid as to be almost staggering. The learning process can never be said to end.

Knowledge and experience have given the middle adult advantages that were beyond reach as a young adult. Wisdom in dealing with the personal self and the surrounding world has been acquired. The right to feel confident and secure has been established, but the middle adult must learn to profit from experience. Wisdom should be used as a guide rather than a straightjacket.

**Emotional tasks**  Peck's stages of emotional development are broad concepts that apply to growth in the middle years. Within these stages are four emotional tasks that help the middle adult successfully cope with the emotional development of the middle years. These are increasing self-esteem through self-awareness, separating from parents and children by becoming independent, reviewing one's own value system and changing or reinforcing it, and initiating plans for the future that take into account the aging process.[24]

**Increasing Self-esteem Through Self-awareness** Middle adults who do not use the middle years to deepen their sense of self-esteem often complain that life is growing boring and dull. They lack the awareness that this is a time for new growth. The responsibilities of child-bearing and child-rearing are behind them, and they may have new economic security as well as time for self-development. To fail to take advantage of these opportunities to reinforce the sense of worth may leave the adult despondent or depressed as failing powers, changes in appearance, or shrinking social horizons that accompany aging are first recognized.

Self-esteem is enhanced through a process of increasing self-awareness. This may involve examining assets and limitations, seeking out a close relationship, or developing or strengthening a love relationship. The process can be painful and may involve developing some significant insights. It may be time for a new career or a business of one's own, returning to school, or taking the summer off and touring the country. It can be a disturbing time in love relationships and often brings crises and separations. Sharing these problems may be a way for both partners to grow.

Learning more about one's self and discovering one's assets can involve periods of pain and joy. The nurse who is aware of the importance of this task can support middle adults as they increase their self-esteem through developing self-awareness.

**Separating from Parents and Children by Becoming Independent** The middle adult, in Eda LeShan's words, sometimes feels "caught between his children and his parents."[25] Some adults feel guilty at making a decision that their parents do not approve of, particularly when they reflect that their parents are growing older and may not have much longer to live. Other adults are overanxious to please their children, and adolescent children may make excessive, unrealistic demands on the parents. Frequently, older children are not grateful for what seems to them to be overprotectiveness and may resent it bitterly. Nor should they be grateful, since they are in the process of establishing their own independence. The middle adult needs to be able to say to the child, "we've done our best, now it's time for you to assume responsibility for your life and your decisions." To be trapped as a buffer between the demands of aging parents and the needs of young adults can only lead the middle adult to decreased self-esteem and increased dissatisfaction with life. Slowly and without guilt or regret, the adult in these middle years must separate from parents and children by emphasizing independence.

Frequently this is accomplished through a series of family events and interactions in which decisions are made for and by oneself. Middle adults begin to make purchases, plan trips, or organize their own social calendar considering *their* needs first. It can be a difficult time when separating from one's parents since role reversal with aging parents may become necessary. The middle adult needs to accomplish this without active domineering. Achieving independence is a life-long process beginning with adolescence and young adulthood, but the middle adult must focus on it to achieve satisfaction in later life.

The nurse who is personally uninvolved may help to reduce the pain that is involved for all generations by providing support to middle adults as they separate from their children, take pride in their accomplishments, or accept their friends and mates. The nurse can also become actively involved when middle adults interact with their parents.

**Reviewing One's Value System** Middle adults need to feel secure about the foundation on which their values are based. Values change along with everything else, sometimes too rapidly to be evaluated during years that are filled with parenting or pursuit of a career. Middle adulthood is a period that allows time to go back and reexamine values. Some middle adults, now freed from their parental roles, experiment in new social behaviors. The common result is that some values are discarded, others are retained, and confidence is enhanced for one's having taken stock.

The nurse should support middle adults and encourage them to look closely and carefully at their values, especially those established in adolescence and young adulthood. There is potential for growth in an examination of what to discard, what to alter, and what to hold as meaningful, and the nurse has a responsibility to help the middle adult recognize that potential.

**Initiating Plans for the Future by Anticipating Aging** For the middle adult, the future means retirement and old age. Retirement is a complex issue, with financial, social, and geographic implications, and it needs to be prepared for early. This task involves anticipating and planning for the next stage of growth, older adulthood. Frequently such planning is based upon current abilities and interests.

As stated earlier, physical powers decline during the aging process. The first signs of aging are usually losses in sense acuity. Thus, any plans the middle adult makes for retirement and old age should allow for these physical changes.

It is important for the middle adult to give thought to developing new sources of enjoyment, since it is inevitable that some current interests will disappear as one ages (Fig. 3-4). Because it is impossible to know which physical abilities will begin to diminish first, it is of value to cultivate a variety of activities involving all of the senses: music for hearing, painting and reading for sight, knitting or carpentry for touch, cooking for taste, and flower or herb gardening for smell. Much of what is dreaded about old age can be minimized, and much of what is happily anticipated can be increased if the middle adult begins to prepare for retirement and old age early. Nurses have a responsibility to clients in the middle years to encourage them to look to the future realistically.

### Sexuality*

Most middle-aged Americans are victimized by a sexual stereotype that is culturally induced and perpetuated by commercialism. In Western society, body beauty and physique tend to be equated with sexual desire and potency. Generally, it is acceptable to be chronologically old if one looks young, and to be sexually active if one looks attractive. Conversely, the aging body may be considered by some to be repulsive or even obscene.

The advertising media have played a major role in perpetuating this myth. Models are generally either "beauties" or "uglies." The uglies often promote paper towels and drain cleaners while the beauties promote cigarettes, liquor, cosmetics, and new cars. The beauties are generally slim, sleek, impeccably groomed and garbed, and almost always young. Many ads imply that the person who chooses "brand A" is discriminating in taste, successful in business, cultured, refined, and a tiger in the bedroom.

Bombarded daily with these messages, it is little wonder that the middle-aged adult with thickening midriff, partial dentures, thinning hair, or sagging breasts may discount the possibility of

* From Sheila Dresen, "Sexuality," in *Primary Health Care of the Well Adult,* Nancy Diekelmann (ed.), McGraw-Hill, New York, 1977, by permission.

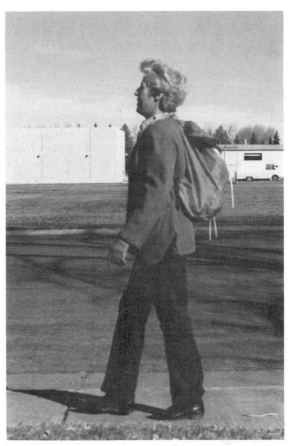

**FIGURE 3-4**
Middle adulthood is often a time to develop new interests.

offering continuing sexual attraction to a significant other. Is loss of libido inevitable or circumstantial for those in the middle years? A review of the research on the physiological effects of aging and reported changes in interest and involvement in sexual activity will provide the nurse with important information to help care for middle-aged clients.

One of the most enlightening reports about middle-aged sexuality comes from Duke University's longitudinal studies on aging. Pfeiffer and Davis obtained information about the sexual behavior of 502 whites aged 45 to 69 years, mainly of middle and upper socioeconomic status.[26] They concluded that the most significant contributing factor to current sexual functioning (including interest in, frequency of, and enjoyment of sexual relations) was previous sexual experience. Income, social class, objective physical function rating, and expectation of future life satisfaction were positively correlated with current sexual function. For women, intact marriages and being employed were also positively correlated with present sexual function. Furthermore, the enjoyment rather than the frequency of sexual relationships in younger years seems to be of particular importance in determining a middle-aged woman's current interest in and frequency of sexual intercourse.

Hunt's study of sexual behavior in the 1970s concludes that the greatest sexual liberation occurred among married people. Coital frequency has increased and is more egalitarian as to which partner initiates and which refuses. (The highest increase was found in those aged 56 to 60, who reported a frequency of once a week, as compared with once every other week reported by the Kinsey sample.) There is increased freedom to vary sexual positions and behaviors, with large increases in mouth-breast activity, manual manipulation of the penis, and oral techniques. Over 70 percent of those who found married sex very pleasant have a close relationship; very few have good sex and a poor marital relationship. This seems to indicate a reciprocal relationship between the two variables that is worth emphasizing.[27]

**Common sexual patterns for married middle-aged adults** Assuming that the desired family size has been achieved, procreation for the middle adult is probably the least desirable and most unexpected outcome of sexual intercourse. Yet the act itself continues to remain important as an expression of tenderness, trust, and love. Indeed, the multiple pressures of daily living experienced by middle-aged adults, as well as the irrefutable evidence of physical aging, may increase their desire for physical intimacy and for personal reassurance of their continuing sexual attractiveness and competency. Mace estimates that the entire time occupied in sexual intercourse by the average married couple adds up to the equivalent of about one weekend, or approximately 72 hours, a year.[28,29] Clearly, this is not enough. Hopefully, throughout their marriage the partners have remained lovers who could excite one another, not always easy while working hard at being devoted parents. Because the sexual side of their relationship may now take on added importance, the couple should be encouraged to work at the relationship, to discuss their likes and dislikes regarding techniques, positions, and sex play. Freed from responsibilities to children, they might consider spending a weekend together away from their normal environment, or experimenting with some sensual activities, such as showering together and body massage with warmed oil and fra-

grant lotions. The nurse can facilitate the couple's consideration of these activities as a celebration of their love and affection, rather than something frivolous and unimportant.

Incompatibility of sexual drive may appear for the first time during the middle years. It is not uncommon for the woman's libido to increase after menopause, when she no longer fears pregnancy. However, if she devalues herself because of losses related to role change, she may require a lot of her mate's energy to support her, leaving both with depleted reserves to invest in their sexual experience and predisposing either or both to develop sexual dysfunction. In contrast to women, middle-aged men tend to experience a gradual decline in their sexual interest and activity. Unresolved differences in sexual drive may generate much stress between the partners, and cultural inhibitions unfortunately often result in avoidance of a discussion of these difficulties either between the partners or with health care professionals. Obtaining a good health history continues to be an excellent tool for the nurse both to teach about normal behavior and to gather diagnostic information. Couples who do not intuitively understand that the need for sexual intimacy can be met in a variety of ways may not feel comfortable with anything short of vaginal intercourse unless they are specifically told that options such as mutual masturbation are normal and healthy and not indicative of a "poor" sexual relationship. Nurses can provide this kind of sex education.

The developmental stage of their family life causes middle-aged adults to be vulnerable to prolonged periods of separation from their partners. Business trips, visits to adult children, and responsibilities for ailing parents living in other areas are common realities for many middle-aged couples. The increase in sexual tension during their separation may be problematic for both partners unless they have previously learned how to cope with it. Nurses are in an unique position to detect this stress and to assist in exploration of alternative coping behavior.

Women apparently tolerate periods of little or no sexual activity better than men.[30] There is still a general belief that men engage in extramarital affairs more frequently than women. However, one recent study found that 26 percent of married women interviewed, as compared with 25 percent in the Kinsey study, had experienced at least one extramarital affair.[31] It is likely that there will be considerable leveling of these differences between the sexes in the next decade or two.

**The single middle-aged adult** Relatively little is actually *known* about the sexual behavior of single middle-aged adults, although there are plenty of myths. Divorcees are frequently feared and avoided by married women because they are perceived as seductive, promiscuous, and a threat to their marriage. Adults who lose a spouse due to death are frequently "neutered" by family and friends who are unable or unwilling to acknowledge their continuing need for physical and emotional intimacy. Women who choose to remain single are labeled as "marital rejects" with little or no sexual drive. Men who choose to remain single are perceived as "swingers" with high sex drives requiring a variety of partners. Two middle-aged men who live together are presumed to be homosexual, although it has traditionally been a matter of little interest or speculation for two women to live together.

The only statement about the sexual needs of the single middle-aged adult that can be made with any degree of certainty is that they clearly exist. Whether the individual deals with them by sublimation, fantasy, cold showers, masturbation, and homosexual or heterosexual activity is a matter of chance, choice, availability, and timing.

Research indicates that nearly all divorced females resume sexual activity following the divorce, as compared with about 50 percent of widows. Widows are usually more financially secure, have feelings of loyalty to the deceased husband, and are subtly inhibited through continuing bonds with in-laws from engaging in sex with other men.[32]

It is essential that nurses acknowledge sexuality as a continuing human drive in all adults. The nurse's listening skills are vital in picking up subtle clues that indicate clients' needs to discuss their sexuality, and the nurse's own behavior will establish a climate which either encourages or discourages tentative efforts to explore this sensitive area.

It seems highly unreasonable to assume that the termination by death, divorce, or separation of a satisfying sexual relationship will not place stress on the person involved. Nurses are becoming increasingly skilled at enabling clients to handle their grief, but the sexual needs of the "survivor" frequently are assigned a very low priority or are conspicuous by their absence from nursing-care plans. Nurses, as well as other members of a community, are frequently punitive towards single parents who acknowledge and deal with their sexual drive. Somehow the behavior, no matter how discreet, is interpreted as an affront to the memory of the previous spouse, the moral environment of the children,

and respectability of the neighborhood. The client has a right to be treated with respect, and the nurse has absolutely no responsibility either to condone or reject whatever decisions have been made. The nurse can help the client to look at all available options and their outcomes as well as available resources and can support the client in taking responsibility for making an informed choice.

This type of problem solving may bear little relationship to the nurse's formal education. For example, if the problem is inadequate space and/or privacy, the nurse may help the client explore the possibility of making an arrangement with another single parent to swap periodic overnight or weekend child-care responsibilities. For the nurse who gets "rattled" by this type of discussion, it may be helpful to consider it a kind of contingency planning designed to promote and safeguard the health and welfare of both the parent and the child. It is also important for the heterosexual nurse to be aware that previously married individuals do not always remain heterosexual in their preference. The nurse will avoid embarrassment for all concerned by not making unwarranted assumptions.

Aside from the adult's own reputation, the major concern about extramarital relationships is usually their effect on the children. The issue becomes more complicated when the parent has a homosexual preference. The developmental stage of the child will determine what he or she understands about the nature of a parent's relationship with another adult, and the impact of that relationship on the parent-child dyad. It is not the purpose of this book to consider childhood experiences in depth, but only to acknowledge that most parents take very seriously the potential effect of their personal behavior on their children. Having adult children may increase rather than decrease the anxiety about engaging in an extramarital relationship, since adult children can be critical and punitive— ostensibly because of loyalty to the other parent, but frequently because of their own hang-ups. The prerequisite for any attempt by an adult to explain the nature of an intimate relationship to a child is honesty, honesty with self, with the partner, and with the child (dependent upon the ability of the child to understand). Beyond that, nurses can offer no recipe, since each family situation is unique.

In situations where sexual partners are not available, or available partners are unacceptable, many single middle-aged adults use masturbation to relieve sexual tension. The women's movement and the appearance in "respectable" bookstores of a variety of publications on "self" and "other" pleasuring have "legitimized" masturbation as an acceptable sexual outlet for both men and women. It can be a highly gratifying experience, in spite of its common association with a sense of guilt. Nurses can be helpful by acknowledging that masturbation is a perfectly normal, universal phenomenon. Nurses, however, may tend to be sensitive to their own biases, particularly as they relate to "gimmicks" and "devices" such as body oil and vibrators. Advice should be limited to matters of safety only, such as the danger of using an electric vibrator in the bathtub or shower stall.

Another obvious alternative for single adults to meet their sexual needs is to engage in a homosexual relationship. Statistics about the number of American adults having a homosexual preference remain unreliable. One should note that there is a degree of commitment and permanence in many homosexual relationships equal to or greater than that found in many heterosexual marriages, particularly if one considers the rising incidence of serial monogamy. Indeed, the existence of long-term homosexual relationships is a phenomenological wonder, considering how many social forces are arrayed against the homosexual couple as compared with the social supports that tend to shore up faltering heterosexual marriages. Therefore, to consider homosexual behavior as a practice engaged in only by single adults is to discount the reality of many homosexual couples' life experiences. Again, the women's movement may exert a significant influence on the future prevalence of lesbianism in middle-aged women. Today's young adult women are more likely than their mothers to accept and value a warm, loving, and perhaps sexual relationship with another woman. Considering the differences in life expectancies and the resulting male-female ratio in adult groups, a lesbian relationship may be an increasingly viable option for some single middle-aged women who cannot or prefer not to engage in an intimate relationship with a single male or with someone else's husband.

Some of the concerns of aging in the middle years are common to both heterosexual and homosexual adults. Many homosexual men verbalize an awareness of the significance of youth and body beauty in their partners, and a fear of the effects of aging on their ability to attract and retain a "significant other." Middle-aged homosexual men may seek out youthful partners to maintain their own illusion of youth. While some young homosexual men prefer the maturity and experience of a middle-aged lover, others may find the visible signs of aging abhorrent in their partners because it confronts them with their own inevitable aging. Regardless of their personal opinions, it is important for nurses to be aware that the homosexual culture imposes the same kinds of stereotypes on its community as does the "straight" society.

Generally speaking, no sexual practices are unique to a homosexual experience. Consequently, there is no specific additional information which nurses need to have when dealing with a homosexual client. Sexual behavior, regardless of the gender of one's partner, is as rich and varied as the involved individuals wish it to be.

One final option for the single adult deserves attention. While it may no longer be fashionable to be a virgin, there remain some people who choose celibacy as a way of life. They have a right to that choice, yet because it constitutes a deviation from the accepted norm, it may be perceived as somehow threatening. Many people harbor a good deal of resentment against celibates, especially avowed ones like priests and nuns, and deal with that resentment by making crude jokes, uninformed guesses, or outright statements of disbelief. Just as nurses must avoid the temptation to judge other life-style options, they need to guard against a prejudicial approach to celibates.

It is the nurse's responsibility to detect and encourage discussion of clients' stress related to sexuality. Young nurses need to consider their feelings and attitudes about human sexuality in middle age, particularly when a client is their parents' age. Professional training allows nurses to inform clients about the various choices and their consequences; clients make their own decisions.

## Male and Female Menopause*

*Change of life* is a term that, as it is commonly used, roughly equates menopause and the climacterium and tends to disregard the male altogether. Properly speaking, menopause is an event that occurs only in women and involves the cessation of the menses. Climacterium occurs in both men and women and denotes the loss of ability to reproduce. In women, menopause and climacterium occur together, between the ages of 45 and 60. In the male, climacterium occurs 20 or 30 years later, between the ages of 70 and 90. Also hidden by the popular use of the term is the fact that men do experience a primarily psychosocial reaction that re-

---

* From Nancy Diekelmann and Sheila Dresen, "Menopause," in *Primary Health Care of the Well Adult*, Nancy Diekelmann (ed.), McGraw-Hill, New York, 1977, by permission.

sembles those experienced by women at menopause and occurs at about the same time as the female menopause. This has been referred to as a pseudoclimacterium or male menopause.

Overall, menopause has received little attention in the nursing literature. Perhaps it is felt that because menopause is not a health problem, nurses need not be concerned with it. Possibly we along with others believe that the physician is best prepared to deal with it, or perhaps it it felt that nothing can be done about it and that there is no sense dealing with it. The fact is that menopause is one of the fundamental landmarks of the middle years, and to ignore it is to leave ourselves unprepared to counsel clients who come to us with questions or menopausally related problems.

**Physiological changes of the female menopause** The emphasis in this section is that menopause is a normal physiological event, not a pathological state. It represents a transitional phase of a woman's life, a period of adjustment to the waning potential of the ovary which takes place over a period of about 15 years, between 45 and 60 years of age, and is the counterpart of puberty in the adolescent. A premature menopause, one that takes place before age 40, occurs in only about 8 percent of women.[33]

During this time, the woman is neither predictably sterile nor frigid. The key physical change is permanent and irreversible atrophy of the ovaries, accompanied by a corresponding decline in estrogen and progesterone production. With the cessation of ovulation, it has been established that estrogenic production in the human female does not completely disappear. Studies of vaginal smears have shown an estrogenic effect to persist for a decade or more beyond the menopause in nearly 80 percent of all postmenopausal women.[34,35] One study found that 40 percent of postmenopausal women maintain moderate levels of estrogenic activity during the remaining years of life. This residual estrogen is produced by the adrenal gland, the ovarian stromal cells which have the capacity for steroidogenesis, and perhaps from an unknown source.

Because an individual's potential for functioning in a satisfactory sexual relationship is so closely involved with the perception of one's body as sensuous and attractive, it is important to consider the visible effect on the body of the gradually diminishing ovarian function. Some signs precede menopause. For example, the breasts may become turgid and tender, and even increase in size, probably as a result of the unmodified effect of the estrogen during anovulatory cycles, and also, it is thought, because of increased pituitary stimulation. At this time, cystic mastitis or other fibrocystic conditions of the breasts may develop or grow worse.[36] Following menopause, buttocks and breasts shrink and droop as fat, glandular tissue, and tone decrease. The nipples become smaller and lose their erectile character.

The hot flush or flash is the sure sign of the menopausal syndrome, as it occurs only in this instance. Hot flashes may occur over a period of from 1 to 10 years and in some women appear before the menopause is definitely established, during the time when the estrogen levels are known to fluctuate. They gradually begin as a sensation of warmth over the upper part of the chest and characteristically spread, wavelike, over the neck, face, and upper extremities. They come on with unpredictable suddenness, and are often followed by profuse perspiration and chills. They are especially disturbing at night, interfering with sleep, and the perspiration may be so drenching as to require a change of bedclothes. The frequency and severity are subject to wide variation. Flushes and sweats are usually more severe in anxious women and are intensified by excitement or stress. Other vasomotor symptoms include numbness and tingling, cold hands and feet, vertigo, and palpitations. The precise mechanism for the vasomotor symptoms is uncertain, but evidence points to a disturbance in the equilibrium between the hypothalamus and the autonomic nervous system, both of which apparently become conditioned to a high estrogen level and then react to its decline.

Atrophic vaginitis occurs more commonly some years after menopause begins. As a result of estrogen insufficiency, the vaginal epithelium eventually becomes pale and dry due to decreasing vascularity and atrophy of the mucous membrane. The loose purple rugae of the vaginal walls become thin, pale, and fragile and "sweat" less lubricant during sexual arousal, especially if the woman neither masturbates nor has intercourse more than once or twice a month. There may be pain on penetration, and the vaginal mucosa is easily eroded, may bleed, or develop adhesions. The normally acidic vaginal secretions become alkaline or only slightly acidic, thus increasing susceptibility to infection, even by organisms of normally low virulence. The predominating symptoms of senile vaginitis reported by women clients are discharge, itching, burning, and dysparunia or painful intercourse.

Many women do not realize that these changes

are normal and that the problems that can result can be remedied with medication. Thus if the nurse prepares the premenopausal woman for these changes, especially the possibility that she may experience painful intercourse, the client will not blame herself for not being able to respond to her partner, nor will she feel that she is frigid or incapable of being sexually active anymore. She will be alert to the probable cause and will seek out medical advice at that time.

Atrophic changes due to estrogen deficiency also cause the supporting structures of the uterus, bladder, and rectum to lose tone and strength, favoring the development of uterine prolapse, cystocele, and rectocele, especially in women who have borne children. Urinary symptoms such as frequency, urgency, burning on urination, and defective bladder control may send women to consult their doctors. Since menopausal women are particularly susceptible to bladder infections, it is important for the nurse to review good personal hygiene, so that bladder infections are avoided whenever possible.

During menopause, menstruation generally involves decreased flow and may vary in frequency, at times skipping 1 or more months. However, all kinds of menstrual disturbance—menorrhagia, metrorrhagia, hypomenorrhea, polymenorrhea, and oligomenorrhea—may herald the menopause. Of major concern to sexually active women is the question of how long following the cessation of menstruation is it safe to discard birth control. Pregnancy has occurred up to age 50.[37] Occasionally an ovulatory cycle will occur while the woman is still menstruating. Taking oral contraceptives will not postpone the beginning of menopause, which is genetically determined, but will simply mask it. If on the pill, a woman will not menstruate if she is menopausal when the drug is stopped. One gynecologist recommends that women discontinue the pill at age 44. If normal menses resume spontaneously within 3 months, the woman would resume taking the pill for another 9 months. She then goes off the pill for 3 months and repeats the cycle. If no menstrual period occurs during this time, she is assumed to be menopausal.[38] A reasonably safe time to discontinue birth control is 6 months after the cessation of menstruation. Most gynecologists recommend the use of some form of birth control other than oral contraceptives during these months as an extra precautionary measure. It is important that unwanted pregnancies be avoided for the sake of both mother and child. The 40-year-old mother is considered to be high risk on the basis of age, and there is

a high incidence of abnormal births, particularly children with Down's syndrome, among women in this age group.

The physiological signs of aging may be very difficult for a woman to accept, especially in view of today's emphasis on youth and the competition which she may feel from younger members of her sex. For a woman who cannot accept fading physical allure and youthfulness, and whose sense of self-worth is derived from a need to have her body admired, a sense of loss will inevitably follow as the aging process begins to become more visible and public. Similarly, the loss of the power of generativity which accompanies menopause may precipitate a full-blown grief reaction in the woman whose sense of femininity is intimately tied to her fertility, regardless of her marital status.

**Psychosocial aspects of menopause** If we think of this period as it has been defined, as a transition from one period of life to another and the counterpart of puberty, it is easy to see that many women may find difficulties in making the adjustment. The physiological signs of aging may be very difficult for many women to accept, particularly a woman who is influenced by the exaggerated American emphasis on youth and has become accustomed to having her body admired. For any woman, the recognition that she has lost her power of generativity is bound to be a milestone, especially if she feels it is the essence of her femininity. If she has devoted the major share of her energy to efforts to stay young and physically attractive, instead of looking forward to the challenges, services, and rewards which inevitably accompany maturity, the transition may be especially difficult. The nurse can do much to help her clients make this transition with grace.

Some women, overwhelmed by menopause as a sign of their own mortality, may feel cheated and angry as they realize that they have given a large portion of their lives to child-bearing and child-rearing, and that their children are now at the point of leaving home to live their own lives. For such a woman, the adjustment of being "alone together" with her husband may require as much effort as did the initial adjustment to marriage. Not only can the nurse help to show her that she has much to look forward to in the new situation, but the nurse can also help the husband to understand and be sympathetic to his wife's point of view. The husband should be aware that during menopause his wife may need more recreation, amusement, and rest than usual. She may need to be told more that she's loved and appreciated and that she is sexually satisfying. It may be helpful for the husband to show more interest in birthdays and anniversaries. Sometimes, when she is feeling "blue" it may be helpful to go to a movie or to pitch in to do the household chores together. A long-wished-for trip might also help the wife better cope with menopause.

In a study by Neugarten[39] of 100 women between the ages of 45 and 55, in which the participants were asked to list the fears they had of middle age, menopause did not rank very high. Of greatest concern was widowhood. Generally, women feared "getting older," "lack of energy," and "poor health or illness." The best aspects of menopause were seen to be not worrying about pregnancy and not having to bother with menstruation; the worst aspects were not knowing what to expect, the pain and discomfort, and the indication that they were growing older. A most significant finding of this study was that the women concerned were extremely eager to discuss menopause and were very curious about it. We give little social support to menopausal women as compared with the very great amount we give to pregnant women.

Many women are reluctant to bring up menopause with their doctor because they are afraid he will brush the topic off as unimportant. They will talk much more freely with the nurse, who should be an attentive, careful, encouraging listener. A listening attitude is very important because many times the client is validating that what she is experiencing is normal. Nurses can give this assurance, and they can also encourage the woman to relax and go along with, rather than fight, changes in body rhythms. Many women in the menopause feel bursting with energy one day, and as if they were getting over a bad flu attack the next; the nurse can suggest some rearrangement of their schedules so that they can tackle heavy jobs on the former and rest on the latter. Since insomnia is common in this period, patients should be advised to get up in the night and do something such as writing letters or reading, instead of tossing and turning. For many clients, menopause is an excellent time to develop some outside activities, such as shopping or luncheon engagements with friends, volunteer work, concerts, or short trips, though these should be well planned to avoid overexertion. The advantages of taking naps when they feel like it and have the chance should also be pointed out.

One myth of menopause the nurse should dispel is that it ends a woman's interest and participation in a regular sexual relationship. In fact, the function of the ovary has little to do with either libido or orgasm. It is true that a woman's view of herself as a lovable, sexually desirable partner may depend on her own body image or sense of self-esteem, and if either of these is diminished, her libido is bound to be affected also. Pfeiffer also suggests that the extent of an aging woman's sexual activity and interest depends heavily on the availability of a socially sanctioned, sexually capable partner.[40] Physiologically, there is no reason why a woman may not engage in sexual activity well into her advanced years. Opportunity for regular sexual expression, at least once a week, is important to maintain lubrication and distensibility, and the vagina is not discriminatory as to the source of that stimulation, whether it be self or other-initiated. If there is genital discomfort and/or senile vaginitis, local application of estrogen cream or suppositories will restore the vaginal epithelium to its former thickness and alleviate the symptoms. Positive feelings about oneself, the opportunity to be sexually active, and habit are the key to sexual satisfaction.

**Physiological changes of male menopause**
A differentiation should be made between what happens to a man in his fifties and what happens to a man in his seventies. Testosterone levels reach their peak about age 20 in the male, after which they begin dropping, though there is a plateau between the ages of 40 and 60. After 60, they continue to drop until about age 70, when they become so low as to cause a serious decline in libido, sexual capacity, muscular strength, and aggressiveness. At this time, climacterium, the man may experience hot flashes, sweating attacks, anxiety, depression, and nightmares. He may even forget where he is or what he is doing. Since this occurs 20 years later than in the female and the individual is usually in his seventies, the forgetfulness is often times just attributed to hardening of the arteries. While this may be a factor, it may not account for all the forgetfulness.

There is disagreement among the "experts" as to whether or not there is a discrete phenomenon known as *male menopause*. The middle-aged man may experience a gradually diminishing virility and a slackening of his ability to perform sexually, a syndrome particularly distressing to men who have depended on sexual prowess to sustain their sense of masculinity and youthfulness. Change in the sexual response cycle reflects the general slowing-down effect of normal aging on other parts of the musculoskeletal system. The sex flush decreases, erection takes longer to achieve, ejaculation is less forceful and shorter in duration, and the refractory period may increase. However, with regular sexual expression and a stimulating sexual climate, a healthy man's sexual capacity may extend well into his eighties. Again, it is critical to remember that there is much individual variation. A 47-year-old may enjoy a ½-hour refractory period while a 32-year-old may require 8 to 12 hours. There is no national norm against which all men can measure their sexual behavior.

However, those symptoms which are associated with male menopause, such as moodiness, impatience, worry, touchiness, headaches, and hypochondria, are often attributed to the fact that the middle-aged man is worried about competition from younger men, decreasing opportunities for job changes and/or advancement, and pressure to provide for retirement while maintaining the present standard of living.

Whether or not a man is diagnosed and treated for male menopause depends on the physician from whom he seeks care. Borderline testosterone titers are associated with decreasing libido, but the titer is also known to fluctuate according to increased stress and loss of self-esteem.

Nathaniel, age 52, has been feeling generally rundown. He is aware that his sexual drive has decreased markedly over the past year. Once or twice he has been impotent. He is feeling depressed because he has reached his maximum earning potential as a semiskilled laborer, and he worries about financing his daughter's upcoming wedding. There is a history of adult-onset diabetes in Nathaniel's family.

Given that the findings on his medical exam and lab tests are within normal limits, except for a borderline testosterone level, Nathaniel may be seen as premorbid in whatever area of specialization his physician practices. For example, a psychiatrist may interpret reduced libido as a part of depression due to his life experiences and prescribe psychotherapy. An internist may see it as a precursor of diabetes and prescribe diet modification and weight loss. An endocrinologist may prescribe testosterone to elevate the libido. In all probability, any intervention that improves Nathaniel's general state of health and induces a sense of well-being will be effective in causing an increased libido, because men are vulnerable to suggestion of sexual failure and are easily locked into a spiral of self-defeat. The important thing for nurses to be aware of is the complexity of the syndrome and the variety of approaches to treatment. Testosterone can be prescribed for symptomatic purposes; however, it is not usually prescribed for prolonged periods since it tends to accelerate atherosclerosis or heart disease.[41] Nurses need to bear in mind that there are expectations related to socioeconomic status and culture that may exacerbate a client's problem. Studies show it is not uncommon for blue-collar workers of all ages to expect to be sexually very active and to perceive any reduction or interruption in that activity as a serious threat to their health.[42] Nurses need to be alert and responsive to this type of concern.

**Psychosocial aspects of male menopause**
After the age 50, depression and self-destructive behavior significantly increase in males; 25 percent of all divorces and remarriages involve middle-aged males.[43] At this time many men desire and feel that they need greater stimulation in all areas of their lives, including sex, and seek out younger partners to experience it. The man often is not aware that his desire may be the result of a normal reduction, at his age, in his ability to see, hear, smell, and experience sexual and sensual stimulation. It is equally important for the man to understand these changes, and for his wife to understand him. This is often asking a good deal. The wife may also be experiencing menopause and be in need of understanding and support. It is not only possible, but easy, for great misunderstandings to arise between them; the nurse may do much to dispel these misunderstandings if she is sympathetic with both husband and wife in this situation.

We have already pointed out that the nurse can help to show the woman that middle age is not an end, but a new beginning. She can do the same thing for the man. Something has been lost, yes, but lost normally and inevitably in the process of moving toward potential gain. At this time, a man may naturally take stock of what he has accomplished with his life, and he may not feel satisfied. He may perceive new horizons and want to do his own thing. An understanding wife can sympathize and encourage. A man may turn to alcohol or to hypochondria. Again, an understanding wife can try to distract her husband from these undesirable outlets by providing variety and excitement, perhaps in bed. In each case the nurse can help in explaining the normal, physiological reasons underlying a man's behavior. Our society teaches women how to satisfy their husbands' appetites at the dinner table, but not in bed; the nurse may help an uninstructed wife here, as well. She can certainly point out the importance of giving the husband compliments rather than criticism, a sympathetic ear rather than an angry voice, at this period of his life. For example, if the husband falls asleep in front of the TV after dinner, the wife should not make a scene about it but understand that he may simply need a nap. At this time of life, some men panic, but there is no more need for a man to panic because he has reached an inevitable and normal change-of-life stage than there is for a theater audience to get up and go home when the curtain falls after the first act. There is much for him to look forward to as it rises on a new stage set.

Since we are all human, we all deal in different ways with the change of life, and with varying degrees of success. The nurse by providing anticipatory guidance can help her clients successfully cope with menopause. She can listen, provide suggestions, and reassurance. Some people choose to deal with the change of life by denying it and turning their attention to other things. This method might be quite successful, as in the case of a teacher who decides it is the right time to write a book on a subject of long-term interest. It might be unsuccessful, as in the case of a man who overcompensates by sexual conquests and thereby breaks up a long-standing, happy marriage at the cost of great pain to wife and children; or of a woman who feels a compulsion to spend large amounts of money on surgery to restore the youthful appearance it is impossible for her to maintain. Other ways of coping include decompensation, depression, anxiety, alcoholism, and hypochondriasis. Intervention and referral may be appropriate by the nurse in each situation.

Many middle adults can be helped to see the change of life for what it is: inevitable and hopeful. It can be the opportunity to make progress in freeing oneself from childish self-centeredness; the opportunity to grow not old, but mature, wise, and happy; the opportunity to become interested in, and to serve others.

### Life-styles

As the middle adult changes physically and emotionally, so alterations in life-style occur, not necessarily as a consequence of the physical and emotional changes but as an integral part of the aging experience. Life-styles are affected by changing societal roles, cultural influences, economic factors, and family structure.

**Societal influences**  In our American society, the young adult is likely to set as goals such things as job security, owning a house, and establishing a good nest egg in the bank. These are likely to be attained by age 40. What then? More of the same? What for? Life is bland without the savor of something for which to work.

Leisure is increasing in American life, and middle-aged men and women may find time hanging heavily on their hands. People do not allow jobs to cut into their personal time as much as in times past; smaller families mean less time devoted to household chores. Nurses can at least encourage their clients to enlarge their interests and develop new hobbies and activities which will be satisfying and enjoyable. The needs of the middle adult for exercise, particularly of the heart, should not be overlooked. Jogging, swimming, and bicycling, judiciously practiced in the middle years, will actually retard the aging process and can continue to be a source of enjoyment for a long time.[44] Also, clients can be encouraged to find ways to become contributing members of the community; volunteer workers are always in demand, and this is often a rewarding way of spending time.

Many middle-adult workers enjoy the success, prestige, authority, autonomy, and income they have. Others, also trained and experienced, find themselves in less satisfying jobs. Many factors contribute to successful vocational adjustment, some of which are congenial relationships with co-workers, opportunities for self-actualization on the job, and satisfaction on the part of family members (especially the spouse) with the worker's vocational achievements. Other factors influencing positive adjustment include satisfaction with the treatment received from management and direct superiors; satisfaction with the provisions made by management for illness, vacations, disability, retirement, and other fringe benefits; and feelings of security about the job, that is, not being forced to relocate to hold a job, advance in it, or get a new job.[45]

**Cultural influences**  Various cultures cope with the experience of aging differently. In many cultures developmental "milestones" are marked with special rituals and celebrations. Western societies, however, tend to treat developmental stages casually. This lack of ritual leaves people without a clear sense of where they are, and this is especially true in middle adulthood. Once the status of adulthood is attained, developmental changes are virtually ignored until retirement. This often leaves middle adults torn between two generations, as they see part of themselves in their aging parents and part in their children. One generation considers them old and the other young. Without clear rituals to help them enter a different life stage, middle adults must rely on other cues within the culture. At home their children are growing up, leaving home, marrying; at work younger workers are asking advice. In Western societies, this transition to middle adulthood is made more difficult by the status attributed to it. While it is the middle adult who is deemed most powerful, the fact of aging is held in a negative light. The nurse can be supportive of the middle adult's feelings of competence and ability and emphasize the joy of these years of productivity. Middle adults who are unhappy with life decisions should be encouraged to explore new outlets for their energy. The decision that it is "too late to change" in middle adulthood will only make the inevitable dissatisfaction more difficult to cope with in late adulthood.

In a discussion of cultural influences it is convenient to speak of "Western societies." However, variations in the aging experience exist between the various cultures found in the West. Unfortunately, little has been written to help nurses understand the European middle adult as opposed to the black middle adult or Japanese Americans.

**Economic influences** According to statistics, middle adults are in the fortunate position of having more money in savings accounts and proportionally less debt than any other age group. Yet they can easily be overwhelmed by extraordinary expenses, to which their position of responsibility to both younger and older generations makes them very vulnerable. Many American parents start a college fund early for each child, but the explosive increase in the cost of a college education in recent years often makes these funds seem pitifully small. Sky-rocketing medical costs (especially when elderly parents are vulnerable) can completely impoverish persons considered well-to-do. Too often health insurance is not adequate to offset unusual expenses.

Economic instability can mean job loss for many middle-aged men. It is not easy for a man of 50 to start a new career, nor is it easy for a woman who has not worked outside her home for 20 years to go back into a field which has changed significantly since she left it. Often it is difficult for either a man or a woman to find any job at all. Even for those who maintain their jobs, current economic conditions may put customary life-styles beyond the means of the average wage earner. For all of these situations, the nurse can be a source of encouragement and support, and can help clients to see that making the best of all the changes with which they are faced is an opportunity for personal growth.

**Family influences** For middle adult parents this is a time when children leave home to make their own lives. While this frees the parents from financial responsibility, it also diminishes their roles as parents. In coping with this role change, women commonly experience more difficulty than men, since the father's role traditionally has been less time and energy consuming than the mother's. Men can also compensate for this loss by deriving added satisfaction from their work. Some middle-aged couples experience difficulty if they expect to have the same parent-child relationship that existed before the child's marriage, or if they anticipate that their relationship with a son-in-law or daughter-in-law will be the same as the relationship with their own children.

This sense of loss is exacerbated by our new social mobility. The continuity that existed when a son took over the family farm no longer applies. Today, to an unprecedented extent, the children of blue-collar workers go to college and develop tastes or interests unfamiliar or unavailable to their parents. The farmer's son, for instance, gets a Ph.D. in biochemistry, marries, and settles down in a big city as a faculty member of a large university. The son of a maintenance man becomes a professional violinist who plays with a large metropolitan symphony. Second generation families have moved away from their parents; they have different occupations, different recreations, different friends, different interests, and different life-styles.

Another change in this period is in the relationship between husband and wife. When they were in their twenties, they were raising their children, working hard for career or business advancement, and too much occupied to give time or thought to self-analysis. With the children now gone, and often faced with decreasing job pressure, they are conscious of empty time. They look at each other and perhaps see the face of a stranger. Sadly, the divorce and suicide rates are very high among middle adults. It may be possible for the nurse to help by suggesting that that period of life need not imply a rift between spouses, but an opportunity to form a new and stronger relationship, a second "coming together."

Still another change in the family is the relationship of middle adults to their own parents. For most, parents now are elderly, and this can present problems even more difficult and painful than those involving children. Again, the most successful way to deal with these problems is by facing them early, before they become so acute as to call for extreme measures which often result in great unhappiness, bitterness, and feelings of guilt.

While elderly parents are still in good health, self-reliant, and able to make decisions adapted to the variety of situations that may arise, middle-aged children should discuss future possibilities with them. If it has not occurred to them to do so, the nurse will do well to suggest this type of assessment. Even with careful planning, a situation in which elderly parents need help can be a difficult one (Fig. 3-5). To force elderly parents to leave their own home against their wishes, as is often the case with a recent widow or widower, intensifies the pain and suffering of the parent. These situations are distressing for any sympathetic child and often produce a keen sense of guilt. But on the whole, difficulties are lessened if conditions are explored together by middle-aged children and elderly parents before a crisis arises.

Potential obstacles for successful social and personal adjustment of the middle adult in terms of family life are a child's growing up and marrying, the necessity to establish satisfactory interpersonal relationships with the spouse, changing sexual capabilities, the problems of elderly parents, the potential for divorce, and the prospect of remarrying. The nurse, aware of these hazard areas, can provide anticipatory guidance to these "at-risk" middle adults.

In spite of all the changes and problems that we have cited, it is always to be remembered that middle adults, as a group, have the basic power and importance to provide leadership. They furnish significant influence in business, education, and all social activities. Like Atlas in the Greek myth, they hold up our world. Society depends on them.

## THE OLDER ADULT

Just as every person changes as he grows up,
he will continue to change as he grows old.
But aging will not destroy the continuities
between what he has been, what he is,
and what he will be.

B. L. Neugarten

All nurses will at one time or another care for an older adult, and for many the majority of their patients will be over age 65. This twentieth-century

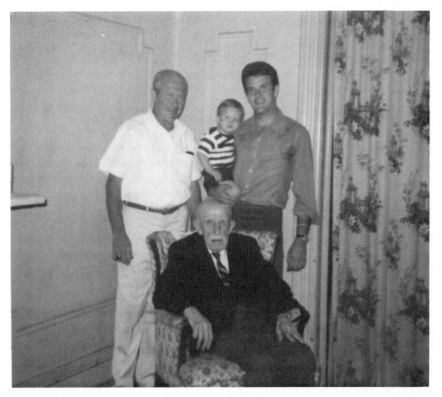

**FIGURE 3-5**
The middle adult often develops new relationships with parents and children.

phenomenon is caused by the increasing number of people living to old age. Increased longevity has resulted from improvements in maternal-child and infectious disease care rather than advances in the basic mechanisms of aging or cures for degenerative diseases. The normal maximum human life span remains at 90 to 100 years with most older adults in the United States demonstrating the clinical signs of aging and having one or more degenerative health problems by the age of 70 to 75 years.[46]

Today 10.4 percent of the total population of the United States is 65 years old or older in comparison to 4.1 percent in 1900. Projected population figures show the older adult portion of the population stabilizing at 11.7 percent, if the birth rate remains low, but the number of persons over 75 increasing disproportionally.[47] At this time, the over-75 age group accounts for a majority of the feeble aged, a fact which has important implications for health practitioners.[48]

Before considering the known or presumed facts about aging, it is important to consider what you as a person and as a practitioner believe about aging. The nurse's basic view of aging will have a great impact on what is observed, treatment modalities used, and evaluation of the care given. Basically there are two prominent views of aging. One considers aging a matter of *irreversible decrement* while the other focuses on *adaptation.* Until recently most people accepted the irreversible-decrement view in which it is felt that aging is merely a progressive decline in functioning ability which can not be stopped, modified, or reversed. The adaptation view, on the other hand, recognizes that decline occurs with age but attempts to discover whether the decline is intrinsic or environmental in origin. The health-care practitioner then intervenes to help the older adult overcome or modify these changes in order to remain functionally independent. For example, the practitioner who believes in the irreversible-decrement model of aging will tell the aged client complaining of stiff fingers that it is part of old age and nothing can be done about it, while the believer in the adaptation model will teach the client exercises to increase joint flexibility. This difference in practice pervades all levels of decision making. The most important homework you as a nurse can do is to explore your own beliefs on aging and recognize the impact that those beliefs have on the care you plan and deliver. It is ironic that nurses have been found to have a more positive attitude toward death than old age.[49]

Just what is old age? Is it a state of mind, a chronological age, a mental age, or a certain level of physiological functioning? When observing a group of older adults one can certainly list some common characteristics—wrinkled skin, gray or white thinning hair, and a flexed posture—but the differences between older individuals are more striking. One person has difficulty hearing you while the next says "don't shout at me." Some older adults are going on a 5-mile nature hike and others can't walk a block comfortably. As one grows older one has more diverse life experiences that make the older adult the most heterogeneous age group with whom you will work. This is not to say that commonalities within groups of older adults and among all aged are nonexistent. There are biological changes and experiences that will happen to all humans if they live long enough. At what age these changes occur varies among individuals. Some people are old physically and mentally when their chronological age is 40 while some 70-year-olds are still in the prime of middle age.

Since one's total life experiences have a great impact on the way old age is experienced, the information social scientists have gathered can be generalized only to the existing generation of older adults. The next generation is likely to be better educated, healthier, and more experienced at coping with lesiure time, and to have a more adequate pension than the present older generation. Changes in these values may be translated into different patterns of behavior such as an easier transition into retirement, more active health-care seeking, or political activities.

One of the first concepts nursing needs to accept and practice is treating clients as unique individuals rather than viewing them through the blur of a stereotype. The purpose of this section is to introduce changes and problems which commonly occur with advanced age in our society. When developing a data base, this information will serve as a guide but should not be considered a blueprint.

**Physical Dynamics**

There are several biological theories of aging, all of which can demonstrate a relationship to the aging process, but none of which prove the presence of a universal mechanism. Popular theories include *limited cell replication, autoimmune,* and *genetic theories.* The limited-cell replication theory posits that a cell can only divide a certain number of times. Hayflick has shown that embryonic cells will divide 50 times in culture, while adult cells will only divide 20 times before there is a decline in mitotic activity. An immune reaction to one's own tissues leads to cell dysfunction and death according to the autoimmune theory. The genetic theories generally focus on mutational changes in the cell, particularly related to DNA and RNA.[50] While these theories are interesting, they have little impact on current accepted gerontological health practices. Therefore, this section will emphasize the physical changes that are associated with aging and their implications for nurses.

The aging process is not uniform. Individuals, as well as organs in individuals, age at their own rate based on genetic heritage and environmental factors. For this reason information on the biologi-

cal changes which commonly occur will be given. Again, these should be used as a guide in developing a data base about a particular client; don't expect to find all of these changes in any one client. Because it is not possible to consider all changes, Table 3-3 is provided as a guideline when assessing and meeting the needs of the older adult.

**Cellular changes** The cellular changes that began in young adulthood and first evidenced themselves in the middle adult become obvious to greater and lesser degrees in the aged (Fig. 3-6). Changes in connective tissue as a result of age-

**TABLE 3-3**
AN OVERVIEW OF PHYSICAL CHANGES COMMONLY FOUND IN THE ELDERLY*

| Organ or System | Important Physical Symptoms | Cause of Symptoms |
|---|---|---|
| General | (1) Diminished pain sensation, (2) lack of febrile response to disease, (3) confusion | (1) Normal changes in autonomic nervous system; (2) normal change in thermoregulatory response; (3) general symptom meaning "something is wrong," e.g., hypoxia, infection, dyspnea, drug toxicity, sensory deprivation, overstimulation, etc. |
| Skin | (1) Loss of elasticity, (2) dryness, poor indicator of hydration status, (3) pressure areas, (4) breast lumps | (1) Normal age changes in connective tissue, (2) oil gland atrophy, (3) poor circulation, (4) neoplasms, cystic disease |
| Eyes | Decreased visual acuity | Normal aging change, senile mascular changes (vascular), cataracts, glaucoma, retinal detachment |
| Ears | (1) Gradual decreased auditory acuity, (2) sudden hearing loss | (1) Normal aging changes or presbycusis, wax accumulation, (3) decreased blood supply to the organ of Corti, neurological diseases |
| Mouth-throat | Hoarseness | Laryngeal pathology |
| Head-Neck | (1) Rigidity, (2) lymphadenopathy, (3) elevation of left jugular pulse, (4) arterial bruits | (1) Cervical spondylosis, Parkinson's disease, arthritis, (2) infection, (3) elongated aortic arch and obstruction, (4) obstruction in carotids, heart murmurs |
| Cardiovascular | (1) Irregular radial pulse, (2) increased systolic and diastolic pressure, (3) systolic and (4) diastolic murmurs | (1) Ectopic beats, atrial fibrillation, (2) arteriosclerotic changes in arterial system, (3) usually ejection type and not pathological, (4) significant cardiac pathology |
| Respiratory | (1) Breathing pattern disturbance, (2) deviation of trachea, (3) limited expansion | (1) Lung pathology, neurological disease, (2) kyphosis, scoliosis, (3) normal age changes in rib cartilage |
| Gastrointestinal | (1) Changes in bowel habits, (2) nonrigid peritoneum in acute abdomen | (1) Normal age changes in connective and muscle tissues, drugs, infection, organic brain disease, depressive illnesses, diverticulitis, cancer, diet changes, (2) weak abdominal muscles |
| Genitourinary | (1) Frequency, (2) dysuria, (3) incontinence | (1), (2), (3) Capacity of bladder decreases to about 250 ml, BPH, cancer, drugs, habitual overdistension, (3) neurological disease, weakened pelvic muscles |
| Musculoskeletal | (1) Slightly flexed posture, (2) enlarged, stiff joints with crepitation, (3) fractures, (4) tremors, (5) gait changes | (1) Normal aging change, (2) osteoarthritis, (3) osteoporosis, falls, demineralization, (4) infections, lung disease, Parkinson's disease, neurological disease, drug induced, (5) corns, calluses, fractures (hip), neurological disease |
| Central nervous system | (1) Sudden onset of symptoms, (2) progressive, slow onset | (1) Vascular or epileptic diseases, (2) degenerative or neoplastic diseases |

* Developed by Deborah Downey, R.N., M.S.

With age there is also a decrease in the number of sweat glands found in the skin. This causes the aged a twofold problem. With decreased sweating the skin becomes dry, but this often can be alleviated through the use of moisturizing creams. Bath oils should be avoided because they may cause cystitis. Of greater concern is the decreased ability to eliminate body heat through evaporation. Because of this the elderly are prone to heat stroke and should be taught to avoid situations where they would be excessively exposed to the sun.

The loss of pigment in the skin and hair which began in middle age, in general, becomes quite prominent in the aged. Caucasians become whiter and the hair of all racial groups turns gray. Hair loss for both men and women may be very noticeable. Because of hormonal changes, women often develop facial hair for the first time; although this can be quite distressing, depilatories or shaving can be helpful.

### Changes in perception and coordination

The brain is vital to normal perception and coordination. With age there is a 44 percent cell loss from all parts of the brain with marked losses in the cerebral cortex, particularly in the temporal and frontal areas. In general this shrinkage causes only minor functional changes. The effects are individual and are often related to concurrent hypertensive disease.

An outstanding characteristic of the aged is *slowness.* This slowness, particularly in their *reaction time,* is a pertinent safety issue for the aged when they are driving a motor vehicle. Most drivers compensate by driving slower and using low density roads, but some aged must be helped to recognize that they should give up driving and use alternative modes of transportation. When working with older adults, particularly when they are ill, the nurse should provide a relaxed atmosphere which means slowing of one's own activities to meet the level of the patient.

The older adult's reaction time is slowed in terms of their internal as well as their external mileu. Under normal circumstances, the aged have no difficulty meeting physiological needs. During stress, however, the recognition of the stressor and relaying of the information to the hypothalamus to stimulate an endocrine response is slowed, thus delaying the body's overall response to the stressor. This is true whether the stress is a result of such diverse stressors as a glucose tolerance test, traumatic shock, cold temperatures, an argument, or relocation from one institution to another. Hospi-

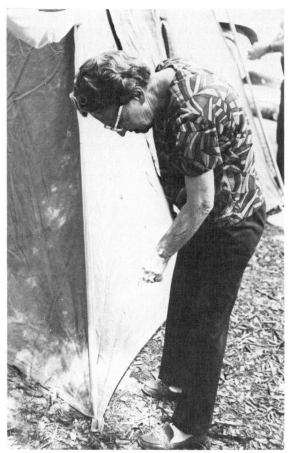

**FIGURE 3-6**
The physical changes associated with age do not prevent an active life style.

related changes in collagen and ground substance, are often obvious. The shrinkage of the intravertebral disks and curvature of the thoracic region of the spine will cause a height loss of ½ to ¾ inch by the time old age is reached. Thinning of the epithelium and a decrease in subcutaneous fat cause the skin to appear translucent, and blood vessels become more prominent and tortuous. The skin becomes less elastic and therefore wrinkled. The amount of wrinkling also varies according to the amount of exposure to the sun. Pigmentation is also a factor; people with yellow and especially black skin will wrinkle much less with age than white and light-skinned individuals. The decrease in cutaneous fat lessens the skin's insulating ability, making the aged susceptible to temperature extremes. The aged's thin, inelastic skin is very susceptible to breakdown, and nurses should be aware of this when planning care.

talization itself is stressful and can cause confusion or disorientation. This altered response to stress has many nursing implications; the hospitalized elderly should be protected from unnecessary stress, and the emergency room nurse should be aware that an aged accident victim is more likely to go into a state of shock than a younger person.

A significant perceptual change that occurs with aging is a *reduction in pain sensation.* Pain acts as a defense mechanism and warns the body of injury before it becomes severe. The aged should be cautioned to compensate for this loss. Feet should be examined regularly for sores resulting from pressure. Hot packs and heating pads should be watched carefully when in use. Smokers need to be especially careful and should always sit up when smoking. The elderly need to train their eyes to see what they cannot feel. Nurses must also obey that rule because the older adult will not demonstrate the same level of pain as younger age groups. This, combined with the fact that the elderly rarely have a strong fever defense reaction, can mean that problems like bowel obstructions or pneumonia may be present with few outstanding symptoms.

One problem often associated with the older adult is *difficulty in sensory perception.* Many age-related changes gradually occur in the eye beginning in middle age. The crystalline lens has a gradual accumulation of inert tissue, dehydration, yellowing, and loss of elasticity. The optic nerve narrows, retinal reflexes weaken, and there is a loss of retinal pigment. These changes lead to *tunnel vision* and *light transmission impairment* (only one-third of the light reaching a 30-year-old's retina reaches that of a 60-year-old). Tunnel vision can be compensated for by turning the head. It is also helpful to approach the patient from the front. The decrease in light transmission can be aided by increasing nonfluorescent lighting in areas frequented by the elderly. Difficulty adjusting to glare and light changes and an increase in night blindness also occur. Night lights should be used consistently to prevent injury. Large print and bright warm colors are useful because they are easier for the aged to read. As with slowed reaction time, these vision changes have special implications regarding driving and pedestrian safety. Periodic vision tests should be taken, and driving may have to be limited to the daytime.

Hearing also undergoes change with age. Most changes occur before age 50. *Otosclerosis* originates in young or middle age and causes an increased hearing loss until treated. *Presbycusis* is the true hearing problem of the aged. It begins at a young age with loss of high frequency tones, and by old age there may be a gradual loss of middle tones where most speech sounds are located. Finally even low tones are lost. Distortion caused by an imbalance of auditory tones can affect the ability to understand speech. Discrimination is poorest for consonants with high-frequency components in their acoustic patterns, that is, s, e, t, f, g. Consonants lack the acoustical power of vowels, so noisy environments tend to mask them.

These difficulties, plus transmission changes in the central nervous system due to neuronal loss, lead to *phonemic regression,* a combination of slowed processing and perceptual distortion which prevent the older adult from extracting meaning from the words they hear. An analogy would be beginning Spanish language students trying to comprehend a conversation with a native Spaniard speaking at a normal rate of speech. In order to overcome this problem, one should speak slowly, increasing the time it takes to say a word, not the time between words. Voice should be projected without shouting, speech should be distinct, and the older adult should be faced so lip reading cues are available. Because of the various causes and levels of hearing loss, the nurse should recommend an audiology consultation before the purchase of a hearing aid. When a hearing aid is purchased, the ear mold should be made specifically for the user.

Changes in *musculoskeletal integrity* affect coordination. Muscle mass can increase until about age 50. After that collagen begins to replace some muscle fibers and the muscle's ability to store ATP and rid itself of lactic acid diminishes. These changes decrease the size and tone of muscles and result in decreased strength and earlier fatigue, with longer periods of time needed to recover from fatigue. This does not mean, however, that the older adult is relegated to a rocking chair. These changes occur over a long period of time and the older person can remain relatively active, not at the level he or she performed 30 years ago, but well enough to participate in most activities. The true loss of mobility in aging occurs from disuse. Older people need to routinely participate in body conditioning activities. Regular exercise can maintain range of motion, improve muscle tone, ventilatory ability, and cardiac functioning.

As a person ages, the bones become more porous, a condition called *osteoporosis.* This makes them brittle and more easily broken. Care should be taken to prevent accidents both in the hospital and at home. Coordination is especially affected by *joint changes.* Cartilage becomes less pliable with rough articulating surfaces. Connective tissue also becomes inflexible leading to stiffened joints. This may affect the older person's ability to perform unaccustomed fine movements, a point that should be taken into consideration when teaching new skills such as the use of an insulin syringe. The nurse should realize that more time will be needed to accomplish the task.

Consistent exercise will improve joint movement, but in some cases alternative methods may be used. Immobility enhances joint stiffness, and bed rest should never be prescribed for the older adult without first seriously contemplating the effects. The importance of active range of motion exercise should be impressed upon the elderly and passive exercises should be done consistently when necessary. Older adults engaged in active sports should be advised of the importance of warm-up exercises.

**Metabolic changes** Before metabolism can occur an individual must consume and digest food. Both of these areas can be affected by age. Missing or absent teeth are a problem for some elderly, while others have ill-fitting dentures. Clients may need to be reminded that dentures must be relined when gum atrophy occurs. Digestion of food is less efficient with age because of atrophy of the salivary glands and change in the pH of stomach acids. The latter may also lead to vitamin $B_{12}$ deficiency. The main reason for malnutrition among the elderly is lack of eating and/or eating snack foods rather than regular meals. This is a particular problem for the older adult who lives alone. These people should be encouraged to attend congregate meals if they are available. If they are not available, perhaps a meal club can be started where everyone meets at a different home everyday for a meal. This will provide the mechanism for having a well-balanced meal and also improve nutrient metabolism. Older adults generally lack knowledge of nutrition, which makes them susceptible to dietary fads such as megavitamin therapy. At the same time older adults have well-established food patterns which the wise nurse may attempt to modify if necessary, but should not try to radically change. A man who has not eaten a salad in 76 years probably won't begin to eat "rabbit food," but he may be willing to have bran muffins for breakfast. Additional bulk and liquids are often a dietary need of the elderly because of slowed peristalsis and less sensitivity to thirst. This combination often leads to constipation. Dietary modifications are the optimal method for relieving this problem because dependency on laxatives, cathar-

tics, and enemas is easily established. Difficulty in defecation can be helped by having older adults put their feet on a low stool when sitting on the toilet. This modified squatting position promotes the passage of stool.

In general there is a reduction of *overall body metabolism* as evidenced by a progressively decreasing basal metabolic rate. The body is sluggish in its ability to produce heat. This leads to a lower response to infections, fever, and changes in the external environment. The decrease in basal metabolism combines with decreases in muscle contractibility and loss of fat pads to make the elderly susceptible to cold. Environments should be adequately heated and free of drafts. Proper clothing plus extra layers such as sweaters should be available and additional blankets used at night. The loss of glycogen deposits, because of increased inert tissue and unavailability of collagen glycogen stores, creates the need to eat frequently. The elderly should be counseled not to skip meals and to supplement their feeding with a bedtime snack.

Hormones play an important role in the body's *metabolic response to stress*. Table 3-4 summarizes the hormonal changes associated with aging. It is not known if there is a decrease in the secretion of, cellular response to, or metabolism of hormones, but the end result is an inefficient response to stress. For example, the older adult's normal fasting blood sugar is within the parameters of a young adult's, but it takes 5 hours rather than 3 for the aged person's blood sugar to return to normal after a glucose tolerance test. It is important to be aware of bodily reserves and to minimize stress whenever possible.

**Changes in oxygenation** The age-related changes in oxygenation are found primarily in the heart, vessels, and lungs. Cardiac output decreases with age. The *myocardium* shows a delay in recovery of contractibility and irritability, and the valves become rigid. Over the years fat often accumulates around the heart. Under normal conditions these changes result in little functional difficulty; however, under stress, the heart reacts poorly. Stress often leads to tachycardia, and this can precipitate heart failure.

*Respiratory status* is also affected and vital capacity is reduced by 40 percent in the aged. This is a result of decreases in the elasticity and number of alveoli, rigidity of the chest wall, and poor posture. The lower lobes, especially, are poorly ventilated; consequently this is the usual site of pneumonia in old age. The rate of $O_2$ uptake gradually decreases from 4 liters/min in 20-year-olds to 1.5 liters/min in 75-year-olds. Not only is oxygen exchange less efficient, but the energy required to breathe is 20 percent more at 60 years of age than it was at 20. Other important changes are a sluggish recognition of increases in $O_2$ and $CO_2$ concentrations in the blood and an impaired cough reflex causing diminished cleansing ability of the lungs. Again, under normal conditions these changes are not remarkable, but on exertion, however, dyspnea often develops. Regular moderate exercise should be encouraged and activities paced to the capacity of the individual.

The most striking of the *vascular changes* is the

**TABLE 3-4**
KNOWN HORMONE CHANGES WITH AGE*

| Hormones, Endocrine Glands, and Controlling Factors | Normal Action | Age Change |
|---|---|---|
| ADRENAL CORTEX<br>Cortisol<br>ACTH | Stimulates protein catabolism, stimulates liver uptake of amino acids and their conversion to glucose, is permissive for stimulation of gluconeogenesis by other tissues, inhibits glucose uptake and oxidation by many body cells | Secretion somewhat decreased in proportion to decreased muscle mass |
| Aldosterone<br>Angisterin plasma $K^+$ concentration | Stimulates $Na^+$ reabsorption, specifically by distal tubules, stimulates transport of $Na^+$ by other epithelial cells in the body, e.g., sweat glands, is an "all-purpose" stimulator of $Na^+$ retention | Young people have been found to have secretion rates for aldosterone that are more than twice as high as those of elderly subjects; metabolic clearance rates and calculated plasma concentrations of aldosterone are also decreased |
| GONADS<br>Ovaries<br>  Estrogen<br>  FSH<br>  LH | Maintains the entire female genital tract and the breasts, is responsible for body hair distribution and the general female configuration, is required for follicle and ovum maturation, permits ovulation, and onset of menses | Loss of germinal cells causes decrease in levels of estrogen, which is associated with increase in pituitary activity and a decrease in estrogen levels; source of estrogen in postmenopausal women, adrenal cortex (primarily) |
| Progesterone<br>FHS<br>LH | Present only in significant amounts during luteal phase of menstrual cycle, has an effect on the endometrium, breasts, oviducts, and uterine smooth muscle | A decrease of 50% of pregnanediol (a by-product of progesterone breakdown) in urinary excretion of women between 30 to 80 |
| Testes<br>  Testosterone<br>  LH | Spermatogenesis, needed for the morphology and function of the entire male duct system, development and maintenance of normal sexual drive and behavior in men, development of secondary sexual characteristics | Is not as abrupt or sudden as in female; loss of geminal cells also occurs when pituitary is functioning at high level |
| PANCREAS<br>Insulin<br>Plasma glucose concentrations | Stimulates the facilitated diffusion of glucose into certain cells (muscle and adipose), stimulates protein synthesis | Response of elderly person to insulin is decreased |
| KIDNEYS<br>Renin | Catalyzes the reaction in which angiotensiogen becomes angiotensin | Suggested slower response but no evidence |
| Angiotensin | Profound stimulator of aldosterone, secretion is the primary input into the adrenal gland, which produces aldosterone | Suggested slower response but no evidence |
| Erythropoietin | Stimulates erythrocyte and hemoglobin synthesis | Suggested slower response but no evidence |
| POSTERIOR PITUITARY<br>ADH<br>  Blood volume<br>  Blood pressure<br>  Electrolyte levels | Antidiuretic effect on kidney, keeps water permeability of latter nephron segments up, so $H_2O$ reabsorption is able to keep up with $Na^+$ reabsorption | Kidney (increased) response time |
| THYROID GLAND<br>Thyroxine<br>TSH | An iodine containing amino acid, influences metabolic rate, $O_2$ consumption, and heat production in most body tissues | From 25 years onward there is a slow gradual decline in thyroid activity (until eighth decade) |

* Developed by Catherine Kapac, R.N., M.N.[51,52,53]

loss of elasticity in the walls of the larger arteries. This inelasticity and calcification of the aortic arch results in an increased systolic blood pressure and possibly an increase in diastolic pressure. A little hypertension is considered an old folks friend because it improves cerebral circulation. Many medical gerontologists do not believe blood pressures up to 180/100 should be treated unless accompanied by clinical signs of organic damage such as right-sided heart failure. Presently atherosclerosis is again believed to be a normal part of aging and thus contributes to the structural changes in the arterial system. Decreases in capillary permeability result in sluggish exchange in the capillary beds. There is also an increased lability of the vasopressor control mechanism, and orthostatic hypotension often develops. The elderly should compensate for dizziness upon standing by rising slowly to give their bodies time to adjust to the new position.

### Changes in fluid and electrolyte balance

Fluid and electrolyte balance is affected by various changes in the kidney. There is an overall loss of nephrons and the remaining nephrons are functionally impaired. Blood flow to the kidney is also decreased with age. Under normal conditions the kidneys function at a marginal level with impairment of excretory and reabsorptive capacities. For example, glucose reabsorption is 350 mg/min at ages 50 to 60 and 220 mg/min after 80. There are also increased numbers of casts and red blood cells in the urine of older adults and the specific gravity decreases. This lowered kidney efficiency makes the elderly more vulnerable to drug toxicity. Drugs eliminated in the urine should be used cautiously with recognition that their half-life is prolonged.

With impaired kidney function fluid and electrolyte imbalances can occur. The elderly are vulnerable to this in normal circumstances, but become even more so under stress conditions where the kidneys are inadequate to the task. They are less responsive to the antidiuretic hormone and are less capable of quickly excreting acid or base to maintain balance. Fluid balance needs to be monitored in the elderly and the importance of adequate intake impressed upon them.

### Changes in sleep patterns

Older adults often complain about inability to sleep through the night. This is an age-related phenomenon, as older people have less deep sleep (stage four) and dream less than younger persons. Spontaneous awakenings are rare in children, in young adulthood they are brief, but by the forties the awakenings are longer and the time awake in bed begins to increase. By old age the frequency and duration of awakenings are increased so that the older adult appears to be an insomniac, often awakening every hour and in some instances having no stage-four sleep.

The aged adapt to this problem by spending more time in bed in order to get an amount of sleep equivalent to that experienced in younger years; this often includes naps. The nurse should reassure the older adult that this sleeping pattern is not unusual and discourage the use of hypnotics since they will further reduce dreaming. A frequent cause of insomnia is overfatigue. In such cases naps are a recommended remedy. The nurse might also recommend warm milk at bedtime or avoidance of caffeine-containing drinks in the evening.

## Personality Dynamics

Intrapsychic dynamics are a part of old age, as well as any other period of the life cycle. As mentioned earlier, most personality and developmental theorists tend to end their theoretical constructs with early adulthood with the assumption that the rest of life is characterized by stability. For example, Kohlberg's theory of morality explicitly stated that change did not occur after early childhood. He has since modified his stance to say that changes are possible if a person is exposed to an intense situation which leads to questioning of one's basic beliefs, e.g., exposure to war.

Among the few theorists who have developed life-span theories, it is rare to find any who have tested or done clinical observations related to the older adult portion of the theory. Therefore, one must consider the theories that relate to the older adult to be exercises in logic. However, if one considers that theories are, in reality, conceptual frameworks which make ideas available for testing in a systematic manner, they can be valuable aids in thinking about the aging process and the aged. In any case, one should never equate theory with truth.

The major life-span theorists discussed here are Erikson and Buhler. Relevant adult developmental theories of Peck, Neugarten, and Havighurst are also covered. These theorists reflect the practices of our culture; therefore, they often state what *is* rather than what *could* or *must* be.

### Emotional development

*Erikson* developed a life-span development theory but concentrated his efforts on the adolescent period. His eighth stage, which encompasses old age, is *ego integrity vs. despair.* Erikson's short essay on this stage is vague, but implies an objective life review that includes pride in the life led, acceptance of death as inevitable, and an ability to be a follower as well as a leader. The older adult must be able to voluntarily (or at least gracefully) give up many of the hopes and activities which previously gave life importance, i.e., take pride in what they were rather than what they are or will be. Wisdom provides the stabilizing force in the development and operationalization of a set of human values based on one's life experiences.

Erikson's stages are forced, meaning that one does not move from one stage to another after having achieved competency, but because one reaches a certain age. Therefore, individuals arrive at each stage with a different level of growth and varying reactions and abilities to resolve the new developmental problems. In reality, the only study testing Erikson's stage sequence found that passage through the stages was invariant, but the age at which an individual began to focus on the developmental problems prominent in a particular stage varied.[54]

*Peck* attempted to elaborate Erikson's adulthood stages. He felt that the eighth stage encompassed the last 40 to 50 years of life and therefore should be divided into two substages which are further broken down into specific issues relevant to the age period. The issues for old age are: ego differentiation vs. work-role preoccupation, body transcendence vs. body preoccupation, and ego transcendence vs. ego preoccupation.

*Ego differentiation vs. work-role preoccupation* speaks directly to the crisis of retirement. Peck saw this primarily as a male issue, but studies of retirement have found this to be a crisis for all people whose life orientation revolves around their work role. In order to successfully adapt to this problem, it is important to develop various values, activities, and attributes that are not directly connected with employment. These could vary from being the expert in regional history, to painting, to being a volunteer for a community organization. The important aspect is having self-worth which is not dependent upon employment.

*Body transcendence vs. body preoccupation* is concerned with the acceptance of the physical changes which occur with aging, not just visually but functionally. In order to meet this crisis older adults look outside of their physical activities and gain pleasure and satisfaction from mental and social activities. Persons who do not adapt to the inevitable physical changes of aging become increasingly obsessed with body monitoring.

Throughout the life cycle there is always need to gain satisfaction and worth from intangibles rather than physical attributes, and this issue is the ultimate test of whether a person has been able to accomplish body transcendence.

The third issue of old age, *ego transcendence vs. ego preoccupation,* is concerned with facing the inevitability of one's death. The successful resolution of this issue is marked by a continuing involvement with other persons and activities and an orientation towards the present and future. Realistically these older adults know their personal future is limited, but their interest includes improving the future for younger generations. Unsuccessful adaptation is demonstrated by the aged persons who have interest only in themselves; because death is near, their world revolves only around themselves and their interest is in self-gratification.

*Buhler's* life-span theory emphasized the self. In order to maintain and develop the self one uses four basic tendencies toward one's fulfillment: need satisfaction, self-limiting adaptation, creative expansion, and upholding of internal order. All four tendencies are present in activities which are goal directed.

Buhler divides the life span into five phases based on the assumption that biological changes are predictable, but psychological changes are not. The fifth phase, which begins approximately at age 65 to 70, is a period of further biological decline following loss of reproductive ability.

Using biographical materials and clinical studies Buhler has developed life goals for each self-determination phase. During the fifth phase she believed that most people rest from self-determining and goal setting. At this period one experiences life as fulfillment, resignation, or failure. The older adult gradually, through a life review, evolves an awareness of past life as a whole and judges it. Because older adults have retired from goal setting, they accept the status quo rather than develop and implement changes to improve their opinion of their life.

*Havighurst's* developmental tasks are based on social roles. Each period of life has a series of tasks for which one must achieve competency. Throughout life, learning is occurring, according to this theory. The developmental tasks of later maturity differ from other periods of life because there is an enforced separation from some of the active roles of middle age. The older adult must decide whether to take on new roles, e.g., volunteer, grandparent, etc., or to accept an increased separation from active segments of society.

Some of the tasks outlined by Havighurst are discussed earlier in this section. These include adjusting to decreasing physical strength and health, retirement, reduced income, and the death of a spouse. His fourth task involves establishing an explicit affiliation with one's age group. Havighurst believed that one must accept the role of elder and become an active participant in constructive activities with others of one's age group. He believed it is too difficult physically, psychologically, and economically to keep up with the middle aged, and the effect of the older adults banding together could lead to political, economic, and social benefits.

The fifth task is adoption of and adaptation to social roles in a flexible way, another task which relates to retirement and increased time for recreational activities. One must develop roles which will loosely organize and structure one's life so that it is not an "empty" time, while maintaining a leisurely pace. Patterns of activity include increasing one's investment in family and housekeeping activities, community activities, and hobbies or interest areas.

The sixth activity is the establishment of satisfactory physical living arrangements. The scope of this task may be as broad as relocation to a favorable climate or as narrow as living in a place that you have the energy and financial resources to keep up and allow for easy movement, e.g., a house all on one level, close to shopping areas, etc.

*Neugarten,* working within an ego psychology orientation but considering sociological and cultural data, developed a series of adult age-relevant issues. These issues are appropriate for a Western culture, and it is not known if they can be universally applied to all aged persons. According to Neugarten, old age presents three specific issues with which one must cope. First, the older adult must relinquish a sense of competency and authority. In one sense this refers to retirement, but in a broader sense it reflects society's inclination to put older adults and their contributions in the background. Society frequently forces older adults to give up their position in both work and social spheres. Elderly persons holding leadership positions are often rare except in age-segregated groups or congressional committees.

The second issue to be resolved is gaining a sense of integrity about what one was rather than what one is now. The young adult is valued for what he or she will become, the middle aged for what they are, but the old must take pride in what they were. The older adult's future rarely includes maintenance of a position that is valued in our society. If one can not take pride in what one was, one tends to continue striving for life goals which will be gratifying or become depressed because of the feeling that one's life was fruitless.

Neugarten's third issue is reconciliation with family members. Traditionally, the family is the primary support system in our society. Children generally meet the dependency needs of their older parents, and older persons without children tend to rely on siblings. When reminiscing about their life, older adults realize, on an intrapsychic level, the value of the family and perhaps want to make up for past wrongs, either real or imagined. In essence, Neugarten believed well-adjusted older adults maintain the continuity of their personality by using the passive coping strategies of introspection and decreasing their emotional investments outside of their primary support system.

**Emotional behavior** Emotional behavior in old age, for the most part, can be predicted by a person's previous behavior. Because the emotionally stable older adult has had a lifetime of experiences in which there was continuous adjustment to change and the development of a stable feeling of self, most aged persons are able to use the wisdom accumulated from these past experiences to confront the problems of old age. Coping or adaptive mechanisms previously used successfully tend to continue to be used. When these mechanisms are used inappropriately or too rigidly, maladaptive behavior results. Generally this behavior occurs during periods of stress or crisis, and the nurse should be aware of the older patient's typical mode of adaptation in order to be able to help the older adult use more appropriate coping mechanisms and/or recognize the possible origin of the behavior.

**Life perspective** A normal psychological phenomenon of old age is the *life review.*[55] This has been alluded to in the discussion of developmental theories of old age. Butler believed the life review occurred in all persons during the final years of life. This review has often been confused with unselective nostalgia and reminiscence, and, therefore, considered by health professionals as proof of an unhealthy preoccupation with the past. Nothing could be farther from reality. Rather, it is a progressive return to the consciousness of past events which, among other things, allows the individual to grapple one more time with unresolved conflicts and to place these conflicts and other important events in proper perspective.

Many older persons are able to remember early

life events with accuracy and clarity. The life review process, however, is not without pitfalls. For some older adults remembering past events is a painful experience. Regret over previous actions can lead to emotional reactions ranging from mild depression or guilt to inner rage or suicide. An example of such feelings is one very depressed elderly woman who expressed regret over an event which had occurred 50 years earlier. She allowed her daughter to be brought up by her ex-husband's family because she had no money or job prospects. Today she wonders what happened to her child and if that decision was the right one or just situationally the easiest at the time. Mrs. M.'s depression was partially relieved when she was able to discuss her problem with the nurse, who consoled her with the thought that that was a difficult decision in which she as a mother did what she thought was best for her child.

**Time perspective** Time perspective can be approached from two different views, the total life cycle and day-to-day functioning. The older adult, because of longevity, has a recognition of both the past and the future. Only by being old can one have a recognition of what it means to be old, and, with few exceptions, the elderly have given up the fear of growing old so commonly seen in middle age. The elderly develop a sense of inner self which is necessary for comprehending the final developmental task—death. The change in time or life perspective is not a concept which is found only in Western cultures. The Indians believe that the second half of life is spent in developing an inner sense of self and guiding others to find it. Adults who do not develop this perspective have a difficult time facing death.

The older adult's time perspective tends to change from "time lived" to "time left." The older person has a fairly realistic view of the number of years left to accomplish what he or she wishes to accomplish in life. For example, a 60-year-old male, knowing that males in his family have generally died by age 70, plans what he can do in the 10 years left in his life. For the 30-year-old, life seems to loom endlessly on, and time is marked by past events rather than a future termination point.

On a daily basis one's time perspective gradually changes as one ages. For the child time passes very slowly, but with age the momentum picks up until time, perhaps because it has become so precious, passes very rapidly. Because the time left is short, in comparison to younger age groups, Kastenbaum describes the older adult as developing a feeling of immediacy. They can not easily wait months or years for gratification but look only to the present. They consider today or the week but rarely next year, or if they do, they generally add a conditional "if I'm still here." For those elderly who have developed a "oneness" with themselves and life, the simple elemental aspects of life, such as a flower, a picture, colors, touching, a sunrise, will gain in significance and ability to give pleasure.

**Change in self-image** Generally the acceptance of being old is linked to loss of one's functional capabilities rather than chronological age. Healthy older adults rarely think of themselves as old, and even persons in their eighties will state they are middle aged if they feel well. A 76-year-old woman told me that her view of herself had not changed since she married at 19. She knew physically she looked different, but her self-concept in essence had not changed.

However, when a person's level of activity is curtailed, particularly if a valued activity is lost, the older adult will then conclude old age has arrived. For example, an 82-year-old woman recently confided she was now old. When asked why she had made this decision, she stated she could no longer make a garden because she couldn't tolerate the heat. This exemplifies the gradual loss in functional capability that allowed her to accept her diminished ability to tolerate heat and, therefore, demonstrate calm recognition of the fact. Many people, however, have loss of functional abilities linked to disease processes. The loss may be abrupt, and the older adult may have to work out acceptance in the alien environment of the hospital. Reactions may range from denial to grieving over one's loss of health and stamina. It is not easy under any circumstances to consider oneself old in a youth-oriented society, and it is twice as difficult when one must also accept a chronic illness or disability. The nurse must recognize the implications surrounding the loss of functional capability both in terms of supporting the patient through this crisis and helping the patient to recognize and capitalize on remaining strengths so that their life-style is not greatly affected.

**Death and dying** Death is a universal phenomenon of life. It has been described as a crisis, a decision-making process, and a natural part of life. Death is more imminent for the older adult, but death and the process of dying is not unique to the aged. This discussion is applicable to any dying person.

*Attitudes* both of society and of health professionals can greatly influence the process of dying. Society fears death, so much so that it has institutionalized and sterilized it. People no longer die at home surrounded by their families. About 80 percent of deaths occur in a hospital or nursing home. All too frequently this means the person dies alone.

Health professionals often refuse to accept death. It is the antithesis of everything they believe. As a result, death often occurs in an arena of machines, tubes, and technicians. The dying patient often becomes an object of intense effort and loses the "right to die." Increasingly, people are beginning to recognize this right and the "living will" is becoming popular. In it people formally request that if recovery is not reasonable, they do not wish to be kept alive by heroic or mechanical means.

Patients also have a "right to know." Physicians or family members, unable to accept the fact of dying, may choose not to tell a patient he or she is dying. The imprudence of such a decision has been documented repeatedly. In most instances, the patient is aware of impending death but is robbed of the opportunity to face it normally. Nurses should recognize their role in helping physicians and family members to face death with the patient.

Attitudes of nurses toward death can greatly affect the care they give dying patients. Nurses should work to view death not as a defeat but as the final culmination of life. Perhaps the first step to be taken to understand one's own attitude toward death is to review one's earliest memories of death and share them with others.[56] Openly looking at past experiences and exploring their meaning can help in understanding reactions to present experiences.

People experience a *loss* when they are deprived of something they once had. When the loss is a love-object, grief results. *Grief* is the normal and appropriate emotional response to a significant loss, and usually occurs directly after the loss. A person can experience *anticipatory grief;* that is, he or she can grieve before the actual loss occurs. This is a frequent occurrence when a loved one is terminally ill. Grief, however, can be premature if the family grieves for and separates from the dying person before death actually occurs.

Death is often viewed as the ultimate loss. It involves the loss not only of *all* significant relationships, but the loss of oneself. There are four types of death: *physical death,* in which the brain and heart stop functioning; *intellectual death,* in which a person is unable to cognitively function; *psychological death,* in which one feels there is no longer a reason to be alive; and *social death,* where others no longer think of the person as being alive. Psychological and social death may occur when a person enters a nursing home. Nurses can play a vital role in preventing "inappropriate" death, and should realize that families should be included in patient care. Nursing home personnel should be particularly sensitive to the patient's and the family's needs. Affective contact should be maintained within the limits of reasonable family resources even when the patient is unable to respond.

Dying is the final developmental step in the human life-span. It generally involves the process of grieving. Kubler-Ross has identified steps in this grieving process that patients seem to go through.[57] All people do not grieve by following the steps sequentially. Some move back and forth from one stage to another, while others experience several steps at once. It is not productive for nurses to get deeply involved in identifying which stage their patients are going through. This often "intellectualizes" the dying process and relieves the nurse of a deeper involvement. Yet, an understanding of the steps in the grieving process can contribute to a better understanding of the dying patient.

When patients first become aware of the fact that they are dying, a frequent response is shock and *denial.* This is quickly followed by *anger.* The angry patient is often irritable and difficult to please. The patient then begins the *bargaining* stage. Patients are generally looking for temporary reprieves, for example, "just until my son's wedding." As the patient begins to fully acknowledge the impending death, the sense of loss is acutely felt and *depression* occurs. The grief work is most difficult in this stage. As the patient works through depression, the many lost relationships are realized and slowly the patient separates from others. As depression is resolved, *acceptance* replaces it. At this final stage the patient has often separated from all but one or two close persons.

The nurse's role in death and dying focuses on the patient and the family. As patients go through the grieving process, they need support. This nurse-patient relationship requires an intimacy the nurse must be able to tolerate. Because of this, support systems for nurses and other health personnel should be available. Nurses should communicate to their patients a willingness to talk. Issues should not be avoided. At the same time, the patients' coping mechanisms should be respected. Rejection of any references to death is likely in the denial stage. The patient will need a good listener to ventilate hostilities when angry. During depression, the most difficult stage for both the nurse and the patient, discussions should be realistic without negating all hope. The patient will need to "talk through" life decisions and may need confirmation that decisions made were the best at the time. As acceptance emerges, the patient will seek out the nurse who was willing to establish a relationship, and lengthy discussions often ensue.

Nurses, too, can be instrumental in encouraging patients to die at home. The feasibility of this should be explored and available community resources brought to the patient and family's attention. Hospices have recognized the needs of dying patients and have tried to provide an environment where physical as well as psychosocial needs are met. The emphasis is on living and the patient is surrounded by family.

Nurses should be aware that the family of the dying patient often needs help in working through their own grief and in understanding the dying patient's behavior. Family members should be helped to understand the separation of the patient from all but one or two members so that they do not interpret it as rejection. Grief of family members is often accompanied by guilt and the nurse should offer encouragement and support. Including the family in the physical care often allows them to "pay back" and, therefore, work through guilt feelings.

When the family is first told of the death, the sense of loss may be accompanied by physical symptoms such as tightness in the throat, choking, an empty feeling, vomiting, or fainting. The family often feels shock and disbelief. These may be accompanied by anger or bitter accusations. A sensitive nurse will provide a quiet place for the family to work through these initial reactions and regain their composure.

The rituals associated with death which allow the family to share their feelings and openly express them help the family to recover. These rituals vary according to culture, and recently, American rituals have come under fire because funerals have become "big business" and families make arrangements at a time when they are vulnerable. The person who knows death is imminent should be allowed to discuss funeral arrangements and make plans in advance.

Normal grieving often takes 6 months to 1 year. Generally, grieving that continues beyond 1 year is pathological and the person should be encouraged to seek help. Part of grieving involves talking about the loss. Stories of the deceased person may be repeated. The loss may be exaggerated and the loved

one fantasied into someone greater than he or she was.

For both the *widow* and the *widower* there is a change in life-style. It takes about a year to adjust to a change of this magnitude, and people should be advised not to make any drastic alteration in their life-style during the first year. The loneliness of widowhood is often a problem. Some people begin to stay up quite late because they have difficulty sleeping. Widowers, especially, may have difficulty developing social contacts. Young widows may find the loss of a partner excludes her from previously enjoyed social affairs. In all cases the nurse should consider that the widow or widower will need support, not only in coping with being alone, but in coping with activities of daily living previously handled by the lost spouse.

**Cognitive development**  Given adequate health, environmental factors, sensory ability, and motivation, intelligence and learning ability are not noticeably affected by aging. For many years it was generally believed, however, that as one grew older one's intelligence and potential for learning declined. Not only is this demonstrated in our folklore by sayings such as "you can't teach an old dog new tricks," but this belief is a basic tenet of the irreversible-decrement model. Another reason for the belief in intellectual decline was that until recently most studies of intellectual functioning were cross-sectional studies, and therefore, did not take into consideration generational differences. Also, these studies chose their older adult sample from homes for the aged and nursing homes, while the comparative younger adult sample usually was the college sophomore. Each group represented opposite extremes for their generation.

Much research has been done to establish a causal link between age-related neurobiological changes and intellectual performance. Results of postmortem studies showed some structural changes with age. Correlation between structural changes and behavior applied only to institutionalized aged with a chronic brain syndrome diagnosis and not to other institutionalized or community-based aged.[58] EEG studies are based on the hypothesis that age differences in behavior could be related to differences in the duration of the alpha cycle. Many elderly have slowed alpha waves as compared to young adults. It has been demonstrated, however, that by using biofeedback techniques an older adult can control the speed of the alpha wave.[59] Studies comparing institutionalized and community-based elderly showed a correlation between slowed alpha waves and intelligence test scores only for the institutionalized aged.[60] These studies tend to indicate that, in the absence of an organic brain syndrome, changes in the central nervous system and behavior are not strong enough to cause irreversible functional changes. The effects of other factors, such as general health status, type of living arrangement, and biofeedback training, appear to be more pertinent.

Poor health or nearness to death does have an effect on the cognitive ability of older adults. The few studies using healthy older males showed a decline in the speed of performance only, which has been a fairly consistent age-related finding.[61] However, a group of studies comparing aged persons with and without cardiovascular disease symptoms found that the typical picture of intellectual decline with aging may be secondary to a pathological process rather than a normal aging process.[62] Somatic problems in the elderly are often first demonstrated by a change in behavior. Some of the problems which can lead to behavioral changes include malnutrition, hypoxia, lowered sex hormone levels, and adverse effects of medication. Emotional pathology, such as depression or psychosis, also has a detrimental effect on cognitive functioning.

Recently there have been studies indicating that nearness to death may be the prime factor in intellectual decrement. Longitudinal studies show stable cognitive performances for long-term survivors, but a sudden drop in the scores of nonsurvivors in a period up to 5 years before death.[63] This would mean that it is not growing old, but having pathological conditions which are terminal, that inevitably leads to a decline in cognitive ability.

Besides health status, environmental factors, both immediate and long-term, have been found to have an effect on the cognitive performances of the older adult. Studies done in this area have also been pivotal in demonstrating that cognitive losses not caused by terminal pathology are potentially reversible. Changes in the immediate environment of institutionalized persons, either from a custodial to therapeutic focus or entry into the institution, improve their cognitive functioning.

Correlations between the older adult's general life-style and cognitive performance are often found. Those cognitive skills needed in one's occupation or hobbies remain functionally high, while those skills least used tend to atrophy with age. This type of information tends to make one consider that the reason the older adult does not perform at the same level as the college sophomore is that the problems posed on the intelligence tests are both artificial and unfamiliar. For example, many older adults have not taken any type of test for at least 20 years or more and some have never taken a multiple choice test. The college student, on the other hand, in order to demonstrate competency in academia must be an astute test taker. In fact, orienting the older subject to the skills and requirements of test taking will dramatically improve their test scores.

In order to place this information in a utilitarian perspective we will discuss how it can be used in modifying health teaching interventions aimed at the older adult population. In the initial assessment the nurse should explore several facets pertinent to the learning situation. When the client last had a structured learning experience and how successful they felt about it should be elicited. If necessary, materials and exercises on how to learn should be incorporated into the teaching plan. The elderly's sensory ability should be determined and the necessary adjustments made. Adequate lighting, clear speech, and large print are a few examples. The older adult's motivation to learn must not be overlooked. Too often, time is not taken to "win the client over to learning" before the teaching begins. The aged may want to understand the relevance of the learning before giving it their time and energy.

A common characteristic of the elderly is a slowing of behavior, and because of this more time must be given for learning to occur. In order to provide a feeling of success, it is better to offer smaller amounts of information at one time to compensate for this. Printed materials are also useful as supplements.

## Sexuality

Sexuality can be considered from two perspectives. In broad terms it can be related to social identity. In a more narrow sense it can refer to sexual intercourse. Both are appropriate ways of looking at sexuality in the aged population.

As a young child we learn to identify with a particular sex and internalize our culture's values and beliefs concerning gender differences. Our personal identity is, in part, our sexual identity. In other words, our sexual behavior is an ingrained way of looking at ourselves and behaving toward others, which essentially does not change over time. Between generations a slightly different system of values or behavior may be evident, but on an intra-individual level one is consistent over a lifetime. The effect of heterosexuality can be seen in the different behaviors exhibited when aged persons are in an own-sex versus a heterosexual environment.

When in the latter environment grooming immediately improves, the men's language is more socially acceptable, and there tends to be less bickering among women.

Unfortunately, younger generations tend to believe that the elderly are neuter and expect their behavior to be sexless. When an elderly woman acts in a warm feminine manner to a man there are comments like "why doesn't she act her age" or nervous laughter. In fact, the elderly are so neutered that affection between the same sex, especially women, is acceptable. Homosexuality in the aged is thought to be unthinkable. How many "dirty old men" just behave naturally towards friendly or even flirtatious behavior? One example could be a young nurse's aide working in a nursing home who slips into an elderly man's room and straightens her hose and slip. When the man makes a pass at her, she is shocked and he is surprised, since he is responding appropriately to her actions.

One reason for the "sentence of sexlessness" after 60 is our society's time frame for activities. In the past few years there have been programs on television dealing with romance among the elderly, each treating the topic as a comedy. Ironically, "shacking up" among the elderly is fairly easy to pass off because the younger generations have difficulty viewing the elderly as sexually desirable, wanting or being capable of sexual intercourse, and of openly expressing their desires. Therefore, elderly couples living together is often viewed more as a roommate arrangement. The appropriateness of sexual behavior may in a few generations extend into old age, but our youth-oriented society views courting and mating as activities of the young. Today's children accept the fact that their parents have intercourse, but are they ready to believe their grandparents and even greatgrandparents do also?

If we look at the activities related to sexuality we realize that when one is assigned a sexless role much more is lost than actual sexual intercourse, particularly for persons in institutions or living without a partner. They also lose physical closeness and physical contact. They are not touched! Caressing, hugging, and holding hands are part of our normal world until we grow old and are alone. Nothing makes one feel so alone as the lack of physical closeness and contact. The next time an older adult in a nursing home holds onto your hand longer than the second considered socially acceptable you are receiving two messages—"I want you to stay with me" and "I want to be touched." Observational studies in nursing homes have demonstrated that guests are rarely touched except for necessary activities, and almost all touching is instigated by employees.

Are older adults interested in sexual activities? Like most other areas of activity this depends on the level of interest in sex they have had throughout life. People who were not particularly interested in sex tend to give up the activity when it is socially acceptable. On the other hand, people who have had an active enjoyable sex life in young and middle adulthood will continue to have sexual relations. The few studies done on sexual activities of the elderly make this point. For those elderly who are desirous of sexual intercourse there is rarely a physiological barrier to fulfillment. For both males and females the disuse principle is in force.

The basis for most information on the physiological capabilities of the elderly is from Masters and Johnson.[64,65] While their sample was small, the data are consistent with that collected indirectly by Kinsey, as well as the Duke study. Because of the more rapid decline in estrogen, women show more anatomical changes with shrinkage and decrease in the size of all secondary sex organs. The vaginal walls thin, the length shrinks, and there is less lubrication. Estrogen replacement therapy slows this process for women who do not compensate with sufficient increased gonadotrophic production. Lubrication and flexibility of the vaginal barrel is better in women having regular coital experiences, at least one a week, in comparison to women having infrequent intercourse, once a month or less. Estrogen creams are very helpful. Physiologically, clitoral stimulation is effective, but more time is required for a response. The phase of excitement is shorter, the plateau phase may be longer, and orgasm and resolution are shorter in duration. Factors related to continued sexual activity for women who are over 70 are a sanctioned partner who wishes to be sexually active and good past sexual experiences. Loss of sexual capacity was generally related to problems caused by disuse. For some women over 60 the uterine contractions occurring during orgasm become very painful, causing them to avoid intercourse.

For males, the gradual decrease in testosterone leads to some atrophy of the testes, a decline in spermatogenesis, and an increase in abnormally shaped and sized sperm. However, fertility generally remains through the eighties and nineties. Physiologically, it takes longer for older men to reach an erection, but once erection has been reached, it can be maintained for a longer period of time before orgasm. Orgasm occurs in one stage with ejaculation, and the period of resolution is shorter. Greater time is required before another erection can be reached. The Duke studies showed that the combination of feeling youthful, having good health and enjoyable past sexual experiences, and a feeling of competency as shown by having a respected position in one's society were present in sexually active men over 70. Loss of sexual capacity can result from factors other than the aging process such as disuse, excessive alcohol intake, drugs (particularly tranquilizers and barbiturates), diabetic neuropathy, and depression. Some men fear that intercourse may be too rigorous an activity for them; however, the rule of thumb for capability (being able to walk up two flights of stairs without dyspnea) still holds true for this age group.

Sexuality is a part of one's life activities and like most activities needs regular practice in order to maintain the necessary physical status. The nurse can play a vital role in bringing sex "out of the closet" for the aged. Many elderly are well conditioned by our culture and have come to believe that they are no longer capable of sex. When questions regarding sexual activity first arise, they should be answered honestly and openly. The importance of regularity in sexual encounters should be emphasized. Couples should be encouraged to discuss techniques that are satisfying to them, and the use of lubricants should be advised. The woman should discuss sexual function with her doctor who may prescribe estrogen creams or the like. Health centers should make counselors available to couples experiencing specific difficulties.

Sexual connotations during social events should be encouraged as they are with any age group. This is especially pertinent in nursing homes and housing for the elderly. Meals should be taken together and events, dances, lectures, etc., should include both sexes. Married couples should be allowed to room together and privacy given. The same should apply to homosexual couples, although "gay liberation" is a relatively new movement and the present aged homosexual is often hidden. The aged should be supported in their attempts to establish relationships. This again applies to homosexuals, as well as heterosexuals.

### Life-styles

As older adults evolve through a variety of physical and emotional changes, their life-styles are altered. While influenced by the physical and emotional aspects of aging, the older adult's life-style is greatly affected by societal, cultural, economic, and familial factors.

**Societal influences** Society influences behavior by creating external pressures. The source of these pressures may be governmental or from the expectations of significant others. Internal pressures are those behaviors and beliefs we have been socialized to accept since birth. People generally behave as they and their social circle expect them to behave. Neugarten has demonstrated the existence of a social clock that indicates the appropriate time of life for certain events and behaviors to be normal.[66] To begin the discussion on the societal view of aging, four sociological theories will be examined: activity, disengagement, social reconstruction, and social exchange. The first two theories are an integral part of the professional and governmental view of aging and, therefore, have been translated into practice and policy. The latter two theories are relatively new and untested. Again, remember these are theories, not fact; they do, however, influence our attitudes and behavior.

**Behavioral Theories** The *activity theory* was not developed by any one person, but is a concept that has been used for many years by persons who believe that there is a positive relationship between how active older adults remain and their morale (Fig. 3-7). This belief has been translated into such programs as senior citizen clubs, activity centers in apartment complexes for the aged, and recreation therapy departments in nursing homes. The activity theory does not have a given set of principles or concepts to be tested, but has gained acceptance from the observation that people who are not active are generally not happy. However, research in this area has not demonstrated a causal relationship between the level of activity and an older adult's life satisfaction. Some older adults are happier when active; however, increased activity does not always equal increased morale. Using this knowledge the nurse should assess the life-style and preferences of the individual older adult client rather than assuming that every aged person needs to be involved in an activity every minute or even every day.

Cummings and Henry developed the *theory of disengagement* based on data from an extensive University of Chicago study of the middle aged and aged in Kansas City. Originally disengagement was considered to be the universal explanation of how society and the older adult, through a process of mutual withdrawal, prepared for the older adult's eventual death. There are two ways disengagement can be initiated: the individual can withdraw from activities involving society or society can close off avenues of involvement, e.g., retirement. In some cases, both the individual and society seek disengagement, and in such cases disengagement is a simple process. If society and the individual have differing opinions, the wishes of society supersede those of the individual.

Disengagement does not mean total withdrawal from all social contacts, but it is a gradual process in which relationships contract to only family members and close friends. Disengaging persons do not want to make new friends or engage in new activities, but are actually giving up peripheral friends and activities which no longer interest them. One still has social roles, but they have altered in quality and quantity. The family members and friends remaining have the responsibility for meeting all the social needs of the disengaging older adult.

The nurse must be able to make a differential diagnosis—is the older adult disengaging or depressed? If the former, the nurse does not plan activities but accepts the disengaged person's wishes and helps the family and close friends cope with the increasing social dependence that is being exhibited. If the latter, appropriate psychological and medication therapy should be instituted.

The *social dysfunction theory* as suggested by Bengston is a social interaction theory which suggests that the older adult is labeled as incompetent by society. This creates a vicious cycle in which the person actually does become incompetent. First when one retires or grows old one is considered to be unable to fulfill a societal role. Older persons internalize this and begin to believe themselves sickly, incompetent, and perhaps senile. This leads to social, if not physical, death. Bengston suggested that we must change our view of the elderly and also provide coping mechanisms which will help the person to remain competent. Society should provide alternatives in which the elderly can be in control of aspects of their life that they are strongly interested in, such as running a home for the elderly or being on the board of service agencies involved in providing services to the elderly. This change in attitude and behavior towards the elderly would in turn lead to a social reconstruction syndrome, rather than the social breakdown syndrome we have at the present time.

The *social exchange theory* posited by Black suggests the aged behave as they do because they have no power; there is an unequal power ratio, with society being in control. Societal norms are seen as the rules for the older adult's behavior. As Blau stated, the mellowness of old age is nothing more than a manifestation of compliance which the

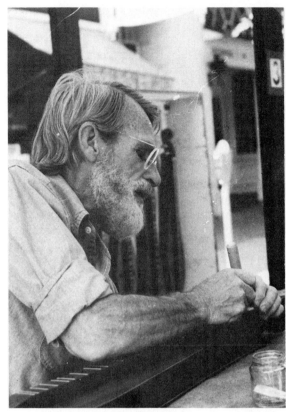

**FIGURE 3-7**
For some older adults staying active is part of a happy life.

older person resorts to in order to gain social acceptance.[67] According to this theory the nurse should look to the community to find the parameters of behavior allowed the elderly. If the parameters reflect a narrow viewpoint, work should be focused on changing the total community's viewpoint as well as the behavior of an individual. The *Gray Panther movement* is one group that is trying to change society's view of the aged, as well as gain political and economic strength for older adults.

**V**iews of the Aged  Society tends to label the elderly as inadequate because they are no longer productive members of society. Unimportant or unproductive members of our society are allowed more deviant behavior; therefore, eccentricity for the aged is permissible. Perhaps our present view of the aged can best be summed up by the parodies of television comedians such as Carol Burnett and Johnny Carson. The older adult is at high risk of being labeled senile, a diagnosis which is neither specific nor scientific. Treatments for mental illness in the aged often reflect the view that professionals consider deviant behavior an incurable part of being old.

Some young people equate the aged with death, and their fear of death tends to make them avoid the elderly. This is often made easy by the fact that many suburbs are, in fact, age-segregated, so interacting with older people is an uncommon event. The college age adult is the one most likely to allow a great deal of latitude in what is acceptable behavior for the older adult, with the middle age and aged more narrow in these perspectives.

With an increasing number of elderly in our society, along with a decreasing birth rate, the older adult will make up a sizeable proportion of the total population. Can we afford the luxury of considering over 18 percent of our population as unproductive and capable only of waiting for death? Or will we change our view of the older adult, which according to Bengston and Black, will change the aged's concept of themselves and their behavior?

Although society's view of the aged is a strong influence on both governmental policy and the belief systems we internalize, the most significant influence on the individual older adult is the expectations of significant others. Aged persons often can tolerate society's expectations that they have little to offer but become upset if their significant others label their behavior as inappropriate. The nurse should be aware that certain behavior may be the result of censorship by significant others. The stress of having to decide between the wishes of one's family and friends and one's personal wishes can be very difficult. Empathetic listening is often helpful in this situation, as well as encouraging the significant others to become more understanding and less judgmental.

**S**ocial Losses  Coping with social losses is a common problem for older adults. They must accept cultural devaluation and loss of job and income, as well as a contracting social circle. Later they face the problems of decreasing independence and the need to accept help from others. Many of these losses have been discussed in earlier sections. Therefore, the loss explored here will be that of decreasing independence. Many older adults have a greater fear of dependency than death, particularly fearing the need to depend on others to fulfill the activities of daily living. For example, the nurse must be sensitive to the impact giving up one's driver's license has on one's life. The older adult, particularly if living in an area not serviced by mass transportation, suddenly is dependent on others to get to the grocery store, doctor, social activities,

etc. Generally, this creates a decrease in social contacts and the elderly must wait to be visited rather than initiating a social call. Since they must depend on others for transportation, they tend to limit trips to essential ones. Exploring alternative means of transportation such as the Older Adult Transportation Service, which is becoming increasingly available in all communities, or adult tricycles for shopping would be ways the nurse could soften the blow for those who must give up driving. On a community level the nurse should work with agencies interested in the older adult's welfare to develop alternative transportation schemes.

The greatest contribution the nurse can make is to help the older adult remain independent in activities of daily living. In many instances this means long-term planning. When planning a retirement home or doing remodeling, counseling should include energy-conserving floor plans, showers with seats, and easy interior and exterior maintenance. The older adult should be made aware of the disuse phenomenon and helped to develop an exercise regimen that promotes vigor. The nurse needs to be familiar with the community services available to clients and to work to develop energy-saving services such as errand, laundry, meal, and housekeeping services.

When an older adult becomes dependent on others for daily living activities, the nurse should provide support to both the patient and the caretaker. In many cases the caretaker is the spouse or a child. They should be counseled to keep the level of dependency at a minimum. The nurse also can be a person to whom both client and caretaker can safely ventilate feelings and who will suggest methods of coping for each.

**Cultural influences**  Ethnic influences do not change with old age, and the effect of society, particularly prejudice, may be compounded. To be old and a member of a minority group is "double jeopardy." Add to this being a woman, and the situation is worsened. Particularly important are economic problems, since minority workers often have the lower paying jobs which in turn mean low social security payments and the residue of a life of poverty: more health problems, little or no savings, and poor living conditions. For blacks the probability of living to old age is less than it is for whites, with women being more likely to live longer. Black aged women tend to be without a spouse more frequently than white elderly women. Minority women have often worked in low paying jobs which were not covered by social security payments. Most

American Indians have shorter life-spans, inadequate living and health care facilities, and poverty.

The older adult population has a greater proportion of immigrants than other age groups. The nurse working with older adults having a strong ethnic influence should consider the traditions and beliefs of their culture. For example, it was noted that few Mexican-American older adults in Texas lived in low-cost apartments for the aged, although they made up a sizeable proportion of the population. Viewed superficially, it appeared that the problems were that housing were not located in their neighborhoods and not built in the Spanish style. An apartment building built to meet this criteria still did not attract the Mexican-American elderly. Further research revealed that it is considered the children's responsibility to provide for their parents, and any parents living alone were acknowledging that their family life was inadequate.[68] In such a situation it would be more reasonable to develop services to support the children caring for the parents, rather than providing governmental support to the elderly to remain independent.

For many elderly immigrants, whether European, Asian, or Mexican, this is a stressful time because they are witnessing a breakdown in their traditional social system. Their grandchildren do not remain in the ethnic neighborhoods or towns and have taken on American life-styles. Often urban, ethnic neighborhoods are changing in character or are obliterated by urban renewal. The nurse needs to help the older adult make sense of the alien environment and if relocation is required, help find an area having the stores, religious facilities, and people most compatible with their origins. As with any client age group, the nurse should provide care within the context of the client's cultural beliefs and practices.

**Economic influences** The elderly are at high risk for being poor because of forced retirement and illness expenses. Those who have had a marginal income find themselves with an inadequate income in old age, but persons with good incomes also find themselves among the poor when they must live entirely on a pension. Income often takes a sharp decrease when the principal breadwinner dies, because union or other nongovernmental pensions end upon the earner's death. Retirement and ill health have important economic implications for the elderly.

One must remember that retirement does not have any rational purpose in terms of aging, but rather is an answer to technological and demographic changes. There are not enough jobs available for all persons. Society has increased the educational standards needed to obtain jobs, keeping the younger person in school longer and not available to the job market. Insufficient jobs often force older people to retire. The retirement age of 65 was set arbitrarily for political expediency, not for physiological, psychological, or social reasons.

Retirement is a social phenomenon. What effect does it have on the individual retired person? It has been found that retirement is not the traumatic event that it was once considered to be. If a person knows when he or she is going to retire and makes preparations, it is more frequently accepted and even anticipated. For the person who retires unexpectedly, the event becomes traumatic. Take, for example, the man who is called into the office and told that there is a need to cut the work force and, therefore, he is going to be retired a year or two before he planned. Inevitably, he will react to this event in a negative manner. On the other hand, the man who knew he was going to retire at 65 and has known for a period of time generally accepts retirement well. After retirement, people often begin special activities which take about 6 months to accomplish. For example, they may take a trip around the United States or visit with family and friends. After this, however, there is often a difference in how they view retirement. Most people who have an adequate income to pursue hobbies or plans that they have made usually enjoy retirement, while the person who does not have the income will find retirement frustrating. Generally, two things that a person must have in order to really enjoy old age are adequate income and good health.

Unfortunately, today's elderly do not always find that retirement brings an adequate income. Society may not be able to do anything about a person's health, but they should be able to provide an income adequate to meet the needs of their citizens. For the first time in their lives many elderly find themselves at the poverty level. These are generally people who have only social security to fall back upon. In most cases income at least takes a rapid drop after retirement. According to the 1975 census, 15.3 percent of all persons over 65 are below the poverty level.

If older adults retiring at 65 meet the requirements for social security benefits, which in 1976 was 6¼ years of coverage, they will receive per month a minimum of $101.40 and a maximum of $378.80 if a woman and $364.00 if a man. Beginning in 1978 there are no differences in payments based on sex. If retiring at 62, this payment scale goes down to a range of $81.20 to $291.20. Payments to couples are higher. For example, when both are 65, $152.10 to $568.20 is the range of payment.[69] It is obvious that these amounts would be difficult to live on without other financial support. Besides the individuals and families who are below or near the poverty level, there are many whose retirement has dropped them far below their previous income. Two surveys show that one-fifth to one-third of the respondents felt their retirement standard of living was below their previous standard. One study asked the retired person to estimate their retirement to preretirement income ratio and found 60 percent thought it was one-half or less.[70] Although the majority of the elderly own their own homes, they were generally purchased 30 to 40 years ago and probably will be in need of extensive repairs. The nurse who is asked to help an older adult balance a budget will find it is a difficult task. Most, if not all, of their money must be spent on essentials. It is a myth that older people need less; actually they do without many items because they cannot afford them.

One of the older adult's greatest expenses, in comparison to other age groups, is health care. A greater proportion of their budget goes for health care services, medications, and equipment than any other age group. Many people have the mistaken idea that Medicare frees the elderly of concerns about health-related expenses. Nothing could be farther from the truth. Medicare meets only an approximate 45 percent of the health-related expenses. It does not pay for health maintenance activities, glasses, dentures, hearing aids, special foods, or outpatient medications. In order to have hospital benefits the older adult must have an initial sum of over $100 and after 60 days pay a substantial amount for each hospital day. The older adult must have some money in order to begin to receive benefits from Medicare and then has 60 days to get well or die! Medical expenses also require an initial outlay by the client, effectively preventing the old from using health-care resources. The amount of initial outlay required before services are given under Medicare changes each year based on the cost of services. The cost for both hospital and physician coverage has increased in terms of insurance cost as well as the initial expenses for which a client is responsible.

In 1975 the federal government began to monitor the services provided to the aged based on the participants' monetary worth. This includes the administration of a ''means'' test to decide who may participate in the congregate meal plan or use the senior centers. This is unfortunate since many older adults will not accept services that they consider to be charity or mark them as indigent. Programs that are based on the needs of the elderly for social contact, activities, and good nutrition should not be viewed as programs for the poor. These are basic needs of all aged persons, and ones for which our society has not adequately provided. The nurse, as a citizen and a health professional, should actively fight to eliminate the criterion of financial need for participation in programs for the elderly.

**Family influences** In evaluating the family life of the older adult, consideration will be given to the members of the nuclear family or persons in residence and also to the existence and functioning of the modified extended family. Relationships between family members are discussed here, with particular emphasis on the parent-child relationship.

The older adult nuclear family generally consists of a husband and wife or a single person. Occasionally a child is also present, often one who is dependent on the parents. In other cases one child remains at home to help the parents cope. This is particularly true if the parent was widowed before a child married. The elderly couple has two important developmental tasks to accomplish—coping with retirement and combating failing health. To help them meet their tasks they often rely on companionship, long-term knowledge of each other, stable, loving family and friends, and a secure community relationship. When any of the strengths are lacking, it becomes more difficult for the family to complete these tasks.

When one or both members of the family retire, their life habits change drastically. It is generally been the husband who retires and the wife who has remained at home. In the future, this will probably not be true. This often creates problems, as one or both spouses must redefine their social roles. Those who have retired no longer leave the house early in the morning and return late in the afternoon. They must find something to do with those hours. In one study, it was found that the male union workers used the retirement center much more than the female members.[71] The researcher concluded that most often this was so because the male needed to have a place to go to, to leave the house in the morning, to spend the day with other males, and then come home. Often, a man, and perhaps his wife, consider that the husband is invading what is essentially a female territory when he remains at home. A woman may have developed social contacts that she keeps up during the day that are generally of a female nature; her life revolves around tasks that many men would consider of "feminine orientation." Males generally have not developed the skills of finding friends and maintaining friendships outside of the work situation. It has generally been a female role to organize and maintain a couple's social life. Therefore, elderly males do not have places to go and people to be with unless someone has organized these events for them. Most couples are able to cope with retirement and to develop new, compatible social roles. In some cases, however, marriages which have been under a great deal of strain cannot tolerate the extra strain of this development, and one or both persons will seek outside help. The couple who found that they had nothing to discuss and no common interests after their children left home will find being together 24 hours a day makes living together even more difficult. The nurse should refer the couple to a marriage counselor and encourage them to work to improve their marital situation.

A second, more difficult problem for the older adult couple is adjusting to the failing health of one or both members. Women have had a tendency to marry men who are older than they are, and at the same time men have a tendency to die younger than women. It is often the wife who has, in the later stages of a marriage, become the nurse to her husband. No matter who becomes the invalid, it creates problems for both members of the family. The more common example will be used, but the situation is the same if the sexes are reversed. The man often feels guilty that he is taking up the wife's energy and time caring for him. On the other hand, he may also feel that if she does not show complete devotion she no longer loves him. The wife feels that she should be happy to take care of her husband, but over a period of time begins to feel resentment because she is unable to participate in her normal social activities. She may even begin to daydream about how life will be different once he dies. The wife is shocked to find that she is thinking these things. "It is not right—after all this is the man that I have been married to for 50 years. We have shared a lot, I should want to take care of him." This guilt is often increased when the husband dies or when it is necessary for him to go to a nursing home because the wife can no longer adequately care for him. The nurse needs to support the older adult with the responsibility for caring for a spouse. Often there are services available that will allow the older adult placed in this role to have some free time. Support should be provided to help those in this position

cope with guilt when the ill spouse is institutionalized or dies. A third area of support is providing information to help the older adult finance medical care in case of illness. The elderly should understand their rights and be referred to agencies able to help them as soon as possible. This remains true after the death of a spouse because often the majority of any savings and equity will be gone. The financial problem is compounded for a wife because she often is not eligible for her husband's job-related union pensions; therefore monthly income is curtailed. All of this sounds very depressing, but not all elderly couples are faced with this type of situation during the growing-old period. Many find this to be a time of companionship to know each other better, develop new interests together, and enjoy expanding, rather than contracting, horizons.

With increasing age, many marriages end with the death of one spouse, generally the male. Aside from the economic problems, the surviving spouse must now cope with *loneliness*. Part of what new widows or widowers must face is the development of a life alone. Others may be available for social contact, but it is not the unique social contact they shared with their spouse. In the discussion of death and dying, the problems of new role alignment for the elderly were explored. However, combating loneliness can also be a major problem for persons who were close to their spouse or who are dependent on others for developing social contacts. Often they need to be sought out and brought to such activities as senior citizens meetings or congregate meals. They will not venture out and try something new without a person who will provide entree. This fear of new social contacts and environments can create financial problems when widowed persons cling to homes that are too expensive for their present income. Many people live in quite desperate straits because they will not leave a home they have lived in all of their life. This may be for sentimental reasons or because the prospect of moving to a new area, discovering new facilities, and adjusting to new people and a new environment are just too overwhelming. The nurse who recognizes this problem can be an aid in helping the elderly person become familiar with a new area before a move is made and perhaps in helping them to make the decision to move to a more economically feasible area.

Older adults are often eager to help others. The nurse can direct this desire to help by suggesting that older persons become involved in volunteer organizations as hospital volunteers, or members of RSVP groups or other local organizations. The elderly in a nursing home could act as phone volunteers and call other elderly people who live in the community, thereby providing communication that is very important to those living alone. Many older adults fear that something will happen to them and no one will know about it for hours or even days. Therefore, this service provides some ease of mind and allows some elderly to remain in their homes when they would have otherwise moved into a sheltered environment.

While the individual and the couple are important family units, they are not the only family unit relevant in old age. The nuclear family is not as common as sociologists once believed. Instead, industrial societies have developed a *modified extended family structure* in which parents live independently of their children as long as possible, but all family members carry out an intradependent relationship (Fig. 3-8). Most older adults have living children or siblings. If they have children, they have a mutually dependent relationship with them; if not, they develop such a relationship with their siblings. Shanas et al. found about 82 percent of the aged surveyed have at least one living child, most have three or more. Of those having children, 93 percent have grandchildren and 40 percent have great-grandchildren. Most older adults communicate with at least one child weekly and often live within 10 minutes of one of their children. While children may not provide economic support to their parents,

they usually provide services which help their parents cope with independent living. When independent living is no longer feasible, the parents are usually taken into one of the children's households. Children provide more services to their parents than those provided by the community. Of the 2 percent community-living bedfast elderly, 80 to 90 percent get the majority of their help from their families. Community services provided do not substitute for children's services and rarely are family support services provided. Only when the children find it physically or psychologically impossible to continue to care for their parents is institutionalization of the parent(s) considered.[72]

Children often feel that they are abandoning their parents when they put them in a nursing home, and usually have guilt feelings. These guilt feelings are evidenced in many ways. Sometimes the child stays away from the nursing home, does not visit the parent, and seems to show no interest at all. Other children are always at the nursing home, are critical of the care being given, and wish everything to be done for their parents. These are, of course, two extremes; however, they do exist. Nurses can be helpful to children by behaving in a nonjudgmental manner, providing individual or group counseling for children that would allow them to express their feelings of guilt and recognize that institutionalization is an acceptable manner of coping, and make them aware that other

**FIGURE 3-8**
In a modified extended family structure, elderly parents are often included in family outings and vacations.

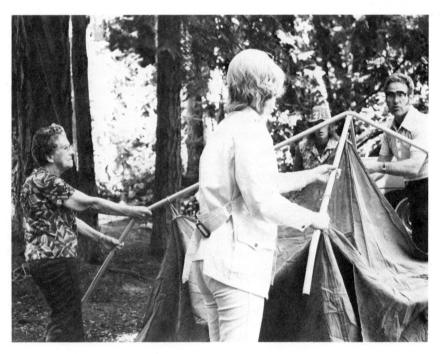

children have the same problems they do. The nurse can also work to develop family support services so that parents do not have to be institutionalized, for example day care centers in which elderly people are cared for during the day and go home at night. This provides relief for family members, allowing them to go out and do other activities. Another alternative is providing services to the older adult's or child's home such as chore or laundry service, meals on wheels, or nursing care. Temporary full-time care, in the home or institution, would also allow children more free time.

The parent-child relationship remains a strong force throughout life. The nurse needs to be aware of the developmental stage coined by Margaret Blenkner called *filial maturity,* a stage coming after Freud's last stage of genital maturity in which the relationship between aging parents and their children is optimal. Children, in order to successfully reach this stage, must become independent of their parents and view them as human beings capable of having faults, as well as good points. Parents must recognize their children as adults and also recognize their dependency on their children. When the dependency needs of aging parents become apparent to middle-age children, a "filial crisis" occurs in which the child works through a new relationship with parents and develops a mature understanding. The child can be depended on to meet parental needs while recognizing that parents are adult individuals with rights, faults, needs, and life histories. Parents do not become children and children do not become parents, as believed by role reversal advocates. Rather, children meet the dependency needs of the parents by helping in areas that need help, and not helping in other areas where elderly parents are competent. Of course, the nurse comes in contact with family situations which are not ideal and should begin an intervention to prevent family strain during the period of filial crisis. Family or individual counseling may be helpful, particularly for families in which children do not accept their elderly parents as still being human beings or who have hostile or unresolved conflicts concerning their parents. Parents may also need help in being gracious receivers. This preventative work can make life more bearable for parents and children. When the nurse receives controlling instructions from the children such as "I don't want the following people to be allowed to visit my mother," the nurse should ask the parent if that is to be so; if it is not, the nurse should encourage the children and the parent to resolve the problem. The nurse should attempt to help the child see the parent as an adult, but in any case be consistent in behavior and acknowledge the older adult's rights.

**G**randparenthood Grandparenthood is not the major task of late adulthood. Most older adults enjoy being grandparents, but usually not to the exclusion of their social activities, volunteer activities, and personal relationships with persons of their generation and other family members. This is not to give the impression that older adults don't like having and being with grandchildren, but generally they wish to do so on a selective basis. They do not wish the responsibility of raising a child or having regular baby-sitting duties, but like to be with grandchildren for "fun" occasions. They want to take the children to the park or fishing, not do their laundry or be responsible for discipline. This can cause problems in the families where the young adults consider grandmother the perfect baby-sitter while both the husband and wife work. Grandparents may find this too restrictive and perhaps too much of a physical strain. The nurse should counsel both parents and grandparents that this will probably not be a long-term practical solution, and that the parents should seek alternative solutions. Some grandparents feel that their feelings are selfish or unnatural and they need an objective person, such as the nurse, to tell them that their feelings are normal.

## SUMMARY

Persons in all age groups encounter health problems and seek health care. A young, middle, or older adult may experience similar health problems, but, because of physical development, personality dynamics, differences in sexuality, and variations in life-style, responses to these health problems can differ greatly. A thorough understanding of age-related phenomena is essential for the nurse to adequately care for and help patients as they interact with their environment.

## REFERENCES

1  Alexander Leaf, *Youth in Old Age,* McGraw-Hill, New York, 1975, p. 144.
2  Nancy L. Diekelmann, "The Young Adult: The Choice is Health or Illness," *Am J Nurs,* **8:**1272–1277, August 1976.
3  *Ibid.,* 1275.
4  *Ibid.,* 1276.

5 Maxwell M. Wintrobe, George W. Thorn, et al. (eds.), *Harrison's Principles of Internal Medicine,* 7th ed., McGraw-Hill, New York, 1974, p. 1433.

6 D. B. Bromley, *The Psychology of Human Aging,* 2d ed., Penguin, Middlesex, England, 1974, pp. 179–180.

7 *Ibid.,* 211—217.

8 Erik Erikson, *Childhood and Society,* 2d ed., Norton, New York, 1963, pp. 263–264.

9 Norma Haan, "Personality Development from Adolescence to Adulthood in the Oakland Growth and Guidance Studies," *Sem Psychiatry,* **4:**399–414, 1972.

10 John Nash, *Developmental Psychology: A Psychobiological Approach,* Prentice-Hill, Englewood Cliffs, N.J., 1970, p. 176.

11 Gail Sheehy, *Passages: Predictable Crises of Adult Life,* Dutton, New York, 1974, p. 36.

12 Daniel Yankelovich, *The New Morality: A Profile of American Youth in the 70's,* McGraw-Hill, New York, 1974, p. 4.

13 *Report of the White House Conference on Youth,* publication 4000-0267, April 1971, p. 248.

14 Theodore Roszak, *The Making of a Counter Culture,* Doubleday, New York, 1965.

15 *Report of the White House Conference on Youth,* publication 4000-0267, April 1971, p. 246.

16 Kenneth Keniston, *The Uncommitted: Alienated Youth in American Society,* Dell, New York, 1965, p. 14.

17 Anne W. Simon, *The New Years: A New Middle Age,* Knopf, New York, 1968, p. 170–171.

18 David W. Smith and Edwin L. Bierman, *The Biologic Ages of Man from Conception Through Old Age,* Saunders, Philadelphia, 1973, p. 154.

19 Clark Tibbits, and Wilma Donahue (eds.), *Aging in Today's Society,* Prentice-Hall, Englewood Cliffs, N.J., 1960, p. 44.

20 *Statistical Bulletin,* Metropolitan Life, New York, September, 1975.

21 Elizabeth B. Hurlock, *Developmental Psychology,* 4th ed., McGraw-Hill, New York, 1975, p. 270.

22 Ruth Murray and Judith Zentner, *Nursing Assessment and Health Promotion Through the Life Span,* Prentice-Hall, Englewood Cliffs, N.J., 1975, p. 264–265.

23 B. L. Neugarten, "Adult Personality: Toward a Psychology of the Life Cycle," in B. L. Neugarten (ed.), *Middle Age and Aging: A Reader in Social Psychology,* University of Chicago Press, Chicago, 1968.

24 N. Diekelmann, "Emotional Tasks of the Middle Adult," *Am J Nurs,* **75**(6):997–1001, June 1975.

25 Eda LeShan, *The Wonderful Crisis of Middle Age,* McKay, New York, 1973.

26 Eric Pfeiffer and G. C. Davis, "Determinants of Sexual Behavior in Middle and Old Age," *J Am Geriat Soc,* **20:**151–158, April 1972.

27 Morton Hunt, *Sexual Behavior in the 1970's,* Playboy, Chicago, 1974.

28 David Mace and Vera Mace, "The Joy of Human Sexuality in Marriage," *J Sex Educ Ther,* **2:**35–41, Fall-Winter 1975.

29 Paul H. Gebhardt, "Heterosexual Behavior," lecture delivered at Institute for Sex Research, University of Indiana, Bloomington, June 19, 1974.

30 Wardell B. Pomeroy and Cornelia V. Christenson, *Characteristics of Male and Female Sexual Responses,* Study Guide 4, SIECUS, New York, 1967.

31 Robert Athanasion, "Questionnaire," *Psychology Today,* **4:**37–52, July 1970.

32 Gebhardt, *op. cit.*

33 Robert W. Cali, "Management of the Climacteric and Post-Menopausal Woman," *Med Clin North Am,* **56**(3):789–800, May 1972.

34 T. Masukawa, "Vaginal Smears in Women Past 40 Years of Age with Emphasis on Their Remaining Hormonal Activity," *Obstet Gynecol,* **16:**407–413, October 1960.

35 M. T. McLennan and C. E. McLennan, "Estrogenic Status of Menstruating and Menopausal Women Assessed by Cervico-vaginal Smears," *Obstet Gynecol,* **37:**325–331, March 1971.

36 *A Clinical Guide to the Menopause and the Post-Menopause,* Ayerst Laboratories, New York, 1968.

37 A. D. Claman, David Swartz, R. A. H. Kinch, and N. B. Hirt: "Panel Discussion: Sexual Difficulties After 50: General Discussion," *Can Med Assoc J,* **94:**215–217, January 29, 1966.

38 S. Bender, "Is Your Menopause Really Necessary," *Nursing Mirror,* **133**(1):30–31, July 2, 1971.

39 Bernice L. Neugarten, "The Awareness of Middle Age," in Robert Owne (eds.), *Middle Age,* British Broadcasting Corporation, London, 1967.

40 Eric Pfeiffer, Adriaan Verwoerdt, and Glenn C. Davis: "Sexual Behavior in the Middle Life," *Am J Psychiatry,* **128**(10):1262–1267, April 1972.

41 G. Allen, "Do Men Go Through a Change of Life," *Family Health,* **4:**20–23, November 1972.

42 E. E. LeMasters, *Blue Collar Aristocrats,* University of Wisconsin, Madison, 1975.

43 Allen, *op. cit.*

44 Kenneth Cooper, *The New Aerobics,* Bantam, New York, 1970.

45 Elizabeth B. Hurlock, *Developmental Psychology,* 4th ed., McGraw-Hill, New York, 1975.

46 D. W. Smith, and E. L. Bierman, *The Biologic Ages of Man,* Saunders, Philadelphia, 1973.

47 U.S. Department of Health, Education, and Welfare, Office of Human Development, *Facts About Older Americans 1975,* publication OHD 75-20006, 1975.

48 E. Shanas, "Measuring the Home Health Needs of the Aged in Five Countries," *J Gerontol,* **26:**37–40, 1971.

49 L. Lowy et al., "Attitudes of Nurses and Social Workers Toward Aging and Their Relationship to Life Satisfaction of Patients and Clients," unpublished study available at Mugar Library, Boston University, Boston, 1974.

50 P. S. Timiras, *Developmental Physiology and Aging,* Macmillan, New York, 1972.

51 O. H. Robertson, *Endocrines and Aging,* MSS Information Corporation, New York, 1972.

52 P. S. Timiras, op. cit.

53 Arthur J. Vander, et al.: *Human Physiology: The Mechanisms of Body Function,* McGraw-Hill, New York, 1975.

54 R. F. Peck and H. Berkowitz, "Personality and Adjustment in Middle Age," in B. L. Neugarten (ed.), *Personality in Middle and Late Life,* Prentice-Hall, Englewood Cliffs, N.J., 1964.

55 R. N. Butler, "The Life Review: An Interpretation of Reminiscence in the Aged," *Psychiatry,* **26:**65–76, 1963.

56 Charlotte Epstein, *Nursing the Dying Patient,* Reston, Reston, Virginia, 1975.

57 E. Kubler-Ross, *On Death and Dying,* Macmillan, New York, 1969.

58 H. Brody, "Structural Changes in the Aging Nervous System," in H. T. Blumenthal (ed.), *The Regulation Role at the Nervous System in Aging,* Karger, Basel, 1970.

59 D. S. Woodruff, "Biofeedback Control of the EEG Alpha Rhythm and Its Effect on Reaction Time in the Young and Old," University Microfilms, no. 72-33, 1833, Ann Arbor, Michigan, 1972.

60 Q. S. Obrist, E. W. Busse, C. Eisdorfer, and R. W. Kleemeier, "Relation of Electroencephalogram to Intellectual Function in Senescence," *J Gerontol,* **17:**197–206, 1962.

61 S. Granick, "Psychological Test Functioning," in S. Granick and R. D. Patterson (eds.), *Human Aging, II,* U.S. Department of Health, Education, and Welfare Publication HSM 71-9037, 1971.

62 C. Eisdorfer, and F. Wilkie, "Intellectual Changes with Advancing Age," in L. F. Jarvik, C. Eisdorfer, and J. C. Blum (eds.), *Intellectual Functioning in Adults,* Springer, New York, 1973.

63 K. F. Riegel, and R. M. Riegel, "Development Drop and Death," *Dev Psychol,* **6:**306–319, 1972.

64 W. H. Masters and V. E. Johnson, *Human Sexual Inadequacy,* Churchill, London, 1970.

65 W. H. Masters and V. E. Johnson, *Human Sexual Response,* Little, Brown, Boston, 1966.

66 B. L. Neugarten, J. Wand Moore, and J. C. Lowe, "Age Norms, Age Constraints, and Adult Socialization," in B. L. Neugarten (ed.), *Middle Age and Aging,* University of Chicago Press, Chicago, 1968.

67 Z. S. Blau, *Old Age in a Changing Society,* New Viewpoint, New York, 1973.

68 F. Carp, "New Housing Developments for the Older Citizen Must Make Allowances for Cultural Differences," *Geriatric Focus,* **9:**2–9, 1970.

69 *Your New Social Security and Medicare Fact Sheet,* pamphlet of the National Retired Teachers Association, American Association of Retired Persons, Washington, D.C., 1976.

70 J. H. Schulz, *Background and Issues: Retirement,* White House Conference on Aging, 1971, pp. 12–13.

71 A. Pallak, P. Sagin, and E. P. Friedman, *A Utilization Study of a Senior Citizen's Center,* Administration on Aging, Washington, D.C., report 33, 1970.

72 E. Shanas, P. Townsend, D. Wedderburn, H. Frus, P. Milhoz, and J. Steinhouwer, *Old People in Three Industrial Societies,* Atherton, New York, 1968.

## BIBLIOGRAPHY

### The Young Adult

Bahra, Robert J.: "The Potential for Suicide," *Am J Nurs,* **10:**1782–1788, October 1975.

Buhler, Charlotte: *Psychology for Contemporary Living,* Hawthorn, New York, 1968.

Erikson, Erik: *The Challenge of Youth,* Doubleday, New York, 1965.

Fleshman, Ruth: "The Young Adult in Today's World," *Nurs Clin North Am,* **1:**1–104, March 1973.

Goodman, Paul: *Growing Up Absurd,* Random House, New York, 1960.

Gould, Roger L.: "The Phases of Adult Life: A Study in Developmental Psychology," *Am J Psychiatry,* **129:**521–531, 1972.

Guyton, Arthur C.: *Medical Physiology,* 2d ed., Saunders, Philadelphia, 1964.

Havinghurst, Robert: *Developmental Tasks and Education,* McKay, New York, 1965.

Hunt, J. McVicker (ed.): *Human Intelligence,* Rutgers University, New Brunswick, 1972.

Lidz, Theodore: *The Person,* Basic Books, New York, 1968.

Master, William H. and Virginia E. Johnson: *Human Sexual Response,* Little, Brown, Boston, 1966.

Reich, Charles A.: *The Greening of America,* Random House, New York, 1970.

Toffler, Alvin: *Future Shock,* Random House, New York, 1970.

Vaillant, George E. and Charles C. McArthur: "Natural History of Male Psychologic Health. I. The Adult Life Cycle From 18–50," *Semin Psychiatry,* **4:** 417–429, 1972.

**The Middle Adult**

Bischof, L. J.: *Adult Psychology,* Harper and Row, New York, 1969.

Erikson, Erik H.: *Childhood and Society,* 2d ed., Norton, New York, 1963.

Galloway, Karen: "The Change of Life," *Am J Nurs,* **75**(6):1006–1011, June 1975.

Marmor, J.: "The Crisis in Middle Age," *RN,* **30**(11): 63–68, 1967.

McEwan, J. A.: "Menopause: Myths and Medicine," *Nurs Times,* **69:**1483–1484, November 8, 1973.

Peck, R. C.: "Psychological Developments in the Second Half of Life," in B. L. Neugarten (ed.), *Middle Age and Aging: A Reader in Social Psychology,* University of Chicago, Chicago, 1968, pp. 88–92.

Rubin, T.: "Male Menopause," *Ladies Home Journal,* **88:**52, November 1971.

Sutterley, Doris Cook and Gloria Ferraro Donnelly: *Perspectives of Human Development: Nursing Throughout the Life Cycle,* J. B. Lippincott, Philadelphia, 1973, pp. 50–53.

The Retirement Council: *Better Health After Fifty,* American Heritage, New York, 1964.

**The Older Adult**

Bengtson, V. L.: *The Social Psychology of Aging,* Bobbs-Merrill, Indianapolis, 1973.

Blumenthal, H. T., (ed.): *The Regulatory Role of the Nervous System in Aging,* Karger, Basel, 1970.

Brockelhurst, J. C.: *Textbook of Geriatric Medicine and Gerontology,* Churchill-Livingstone, London, 1973.

Brody, E. M.: "The Etiquette of Filial Behavior," *Aging and Human Development,* **1:**87–94, 1970.

Brotman, H.: "The Fastest Growing Minority: The Aging," *Am J Public Health,* **64:**249–252, 1974.

Buhler, C.: "The Developmental Structure of Goal Setting in Group and Individual Studies," in Buhler, C. and F. Massarik (eds.), *The Course of Human Life,* Springer, New York, 1968.

Burnside, L. M., (ed.): *Sexuality and Aging,* University of Southern California, Los Angeles, 1975.

Butler, R., and M. Lewis: *Aging and Mental Health,* Mosby, St. Louis, 1973.

Cartwright, A., L. Hockey, and J. L. Anderson: *Life Before Death,* Routledge and Keyan Paul, Boston, 1973.

Chen, Y.: *Background and Issues: Income,* 1971 White House Conference on Aging, 1970.

Chinn, A. B. (ed.): *Working with Older People, A Guide to Practice,* vols. I–IV, U.S. Department Health, Education, and Welfare, 1971.

Corso, J. F.: "Sensory Processes and Age Effects in Normal Adults," *J Gerontol,* **26:**90–105, 1971.

Cottrell, F.: *Aging and the Aged,* William C. Brown, Dubuque, Iowa, 1974.

Craven, J., and F. S. Wald: "Hospice Care for Dying Patients," *Am J Nurs,* **75:**1816–1822, October 1975.

Cumming, E., and W. E. Henry: *Growing Old,* Basic Books, New York, 1961.

deVries, H. A.: "Physiological Effects of an Exercise Training Regimen Upon Men Aged 52 to 88," *J Gerontol,* **25:**325–336, 1970.

Eisdorfer, C.: "Discussion: Mind and Body," in L. F. Jarrick, C. Eisdorfer, and J. C. Blum (eds.), *Intellectual Functioning in Adults,* Springer, New York, 1973.

Eisdorfer, C., and M. P. Lawton (eds.): *The Psychology of Adult Development and Aging,* American Psychological Association, Washington, D.C., 1973.

Eisele, F. K. (ed.): "Political Consequences of Aging," *Annals,* **415:**1–212, 1974.

Erikson, Erik H.: *Childhood and Society,* 2d ed., Norton, New York, 1963.

Glaser, B. G., and A. L. Strauss: *Awareness of Dying,* Aldine, Chicago, 1965.

Granick, S., and R. D. Patterson (eds.): *Human Aging II,* National Institute of Mental Health, U.S. Department of Health, Education, and Welfare, publication HSM 71-9037, 1971.

Harris, R.: "The Management of Geriatric Cardiovascular Disease," *Gerontologist,* **11:**253–256, 1971.

Havighurst, R. J.: *Developmental Tasks and Education,* 3d ed., McKay, New York, 1972.

———: "Social Class Perspective on the Life Cycle," *Hum Dev,* **14:**110–124, 1971.

Hodkinson, H. M.: *An Outline of Geriatrics,* Academic, New York, 1975.

Howell, S. C., and M. B. Loeb: "Nutrition and Aging— Special Edition," *Gerontologist,* **9:**7–73, 1969.

Howell, T. H.: *A Student's Guide to Geriatrics,* Thomas, Springfield, 1970.

Kastenbaum, R.: "The Foreshortened Life Perspective," *Geriatrics,* **24:**126–133, 1969.

Kohlberg, L.: "Continuities in Childhood and Adult Morale Development Revisited," in P. B. Baltes and K. W. Sehaie (eds.), *Life Span Developmen-*

*tal Psychology: Personality and Socialization,* Academic, New York, 1973.

Meyerson, M. D.: "The Effects of Aging on Communication," *J Gerontol,* **31:**29–38, 1976.

Miller, M. B.: "Iatrogenic and Nurisgenic Effects of Prolonged Immobilization of the Ill Aged," *J Am Geriatr Soc,* **23:**360–369, 1975.

Miller, S. M.: "Rx for the Aging Person: Attitudes," *J Gerontol Nurs,* **2:**22–26, 1976.

Morison, R. S.: "Dying," in *Life and Death and Medicine, Readings from Scientific American,* Freeman, San Francisco, 1973.

Neugarten, B. L.: "Continuities and Discontinuities of Psychological Issues Into Adult Life," *Hum Dev,* **12:**121–130, 1969.

Panicucci, C., P. Paul, J. Symonds, and J. Tambelline: "Expanded Speech and Self-Pacing in Communication with the Aged," master's thesis, Boston, University, 1967.

Peck, R. C.: "Psychological Developments in the Second Half of Life," in B. L. Neugarten (ed.), *Middle Age and Aging,* University of Chicago, Chicago, 1968.

Schaie, K. W., G. V. Labouvie, and B. U. Buech: "Generational and Ontogenetic Components in Adult Cognitive Functioning: A Fourteen Year Study of Independent Samples," *Dev Psychol,* **10:**305–320, 1974.

Sherwood, S.: "Gerontology and the Sociology of Food and Eating," *Aging and Human Development,* **1:**61–85, 1970.

Spirduso, W. W.: "Reaction and Movement Time as a Function of Age and Physical Activity Level," *J Gerontol,* **30:**435–440, 1975.

Steib, G., and C. J. Schneider: *Retirement in American Society,* Cornell University, Ithaca, New York, 1971.

Townsend, P.: *The Family Life of Old People,* Penguin, Baltimore, 1963.

Weinberg, J.: "Geriatric Psychiatry," in A. M. Freedman, H. I. Kaplan, and B. J. Sadock (eds.), *Comprehensive Textbook of Psychiatry,* vol. II, 2d ed., Williams and Wilkins, Baltimore, 1975.

Weisman, A. D.: *The Realization of Death,* Aronson, New York, 1974.

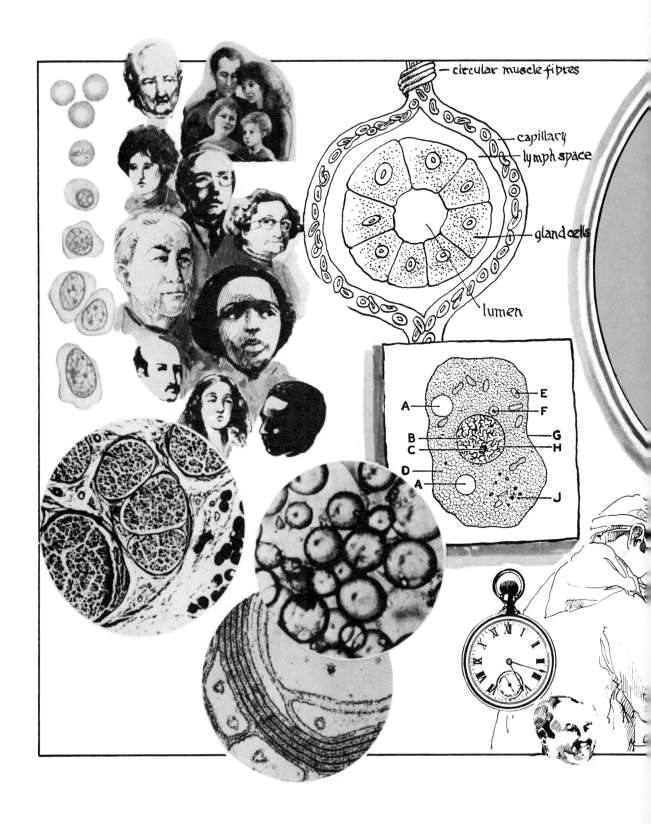

circular muscle fibres

capillary

lymph space

gland cells

lumen

A

B

C

D

A

E

F

G

H

J

# PART 2

## CELLULAR GROWTH AND PROLIFERATION

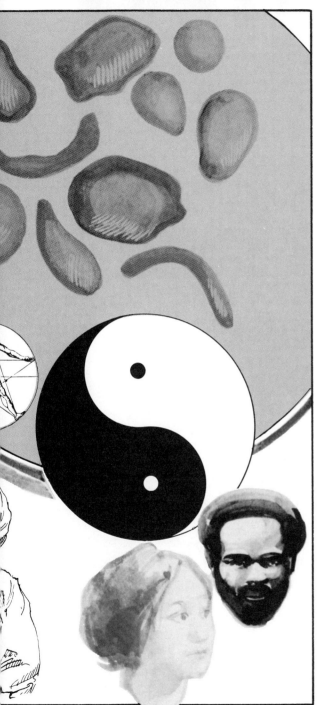

# 4
# THE CONCEPT OF CELLULAR GROWTH AND PROLIFERATION*

Claire Ford Dunbar
Thomas H. Cook

**M**an and the surrounding environment share the same basic structural unit: the *cell.* Normal cellular growth and proliferation is dependent on a healthy internal and external exchange of nutrients and wastes, the functioning of internal growth regulators, and the absence of external factors such as pathogens or injury. The emphasis of this chapter is upon the structure and function of the cell, adaptive cellular growth, and body structures that are especially pertinent because of ongoing cellular growth and proliferation (breast and reproductive tissue). Physical assessment is directed toward detectable and normally undetectable cellular growth, such as that found in the lymph nodes, uterus, and prostate.

## THE NORMAL CELL

The normal cell is composed of *protoplasm,* which is 75 to 85 percent water and has a protein content of 10 to 20 percent, a lipid content of 2 to 3 percent, and carbohydrate and inorganic solute composition of 1 percent each.[1] The cell is divided into two basic parts, the nucleus and the cytoplasm (Fig. 4-1), and is surrounded by a semipermeable cellular membrane; the nucleus and cytoplasm are separated by a *nuclear membrane* (Fig. 4-1).

The functions of the cell are carried out by *organelles* found within the cytoplasm. The major organelles are the mitochondria, the endoplasmic reticulum (ER), the Golgi apparatus, lysosomes, and centrioles. Each of these structures is surrounded by its own membrane; these membranes are similar in composition to the nuclear and cellular membranes mentioned previously.

### Membrane Structure

A new theory of membrane construction holds that the membrane is composed almost entirely of lipids (primarily phospholipids) in which protein appears to be dispersed, forming a mosaic of lipids and globular protein.[2] The proteins seem to contribute to the strength and elasticity of the membrane, promote chemical reactions by acting as enzymes, function in the transport of substances, and provide breaks in the lipid portion of the membrane (*pores*).[3] The proteins acting as *enzymes* are believed to assist in the transport of substances through the cell membrane. The *pores* are thought

* The section on Cellular Growth and Proliferation was written by Claire Ford Dunbar, and the Physical Assessment of Cellular Growth and Proliferation section by Thomas H. Cook.

to be responsible for the passage of lipid-insoluble substances, such as water and urea.

The *nuclear membrane* differs slightly from the other membranes (Fig. 4-1). A most important difference is the presence of much larger pores. The pores are believed to be enlarged to permit easy passage of substances between the nucleus and the cytoplasm.

### Cytoplasm

Cytoplasm is the viscous protoplasm found outside the nucleus of the cell. As mentioned previously, it contains all the organelles. Each of these structures is considered in a brief discussion focusing on its contribution to cellular function.

**Mitochondria** Mitochondria may be found in all aerobically respiring cells. They function in the conversion of energy from nutrients and oxygen to *adenosine triphosphate* (ATP). This oxidation of nutrients is accomplished by dissolved enzymes in the "matrix" of the mitochondria, in conjunction with oxidative enzymes found on the "shelves" formed by infoldings of the mitochondrial membranes (*cristae*) (Fig. 4-1).

**Endoplasmic reticulum** Within the cytoplasm is a network of tubular and vesicular structures known as *endoplasmic reticulum* (ER). There are two types of ER, smooth or agranular (SER) and rough or granular (RER) (Fig. 4-1). *Agranular endoplasmic reticulum* is involved in lipid synthesis (especially triglycerides), conjugation of bile pigments, glycogenolysis, and drug detoxification. In striated muscle it is referred to as *sarcoplasmic reticulum* and functions in the conduction of contractile impulses. *Granular endoplasmic reticulum* gets its name from the particles or granules attached to its outer surface. These granules, referred to as *ribosomes,* are composed primarily of ribonucleic acid (RNA) and function in protein synthesis. Hepatocytes and plasma cells are examples of cells with a large quantity of RER and a major role in protein synthesis (plasma proteins and immunoglobulins). Ribosomes may also be present as

**FIGURE 4-1**
The cell and its organelles.

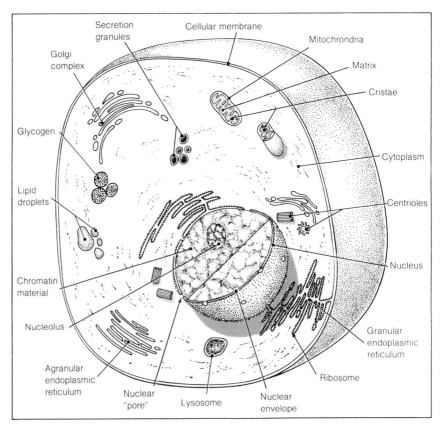

clusters in the cytoplasm called *polyribosomes,* which also function in the synthesis of protein.

**Golgi apparatus** The Golgi apparatus or complex may actually be a specialized form of ER and seems to be connected to it. The Golgi apparatus is especially apparent in secretory cells and participates in the "segregation, aggregation, and exportation" of products formed by the cell.[4] It also has a role in carbohydrate synthesis and the subsequent formation of glycoproteins. Glycoproteins compose the secretory substances of many cells, such as mucus, insulin, and the ground substance of bone and cartilage. The Golgi apparatus also functions in the formation of *lysosomes,* which are cellular structures filled with hydrolytic enzymes. These enzymes are utilized in the digestion and removal of dead or damaged tissue or foreign substances, such as microorganisms.

**Centrioles** Two pairs of centrioles are present in the cytoplasm of each cell. These cylindrical structures are situated near the nucleus and play an active role during cell division (*mitosis,* discussed in detail later in this chapter).

**Other cytoplasmic structures** Other structures found in cellular cytoplasm include microtubules, secretory granules, and specialized structures such as myofibrils. *Microtubules* are fine tubules present in cells such as sperm and cilia. *Secretory granules* are probably all formed by the Golgi apparatus. They store special substances such as pancreatic enzymes for secretion as needed. *Myofibrils* are specialized structures found in muscle cells that function in muscle contraction (Chap. 31).

**The Nucleus**
The nucleus of the cell is responsible for the control and integration of all the activities of the cell. It contains large amounts of *deoxyribonucleic acid* (DNA). DNA is especially important in cellular reproduction (mitosis), and it also controls activities of the cytoplasm. The interphase nucleus (nondividing nucleus) contains DNA in the form of clumps or filaments of *chromatin material,* which later becomes part of the chromosomes during mitosis. Nuclei also possess one or more *nucleoli.* Nucleoli are composed of *ribonucleic acid* (RNA) and are functionally active in the synthesis of ribosomal RNA.

**Cellular Function**
Many of the functions of the cell have already been mentioned in the discussion of each organelle. Cellular ingestion, protein synthesis, and cellular growth and reproduction (the cell cycle), however, involve the entire cell and are now presented in more detail.

**Ingestion** Ingestion is necessary in order for the cell to obtain nutrients and other substances necessary for growth and reproduction. These substances are obtained through diffusion, active transport, and pinocytosis.

*Diffusion* involves the random movement of particles among other particles. This movement is maintained by the kinetic energy generated when one molecule approaches another molecule, is repelled, and moves away. Dissolved substances and water molecules are all in constant motion and therefore participate in diffusion. Substances (solutes) diffuse from areas of high concentration to areas of low concentration. Small molecules diffuse more rapidly than large ones. Molecular motion is increased by heat, as is the rate of diffusion.

Substances pass into the cell via one of two methods of diffusion. First, they may become dissolved in the lipid substance of the cellular membrane and pass quickly through; oxygen is an example of such a substance. Other particles, such as glucose, attach themselves to a carrier, in this case insulin, and then pass through the lipid matrix of the membrane. This latter process is referred to as *facilitated diffusion.* The second method of diffusion is through the pores of the cellular membrane. Urea, ions, and water are examples of substances that diffuse freely through the pores of cells. Water is the substance which diffuses in the largest quantities, in response to a concentration difference on either side of the cellular membrane. If water moves into the cell, it swells; if water moves out, the cell shrinks. This movement is referred to as *osmosis.* Excessive swelling can cause cellular rupture or *hydrolysis,* and extreme shrinking of a cell results in a state called *crenation.*

The movement of substances (particularly ions, some sugars, and amino acids) against the concentration gradient is referred to as *active transport.* The mechanism to achieve active transport requires that the substance be bound to a carrier, that energy be utilized (usually in the form of ATP), and that enzymes be present to act as catalysts. An example of active transport in the body occurs when sodium is transported to the outside of the cell

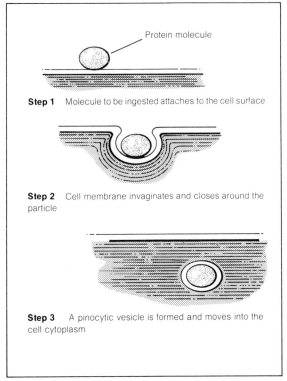

Step 1  Molecule to be ingested attaches to the cell surface

Step 2  Cell membrane invaginates and closes around the particle

Step 3  A pinocytic vesicle is formed and moves into the cell cytoplasm

**FIGURE 4-2**
Pinocytosis (*Adapted from Guyton, Arthur C., Textbook of Medical Physiology, W. B. Saunders Company, Philadelphia, 1976.*)

while potassium is transported inside; active transport is necessary in these instances because sodium is normally high in concentration outside the cell, as compared to inside, with the opposite being true of potassium (see Chap. 11).

*Pinocytosis* is the third process involved in cellular ingestion. It is used primarily for protein molecules and strong electrolyte solutions that are incapable of passing into the cell by either diffusion or active transport. The process is illustrated in Fig. 4-2. Briefly, it involves the following steps:

1   The molecule to be ingested attaches to the surface of the cell.

2   The cell membrane invaginates and closes around the particle.

3   A pinocytic vesicle forms, breaks away from the cell surface, and moves into the cytoplasm.

Once the pinocytic vesicle is free in the cytoplasm, it is approached by lysosomes. The lysosomes attach themselves to the vesicle and deposit their

enzymes within it. Digestion takes place, and substances such as amino acids and glucose are released into the cytoplasm. The vesicle's "residual body" is then dissolved or excreted.

**Protein synthesis**  Protein synthesis, in large part, controls the structure, growth, and function of cells. It, in turn, is determined and controlled by DNA. As mentioned previously, DNA is found in the nuclei of human cells; the exact amount per nucleus is not known.

Each DNA molecule exists in the form of a long, double-stranded helix composed of phosphoric acid, deoxyribose (a sugar), and four nitrogenous bases (*adenine* and *guanine,* which are purines, and *thymine* and *cytosine,* which are pyrimidines). Phosphoric acid and deoxyribose form the two strands, and the bases connect them (Fig. 4-3).[5]The arrangement of the bases is the mechanism determining the so-called *genetic code.* It is this code which controls the formation of substances within the cell. When the two strands of the DNA molecule are separated, the interior bases are exposed. These exposed bases have been found to be arranged in groups of three (triplets). Each grouping of three bases (e.g., guanine, guanine, and cytosine, or GGC) is called a *code word.* These code words cause amino acids to be arranged in a particular sequence in a protein molecule during its synthesis. They also control the quantity of a certain protein that is formed.

Protein synthesis in the cytoplasm is controlled by *ribonucleic acid* (RNA), which is formed under the direction of DNA in the nucleus. RNA is synthesized from one of the strands of DNA. Its structure differs in that the sugar used in its formation is *ribose* instead of deoxyribose, the base *uracil* replaces the base thymine, and the final molecule exists as only one strand.

There are three types of RNA: messenger RNA (mRNA), transfer RNA (tRNA), and ribosomal RNA. Each has a specific role in the synthesis of protein. *Messenger RNA* obtains the genetic code from DNA in the nucleus and carries it to the cytoplasm. This process of transference of the code from DNA to mRNA is called *transcription.* In the cytoplasm, the strands of mRNA find their way to the ribosomes where protein molecules are formed.

Protein molecules are formed from chains of amino acids. *Transfer RNA* transfers these amino acids to the protein molecules. Each type of tRNA seems to be specific for a particular type of amino acid and acts as a carrier of that amino acid to the ribosomes where protein molecules are synthesized. The amino acids carried into the ribosome by tRNA are lined up in a chain according to the genetic code word carried by mRNA. As amino acids are deposited in their appropriate place along the chain, the protein molecule is formed.

The third kind of RNA that participates in this process is *ribosomal RNA.* Ribosomal RNA composes about half of the ribosome and exists as particles of two sizes. The smaller of these joins with tRNA and its amino acid. The larger particle contributes enzymes that assist in the formation of linkages between the amino acids on the protein chain.

The entire process of protein synthesis in the ribosomes is referred to as *translation.* Summarized, the sequence is as follows:

1   mRNA brings the genetic code from DNA in the nucleus to the cytoplasm.

2   The smaller ribosomal RNA particle joins with tRNA and its amino acid in the ribosome.

3   mRNA comes in contact with a ribosome and proceeds to travel through it.

4   Amino acids are released by tRNA and lined up according to the sequence determined on mRNA (the tRNA returns to the cytoplasm for another amino acid).

5   Predetermined starting and stopping points are located on the mRNA. When the "stop" point on the chain is reached, the protein molecule is released to the cytoplasm.

**The cell cycle**   Cellular reproduction, or *mitosis,* is necessary, as cells are constantly lost through damage and death. The process begins in the nucleus of the cell, and the entire period from reproduction to reproduction is referred to as the *cell cycle.* Some cells, such as those in the bone marrow, complete a cycle in 10 hours, while others, such as nerve cells, have a cycle that persists for a lifetime without further reproduction.

The cell cycle has two periods, the period of interphase and the period of mitosis[6] (Fig. 4-4). *Interphase* is the period of cellular growth that occurs between divisions. *Mitosis* is the relatively short period in the cycle during which cellular division or reproduction takes place.

Interphase is a vital period to the cells, for it is during this time that DNA replication takes place. The interphase period has been divided into three phases, $G_1$, S, and $G_2$ (Fig. 4-4).

The $G_1$ *phase* appears to be the period of greatest variability in length. It is the time of initial

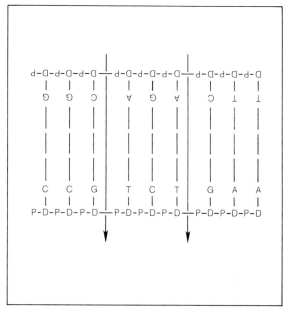

**FIGURE 4-3**
DNA structure. Phosphoric acid and deoxyribose form the two strands connected by the four bases arranged in groups of three (code word).

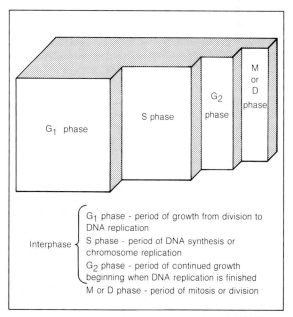

**FIGURE 4-4**
The cell cycle with phases as defined by Howard and Pelc.

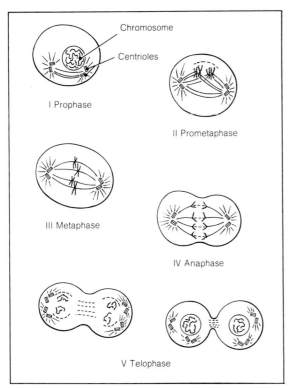

I Prophase

Chromosome

Centrioles

II Prometaphase

III Metaphase

IV Anaphase

V Telophase

**FIGURE 4-5**
Stages of mitosis (*Adapted from D. Mazia, Scientific American,* **205**:*102, 1961 and D. Mazia, Scientific American,* **230**:*56–57, 1974.*)

cellular growth following division and tends to be the longest of the phases in the cycle. Because of this, the rate at which cells multiply seems to be determined by the length of the $G_1$ phase.[7]

The *S phase* begins with the replication of DNA. In this phase DNA duplicates, resulting in two exact sets, which will eventually occupy the nuclei of the two daughter cells formed during mitosis. In human beings, DNA is normally contained within 46 chromosomes (23 pairs). As the DNA replicates, so do the chromosomes, forming 46 *pairs* of chromosomes.

The completion of DNA synthesis marks the beginning of the $G_2$ *phase.* This is a period of continued growth during which the cell doubles in size or reaches its "critical mass."[8] If protein synthesis, and therefore growth of the cell, is somehow interfered with so that this critical mass is not reached, mitosis will not take place.

Mitosis, the *M or D phase,* is the period of cell division. It begins when the cell has doubled in size or has reached its critical mass. The stages of mitosis are illustrated in Fig. 4-5. Before they begin, at the end of interphase, the *mitotic apparatus* forms[9] as two pairs of centrioles in the cytoplasm move apart and line up near opposite poles of the nucleus. They are connected by a set of protein microtubules known as the *spindle.* The centrioles plus the spindle constitute the mitotic apparatus.

*Prophase* is the first stage in mitosis and is marked by the shortening or "condensing" of the chromosomes into well-defined threads. This is followed by *prometaphase,* during which the nuclear membrane disappears and the chromosomes become attached to the microtubules at a point on the chromosome called the *centromere.* As the centrioles are pushed farther apart by the spindle, the chromosomes line up at the center of the cell during *metaphase. Anaphase* is the stage in which each pair of chromosomes is broken apart. This results in 46 daughter chromosomes being pulled toward each pole of the spindle. The final stage of mitosis is *telophase.* It is during this time that the chromosomes become completely separated: nuclear membranes form around each new set of chromosomes, and the two cells divide at a point halfway between the two nuclei. Each of these stages is visually represented in Fig. 4-5.

The exact mechanism for the regulation of cellular growth is not known. It is believed, however, that control substances may be produced by cells and exert a feedback effect to stop or slow growth when necessary. Cellular reproduction and growth of many cells occurs in response to demand, for example, regeneration of liver cells. Some cells, such as epithelial and hematopoietic cells, grow and divide constantly. Others, such as muscle cells, may take years to reproduce, and some, such as neurons, never do.

*Meiosis* is the specialized division that takes place in human germ cells (sperm and ovum). In this process, the 46 chromosomes (diploid number) divide to give each daughter cell 23 chromosomes (haploid number). This is known as *reduction division* and is followed by the regular steps in mitotic division. The mature haploid germ cell of the male (sperm) then joins with the mature germ cell of the female (ovum) at fertilization, forming a zygote with its full complement (46) of chromosomes (DNA or genes).

## Adaptive Cellular Growth and Proliferation

Cells respond to changes within their environments by various processes of normal adaptation. These processes include hypertrophy, atrophy, hyperplasia, metaplasia, and dysplasia. Each of these may actually interfere with normal body functioning and could therefore be termed "maladaptive" at times. However, they serve primarily protective and reparative functions and hence are considered adaptive for the purposes of this discussion.

Hypertrophy and atrophy are changes related to alterations in cellular growth rather than proliferation. *Hypertrophy* is enlargement of the structural portion of cells in response to an increased workload, for example, in striated muscle cells. This process can also occur in muscular organs such as the heart. *Atrophy* is characterized by a loss of cellular substance with subsequent shrinking of the cell. It occurs as a result of disuse, the aging process, poor nutrition, a diminished blood supply, or a loss of endocrine or nervous stimulation. The heart, brain, skeletal muscles, and external genitalia are frequently affected.

*Hyperplasia* is an increase in the number (proliferation) of cells in a particular organ or tissue. It occurs only in those cells which undergo mitotic division, e.g., hematopoietic cells. Hyperplasia occurs in response to stress or an increased body need, for example, in the presence of blood loss. It may also result from endocrine stimulation, as in breast enlargement at puberty and during pregnancy. Goiter is an example of "pathologic" hyperplasia in response to iodine deficiency.

Epithelial and mesenchymal cells are capable of a reversible change known as *metaplasia*. This change involves replacement of one adult cell type by another cell type. For example, squamous metaplasia takes place in the respiratory tract as a result of chronic irritation or inflammation. In this situation, stratified squamous epithelium replaces the more fragile ciliated columnar epithelium normally present. While this is not a completely desirable change because of the loss of mucus production, it is protective in the presence of adverse and stressful conditions. Mesenchymal cells can also undergo metaplasia; they do so, for example, at the site of a soft-tissue injury. Bone or cartilage may be produced where it is not ordinarily found as fibroblasts are replaced by osteoblasts or chrondroblasts.

*Dysplasia* is a third cellular response that may occur. This is also frequently the result of chronic irritation, as in the cervix following cervicitis. Adult cells, in this situation, vary from their normal development in terms of size, shape, and organization. The process may reverse itself or may progress to a cancerous state.

## THE BREAST

Breast tissue remains relatively dormant in the male but at puberty undergoes dramatic cellular proliferation in the female. After puberty, breast growth and function increase in response to the menstrual cycle, pregnancy, and lactation. This growth and development of breast tissue occur in response to estrogen, progesterone, and growth-hormone stimulation.

The young female adult's breasts are located on the anterior chest wall, covering an area extending from the second to the sixth rib bilaterally. Each breast is bounded medially by the lateral border of the sternum and laterally by the anterior axillary line (Fig. 4-6). It is contained between the deep and superficial layers of the superficial fascia of the chest wall. Near the center of each breast is located an area of deeper pigmentation (varying in color according to the person's skin coloring) known as the *areola*. The areola contains smooth muscle that upon contraction causes the nipple to become erect and firm. The muscle fibers are stimulated by touch, as in the sucking of an infant.

Fibrous tissue and subcutaneous fat form the stroma and give the breast its shape and mass. The mammary parenchyma is composed of the ductile system, lobules, and alveoli.

Glandular tissue in the parenchyma is arranged in a series of *lobes,* which are further divided into *lobules* and are located in a circular fashion around the nipple. Each lobe has its own series of excretory ducts draining the lobules and opening on the surface of the nipple. Within the lobules these ducts terminate in structures called *alveoli.* The alveoli contain the secretory cells of the breast and function during lactation. The ductile system grows and enlarges in response to the stimulation of estrogen. Lobules and alveoli need the additional stimulation of progesterone.

Because of lymphatic drainage of the breast into the axillary and internal mammary lymph nodes, these structures are vital in assessing cellular changes. Evaluation of these nodes is described later in this chapter.

## THE FEMALE REPRODUCTIVE TRACT

The female reproductive or genital tract is composed of both external and internal organs. The growth and function of these organs are regulated by hormones. Because of its ongoing role in cellular growth and proliferation, the female genital tract

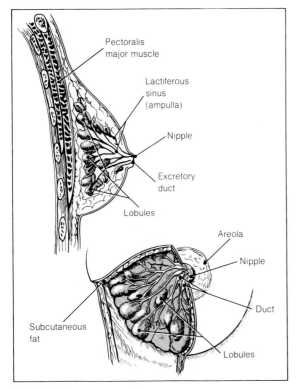

**FIGURE 4-6**
The breasts, or mammary glands.

is discussed in terms of external and internal genital organs and endocrine control.

### External Female Genital Organs

The external female genital organs are collectively known as the *vulva,* or *pudendum.* Specifically, they include the mons pubis, the labia majora and labia minora, the clitoris, the vaginal vestibule, and the vestibular glands (Fig. 4-7a).

The *mons pubis* is composed of fatty tissue and is located in front of the pubic symphysis. This rounded area becomes covered with hair at puberty. The *labia majora* are two folds of skin covered by hair on their external surface and containing sebaceous follicles on their smooth inner surface. Between the labia majora are the labia minora and the urethral and vaginal orifices. The *labia minora* extend from the clitoris to the frenulum. Their surfaces contain many sebaceous follicles. The *clitoris* is composed of erectile tissue and is located at the anterior end of the labia minora. It is homologous with the male penis and becomes erect and more prominent upon stimulation. The *vaginal vestibule* is the name given to the area behind the clitoris and between the labia minora. It contains the vaginal

and urethral orifices and the openings of the ducts of the vestibular glands. The *greater vestibular* or *Bartholin's glands* are located on either side of the vaginal orifice. These glands secrete a lubricating substance during sexual excitation.

A final area that deserves mention is the *perineum.* This is the space between the vagina and the rectum. It is in this area that episiotomies are made to facilitate childbirth.

### Internal Female Genital Organs

The internal female genital organs are located within the pelvis and are illustrated in Fig. 4-7b. They are the ovaries, the fallopian tubes, the uterus, and the vagina.

There are two *ovaries,* one located on either side of the uterus. They are grayish pink in color, and their surface is composed of germinal epithelium. The stroma or framework is formed from connective tissue and contains the *ovarian follicles.* Each follicle contains a single ovum; as the ovum grows, follicular cells proliferate by mitosis until many layers are formed. The mature follicle contains a large amount of fluid and bulges outward on the surface of the ovary. In the presence of hormonal stimulation the follicle ruptures and the ovum is released to the fallopian tubes. The follicular cells that remain appear yellow, and the empty follicle is called the *corpus luteum.*

The *uterine* or *fallopian* tubes are bilateral; they are attached to the superior lateral angle of the uterus on one end and terminate in funnel-shaped, fibriated portions over each ovary (Fig. 4-7b) on the other end. The tubes function in transporting the ova from the ovaries to the uterus; this is accomplished by cilia that line the tubes. Fertilization of the ovum by the sperm is also thought to take place in the tubes; afterward the fertilized ovum continues its passage into the uterus.

The *uterus* is a pear-shaped, hollow organ located between the bladder and rectum, within the pelvis. It is composed of a body, or fundus, that narrows at a point midway between its two ends called the *isthmus.* The portion of the uterus between the isthmus and the vagina is called the *cervix.* The uterine orifice opens through the cervix into the vagina. It is referred to as the *internal os* on the uterine side and the *external os* on the vaginal side. Like the fallopian tubes, the uterine wall has three layers: an external or serous layer (*perimetrium*), a middle or muscular layer (*myometrium*), and an internal or mucous layer (*endometrium*). The muscle layer forms the major bulk of the uterus, becoming greatly enlarged during preg-

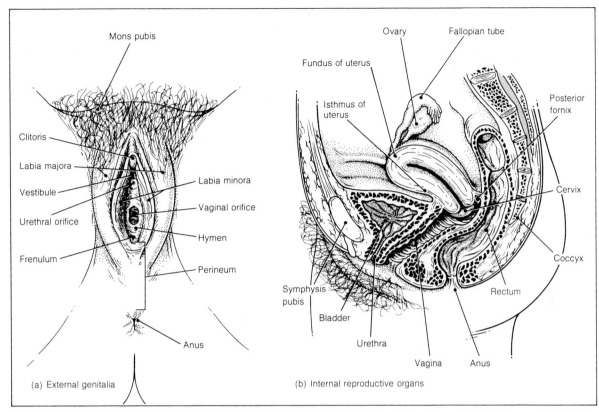

Mons pubis

Clitoris

Labia majora

Vestibule

Urethral orifice

Frenulum

Labia minora

Vaginal orifice

Hymen

Perineum

Anus

(a) External genitalia

Ovary

Fallopian tube

Fundus of uterus

Isthmus of uterus

Posterior fornix

Cervix

Coccyx

Rectum

Symphysis pubis

Bladder

Urethra

Vagina

Anus

(b) Internal reproductive organs

**FIGURE 4-7**
The female reproductive tract.

nancy. The endometrium is of special significance because of the cyclical changes it undergoes after puberty. These periodic endometrial changes, referred to as the *menstrual cycle,* are discussed in more detail under Endocrine Control.

The *vagina* extends from the uterine cervix to the exterior of the body at the vaginal orifice. It is a muscular structure that is lined with mucous membrane. The mucous membrane is arranged into many ridges, or rugae, that allow for expansion. The vagina extends up to and around the cervix, forming a *posterior fornix* or recess on the dorsal portion of the cervix and *anterior* and *lateral fornices* on the ventral and lateral portions (Fig. 4-7*b*).

### Endocrine Control

Development and function of the female reproductive organs are controlled by the interaction of the central nervous system with hormones secreted by the ovary and the anterior pituitary gland. The major hormones of the ovary are *estrogen* and *progesterone;* the influencing hormones of the anterior

pituitary are *follicle-stimulating hormone* (*FSH*) and *luteinizing hormone* (*LH*), otherwise known as the *gonadotrophic hormones*. The release of these hormones at regular intervals determines the cyclic variation in reproductive activity and organ function. This *female sexual cycle* or *menstrual cycle* is characterized by the maturation of an ovarian follicle, the release of an ovum, and the preparation of the uterus for implantation of the fertilized ovum. Should conception and implantation not take place, the cycle is repeated on the average of once every 28 days (Fig. 4-8).

**The menstrual cycle**   The release of the gonadotrophic hormones (FSH and LH) begins at about the age of 8 years in the female. Between the ages of 11 and 15, the menstrual cycle begins. This cyclic onset is termed *puberty.*

*FSH* initiates the cycle by causing one of the ovarian follicles to mature. As it grows, the follicle produces estrogen. The estrogen, in turn, causes proliferation of the glands and blood vessels of the endometrium. This follicular maturation is referred to as the *proliferative phase* of the female sexual cycle.

The ovarian follicle continues to mature and finally ruptures, releasing an ovum (*ovulation*). This event occurs about halfway through the cycle (Fig. 4-8). Luteinizing hormone causes the ruptured follicle to develop into the corpus luteum. The cells of the corpus luteum secrete progesterone (as well as estrogen), which causes the enlarged endometrium to grow even more and to become twice as thick. The endometrial glands become markedly secretory, containing large quantities of stored nutrients, in preparation for the implantation of a fertilized ovum. This second stage of the cycle is referred to as the *secretory* (progestational or progravid) phase.

Should conception not take place, the corpus luteum begins to degenerate and the levels of estrogen and progesterone decrease rapidly. The endometrium shows deterioration and necrosis of tissues and blood vessels; the outer layers separate; and uterine contractions that expel the tissue and blood (*menses*) are initiated. This final stage of the cycle is referred to as the *menstrual phase*. Menstruation normally continues from 3 to 7 days, followed by the beginning of a new cycle (Fig. 4-8).

**Other effects of estrogen**   Estrogen is secreted in small amounts by the adrenal glands as well as by the ovary. In addition to its effects upon the reproductive organs, estrogen can cause renal retention of $Na^+$ and $Cl^-$, promote protein anabolism, and affect skeletal growth. The female secondary sex characteristics, including fat distribution, skeletal size, and hair distribution, are also the result of estrogen secretion.

## THE MALE REPRODUCTIVE TRACT

The male genital organs are the testes, the vas deferens, the seminal vesicles, the ejaculatory duct and the penis. Accessory structures include the prostate and the bulbourethral glands. As in the female, growth and functioning of these organs are controlled by hormonal stimulation. Their major functions are spermatogenesis, production of hormones, and performance of the male sexual act.

**FIGURE 4-8**
The female sexual cycle.

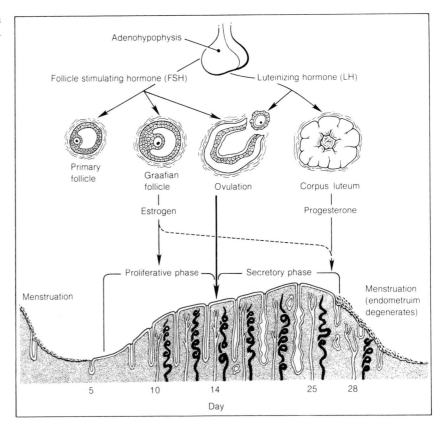

## Genital Structure

The *testes* are oval organs that are suspended in the *scrotum* by the spermatic cords. It is in the testes that *sperm* are formed. The scrotum is divided into two lateral portions by a ridge or "raphe," each containing one testis. The left side of the scrotum hangs lower than the right because of the greater length of the spermatic cord on that side. Ambient temperature further alters the appearance of the scrotum; increased warmth causes it to become elongated and flaccid, permitting the testes to be suspended farther away from the body; colder temperatures cause it to contract, appearing corrugated and drawing closer to the testes and the body. The purpose of this environmental adaptation is to maintain an optimal temperature for spermatogenesis (about 5°F lower than body temperature).

Each testis is composed of seminiferous tubules and interstitial tissue (*cells of Leydig*). The seminiferous tubules are arranged in a pattern of convolutions and loops; they connect with excretory ducts that eventually carry the seminal fluid from the testis to the epididymis (a coiled duct located

on the surface of each testis), as illustrated in Fig. 4-9. Between the seminiferous tubules are the interstitial cells of Leydig, blood vessels, nerves, and lymphatics. Leydig cells function in the synthesis of androgens, the most important of which is testosterone.

The *vas deferens*, or *seminal duct*, is the excretory duct of the testes. It begins at the "tail" of the epididymis and ends by joining with the duct of the seminal vesicles to form the *ejaculatory duct.*

Between the fundus of the bladder and the rectum are located the *seminal vesicles*, which secrete a mucoid fluid that is high in fructose and other nutrients. The seminal vesicles empty shortly after the vas deferens empties its sperm during ejaculation. The bulk of the ejaculated semen is thus increased, and the sperm are provided with nutrients until fertilization takes place.

The *prostate gland* is located immediately below the internal urethral orifice at the beginning of the urethra. It is ventral to the rectum and its base is continuous with the surface of the bladder (Fig. 4-9). The two ejaculatory ducts enter the posterior portion of the prostate and open into the

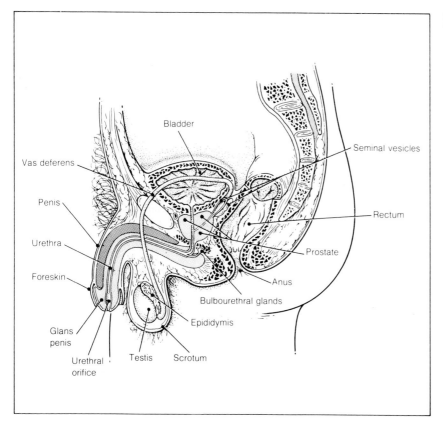

**FIGURE 4-9**
The male reproductive tract.

prostatic urethra. A thin, milky, alkaline fluid is secreted by the prostate and added to the semen. The alkaline nature of this fluid is believed to be helpful in neutralizing the acidity of other fluids, thus providing for maximum motility and fertility of the sperm.

The *penis* is a cylindrical organ that is attached to the front and sides of the pubic arch. It is the male organ for ejaculation of semen as well as voiding of urine. Three cylindrical masses of cavernous tissue held together by fibrous bands (trabeculae) and covered by skin form its basic structure. The two lateral masses are called the *corpora cavernosa;* the ventral cylinder, which contains the urethra, is called the *corpus spongiosum.* They are divided into many compartments or blood sinuses. When there is cerebral or spinal stimulation, arterial blood to the sinuses increases and the penis becomes erect because of mechanical engorgement. Penile skin is thin, dark, and loosely connected to the deeper parts of the organ to allow for expansion. The distal portion of the penis, at which the urethral meatus is located, is called the *glans.* In the uncircumcised male, the glans is covered by a folding of skin called the *prepuce,* or *foreskin.*

The *bulbourethral* or *Cowper's glands* are two pea-sized structures that empty into the urethra. Parasympathetic impulses cause them to secrete mucus during sexual stimulation. During intercourse, the mucus travels the length of the urethra to help provide lubrication during coitus.

### Spermatogenesis

Spermatogenesis (development of sperm) occurs in the seminiferous tubules of the testes. The process is initiated by FSH and LH, which are secreted by the adenohypophysis beginning when the male is about 13 years old. Under the stimulation of these hormones as well as testosterone, germinal epithelial cells called *spermatogonia* proliferate and develop into *spermatozoa.* The sequence is as follows:[10]

Spermatogonia $\xrightarrow{\text{growth}}$ primary spermatocytes $\xrightarrow{\text{meiosis}}$ secondary spermatocytes $\xrightarrow{\text{mitosis}}$ spermatids $\xrightarrow[\text{metamorphosis}]{\text{undergo}}$ spermatozoa (containing 23 chromosomes)

The spermatozoa pass from the seminiferous tubules to the epididymis, where they mature and develop motility. Fluid secreted by the epididymis is high in nutrients thought necessary for this maturation. Some sperm is stored in the epididymis, but most is stored in the vas deferens until ejaculation.

### Other Hormonal Effects

FSH and LH also stimulate the cells of Leydig to secrete androgens, principally testosterone; androgens are produced by the adrenal gland as well. In addition to spermatogenesis, testosterone is responsible for secondary male sex characteristics, increased bone size and strength, increased basal metabolism and protein synthesis, and increased sodium reabsorption from the kidneys.

## PHYSICAL ASSESSMENT OF CELLULAR GROWTH AND PROLIFERATION

Normally, various cells throughout the body undergo some degree of cellular growth and proliferation. Therefore, physical assessment should include evaluation of all body parts and organ systems, to distinguish abnormal from normal cellular growth.

Because of its common association with the spread of cancerous cells, the lymphatic system should be given special attention. Both male and female reproductive systems have a unique relationship to cellular growth and proliferation and should also be carefully evaluated.

All physical assessment should be preceded by a history relevant to the area of the body to be examined. The *health history* is thoroughly discussed in Chap. 2. Those sections of the history which reveal abnormal cellular growth include cancer's seven warning signals, individual and family history of abnormal growths whether benign or malignant, environmental factors, and the regular use of medications and food products that are thought to have carcinogenic properties. This information may reveal abnormal cellular growth or arouse suspicion of abnormal cellular growth. Terms that may appear throughout this section are defined in Table 4-1.

### Inspection

Normal versus abnormal cellular growth may reveal itself during a systematic inspection by the nurse. To be truly effective, this inspection must be knowledgeable looking, not merely observation.

All body parts should be inspected for size, symmetry, contour, masses, and sores. Findings should be compared with the part's normal structural appearance. Bilateral parts (breasts, extremities, etc.) need to be evaluated for similarities and differences.

**Head and neck** The head and neck should be carefully inspected for the appearance of masses which distort normal physical symmetry. Any abnormal structure needs to be described in relation to its exact location, size, and appearance.

The mouth should be carefully inspected, particularly in those patients who have a history of oral cancer, smoking, or high alcohol consumption.[11] The mucous membrane of the mouth is normally moist, pink, and smooth. Any lesion of the oral cavity which is asymptomatic, unilateral, and friable should be suspected as malignant, especially in high-risk persons.[12]

The neck must be carefully inspected for the appearance of enlarged lymph nodes (Fig. 4-10), deviations of the trachea, and the presence of an abnormally large or small thyroid gland. *Lymph nodes* are normally not visible. The node itself is a rounded body made up of lymphatic tissue which filters circulating lymph, retaining foreign particles. In the presence of disease, the nodes may become enlarged and visible. Their size diminishes gradually as the disease lessens. Observation of the neck for *deviations of the trachea* should include a description of the abnormality. For inspection of the *thyroid gland,* the patient should be instructed to hold a small amount of water in the mouth and to swallow when asked. The symmetry of the gland will be apparent as the patient swallows. Inspection of the thyroid gland depends greatly on the patient's physical makeup: excessive thinness or a short, stocky neck hinder adequate inspection.[13]

**Breasts** Inspection of the breasts of both men and women should be done first with the patient sitting, with hands by the sides of the body and pressed against the hips; then with the patient's hands resting on the top of the head; and lastly with the patient supine.

The breasts should be inspected particularly for symmetry and appearance. *Asymmetry* in one breast may be the result of infection or of the development of a growth requiring further investigation. The nipples should both point in the same direction.[14] Any abnormality as to position, size, and appearance of the breasts and nipples should be described.

Breasts and nipples must also be inspected for *dimpling* or *observable skin lesions.* The nipples should also be observed for dryness, cracking, and any discharge. Because of their close proximity to

**TABLE 4-1**
TERMS FREQUENTLY ASSOCIATED WITH PHYSICAL ASSESSMENT OF CELLULAR GROWTH AND PROLIFERATION

*Bleb:* A blister.
*Macule:* A circumscribed area of color change.
*Mass:* A grouping of cells within or attached to an organ system which unite or adhere to each other. The grouping may be soft or quite hard, fixed or movable.
*Nodule:* An aggregation of cells.
*Papule:* A small palpable mass, generally above the skin surface.
*Primary lesion:* The original pathologically altered tissue occurring within a localized area. Primary lesions include macules, papules, blebs, wheals, and tumors.
*Secondary lesion:* Pathologically altered tissue resulting from a primary lesion. Secondary lesions include crusts, fissures, scales, scars, and ulcers.
*Tumor:* A growth of tissue that becomes an abnormal mass performing no physiologic function. Depending on its location, it may interfere with normal physiologic functioning.

the breasts, axillary lymph nodes need to be inspected for visible masses.

**Male genitalia** The skin of the penis and scrotum should be inspected for the presence of any lesions, masses, or areas of inflammation. If the foreskin is present, it must be retracted in order to look for lesions on the glans.

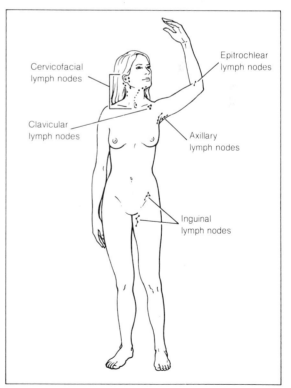

**FIGURE 4-10**
Location of clinically palpable lymph nodes.

**Female genitalia** To adequately inspect the female genitalia, the patient must be placed in the lithotomy position with the thighs flexed and abducted and the feet resting in stirrups attached to the examining table.[15] The external genitalia should be inspected first for the presence of masses or lesions. Wearing gloves, the examiner next separates the labia and inserts two fingers of one hand into the introitus. Then, with the other hand, a closed, warm-water-lubricated speculum is introduced sideways and downward, at a 45° angle, into the vagina (Fig. 4-11). The examiner's fingers are removed from the vagina, the blades are rotated from a vertical to a horizontal position, and the speculum is opened to make the cervix visible. Once the speculum is secured in the open position, the cervix should be inspected for color, lesions, masses, and discharge. Specimens may be taken of the cervix, its opening, and the vaginal walls. The mechanical tension on the speculum is then released and the instrument is removed slowly. This slow removal permits inspection of the vaginal mucosa for lesions, discoloration, inflammation, and discharge.[16]

**Rectal-anal region** The anal canal is normally closed; it can be distinguished from surrounding skin by its moist, hairless appearance.[17] The anal region should be inspected for skin lesions, masses, and scars. Gluteal-cleft inspection will determine the presence of any pilonidal inflammation or open sinus drainage. Hemorrhoids and anal fistulae, if present, will be apparent at the anal opening as the patient "bears down."[18]

## Palpation

Any observable mass or lesion should also be palpated. The mass or lesion may then be described in terms of its location, consistency, size, and movability. Tenderness upon palpation is also important to note, according to degree and the position of the body part when the discomfort is felt.

**Head and neck** A careful *oral* examination should include palpation of the parotid areas for masses, as well as the floor of the mouth, especially under the tongue. The neck should be palpated for masses associated with the thyroid gland and the lymphatic system.

*Cervicofacial nodes* (Fig. 4-10) are palpated from either the anterior or posterior approach. The examiner using the *anterior* approach is positioned in front of the patient. The nonexamining hand is used to steady the head, while the examining hand is used to palpate for the presence of nodes on both sides of the head and neck. With the *posterior* approach, the examiner is positioned behind the patient; the head is flexed and the examiner uses both hands to palpate for nodes simultaneously.

**Lymph nodes** Lymph nodes are normally not palpable; Fig. 4-10 illustrates the primary sites for lymph node palpation should abnormality exist. The middle three fingers are employed to palpate the nodes. Slow, gentle movements are used in a rotary motion around the node and in an up-and-down, back-and-forth motion across the node. Lymph nodes, if palpable, should be described in terms of bilateral symmetry, location, size (in centi-

**FIGURE 4-11**
Inspection of the cervix and vagina. (A) Speculum blades are held obliquely to enter the vagina.
(B) Blades are placed in a horizontal position upon passing the introitus. (C) Blades are separated to allow viewing of the cervix. (*Adapted from Richard D. Judge and George G. Zuidema (eds.), Methods of Clinical Examination: A Physiologic Approach, 3d ed., Little, Brown, Boston, 1974, p. 321.*)

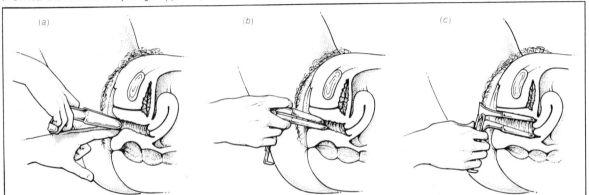

meters or descriptive terms such as pea, bean, or almond), movability (fixed, matted, movable), and texture (hard, soft, firm). Lymph nodes are described as "shotty" if they are firm, freely movable, nontender, and from 0.5 to 1 cm in diameter.[19]

**Breast** When palpating the breast for abnormal cellular growth and proliferation, normal tissue must be distinguished from abnormal tissue. The breast should be mentally divided into four quadrants or sections, using horizontal and vertical lines, with the nipple as the central point.[20] To examine in the supine position, a small pillow is placed under the patient's shoulder on the side of the breast to be examined. Using the pads of the middle fingers, the breast tissue should be gently depressed against the chest wall, in each quadrant. It is usual to begin with the left breast, to start palpation in the upper lateral quadrant, and to continue in a clockwise direction. Palpation should be light initially and become deeper as necessary, for example, in the presence of massive breast tissue. The patient is examined with arms by the sides and overhead and while in supine and sitting positions. Special attention should be given to palpation of the areolar area in the male breast.

The axilla is examined next, to detect the presence of any lymphatic enlargement or masses. With the patient in either a supine or sitting position, arm supported, the examiner reaches up toward the axillary apex with slightly cupped hand. The hand is then used to palpate down the chest wall several times, to detect the presence of any enlarged pectoral, subscapular, or lateral nodes.[21] It has been suggested that the patient move each arm in a full range of motion while each axilla is examined. However, the arm should not be abducted to the point of putting tension on the axillary skin and muscles, as this may interfere with deep palpation.

When making this examination, it is important to remember that breast tissue consistency varies with age, obesity, stage of the menstrual cycle, and pregnancy.[22] Normal breast tissue is distinctly but vaguely nodular.[23] Only experience permits differentiation of normal from abnormal breast masses. For this reason, a patient should be referred to a physician for evaluation at the slightest indication of a breast lesion.

**Female genitalia** Palpation of the female genitalia is generally limited to any observable mass of the external genitalia and bimanual exam of the cervix, uterus, and adnexa. A gloved hand should be used to palpate the external genitalia, particu-

larly the labia and the area of the Bartholin's glands, with the index finger and thumb.

The *bimanual examination* starts with the insertion of the lubricated index and middle fingers of the gloved hand into the vagina (Fig. 4-12). The cervix is palpated, noting any mass or tenderness. The opposite hand is placed on the abdomen at the midline, approximately three-fourths of the way toward the umbilicus. As a point of reference, the cervix usually points in a direction opposite to the fundus of the uterus.[24] The normal uterus may be at the midline in the lower abdominal quadrants or minimally anteflexed or retroflexed. While the intravaginal hand gently restrains the uterus from moving downward, the abdominal hand palpates it for size, contour, and mobility. Any bulging, tenderness, or masses of the cul-de-sac region should be noted with the intravaginal fingers. The abdominal hand is then placed on the right lower quadrant and the pelvic hand in the right lateral fornix; the abdominal hand is moved downward toward the examiner. Using the pelvic, or intravaginal, hand, the right ovary is palpated for any mass (Fig. 4-12). This procedure is repeated on the left side, remembering to use only enough pressure to identify the ovary and any mass associated with it.

A rectovaginal examination should then follow for the female patient (Fig. 4-13). The examiner's gloves should be changed and the middle and index fingers (of the same hand) lubricated. The index finger is inserted into the vagina and the middle finger into the rectum (Fig. 4-13). The maneuvers of the bimanual examination are then repeated. While the middle finger is within the rectum, special note should be taken of the sphincter tone of the anus and any node or palpable mass along the rectal wall. If sphincter tone is poor or absent, the constricting sensation normally felt around the examiner's finger will be diminished or absent.

**R**ectal-Anal Region For a separate rectal examination, the patient is placed in the lateral position and the gloved, lubricated index finger of the examiner is inserted into the rectum. Sphincter tone is noted and the rectal walls palpated for any nodes or masses. After withdrawal of the finger, any stool should be examined for the presence of occult blood.

**Male genitalia** During examination of the male genitalia, any observable lesion should be palpated with a gloved hand. The tenderness, induration, size, and consistency of any mass should be noted.

**FIGURE 4-12**
Bimanual pelvic examination. (a) Palpation of the uterus. (b) Palpation of the right ovary. (*Adapted from Richard D. Judge and George D. Zuidema (eds.), Methods of Clinical Examination: A Physiologic Approach, 3d ed., Little, Brown, Boston, 1974, p. 323.*)

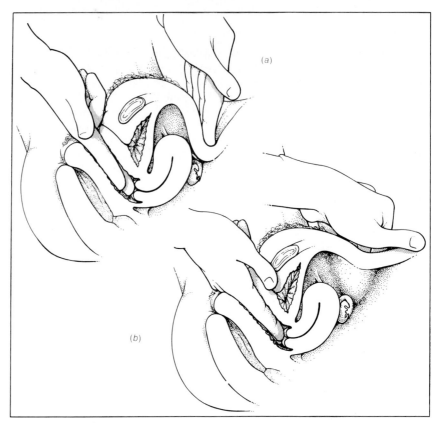

**FIGURE 4-13**
Rectovaginal examination. One finger is inserted into the vagina and one into the rectum. (*Adapted from Richard D. Judge and George Zuidema (eds.), Methods of Clinical Examination: A Physiologic Approach, 3d ed., Little, Brown, Boston, 1974, p. 325.*)

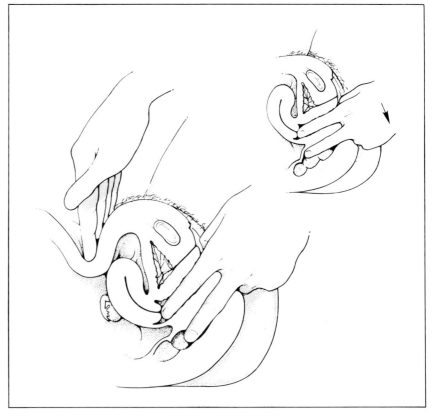

Each testis and epididymis should be palpated between the thumb and the index and middle fingers;[25] their size, shape, and consistency and the presence of any tenderness should be described. It is important to remember during the examination that the testes are tender to anything other than light palpation.

**R**ectal-Anal Region   The male rectum can be palpated with the patient in a lateral position or standing, hips flexed, and leaning over a table (Fig. 4-14). The rectum is palpated for any mass or unusual tenderness with a gloved, lubricated index finger. The rectal examination is carried out in a systematic manner, that is, beginning with the right lateral surface and, then proceeding to the posterior, left lateral, and anterior surfaces. While examining the anterior rectal surface, the lobes of the prostate and the median sulcus separating them should be palpated for size, smoothness or nodularity, and tenderness (Fig. 4-14).[26] The normal prostate is approximately $2 \times 4 \times 3$ cm and is enclosed in a smooth capsule. After withdrawal of the gloved finger, any stool should be examined for occult blood.

## Percussion

Percussion, or systematic tapping, has the potential of revealing the solidity of or the presence of air or fluid in underlying structures. It may yield pertinent findings, in terms of cellular growth and proliferation, when associated with the left border of the heart and superficial masses in the chest or abdomen. Masses close to the surface in the chest and abdomen produce a flat or dull sound—vibration rather than resonance. Abnormal cellular growth cannot be assessed on the basis of percussion alone: percussion vibrations penetrate only 5 to 7 cm and therefore cannot reveal deep-seated lesions. Percussion may, however, be of assistance following a health history, inspection, and palpation of the system involved.

## Auscultation

Auscultation, or listening to an organ system, would not of itself be helpful in the assessment of abnormal cellular growth and proliferation—that is, except for large masses which may obstruct the functioning of the organ system and interfere with normal sounds (for example, bronchial obstruction), which are diminished or absent over the mass.

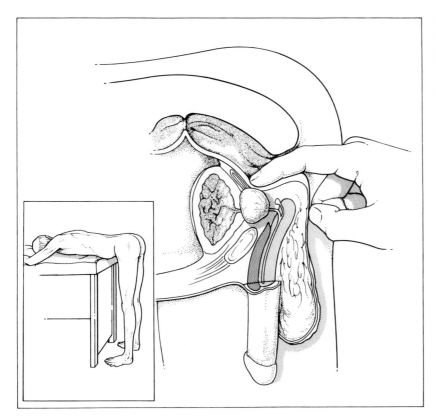

**FIGURE 4-14**
Examination of the lobes of the prostate gland during the male rectal exam. Optimum position for this examination is shown in the insert. (*Adapted from Richard D. Judge and George Zuidema (eds.), Methods of Clinical Examination: A Physiologic Approach, 3d ed., Little Brown, Boston, 1974, p. 325.*)

## REFERENCES

1   Stanley L. Robbins, *Pathologic Basis of Disease,* Saunders, Philadelphia, 1974, p. 2.
2   *Ibid.,* p. 3.
3   Arthur Guyton, *Textbook of Medical Physiology,* 5th ed., Saunders, Philadelphia, 1976, p. 14.
4   Robbins, *op. cit.,* p. 9.
5   Guyton, *op. cit.,* p. 28.
6   Daniel Mazia, "The Cell Cycle," *Sci Am,* **230:**54–64, January 1974.
7   Lord Florey, *General Pathology,* 4th ed., Saunders, Philadelphia, 1970, p. 634.
8   Mazia, *op. cit.,* p. 56.
9   Guyton, *op. cit.,* p. 37.
10   Howard Balin and Stanley Glasser, *Reproductive Biology,* Excerpta Medica, Amsterdam, 1972, p. 147.
11   Laureen V. Ackerman and Juan A. del Regato, *Cancer,* 4th ed., Mosby, St. Louis, 1970, p. 183.
12   Mary H. Browning and Edith P. Lewis, "Nursing and the Cancer Patient," *American Journal of Nursing,* New York, 1973, p. 183.
13   Barbara Bates, *A Guide to Physical Examination,* Lippincott, Philadelphia, 1974, p. 47.
14   *Ibid.,* p. 155.
15   *Ibid.,* p. 190.
16   *Ibid.,* pp. 191–193.
17   *Ibid.,* p. 205.
18   Henry U. Hopkins, *Leopold's Principles and Methods of Physical Diagnosis,* Saunders, Philadelphia, 1965, p. 347.
19   Richard D. Judge and George D. Zuidema (eds.), *Methods of Clinical Examination: A Physiological Approach,* 3d ed., Little, Brown, Boston, 1974, p. 269.
20   Bates, *op. cit.,* p. 146.
21   *Ibid.,* p. 153.
22   Judge and Zuidema, *op. cit.,* p. 264.
23   *Ibid.,* pp. 266–267.
24   *Ibid.,* p. 279.
25   Bates, *op. cit.,* p. 181.
26   *Ibid.,* p. 208.

## BIBLIOGRAPHY

Ackerman, Laureen V., and Juan A. del Regato: *Cancer,* 4th ed., Mosby, St. Louis, 1970.

Balin, Howard, and Stanley Glasser: *Reproductive Biology,* Excerpta Medica, Amsterdam, 1972.

Bates, Barbara: *A Guide to Physical Examination,* Lippincott, Philadelphia, 1974.

The Boston Women's Health Book Collective: *Our Bodies Ourselves,* Simon & Schuster, New York, 1973.

Browning, Mary H., and Edith P. Lewis: "Nursing and the Cancer Patient," *American Journal of Nursing,* New York, 1973.

Gallager, H. Stephen: *Early Breast Cancer,* Wiley, New York, 1975.

Gray, Henry, and Charles Goss: *Anatomy of the Human Body,* Lea & Febiger, Philadelphia, 1973.

Haagensen, C. D.: *Diseases of the Breast,* 2d ed., Saunders, Philadelphia, 1971.

Heidenstam, David (ed.): *Man's Body,* Diagram Visual Information, 1976.

Hopkins, Henry U.: *Leopold's Principles and Methods of Physical Diagnosis,* Saunders, Philadelphia, 1965.

Judge, Richard D., and George D. Zuidema (eds.): *Methods of Clinical Examination: A Physiologic Approach,* 3d ed., Little, Brown, Boston, 1974.

Rubin, Philip (ed.): *Clinical Oncology for Medical Students and Physicians,* 4th ed., American Cancer Society, New York, 1974.

Schwartz, Seymour I.: *Principles of Surgery,* 2d ed., McGraw-Hill, New York, 1974.

Seedor, Marie M.: *The Physical Assessment,* Teachers College, New York, 1974.

Seidman, Herbert: *Cancer of the Breast,* American Cancer Society, New York, 1972.

Selkurt, Ewald E.: *Physiology,* 4th ed., Little, Brown, Boston, 1976.

Shapiro, Sam, Philip Strax, and Louis Venet: *Periodic Breast Cancer Screening in Reducing Mortality From Breast Cancer.* American Cancer Society, New York, reprinted from *JAMA,* **215:**1777–1785, 1971.

Sherman, Jacques, and Sylvia Kleiman Fields: *Guide to Patient Evaluation,* Medical Examination Publishing, Flushing, New York, 1974.

Thomas Clayton: *Taber's Cyclopedic Medical Dictionary,* 12th ed., Davis, Philadelphia, 1973.

# 5
# NEOPLASTIC PROCESSES

Susan P. Molloy Hubbard

Cellular growth and proliferation are influenced by many factors within the cell's environment. *Neoplasms* (new growths) are characterized by uncontrolled cellular growth that fails to conform to the normal pattern of growth for a particular tissue. These neoplasms or tumors may be initiated by circumstances in the organism's external or internal environment. They may be *malignant* (capable of metastasizing, etc.) or *benign* (non-metastasizing). Malignant neoplasms, commonly referred to as *cancers,* are the focus of this chapter.

## PATHOPHYSIOLOGY

Knowledge of the behavior and characteristics of normal living tissue is essential in order to understant the complex nature of neoplastic processes and the rationale on which treatment is based. The basic unit of all plant and animal life is the cell (see Chap. 4). Of critical importance is the fact that all living cells have the inherent capacity to multiply. Regulation of this reproduction is necessary. For example, bacteria and other unicellular organisms multiply until they outstrip the available supply of nutrients or until toxic waste products accumulate in their environment. In more complex, multicellular organisms, each cell type performs different functions to sustain life; unrestricted multiplication of any one of these cells would be detrimental to the welfare of the community of cells. Control is provided by a cellular "brake" which inhibits growth as cells reach a critical mass and begin to crowd one another.[1] This surveillance system is not well understood but is thought to be a feedback mechanism resulting from contact with other cells (contact inhibition).[2] A normal cellular brake is critical. When it is set, the brake prevents overgrowth. When cells are injured or destroyed, the feedback mechanisms release the brake for a specific period during which multiplication and regrowth may occur. Wound healing and regeneration of hepatic cells following injury are examples of a normal release of the cellular brake, since the tissues cease multiplication appropriately when the damage is repaired.[3] Neoplasms represent an abnormal release of the cellular brake.

### The Cell Cycle and Tumor Growth

A brief discussion of the cell cycle is essential for an understanding of fundamental principles of tumor growth. The phases of a normal cell cycle are depicted in Fig. 5-1 using the G (Gap) terminology. At

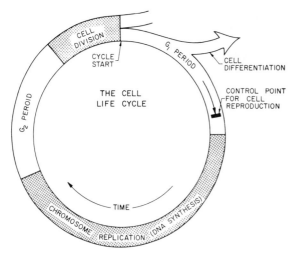

**FIGURE 5-1**
The phases of the cell cycle. (*From R. A. Bender and R. L. Dudrick, "Cytokinetic Aspects of Clinical Drug Resistance," Cancer Chemotherapy Reports 59, p. 805, 1975, U.S. Department of Health, Education, and Welfare.*)

the completion of cell division (mitosis), cells undergo a "resting" period referred to as *Gap 1* ($G_1$ phase), during which DNA synthesis ceases except for repair of damaged DNA, but RNA and protein synthesis continue actively.[4] At a critical point

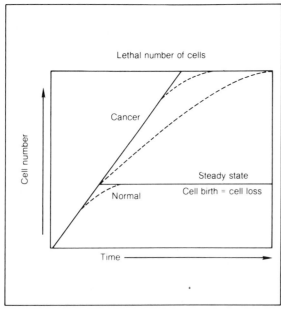

**FIGURE 5-2**
Graphic comparison of normal and cancerous growth. (*From V. T. DeVita, "Cell Kinetics and the Chemotherapy of Cancer," Cancer Chemotherapy Reports, vol. 2, p. 24, 1971, U.S. Department of Health, Education, and Welfare.*)

late in the $G_1$ period, the decision for a cell to divide occurs and is signaled by a burst in RNA synthesis. Following this burst the cell is doubled in preparation for mitosis; RNA and protein synthesis continue at normal rates.[5] Data suggest that S phase for both normal and malignant cells is relatively similar and constant (8 to 30 hours).[6] Following DNA replication, the cell enters *Gap 2*, or $G_2$ *phase,* a premitotic period when DNA synthesis ceases, which is followed by mitosis (the M phase), during which daughter cells are formed and separate (see Chap. 4 for more detailed discussion).

Individual tumor cells do not grow faster than normal cells, but tumor masses often have shorter *doubling times* (time required to double in size) related to other variables. Mendelsohn hypothesized that only a fraction of cells undergoes mitosis at any one time.[7] His experiment demonstrated that a portion of viable cells, with the capacity to divide, remains in the resting phase for prolonged time periods. The *growth fraction* in a tumor (the ratio of dividing cells to resting cells) varies at different times and accounts for the changes in doubling time and tumor volume. In a given cell cycle, a tumor with a large growth fraction will double faster than a tumor of the same size with a small growth fraction, if loss of cells through death and metastases remains constant. A high rate of cell loss can account for a long doubling time even in tumors with large growth fractions. Cells in a prolonged $G_1$ period may be considered in suspended animation, or $G_0$ *phase.* This is an important concept to understand, for these cells, not actively synthesizing DNA, are far less vulnerable to damage from irradiation or drug therapy. Recruiting resting tumor cells from $G_0$ into the cell cycle is a key to the eradication of viable cancer cells.

**Cell kinetic considerations in malignant growth** *Cancer* is a growth which fails to obey the normal biologic controls over cell proliferation. An operational definition of cancer is depicted in Fig. 5-2, which compares the growth characteristics of normal and cancerous cells. The initial slope of the rising solid line represents the tremendous exponential growth that is characteristic of early growth in the embryo or in rapidly growing tumors. The horizontal line represents the steady state of equilibrium that is normal in most mature living tissues; this equilibrium occurs because cell birth equals cell death. In cancer, cell birth exceeds cell death, as represented in Fig. 5-2 by the continued rising line. Cells continue to multiply despite overcrowding, violating the feedback mechanism of contact inhibition. Failure of the cellular brake to control growth would be rapidly lethal to the host if growth were to continue on an exponential basis. However, *slowing* of the growth rate occurs in cancer as the tumor mass increases in volume. This is depicted by the dotted lines on the graph (Fig. 5-2), which show a prolongation in the time required to double the tumor mass (doubling time) as the tumor increases in size. Changes in doubling time are related to (1) the duration of the cell cycle time (the time from one mitosis to another), (2) the fraction of cells undergoing mitosis, and (3) the rate of cell loss from the mass.[8]

All these biologic considerations have clinical significance. Knowledge about tumor cell kinetics has provided critical information about the failure of specific treatments to effectively control cancers and about the development of resistance. An understanding of the kinetics of growth in both normal and cancerous tissue is the foundation for the development of successful treatment, which is often designed to exploit these differences.

The individual cells in a given tumor mass may be described as residing in one of three general compartments shown graphically in Fig. 5-3. Cells in *compartment A* are the most susceptible to injury, because the cells are actively replicating. *Compartment B* consists of cells in the $G_1$, or resting phase. These cells are relatively insensitive to modalities which interfere with cell division or the synthesis of essential proteins required for successful division. Cells can usually move freely between compartments A and B and are always considered mitotically competent. Cells in *compartment C* are like static cells; they have lost their ability to divide and contribute only mass to the tumor.

The entire course of a tumor from inception until it reaches a volume of cells which is lethal in man requires only 40 doublings over variable time periods. A tumor is often undetectable by current diagnostic techniques until it has gone through two-thirds of its growth, usually about 27 doublings. Figure 5-4 correlates the number of doublings with tumor size and approximate cell volume. The earliest point at which a tumor mass can usually be visualized by x-ray is at a mass of 0.5 cm³; the smallest palpable mass is approximately 1 cm³ (approximately 30 doublings) and actually represents more than 1 billion ($1 \times 10^9$) cancer cells. With as few as five additional doublings, the tumor mass could, as an aggregate, be as large as 1 foot in diameter. An additional five doublings can increase tumor volume to approximately $1 \times 10^{12}$

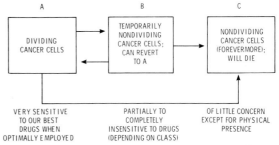

**FIGURE 5-3**

Schematic representation of cell types within an individual tumor mass. (*From V. T. DeVita, "Cell Kinetics and the Chemotherapy of Cancer," Cancer Chemotherapy Reports, vol. 2, p. 26, 1971, U.S. Department of Health, Education, and Welfare.*)

cells (1 trillion), or 1 kg, and is usually sufficient to kill the host.[9]

In effect then, cancers are "advanced" when they are large enough to be diagnosed by current techniques. Up to a billion tumor cells ($1 \times 10^9$) may be scattered throughout the body and be undetectable by careful physical examination. The great majority of patients with clinically detectable cancer have tumors which are in the late stages of biologic growth. In most cases these tumors are shedding cells throughout the body, and many patients have microscopic disease at diagnosis even when the tumor is small and apparently localized. In cancers which are "cured" by surgery or radiation, normal defense mechanisms can theoretically eradi-

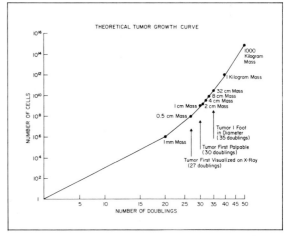

**FIGURE 5-4**

Theoretical tumor growth curve, illustrating the number of tumor doublings in relation to the number of tumor cells and the level of clinical detectability. (*From V. T. DeVita, R. C. Young, G. P. Canellos, "Combination versus Single Agent Chemotherapy: A Review of the Basis for Selection of Drug Treatment of Cancer," Cancer, 35:101, 1975.*)

cate these small foci of tumor cells. Conversely, cancers known to recur even after what is thought to be curative surgery may have multiple foci of clinically undetectable cancer which contain millions of viable cells and regrow as metastatic disease to kill the host. This is an important concept and one that will be considered at length in the discussion of clinical staging and management decisions.

## Malignant vs. Benign Neoplasms

All neoplasms are *not* malignant. *Benign neoplasms* can occur and, while such growths are abnormal, they are rarely lethal to the host. The cells of benign lesions are *well differentiated* and closely resemble the tissues from which they arise. Such growths are usually encapsulated, grow slowly, and remain truly localized, rarely infiltrating adjacent tissues. Destruction in surrounding tissues is generally minimal. Benign tumors, such as most primary brain tumors, can cause death if they produce pressure on a vital organ. In general, such lesions can be removed surgically and tend not to recur. Certain benign lesions, such as moles and intestinal polyps, can undergo malignant transformation. These are classified as *precancerous* lesions and should be watched carefully.

The cells of a *malignant tumor* have an *immature,* or *poorly differentiated,* appearance, with profound nuclear and cytoplasmic abnormalities. Large, irregular nucleoli are often present and may be numerous. Growth of a malignant tumor mass is generally more rapid than its benign counterpart, and many mitotic figures may be seen under the microscope. Malignant growths infiltrate surrounding tissues, causing *dysplasia* and fibrosis and often making complete surgical removal difficult. Extensive *tissue necrosis* may also occur, resulting in hemorrhage or infectious complications. When surgically removed, malignant tumors tend to recur, either locally from residual tumor cells left behind at surgery or from secondary satellite growths occurring in other sites.

## Metastasis

The capacity to form satellite tumors, or *metastases,* at distant sites is a characteristic of malignant neoplasms. Metastases originate when viable tumor cells are shed by the growing malignant growth. Some of these cells are destroyed by the host or have lost their mitotic capacity. Others have the ability to establish new colonies and can grow when the primary lesion has been surgically re-

moved. These metastatic lesions are, therefore, of the *same cell type* as the *primary* lesion. Metastatic spread of cancer is facilitated by the invasive nature of malignant growth. Even the smallest microscopic cancer may infiltrate adjacent tissues. The pattern of metastatic spread varies and is influenced by the type of tissue invaded by tumor cells. Generally, cancers spread in one or more of the following manners: direct invasion, hematogenous spread, lymphangitic spread, or serosal seeding.

**Direct invasion** *Direct extension* of the tumor into surrounding local and regional tissue is thought to be related to several mechanisms. It has been postulated that enzymatic or lytic substances are produced and released by tumor cells. Tissues vary in their susceptibility to such involvement. Dense, elastic, or fibrous tissue such as cartilage, ligaments, and tendons is relatively resistant to direct tumor invasion, in contrast to soft tissue and muscle. Arteries are less susceptible than veins, which is thought to be related to the elastic tissue in the arterial walls.

The ability of malignant cells to achieve locomotion is another factor contributing to direct invasion. It has been demonstrated that tumor cells have *motility,* much like leukocytes, and actively migrate throughout the body. This motility is increased by their relative lack of cohesiveness in comparison to normal cells.[10]

**Hematogenous spread** Hematogenous spread of cancer occurs as malignant cells invade the vasculature and migrate to distant sites. Development of metastatic foci in highly vascular organs and the bone marrow is common. Tumor cells may be released directly into blood vessels during surgical biopsy or excision. Then tumor cells may adhere to the vascular lining or endothelium of small veins and subsequently penetrate perivascular connective tissue, because of alterations in endothelial properties. It has also been postulated that other factors, including hormonal alterations, temperature, histamine levels, coagulability, and numbers of viable tumor cells shed from the primary tumor, may affect the development of hematogenous metastases.[11] These factors may alter vascular permeability and act as mediators for tumor cell invasion. It has been demonstrated that tumor cells readily proliferate within perivascular connective tissue. It has also been shown that new blood vessels develop from preexisting venules near the new tumor nodule. Venous invasion by tumor cells is recognized in about 80 percent of resected gastric cancers, 70 percent of lung cancers, and 40 percent of colorectal cancers.[12] The predilection for early, widespread dissemination of small primary lesions may be related to early vascular invasion.

**Lymphangitic spread**  Malignant cells can invade lymph vessels, develop metastatic foci in lymph nodes, and disseminate throughout the lymphatic system. However, the role of the lymphoreticular system in the growth and dissemination of cancer is complex. The relationship of *immunocompetence* and *immune surveillance* to the development of cancer is the subject of intensive research. Initially, the lymph nodes function as an effective filter where metastatic tumor cells are trapped and destroyed.[13] However, when lymph nodes themselves become involved with tumor, they serve as a gateway for dissemination throughout the body. Lymphatic invasion may be related to the thin, delicate walls of the lymphatic tissue. Lymphangitic spread may also be enhanced by physiologic communication with small blood vessels. The reason nodes lose their ability to trap and destroy tumor cells is not clear. Factors such as the intensity and duration of challenge by tumor cells seem important to the development of nodal involvement. The immunologic integrity of lymphatic tissue in general and the immunocompetence of cells of the lymphocytic series are critical factors. In breast cancer, it is known that patients with lymph nodes which are negative for tumor involvement at the time of mastectomy have a more favorable prognosis. The same is true in cervical and gastrointestinal malignant disease. Increasing numbers of positive lymph nodes are associated with a poorer prognosis in terms of the likelihood of developing systemic metastases and therefore of survival.

**Serosal seeding**  Cancers can metastasize if viable tumor cells rupture into the intraperitoneal or intrapleural cavities and implant on serosal surfaces where they can grow. *Seeding* into a body cavity as a mode of dissemination frequently occurs in adenocarcinomas arising from tissues of epithelial origin. Ovarian cancer is frequently metastatic to the serosal surfaces of the liver and diaphragm.[14] Microscopic tumor implants frequently stud the mesentery and dependent portions of the pelvis, especially the peritoneal surfaces of the bowel and the dome of the bladder. Ascites, due to lymphatic obstruction, is commonly the presenting sign in patients with diffuse seeding.

## Classification of Malignant Neoplasms[15]

Neoplasms are classified according to their cellular origins. *Carcinomas* are malignant tumors which are derived from tissues of epithelial origin. Carcinomas are further classified and named by the organ site in which the tumor arises and the type of epithelial cell involved. While *adenocarcinomas* appear glandular, *squamous cell carcinoma* resembles cells of the basal epithelium. *Sarcomas* and *lymphomas* are malignant growths of mesenchymal origin. Sarcomas include tumors of soft tissue, bone, muscle, and stromal elements such as connective tissue. Sarcomas are commonly designated by the predominant cell type found within the tumor. Lymphomas are malignant neoplasms of the lymphoreticular system. As a broad classification, lymphomas include Hodgkin's disease and the non-Hodgkin's lymphomas. *Leukemia* is a malignant disease of the blood-forming organs which occurs in both acute and chronic forms. Leukemias are named according to the dominant cell type. Other malignant diseases of the blood-forming organs include multiple myeloma and plasma cell dyscrasias.

Carcinomas, as a group, tend to spread via the lymphatics early, with hematogenous spread occurring as a result of involvement of local or regional nodes. Sarcomas, in contrast, frequently establish huge local tumors without nodal metastases and are characterized by blood-borne metastases to vascular organs such as the lung and liver. Lymphoma is commonly localized in Hodgkin's disease, but local presentations are rare in the non-Hodgkin's lymphomas, which are generally disseminated at diagnosis, involving multiple extranodal sites. Leukemia, by definition, is a systemic disease manifested by diffuse involvement of the bone marrow.

## The Etiology of Cancer

A number of theories have been proposed to explain which events, interactions, or circumstances predispose a cell to malignant transformation. Etiologic factors which have been suggested in carcinogenesis include hereditary susceptibility, chromosomal disruption, failures in immunologic surveillance, and environmental factors such as exposure to radiation and chemical or viral carcinogens. At present, no single unifying theory can provide a clear, coherent explanation for the evolution of all neoplasms. However, epidemiologic studies and genetic research have identified populations which have an increased risk of developing cancer.

Substantial evidence exists that the clinical expression of neoplastic transformation is influenced by the interrelationships between the genetic material of the host and influence of the environment.

**Hereditary factors** Certain congenital and genetically abnormal ties are associated with the inheritance of specific neoplasms or a significant increase in the incidence of cancer. Inherited malignant diseases may occur in a constellation of developmental anomalies or as the only manifestation of a genetic defect. The syndromes are transmitted and expressed as autosomal or recessive traits consistent with Mendelian inheritance patterns.[16] The coexistence of congenital birth defects and early development of cancers in patients with some of these syndromes presents strong evidence that a common etiologic mechanism exists during embryonic development. The genetic defects may be produced by chromosomal breakage, translocations, or deletions. The syndromes are frequently associated with cytogenetic abnormalities. Retinoblastoma and Wilms' tumor are two examples of hereditary neoplasms seen in children which are associated with deletions from a chromosomal arm and multiple birth defects. Pheochromocytomas and medullary thyroid carcinoma occur as an inherited syndrome, characterized by the simultaneous development of multiple tumors in both adrenals and the thyroid in young adults.[17]

Other genetic disorders are considered "premalignant lesions" because they are associated with a significant increase in the incidence of specific tumors. Down's, Bloom's, and Fanconi's syndromes, autosomal recessive dermatoses such as albinism and xeroderma pigmentosum, and congenital immunodeficiency syndromes are all associated with a twenty- to fifty-fold increase in the risk of developing acute leukemia. The incidence of lymphoreticular malignant neoplasms with immunodeficiency states such as ataxia-telangectasia and Wiskott-Aldrich syndrome is extremely high.[18]

**Familial susceptibility** It has been determined empirically that a familial predisposition also exists for the development of some of the more common cancers. Susceptibility is influenced by many variables, including environmental factors. Significantly higher incidence rates of some types of cancer, such as breast cancer, have been documented among close relatives.[19] It is unclear how common genetic and environmental mechanisms interact. However, it is known that familial cancers may

occur even when geographic and environmental differences exist.

**Acquired diseases** Certain *acquired disorders* are known to predispose individuals to the development of specific cancers. Screening and careful follow-up of such high-risk individuals are crucial for early detection. Screening studies may identify common etiologic factors in highly susceptible individuals and may provide key information about factors involved in carcinogenesis. The goal of such studies is to define causative factors and ultimately to control risk factors and prevent the development of cancer in high-risk groups through medical and nursing intervention.

Pernicious anemia, ulcerative colitis, and regional enteritis (Crohn's disease) are conditions which are clearly associated with an increase in the incidence of gastrointestinal cancers.[20] Autoimmune disorders such as Sjögren's syndrome and Hashimoto's disease are associated with the development of malignant lymphomas.[21] Cirrhosis and hepatitis have been related to an increased incidence of hepatocellular cancer.[22] Obesity as well as nutritional disorders, including those associated with alcoholism, have also been implicated as etiologic factors in the development of cancer.[23]

**The role of viruses** The possibility that *viruses* play a significant role in the development of cancer in human beings is now under investigation. Viruses infect many living organisms, including plants, bacteria, animals, and human beings. The study of viruses has been difficult because of their small size and the fact that they proliferate only within living organisms and because human viruses are often difficult to grow in animals.

Bittner, in his studies of strains of inbred mice which spontaneously develop breast cancer, found that multiple factors, including a virus, were necessary for consistent development of mammary tumors.[24] The identification of this virus has stimulated scientists to study how viruses interact with cells and whether such viruses can cause tumors in man. To date, little direct evidence exists implicating viral infection in familial cancer. Exact information about how they influence predisposition toward or protection from cancer is unclear.

At present, only the Epstein-Barr virus is strongly associated as an etiologic factor in the development of human malignant disease.[25] Evidence exists that this virus plays a major role in the pathogenesis of infectious mononucleosis. The virus or antibodies to the virus are also demonstrable in all patients with African Burkitt's lymphoma.[26,27] It should be emphasized that the virus might grow well in lymphoid cells and that the proliferation of these lymphoid cells would stimulate production of virus as well as antibody. In effect this would mean that the virus represents "a passenger rather than an inducer" of the disease.[28]

**Environmental factors** A great number of *environmental factors* or agents have been implicated in carcinogenesis. These factors include both natural and synthetic chemicals, tobacco, alcohol, ionizing radiation from a variety of sources, occupational hazards, certain social customs, and personal habits. Beginning research on personality types and their response to stress may also yield significant results about the prediction and prevention of specific types of cancer.

**Tobacco and Alcohol** A well-established relationship exists between tobacco smoking and the development of lung cancer. Studies have shown a close relationship between the duration and amount of smoking and lung cancer mortality. The preventability of lung cancer is demonstrated by the markedly decreased incidence of lung cancer among nonsmokers. Use of pipes, snuff, and chewing tobacco also constitute etiologic factors in the development of oral cancer.[29]

Evidence suggests that alcohol acts as a co-carcinogen enhancing the carcinogenic effect of other agents. The impact of smoking as a carcinogen is significantly increased when associated with a heavy intake of alcoholic beverages.[30] Alcoholism alone is known to predispose to the development of cancer. Despite indisputable evidence that smoking and alcoholism are synergistic and significantly increase the risk of cancer, the prevalent use of these carcinogens continues to represent a major healthcare problem in our society.

The carcinogenicity of alcohol may be related to compounds present in the beverage which are contaminants and irritants to mucous membranes.[31] Studies have demonstrated that increased incidence of oral and liver cancers is associated with alcohol consumption. Since alcoholics can be identified as high-risk individuals, they should be screened for cancer, especially cancers of the head and neck.

**Radiation** Radiation has been implicated as having leukemogenic as well as carcinogenic effects. A long latent period may exist between the initial exposure and the development of clinical cancer. In-

dividuals exposed to radiation in the atomic explosions at Hiroshima and Nagasaki demonstrate clearly the carcinogenic effects of radiation, as well as relationships between the dose received and the time of appearance of clinical leukemia. An increase in acute leukemia was first documented in 1948 in survivors exposed to large doses of radiation, and the leukemia rate has continued to remain significantly higher as late as the 1970s among survivors exposed to doses of 100 rads or more.[32] Carcinomas, as opposed to leukemia, were noted to have increased after 1960 among Japanese survivors of the atomic explosions.[33]

Children irradiated in utero during diagnostic x-ray procedures given to pregnant women have also demonstrated an increased incidence of acute leukemia and other cancer. Non-ionizing radiation such as that produced by ultraviolet light is associated with an increase in skin cancers and malignant melanomas. This correlates with data demonstrating that DNA in epidermal cells is particularly sensitive to damage from ultraviolet radiation.[34]

**Occupational Hazards** Factors involved in occupational carcinogenesis are not easily defined, because a relatively long latent period often exists between exposure and the clinical development of cancer. Occupational changes and geographic mobility compound the difficulty in identifying common etiologic agents.[35] Agents identified thus far include aromatic hydrocarbons, certain inorganic compounds, fibers and dusts of leather, wood, and heavy metals, and other chemicals such as vinyl chloride. Latent periods are always long, and the development of clinical cancer is related to the degree of exposure and individual sensitivity. Epidemiologic studies continue to identify carcinogenic hazards in occupational environments.

**Drugs** A variety of drugs have been implicated in human cancer. Among them are immunosuppressive agents, cytotoxic drugs, synthetic estrogens, and androgenic-anabolic steroids. Additional drugs in clinical use which are under suspicion include chloramphenicol, phenytoin, reserpine, and coal tar ointments.[36] A number of these agents have been withdrawn from clinical use because of their carcinogenicity in animal systems. In special clinical situations where the therapeutic benefit outweighs the potential risk, however, continued use of these drugs is warranted.

*Immunosuppressive drugs,* utilized to prevent rejection in organ transplantation, increase the risk of developing malignant lymphoma. This increase is thought to be a result of alterations in the immune system induced by the agents, although the exact mechanisms have not been defined.[37] Cancer chemotherapy frequently involves treatment with drugs which are known to be carcinogenic in animal systems and are both immunosuppressive and cytotoxic. Significant increases in survival as well as improvement in the quality of life of successfully treated cancer patients outweigh the increased risk of a second malignant growth.

**A**ge  The effect of age at exposure on the carcinogenicity of any substance has also been demonstrated. Animal studies have provided evidence that exposure to a carcinogen early in life can increase the risk of tumor development.[38] Recently it has been shown that the female offspring of women treated with *diethylstilbestrol* (DES) during early pregnancy have a high incidence of vaginal carcinomas. This lends strong support to the idea that environmental hazards to which the young can be exposed should always be minimized. Other agents seem capable of affecting different organ systems during different ages of life. Clearly, variables such as age at onset of exposure and duration of exposure are important factors in these relationships.

**A**ir Pollution  Chemical carcinogens harbored in polluted air may represent a significant environmental cancer risk for modern city dwellers. Evidence of such a substance in polluted air has been identified in areas where *coal* is used extensively. Incomplete combustion results in the release of large amounts of aromatic hydrocarbons into the air; these have been identified as chemical carcinogens.[39] Other pollutants, such as substances found in smog, may also be involved in carcinogenesis.

**D**iet  Diet may play a potential role in introducing carcinogens into man's environment. A well-known example of a documented carcinogen in food is *aflotoxin,* a fungal contaminant which grows on grain under conditions of sustained high humidity and is an etiologic factor in the development of liver cancer.[40] Other possible carcinogens include nitrosamines, dyes, and polycyclic aromatic hydrocarbon additives, which are found frequently in prepackaged foodstuffs.[41] Other dietary factors which may contribute to carcinogenesis are alcoholism, obesity, high animal protein intake, and the absence of proper fiber in the diet. Cancers of the large bowel, breast, prostate, endometrium, and ovary seem to be associated with affluence and a high intake of refined carbohydrates, high fat, low fiber, and high animal protein.[42]

## FIRST-LEVEL NURSING CARE

Cancer constitutes one of the major health and social problems facing society today. Each year approximately 675,000 new cases are diagnosed in the United States and 370,000 persons die from cancer.[43] While cancer was ranked seventh in 1900 as a cause of death, today it is second only to cardiovascular diseases. Cancer can develop at any age, although it occurs more frequently in people over 40. In children under 15 years of age, only accidents surpass cancer as a cause of death. Table 5-1, compiled annually by the American Cancer Society, lists cancers by site of origin and by sex as well as by estimated annual incidence and death rates. In men, lung cancer is the leading site, followed by prostatic, colorectal, bladder, and stomach cancers. In women, breast cancer is the most common, followed by colorectal, uterine, lung, and ovarian cancers. In this table, for the most part, the prognosis for prolonged survival is closely related to the proportion of patients diagnosed with localized disease. Cancers such as carcinoma of the lung and pancreas, in which the annual death rate approaches the number of new cases (incidence), are rarely diagnosed in localized stages. The correlation between localized disease and a favorable prognosis has made it critical to determine whether the cancer has involved other tissues.

How genetic and environmental factors affect susceptibility to cancer is not well understood. Latent periods between the carcinogenic event and the development of clinical cancer are often prolonged. Nonetheless, it is not always necessary to understand the exact role etiologic factors play in human cancer in order to take preventive action. Certainly no known measure would have a greater role in cancer control and prevention than the elimination of cigarette smoking; the reduction in the incidence of lung cancer would be striking. Moreover, the beneficial effects of such a preventive action would not be restricted to cancer alone. The incidence and morbidity of cardiovascular and pulmonary diseases induced by tobacco use would also be significantly reduced. Clearly, any discussion of etiologic considerations must do more than define risk factors. *Prevention* must be focused on *health education* and *early detection.*

### Health Education

Health education remains one of the most important areas of health care. As a profession, nursing has an obligation not only to provide care for the sick but also to teach and motivate well individuals to protect and maintain their health. Health education related to cancer must be designed to inform and educate the public about treatable forms of cancer. These programs should provide information to the public about effective therapy that is available, so that fear will not inhibit people from seeking early medical assistance. *Fear* remains the largest single obstacle that complicates and compromises early detection efforts. It is difficult, if not impossible, to convince people to participate in screening programs for early detection or to seek medical attention for suspicious but tolerable

**TABLE 5-1**
ESTIMATED NEW CASES OF CANCER
AND CANCER DEATHS BY SITE AND SEX IN 1976

| Site | Estimated Deaths | | | Estimated New Cases | | |
|---|---|---|---|---|---|---|
| | Total | Male | Female | Total | Male | Female |
| ALL SITES | 370,000 | 202,000 | 168,000 | 675,000 | 339,000 | 336,000 |
| BUCCAL CAVITY & PHARYNX (ORAL) | 8,300 | 5,900 | 2,400 | 23,800 | 16,900 | 6,900 |
| Lip | 225 | 200 | 25 | 4,100 | 3,800 | 300 |
| Tongue | 2,000 | 1,400 | 600 | 4,500 | 3,100 | 1,400 |
| Salivary gland | 650 | 400 | 250 ⎫ | | | |
| Floor of mouth | 525 | 400 | 125 ⎬ | 8,600 | 5,100 | 3,500 |
| Other & unspecified mouth | 1,250 | 800 | 450 ⎭ | | | |
| Pharynx | 3,650 | 2,700 | 950 | 6,600 | 4,900 | 1,700 |
| DIGESTIVE ORGANS | 101,900 | 53,800 | 48,100 | 169,000 | 88,200 | 80,800 |
| Esophagus | 6,600 | 4,800 | 1,800 | 7,500 | 5,600 | 1,900 |
| Stomach | 14,400 | 8,500 | 5,900 | 22,900 | 14,000 | 8,900 |
| Small intestine | 700 | 350 | 350 | 2,200 | 1,200 | 1,000 |
| Large intestine (colon- | 38,900 | 18,000 | 20,900 | 69,000 | 31,000 | 38,000 |
| rectum) | 10,300 | 5,700 | 4,600 | 30,000 | 17,000 | 13,000 |
| Liver and biliary passages | 9,800 | 4,800 | 5,000 | 11,800 | 5,800 | 6,000 |
| Pancreas | 19,600 | 10,900 | 8,700 | 21,700 | 12,000 | 9,700 |
| Other & unspecified digestive | 1,600 | 750 | 850 | 3,900 | 1,600 | 2,300 |
| RESPIRATORY SYSTEM | 88,450 | 68,900 | 19,550 | 104,700 | 82,700 | 22,000 |
| Larynx | 3,250 | 2,800 | 450 | 9,200 | 8,100 | 1,100 |
| Lung | 83,800 | 65,200 | 18,600 | 93,000 | 73,000 | 20,000 |
| Other & unspecified respiratory | 1,400 | 900 | 500 | 2,500 | 1,600 | 900 |
| BONE, TISSUE, AND SKIN | 8,500 | 4,850 | 3,700 | 15,700 | 7,900 | 7,800 |
| Bone | 1,900 | 1,100 | 800 | 1,900 | 1,100 | 800 |
| Connective tissue | 1,650 | 850 | 800 | 4,500 | 2,400 | 2,100 |
| Skin | 5,000 | 2,900 | 2,100 | 9,300 | 4,400 | 4,900 |
| BREAST | 33,100 | 300 | 32,800 | 88,700 | 700 | 88,000 |
| GENITAL ORGANS | 43,200 | 20,400 | 22,800 | 128,800 | 60,600 | 68,200 |
| Cervix, invasive ⎫ uterus | 7,700 | — | 7,700 | 20,000 | — | 20,000 |
| Corpus uteri ⎭ | 3,300 | — | 3,300 | 27,000 | — | 27,000 |
| Ovary | 10,800 | — | 10,800 | 17,000 | — | 17,000 |
| Other female genital | 1,000 | — | 1,000 | 4,200 | — | 4,200 |
| Prostate | 19,300 | 19,300 | — | 56,000 | 56,000 | — |
| Other male genital | 1,100 | 1,100 | — | 4,600 | 4,600 | — |
| URINARY ORGANS | 16,600 | 11,100 | 5,500 | 44,700 | 31,200 | 13,500 |
| Bladder | 9,500 | 6,600 | 2,900 | 29,800 | 22,000 | 7,800 |
| Kidney & other urinary | 7,100 | 4,500 | 2,600 | 14,900 | 9,200 | 5,700 |
| EYE | 400 | 200 | 200 | 1,700 | 800 | 900 |
| BRAIN & CENTRAL NERVOUS SYSTEM | 8,600 | 4,800 | 3,800 | 10,800 | 5,900 | 4,900 |
| ENDOCRINE GLANDS | 1,650 | 650 | 1,000 | 9,100 | 2,700 | 6,400 |
| Thyroid | 1,150 | 350 | 800 | 8,100 | 2,200 | 5,900 |
| Other endocrine | 500 | 300 | 200 | 1,000 | 500 | 500 |
| LEUKEMIA | 15,000 | 8,400 | 6,600 | 21,300 | 12,000 | 9,300 |
| LYMPHOMAS | 19,000 | 10,100 | 8,900 | 29,500 | 16,000 | 13,500 |
| Lymphosarcoma & reticulosarcoma | 7,500 | 4,000 | 3,500 | 10,400 | 5,600 | 4,800 |
| Hodgkin's disease | 3,200 | 1,900 | 1,300 | 7,200 | 4,200 | 3,000 |
| Multiple myeloma | 5,300 | 2,700 | 2,600 | 8,000 | 4,100 | 3,900 |
| Other lymphomas | 3,000 | 1,500 | 1,500 | 3,900 | 2,100 | 1,800 |
| ALL OTHER & UNSPECIFIED SITES | 25,250 | 12,600 | 12,650 | 27,200 | 13,400 | 13,800 |

symptoms if they think a diagnosis of cancer signifies a painful and relentless progression toward death. Nurses and other health professionals must recognize that powerful social and cultural customs must often be overcome. A didactic education program which is not adapted to the particular attitudes of a specific audience, at their level of understanding, is likely to have little impact. Clearly one of the most important goals of public education is to motivate individuals to change patterns of behavior and to convince them of the benefits of taking precautions against unnecessary risks.

Medical professionals and patients may be placed at greater risk of developing cancer if inadequate precautions are taken during routine use of diagnostic and therapeutic radiation. It is critical in cancer control and prevention to limit radiation exposure as much as possible and to follow patients who have been exposed to significant amounts of radiation for prolonged periods to screen for cancer and to assess mortality related to radiation exposure.

When a potentially carcinogenic drug can be replaced by an equally effective and safe agent, the alternate drug should be utilized. Patients exposed to known carcinogenic drugs should be followed closely, and information about the increases in true incidence following drug exposure should be documented systematically.

While the mass media have the advantage of reaching large numbers of people, the power of person-to-person education must not be underestimated. Well-informed and motivated health professionals have the greatest potential for influencing individuals.

### Early Detection

A logical outgrowth of knowledge about etiologic factors in carcinogenesis is surveillance of those at high risk. Routine surveillance is useful for several purposes. First, it permits early diagnosis of treatable cancers, which is an important factor influencing the prospects for cure. Examples of screening programs that are presently available include chest x-rays and cytological examinations of bronchial secretions for lung cancer, urine cytologies for bladder cancer, liver function studies and scans for liver cancer, periodic blood counts for workers exposed to benzene, and vaginal examinations for children of women treated with DES during pregnancy. One of the most successful screening programs involves the routine use of soft-tissue breast x-rays (mammograms) for women over age 50, and for those below 50 with known risk factors.

Screening is also valuable for the identification of previously unrecognized health problems in the setting of multiple environmental hazards. Identification of industrial risk factors has provided the opportunity to reduce the incidence of cancer for workers by curtailing or eliminating carcinogenic exposure.

Prospective screening studies of high-risk groups offers the opportunity to define changes which occur prior to the development of clinical signs and symptoms. Papanicolaou smears to detect early cervical cancer have been utilized extensively and have resulted in a dramatic decrease in mortality from this disease due to early disease identification in asymptomatic patients.

The success of voluntary screening programs in high-risk groups or in the general population is clearly dependent on the awareness which motivates people to participate. It is imperative that health educators emphasize the need for regular routine testing.

Nurses can be extremely persuasive in influencing people to be screened for cancer. They are often more readily accessible than physicians. Community health nurses, as well as those specializing in school or industrial nursing, may initiate intervention in the community before the physician has any contact. Nurses may also perform pertinent health history and physical examinations in screening clinics, may counsel, teach, and make appropriate referrals, and may be the primary health professionals involved in follow-up. Nurses have been active participants in breast cancer screening as well as other research projects. In New York City a study showed a 30 percent reduction in mortality due to early case findings in women with breast cancer.[44] Strax has emphasized mobile vans and neighborhood-based examining centers, staffed by nurses, as a means of doing periodic screening for breast, cervical, and lung cancers.[45]

## SECOND-LEVEL NURSING CARE

Any person who seeks medical attention for a specific complaint may have cancer. Cancer is a great imitator, producing acute and chronic symptoms which mimic a variety of common disorders.

### Nursing Assessment

A thorough *health history* should be obtained from the patient. Presenting tumor manifestations are due to the *local mechanical effects* as well as the *systemic effects* of the primary or the metastatic tumor. Specific signs and symptoms depend on the anatomic and functional characteristics of the organ or structure involved with the cancer. Nurses must understand these effects and constantly assess patients for their presence.

**Local effects**  Local mechanical effects are related to the area that a neoplasm occupies. As a tumor grows, it accumulates greater mass and occupies more space. The appearance of signs and symptoms will depend on the ability of the involved organ or space to accommodate tumor growth without exerting *pressure* on surrounding tissues or functionally impairing the tissue. For example, an ovarian cancer may be of considerable size before affecting the function of surrounding organs because the abdominal cavity is distensible. Clinical manifestations of cancers in such locations may be vague and nonspecific or completely absent until the tumor is large enough to compromise the abdominal organs. In contrast, a tumor originating in bone will cause pain early in its growth, since rigid bony walls allow for little expansion. Consequently, signs and symptoms of the tumor occur early, as local pressure is exerted on sensory nerves. Large tumor masses may be observable on inspection or be directly palpable.

Another mechanical effect of tumors results from *inlet or outlet obstruction* caused by compression of tubular structures such as the esophagus, ureters, bronchi, or bowel, as well as ducts, blood vessels, and lymphatic channels. Symptoms are related to interference with the passage of normal contents (e.g., chronic constipation, inability to swallow, etc.) and dilatation of the structures proximal to the site of obstruction. Chronic obstruction may cause stasis and frequently results in infection and, eventually, organ failure.

In addition to interfering with the functional capacity of local structures or organs, a tumor mass may *compromise the blood supply* to normal surrounding tissue. This occurs directly, as a result of external compression of normal vessels, or indirectly, as the normal blood supply is diverted into a highly vascular tumor mass. Unless collateral blood vessels restore adequate circulation, tissue oxygenation and nutrition will be compromised. If the impairment is prolonged and severe, *necrosis* and *ulceration* of involved tissue will occur, predisposing the area to *hemorrhage* and *infection.* If tumors outgrow their own blood supply, the same effects will be observed, with eventual necrosis of the tumor.

**Systemic effects**  Malignant tumors are also distinguished from benign tumors by the systemic effects of the cancer on the host. Profound abnormalities in organ functioning can occur as a result of the growth and metabolic effects of the cancer. Systemic manifestations of malignant tumors may represent the effect of invasion and subsequent replacement of normal tissue by the primary tumor or metastatic tumor cells. Any organ system can be affected. Tumor infiltration may occur diffusely throughout the organ or as solitary lesions.

*Cachexia* may occur even with small tumors and is characterized by anorexia, weakness, wasting, metabolic disturbance, hormonal aberrations, and electrolyte and fluid abnormalities.[46] Patients often appear chronically ill and emaciated; apathy, detachment, and anxiety may contribute to the problem. The cause of cachexia is not well-defined: malabsorption secondary to intestinal infiltration by the tumor may cause malnutrition, or anorexia may be present from poorly understood metabolic causes. When considering cachexia, the relative autonomy of cancerous growth must be remembered. Metabolically, this autonomy is represented by the tumor's priority for nutrients at the expense of normal tissue. Clearly, a normal caloric intake may be insufficient to support the tumor and the host.

The production of certain pharmacologically active substances or hormones by the tumor also exerts a systemic effect on the host.[47] Even tumors which do not involve organs of the endocrine system may produce such substances and are characterized by a lack of normal feedback regulation. When this occurs, signs and symptoms similar to excess hormone production are observed. *"Ectopic hormone"* production by tumor cells includes syndromes in which there is inappropriate production and release of antidiuretic hormone (ADH), adrenocorticotropic hormone (ACTH), thyroid-stimulating hormone (TSH), or parathyroid hormone (PTH), as well as ectopic gonadotropins and insulin. The clinical manifestations of such syndromes are complex and are discussed fully in Chaps. 12 and 21.

**Seven danger signals**  The preceding local and systemic effects have been condensed by the American Cancer Society into *seven danger signals* that may indicate a malignant disease. Assessment of patients for these should be performed routinely in every area of nursing practice.

The seven danger signals are (1) any sore that does not heal, (2) a lump or thickening in the breast or elsewhere, (3) persistent indigestion or difficulty in swallowing, (4) any change in a wart or mole, (5) unexplained bleeding or discharge, (6) persistent hoarseness or cough, and (7) any change in bowel habits.

### Nursing Problems and Intervention

The clinical manifestations discussed above are not diagnostic of cancer, nor do they always represent early or localized cancer. However, when the nurse identifies problems that include *unexplained pain, weight loss, lumps,* or *disorders in gastrointestinal, respiratory, neurologic,* or *genitourinary function of 2 or more weeks' duration,* a workup for cancer is indicated. The nurse who finds any of the local or systemic symptoms of a tumor should immediately *refer* the patient to an appropriate diagnostic facility for a complete medical workup.

### THIRD-LEVEL NURSING CARE

Patients with cancer may be hospitalized for definitive diagnosis and staging, therapeutic intervention, or terminal care. Nursing assessment, on this level, is directed toward common manifestations of cancer, despite the primary site. This is followed by delineation of major nursing problems in caring for the patient with cancer and therapeutic interventions.

### Nursing Assessment

The person with cancer who enters the hospital may or may not be aware of the diagnosis. The *health history* should determine the patient's knowledge of the disease. It should also elicit any subjective symptoms of the tumor's presence, e.g., pain, bleeding, altered bodily function, etc.

*Physical assessment* of the patient with cancer may reveal pallor, weight loss, and weakness. There may be dyspnea on exertion if the patient is severely anemic, as well as increased pulse and respiratory rates.

Bleeding is a frequent finding if the tumor involves pressure on a mucous membrane or affects normal liver function. All possible bleeding sites should be evaluated: gums, stools, gastric secretions, skin, and urine. Vital signs, including the neurologic examination, may reveal nonvisible signs of internal bleeding.

Obvious signs of infection may be present in visible tumors. A foul odor, increased body temperature, and signs of inflammation all signal an area of infection.

The presence of a lump may be revealed during breast, abdominal, or lymph node examinations. Close observation may reveal guarding when a particular area of the body is touched or moved. Patients should be asked about the presence of pain and its location, duration, and severity.

Anxiety may be manifested by withdrawn *or* demanding behavior, crying, quick nervous gestures, or stoic cheerfulness. Nurses should be particularly alert in assessing the behaviors that may be indicative of a patient's coping patterns.

**Diagnostic procedures** Proof by *biopsy* of a malignant neoplasm is of critical importance even in the presence of convincing clinical and laboratory evidence. Biopsies may be *excisional, incisional,* or *needle. Excisional* biopsy removes the entire tumor with the specimen. Excisional biopsies are used for small, discrete masses.

*Incisional* biopsy removes a part of a tumor mass. It is used during bronchoscopic, cystoscopic, esophagoscopic, and proctoscopic examinations. Biopsies are usually incisional when tumor masses are too large to be removed entirely. There is some danger of surgical "seeding" (systemic spread) of tumor cells, however; the physician weighs this objection against the need for histologic information to determine therapy.

*Needle* biopsy involves aspiration of cells from subcutaneous masses, muscle masses, and internal organs such as the liver. It is also used for obtaining bone marrow for examination. Needle biopsy may not be definitive and may require confirmation by incisional or excisional biopsy.

*Exfoliative cytology* is a fourth method of obtaining cells for examination. The cervical smear is the most common example of this method. However, exfoliative cytology may be used on any epithelium-lined body cavity or orifice. Scraping to remove specimens may be done on mucous membranes of the mouth, vagina, bronchus, etc.

Other diagnostic procedures include x-ray (barium and dye studies) and blood and urine examinations. These indirect examinations have their limitations, making biopsy the major diagnostic method to establish tumor classification (described earlier) and staging.

**C**linical Staging  Clinical staging establishes the presence and extent of a tumor according to its degree of spread or metastasis. The curative potential of any treatment modality is dependent on accurate determination of the extent of the disease (localized vs. systemic) and correlation of this staging data with the *natural history.*

The *natural history* of a cancer describes the individual biologic, physiologic, and biochemical features, patterns of spread, and typical behavior which characterize the disease and its progression. Therapeutic alternatives will vary according to the pathologic type of tumor as well as the presence or absence of metastatic disease. Knowledge about the natural history of the neoplasm often provides key information about where metastases are likely to occur.

The International Union Against Cancer (UICC) has standardized the clinical staging of carcinomas with the development of the TNM system.[48]

---

T—Primary Tumor; N—Regional Lymph Nodes; M—Distant Metastases

These may be extended by the following designations:

| | |
|---|---|
| Tumor | T0—No evidence of primary tumor<br>TIS—Carcinoma in situ (no evidence of invasion)<br>T1, T2, T3, T4—Ascending degrees of tumor size |
| Nodes | N0—Regional nodes not demonstrable<br>N1a, N2a—Demonstrable regional lymph nodes; metastases not suspected<br>N1b, N2b, N3b—Demonstrable regional lymph nodes; metastases suspected<br>Nx—Regional lymph nodes cannot be assessed clinically |
| Metastases | M0—No evidence of distant metastases<br>M1, M2, M3—Ascending degrees of metastatic involvement, including distant nodes |

---

This system is applicable to most organ sites and encompasses the evolution of a lesion from carcinoma in situ to widely disseminated metastatic disease. Although the TNM method is applicable to all tumors, additional staging systems have been established and are discussed in detail in Chaps. 6 and 7. The procedures employed in the staging of cancers are to some degree influenced by what is already known about their individual natural histories. Staging procedures are designed to examine areas that would be likely sites for metastatic disease. These sites are defined by the high incidence of known metastases in these areas, historically documented by a series of patients with disseminated disease or by collected autopsy results. Staging workups should also include a careful and detailed medical and family history and documentation of significant weight loss or fever. Immunologic evaluations should be performed to evaluate cell-mediated and humoral immunocompetence (see Chap. 8 for discussion).

The physician's *staging workup* of patients with cancer includes assessment of the following: (1) *all lymph node areas*—especially supraclavicular nodes commonly involved early in cancers which originate in the abdomen, breast, lungs, gonads, and head and neck area; (2) *skin*—examining the body surfaces for subcutaneous as well as cutaneous metastases, which are often seen in melanomas and carcinomas of the lung, kidney, and breast; (3) *pelvic area*—including bimanual pelvic examination for unsuspected masses and Papanicolaou smear in all females; (4) *rectum*—digital examination of the rectum, followed by proctoscopy or sigmoidoscopy if suspicious lesions are found; (5) *lungs*—radiologic examinations, including chest x-ray (tomography in selected patients), and diagnostic thoracentesis if pleural effusions are present; (6) *bones*—skeletal surveys with x-rays and bone scans routinely; (7) *liver and spleen*—physical examination for hepatosplenomegaly, biochemical studies of hepatic function, hepatic scans, and biopsy if suspicious lesions are found; (8) *hematologic evaluation*—complete blood count (CBC) with differential cell count; bone marrow aspiration and biopsies, especially in leukemia, lymphomas, neuroblastoma, and breast cancer, with known predilection for bony metastases; (9) *abdomen*—physical examination for discrete tumor masses, nodal enlargement, hepatosplenomegaly, or paracentesis in the presence of ascites; and (10) *central nervous system*—examination for evidence of increased intracranial pressure, motor and sensory abnormalities, visual disturbances, headaches, or cranial nerve abnormalities, with lumbar punctures and brain scans.

The *role of the nurse* in the diagnostic workup is twofold: (1) to provide the patient with psychological support and information regarding necessary staging procedures, and (2) to assist in or perform procedures when appropriate.

Cancer terminology should, after classification and staging, indicate the site of origin, predominant cell type, and extent of spread. Nurses must inform themselves about these terms and their meanings.

Data accumulated during the clinical and pathologic staging provide information about variables affecting prognosis and the choice of primary therapy. It is imperative that all members of the medical team, including the patient, know why a procedure is being done, what the benefits and risks are, and what new information will be gained for all patients. Informing the patient (obtaining informed consent or permission to proceed with the procedure or clinical trial) is the physician's responsibility. However, informed consent is a continuing process, a learning experience for patients. Nurses participate in the process of informed consent and frequently are the focal persons who keep patients informed about the progress of the studies.

### Nursing Problems and Interventions

*Anemia, hemorrhage, infection, malnutrition, pain,* and *anxiety* are problems common to most cancers. Each poses unique nursing challenges, and each may be very threatening to the patient's survival.

**Anemia**  Anemia can be documented in the majority of patients with advanced cancer and may be the presenting symptom. Anemia may be caused by hemolysis, bleeding, poor nutrition, inadequate red blood cell production secondary to metastatic involvement of marrow, or drug-induced myelosuppression. Rest, an iron-rich diet, supplemental iron, and red blood cell transfusions are prescribed as necessary.

**Hemorrhage**  Hemorrhage may be caused by thrombocytopenia, clotting factor deficiency, disseminated intravascular coagulation, or erosion of blood vessels by a tumor. When platelets fall below 20,000/mm³ of blood, life-threatening hemorrhage may occur. Prophylactic platelet transfusions have reduced the incidence of fatal hemorrhage by more than 50 percent. Random donor platelets are commonly used for short-term platelet support. When prolonged thrombocytopenia is expected, histocompatible platelets should be administered from specially typed, specifically matched donors.

**Infection**  Cancer itself may compromise the host's ability to prevent or fight infection by decreasing the effectiveness of normal cells to destroy organisms or by impairing cell-mediated and humoral immunity. Chemotherapy can also contribute to the development of infection by suppressing bone-marrow production of white blood cells. Corticosteroids not only impair phagocytosis but also inhibit normal febrile reactions to infection. Immunosuppressed and leukopenic patients are frequently unable to demonstrate classic signs and symptoms of infection such as fever and abscess formation. Infections in these patients often disseminate rapidly and kill within a matter of hours. Nurses evaluate patients for (1) sudden changes in vital signs, (2) alterations in consciousness such as lethargy or confusion, (3) acute abdominal pain, (4) changes in the appearance and temperature of the skin or development of skin lesions, and (5) decreased urinary output.

Any one of the above signs may indicate impending sepsis from an uncontained localized infection which has disseminated. Intervention must be prompt and entails the culturing of blood, skin, orifices, and excreta. Broad-spectrum antibiotic therapy is instituted quickly, even though the source and organism are not yet identified.

Granulocyte transfusions are valuable in septic patients who remain profoundly leukopenic for more than 2 weeks. However, white cells must be given daily in order for a patient to derive any significant benefit, since the life span of white blood cells (granulocytes) is less than 12 hours. White blood cells are obtained from compatible family members, using blood cell separators or filtration leukopheresis.

**Malnutrition**  Maintenance of good nutritional status in patients with disseminated cancer is a difficult problem. Patients with cachexia should be given nutritional supplements to augment poor caloric intake. Parenteral hyperalimentation (high caloric intravenous feedings) may be valuable for patients who are unable to maintain an adequate intake.

**Pain**  Pressure caused by the tumor frequently results in severe pain for the patient. The extent of the disease and the patient's level of consciousness are frequently used as guides in the prescription and administration of narcotics and analgesics.

There is much debate over the question of addiction; some feel it is warranted if comfort results for the patient; others view it as harmful under any circumstances. Much of the decision making in this area must be individual to the persons involved, the patient and the family, the physician and the nurse.

It is a nursing responsibility to alleviate as much of the patient's pain as possible. This includes assessing for nonverbal cues in the stoic patient, as well as answering the call bell of the patient who rings incessantly. Position changes, conversation, massage, and diversion, in addition to medication, may aid in pain relief and the provision of comfort.

**Anxiety**  Patient fears and anxieties originate from many sources. These include family concerns, finances, the actual diagnosis, the therapy, and the future—or lack of future. Frequently the nurse can act as a perceptive and supportive listener. Occasionally a nursing referral to another agency will result in a problem solved. Mostly, it is the presence of this other caring person that is beneficial.

**General therapies**  One of the key considerations in the treatment of cancer is the therapeutic intent. When aggressive therapeutic intervention is potentially curative, it is not only warranted but totally justifiable, even if the therapy is associated with potentially serious side effects. If one expects only palliation, however, such morbidity may be unacceptable. It is critical, therefore, to consider all therapeutic alternatives. When cure is the goal, the initial management of the patient is usually the critical step determining the ultimate outcome. The construction of a treatment plan for the overall care of a patient must take into consideration the following factors: (1) the natural history of the specific cancer, (2) the extent of dissemination as determined by staging, and (3) the therapeutic potential of *surgery, radiotherapy, chemotherapy,* and *immunotherapy* to remove or kill all viable tumor cells in the specific cancer.

Surgery and radiotherapy alone may be curative in truly localized stages of disease. Chemotherapy, in contrast, may be curative when widespread disease is present. Each major modality has its shortcomings. When used alone, surgery and radiation may leave behind viable tumor cells which are capable of regrowing and killing the host. Chemotherapy and immunotherapy may eradicate systemic foci but leave viable cancer cells if a bulky tumor mass is present. Modern treatment programs are designed to maximize the curative potential of each modality by utilizing each to exploit the different biologic characteristics of a variety of cancers.

**S**urgery Until the turn of the century, surgery represented the only effective form of treatment for cancer. In the early 1900s radiation was recognized as a potentially powerful tool in cancer treatment. During the next 50 years, survival rates for cancer patients improved tremendously as sophisticated surgical and radiotherapeutic techniques and equipment became available, and the morbidity associated with treatment fell dramatically. Nonetheless, the improvement in survival began to level off during the 1950s despite continued technological development. This plateau occurred because, as discussed earler, cancers believed to be localized proved to have undetectable micrometastases not controlled by either surgery or radiotherapy.

Table 5-2 lists the current role, whether primary, alternate, or investigational, of each of the major treatment modalities in the management of localized or regional cancer. Surgery remains the primary treatment of choice in most local tumors, although many, such as pancreatic, colon, and head and neck cancers, are operable but not completely resectable. Surgical techniques are also valuable when management decisions depend on histologic proof of metastatic tumor and for differentiation of tumor from an infectious or nonmalignant process.

*Curative surgery* When considering the reason for treatment failure with any therapeutic modality, it is helpful to think of a tumor as having three separate and biologically important compartments, as expressed in the TNM classification: the primary tumor (T), regional node metastases (N), and distant metastases involving an organ system (M).

When a cancer is localized, or contained within the T compartment, surgery is *curative* if it is anatomically possible to resect the entire tumor mass. Surgical treatment of patients will vary with the site of the primary lesion. The extent of curative surgery will depend not only on the volume of tumor but also on the nature and degree of direct invasion of surrounding tissues or structures.

Treatment failures of truly localized cancer (T compartment) are related to inability to surgically resect all neoplastic tissue because the primary lesion is inaccessible or because resection would unduly compromise a vital structure. Historically, surgeons have devised more extensive procedures to improve the cure rate in apparently resectable cancer. In breast cancer, for example, radical mastectomy represents an attempt to prevent locally recurrent disease by resection of the breast and all regional lymph nodes (N compartment).

M compartment failures, even with radical surgical techniques, are common in what appears to be completely resected cancer. The reason for failure is now clear: clinically undetectable cancer cells are left behind and are eventually manifested as recurrent disease.

Indications for radical procedures should be considered carefully by physicians and patients before a recommendation is made. Radical surgery is useful in the management of localized but bulky tumor masses or locally recurrent tumors when no effective systemic therapy is available. Patients must understand the nature, degree, and permanence of the mutilation involved as well as the possible complications.

Table 5-3 presents a combined-modality strategy for 16 visceral neoplasms which traditionally have been approached initially with surgery and/or radiotherapy. The options are ranked in priority on the basis of current knowledge about the curative potential of available treatment programs and an understanding of how and why treatment failures occur.

*Palliative surgery* Surgical procedures are often employed when *hormonal manipulation* has proven therapeutic value. The most common operation is *oophorectomy,* which is employed for premenopausal women with metastatic breast cancer. Thirty percent of patients, notably those with skeletal and soft tissue metastases, have objective evidence of tumor regression following hormonal ablative surgery. *Orchiectomy* can produce prolonged tumor regression in patients with prostatic cancer. Other ablative procedures, including *adrenalectomy* and *hypophysectomy,* are chiefly utilized in advanced breast cancer. Responses to endocrine ablation vary with age, menopausal status, and dominant sites of metastatic disease.[49]

*Obstructive symptoms* produced by tumor masses can be successfully managed with surgical intervention. Small bowel and ureteral obstruction are not uncommon in the clinical course of ovarian cancer or other pelvic cancers. While surgical bypass and decompression have no intrinsic therapeutic effect, they may provide considerable relief, improve performance status, and facilitate definitive treatment with radiation or chemotherapy.

Surgery may have a more important role in the management of patients with *bulky metastatic cancer* in the future. Surgical procedures which remove bulky tumor masses may enhance the effectiveness of treatment with other therapies. Surgery has also been valuable when removal of a solitary life-threatening metastasis, such as a single brain lesion, is necessary. Finally, neurosurgical proce-

**TABLE 5-2**
CHOICE OF TREATMENT PRESENTLY EMPLOYED
IN THE THERAPY OF LOCALIZED AND REGIONAL CANCERS

| Diagnosis | Surgery | Radio-therapy | Chemo-therapy | Immuno-therapy |
|---|---|---|---|---|
| CARCINOMAS | | | | |
| Melanoma | P | Adj | T | T |
| Other skin cancers | P | P | P | P |
| Breast | P | Alt/adj | T | T |
| Ovary | P | Alt/adj | T | — |
| Uterine body | P | Alt | T | — |
| Uterine cervix | P | P | T | — |
| Choriocarcinoma | Alt | — | P | T |
| Lung | P | Alt | T | — |
| Stomach | P | — | T | — |
| Pancreas | P | — | T | — |
| Large bowel | P | — | T | T |
| Thyroid | P | Alt | T | — |
| Head and neck | P | P | T | T |
| Bladder | P | Alt | T | — |
| Kidney | P | — | — | — |
| Testis | P | Alt | Alt/adj | — |
| Prostate | P | P | T | — |
| Sarcomas | P | T | T | T |
| CHILDHOOD TUMORS | | | | |
| Wilms' tumor | P | P | P | — |
| Neuroblastoma | P | Alt | Alt | — |
| Embryonal rhabdomyosarcoma | P | P | P | — |
| Ewing's sarcoma | P | P | P | — |
| LEUKEMIAS AND LYMPHOMAS | | | | |
| Leukemia | | | | |
|     Acute myeloblastic | — | — | P | T |
|     Acute lymphoblastic | — | Adj | P | T |
|     Chronic granulocytic | — | Alt | P | — |
|     Chronic lymphocytic | — | Alt | P | — |
| Hodgkin's disease | Alt | P | T | T |
| Lymphocytic lymphoma | Alt | P | Alt/T | T |
| Histocytic lymphoma | Atl | P | Alt/T | T |
| Mycosis fungoides | — | P | P | T |
| Multiple myeloma | Atl | Alt | P | — |
| Polycythemia vera | — | Alt | P | — |

P = primary method of treatment
Alt = alternative method of treatment or therapy of choice in special situations
Adj = primary method of therapy utilized in adjuvant situations
T = treatment currently under investigation as adjuvant therapy
— = no data available

| Tumor | Cell-kill Potential as Determined in Patients with Advanced Disease | Cure Potential from Initial Surgical or X-ray Therapy with Local or Regional Disease | Incidence or Impact of Tumors |
|---|---|---|---|
| 1. Breast | Very high: ≅60% response rate with combinations; good durations of remission; significant rates of complete remissions; many active drugs | Excellent: almost all patients are eligible to receive treatment of curative intent, i.e., the primary tumor is removed; criteria exist for separating good and poor risk for cure | Most common cause of death in women |
| 2. Ovary | High: single agents can give 50% response rates and 20% complete remissions; several agents active; combinations poorly tested | Generally poor: overall 5-year survival 20–25%; 36–50% of women inoperable when first diagnosed | High incidence; attacks relatively young women |
| 3. Colon | Poor but recently improved: several "active" agents but none exceeds 20% response rate; recent identification of more effective combination of 5-FU and MeCCNU | Good: ≅75% of patients amenable to curative resection; cure rate ≅50% in those undergoing curative resection | Second leading cause of death from cancer for both sexes; highest incidence for both sexes |
| 4. Stomach | Poor–fair but recently improved: several active drugs but none highly active; successes with combinations, e.g., BCNU + 5-FU, offer some hope of useful adjuvant treatment | Fair–poor: 25% of patients resectable for cure; 25% of resected patients live 5 years; overall 5-year survival 12% | Although incidence dropping, still ranks 6 as a cause of death in United States; 21,000 new cases yearly with 15,000 deaths |
| 5. Sarcoma | Fair–good: some degree of activity for the few drugs tested; combinations give 40–50% response rates; complete remissions possible in advanced disease | Variable, depending on the many histologic types | Generally rare |
| 6. Pancreas | Poor: two or three minimally active drugs with little impact on survival | Dismal: overall only 7–10% amenable to curative resection with high surgical mortality rate and minimal survival (5–10%) | Ranks 4 among cancers in terms of mortality; incidence rising dramatically |
| 7. Lung | Small cell—fair, adenocarcinoma and large cell—poor, epidermoid—poor; response rates reasonably high but impact on survival (small-cell) minimal | Poor: only 25% operable for cure; 5-year survival for those undergoing surgery is 25% | The single and most important cause of death from cancer in the United States |
| 8. Bladder | Recently improved: some activity for adriamycin, 5-FU and alkylating agents, no good data for other drugs; poorly studied tumor | Fair–good: 56% overall 5-year survival | 24,000 new cases yearly with 7,000 deaths |
| 9. Melanoma | Fair–poor: only a few active drugs with none greater than 20% response rate; no successful combinations to date | Good: 61% overall 5-year survival | 5,200 estimated yearly deaths |
| 10. Prostate | Little information available on chemotherapy; poorly studied tumor | Generally good, dependent on stage; 51% overall 5-year survival | 45,000 new cases yearly with 18,000 deaths |
| 11. Cervix uteri | Fair–good: several active agents, many not tried; no combination data; poorly studied tumor | Good—cure rate dependent on stage: IA—100%, IB—90%, IC—70%, II—50%, III—30%, IV—5%; both surgery and x-ray curative, 60% overall 5-year survival | 57,000 new cases yearly with 9,000 deaths |
| 12. Testicular | Excellent: curative potential against metastatic disease; highly active combinations | Good: both surgery and x-ray cure | Rare overall, but most common tumor in young men age 28–32 |
| 13. Head and neck | Appears good (data somewhat scarce): several active agents MTX with 50% response rate when optimally used; most drugs not studied; almost no combination data | Good: both surgery and radiotherapy curative; 50% overall 5-year survival—varies with location of primary lesion | 31,000 new cases yearly with =10,000 deaths |
| 14. Brain | Poor: one active class of drugs with minimal impact on survival; most drugs not studied; no combination data | Depends on histologic type in Grade III or IV glioma, no curative potential with surgery or x-ray alone; overall survival at 5 years of all types is 28% | 8,000 estimated yearly deaths from all types; attacks the young |
| 15. Kidney | None—most drugs not tested | Fair: 36% overall 5-year survival | Estimated 9,000 deaths per year |
| 16. Esophagus | None | Dismal | Relatively uncommon |

dures can provide *pain relief* for patients whose pain cannot be controlled with analgesics and narcotics.

*Cancer cell seeding during surgery* There is always the risk of disseminating cancer cells during an operative procedure. This may occur if cancer cells (from the tumor, involved lymph nodes, contaminated gloves and instruments, or cut lymphatics and blood vessels), enter the wound. Preventive measures include plastic drapes, changing instruments after biopsy, cauterization of tumor edges (if tumor is incised), and wound irrigation with cytotoxic solutions. Vascular dissemination of tumor cells may be prevented by *minimizing manipulation of tumor masses.* This principle of "no touch" is also applicable during physical examination procedures.

*Nursing intervention* Nursing intervention for patients in the preoperative period should focus on preparation for surgery, teaching about the postoperative period, and any additional therapy. Preparation of the patient includes both physical and emotional factors. Many cancer patients are malnourished and anemic and suffer from vitamin deficiencies and defects in blood coagulation. These deficiency states must be corrected with high protein diets (frequently hyperalimentation), blood transfusion, and vitamin supplements. Failure to achieve the patient's optimal physical condition increases the chance of surgical mortality.

Emotional factors affecting the patient frequently include fear of the operative procedure and misunderstanding about the diagnosis. Before doing elaborate teaching, the nurse must assess the patient's readiness for and ability to comprehend information about the cancer. Often a family member will be able to help the patient understand; it is therefore useful to include this person in teaching sessions.

Patients should be instructed about the immediate postoperative period, including deep-breathing techniques, care of ostomies or tubes, and a general description of what may be expected after the operative procedure. This is particularly important if the surgery is disfiguring, alters normal body function, or affects sexual identity. The surgeon must explain the effects of the surgery, but the nurse may clarify any questions and assess the patient's level of understanding.

Nursing intervention during the postoperative period is directed toward assisting the patient with an uncomplicated recovery. Anticipation of compli-cations is critical, as is early intervention. Important considerations include (1) maintenance of vital physiologic functions, protection of operative sites, and accurate monitoring, interpreting, and reporting of pertinent observations about changes in the patient's condition; (2) prevention of infection through aseptic management of surgical sites, maintenance of respiratory function, and passive exercises; (3) assistance in early ambulation; (4) appropriate management of pain with analgesics; (5) maintenance of optimal nutritional status; (6) involvement in total rehabilitation, both physical and psychosocial; and (7) preparation of patients for further therapy such as radiation or chemotherapy.

**R**adiotherapy Radiation is a phenomenon which occurs naturally throughout the universe and is a normal component of the human environment. It was not recognized, however, until 1895, when Wilhelm Conrad Roentgen discovered x-rays (rays of unknown origin). X-rays are emitted when electrons within an atom are excited, accelerate to high speed, and strike an appropriate excitable metal target. X-rays can penetrate material which is opaque to normal light, produce fluorescence of certain materials, and blacken silver emulsion on a photographic plate. These properties are invaluable in radiology, where they are utilized to produce diagnostic x-rays. The effects of radiation are the result of the absorption of the energy carried and released by the rays. Radiotherapy is used in high doses to exploit the lethal qualities of this energy to kill cells.

Two types of radiation are employed in the treatment of cancer: *electromagnetic radiation* (x-rays and gamma rays) and *particulate radiation* (beta and alpha particles and neutrons). The common characteristic of all radiation energies is the capacity to ionize atoms within the tissues penetrated.[50] Exposure to radiation is measured in *roentgens.* Energy output is calibrated in roentgens per minute for a specified distance. Actual absorption of radiation by tissue, a measurable factor in determining biologic effect, is measured by *rads.*

*Electromagnetic radiation* Electromagnetic radiation can be produced within a vacuum tube in which electrons are excited by applying an electric current across the tube. This type of man-made apparatus is used in x-ray machinery. Radium, a naturally occurring radioactive element, is a source of x-rays called gamma rays, which are produced by nuclear disintegration. Radioactive substances such as cobalt-60 may be created from non-radio-active elements. X-rays and gamma rays share many of the physical characteristics of visible light and infrared rays: they have short wavelengths, and they penetrate water and tissue, which are low in atomic weight, but cannot penetrate material such as lead, which has a high density.

The mechanism by which electromagnetic radiation exerts its biologic effect is a complicated process consisting of many interactions. Basically, a quantity of energy collides with an orbital electron in an atom of the tissue, knocking it out of position and producing an ion or electrically charged particle, which in turn ionizes or excites molecules within the surrounding tissue. As a result of this energy transfer, charged particles and other ionizing agents are formed within the cell. These products interact with cellular DNA and produce widespread disruption and damage to DNA molecules. While the exact nature of the lethal lesion is undefined, the loss of the DNA molecule's integrity results in faulty transcription of genetic information, defective DNA repair, and, eventually, death of daughter cells during future cell division.[51]

*Particulate radiation* Natural and artificial atomic reactions also produce a variety of *particulate radiations.* Particulate radiations have physical characteristics which are substantially different from electromagnetic radiations. Ionization occurs as a result of the direct collision of energized particles with orbital electrons of the nuclei in irradiated tissue. The biologic effect of particulate radiation is a function of the particular mass and charge of the energized particles (electrons, mesons, positrons, neutrons, protons, deuterons, and alpha rays). The depth to which these particles can penetrate is a function of the energy with which they are propelled and the mass of the particle. Alpha particles are unable to penetrate paper; beta particles penetrate paper but not wood. Particulate radiations have denser ionizing beams, transfer energy to a narrower area, and can therefore be directed into localized areas of tissue. Particulate radiation produces more damage to tissue per rad dose than x-rays or gamma rays.[52]

Tumor masses contain a fraction of cells which are deficient in oxygen and less sensitive to the effects of radiation. Part of the greater biologic effect of particulate radiation occurs because the heavy particles are equally effective in killing *both* hypoxic and well-oxygenated cells. X-rays and gamma rays can be made more effective in killing hypoxic cells by *fractionating* (dividing) the total dose to permit reoxygenation of tumor cells between treatments.

*Tumor sensitivity* Tumors can be defined as *sensitive* or *resistant* to radiotherapy. For clinical purposes, sensitivity to irradiation of all types is defined by the dose that will kill all tumor tissue in the irradiated field and still allow recovery of normal irradiated tissues. Most tumor tissue can be destroyed by radiation, but the dose required in some cancers is too toxic to normal tissue in the radiation fields. These cancers are designated *radioresistant.*

Tumor cells and normal cells that are in active mitosis are more sensitive to radiation. Also, radiosensitivity of malignant tumor cells is usually commensurate with the radiosensitivity of their cell of origin. Epithelial cells, hair follicles, hematopoietic cells, and germinal cells are highly radiosensitive because they are rapidly dividing. One can see this exemplified in the toxic effects of radiation described later in this chapter.

*Treatment schedules Fractionation* of the total dose of radiation over time is designed to allow maximal repair of sublethal damage in normal tissue. This also helps to overcome the protective effect that hypoxia creates for tumor cells and minimizes radiation sickness. The total dose of radiation should be stated as to time and daily dosage parameters (e.g., 4000 rads at 200 rads/day for 5 days/week over 4 weeks).

*Radiation equipment* Different types of equipment are utilized to generate suitable radiation for the treatment of particular cancers. Radiation energy is measured in electron volts (eV); low energy is measured in thousands of electron volts or kilovolts (keV), and high energy is measured in millions of electron volts, or megavolts (MeV). Radiation equipment which generates energy in the range of 40 to 140 keV (40,000 to 140,000 volts) is utilized for the treatment of superficial lesions of the skin. At this voltage the x-rays generated can penetrate only short distances before all their energy is released and absorbed. Tissues beyond a specific distance receive little or no radiation damage.

When deeper penetration of x-rays is required, more powerful equipment must be utilized. Radiation energy which is generated in the range of 200 to 300 keV is referred to as *orthovoltage radiation.* Since greater penetration is achieved, treatment of deeper areas, such as the entire tissue of the breast, is possible. The maximum dose of radiation still occurs on the skin surface; the degree of skin toxicity encountered depends on the dose of radiation and the sites irradiated. In areas such as the groin and axilla, where skin is moist and in apposition to other skin surfaces, the reaction may be severe, limiting the dose that can be tolerated. The patient must be rotated in order to administer the total dose to the area from different directions and thus reduce skin toxicity. Although orthovoltage equipment is still widely used, it is generally considered obsolete and should no longer be used for the definitive treatment of cancer (other than skin cancer).

As the energy of the equipment increases, radiation emitted becomes more penetrating and is referred to as *supervoltage radiation.* The percentage of radiation delivered to a specific depth as compared to the dose at the skin surface increases as the radiation energy is increased. The *cobalt-60 unit* is the most common supervoltage unit in use today. Cobalt-59 is placed inside a nuclear reactor, where the nucleus captures a neutron. Cobalt-60, an unstable radioactive material with a half-life of 5¼ years, is produced and, when placed in a shielded x-ray unit, serves as the radiation source. The energy produced by the gamma ray emissions is equal to the energy of a 3-million-volt x-ray machine. Supervoltage radiation is also produced by powerful machines such as linear accelerators, which produce energy in the range of 4 to 10 MeV (4 to 10 million volts). Linear accelerators produce high-intensity x-ray beams by accelerating low-energy electrons on electromagnetic waves in wave guides. The electrons strike a target and produce x-rays. Such equipment produces powerful beams of radiation which can penetrate deeply and can be utilized in the treatment of deep-seated tumors such as lymphomas and cancers of the uterine cervix and bladder. With supervoltage therapy, only 10 to 20 percent of the maximum dose of radiation is deposited in skin, so there is less toxicity at the site of entry. However, the energy of these rays is so powerful that the skin within the exit field may still receive a high dose of radiation and develop evidence of toxicity. Linear accelerators can deliver several hundred rads per minute, and patient discomfort is minimized by short treatment times.

Supervoltage units have three characteristics which make them particularly desirable. First, high-energy transfer reduces radiation scatter to normal tissues outside the treatment field. This reduces the incidence of radiation sickness, which is related to the volume of body tissue that receives significant radiation. Secondly, the amount of energy absorbed by bone is reduced; and finally, superficial tissue, notably skin, is spared. Supervoltage radiation is almost always employed for deep-seated lesions.

Modern radiotherapy equipment such as the linear accelerator is capable of generating energy in the *megavoltage* range (in excess of 10 million electron volts) as well as supervoltage radiation. The *betatron* can produce radiation up to 18 MeV by exciting electrons in a circular magnetic field. Betatrons have the same treatment characteristics as linear accelerators. Particulate radiation units are not widely available, since they require cyclotrons to generate the beam. However, clinical trials with fast-neutron generators and pi-meson particles have begun in the United States and elsewhere.

*Curative radiotherapy* Cancers which are amenable to cure by radiotherapy are those which tend to remain relatively localized and are *radiosensitive.* The pattern of metastasis must be predictable and, in general, limited to regional nodes relatively close to the primary lesion. Such cancers include Stages I and II Hodgkin's disease, localized lymphocytic and histiocytic lymphomas, cancer of the uterine cervix, seminomas of the testis, and a variety of head and neck tumors. Radiotherapy to the brain and spinal cord may be used in acute leukemia to kill malignant cells not effectively treated with chemotherapy.[53,54]

Postoperative radiotherapy is frequently administered when the local tumor is inoperable because of its anatomic location, when a tumor is operable but not completely resectable and nodal metastases are suspected, or with excisional surgery to avoid a more extensive procedure (e.g., "lumpectomy" or simple mastectomy plus radiation instead of radical mastectomy).[55]

Preoperative radiation may increase the curative potential of surgery in rectal cancer and in head and neck tumors. Relatively low doses of radiation are employed to kill tumor cells without compromising the integrity of normal tissue. In this way, preoperative irradiation permits the use of less extensive surgery.[56]

Prophylactic radiotherapy has been used successfully to treat the brain and spinal cord before clinical evidence of disease has developed. This is a standard part of the therapeutic program for children with acute lymphocytic leukemia (see Chap. 7).

*Radioactive implants* permit the delivery of high doses of radiation to localized areas in specific tissues. The rationale for using radioactive implants is that the dose of radiation decreases rapidly as the distance from the source increases. Considerations for use of local radiation include (1) a relatively well-defined tumor, (2) a need for a larger dosage than can be administered by an external source, (3) a critical need to restrict the amount of normal tissue receiving radiation, and (4) accessibility of the site for introduction of the radiation source. Radium and cobalt are the most common sources of radiation used in local implants. Implants may be placed permanently or may be temporary applications to achieve a specific therapeutic dose. The source of radiation is placed in sealed containers, such as molds, which can be inserted into body cavities such as the mouth or vagina (*intracavitary radiation*) or applied to body surfaces such as the skin or lip. In addition, the radioactive source may be inserted directly into malignant tissues within needles or seeds which are implanted during surgery at calculated distances (*interstitial radiation*).[57]

*Palliative radiotherapy*  Radiotherapy is frequently useful for local palliation of uncontrolled symptomatic metastases, especially in lymph nodes, soft tissue, and bone. Indications for use of radiation are (1) pain, (2) threatened ulceration, (3) compression of vital structures such as the brain, spinal cord, or superior vena cava, and (4) bony metastases which are likely to develop pathologic fractures, especially lesions in weight-bearing areas such as the femur or a vertebral body. Generally, patients in these situations have widespread disease and require systemic treatment to achieve true tumor control. Treatment schedules should be planned, when possible, so that they do not compromse the delivery of systemic therapy.

*Nursing intervention*  It is difficult to accurately predict the exact severity of any of the side effects associated with radiotherapy. A dose of radiation which is tolerated in one patient may produce severe toxicosis in another. Radiation-induced toxicosis may be *localized,* affecting only tissues within the radiation field, or *generalized,* causing radiation sickness.[58] Radiation dosages and schedules are fractionated to produce minimal side effects.

The incidence and severity of generalized *radiation sickness* is related to the volume of body tissue which receives significant amounts of radiation. Radiation sickness occurs most frequently when large fields are irradiated, particularly the upper abdomen; it is manifested by nausea, vomiting, and anorexia. The cause is thought to be related to toxic products produced by the destruction of tumor cells within irradiated tissue, as well as the effect of radiation on the mucous membrane of the gastrointestinal tract. Nursing intervention should include the liberal administration of antiemetics and adequate hydration. If nausea is severe enough to cause dehydration, administration of intravenous fluids should be instituted.

*Skin toxicosis* is commonly encountered within radiation fields. This is thought to be due to the fact that epithelial cells are constantly dividing and are in the direct path of the radiation. The dose of radiation received by skin surfaces can be minimized with the use of modern supervoltage equipment (such as the cobalt-60 unit and the linear accelerator). Moist skin in areas like the axilla, perineum, and groin, where skin surfaces are in apposition, tolerates radiation less well, and doses must be reduced to avoid severe toxicity. Skin toxicosis resembles damage from heat burns and ranges from mild erythema and hair loss to blistering and desquamation of skin. More extensive damage to skin represents an overdose of radiation and can, like third-degree heat burns, require skin grafting. In addition to causing burnlike damage, radiation can cause permanent skin pigmentation and dysplastic reactions. Physical injury to irradiated skin may cause painful ulcerations which heal slowly because of fibrotic changes and impaired circulation.

Nursing intervention for radiation-induced skin toxicosis consists of the following measures:

1    Vigorous washing should be avoided to prevent removal of markings which define the field and to reduce irritation. Skin should be kept dry and clean with baby powder or cornstarch, which absorbs perspiration and contains no irritants. Powders containing heavy metals (e.g., zinc oxide), which produce radiation scatter on skin surfaces within radiation fields, should be avoided.

2    All friction should be minimized. This includes shaving, tight constricting clothing, belts, straps, and stiff collars. If a male must shave, an electric razor should be used.

3    Patients should avoid strong sunlight and should protect irradiated skin from extremes of temperature and wind.

4    Patients should avoid synthetic fibers, such as nylon, which are not porous and do not let skin breathe.

5    Nonadherent dressings and paper tape should be used if desquamation occurs. Application of ointments or lotions should be ordered specifically by the radiotherapist to avoid irritants or contaminants that contain heavy metals.

When the radiotherapy is completed, the time period that must elaspse before normal skin care may be resumed will depend on the severity of the reaction encountered. Generally, patients can wash treated areas within 3 weeks but should use bland soaps. When toxicosis occurs, the skin will be hypersensitive for some months after the completion of therapy.

*Mucositis* is a radiation-induced toxicosis that is frequently encountered when tissues lined with mucous membrane lie within the radiation fields. The tissues commonly affected are the oropharynx and esophagus, intestinal mucosa (small and large bowel and rectum), and the vagina. Mucositis is characterized by tenderness, erythema, and dryness, which may progress to patchy inflammation of irradiated membranes, becoming confluent. Areas of *ulceration* may exist underneath the inflamed membranes, and a serosanguineous exudate can be seen. Attempts to debride damaged tissues can frequently induce frank bleeding. These areas may persist for several weeks. Healing of the ulcerated mucosa beneath the membrane must occur before the inflammatory reaction subsides. Complete healing may take 1 to 2 months, during which sensitive tissues must be kept meticulously clean and protected from further damage.

Radiation toxicosis to the oropharynx is compounded by damage to the salivary glands and the loss of *saliva*. Saliva is a natural lubricant which facilitates the chewing, digestion, and swallowing of food; it also has bacteriostatic properties. The absence of saliva promotes tooth decay and allows thick, tenacious mucus to develop, predisposing damaged tissues to infection. Lack of saliva contributes to the dysphagia experienced by patients with mucositis and the compromise of optimal hydration and nutrition. Nursing measures consist primarily of meticulous hygiene. Oral ulcerations should be irrigated with mild solutions and oxidizing agents. Prophylactic measures such as the use of an antifungal mouthwash can reduce the incidence of opportunistic infections caused by organisms such as *Candida*. The patient's diet should be served at moderate temperatures and should be bland and soft in texture or blenderized, to reduce irritation to sensitive tissues. Gravies and sauces facilitate the swallowing of solid foods when saliva is reduced or lost. Nutritional supplements should be used to augment the caloric intake. Analgesics should be administered liberally so that nutrition is not compromised by pain. The nurse assists patients in the proper use of topical anesthetics such as Xylocaine or anesthetic sprays.

Similar toxicosis of mucous membranes of the intestine and rectum occur, characterized by *pain* and *diarrhea,* which may be profuse and bloody. Intravenous fluid replacement may be required. The toxic condition may persist for several weeks before improvement is seen. Severe radiation damage may cause chronic or recurrent symptoms which persist for years.

*Respiratory dysfunction* occurs when pulmonary tissue is irradiated; severe inflammation may occur and is manifested clinically as an *interstitial pneumonitis*. Acute respiratory distress may result if a significant volume of lung is irradiated. *Pulmonary fibrosis* occurs when damaged tissues heal, causing pulmonary compromise that may be permanent. Nursing care is symptomatic and adjusted to the degree of damage.

Reproductive organs are highly sensitive to the effects of radiation, and *sterility* is frequently produced. The effects of radiation on reproductive capacity must be explained to patients of childbearing age who are likely to be cured of their disease.

Frequently radioactive implants are used to treat tumors of the reproductive system, especially the cervix. Intracavitary and interstitial implants with radioactive substances can cause toxicity to surrounding local tissues. Nurses must know what type of radiation is emitted by the radiation source. Beta rays are effectively blocked by the patient's body or heavy plastic, but shielding from gamma-ray emissions must be provided by lead. The nurse must therefore be aware of the need to limit exposure and to maximize distance between the patient and the professional or the family. Careful handling of urine, feces, and drainage is required and is carried out according to hospital policy. *Psychological support* of the patient in total or semi-isolation is necessary to maintain emotional well-being and requires ingenuity on the part of the entire nursing staff (see Chap. 6 for further discussion).

*Myelosuppression* (depression of white blood cells and platelets) caused by radiation to marrow-bearing areas may cause life-threatening or fatal toxicosis. It is important to monitor hematologic status and to interrupt therapy if profound myelosuppression occurs. The effects of radiation on bone marrow are related to the dose and volume of marrow irradiated. Patients may be placed on "reverse isolation" to protect them from exposure to infectious agents. They may also receive transfusion of needed blood components.

*Other radiation effects* may include permanent

damage to tissues of the kidneys, liver, spinal cord, and lens of the eye. Fortunately, severe complications, such as *radionecrosis* (radiation-caused tissue death), are not common. However, nurses caring for irradiated patients must be aware of any signs or symptoms indicating particular organ damage, so that appropriate intervention can be instituted.

**C**hemotherapy   The chemotherapy of cancer has its roots in the development of successful drug therapy for infectious diseases. Evidence of the antitumor potential of chemicals was documented as long ago as 1865, when potassium arsenite produced remissions in chronic leukemia patients. In 1919, autopsies of soldiers exposed to fatal doses of mustard gas demonstrated evidence of selective atrophy of lymphoid and bone marrow tissues.[59] In the 1940s investigators began to study a derivative of mustard gas in mouse lymphosarcoma and noted that the agent produced tumor regression. In 1946, dramatic though short-lived tumor regression with nitrogen mustard was reported in patients with advanced Hodgkin's disease, lymphosarcoma, and chronic leukemia that had been unresponsive to conventional therapy.[60]

*Therapeutic concepts*   Figure 5-5 depicts the reduction in tumor size observed during chemotherapy with single agents and combination programs. Reduction in tumor size depends on the rate of cell destruction, the rate of cell removal, and the rate of regrowth of both sensitive and resistant tumor cells. It is known that antibiotics kill a constant fraction of susceptible organisms rather than a fixed number. This concept is known as *first-order kinetics* and is applicable to the destruction of tumor cells by chemotherapeutic agents.[61] Simply stated, this means that a given dose of drug will kill a specific percentage of cells. If the drug destroys 99 percent of the tumor cells, it will reduce 1,000,000 tumor cells to 10 cells and 100,000 cells to 1 cell. It is also crucial to remember that a single surviving cancer cell can and will multiply and kill the patient if not destroyed by therapy or by the host defenses.

Both single drugs and combinations kill at constant rates, but effective combinations destroy a greater fraction of tumor cells. In addition, combinations prevent regrowth of tumor cells because they cause multiple cellular lesions which are less effectively repaired. As a result, consecutive doses of combination therapy are maximally effective because the tumor burden is markedly reduced with

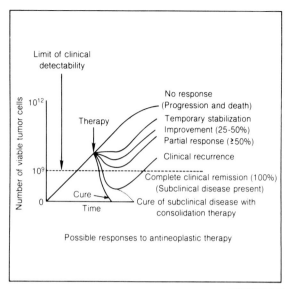

**FIGURE 5-5**
Possible responses to neoplastic therapy.

each successive course of medication. It is important to remember that the *level necessary for clinical detection is a volume of 1 billion cells (1 × 10⁹).* Below this "level of clinical detection" there are large numbers of cells which can be thought of as *subclinical disease.* The major difficulty in all cancer therapy is inability to measure residual subclinical disease (Fig. 5-5).

In the past twenty-five years over 40 drugs with antitumor activity have been identified, and 25 are now commercially available. Agents can be grouped into six major categories: alkylating agents, antimetabolites, plant alkaloids, antibiotics, steroid hormones, some miscellaneous agents which are not easily classified, and immunologic stimulants.[62-67] Table 5-4 lists chemotherapeutic agents by class, and Table 5-5 lists various hormonally active agents. The tables present active drugs, indications, dosage, schedules, and major toxicities. Figure 5-6 depicts the mechanisms of action of anticancer drugs at a cellular level.

*Alkylating agents*   Alkylating agents are a class of drug which interferes with the structure of DNA, the carrier of the genetic material of the cell. They are able to substitute an alkyl group for hydrogen atoms, causing breaks in the molecule and cross-linking of the DNA strands. Because synthesis of other cellular components continues, growth becomes unbalanced and cell death results. The antitumor activity of alkylating agents is *not* cell cycle–specific. This means that they are effective in killing

**TABLE 5-4**
CHEMOTHERAPY AGENTS IN CLINICAL USE CLASSIFIED BY MECHANISMS OF ACTION

| Commercially Available Drugs | Dose, Route, and Schedule | Acute Toxicity | Bone Marrow Suppression 1+ (mild) to 4+ (severe) | Other Toxicity | Comments and Nursing Implications |
|---|---|---|---|---|---|
| **ALKYLATING AGENTS** | | | | | |
| Mechlorethamine (nitrogen mustard, Mustargen) | 0.4 mg/kg IV q 3–4 wk | Severe nausea and vomiting (N & V) in ½–2 h | 4+ | Powerful vesicant; avoid eye, skin contact | Rapid alkylating action; direct instillation can control malignant effusion |
| Cyclophosphamide (Cytoxan, CYT) | 500–1500 mg/m² IV q 3–4 wk 60–120 mg/m² po qd continuous | N & V is dose-related; occurs in 4–12 h post IV admin. | 3+ | Alopecia in 50%, occurs in 3 wk; hemorrhagic cystitis; hepatotoxicity | Force fluids to 3 liters with high doses IV to prevent cystitis |
| Chlorambucil (Leukeran) | 0.1–0.2 mg/kg po qd | Rare N & V at high doses | 3+ | | Continuous daily oral administration |
| L-Phenylalanine mustard (melphalan, l-PAM) | 0.2 mg/kg po qd × 5 q 4–6 wk | Minimal N & V | 3+ | With prolonged administration, can cause persistant thrombocytopenia | Used in 5-day courses in adjuvant therapy |
| Busulfan (myleran) | 0.05–0.2 mg/kg po qd | Rare N & V | 3+ | Hyperpigmentation of skin; pulmonary fibrosis ("busulfan lung"); gynecomastia | Continuous daily oral administration, renal excretion; check kidney function |
| Triethylene thiophosphoramide (TSPA, thiotepa) | 0.8 mg/kg IV q 3–4 wk | Rare N & V | 3+ | Can cause allergic reactions; dermatitis, headache, fever | Can be given intramuscularly; intracavitary installation for control of malignant effusions |
| **ANTIMETABOLITES** | | | | | |
| 5-Fluorouracil (5-FU) | 7.5–12 mg/kg IV qd = 5d, then qod to toxicity or q wk | Occasional N & V | 3+ | Chronic N & V after prolonged administration; stomatitis, diarrhea, ataxia, photophobia, alopecia | Oral administration of IV preparation possible but seems less effective |
| 6-Thioguanine (6-TG) | 2 mg/(kg)(day) po qd, IV preparation under investigation | Occasional N & V | 3+ | Diarrhea, stomatitis | Hepatic metabolism, urine excretion; use at reduced doses in patients with renal or hepatic dysfunction |
| 6-Mercaptopurine (6-MP) | 2.5 mg/(kg)(day) po | Occasional N & V | 3+ | Stomatitis; hepatotoxicity | Allopurinol delays degradation of 6-MP and increases toxicity; concurrent use of both drugs requires decrease of 6-MP dose to only 30% of normal dose for therapeutic effect with tolerable toxicity |
| Arabinosyl cytosine (ara-C) | 200 mg/m² IV qd × 5 q 2–3 wk; can be given subcutaneously | Dose-related N & V | 4+ | Stomatitis, diarrhea, alopecia, hepatotoxicity | Intrathecal administration for CNS disease; hepatic metabolism, renal excretion |
| Methotrexate (MTX) | 20–80 mg/m² IV, IM, po, q wk | Mild N & V | 3+ | Stomatitis, GI ulceration, hepatotoxicity | Renal excretion; nephrotoxic at high dose; decreased effect with salicylates |
| | 15 mg/m² intrathecal q wk | None | 1+ | Arachnoiditis, neurotoxicity | Intrathecal dose should replace systemic dose in leukemic patients or be given with leucovorin rescue |

| Drug | Dose | Nausea & Vomiting | | Toxicity | Comments |
|---|---|---|---|---|---|
| | "High-dose" MTX 2–10 mg/m² IV over 6 h q 3–4 wk; calcium leucovorin rescue mandatory | Moderate N & V | +/– | Renal failure at high doses due to crystallization of drug in kidneys | Urine should be alkyline to prevent crystallization; high doses lethal without rescue with leucovorin |
| **PLANT ALKALOIDS** | | | | | |
| Vincristine (VCR, Oncovin) | 0.5–2 mg/m² IV q wk | Rare N & V | 1+/– | Paresthesias, weakness, areflexia, motor weakness, constipation, abdominal or jaw pain, alopecia, hoarseness; tissue necrosis if extravasated | Neurotoxicity increased in elderly and immobilized patients; paralytic ileus; increased neurotoxicity and myelosuppression in patients with severe hepatic damage owing to hepatic metabolism and excretion |
| Vinblastine (VLB) | 0.1–0.3 mg/kg IV q wk | Occasional N & V | 3+ | Headache, minimal neurotoxicity, alopecia, cumulative myelotoxicity; diarrhea, stomatitis; tissue necrosis if extravasated | Decrease dose with hepatic dysfunction; myelosuppression severe compared to vincristine |
| **ANTIBIOTICS** | | | | | |
| Actinomycin D (bactinomycin, Cosmegen) | 0.015 mg/(kg)(day) × 5 IV q 3–4 wk | Severe N & V in 4–5 h | 3+ | Alopecia, stomatitis, diarrhea; anorexia lasting days to weeks; tissue necrosis if extravasated | Severe skin reactions in previously irradiated areas |
| Mithramycin | 0.05 mg/kg qod IV to toxicity | Moderate N & V in 6 h | 3+ | Fever, stomatitis, facial flush, CNS alterations, azotemia, hemorrhage due to drug-induced clotting abnormalities and severe thrombocytopenia; hypokalemia, hypocalcemia, neuromuscular hyperexcitability | Stop drug if rise in BUN or LDH; causes hypocalcemia—useful in treatment of tumor-related hypercalcemia |
| | 0.025 mg/kg dose for hypercalcemia | None | 0 | | |
| Adriamycin (Adria, Doxorubicin) | 45–60 mg/m² IV q 3–4 wk | Moderate to severe N & V | 4+ | Stomatitis, diarrhea; tissue necrosis if extravasated; alopecia and loss of all body hair in 20% of patients; hepatotoxicity | Cardiotoxicity may be irreversible and fatal; total dose limitation of 550 mg/m²; urine may turn red from excretion of metabolites |
| Daunorubicin (Daunomycin, Rubidomycin) | 30 mg/m² IV qd × 3d q 3–4 wk | Moderate to severe N & V | 4+ | Stomatitis, alopecia, skin rash; tissue necrosis if extravasated; anaphylactic reactions can occur | Cardiotoxicity, total dose limitation 550 mg/m²; urine may turn red from excretion of metabolites |
| Bleomycin (Blenoxane, Bleo) | 15 units/m² IV, IM, subcutaneous (SC) q wk; 5 units/m² IV, IM, SC 2/wk | Minimal N & V | 1+ | Anaphylactic reaction, fever and hypotension frequent; macular rash can progress to ulcerations of skin; hyperpigmentation, alopecia, stomatitis | Administration of Benadryl and Tylenol to reduce febrile reactions; pulmonary fibrosis, common at 300 m/m², can occur at low doses —may be lethal but is often reversible with steroid therapy |
| **NITROSOUREA COMPOUNDS** | Probably activated by alkylation | | | | |
| BCNU (carmustine) | 200 mg/m² IV q 4–6 wk | Severe N & V in 6–12 h | 4+ | Brown spots on skin if direct contact occurs; bone marrow suppression delayed to 4–6 wk | Sensation of burning on vein and generalized flushing due to alcohol diluent; crosses blood-brain barrier |
| CCNU (Lomustine) | 130 mg/m² po q 4–6 wk | Moderate to severe N & V in 2–6 h | 4+ | Delayed marrow toxicity at 4–6 wk; cumulative marrow suppression | Should be taken on empty stomach; crosses blood-brain barrier |
| Methyl CCNU (Semustine) | 200 mg/m² po q 4–6 wk | Moderate to severe N & V | 4+ | Delayed marrow suppression at 4–6 wk; more pronounced thrombocytopenia | Take on empty stomach |

**TABLE 5-4**
CHEMOTHERAPY AGENTS IN CLINICAL USE CLASSIFIED BY MECHANISMS OF ACTION (*Continued*)

| Commercially Available Drugs | Dose, Route, and Schedule | Acute Toxicity | Bone Marrow Suppression 1+ (mild) to 4+ (severe) | Other Toxicity | Comments and Nursing Implications |
|---|---|---|---|---|---|
| Streptozoticin | 500 mg/m² IV qd × 5d q 3 wk; 1500 mg/m² IV q wk | Moderate N & V | 0 | Renal tubular acidosis; can cause anuria—prevent with infusion of 1–2 liters normal saline; hepatotoxicity; reactive hypoglycemia; rapid infusion causes localburning | No marrow toxicity; diabetogenic —test urine for glucose and proteinuria prior to each dose, discontinue if grossly positive |
| **MISCELLANEOUS COMPOUNDS** | | | | | |
| Procarbazine (Mutulane, methylhydrazine) | 100–200 mg/kg po qd; continuous oral admin.; IV admin. investigational | Moderate to severe N & V subsiding with daily doses | 3+ | CNS alterations: somnolence. hyperexcitability; rare psychosis; postural hypotension, allergic skin rash; alcohol ingestion can result in Antabuse effect | Potentiates effects of phenothiazines; inhibition of monoamine oxidase; tyramine-rich foods can cause hypertensive crises (beer, wine, ripe cheese); CNS toxicity in large IV doses |
| L-Asparaginase | 1–5,000 IU/(kg)(day) × 14–28 | Severe N & V in 50% | 0 | Fever, hepatotoxicity, acute pancreatitis; anaphylactic reactions; CNS toxicity; azotemia; hyperglycemia, coagulation abnormalities | Physician should be present during infusion because anaphylactic reactions may occur; desensitization can be done with test doses |
| Hydroxyurea (Hydrea) | 25 mg/kg po qd continuous; 100 mg/kg IV push q3d | Minimal N & V | 3+ | GI ulcerations, skin rash, alopecia | Rapid reduction of high blast counts when given IV; marked effect seen in 24–48 h |
| Hexamethylmelamine | 6–10 mg/kg po qd continuous | Severe N & V | 1+ | Peripheral neuropathy, motor weakness, dysphasia, somnolence, depression, hallucinations, diarrhea | Exacerbation of VCR neuropathy, N & V may require discontinuation of drug |
| Imidazole carboxamide (DTIC) | 250 mg/m² IV × 5d q 3 wk | Severe N & V | 3+ | Flu-like syndromes, headache, myalgias, malaise, mild hepatotoxicity; local venous burning at infusion site | Protect from light when administered |
| O, p'DDD (mitotane, lysodren) | 2–10 g/qd po continuous | Severe N & V | 0 | Skin rash, motor weakness, confusion, depression, diplopia, vertigo, diarrhea | N & V may require discontinuation of drug; hypoadrenocorticism may be permanent |
| **IMMUNE STIMULANTS** | (10⁶–10⁸ viable organisms) | | | | |
| BCG (bacillus Calmette-Guerin) substrains; Pasteur, Connaught, TKE, GLAXO, | Intradermal, scarification, intralesional, in multiple-sites q 1–4 wk | Flu-like syndrome with variable N & V | 0 | Local inflammation, necrosis, fever, flu-like syndrome, myalgia, regional lymphadenopathy, hepatotoxicity | Systemic BCG infection if live organisms are used rather than attenuated organisms; anaphylactoid reactions |
| MER (methanol-extracted residue of BCG) | 0.5–1 mg in multiple sites q 3–4 wk intradermal | Flu-like syndrome with variable N & V | 0 | Local inflammation & ulceration, regional lymphadenopathy, fever, malaise | Investigational |
| Corynebacterium parvum | 2.5 mg/m² IV, subcutaneous q 1–4 wk | Flu-like syndrome with variable N & V | 0 | Local pain, ulcerations, flu-like syndrome, fever | Investigational |

resting cells as well as cells which are dividing or preparing to divide.

*Antimetabolites* An antimetabolite is a chemical analogue, a drug which resembles an essential metabolite so closely that it enters the essential metabolic pathways. An antimetabolite, however, interferes with or blocks normal biosynthesis of nucleic acids necessary for synthesis of DNA and RNA. Antimetabolites are *cell cycle–specific.* Their antitumor activity is exerted when cells are in the *synthetic phase* of the cell cycle (S phase). Antimetabolites can be subdivided into purine, pyrimidine, and folic acid antagonists. Several antimetabolites are dependent on adequate hepatic function for degradation or inactivation of the drug. Severe liver abnormalities therefore make dose reduction necessary to prevent increased toxicity.

*Plant alkaloids* Certain antitumor agents are prepared from plants. The two most common are vin-

cristine and vinblastine, which are derived from the periwinkle plant. These agents cause *metaphase arrest* by inhibiting spindle formation during cell mitosis. Although the two have very similar structure, mechanism of action, and metabolism, their dosage, toxicity, and antitumor spectrum are different. While vincristine causes little bone marrow toxicity, this is the major side effect of vinblastine. Neurotoxicity, which is probably related to binding of both agents to spindle proteins, is the major toxicity with vincristine administration but is minimal with the use of vinblastine. Both agents are metabolized by the liver and excreted into the bile. Inordinate toxicity is observed in patients with severely compromised hepatic function and also in elderly patients.

*Antitumor antibiotics* Antibiotics effective against cancer are a heterogeneous group of compounds produced by various bacterial and fungal organisms. Most antibiotics are *not* cell cycle–specific.

**TABLE 5-5**
HORMONAL AGENTS IN CLINICAL USE IN CANCER THERAPY

| Drug | Dose, Route, and Schedule | Side Effects | Indications for Use |
|---|---|---|---|
| ADRENAL CORTICAL STEROIDS | | | |
| Prednisone (Deltasone) | 40–60 mg/m² po qd | No acute toxicity | Leukemia, Hodgkin's disease, non-Hodgkin's lymphomas, multiple myeloma (used frequently in drug combinations) |
| Prednisolone (Delta Cortef) | 40–60 mg/m² po IM | Immunosuppression: infection, gastrointestinal bleeding, ulcers, hypertension; moon facies, edema, diabetes, hyperglycemia, electrolyte disturbances; potassium loss; adrenal atrophy, possible osteoporosis; euphoria, emotional lability, psychosis | |
| Methyl prednisone (sodium succinate (Medrol) | 10–125 mg/day IV, IM, po | | |
| Hydrocortisone (Cortef po, IM) (Solu-Cortef IV, IM) | 100–500 mg/day IV | | |
| Dexamethasone (Decadron) | 0.5–16 mg/m² po | | |
| ANDROGENS | | | |
| Testosterone propionate | 50–100 mg 3/wk | Acute toxicity: nausea; varying degrees of masculinization, stimulation of erythropoiesis, hepatotoxicity, fluid retention, hypercalcemia (calusterone: less masculinization) | Breast cancer in postmenopausal women |
| Fluoxymesterone | 10–20 mg po qd continuous | | Aplastic anemia |
| Testolactone | 100 mg po 3/wk | | |
| Calusterone | 0.3 mg/(kg)(day) po continuous | | |
| ESTROGENS | | | |
| Diethystilbesterol | 1–15 mg po qd | Feminization, muscle weakness, uterine bleeding, fluid retention, increased mortality from cardiac disease, hypercalcemia | Prostatic cancer |
| Ethinyl estradiol (Estinyl) | 0.1–3 mg po qd | | Breast cancer in postmenopausal women |
| PROGESTINS | | | |
| Hydroxyprogesterone | 0.5–1 g 2/wk or 1/wk | No acute toxicity; fluid retention, occasional hypercalcemia, thrombocytosis, thrombotic disorders (pulmonary emboli, cerebral vascular accidents) | Endometrial cancer, renal carcinoma, ovarian carcinoma |
| Medroxyprogesterone acetate (Provera—oral use) Depo-Provera—IM use) | 100–200 mg/d 200–600 mg 2/wk | | |

In general, antibiotics inhibit DNA synthesis by binding with DNA at various points and preventing dependent RNA synthesis.

*Nitrosoureas* Several related *nitrosourea* compounds have been developed which have activity in a variety of neoplasms. The various agents and their indications are listed in Table 5-4. Some are useful both orally and parenterally. Others are available in only one form. Their antitumor spectrum includes Hodgkin's disease, colon and other gastrointestinal cancers, melanoma, multiple myeloma, and brain tumors. Their effectiveness in brain tumors is related to lipid solubility, which permits them to cross the blood-brain barrier with systemic administration. The mechanism of action of nitrosoureas is unclear but resembles alkylating activity in some respects. The most impressive toxicity of this class is delayed bone marrow toxicity, which develops 3 to 4 weeks after administration. As a result, the interval between treatments is usually 6 weeks.

L-*Asparaginase* This compound is the first enzyme to be successfully used in cancer chemotherapy. It

**FIGURE 5-6**

Mechanisms of action of anticancer drugs at a cellular level. (*Reproduced with permission from I. H. Krakoff, "Cancer Chemotherapeutic Agents," Ca–A Cancer Journal for Clinicians, May–June 1977, p. 140.*)

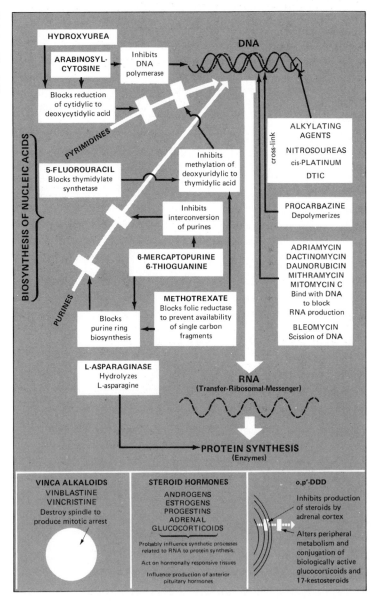

is prepared from various sources, including guinea pig serum, yeast, and *Escherichia coli* bacteria. The enzyme converts L-asparagine, an essential amino acid involved in protein synthesis, to L-aspartic acid. Many leukemic and some lymphoma cells require exogenous L-asparagine stored in body tissues, while normal tissues can independently synthesize this amino acid. Resistance to this drug may be related to an increased production of cellular L-asparagine synthetase, which converts L-aspartic acid to L-asparagine. It is effective in inducing remission of acute lymphoblastic leukemia. Its major life-threatening toxicity is anaphylaxis, which occurs in approximately 15 to 30 percent of patients and may be related to endotoxin contamination. Myelosuppression is rare, but hemolytic anemia, liver dysfunction, severe nausea, and coagulation abnormalities are not uncommon. Acute pancreatitis and hypoglycemia (related to depressed serum-insulin levels) also occur and are dose-related.[68]

*Miscellaneous agents* A variety of other drugs exist whose mechanism of action is unknown or which cannot be classified in any of the groups listed above. Although little is known about their mechanisms of action, the toxicity of many is well documented and should be understood by nurses administering them in cancer treatment (see Table 5-4).

*Immune stimulants and immunotherapy* *Immunocompetence* of the host may be an important surveillance mechanism which prevents the development of neoplasms.[69] Theoretically, the body should recognize tumor-specific or tumor-associated antigens produced on the surface of the cancer cell as foreign. Once the host has recognized this foreign antigen, the immune system attempts to destroy the abnormal cells. Experimental evidence suggests that a normal immune response may continually kill abnormal cells which are formed and which could develop into clinical cancer. It is unclear whether a failure in *immune surveillance* is always involved in tumor initiation. However, it is known that persons with immunodeficiency diseases and those whose immune system is suppressed for prolonged periods (as after renal transplants) have an increased incidence of cancer. Evidence exists to show that an active immune system may be involved in controlling the growth of cancer as well as keeping the process localized. Data suggest that patients whose immune system is intact achieve more complete responses to therapy and that patients who have rapidly progressive disseminated

cancer have impaired or depressed immune responses.

Immunotherapeutic agents are optimally effective when maximal tumor cell removal or destruction is achieved with surgery, radiation, or chemotherapy. The basic rationale for immunotherapy is that certain biologically active substances can generally stimulate the host immune system to destroy the last residual cancer cells, producing a permanent cure. Since radiation and chemotherapy produce immunosuppression, patients should be evaluated for immune reactivity before the institution of immunotherapy.

Immunotherapy can be divided into active and passive categories. An example of *passive immunotherapy* is the transfer of sera containing antibodies to the patient with cancer. *Active immunotherapy* involves the stimulation of the patient's own immune system and can be *specific* or *nonspecific* in nature. Active, nonspecific immunotherapy involves the use of substances which augment cellular and humoral immunity. The three most common agents in clinical use are *bacillus Calmette-Guérin* (BCG), the *methanol-extractable residue of BCG* (MER), and *Corynebacterium parvum* (*C. parvum*). Clinical studies with BCG and MER have shown tumor regressions in patients with cutaneous melanoma after intralesional injections of BCG. When given by scarification, these agents may prevent or delay the development of recurrent disease in surgically resected melanoma patients. BCG and MER are also in use as maintenance therapy in acute myelocytic leukemia after remissions are achieved with combination cheomtherapy. Studies thus far have not demonstrated the clinical value of *C. parvum*.

Active, specific immunotherapy involves immunization of the patient with tumor cells or tumor extracts. Vaccines are prepared from the patient's own tumor cells or from a similar tumor, in an attempt to produce cytotoxic antitumor antibodies which can destroy the patient's tumor.

*Steroid hormones* Adrenal corticosteroids can be administered in large nonphysiologic doses to alter the hormonal balance and to modify the growth of neoplasms. *Prednisone* is the most commonly used steroid hormone. The mechanism of action of corticosteroids is not clearly defined. It is thought that they may interfere at the cell membrane and inhibit the synthesis of RNA to protein. Corticosteroids are known to inhibit mitosis and have the capacity to destroy lymphocytic elements. Corticosteroids are active in a variety of neoplasms. As a single agent, prednisone can induce complete but short remissions in 60 percent of children with acute lymphocytic leukemia.[70] It is also active in lymphomas, multiple myeloma, and breast cancer. Prednisone is commonly used in combination chemotherapy because of its lack of bone marrow toxicity. However, corticosteroids are potent immunosuppressive agents. Steroids also have anti-inflammatory activity, which is useful in the management of cerebral edema; however, this anti-inflammatory property has the disadvantage of disguising the cardinal signs and symptoms of infection.

*Endocrine manipulation*  Tissues which are normally dependent on or responsive to endogenous physiologic hormones are often responsive to endocrine manipulation when the tissues develop neoplasms. Frequently this hormonal dependence can be exploited as therapy. Neoplasms responsive to endocrine manipulation are carcinomas of the breast, endometrium, prostate, and thyroid.

Surgical management of breast cancer has historically used *endocrine ablation* to achieve regression of the disease. *Castration* (oophorectomy) is known to be beneficial in premenopausal women who have experienced tumor recurrence following mastectomy. Failure to respond to castration is now thought to be related to the absence of steroid-binding receptor proteins.[71] Patients who do not respond to ablative endocrine manipulation, such as castration, are unlikely to respond to additional endocrine manipulations and should receive active chemotherapeutic agents. However, 50 percent of patients who respond objectively to castration and then relapse will respond to *adrenalectomy* or to *hypophysectomy*. Such procedures are also successful in the treatment of postmenopausal women who have responded to exogenous estrogen administration. Castration also produces a high response rate (70 percent) in male breast cancer;[72] and in prostatic carcinoma, response to orchiectomy often lasts 2 to 3 years.[73]

*Exogenous estrogen therapy* will produce responses in 35 percent of postmenopausal women with breast cancer without regard to hormone-binding proteins. Estrogens are metabolized in the liver and excreted in urine. In males with recurrent prostatic cancer following orchiectomy, administration of estrogens is beneficial, although there is some risk of cardiovascular complications.[74] *Androgens* produce tumor regression in 20 percent of women with metastatic breast cancer. The best responses are seen in postmenopausal women with osseous disease.[75] *Progestins* are compounds re-

lated to progesterone and are useful in the treatment of metastatic endometrial, breast, and possibly renal cell carcinomas.[76] Remissions in endometrial cancer with the use of progestins occur in 30 percent of patients and may last several years, especially in those women who have experienced a long disease-free interval between primary resection and recurrent disease or who have well-differentiated tumors. Major hormonal agents are described in Table 5-5.

The growth of some papillary thyroid adenocarcinomas may be controlled by *thyroid hormones,* which act by inhibiting the secretion of thyroid-stimulating hormone (TSH) by the pituitary. Control with thyroxine is limited to tumors responding to the normal TSH feedback mechanism.

*Combination chemotherapy*  Treatment of advanced cancer, where the tumor burden is large, is frequently most successful with *combination chemotherapy*. Potentially curative dosages of a single agent may be so high that life-threatening or fatal toxicity precludes its use. Furthermore, repeated administration of tolerable dosages over prolonged time periods can result in the development of resistant tumor cell lines. Various mechanisms for drug resistance to chemotherapeutic agents have been proposed, including rapid repair of drug-induced DNA damage (alkylating agents), development of alternate metabolic pathways (antimetabolites), inadequate uptake of the drug by tumor cells (methotrexate), inadequate drug activation (antimetabolites), and increased inactivation of drugs (arabinosyl cytosine).[77,78]

The development of resistance to single drugs has stimulated the development of treatment programs using drug combinations to circumvent the mechanisms of resistance and to achieve reduction of the tumor cell population to a number that can be destroyed by the host's own defense mechanisms. The success of any therapy in achieving cure is indicated by the length of time a patient remains free of disease after all therapy is discontinued.

Evaluation of a patient's response with combination chemotherapy is complicated because in many cases it is difficult to document the presence or absence of disease. A combination of objective and subjective changes is considered in the *evaluation of a response.*

*Complete remission* (CR)  Complete regression of all evidence of cancer by all criteria (physical, radiologic, biochemical) and a return to normal performance status (all residual symptomatic abnormalities must be related to side effects of therapy). The duration of complete remission must exceed 1 month (remissions are always expressed in terms of duration).

*Partial remission* (PR) Objective regression of 50 percent of measurable disease without any other evidence of progression and with subjective improvement. The duration of partial remission should be expressed in months. The appearance of any new lesion or increase in the size of residual lesions terminates the remission.

*Improvement* (I) Objective tumor regression of 25 to 50 percent with subjective improvement. (In some studies improvement means *no* objective regression but significant subjective improvement or regression of some, but not all, measurable lesions.)

*No response* (NR) Objective change in the tumor mass is not seen or represents less than 25 percent regression without significant subjective improvement.

*Progression* (P) This indicates growth of objective disease or appearance of new metastases.

Table 5-6 lists 11 neoplasms in which combination chemotherapy can *cure* a significant percentage of patients with metastatic disease. Excluding skin cancer, which is localized and rarely fatal, the statistical impact of these successful therapies is small, since the neoplasms listed make up only 8 percent of cancers and 7 percent of all cancer deaths. Although these cancers do not represent the most common cancers, they occur in a relatively youthful population, and the economic and social impact of cure is great. While in some cases (choriocarcinoma and Burkitt's lymphoma) cures have been seen with highly effective single-agent chemotherapy, most often cures are achieved using combinations. In Hodgkin's disease, acute lymphoblastic leukemia of childhood, and diffuse histiocytic lymphoma, unmaintained remissions following combination chemotherapy extend beyond 10 years.[79]

Table 5-6 also lists cancers which make up 26 percent of all cancers and 26 percent of cancer deaths and in which combination chemotherapy can *prolong* life. Complete remissions are less frequent, however, and only a small fraction of patients remain disease-free for prolonged periods of time. Administration of chemotherapy earlier in the course of the disease may have a great potential for improving cure rates in these diseases, since available drugs are clearly active in patients with advanced disease.

*Calculation of dosage* In Table 5-4 the dosage of agents is presented in terms of body weight or body surface area. Body-weight dose calculations are expressed as milligrams per kilogram of weight. Body-surface dose calculations, the preferred unit of measure, are expressed as milligrams per square meter of body-surface area. Dosage calculated in terms of body-surface area (also known as BSA) minimizes the variation in total dose between fat and thin persons and provides comparable dosages for adults and children.

*Nursing intervention* Nurses assuming responsibility for patients receiving chemotherapeutic agents must have a thorough understanding of the clinical pharmacology of the drugs. This understanding must include (1) appropriate routes of administration; (2) mechanisms of action and excretion; (3) conventional vs. investigational dosages; (4) expected side effects, especially serious or life-threatening toxicity, which requires dose reduction or discontinuation; and (5) recognition of drug incompatibilities and chemical interactions which alter the normal activity of drugs taken concomitently with chemotherapy, decrease antitumor activity, or increase drug-related toxicity.[80]

Side effects of commonly used chemotherapeutic agents are listed in Tables 5-4 and 5-5. Several will be highlighted because of the frequency of their occurrence and the discomfort they cause for the patient.

*Nausea and vomiting* may occur shortly after drug administration or may be delayed by 8 to 12 hours. Symptoms can often be ameliorated with antiemetics such as phenothiazines or sedatives. Patients should be medicated prior to chemotherapy administration and encouraged to use antiemetics as needed. If intractable nausea and vomiting occur, patients should be assessed and treated for dehydration. Dose reduction or drug withdrawal should not occur without the physician's order.

*Stomatitis,* manifested as erythema, pain, and ulceration of the oropharynx, primarily occurs with antimetabolites and antitumor antibiotics. It is an indication for stopping the drug until the toxic effect has cleared and lowering the dosage level when therapy is reinstituted.

Mucosal ulcerations may extend throughout the intestinal tract and are associated with watery *diarrhea* and occasional evidence of bleeding from ulcerations. Drug administration should be stopped

**TABLE 5-6**
METASTATIC CANCERS WHICH ARE RESPONSIVE TO ANTITUMOR THERAPY

| Cancer | Active Drugs | Current Status |
| --- | --- | --- |
| CURES IN A SIGNIFICANT FRACTION OF PATIENTS OR PROLONGED DISEASE-FREE SURVIVAL POSSIBLE | | |
| Acute lymphoblastic leukemia of childhood | Combination chemotherapy and CNS radiations; MTX, corticosteroids, VCR; L-Asparaginase, antimetabolites, adriamycin | 80% complete remission (CR) rate lasting 2–3 yr; 20–50% free of disease at 5 yr with combinations (50% cured) |
| Ewing's sarcoma | CYT, VCR, Adria and radiation | 74% of patients free of disease at 4 yr |
| Wilms' tumor | CYT, VCR, actinomycin and radiation | 92% CR rate with long disease-free survivals |
| Burkitt's lymphoma | CYT, MTX, VCR | 40% cured all stages, cures in 60% early stages with CYT alone |
| Choriocarcinoma | MTX, CYT, 6-MP, actinomycin D | 75% cures in advanced disease, 90% cures in early stages with MTX alone |
| Hodgkin's disease | Alkylating agents, Bleo, Adria, procarbazine; nitrosoureas, DTIC, plant alkaloids | 80% CR with combinations; 50% disease-free at 10 yr with combination chemotherapy |
| Histiocytic lymphoma | Alkylating agents, plant alkaloids, procarbazine, nitrosoureas, high-dose MTX | 40% CR with combination chemotherapy; disease-free survival 2–10 yr |
| Skin cancer | Topical 5-FU, dinitrochlorobenzene (DNCB) | 70% controlled effectively with topical therapy |
| Testicular carcinoma | Alkylating agents, antibiotics, MTX | 15–30% CR rate; 7% long-term disease-free survival (cured) |
| Embryonal rhabdomyosarcoma | Chemotherapy, surgery and radiation, Cytoxan, VCR, actinomycin D | 76% CR up to 4 yr |
| Neuroblastoma | Alkylating agents, antibiotics, corticosteroids | 5% cured in advanced disease |
| PALLIATION WITH PROLONGATION OF SURVIVAL | | |
| Ovarian carcinoma | Alkylating agents, antimetabolites, adriamycin, progestins | 40–60% objective response, 20% achieve CR, 10% with disease-free survival up to 10 yr |
| Breast carcinoma | Alkylating agents, antimetabolites, hormonal agents, VCR, adriamycin; combination chemotherapy | Clinical CR in 20–40% lasting 2 yr |
| Acute myelogenous leukemia | Antimetabolites, Daunomycin, alkylating agents, combination chemotherapy; immunotherapy | 50% CR rate with combination therapy; 10% prolonged disease-free for 10 yr |
| Multiple myeloma | Alkylating agents; corticosteroids, nitrosoureas | Survival improved, 35% objective response, but disease-free survival uncommon |
| Endometrial carcinoma | Progesterones | 25% overall responses, CR in 10%, some 5-yr disease-free survivals |
| Prostatic carcinoma | Estrogens, Cytoxan, 5-FU; adriamycin | 70% respond with good disease control |
| Adrenal cortical carcinoma | op'-DDD, 5-FU | Palliation of symptoms, occasional CR |
| Malignant insulinoma | Streptozoticin | CR in 25% lasting more than 1 yr |
| Oat-cell carcinoma of lung | Procarbazine, antimetabolites, VCR, alkylating agents, adriamycin, combination chemotherapy | CR in 20–60% with improved survival; some disease-free at 2–3 yr |
| Soft tissue sarcomas, osteogenic sarcomas | Combination chemotherapy with adriamycin, DTIC, actinomycin D, high-dose MTX | CR in 20% |

until toxicity has cleared. Antidiarrheal drugs may be useful to relieve symptoms.

*Local tissue damage* may occur when there is leakage (extravasation) of intravenously administered chemotherapy from the vein into surrounding tissues. Nurses who administer intravenous chemotherapeutic agents must be careful that the placement of the needle in the vein is correct. Despite precautions, extravasation does occur, and the infusion should be terminated immediately. Ice packs should be applied for several hours to induce vasoconstriction and minimize local tissue damage. This should be followed by warm compresses to alleviate discomfort.

When rapid lysis of large volumes of tumor cells is produced by chemotherapy, high levels of uric acid (*hyperuricemia*) develop and crystals can obstruct renal tubules and cause permanent kidney damage. Prophylactic use of allopurinol, a drug which prevents uric acid production, along with hydration and alkalinization of urine, can prevent the development of this renal toxicity.

**C**ombined Modalities and "Adjuvant Treatment" Programs  The rationale for utilizing a combination of treatments is based on the fact that the volume of residual cancer cells is a critical factor in the failure of any single treatment modality. Combined-modality treatment programs utilize surgery, radiation, chemotherapy, and immunotherapy in specific sequences to maximize the curative potential of each.[81] Adjuvant therapy is under investigation in patients who are at great risk of dying from recurrent cancer following apparently curative surgical removal. Adjuvant programs employ additional local or systemic therapy prophylactically in an attempt to destroy occult disease.[82] Only therapy which has proven effectiveness in patients with advanced metastatic tumor should be administered. The short- and long-term complications of treatment are weighed against the potential benefits. Since all measurable evidence of disease is absent when therapy is administered in adjuvant situations, controlled trials are necessary to document any improvement in the disease-free survival of treated patients compared to untreated patients. The effectiveness of adjuvant therapy in preventing tumor recurrences has generated enthusiasm for utilizing a combination of treatment modalities in early, localized cancers. The use of effective chemotherapeutic programs to eradicate residual cancer cells following surgery or radiation may permit the use of less extensive techniques.

Table 5-3 lists facts which must be considered in the development of adjuvant therapy in the common neoplasms. For those cancers potentially curative by surgery or radiation and for which effective chemotherapy is available, evidence strongly indicates that adjuvant treatment programs may be highly beneficial.

**P**sychological Considerations  As in all human interactions, the nature and quality of professional relationships between nurses and their patients is related to their personal attitudes. The development of a therapeutic relationship is dependent on the generation of mutual trust. Demonstration of true concern for cancer patients must be accompanied by a demonstration of professional competence and knowledge about the specific neoplasm, available effective therapies, side effects associated with treatment, and ultimately the prognosis for survival. A nursing assessment of the *patient's* interpretation of the meaning of the diagnosis is critical if patient perceptions or misconceptions are to be understood. Nurses have traditionally seemed more approachable to many patients, and this allows a nurse to explore the patient's fears and encourage the expression of anxiety so that helpful and informative discussions can take place. Nurses should talk in terms of probabilities rather than absolutes. It is important to keep future options open and to provide relative hope while preparing patients for difficult realities.

## FOURTH-LEVEL NURSING CARE

*Rehabilitation* is designed to meet the ongoing emotional, social, and physical needs of patients. It is an essential part of the treatment program for patients who may be cured of their cancers as well as for those who have long-term, chronic illnesses. The quality of a patient's life should be as important a consideration as the duration of survival. Physical, emotional, and sexual adjustments necessary within the home setting are often formidable following mutilating surgery. Prolonged periods of therapy may entail serious or incapacitating side effects with which the patient and family must cope.

*Physical therapy* is an instructive example of the overall rehabilitation process. It provides graded physical activities which are designed to restore maximal strength and function as soon as possible. Physical therapy is often started when the patient can only cooperate or passively participate in the physical activity. The reason for this is twofold. The difficulty that the patient will encounter upon resumption of physical activity is minimized by maintaining range of motion and muscular tone. Secondly, the patient is stimulated to become actively involved early in the rehabilitation process and sees tangible evidence that a return to normal activity is possible. The goal is for the patient to regain control and assume primary responsibility for all physical needs.

The philosophy of physical therapy is applicable to the entire *emotional, sexual, vocational,* and *socioeconomic* rehabilitation of the patient with cancer. The psychological shock and physical stress experienced during the diagnosis and definitive treatment may induce dependency and subsequent reluctance or fear of relinquishing this dependence. The nurse's responsibility is to assess the patient's needs and to provide the necessary physical and emotional support, while always encouraging the patient's return to self-control and independence. Application of this philosophy promotes the earliest recovery of patients while protecting them from any additional morbidity due to potential complications.

*Goals* of rehabilitation fall into three categories: restorative, supportive, and palliative.[83] *Restorative* efforts are directed toward patients expected to recover completely with little or no residual disability. *Supportive* efforts relate to patients for whom permanent disability will persist. Rehabilitation can enable such patients to return to a normal status with some adjustments in life-style. *Palliative* goals apply to patients with progressive cancer and are directed toward assisting them to maintain maximal independence and comfort in their daily living. Rehabilitation in an individual patient may shift with response to goals during the course of the clinical illness based on the response to treatment. For this reason, rehabilitation goals are dynamic and open-ended to meet changing patient needs.

Patients who are in all probability cured of cancer may encounter emotional difficulties as they resume responsibility for their lives and return to the community as normal healthy individuals. Such patients may require a significant amount of support and reassurance to overcome dependent behavior related to their fears of recurrent disease.

When any patient's physical, emotional, or financial needs are great, skilled nursing care involves the coordination of the services of health professionals who can provide necessary resources and assistance to patients and their families. Thorough discharge planning which facilitates patient adjustment and continued recovery is an important facet of patient rehabilitation. Referrals to visiting or public health nurses can ensure appropriate supervision, reinforcement of the patient's efforts, and medical intervention if problems occur.

To provide real support throughout many adjustments, nurses, medical staff, family, and friends must attempt to develop insight into the nature of the patient's experience. Most patients are acutely aware of the gravity of their disease and are desperately concerned with survival and comfort for as long as possible. Fears about disfiguration, pain, emotional and financial burdens to loved ones, abandonment, and dying can impair patients' ability to redirect and focus their physical and emotional energies productively. An understanding of these fears can provide insight into the meaning of upsetting or unexplained behavior. This implies the ability and willingness to answer or discuss difficult questions. Nurses must examine their personal attitudes toward these questions in order to become comfortable discussing them with the patient. The nurse to whom death is personally frightening will be threatened by the patient's needs and be able to offer little more than false bravado. Mastery of one's own feelings of impotence to change the course of the disease and of the sense of personal loss when patients die is a painful process, and nowhere is this successful mastery more evident than when reflected in empathetic and realistic support. *Openness* is essential, since the future is uncertain and patients need help in preparing for all possible alternatives. *Honesty* will always be of greater value than kind empty words and should convey the truth while maintaining realistic hope. This encourages continued communication, since the patient is guaranteed meaningful information.

The series of emotional reactions experienced by patients with an incurable disease have been described in detail by Elizabeth Kubler-Ross as *denial, anger, bargaining, depression,* and finally *acceptance* of the inevitable. On the basis of five years of interviews with dying patients, she provides valuable insight into cultural and personal attitudes toward death. The emphasis is on the meaning of death from the patient's point of view, how our responses affect patients, and their progress toward the point of acceptance or resignation to death. Clearly, nurses must recognize these reactions in order to understand and support patients and their families. This means taking time to sit and listen. All too often patients are reluctant to impose on others problems and conflicts which seem virtually unsolvable.

Physical and emotional rehabilitation must involve family members so that they can discern and understand the patient's needs and learn to interpret and cope with behavioral changes. Nurses can guide and teach family members to participate in patient care and encourage them to maximize the patient's sense of independence and personal responsibility. Likewise, emotional support is extended to family members who share many of the same uncertainties and often must bear the financial burden, which can be significant when the disease is prolonged and chronic in nature. The nurse is often the person to whom such concerns are expressed. By coordinating available resources and social services for the cancer patient, invaluable support for the entire family unit can be provided.

Rehabilitation may not be easy, nor is it always completely successful. Nonetheless, it is tangible evidence for patients that there is ongoing hope and help available. Throughout the patient's rehabilitation, teaching is incorporated into the nursing care plan so that the patient will have the necessary knowledge and skills to take responsibility for personal needs. A warm, relaxed relationship based on mutual trust and respect is important throughout the entire course of a patient's illness and is implicit in rehabilitation.

## REFERENCES

1   M. Abercrombie, "Contact Inhibition: The Phenomenon and its Biological Implications," *Natl Cancer Inst Monogr,* **26:**249, 1967.
2   V. T. DeVita, "Cell Kinetics and the Chemotherapy of Cancer," *Cancer Chemother Rep,* **2:**23–31, 1971.
3   R. J. Goss, "The Strategy of Growth," in H. Teir and T. Rytoma (eds.), *Control of Cellular Growth in Adult Organisms,* Academic, New York, 1967, pp. 3–27.
4   DeVita, op. cit., p. 25.
5   R. Baserga, "The Relationship of the Cell Cycle to Tumor Growth and Control of Cell Division: A Review," *Cancer Res,* **25:**581–595, 1965.
6   G. G. Steel, "The Cell Cycle in Tumors: An Examination of Data Gained by the Technique of Labelled Mitoses," *Cell Tissue Kinet,* **5:**87–100, 1972.
7   M. L. Mendelsohn, "Autoradiographic Analysis of Cell Proliferation in Spontaneous Breast Cancer of C3H Mouse. III. The Growth Fraction," *J. Natl Cancer Inst.,* **28:**1015–1029, 1962.
8   DeVita, op. cit., p. 25.
9   V. T. DeVita, R. C. Young, and G. P. Canellos, "Combination Versus Single Agent Chemotherapy: A Review of the Basis for Selection of Drug Treatment in Cancer," *Cancer,* **35:**98–110, 1975.
10  S. Wood and P. Strauli, "Tumor Invasion and Metastasis," in J. Holland and E. Frei (eds.), *Cancer Medicine,* Lea & Febiger, Philadelphia, 1973, pp. 140–151.
11  S. Wood, Jr., E. D. Holyoke, and J. H. Yardley, "Mechanisms of Metastasis Production from Bloodborne Cancer Cells," *Can Cancer Conf,* **4:**167, 1961.
12  W. H. Cole, G. O. McDonald, S. S. Robert, and H. W. Southwick, *Dissemination of Cancer, Prevention and Therapy,* Appleton-Century-Crofts, New York, 1961.
13  P. Strauli, "The Barrier Function of Lymph Nodes: A Review of Experimental Studies and Their Implications for Cancer Surgery," in F. Saegesser and J. Pettavel (eds.), *Surgical Oncology,* Hans Huber, Bern, 1970, pp. 161–176.
14  C. M. Bagley, R. C. Young, P. S. Schein, B. A. Chabner, and V. T. DeVita, "Ovarian Carcinoma Metastatic to the Diaphragm: Frequently Undiagnosed at Laparotomy," *Am J Obstet Gynecol,* **116:**397–400, 1973.
15  L. V. Ackerman and J. Rosai, "The Pathology of Tumors: Grading, Staging and Classification of Neoplasms," *Ca,* **21:**368–378, 1971.
16  J. J. Mulvihill, "Congenital and Genetic Diseases," in J. F. Fraumini (ed.), *Persons at High Risk of Cancer: An Approach to Cancer Etiology and Control,* Academic, New York, 1975, pp. 3–38.
17  A. G. Knudson and L. C. Strong, "Mutation and Cancer: Neuroblastoma and Pheochromocytoma," *Am J Hum Genet,* **25:**514–532, 1972.
18  Mulvihill, op. cit., pp. 9–14.
19  D. E. Anderson, "A Genetic Study of Human Breast Cancer," *J Natl Cancer Inst,* **48:**1029–1043, 1972.
20  M. T. Macklin, "Inheritance of Cancer of the Stomach and Large Intestine in Man," *J Natl Cancer Inst,* **22:**927–951, 1960.
21  C. G. Anderson and N. Talal, "The Spectrum of Benign to Malignant Lymphoproliferation in Sjogren's Syndrome," *Clin Exp Immunol,* **10:**199–221, 1972.
22  J. Higginson, "The Epidemiology of Primary Carcinoma of the Liver," in G. T. Pack and A. H. Islami (eds.), *Tumors of the Liver: Recent Results in Cancer,* vol. 26, Springer-Verlag, New York, 1970, pp. 15–37.
23  K. J. Rothman and A. Z. Keller, "The Effect of the Joint Exposure to Alcohol and Tobacco on Risk of Cancer of the Mouth and Pharnyx," *J Chronic Dis,* **25:**711–716, 1972.
24  D. H. Moore, et al., "Search for a Human Breast Cancer Virus," *Nature,* **229:**611–614, 1971.
25  M. A. Epstein, B. G. Achong, and Y. M. Barr, "Virus Particles in Cultured Lymphoblasts from Burkitt's Lymphoma," *Lancet,* **1:**702–703, 1964.
26  P. H. Levine, C. T. O'Conor, and C. W. Berard, "Antibodies to Epstein-Barr Virus (EBV) in American

Patients with Burkitt's Lymphoma," *Cancer,* **30**:610–615, 1972.

27 P. H. Levine, et al., "The American Burkitt Lymphoma Registry: A Progress Report," *Ann Intern Med,* **83**:31, 1975.

28 F. J. Rauscher and T. E. O'Conor, "Virology," in J. Holland and E. Frei (eds.), *Cancer Medicine,* Lea & Febiger, Philadelphia, 1973, pp. 15–44.

29 E. L. Wynder and K. Mabuchi, "Etiological and Preventive Aspects of Human Cancer," *Prev Med,* **1**:300–334, 1972.

30 A. H. Conney and J. J. Burns, "Metabolic Interactions between Environmental Chemicals and Drugs," *Science,* **178**:576–586, 1972.

31 M. Kuratsune, "Test of Alcoholic Beverages and Ethanol Solutions for Carcinogenicity and Tumor Promoting Activity," *Gann,* **62**:395–405, 1971.

32 A. Brill, M. Tomonaga, and R. M. Heyssel, "Leukemia in Man Following Exposure to Ionizing Radiation: Summary of Findings in Hiroshima and Nagaski, and Comparison with Other Human Experience," *Ann Intern Med,* **56**:590–609, 1962.

33 S. Jablon, et al., "Cancer in Japanese Exposed as Children to Atomic Bombs: Radiation Research," *Lancet,* **1**:927–932, 1972.

34 J. Jagger, "Ultraviolet Effects," in G. V. Dabrymple, M. E. Gaulden, G. M. Kollmorgen, and H. H. Vogel (eds.), *Medical Radiation Biology,* Saunders, Philadelphia, 1973.

35 B. McMahon, "Overview: Environmental Factors," in *Persons at High Risk of Cancer: An Approach to Cancer Etiology and Control,* Academic, New York, 1975, pp. 285–293.

36 J. A. Miller, "Carcinogenesis by Chemicals: An Overview," *Cancer Res,* **30**:559–575, 1970.

37 R. Hoover and J. F. Fraumeni, "Risk of Cancer in Renal Transplant Recipient," *Lancet,* **2**:55–57, 1973.

38 A. L. Herbst et al., "Clear Cell Adenocarcinoma of the Vagina and Cervix in Girls: Analysis of 170 Registry Cases," *Am J Obstet Gynecol,* **119**:713–724, 1974.

39 M. C. Pike et al., "Air Pollution," in *Persons at High Risk of Cancer: An Approach to Cancer Etiology and Control,* Academic, New York, 1975, pp. 225–240.

40 F. G. Peers and C. A. Linsell, "Dietary Aflotoxins and Liver Cancer: A Population Based in Kenya," *Br J Cancer,* **27**:473–484, 1973.

41 M. J. Hill, G. Hawsworth, and G. Tattersal, "Bacteria, Nitrosamine and Cancer of the Stomach," *Br J Cancer,* **28**:562–567, 1973.

42 J. W. Berg, *Diet in Persons at High Risk of Cancer: An Approach to Cancer Etiology and Control,* Academic, New York, 1975, pp. 201–222.

43 *1976 Cancer Facts and Figures,* American Cancer Society, New York.

44 S. Shapiro, P. Strax, and L. F. Venet, "Periodic Breast Cancer Screening," *Arch Environ Health,* **15**:547–555, 1967.

45 S. Shapiro, P. Strax, and L. Venet, "Periodic Breast Cancer Screening in Reducing Mortality from Breast Cancer," *JAMA,* **215**:1777–1785, 1971.

46 G. Costa, "Cachexia and the Systemic Effects of Tumors," in J. Holland and E. Frei (eds.), *Cancer Medicine,* Lea & Febiger, Philadelphia, 1975, pp. 1035–1044.

47 Ibid., p. 1040.

48 International Union Against Cancer, *Illustrated Tumor Nomenclature,* Springer-Verlag, Berlin, 1965.

49 S. G. Taylor, "Endocrine Ablation in Disseminated Mammary Cancer," *Surg Gynecol Obstet,* **115**:443, 1962.

50 M. M. Kligerman, "Principles of Radiation Therapy," in J. Holland and E. Frei (eds.), *Cancer Medicine,* Lea & Febiger, Philadelphia, 1973, pp. 541–565.

51 L. M. Van Putten and R. F. Kallman, "Oxygenation Status of a Transplantable Tumor during Fractionated Radiation Therapy," *J Nat Cancer Inst,* **40**:441–463, 1968.

52 Kligerman, op. cit., p. 548.

53 Kligerman, op. cit., pp. 553–555.

54 F. Buschke and R. G. Parker, *Radiation Therapy in Cancer Management,* Grune & Stratton, New York, 1972.

55 G. Fletcher, *Textbook of Radiotherapy,* Lea & Febiger, Philadelphia, 1973.

56 Kligerman, op. cit., p. 558.

57 Buschke and Parker, op cit., pp. 18–20.

58 T. J. Deely, *A Guide to Radiotherapy Nursing,* Livingstone, London, 1970.

59 E. B. Krumbhaar and H. D. Krumbhaar, "The Blood and Bone Marrow in Yellow Cross Gas (Mustard Gas) Poisoning: Changes Produced in the Bone Marrow of Fatal Case," *J Med Res,* **40**:497–501, 1919.

60 L. Goodman et al., "Use of the Methyl-bis (B-chloroethyl) Amine Hydrochloride for Hodgkin's Disease, Lymphosarcoma, Leukemia and Allied and Miscellaneous Disorders," *JAMA,* **132**:126–132, 1946.

61 DeVita, op. cit.

62 B. A. Chabner, C. E. Myers, N. C. Coleman and D. G. Johns, "The Clinical Pharmacology of Antineoplastic Agents," *N Engl J Med,* **292**:1107–1113, 1159–1168, 1975.

63 E. B. Marino and D. H. LeBlanc, "Cancer Chemotherapy," *Nursing,* **5**:22–33, 1975.

64 J. C. Marsh and M. S. Mitchell, "Chemotherapy of Cancer I, II, III," *Drug Ther,* 1–30, 1974.

65  I. H. Krakoff, *Cancer Chemotherapeutic Agents,* American Cancer Society, New York, 1973, pp. 1–20.

66  P. B. Bergevin, D. C. Tormey, and J. Blom, "Guide to the Use of Cancer Chemotherapeutic Agents," *Mod Treatment,* **9**(2):185–273, 1972.

67  E. S. Greenwald, *Cancer Chemotherapy,* Medical Examination Publishing Company, New York, 1973, pp. 80–162.

68  Greenwald, op. cit., pp. 263–265.

69  R. C. Bast, B. Zbar, T. Borsos, and H. J. Rapp, "BCG and Cancer," *N Engl J Med,* **290:**1413–1420, 1458–1469.

70  E. S. Henderson, "Treatment of Acute Leukemia," *Semin Hematol,* **6:**271–301, 1972.

71  E. V. Jensen, "Estrogen Binding and Clinical Response in Breast Cancer," in J. Holland and E. Frei (eds.), *Cancer Medicine,* Lea & Febiger, Philadelphia, 1973, pp. 900–906.

72  N. Treves, "The Treatment of Cancer, Especially Inoperable Cancer of the Male Breast by Ablative Surgery and Hormone Therapy," *Cancer,* **12:**820–825, 1959.

73  Veterans Administration Cooperative Urological Group, "Treatment and Survival of Patients with Cancer of the Prostate," *Surg Gynecol Obstet,* **124:** 1011– 1022, 1967.

74  Ibid.

75  I. S. Goldenberg and A. Segaloff, "Androgens," in J. Holland and E. Frei (eds.), *Cancer Medicine,* Lea & Febiger, Philadelphia, 1973, pp. 929–932.

76  R. Kelley, "Progestins," in ibid., pp. 923–929.

77  R. Bender and R. L. Dudrick, "Cytokinetic Aspects of Clinical Drug Resistance," *Cancer Chemother Rep,* **59:**805–809.

78  DeVita, Young, and Canellos, loc. cit.

79  Ibid.

80  S. P. Hubbard and V. T. DeVita, "The Chemotherapy Nurse," *Am J Nurs,* **76:**560–656, 1976.

81  J. Holland, "Principles of Management," in J. Holland and E. Frei (eds.), *Cancer Medicine,* Lea & Febiger, Philadelphia, 1973, pp. 489–498.

82  E. A. Gehan and M. A. Schniederman, "Experimental Design of Clinical Trials," in ibid., pp. 499–520.

83  J. Healey, R. Villaneuva, and E. Donovan, "Principles of Rehabilitation in Cancer Medicines," in J. Holland and E. Frei (eds.), *Cancer Medicine,* Lea & Febiger, Philadelphia, pp. 1917–1930, 1973.

## BIBLIOGRAPHY

Ackerman, V., and J. Del Regato: *Cancer Diagnosis, Treatment and Prognosis,* Mosby, St. Louis, 1970.

Behnke, H. D. (ed.): *Guidelines for Comprehensive Nursing Care in Cancer,* Springer, New York, 1973.

Deely, T. J., E. J. Fish, and M. A. Gough: *A Guide to Oncological Nursing,* Livingstone Nursing Texts, London, 1974.

Frei, E., and J. Holland (eds.): *Cancer Medicine,* Lea & Febiger, Philadelphia, 1973.

Greenwald, E. S.: *Cancer Chemotherapy,* 2d ed., Medical Examination Publishing Co., Flushing, N.Y., 1973.

Kubler-Ross, E.: *On Death and Dying,* Macmillan, New York, 1969.

Kubler-Ross, E.: *Questions and Answers on Death and Dying,* Collier, New York, 1974.

Rubin, P.: *Clinical Oncology for Medical Students and Physicians: A Multidisciplinary Approach,* 4th ed., American Cancer Society, New York, 1974.

# 6 SOLID NEOPLASMS*

Linda Hannawalt Rickel
Pamela Gaherin Watson
Barbara Sigler

**S**olid neoplasms or solid tumors that form perceptible masses may occur in almost any organ or tissue of the body. General characteristics of all neoplasms and causative factors in the environment are discussed in Chap. 5. Those characteristics apply to the neoplasms discussed in this chapter; but the special characteristics of *breast, genital, bladder, head and neck,* and *skin* tumors are discussed here in more detail. Lung tumors are briefly discussed in Chap. 30; hepatic, pancreatic, and gastrointestinal neoplasms in Chap. 17, 18, and 19; renal tumors in Chap. 14; and tumors arising from nervous tissue in Chap. 35.

## BREAST NEOPLASMS

Breast neoplasms may be malignant or benign. Breast cancers (*malignant neoplasms*) are the leading cause of death in women 40 to 44 years old and the most frequently occurring cancer in women over 40.[1,2] In 1976 an estimated 89,000 new cases were diagnosed, including 33,000 eventual deaths.[3] Of every 100,000 women, 100 will have cancer of the breast in any given year; the male to female ratio is 1:100.[4] *Benign* tumors of the breast are very common. Almost all women develop some degree of chronic cystic mastitis at some time in their lives.

### Benign Breast Neoplasms

Many conditions of the breast, although benign, are nevertheless of great concern. When they occur, the breasts should be thoroughly examined and complete follow-up care given. Almost all women have sufficient breast symptoms to consult a physician or nurse practitioner at some time in their lives.[5] The discovery of any lump in the breast causes anxiety and fear, and prompt medical attention should be sought to alleviate unnecessary concern.

**Pathophysiology** *Fibrocystic disease* is the most common cause of a lump in the breast in women aged 30 to 50. These masses most frequently appear after adolescence and usually disappear after menopause. It is thought that their appearance is related to hormonal stimulation during the menstrual cycle. Indeed, the masses become more

---

* The sections Breast Neoplasms, Neoplasms of the Female Genital Tract, and Neoplasms of the Skin were written by Linda Hannawalt Rickel; Neoplasms of the Male Genital Tract and Urologic Neoplasms by Pamela Gaherin Watson; Neoplasms of the Head and Neck by Barbara Sigler.

prominent and tender just before the onset of each menstrual period.

Although fibrocystic disease is divided into three types—*fibrosis, cystic disease,* and *adenosis*—actual lesions may show evidence of all three. *Fibrosis* of the breast is characterized by the proliferation of fibrous connective tissue. *Cystic disease* involves both stromal and epithelial hyperplasia; the cysts are usually multifocal and may be filled with fluid. *Adenosis* tends to involve glandular epithelium and is sometimes difficult to distinguish from carcinoma. Fibrocystic disease may be a precursor to cancer and should therefore be followed closely.

Another common mass found in breast tissue is a *fibroadenoma.* This is a solid lump most often seen in women in their teens and early twenties. Fibroadenomas contain normal breast elements (fibrous and glandular tissue) surrounded by a capsule, making the mass relatively movable.[6]

A *benign papilloma* (intraductal papilloma) is a small, harmless growth in a duct, usually near the nipple. The majority of these benign papillary lesions present as a solitary nodule; multiple benign papillomas are infrequent. The presence of a papilloma is often frightening to the patient because the predominant symptom is a discharge from the nipple, which is frequently bloody.

An injury to a breast can cause a *hematoma,* which is associated with bleeding under the skin. Mammography is useful in following the progress of such an injury and making sure no other abnormal conditions are present.

## Malignant Breast Neoplasms

A malignant breast neoplasm, or cancer of the breast, may originate from either ductal or lobular epithelium. It may be either infiltrating (penetrating the limiting basement membranes) or noninfiltrating (not penetrating the limiting basement membranes). The classification of breast carcinomas is shown in Table 6-1.

**Pathophysiology** All forms of breast cancer spread locally by invasion. They tend to adhere to the pectoral muscles or deep fascia of the chest wall beneath the breast and to the skin overlying the breast. The skin adherence causes an appearance of dimpling or retraction.

Redness, tenderness, and swelling of a tumor-containing breast indicates rapid cancer spread. This rapid growth incites an acute inflammatory response referred to as *inflammatory carcinoma.*

**Metastasis** Unfortunately, more than half of all patients with carcinoma of the breast present with or develop systemic metastasis. The usual spread extends from the breast to the axillary nodes, the internal mammary nodes, and the supraclavicular nodes. Wider dissemination is predominantly hematogenous, with the most common sites of distant

**TABLE 6-1**
CLASSIFICATION OF BREAST CARCINOMA

| Origin | Effect on Basement Membranes | Type of Cancer | Percentage of Breast Cancers | Description |
|---|---|---|---|---|
| Ductal epithelium | Noninfiltrating | Comedocarcinoma or intraductal carcinoma | 1% | Tumor tissue fills ducts and can be expressed from the nipple without invading the ductal basement membrane |
| | Infiltrating | Scirrhous carcinoma | 75–78% | Invades breast widely, hard in consistency |
| | | Medullary carcinoma | 4% | Soft, fleshy, large tumors |
| | | Colloid (mucinous) carcinoma | 2% | Soft, bulky tumors that produce intracellular and extracellular mucin |
| | | Paget's disease | 1% | Involves the main excretory ducts, the nipple, and the areola; frequent inflammation and ulceration |
| | | Infiltrating comedocarcinoma | 5% | Fills large mammary ducts with cords of cancer cells that eventually invade the basement membranes |
| Lobular epithelium | Noninfiltrating | In situ lobular carcinoma | — | Tends to be bilateral; often multicentric, involving glandular epithelium |
| | Infiltrating | Lobular carcinoma | 9% | |

SOURCE: Stanley Robbins and Marcia Angell, *Basic Psychology*, 2d ed., Saunders, Philadelphia, 1976, pp. 588–589; and Seymour Schwartz, *Principles of Surgery*, 2d ed., McGraw-Hill, New York, 1974, pp. 539–540.

metastasis being the lymph nodes, lungs, bone marrow, liver, and bone.[7]

Fifty percent of those who have had a lump for 1 month already have positive axillary nodes; at 6 months, 68 percent have positive axillary nodes. If not seen by a physician, biopsied, and treated immediately, the chance of more advanced disease continues to increase. Cancer in the male breast seems to have early diffuse lymphatic and nodal involvement, which leads to a poorer prognosis.

**Causative Factors**  Research continues to focus on the causative factors in breast cancer, although as yet no common etiology has been determined. Factors such as hormonal mechanisms, viral agents, and immunologic processes are being explored. The hormonal mechanisms remain in question. The fact that breast cancer is not observed in prepubertal females suggests that prior conditioning of the breast tissue by endogenous steroids may be essential for neoplastic development. Many breast cancers have been found to be hormone-dependent. The part that hormones play in breast cancer is not clearly understood, but hormonal balance or imbalance may be the key. There is no convincing evidence that birth-control pills contribute to or induce cancer of the breast.

Lactation does not have a notable protective effect against breast cancer for the nursing mother, but breast cancer appears less frequently in societies where infants are nursed rather than artificially fed.[8]

Data suggest that a continuing immunologic competence and activity may ordinarily operate as a surveillance mechanism to recognize and destroy incipient neoplasia. Immune-system suppression or failure may therefore serve as an etiologic factor.

Viral studies have explored a type B virus found in mice that is known to be a causative factor in mouse mammary tumors. The discovery in human milk of type B virus particles resembling the mouse mammary tumor has led to increased interest in and investigation of a possible viral etiology in human mammary cancer. Isolation of a C-type virus associated with an adenocarcinoma of the breast in a rhesus monkey has further kindled the search for a viral etiology in human breast cancer.[9]

Low rates of breast cancer correlate with (1) pregnancy prior to the age of 20 years, (2) multiple pregnancies, (3) castration prior to age 37, (4) prolonged lactation, (5) low economic status, and (6) non-Caucasian racial origin.[10]

Unfortunately, there has been a lack of significant improvement in survival in the last thirty years.[11] The median survival following metastasis is less than 2 years, and the survival rate in all cancers of the breast at 10 years remains less than 50 percent.

### First-level Nursing Care

Carcinoma of the breast can develop in anyone. It usually occurs at an age when many women are living their fullest lives. Their children are frequently in high school or college. Their careers or their husbands' are peaking. The risk of developing breast cancer increases after age 35 and is higher in the United States for whites than for nonwhites. It is also higher for women who have never had a child, have had a first child after the age of 25, have had an early menarche, have had menses for more than 30 years, have a family history of mammary cancer, or have already had cancer in one breast.[12,13]

**Prevention and early detection**  Because the etiology of mammary carcinoma is unknown, it is difficult to formulate a program for prevention. Early detection is the one strong ally in preventing this disease from killing. The malignant disease must be found *before* an obvious lump is discovered by the victim.

The American Cancer Society and the National Cancer Institute have jointly funded Breast Cancer Detection Demonstration projects across the nation to demonstrate the value of modern diagnostic technology in finding early breast cancers in asymptomatic women. This project has resulted in the discovery of cancers in six women per 1,000, 77 percent of whom have had negative axillary lymph nodes at the time of surgery. The significance of this is more apparent when compared to the general population, in which only 45 percent have negative axillary lymph nodes at surgery. Detection prior to distant nodular metastasis increases the chance of 5-year survival to 84 percent.[14] Women should familiarize themselves with the Breast Cancer Detection Demonstration project screening center in their geographic area. The standard examination consists of four parts:

1  Interview (health history related to breast)

2  Palpation (physical examination of each breast)

3  Mammography (low-dose x-ray study of the structure of the breast to pinpoint any abnormality)

4  Thermography (photograph which shows skin-surface heat pattern of the breast)

In addition, all women are taught the breast self-examination.

**B**reast Self-examination (BSE)   The importance of self-examination of the breast cannot be overemphasized. The breasts are located in an area that allows for frequent and regular examination.

Nurses in all phases of practice have the responsibility of teaching BSE to all persons with whom they come in contact. A film prepared by the American Cancer Society is available for loan from local chapters. Men as well as women should know how to perform BSE, both for themselves and for their loved ones.

BSE should be done *monthly,* following a regular procedure. The best time to check the breasts is about a week after the conclusion of the menstrual period; this prevents confusion of normal premenstrual glandular enlargement with abnormal masses. Postmenopausal women should check their breasts on a particular day, such as the first day of the month. The American Cancer Society recommends the following steps, illustrated in Fig. 6-1:

*Step 1 (in the shower)*   Examine the breasts during a bath or shower—hands glide more easily over wet skin. With the fingers flat, move the hand gently over every part of each breast. Use the right hand to examine the left breast and the left hand for the right breast. Check for any lump, hard knot, or thickening.

*Step 2 (before a mirror)*   Inspect the breasts with the arms at the sides and then raise both arms high overhead. Look for changes in the contour of each breast, swelling, dimpling of the skin, or changes in the nipple. Rest both palms on the hips and press firmly to flex the chest muscles and observe for any differences.

*Step 3 (lying down)*   Put a pillow under the shoulder on the side of the breast to be examined and place the hand on that side behind the head. With the opposite hand, fingers flat, press gently in small circular motions around an imaginary clock face. Begin at the outermost top of the breast for 12 o'clock, then move to 1 o'clock and continue around the circle back to 12. Move in an inch closer to the nipple and repeat the circle again (at least three circles). Repeat the procedure for the other breast. Palpate both breasts a second time, using a firmer pressure to evaluate changes. Squeeze the nipple of each breast gently between the thumb and index finger; any discharge should be reported to a physician.

**M**ammography and Thermography *Mammography* is a soft-tissue roentgenographic examination of the breast without injection of a contrast medium. It can be used to detect lesions before they can be palpated. "It's primary purpose is to demonstrate the absence or presence of a breast lesion and if one is present, the benignity or malignancy of the lesion."[15] Regular annual mammography is specifically indicated in patients with

Signs and symptoms of breast disease

Previous breast biopsy

Familial history of breast cancer

Need for survey of opposite breast after mastectomy

Lumpy or large pendulous breasts, difficult to examine

Cancerophobia

Adenocarcinoma, site undetermined[16]

A low-energy x-ray beam is required to delineate the breast structure on a mammogram. Compression of the breast is necessary to reduce its thickness so that lesions can be better defined. Usually three main roentgenograms are taken, one of the axilla and two of the breast. The three positions are the craniocaudal view, the mediolateral view, and an axillary view.

*Thermography* is a procedure in which a thermograph records the infrared radiation emitted from the breast, thus mapping out any variations in surface temperature. Although the procedure is helpful in determining asymmetry of the thermic pattern and the pattern of the subcutaneous veins, many investigators feel its value as a diagnostic tool is limited: many patients with mammary cancer have a normal thermogram, and false-positive results are common. The smaller the tumor, the less reliable is thermography.[17]

Educating the public to the benefits of early detection of breast cancer must be stressed. Too often fears deprive the patient of early treatment that can be lifesaving. Publicity should focus on the statistics related to patients with cancer of the breast who have sought out and received medical treatment and intervention early.

## Second-level Nursing Care

A lump or mass found in the breast, whether accidentally, by BSE, or at the time of an annual physical examination, arouses fear in anyone. Although most lumps are not malignant, a biopsy and patho-

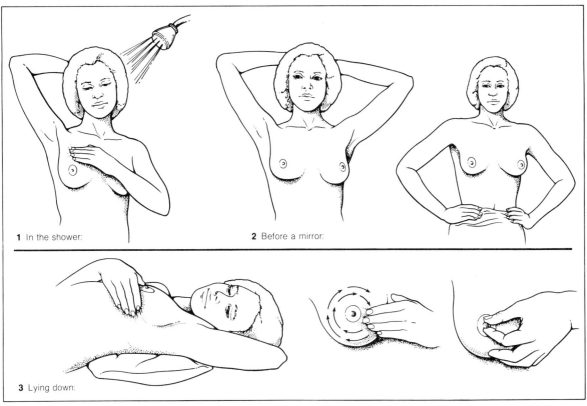

**1** In the shower.

**2** Before a mirror:

**3** Lying down:

**FIGURE 6-1**

Breast self-examination: (1) in the shower, check for any lump or thickening; (2) before a mirror, look for changes in contour of breasts, a swelling or dimple in the skin; (3) lying down, put pillow under shoulder, with fingers flat examine that breast, press in circular motion; squeeze nipple to check for discharge; repeat for other breast. (*How To Examine Your Breasts,* American Cancer Society, Inc.)

logic diagnosis must be made before definitive information can be given. Because of the fear of cancer, many women delay seeking medical attention and thus greatly increase their risk of more advanced disease.

**Nursing assessment** Cancer of the breast often is first apparent as a nonpainful lump in the breast which may be discovered by the victim or spouse. In the early stages this lump is usually isolated, movable, and painless. Over 50 percent occur in the upper outer quadrant of the breast, with 20 percent each in the central and medial half and 10 percent in the lower outer quadrant (Fig. 6-2).[18] Slightly more cancers are found in the left than in the right breast. The nursing assessment at this time must include a complete *health history.* Questions should explore any family history of breast cancer, other breast problems, menstrual patterns, pregnancies and lactation, and use of oral contraceptives. The subjective evidence of a lump should be docu-

mented objectively by *physical assessment,* noting the location and physical description. A hard, circumscribed mass which is *not* freely movable is a suspicious lump suggesting malignancy. Fixation to the skin, nipple retraction, skin edema, or deep fixation is further evidence pointing to cancer. These lesions are usually painless. Benign cysts are soft, movable, and frequently have a discrete spherical shape. They may appear bilaterally, may be multiple, and may change in size during the menstrual cycle.

**Diagnostic Tests** Once a lump or mass is noted, diagnostic procedures must be done to rule out malignancy. Many of these procedures do not necessitate hospitalization, as some fears of malignancy can be allayed through examinations such as aspiration, mammography, and needle biopsy.

As previously mentioned, fibrocystic disease of the breast accounts for the majority of mammary masses. These cysts are frequently filled with fluid

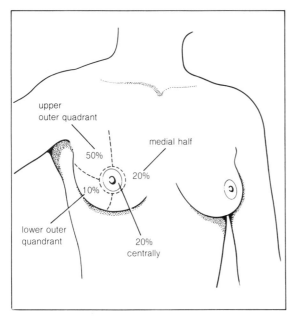

**FIGURE 6-2**
Incidence of breast cancer according to involved area.

that can be aspirated. *Aspiration* of a lesion with disappearance of the mass after evacuation, coupled with thermography that shows no localized heat over the cyst, is highly suggestive of a benign cyst.[19]

On *mammography,* benign tumors tend to have sharp margins, are homogeneous in density, and are frequently surrounded by a radiolucent halo of fat. In contrast, malignant tumors are poorly circumscribed and exhibit tentacle-like infiltrations into surrounding tissue.[20]

Benign lesions push breast tissue aside as they expand, while malignant lesions invade the surrounding breast tissue (Figs. 6-3, 6-4, and 6-5). A benign lesion has a round, oval, or lobulated shape with a regular, smooth, well-circumscribed border. The size is usually the same as that palpated during the physical examination. The density is homogeneous, and the surrounding tissue is displaced but not invaded. The malignant lesion has a variable, ragged, spicular, tentacled space that is irregular and poorly circumscribed. It is often smaller than the palpable mass and is nonhomogeneous. The surrounding tissue is infiltrated and retracted.

*Needle biopsy* is a term used to designate the removal of cylinders of tissue for histopathologic examination. Some feel that this should be reserved only for masses strongly suspected to be nonmalignant, as it carries the risk of spreading the tumor.[21]

**Nursing problems and interventions** When x-ray and clinical examinations indicate even a small possibility of malignancy, patients may still fail to seek out further medical care. It is often the

**FIGURE 6-3**
Mammogram: left normal; right shows benign lesion (fibroadenoma).

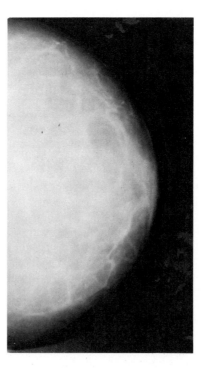
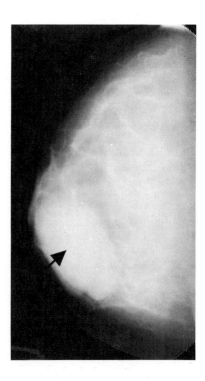

nurse from whom the patient seeks advice. Nurses must encourage and *refer* the patient for a definitive diagnosis. It is also important to emphasize to patients with a negative checkup that continued monthly BSE examinations and annual or semi-annual physical examinations are still essential.

Patients often fear the worst. They may worry about the possible loss of a breast, their own sexuality, or their spouse's reaction. Some patients may begin to grieve prematurely. Nurses should be aware of these feelings and permit the patient to ventilate them. Realistic reassurance that provides information and direction to the patient must be given.

A positive finding makes it necessary for the already frightened patient to leave her home and often the community to enter the hospital for more definitive procedures. Full emotional support begins at this important time.

### Third-level Nursing Care

When it becomes necessary for the patient with a suspected malignant tumor to enter the hospital, continued assessment by the nurse is vital. The nurse must be aware of the patient's emotional stability, family ties, religious beliefs, financial situation, and what the patient has been told by the medical personnel.

**Nursing assessment** Nursing assessment of the lesion at this time is crucial. The *health history* should include the elements discussed under second-level nursing care. During the *physical assessment,* the findings may range from a barely palpable lump to a visibly ulcerated, discolored mass. If the tumor is fixed to underlying tissue, there will be dimpling of the skin, and retraction of the nipple may be evident. The nurse should thoroughly examine the breast (see Chap. 4). Attention must be given to both breasts and axilla and any edema, dimpling, retraction, or ulceration should be noted, as well as the color and mobility of the mass. Severe edema, ulceration, or discoloration and palpable axillary nodes are highly suspicious indications of advanced malignancy.

Since the physical signs and symptoms at this time most often consist of an isolated mass discovered by one of the previously mentioned diagnostic means, a suspicion that a lesion is malignant makes mandatory a thorough search for other involvement. During the physical examination, special attention should be given to the lymph nodes, particularly those of the axillae and the supraclavic-

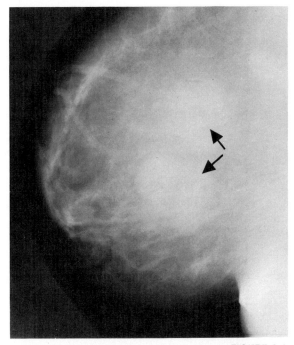

**FIGURE 6-4**
Mammogram: Two lobulated, fuzzily outlined masses (medullary carcinoma).

lar areas. Radiographic and radioisotope studies to rule out pulmonary, bone, or liver metastasis should be made. After a thorough history, physical examination, and diagnostic workup, suspected malignant tumors must be surgically biopsied. Any lump in the male breast demands immediate biopsy.

**Nursing problems and interventions** The major nursing problems encountered in caring for a patient with a breast neoplasm are the *mass* and any *effects related to the mass,* as well as the psychological problems of *fear* and *anxiety.* The intervention of choice is *curative surgery;* however, *palliative surgery, radiotherapy, chemotherapy,* and *hormonal therapy* are also used.

**S**urgery The woman who faces breast surgery often develops extreme anxiety from fear of mutilation, suffering, and death. She is also faced, at the time of the biopsy, with the *fear of the unknown.* Since the general practice is to make a microscopic diagnosis by frozen section and, if it is positive, to do an immediate mastectomy, the patient must be fully prepared for this possibility. Nursing intervention at this time will establish a rapport that will be

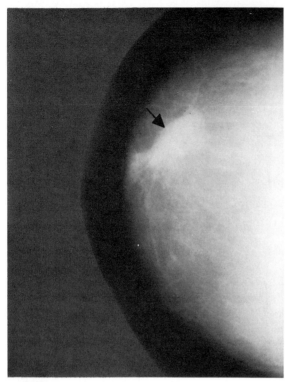

**FIGURE 6-5**
Spiculated mass beneath areola with infiltration to the nipple area along the ducts (scirrhous carcinoma).

needed through a long postoperative rehabilitative period.

Much emphasis is placed on the female breast in our culture as a symbol of attractiveness. The *fear* of losing this symbol becomes almost intolerable, especially to a woman who feels that her attractiveness is the reason she is held in esteem by others. In order to offer the emotional support so necessary at this time, the nurse must be fully conscious of how the patient views herself as a woman and what values rest on her *body image.* The nurse must also know her own feelings toward breast amputation.

Too often a woman is taken to the operating room for a "minor biopsy" only to wake up with a breast missing. The woman facing breast surgery has a special need to be accepted and understood by those around her.

Upon admission to the hospital, a conference should be held with the patient, her family, the nurse, and, whenever possible, the surgeon. This conference should concentrate on the patient's needs and open a pathway of communication to

discuss treatment alternatives if malignancy is present. At the same time, arm exercises, breast prosthesis, clothing, sexual relations, and any other subjects that concern the patient can be explored. This planned preoperative meeting can assist the nurse in assessing not only the patient's fears but also her strengths. Making a patient who is scheduled for a biopsy wait for answers to her questions until "we know for sure" is jeopardizing the psychological rehabilitation that will remain so important to her care.

*Preoperative care* The preparation for surgery is similar in many ways to any operative procedure. All procedures should be explained. Because of the stress the patient is under, the simple act of shaving and preparing the skin can become of major concern if the patient is not forewarned.

The fear of the unknown often hinders a patient's cooperation. A histologically positive biopsy may be immediately followed by more extensive surgery. The patient must be told of this possibility and prepared for what she may experience postoperatively. When possible, she should be informed of the surgical choices by the physician and given a voice in the final decision.

Preoperative teaching includes information about dressings, the possibility of a catheter attached to suction, and the shoulder imbalance that the patient may feel if a breast is removed. She should understand that her arm will be exercised and positioned and that she will start ambulating as soon after surgery as possible.

A thorough workup is necessary to determine the exact extent of the cancer in order to stage the patient accurately (Table 6-2). Complete clinical evaluation of the tumor and regional nodes, with pathologic evaluation of resected nodes, is needed. Radiographic, radioisotopic, hematologic, and hormonal studies are made and evaluated.

Radical mastectomy may be contraindicated if distant metastasis is present. Extensive edema of the breast or arm, inflammatory carcinoma, and fixation of the tumor or nodes to the chest wall may also contraindicate surgery. If surgery is not considered as a treatment modality, alternatives such as radiation therapy and chemotherapy may be instituted. These are discussed later in this section.

A long-standing controversy concerns the extent of the surgical procedure. Clinical Stage I, in which the primary tumor is less than 2 cm in its greatest dimension and where there are no regional lymph nodes that contain tumor, and clinical Stage

II, which is a primary lesion less than 5 cm in dimension with movable homolateral axillary nodes, are the stages in which this discussion has flourished.

*Radical mastectomies* involve removal of the entire mammary fat pad, both pectoral muscles, and the lower, middle, subclavicular, and axillary nodes. Some even include removal of the internal mammary nodes. *Simple mastectomies* include only a portion of the mammary fat pad and commonly remove a few of the lowermost tier of axillary nodes directly adjacent to the breast.[22]

Another procedure that avoids many of the dis-

**TABLE 6-2**
CLINICAL STAGING SYSTEM FOR CARCINOMA OF THE BREAST

### DEFINITIONS OF T, N, AND M CATEGORIES

#### T PRIMARY TUMORS

| | |
|---|---|
| TIS | Preinvasive carcinoma (carcinoma in situ), noninfiltrating intraductal carcinoma, or Paget's disease of the nipple with no demonstrable tumor |
| | Note: Paget's disease associated with a demonstrable tumor is classified according to the size of the tumor |
| T0 | No demonstrable tumor in the breast |
| T1* | Tumor 2 cm or less in its greatest dimension |
| | T1a With no fixation to underlying pectoral fascia and/or muscle |
| | T1b With fixation to underlying pectoral fascia and/or muscle |
| T2* | Tumor more than 2 cm but not more than 5 cm in its greatest dimension |
| | T2a With no fixation to underlying pectoral fascia and/or muscle |
| | T2b With fixation to underlying pectoral fascia and/or muscle |
| T3* | Tumor more than 5 cm in its greatest dimension |
| | T3a With no fixation to underlying pectoral fascia and/or muscle |
| | T3b With fixation to underlying pectoral fascia and/or muscle |
| T4 | Tumor of any size with direct extension to chest wall or skin |
| | Note: Chest wall includes ribs, intercostal muscles, and serratus anterior muscle but not pectoral muscle |
| | T4a With fixation to chest wall |
| | T4b With edema (including peau d'orange), ulceration of the skin of the breast, or satellite skin nodules confined to the same breast |
| | T4c Both of above |

* Dimpling of the skin, nipple retraction, or any other skin changes except those in T4b may occur in T1, T2, or T3 without affecting the classification.

#### N REGIONAL LYMPH NODES

| | |
|---|---|
| N0 | No palpable homolateral axillary nodes |
| N1 | Movable homolateral axillary nodes |
| | N1$_a$ Nodes not considered to contain growth |
| | N1$_b$ Nodes considered to contain growth |
| N2 | Homolateral axillary nodes considered to contain growth and fixed to one another or to other structures |
| N3 | Homolateral supraclavicular or infraclavicular nodes considered to contain growth or edema of the arm* |
| | Note: Edema of the arm may be caused by lymphatic obstruction; lymph nodes may not be palpable |

#### M DISTANT METASTASIS

| | |
|---|---|
| M0 | No evidence of distant metastasis |
| M1 | Distant metastasis present, including skin involvement beyond the breast area |

* Homolateral internal mammary nodes considered to contain growth are included in N3 for surgical evaluative classification and postsurgical treatment classification.

### CLINICAL STAGE GROUPING IN CARCINOMA OF THE BREAST

| | | |
|---|---|---|
| TIS | Carcinoma in situ | |
| Invasive carcinoma: | | |
| State I | T1a N0 or N1$_a$ | } M0 |
| | T1b N0 or N1$_a$ | |
| Stage II | T0 N1$_b$ | |
| | T1a N1$_b$ | |
| | T1b N1$_b$ | } M0 |
| | T2a or T2b; N0, N1$_a$ or N1$_b$ | |
| Stage III | any T3 with any N | |
| | any T4 with any N | |
| | any T with N2 | } M0 |
| | any T with N3 | |
| Stage IV | any T; any N with M1 | |

figuring effects of mastectomy is the *"lumpectomy."* This procedure removes a one-fourth to one-third segment of breast tissue. It is useful in only occasional selected patients who have small, peripheral lesions detected in the very early stages. There is much discussion and disagreement among professionals concerning the long-term therapeutic effectiveness of this type of surgery. It may, however, offer the patient some alternative to total breast removal when the criteria for its use are met.

A more common surgical practice today is the *modified radical mastectomy,* which leaves both pectoral muscles in situ along with the interpectoral lymph nodes. The axillary extension of the breast and the lower and mid portions of the axillary fat pads, with its lymph nodes lying below the pectoralis minor, are removed en bloc. This may or may not involve skin grafting.

Studies as yet have not proved that simple mastectomy is better than or equal to radical surgery, and the controversy continues. Since adequate conclusions have not been reached in regard to the surgical procedure, the patient should be allowed a voice in the decision.

*Postoperative care*  A tremendous physical and emotional adjustment is ahead for the patient following a mastectomy. When she is told that a breast has to be removed, realistic *hope* must be conveyed. A reassurance that there is a possibility for complete and permanent cure should be emphasized, and the patient can be assured of maximum functional ability through proper follow-up exercises. She should be reassured by all members of the health team and her family that she can expect to return to her daily activities shortly and, with proper prosthetic fittings, have a normal appearance.

Postoperatively, the patient will experience *grief* at the loss of a body part. In order to cope with this grief, she will utilize many coping mechanisms. This crisis period is essential and may include denial, hostility, anger, guilt, and depression before reaching acceptance.

Acceptance and understanding of the need for this meaningful expression of feelings are paramount. The nurse may observe the patient striking out verbally at the hospital staff, her husband, and family. She may refuse to move and bathe, visit with her family, or take medication that is ordered. She may withdraw and become nonverbal or deeply depressed. An understanding but realistically hopeful attitude by the nurse should prevail. A time to share these feelings with the nurse should be allowed and

encouraged. Each woman will work through the grief process at her own rate and can be assisted in this task by medical personnel, clergy, and the American Cancer Society's Reach-to-Recovery volunteers.

*Pain control* is one of the first considerations during postoperative rehabilitation. The pain immediately after surgery is due to trauma during the operative procedure. Analgesic agents should be used as necessary to enable the patient to attain maximum mobility as soon as allowed. Nerve irritation, muscle spasm, or strain may account for pain in the late convalescent period.

Immediately after surgery the dressings should be observed for excessive *drainage* or bleeding. Frequently a catheter is inserted at the operative site to facilitate proper drainage. This is often connected to a source of negative suction such as the Hemovac. The drainage unit should be emptied and cared for in accordance with instructions accompanying the apparatus. The catheter is often left in place for 3 to 5 days or until the amount of drainage is minimal (less than 100 ml/24 hours).

One of the problems following mastectomy is *edema* of the affected arm due to disruption of lymph drainage. There are two types of edema. *Acute edema* may be transient and mild, immediately postoperatively; transient and painful, 2 to 6 weeks postoperatively; or recurrent, painful, febrile, and erysipeloid, occurring at any time, usually in the chronically edematous arm. *Insidious edema,* which is painless and persistent, may develop weeks or even years after surgery.[23]

Acute edema of the affected arm appears to be associated with trauma to the axillary vessels during surgery. The etiologic factors are unclear, but an infectious etiology often cannot be ruled out postoperatively. Infections are often signaled by localized induration and may occur even years later as a result of burns, cuts, insect bites, severe bruises of the hand, arm, or forearm, intravenous or hypodermic injections, or vaccination. The mechanisms producing lymphedema are essentially the same, regardless of the etiology. An increase in hyperstatic pressure is caused when the lymph flow from the extremity is blocked because of surgical interruption. This leads to dilated vessels and incompetent lymph valves. A lymphedematous extremity is an excellent culture medium for bacteria. Infections that may result lead to thrombosis of the lymph vessels and further blocking of lymph flow. Fibrosis can also occur following radiation therapy.

Immediately after surgery the affected arm should be elevated, with the elbow at the level of the right atrium and the hand above the elbow to minimize the development of edema. In addition, the arm should be compressed with an elastic bandage. These measures facilitate drainage, prevent the accumulation of fluid in the interstitial spaces, and aid in the regeneration of lymphatic pathways. Postoperatively and at the time of discharge, a list of instructions should be given to the patient which will minimize complications. They are shown in Table 6-3.

*Exercise* instructions should begin the first postoperative day, when hand, wrist, and elbow flexion and extension are encouraged. These exercises help to maintain function and prevent further fluid accumulation. Full exercises occur after consideration of factors such as wound healing, grafts, drainage tubes, and the patient's level of tolerance. The exercises are progressive. They begin in the hospital and continue throughout the patient's rehabilitative period. The arm used in all exercises is that on the side of the operation unless otherwise stated.

The *hair-brushing* exercise can begin in the hospital. The patient should be sitting at a table with her elbow elevated on a few books to rest the arm. She can begin brushing her hair, with hand erect, progressing slowly until all areas have been reached (Fig. 6-6). Rest periods should be taken whenever the need is felt. The *paper-crumpling* exercise can be done by placing ten sheets of newspaper in a flat pile. With the forearm resting on a table, the sheets are crumpled one at a time and discarded, starting at one corner of the pile.

For all standing exercises, flat shoes should be worn or feet may be bare. The patient should stand relaxed with head erect, chin in, arms at her sides, weight on the balls of the feet, knees slightly bent, and feet apart the width of the hips. The *rubber-ball* exercise can begin in the hospital. The patient holds a rubber ball in the affected hand, alternately squeezing and relaxing (Fig. 6-7). By attaching elastic to the ball and looping it around a finger, the ball can be thrown easily in any direction. Throwing it farther and farther each day and reaching for it strengthens the shoulder and arm.

*Wall-reaching* exercises can be done by having the patient stand close to the wall, feet apart, and begin "crawling" and reaching with both hands, moving up the wall slowly. This should be done several times a day until the arms are extended full length with elbows straight (Fig. 6-8).

The *rope* exercise can be done by attaching one end of the rope to a doorknob, inserting a tongue depressor in the other loop, and grasping

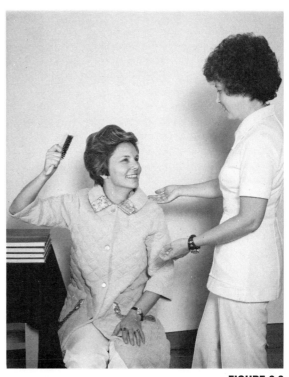

**FIGURE 6-6**
Hair-brushing exercise is done with encouragement from the nurse. Brush is held in the hand on operative side.

**TABLE 6-3**
HAND AND ARM CARE (POSTMASTECTOMY)

1  Avoid vaccinations, injections, or having blood drawn from the affected arm; have blood pressure taken on the unaffected side.

2  Housework is healthful, but ask for help when it comes to lifting heavy things and moving furniture. Be wary of burns while cooking; use a mitt to cover your hand and arm in the oven.

3  In manicuring, do not cut the cuticle on the affected hand. Lanolin-based cream will help keep the cuticle soft.

4  Take care of cuts and scrapes immediately by washing and covering them with a protective dressing.

5  Try to carry your purse on the unaffected side.

6  Gloves should always be loose-fitting. Do not wear anything that constricts the hand or arm, such as jewelry or tight sleeves.

7  When gardening, wear strong work gloves; when sewing, use a thimble and watch out for pinpricks; when washing, avoid harsh detergents; and wear gloves when hands must be in water for long periods.

8  Keep the arm at least shoulder high as much as possible (to help prevent swelling). When seated, rest it on the back of a chair or sofa.

9  Excessive sunburn may result in swelling.

10  Any skin that has had x-ray treatment should be shielded from the sun.

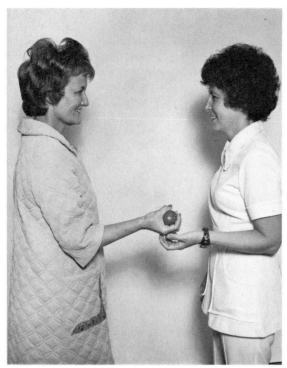

**FIGURE 6-7**
Nurse teaches patient rubber ball exercise to extend and flex fingers and hand.

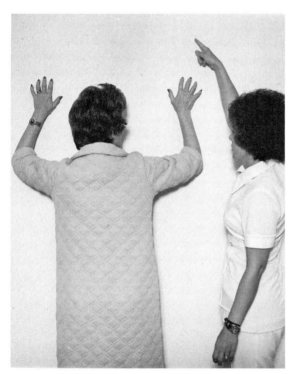

**FIGURE 6-8**
Nurse assists patient with "wall climbing."

it with the affected hand. The patient stands alongside the rope at right angles, looking straight ahead, with the other hand on the hip, feet apart and knees relaxed. She should then make circles with the rope, moving the entire arm from the shoulder. Movement progresses from small to larger circles, pausing when discomfort occurs, then resuming the exercise. The rope can then be thrown over a door, screen, or shower rod to make a pulley. Have the patient sit erect under the pulley, grasp each end with the hands, and pull slowly. Keep the pulley close to the patient's nose; in this way the arm will be brought up with elbows straight, close to the ears (Fig. 6-9).

All exercises, including household activities such as hanging clothes and washing windows, should be done slowly, resting when tired and pausing when discomfort occurs. Some discomfort or pain should be expected and is *not* a reason to stop the exercise.

**R**adiation Therapy   Radiation therapy is used in different stages of mammary carcinoma:

1   Following mastectomy, when the axillary lymph nodes are found to contain tumor. Doses are usually 4500 to 5000 rads to nodal sites.[24]

2   As primary therapy in *clinical Stage III* (T3, N4 & N2, N3):

    *a.* T3 treated with simple mastectomy plus McWhirter's technique (treating chest wall and all surrounding nodal drainage with tangential radiation fields to avoid lung tissue). Residual breast tumor can be treated with implants of radioactive substances.

    *b.* If no surgical intervention is done because the tumor is fixed to the chest wall (T4) or there is extensive skin metastasis, radiation therapy is employed alone with doses of 7000 to 9000 rads.[25]

3   In *clinical Stage IV,* as part of a multiagent approach that may use palliative surgery or chemotherapy.

The ideal in radiation therapy of any malignant disease is to completely eradicate the tumor without injury (either structural or functional) to surrounding normal tissue. This effect is infrequently obtained with breast cancer.

The objective of radiotherapy is either *curative* or *palliative.* In cancer of the breast it may be administered *externally* or *internally.* The patient needs an adequate explanation of what to expect both during and after treatment; the fear of unpleasant effects, such as nausea and skin burns, is usually great. With modern advances in the equipment used for external radiotherapy, the side effects have been much reduced and the patient should be made aware of this.

The patient needs to be informed that during therapy she will be placed on a table in a room by herself with equipment somewhat like x-ray machinery, although sometimes larger and more complicated. The therapist will be positioned outside the room to observe and communicate with the patient. The patient should be specifically informed that there is no pain associated with external radiation therapy to the breast. (Radiotherapy procedures and techniques are discussed in Chap. 5.)

External radiation must pass through the skin in order to reach the tumor. With the use of high-energy beams, the effects on the skin have been greatly minimized along with the surface area of skin exposed. The nursing care of the skin during radiation therapy of the exposed areas should be outlined by the individual therapist. Postradiation skin conditions such as dryness should be treated symptomatically.

Irradiation of the tumor site will involve the body hair growing in that area. Although this should not be of great concern to the female receiving breast irradiation, it should be mentioned so that she will understand the process. Often the loss of body hair is of greater concern to the male patient, and the psychological problems that arise must be recognized and individual action taken.

Because the gastrointestinal tract is not included in the area of primary breast irradiation, nausea, vomiting, and anorexia should not be problems. Patients who are not informed of this fact often experience the side effects that they expect to have. Preliminary orientation to radiotherapy, including its administration, side effects, and hoped-for results, should be given by the therapist and the nurses responsible for the patient's care.

When *internal* breast radiation is employed, the time spent with the patient should be restricted, depending on the amount of radioactive material used, its location, and the kinds of rays being emitted. The patient should be informed about these precautions, and every effort should be made to spend the total allotted time with the patient to alleviate any feelings of isolation.

**C**hemotherapy Medical oncologists have been treating the *failures* of primary therapy (surgery and radiotherapy) for years. Less than 5 percent of all patients with cancer of the breast received systemic

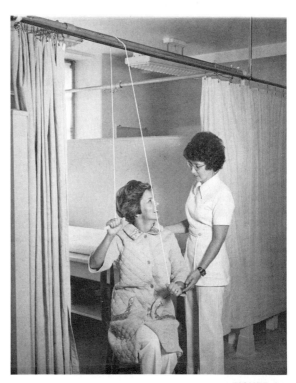

**FIGURE 6-9**
Nurse assists patient with arm exercises using pulley.

treatment as part of their primary care before 1969, and there has been a lack of significant improvement in survival rates in the past thirty years.[26] The Breast Cancer Task Force has stressed the importance of new approaches, particularly in the use of combined surgery and chemotherapy.

Chemotherapy is used in three major situations: (1) as adjuvant therapy (early combined approach at the time of diagnosis), (2) at the time of recurrence, and (3) when metastasis is present at diagnosis.

*Adjuvant chemotherapy* The use of adjuvant chemotherapy following surgical treatment in operable cases of breast carcinoma with positive axillary nodes has in recent years become the treatment of choice. Postoperative oophorectomy or a radiologic castration has been tried. This prophylactic endocrine therapy prolonged the disease-free period in some cases but failed to improve the overall survival.[27] The high correlation between positive axillary nodes and relapse rate and the frequent appearance of cancer cells in the circulating blood of patients during operative procedures provides the rationale for using adjuvant systemic treatments.

Studies have shown that premenopausal patients with positive axillary nodes at the time of mastectomy who were treated with adjuvant chemotherapy (phenylalanine mustard—L-Pam) experienced a longer disease-free interval than those who were not.[28] Those patients with operable breast cancer and with positive lymph nodes at the time of mastectomy show a statistically significant reduction in recurrence rate during the first 27 months after radical mastectomy when treated with cyclic prolonged combination chemotherapy.[29]

Patients with one to three positive nodes have an average recurrence time of about 5 years; with four or more nodes the average time is 18 months.[30] Patients with negative nodes have approximately a 25 percent failure rate and a 75 percent survival, while those with positive nodes have almost the reverse—75 percent failure and 25 percent survival.[31]

Response rates to single-agent drugs range from 10 to 60 percent.[32] These drugs are adriamycin, cyclophosphamide, methotrexate, fluorouracil, and vincristine. Combination chemotherapy has fast become useful, with response rates approaching 80 percent.[33]

Many cancer study groups throughout the world are using drugs in treating patients with advanced mammary cancer. In the majority of these patients, all other treatment modalities—surgery, radiotherapy, and hormonal therapy—have already been tried. Because of the different types of drug action, it is possible to combine drugs that individually have been known to exhibit activity against breast cancer cells. Such combinations may include Cytoxan (CTX), methotrexate (MTX), 5-fluorouracil (5-FU), adriamycin, vincristine (VCR), or prednisone. Two or more drugs constitute a combination. A 5-day regimen using CTX, VCR, MTX, 5-FU and prednisone showed a response rate of 70 to 90 percent.[34] Other combinations with adriamycin may improve this, since adriamycin alone has a response rate of approximately 40 percent.[35]

Combinations are possible with nearly a full therapeutic dose of the individual drugs, since the toxicity is not additive if the drugs have different mechanisms of action. For instance, CTX and adriamycin are not cell cycle-active drugs, which are suited to breast cancer in which a large fraction of cells are not in S phase at any one time. Methotrexate is a cell cycle-active agent that works by competitive binding of dehydrofolic reductase. 5-FU binds thymidylate synthetase. Both 5-FU and MTX interfere with DNA synthesis.

The *nursing problems* related to chemotherapy involve two areas: the side effects of the drugs and emotional support. *Side effects of antineoplastic drugs* can be classified in five general areas, with the addition of specifics for each individual drug. The general areas are (1) bone marrow depression, (2) gastrointestinal disturbances, (3) fluid retention, (4) neuropathies, and (5) alopecia. It must be understood that all antineoplastic drug agents *do not* carry each and every one of the side effects. Conscientious nursing care cannot be given unless the nurse takes upon herself the responsibility of knowing the drug action, side effects, and toxic signs of the specific drug or drugs that the patient is receiving. Details of these side effects are discussed in Chap. 5.

**H**ormonal Therapy    The oldest and best hormonal therapy for advanced carcinoma of the breast in premenopausal women and in men is *castration,* either surgically by oophorectomy (or orchiectomy in male patients) or medically by irradiation. For years, this treatment has produced objective regression of lesions in all metastatic sites, sometimes for long periods of time. Because of such promising results, castration was suggested as an adjuvant to the surgical or irradiation treatment of primary breast cancer. Most studies found only small differences in the patient's outcome, with no difference in survival rates.[36]

If the patient responds to *oophorectomy,* the tumor is said to be hormone-responsive; therefore, when the inevitable progression of tumor begins, other forms of hormonal therapy may be sought. This is usually given in the form of potent *estrogens* or *androgens.* The unpleasant effects of androgen therapy are virilization and increased libido. The most unpleasant side effect of estrogen is stress incontinence, which is very distressing to most women and often causes them to discontinue their hormonal therapy. Other side effects are salt retention and hypercalcemia. Some patients experience nausea and vomiting.

Women who are more than 5 years postmenopausal are often given the estrogen or androgen therapy. When a relapse occurs while on these hormones, an additional response period may occur at the cessation of therapy.[37] *Androgens* are usually used in premenopausal women and in women less than 10 years postmenopausal; *estrogens* are usually more effective in elderly women or those 10 or more years postmenopausal. Estrogens are contraindicated in those women in whom estrogen dependence has not been excluded.[38]

Many physicians advocate the use of further hormonal ablation by adrenalectomy and hypophysectomy, in patients who have evidence of an endocrine-dependent tumor with progressive metastatic disease, particularly bone metastasis. The adrenal cortex becomes the chief source of estrogen and androgen once ovarian or testicular function has been destroyed or suppressed. This fact is the basis for the use of *adrenalectomy* in advanced breast cancer. An adrenalectomy reduces estrogen excretion; it does not always eliminate it. Postoperatively the patient will be placed on cortisone replacement therapy.

The need for hormonal replacement should be explained carefully prior to surgery. The nurse, patient, and family should be aware of symptoms that indicate inadequate cortisone replacement, such as anorexia, progressive weakness, lethargy, nausea, vomiting, and eventual prostration. The patient should be aware that during times of stress these symptoms may also appear, signaling the need for increased therapy. Nursing care of the patient with inadequate adrenal function is discussed in Chap. 21.

*Hypophysectomy* (the surgical removal of the pituitary gland) is done in patients with advancing carcinoma of the breast to remove adrenocorticotrophic hormone (ACTH) and somatotrophic hormone (STH) (see Chap. 21). Patients undergoing both these surgical procedures have had previous extended treatments, and continuing emotional and physical support is essential. The patient facing a hypophysectomy has an additional fear of brain injury. Any operative procedure involving the brain carries with it the natural fear of loss of intellectual capacity and personality characteristics. A careful explanation of the procedure by the surgeon can help overcome this fear.

Because the source of ACTH has been removed, the hypophysectomy patient will require corticosteroid replacement. Since the thyroid-stimulating hormone (TSH) from the pituitary gland is also absent, thyroid hormone replacement will be required. Dryness of the skin, cold intolerance, constipation, and mental apathy may mean that additional thyroid medication is needed.

Immediately following the surgery, secretion of the antidiuretic hormone (ADH) may be disrupted, necessitating accurate monitoring of intake and output. The placement of a Foley catheter helps in measuring the exact urinary output. Fluid intake must be increased to meet the urinary output. The patient should be an active participant in recording her intake and output. Excessive urinary output (exceeding 1000 ml/hour) should be reported to the physician so that Pitressin can be administered to control *diabetes insipidus.* Pitressin may be given intramuscularly or in the form of a nasal "snuff."

*Estrogen receptors*　New research into estrogen receptors has permitted prediction as to which patients will benefit from hormonal therapy.

In estrogen target tissues and hormone dependent tumors, the steroid enters the cells and binds to a cytoplasmic protein called the estrogen receptor (ER). The steroid-receptor complex then migrates to the nuclei, where it initiates the biochemical events characteristic of estrogen stimulation.[39]

Clinical trials have clearly shown that if the patient's tissue does not contain ER there is little chance that tumor regression will occur following endocrine ablative therapy. Many patients could be spared unnecessary procedures if ER assays were performed routinely when an estrogen-dependent tumor is suspected. If the ER assay is positive, 55 to 60 percent will respond to endocrine therapy.[40]

**M**etastatic Disease　Unfortunately, until present treatment effects a "cure" or early diagnosis gains time that ensures a cure, there will remain a percentage of patients with carcinoma of the breast who have or will develop widespread metastatic disease. The four main sites of metastasis are (1) bones, (2) chest and soft tissue, (3) brain, and (4) viscera; nursing care is discussed in relation to these areas.

With *bone metastases,* the primary problem is *pain* that is aggravated by moving. Patients who have pain when moving about often do little to improve their personal appearance, preferring to lie in one position without moving. Pain medication in large amounts is often essential to enable the patient to maintain interest in her personal needs and to continue ambulation. Analgesics should be used on a regular basis once the lesion has been identified and radiation therapy begun. Medications given as needed are often not effective because the pain becomes too great before relief is gained. Pain medication should be given on a 3- to 4-hour schedule, later lengthened as therapy becomes effective. Patients have stated that they could handle the progression of their disease, but "could not handle the pain as a constant reminder that death was inevitable."[41]

Patients with bone metastasis should be cautioned against falling, reaching, twisting, or lifting heavy objects, as pathologic fractures may occur. Things should be kept within easy reach and their needs anticipated. Sexual intercourse should be encouraged if desired, as long as a comfortable position can be found.

*Brain metastasis* symptoms vary widely, depending on the area involved. They may include headache, papilledema, visual disturbances, difficulty in walking, loss of memory, and convulsive seizures.

Most patients are aware of the lessening of their functional abilities and realize that they are becoming more dependent. Independence and self-care should be encouraged as long as possible. The nurse must allow the patient to work at her own pace and must be alert to her special problems, such as difficulties in ambulation, swallowing, eating, talking, or incontinence.

*Visceral* (liver) *metastasis* is usually accompanied by ascites requiring diuretics or paracentesis. Electrolyte imbalances occur secondary to digestive disturbances, and accurate intake and output and daily weights should be recorded.

The major symptoms of *chest and soft tissue lesions* are lymphedema, ulceration, and pleural effusions which cause pain, shortness of breath, and coughing. Repositioning the patient frequently will contribute to comfort and relief of pressure areas.

The nurse must examine and evaluate her own feelings toward caring for the patient with advanced disease and set her goals in a realistic manner. Planning should be aimed at providing comfort for the patient in terms of pain relief, recreation, ambulation, odor control, skin care, and emotional support. Providing for nutrition and hydration in the face of nausea, vomiting, and problems of elimination becomes a challenging aspect of cancer-care nursing. Ambulation should be continued as long as possible, with recreational activities provided to keep the patient occupied and functioning.

## Fourth-level Nursing Care

*Rehabilitation* begins when the patient first enters the health-care system. In order for the mastectomy patient to return to equilibrium, she must

Accept the loss of her breast by fully mourning for that loss. This necessarily includes grief around the fear that she may lose a husband or even ultimately her life.

Reintegrate a self-image worthy of love and the rewards of life.

Begin to make peace with the albatross of potential recurrence.[42]

*Discharge planning* for the mastectomy patient must begin immediately upon the patient's arrival at the health-care facility. Attention should be paid to a continuing exercise program, vocational problems and planning, breast prosthesis, arm and hand care, and follow-up examinations and care. (Refer to Table 6-3 regarding hand and arm care.)

If possible, the mastectomy patient should be visited by an attractive woman who has undergone a mastectomy. The Reach-to-Recovery Program sponsored by the American Cancer Society will meet that need if such services are available in the area and are requested by the attending physician.

Costello, at the First National Conference on Cancer Nursing, presented the following steps which seem necessary for a patient dealing with surgically created alterations in body image. The patient

Accepts the importance of viewing the operative site

Touches and explores the operative site

Accepts the necessity of learning to care for the defect

Develops independence and competence in daily care

Reintegrates the new body image and adjusts to a possibly altered life-style.[43]

The challenge to nurses is to assist the patient in meeting these goals by accepting the patient and her altered body image and allowing her to express her feelings in this area. At the time of altered body image, the nurse is essentially providing crisis intervention for both the patient and her family. The patient and family must be made members of the team and co-managers of her care. If the patient is allowed to set goals, motivation is less of a problem.

Besides the cosmetic effect of a mastectomy, a woman's (or man's) sexuality is continually bombarded from the moment of diagnosis. Breast cancer is a visual assault to the female body. The significance of the female breast is far greater than its physiologic function, because men and women alike have associated sexual attractiveness of females and femininity with breast size.

"The most important single factor in a woman's response after mastectomy is the reaction of the male with whom she is most intimately—often sexually—involved."[44] Many men are supportive, but some are not. Since one in three marriages are under enough stress to end in divorce, the added stress of illness or mastectomy may push a marriage over the brink.

The supportive male should be helped in this area. The nurse who deals with the patient and family must be observant and allow *him* to acknowledge his feelings and express himself. The patient will need the reassurance of his love, his support, his faith in her and the future. Some Reach-to-Recovery chapters have couple volunteers who work with couples undergoing the crisis of mastectomy.

It is not until after the patient has met some of her own emotional needs and has begun to accept her diagnosis that she will be motivated enough to exercise and work at recovery. Many patients "cured" of mammary cancer are incapacitated and cannot maintain pretreatment activities. The two main problems are limitation of shoulder movement, which can result from surgery or radiation fibrosis, and lymphedema. Early postoperative instructions on exercise with total involvement and cooperation can reduce these complications to a minimum. An exercise program endorsed by the American Cancer Society has been discussed previously (Figs. 6-6 through 6-9).

A breast form (*prosthesis*) is often of major concern for the mastectomy patient. A temporary breast form can be inserted inside the bra until the physician gives permission for the fitting of a permanent form. There are many types, and the choice should be the patient's. The nurse can refer the patient to a good corsetiere in a local department store or specialty shop. The American Cancer Society, through the Reach-to-Recovery volunteer, can supply the patient with a list of types of prostheses and where to purchase them. The prostheses may be soft, fluid-like, filled, weighted forms to balance the opposite side, rubber, air-filled, or combinations. Sheepskin pads can be worn to absorb perspiration. A properly fitting, comfortable breast prosthesis can make the difference in a woman's attitude toward recovery.

*Health counseling* is an ongoing process with patients and their families. Since the tendency for breast cancer seems to be higher in women who have a family history of breast cancer, counseling must include extended-family members—grandchildren, sisters, etc.

The patient and family should be reassured that, according to available knowledge, breast cancer is not transmitted by direct contact. The cancer patient who is ill-informed often imposes isolation on herself.

The cancer patient and her family should be encouraged to resume all previous activities as soon as the initial healing process has taken place and physical toleration has developed.

*Follow-up care* is a must for patients with a known cancer of the breast, since cancer in the opposite breast occurs in 4 to 10 percent of all cases.[45] These women must be examined semiannually both clinically and by mammography.

A 5- or 10-year survival does not assure a "cure." Progressive cancer can recur as long as 20 years after the initial surgical treatment.[46] Even with present treatment modalities, including surgery, radiation, chemotherapy, hormonal therapy, and immunotherapy, over half of those with cancer of the breast develop metastases.[47] As with early primary diagnosis, recognition of metastases while their tumor-cell mass is relatively small may increase the probability of remission with combination therapy and possibly produce a longer survival period.

The patient with mammary carcinoma is subjected to many forms of therapy for her illness. She often has faced the loss of a body part or parts, has had to deal with an altered body image, and has met with the sociocultural stigma of having cancer. Her survival is being extended through early diagnosis and more advanced systemic therapies. At the time of diagnosis, she still has only a 50 percent chance of living 10 years but has one essential for survival—the hope that more sophisticated therapies will be discovered to completely eradicate the ever-threatening cancer in her body.

## NEOPLASMS OF THE FEMALE GENITAL TRACT

Neoplasms of the female genital tract comprise one-fifth (22 percent) of all cancer in women. These cancers, with the exception of ovarian and tubal neoplasms, are easily accessible and thus amenable to early diagnosis and treatment. Over the last three decades a marked reduction in mortality has occurred in carcinomas of the uterus and cervix. This has been due to the wide use of cytologic screening, radical surgery, and effective radiotherapeutic techniques. Even so, the American Cancer Society estimated that there would be 11,000 deaths in the United States in 1976 from cancer of the uterus and cervix. The use of chemotherapy has completely changed the treatment of trophoblastic neoplasia by putting this once fatal choriocarcinoma into the category of curable diseases. Chemotherapy has also added an effective means of palliation in ovarian tumors. The use of progestational hormones in adenocarcinoma of the uterine corpus has provided palliation and demonstrated the susceptibility of neoplasms to endocrinologic effects.

Modern research gives hope that even more promising results will be forthcoming through integration of the three therapeutic modalities, surgery, radiation, and chemotherapy, with the adjuvant use of immunotherapy.

### Benign Uterine Neoplasms

*Myomas* or *fibroid tumors,* which affect approximately 20 percent of all women over 30 years of age, are benign tumors of the uterus. They rarely become malignant, and at the advent of the menopause may tend to disappear spontaneously. Menorrhagia is the most common symptom. The bleeding is due to both the hormonal effects and the increased surface available to bleed. Low backache, abdominal pressure, constipation, dysmenorrhea, and urinary retention are results of pressure by the tumor mass.

The treatment of benign tumors depends on the patient's age, whether or not she desires children, and how near she is to the menopause. A *myomectomy* (surgical removal of the tumor) may be performed if the tumor is near the outer wall of the uterus. *Hysterectomy* is necessary in cases of severe bleeding, pressure symptoms, or obstruction. If the patient is nearing the menopause or surgery is contraindicated, *x-ray therapy* or *radiation* may be used to reduce the size of the tumor or to stop bleeding.

### Malignant Uterine Neoplasms

Malignant neoplasms of the uterus and cervix are generally squamous-cell carcinomas or adenocarcinomas. Adenocarcinoma of the endometrium accounts for 90 percent of all *endometrial neoplasms.* Sarcomas, mesodermal tumors, and leiomyosarcoma of the endometrium are occasionally seen. Squamous-cell carcinoma accounts for about 95 percent of all primary *cervical cancers,* with adenocarcinoma making up 4 to 5 percent.[48]

**Pathophysiology** *Metastasis* or spread of carcinoma of the cervix and uterus depends on the area of primary involvement. Those cancers which begin in the cervix usually spread by *direct extension* into the parametrium laterally. Invasion of the vagina may occur, which worsens the prognosis. Anteroposterior extension into the bladder or rectum drastically lowers the survival rate. Extension

into these areas frequently results in fistula formation. Metastasis occurs in three lymph-node groups: the external iliac lymph-node chain, the hypogastric lymph-node chain, and the para-aortic lymph nodes. Metastases are rarely blood-borne. The incidence of pulmonary metastasis is 5 percent; bone metastasis occurs even less frequently.

Cancer of the uterine body remains localized in the vast majority of cases. As a result, the 5-year survival rate is high. If invasion occurs, spread is usually to the myometrium or to the cervix. If the myometrium and lymphatics are involved, spread may be via the upper broad-ligament channels, to the ovary, then to the para-aortic nodes, as the first lymph-node station outside the pelvis. If the cancer spreads downward to the cervix, the subserosal plexus of lymphatics may disseminate it through the parametrium to the deep pelvic lymph nodes.

Both cancer of the cervix and cancer of the uterine body can be "cured," if diagnosed at an early stage, with adequate surgical treatment. Surgical treatment of intraepithelial (in situ) carcinoma of the cervix has a 5-year survival rate of almost 100 percent. Early carcinomas of the uterine body have a 5-year survival rate of more than 90 percent with combination treatment by surgery and irradiation. Early diagnosis must be increased to reduce the mortality and morbidity from these potentially curable neoplasms.

**Clinical staging** The staging of the disease in carcinoma of the uterus is important both for prognosis and for determining the treatment program. The *international staging* for clinical classification of *endometrial* cancer is as follows:

*Stage I:* Carcinoma confined to the corpus

*Stage II:* Carcinoma involves the corpus and the cervix

*Stage III:* Carcinoma extends outside the uterus but not outside the pelvis

*Stage IV:* Carcinoma extends outside the true pelvis or obviously involves the mucosa of the bladder or rectum[49]

The staging schema is useful for the reporting of comprehensive series but is not widely accepted in the management of endometrial tumors. They are also classified according to (1) size, (2) differentiation of the tumor, and (3) cervical involvement. The pathologic staging of carcinoma of the endometrium usually include TNM (tumor, nodes, and metastasis), a classification much like that used for cancers of the head and neck and of the breast. The international staging for carcinoma of the *cervix* is shown in Table 6-4.

Diagnosis at an early stage in uterine cervical cancer increases the survival rate. If diagnosed in Stage 0 (carcinoma in situ), the 5-year survival rate approaches 100 percent. Stage I diagnosis offers an 80 to 85 percent chance of 5-year survival. A later diagnosis, made at a time when the disease has progressed to Stage II, reduces the 5-year survival to 50 to 75 percent. In more advanced stages, the likelihood of a 5-year survival with the present modalities of treatment is reduced to less than 30 percent. In addition, the quality of survival is poor: the patient is in pain and dependent on others, with urinary and bowel complications, as a result of extension of the disease or of therapy.

### First-level Nursing Care

*Cervical cancers* are epidemiologically linked with socioeconomic factors. These include low income, early marriage and coitus, sexual intercourse with multiple partners, venereal disease, inadequate pre- and postnatal care, and infrequent medical examinations and Pap tests. Endometrial cancer is not linked with any of these factors except the last.

A large proportion of women who have *endometrial cancer* are obese, multiparous, hypertensive, and have a history of diabetes. Endometrial cancer usually develops after menopause, in contrast to cervical cancer, which develops more often in premenopausal women. Recently, prolonged estrogenic stimulation in high doses has been suggested as a causative factor.[50]

Annual examination with a Pap smear provides for detection at an early and curable stage. Nurses should encourage annual Pap smears in all women over 20 years of age, those younger women who are sexually active, and those who take oral contraceptives. The remarkable decrease in deaths from uterine cancer in the last 40 years has been attributed to early diagnosis as a result of screening with the Pap test.

A major program of the American Cancer Society aims to encourage every woman over 20, and those younger who are at risk, to have Pap tests. Nurses who work as primary health-care providers and in community health should be actively participating in this program.

### Second-level Nursing Care

Persons seen in community clinics, doctors' offices, and outpatient departments may have a Pap smear as part of a routine examination. Nurses may perform or assist in such assessments.

**Nursing assessment** The initial assessment of the patient presenting for routine Pap smear or with problems associated with "female" complaints should include a thorough *health history,* including menses, hormonal ingestion, sexual activity, pregnancy, and pre- and postnatal complications. Bleeding not related to menses is the most common presenting complaint of females with "suspect" tumors of the uterus.

No symptoms may be associated with early cancer of the *cervix.* However, symptoms which demand diagnostic studies include postcoital spotting, unexplained vaginal spotting or bleeding, and vaginal discharge. Pelvic pain, leakage of urine or feces, weight loss, and anorexia are often indicative of advanced disease.[51]

The typical presentation of cancer of the *endometrium* in the menopausal or postmenopausal female is unexplained vaginal bleeding. A "bloody menopause" is often the history given by patients with adenocarcinoma. Low-back pain and abdominal pain may be present. Even with advanced disease, such women are rarely debilitated. Hypertension, diabetes, and obesity are frequently associated with endometrial carcinoma and should be evaluated.

**D**iagnostic Tests The *Papanicolaou smear* (Pap smear) was named after George Papanicolaou, who developed this accurate and effective cancer-screening technique. The Pap smear is based on the principle that the uterus is an exfoliating organ and that cells (tumor as well as normal) from the fallopian tubes, uterus, and vagina exfoliate and pass into the cervical and vaginal secretions.

**TABLE 6-4**
INTERNATIONAL CLASSIFICATION FOR STAGING CARCINOMA OF THE CERVIX

| | |
|---|---|
| Stage 0 | Carcinoma in situ, intraepithelial carcinoma |
| Stage I | Carcinoma strictly confined to the cervix |
| Stage II | Carcinoma extends beyond the cervix but has not extended into the pelvic wall; carcinoma involves the vagina, but not the lower third |
| Stage III: | |
| Stage IIIa | Tumor involves the lower third of the vagina but has not extended into the pelvic wall |
| Stage IIIb | Carcinoma has extended into the pelvic wall; on rectal examination there is no cancer-free space between the tumor and the pelvic wall |
| Stage IV | Carcinoma has extended beyond the true pelvis or has involved the mucosa of the bladder or rectum |

When these excretions and scrapings from the cervical, vaginal, and endocervical areas are collected and smears made and examined by a pathologist, the cellular changes may be detected early, before the lesions are seen or become symptomatic. (The procedure for Pap screening is described in Chap. 4.) Deaths from cervical cancer have decreased by over 50 percent in the last 15 years, and that percentage of decrease is expected to increase as education of the public concerning the need for regular Pap smears becomes more widespread. The World Health Organization has classified cancer of the cervix as a preventable disease. The patient should be told of the routine system used to notify patients with the reassurance that notification of the need for a repeat smear does not indicate that malignancy is present.

The Papanicolaou classification for uterine cervical changes is complicated, but the usual readings are given in four or five classes. More recently, pathologists have avoided the "numbers game" and reported the abnormality by a description of the findings:

*Negative* or *Class I:* Only normal cells seen

*Inconclusive* or *Class II:* Smear contains cells with atypical features but not suggestive of malignant cells

*Suspicious* or *Class III:* Smear contains cells with abnormalities suggestive of but not definitive for malignant cells

*Positive* or *Class IV:* Smear contains cells with abnormalities definitive for malignant cells

*Positive* or *Class V:* Smear contains malignant cells as above with changes more advanced than in Class IV[52]

The nurse should be able to interpret to patients the meaning of the test result and the need for and availability of diagnostic and definitive care (see Fig. 6-10). Aggressive management is indicated when an abnormal smear is found.

*Dysplasia* is a deviation from normal that may be found in the epithelium of the uterine cervix. It is thought to be the beginning stage in the spectrum of developing squamous-cell carcinoma. In one clinic, one out of three women with severe dysplasia went on to develop carcinoma in situ.[53] Women with dysplasia should have frequent Pap smears, and if their desire for childbearing is past, a hysterectomy on those with severe dysplasia is recommended.[54]

The widespread use of *colposcopy* (examination of the cervical and vaginal tissues by specially designed microscopic equipment) has made possible examination and direct cervical biopsy on an outpatient basis. Colposcopy is indicated for study and diagnosis when inconclusive Pap smears do not revert to negative after treatment for specific or nonspecific cervicitis and when the Pap smear is suspicious or positive.

The *Schiller stain* continues to be of some value, especially when colposcopy is not available. The Schiller test is performed by staining the cervix and upper vagina with an iodine solution in order to define the abnormal area for biopsy. This test is based on the presence of glycogen in the normal cervical and vaginal mucosa. Any type of cellular abnormality frequently produces a dilution of glycogen which prevents the solution from staining.

*Conization* of the cervix is indicated when the entire transformation zone between the squamous and columnar epithelium cannot be visualized by colposcopy. This procedure usually requires hospitalization and is discussed under third-level care.

**Nursing problems and interventions** The major nursing problem is the *finding of a neoplasm or cellular abnormality.* Intervention is directed toward *referral* of the patient to a medical facility for further diagnosis and evaluation. A negative finding requires that the nurse continue to encourage the patient to follow through with regular examinations.

### Third-level Nursing Care

Following a positive Pap smear, a suspicious lesion seen at the time of examination, or undiagnosed physical complaints, entry into a hospital is usually necessary for a more complete and comprehensive workup.

**Nursing assessment** Development of rapport during assessment of the patient is crucial. The patient possibly faces invasive diagnostic tests, a positive diagnosis of cancer, radical surgery, or, with symptoms of advanced disease, impending death.

**H**ealth History  Some patients seek further medical attention solely because of a positive Pap smear; others may give health histories that signal the presence of advanced disease. Early indications of disease include watery, foul-smelling vaginal discharge and bleeding. The patient may describe spotting or minimal bleeding that has become

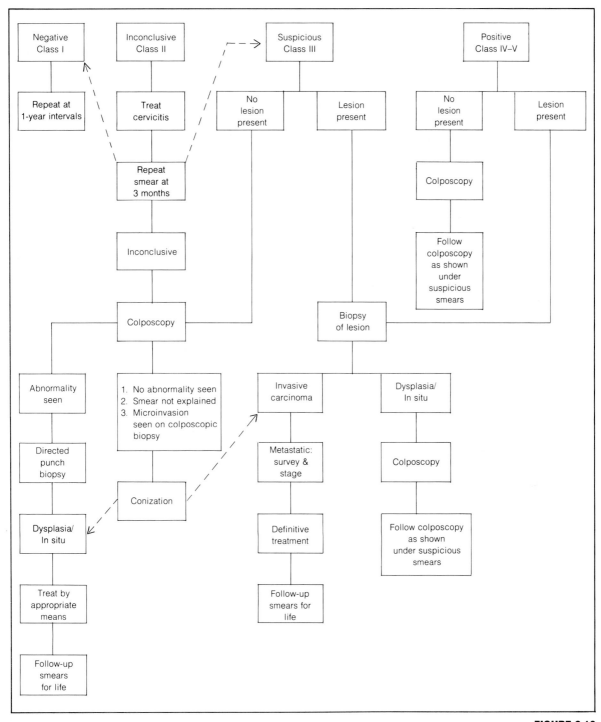

**FIGURE 6-10**
Cervical smear flow chart.

heavier over time. This bleeding is particularly noticeable to postmenopausal women. Premenopausal women may describe their menstrual periods as prolonged and unusually heavy or may experience bleeding between periods.

Pain is usually a later symptom and denotes pressure on and involvement of sensory nerve endings. Other complaints associated with advanced disease include feelings of lower abdominal pressure, constipation, rectal discharge, and difficulty voiding. Systemic manifestations often include weakness, loss of appetite, and weight loss.

**P**hysical Assessment   The patient who is hospitalized because of a positive Pap smear may have no other physical symptoms. In contrast, a patient with an advanced or invasive tumor may appear cachectic, pale, and weak. An abdominal mass may or may not be palpable; she may describe pain upon movement or manipulation. The presence of a gastrointestinal obstruction may be evidenced by vomiting or distention (see Chap. 18). Vaginal bleeding may be severe, to the point of hemorrhage, and be reflected in an increased pulse rate and decreased blood pressure. Severe hemorrhage or intestinal obstruction requires immediate medical intervention.

**D**iagnostic Tests   The diagnostic tests used to evaluate a patient with a positive Pap smear include colposcopy, Schiller test, biopsy to determine cell type, cone biospy, examination under anesthesia (EUR), and dilatation and curettage (D and C).

The *colposcopy* has been used for many years to assist in the diagnosis of cervical cancer. It provides a well-lighted, magnified, stereoscopic view of the cervix. Cervical intraepithelial neoplasia begins in the transformation zone, that area of the cervix in which columnar epithelium is replaced by squamous epithelium. The colposcopic evaluation of the transformation zone and of the endocervical canal is a useful procedure in the evaluation of the patient with an abnormal cervical smear. During colposcopy, the cervix is bathed with a 3% acetic acid solution to accentuate the topographic and vascular alterations which are found in neoplastic epithelium and serve to differentiate it from the normal metaplastic areas. Colposcopy can detect the location of the abnormality to determine whether conization is necessary.

A *biopsy* is necessary to confirm by tissue diagnosis the histology and extent of the lesion. If the target site for biopsy is predetermined by the

Schiller test or colposcopy, a tissue sample is taken of that area. Four-quadrant cervical biopsies will give a 96 percent accurate diagnosis and will eliminate the morbidity occasionally associated with cone biopsy.[55] This technique for the most part has been replaced by colposcopically directed biopsies.

A *cone biopsy* (conization) is often performed when a target lesion is not evident or when the transformation zone is not adequately visualized. This provides a cone-shaped section of the cervix in one particular area that contains more tissue for examination. If the diseased portion of the cervix can be completely localized in the removed section, conization may be the only procedure required. Patients should be told of the likelihood of a vaginal discharge for a few days following the procedure.

*EUA* (examination under anesthesia) allows the physician to perform a more thorough pelvic examination for abnormalities on a totally relaxed patient. This procedure is done in the operating room and may include a biopsy.

*Dilatation and curettage* (D and C) is a surgical procedure that requires anesthesia and consists of dilatation of the cervix and curettage (scraping) of the endometrial lining of the uterus. This is used for diagnosis of lesions other than those limited to the cervix.

Psychological and physical preparation for this procedure is similar to that given to anyone undergoing general anesthesia. The preparations necessary, such as enemas, douches, shaving of the pubic and perineal area, and insertion of an indwelling urinary catheter, should be thoroughly explained to the patient.

A *fractional D and C* is done by keeping the fragments from the endocervix and endometrial cavity in separate specimen containers in order to enable the pathologist to locate the abnormal tissue.

It is often during the diagnostic period that additional tests are done to "stage" a patient who has been found to have invasive disease. These may include sigmoidoscopy, intravenous pyelograms, and other tests to determine the extent of the disease.

An abnormal cervical smear report on a pregnant patient should not preclude immediate investigation to make a definitive diagnosis with the same determination as in the nonpregnant patient.[56] The class of the smear and length of the pregnancy determine the aggressiveness of the treatment. Colposcopy is not usually contraindicated. Conization usually is contraindicated until after delivery. In those patients with positive findings, a cesarean section is usually performed as soon as it is safe for the mother and child.

The stress factor in the patient's life may be high. An unfamiliar environment, unfamiliar procedures, and fear and apprehension of the results may all contribute to anxiety. Each procedure should be explained in detail, allowing the patient to express her feelings. Many women face a period in which they feel guilty for what has happened to them. Hostility is often exhibited as a mechanism of expressing fear.

Occasionally the patient completely withdraws and experiences a time of depression or denial. All these coping mechanisms must be accepted by the nurse as a necessary part of the patient's working through a difficult situation. A positive, realistic approach by the nurse can help the patient to cope with this time of crisis.

**Nursing problems and interventions** Nursing problems most readily identified during this time are *emotional stress, bleeding, pain,* and *vaginal discharge.* Each woman will have a unique response to the diagnosis of a cancer of the reproductive tract. How a woman views herself, her relationship to her family, and how she reacts to the medical personnel will help the nurse recognize her response to the diagnosis. A young woman who desires to have children may react more violently than a woman who has already raised her family. Her feelings may stem from feeling "undesirable" to her husband or her inability to offer him a "complete woman." If she has a strong feeling of her own value as a contributing family member, the reaction to loss of her ability to have children may be lessened. When cancer of the uterus or cervix is diagnosed at an early stage, an optimistic outlook is realistic even in the face of major surgery and radical treatment modalities.

*Bleeding* is a major factor during both the diagnostic workup and the postoperative period of care. Nursing observation and accurate recording of blood loss is essential. Whether the blood loss is part of the presenting picture or a result of biopsy, D and C, or radical surgery, the amount of blood lost must be continually monitored, recording the amount in estimated milliliters, documenting the numbers of perineal pads used each 24 hours (a blood loss of at least 60 ml is required to saturate a perineal pad), and paying particular attention to the red blood count so that anemia from blood loss can be corrected before it becomes severe.

*Pain* should be assessed adequately to determine the site, frequency, and cause. Analgesics should be ordered and offered in doses and frequencies that will enable the patient to continue the activities of daily living without being hampered by intolerable pain. Pain is often a factor following surgical procedures and in advanced disease but is not always due to the cancer. Analgesics are often given to patients with cancer without complete investigation. Cancer is not always painful; the pain may result from a problem that can be corrected by change of position, laxatives, or catheterization.

*Vaginal discharge* is often one of the most distressing symptoms for the female patient. Odor and irritation can become a disturbing factor. Bathing the perineal area with soap and water several times a day may offer relief. If the discharge is caused by infection, specific treatment should be aimed at eliminating it.

**S**urgery Unlike many other cancers, cancer of the uterus can be cured. Palliation is necessary in those patients with distant metastasis. Therapy aims to "cure," whether it be surgery, radiotherapy, hormonal therapy, chemotherapy, or a combination of these. Nursing problems can be greatly minimized by patient education. A patient who is well informed is better equipped to cooperate in the planned therapy. The constant reminder that cure is the goal will enable the patient to maintain an optimistic outlook even during times when radical treatment may be necessary.

*Radical hysterectomy* includes removal of the uterus and cervix, fallopian tubes, ovaries, and pelvic lymph nodes. This procedure is appropriate in selected patients whose tumor has deeply penetrated the myometrium or has invaded the cervix and taken the parametrial route of spread toward the pelvic lymph nodes.

Cancer of the endometrium will require not only removal of the uterus by an abdominal hysterectomy but a bilateral salpingo-oophorectomy as well, for although the thick wall of the myometrium serves as a barrier to early spread and invasion, the ovaries may become involved by direct extension; the majority of women in such cases are postmenopausal and are less severely affected by the alteration in the hormonal state.

*Pelvic exenteration* for advanced carcinoma includes radical hysterectomy, pelvic node dissection, cystectomy, vaginectomy, and rectal resection. Such radical surgery is done only on far-advanced pelvic malignancies with extensive invasion. The patient having this procedure will have both urine and feces passing from the body through openings in the abdominal wall. Urine is eliminated through an ileal conduit, discussed later in this chapter, and feces pass through a colostomy, discussed in Chap. 18. After a pelvic exenteration, the patient will not be able to bear children or have sexual intercourse, and symptoms of the menopause will begin.

*Nursing problems after surgical intervention* The relevant nursing problems are of two kinds: those similar to the problems after any abdominal operative procedure and those specific to cancer. With *abdominal hysterectomy,* the routine postoperative care is the same as with any abdominal surgery. Special consideration should be given to coughing, deep breathing, and leg exercises. When extensive procedures are done, such as radical hysterectomy or exenteration, there is a predisposition to femoral thrombophlebitis. Measures to preserve optimum circulation are helpful. Occasionally elastic stockings and anticoagulant therapy are ordered. Symptoms of phlebitis, such as local or systemic pain, redness, swelling, and fever, should be observed for and reported to the physician.

*Abdominal distention* and, occasionally, paralytic ileus may follow extensive surgery (see Chap. 18). Reestablishment of normal peristalsis and bowel function is necessary. Early ambulation and proper diet are helpful in eliminating this complication.

*Urinary retention* is frequently a complication after extensive lower abdominal surgery, and Foley catheters are often used. Directly after surgery or following removal of a Foley catheter, the patient may be unable to void and should be observed closely for retention. The patient who has not voided for 8 hours should be catheterized.

With any type of surgical procedure, whether it be a wide conization or a pelvic exenteration, the patient is going through a *crisis period.* The patient with cancer must also deal with the fact that she has a malignant disease. In addition, she may be concerned about her femininity and possible changes in secondary sex characteristics.

Postoperatively, women usually experience a few days of depression. This is apparently due to two factors: a change in hormonal balance and a psychologic reaction. The patient may cry, feel depressed, and not be able to express the reason. She must often go through the grief process associated with the loss of a body part or parts.

Continuing activities such as using makeup, arranging her hair, and dressing in her own clothes as soon as possible after surgery will help her retain her feeling of femininity. Except for the patient who has had pelvic exenteration, sexual intercourse may be resumed several weeks after surgery.

**R**adiation Therapy Radiotherapy is a common treatment modality for carcinoma of the cervix and endometrium. It is used both externally and internally. *External* radiation can be used to reduce the tumor mass to make it more amenable to radium implant or surgery or to destroy microscopic implants following surgery. This is discussed more fully in Chap. 5.

The form of radiation therapy most commonly used is the *internal implantation* of radium. Radium is a naturally occurring element that emits gamma radiation. Since the uterine cavity is easily accessible, the radium can be placed in special containers to conform to uterine and vaginal contours. The nurse, the patient, and her family should work together in a team effort with the radiotherapist and physician. The well-informed patient and family who understand the basis of this form of radiotherapy will be better able to accept the restrictions on the nursing staff and family to prevent their exposure to radiation by close contact. *Needless* time should not be spent with the patient, but physical isolation is not necessary. The medical team and family should receive specific instructions as to the amount of time permitted with the patient and the safe distances.

Once the containers are placed in the cervix or uterus and placement is verified by x-ray, the radium is loaded while the patient is in the radiation therapy unit. The patient then returns to the nursing unit at the completion of the procedure and remains on bed rest during the course of therapy. Total insertion times vary from 48 to 144 hours. Extended times are divided into two applications 2 to 3 weeks apart.

During therapy, a urinary catheter is used to avoid contamination of the urine. Close observation is necessary to assess problems early. Since perineal care is not permitted during treatment, the discharge usually accompanying treatment may be distressing to the patient. After the radium, applicators, and packing are removed, a douche under low pressure may be used.

Throughout therapy, the nurse must be accessible to the patient to make her feel as little isolation as possible. Brief visits at safe distances should be made frequently to alleviate her fears and apprehension. (Full discussion of the care of the patient with a radiation implant is found in Chap. 5.)

**C**hemotherapy   Since cancer of the endometrium and cervix are best treated with surgery for cure, chemotherapy is usually reserved for advanced disease and widespread metastasis. Alkylating agents have been used with a 25 to 30 percent palliation rate for endometrial carcinoma.[57] Hormonal therapy with progestins is accompanied by fewer complications than therapy with the alkylating agents. Delalutin given by weekly injections causes local discomfort but no untoward side effects. Some long-term regressions have been produced with this therapy.[58]

**Fourth-level Nursing Care**

The plan for *rehabilitation* is determined by many factors. These include the extent of the operative procedure, the patient's prognosis, the patient-family interaction, and the emotional level and stability of the woman regarding her altered body image and sexuality.

The level of emphasis on postoperative rehabilitation is directly related to the extent of the operative procedure. After total hysterectomy with or without salpingo-oophorectomy or after a less extensive procedure, little, if any, change would require extensive physical rehabilitation. A patient who has undergone a pelvic exenteration, however, must be rehabilitated for body function, including altered urinary and fecal passages. Rehabilitation should begin before surgery so that the patient will have some understanding of the procedure. Full rehabilitative services should be offered to the patient and her family regarding care of the colostomy and ileal bladder (or other form of urinary diversion).

The nurse has a major role in motivating the patient to work toward her own recovery in order to reach her optimal level of function. The goal can be accomplished by allowing the patient to enter into decisions concerning her care and encouraging self-care whenever possible. The patient must regain pride in herself as a woman by fixing her hair, applying makeup, and dressing in her own clothes. In any rehabilitation program, the nurse must nourish and support a hopeful atmosphere. From the time the patient enters into the health-care system, the nurse must work toward the goal of patient independence. It is at the onset that plans must be made for *follow-up care and health counseling.*

A woman who has been treated for a cancer of the genital tract, even though cured, must appreciate the necessity for continuing annual or semiannual physical examinations. Health counseling of the patient should focus on the prevention of complications, the resumption of sexual function, and hormone replacement therapy.

*Complications* following therapy for cancer of the female genital tract may be due to the basic disease or to the treatment modality. Fistulas may result from invasion by the disease, destruction of tissues by radiation, or poor healing after surgery. Treatment of a fistula by primary surgical repair or by other means that may result in spontaneous closure depends on multiple factors. Regardless of the type of treatment, nursing care should be aimed at three goals: (1) maintenance of nutrition and hydration, (2) protection of the skin, and (3) prevention and control of infection. Incontinence may also be a problem. The cause must be determined: if it is related to the treatment (chemotherapy, radiation, or hormone therapy), an adjustment of therapy may be helpful.

*Sexual function* is an important part of most people's lives. Sexuality and the expression of that sexuality is a highly individualized aspect of one's personality. Sexual expression is both a biologic function and a form of communication. Often a woman's sexual expression is altered because of emotional problems related to the diagnosis. She may blame the cervical cancer on herself, her mate, or her sex life. It often takes longer for the emotional wounds of an altered body image to heal and problems related to sexuality to resolve themselves. The nurse must be aware of such feelings and allow the patient to express them throughout her illness and convalescence so that full rehabilitation can be achieved. In all but total pelvic exenteration, sexual intercourse can be resumed following healing of the surgical site. After hysterectomy, for some women, sexual expression may even be more satisfactory as a result of the elimination of the fear of pregnancy.

Removal of the reproductive organs alters the normal interrelationship between the endocrine glands. Oophorectomy in a premenopausal woman produces an *artificial onset of menopause.* The patient may experience flushing of the head, neck, and thorax with sweating (hot flashes). Later, atrophy of the genital tract, breasts, and skeletal structures may develop.

Often physicians recommend estrogen replacement therapy to suppress the hot flashes, vascular phenomena, and other estrogen-deprivation symptoms. Dyspareunia may be caused by thinning and atrophy of the vaginal mucosa resulting from low estrogen levels. Estrogen creams used as a local treatment in the vagina may be helpful. Patients should be cautioned not to apply the cream before intercourse, as it may have a negative effect on the male partner.

## Ovarian Cancer

Ovarian cancer is the fourth leading cause of cancer deaths in American women, following tumors of the breast, colon, and lung.[59] The silent, insidious onset and lack of accessibility contribute to the mortality rate. Over one-half of all malignancies of the ovary are inoperable and have metastasized at the time of diagnosis. Recently the incidence has increased without an improvement in therapeutic approaches. Careful examination at the time of an annual physical examination may detect the tumor before it becomes symptomatic. A palpable ovary in a postmenopausal woman is considered abnormal and cause for exploratory surgery. Symptoms usually signal metastatic disease. Many believe that ovarian cysts should be vigorously treated, as they may be precursors of malignant disease.

Presenting complaints usually include lower abdominal pain and pressure or abdominal enlargement. Unfortunately, these may represent a tumor mass that is enlarged or has metastasized.

Surgical removal of the tumor and the ovary is the treatment of choice whenever possible. Total hysterectomy with bilateral salpingo-oophorectomy is advocated. Often surgery is followed by deep x-ray therapy, but the role of postoperative radiotherapy is ill-defined.

Chemotherapy has been used for many years as systemic therapy in advanced ovarian carcinoma. The alkylating agents (nitrogen mustard, chlorambucil, triethylene thiophosphoramide, cyclophosphamide, melphalan, mitomycin C, and triethylene melamine) have been tried, with objective response rates of 17 to 40 percent.[60] The use of antimetabolites and the vinca alkaloids has been even less promising.

Because of the poor prognosis and response to treatment, supportive care is the main function of the nurse. The disease usually progresses to a protracted terminal phase complicated by nausea, vomiting, abdominal distention, ascites, bowel obstruction, anemia, and pleural effusion. Appropriate supportive care is indicated for complications. Empathy is essential in giving conscientious care.

## Fallopian-tube Cancer

Cancer of the fallopian tubes is rare and accounts for less than 0.5 percent of all primary cancers of the female genital tract. Relative infertility has been associated with tubal cancer in about one-half of all cases, engendering the belief that preexisting tubal infections might play a role in carcinogenesis. In view of its rarity and the frequency of chronic salpingitis, however, this seems unlikely.

Like ovarian cancers, tubal masses remain relatively asymptomatic during the early stages. Carcinomas constitute 95 percent of these neoplasms, with rare tumors such as mesodermal sarcomas, leiomyosarcomas, choriocarcinomas, and lymphomas making up the remainder.[61] About 50 percent of the patients present with abnormal vaginal bleeding. Diagnosis is seldom made before laparotomy. Treatment, like that of ovarian tumors, is with hysterectomy and bilateral salpingo-oophorectomy. Postoperative radiotherapy usually includes the lymph nodes in the inguinal area, pelvis, and aortic chain, because of the frequency of lymphnode involvement. Alkylating agents are also being used.

## Choriocarcinoma

Unlike cervical or endometrial cancer, chemotherapy is the primary treatment for *gestational choriocarcinoma*—a tumor that arises from the products of conception. Its incidence is low in the United States but relatively high in Asian countries. Treatment with methotrexate and actinomycin D produces a "cure" rate approaching 100 percent for this rare tumor. Because of the high dose levels of drugs used in the treatment of choriocarcinoma, the nursing care becomes extremely challenging. The nurse must be alert to the side effects and must be able to improvise to meet the needs of the patient. The side effects of chemotherapy are discussed in Chap. 5.

## Vaginal Cancer

Primary cancer of the vagina constitutes only 1 to 2 percent of all cancers of the female genital tract. The majority of vaginal neoplasms are of the squamous-cell type. The average age is 50 or over. Clear-cell adenocarcinoma in young girls has aroused considerable interest, since it appears to be correlated with prenatal ingestion of diethylstilbesterol (DES) by the mother. Synthetic estrogens such as DES have been used in threatened abortions, so children born after such an occurrence should be carefully monitored. Colposcopy can add an important diagnostic tool.

The most common symptoms are bladder pain and frequent voiding, which seem to be a result of tumor pressure. Vaginal tumors can be detected easily at the time of pelvic examination by cytologic examination. Earlier diagnosis would result if the vagina were examined during the routine pelvic examination or whenever a cytologic smear of the cervix is taken. Careful follow-up is needed for patients with diagnosed and treated cervical cancer and patients undergoing hysterectomy for a benign condition.

Treatment should be individualized. In situ lesions of the vagina are treated surgically. Surgical procedures, in the more advanced stages, are often radical and mutilating. The proximity of the bladder and rectum complicate the treatment. External irradiation in advanced stages is used alone or in combination with surgical exenteration.

Intravaginal radium is most commonly used for moderately advanced lesions, because treatment can be delivered directly to the lesion without first traversing normal tissue and therefore a higher dose can be delivered to a localized area. Early identification and improved therapy have resulted in improvement of the prognosis of vaginal cancers.

## Cancer of the Vulva

Vulvar carcinoma occurs most often in women over 60 years of age, with a large percentage over 70. It has been reported in association with leukoplakia, diabetes, syphilis, and granulomatous disease.

*Chronic leukoplakia* is a precancerous condition of the vulvar skin, which appears white and thickened. Itching which exacerbates the condition is frequent. A *vulvectomy* (surgical removal of the vulva) is advocated in women over 60 who do not respond to more conservative treatment.

The most frequent presenting symptoms are *pruritus, bleeding,* and a *vulvar mass.* Delay in diagnosis is a major problem, with many women waiting months before seeking medical help after the lesion has appeared. Because of the older age group involved, many are not accustomed to and resist examinations.

A histologic examination of the tissue is the basis for a definitive diagnosis. All tumors removed from the vulvar area should be subjected to microscopic examination even though the clinical diagnosis is furuncle or cyst, dermatitis, or allergic disturbance.

The treatment of choice is usually surgery, the

extent depending on the patient's age and the stage of the disease. Small, localized lesions, particularly in sexually active women, have been treated with wide excision and close follow-up. A vulvectomy alone somewhat abbreviates the external genitalia, but the vaginal introitus remains functional. There may be loss of some sensation, and emotional distress occurs as a result of the altered anatomy.

For more extensive local disease a radical vulvectomy and inguinal lymphadenectomy are performed. Surgery often includes the vulva, mons pubis, terminal portions of the urethra, vagina, and other vulvar organs, portions of the round ligaments, and the saphenous veins. Reconstruction of the vaginal wall and the pelvic floor are usually performed. Because of the extensiveness of this procedure and the age group of the patients, this radical procedure is modified according to the situation of the individual patient.

Tumors confined to the vulva respond well to surgical treatment and may have a good prognosis. Once the disease spreads outside the vulva, prognosis declines.

The management of patients undergoing vulvectomy is similar to that of all pre- and postoperative patients. Emotional support relating to alteration of body image, alteration of sexuality, and the diagnosis of cancer is vital.

## Endometriosis

When endometrial cells that normally line the uterus are seeded throughout the pelvis, the condition is called *endometriosis.* The exact etiology is not known. Theories include the congenital presence of endometrial cells out of their normal location, the extragenital transfer of such cells by the vascular or lymphatic system, and the reflux of menstrual fluid containing endometrial cells from fallopian tubes into the pelvic cavity. The endometrial cells are hormonally stimulated during the menstrual cycle and may bleed into the surrounding tissue or peritoneal cavity, thus resulting in further spread.

Endometriosis usually progresses slowly. The patient may not become symptomatic until the fourth or fifth decade of life. Pain with menstruation is the most common complaint. Other symptoms may be a feeling of fullness in the lower abdomen, dyspareunia, and generally poor health. Infertility accompanies endometriosis in about one-half those affected.

Young women with endometriosis who desire children are encouraged to have a family without delay, because the fertility rate is low and sterility due to adhesions is high. In severe cases, hysterectomy, oophorectomy, and salpingectomy may be offered as therapeutic measures.

## NEOPLASMS OF THE MALE GENITAL TRACT

Prostatic neoplasms are the most prevalent type of tumor found in the male genital tract. Lesions of the penis and scrotum also occur and are discussed briefly.

### Prostatic Neoplasms

Neoplasms of the prostate may be either benign (hyperplasia) or malignant (carcinoma). Assessment and interventions are largely the same for both, although their growth characteristics are quite different.

**Hyperplasia** *Benign prostatic hyperplasia* (BPH) is a common pathologic condition. Although fre-

quently described as prostatic hypertrophy, the process which occurs is actually an example of controlled cellular proliferation resulting in mild to moderate enlargement of the gland. Functionally the prostate is not altered by the process of hyperplasia. When hyperplasia takes place, there is an overgrowth of glandular and fibromuscular tissue in varying degrees. The proliferating cells form large, soft *nodules* within the prostate. The nodules are not encapsulated but are well demarcated. Recent work on the morphogenesis of prostate hyperplasia indicates that most nodules are composed of proliferating glandular and fibromuscular tissue in varying proportions.[62] The nodules are found in the median and lateral lobes which form the inner periurethral part of the prostate. The mass formed by the nodules is generally believed to compress the outer prostate into a false capsule known as the *surgical capsule* (Fig. 6-11). This occurrence permits the nodular mass to be shelled out at surgery, leaving the functioning prostate or surgical capsule intact.[63]

**FIGURE 6-11**
Prostatic hyperplasia. (*Reproduced with permission from Donald R. Smith, General Urology, 8th ed., 1975, Los Altos, California, Lange Medical Publications.*)

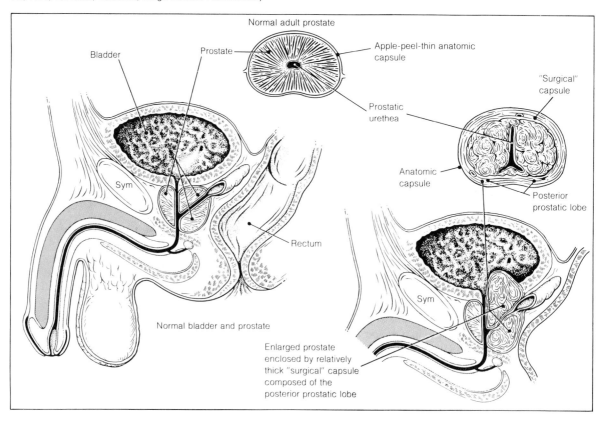

Normal adult prostate

Bladder

Prostate

Apple-peel-thin anatomic capsule

"Surgical" capsule

Prostatic urethea

Anatomic capsule

Posterior prostatic lobe

Sym

Rectum

Sym

Normal bladder and prostate

Enlarged prostate enclosed by relatively thick "surgical" capsule composed of the posterior prostatic lobe

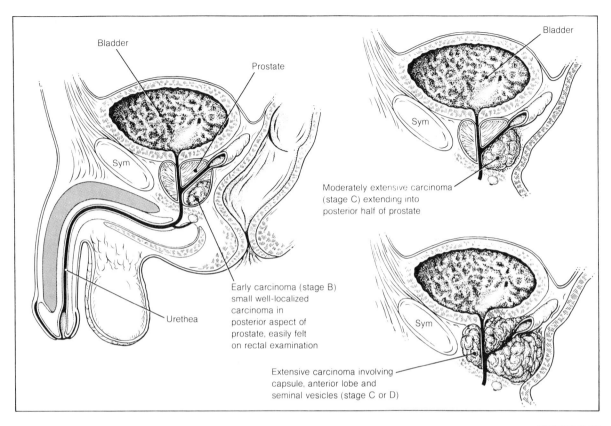

Bladder

Prostate

Sym

Early carcinoma (stage B)
small well-localized
carcinoma in
posterior aspect of
prostate, easily felt
on rectal examination

Urethea

Bladder

Sym

Moderately extensive carcinoma
(stage C) extending into
posterior half of prostate

Sym

Extensive carcinoma involving
capsule, anterior lobe and
seminal vesicles (stage C or D)

**FIGURE 6-12**
Prostatic carcinoma. (*Reproduced with permission from Donald R. Smith, General Urology, 8th ed., 1975, Los Altos, California, Lange Medical Publications.*)

**Malignant neoplasms** In contrast to prostatic hyperplasia, cancer of the prostate is an example of uncontrolled abnormal cellular proliferation. Benign prostatic hyperplasia and cancer of the prostate frequently occur together. Until recently this phenomenon had been considered coincidental, but in 1974 a study demonstrated an incidence of prostatic cancer 3.7 times greater in men with benign prostatic hyperplasia than in a controlled group. The methodology and conclusions of this study were subsequently challenged, so the causal relationship of prostatic hyperplasia and cancer of the prostate remains controversial. Cancer of the prostate usually originates in the posterior lobe, located in the peripheral portion of the gland, away from the prostatic urethra (Fig. 6-12). The cancerous nodules are firm or hard and gritty in consistency. Ninety-seven percent of prostatic tumors are *adenocarcinomas* with varying degrees of differentiation. Three percent are rare sarcomas and squamous carcinomas. Squamous carcinomas are thought to originate in the prostatic urethra.[64] Mic-

roscopically the identification of prostatic carcinoma is based on anaplasia and invasion. Morphologic identification of prostatic cancer is frequently difficult. On occasion the tumor may blend into the background of the gland, making it difficult to distinguish carcinoma of the prostate from nodular hyperplasia.

**M**etastasis  The principal difference between prostatic hyperplasia and cancer of the prostate is that the neoplastic cancer cells have the power to invade and destroy other tissue, while the hyperplastic process remains confined to the area of the prostate in which it develops. As the hyperplastic process progresses it may compress structures such as the urethra and surrounding prostatic tissue, but it cannot invade.

Carcinoma of the prostate gradually spreads in the posterior lobe and may eventually involve the entire prostate. It can then invade the seminal vesicles. Further extension may include the urethral mucosa or bladder wall and external sphincter. The rectum may also become involved. The perineural lymphatics account for metastasis to pelvic, sacral, external iliac, and lumbar lymph nodes. Venous involvement enables the tumor to metastasize to the bones of the pelvic region and the lumbar spine. Bone-marrow infiltration is also seen, as is metastasis to the skull, lungs, and liver. Factors which determine the pattern of dissemination are unknown.[65] Both hyperplasia and carcinoma of the prostate most often remain essentially dormant and are found incidentally at autopsy. In other instances, however, the disease processes are active, produce symptoms, and eventually kill the host if the proliferating cells are malignant.

**C**ausative Factors  The reasons for the development of prostatic hyperplasia and cancer of the prostate are largely unknown. Various *hormonal theories* have been advanced to explain both conditions. One theory suggests that prostatic cancer and hyperplasia are influenced by, or result from, alterations in the ratio of circulating estrogenic and androgenic gonadal hormones.[66] It has also been suggested that the main part played by hormones is the proliferation of prostatic epithelium, so that a sufficient number of cells are present in which malignant changes can occur.[67] Conclusive evidence has not been found to support these hormonal theories, but hormonal imbalance is considered a logical explanation.

**E**ffects on Patient  In both prostatic hyperplasia and cancer of the prostate, it is the *urinary-tract obstruction* which produces the initial undesirable effects most often causing the patient to seek medical attention. In persons with prostatic cancer, the disease is usually in an advanced state when it produces urinary-tract symptoms. The obstructive process is similar in both conditions. The prostatic urethra becomes distorted or obstructed. In an effort to empty the bladder through the narrowed urethra, the detrusor muscle becomes hypertrophied. Eventually the urethral effects of the prostatic enlargement exceed the bladder's ability to produce adequate voiding pressure for urinary flow. Subsequent *bladder decompensation* occurs, and *chronic urinary retention* results. Residual urine in the bladder predisposes to urinary-tract infection and calculus formation. *Vesical-sphincter incompetence* may develop. Progressive *proximal ureteral dilatation* occurs as it becomes more difficult for the ureters to deliver urine into the decompensated bladder. *Ureterohydronephrosis* and impaired renal function eventually result. In addition

to the obstructive process, ruptured dilated blood vessels or cancerous invasion of adjacent structures may cause bleeding.

The effects of prostatic cancer on the host are most accurately evaluated by a process of *grading and staging. Grading* assesses the degree of morphologic departure from normal cells; the tumors are graded from I to III on the basis of cellular differentiation. The extent to which the tumor is undifferentiated is believed to reflect the degree of malignancy. The *staging* system assigns a prostatic tumor to one of four categories according to the extent of spread. In *Stage A,* clinical manifestations of the tumor are absent. A *Stage B* tumor consists of a palpable, discrete nodule which is confined within the prostatic capsule. *Stage C* indicates that the tumor has extended beyond the prostatic capsule; it may include pelvic nodes, seminal vesicles, and the base of the bladder. *Stage D* indicates a metastatic tumor with bony or extrapelvic involvement.[68]

**First-level nursing care**  Some degree of prostatic hyperplasia is probably part of the normal process of aging. It is also possible that occult carcinoma of the prostate may be found to be a normal phenomenon. A majority of men have palpable evidence of prostatic hyperplasia by age 60; it rarely produces symptoms before age 50. Cancer of the prostate is the most common cancer in men; it remains second only to cancer of the lung as a cause of death from cancer in the male population of the United States.[69] A few cases of carcinoma of the prostate have been reported in young men, but it is a rare occurrence. In the United States, black males have the highest reported death rate from prostatic carcinoma.[70] There is no apparent reason for the development of either hyperplasia or prostatic cancer in some men and not in others.

**P**revention  No means of preventing the development of either hyperplasia or cancer of the prostate is known. However, the nurse can play an important community role in both disease entities. Perhaps most important is health teaching concerning the need for regular physical examinations which include a *digital rectal examination.* In addition, it should be noted that certain drugs may produce further bladder problems in men who already have compensatory bladder changes secondary to obstructive prostatic hyperplasia. For example, the drug diazepam may lead to vesical atony. Ganglionic blocking agents and parasympatholytics, used in the treatment of hypertension and peptic ulcer, may weaken detrusor contraction, causing symptoms similar to bladder-neck obstruction.[71]

**Second-level nursing care** Frequently nurses will make the initial patient assessment in an office or outpatient situation. Alertness to the sometimes subtle signs of beginning urinary obstruction is vital to the early diagnosis and treatment of prostatic lesions.

Nursing Assessment In some men a prostatic problem is discovered during the course of a routine *physical examination;* more often, medical attention is sought for a variety of voiding problems. The *health history* discloses symptoms ranging from *frequency* and *nocturia* to acute urinary retention. Other common complaints include *dysuria,* a *decrease* in volume and force of the urinary stream, a sensation of *incomplete* bladder emptying, burning on urination, and *gross hematuria.* *Pain* may be experienced along with the voiding problems. Perineal aching may occur with a hyperplastic prostate. Back pain may be associated with metastatic prostatic cancer.

*Physical assessment* In cases of *acute urinary retention* the patient is extremely uncomfortable. The bladder may be at the level of the umbilicus and will be very tender to palpation. *Chronic urinary retention* may result in a flabby, atonic bladder which is difficult to identify.

On rectal examination, the hyperplastic prostate is characterized by a smooth, soft to firm enlargement of the gland. A cancerous prostate is usually hard to stony on palpation, and it may or may not be enlarged. The prostate is not usually tender in either condition.

*Diagnostic tests* A urine specimen for *urinalysis* should be obtained before prostatic massage and analyzed for the presence of pus and bacteria. *Seminal fluid* is obtained by prostatic massage and urethral milking and is examined to rule out the presence of prostatitis. The *phenolsulfonphthalein test (PSP)* is done to evaluate renal function and as an indirect measure of residual urine. Ability to excrete the dye indicates the level of kidney function and the degree of obstruction.

*Blood urea nitrogen (BUN) and serum creatinine* tests are done to evaluate the extent to which kidney function has been impaired from chronic urinary-tract obstruction. *Acid phosphatase* is an enzyme excreted by the prostate. In advanced prostatic cancer the acid phosphatase level is usually markedly elevated. However, other factors such as a routine rectal examination can cause a similar elevation. *Alkaline phosphatase* is an enzyme that may be indicative of bony metastasis when it is elevated. The enzyme is a measure of osteogenic activity occurring in the body. A *complete blood count* is also done. The hemoglobin is evaluated to check for the presence of anemia as an indication of bone-marrow metastasis from prostatic cancer. A white blood cell count is used to check for secondary urinary-tract infection.

A *plain abdominal film* may be utilized to observe for complicating calculi or ureterohydronephrosis. An *excretory urogram* visualizes the renal parenchyma, calcyces, pelves, and ureters. It may demonstrate ureteral hydronephrosis secondary to urinary-tract obstruction caused by the diseased prostate. Having the patient void following the urogram permits bladder visualization (excretory cystogram). A postvoiding film is then taken to demonstrate residual urine in the bladder.

As a diagnostic tool, *bladder catheterization* with a straight catheter is done immediately after voiding in order to measure the amount of residual urine left in the bladder. In instances of acute retention, catheterization is employed to empty the bladder and relieve distress. The ability to void spontaneously within approximately 8 to 10 hours is then evaluated. If the patient is unable to void spontaneously, an indwelling catheter is inserted and left in place for a few days. Often this will restore normal voiding patterns.

Nursing Problems and Interventions The major nursing problems encountered at this level are *voiding difficulties.* Intervention may begin on an outpatient basis, but hospitalization is usually required at some point.

*Conservative treatment* may be employed with prostatic hyperplasia. Prostatic congestion may be decreased through regular sexual intercourse or prostatic massage. Bladder tone can be protected by teaching the patient to avoid excessive intake of fluids over a short period of time. If the patient is sent home with an indwelling catheter, he and his significant others must be taught how to take care of it. The teaching plan for *catheter care* should include the following information given verbally and reinforced in writing:

1   Adequate *anatomical explanations* concerning catheter placement and the need for maintaining a sterile closed system for urinary drainage.

2 A demonstration of the mechanical manipulation of *collecting devices,* methods of anchoring tubing, and the procedure for changing from one collection device to another. The use of a leg bag during the day should be encouraged. The importance of nighttime bedside *gravity drainage,* to avoid vesicle reflux problems, should be emphasized.

3 *Fluid intake* of approximately 3000 ml/day should be recommended.

4 *Problems* warranting the attention of a physician —e.g., pain, decreased output, loss of the catheter, and leakage—need to be identified.

5 The importance of a *hygiene routine,* including cleaning the meatus and showering regularly, should be emphasized.

The conservative interventions described above may be sufficient to relieve symptoms and post-pone surgery for the man with prostatic hyper-plasia. When prostatic cancer is suspected, the patient is always referred to a hospital for further diagnostic work-up.

**Third-level nursing care** The health history and physical examination for the third level are largely as described for the second level. However, hos-pitalization presents new situations and opportu-nities for perceptive nursing assessment.

**N**ursing Assessment Men who enter a hospital be-cause of prostatic disease may be in various states of general health. Usually those with prostatic hyperplasia are not physically ill. During the *health history* they describe only uncomfortable urinary symptoms. This may also be the case for men with early prostatic cancer, who may not have any symp-toms. Conversely, one may see a man with ad-vanced prostatic cancer who is quite debilitated. Not infrequently, patients hospitalized for other problems involving immobility develop urinary-tract symptoms related to prostatic hyperplasia and thus unexpectedly become urologic patients. The *physical assessment* findings will be similar to those discussed for level two and will depend on the extent of involvement.

*Diagnostic tests* The patient's basic health status is important in terms of formulating the hospital plan of care. Frequently the stress imposed by the diagnostic tests is overlooked. The nurse should try to ensure that the scheduling of diagnostic proce-dures allows periods of rest for the patient. In addi-tion, the nurse is in the best position to monitor the patient's hydration and nutritional status during this time, when he will often not be receiving fluid or food by mouth because of diagnostic tests. The hospital plan of care will range from treatment aimed at cure to that directed at palliation. In al-most all instances the patient will return to the com-munity. Plans for the patient's eventual discharge should be considered at the time of the initial assessment.

During the endoscopic examination, use of the *cystoscope* and *panendoscope* permit visualiza-tion of the bladder and urethra, respectively. This is an extremely useful procedure for evaluating pros-tatic enlargement, urethral distortions, bladder changes, and obstruction caused by prostatic hy-perplasia. It is not considered particularly useful as a specific diagnostic tool in prostatic carcinoma unless bladder invasion has occurred. Following cystoscopy, it is necessary to evaluate the patient's ability to void spontaneously within 8 to 10 hours after the procedure. Hematuria is normal only for the first few voidings.

In order to positively establish a diagnosis of prostatic cancer, tissue analysis by *prostatic biopsy* is required. A variety of biopsy techniques are em-ployed. The techniques most often used are trans-rectal or perineal biopsies. The rectal method is generally considered the safest. With any method there is the possibility of seeding tumor cells along the biopsy tract.[72] The patient who has had a rectal biopsy should be checked for rectal bleeding, which is an abnormal occurrence. Pain other than minimal discomfort should always be investigated.

It is necessary to survey the skeletal system in order to detect bony metastases which may or may not be suspected. This is accomplished with a *roentgenographic bone scan.* The majority of pa-tients with prostatic carcinoma are said to have osseous involvement at the time of initial diagnosis. Information concerning bony metastases is ex-tremely important in selecting appropriate treat-ment.

Though controversial, *lymphangiography* is being used with increasing frequency to detect metastasis to pelvic nodes. A number of problems concerning interpretation have led some to believe that lymphoangiograms have limited clinical use.

**N**ursing Problems and Interventions The primary concerns of the nurse center on identifying any *physical, cognitive,* or *psychological* problems the patient may present regarding the diagnostic and therapeutic procedures he will undergo. The *pos-*

*sibility or presence of pain* is usually uppermost in every patient's mind. Certain aspects of many procedures involve discomfort, and every patient has a right to know if this may occur. For example, the injection of local anesthesia for a transrectal needle biopsy may be quite painful, and the intravenous injection of contrast media for x-ray procedures is often painful. Remaining in one position for long periods of time may be an ordeal for some patients.

The next issue of major concern to most patients is the *nature of the procedure itself:* what it is expected to show and how long it will take to complete. The nurse must be prepared to explain the procedure. Patients need to know whether foods or fluids will be withheld and for how long. Patients should be informed whether cathartics or enemas are to be administered and should be consulted concerning the most convenient time for these interventions to take place. A discussion of the immediate postprocedure period is an important part of preparation, including such facts as when the patient may eat, whether he is likely to feel pain, when he should void, and whether his urine will be hematuric.

Emotional preparation for diagnostic procedures requires that the nurse explore the patient's *feelings concerning what is about to happen to him.* It is well known that any hospitalization is a stressful situation. Patients faced with the possibility of cancer, surgery, and general uncertainty concerning the future will have many fears and worries. The nurse plays a crucial role in helping patients to deal with these problems. Patients with *acute retention* admitted for diagnostic workup are sometimes placed on a schedule of intermittent catheterization, usually at 8- to 10-hour intervals, with a straight catheter. Strict aseptic technique is required. The bladder should be completely emptied at each catheterization. Those patients who have an indwelling catheter should follow a routine similar to that described for the patient at home.

*Surgery* The general considerations governing the selection of an appropriate surgical procedure for the removal of the prostate include the patient's general health, the extent of the prostatic disease, the technical advantages and disadvantages of each procedure, and the skill of the surgeon. The following procedures are used most often in the correction of prostatic disease:

*Transurethral resection* (TUR) is the most common procedure in the treatment of prostatic hyperplasia. It may also be used as a palliative measure in meta-static cancer of the prostate, in order to maintain a patent urethra. An external incision is not made. A visualizing instrument is inserted up through the urethra. The hyperplastic tissue is completely enucleated by the use of an electric wire loop passed into the telescopic instrument. This procedure requires a skillful surgeon. The incidence of impotence is low. There is some possibility of incontinence secondary to sphincter-mechanism trauma during surgery.[73]

*Suprapubic prostatectomy (transvesical)* is carried out by a lower abdominal incision into the urinary bladder. The hyperplastic prostatic tissue is removed by the surgeon, reaching into the bladder. The incidence of impotence and incontinence is low.

*Retropubic prostatectomy* is accomplished by a lower abdominal incision below the urinary bladder. The anterior prostatic capsule is opened to remove the hyperplastic tissue. Impotence and incontinence occur infrequently.

*Perineal prostatectomy* is used most often in cancer of the prostate. An incision is made through the perineum. It is a difficult surgical procedure which carries with it a high incidence of impotence, incontinence, and rectal injury.[74] If cancer is present, the procedure is often radical, including removal of all prostatic tissue as well as pelvic node dissection.

*Cryosurgery* is a procedure sometimes performed on patients who are poor risks for major surgery. An instrument is passed through the urethra and the tumor mass is destroyed by freezing.

The *preparation of the patient for surgery* is similar to that described for diagnostic procedures. Every aspect of the 24 hours preceding surgery should be explained in detail. This includes explanation of further diagnostic procedures or laboratory tests, the physician's examination, the anesthesiologist's assessment, bowel preparation, medications, food and fluid restrictions, morning care routine prior to surgery, care of belongings, attire to be worn to the operating room, denture removal, operating-room escorts, recovery-room care, and a description of the immediate postoperative period, including catheters and drainage tubes. The time element is of particular importance to most patients; time approximations should always be given. Once pertinent information has been imparted to the patient, he must be provided with the opportunity to ask questions and to talk about his fears. The nurse should be prepared to explore feelings with the patient. Discussing the possibility of sexual dysfunction or incontinence should be part of preoperative preparation. The surgeon is responsible for providing the patient with the facts concerning the likely outcome of surgery. The term *impotence* is best avoided unless it is an absolute certainty; it is well known that its mention may function as a self-fulfilling prophecy. False encouragement should not be given. The patient should be advised that it may take time for normal sexual functioning to be restored, so that he will not assume that early failures to achieve erection mean that he is impotent.

Following surgery, the patient who has had a prostatectomy will have an *indwelling urethral catheter.* One who has had a suprapubic prostatectomy will also have a *suprapubic tube* inserted through the abdomen into the bladder and may also have a *penrose drainage tube* inserted through the suprapubic incision and lying anterior to the bladder. Following a perineal prostatectomy a drain is usually inserted into the perineum. Drains are managed by the use of dry sterile dressings or disposable ostomy appliances.

*Catheter care* is of particular importance. The urethral catheter is frequently a three-way indwell-ing catheter connected to constant closed bladder irrigation with normal saline (Fig. 6-13). This method of irrigation considerably reduces catheter blockage from clot formation. Special attention should be paid to the irrigating-fluid drip, to make sure it flows *continuously* and at a constant rate. Output from a urethral catheter must be carefully monitored to be sure that the catheter is draining adequately. The patient's bladder should also be palpated and the patient questioned concerning a sensation of fullness. Urine will be *hematuric* for the first few days following surgery. Should the catheter fail to drain properly, it may become necessary to irrigate it by hand. Specific instructions should be provided by the surgeon concerning hand-irrigation procedures. Ball syringes should not be used, as they exert too much pressure on the mucosa of the bladder wall. A piston-type syringe is most effective. Often it is necessary to deflate the catheter balloon in order to establish normal drainage. This should be done by the surgeon. Inadvertent loss of a urethral catheter is a dreaded event, especially with the more involved open prostatectomy procedures. If the catheter falls out, it is usu-

**FIGURE 6-13**

Constant closed bladder irrigation.

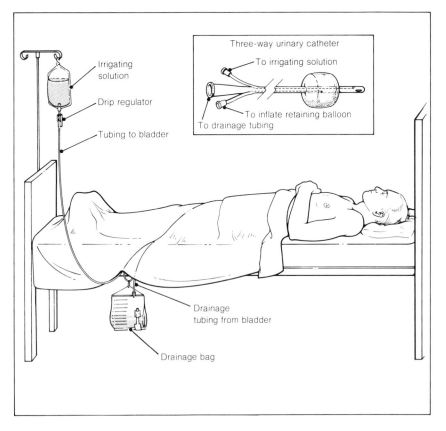

Irrigating solution

Drip regulator

Tubing to bladder

Three-way urinary catheter

To irrigating solution

To inflate retaining balloon

To drainage tubing

Drainage tubing from bladder

Drainage bag

ally not reinserted if the patient is able to void spontaneously. For the patient who is unable to void, procedures employed to reestablish urinary drainage can be very painful and traumatic to tissue. Closed bladder drainage tubing and bags should be changed frequently, particularly while urine is hematuric.

Rules governing the removal of a urethral catheter vary. Urethral catheters are known to cause bladder spasms, which sometimes prompts early removal. With a simple transurethral resection the catheter is usually removed when the urine remains clear, on the second or third postoperative day. With a perineal prostatectomy, the catheter usually remains in place for 12 to 14 days.

Prostatectomy patients should be encouraged to drink large amounts of fluid while the catheter is in place. Early ambulation should be encouraged. Bladder spasms frequently make patients quite miserable. An anticholinergic medication should be administered to alleviate this problem if the catheter cannot be removed. After the catheter is removed, the patient may experience urgency and some dribbling, usually due to the hypertrophic changes which have taken place in the bladder. In most situations voiding ability will return as the bladder reverts to normal.

*Radiotherapy*   Radiation in the treatment of cancer of the prostate may be used (1) *preoperatively* to reduce tumor size, (2) as a *cure* in itself for patients with locally extensive disease, and (3) as a *palliative measure* to reduce the incidence of metastatic problems such as pathologic fractures. Supervoltage radiation (cobalt, betatron) and interstitial radiation are both employed. A number of complications are associated with radiation therapy, such as *rectal bleeding, impotence,* and *fistula development.* Side effects such as *diarrhea* and *cystitis* may also occur.[75]

Many fears are associated with receiving radiation therapy. The patient will require a thorough explanation of the therapy plan, including the number of treatments he will receive. A pretreatment visit to the radiation therapy department may help to reduce anxiety. The patient must be informed that the treatment will not be painful. *Skin markings* should be explained, along with discussion of a *skin care* routine which will not eradicate the markings. Soap should be avoided. Factual information concerning possible *side effects* should be included. Patients must be afforded an opportunity to express their feelings about radiation therapy.

*Endocrine therapy and chemotherapy*   The major principle of hormonal therapy in the treatment of prostatic cancer is suppression of prostatic stimulation by androgenic hormones. This is based on the fact that prostate growth and function are regulated by the androgenic hormones. The major programs include

1   *Bilateral orchiectomy or oral estrogen therapy.* Recent data indicate that orchiectomy and estrogen (3 mg diethylstilbestrol/day) are equally effective in controlling symptoms from metastatic cancer of the prostate. Additional therapeutic effects are not achieved by combining the two treatment modalities, as bilateral orchiectomy by itself eliminates 90 percent of the circulating testosterone.[76] Diethylstilbestrol has recently been implicated as the cause of various venous and cardiopulmonary problems. It produces feminizing effects such as gynecomastia, which is often painful. Voice changes and loss of body hair are also observed with its use.

2   *Antiandrogen therapy.* This treatment mode is aimed at blocking the effects of androgens on the prostate by interfering with pertinent intracellular events. Cyproterone acetate and flutamide are antiandrogens currently being used on an experimental basis.[77]

3   *Andrenalectomy and hypophysectomy.* These major surgical procedures are sometimes performed when there is a reactivation of symptoms following orchiectomy or estrogen therapy but are not generally advocated. The relief of symptoms they provide is not considered significant enough to warrant their use.

4   *Cortisone therapy* is often employed to reduce pain, particularly when estrogen therapy is no longer effective.

5   *Chemotherapy* using alkylating agents or 5-fluorouracil is advocated by some. Data concerning their effectiveness are not conclusive.

The goal of endocrine therapy and chemotherapy is to increase the length and quality of the patient's life. Use of these treatment modalities is not without cost to the patient's intact body image. *Orchiectomy* involves the amputation of sexual organs. *Estrogen,* with its distressing feminizing effects, may threaten the sense of self. *Chemotherapeutic agents* produce undesirable side effects such as alopecia, loss of appetite, nausea, and diarrhea. *Cortisone* use involves a number of problems such as salt and water retention, redistribution of body fat, and emotional lability. The patient who undergoes *adrenalectomy* or *hypophysectomy* will have additional problems associated with the need for lifelong replacement drug therapy (discussed in greater detail in relation to breast cancer).

Patients receiving endocrine therapy and chemotherapy require considerable *emotional support*. They may often become quite depressed because of disease progression compounded by undesirable side effects of drug therapy. Frequently therapy is initiated in the hospital and continued while the patient is at home. Before the patient leaves the hospital, it is imperative that members of the health team meet with him and his significant others in order to review the treatment plan. Specific written instructions covering all aspects of treatment, including side effects and miscellaneous problems along with methods for alleviating them, should be provided.

**Fourth-level nursing care** A number of sequelae associated with the treatment of prostate disease may inhibit a patient's ability to achieve *rehabilitation* goals. The psychosocial implications of postprostatectomy *urinary incontinence* may be profound. A person experiencing this problem may withdraw from society because of inability to remain dry. The *alopecia* and *feminizing effects* of drug therapy are often a tremendous source of embarrassment, preventing the patient from resuming normal social roles. *Sexual dysfunction* may be an extremely depressing experience for the person who is sexually active. The nurse plays a vital role in facilitating rehabilitation by approaching these issues in a direct manner and providing the patient with emotional support.

Certain interventions are available to correct some of the problems discussed above. Alopecia may be concealed by use of a wig. *Sphincter exercises* can be taught to patients with postprostatectomy urinary incontinence. The exercises should be done 20 to 30 times each waking hour. The patient is instructed to relax all muscles and concentrate on squeezing the rectal sphincter while keeping both hands on the abdomen. If abdominal muscles tighten or a Valsalva maneuver becomes apparent, the exercise is not being done correctly.[78] It may be helpful to have the patient repeat the words "squeeze—release" or "contract—relax" while performing the exercise. Relaxation exercises are also helpful in teaching the patient how to relax. A regular routine should be established for doing the exercises. In addition, the nurse should guide the patient through the exercises while he is stand-

ing. A positive supportive approach is necessary in encouraging the patient to continue the exercises indefinitely. In addition to sphincter exercises, surgical procedures are also available to correct incontinence. Recent techniques involve increasing urethral resistance just below the external sphincter by placing a prosthetic device under the urethral bulb.

For some patients a surgical procedure to correct *postprostatectomy impotence* may be feasible. One type of surgery involves the implantation of an inflatable erectile prosthetic device. In a less complicated surgical procedure, silicon prostheses are inserted bilaterally along the shaft of the penis. Patients for whom surgery is not advisable should be counseled concerning other types of mutually satisfying sexual activity.

One of the most important aspects of the rehabilitation phase is the provision of a smooth transition from hospital to community. Contact should be made with appropriate community health agencies to provide for follow-up health-care visits in the home. Every patient should be provided with detailed written instructions concerning all aspects of treatment that will carry over into the community. The instructions should include a list of signs or symptoms which warrant medical attention. The importance of continuing health care cannot be overemphasized. Appointments for follow-up physical examinations should be made before the patient is discharged from the hospital. The patient should return to the community equipped to care for himself to the extent possible within the limits of the disease process.

**Penile Neoplasms**

A number of genital-tract disorders are manifested by visible, often painless, lesions on the surface of the penis. Penile neoplasms are classified as *benign, premalignant,* or *malignant*. Condyloma acuminatum is an example of a virus-caused benign papillomatous lesion. Several premalignant lesions occur, the most common being leukoplakia. Leukoplakia may progress to squamous-cell carcinoma of the penis; most malignant neoplasms of the penis are squamous-cell carcinomas.

The incidence of penile cancer increases with age; it is rare in men who have been circumcised in infancy. The development of penile neoplasms is related to poor hygiene, except for condyloma acuminatum. Chronic irritation from clothing and sexual intercourse tends to aggravate precancerous lesions and may play a role in their transformation to malignant neoplasms. Syphilis, phimosis, and balanoposthitis are also thought to play important predisposing roles.[79]

Health teaching regarding circumcision and good hygiene seem to be the most significant preventive measures. In addition, seeking medical attention at the first appearance of any lesion should be emphasized. Positive diagnosis is established through tissue biopsy.

Small neoplasms are locally excised or treated by radiation therapy. More extensive lesions often require amputation of the penis with subsequent irradiation of lymph nodes.

A person entering the health-care system for treatment of a penile neoplasm is likely to be self-conscious and fearful about the condition. A body-image assault of the most extreme nature is associated with penile amputation. The nurse must assume a particularly supportive role in assisting the patient to cope with this mutilating experience. Usually the external urinary sphincter is preserved, and voiding takes place through a fistulous opening in the perineum. Depression is common and may significantly inhibit the rehabilitation process.

### Neoplasms of the Epididymis

Neoplasms of the epididymis are rare, and most are benign. They arise from epithelial or connective tissue.[80] Health care is usually sought when a painless enlargement in the scrotum is noted by the patient.

The epididymis is surgically excised if the neoplasm is benign. Malignant neoplasms require orchiectomy followed by radiation therapy to regional lymph nodes.

Embarrassment concerning a problem in the genital area may be experienced by the patient. A direct supportive approach by the nurse can help to alleviate this situation. For many patients surgery in the genital area carries with it the fear of sterility or impotence. The nurse should explore such fears with the patient and offer reassurance based on factual information.

Considerable postoperative pain is associated with scrotal surgery. Ice packs and an athletic support may be helpful in alleviating discomfort.

### Neoplasms of the Scrotum

Neoplasms of the scrotal skin are uncommon. Because of its rare occurrence, cancer of the scrotum has often been overlooked in its early curable stages. Most scrotal-skin neoplasms arise from occupational exposure to various carcinogens such as soot, tars, creosote, and petroleum products.[81] Wide surgical excision of a malignant neoplasm is generally performed. Lymph-node dissec-

tion may be included. The *body-image disturbance* associated with extensive scrotal-sac excision may be quite marked because of the disfiguring surgical intervention. Subsequent skin grafting may be required. Considerable pain and discomfort are experienced in the postoperative period. Sexual dysfunction may result from radical surgery which includes lymph-node dissection.

### Neoplasms of the Testis

Neoplasia in the testis, with rare exception, represents uncontrolled malignant cellular proliferation. Almost all the neoplasms are of germ-cell origin. The most common are seminoma, embryonal carcinoma, teratoma, and teratocarcinoma. Choriocarcinoma is also found, although infrequently. Seminomas are the least malignant. The other tumors tend to be poorly differentiated and highly malignant.[82]

Metastasis most often occurs via regional lymph nodes and frequently spreads to the lungs. Cerebral metastasis may be observed as well. A system of staging is used as a guide in establishing a treatment plan and predicting outcomes.[83] *Stage IA* identifies a tumor confined to one testis without evidence of further spread. *Stage IB* refers to a tumor that is accompanied by lymph-node involvement. *Stage II* indicates lymph-node metastasis below the level of the diaphragm. *Stage III* signifies a tumor which has metastasized above the level of the diaphragm or to distant body organs.

A number of theories have been put forward to explain the development of testicular cancer. Among the more common explanations are *endocrine abnormality* involving androgenic activity, *genetic factors,* and a *viral infection* which triggers carcinogenesis. Young men between the ages of 20 and 35 are most commonly affected. It is a common form of cancer in this age group. The incidence is higher in males with a history of an undescended testicle.

The nurse can play an important role in preventive health teaching. *Self-examination* of the scrotum and testes should be practiced. The examination should be performed in a standing position. Size, heaviness, and consistency of each testicle should be noted. *Early medical attention* for any abnormality is essential in order to avoid the somewhat common situation in which health care is not sought until the disease is in an advanced stage.

In most instances the only sign presented by a testicular neoplasm is a painless swelling of a testis, sometimes accompanied by a sensation of heaviness in the scrotum. Gynecomastia may be present if the tumor is a choriocarcinoma. Urinary levels of chorionic gonadotropins are measured to determine the presence of choriocarcinoma. Any suspicious lesion requires surgical intervention to establish a positive diagnosis. Biopsy is contraindicated with testicular neoplasms, as it is associated with tumor-cell seeding and a poor prognosis.[84]

Surgical intervention for a testicular neoplasm consists of *radical orchiectomy.* Patients with non-seminomatous germ-cell tumors are treated with orchiectomy, lymphadenectomy up to the level of the diaphragm, and removal of metastatic lesions beyond the retroperitoneum.[85]

Prior to testicular surgery a patient will probably experience considerable fear and apprehension concerning the outcome of the surgery and his future. False reassurance should not be offered to the patient and his significant others. A direct, empathetic, supportive approach is most helpful. The patient should be provided with detailed information concerning preoperative routines. A description of the immediate postoperative period must also be included. Some patients may have difficulty voiding in the immediate postoperative period. As a rule an indwelling catheter is not necessary. *Pain* is nearly always a problem. In addition to analgesics, the use of an athletic support in a large size may be helpful in relieving discomfort. If the diagnosis is unfavorable, the patient is apt to become quite *depressed* during the postoperative period. The nurse should continue to maintain a supportive approach, providing an environment in which the patient will feel free to verbalize his feelings. It is important to bear in mind that the patient will be responding to the loss of a testis, as well as the threat to survival imposed by cancer.

*Supervoltage radiation therapy* is administered to lymph-node areas after surgical treatment of testicular neoplasms. Irradiation may be used for cure or palliation. *Chemotherapy* is most commonly employed for patients with Stage II nonseminomatous tumors. The choice of appropriate chemotherapy is a controversial issue. A combination program consisting of methotrexate, chlorambucil, and dactinomycin has been recommended; a number of other agents are also used.

For the patient with a seminoma, the prognosis is generally favorable. For all other testicular tumors the prognosis is considerably less optimistic. Follow-up health care is extremely important in order to search for any indication of metastases. The patient who has undergone a retroperitoneal lymphadenectomy may be unable to ejaculate. A recent study indicates that the incidence of this complication has been overemphasized; however, a decrease in semen volume is likely to occur.[86] In any event the person who has undergone treatment for a testicular tumor may experience considerable anxiety in relation to sexual function. *Sexual counseling* should be provided. If the prognosis is favorable the patient will usually be fully rehabilitated. For the patient with an unfavorable prognosis a downhill course may be fairly rapid, producing an extremely distressing situation for the patient and the family.

## UROLOGIC NEOPLASMS

Urethral, bladder, and ureteral tumors constitute the urologic neoplasms. Because of their frequency, bladder neoplasms are discussed in detail; urethral and ureteral tumors are examined more briefly.

### Bladder Neoplasms

Neoplasms of the bladder are described as *papillomatous* or *nodular* (*solid*), depending on their pattern of growth. They may be benign or malignant, noninvasive or infiltrating. The majority of vesical neoplasms grow in papillomatous formations into the lumen of the bladder. Many consider all bladder papillomas to be either precancerous or malignant. *Nodular neoplasms* occur less frequently and tend to grow into the bladder wall. *Papillary carcinoma* often also invades the bladder wall. The cellular proliferation which takes place usually involves cells of transitional epithelial origin. In rare instances, squamous or glandular (adenocarcinoma) cells proliferate.

**Pathophysiology**    The degree of malignancy and depth of invasion of bladder neoplasms are assessed by systems of *grading* and *staging.* Most *Grade I tumors* resemble benign papillomas except for some atypical cellular characteristics. For this reason they are called atypical transitional-cell papillomas, or transitional-cell carcinomas.[87] *Grade II tumors* are clearly transitional-cell papillary carcinomas. They are larger than Grade I tumors and have a broader attachment to the bladder wall. *Grade III and Grade IV tumors* are poorly differentiated. They are usually solid (nodular) rather than papillary.

A number of *staging methods* are also used. The most common system combines two methods.[88] *Stage 0 (T1S)* identifies a papillary tumor which has not invaded the mucous membrane. *Stage A (T1)* tumors have invaded the mucous membrane but not the bladder-wall musculature. *Stages B₁ and B₂ (T2 and T3)* tumors show invasion of superficial and deep muscles, respectively. *Stage C (T3)* tumors have extended into perivesical fat or the overlying peritoneum. *Stage D (T4) tumors* have invaded adjacent organs or show evidence of metastases.[89] Examples of various grade and stage transitional-cell carcinomas of the bladder are shown in Fig. 6-14.

**C**haracteristics  Most neoplasms of the bladder are malignant. Seventy percent of them occur in the lateral and posterior walls near the base of the bladder. They are usually discovered early and are amenable to treatment.[90] Tumors occurring elsewhere in the bladder tend to be invasive. The most prominent characteristic of bladder neoplasms is the tendency, following removal, to new growth or recurrence with increased aggression.

**M**etastasis  Vesical neoplasms commonly metastasize to regional lymph nodes. *Bony metastasis* may occur, most often affecting the pelvis, ribs, and vertebrae. *Visceral metastasis* usually involves the kidney, adrenals, liver, and lungs. *Local extension* to neighboring organs may take place. The bladder may also be a target for metastasis from other primary cancer sites, such as adjacent organs, the stomach, and the lungs.

**C**ausative Factors  A summary of the possible causes of bladder cancer by Morrison and Cole[91] suggests that although *occupational exposures* in the dye, rubber, and leather industries can cause bladder cancer, the offending carcinogens may be commonplace in the environment. A causal relationship between *smoking* and bladder cancer has not been established, but smoking is known to be associated with an increased risk of bladder cancer. *Tryptophan metabolites* may be involved in bladder cancer. Morrison and Cole report, however, that recent work indicates that aberrations of tryptophan metabolism are probably not specific to bladder cancer. *Schistosomiasis* has been men-

**FIGURE 6-14**
Carcinoma of the bladder. (*Reproduced with permission from Donald R. Smith, General Urology, 8th Edition, 1975, Los Altos, California, Lange Medical Publications.*)

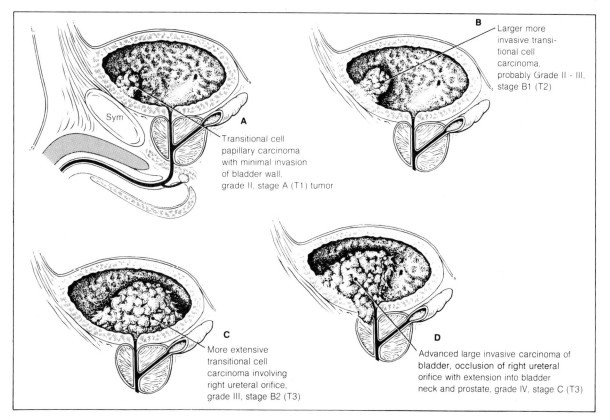

tioned in relation to an increased risk of bladder cancer. *Pelvic irradiation, coffee drinking,* and a large intake of analgesics containing *phenacetin* have also been proposed as possible causes of bladder cancer.

**E**ffects on Patient   Bladder tumors frequently *ulcerate, bleed,* and cause *bladder infections.* Tumor-related *obstruction of ureteral orifices* on the bladder neck may occur, producing flank pain and eventually causing renal impairment. It is now generally believed that the effects of bladder cancer are largely governed by the immune mechanism. In the presence of an impaired immune response, growth and spread of the tumor is assured. This finding has led some to challenge irradiation and chemotherapy as modes of treatment, since both may impair the immune response of the host.[92]

**First-level nursing care**   Cancer of the bladder is the second most common cancer of the genitourinary tract. The incidence of bladder tumors is greater in men than in women. For men the risk of bladder cancer increases with age. The greatest incidence is in *men over 50.* It has been found consistently that *urban dwellers* have a greater risk of bladder cancer.[91] The population at risk includes people regularly exposed to known industrial carcinogens. Cigarette smokers and coffee drinkers may also be at risk.

**P**revention   A thorough psychosocial and urologic assessment provides the nurse with pertinent information indicating whether a person is at risk of developing bladder cancer. Appropriate health-care teaching concerning exposure to known carcinogens is essential. It has been suggested that persons at risk be *screened* through the use of cytologic urinalysis. Persons employed in the dye, rubber, and leather-refining industries should be cognizant of the risks involved so that they may limit their length of employment to a recommended 3-year period of time.[93] *Legislation* may be needed to restrict the use of known carcinogens in industry. The use of *ascorbic acid* for persons found to have carcinogens in the urine has been proposed, as it reportedly neutralizes the urinary carcinogens.[94]

**Second-level nursing care**   Early signs of bladder cancer are vague and often subtle. Nurses should, therefore, be particularly astute in assessing its symptoms in susceptible persons.

**N**ursing Assessment   During the *health history,* the most common and often the only difficulty re-

ported by the patient is *hematuria. Frequency* and *urgency* may also be present. Complications related to the presence of a tumor may produce other symptoms, such as *flank or pelvic pain* secondary to upper urinary-tract obstruction or metastasis, and *burning on urination* and other symptoms of cystitis brought on by an infected bladder tumor. Questions should be asked about drug use, smoking, and exposure to carcinogens. *Physical assessment* usually does not reveal any abnormal findings. Occasionally a vaginal or rectal examination may indicate a possible mass.

During the initial diagnostic workup, a *hemoglobin test* will usually show anemia if hematuria is present. The routine urinalysis may reveal grossly to microscopically bloody urine. Bacteria and pus will be present in the urine if the bladder is infected.

**N**ursing Problems and Intervention   The presence of *hematuria* demands a definitive diagnostic evaluation, which requires a *referral* for hospitalization. Patients should be informed of any findings and the reasons for further testing.

**Third-level nursing care**   For one whose only symptom is *hematuria,* the need for hospitalization is generally quite unexpected, as the patient appears essentially healthy. The *health history* may reveal *flank pain, dysuria,* and a variety of symptoms of obstruction or renal impairment. On *physical assessment,* persons who have been experiencing additional symptoms for varying periods of time may be *emaciated* and *anemic* and appear *chronically ill.*

**D**iagnostic Tests   The three procedures which constitute the major means of diagnosing bladder cancer are the *bimanual examination, cystoscopy,* and *tumor biopsy.* With the patient under general anesthesia, the bladder wall is palpated by abdominorectal or abdominovaginal means. This permits estimation of the size and extent of the tumor. The bladder and urethra are then observed through a transurethrally inserted cystoscope. At this time biopsies of the tumor and underlying bladder wall are obtained. A bimanual examination is repeated after the biopsies are taken.

*Cystoscopy* is done in the operating-room suite. Food and fluids will be omitted after the midnight before the procedure. Following cystoscopy, spontaneous voiding should occur in 8 to 10 hours. *Hematuria* is often increased in the first few voidings. Symptoms of bladder irritability are common. *Low back pain* is often experienced. Fluids should be encouraged and mild analgesics administered to reduce discomfort. Sharp abdominal pain, fever, or chills are abnormal problems requiring immediate attention.

The *excretory urogram* permits visualization of the renal pelvis and ureters through the use of an injected contrast medium. Tumor-related upper-urinary-tract abnormalities can be detected with this diagnostic study. *Retrograde and fractionated cystograms* are sometimes performed. They are of limited value in the definitive diagnosis of bladder cancer. *Pelvic arteriography* and *lymphangiography* are occasionally used as a supplementary means of diagnosing bladder tumors, muscle invasion, and nodal involvement.

**N**ursing Problems and Interventions A person entering the hospital for diagnostic studies and definitive treatment of a bladder neoplasm is likely to be quite *apprehensive.* The presence of hematuria in itself can be frightening. The prospect of *unfamiliar diagnostic procedures* is a worrisome situation for the patient. Thorough explanations about all diagnostic procedures should be given. The patient should know the nature of a procedure and whether it is likely to be painful or uncomfortable. In addition, preparatory routines and pertinent postdiagnostic procedures should be discussed.

It is imperative for the nurse to be available and supportive to patients during the diagnostic evaluation period. During this time patients are often overlooked because they are relatively independent and frequently away from their room for the various diagnostic procedures.

The counseling role of the nurse is most important. The patient should be provided with the opportunity to verbalize feelings and ask questions. It is during this phase of hospitalization that a meaningful nurse-patient relationship can be established, which will facilitate the process of rehabilitation.

*Surgical procedures Fulguration* is usually used to destroy papillomas and noninvasive papillary carcinomas. This is a simple procedure in which a wire electrode is passed through a transurethrally inserted telescopic instrument. Electronic current is then applied while the electrode is in contact with the growth. The patient generally returns from surgery with an indwelling catheter connected to closed bladder irrigation. The catheter remains in place until the hematuria clears. As soon as the patient is fully awake, ambulation is permitted and oral intake is resumed. Discomfort similar to that experienced following diagnostic cystoscopy is common. Discharge from the hospital usually takes

place as soon as the indwelling catheter is removed and normal clear voiding resumes.

*Open-cystotomy fulguration* is used when diffuse papillomas or noninvasive papillary carcinoma are present. This type of fulguration is carried out through a lower abdominal incision into the bladder. With the exception of the incisional pain and healing process, the postoperative course is similar to that described for the closed fulguration procedure. The hospitalization period is usually about 7 days.

*Partial cystectomy* permits the excision of malignant bladder tumors which do not lie at the base of the bladder. However, few bladder tumors are amenable to this method of treatment. Half the bladder may be removed, drastically reducing bladder capacity for several months until some regeneration of bladder tissue occurs. The bladder is segmentally resected through a lower abdominal incision. A *cystotomy tube* and an *indwelling urethral catheter* are used during the postoperative period. The presence of two drainage tubes in the remaining portion of the bladder causes bladder spasms which are often extremely uncomfortable. Antispasmodics help to alleviate this problem. Early ambulation should be encouraged. Care must be taken to avoid obstruction of the drainage tubes. When both drainage tubes are discontinued, the patient will become acutely aware of the markedly diminished capacity of the bladder. Often the need to void seems continuous. Adequate hydration must be maintained. This can best be achieved by establishing a schedule for drinking fluids at convenient times when a bathroom is readily available. The nurse should be supportive in reassuring the patient that bladder capacity will increase to some extent.

*Total cystectomy* is used to treat invasive carcinoma and noninvasive papillary carcinoma with frequent diffuse recurrence. In men, the prostate and seminal vesicles are usually also removed. The surgery generally includes pelvic lymph-node dissection and urethrectomy when the carcinoma is invasive. *Permanent supravesical urinary diversion* is required. Frequently the surgery is done in two stages. Diversion of the urinary stream is followed by a course of irradiation and total cystectomy 6 weeks after irradiation.

*Supravesical urinary diversion Ureterosigmoidostomy* and *ureteroileosigmoidostomy* are two methods of diverting the urinary stream so that urine is voided through the rectum. The major advantage for the patient is that no abdominal stoma is involved. As shown in Fig. 6-15*a* and *b*, the ureters are implanted either directly into the sigmoid colon or into an isolated segment of ileum which is anastomosed to the sigmoid colon. The use of the ileal segment (ureteroileosigmoidostomy) is said to buffer intraluminal ureteral and colonic pressure differences, thus reducing the hazards of renal problems secondary to ureteral reflux and upper-urinary-tract infection.[95] A reduction in hyperchloremic acidosis and other electrolyte problems, commonly associated with ureterosigmoidostomy, is also claimed for the ureteroileosigmoidostomy. Both procedures continue to be associated with *electrolyte imbalance, pyelonephritis, hydronephrosis,* and *daily management problems.*

The *ileal conduit* is the most widely used method for permanent supravesical urinary diversion. The ureters are implanted in the posterior end of an isolated piece of ileal segment, as illustrated in Fig. 6-15c. In some instances a piece of jejunum or sigmoid colon may be used as a conduit. Peristalsis in the ileal segment avoids residual urine. Urine exits through an abdominal stoma, requiring the use of an ostomy appliance at all times. The major disadvantage of the ileal conduit is the presence of a stoma which constantly drains urine. Complications associated with the procedure include *urinary-tract infections, ureteral leaks* or *obstruction, ileal-loop necrosis, intestinal obstruction, fistulas, stomal stenosis, parastomal hernia, hyperchloremic acidosis, pyelonephritis, calculi, hydronephrosis,* and *uremia.*[96] In addition, stoma-related problems may occur such as *peristomal skin irritation, stomal encrustation,* and *stomal ulceration.*

*Cutaneous ureterostomy* (bilateral ureterostomy, transureteroureterostomy) can also be used to accomplish supravesical urinary diversion. This is done by implanting the ureters directly into the abdominal wall (see Fig. 6-15d). This procedure is usually employed in the patient who is not considered a good candidate for major surgery. If possible, one ureter is usually anastomosed to the other so that only one ureter is brought out to the skin (transureteroureterostomy). Urine drains continuously through the ureterostomy. An ostomy appliance is used to collect the urine.

*Nephrostomy tubes* can be inserted into the renal pelves to allow for urinary drainage. This is a palliative measure generally used for patients with advanced disease when other methods of urinary diversion are not feasible. A surgical incision is required to insert a nephrostomy tube (as shown in Fig. 6-15e). Balloon- or mushroom-tipped catheters are used as drainage tubes. Urine drains continuously into collecting devices. Kidney infection is common with a nephrostomy.

Any surgery which diverts the urinary stream, permanently altering a lifelong pattern of elimination, is a tremendous assault on the intact *body image.* Thorough supportive *preoperative preparation* is extremely important for any patient about to undergo a urinary-diversion procedure. The patient's family should be included in the preparatory process. Preoperative teaching should begin with a description of the surgical procedure and general information about the immediate pre- and postoperative periods, including skin preparation, fluid restrictions, medications, operating-room routine, postoperative pulmonary integrity, activity, pain, and intravenous-fluid therapy. A bowel-cleansing regime is ordered for patients undergoing diversions involving the sigmoid colon. Generally this includes a low-residue to clear liquid diet, cathartics, enemas, and bowel-sterilizing antibiotics. The patient undergoing ureterosigmoidostomy may be given enemas in amounts from 50 to 250 ml to develop *sphincter control* as well as an awareness of rectal-pressure sensations to be expected postoperatively.[97] The ureterosigmoidostomy patient should be informed that a *drainage tube* will be inserted in the rectum during the early postoperative period. When the tube is removed, *rectal voiding* must take place frequently in order to minimize reflux and electrolyte problems. The patient must be prepared for the new pattern of elimination. *Flatus* will be a lifelong problem for the ureterosigmoidostomy patient. In addition, the patient must learn that gas should only be expelled into a toilet, to avoid soiling of clothing and subsequent embarrassment. Dietary discussions concerning gas-forming foods should be started in the preoperative period.

If the patient is to have an ileal conduit, sigmoid conduit, or cutaneous ureterostomy, a site for *stoma placement* should be marked preoperatively. Since the location of a stoma is crucial in terms of successful postoperative management, it is imperative that the nurse discuss this subject with the surgeon. Selection of a cutaneous ureterostomy site may be limited by the length of ureter available. Figure 6-16 illustrates a convenient method for establishing an appropriate stoma site. Although the right lower quadrant of the abdomen is the most desirable location, the left lower quadrant may be used if it provides a better fit for an ostomy appliance.[98] The most important consideration is that adequate room be available for the appliance face plate to adhere to the abdomen. The stoma should be away from the belt line, scars, fat folds, bony prominences, and the umbilicus. In order to accurately determine an ideal stoma location, the pa-

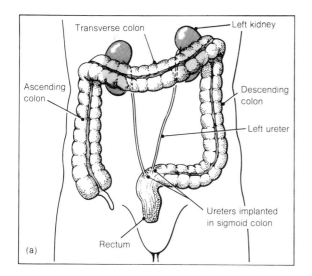

(a)

Transverse colon

Left kidney

Ascending colon

Descending colon

Left ureter

Ureters implanted in sigmoid colon

Rectum

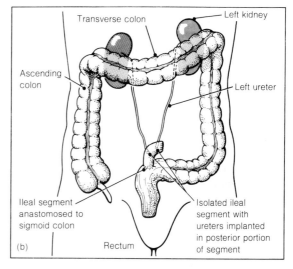

(b)

Transverse colon

Left kidney

Ascending colon

Left ureter

Ileal segment anastomosed to sigmoid colon

Isolated ileal segment with ureters implanted in posterior portion of segment

Rectum

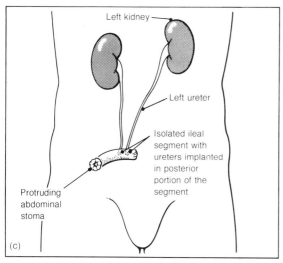

(c)

Left kidney

Left ureter

Isolated ileal segment with ureters implanted in posterior portion of the segment

Protruding abdominal stoma

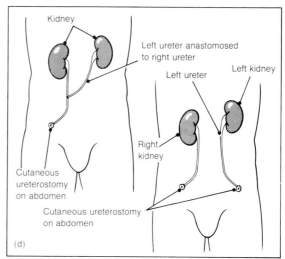

(d)

Kidney

Left ureter anastomosed to right ureter

Left ureter

Left kidney

Right kidney

Cutaneous ureterostomy on abdomen

Cutaneous ureterostomy on abdomen

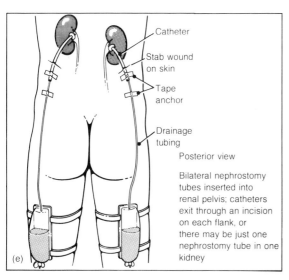

(e)

Catheter

Stab wound on skin

Tape anchor

Drainage tubing

Posterior view

Bilateral nephrostomy tubes inserted into renal pelvis; catheters exit through an incision on each flank, or there may be just one nephrostomy tube in one kidney

**FIGURE 6-15**

Methods of urinary diversion: (*a*) ureterosigmoidostomy; (*b*) ureteroileosigmoidostomy; (*c*) ileal loop (or ileal conduit); (*d*) ureterostomy (transcutaneous ureterostomy and bilateral cutaneous ureterostomies); (*e*) nephrostomy.

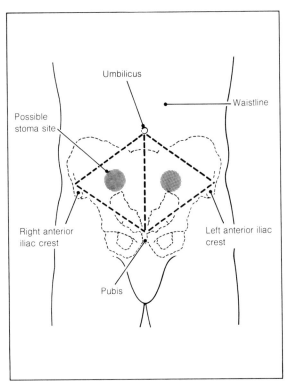

**FIGURE 6-16**

Marking stoma site with patient lying flat

1  Patient's waistline is marked.
2  Triangle is drawn on right or left lower quadrant from umbilicus to anterior iliac crest to symphysis pubis. Have patient sit, stand, bend, and flex hip, and observe for folds and creases in skin.
3  Stoma should be located within triangle two inches below belt line and far enough from inguinal fold so that exercise will not dislodge an appliance.

*(Courtesy of Katherine Jeter, Squier Urology Clinic, Columbia Presbyterian Hospital, New York, N.Y.)*

tient must be viewed standing, sitting, and lying down. Once selected, the site can be marked by intradermal injection of a dye such as methylene blue or the use of an indelible marker. Ostomy appliances should be demonstrated at the time the stoma site is marked. In addition, an accurate drawing or model of a stoma should be shown to the patient and family. Ileal- and sigmoid-conduit stomas should protrude from the skin. This provides for more effective ostomy management by the patient.

During the preoperative period many patients and families benefit from a visit by a rehabilitated person who has undergone urinary diversion. The United Ostomy Association, with its many chapters, provides this service. The nurse should discuss with the patient and family the possibility of an Ostomy Association visitor. A visit can occur any time during hospitalization or when the patient goes home.

For men, a cystectomy is frequently associated with *sexual dysfunction.* Thus the body-image assault imposed by a urinary diversion may be compounded by the threat of *impotence.* The surgeon has a responsibility to discuss this issue with the patient prior to surgery. The nurse should then engage in informative and supportive counseling with the patient. Helpful pamphlets containing information about sex are available from the United Ostomy Association and should be given to patients having ostomy surgery.

Patients who have undergone permanent urinary diversion are acutely ill in the immediate postoperative period. The insertion of bilateral nephrostomy tubes is a less complicated procedure, but the patient undergoing this procedure is usually suffering from advanced disease which may make the postoperative period difficult. A clear, disposable urostomy appliance connected to gravity drainage should be in place when the patient returns from surgery. Although it is usually possible to observe the stoma through the appliance, the appliance should be removed during the first 24 hours to carefully examine the stoma and peristomal skin. The stoma usually appears somewhat *edematous.* A dusky or cyanotic appearance should be reported to the surgeon. In some cases small ureteral stints may be seen protruding from the stoma. These are a temporary measure to assure ureteral patency. They will be removed before the patient is discharged from the hospital. The nurse must carefully monitor the patient's intake and output. It is most important to provide for adequate fluid intake. Any decrease in urinary output should be reported.

*Depression* in the postoperative period should be anticipated as a normal response. The patient must be allowed to grieve in order to make a successful adaptive response to the loss of a normal pattern of elimination and the presence of a stoma.

As soon as possible the patient should begin to participate in stoma care. A properly fitting ostomy appliance which does not leak facilitates adjustment to the stoma. Many products are now available for stoma care. Healthy peristomal skin is crucial. The use of a skin barrier such as Stomahesive or Reliaseal is frequently recommended. The appliance used must be one specifically designed for a *urostomy.* It must be open-ended, with a *valve-type adaptor* which can be opened for connection to closed gravity-drainage tubing, or closed, permitting the urine to collect in the appliance pouch. Each time the appliance is removed, the stoma and *peristomal skin* should be examined and washed with plain water. The peristomal skin must be dried thoroughly. A wick made of gauze or tissue should be placed over the stoma to prevent urine from draining onto the newly dried skin. An opening just slightly larger than the stoma is cut into the skin barrier. A hole approximately $1/16$ inch larger than the stoma is cut into the face plate of the appliance. The skin barrier is then applied over the stoma, followed by the appliance. The opening at the bottom of the appliance should be toward the patient's feet, so that urine can drain adequately when the patient is lying on either side. The appliance should be pressed down around the stoma, creating a seal. Micropore tape is used along the four sides of the appliance in a picture-framing effect to help hold the pouch in place. Frequent turning and early ambulation are essential. As soon as possible, stoma care should take place in the bathroom. During the day, urine should collect in the appliance when the patient is out of bed. *Continuous drainage* is used when the patient is in bed and at night. The patient should be taught how to empty the appliance early in the postoperative period. The pouch should be emptied before it gets heavy with urine and compromises the appliance seal.

All patients must be closely observed for signs of *complications.* Persistent *stomal bleeding* or *hematuric urine* should be reported. *Abdominal pain, fever, loss of bowel sounds,* and *cloudy or foul-smelling urine* all require careful investigation.

Following ileal-conduit surgery, a *nasogastric tube* connected to intermittent suction will be in place. The patient will not receive fluids by mouth for approximately 3 to 5 days. When the nasogastric tube is removed and peristalsis has resumed, clear liquids are started. A low-residue diet is then ordered. The patient usually remains on a low-residue diet until the intestinal anastomosis is healed. The patient should be eating a regular diet before discharge from the hospital. Large amounts of fluids are recommended. Measures to keep the urine acid are prescribed. Cranberry juice and ascorbic acid tablets are often used for this purpose. Once the patient is well enough to get out of bed independently, he or she should be encouraged to dress in street clothes. This provides an opportunity for the patient to practice stoma emptying as it will be done at home. In addition, street clothes enable the patient to observe that an appliance is not visible underneath clothing. Socialization with other patients should be encouraged.

*Radiation therapy*    Irradiation is an accepted form of treatment for bladder cancer. However, there is lack of agreement concerning the most judicious use of this mode of therapy. *Intracavitary radiation* has been advocated in the treatment of superficial low-grade tumors and carcinoma in situ.

*External radiation* may be employed in a number of different ways. *Supervoltage radiation* therapy has been used alone, but its success in treating bladder cancer is considered disappointing. When administered in favorable situations, radiation therapy combined with surgery is thought to cure the disease.[99] Radiation therapy can be interposed between the creation of a urinary diversion and the removal of the bladder. *Postoperative irradiation* is usually considered when there is known residual disease following surgery. A combined course of supervoltage radiation and 5-fluorouracil as an *adjuvant* to surgery has been suggested. Irradiation has also been proposed as a *palliative measure* in selected patients with bladder cancer.

The patient undergoing radiation therapy is likely to be apprehensive and fearful. Thorough explanations of all aspects of the treatment program must be given by the nurse. If intracavitary radiation is used, the patient will be placed on radiation precautions, and every effort must be made to reduce the patient's sense of isolation during this time when contact with people is strictly limited. Patients often consider radiation therapy to be a last-resort therapy. *Depression* is not uncommon. The nurse must provide the patient with the opportunity to verbalize feelings about the radiation-therapy experience.

*Bladder irritability,* characterized by frequency, urgency, dysuria, and nocturia, is a common side effect of radiation therapy. Increased amounts of fluids, antispasmodics, and urinary-tract antiseptics are given to alleviate bladder symptoms. *Diarrhea* may also occur. Agents which decrease intestinal motility should be used to relieve this problem.

*Chemotherapy*    The effects of chemotherapy in the treatment of bladder cancer are not considered impressive. 5-Fluorouracil has been commonly used in the treatment of advanced bladder cancer. In one study, however, 5-fluorouracil was not found to be any more effective than a placebo.[100] Mitomcyin-C, adriamycin, bleomycin, and other agents have also been tried with varying degrees of success.

Despite the uncertain response to chemotherapeutic agents, this treatment modality is often offered to patients in an effort to prolong life. The patient receiving chemotherapy and the family should be informed verbally and in writing of the nature of the drug being used, the desired outcome, the route and schedule of drug administration, the duration of treatment, and the common side effects, with a regimen for alleviating them.

The *side effects* of chemotherapeutic agents, such as alopecia, diarrhea, and nausea, are distressing and frequently a cause of depression in patients. In addition to careful assessment of *toxic effects,* which may warrant cessation of treatment, the nurse must provide a supportive milieu in which the patient is able to *verbalize feelings* about chemotherapy and the disease process involved.

**Fourth-level nursing care** Treatment of the person with a bladder neoplasm is directed at curing the disease or holding it in abeyance. In either case, every effort should be made to assist the patient to maintain a maximum level of independence within the limits of the disease. Family participation is known to be a crucial factor in successful rehabilitation.

A smooth transition from hospital to community can best be provided through contact with a Visiting Nurse Association or other community agency in the patient's home area. All patients should be visited at least once in their homes after hospital discharge. This enables the nurse in the community to assess the home situation and determine whether further home visits are necessary.

The person with a urinary diversion of any kind needs home-care follow-up for varying periods of time. Before leaving the hospital, the patient must be carefully and thoroughly prepared for discharge. At the time of discharge the patient should be showing indications of accepting the presence of the stoma or other means of urinary diversion. If the patient does not appear to be making a *positive adaptive response,* this fact should be reported to the surgeon. Plans should be made for dealing with psychosocial problems before the patient leaves the hospital. Sexual functioning should be discussed and clarified.

For the person with a stoma, the issue of disposable versus reusable equipment should be broached. The names and addresses of appliance suppliers ought to be given, and a *discharge kit* should be assembled for the patient, containing an adequate supply of skin barriers, disposable appliances, night drainage equipment, skin remedies, and detailed written information concerning stoma care, equipment being used, normal changes in stoma size, regimen to follow for skin problems, and the name and number of the local United Ostomy Association chapter. Pertinent ostomy literature for patients should also be included.

The person with a urinary diversion will need to know how to set up *night drainage.* In general, constant drainage is recommended for nighttime use, as it avoids the potential dangers of retention and reflux. For the person with a ureterosigmoidostomy, this means that a rectal tube must be inserted and attached to a closed drainage system. Some ureterosigmoidostomy patients sleep in a semi-sitting position instead of using the tube. Instructions should be given for dealing with common problems and complications associated with the various methods of urinary diversion. One should emphasize the need to contact a physician or nurse immediately when complications occur.

Adequate follow-up health care is essential for the person with a bladder neoplasm. New papillomas may appear, and tumors may recur. *Periodic cystoscopy* and *urinary cystologic examination* are necessary for several years. Bladder neoplasms are known for their tendency to recur. Some patients may need to be admitted at intervals for repeated fulguration procedures. Eventually more aggressive surgery may become necessary.

For the person with bladder cancer, the threat of recurrence is often a nagging problem. Patients and their families will require a supportive, empathetic approach by the nurse in the community. Every effort should be made to reintegrate the patient into society.

### Urethral Neoplasms

*Benign urethral caruncles* occur fairly often in women between the ages of 40 and 65. These neoplasms develop at the meatus and are said to be caused by chronic irritation. *Papillomatous neoplasms* appear more frequently in men. They may occur anywhere within the urethra. *Malignant urethral neoplasms* occur more frequently in women than in men. However, carcinoma of the urethra is not common in either sex. The most prevalent tumors of the female urethra are *epidermoid carcinoma* and *adenocarcinoma.* In men, *squamous-cell* and *transitional-cell carcinomas* occur most frequently. The tumors may metastasize to regional lymph nodes. In women, the vulva and vagina may become involved. Distant metastasis is usually to the lung, liver, bone, and brain.[101]

Both benign and malignant urethral neoplasms may produce symptoms of *dysuria, urinary obstruction,* and *bleeding.* Diagnosis is by *biopsy* of the neoplasm. Transurethral electrocoagulation cures the benign neoplasms; *recurrence* is uncommon. Radical surgery is generally required to treat the malignant tumors. Amputation of the penis, accompanied by radical groin dissection and urinary diversion, is often indicated. In women, *urethrocystectomy* with urinary diversion may be necessary.

*Pelvic exenteration* is performed in some instances. Interstitial, intracavitary, and external supervoltage radiation may be used alone or in conjunction with surgery.

Patients with benign urethral neoplasms undergo relatively minor surgery, but the patient is likely to experience considerable apprehension until such time as a biopsy establishes the neoplasm as benign. After surgical removal of the neoplasm, early voidings are painful. *Sitz baths* may reduce discomfort and meatal swelling.

The patient with a malignant urethral neoplasm may be faced with the prospect of extremely mutilating surgery. The body-image assault imposed by amputation of the penis or the vulva and vagina is immeasurable. The nurse will be called upon to play a most challenging role in assisting the patient to make a *positive adaptive response* to this devastating situation. Elimination problems are similar to those of the patient with bladder cancer who undergoes a urinary-diversion procedure. When a cystectomy is not performed, the external sphincter is preserved and a perineal orifice is created for the elimination of urine. The *perineal area* may be quite painful in the early postoperative period, particularly after extensive lymph-node dissection. The patient will need help to change positions frequently. Analgesics should be administered to relieve pain. Some patients may become very *depressed* and *withdrawn*. The nurse should be alert to the need for psychiatric assistance in such situations.

### Ureteral Neoplasms

Carcinoma of the ureters is uncommon. When it occurs, *papillary transitional-cell carcinoma* predominates. It is often secondary to cancer of the prostate, bladder, and renal pelvis. Bilateral ureteral involvement is not common. *Elderly men* are most frequently affected. The cause of malignant ureteral neoplasms is unknown. *Carcinogens* implicated in bladder cancer may be involved. Phenacetin has been suggested as a possible causative agent.[102] Ureteral neoplasms may metastasize to regional lymph nodes, lungs, and liver. *Hematuria* is the most common symptom. Ureteral or renal pain may be present if obstruction has occurred. Diagnosis is by *cystoscopy* and *excretory urograms.* Urine cytologic studies are usually performed.

Appropriate surgical treatment of ureteral neoplasms is a controversial issue. A case has been made for local excision of the neoplasm instead of the customary nephroureterectomy with removal of a cuff of bladder around the ureteral orifice. A total cystectomy with urinary diversion may be employed in some instances as a palliative measure to relieve pain and obstruction. Radiation therapy and chemotherapy are not effective.

Any person with hematuria should be referred for further diagnostic evaluation, which takes place in the hospital. Adequate physical and psychological preparation of the patient for all diagnostic procedures is mandatory.

The patient about to undergo surgery for the removal of a ureteral tumor is likely to be very apprehensive. The surgical procedure must be carefully explained. All preoperative routines should be discussed. Sufficient opportunity must be provided for questions and verbalization of feelings. Nursing problems in the pre- and postoperative period are similar to those of the patient undergoing partial cystectomy and nephrectomy.

The outlook for rehabilitation is excellent when the neoplasm is benign. It is considerably less optimistic for malignant lesions. Follow-up health care is essential. Patients who have had a nephrectomy must be particularly vigilant about any urinary-tract problems.

## NEOPLASMS OF THE HEAD AND NECK*

Cancer of the head and neck constitutes approximately 5 percent of all cancers. Because of the marked cosmetic and functional deformities associated with these tumor types, patients diagnosed with this disease provide a special challenge to health-team workers. Tumors of the head and neck can be divided into five main categories: nose, nasopharynx, and paranasal sinuses; oral cavity; oropharynx; laryngopharynx; and salivary glands. Each tumor group produces different symptomatology requiring unique treatment modalities and nursing intervention. The primary goals of the health team providing care to patients with head and neck cancer, as with all malignant disease, are prevention, early detection, and cure of the disease.

### Cancer of the Larynx

Cancer of the larynx appears to be the most widely discussed type of head and neck neoplasm, although oral-cavity tumors are more common. These tumors affect any part of the anatomic struc-

* The author wishes to express appreciation to Eugene N. Myers, M.D., Chairman of the Department of Otolaryngology at Eye and Ear Hospital in Pittsburgh and the University of Pittsburgh, for his help in reviewing the manuscript of this section.

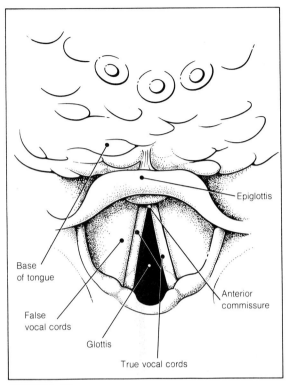

**FIGURE 6-17**
Normal indirect view of larynx.

ture known as the larynx and include cancers of the true or false vocal cords, epiglottis, aryepiglottic folds, laryngeal ventricle, and laryngeal cartilages (Fig. 6-17).

**Pathophysiology**   The laryngeal cavity is lined with mucous membrane that is continuous with the pharynx superiorly and with the trachea inferiorly. The area extending from the tip of the epiglottis to the laryngeal tubercle and the area of the vocal cords is lined with stratified columnar epithelium, while the remainder of the larynx shows pseudo-stratified ciliated columnar epithelium. Both types of cell lining give rise to the most commonly seen laryngeal cancer, *squamous-cell carcinoma.* Ballenger has stated that approximately 95 percent of all laryngeal tumors are of the squamous-cell variety.[103] These tumors can range from poorly differentiated to well-differentiated types, with moderately well-differentiated squamous-cell carcinomas being the most common.[104] Metastatic spread of laryngeal tumors may be by direct mucosal or submucosal extension, lymphatic or vascular involvement, or perineural invasion. The potential for metastasis of laryngeal tumors depends on the degree

of differentiation, the size and location of the primary lesion, and the evidence of nerve-sheath invasion.[105]

**C**ausative Factors   Although there are no definite causative agents in carcinoma of the larynx, several factors have been indicated as related or probable *contributing factors.* The primary etiologic factor appears to be *heavy cigarette smoking.* Cigarette smokers exhibit excessive keratinization of the true vocal cords, epithelial hyperplasia of the true and false vocal cords and the subglottic area, squamous metaplasia, edema, and chronic submucosal inflammation.[106] It was recently stated in an article on prevention of laryngeal cancer that cigarette smoking was "the principal risk factor in glottic and supraglottic laryngeal cancer. The more the individual smokes, the greater is that person's risk for developing cancer of the larynx."[107]

Another factor often discussed in relation to cancer of the larynx is *heavy alcohol consumption.* There is still much discussion as to the relationship of increased alcohol intake and laryngeal cancer, but two of the theories point to nutritional deficiencies associated with alcohol consumption and the combination of heavy cigarette smoking with increased alcohol intake.[108] Other related factors may include air pollution, viral invasion, and chronic upper and lower respiratory-tract infections. The exact relationship of these factors is still controversial, and no linkage has been proved.

Although not a causative agent, *leukoplakia* is classified as a premalignant state. Leukoplakia is a white, plaquelike lesion that can be seen on mucosal surfaces. The characteristic feature of leukoplakia is marked hyperplasia of the epithelium with hyperkeratosis. It is most commonly caused by excessive smoking.[109]

**C**lassification   Malignant tumors of the larynx are divided according to specific anatomic zones. These zones exhibit different symptomatology, progression of the disease, and patterns of metastatic spread and require a variety of treatment modalities. Those primary lesions affecting the true vocal cords, *glottic tumors,* make up the first division. Tumors originating on the true vocal cords tend to be diagnosed earlier and remain localized for a longer period of time than lesions beginning elsewhere in the larynx. Because the lymphatics of the true vocal cord are sparse compared to the other areas, regional metastasis usually does not occur until late in the disease or after the cancer extends beyond the area of the true cord. The earliest symptom of a glottic tumor is hoarseness, which may be intermittent or constant. With the increased public knowledge of persistent hoarseness as one of the American Cancer Society's warning signals, early investigation of this manifestation can be undertaken. Other symptoms that may be associated with carcinoma of the true vocal cords are: dyspnea, which occurs when enlargement of the tumor decreases the glottic space and thus the airway; the sensation of a lump in the throat, which is also described as a foreign-body sensation; otalgia; and pain, which is usually an indication of extension of the disease and infiltration of nerve fibers.

The second classification of tumors of the larynx comprises *supraglottic lesions,* which are located in the region from the false vocal cords to the tip of the epiglottis. These tumors do not involve the true vocal cords as part of the primary site. Supraglottic laryngeal tumors are more aggressive than glottic tumors. They invade the surrounding structures more rapidly and tend to metastasize to the regional lymph nodes earlier in the disease process, because of the rich lymphatic drainage through the thyrohyoid plexus to the cervical lymph nodes. Symptoms of supraglottic lesions are subtle and usually seen late in the progression of the disease. Hoarseness or dyspnea may be present with invasion of the glottis or with recurrent laryngeal-nerve involvement; sore throat, primarily on swallowing, may occur with superior extension, while actual difficulty in swallowing appears even later in the disease.

*Infraglottic tumors* are those lesions extending from the inferior margin of the vocal cords to the inferior border of the cricoid cartilage. Primary tumors in this area are relatively rare and are more difficult to diagnose, as early infraglottic or subglottic tumors are less accessible to visualization by the usual office technique of indirect mirror examination. Because of this, many are not diagnosed until extension to the vocal cords or obstruction of the airway has occurred. The infraglottic lymphatics begin as a network in the mucous membrane on the inferior border of the vocal cords. These channels terminate in the lower deep jugular chain or the prelaryngeal (Delphian) node, which further drains into the pretracheal and supraclavicular nodes.[110] Early symptoms of infraglottic tumors are not common, but in later progression of the disease the patient may exhibit stridor, dyspnea, and hoarseness.

Tumors which extend across or involve the laryngeal ventricle are classified as transglottic. *Transglottic tumors* have the highest rate of regional lymph-node metastasis and produce a variety of symptoms, as they usually involve two or more of the areas previously discussed.

*Staging of tumors* A uniform classification of tumors is important for comparison of end results and for selection of treatment in cancer of the head and neck. The systems developed by UICC and the American Joint Committee on Cancer Staging utilize the *TNM classification.* T represents primary tumor and may range from T1S (carcinoma in situ) to T3 or T4, which is a large primary tumor usually involving other anatomical structures by direct extension. N represents regional lymph-node involvement. N0 indicates no regional lymph-node involvement; the scale continues to N3, meaning lymph nodes fixed to deeper structures with other metastasis suspected. Distant metastasis is noted by use of the letter M. M0 indicates that there is no evidence of distant metastasis; M1 indicates clinical or laboratory evidence of metastasis to areas other than the cervical lymph nodes.[111] Each area of the head and neck has a slightly different staging system, and it is important for the nurse to compare the various systems and understand that identical terms do not necessarily mean identical stages.

**First-level nursing care** As stated earlier, the definite causative factors of head and neck carcinoma have not been identified, but smoking and alcohol consumption are certainly indicated. A history of many years of cigarette smoking tends to be the most common historical fact in laryngeal carcinoma. *Cigarette smoking* causes changes in the lining cells of the larynx, as well as chronic irritation to these membranes. The risk is directly related to the number of cigarettes smoked per day and the number of years of smoking. The majority of patients who develop cancer of the larynx are male, but this trend is changing with the recent increase in women smokers.[112] A comparative study of male and female patients with laryngeal cancer in 1956 showed a 14.9:1 ratio, while a similar study in 1972–73 showed a ratio of 4.6:1.[113]

*Alcohol consumption* is another related factor in laryngeal carcinoma. It is unknown at this time whether the increased risk is related to the intake of alcohol per se or to the associated manifestations of alcohol intake. Some researchers in the epidemiology of cancer of the head and neck believe that the correlation may be with the nutritional deficiencies, especially protein depletion, that accompany heavy alcohol use. Wydner believes the relationship to be based on a combination of heavy cigarette smoking and heavy alcohol use. His data revealed an increase in the risk of developing laryngeal cancer with the smoking and alcohol combination but no significant increase in risk with alcohol consumption in the absence of smoking.[114]

Persons with one primary carcinoma in the head and neck region have an increased incidence of developing a second primary tumor in the same region. It is believed to be more common in patients who have continued the same patterns in relation to smoking and drinking.[115] If these factors are indeed the causative ones, it is a health-team responsibility to educate the public regarding them. Nurses should join with other health workers and with community agencies such as the American Cancer Society and the National Cancer Institute in promoting smoking-control clinics as well as anti-smoking legislation. The National Cancer Institute has developed cancer-control task forces for the leading primary-cancer sites, with head and neck cancer forming one section. The aim of these groups is control of cancer through screening for early diagnosis and early treatment. Educational programs have been developed for physicians, dentists, and nurses to reinforce the techniques of screening for cancer of the oral cavity and larynx, with the objective of setting up programs in high-risk population areas and in rural districts, conducted by physicians and nurses, with screening and public education as the main priorities. The head and neck cancer task force will also combine efforts with the lung cancer task force to support *smoking-control clinics,* as this is an area of prevention for both types of cancer. The ultimate goal of these groups is prevention, with early detection and treatment as the second objective.

Consumer education appears to be the area of greatest neglect in the prevention of laryngeal carcinoma. The nurse is a key factor in primary prevention by educating the public.

**Second-level nursing care** This level of nursing care centers on the early onset of the disease and, most important, its early detection. It may first be detected by an astute nurse completing a detailed nursing assessment.

**N**ursing Assessment A thorough *health history* should be taken at the time the patient first presents in any health-care setting. The nurse can identify existing as well as potential problems in the area of the head and neck by completely assessing the *physical* and *psychosocial aspects* of the patient. Questions should be directed to problems the patient has had in the past as well as the present.

Symptoms associated with laryngeal carcinoma should be followed by a thorough examination of the area.

*Health history* A more detailed description of the health history is found under Third-level Nursing Care; its content and principles apply here as well.

*Hoarseness* usually causes the patient to seek medical attention. It may be caused by inflammation, a benign tumor such as a polyp, vocal-cord paralysis, a primary lesion on the true cord, or a primary tumor extending to the area of the true cord. This symptom, intermittent or continuous, should prompt a mirror examination of the laryngopharynx.

Another symptom requiring further investigation is the sensation of a *lump* or foreign body in the throat. This symptom also may be intermittent or persistent.

Some patients will describe a *sore throat* as their only discomfort. (This symptom is often inadequately treated with a prolonged course of antibiotics if the area is not thoroughly investigated.) A persistent sore throat may indicate a tumor of the pharynx or larynx.

The patient may indicate a *change in eating habits* over time, with or without an associated *loss of weight.* A change in the type of food as well as a change in the consistency of foods tolerated should alert the nurse to delve further into this area. Many patients progress from general foods to soft or pureed foods to liquids before seeking medical attention.

*Pain on swallowing, aspiration of food* secondary to tumor bulk, and *bleeding* may also be present prior to the first medical consultation. With these complaints of obstruction, the nurse should be aware of the possibility of pressure being exerted on the pharynx or even the esophagus by a bulky tumor.

*Airway obstruction* and *dyspnea* are generally symptoms occurring with more advanced tumors. They are not usually apparent until the tumor reaches a large size, resulting in encroachment or narrowing of the lumen of the airway.

*Pain* and a *mass* in the neck are also relatively late symptoms of cancer of the larynx. Pain may be felt at the site of the lesion or, more commonly, may be referred to the ear. A mass in the neck indicates regional cervical lymph-node metastasis. As indicated earlier, cancers of the various parts of the larynx tend to metastasize at different rates, depending on the degree of lymphatic drainage from the particular site. A lump in the neck may be the patient's only presenting symptom. The mass may be on the same side as the lesion, the opposite side, or both sides of the neck, depending on the location and extent of the primary lesion. Any patient presenting with a lump in the neck requires a thorough examination of the head and neck area to locate the primary site. Neck disease cannot be treated without first diagnosing and treating the area causing the metastasis.

*Psychosocial assessment*  In addition to investigating and obtaining physical symptomatology, efforts should be made to evaluate *psychosocial aspects.* It is important to determine the life-style of the patient, including work habits and environment. Does the patient have a job requiring excessive use of the voice, which may put stress on the vocal cords, e.g., work in a noisy factory where straining the voice is essential in order to be heard? Is there evidence of exposure to noxious fumes or heavy pollution over a period of time that could have caused irritation of the mucous membranes lining the head and neck area? The cultural background of the patient should be investigated as well as the family history. Is there a history of cancer, especially head and neck cancer, in the extended family? Has a cancer in any other body part ever been diagnosed? Investigate the client's health patterns, including regular medical examinations and daily health habits such as oral hygiene and nutrition. Initiate discussions related to the patient's use of tobacco (in any form), alcohol (amount consumed, with special attention to changes in this pattern recently), and drugs.

*Physical assessment*  The nurse should give the patient and family thorough explanations of all procedures being performed in order to allay some of the anxiety associated with fear of the unknown. Physical assessment of the head and neck area begins with the oral cavity. If the patient wears dentures, they should be removed prior to the examination. The tongue, buccal mucosa, pharyngeal wall, and soft and hard palate are *inspected* for sores, masses, leukoplakia, and areas of erosion or chronic irritation. A small nasopharyngeal mirror is next used to inspect the area of the nasopharynx. A mirror examination is necessary for examining the laryngopharynx. During this examination, the tongue is extended and held and a laryngeal mirror is inserted. The patient is instructed to breathe through the mouth to prevent gagging. The examiner can visualize the area from the epiglottis to the vocal cords by this examination (Fig. 6-17).

The neck is *palpated* for any lymphadenopathy or masses. Positive findings should be indicated by drawings and descriptions showing approximate anatomic location and size. Other types of evaluation, such as biopsy and x-ray studies, are usually delayed until hospitalization can be arranged.

**N**ursing Problems and Intervention  The *presence of a mass* or any of the previously described *suspicious findings* are the problems of importance at this level. Any suspicious finding in the initial assessment should be noted and the patient should be *referred* to an otolaryngologist for further investigation. If biopsy or x-ray examinations have been performed, the slides and reports of the studies should be forwarded to the consultant for review. The patient and family should be prepared for the consultation and given any information discovered on the initial evaluation. *Health teaching* is also given during this assessment in relation to general health habits and follow-up. In addition, referrals to smoking-cessation clinics can be made and encouragement given both to the patient and to any family members present.

**Third-level nursing care**  Admission to the hospital for further diagnostic procedures or for treatment of a laryngeal carcinoma can be a frightening experience for the patient and family. The anticipation of what will be found as well as the fear of mutilating surgery will alter the normal life pattern.

**N**ursing Assessment  The nursing assessment is the first step toward getting to know the patient. By conducting an interview with the patient, the nurse can develop a data base and initiate the patient problem list. The nursing assessment should be completed within several hours of admission. This is the nurse's opportunity to gather the information necessary to develop a plan of care for the patient while hospitalized and during rehabilitation, as well as a time to show sincere interest in the patient as a person and to begin to develop rapport. Areas that should be investigated vary with the health-care agency, but some aspects that are essential do not change. Most nursing assessments begin with an investigation of the chief complaint.

*Health history*  The nurse should inquire what caused the patient to initially seek medical attention and what other associated manifestations of head and neck cancer the patient has experienced, how long the patient has had the symptoms, and what has been done at home to aggrevate or alleviate them. Some examples are the type, degree, location, and character of any *pain* and what methods have been tried, with or without success, to relieve the pain, for example, medication (type, dosage, and frequency), relaxation techniques, imagery; any *breathing difficulty,* i.e., dyspnea on exertion or at rest, and positions or techniques used to make breathing easier; *swallowing ability,* i.e., what types of food the patient is now able to eat, how long the swallowing problem has existed, and the degree of related weight loss.

By *observation* the nurse can gain information from nonverbal cues such as facial grimaces, the position the patient assumes during the interview, any breathlessness exhibited while talking, the condition of the skin, and the general nutritional state. The nurse should also assess the patient's and the family's knowledge of the disease condition by determining what information has been given by the physician prior to hospitalization in regard to the diagnosis and the anticipated treatment. Experience indicates that the patient does not always hear what is said after the term "cancer" is used and more often understands even less. Health-care workers are accustomed to the medical terms used to indicate carcinoma, but it must be remembered that medical terminology is not part of the patient's daily vocabulary, as the following account shows:

A 46-year-old male and his wife presented at the office of an otolaryngologist with the chief complaint of intermittent hoarseness for the past six months. After thorough examination, the diagnosis of a $T_2$ lesion of the supraglottic larynx was made.

The patient was admitted to the hospital and a biopsy was performed to confirm the suspicion of squamous cell carcinoma. Explanations were given by the physician to the patient and his wife about the presence of a malignant tumor and the required surgery. Later the nurse entered the room to reinforce previous explanations and found the patient and his wife crying. Mrs. J. apologized for crying but clarified her reaction by saying, "We are so happy and relieved that the tumor is only malignant and not cancer."

It is important for health-care workers to be alert to the need of patients and their families for thorough and basic explanations.

After investigating the disease condition, the nurse must devote the remainder of the assessment to the patient as an individual. The nurse must examine the patient's past medical history. What other disease process may have been experienced? What other conditions have required hospitalization, and what effect did the hospitalization have? What coping mechanisms were employed to deal with the stress incurred because of the hospital stay and illness? Each individual draws upon previously used defense systems.[116] By investigating the patient's past experiences with disease and treatment, the health-team member may gain some insight into how the patient will deal with the present situation.

Investigation of the work situation can reveal such things as exposure to pollutants, noxious fumes, and radiation. It is important to determine the amount and duration of the exposure. Information should be elicited regarding contacts with other people and the degree of voice use required in order to fulfill job requirements.

Also important to determine are the *support systems* available to the patient. What is the relationship of the family members? Is the patient the one who is usually the "tower of strength," the one who gives the needed support to the family? Are the family members dependent on the patient for decision making, or will they be capable of handling everyday activities while the patient is hospitalized? Because of the age-group and male-sex predominance of laryngeal cancer, this can pose a threat to patient and family. The absence of a person who is the dominant figure in the home can add great stress to the family situation. The patient can sometimes be burdened with daily problems in the home in addition to dealing with the hospital and the disease. It is essential for the nurse to recognize this situation and to identify other family members who can be utilized in the support system.

The patient's *personal habits* may be another area to include in the health history. Those of primary interest are the use of cigarettes and other tobacco products, including the amount smoked and the duration of the habit; the amount of alcohol consumed on a daily basis and the duration of this pattern; and the use of drugs, with emphasis on the type used and the length of time they have been utilized. The areas of alcohol intake and drug usage have implications for hospitalization, especially during the first few days. Withdrawal symptoms, if anticipated, can be avoided or treated. If the use of alcohol or drugs is not recognized, severe problems in management may occur.

The initial interview is the ideal method of gathering the information required to provide optimal patient care, and it is also a perfect time to permit patient verbalization. There may be many fears or thoughts going through the patient's mind that could be resolved if expressed and clarified.

*Physical assessment* Examination of the patient reveals findings as described under Second-level Nursing Care. Inspection and palpation are the major techniques used to determine abnormalities. Far-advanced disease may present with obvious masses, ulceration, bleeding, and obstruction. The obstruction may result in breathing difficulties and pain.

Widespread dissemination of the cancer or interference with nutrition may result in weight loss. The patient may appear cachectic and pale. Ideally, the patient's weight should be compared to a previous weight record.

Some patients will seek medical attention for earlier symptoms, such as hoarseness or chronic sore throat. All these symptoms require further investigation with diagnostic tests during hospitalization.

Several special diagnostic procedures may be required to diagnose the presence of cancer of the larynx. The exact location of the lesion, the extent of involvement of the tumor, and the possibility of regional or distant metastasis must be evaluated.

The major *diagnostic techniques* include radiographic studies and direct laryngoscopy with biopsy. The *laryngogram* is a contrast-dye study of the larynx. A contrast material is dripped into the laryngopharynx during fluoroscopic examination, and films are made on inspiration, on phonation, and during the Valsalva maneuver.[117] Several different views are taken to assess the function of the laryngeal structures. The laryngogram is helpful in delineating the exact location of the tumor, as well as the extent of tumor involvement.[118] Patient preparation for this examination is usually a joint effort of the physicians performing the study and the nursing staff on the patient unit. The patient is usually allowed nothing by mouth from the midnight preceding the procedure and is premedicated with a sedative and atropine to reduce secretions. The study is done in the radiology department, and the patient should be prepared for a few hours' absence from the patient unit. Other radiographic studies performed include *polytomography,* lateral soft-tissue films to "emphasize the soft tissue–air contrast and the pattern of calcification of the laryngeal cartilage," barium swallow, and chest x-ray to determine tumor extent and evidence of metastasis.[119]

Probably the most important of all preliminary diagnostic procedures is *direct laryngoscopy with biopsy.* Indirect laryngoscopy, or mirror examination of the larynx, discussed earlier, is important for initial inspection, but because of inability to visual-ize the entire area and the severe gag reflex of some patients, it cannot be considered a conclusive technique. Direct laryngoscopy is done under local or general anesthesia, depending on the patient and the physician's preference. It is utilized for a more thorough evaluation of the tumor and to biopsy the suspected area. Patient preparation should include nothing by mouth for 8 hours prior to the procedure, preoperative sedation, and a medication to decrease secretions. The procedure is usually a short one involving insertion of a laryngoscope to visualize the area and to obtain an adequate specimen for pathologic diagnosis. The patient may require a tracheotomy at the time of the laryngoscopy, especially if the tumor is large and is causing airway distress. The patient returns to the room after recovering from the anesthesia and is placed on voice rest. After the effects of anesthesia have subsided, fluids can be started.

Depending on the health-care agency and related policies, the patient may be discharged following the laryngoscopy or may remain in the hospital to await the results of the biopsy. Only after pathologic diagnosis will explicit plans for treatment be initiated.

**N**ursing Problems and Interventions *Respiratory interference, speech impairment, facial disfigurement,* and the *diagnosis of cancer* are among the major problems encountered in caring for a patient with laryngeal cancer. Interventions center around surgery and radiation, with rehabilitation being a large part of posttreatment care.

Patient *referrals* are a vital part of the early hospital period for the patient with cancer of the larynx. The social service department should be involved with the patient from the time of entrance to the hospital through discharge planning. Social workers can help the nursing staff in the counseling phase, can assist in gathering pertinent information about support systems and the availability of helping family members and friends for the discharge plans, initiate visiting-nurse and vocational-planning referrals, and help to determine financial burdens. The patient will benefit from early involvement of the social service department. It is impossible for any health-team member to act effectively if not included in the planning phase at the time of hospitalization.

The speech pathology department is another part of the health team that requires early referral. One of the patient's biggest adjustments as a result of laryngeal cancer involves loss of the ability to communicate. The speech pathologist, who should begin working with the patient while he or she still has the ability to communicate, will make a preoperative speech evaluation to determine the anatomic structures used in communication and the special accents or dialects the patient uses, as well as counseling the patient about speech after laryngectomy.

The third early referral that should be made is to the maxillofacial prosthetics department. This department is concerned primarily with intraoral and extraoral devices that can be used in the reconstructive phase of care of a patient with head and neck cancer. Impressions must be made prior to surgical intervention in order to duplicate the missing structures as closely as possible. The maxillofacial department is involved more with other phases of head and neck cancer than with those persons having cancer of the larynx.

All treatment of laryngeal carcinoma is aimed at eradication of the disease while maintaining a reasonable quality of life. The type of treatment suggested to the patient will be based on this philosophy, with the location and extent of tumor involvement providing the main criteria.

*Radiation therapy*　Radiation therapy may be used alone as the treatment of choice, depending on the location and size of the lesion. Small lesions of the larynx respond equally well to either radiation or surgery, with radiation being chosen more often for the sake of maintaining the normal function of speech. As lesions increase in size, treatment may combine radiation and surgery, with an improvement in cure rates. Radiation therapy destroys the actively dividing tumor cells. As tumors enlarge, the center or core of the tumor is less oxygenated and receives less blood supply, therefore the cells divide more slowly. These cells are not usually radioresponsive; the treatment in these cases shrinks the tumor to a size more accessible to surgical intervention. Patients receiving radiation therapy as total or partial treatment for cancer of the larynx require careful explanations of the procedure that will be followed as well as side effects that may occur.

The radiation oncologist begins the consultation with a thorough examination of the patient. After determining the location and size of the lesion, a dosage schedule is developed and the portals of entry necessary to destroy the tumor are located. The therapeutic effects of radiation can be delivered in a daily dose until the maximum number of rads is reached or, in "split-course" therapy, a higher amount may be given in each treatment, with a rest period between courses. Radiation given with curative intent delivers a higher dosage than that used in combination therapy.

There is still much controversy regarding the efficacy of preoperative vs. postoperative radiation in conjunction with surgery. Preoperative radiotherapy has three main objectives: to reduce the incidence of metastasis by destroying the well-oxygenated cells at the periphery of the tumor, to shrink the size of the tumor to permit surgical resection, and to treat the regional lymph nodes that may or may not be included in the surgery.[120] The plan to use preoperative radiotherapy requires a collaborative effort between the radiation oncologist and the surgeon. The dosage given is less than that given as a curative procedure, and the patient requires a 4- to 6-week period of rest between completion of the initial therapy and surgical intervention.

Postoperative irradiation is used in some cases where adequate surgical resection is not successful or in cases of tumors with a high incidence of lymph-node involvement. Radiation oncologists prefer treatment prior to surgery, as the surgical intervention decreases the blood supply to the tumor site, making the tumor cells more radioresistant.[121] Surgeons generally recommend postoperative radiation because of the possibility of decreased healing in previously irradiated tissues.

Nursing intervention for the patient receiving radiotherapy for a laryngeal cancer involves patient education and care regarding side effects. The nurse should be cognizant of the procedures in the radiation-therapy clinic in order to reinforce and re-explain the physician's information to the patient. Side effects, if explained and anticipated, will be handled with much less anxiety by the patient. Radiation side effects in the head and neck are relatively common. Dryness of the mucous membranes and resulting *mucositis* is one common result of radiation therapy. Because of the portals of entry, the salivary glands are usually involved in the beam of radiation. With the combination of decreased saliva and damaged mucosa, the patient may complain of dryness and a resultant *difficulty in eating.* Good oral hygiene is the primary treatment for this symptom. Hydrogen peroxide and water or saline mouth rinses used frequently during the day will aid in providing comfort by cleansing the intraoral tissue and lubricating the membranes.[122] Adequate fluid intake is essential to maintain fluid balance and will temporarily overcome the sensation of dryness. The use of tobacco and alcohol causes increased irritation of the already inflamed mucous membranes and should be discontinued before radiotherapy.

Radiation caries are a frequent occurrence in postirradiation patients because of the decreased saliva and altered pH.[123] Fluoride carriers should be used several times a day as a protection against this decay. The patient should be instructed in the use of these carriers prior to initiation of radiotherapy. Consultation with a dental hygienist for prophylactic oral hygiene, with further therapy by a prosthodontist, is also helpful.

*Inadequate nutrition* is another related effect of radiation treatment. The dryness described above plus discomfort and a loss of the sense of taste result in decreased food intake. Any feasible method of improving the patient's nutritional status should be used. Small, frequent meals with soft or liquid foods are tolerated better than a regular diet. Blenderized diets provide an adequately balanced yet well-tolerated variety of foods. These related side effects generally subside after therapy is discontinued but may remain for an indefinite time in some patients.

*Surgical intervention* Surgical intervention for laryngeal cancer, as with radiation therapy, depends primarily on the site of the lesion and the extent of tumor involvement. Operative procedures for primary cancer of the larynx include supraglottic laryngectomy, hemilaryngectomy, and total laryngectomy. With all procedures, radical neck dissection may be done if there is suspicion of regional lymph-node metastasis.

A *supraglottic laryngectomy* excises all or nearly all of the larynx above the vocal cords and is performed for primary lesions of the supraglottis (the area from the false vocal cords to the epiglottis). Patients must be carefully evaluated prior to this procedure, primarily in regard to pulmonary function. The epiglottis, a fibroelastic cartilage that protects against aspiration on swallowing, is removed during the operative procedure, providing an easy passage for food and fluids to enter the airway. The patient's pulmonary status must be adequate to permit swallowing without aspiration in the postoperative period. The positive aspect of this procedure is the preservation of the vocal cords and a normal speaking voice.

*Hemilaryngectomy* involves the removal of part of the larynx. It is used where there is involvement of one vocal cord or one true cord with minimal extension to the vocal process, across the anterior commissure or slight subglottic extension.[124] Ballenger states that these tumors, because of their potential for recurrence, respond more favorably to hemilaryngectomy than to radiation therapy.[125] This procedure also effectively preserves the patient's speaking voice.

*Total laryngectomy* is the treatment of choice for all laryngeal tumors that do not fit into the categories previously described and for patients who cannot tolerate partial surgery. Cancer of the vocal cords, cancer of the glottis with fixation of the true cords, or persistent tumors of the larynx after attempts with other treatment modalities are handled with a total laryngectomy.[126] This procedure removes the entire larynx and thus the normal speaking voice of the patient.

*Radical neck dissection* is used when there is metastasis to the cervical lymph nodes and structures of the neck. It involves surgical removal of involved structures and is discussed in more detail later in this chapter.

Nursing intervention beginning in the *preoperative period* is essential for all patients requiring surgical procedures for cancer of the larynx. Preoperative teaching and support require skill in the physical and psychological aspects of nursing care. Both the patient and the family members should be included in the teaching sessions, which will require reinforcement throughout the presurgical period.

The *physical aspects of the preoperative teaching* should include a detailed discussion of changes and procedures that will occur before and after surgery. Fear of the unknown continues to be the leading cause of anxiety, and it is a nursing responsibility to attempt to alleviate it.

*Oral hygiene* is an area of concern prior to surgery. The patient should be instructed in the use of hydrogen peroxide and water mouth washes frequently during hospitalization. Carious teeth should be removed prior to surgery, as the oral cavity is an area of contamination in the postoperative stage of care. It is important to have the mouth as clean as possible to prevent postoperative problems.

Detailed explanations are given regarding the change in the patient's airway. Diagrams are useful in showing the patient the alterations that are made during surgery. It will be important to distinguish between a temporary and permanent tracheotomy at this point. If the surgical procedure anticipated is a supraglottic laryngectomy or a hemilaryngectomy, a *tracheotomy tube* will be used temporarily to prevent respiratory distress due to edema in the immediate postoperative stage. The tracheotomy is an incision made into the trachea at a level below the vocal cords. The vocal cords in these two procedures are not removed, so the patient will have a near-normal speaking voice after surgery. While the tube is in place, the patient will require the same care as described later for a total laryngectomy. Communication by talking will not be possible until the edema has subsided and the tube is removed. While the tracheotomy tube is in place, inhaled and exhaled air bypasses the vocal cords, preventing vibration of the cords to produce speech. Later in the postoperative stage it is possible to cover or plug the opening of the tracheotomy tube to permit the patient to speak.

The teaching for a total laryngectomy patient must describe a permanent alteration of the airway. The total larynx is removed and the trachea is sutured to the neck, creating a permanent tracheostoma. The vocal cords are absent following this procedure, and the normal method of speech production is gone.

For all patients with a tracheotomy, it is imperative for the nurse to explain methods of communication following surgery. One of the biggest fears expressed by patients is that of not being able to tell anyone what they need after surgery. If this is discussed fully in advance, the patient can adjust to the change. Communication in the immediate postoperative period will be by writing. The use of a magic slate has been found the best mechanism for written communication with others. It obviates the need for reams of paper at the patient's bedside, as well as giving the privacy of being able to erase a message after it has been read. If the patient cannot write or has difficulty communicating in this manner, flash cards can be devised to indicate those things the patient may require in the immediate postoperative period. If flash cards will be used, it is essential to review them with the patient prior to the time they must be relied upon.

The postlaryngectomy patient has no connection between the nose, mouth, and trachea, while supraglottic and hemilaryngectomy patients continue to have this area intact. It is essential for the nurse to know the differences between total laryngectomy and partial laryngectomy in order to adequately teach the patient as well as provide nursing care following surgery.

Explanations of the procedures performed in the postoperative period must be given. It is beneficial to have a teaching tray designed for this phase of instruction. If the patient can see the equipment used, handle the equipment, and ask questions, understanding of what to expect will be greater. The patient must be forwarned of the presence of

tracheotomy tubes and the need to suction the area frequently after surgery to remove mucous secretions and prevent respiratory complications. Oxygen mist will be given by nebulization after surgery to maintain moisture content and prevent drying of the tracheal mucosa. It may be beneficial to refer to the surgical diagram in order to demonstrate how the nose is bypassed in breathing directly through the tracheotomy tube. The nose is the normal humidifier of inspired air, and this humidification is absent as long as the patient breathes through a tracheostoma.

The patient will be allowed nothing by mouth from the midnight preceding surgery through 7 days (plus or minus a few days) after surgery. Since it is important to keep the surgical area as free of contamination and pressure as possible, the nurse should instruct the patient not to swallow and explain the presence of a nasogastric tube for nourishment. The nasogastric tube is inserted, following the surgical procedure, in a manner that avoids trauma to the suture line. Intravenous therapy will be maintained for 24 to 48 hours postoperatively or until bowel sounds are heard.

Dressings and neck drainage tubes will be used postoperatively, especially if a radical neck dissection is performed. The presence of the dressings will result in a flexed position of the head and some discomfort. The neck drains will be attached to a source of negative pressure, such as a Hemovac or a wall suction tube.

A Foley catheter is usually inserted in the operating room prior to the long surgical procedure. It may be removed the first postoperative day, depending on the individual patient and the physician's preference.

Deep breathing and coughing are as important to the patient having laryngeal surgery as with any other major surgical procedure. These procedures are explained and practiced prior to the time they are required. Intermittent positive-pressure breathing treatments, ultrasonic nebulization, and chest physiotherapy are additional techniques that can be used to prevent postoperative pulmonary complications. Because of the typical pattern of heavy cigarette smoking leading to laryngeal carcinoma, one can expect some pulmonary dysfunction, and every measure should be taken to prevent further compromise of the situation.

Early ambulation is a primary objective in caring for a patient with head or neck cancer. The patient is usually allowed to sit on the side of the bed the night of surgery and allowed out of bed the first postoperative day. The patient should be aware of this procedure prior to surgery.

Depending on the extent of tumor involvement and the reconstruction anticipated by the surgeon, skin grafts or skin flaps may be used. Skin *grafts* are sections of tissue completely removed from their blood supply that can be used to line various surgical areas where diseased tissue has been removed. A *flap* is a segment of skin, subcutaneous tissue, and fascia raised to cover a defect. A flap maintains its original blood supply at the proximal portion of the segment. Flaps are raised from an area of good blood supply, such as the forehead, the nape of the neck, the chest, or the deltopectoral region. The distal end of the flap is inserted into the area of reconstruction. The flap maintains this position for two or three weeks or until adequate circulation is established at the area of insertion. At this time the flap is transected and the carrier portion is returned to its original site. If a skin graft or flap is anticipated, surgical soap scrubs to the area are instituted a few days prior to surgery.

*Psychological preparation* of the patient is an integral part of all preoperative teaching. It is separated here for convenience and clarity but is integrated throughout the entire instruction phase. The way the patient views the anticipated surgery and the alterations in body image must be investigated. The nurse should have established good rapport with the patient by this stage and can encourage verbalization of feelings. The fears expressed are as individual as each patient, but they usually center around fear of the disease itself, fear of undergoing the surgical procedure, and fear of mutilation and its effect on future interpersonal relationships.

One method of possibly alleviating some of the fear is having the patient talk to other patients who have had the same or a similar surgical procedure. Some patients find it beneficial to ask questions of someone who has already gone through the experience. A member of the local Lost Chord Club can be contacted to spend time with the patient to give the "inside story" of what it is like to have a laryngectomy. This area is still controversial and depends on the patient's as well as the attending physician's views.

Fear of the disease itself is dealt with on an individual basis. To many people, the word "cancer" is synonymous with death. It is a nursing responsibility to help overcome this misconception, but until it is overcome, it must be managed with each patient. The nurse must instill hope without presenting unrealistic expectations that will not be achieved. Investigation of the patient's previous exposure to cancer patients may aid the nurse in uncovering the underlying fear. Past experiences, if negative, can leave a lasting impression.

Fear of having surgery can best be managed by a team effort. Assistance in the preoperative teaching by operating-room and recovery-room personnel can give the patient some awareness of what to expect after leaving the familiar area of the nursing unit. Obtaining the help of personnel from other areas to which the patient will be exposed will also provide an opportunity to meet those health-care workers who will be providing care off the patient unit. A familiar face in a strange place will help relieve some of the anxiety of the situation.

Donovan and Pierce describe *body image* as "the sum total of the feelings and perceptions an individual has about his body."[127] The patient's response to alterations in body image will depend largely on the degree to which the sense of security is based on the integrity of a particular body part, as well as the effect of its loss on patterns of daily living.[128] Changes in the body image of patients with cancer of the head and neck cannot be denied. This area is the only body part usually exposed in day-to-day contact. The face is the portion of the body most closely identified with the personal entity one calls "self." Nursing intervention lies primarily in helping the patient cope with the changes rather than preventing them from happening. The nurse can offer support by emphasizing the patient's strengths. Mobilizing family resources in helping the patient deal with the anticipated loss and an attitude of acceptance by staff members and family will assist in resolving some of the anxiety. It is important to stress that the patient's worth and acceptability to those significant others does not rely solely on physical attributes.[129] Many patients do not express anxiety in the area of body-image alterations until the postoperative period. They are more concerned about eliminating the cancerous growth, and living, than with how they will look. Whether the subject is encountered before or after surgery, the nurse must exhibit an accepting and understanding attitude in order to help the patient express and resolve feelings.

The surgical procedure and anesthesia recovery time are usually long, especially for the family members awaiting the patient's return. This time should be spent with the family, keeping them current on the activities in the operating room. To avoid unnecessary anxiety about the long wait, they should be made aware of the long duration of the surgical procedure. Reinforcement may also be required in preparation for the patient's physical appearance after surgery.

While the patient is in surgery, the nurse begins preparing the postoperative room. If the patient returns to the original unit rather than to a special head-and-neck unit or intensive-care area, he or she should be placed in a room near the nurses' station. If an intercom call system is used, the area over the patient's door should be marked to indicate the loss of speech.

Attention is focused on *maintaining a patent airway* in the immediate postoperative period. The patient may return with a tracheotomy tube made of either plastic or metal. Most patients with a temporary tracheotomy tube will have a cuffed tube during the first few days after surgery (Fig. 6-18). Cuffed tubes are used to prevent aspiration of blood, food, and secretions and for assisted or controlled ventilation. By inflating the cuff around the tube, substances that may be aspirated into the lungs are kept at the level above the cuff, preventing entrance into the trachea. The use of a cuff also provides a seal between the tracheotomy tube and the trachea which produces a closed system, preventing air escape around the tube. This closed system is essential with any type of ventilatory assistance, as air tends to take the path of least resistance, which would be back out around the tube instead of into the lungs.

The routine procedures necessary to care for the patient with a cuffed tracheotomy tube involve *inflating and deflating the cuff.* The cuff must be deflated for 5 minutes every hour to prevent damage to the tracheal mucosa, as the pressure applied by the cuff decreases the circulation to the area and can result in tracheal ischemia or necrosis. Prior to cuff deflation, the tube and oropharynx should be suctioned to prevent aspiration of any secretions during the procedure.[130] While the cuff is being deflated, further suctioning should be done or the patient should be instructed to cough in order to expel any material that may have pooled in the area above the cuff. The cuff should be deflated during exhalation, again to prevent aspiration of any secretions. If the patient has a tendency to aspirate, the nurse should remain at the bedside until inflation is completed. The tracheotomy-tube cuff is inflated during inspiration with a specified amount of air, the amount depending on the cuff and tube size as well as the size of the patient's trachea. Only the minimum amount of air needed to seal the area round the trachea should be injected. This point is

reached if no air is felt leaking around the area of the tube or mouth. The amount of air needed to inflate the cuff should be noted in the patient-care plan, and any change in this amount should be documented in the chart. After the initial aspiration-danger period is over and ventilatory assistance is intermittent, the cuff remains deflated until needed. This need arises if the patient receives intermittent positive-pressure breathing treatments and during feedings by nasogastric tube. The cuff should be inflated at these times and remain inflated for 20 minutes after the procedure.

*Suctioning* the patient with a tracheotomy tube is an important procedure following surgery to keep the airway free of secretions. The frequency of the procedure depends on the patient and can range from every 15 minutes to every few hours. It is a nursing responsibility to assess the patient's condition to determine the need to suction. The suctioning procedure should be performed under aseptic conditions, in order to limit the introduction of microorganisms into the tracheobronchial tree. The equipment needed for this procedure is a source of negative pressure, the suction kit containing a sterile basin, a sterile suction catheter, sterile glove, and sterile saline or water. Explanations of suctioning as they were initially discussed in the preoperative teaching are reinforced. The technique can be outlined as follows:

1   Evaluate breath sounds to assess the need for suctioning.

2   Open suction container.

3   Apply sterile glove to one hand. This hand will handle all sterile equipment and guide the catheter into the lungs.

4   Attach catheter to source of negative pressure.

5   Fill basin with sterile water or saline.

6   Moisten catheter with water or saline and check patency of equipment by applying suction.

7   Insert catheter into tracheotomy tube, *without* suction, 4 to 5 inches or until resistance is felt. At this point, withdraw the catheter slightly, as resistance may indicate that the catheter is resting at the carina.

8   Apply suction and withdraw the catheter in a rotating manner.

9   Suction no longer than 10 to 15 seconds, as this is the patient's only airway and the catheter is causing obstruction.

10 Rinse catheter and reinsert until the airway sounds clear.

It must be remembered that during the suctioning procedure one is removing not only excess secretions but also oxygen that is vital to the patient. Pre- and postoxygenation have been recommended to prevent hypoxia from the procedure. If the patient has been hyperoxygenated with high concentrations of oxygen for 1 minute prior to suctioning, the fall in arterial $pO_2$ may not reach hypoxic levels.[131] Following the procedure, the nurse should document the patient's tolerance of the procedure as well as the amount and appearance of the aspirate.

The inner cannula of the tracheotomy tube is cleaned, using clean or aseptic technique, after suctioning as well as at other times as needed throughout the day. The author recommends aseptic technique when it is done as a nursing procedure and clean technique when it is being taught to the patient and family. In the aseptic technique, the tube is removed with a gloved hand and placed in a solution of sterile water and hydrogen peroxide to loosen the mucus. The cannula is then held with the gloved hand while a small tracheotomy brush is used to remove the collected secretions. The tube is next placed in a basin of sterile water for rinsing; the excess water is shaken from the tube and it is reinserted into the outer cannula. In the clean technique, the inner cannula is placed under running water while the accumulated secretions are brushed from the inside of the tube. It is rinsed under running water and reinserted as described above. Care should be taken to avoid contamination of the tube during this procedure, but strict asepsis is not required.

Humidification by oxygen nebulization is another aspect of the postoperative care of the patient. Supplementary humidification is required to prevent dryness and crusting of the tracheal mucosa. Continuous nebulization is usually ordered for the first 24 to 48 hours, after which it can be given several times during the day. If the patient is using a tracheotomy tube without an inner cannula, it is imperative to have continuous nebulization until the tube is changed. Without an inner cannula, any collection of mucous secretions will remain in the outer cannula, which cannot be removed for cleaning. This collection of mucus can result in partial or total obstruction of the airway.

Pressure dressings and neck drainage catheters may be present, depending on the surgical pro-

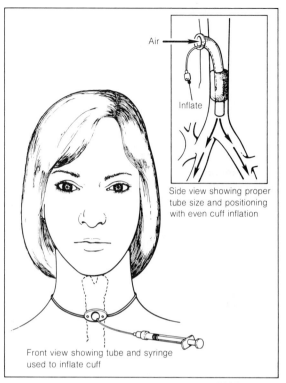

Side view showing proper tube size and positioning with even cuff inflation

Front view showing tube and syringe used to inflate cuff

**FIGURE 6-18**
Cuffed tracheotomy tube placement.

cedure and physician's preference; both are used to keep the neck flaps flat or to reduce the accumulation of blood or serum beneath the skin flaps. Maintaining the viability of flaps is of the utmost importance in postoperative patient care. If catheters are used, they are inserted into the wound at the completion of the operative procedure. When the patient returns to the room, the drains are attached to a source of negative pressure, either wall suction set at 100 to 120 mmHg or a Hemovac container. The drainage is measured on a daily basis; removal is indicated when the amount is minimal. Aspirating neck drains is one procedure recommended to mobilize the secretions that tend to accumulate in the small catheters. The catheters are clamped about 3 inches from the point of insertion with rubber-tipped hemostats. Using strict aseptic technique, the catheters are removed from the connector and cleaned. A size-18 angiocatheter is inserted into the end of the drain and the hemostat is removed. The drain is aspirated and is reclamped until the procedure is repeated on the second one. The drains are reattached to the source of negative pressure, and the hemostats are then removed. This procedure will prevent clotting of blood or serum in the catheter, which will eventually obstruct the drainage.

*Nutrition* in the postoperative time can be a challenge to health-team members. Intravenous therapy is maintained for 24 to 48 hours or until bowel sounds return. Initially, the nasogastric tube is connected to intermittent suction to prevent vomiting. Once the patient can tolerate fluids, they are introduced by tube. Tube feedings progress from clear liquids to high-calorie, high-protein liquids as soon as possible. Specially prepared diets can also be used, depending on the individual patient's nutritional status. Supplemental high-calorie feedings are frequently recommended. The nurse begins teaching the procedure used in the feedings as soon as the patient is able to perform the activity. This is usually the first step in returning the patient to independence. Accurate intake and output measurements are recorded until the nutritional status of the patient stabilizes.

*Care of the wound* begins with astute observation of the incisional area, with special attention devoted to color and temperature of skin flaps to assure viability. Surgical incisions should be cleansed several times a day with hydrogen peroxide to remove accumulated secretions. Antibiotic ointment is then applied. Antibiotic ointment will aid healing without superficial infection and keep the incision line soft. Dressings should be specifically ordered by the surgeon, as different types of incision may require different types of dressing. Care must be taken when applying any dressing to a patient who has had regional-flap reconstruction, to avoid applying pressure to the flap with resulting compromise of circulation.

Graft donor sites also require special attention in the postoperative period. Most donor sites are covered with surgical silk and an outer dressing of stretch bandage. The outer dressing is removed the first postoperative day and the inner silk dressing is exposed to the air. Once the outer protective dressing is removed, the donor site should be protected from pressure of clothing or bed linens by cutting away the clothing and using a bed cradle.

A few days of exposure to the air will produce some dryness and healing of the donor site. A heat lamp can be used, with close supervision, to hasten this process. The silk is removed as it loosens. If it is not loosening after sufficient healing has occurred, the patient may soak the area in the bathtub to help remove the dressing. A proteolytic-enzyme ointment may also be ordered to help remove the crusted areas which delay the healing process.

Prevention of *pulmonary complications,* mentioned in the preoperative teaching sessions, cannot be overemphasized. Early ambulation, in conjunction with deep-breathing and coughing exercises planned specifically for each patient, is usually sufficient to prevent the common pulmonary problems that may occur in a patient with near-normal lung function. In patients with an already compromised pulmonary reserve, more intense pulmonary programs should be planned. Intermittent positive-pressure breathing treatments, ultrasonic nebulization, and chest physiotherapy followed by good coughing technique or deep tracheal suctioning can further reduce the risk of postoperative difficulties.

*Pain* in the postoperative period tends to be minimal compared to that experienced prior to surgery. Severing of nerve fibers during the operative procedure results in a relatively low level of pain afterward. Most patients complain more of discomfort from skin-graft donor sites and from positioning than from the operative site.

*Adjuvant chemotherapy and immunotherapy* Areas of recent study in the treatment of head and neck carcinoma are adjuvant chemotherapy and immunotherapy. The Eastern Cooperative Oncology Group recently activated a study to determine whether the use of immunotherapy will prolong the tumor-free interval in patients with head and neck cancer after maximum cell destruction by surgery or radiation plus chemotherapy. Skin testing of patients with known head and neck tumors is being carried out to determine the degree of immune response. The goal of immune therapy is to improve host recognition of tumor-cell antigens in order to destroy them. Other objectives of this study concern the use of either adjuvant methotrexate therapy or *Corynebacterium parvum* alone after primary treatment and the correlation of the therapeutic effect of treatment with changes in the patient's immunologic response.[132] The study data are not yet available.

**Fourth-level nursing care** After the acute phase of postoperative care, the nurse focuses attention on restoration of the patient's independence and preparation for discharge. After the first few days of more intensive care, the patient begins performing the activities of daily living with slight supervision.

Teaching the patient the correct procedure for administering nasogastric tube feedings is usually the first step toward independence. The nurse continues to supervise the procedure, but the main responsibility lies with the patient. Once adequate healing has occurred and oral feeding has been instituted, the nurse's major role is to provide support to the patient. Patients with a total laryngectomy seldom have any difficulty swallowing unless a fistula has developed. If this occurs, the nasogastric tube is reinserted until the area heals. Patients who have had a supraglottic laryngectomy will usually require more time to relearn the swallowing process. The supraglottic laryngectomy procedure removes the epiglottis, which is the anatomic area that normally prevents aspiration when swallowing. Following this procedure the patient must develop a technique that will permit the food to enter the esophagus rather than the trachea. Patients will usually devise their own methods, which range from different eating positions to throwing the head back in order to have the food enter the esophagus. Closure of the glottis by producing a Valsalva maneuver will prevent aspiration, with the patient coughing to expel the substances collected by the vocal cords. The majority of patients tolerate pureed or soft foods with a thicker consistency better than liquids. Most patients can develop the ability to swallow and maintain a normal eating pattern if they are well motivated and have good pulmonary function.

Care of the tracheotomy tube is the second thing taught to the patient. The nurse performs the routine tracheotomy care until the pressure dressing is removed and the patient is able to learn the procedure. The patient is initially taught how to remove and clean the inner cannula a few days after surgery. A mirror must be used to enable the patient to see how and where to place the tube. At this time, tracheotomy care is performed using clean technique. The inner cannula is rinsed under running water, as previously described, using a brush to mobilize secretions. Most patients master this procedure easily and assume the responsibility of cleaning the cannula several times a day. Nursing supervision must continue to ensure proper technique.

Suctioning the tracheotomy tube is a patient procedure in some institutions. It is the author's feeling that if suctioning is required in the intermediate postoperative phase, it is due to potential or present pulmonary complications, and the nurse should therefore continue to perform the procedure. Later in the hospitalization and at home, the suctioning procedure can be the responsibility of the patient and family.

Psychological support of the patient concerns the patient's feelings about surgery and about returning to normal activities. Most patients appear to accept the treatment with little difficulty until the third or fourth postoperative day. At this time the patient begins to realize the effects of surgery and becomes depressed. The health team should spend time with the patient to permit expression of any concerns. The nurse must be aware of the patient's method of communication and plan to spend the time it takes to express oneself in writing. The fears and concerns may be in the areas of communication, body image, acceptance, return to normal activities, and many more. Each one must be handled individually, utilizing the resources of all members of the health-care team. The patient should be reassured and progress explained to help alleviate concerns in the postoperative period. Family involvement is also essential. The family must be an integral part of all phases of care of the head and neck cancer patient. They must be prepared for receiving the patient back into the home situation.

**D**ischarge Teaching   Discharge teaching begins when the patient is first admitted to the hospital. All efforts are directed toward preparing the patient to return to a life of acceptable quality. Teaching continues until the patient masters any procedures.

The total-laryngectomy patient is taught complete care of the tracheostoma. Changing the entire tracheostomy tube is not a difficult procedure once cleaning of the inner cannula has been mastered. The pieces of bias tape that hold the tube in place are cut and the entire tube is removed. The area around the stoma is cleansed with soap and water, and ointment is applied if the area appears irritated. The obturator or guide is inserted into the outer cannula and a thin layer of water-soluble jelly is applied to the outside of the cannula and obturator. Once the tube is in the neck, the guide is removed, as it obstructs the outer-cannula opening. The tapes are tied at the back of the neck to hold the tube in place. Insertion of two fingers under the tapes when tied will indicate when the tube is tight yet comfortable to the patient. The used tube is disassembled and placed in hydrogen peroxide for several minutes to loosen secretions. The same procedure used to clean the inner cannula is followed to finish cleaning the tube. It is placed under running water, and a brush, similar to the percolator brush used to clean a coffee-pot spout, is used to remove the loosened mucus. Once the tube is cleaned, it should be placed in a pan of water and boiled for 20 minutes to ensure sterility. It may then be wrapped in a freshly ironed handkerchief and stored until needed for the next daily change. The patient will usually wear a tube for a few months after surgery, but the exact length of time will depend on the individual surgeon's preference and the size of the tracheostoma.

The teaching plan should include content related to avoiding the introduction of water into the stoma. Showers are permitted if the water stream is aimed low on the trunk or if a special shield is used to protect the area. A humidifier at the bedside is important to prevent drying and crusting with resultant bleeding of the tracheal mucosa. If drying occurs and the airway becomes obstructed, the patient may be taught to instill a few drops of normal saline solution into the stoma to loosen the crust and promote coughing. In a patient with a tracheotomy tube, the tube should be removed prior to instilling the saline, as the crusted mucus may be too large to be coughed through the lumen of the tube. Crusting of the mucosa is seen more in the winter season with the decreased humidity. The patient should be aware of this to prevent anxiety.

The patient should be taught to prevent the entrance of dust and foreign bodies into the tracheostoma by wearing a crocheted bib or a moistened 4x4 gauze sponge around the neck. The moistened gauze will also aid in humidifying the air breathed. Ways to avoid drawing attention to the stoma should also be demonstrated. Women can wear scarves or beads, and men can continue to dress as before but avoiding the use of constricting necklines.

The patient who has had a supraglottic laryngectomy or a hemilaryngectomy will usually have the tracheotomy tube removed prior to discharge. The area is cleansed and a small dressing is taped over the stoma to promote healing. The incisional area is generally healed by discharge or shortly afterward, so the discharge teaching centering around care of the stoma is eliminated for these patients.

Routine follow-up visits to the physician must be encouraged. The physician can give the support required by the patient in the transition stage from hospital to home, as well as evaluate the healing process and check for recurrence and second primary-tumor sites. Return visits to the physician should be an ongoing process once the initial diagnosis has been made.

Referral patterns set up early during hospitalization are continued through discharge. The one additional referral that is important is to the Visiting Nurse Association. Patients who need more supervision or who may require dressing changes at home will benefit from having a nurse available in the home. Special detailed instructions should be written. If care other than routine is necessary, the VNA nurse may visit the patient in the hospital and observe the care that will have to be continued in the home. This referral should be made as early as possible to ensure availability of the service at discharge.

The social service department has been mentioned previously as an important early referral. It plays a vital role in assessing the patient and family situation, which is important at discharge. The social worker can assist the rest of the health team in evaluating the home situation and preparing the patient and family for the initial transition phase. If disposition of the patient after hospitalization appears to be a problem, the social worker can begin to help the team make arrangements early, in order to prevent a delay when the patient is discharged and to help provide needed follow-up care.

*Speech therapy* will be started after sufficient healing has occurred. The time period after surgery is individual, but the patient is informed of the opportunity to learn a new method of communication. Having made an initial speech evaluation in the preoperative period, the speech therapist is able to recommend the appropriate rehabilitation when needed. Esophageal speech is one possible method of speaking after a total laryngectomy. Air is trapped in the esophagus and forced back into the mouth. The pulsating air, in combination with the other structures of the mouth, permits the patient to form words. This method of speaking can be taught by a speech therapist or by another laryngectomy patient who has mastered the procedure. An electronic larynx can also be used by the laryngectomee. This vibrating device produces a mechanical voice and can be used by the patient prior to developing esophageal speech or for those patients unable to master the alternate method.

Returning the patient to employment, retirement, or home activities is one major goal of the health team working with the patient with cancer of the head and neck. This objective requires a multidisciplinary team approach with patient and family participation. If the patient's occupation involves exposure to pollution, it may be necessary to recommend a vocational change. The Bureau of Vocational Rehabilitation is a good resource to help the health team deal with these changes. Encouragement by the family as well as the health team may be the essential ingredient in returning the patient to the quality of life experienced in the premorbid period.

## Tumors of the Oral Cavity

The oral cavity includes the lip, anterior portion of the tongue, floor of the mouth, buccal mucosa, gingiva, and hard palate. Since carcinoma of the lip and tongue are the most frequent cancers seen in this area, these two types of head and neck cancer are discussed here.

**Tumors of the lip** Carcinoma of the lower lip is the most frequent tumor found in the anatomic structure known as the oral cavity, constituting approximately 15 percent of head and neck tumors.[133] Lip cancer is primarily epidermoid in nature, with only a small percentage of the tumors being of the basal-cell, minor-salivary-gland, or melanoma variety. Etiologic factors associated with cancer of the lip include chronic irritation, excessive exposure to actinic radiation, and syphilis.[134] Patients presenting with early carcinoma of the lip will usually complain of a painless ulcer that does not heal. Larger, more advanced lesions may demonstrate invasion of the underlying structures, including the skin. Metastasis to the regional lymph nodes occurs late in the disease process, with the spread going first to the submental and facial nodes and terminating in the jugular chain.

Treatment for early carcinoma of the lip can be either surgery or radiation therapy, with equally successful cure rates. Depending on the size of the lesion, surgical intervention is aimed at wide excision of the tumor with either a primary closure or a small rotational flap to cover the defect. Nursing intervention for patients with primary lesions of the lip is in prevention and early detection. The nurse is in a unique position to be influential in this first level of care. Treatment of patients with early tumors in this area results in little cosmetic deformity and minor changes in the life-style. This can be determined only by a thorough nursing assessment, as described earlier.

**Tumors of the tongue** Embryologically the tongue is a pharyngeal derivative, with the anterior portion being ectodermal and the base entodermal, which accounts for the difference in tumors arising from these two sites.[135] The anterior two-thirds of the tongue, the oral or mobile portion, is the most frequent site of a primary tumor of this organ. Other structures of the oral cavity may become involved through direct extension of the primary lesion, depending on its exact location. Factors predisposing to this malignancy include chronic use of tobacco and alcohol, poor oral hygiene, long-term dental trauma, syphilis, and Plummer-Vinson syndrome.

Well-differentiated *squamous-cell carcinoma* is the most frequent pathologic diagnosis of tumors of the tongue. They present as either exophytic masses or infiltrative tumors, with the infiltrative type demonstrating a more rapid growth and a greater tendency for recurrence and metastasis (Fig. 6-19).[136]

Patients with carcinoma of the tongue tend to

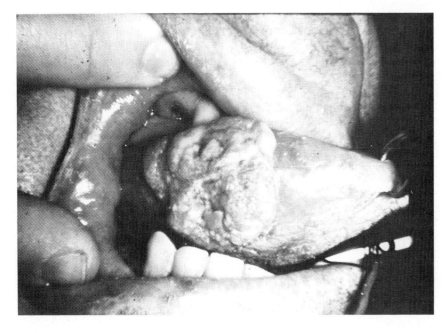

**FIGURE 6-19**
Squamous-cell carcinoma of lateral aspect of tongue.

seek medical attention late in the course of the disease. This may be due to fear or it may be caused by failure to have routine medical or dental evaluations. The earliest symptoms of cancer of the tongue are leukoplakia and a painless ulcer that fails to heal. *Leukoplakia,* a term that means "white patch," is produced by hyperkeratosis of the lining epithelium of the oral cavity (Color Plate 6-1). Leukoplakia has been classified as a premalignant change in the mucosa and cannot usually be differentiated from areas undergoing malignant alteration without investigation of anaplastic microscopic changes in the epithelium.[137] Other symptoms the patient may demonstrate are found in more advanced situations and include local or radiating pain, otalgia, dysphagia, weight loss, and neck masses.

Tumors affecting the tongue metastasize to the floor of the mouth or to the muscles affecting the tongue and their insertions in the hyoid bone, the mandible, or the styloid process.[138] Regional lymph-node metastasis is found relatively early in the disease, with the collecting channels terminating in the submental, submaxillary, and jugulodigastric nodes.[139]

Staging of tumors of the oral cavity is similar to that described for laryngeal carcinoma. The TNM classification describes the primary tumor size and infiltrative characteristics, the evidence of regional lymph-node involvement, and distant metastasis. Treatment modalities are dependent on the classification of the tumor by the primary physician.

Tumors of the tongue are diagnosed initially by visualization and palpation. Early exophytic tumors can be easily recognized by a thorough oral examination, but infiltrative tumors of the oral portion of the tongue and more importantly the base of the tongue cannot be seen and therefore must be palpated to determine their presence and extent. As with tumors affecting the larynx, a palpable lymph node requires thorough investigation of the head and neck to determine the site of the primary lesion.

The treatment modality suggested to the patient will depend on the extent of the tumor. As with other head and neck tumors, early lesions can be treated effectively with either surgical excision or radiation therapy. Radiation can be administered by external beam or by radiation implants. Radiation therapy may be the curative treatment for small lesions or it may be used in combination with surgery for larger tumors. Regardless of the reason for treatment by radiation, the patient must be prepared for the therapy. Adequate nutrition, alleviation of side effects, and thorough explanations of the procedure are essential nursing measures. Patients presenting with tumors of the tongue should be thoroughly evaluated in relation to their nutritional status. A painful, immobile tongue can drastically reduce the oral intake prior to the time the patient seeks medical attention. Supplemental nutritional therapy may require the insertion of a nasogastric tube or parenteral hyperalimentation. These patients require an accurate record of intake and output as well as frequent blood-chemistry evaluations. Explanations of the side effects as well as the procedure are imperative to reduce anxiety.

Surgical intervention requires the same initial evaluation of the patient as described for laryngeal tumors. The exact procedure anticipated will depend on the extent of the tumor. Local wide excision with minimum functional or cosmetic deformity is the treatment for small localized lesions. Unfortunately, few patients present with tumors that can be treated in this manner. The patients discussed in the remainder of this section are those who require more extensive surgery for removal of the cancer.

*Partial glossectomy* and *total glossectomy,* with or without partial removal of the mandible and *radical neck dissection,* are the most widely accepted treatments for patients with a large carcinoma of the tongue. These patients tend to respond less favorably to radiation therapy because of the condition of the mucous membrane of the oral cavity from chronic use of tobacco and alcohol plus poor nutritional status.[140]

Prior to surgical intervention, the patient must be thoroughly evaluated. In addition to the tumor size and nutritional status already discussed, the degree of pulmonary function must be investigated. If a total glossectomy is anticipated, the patient will be faced with difficulty in swallowing. Many surgeons advocate a total laryngectomy with the glossectomy, while others feel that this additional procedure is unnecessary if the pulmonary function is adequate to produce a good cough in order to prevent aspiration. Myers, in a recent study, stated that total glossectomy without laryngectomy is most useful in treating cancers that infiltrate and destroy the oral portion of the tongue, if the patient has good pulmonary reserve.[141]

Another area in need of evaluation is the patient's psychological status. Following the surgical procedure, the remainder of the rehabilitation is dependent on the patient. The patient must believe that the handicaps associated with removal of the tongue can be overcome.

The exact surgical procedure performed varies.

In general, extraoral incisions are made in order to have full access to the tumor. Patients requiring partial removal of the tongue, with or without partial removal of the mandible and regional lymph nodes, face minor adjustments in the postoperative and rehabilitative period. The area is usually reconstructed at the time of the primary surgery and generally requires a skin graft or flap to cover the area. With part of the tongue still remaining, the patient can regain the ability to swallow and talk with minimal effort.

Tumors that cannot be adequately resected with partial glossectomy require total removal of the tongue. If the entire tongue is involved, one generally finds additional involvement of the floor of the mouth, part of the mandible, and regional lymph nodes in the neck. These patients present more of a challenge to the health-care team in terms of reconstruction and rehabilitation. Initially the goal of the patient is to be pain-free and tumor-free. Following surgery, this goal changes to one of returning to a normal life. The first goal can be accomplished only by the surgical team, while the second requires a multidisciplinary team effort centering around the individual patient.

Nursing intervention involved in providing care to patients with cancer of the tongue is essential. An initial nursing assessment is invaluable. The nurse can, at this time, assess not only the patient's physical status but also the psychological status of the patient and family. Thorough explanations provided by the physician must be reemphasized throughout the pre- and postoperative periods of hospitalization. A return to an acceptable, pain-free quality of life is the primary objective in this form of treatment, but the patient must be aware early in the discussion of therapy that rehabilitation is largely dependent on a desire to overcome any disability, with frustration in the rate of improvement being one of the most common areas of discouragement. The patient must be prepared for a long rehabilitation period, both in the hospital and following discharge. It has been the author's experience and the experience cited by Myers that if the patient has the power to continue to overcome periods of frustration, swallowing, speaking, and a reasonably good quality of life can be achieved.[142]

Preoperative preparation of the patient requires measures similar to those described for the patient presenting for laryngeal surgery. Placement of a temporary tracheotomy tube for potential airway difficulties, dressings, neck drainage catheters, and pulmonary hygiene are the same as with other head and neck cancer patients.

Preoperative consultations with the social service department, speech pathology department, and maxillofacial prosthetics department are also essential. The maxillofacial referral is especially important if reconstruction is a goal at the time of surgery. If part of the mandible will be removed in conjunction with the tongue, preoperative impressions must be made in order to design a mandibular replacement.

The initial *postoperative concerns* are maintaining a patent airway and observation of the surgical area. When sufficient healing has occurred, the nursing responsibility is concerned with rehabilitation of the patient's *swallowing* and *communication* abilities. It is essential for the nurse to understand normal swallowing mechanisms in order to realize the changes that surgical intervention produces in this vital function.

Swallowing is divided into three main phases: the voluntary oral phase, the involuntary pharyngeal stage and the esophageal stage. The *oral-hold phase* permits one to hold the food in the mouth and is followed by raising the soft palate to enlarge the size of the oral cavity and seal off the nasopharynx. The tongue then produces a stripping wave-like motion to move the bolus of food back toward the pharynx.[143]

For patients with a total glossectomy, this oral phase of swallowing is eliminated. As soon as food enters the mouth, it begins its movement toward the pharynx. Normally, as food enters the *pharynx,* there is closure of the epiglottis to prevent aspiration of the food into the larynx. Following surgery, the muscles that permit this action are detached, which prevents the epiglottis from closing. One method of retraining for swallowing involves teaching patients to take small amounts of liquid in a small medicine glass. The liquid is placed in the mouth, the head tilted backward, and a gulping mechanism is used to swallow. Later, soft foods or blenderized diets are introduced, using the mechanism previously described, then using a spoon. Many patients devise their own methods of swallowing, while others utilize either a syringe or a nasogastric tube to provide supplemental nutrition until they are able to swallow a nutritionally suitable diet. The swallowing technique will be learned by patients who are well motivated and who receive maximum support and encouragement from the family, surgeon, and nursing staff.

Restoring the power of communication is another vital area of rehabilitation facing the patient after total glossectomy. After a thorough preoperative speech evaluation, the speech patholo-gist can begin working with the patient's remaining strengths. Although some sounds are impossible to make, most attempts at verbal communication are intelligible following total glossectomy.

### Regional Lymph-node Metastasis

Regional lymph-node metastasis and *radical neck dissection* are two terms that have been used fre-quently in discussing tumors of the head and neck. The lymphatic system consists of lymph capillaries, vessels, ducts, and nodes. Lymph *nodes* are small oval bodies of lymphatic tissue found at intervals along lymphatic vessels, which have as one func-tion the filtering of lymphatic fluid passing through them. One important feature of the lymphatic sys-tem is its relationship to tumor spread. Lymphatic drainage from primary tumor sites may carry with it small tumor emboli which implant and grow in the regional lymph nodes. As these tumor emboli grow, they develop the cellular structure and character-istics of the mother cell. The positive feature of this system within the head and neck area is the close proximity of the cervical lymph nodes, which may produce an initial check system against early dis-tant metastasis.

Treatment of regional lymph-node metastasis in the head and neck can be by radiation therapy or surgical intervention by way of a radical neck dis-section. These treatments may be instituted with or without clinically palpable nodes, depending on the site of the primary lesion. Patients presenting with a primary tumor in an area of sparse lymphatics, such as the true vocal cords, will not usually require any treatment to the neck, while other locations (supra-glottic larynx or tongue) may necessitate prophy-lactic treatment because of the high incidence of regional metastasis associated with them.

Radiation therapy to the neck nodes and the necessary patient teaching are the same as pre-viously described. Radical neck dissection is the surgical treatment for patients with regional lymph-node involvement. The classic radical neck dissec-tion, known as *en bloc resection,* removes the afferent and efferent lymphatic channels from the lateral and anterior aspects of the neck. This opera-tive procedure also necessitates removal of the sternocleidomastoid muscle, the omhyoid muscle, the spinal accessory nerve, the internal and external jugular veins and their tributaries, the cervical cuta-neous plexus, and local subcutaneous tissue.[144] The essential transit system for the metastatic spread of cancer in this area is thus removed.

Nursing measures for patients following a radi-cal neck dissection employ many of the techniques included earlier in this section. A recent article by Ardis O'Dell reviewed the objectives for care of a patient with a radical neck dissection, grouping them in four main areas:

1 To keep the patient free of complications

2 To minimize pain and discomfort

3 To reduce fear and anxiety

4 To prepare the patient for post-hospitalization[145]

Maintaining the patient free of complications in-cludes care of the wound as discussed for patients with cancer of the larynx. The incisional area must be frequently observed for the condition of the flaps. Temperature and color are good indicators of adequate circulation to the area. Measurement of neck catheter drainage and observation of the con-sistency of the drainage will provide the nurse with information about what is happening under the flaps. An increase in the amount of bloody drainage may indicate formation of a hematoma, an increase in the amount of serous drainage may demonstrate the presence of a seroma, and an increase in drain-age of a milky, opaque fluid indicates the presence of a chylous fistula. A *chylous fistula* results from a leak in the thoracic duct which begins at the cis-terna chyli, the area where the lacteals of the small intestine inject their contribution to the lym-phatic system. An increase in chyle is usually noted following meals, as the fluid is increased during digestion and absorption of fat. The amount of drainage in all instances must be recorded to serve as an indicator for removal of the catheters. Scru-pulous care in the managing of dressings and cleansing of the wound are essential to prevent postoperative wound infections. Strict aseptic tech-niques must be practiced by every health-team member who has direct contact with the surgical site.

The head of the bed should be elevated to 45° following surgery to allay discomfort from the posi-tioning and the dressings, to decrease facial edema, to decrease bleeding, and to improve lymphatic and venous drainage. It must be remembered that both lymphatic and venous drainage systems are re-moved with this surgical procedure, and a certain degree of facial edema is anticipated in the early postoperative period until a collateral drainage sys-tem is developed.

Actual pain in the postoperative phase is not common. Medications should be available to the patient to relieve discomfort from positioning and dressings, but a mild analgesic is usually sufficient. Time spent with the patient to reinforce teaching and explain the progress will usually give more relief than a medication.

Limitations following discharge are related to dysfunction of the shoulder resulting from removal of the spinal accessory nerve. Many patients complain of weakness in the arm of the affected side, with resultant inability to lift the arm appreciably. Many physicians utilize the department of physical medicine and a physical therapist to evaluate the deformity and recommend an exercise routine, similar to those performed after radical mastectomy, to improve function. Cosmetic deformity following a radical neck dissection is related mainly to the change in the contour of the neck from the removal of the muscles. This problem with cosmesis may be overcome with clothing that conceals the defect.

### Tumors of the Maxillary Sinus

The maxillary sinus is the largest of the paranasal sinuses and is located in the maxilla. It is an air-filled cavity lined with mucous membrane continuous with that of the nasal cavity. Anatomically the medial wall or base of the sinus is related to the lateral wall of the nasal cavity, the apex extends into the zygomatic process, the anterior portion is the cheek, the posterolateral part is the infratemporal space, the roof of the antrum forms the floor of the orbit, and the inferior portion forms the alveolar process of the maxilla in the area of the molars.[146] Tumors of the maxillary sinus form about 3 percent of tumors of the head and neck, with predisposing factors being inconclusive at this time.[147] There is an increased incidence of squamous-cell carcinoma of the antrum in patients with chronic sinusitis, thought to be related to metaplasia of the respiratory epithelium lining the sinus cavity.[148] Presenting symptoms of the patient with an early cancer are usually vague and will vary according to the exact location of the primary tumor. Many patients and physicians diagnose chronic sinusitis, as the symptoms of local pain and drainage mimic those of sinusitis. For this reason, diagnosis is usually delayed until more definite symptoms resulting from tumor extension are demonstrated. Symptoms of maxillary-sinus carcinoma include epistaxis and nasal obstruction with medial extension, proptosis and diplopia from superior extension, paresthesias and anesthesias of the cheek and upper lip with infraorbital-nerve involvement, oral mass or loosening of the teeth with inferior

extension, and ulceration of the skin over the cheek with late anterior tumor masses. Other late symptoms include decreased hearing and otalgia as a result of invasion of the nasopharynx and trismus resulting from extension to the mandibular branch of the trigeminal nerve or pterygoid muscle.[149]

Tumors of the maxillary sinus are classified according to the TNM system, with an additional prognostic classification made by dividing the area with a line from the angle of the mandible to the inner canthus of the eye. This division, known as Ohngren's line, defines tumors of poor prognosis as those lying behind the line, because of the close proximity to the base of the skull.[150]

These tumors are best treated by combined radiotherapy and surgery. Preoperative radiation is usually the treatment of choice, because the increased oxygenation of a preoperative tumor provides a more radiosensitive site and decreases the size of the tumor, making it more easily resectable. The surgical procedure requires removal of the maxillary sinus, including part of the palate, plus any other structure involved with the tumor, such as the skin and orbit (Fig. 6-20).

Nursing intervention after initial assessment of the patient is the institution of early referral patterns. The maxillofacial consultation is of prime importance for patients with carcinoma of the maxillary sinus. Preoperative impressions are essential in order to develop a surgical splint and maxillary obturator. A split-thickness skin graft is used to line the maxillary cavity after tumor removal, with a bolus of packing inserted afterward. The surgical splint is applied to protect the surgical area and hold the bolus of packing in place. With the use of this splint, the patient can begin taking oral feedings a few days after surgery. Once the packing is removed, the first obturator can be used. This device resembles an upper denture with a built-up area constructed to fill the defect (Fig. 6-21). It is used to prevent food from entering the surgical defect and flowing through the nose. As edema subsides, the obturator is adjusted to fit as an upper denture, protecting the cavity and allowing normal eating and swallowing to occur (Fig. 6-22).

Oral hygiene is of prime importance following a maxillectomy. The skin graft lining the surgical defect must remain clean in order to heal. Oral-hygiene measures are carried out with a catheter and syringe or a Water Pik. A solution of hydrogen peroxide and water is introduced into the cavity several times a day, especially after meals, to ensure thorough cleansing. Removal of any crusted material is also essential to assure adequate healing of the underlying tissue.

Physical deformity of the patient following this procedure depends on the extent of the surgical procedure necessary to eradicate the tumor. Excision of the skin can result in a surgical defect if early attempts at reconstruction are not made. Regional or distant flaps can be utilized to cover the defect, or if this is not possible, an extraoral prosthetic device can be used. Surgical removal of the eye in addition to the maxillary sinus necessitates an ocular prosthesis. Following reconstruction, either by flaps or by prosthetic appliances, the patient is returned to a near-normal cosmetic state with freedom from pain and discomfort.

### Malignant Tumors of the Parotid Gland

Tumors of the parotid glands constitute a minor proportion of all cancers and only about 2 percent of those affecting the head and neck.[151] The pair of parotid glands are classified as major salivary glands and are anatomically surrounded by the masseter muscle, ramus of the mandible, and internal pterygoid muscle anteriorly, the mastoid process and sternocleidomastoid muscle posteriorly, and the external auditory meatus and temporomandibular joint superiorly.[152] The gland is made up of two lobes, a larger superficial lobe and a smaller deep lobe, with the facial nerve passing through the isthmus between these sections. Histologically, malignant tumors of the parotids tend to be of mixed-tumor or mucoepidermoid origin, with squamous-cell carcinomas and adenocarcinomas forming the remaining small percentage (Fig. 6-23).[153]

The patient with an early tumor of the parotid gland usually complains of a small mass which is firm and generally fixed in position. Benign and malignant tumors begin with the same symptoms, and accurate diagnosis is impossible without excision of the mass and pathologic examination of the specimen. Benign tumors of this area tend to be slower-growing and freely mobile, with minimal extension to the underlying structures. Malignant tumors, if untreated, may present as large masses, with facial weakness or paralysis and pain.

Preoperative preparation of the patient includes many of the areas previously discussed: nursing assessment, reclarification of the physician's instructions, and deep-breathing and coughing exercises. Complications of the surgery are rare, but temporary symptoms are frequently exhibited. Because of manipulation of the facial nerve during surgery and possible sacrificing of this structure, facial paralysis or a temporary facial weakness may be noted after surgery. The extent of this cannot be determined until after the surgery, but the patient and family must be aware of the possibility.

Following the operative procedure, the patient will return with a pressure dressing and possibly drainage catheters in place. These remain in place approximately 48 hours or until the drainage sub-

**FIGURE 6-20**
Palatal defect following maxillectomy.

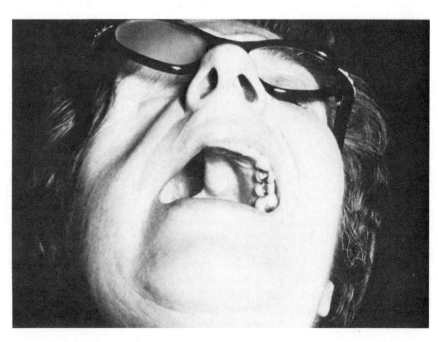

sides. Placing the patient in a semi-Fowler's position will alleviate some of the discomfort caused by the dressings and minimize facial edema. A liquid diet is ordered for the first few meals, especially if manipulation of the area has resulted in a degree of trismus. Observation of the patient is one of the main responsibilities of the nurse. The dressing must be examined frequently and the degree of drainage evaluated.

The nurse must routinely assess any facial weakness or change in the degree of weakness exhibited by the patient. This is best accomplished by instructing the patient to move those areas innervated by the facial nerve, e.g., wrinkle the forehead, show the teeth, purse the lips, smile, protrude the tongue. The patient's ability to perform these movements is documented in the chart.

If the patient demonstrates a facial weakness, nursing care is directed to preventing complications in the affected areas. The patient may exhibit ocular symptoms, with an inability to completely close the eye. If this is a problem, normal-saline eye drops are administered hourly to prevent drying of the cornea with resultant abrasions or infections. Taping the eyelid closed when the patient is sleeping will also prevent damage to the sensitive cornea. If the problem appears to be long-term, some physicians recommend a tarsorrhaphy to suture the eyelids closed.

Patients with facial paralysis may also complain of constant drooling of secretions from the

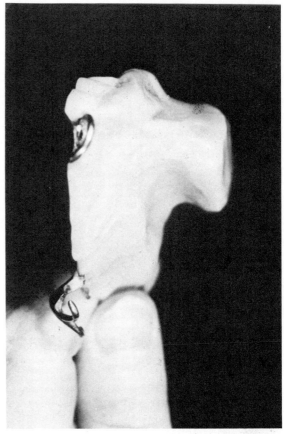

**FIGURE 6-21**
Permanent maxillary obturator.

**FIGURE 6-22**
Obturator occluding defect.

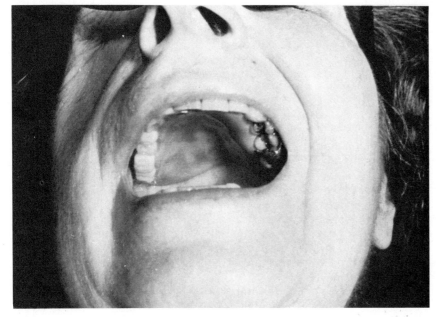

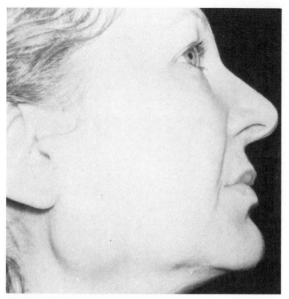

**FIGURE 6-23**
Malignant tumor of the parotid gland.

mouth on the affected side. A small piece of gauze can be placed in the mouth to prevent this irritating problem, but it must be replaced frequently. The nurse should instruct the patient, when eating, to place food in the unaffected side of the mouth to prevent drooling or lodging of food in the affected portion. Good oral hygiene and inspection of the oral cavity after meals provides the nurse with an opportunity to detect food that may remain and any irritation caused by eating, of which the patient may be unaware.

*Auriculotemporal syndrome,* also known as *Frey's syndrome* or *gustatory sweating,* may be a source of annoyance to the patient 6 to 12 months following a parotidectomy. This syndrome is related to abnormal reanastamosis of sympathetic and parasympathetic nerve fibers after injury to the auriculotemporal nerve.[154] The patient will notice a flushing of the face and sweating in the area above the incision while eating. This complication is not unusual or harmful but can be bothersome to the patient.

Care of the surgical wound is a nursing responsibility while the patient is hospitalized and an area of discharge teaching when the patient is prepared to return home. The area should be cleansed with hydrogen peroxide and water and antibiotic ointment applied three or four times a day. This procedure is usually taught to a family member, as it may be an awkward one for the patient to perform because of the anatomic location.

Return to normal daily activity is relatively rapid for most patients following a parotidectomy. After the posthospitalization recovery period, the patient should be capable of returning to the usual pattern of activity. One addition to normal routines will be monthly follow-up visits to the physician. The necessity of periodic examinations of the head and neck area must be reinforced, even if no problems are evident to the patient.

## NEOPLASMS OF THE SKIN

Skin cancer is the most common human cancer. It is estimated that 40 to 50 percent of all people who live to 65 will have at least one skin cancer in their lifetime. Cancers of the skin occur on exposed surfaces of the body 90 to 95 percent of the time, usually resulting in early, accurate diagnosis. Skin cancer has a cure rate of over 90 percent, except for malignant melanoma, which is discussed separately below.[155]

### Pathophysiology

The skin is the largest organ in the human body. It is divided into three main parts: the epidermis or epithelium, the dermis, and the subcutaneous tissue. The *epidermis* is further divided into four layers: the basal-cell layer, the prickle-cell layer, the granular-cell layer, and the cornified layer. The *dermis* is the connective-tissue layer of the skin that supports the epidermis and separates it from the cutaneous adipose tissue. Skin tumors usually spread locally by multiplication of their cells. Tumors may spread outward, leading to a vegetating growth with eventual destruction of the epidermis and ulceration; laterally, producing a plaquelike lesion; or downward, to produce a tumor. The more malignant tumors may spread in all three directions.

According to the American Cancer Society, risk is highest for farmers, sailors, and those in other outdoor occupations requiring frequent and protracted exposure to sun. Workers who deal with coal, tar, pitch, or creosote are also at risk, as are those with fair complexions who have excessive exposure to sun. Sunlight, xeroderma pigmentosum, prior irradiation, chronic exposure to chemicals, and scars of severe burns have been implicated as possible etiologic factors.

Skin lesions may be premalignant or may be squamous-cell or basal-cell carcinomas.

**Premalignant lesions** *Actinic keratosis* is a premalignant lesion of the surface epidermis caused by ultraviolet radiation (usually sunlight). It begins in an area containing dilated capillaries on which white or slightly pigmented scales gradually appear (Fig. 6-24). The lesions are usually discrete, and their scaliness varies from that which can be delineated only by touch to a consistency so hyperkeratotic that the lesions appear as cutaneous horns (Fig. 6-25).

Other premalignant lesions include arsenical keratoses, xeroderma pigmentosum, and radiation dermatitis. All premalignant lesions of the epidermis are precursors of squamous-cell carcinoma.

**Squamous-cell carcinoma** Squamous-cell carcinoma of the skin can remain fairly indolent or become rapidly progressive and fatal. Most squamous-cell carcinomas of the skin arise from a sun-damaged skin area or from a precancerous lesion. These tumors usually develop from suprabasal layers of the epidermis. They may grow slowly with little invasion and no metastasis or may spread rapidly, becoming deeply invasive, with early onset of distant metastasis (Figs. 6-26 and 6-27).

**Basal-cell carcinoma** Basal-cell carcinomas are epithelial tumors of the skin probably arising from primitive germ cells and often resembling skin appendages. They develop almost exclusively on hair-bearing skin; they are usually on the face, although some have been reported on other areas. They do not develop on mucous membranes (Figs. 6-28 and 6-29).

Basal-cell carcinomas present in four common forms: (1) nodular-ulcerative, (2) pigmented, (3) sclerosing, and (4) superficial. The *nodular-ulcerative type* is the most common and usually begins as a firm, waxy papule which enlarges slowly and may ulcerate. A crust forms over the ulceration and requires care to avoid dislodging it, which may bring on hemorrhage. The *pigmented* type is the same as the nodular-ulcerative except that it contains pigment. *Sclerosing basal-cell carcinomas* are less common and are difficult to see, as their appearance differs only slightly from normal skin, although they are palpable. *Superficial basal-cell carcinomas* appear most commonly on the trunk and have an overall appearance of patchy pigmentation. Basal-cell carcinomas rarely metastasize.

### Management

The primary goal in treating skin cancer is *cure.* Early treatment helps eradicate small tumors before extensive cosmetic repair is necessary.

*Curettage and electrodesiccation* or electro-

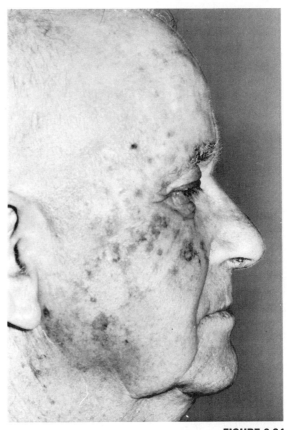

**FIGURE 6-24**
Actinic keratosis.

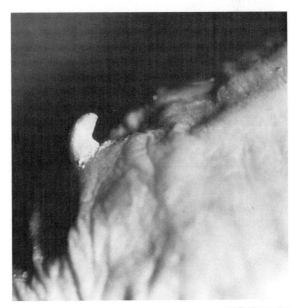

**FIGURE 6-25**
Cutaneous horn.

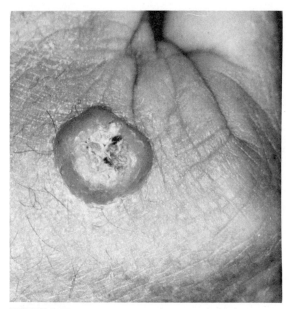

**FIGURE 6-26**
Squamous-cell carcinoma of the hand.

surgery is a combination of surgical removal and a physical modality. The area is cleansed and anesthetized. A curet is used to remove the bulk of the lesion, and this sample is submitted for pathologic examination. This is followed by vigorous curetting (cutting away) until the base of the lesion is reached and all the soft tumor tissue removed. After curettage, electrodesiccation is used to destroy any ab-

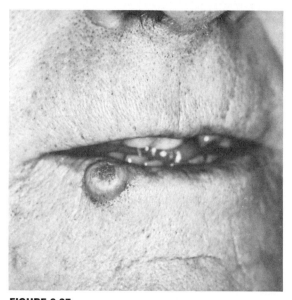

**FIGURE 6-27**
Squamous-cell carcinoma of the lip.

normal cells remaining at the base or sides of the operative site and to provide hemostasis—a modality whose effectiveness stems from the action of radiofrequency waves that render living tissue devitalized and amorphous. The procedure is usually repeated. This form of treatment is effective for tumors of less than 5 mm regardless of anatomic site; deep tumors should not be treated with this method.[156] Larger lesions (up to 4 cm) may be treated with electrosurgery, depending on the skill of the operator and the depth and penetration of the lesion.

*Excisional surgery* is often the treatment of choice. For small lesions, less than 2 cm, complete excision of the lesion together with a margin of 0.5 to 1.0 cm is frequently the definitive therapy. Large lesions can be treated with surgery and closed by sliding flaps or covered with grafts. Cosmetic plastic surgery can follow if necessary.

*Chemosurgery* is an accepted technique valuable in certain persistent tumors; it avoids unnecessary destruction of tissue in removing the tumor completely. A zinc chloride fixative paste is applied to the tumor for several hours to destroy the upper layer. The undersurface is diagramed, and the pathologist can map the remaining tumor. Zinc chloride paste is reapplied until the pathologist can no longer find tumor cells. The cure rate is 99 percent, and the cosmetic results are satisfactory.

*Chemotherapy* has had much therapeutic success in the treatment of skin neoplasms and precancerous lesions. The topical administration of 5-fluorouracil (5-FU) and other antimitotic agents inhibits DNA synthesis, but the mechanism of its action on keratosis is unknown. The reaction to topical 5-FU normally starts 5 to 20 days after application and usually progresses from erythema to vesiculation, erosion, ulceration, necrosis, and healing. *Cryosurgery* is the topical application of liquid nitrogen to superficial cutaneous neoplasms to destroy them. *Radiation therapy* is used in some cutaneous cancers and is especially helpful in areas such as the nose, eyes, and lips.[157]

*Immunotherapy* is fast becoming a major form of treatment. Many skin cancers have been eradicated by control of immune factors. Immunotherapeutic approaches have included inducing a delayed hypersensitivity to an organic chemical such as 2,4-dinitro-3-chlorobenzene (DNCB) or triethylene-iminobenzoquinine (TEIB) in order to induce a cell-mediated immune reaction, resulting in therapeutic effects on the tumor.

The nursing care in skin cancer begins with prevention. The nurse in any setting can instruct people, especially teenage girls, about the ill effects of excessive sunning. Those whose work requires them to be in the sun should be advised as to proper screening and the advantage of wearing wide-brimmed hats. The nurse is also instrumental in recognizing lesions of the skin during her physical assessment of any patient. All abnormal or changing areas of the skin require further investigation.

Care of lesions during the treatment phase should be explained in detail to the patient, with full regard to the instructions given by the individual physician or therapist. Nurses must constantly reinforce the need for frequent follow-up of all lesions. Most skin cancers are curable if diagnosed and treated early and if recurrences are treated immediately.

## Mycosis Fungoides

Mycosis fungoides (MF) is an uncommon, chronic fatal disease which originates in the reticuloendothelial system of the skin. It primarily and predominantly affects the skin but is known to invade the lymph nodes and internal organs. The etiology is unknown. MF progresses through three stages: *erythematous* or *premycotic* stage, *plaque* or *infiltrative* phase, and *tumor, fungoid, or mycotic* phase. Treatment does not seem to increase life expectancy[158] but is given to control symptoms. Immunotherapy, chemotherapy, and ionizing radiation are effective in some patients, and further investigation into more effective therapy is going on.

## Malignant Melanoma

Malignant melanoma is a tumor derived from pigment-producing melanocytes. Although it is generally located in the skin and frequently occurs as a change within a nevus, its spread is hematogenous, and widely disseminated metastases characterize the advanced stage of the disease.

The most important etiologic factors are skin pigmentation and exposure to ultraviolet light. The risk of melanoma rises with age. Over 50 percent of patients with melanoma give a history of a pre-existing nevus at the primary site.[159]

The diagnosis of malignant melanoma is based on the history and clinical appearance of the lesion and must be confirmed by microscopic examination after surgical excision (Fig. 6-30).

Malignant melanoma should be suspected if any of the following changes occur:

Change in size: Spread to a larger area.

Change in elevation: Flat lesion becomes elevated or a nodule develops within the tumor.

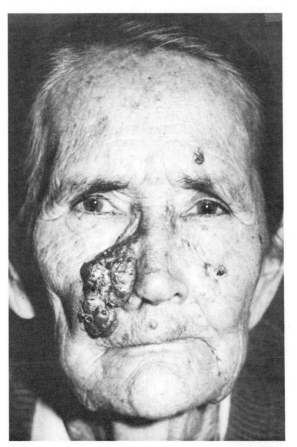

**FIGURE 6-28**
Basal-cell carcinoma.

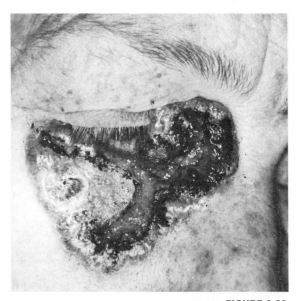

**FIGURE 6-29**
Advanced basal-cell carcinoma.

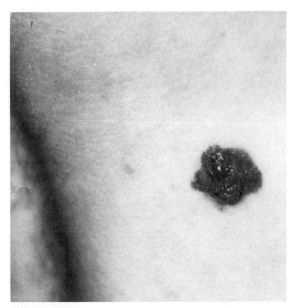

**FIGURE 6-30**
Malignant melanoma.

Change in color: A brown mole becomes black. Change in pigmentation may not be uniform, producing all shades of brown, blue, gray, black, and pink or amelanosis.

Change in surface characteristics: A previously smooth surface becomes rough and scaly. Serous discharge or bleeding after mild trauma.

Change in surroundings: Pigmented or amelanotic satellite tumors develop in the immediate vicinity of an advanced melanoma.

Change in sensation: A mole begins to itch or tingle.[160]

The primary treatment for melanoma is local excision followed by wide excision and adjacent lymph-node resection. The aggressiveness of the surgical intervention is dependent on the stage and location of the disease. Patients with more advanced local disease may have to undergo extensive surgery requiring skin grafts or amputation of extremities, depending on the tumor location.

Combination-drug isolation perfusion may be done when the lesion is located on an extremity. The advanced disease with distant metastasis is treated with a combination of modalities usually involving chemotherapy, immunotherapy, and palliative surgery.

Several drugs have been used as single agents in systemic chemotherapy, with response remaining unsatisfactory. One agent, dimethyltriazeno

imidazole carboxamide (DTIC), has produced 20 to 30 percent response rates.[161] This had led many clinical investigators to continue studying this drug in combination with other chemotherapeutic agents as well as immunotherapeutic agents.

Human melanoma cells contain antigens not shared by normal host cells that result in the production of both cellular and humoral immunity on the part of the host. The evidence of spontaneous remissions and more favorable responses in those patients whose lesions show lymphocytic infiltration (homograft response) has kindled interest in immunotherapeutic agents in the treatment of melanoma.[162]

The use of nonspecific immunostimulants such as BCG (bacillus Calmette Guérin) is being studied. BCG is sometimes used by direct injection into the tumor, with regression of the injected lesion and occasional regression in remote noninjected tumors.[163] Many investigators are using BCG and other immunotherapeutic agents in the treatment of both early and advanced disease. BCG can be given by the subcutaneous route, by direct injection into the tumor, by scarification, or by the tine technique. It is too early to determine results, but immunotherapy appears promising in the treatment of malignant melanoma.

The *nursing intervention* in malignant melanoma involves all levels of nursing care. A suspicious skin lesion or changing nevus found during the physical assessment of the patient should alert the nurse to investigate further. The earlier the stage of the disease at diagnosis, the better the prognosis. Malignant melanoma frequently metastasizes, and supportive nursing care is needed during all stages, including diagnosis, treatment, and terminal care. Over 20 percent of malignant melanomas recur after 5 years, so lifelong follow-up is necessary.[164]

## REFERENCES

1   American Cancer Society, '76 *Cancer Facts and Figures,* New York, 1975.
2   Phillip Rubin (ed.), *Clinical Oncology for Medical Students and Physicians,* American Cancer Society, New York, 1974.
3   American Cancer Society, op. cit.
4   Rubin, op. cit.
5   Phillip Strax, *Early Detection: Breast Cancer Is Curable,* New American Library, New York, 1975.
6   Ibid.
7   James E. Holland and Emil Frei, *Cancer Medicine,* Lea & Febiger, Philadelphia, 1974.
8   Ibid.

9   Ibid.

10   Ibid.

11   Paul Carbone, "The Role of Chemotherapy in Treatment for Breast Cancer," *Cancer Chemotherapy: Fundamental Concepts and Recent Advancements,* Year Book, Chicago, 1975, pp. 311–322.

12   American Cancer Society, op. cit.

13   Rubin, op. cit.

14   American Cancer Society, op. cit.

15   Robert L. Egan, "Mammography," *Am J Nurs,* **66:** 108–111, January 1966.

16   Ibid.

17   N. Bjurstam, K. Hedberg, K. A. Hultborn, M. T. Johansson, and S. Johnson, "Diagnosis of Breast Carcinoma: An Evaluation of Clinical Examination, Mammography, Thermography and Aspiration Biopsy in Breast Disease," *Prog Surg,* **13:**2–65, 1974.

18   Rubin, op. cit.

19   Holland and Frei, op. cit.

20   Ibid.

21   Bjurstam et al., op. cit.

22   Holland and Frei, op. cit.

23   Aurora Mamaril, "Preventing Complications after Radical Mastectomy," *Am J Nurs,* **74:**2000–2003, November 1974.

24   James Nelson, H. Averette, and R. Richard, *Dysplasia and Early Cervical Cancer,* American Cancer Society Professional Education Publication, New York, 1975.

25   Rubin, op. cit.

26   Carbone, op. cit.

27   Margaret Ruth McCorkle, "Coping with Physical Symptoms in Metastatic Breast Cancer," *Am J Nurs,* **73:**1034–1038, June 1973.

28   B. Fisher, P. Carbone, S. Economoir, R. Frelich, A. Glass, H. Lerner, C. Redmond, M. Zelen, P. Band, D. Katrych, N. Wolmark, and E. Fisher, "L-Phenylalanine Mustard (L-Pam) in the Management of Primary Breast Cancer," *N Engl J Med,* **292:**117–122, January 1975.

29   Gianna Bonadonna, E. Brusamolino, E. Valagussa, P. Rossi, Anna Brugnatelli, L. Brumbilla, C. DeLena, M. Tonuni, G. Boyetta, E. Musumeci, and R. Veronesi, "Combination Chemotherapy as an Adjuvant Treatment in Operable Breast Cancer," *N Engl J Med,* **294:**405–410, February 1976.

30   Rubin, op. cit.

31   Carbone, op. cit.

32   Rubin, op. cit.

33   Ibid.

34   Ibid.

35   Ibid.

36   A. Segaloff, "Hormonal Therapy in Breast Cancer," *Cancer,* **30:**1541–1542, December 1972.

37   Rubin, op. cit.

38   Holland, and Frei, op. cit.

39   William McGuire, "Current Status of Estrogen Receptors in Human Breast Cancer," *Cancer,* **36:** 638–644, August 1975.

40   Ibid.

41   McCorkle, op. cit.

42   Roberta Klein, "A Crisis To Grow On," paper presented at the Second National Conference on Breast Cancer, Los Angeles, Calif., May 1971.

43   Alice Costello, "Supporting the Patient with Problems Related to Body Image," *Proceedings of the National Conference on Cancer Nursing,* American Cancer Society, New York, 1974.

44   M. Donovan and S. Pierce, *Cancer Care Nursing,* Appleton-Century-Crofts, New York, 1976.

45   Bonadonna et al., op. cit.

46   Ibid.

47   Rubin, op. cit.

48   Holland and Frei, op. cit.

49   Ibid.

50   Ibid.

51   Rubin, op. cit.

52   Bjurstam et al., op. cit.

53   Holland and Frei, op. cit.

54   Ibid.

55   Rubin, op. cit.

56   Holland and Frei, op. cit.

57   Ibid.

58   Iibd.

59   Ibid.

60   Iibd.

61   Ibid.

62   B. K. Pradhan and K. Chandra, "Morphogenesis of Nodular Hyperplasia: Prostate," *J Urol,* **113:**210–213, February 1975.

63   F. K. Mostofi and R. V. Thompson, "Benign Hyperplasia of the Prostate Gland," in M. F. Campbell and J. H. Harrison (eds.), *Urology,* 3d ed., Saunders, Philadelphia, 1970, p. 1065.

64   David C. Utz and M. Farron, "Pathologic Differentiation and Prognosis of Prostatic Carcinoma," in Phillip Rubin (ed.), *Cancer of the Urogenital Tract,* Part II, "Prostate and Testes," American Cancer Society, New York, 1970, p. 7.

65   Willet Whitmore, Jr., "The Natural History of Prostatic Cancer," in *Proceedings of the National Conference on Urologic Cancer,* American Cancer Society, New York, 1973, pp. 1104–1111.

66   M. F. Campbell and J. H. Harrison, (eds.), *Urology,* 3d ed., Saunders, Philadelphia, 1970, p. 1145.

67   L. M. Franks, "Etiology, Epidemiology and Pathology of Prostatic Cancer," in *Proceedings of National Conference on Urologic Cancer,* American Cancer Society, New York, 1973, p. 1092.

68 George R. Prout, "Diagnosis and Staging of Prostatic Carcinoma," in ibid., p. 1096.

69 Martin J. Resnick and John T. Grayhack, "Treatment of Stage IV Carcinoma of the Prostate," *Urol Clin North Am,* **2**(1):141, February 1975.

70 Ibid.

71 Donald R. Smith, *General Urology,* 8th ed., Lange Medical Publications, Los Altos, Calif., 1975, p. 272.

72 William L. Valk and Winston Mebust, "The Management of the Prostatic Nodule," in Phillip Rubin (ed.), *Current Concepts in Cancer: Multidisciplinary Views,* Part II, "Cancer of the Urogenital Tract," American Cancer Society, New York, 1970, p. 3.

73 David A. Culp, "Benign Prostatic Hyperplasia," *Urol Clin North Am,* **12**(1):29–48, February 1975.

74 Ibid., p. 45.

75 Rubin Flocks, "Radiation Therapy for Prostatic Cancer," *Urol Clin North Am,* **2**(1):183, February 1975.

76 Patrick Walsh, "Physiologic Basis for Hormonal Therapy in Carcinoma of the Prostate," *Urol Clin North Am,* **2**(1):125–139, February 1975.

77 Ibid., p. 134.

78 Dennis J. Krauss, Gary J. Schoenrock, and Otto M. Lilien, "Reeducation of Urethral Sphincter Mechanism in Postprostatectomy Incontinence," *Urology,* **5**(4):533–535, April 1975.

79 Stanley L. Robbins and Marcia Angell, *Basic Pathology,* 2d ed., Saunders, Philadelphia, 1976.

80 Smith, op. cit., p. 286.

81 Ibid.

82 Robbins and Angell, op. cit., p. 550.

83 Anthony A. Borski, "Diagnosis, Staging and Natural History of Testicular Tumors," in *Proceedings of the National Conference on Urologic Cancer,* American Cancer Society, New York, 1973, p. 1205.

84 F. K. Mostofi, "Testicular Tumors," in ibid., p. 1187.

85 William Staubitz, Kendall S. Early, Irma V. Magoss, and Gerald P. Murphy, "Surgical Treatment of Non-Seminomatous Germinal Testes Tumors," in ibid., p. 1206.

86 R. B. Bracken and D. E. Johnson, "Sexual Function and Fecundity after Treatment for Testicular Tumors," *Urology,* **7**(1):37, January 1976.

87 Robbins and Angell, op. cit., p. 451.

88 Smith, op. cit., p. 286.

89 Hugh J. Jewett, "Cancer of the Bladder, Diagnosis and Staging," in *Proceedings of the National Conference on Urologic Cancer,* American Cancer Society, New York, 1973, pp. 1072–1074.

90 Meyer M. Melicow, "Tumors of the Bladder: A Multifaceted Problem," *J Urol,* **112**:476, October 1974.

91 Alan S. Morrison and Philip Cole, "Epidemiology of Bladder Cancer," *Urol Clin North Am,* **3**(1):13–27, February 1975.

92 Melicow, op. cit., p. 474.

93 Smith, op. cit.

94 J. U. Schlegel, et al., "The Role of Ascorbic Acid in the Prevention of Bladder Tumor Formation," *J Urol,* **103**:266, 1970.

95 Bernard Pinck, Steven Alexander, and Saul Siegendorf, "Ureteroileosigmoidostomy," *Urology,* **5**(5):595–598, May 1975.

96 Richard V. Remigailo, Ernest L. Lewis, John R. Woodward, and Kenneth N. Walton, "Ileal Conduit Urinary Diversion: Ten Year Review," *Urology,* **3**(4):343–348, April 1976.

97 Rosemary C. Watt, "Urinary Diversion," *Am J Nurs,* **74**(10):1805–1811, October 1974.

98 Ralph A. Straffon, "Urinary Diversion by Cutaneous Ureterostomy," in Russell Scott (ed.), *Current Controversies in Urologic Management,* Saunders, Philadelphia, 1972, p. 300.

99 Joseph J. Kaufman, "Adjunctive Radiotherapy in the Treatment of Invasive Carcinoma of the Bladder," in ibid., p. 61.

100 Martin J. Cline and Charles M. Haskell, *Cancer Chemotherapy,* 2d ed., Saunders, Philadelphia, 1975, p. 104.

101 Harry Grabstald, "Tumors of the Urethra in Men and Women," in *Proceedings of the National Conference on Urologic Cancer,* American Cancer Society, New York, 1973, p. 1249.

102 Smith, op. cit., p. 261.

103 John Jacob Ballenger, *Diseases of the Nose, Throat and Ear,* Lea & Febiger, Philadelphia, 1971, p. 427.

104 William S. Maccomb and Gilbert H. Fletcher, *Cancer of the Head and Neck,* Williams & Wilkins, Baltimore, 1971, p. 253.

105 John G. Batsakis, *Tumors of the Head and Neck,* Williams & Wilkins, Baltimore, 1975, p. 140.

106 Ibid., p. 145.

107 Ibid., p. 135.

108 Ernst L. Wydner, "Toward the Prevention of Laryngeal Cancer," *Laryngoscope,* **85**:1190, July 1975.

109 Ibid.

110 Ballenger, op. cit., p. 229.

111 Rubin, op. cit., p. 305.

112 Ibid., p. 328.

113 Wydner, op. cit., p. 1192.

114 Ibid., p. 1190.

115 Myers, Eugene N., personal communication.

116 Ronald H. Rosillo, Mary Jane Welty, and William P. Graham, "The Patient with Maxillofacial Cancer: Psychological Aspects," *Nurs Clin North Am,* **8**:155, March 1973.

117 Ballenger, op. cit., p. 431.
118 Maccomb, op. cit., p. 267.
119 Ibid., p. 265.
120 Leonard R. Prosnity, "Radiation Therapy: Treatment for Malignant Disease," *RN,* March 1971, p. 5.
121 Ibid.
122 Janet E. Trowbridge and William Carl, "Oral Care of the Patient Having Head and Neck Irradiation," *Am J Nurs,* **75:**2146, December 1975.
123 Ibid., p. 2148.
124 Ballenger, op. cit., p. 432.
125 Ibid., p. 434.
126 Ibid., p. 432.
127 Donovan and Pierce, op. cit., p. 205.
128 Rosillo, Welty, and Graham, op. cit., p. 154.
129 Donovan and Pierce, op. cit., p. 211.
130 Helen White, "Tracheostomy: Care with a Cuffed Tube," *Am J Nurs,* **72:**75, January 1972.
131 Robert R. Demers and Meyer Saklad, "Minimizing the Harmful Effects of Mechanical Aspiration," *Heart and Lung,* **2:**543, July–August 1973.
132 Eastern Cooperative Oncology Group, *Adjuvant Chemotherapy and Immunotherapy in Head and Neck Carcinoma: A Research Proposal,* 1976, pp. 1–2.
133 Rubin, op. cit., p. 317.
134 Ibid.
135 Ballenger, op. cit., p. 456.
136 Maccomb, op. cit., p. 114.
137 Stanley L. Robbins, *Pathologic Basis of Disease,* Saunders, Philadelphia, 1974, p. 884.
138 Maccomb, op. cit., p. 98.
139 Ibid.
140 Ibid., p. 118.
141 Eugene N. Myers, "The Role of Total Glossectomy in the Management of Cancer of the Oral Cavity," *Otolaryngol Clin North Am,* **5:**345, June 1972.
142 Ibid., p. 355.
143 Ibid., p. 351.
144 Mary Jane Welty, William P. Graham, and Ronald H. Rosillo, "The Patient with Maxillofacial Cancer: Surgical Treatment and Nursing Care," *Nurs Clin North Am,* **8:**140, March 1973.
145 Ardis J. O'Dell, "Objectives and Standards in the Care of the Patient with a Radical Neck Dissection," *Nurs Clin North Am,* **8:**160, March 1973.
146 Rushdy Abadir, "Carcinoma of Maxillary Antrum," *Eye Ear Nose Throat Mon,* **52:**38, December 1973.
147 Rubin, op. cit., p. 312.
148 Batsakis, op. cit., p. 117.
149 Abadir, op. cit., p. 444.
150 Ibid., p. 445.
151 Norman E. Hugo, Peter McKinney, and B. Harold Griffith, "Management of Tumors of the Parotid Gland," *Surg Clin North Am,* **53:**105, February 1973.

152 Maccomb, op. cit., p. 359.
153 Hugo, op. cit.
154 Eugene N. Myers and John Conley, "Gustatory Sweating after Radical Neck Dissection," *Arch Otolaryngol,* **91:**534–542, June 1970.
155 Rubin, op. cit.
156 Holland and Frei, op. cit.
157 Ibid.
158 Ibid.
159 Ibid.
160 Neville G. Davis, Roderick McLeod, G. L. Beardmore, J. H. Little, R. L. Quinn, and J. Holt, "Primary Cutaneous Melanoma; A Report from the Queensland Melanoma Project," *CA,* **26:**80–107, March/April 1976.
161 Holland and Frei, op. cit.
162 Ibid.
163 Ibid.
164 Ibid.

## BIBLIOGRAPHY

Anderson, W. A. D. (ed.): *Pathology,* Mosby, St. Louis, 1971.

Armenian, Haroutune K., Abraham M. Lilienfeld, Earl L. Diamond, and Irwin D. J. Bross: "Relationship Between Benign Prostatic Hyperplasia and Cancer of the Prostate," *Lancet,* **2** (20 July, 1974): 115–117.

Bates, Barbara: *A Guide to Physical Examination,* Lippincott, Philadelphia, 1974, pp. 8–16, 145–157, 188–204.

Behnke, Helen (ed.): *Guidelines for Comprehensive Nursing Care in Cancer,* Springer, New York, 1973.

Blumenschein, G.: "Chemotherapy in the Management of Breast Cancer," *Cancer Chemotherapy: Fundamental Concepts and Recent Advancements,* Year Book, Chicago, 1975, pp. 403–415.

Bouchard, Rosemary, and Norma F. Owens: *Nursing Care of the Cancer Patient,* Mosby, St. Louis, 1972.

Burbick, Daniel: "Rehabilitation of the Breast Cancer Patient," *Cancer,* **36:**645–648, 1975.

Caldwell, William L.: *Cancer of the Urinary Bladder,* Warren H. Green, St. Louis, Mo., 1970.

Caldwell, William L.: "Radiotherapy: Definitive, Integrated and Palliative Therapy," *Urol Clin North Am,* **2:**1, February 1976.

Chiu, Ching L., and David L. Weber: "Prostatic Carcinoma in Young Adults," *JAMA,* **230**(5):724–726, Nov. 4, 1974.

Committee on Professional Education of UICC (ed.):

*Clinical Oncology,* Springer-Verlag, New York, 1973, pp. 111–120, 207.

Conley, John: "Radical Neck Dissection," *Laryngoscope,* **85:**1344–1352, August 1975.

Conner, George H., Dorothy Hughes, Martha J. Mills, Barbara Rittmanic, and Lisa V. Sigg: "Tracheostomy: When It Is Needed: Postoperative Care," *Am J Nurs,* **72:**68–74, January 1972.

Culp, Ormond S., and James J. Meyer: "Radical Prostatectomy in the Treatment of Prostatic Cancer," in *Proceedings of the National Conference on Urologic Cancer,* American Cancer Society, New York, 1973, pp. 1113–1118.

Drill, V. A.: "Oral Contraceptives: Relation to Mammary Cancer, Benign Breast Lesions and Cervical Cancer," *Annu Rev Pharmacol,* **15:**367–383, 1975.

Emmett, John L., and David M. Witten: *Clinical Urography,* 3d ed., Saunders, Philadelphia, 1971, vol. I.

Fitzpatrick, Genevieve: "Care of the Patient with Cancer of the Cervix," *Bedside Nurse,* January–February 1971.

Frazell, Edgar L., Elliott W. Strong, and Barbara Newcombe: "Tumors of the Parotid," *Am J Nurs,* **66:**2702–2708, December 1966.

Freeman, R. G., and C. Knox, Jr.: *Treatment of Skin Cancer: Recent Results in Cancer Research,* Springer-Verlag, New York, 1967.

Gibson, Thomas E.: "Treatment of Transitional Cell Carcinoma of the Upper Urinary Tract by Local Resection," in Russell Scott (ed.), *Current Controversies in Urologic Management,* Saunders, Philadelphia, 1972.

Golumbu, Mircea, and Pablo Morales: "Electrolyte Disturbances in Jejunal Urinary Diversion," *Urology,* **1**(5):432–438, May 1973.

Haagensen, C. D.: *Disease of the Breast,* Saunders, Philadelphia, 1971.

Healey, John E., Jr.: "Role of Rehabilitation Medicine in the Care of the Patient with Breast Cancer," paper presented at the Second National Conference on Breast Cancer, Los Angeles, May, 1971.

Hewitt, Clarence B.: "Transitional Cell Carcinoma of the Upper Urinary Tract" in Russell Scott (ed.), *Current Controversies in Urologic Management,* Saunders, Philadelphia, 1972.

Hilkemeyer, Renilda: "Nursing Care of the Patient with Head and Neck Cancer," *Neoplasia of Head and Neck,* Year Book, Chicago, 1971, pp. 303–310.

Hollander, Lawrence, and Myles P. Cunningham: "Management of Cancer of the Parotid Gland," *Surg Clin North Am,* **53:**113–121, February 1973.

Jacob, Stanley, and Clarice Ashworth Francone: *Structure and Function in Man,* 3d ed., Saunders, Philadelphia, 1974.

Keough, Gertrude, and Harold N. Niebel: "Oral Cancer Detection: A Nursing Responsibility," *Am J Nurs,* **73:**684–686, April 1973.

Landa, Stuart J. F., and Harvey A. Zaren: "Cancer of the Floor of the Mouth and Gingiva," *Surg Clin North Am,* **53:**135–147, February 1973.

Lasser, Terese: *Reach to Recovery,* American Cancer Society, New York, 1974.

Lawless, Carolyn A.: "Helping Patients with Endotracheal and Tracheostomy Tubes Communicate," *Am J Nurs,* **75:**2151–2153, December 1975.

Leadbetter, Guy W., and Paul M. Morrisseau: "Urology," in George L. Nardi and George D. Zuidema, *Surgery: A Concise Guide to Clinical Practice,* 3d ed., Little, Brown, Boston, 1972.

Litton, Ward B., and Charles J. Krause: "Surgical Management of Carcinoma of the Oral Cavity," *Otolaryngol Clin North Am,* **5:**303–320, June 1972.

Mahoney, E. M., E. T. Weber, and J. H. Harrison: "Post-diversion Pre-cystectomy Irradiation for Carcinoma of the Bladder," *J. Urol,* **114:**46–49, July 1975.

Marino, Elizabeth, and Donna LeBlanc: "Cancer Chemotherapy," *Nursing '75,* November 1975, pp. 22–23.

Mehm, M. C., Jr., T. B. Fitzgerald, M. Lane Brown, J. W. Raker, R. A. Malt, and J. S. Kaiser: "Early Detection of Primary Cutaneous Malignant Melanoma," *N Engl J Med,* **289:**989–996, November 1973.

Murphy, Gerald P.: "The Diagnosis of Prostatic Cancer," *Cancer,* **37**(suppl):589–596, January 1976.

Nardi, George L., and George D. Zuidema (eds.): *Surgery: A Concise Guide to Clinical Practice,* 3d ed., Little, Brown, Boston, 1972.

Nicholson, Elsie M.: "Personal Notes of a Laryngectomee," *Am J Nurs,* **75:**2157–2158, December 1975.

Pearlman, Alexander W., and Rushdy Abadir: "Carcinoma of the Maxillary Antrum: The Role of Preoperative Irradiation," *Laryngoscope,* **84:**400–409, March 1974.

Pugh, R. C. B.: "The Pathology of Cancer of the Bladder," in *Proceedings of the National Conference on Urologic Cancer,* American Cancer Society, New York, 1973.

Rickel, Linda: Human Values and the Quality of Survival, *J Ark Med Soc,* **70**(6):210–213, November 1973.

Robbins, Stanley L., and Marcia Angell: *Basic Pathol-*

*ogy,* Saunders, Philadelphia, 1976, pp. 588–592.

Roman-Lopez, Juan: "Colposcopies: Evaluation of Abnormal Cervical Cytology," *J Ark Med Soc,* **70**(6):200–203, November 1973.

Rozen, Richard D., Doris E. Ordway, Thomas A. Curtis, and Robert Cantor: "Psychosocial Aspects of Maxillofacial Rehabilitation: Part I, The Effect of Primary Cancer Treatment," *J Prosthet Dent,* **23:** 423–428, October 1972.

Rubin, Philip (ed.): *Cancer of the Urogenital Tract,* Part 2, "Prostate and Testes," American Cancer Society, New York, 1970.

Sartwell, P., F. Arthur, and J. Tonascia: "Epidemiology of Breast Lesions: Lack of Association with Oral Contraceptives," *N Engl J Med,* **288:**551–554, March 1973.

Saunders, W. H., and E. W. Johnson: "Rehabilitation of the Shoulder after Radical Neck Dissection," *Arch Otolaryngol,* **84:**812–816, December 1975.

Scardino, Peter T., Demetrius H. Bagley, Nasser Javadpour, and Alfred S. Ketcham: "Sigmoid Conduit Urinary Diversion," *Urology,* **6**(2):167–169, August 1975.

Schmidt, Joseph D.: "Chemotherapy of Prostatic Cancer," *Urol Clin North Am,* **12**(1):185–195, February 1975.

Schmidt, Joseph D.: "Cryosurgical Prostatectomy," in *Proceedings of the National Conference on Urologic Cancer,* American Cancer Society, New York, 1973.

Schmidt, Joseph D., and Stephen H. Weinstein: "Pitfalls in Clinical Staging of Bladder Tumors," *Urol Clin North Am,* **3:**1, February 1976.

Scott, F. Brantley, William E. Bradley, and Gerald W. Timm: "Management of Erectile Impotence," *Urology,* **2**(1):81–83, July 1973.

Scott, Russell, Jr. (ed.): *Current Controversies in Urologic Management,* Saunders, Philadelphia, 1972.

Shedd, Donald P., Peter M. Calaniel, Norman G. Schaaf, and Janet E. Trowbridge: "The Nurse's Role in Rehabilitation of Cancer Patients with Facial Defects," American Cancer Society Professional Education Publication, 1974.

Smith, Mary L.: "Parotidectomy," *Am J Nurs,* **76:**422–426, March 1976.

Smith, Ray, Franklin O. Black, and William S. Teachey: "Large Rotational Flaps for Neck Dissection and Facial Skin Replacement," *Arch Otolaryngol,* **99:** 122–124, February 1974.

Southwick, Harry W.: "Cancer of the Tongue," *Surg Clin North Am,* **53:**147–159, February 1973.

Stram, John R.: "Topographical Histology of the Oral Cavity," *Otolaryngol Clin North Am,* **5:**201–206, June 1972.

Thomas, Betty J.: "Coping with the Devastation of Head and Neck Cancer," *RN,* October 1974, pp. 25–30.

Trowbridge, Janet E.: "Caring for Patients with Facial or Intra-oral Reconstruction," *Am J Nurs,* **73:** 1930–1934, November 1973.

Westbrook, Kent: "Breast Cancer: Treatment by Chance," *South Med J,* **71**(6):189–192, November 1974.

Yagoda, Alan: "Non-Hormonal Cytotoxic Agents in the Treatment of Prostatic Adenocarcinoma," in *Proceedings of the National Conference on Urologic Cancer,* American Cancer Society, New York, 1973.

Yarbrough, William J., Hrant S. Semerdjian, and Harry S. Miller: "George Washington University Technique for Surgical Correction of Post Prostatectomy Incontinence," *J Urol,* **113:**47–49, January 1975.

Yarrington, C. T., A. J. Yonkers, and G. M. Beddoe: "Radical Neck Dissection," *Arch Otolaryngol,* **98:**306–308, April 1973.

# 7

# THE LEUKEMIAS AND LYMPHOMAS*

Bonny Libbey Johnson
Susan Molloy Hubbard

eukocytes, plasma cells and the reticulo-endothelial system work closely to protect the body from threatening conditions within the external and internal environment. Together they form the components of the human immune system. Disturbances in the production, maturation, or proliferation of these cells result in pathologic conditions of cellular growth. The major disruptive conditions are the *leukemias* (leukocytes), *multiple myeloma* (plasma cells), and the *lymphomas* (lymphoreticular cells). The leukemias and Hodgkin's disease are highlighted here because of their clinical significance; multiple myeloma and other lymphomas are described more briefly.

## LEUKEMIAS

The leukemias comprise a group of primary bone-marrow malignancies which until recently were invariably fatal. The clinical manifestations, course, and response to current therapy vary according to the specific leukemic process, but the principles of pathophysiology and treatment are similar. The normal bone marrow relies upon efficient regulatory mechanisms for appropriate cell proliferation and maturation. In *leukemia,* this control is abnormal, resulting in (1) an abnormal proliferation and accumulation of immature cells, (2) impairment of the cellular maturation process, accounting for many immature cells, and (3) inhibition of the growth or function of the remaining normal marrow elements due to crowding and eventual replacement by leukemic cells or to a poorly understood inhibitory effect of the primary disease.

### Leukemia Nomenclature

Leukemia is described as myelogenous (myelocytic) or lymphatic (lymphocytic) depending on the derivation of the malignant cell. All leukemias arising in cells of myeloid origin fall under the class of *myelogenous leukemia,* e.g., granulocytic leukemia, monocytic leukemia (from the monocyte), or erythrocytic leukemia (di Guglielmo's disease). Eosinophilic and basophilic leukemias are extremely rare. The origin of the malignant cell in the lymphocytic leukemias (acute and chronic) is under investigation. The most apparent difference between the lymphocytic leukemias is the degree of lymphocyte maturity and the presence or absence of lympho-

* Leukemias and Multiple Myeloma written by Bonny Libbey Johnson; Hodgkin's Disease and Other Lymphomas by Susan Molloy Hubbard.

blasts (Color Plate 7-1). This is a factor which correlates with the disease course and prognosis.

The terms *chronic* and *acute* are used in the leukemia nomenclature to describe different clinical courses of the disease. The malignant cells of the *acute leukemias* are immature and rapidly proliferative, while those of the *chronic leukemias* are more mature and tend to accumulate more slowly. Hence, historically, the natural course of the acute leukemias was rapidly fatal, whereas chronic leukemias tended to smolder for years before the accumulation of tumor cells became lethal (Table 7-1). However, current treatment programs have altered the natural course of acute leukemia. The child with acute lymphoblastic leukemia will probably survive longer than the adult with chronic myelogenous leukemia. While these adjectives may become less descriptive in the future, the current and the historical literature apply them to physiologically distinct disease processes.

## Acute Myelogenous Leukemia

Acute myelogenous leukemia (AML) is a neoplastic disease of the myeloid cells arising in the bone marrow. It is also referred to as acute granulocytic (AGL), myelocytic (AML), or nonlymphocytic (ANLL) leukemia. The suffix *-cytic* defines its cellular basis, while *-genous* refers to the site of origin. All the terms are acceptable, although *myelogenous* (originating from myeloid cells) is the most valid description.

**Causative factors** Acute myelogenous leukemia has not thus far demonstrated a unique chromosomal abnormality or congenital defect. Some of the etiologic factors implicated in the disease, however, relate to genetic abnormalities or destruction of cellular DNA.

*Ionizing radiation* and *drugs* which cause chromosomal breakage may be factors and are explained in Chap. 5. The mechanism that results in neoplastic transformation is not known. The dose of radiation appears to be a significant factor, but it is unclear whether oncogenicity relates to the dose applied to the whole body or to the bone marrow.[1] *Cytotoxic drugs* which depress bone marrow function sometimes induce a "rebound hyperproliferation" of normal elements. It is possible that the mechanism for regulation is lost at this point.[2] Benzene, phenylbutazone, and the alkylating drugs phenylalanine mustard and chlorambucil are all associated with an increased risk of developing AML.

*Genetic syndromes* with inherent chromosomal defects have been discussed in Chap. 5. Patients with Down's syndrome, Fanconi's anemia, and Bloom's syndrome tend to be at higher risk of developing AML.

The role of *viruses* in the etiology of AML is the subject of much investigation. While strong evidence has implicated them as causative in animals, studies of human leukemia cells have yet to document this phenomenon. Gallagher and Gallo have defined similar viral particles in the blood cells of a woman with AML.[3] Further investigations of this type on other leukemia cells are necessary to determine whether these particles are causative or merely an expression of transformed leukemic cells.

**TABLE 7-1**
FEATURES OF LEUKEMIA AT PRESENTATION

| | Acute Myelogenous Leukemia | Chronic Myelogenous Leukemia | Acute Lymphoblastic Leukemia | Chronic Lymphocytic Leukemia |
|---|---|---|---|---|
| PRIMARY AGE GROUP | >20 | 40–50 | <15 | 60–70 |
| SURVIVAL WITHOUT TREATMENT | 4–8 weeks | 2–4 years | 4–8 weeks | 7–10 years |
| MEDIAN SURVIVAL WITH TREATMENT | ±12 months | ±4 years | 5 years | 7–10 years |
| CLINICAL FINDINGS Bone marrow | ↑ Myeloblasts, ↓ normal elements | Hyperplasia with few blasts | ↑ Lymphoblasts, ↓ normal elements | ↑ Mature lymphocytes |
| Peripheral WBC | ±50,000 | ±200,000 | ±30,000 | ±50,000 |
| Anemia | | Present | Present | Present |
| Lymphadenopathy | | Rare | Present | Present |
| Splenomegaly | Rare | Present | Present | Present |
| CHROMOSOMAL VARIANT | Nonspecific | 90% Philadelphia chromosome | Nonspecific | None |
| BACTERIAL INFECTION | Present | Absent | Present | Absent |

**Pathophysiology** The actual leukemic cell, or *myeloblast,* is an immature granulocytic precursor which is incapable of normal maturation and function. Compared to normal granulocytes, leukemic cells cannot effectively migrate to areas of inflammation or infection, phagocytize, or destroy bacteria. In addition, although the proliferative *rate* of these cells is actually slower, the percentage of leukemic cells capable of proliferation is increased.[4] The myeloblasts proliferate primarily in the bone marrow and are released into the peripheral bloodstream as the numbers increase and overcrowding occurs.

The erythrocytes and megakaryocytes are also of myeloid derivation. The decrease in number and functional capacity of the red blood cells and platelets in the untreated leukemic patient is attributed both to replacement of the bone marrow by the malignant cells and (perhaps) to defects in the common diseased precursor cells.[5] AML is therefore usually manifested by abnormalities of all blood elements: (1) anemia causing fatigue and malaise, (2) leukopenia and frequent infection, and (3) thrombocytopenia-induced bruising or frank hemorrhage.

The natural course of acute myelogenous leukemia is one of rapid bone-marrow replacement and organ infiltration by myeloblasts. Without treatment, death occurs within weeks of the diagnosis and is usually caused by massive hemorrhage or infection.

The advent of aggressive chemotherapy has lengthened the survival of patients with AML. The immediate goal of cytotoxic therapy is to reduce the number of proliferating myeloblasts. Prior to and during the initial period of therapy, the patient faces the complications of hyperuricemia due to the hypermetabolic state and leukostasis-induced bleeding* due to the enormous number of circulating myeloblasts.

The primary aim of therapy for acute myelogenous leukemia is the induction of a *complete hematologic remission,* defined as a return of normal marrow elements with less than 5 percent myeloblasts in the bone marrow and improvement with eventual disappearance of all subjective signs and symptoms of leukemia.[6] The duration of remission is usually measured in months until the bone marrow becomes repopulated with myeloblasts. Induc-

---

* *Leukostasis* is the most common cause of fatal hemorrhage in AML patients. This is related to high numbers of leukemic cells, which are thought to obstruct capillary bloodflow and infiltrate the walls of blood cells, causing rupture and intracranial bleeding. This can be prevented by chemotherapy to reduce the number of circulating white blood cells.

tion of another remission with chemotherapy may be possible, but further remissions tend to be more difficult to attain, less complete, and shorter in duration. As many as 50 percent of patients with AML stay in the first remission for at least 1 year.[7] In general, however, less than 5 percent of all patients survive longer than 2 years.

*Relapse* is defined as a recurrence of the leukemia at some time after remission has been achieved; it is characterized by progressive infiltration of the bone marrow and extravascular areas, causing bleeding, infection, and anemia. With the advent of effective transfusions of red blood cells and platelets during periods of marrow suppression, infection has become the chief cause of death.

### Chronic Myelogenous Leukemia

Chronic myelogenous (myelocytic, granulocytic) leukemia (CML), like AML, is a malignant disorder of the myeloid cells arising in the bone marrow. CML varies significantly from AML, however, in its insidious onset, natural history, and response to treatment.

**Causative factors** The cause of CML is unknown. The predisposing factors related to all leukemias are implicated, especially those responsible for chromosomal damage. Unique to CML is the "Philadelphia chromosome" (Ph') discovered in 1960 by Nowell and Hungerford of Philadelphia.[8] The abnormal chromosome is formed as the long arms of one of chromosome number 22 are translocated to pair number 9. A screening of patients with CML shows that 90 percent of patients carry this chromosome even before symptoms of the disease occur. In the 10 percent of CML patients without the chromosome, the disease appears to be more aggressive.[9] It is thought that the abnormality is probably an acquired defect, since the Ph' chromosome is not transmitted vertically through normal patterns of inheritance. However, the predisposition to chromosomal fragility or breakage may play an etiologic role in the higher incidence within families. No evidence has yet shown that viral infection is responsible for the chromosomal defect or the onset of the disease in human beings.

**Pathophysiology** CML is unique among all of the leukemias not only for its specific chromosomal variation but also for its two distinct phases of cellular proliferation. These are referred to as the *chronic phase* and the *blast crisis.*

The disease usually presents itself in the *chronic phase,* a period of normal granulocytic hyperplasia or overgrowth which may last for 2 to 3 years. This phase accounts for the longer survival enjoyed by these patients as compared to AML patients and gives the disease its name.

During the chronic phase, the bone marrow is densely packed with normal-appearing cells, but the ratio of myeloid cells to erythroid cells is grossly increased (Table 7-1). While most of the cells are mature and functional, overcrowding by granulocytes impairs the formation and growth of erythrocytes.

In addition to extensive cell proliferation in the marrow, other organs may be involved in making granulocytes; for example, the liver and spleen, sites of embryonic hematopoiesis, become infiltrated and produce granulocytes. It is clear, then, that although the actual rate of cell multiplication is slower than normal (resembling AML), the increased areas participating in granulopoiesis account for an extremely high number of circulating white blood cells in the untreated patient.

The chronic phase undergoes an acute transition to become the *blastic phase.* Other names for this phase are blast crisis, acute transition, blastic transformation, or acute phase. The change occurs abruptly over a 1- to 2-month period. The reason for this transformation is unknown; the Ph' chromosome exists from the beginning of the chronic phase, but other chromosomal aberrations may accompany blastic transformation. *Blastic crisis* is characterized by a sudden rise in the number of myeloblasts, both in the marrow and in the bloodstream, and a fall in the hemoglobin and platelet counts. Some patients will experience a prolonged period of disease acceleration, called the *accelerated phase,* before entering frank blast crisis.

The danger of *leukostasis* is of particular concern in CML. The vessels of the central nervous system are particularly prone to leukostasis-induced rupture and subsequent hemorrhage. Painful enlargement and infarcts of other organs, especially the spleen, occur as a result of massive congestion by myeloblasts.

Progressive failure of normal marrow hematopoiesis is a result of the myeloblastic proliferation, the fibrosis induced in the bone marrow by the disease, and the chronic insult of alkylating chemotherapy. Fibrosis of the myeloid tissue renders patches of the bone marrow completely nonfunctional and devoid of any normal stem cells. As in AML, infection due to granulocytopenia is the most frequent cause of death.

Therapy to return the patient to the chronic phase has been successful in less than 20 percent of cases; attempts to cure the disease by eradicating the Ph' chromosome have been generally unsatisfactory. A major problem is the need for aggressive therapy in a patient with a fibrotic marrow and a resistant malignant cell line. Utilization of potentially lethal therapy at diagnosis has thus far been rejected because of the long periods of chronic but controllable disease.

### Acute Lymphoblastic Leukemia

Acute lymphoblastic or lymphocytic leukemia (ALL) is a malignant disease of proliferating lymphoblasts, or immature lymphocytes, in the bone marrow and lymph nodes. The origin of the malignant cell line is not clearly understood, although it is certain that the myeloid series is not involved. ALL is primarily an acute disease in the bone marrow and lymph nodes which has a well-defined and predictable course.

**Causative factors**   The causative factors of ALL bear close resemblance to those of AML. Again, the common denominator of predisposing or etiologic factors is damage to chromosomes, whether congenital or environmentally induced. Persons with congenital syndromes which demonstrate chromosomal abnormalities are included in the high-risk group, as are identical twins whose counterparts have ALL.

**Pathophysiology**   ALL is characterized by rapid and progressive involvement of the bone marrow, lymph nodes, and extralymphatic areas. Concurrently, the normal elements within the bone marrow are displaced and their growth inhibited. Organ infiltration by lymphoblasts most commonly occurs in areas of embryonic lymphatic tissue: the liver, spleen, and lymphatics. Accumulation of lymphoblasts in these areas causes swelling, pain, and obstruction to normal circulation and function. Not uncommonly, the child with ALL presents with dyspnea and chest pain due to huge mediastinal lymph nodes.

ALL cells are very responsive to current chemotherapeutic agents, and remissions are the rule for the vast majority (90 percent) of children and for 50 percent of adults.[10] The most effective drug combinations employ agents which kill lymphoblasts while generally sparing normal marrow elements. Once the lymphoblasts are cleared, the bone marrow is capable of regenerating a normal population of blood cells. Maintenance therapy utilizing the same drugs at lower dosages for varying periods of time is under investigation.

Currently, 50 percent of children with ALL survive longer than 5 years after initial remission.[11] When relapses do occur, a second and even third remission may be achieved. Studies of cell kinetics show that the lymphoblasts that recur after remission probably grow from the original leukemic stem-cell population.[12] However, as in AML, the first remission is usually of the longest duration, and successive relapses often lead to drug-resistant disease and death.

## Chronic Lymphocytic Leukemia

Chronic lymphocytic leukemia (CLL) is a malignant disease of abnormal and slowly proliferating lymphocytes. These cells vary greatly from the lymphoblasts of ALL, since they are small, mature-appearing cells which grow slowly and are long-lived. Immunologic studies have shown that the neoplastic cell involved is the B lymphocyte, and as a result the humoral immune system is often impaired.[13]

**Causative factors**   The etiology of CLL warrants discussion for its *dissimilarity* to that of the other leukemias. Family clustering, especially among siblings, is seen more often with CLL than with any other leukemia, although only rarely has a specific chromosomal abnormality been detected. The disease is also closely associated with lymphoma and other diseases related to immunocompetence, such as *Sjögren's syndrome,* systemic lupus erythematosus, and autoimmune hemolytic anemia.[14] In contrast to the other leukemias, no evidence is available to correlate CLL with exposure to ionizing radiation or drugs thought to be carcinogenic.

**Pathophysiology**   The onset of CLL is gradual, allowing for up to a year of symptom-free disease. During this period, the small malignant lymphocytes proliferate slowly and accumulate in the bone marrow, lymph nodes, and spleen. It is believed that depression of normal marrow elements, manifested by anemia, leukopenia, and thrombocytopenia, occurs later in the illness, after more than half of the bone marrow has been replaced by lymphocytes.[15] Although the growth rate of CLL cells is generally slow, the longer life span allows for accumulation and pooling in the lymph nodes and spleen.

CLL is generally responsive to antilymphocyte therapy, including radiotherapy and chemotherapy. Most patients enjoy good control of their disease for several years but gradually become resistant to therapy. Progression of CLL causes bone-marrow replacement and inhibition of normal marrow ele-

ments, massive lymphadenopathy, hepatosplenomegaly, and patchy infiltration of other organs. Death occurs usually as a result of infection or disease-related marrow hypoplasia.

### First-level Nursing Care

Prevention of the leukemias will not be possible until exact causative factors are identified. There are, however, identified contributing factors which can be controlled to some extent. Preventive measures include avoidance of unnecessary exposure to ionizing radiation and certain chemical agents (e.g., benzol and phenylbutazone). The nurse should know what populations are at risk of developing leukemia.

AML occurs at all ages but, unlike acute lymphocytic leukemia, is less common in children. The incidence rises with increasing age, with a median age of 49.[16] Considered as a group, nonlymphocytic leukemia is the most common type of leukemia and comprises the largest percentage of leukemia deaths.

CML is a disease of middle to late adulthood, with rare cases reported in children. The incidence ranges from 1/million in children under the age of 10 to 30/million in adults over 60 years of age, with a slightly increased incidence in men.[17]

ALL is primarily a disease of children; 80 percent of all cases in the United States occur in people under the age of 20, with a peak during the fourth year of life. The overall incidence in this country is 2000 to 3000 cases per year.[18]

CLL is a leukemia of middle-aged and older adults. While it is extremely rare in people under the age of 35, it is the most common leukemia found in adults. In fact, 90 percent of all cases occur over the age of 50, and two-thirds of the patients are more than 60 years of age.[19]

### Second-level Nursing Care

During the initial stages of the leukemias, patients are often seen in a community setting. While there are many similarities among the leukemias, significant differences also exist. For this reason, each of the leukemias is discussed separately.

**Acute myelogenous leukemia**   When patients first develop AML, *nursing assessment* often reveals an abrupt onset. During the *health history,* the patient often relates difficulties with infection because of the decreased number of functional leukocytes. The patient may complain of symptoms relating to current infection, particularly fever and cough. The concomitant systemic myeloblastic infiltration may result in gingivitis, bone pain, or abdominal fullness and early satiety due to enlargement of the liver or spleen. Commonly, the patient experiences malaise with anorexia and headaches and undue fatigue or shortness of breath on exertion. Anemia is most often the cause of these complaints and, if severe, can lead to more acute symptoms of high-output congestive heart failure. Further questioning will usually reveal a history of easy bruising or gingival bleeding secondary to thrombocytopenia. Complaints of recent headaches, blurred vision, or episodes of confusion should alert the nurse to the possibility of meningeal leukemia or intracranial leukostasis.

The *physical assessment* of the patient with AML reveals the effects of depressed bone-marrow elements as well as proliferation of myeloblasts. Pallor is the most common manifestation of the anemia; the hypermetabolic state from the myeloid cell proliferation may cause tachycardia and fever as well. Lymph nodes should be palpated; lymphadenopathy is uncommon but may occur and can be generalized or localized. During the abdominal examination hepatosplenomegaly may also be noted.

Ecchymoses and petechiae are usually found on the skin and reflect the low level of circulating platelets. Signs of capillary bleeding can also be detected by examination of the retina and oral cavity. Guaiac-positive stools indicate gastrointestinal bleeding.

**D**iagnostic Tests    Strict attention is immediately directed toward the initial blood picture. The number of *myeloblasts* measured in the peripheral blood may double within a few days and continue to rise at an alarming rate. As a result, the normal marrow elements will progressively decline. Blood studies of hepatic function (enzymes) and renal function (creatinine and urea nitrogen) are critical for evaluation of the extent of disease and its resultant physiologic compromise.

The diagnosis of AML rests on examination of a bone-marrow sample obtained from the sternum or iliac crest. While the nonleukemic marrow contains 0 to 5 percent normal myeloblasts, the marrow of AML is virtually replaced with leukemic cells, with severe reduction of normal erythrocyte and platelet precursors (Table 7-1).

Further workup to evaluate the disease process and its effect on other organ systems includes chest roentgenograms, and scans for measurement of hepatosplenomegaly. In view of current immunotherapeutic investigation, immunologic evaluation

may shed some light on the effect of the leukemic process on the immune system.[20] Skin-test challenges with multiple antigens and in vitro assays of blood may be required.

**Chronic myelogenous leukemia**    The onset of CML is gradual, and by the time the patient seeks medical attention, the disease is usually widespread. Although the patient appears robust and well, careful *nursing assessment* may reveal vague complaints of weakness and malaise during the *health history*. There may also be easy bruising, fever, sweats, and joint pain. Most commonly in CML the patient will complain of satiety after meals and a vague sense of abdominal fullness.

*Physical assessment* will reveal an enlarged and tender spleen during the abdominal examination. Palpable hepatomegaly or lymphadenopathy shows additional involvement. Signs of anemia or bleeding due to thrombocytopenia are less common in CML than AML, occurring in half the patients.[21] In all cases, however, the signs of leukostasis-induced bleeding may occur anywhere in the body. While gingival infiltration leads to diffuse gum bleeding or purpura, CNS bleeding ranges from retinal hemorrhage, causing visual disturbances, to fatal intracranial hemorrhage.

**D**iagnostic Tests    Blood studies reveal white blood counts ranging from 100,000 to 300,000 cells per mm$^3$ (10 times that found in AML), with a vast preponderance of mature granulocytes. Bone-marrow aspiration confirms the diagnosis by showing granulocytes in every stage of maturity, relatively few erythrocytes, and normal or increased numbers of megakaryocytes. Chromosomal studies usually demonstrate the presence of the Ph' chromosome.

**Acute lymphoblastic leukemia**    Although the patient with ALL is usually a child, the *nursing assessment* is similar to that in AML. Careful questioning of the patient or a parent during the *health history* for evidence of fevers and recurrent infections is important. This is the most common reason for seeking medical help. The patient may complain of general weakness and anorexia. Further probing may reveal headaches or visual disturbances.

On *physical examination,* pallor is most commonly present. Thrombocytopenia may be evidenced by diffuse petechiae or ecchymoses. Palpable lymph nodes may be found in any of the lymphatic chains. During the abdominal examination the spleen may be found to be enlarged. Less commonly, ALL may progress to involve other organs such as the heart, lungs, and eyes. Sternal tenderness and dullness at the lung bases may be evident during the chest examination. Retinal hemorrhages may be found during the eye examination.

**D**iagnostic Tests   While the laboratory findings define the extent of leukemic involvement, the diagnosis rests on examination of the bone marrow and the peripheral blood cells (see Table 7-1). Blood studies most commonly show anemia, circulating lymphoblasts, and significant thrombocytopenia. The BUN and uric acid may be elevated because of the hypermetabolic state. The serum lactate dehydrogenase, an enzyme found in lymphocytes, is usually elevated. X-ray studies are helpful in defining mediastinal node enlargement, pleural effusions, or, less commonly, osseous involvement.

**Chronic lymphocytic leukemia**   Initially, 25 percent of all CLL patients will be asymptomatic. Close observation and follow-up *nursing assessment* are essential for *early* detection of infection, lymphadenopathy, or anemia, which are signs of progressive disease. While it is as yet unclear that early treatment prolongs the patient's survival, early therapy designed to relieve the symptoms of disease may improve the patient's quality of life.

The patient who seeks medical help for symptoms related to CLL may describe a *health history* of chronic infections, especially those involving the skin and respiratory tract. Later manifestations include malaise and fatigue or sweating, thought to be part of the infectious processes. Splenomegaly manifests itself in complaints of early satiety and abdominal fullness.

Further inquiry into the patient's past medical history may elicit problems related to immunodeficiency. A family history of cancer or immunodeficiency diseases helps to clarify the epidemiology. Careful documentation of all related or unusual symptomatology along with a social and medical history will alert the nurse to particular areas of concern.

*Physical assessment* will not be remarkable until the patient becomes symptomatic. At that time general or localized lymphadenopathy and splenomegaly can usually be palpated. These masses are generally smooth and nontender. Much less commonly the patient presents with CLL infiltration of the skin, demonstrated by intermittent local rashes of long standing.

**D**iagnostic Tests   The patient will undergo further diagnostic tests so that the exact nature of the disease may be ascertained, especially internal node involvement that may portend complications. Chest roentgenograms will define mediastinal node enlargement, while an intravenous pyelogram (see Chap. 14) may show ureteral deviation or compression due to para-aortic or iliac node involvement. Lymphangiography is useful for determination of subdiaphragmatic nodal abnormalities.

The diagnosis of CLL is based on both the clinical picture and the findings in the peripheral blood and bone marrow. The peripheral blood demonstrates significant lymphocytosis (Table 7-1). While the total leukocyte count ranges between 20,000 and 200,000, the percentage of lymphocytes is usually more than 75 percent of these cells.[22] The absolute number of normal granulocyte cells is most often normal; infection is, therefore, probably more a result of immunologically impaired lymphocytes than of granulocytopenia. Serum levels of immunoglobulin may be low, substantiating the defect in humoral immunity.

Unlike ALL or CML, bone-marrow aspiration in the patient with CLL shows no abnormal blast forms (Table 7-1). Small, mature lymphocytes occur focally or in dense sheets throughout the bone marrow, and, in advanced cases, depression of normal cellular components is evident. Similarly, biopsy of lymph nodes demonstrates replacement of normal structure by these small lymphocytes.

**Nursing problems and interventions**   While the presenting symptoms of the four leukemias may vary, the nursing problems are similar. Current and recurrent *infections, anemia, organomegaly,* and *bleeding tendencies* are the major problems that the nurse in a community setting may encounter. Because these problems almost always require hospitalization, their care is detailed under Third-level Nursing Care.

The most important intervention is *referral* to an inpatient facility for evaluation and care. If the diagnosis has been made on an outpatient basis, the nurse can assist the family to cope with the diagnosis. CML may occasionally be diagnosed in this way and therapy started without the need for hospitalization. If this is the case, the patient presenting with CML may have difficulty realizing the serious nature of the diagnosis, since the presenting symptomatology is not always impressive. Except in cases of initial *blast crisis,* the patient faces a long but uncertain period of normal activity on maintenance chemotherapy (see Third-level Nursing Care). The nurse and physician must carefully present the rationale and details of treatment so that understanding and cooperation may be established. Much of the ensuing medical treatment relies on close follow-up and early detection of disease acceleration or drug toxicity. At the same time, the nurse can promote the self-confidence and independence necessary for the patient to resume a normal life and share the responsibility for health care.

### Third-level Nursing Care

Patients with leukemia are admitted to acute-care settings for diagnostic workups or treatment of exacerbations of their illness. Nursing assessment of the acutely ill leukemic patient reveals symptoms resulting from replacement of bone marrow and organ tissue with abnormal cells. Interventions vary according to the type of leukemia.

**Nursing assessment** The *health history* of the acutely ill leukemic patient is similar to that described under Second-level Nursing Care. The symptoms the patient describes, however, are generally intensified or debilitating. The patient should be asked about bruises and the female patient about any prolonged, excessive menstrual discharges. The presence of severe pain due to splenic infarction or pressure on sensory nerve endings by infiltrated body structures should be explored.

During *physical assessment,* careful attention should be given to any indications of bleeding. The skin should be carefully observed for bruising. Bruises should be outlined with a pen, on the patient's skin, so that changes can be evaluated over time. All orifices should be examined and their excretions tested for blood. Mucous membranes, particularly the gums, may also show signs of bleeding.

Vital signs will reveal a depleted intravascular volume as blood is lost into body spaces. An elevated body temperature and increased pulse may be indicative of infection.

Splenomegaly, hepatomegaly, and lymphadenopathy are other common findings. Central nervous system infiltration may produce a variety of symptoms, including nausea, vomiting, headaches, and seizures.

Obstruction to normal axillary or femoral lymph drainage may result in edema of the dependent extremity. Mediastinal node enlargement may cause dyspnea and progressive impairment of respiratory function, which should be noted and described.

Diagnostic Tests    Blood studies to measure bone-marrow function are repeated frequently during the patient's hospitalization. Bone-marrow aspirates, lymph-node biopsies, x-ray studies, and major-organ function tests may also be readministered to monitor progression of the disease.

**Nursing problems and interventions** Major nursing problems at this level include *infections, bleeding, anemia, hyperuricemia, nausea and vomiting,* and the patient's *impending death.* These nursing problems result from both the pathology and the treatment. Antileukemic drugs kill some normal as well as abnormal cells, and this results in side effects that can be difficult to manage (see Chap. 5). Interventions are described here in terms of general considerations, as well as those therapies specific to the leukemia type.

General Considerations    The aim of treatment in the leukemias is to induce a remission by selectively killing leukemic cells and allowing the normal marrow to recover. Attempts to achieve this have been partially successful utilizing single-drug therapy. By defining the most active single drugs, combinations of chemotherapeutic agents have been developed which attempt to combine synergistic antitumor effects and nonsynergistic toxicities to normal tissue.

The administration of investigational and potentially lethal antileukemic drugs demands in-depth background on the part of the nurse. The specific dose, route, and method of preparation, and expected effects must be clearly understood to assure safe administration and effective patient teaching.

The benefits of *patient teaching* before remission induction can be compared to those achieved by preoperative teaching. Early awareness of the expected outcome and necessary therapeutic maneuvers will serve to decrease anxiety and enable the patient to participate in self-care.

Providing *comfort* is a major objective in the care of the leukemic patient. Pain and nausea often make movement difficult. Analgesics, antiemetics and gentleness can be helpful in this regard. Long periods of time spent in bed can cause much physical and psychological discomfort. Frequent linen changes, back rubs, and attention to the patient's personal hygiene are vital to minimizing these discomforts.

Infection    Infection is a common problem occurring at some point during remission induction, the period of remission, or the terminal phase of virtually every patient with leukemia. Granulocytopenia due to marrow replacement with leukemic cells or to hypoplasia from cytotoxic therapy creates a perfect setting for the introduction and spread of organisms. Other predisposing factors include age, physical condition, and status of the leukemia. Although supportive treatment is usually managed in the hospital setting, careful teaching of the family assures continued observation and early detection by all involved in the patient's care.

The integrity of normal barriers to infection may be compromised by the leukemic and treatment processes. Bacterial invasion may occur from internal or external sources, and nursing measures to prevent, detect, and control infection revolve around consideration of each patient's total physical setting. Determination of temperature and blood pressure levels at regular intervals and early reporting of any physical changes can be lifesaving.

The *oral* and *gastric mucosa,* frequently sites of irritation and ulceration, are portals of entry for normal flora and food contaminants as well as for organisms introduced by such routine and necessary nursing procedures as suctioning, temperature taking, and mouth care. Rectal manipulation of any kind should be avoided, when possible, in the patient receiving cytotoxic therapy. The patient should be carefully observed daily for complaints of oral or rectal pain, gastrointestinal disturbances, and any observable mucosal lesions. If *oral mucositis* occurs, diligent mouth care must be instituted. Maintenance of optimal nutritional status is the first rule of good oral hygiene. Again, early patient teaching reinforces the importance of oral intake for the period during which depression, discomfort, and anorexia may decrease motivation for self-care. Soft foods kept palatable at room temperature and cool fluids may increase the patient's tolerance and willingness to eat and drink.

Frequency of mouth care is an important factor, and early teaching will prepare the patient for the regularity of a task that may become painful and annoying. Careful but forceful irrigation with agents such as hydrogen peroxide or saline, diluted for comfort, prevents the accumulation of oral secretions which harbor pathogenic organisms. Dehydration and frequent cleansing may induce dryness, and sterile emollients help to prevent uncomfortable cracks or tissue sloughs, potential sites for additional infection. If toothbrushing is contraindicated because of bleeding, teeth should be cleansed with gauze swabs and a mouthwash solution.

*Air-borne organisms* are more easily seeded in a patient debilitated by illness whose activity level is minimal. Visitors should be assessed as potential carriers of infection, and masks should be worn when indicated. Early evidence of pulmonary infection such as a cough, rales or rhonchi, or respiratory pain are indications for immediate intervention. Infection from external hospital-borne organisms can frequently be avoided by careful assessment of the patient's immediate environment and early control of any potential environmental sources. Frequent handwashing is implicit. The nurse should examine the patient daily for skin lesions which signal potential systemic infection (Color Plate 7-2). Nursing and medical procedures which invade the physical barriers to infection include needles, oxygen tubing, suctioning, and catheterization of any kind. Strict aseptic technique is mandatory. Any intravenous tubing or plastic intravenous catheters should be changed every 24 hours in the granulocytopenic patient.[23] Procedures such as suctioning or catheterization should be avoided unless absolutely necessary.

Infection to some degree may be unavoidable. Early detection may require routine prophylactic cultures of all portals of entry and environmental sources. At the first sign of fever, the infection should assume the character of an emergency, requiring immediate action by both nurse and physician. The ever-present danger of *septic shock* requires the monitoring of vital signs, a search for the source by cultures, and early institution of empirical antibiotic regimens.[24] Later, identification of the organism by the physician may allow more specific antibiotics to be administered. A rapid response to antibiotic therapy is much more likely in the patient who begins to recover normal granulocytes than in the patient who remains granulocytopenic.[25]

*Fungal infections* are not common in normal adults. However, the immunosuppressed leukemic patient is at great risk of developing infections from these organisms, especially *Candida* and *Aspergillus.*[26] Once the patient is infected, the defense mechanisms may be unable to localize and destroy the fungus, and systemic infection can result. Treatment relies on early detection of suspicious lesions (especially skin and oral), cultures, and specific antifungal agents.[27]

*Prevention, early detection* and *antibiotic therapy* remain the most effective methods of minimizing the incidence of infection. Laminar-air-flow rooms are patient units designed to provide a *sterile environment.*[28] This is accomplished by air flow through a filter into the room which assures that all contaminants are moved continuously "downwind" of the patient. While in the room, the patient receives oral nonabsorbable antibiotics which kill most of the gastrointestinal flora. Any object that enters the room is sterilized, and the patient bathes with sterile water and antibacterial soap. Care is given under strict aseptic conditions and through plastic "arms" constructed into the plastic wall of the room. These rooms are most frequently used to support the patient during periods of bone marrow aplasia induced by chemotherapy or radiotherapy.

*Transfusion of white blood cells* collected from carefully matched donors is being studied as an attempt to replace those functional granulocytes which the patient on aggressive therapy lacks (Chap. 5). *Bone-marrow transplantation* is also a means of repopulating the bone marrow and blood stream with normal marrow elements. However, the incidence of graft rejection and serious side effects from this treatment is a major drawback, since completely compatible nonrelated donors are rarely available.[29]

**Bleeding**  Some degree of *bleeding* occurs in most patients with leukemia. It can be caused as marrow is replaced by leukemic cells or by coagulation abnormalities, or it can be a direct effect of the antileukemic therapy. Since the daily hematologic status of the patient can change dramatically, nursing intervention begins with knowledge of the most recent hematologic values. This provides a base from which to plan care and formulate observational priorities.

In general, leukemic patients rarely develop overt signs of bleeding when their platelet count is over 20,000 per mm$^3$.[30] However, while undergoing remission induction, patients frequently experience life-threatening thrombocytopenia. *Platelet transfusions* derived from normal blood plasma are commonly used as part of the medical regimen and can usually maintain the platelet count at a tolerable level. Since high body temperatures cause lysis of platelets, the febrile patient may derive little or no benefit from transfused platelets. Allergic reactions to platelet transfusions resemble those to red blood cell transfusions: urticaria, pain at the site of infusion, fever, chills, and shock. Premedication with an antihistamine or acetaminophen may be indicated.

Nursing care of thrombocytopenic patients demands close observation. Procedures which require internal manipulation or probing are contraindicated unless determined by the physician to be absolutely necessary. While venipuncture is generally tolerated well, arterial punctures or intramuscular injections are contraindicated, as they allow diffuse extravascular bleeding which may be severe. Invasive procedures such as lumbar punc-

tures, biopsies, and bone-marrow aspirations are done only when absolutely necessary; they may be preceded by platelet transfusions for additional protection against bleeding.

**Anemia**  The leukemic patient undergoing cytotoxic therapy lives with a chronically low level of hemoglobin. Because of this, the tolerance to *anemia* is higher than that of a normal person. However, transfusions of red blood cells are indicated if the patient becomes symptomatic. Pallor, malaise, and weakness are indications for blood transfusions. The overall well-being of the leukemic patient and subsequent tolerance to therapy may be significantly improved by maintaining the hemoglobin at a functional level.

Transfusions carry the threat of incompatibility reactions and hepatitis. Careful and sympathetic teaching and listening can expose fears and alleviate anxiety in relation to transfusions. Before the transfusion is started, the nurse should explain the side effects most commonly seen and the specific reasons for the procedure. Early detection of a reaction is facilitated if the patient is alerted to complain of any unusual sensations.

**Hyperuricemia**  The amount of tumor-cell burden can be estimated in part by the serum uric acid level. *Hyperuricemia* results from (1) the increased metabolism related to rapid cell proliferation and death, and (2) the accumulation of cellular debris produced by effective cytotoxic therapy. The effect of chronic low-grade hyperuricemia is goutlike joint pain; in the setting of acute myelogenous leukemia, however, the rapid onset and severity of hyperuricemia can lead to *renal tubular impairment* and kidney failure. Medical therapy is aimed at counteracting the formation of uric acid and increasing fluid flow through the kidneys. The drug allopurinol is effective in decreasing the serum uric acid level before and during chemotherapy. Increased volumes of fluid may be given orally and intravenously, as tolerated by the patient, and sodium bicarbonate may be added to alkalinize the urine and increase the solubility of uric acid.[31]

**Nausea and Vomiting**  Nausea and vomiting are a direct result of antibiotic, antitumor, or analgesic therapy. Early intervention is usually more effective than intervening after vomiting occurs, and prophylactic antiemetic therapy before the institution of chemotherapy may be indicated. Chronic nausea that accompanies malaise remains a challenge. Frequent small meals of individually chosen palatable foods and antiemetics may help the patient maintain adequate fluid and caloric intake.

**P**ain  Chloromas, or localized accumulations of leukemic cells within organs or tissues, may occur, especially in younger patients or patients with chronic leukemia. *Pain* is usually the most distressing effect for the patient, although splenic or hepatic infiltration may cause obstruction, infarction, and organ failure. These *leukemic infiltrates* generally indicate that systemic therapy has not been successful and are, therefore, a poor prognostic sign.

Palliative treatment consists of low-dose radiation to the specific area.[32] The toxic effects of radiation are usually minimal but relate to the site involved. Irradiation of the spleen, because of its proximity to the gastrointestinal tract, may cause nausea and vomiting. Radiation to marrow-containing areas may induce further hematologic depression. Analgesics and narcotics may be ordered and should be given as directed.

**I**mpending Death  Leukemic patients are almost always hospitalized during the *terminal stages* of their disease. However, preparation for the eventual outcome of the leukemia should begin with the diagnosis. There may be great apprehension on the part of both patient and family. The nurse and other professionals can be of help in creating an open atmosphere of communication. Patients may want to be stoic for the sake of their families; and the family may want only to be able to help in some way. The nurse can demonstrate to family members who wish to participate in the patient's care simple comfort measures, such as bathing, back rubs, and oral hygiene. It is necessary to make sure that families do not feel burdened or obligated but have the opportunity to participate if they wish to do so. (Refer to Chap. 3 for full discussion of the dying patient.)

**S**pecific AML Therapy  The goal of treatment for AML is the successful induction of a complete remission. This is accomplished by the administration of cytotoxic chemotherapy using combinations of effective drugs in schedules designed to maximize their antileukemic effects and minimize toxicity to normal cells. Since, however, the intention is to rid the bone marrow of all leukemia cells, the initial treatment is intensive and is designed to produce ablation, or destruction, of virtually all formed marrow elements. As the hematopoietic stem cells re-

cover and begin to repopulate the marrow, it is anticipated that the malignant cell line will not recur so rapidly and a remission will result.

The current programs of therapy for AML rely on the antimetabolites (cytosine arabinoside, thioguanine, and mercaptopurine) for their cell-cycle specificity and the antibiotics daunorubicin and adriamycin for their effective and rapid action.[33] Pharmacologic details of these drugs are given in Chap. 5. The use of combination chemotherapy from the start may prevent the leukemic population of cells from developing a resistance to any single drug. The drugs used to maintain the patient in remission are usually given in lower doses on a monthly basis, because the number of leukemic or potentially leukemic cells in the body is at its lowest level.

*Consolidation therapy* (readministration of the same drug regimen) is sometimes included at the end of the program of remission induction and just prior to the maintenance drug program. The aim of this therapy is to strengthen the quality of the remission by assuring that any occult myeloblasts have been destroyed even when they are no longer clinically detectable. The drugs involved are usually the same as or similar to those proved effective in remission induction.[34]

During the period of remission induction, the patient is dependent on complex nursing support. Chapter 5 outlines the potentially serious side effects of the antileukemic drugs. Since the drugs are most effective against cells undergoing proliferation, any cell population which has a high growth rate will be affected: bone marrow, oral mucosa, gastrointestinal lining, hair, and germinal cells are all at risk.

The period of intensive induction therapy and recovery may be months in duration. The nurse should observe the patient throughout this period for signs of remission or relapse, unexpected disease, or drug-related complications. The first laboratory indication of remission is usually an overall feeling of well-being, which gradually improves as more normal cells return to the circulation. The ability to fight and avoid infection usually indicates recovery of functional granulocytes. Proof of remission is established by bone-marrow examination.

Failure of normal elements to return usually indicates the need for further antileukemic therapy. The earliest sign of relapse may be a drop in the number of platelets. This is rapidly followed by a rise in myeloblasts in the peripheral blood. These myeloblasts can be visualized by microscopic study of a peripheral blood sample.

**S**pecific CML Therapy  The majority of patients with CML in the *chronic phase* respond to chemotherapeutic management and achieve a remission with oral alkylating agents, especially busulfan. Other drugs, such as chlorambucil, cyclophosphamide, or dibromomannitol, are useful especially when resistance develops to busulfan.[35] As the number of granulocytes returns to normal, the symptoms related to bone-marrow replacement and organ infiltration subside. A remission exists if the blood count can be maintained at a relatively normal level and the patient remains asymptomatic. However, the term *complete* is used with caution, since the patient may remain dependent on intermittent chemotherapy or radiation, and the originally detected Ph′ chromosome remains ever present.

The ability of chemotherapy to maintain the patient's remission and prolong the period before the disease acceleration of blastic transformation has not been proved. However, the *quality* of survival appears to be improved if the number of white blood cells can be kept at a tolerable level.

Two schools of thought currently govern the antileukemic management of the patient with CML. Busulfan is either administered continually, with dose modifications according to the rise and fall in the number of white blood cells, or the drug is instituted only intermittently when the patient shows a rising white blood cell count.

In both cases, nursing assessment of the patient receiving busulfan over a long period of time must consider certain side effects. Although initial myeloid suppression is the desired effect, cumulative drug doses may depress bone-marrow function severely and cause serious thrombocytopenia. Regular evaluation of the patient's blood counts is necessary for appropriate titration of the drug dosage. In addition, chronic busulfan administration can cause pulmonary, adrenal, or ovarian fibrosis and skin hyperpigmentation, which may not be reversible. Early detection is possible by chest x-ray, with follow-up observation and questioning for any respiratory or hormonal changes.

Whether maintenance or intermittent busulfan is used, the patient in this setting remains normally active for 1 to 10 years, with a median survival of 4 years.[36] Continuous assessment is essential to prevent or detect early drug toxicity and disease acceleration.

Management of *blast crisis* has not been as successful as management of the chronic disease. A small minority (10 percent) of patients are able to enjoy a return to the chronic phase of the disease with intensive induction.[37] Splenic irradiation in this setting is purely palliative and has no effect on the steady increase of myeloblasts. For 80 to 90 percent of all patients who enter blast crisis, therefore, nursing and medical treatment are generally supportive. Frequently tremendous numbers of myeloblasts accumulate in organs and cause severe pain. Splenomegaly is common and may be the most debilitating factor. Elective splenectomy during the chronic phase has not significantly facilitated the management of patients during blast crisis.[38] Radiation to the spleen may reduce its size but can cause nausea and vomiting and further bone-marrow depression. Antiemetics and analgesics are liberally used and their effect continually evaluated.

Curiously, the drugs proved effective against the myeloblasts of AML are not as useful against those of CML. This may be due to an intrinsic difference in the leukemic cell and also to the inability of the fibrotic bone marrow to recover from hypoplasia. The most active drugs against CML, to date, are the plant alkaloid vincristine and the corticosteroids.[39] Vincristine and prednisone are given in high doses on a weekly basis and usually induce moderate bone-marrow hypoplasia. Two other drugs which may be used are cytosine arabinoside and thioguanine, which cause severe bone-marrow depression. The waiting then begins, with concurrent supportive therapy, to determine the status of the recovering bone marrow.

The average survival of patients in blast crisis is 1 to 2 months. While maintaining the prescribed plan of medical care, the additional support of companionship is provided as the nurse explains the necessary procedures and listens for expressions of anxiety, fear, anger, and depression. By understanding and interpreting the patient's behavior, the nurse can facilitate acceptance of behavior by both staff and family. Careful insight into the nurse's own feelings is essential for implementing appropriate emotional support.

**S**pecific ALL Therapy  The goal of ALL therapy is identical to that of AML. A complete bone-marrow remission is essential for long-term survival and cure. Remission is defined as the presence of less than 5 percent lymphoblasts in the bone marrow, with a normal peripheral blood picture and disappearance of all leukemic signs and symptoms.[40]

Combinations of chemotherapeutic agents active against lymphoblasts are used to induce a complete remission. The relative selectivity of vincristine and prednisone against lymphoblasts spares normal bone-marrow stem cells and produces less severe marrow hypoplasia and more rapid return of normal blood cells than is seen in AML. In addition, repeated remissions are more likely, presumably because this combination of drugs does not cause so severe a depression of the marrow's reserve of stem cells.

Current programs of induction therapy often combine these two drugs with the antimetabolites methotrexate and 6-mercaptopurine (Chap. 5). These four drugs are given for 5 days and repeated as tolerated until a remission has been achieved. The major cytotoxic effect of the four-drug combination is on the lymphoblasts and normal marrow elements throughout the body, resulting in temporary but severe bone-marrow depression, hyperuricemia, and infection.

The inclusion of high doses of prednisone in the remission-induction program causes certain predictable side effects. Most patients will demonstrate Cushingoid signs and symptoms, a manifestation which clears as the steroids are tapered off and discontinued. Water retention and changes in the pattern of fat distribution cause edema of the extremities, a moon-face appearance, and humped shoulders. Acne, facial hair, and hyperpigmentation may further alter the child's or young adolescent's appearance. The additional problem of alopecia from vincristine or antimetabolite therapy may cause severe embarrassment and anxiety. If the patient and family can be clearly forewarned, the changes induced by treatment may be much more acceptable.

Cytotoxic and steroid chemotherapy render the patient with ALL especially vulnerable to infection during both remission and relapse. Infection during remission is probably due to the chronic immunosuppressive effects of maintenance therapy with antimetabolites or alkylating agents and the use of central nervous system (CNS) irradiation. It is unclear exactly how long this defect in the immune system endures after chemotherapy or radiation therapy is completed, but studies have shown a delay in the return of T-cell function of up to 1 year.[41] Continuous observation for early signs and symptoms of infection is therefore essential in the ongoing assessment of the "well" patient with leukemia.

ALL is the leukemia most likely to sequester malignant cells in "privileged" areas of the body.[42] Because of unique anatomic and physiologic barriers to various chemotherapeutic agents, the CNS and the testicles are two such areas; when the disease recurs in these sites, bone-marrow infiltration and systemic leukemia usually follow. In a few cases, however, local irradiation to these areas may allow the patient to remain in complete remission. In bone-marrow remissions, prophylactic treatment of the brain and spinal cord with radiation therapy or intrathecal methotrexate has been included in programs of induction therapy.[43]

Since therapy to the CNS occurs concurrently with remission induction and maintenance chemotherapy, specific side effects are difficult to isolate. It has been found, however, that children are more apt to experience alopecia, leukopenia, and infection during this stage of therapy.[44] Nursing care includes careful observation for early signs of aseptic meningitis or drug-induced meningeal irritation. Signs and symptoms of headache, nuchal rigidity, nausea, and vomiting also accompany the development of CNS leukemia; a spinal tap is necessary to determine the cause.

**Specific CLL Therapy**   The choice of antineoplastic treatment for CLL is based on the long natural history of the disease and the average age of the patient. Whether chemotherapy or radiotherapy is employed, therapy is generally withheld until symptoms require intervention. As stated above, no study has shown the benefit of treatment for asymptomatic disease in prolonging the actual length of survival. In addition, the patient with CLL is usually older when the disease manifests itself and is generally unable to tolerate aggressive chemotherapy. Experience has shown that in CLL, unlike the acute leukemias, intensive antileukemic therapy is not as effective in clearing malignant lymphocytes from the bone marrow to allow for normal hematologic recovery.

The aim of primary therapy in CLL, therefore, is to relieve the patient's symptoms and, in so doing, to delay the progression of disease in the bone marrow. In most cases the patient will simply be watched for weeks to months; early detection of disease manifestation and progression alerts the nurse and physician to the need for antileukemic therapy. Continual teaching about the disease keeps the patient aware of those clinical signs and symptoms that require reporting and documentation by the medical staff. These include increasing node size or abdominal fullness and progressive fatigue or malaise. Regular follow-up blood studies and collaborative history taking keep the nurse well informed of the patient's health status.

In general, the patient with CLL enjoys good control of the disease symptomatology for a period of months to years. Increasing resistance to current chemo- or radiotherapeutic intervention occurs, however, and progressive anemia, leukopenia, and thrombocytopenia result. Assessment of the patient with progressive disease determines the need for supportive therapy, especially blood-component replacement by transfusions and antibiotic therapy.

The mechanisms behind the development of *anemia* may be complex, and assessment of each individual case is essential in determining appropriate therapy. Bone-marrow replacement by lymphocytes is usually significant when anemia occurs. It has been found, however, that the red cells of the patient with CLL have a shorter life span than normal. This may be exacerbated by an enlarged spleen. Finally, 10 to 15 percent of all patients will have an autoantibody causing hemolysis.[45] Frequently the use of prednisone will decrease this hemolytic effect.

Currently, the therapy considered standard for CLL is the alkylating agent chlorambucil. It is the drug of choice, since patients tolerate the daily low doses well and the drug is absorbed easily by the gastrointestinal tract. Three-quarters of patients achieve a partial remission, with relief of splenomegaly, lymphadenopathy, and systemic symptoms as well as a measurable fall in the peripheral lymphocyte count.[46] Chlorambucil is usually given at higher doses (10 mg/day) initially, to lower the blood count to normal; the patient is then maintained at lower doses on a daily basis. The addition of prednisone to the chemotherapeutic regimen in low doses may increase the killing of abnormal lymphocytes.

The major side effect of this chemotherapeutic program is bone-marrow suppression. While this is generally not severe, regular laboratory determinations of the patient's peripheral blood values are necessary, and excessive leukopenia is an indication for dose reduction. Likewise, nursing teaching and observation is directed toward early detection and management of infection due to leukopenia.

Long-term steroid therapy in older patients has certain well-known side effects. Interference with normal protein synthesis and calcium metabolism causes osteoporosis. The diabetogenic effect of steroids on carbohydrate metabolism and the secretion of insulin can render the patient hyperglycemic. The serum calcium and glucose levels must be evaluated at regular intervals.

Radiation therapy may be used to decrease local accumulations of lymphocytes. This is usually aimed in small ports toward specific nodal groups or the spleen. It is thought that even local radiotherapy may have some systemic effect on the circulating lymphocyte pool, since the malignant cells tend to travel freely throughout the body.[47] Extracorporeal radiotherapy and total-body irradiation are other methods employed to decrease the level of circulating lymphocytes. Extracorporeal radiation is a method by which blood is irradiated outside the body and returned to the circulation. Total-body irradiation is given at doses of 10 to 15 rads/day for 3 to 5 days of each week over 3 to 4 months (100 to 200 rads).[48]

With the advent of deeply penetrating radiation therapy, skin toxicity at sites of local radiotherapy has become uncommon. However, inflammation and fibrosis of underlying mucosal tissue, especially the esophagus or respiratory tract, may occur. Nursing measures to relieve the painful or drying effects on these tissues are presented in Chap. 5.

In general, the toxic effect of systemic radiotherapy (extracorporeal or total-body irradiation) is limited to bone-marrow suppression, especially thrombocytopenia. Close attention to the hematologic status of the patient allows the nurse and physician to document toxicity and provide a rest period from therapy for the patient.

In many instances, the prospect of exposure to radiation may arouse fear in the patient. Careful explanation of the procedure, its expected outcome, and the relative lack of symptomatic side effects should be provided.

The patient frequently demonstrates massive lymphadenopathy and hepatosplenomegaly. Management of *pain* in this setting is a major concern, with analgesic support and careful assistance with exercise and bed positioning. Therapy directed toward shrinking these masses is accomplished by local radiation. These measures are purely palliative, and responses are usually short-lived.

**Fourth-level Nursing Care**

Nursing assessment of the rehabilitative or chronic care needs of patients with leukemia is determined by the individual patient's age, social setting, diagnosis, response to therapy, and ultimate prognosis. Rehabilitation of both patient and family begins with adjustment to the disease and the proposed medical regimen. Comprehensive care must incorporate knowledge about the natural course of each disease into a program of teaching, emotional and physical support, and follow-up care.

It is critical to minimize physical and psychological toxicity whenever possible, but especially during remission induction, when the delivery of full doses of intensive therapy on schedule is a key factor to success. *Hair loss,* for example, is so common a side effect of cancer therapy that physicians and nurses may lose sight of the psychological impact on the patient's body image. Wigs and hats may be suggested to help the patient conceal this loss. Acknowledgment of the significance of this and other sources of emotional trauma can help patients accept such toxicity more easily. Physical effects such as *neurotoxicity,* a common side effect of a regimen containing vincristine, can also present a severe emotional problem for patients. Inability to perform simple tasks for oneself such as buttoning a shirt, climbing stairs, or picking up small objects can be a source of constant frustration. Poor coordination can severely curtail the ability to take care of oneself safely. A nurse who is aware of the implications of such toxicity on the patient's life-style can provide the guidance and direction necessary to assist the patient in carrying out otherwise routine activities. Family teaching as well as occupational-therapist and community-health nurse referrals may provide additional assistance.

Once a patient has been discharged, the degree to which a meaningful life can be resumed, independent of the hospital, depends on the close cooperation of the nurse with the family as well as other necessary professional services. Throughout the entire course of treatment, fears about disease progression or relapse from remission are overriding concerns. It is necessary to understand and accept these fears as normal. Nonetheless, the nurse can promote a hopeful attitude by encouraging "well-oriented" activities and alternative interests and by rewarding healthy, adaptive behavior.

Outpatients remain dependent on physicians and nurses for serial evaluation of response, toxicity, or recurrent disease. Patient- and family-directed teaching is essential to provide careful monitoring of drug toxicity or disease complications, especially infection. Maintenance chemotherapy for the leukemias, usually low doses of antimetabolites on a daily or monthly schedule, keeps the patient in a state of chronic immunosuppression. Systemic infections are not uncommon even during remissions. While the nurse can assist the patient to resume a more normal life-style, teaching must emphasize the importance of avoiding infection, early detection of signs or symptoms such as cough, fever, or pain, and immediate communication of these to appropriate personnel. Maintenance of activity and nutrition, compliance with medical regimens, and prevention of infection are all areas in which the patient and family can participate in rehabilitation.

As discussed in Chap. 5, the psychological and physical stress may encourage emotional dependency and subsequent reluctance or fear to relinquish this dependence. Nursing intervention can provide necessary emotional support while encouraging the patient to regain control and independence. While supportive rehabilitation can assist the patient to cope with disabilities with some adjustments, restorative rehabilitation reinforces self-esteem for those with chronic disease and prepares patients to resume responsibility for a maximum degree of independence.

The prospect of terminal care must be considered at varying points, according to the particular patient and disease. While a limited degree of denial is necessary within the setting of a life-threatening illness, actions regarding long-term family plans or ongoing health responsibilities must be governed by a realistic acceptance of the patient's diagnosis and its implications. Expressions of anger or grief may be subtle, and the nurse can encourage verbalization and self-awareness from both the patient and family members. Careful consideration and respect for privacy, however, is of paramount importance, and the nurse must recognize when the family or the patient desires distance.

A comprehensive discussion of the specific needs of the dying child is not within the scope of this textbook. Questions of importance are those regarding the stage of emotional development, ability to grasp the concepts of separation and death, and degree of family intimacy. The nurse who cares for the well or dying child must not sacrifice health care and needs for "mothering behavior." Close collaboration with the parents enables the nurse to determine the child's needs and formulate a plan for effective medical and emotional care.

During the final stages of illness, the patient's thoughts revolve around fears of pain, abandonment, and dying.[49] Concerns also extend to the family; patients regret the emotional and financial burdens assumed by loved ones and fear adverse effects of their death on the family. Nursing assessment must focus on these areas as the plan for terminal care is established. Much guilt and fear on the part of the family can be minimized by early planning which involves the patient, family, and health professionals. While care in the home setting may be desirable for the patient with a close family and personal attendant, the hospital may provide a more secure base for the older patient whose family members must work. Each patient setting differs, and honest and close communication can provide the optimal conditions of care for the dying patient.

The focus of rehabilitation may be shifted in planning the care for each individual patient, on the basis of changing therapy, environments, and short- and long-term goals. For patients who do not achieve complete remission and will eventually die of their disease, palliative efforts are implemented to maintain independence as long as possible and maximize comfort in daily living. Nursing intervention can assist both patients and family to adjust gradually without depriving them of the hope that has sustained them throughout therapy. By coordinating the services of health professionals for patients and their families, a nurse can provide guidance and support for chronically ill or dying cancer patients. It is imperative that rehabilitation prepare patients with progressive disease as well as those who are apparently in remission to resume responsibility for as independent a life as possible.

## MULTIPLE MYELOMA

Multiple myeloma is a neoplastic disorder of the *plasma cell,* a type of lymphocyte which is capable of secreting immunoglobulin proteins. In theory, the disease results from an abnormal clone of precursor cells in the bone marrow which produces abnormal plasma cells.[50] These cells resemble normal plasma cells but lack the mechanism for regulation of growth and the ability to secrete normal immunoglobulins necessary for effective antibody formation. The abnormal immunoglobulin secreted by the malignant cell is called the *M protein,* referring to its malignant, myeloma, or monoclonal characteristics. The M protein is diagnostic of the disease and can usually be measured in the blood or urine. A high number of myeloma cells in the bone marrow results in low levels of normal plasma cells able to secrete globulins, thus creating a state of reduced humoral antibody production.

Multiple myeloma is a disease of the elderly, with a peak incidence in adults over the age of 50. In fact, 80 percent of people with the disease are more than 40 to 50 years of age. The ratio of men to women who contract multiple myeloma is 2:1 over the age of 60 but more evenly distributed in the younger age group. The annual incidence is 3/100,000.[51]

The etiology of multiple myeloma is unknown, but discovery of chromosomal abnormalities within families of patients implies a genetic predisposition. The role of viruses in the causation is obscure, though viral particles have been detected in both human and animal disease states.[52]

### Pathophysiology

Multiple myeloma is a slow-growing tumor, since only a small percentage of the cells are actually dividing. The disease is characterized by a long prodromal period during which symptoms are not noticeable. Not uncommonly, the disease is diagnosed while the adult is undergoing a routine physical exam. The abnormal plasma cells proliferate and accumulate in the bone marrow and gradually infiltrate bones, causing osteolytic lesions or diffuse osteoporosis and loss of bone integrity. Degeneration of bones leads to high levels of calcium in the bloodstream. Hypercalcemia and hyperuricemia combine with hyperproteinemia to cause renal compromise. Although myeloma is generally responsive to chemotherapy and local radiation therapy, gradual resistance to treatment occurs and the disease progresses.

**Nursing assessment**   The patient with myeloma usually seeks medical attention for complaints of *pain* related to bone lesions. The most common presenting site of bone pain related to myeloma lesions is the back, because of stress on the vertebral bodies. The pain can be elicited by movement or stress and may occur intermittently over time. Pathologic fractures are not uncommon. Symptoms of anemia, bleeding, or weight loss may be present initially.

The degree of symptomatology can give the nurse a clue as to the amount of tumor present. A careful health history can elicit such added symptoms as weight loss, recurrent infections, and subtle personality changes.

The early symptoms of hypercalcemia are subtle, as described in Table 7-2. Complaints of blurred vision or dizziness may indicate a hyperviscosity syndrome. Minor or expected discomforts in elderly patients should not be overlooked. A beginning relationship which is based on sympathetic listening and intelligent probing will supply both the necessary trust for emotional support and the compilation of data important to the physician's diagnostic workup.

The series of laboratory and radiologic tests that ensue require detailed instruction and clarification to the patient, who is faced with the diagnosis of serious illness. In addition, upon completion of the diagnostic workup, the nurse and physician should continue the educational and supportive process by explaining to the patient the clinical picture and plan for therapy.

Diagnostic Tests   Initial laboratory studies reveal a moderate to severe anemia with otherwise normal counts. The high serum-protein level also causes platelet aggregation or clumping, which may induce bleeding in spite of normal platelet numbers. The anemia of multiple myeloma is caused by two mechanisms: (1) excessive protein coating the erythrocytes, impairing their function and shortening their survival; and (2) bone-marrow replacement by plasma cells, inhibiting red cell formation.

Further studies show an elevated serum- or urine-protein level. A concomitant depression of normal immunoglobulins and albumin is apparent on serum electrophoresis. By this method the exact type of immunoglobulin involved in the neoplastic process can be defined. The protein excreted into the urine is called the *Bence Jones protein,* a light-chain protein not found in normal urine. Excretion of excess protein by the kidneys may result in renal compromise, evidenced by a rise in BUN and creatinine.

A complete radiologic metastatic series and isotopic bone scans are necessary to determine the degree of bone involvement. Most commonly, the patient has multiple well-defined osteolytic lesions in the vertebrae, ribs, skull, pelvis, and long bones. X-rays may also show a more diffuse pattern of osteoporosis. Such lysis of bone causes the release of calcium into the bloodstream and subsequent hypercalcemia.

Bone-marrow aspiration shows plasmacytosis, or an increased number of plasma cells relative to normal bone-marrow cells. The degree of plasmacytosis varies from 10 to 95 percent of all cells in the sample. The remaining bone-marrow elements appear normal.

The initial workup of the patient is aimed at confirming the diagnosis and determining the amount of tumor present. This is an important factor in deciding when to begin treatment, since the patient with little symptomatology and low levels of serum or urinary protein may enjoy a long period of subclinical disease. In addition, 10 percent of patients will have a solitary myeloma or plasmacytoma, a lesion curable by local radiation therapy.[53]

**Antineoplastic treatment**   The antineoplastic treatment for systemic multiple myeloma is best achieved with the alkylating agents phenylalanine mustard (melphalan, L-Pam) or cyclophosphamide (Cytoxan). *Phenylalanine mustard* is effective in reducing the number of tumor cells in 40 to 80 percent of all patients. Cyclophosphamide is

thought to be as effective, although studies to confirm this are not complete.[54] The role of nitrosoureas (BCNU) in the treatment of myeloma is under investigation.[55]

Any of these drugs may be used in combination with *prednisone.* They are given orally on a continuous or intermittent schedule according to the tolerance of the individual patient. The schedule of choice for phenylalanine mustard or cyclophosphamide, at present, consists of high doses for 7 to 10 days to lower the plasma cell load, followed by a lower daily maintenance dose. An alternative regimen under study advocates administration of high intermittent doses of either phenylalanine mustard or cyclophosphamide.

The medical objective of antineoplastic therapy is to alleviate the symptoms of anemia and bone pain by decreasing the number of malignant plasma cells. Once the bone marrow and skeletal lesions are cleared of detectable tumor, the hemoglobin and immunoglobulin levels will rise and the bones will recalcify. Unfortunately, resistance to the cytotoxic therapy inevitably occurs and proliferation of plasma cells resumes.

The patient on chronic alkylating and steroid chemotherapy is maintained in a state of moderate leukopenia (200 to 3000 cells per mm³), since the bone marrow is depressed by these agents. Coupled with hypogammaglobulinemia, this produces a predisposition to *infection.* Careful follow-up blood work must be done at regular intervals so that the dose of drug can be monitored according to the degree of leukopenia present. The patient should be encouraged to avoid close contact with obvious sources of infection and to report any signs of infection at once, including fever, chills, areas of skin induration or erythema, and urinary or respiratory symptoms. Consideration must also be given to the diabetogenic and osteoporotic effects of chronic steroid therapy in the elderly patient.

Cyclophosphamide is most frequently used after the patient has become resistant to L-Pam. A side effect unique to cyclophosphamide is sterile

**TABLE 7-2**
SIGNS AND SYMPTOMS OF HYPERCALCEMIA

|  | Renal | Gastrointestinal | Neurologic |
|---|---|---|---|
| Mild | Nocturia | Anorexia | Confusion |
| Moderate | Polyuria, polydypsia | Constipation | Psychosis, somnolence |
| Severe | Dehydration, renal failure | Atonic ileus, abdominal distention | Coma |

hemorrhagic cystitis. This is probably due to the direct effect of a drug metabolite on the bladder epithelium.[56] The patient taking either intravenous or oral cyclophosphamide must be instructed to increase his or her fluid intake up to 2 to 3 liters/day. The degree of vomiting induced by the intravenous drug may necessitate additional IV fluid hydration. By careful questioning, tissue irritation can be detected early and the process reversed by appropriate dose modification and hydration. In addition, cyclophosphamide causes alopecia in half the patients who take it orally and virtually all patients when given intravenously. The nurse must warn the patient of this complication and assess the need for a wig or hairpiece. Loss of hair is often of great concern to the patient, even in the face of serious illness.

**Nursing problems and interventions** Awareness of the life-threatening complications of progressive multiple myeloma is essential as the nurse plans the appropriate objectives and methods of care. Relief of *pain* is of paramount importance to the patient both for comfort and to minimize further complications. Effective preventive and therapeutic nursing maneuvers can lengthen the patient's survival.

The nurse should collaborate with the physician in determining the extent to which the patient may remain active. *Ambulation* must be maintained, and participation in mild exercise should be encouraged. Activity serves to reverse the negative systemic calcium balance induced by the skeletal degeneration and prevent the possibility of spinal-cord compression. Since pain frequently inhibits mobility, an effective regimen of pain medication should be devised. Localized sites of painful lesions may respond to low doses of radiation. Pathologic fractures may require surgical pinning or braces. The nurse can maintain an ongoing assessment of the patient's tolerance to the prescribed pain regimen and the level of activity.

The second nursing objective is to maintain adequate renal function and prevent or manage *hypercalcemia* and *hyperuricemia*. Because the rise of calcium and uric acid in the bloodstream can lead to impaired ability of the kidneys to reabsorb water, the patient may experience an inappropriate diuresis. Ample saline hydration as ordered by the physician serves to both compensate for the extra fluid loss and assist in the excretion of excess calcium and uric acid. If the hypercalcemia is resistant to this maneuver, steroids or the chemotherapeutic agent mithramycin may be indicated to decrease the serum-calcium level. Early detection and nursing care of hypercalcemia (see Table 7-2) is essential for medical therapy to be effective. One-third of patients with multiple myeloma will encounter this potentially fatal complication at some time during therapy.

Excretion of Bence Jones and other proteins further impairs kidney function by causing *tubular obstruction and damage.* Infiltration of the kidney by tumor cells or calcium deposits may induce further obstruction. Again, hydration can be both preventive and therapeutic in maintaining kidney function.

The normal bone marrow elements are depressed as a result of replacement of the marrow by plasma cells and cytotoxic chemotherapy. In order to manage the symptoms of *anemia,* transfusions of red blood cells may be required. In addition, platelet transfusions can reduce the danger of *hemorrhage* in patients whose platelets fall below 20,000/mm³ and may be administered as deemed necessary by the physician. Strict attention must be paid to the signs and symptoms of transfusion reactions. Fever, chills, headache, or the development of pruritis or hives signals an impending reaction.

*Plasmapheresis* is a method by which blood rendered hyperviscous by excessive amounts of abnormal proteins (M protein) is removed from the patient in an attempt to lower the total plasma volume. The syndrome of *hyperviscosity* is usually accompanied by hypervolemia as the high level of proteinemia raises the osmotic pressure of the bloodstream. The syndrome is characterized by increased intravascular resistance with signs and symptoms of heart failure, visual disturbances, confusion, bleeding diatheses, and renal impairment. Again, early detection is critical, and removal of the excess plasma protein load can result in immediate palliation.

Successful treatment of the disease and its complications can allow most patients with multiple myeloma to live at least 3 years.[57] Much of this time is spent with subclinical disease or with a minimal degree of symptoms. However, management is complicated by recurrent infections because of the immunosuppression induced by both the disease and the chemotherapy. Renal failure may accompany the inevitable hypercalcemia, and multiple skeletal lesions provide continual complications. Although the course of the disease may be prolonged, it is invariably fatal as a result of any of the above complications.

## THE LYMPHOMAS

Cancers which originate in lymphoreticular tissues of the body are known as *malignant lymphomas*. This broad classification includes a heterogeneous group of neoplasms which can be distinguished from one another on the basis of histopathologic appearance and different patterns of involvement and spread.[58]

Lymphoid tissues are derived from primitive lymphoreticular cells which have the inherent capacity to differentiate (mature) into highly specialized cell types. Mature cells of the lymphoreticular system include reticular cells, cells of the lymphocyte and monocyte series, plasma cells, and macrophages. The cells of the lymphoreticular system form the anatomical base for the host's immune system. Fully differentiated cells mature along one of two pathways to give rise to either cell-mediated (T cell) or humoral (B cell) immunity.[59] The immunologic origin of the neoplastic lymphoid cells is probably an important factor in determining the biologic behavior of each variant or type of lymphoma and is the subject of intense investigation.

Lymphoreticular cells are widely dispersed throughout the body, populating lymph nodes, thymus, spleen, liver, bone marrow, and the submucosa of the gastrointestinal and respiratory tracts. Microscopic aggregates of lymphoid cells are present in virtually all tissues. Knowledge about the widespread distribution of lymphoid cells is important for a clear understanding of why the malignant lymphomas are frequently systemic rather than localized diseases and of the fact that extranodal presentations can occur in most tissues of the body. Lymphoreticular cells coexist in the bone marrow with hematopoietic elements. It can therefore sometimes be difficult to discriminate certain lymphomas which primarily involve the bone marrow from chronic lymphocytic leukemia with nodal involvement. In actuality, the leukemias and lymphomas represent a spectrum of closely related neoplasms.

At present, malignant lymphomas are divided into two major classifications: Hodgkin's disease and the non-Hodgkin's lymphomas. This section considers them as separate entities for purposes of comparison with regard to presentation, staging, therapeutic alternatives, and survival. Hodgkin's disease and other malignant lymphomas must also be differentiated from nonmalignant, infectious, or inflammatory conditions to which they are similar.

## Hodgkin's Disease

Hodgkin's disease, a progressive and formerly always fatal illness involving the lymph nodes and spleen, was described in 1892 by Thomas Hodgkin and named after him by subsequent investigators.[60] The presence of granulomalike nodules in biopsies of involved lymphoid tissues has, historically, been a source of confusion about the malignant nature of the illness, as granulomas are commonly associated with infections such as tuberculosis. Observers therefore postulated that Hodgkin's disease represented a form of tuberculosis, a transition between infection and a malignant disorder, or an acquired immunologic defect induced by infection.[61]

The *natural history* of Hodgkin's disease is characterized by the proliferation of abnormal cells (recognized as malignant by cytogenetic abnormalities) within lymph nodes. These cells fulfill the criteria for malignancy in terms of the subsequent development of invasive tumor.[62] While there is some variability in the propensity of certain histologic forms of the disease to remain localized for prolonged periods, Hodgkin's disease is invariably fatal if it is left untreated.

**Causative factors**  The cause of Hodgkin's disease, although sought for over a century, is unknown. An infectious etiology has been suspected for several reasons. The histopathologic appearance of lymph nodes involved with Hodgkin's disease frequently is one of marked inflammatory reactions, lymphocytic proliferation, and varying degrees of fibrosis, necrosis, and granulomatous changes.[63] Clinical manifestations of the disease include fevers, night sweats, chills, and leukocytosis, all commonly associated with systemic infection. Epidemiologic studies have suggested that there is geographic clustering of Hodgkin's disease within certain groups in relatively close social contact.[64] However, data are inadequate to prove a common infectious or environmental etiology. To date, no infectious organism, bacterial, parasitic, or viral, has been convincingly implicated in the pathogenesis of Hodgkin's disease. Several studies have also documented the occurrence of Hodgkin's disease in two or more members of the same family.[65] It is thought that the risk of developing Hodgkin's disease in relatives of patients is slightly greater than in the general population.[66] This increased risk may indicate that genetic as well as environmental factors have an etiologic role in the pathogenesis of the disease.

**Pathophysiology** The malignant cell of Hodgkin's disease is called a *Reed-Sternberg cell.* It is a gigantic cell which may be mononuclear, binucleate, or multinucleated or may have multilobulated nuclei. Large inclusionlike nucleoli are present which are larger than the nuclei of normal surrounding lymphocytes.[67]

The diagnosis of Hodgkin's disease must be made by histologic examination of tissue, generally obtained from an enlarged lymph node. The criteria for the diagnosis are the presence of neoplastic cells having the characteristics of the classic Reed-Sternberg cell or a recognized atypical variant, and an appropriate background of inflammatory cells.[68] The presence of both neoplastic and reactive components (inflammatory or reactive changes) is characteristic of this particular type of lymphoma. The morphologic characteristics of Reed-Sternberg cells and the relative number of malignant cells to reactive cells may vary considerably, as may the nature and intensity of the cellular reaction.

Subclassifications of Hodgkin's disease are based on the histopathologic features of both neoplastic and reactive components in the involved tissue. Jackson and Parker devised a classification which subdivided Hodgkin's disease into three categories: paragranuloma, granuloma, and sarcoma.[69] This classification was an attempt to relate histologic features to prognosis. The categories reflect the favorable influence of lymphocytic proliferation on the prognosis. Although this classification separated patients with the most favorable prognosis (paragranuloma) from those with the worst prognosis (sarcoma), nearly 90 percent of cases fell into the granuloma category and had very variable prognoses.[70] In 1965, Hodgkin's disease was reclassified into four histologic patterns by Lukes and associates at the Rye conference on pathology and staging.[71] These four categories, their relationship to the old Jackson-Parker classification, and their relative incidence are shown on Fig. 7-1. The four categories are of clinical value because specific histologic types tend to predict patterns of presentation and dissemination and to have significant predictive value in terms of sites of involvement, tendency to remain localized for prolonged periods, response to therapy, and ultimate survival.[72]

The best prognosis is seen in patients presenting with the lymphocyte-predominant form, followed in order by nodular sclerosis, mixed cellularity, and lymphocyte-depleted varieties. Patients with *lymphocyte-predominant* disease frequently present with limited disease. The *lymphocyte-depleted form* is associated with widespread disease involving virtually all node-bearing areas as well as major organs. Current data strongly suggest that disease progression from lymphocyte predominance to lymphocyte depletion can occur.[73] The proliferation of normal lymphocytes and other reactive cellular components in patients with limited disease and a favorable histologic type suggests that host defense mechanisms, specifically cell-mediated immunocompetence, may be an important factor in determining the course of the disease.[74]

**First-level nursing care** The estimated annual incidence of Hodgkin's lymphoma in the United States is approximately 7200 new cases per year.[75] This represents approximately 25 percent of all malignant lymphomas that are diagnosed. The incidence of Hodgkin's disease has a bimodal age-specific incidence curve, with the first peak between ages 15 and 34 and the second peak after the age of 50.[76] The highest incidence occurs in the third decade of life, with less than 10 percent of patients developing the disease after age 60 or before age 10. Of the cases which are diagnosed yearly, approximately 40 percent have localized disease (Stages I and II) and 60 percent have disseminated disease (Stages III and IV) (refer to Table 7-3). Hodgkin's disease occurs predominantly in males (60 to 65 percent). In children under 10 years of age, 85 percent of the cases are in males.[77] Males generally have a less favorable prognosis, reflecting the increased incidence of a favorable histologic type (nodular sclerosis) in females.

Prevention of Hodgkin's disease is not yet possible, as the cause is unknown. Investigations into viral or altered-immune-system etiologies hold hope that prevention may be possible in the future.

**Second-level nursing care** Patients later diagnosed as having Hodgkin's disease may initially be seen in a variety of outpatient settings. Since nurses may be the first professionals to assess the patient, it is important that they be aware of its manifestations.

**N**ursing Assessment Constitutional symptoms (B category in the staging system) may appear early and be a prominent feature in the *health history* of patients with Hodgkin's disease. These symptoms include (1) unexplained weight loss of more than 10 percent of body weight within the previous 6 months, (2) unexplained fever with temperature about 38°C (100.4°F), and (3) night sweats. Pruritis, fatigue, malaise, and pain in involved lymph nodes following alcohol ingestion are also common in generalized Hodgkin's disease. In mediastinal presentations, the initial symptoms may reflect compression of mediastinal structures and include chest pain and dysphagia. Early satiety can be produced if the stomach is compressed by an enlarged spleen or involved abdominal nodes.

*Physical assessment* generally reveals painless enlargement of peripheral lymph nodes. At the onset of disease the first nodes to become involved are usually the cervical lymph nodes (60 to 80 percent), followed by mediastinal, axillary, and inguinal nodes.[78] Spread of Hodgkin's disease is usually contiguous, extending from one involved lymph-node chain to adjacent nodal areas.[79] Initially, the enlarged nodes are discrete, feel firm or rubbery, and may fluctuate in size. Later, nodes become matted together as invasion outside the node occurs.

Any rashes or skin irritation should be described according to appearance and location. The frequency, duration, and amount of any diaphoresis should also be noted. Any cyanosis or neck edema should be evaluated, as these may indicate mediastinal node enlargement; the enlargement causes pressure on and eventually obstruction of the superior vena cava, thus interfering with its normal drainage functions.

The patient's weight must be evaluated initially and followed at intervals to detect any changes. If anemia is present, the patient may have pallor of the skin and mucous membranes; the pulse and respiratory rates may be elevated.

Periods of fever usually accompany Hodgkin's disease. For this reason, the patient's temperature should be monitored closely for any elevations or subnormal readings. The temperature may be elevated for several days and normal for several; such patterns should be noted.

The abdominal examination may reveal splenomegaly or hepatomegaly. Any signs of jaundice in the skin, sclera, or mucous membranes should be closely evaluated.

Additional physical assessment findings are detailed under Third-level Nursing Care. Since the symptoms of Hodgkin's disease are somewhat variable in occurrence, those findings may also be present on initial evaluation.

*Diagnostic tests*  Blood studies vary greatly; there may be little or no deviation from normal or dramatic abnormalities. Anemia is the most common finding. It is usually moderate and normocytic. The

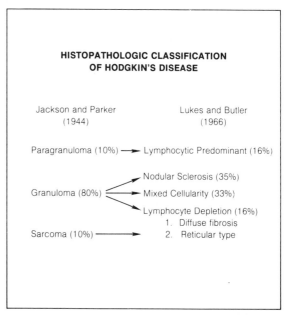

**FIGURE 7-1**
Histopathologic classifications of Hodgkin's disease.

total leukocyte count may be increased, decreased, or normal. Platelets may be abnormal in appearance and increased in number or they may be normal in quantity and appearance. Thrombocytopenia is apparent when there is extensive splenic or bone-marrow involvement.

Lymph-node biopsy is the most definitive diagnostic tool and is usually done within the hospital setting. The node is examined for the presence of Reed-Sternberg cells.

**N**ursing Problems and Intervention  The major nursing problem at this point may be unexplained *lymphadenopathy* or it may be any of the variety of *constitutional symptoms*. When Hodgkin's disease is suspected, however, immediate referral should be made to an appropriate facility for a thorough diagnostic workup. Definitive diagnosis and medical therapy are usually initiated within a hospital setting.

**Third-level nursing care**  Patients with Hodgkin's disease may be hospitalized for diagnosis or because of an exacerbation. Symptoms vary in severity according to the involved body structures.

**N**ursing Assessment  Nursing assessment of the hospitalized patient with Hodgkin's disease may disclose many of the findings described under Second-level Nursing Care. In addition, the patient's *health history* may reveal progressive pain, weight loss, fatigue, and anorexia. Pulmonary involvement may cause chest pain, shortness of breath, and cough. The patient may also report an increased frequency of infections.

*Physical assessment* should be directed toward evaluation of the extent of the disease. Almost all body organs may eventually become involved, and findings are variable.

Dissemination to bone may be apparent in tenderness over the area or on movement; care should be taken during any activity, as spontaneous fractures occur. Compression of nerve roots, if there is extension into the spinal canal, may result in loss of function or sensation. Patients should be assessed thoroughly for neurologic function, particularly in the lower extremities. This would include speed and equality of reaction to touch, command, and pain.

Any stridor, dyspnea, or abnormal breath sounds should also be described. In addition, patients should be continually reassessed for changes in lymph-node size and major-organ function.

*Diagnostic tests*  Blood studies are repeated at intervals to assess any changes. Roentgenographic studies are done to determine the degree of disease dissemination. Finally, lymph-node biopsies are taken to determine cellular abnormalities and the presence of Reed-Sternberg cells. These diagnostic tests form the basis for determination of the *clinical and pathologic staging* of Hodgkin's disease.

The Ann Arbor staging classification, adopted in 1971, divides Hodgkin's disease into four stages based on the extent of anatomical involvement. Each stage is designated by a Roman numeral and is subclassified as A or B, indicating the absence (A) or presence (B) of systemic symptoms. The

staging classification is presented in Table 7-3. Clinical staging (CS) is distinguished from pathologic staging (PS), allowing meaningful comparisons between patients in different manners.[80]

*Clinical stage* is based on the information gathered in the diagnostic workup and includes the following:[81]

1   A detailed history to document the presence and duration of constitutional symptoms

2   A detailed physical examination with inspection of all node-bearing areas and assessment of liver and spleen size

3   Laboratory studies to evaluate hematologic status, renal and hepatic function, and serum-calcium and uric acid levels

4   Radiologic studies, including
   *a.* A complete chest x-ray for evaluation of pulmonary parenchyma and pleural, hilar, and mediastinal nodes, with full chest tomography if suspicious lesions are noted
   *b.* Lymphangiography for evaluation of intra-abdominal nodes
   *c.* A skeletal survey for evaluation of bone involvement

5   Whole-body, liver, spleen, and bone scans with isotopes

6   Evaluation of immunologic status for abnormalities in cell-mediated immune reactivity

The necessity for *pathologic staging* is determined by the information gathered during clinical staging. When equivocal lymph nodes are found on physical examination or lymphangiogram that could change the patient's stage and definitive therapy, additional biopsies may be necessary to document disease involvement. Biopsies of extranodal sites commonly involved with Hodgkin's disease are warranted if suspicious findings are noted during clinical staging.

A controversy exists about the need for exploratory laparotomy and splenectomy in the staging of patients with Hodgkin's disease. The controversy centers around the need to remove the spleen for administration of effective therapy and the need to pathologically document Hodgkin's disease in the intra-abdominal lymph nodes and liver by laparotomy. Current evidence suggests that the staging laparotomy, a major surgical procedure, should not be performed routinely.[82] Such a procedure should be done only if the therapeutic approach, not just

**TABLE 7-3**
STAGING CLASSIFICATION FOR HODGKIN'S DISEASE

| | |
|---|---|
| Stage I | Involvement of a single lymph-node region or a single extralymphatic organ or site ($I_E$) |
| Stage II | Involvement of two or more lymph-node regions on the same side of the diaphragm or localized involvement of an extralymphatic organ or site ($II_E$) |
| Stage III | Involvement of lymph-node regions on both sides of the diaphragm or localized involvement of an extralymphatic organ or site ($III_E$) or spleen ($III_S$) or both ($III_{SE}$) |
| Stage IV | Diffuse or disseminated involvement of one or more extralymphatic organs with or without associated lymph-node involvement. The organ(s) involved should be identified by a symbol.<br>A = Asymptomatic<br>B = Fever, sweats, weight loss > 10% of body weight |

the stage, will be altered by the identification of intra-abdominal disease. Clinically staged asymptomatic patients with localized disease who have normal lymphangiograms and normal-sized spleens do not need pathologic identification of occult Hodgkin's disease in either the spleen or abdominal nodes when the planned radiation therapy is designed to encompass these areas, regardless of the results of laparotomy. Patients who do not have pathologic evidence of Hodgkin's disease at the time of laparotomy may eventually have abdominal involvement. The only situation in which a laparotomy appears justified is when patients have an abnormal lymphangiogram or splenomegaly and no other evidence of disseminated disease. Occult hepatic involvement may occur in 20 percent of patients with this clinical picture.[83] Since patients with liver involvement are not candidates for management with radiotherapy, it is essential to identify this involvement.

A procedure that is just as reliable as laparotomy in the identification of hepatic involvement —peritoneoscopy*—can be done under local anesthesia. Peritoneoscopy is associated with fewer complications than laparotomy and should be the procedure of choice in this situation.[84]

Nursing care of patients undergoing clinical and pathologic staging should focus on the establishment of a good nurse-patient relationship which helps patients understand the rationale for the diagnostic procedures employed and assists them to cope with the diagnosis of a malignant disease. Nursing considerations should include an explanation of each procedure, its technical aspects, and the possible side effects and emotional support during the procedure whenever possible.

**N**ursing Problems and Intervention    Nursing problems are largely defined by the area of the body that is involved with the disease. General problem areas include *lymphadenopathy* and any accompanying *pain* and *interference with bodily function*. *Recurrence* or *exacerbation* is also a problem for those patients already diagnosed. Medical therapy used

to treat Hodgkin's disease frequently causes side effects that require nursing intervention. Because Hodgkin's disease affects a relatively young population, there may be particular *anxieties* and *fears* expressed by the patient with which the nurse can be of help.

*General therapies*    Radiotherapy and chemotherapy are the primary treatment modalities for patients with Hodgkin's disease. The choice of therapy is based on the extent of disease as determined by the staging workup.

Localized stages of Hodgkin's disease are managed with *radiotherapy*. In general, all patients with stages IA, IB, IIA, and IIB should have all lymph node–bearing areas irradiated. This form of treatment, known as total nodal irradiation (TNI), provides the highest cure rate. With less extensive radiotherapy, an increased incidence of recurrent disease is seen, except in certain presentations of nodular sclerosis and lymphocyte-predominant histologies which are known to have favorable prognoses. Figure 7-2 depicts the anatomic areas encompassed when TNI is delivered. Lead shields can be used to protect vital structures such as the lungs, heart, kidneys, liver, and spinal cord from radiation damage.

Disease-free survival at 5 years in accurately staged patients treated with modern techniques of radiotherapy is currently estimated to be 90 percent in stages IA and IIA and 75 percent in stages IB and IIB.[85] Since most relapses of Hodgkin's disease occur within the first 5 years following definitive treatment, freedom from recurrent disease for a duration in excess of 5 years is likely to indicate cure.

Radiotherapy is generally begun in the hospital and continued on an outpatient basis, and patients are encouraged to carry on their normal activities. Complications of TNI include bone-marrow suppression, evidenced by leukopenia and thrombocytopenia, which usually reaches its nadir at the end of the course of treatment. On occasion, therapy must be interrupted for 1 to 2 weeks to allow hematologic recovery. Nursing assessment for signs and symptoms of infection or bleeding is essential.

"Mantle" radiotherapy, as illustrated in Fig. 7-2, often produces a sore, dry mouth and moderate to severe dysphagia. Nursing intervention must focus on teaching the patient meticulous oral hygiene. Treatment with fluoride gel before radiation therapy is started may prevent permanent damage to teeth. Nurses often coordinate the referral of patients to a

---

* Peritoneoscopy is a procedure performed under local anesthesia which permits visualization of the entire upper abdomen through a fiber-optic light source. The abdominal cavity is entered with a blunt needle. Then air is pumped into the abdominal cavity, distending the abdomen and lifting the abdominal wall so that the liver and undersurface of both diaphragms can be visualized. Under direct vision, biopsies can be taken of the liver parenchyma and peritoneal surfaces. After the procedure is completed, the air is expelled from the abdominal cavity through the site of entry. The patient performs a Valsalva maneuver and direct manual pressure is applied over the abdomen. The incision is closed with sutures.

dentist where they can receive such prophylaxis. Temporary alopecia of the lower scalp is a common occurrence in patients receiving "mantle" irradiation. Another complication that can occur after treatment of the mantle field is hypothyroidism, which is seen in 5 to 10 percent of patients (see Chap. 21). Radiation pneumonitis is a potentially severe complication but is uncommon if proper shielding is used. About 10 percent of patients develop symptoms of cough, dyspnea, and fever. Clinical symptoms usually disappear gradually after several months. Radiation pericarditis can also occur. Careful observation of patients is warranted, since progressive accumulation of pericardial fluid can cause tamponade or constrictive pericarditis, necessitating pericardectomy.[86]

During treatment of the "inverted Y" field (Fig. 7-2), patients may experience nausea, vomiting, or diarrhea. Nursing intervention includes teaching patients how to control these symptoms with antiemetic and antidiarrheal medications. Nursing intervention for all patients receiving radiotherapy is discussed in detail in Chap. 5.

While patients with systemic Hodgkin's disease (Stages IIIA, IIIB, IVA, and IVB) respond to intensive radiotherapy, complete remissions are much less frequent and remission durations are often short, with most patients dying within 5 years of developing disseminated disease. Treatment with active *single-agent chemotherapy* can also induce complete remissions in 5 to 27 percent of patients with advanced disease, but remission durations are brief, ranging from 2 to 4 months.[87] Overall survival in these patients is not improved with the administration of any single agent.

The advent of effective *combination chemotherapy,* however, has dramatically increased the percentage of patients achieving complete remission. In addition, these programs have significantly prolonged the duration of the initial remission as well as the survival. The first effective drug combination was developed by DeVita and his colleagues at the National Cancer Institute in the early 1960s and was tested in patients with stage IIIB and IV Hodgkin's disease. The combination, known as *MOPP,* consists of nitrogen mustard (M), Oncovin (O), prednisone (P), and procarbazine (P).[88]

Combinations such as MOPP which have

**FIGURE 7-2**

Schematic diagram depicting the "mantle" and "inverted Y" fields employed in the delivery of total nodal irradiation (TNI). *a.* A two-field technique, with small extension to include the splenic pedicle, used in splenectomized patients; *b.* three-field technique, usually used when the spleen is still present. (*Used with permission from Cancer Medicine, J. Holland and E. Frei (eds.), Lea and Febiger, Philadelphia, 1973, p. 1296.*)

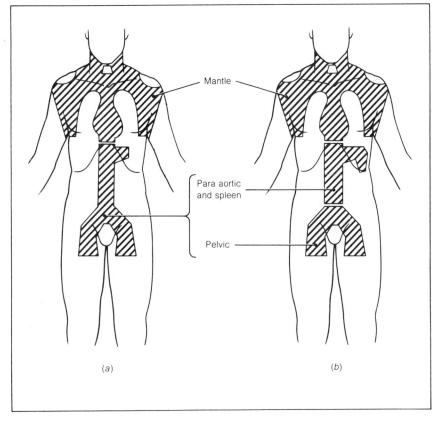

yielded high complete-remission rates exemplify the basic principles of effective combination chemotherapy. Each drug employed in the MOPP combination is active against Hodgkin's disease when used alone. Such selection of independently active agents for use in combination programs is essential to achieve a synergistic antitumor effect. The MOPP combination utilizes four drugs, each with different mechanisms of action and different dose-limiting toxicities. Selection of independently active drugs with different actions creates multiple lesions in tumor cells and prevents their easy repair and regrowth. Furthermore, the use of drugs in combination prevents or delays the development of resistance. With the use of MOPP, the magnitude of tumor kill is greater than could be predicted by adding together responses produced by each drug alone. Different toxicities permit the use of the four drugs at full clinical doses without cumulative toxicity. Because combinations prevent easy regrowth of tumor, therapy may be given intermittently and still achieve progressive tumor kill. The rest periods between cycles of chemotherapy permit normal tissue reparation and immunologic recovery.

Table 7-4 illustrates a single cycle of MOPP therapy. With the use of these four drugs in combination, it is possible to achieve a complete remission in 80 percent of patients (off all treatment), with a median duration in excess of 5 years. The MOPP regimen is administered for a minimum of six monthly cycles. If evidence of residual disease exists at the end of the sixth cycle in a patient who has clearly responded to therapy, additional cycles of MOPP can often produce complete regression of disease.

Side effects of the individual drugs employed in the MOPP regimen are discussed in detail in Chap. 5. In general, side effects encountered include temporary nausea and vomiting, peripheral nervous system toxicity, alopecia, and, most importantly, bone-marrow suppression, which increases susceptibility to infection and bleeding. Patients should be monitored for evidence of leukopenia and thrombocytopenia and drug doses lowered according to a sliding scale on the basis of the peripheral blood counts. The sliding scale is utilized to preserve the integrity of the combination and to ensure that all patients are treated in a standard manner.[89] Side effects are reversible when therapy is stopped.

The results of MOPP chemotherapy in 194 patients treated at the National Cancer Institute (NCI) over an 11-year period have recently been analyzed and confirm that an 80 percent complete remission

(CR) rate has been consistently achieved.[90] Sixty-six percent of all patients achieving complete remission have remained in their initial remission for 5 to 10 years. No patient has relapsed after a remission duration of 5 years. In contrast, all patients who did not attain complete remission have failed to survive for 5 years despite continued therapeutic efforts. The overall survival of all 194 patients at 5 years following the end of treatment is 65 percent and for those achieving complete remission is 82 percent; at 10 years it is 58 percent for all patients and 72 percent for those achieving CR. All deaths between the fifth and tenth year in patients attaining complete remission have been due to other causes.

*Recurrent disease*   The development of *recurrent disease* in areas previously involved with large volumes of tumor remains a significant obstacle to improving the disease-free survival of patients with Hodgkin's disease. Most patients whose disease recurs following total nodal irradiation (TNI) are treated with combination chemotherapy. Only patients with truly localized recurrences in previously uninvolved and untreated lymph nodes can achieve true control with further treatment with radiotherapy. All patients who relapse in previously treated fields, nodes contiguous to treated fields, and extranodal sites usually receive combination chemotherapy. Patients who relapse after TNI tolerate MOPP therapy well. About 75 percent of these patients achieve complete remission with MOPP chemotherapy.[91,92]

Patients who are unable to tolerate combination chemotherapy because of extensive prior radiotherapy or chemotherapy, advanced age, or concurrent physical or emotional illness can achieve significant *palliation* of disease with single-agent therapy. Palliative radiotherapy is also effective in the management of previously unirradiated lymph nodes, skin, or bone. A number of active agents are recommended for use as single agents for the pal-

**TABLE 7-4**
MOPP COMBINATION CHEMOTHERAPY PROGRAM:
OUTLINE OF A SINGLE CYCLE

| Drug (mg/m²) | Days | | | | | |
|---|---|---|---|---|---|---|
| | 1 | 2–7 | 8 | 9 | 14 | 28 |
| VCR | 1.4 | | 1.4 | | | |
| HN₂ | 6 | | 6 | | No | |
| Procarbazine | 100 | ———————— | | | → | therapy |
| Prednisone* | 40 | ———————— | | | → | |

* Cycles 1 and 4 only.

liation of Hodgkin's disease. These include oral alkylating agents (Cytoxan and chlorambucil), vinca alkaloids (vincristine, vinblastine), procarbazine, BCNU, adriamycin, and bleomycin.

Combination chemotherapy programs such as MOPP are started in the hospital but are designed to be administered on an outpatient basis. Outpatient management also gives patients greater control over their lives and frequently allows them to maintain a more normal life-style during the period of remission induction, which entails a minimum of six cycles given over a 6-month period. In an increasing number of clinical settings, nurses are actively involved in drug administration. It is expected that a nurse who administers chemotherapy will exercise judgment in clinical situations where discrimination between drug toxicity and complications of the disease is required. Both patients and physicians depend on the chemotherapy nurse for the safe administration of drugs. Nurses must be knowledgeable about drug interactions and potential incompatibilities. It is essential to know the proper preparation of each drug and to be aware of its stability or lack of stability after reconstitution. The mode of action and side effects and the pattern and timing of the expected antitumor response and toxicity of each drug should be well understood. Such knowledge is a prerequisite for anticipating and amending untoward side effects as well as advising patients and answering their questions.

An experienced and informed oncology nurse may anticipate problems, initiate action, and do patient teaching on the basis of knowledge of the individual patient, the disease and its complications, and the chemotherapy received. Bone marrow toxicity occurs within several days, reaching its maximum between the tenth and fourteenth day, with full recovery by the eighteenth to twenty-first day after administration. Leukopenic patients frequently demonstrate lowered resistance to infection; great care must be taken to identify potential sites of infection in all susceptible patients. A patient with a low white blood cell count who complains of a chill may be manifesting an important signal that the body cannot combat an infection. In such patients, signs of fulminant sepsis may be evidenced within hours.

Increased bruisability and episodes of spontaneous bleeding are clinical signs that platelets have reached dangerously low levels. Careful assessment of the patient is essential to determine risk of severe hemorrhage. Nosebleeds, gum bleeding, petechiae, and blood in stools, urine, or emesis should be reported promptly to the physician. Modification in dosage or withholding of therapy may be required until marrow function returns to an adequate level. When necessary, supportive maneuvers such as platelet transfusions and antibiotic therapy may be employed until marrow recovery occurs. Generally, the toxicity from MOPP is quite tolerable and patients rarely require hospitalization for infectious complications or platelet support for bleeding. *Anemia* is the most common hematologic side effect of therapy requiring treatment. About 17 percent of patients receiving MOPP require red cell transfusions during their course of therapy.[93]

*Pain* Lymph node size is often dramatically decreased with therapy. Before this happens, however, the patient may suffer severe pain and loss of function. Pain relief may be offered in the form of comfort measures such as positioning, massage, and analgesics.

*Interference with bodily function* Nursing intervention for interferences with bodily function depends on the involved area. Vertebral involvement, for example, may cause weakness or impaired mobility. The patient may require assistance in moving from bed to chair or in walking. Families should be taught how to assist with these activities, while encouraging as much patient independence as possible.

Interference with normal erythrocyte activity results in progressive anemia. Patients may receive blood transfusions, iron supplements, an iron-rich diet, or all these. These measures are increasingly ineffective as the disease progresses.

Because of a poorly understood immunologic effect, patients may experience increased susceptibility to infection. They should be advised to avoid exposure to infectious persons, undue fatigue, or an inadequate diet. Extreme situations may require that the patient be placed in protective isolation.

*Fear and anxiety* Patient anxiety may be present for a variety of reasons, including fear of death, knowledge of the effects of therapy, manifestations of the problem, and concerns about family and occupational matters. The nurse must be perceptive of the existence of such anxieties and provide an opportunity for the patient to express them. Referrals, family counseling, or physician consultations may then be appropriate interventions.

**Fourth-level nursing care** Rehabilitation of the patient with Hodgkin's disease is much the same as that described previously for the leukemic patient. Early in the disease the prognosis for survival or cure may be quite good. When this is true, patients should be encouraged to resume their daily lives and be helped to make necessary adjustments.

Because Hodgkin's disease frequently affects a younger age group, there may be many fears about family, occupation, and future abilities. Nurses can assist patients with these concerns by listening and, if necessary, referring them for further professional help.

Teaching about medications and early signs of recurrent disease (e.g., lymph-node enlargement, weakness, fever) are important to ensure early intervention. Family members or significant others should also be involved in this teaching and planning.

## NON-HODGKIN'S LYMPHOMAS

All the malignant lymphomas which do not fulfill the criteria for Hodgkin's disease are classified as non-Hodgkin's lymphomas. This broad classification encompasses a wide spectrum of histologically different diseases with diverse natural histories. As a group, the non-Hodgkin's lymphomas demonstrate several features which distinguish them from Hodgkin's disease. First, *extranodal sites of origin* or presentation are common in the non-Hodgkin's lymphomas, while disease originating in lymph nodes predominates in Hodgkin's disease. Secondly, the *pattern of dissemination* in the non-Hodgkin's lymphomas is unpredictable, while in Hodgkin's disease spread to contiguous lymph nodes or adjacent extranodal sites is characteristic. Finally, in the non-Hodgkin's lymphomas even patients who appear to have localized disease initially actually have *widely disseminated lymphoma.* Less than 20 percent of patients appear to have truly localized disease.[94] In contrast, over 40 percent of patients with Hodgkin's disease have truly localized disease. These striking differences in natural history have a tremendous impact on the staging and treatment of the non-Hodgkin's lymphomas and have stimulated researchers to develop more accurate and clinically useful systems for histologic subclassifications and clinicopathologic staging. While new histologic and staging classifications have been devised in recent years, they are not uniformly utilized throughout the United States or in Europe. Furthermore, these classifications may become obsolete as the origins and predilections of the malignant lymphoid cells are more clearly defined.

### Causative Factors

As in Hodgkin's disease, the cause of non-Hodgkin's lymphomas is not known. Malignant lymphoid tumors occur in many species. In animals, genetic abnormalities, environmental factors (especially ionizing radiation), immunologic defects, and viral factors have been implicated as etiologic agents (see Chap. 5 for detailed discussion). In man a significantly higher incidence of malignant lymphoma has also been reported in patients with a variety of immunologic disorders and also in renal-transplant patients who have undergone immunosuppression for prolonged periods. Various etiologic mechanism are now postulated which suggest that the pathogenesis of malignant lymphoma may relate to a loss of immunocompetence, induction by carcinogenic chemicals, or activation of a latent viral component. To date, however, no conclusive evidence exists to prove any theory.

The incidence of non-Hodgkin's lymphoma is about 14,300 new cases annually. The peak incidence of non-Hodgkin's lymphoma occurs between ages 60 and 69, which is later than that in patients with Hodgkin's disease. About 25 percent of patients develop the disease in their fifties. Children and young adults are also affected, but the incidence is lower and the disease is quite different in behavior. Males develop all lymphomas more commonly than females.[95] Certain lymphomas have a striking predilection for geographic areas. Burkitt's lymphoma, although it occurs in the United States, is most commonly found in tropical climates such as Uganda.[96]

### Pathophysiology

The diagnosis of non-Hodgkin's lymphoma, like that of other cancers, must be made by identification of neoplastic cells in a tissue biopsy. Since these lymphomas commonly present in extranodal sites where the histologic picture may be atypical compared to nodal presentations, the diagnosis may be difficult in many cases. A pathologist specializing in hematologic and lymphoreticular neoplasms must often be consulted to confirm the diagnosis. As in Hodgkin's disease, the differential diagnosis must exclude acute and chronic infections.

At present, non-Hodgkin's lymphomas are divided into lymphocytic and histiocytic types. Each type may appear in a nodular or a diffuse pattern. Both the cellular component and the architectural pattern have clinical significance in terms of patterns of involvement, response to therapy, and prognosis.[97] *Lymphocytic lymphomas* are composed of abnormal small lymphocytic cells which may be well differentiated (mature) or poorly differentiated (immature) in appearance. *Histiocytic lymphomas* are composed of large neoplastic cells which are called *histiocytic* because they resemble reticulum cells or histiocytes morphologically. However, convincing evidence now demonstrates that many of these "histiocytic" cells have T and B cell surface markers and are probably transformed lymphocytes which are malignant, and histiocytic only in appearance.[98] *Mixed lymphomas* also occur and are composed of abnormal small lymphocytic cells and large transformed lymphocytic cells, mistakenly referred to as histiocytic cells. The so-called *"nodular"* lymphomas are characterized by a distinct nodular pattern which can be seen in the involved lymph node or tissues. A *diffuse pattern* is typified by monotonous replacement of tissues by malignant cells which obliterate the normal architecture of the involved tissues. Nodularity is important to note, because patients with nodular forms of lymphoma, regardless of cell type, have a better prognosis. *Undifferentiated* or *stem-cell lymphomas* can occur in nodular or diffuse patterns, although nodularity in this histology is rare.

In the past, only three classifications existed. These categories, lymphosarcoma, reticulum-cell sarcoma, and giant follicular lymphoma, were abandoned because the distinguishing features were vague and there was considerable overlap between the categories. Table 7-5 shows the relationship of the old categories to the present-day histologic classification.

The most common presentation in patients who are diagnosed with non-Hodgkin's lymphoma is *painless lymphadenopathy*. One-third of all patients, however, present with manifestations of extranodal disease which include subcutaneous nodules, bone pain, gastrointestinal masses, or tonsillar masses. Other extranodal sites of involvement occur in the pancreas, pleura, liver (manifested by hepatomegaly), kidney, bone marrow, and central nervous system.[99] Although systemic (A and B) symptoms occur, they are far less common and do not carry the same prognostic significance as in Hodgkin's disease.

**Clinical and pathologic staging** Once the histologic diagnosis of lymphoma is firmly established, patients are clinically staged in a manner similar to the clinical staging of patients with Hodgkin's disease. Patients with minimal adenopathy and seemingly localized lymphoma often have grossly abnormal radiologic examinations on chest x-ray, lymphangiogram, intravenous pyelogram, skeletal films, gastrointestinal series, or sinus films. Nonetheless, patients with extranodal disease may have normal clinical staging evaluations. For this reason, pathologic staging of patients for occult disease in extranodal sites is essential. A staging study conducted at the National Cancer Institute confirmed that disseminated disease, Stages III and IV, could be proved in the vast majority of patients who were consistently staged with routine biopsies of certain extranodal sites.[100] Of particular importance were routine bone-marrow biopsies which revealed Stage IV disease in about 40 percent of 170 consecutive patients. In addition, liver biopsies were abnormal in 50 percent of patients by percutaneous liver biopsy (21 percent) or biopsy obtained during peritoneoscopy (29 percent). In most patients, blood counts were completely normal, and tests for abnormal liver function and enlargement were normal even though one or more sites were positive for lymphomatous involvement.

The use of *peritoneoscopy* to document the presence of lymphoma in the liver parenchyma obviates performance of an exploratory laparotomy in most patients. The non-Hodgkin's lymphomas tend to occur most frequently in patients over the age of 50. The elimination of the need for laparotomy for accurate staging of this group of patients, who have a higher incidence of serious postoperative complications, has significantly improved the morbidity associated with staging evaluations and has reduced the delay between diagnosis and the start of therapy.

Nursing intervention throughout the staging evaluation is directed toward preparing patients for procedures (including explanations of why the procedures are needed), emotional support, and prevention of complications such as infection or hemorrhage.

**TABLE 7-5**
CLASSIFICATION OF THE NON-HODGKIN'S LYMPHOMAS

| | |
|---|---|
| Malignant lymphoma, undifferentiated, Burkitt's type | Burkitt's tumor |
| Malignant lymphoma, undifferentiated, pleomorphic type | |
| Malignant lymphoma, histiocytic type | Reticulum-cell sarcoma |
| Malignant lymphoma, histiocytic-lymphocytic (mixed-cell) type | |
| Malignant lymphoma, lymphocytic type, poorly differentiated | Lymphosarcoma |
| Malignant lymphoma, lymphocytic type, well differentiated | |

## Intervention

The choice of *therapy* in patients with non-Hodgkin's lymphoma is influenced by the extent of disease as determined by a thorough staging evaluation and the histologic classification. Staging is designed to separate those patients with truly localized stages from those with disease which has disseminated to distant lymph nodes or extranodal sites. The capacity to deliver curative therapy depends on the ability of the treatment modality to effectively kill all malignant cells. Curative treatment by both effective treatment modalities, radiotherapy and chemotherapy, is dependent on the exposure of all malignant cells to tumoricidal dosages without producing prohibitive toxicity to normal tissues.

**Radiotherapy** As has been emphasized, the non-Hodgkin's lymphomas are localized in less than 20 percent of all patients.[101] For this reason, cure rates with intensive radiotherapy alone are low compared to those achieved in Hodgkin's disease. Nonetheless, survival of patients treated with radiotherapy for apparently limited disease demonstrates that truly localized lymphoma does exist in a fraction of all patients. It is this group of patients, with Stage I lymphoma presenting in a single nodal or extranodal site, that may be cured with intensive radiotherapy. Conventional radiotherapy to involved lymph nodes entails delivery of 3500 to 4500 rads given over 3 to 4 weeks.[102] Even in patients who are not cured, prolonged survival may be seen in patients with localized *nodular* lymphomas, with median survival in excess of 6 years.[103] In general, patients with *diffuse* histopathologic subtypes, treated with localized radiotherapy, have high recurrence rates and short remissions, presumably because of occult disease outside the field of irradiation.

Truly localized *extranodal* lymphomas can also be treated successfully with localized radiotherapy but may require higher dosages to achieve permanent cures. Tumor doses of 5000 to 6000 rads are given to the involved field over 5 to 6 weeks.[104] In addition, regional lymphatics are usually encompassed within the field of treatment.

Radiotherapeutic management of Stage II lymphoma (extranodal primaries with regional lymph-node involvement or bilateral lymph-node involvement) does not produce good cure rates when employed alone as the primary therapy. When employed with systemic chemotherapy, however, radiation therapy can improve the results of treatment, especially when large tumor masses are present.[105]

Total body irradiation (TBI) is an experimental radiotherapeutic approach which is under investigation in patients who have advanced (Stages III and IV) lymphocytic lymphoma. Data from clinical trials with and without TNI demonstrate that TBI is effective in producing complete remissions in patients with prognostically favorable histopathologic types of lymphoma.

**Chemotherapy** A great number of chemotherapeutic agents are active in the non-Hodgkin's lymphomas. However, as in Hodgkin's disease, complete remissions with single-drug administration are uncommon, occurring in less than 20 percent, and are usually of short duration. As MOPP emerged as an effective drug combination in Hodgkin's disease, combination chemotherapy was devised and put to clinical trial for the non-Hodgkin's lymphomas. At present a great number of clinical trials evaluating a variety of combinations are in progress. The most common agents used in combination include cyclophosphamide, prednisone, vincristine, procarbazine, methotrexate, adriamycin, and bleomycin. Complete remissions can be induced in approximately 50 percent of all patients with advanced disease, varying with histologic subtypes.[106] The impact of chemotherapy on the overall survival of patients with non-Hodgkin's lymphoma is a significant prolongation in life.

Of particular interest and significance are the results of effective combination chemotherapy for the rapidly progressive and fatal histologic types. In these forms of lymphoma, radiotherapy does not exert a favorable effect on survival in the majority of patients. Less than 5 percent achieve complete remissions, and less than 10 percent survive beyond 2 years.[107] Effective drug combinations such as MOPP, however, can produce complete remission rates in the range of 50 percent.[108-111]

## Nursing Problems and Interventions

Patients with Hodgkin's disease and non-Hodgkin's lymphomas may present initially with nursing problems which require special management. These may also occur late in patients whose disease has not been successfully controlled. Early recognition and prompt intervention are essential to prevent severe, life-threatening complications. The reader should refer to the chapters dealing with the involved organ system for specific nursing intervention.

*Ureteral obstruction* from pelvic to periaortic lymphadenopathy can impair renal function. Management with local radiotherapy or systemic chemotherapy is based on the stage of disease and prior treatment. Diffuse lymphomas may also involve the kidneys, causing unexplained renal failure. When renal involvement is suspected, urinary cytology and intravenous pyelography may be employed to identify enlarged kidneys or masses within the kidneys. Nursing assessment of renal function prior to and during treatment with low-dose radiotherapy or systemic chemotherapy is essential.

*Superior vena cava syndrome* can be caused by massive enlargement of mediastinal and paratracheal lymph nodes, obstructing the venous blood flow to the heart. Patients often present with severe respiratory embarrassment, with wheezing, dyspnea, and inability to breathe unless sitting upright, owing to the severity of the obstruction. This syndrome represents a medical emergency and must be managed immediately with radiotherapy or chemotherapy to reduce the lymphadenopathy and relieve the obstruction. Nursing intervention must incorporate knowledge of the course of the disease, prior therapy, and management of patients in acute respiratory distress.

*Pleural effusions* can occur as a result of lymphatic obstruction in the mediastinal area or secondary to pleural or pulmonary involvement with lymphoma. A diagnostic thoracentesis with an examination of pleural fluid or pleural biopsy is warranted. Systemic chemotherapy or intrapleural installation of drugs is utilized for control of the effusions.

*Central nervous system (CNS) involvement* may complicate the course of non-Hodgkin's lymphoma, especially in patients with diffuse histologic patterns. In contrast to Hodgkin's disease, which rarely involves the brain parenchyma, massive lesions may occur. Patients usually present with cranial nerve palsies or evidence of increased intracranial pressure with or without lymphomatous meningitis. As in acute leukemia, even patients in apparent remission may develop CNS involvement. Nursing assessment must include a careful evaluation of patients for headache, nausea and vomiting (unrelated to therapy), and papilledema. Management consists of whole-brain irradiation, corticosteroids, and intrathecal administration of methotrexate.

*Spinal-cord compression* from extradural tumor masses or collapsed vertebrae may also cause neurologic complications. This represents a medical emergency requiring immediate management with surgical decompression (laminectomy) plus radiotherapy or systemic chemotherapy. Compression of peripheral nerves by large tumor masses produces evidence of neurologic damage. Local control may be achieved with radiotherapy. Nursing care must include a careful neurologic evaluation, effective pain management, and preparation for surgical or radiotherapeutic treatment.

Bone is a common extranodal site of disease in the non-Hodgkin's lymphomas. *Hypercalcemia* may occur as a complication of bone involvement. Early intervention to prevent permanent serious renal damage is essential. A detailed description of medical and nursing intervention is included in the discussion of multiple myeloma.

*Bone-marrow involvement* can result in leukopenia, anemia, and thrombocytopenia. In this situation, full doses of chemotherapy are given (despite low blood counts) to treat disease within the bone marrow. Effective chemotherapy generally produces a rise in blood counts rather than more severe depression of marrow elements, as the tumor cells are destroyed and the marrow repopulates with normal hematopoietic elements.

*Anemia* can occur in patients who have lymphoma. The cause of anemia may be hemolysis (due to destruction of cells which are coated with antibody) or hypersplenism (increased sequestration and destruction of cells within an enlarged spleen). Splenectomy is often beneficial for patients who do not achieve control with chemotherapy or radiotherapy.

Nurses are frequently in the position to recognize the many disease- or treatment-related complications that have been described. Early intervention is facilitated when the nurse can pick up early and often subtle signs and symptoms of abnormalities. As already indicated, the cytotoxic action of effective radiotherapy and chemotherapy causes damage to normal tissues, particularly those with a high growth rate such as the cells of the bone marrow and gastrointestinal mucosa and germinal cells. The role of the nurse is to anticipate and ameliorate the toxic effects of the treatment and to teach the patient how to recognize, manage, and report early evidence of toxicity. Good patient teaching can minimize avoidable complications and enable patients to alert both nurses and physicians when nursing or medical intervention is necessary.

# REFERENCES

1 Rose Ruth Ellison, "Acute Myelocytic Leukemia," in J. Holland and E. Frei (eds.), *Cancer Medicine,* Lea & Febiger, Philadelphia, 1973, p. 1231.

2 Ibid., p. 1201.

3 R. E. Gallagher and R. C. Gallo, "Type C RNA Tumor Virus Isolated from Cultured Human Acute Myelogenous Leukemia Cells," *Science,* **187:**350, January 1975.

4 Ellison, op. cit., pp. 1215–1216.

5 Ellison, op. cit., p. 1204.

6 Ellison, op. cit., pp. 1228–1229.

7 K. B. McCredie et al., "The Management of Acute Leukemia in Adults," in *Cancer Chemotherapy,* Year Book, Chicago, 1975, pp. 173–186.

8 T. Caspersson, G. Gahrton, J. Lindsten, and L. Zech, "Identification of the Philadelphia Chromosome as a Number 22 by Quinacrine Mustard Analysis," *Exp Cell Res,* **63:**238, 1970.

9 J. Whang-Peng, C. P. Canellos, P. P. Carbone, and J. H. Tjio, "Clinical Duplications of Cytogenetic Variants in Chronic Myelocytic Leukemia (CML)," *Blood,* **32:**755, 1968.

10 R. Willemze, H. Hillen, C. A. Hartgrink-Groenereld, and C. Haanen, "Treatment of Acute Lymphoblastic Leukemia in Adolescents and Adults: A Retrospective Study of 41 Patients," *Blood,* **46:**823–834.

11 B. D. Clarkson and J. Fried, "Changing Concepts of Treatment in Acute Leukemia," *Med Clin North Am,* **55:**566–567, May 1971.

12 Willemze et al., op. cit., p. 824.

13 D. T. Rowlands, R. P. Daniele, P. C. Nowell, and H. A. Wurzel, "Characterization of Lymphocyte Subpopulations in Chronic Lymphocytic Leukemia," *Cancer,* **34:**1962–1970, December 1974.

14 Ellison, op. cit., p. 1258.

15 W. Williams, E. Beutler, A. J. Ersley, and R. W. Rundles, *Hematology,* McGraw-Hill, New York, 1972, p. 885.

16 Ellison, op. cit., p. 1209.

17 Ellison, op. cit., p. 1236.

18 B. G. Leventhal and S. Hersh, "Modern Treatment of Childhood Leukemia," *Nurs Digest,* July–August 1975, pp. 12–15.

19 Ellison, op. cit., p. 1258.

20 J. U. Gutterman et al., "Chemoimmunotherapy of Adult Acute Leukemia," *Lancet,* 14 December 1974, p. 1406.

21 J. E. Mason, V. T. DeVita, and G. P. Canellos, "Thrombocytosis in Chronic Granulocytic Leukemia: Incidence and Clinical Significance," *Blood,* **44:**483–487.

22 Ellison, op. cit., p. 1266.

23 Malle A. Snider, "Helpful Hints on IV's," *Am J Nurs,* **74:**1981, November 1974.

24 A. S. Levine, S. C. Schimpff, R. G. Graw, and R. C. Young, "Hematologic Malignancies and Other Marrow Failure States: Progression in the Management of Complicating Infections," *Semin Hematol,* **11:**153, April 1974.

25 E. M. Hersh, J. P. Whitecar, K. B. McCredie, G. P. Bodey, and E. J. Freireich, "Chemotherapy, Immunocompetence, Immunosuppression, and Prognosis in Acute Leukemias," *N Engl J Med,* **285:**1211–1216, 1971.

26 Levine et al., op. cit., pp. 157–158.

27 E. M. Hersh et al., "Causes of Death in Acute Leukemia," *JAMA,* **193:**105, 1965.

28 A. S. Levine et al., "Protected Environments and Prophylactic Antibiotics: A Prospective Controlled Study of their Utility in the Therapy of Acute Leukemia," *N Engl J Med,* **288:**477, 1973.

29 E. D. Thomas and R. B. Epstein, "Bone Marrow Transplantation in Acute Leukemia," *Cancer Res,* **25:**1521, 1965.

30 R. G. Graw and R. A. Yankee, "Principles of Hematologic Supportive Care," *Med Clin North Am,* **57:**445, March 1973.

31 Williams et al., op. cit., p. 715.

32 Ellison, loc. cit.

33 McCredie et al., loc. cit.

34 Ibid.

35 G. P. Canellos, V. T. DeVita, P. Schein, B. A. Chabner, and R. C. Young, "The Chronic Leukemias: Current Therapeutic Concepts," *7th National Cancer Conference Proceedings,* Lippincott, Philadelphia, 1973, pp. 351–354.

36 Jean Bernard and Joseph Tanzer, "Chronic Myelocytic Leukemia," in J. Holland and E. Frei (eds.), *Cancer Medicine,* Lea & Febiger, Philadelphia, 1973, p. 1253.

37 W. Crosby, "To Treat or Not to Treat Acute Granulocytic Leukemia," *Arch Intern Med,* **122:**79, 1968.

38 D. C. Ihde, G. P. Canellos, J. H. Schwartz, and V. T. DeVita, "Splenectomy in the Chronic Phase of Chronic Granulocytic Leukemia," *Ann Intern Med,* **84:**17–21, January 1976.

39 G. P. Canellos, V. T. DeVita, J. Whang-Peng, and P. P. Carbone, "Hematologic and Cytogenetic Remission of Blastic Transformation in Chronic Granulocytic Leukemia," *Blood,* **38:**671, December 1971.

40 E. J. Freireich, E. S. Henderson, M. R. Karon, and E. Frei III, "The Treatment of Acute Leukemia Considered with Respect to Population Kinetics," in *The Proliferation and Spread of Neoplastic Cells,* 21st

Symposium on Funadmental Cancer Research, M. D. Anderson Institute for Cancer Research, Williams & Wilkins, Baltimore, 1968, p. 441.

41 E. M. Hersh et al., "Serial Studies on Immunocompetence of Patients Undergoing Chemotherapy for Acute Leukemia," *J Clin Invest,* **54:**401, 1974.

42 B. A. Nies et al., "Persistence of Extramedullary Leukemia Infiltrate during Marrow Remission of Acute Leukemia," *Blood,* **26:**133, 1965.

43 H. O. Husti, J. A. Pur, M. S. Verzosa, J. V. Simone, and D. Pinkel, "Prevention of Central Nervous System Leukemia by Irradiation," *Cancer,* **32:**585–597, September 1973.

44 Ibid., pp. 591–592.

45 Williams et al., op. cit., pp. 885–886.

46 W. H. Knospe, U. Loeb, Jr., and C. M. Huguley, Jr., "Bi-Weekly Chlorambucil Treatment of Chronic Lymphocytic Leukemia," *Cancer,* **33:**555–562, 1974.

47 Williams et al., op. cit., p. 888.

48 R. E. Johnson and U. Ruhl, "Treatment of Chronic Lymphocytic Leukemia with Emphasis on Total Body Irradiation," *Int J Radiat Oncol Biol Physics,* **1:**387–397, March–April, 1976.

49 J. Williams, "Understanding the Feelings of the Dying," *Nurs '76,* pp. 52–56, 1976.

50 R. F. Bakemeier, "The Malignant Lymphomas," in P. Rubin (ed.), *Clinical Oncology: A Multidisciplinary Approach,* American Cancer Society, Rochester, 1974, p. 443.

51 D. E. Bergsagel, "Plasma Cell Neoplasms," in J. F. Holland and E. Frei III (eds.), *Cancer Medicine,* Lea & Febiger, Philadelphia, 1973, pp. 1336–1337.

52 Ibid., p. 1332.

53 E. F. Osserman, "Plasma-Cell Myeloma," *N Engl J Med,* **261:**952–1006, 1959.

54 M. Farhanje and E. F. Osserman, "The Treatment of Multiple Myeloma," *Semin Hematol,* **10:**149–161, April 1973.

55 S. K. Carter, "An Overview of the Status of the Nitrosoureas in Other Tumors," *Cancer Chemother Rep,* **4:**35–46, 1973.

56 P. B. Bergevin, D. C. Tormey, and J. Blom, "Guide to the Use of Cancer Chemotherpeutic Agents," *Mod Treatment,* **9:**218, 1972.

57 Bergsagel, op. cit., p. 1357.

58 C. W. Berard, "Histopathology of the Lymphomas in Hematology," in Williams et al. (eds.), *Hematology,* McGraw-Hill, New York, 1972, pp. 901–912.

59 J. C. Brouet, S. Labaume, and M. Seligman, "Evaluation of T and B Lymphocyte Membrane Markers in Human Non-Hodgkin's Malignant Lymphomata," *Br J Cancer,* **31**(Suppl II):121–128, 1975.

60 T. Hodgkin, "On Some of the Morbid Appearances of the Absorbent Glands and Spleen," *Trans Med Chir Soc Lond,* **17:**68, 1832.

61 Berard, op. cit., p. 902.

62 G. S. Seif, and A. Spriggs, "Chromosome Changes in Hodgkin's Disease," *J Nat Cancer Inst,* **39:**557–560, 1967.

63 B. MacMahon, "Epidemiological Evidence on the Nature of Hodgkin's Disease," *Cancer,* **10:**1045–1054, 1967.

64 N. J. Vianna et al., "Hodgkin's Disease: Cases with Features of a Community Outbreak," *Ann Intern Med,* **77:**169–180, 1972.

65 D. V. Razis, H. D. Diamond, and L. F. Craver, "Familial Hodgkin's Disease: Its Significance and Implications," *Ann Inter Med,* **51:**933, 1969.

66 Ibid.

67 R. J. Lukes and J. J. Butler, "The Pathology and Nomenclature of Hodgkin's Disease," *Cancer Res,* **26:**1068–1081, 1966.

68 R. J. Lukes, "Criteria for Involvement of Lymph Node Bone Marrow, Spleen and Liver in Hodgkin's Disease," *Cancer Res,* **31:**1755–1767, 1971.

69 H. Jackson and F. Parker, *Hodgkin's Disease and Allied Disorders,* Oxford, New York, 1974.

70 S. A. Rosenberg, "Hodgkin's Disease," in J. Holland and E. Frei (eds.), *Cancer Medicine,* Lea & Febiger, Philadelphia, 1973, p. 1278.

71 R. J. Lukes, L. F. Craver, T. C. Hall, H. Rappaport, and P. Rubin, "Report of the Nomenclature Committee," *Cancer Res,* **26:**1311, 1966.

72 A. R. Keller et al., "Correlations of Histopathology with Other Prognostic Indicators in Hodgkin's Disease," *Cancer,* **22:**487, 1966.

73 C. W. Berard et al., "The Relationship of Histopathological Subtype to Clinical Stage of Hodgkin's Disease at Diagnosis," *Cancer Res,* **31:**1776–1785, 1971.

74 R. Brown, et al., "Hodgkin's Disease: Immunologic, Clinical, and Histologic Features of 50 Untreated Patients," *Ann Intern Med,* **67:**271, 1967.

75 *1976 Cancer Facts and Figures,* American Cancer Society, New York, 1975.

76 B. MacMahon, "Epidemiological Considerations in Staging of Hodgkin's Disease," *Cancer Res,* **31:**1854–1857, 1971.

77 Rosenberg, op. cit., p. 1277.

78 P. Rubin, "The Malignant Lymphomas," in *Clinical Oncology for Medical Students and Physicians,* American Cancer Society, Rochester, 1974.

79 H. S. Kaplan, "Contiguity and Progression in Hodgkin's Disease," *Cancer Res,* **31:**1811–1813, 1971.

80 P. Carbone et al., "Report of the Committee on

Hodgkin's Disease Staging Classification," *Cancer Res,* **31:**1860–1861, 1971.

81  R. C. Young and V. T. DeVita, "Hodgkin's Disease," in *Current Therapy,* Saunders, Philadelphia, 1974, pp. 270–277.

82  V. T. DeVita and G. P. Canellos, "Treatment of the Lymphomas," *Semin Hematol,* **9:**193–209, 1972.

83  Ibid.

84  V. T. DeVita et al., "Peritoneoscopy in the Staging of Hodgkin's Disease," *Cancer Res,* **31:**1746–1750, 1971.

85  Rosenberg, op. cit., p. 1295.

86  Ibid.

87  Young and DeVita, op. cit., p. 274.

88  V. T. DeVita, A. Serpick, and P. Carbone, "Combination Chemotherapy of Advanced Hodgkin's Disease," *Ann Intern Med,* **73:**881–893, 1970.

89  Ibid.

90  V. T. DeVita, G. P. Canellos, and S. P. Hubbard, "Chemotherapy of Hodgkin's Disease: A Ten Year Progress Report," *Proc Am Soc Clin Oncol,* 1976, p. 269.

91  J. H. Moxley, V. T. DeVita, and K. Brace, "Intensive Combination Chemotherapy and Y-Irradiation in Hodgkin's Disease," *Cancer Res,* **27:**1258–1268, 1967.

92  T. J. McElwain et al., "Combination Chemotherapy in Advanced and Recurrent Hodgkin's Disease," *Natl Cancer Inst Monogr,* **36:**395, 1972.

93  DeVita, Serpick, and Carbone, loc. cit.

94  P. P. Carbone and V. T. DeVita, "Malignant Lymphoma," in J. Holland and E. Frei (eds.), *Cancer Medicine,* Lea & Febiger, Philadelphia, 1973, pp. 1302–1319.

95  Ibid.

96  J. L. Ziegler, "Burkitt's Tumor," in ibid., pp. 1327–1330.

97  R. C. Braylan, E. Jaffe, and C. W. Berard, "Malignant Lymphomas: Current Classification and New Observations," in S. C. Sommers (ed.), *Pathology Annual 1975,* Appleton-Century-Crofts, 1975, pp. 218–270.

98  Ibid.

99  Carbone and DeVita, op. cit., pp. 1306–1307.

100  B. A. Chabner et al., "Sequential Non-Surgical and Surgical Staging of Non-Hodgkin's Lymphoma," *Ann Intern Med,* **85:**149–154, 1976.

101  Ibid.

102  S. E. Jones, Z. Fuks, H. Kaplan, and S. A. Rosenberg, "Non-Hodgkin's Lymphomas. V. Results of Radiotherapy," *Cancer,* **32:**682–691, 1973.

103  Ibid.

104  J. Newall and M. Friedman, "Reticulum Cell Sarcoma, Part II, Radiation Dose for Each Type," *Radiology,* **94:**643, 1970.

105  V. T. DeVita and P. Schein, "The Use of Drugs in Combination for the Treatment of Cancer: Rationale and Results," *N Engl J Med,* **288:**998–1006, 1973.

106  V. T. DeVita, C. Berard, and R. Johnson, "The Non-Hodgkin's Lymphomas," *Cancer Med* (in press).

107  Ibid.

108  V. T. DeVita, G. P. Canellos, and B. A. Chabner, "Advanced Diffuse Histiocytic Lymphoma: A Potentially Curable Disease," *Lancet,* **1:**248–250, 1975.

109  D. Berd et al., "Long Term Remission in Diffuse Histiocytic Lymphoma Treated with Combination Sequential Chemotherapy," *Cancer,* **35:**1050–1054, 1975.

110  P. S. Schein, et al., "Bleomycin Adriamycin Cyclophosphamide Vincristine and Prednisone (BACOP) Combination," *Ann Intern Med,* **85:**417–422, 1976.

111  A. Skarin, D. Rosenthal, U. S. Moloney, and E. Frei, "Treatment of Advanced Non-Hodgkin's Lymphoma (NHL) with Bleomycin (B), Adriamycin (A), Cyclophosphamide (C), Vincristine (V) and Prednisone (P) (BACOP)," *Proc Am Assoc Cancer Res,* **15:** 133, 1974.

## BIBLIOGRAPHY

Bonadonna, G., R. Zucal, and M. DeLena: "Combined Chemotherapy (MOPP vs. ABVD) Plus RT in Advanced Hodgkin's Disease," *Proc Am Soc Clin Oncol,* 1976.

Coltman, C. A., E. Frei, and T. E. Moon: "MOPP Maintenance Versus Unmaintained Remission of Advanced Hodgkin's Disease: 7.2 Year Follow-up," *Proc Am Soc Clin Oncol,* 1976, p. 289.

Foley, Genevieve, and Ann-Marie McCarthy: "Leukemia," *Am J Nurs,* **76**(7):1109–1114, July 1976.

Freedman, Samuel O.: *Clinical Immunology,* Harper & Row, 1971, New York, p. 15.

Fuks, Z., and H. Kaplan: "Recurrence Rates Following Radiation Therapy of Nodular and Diffuse Malignant Lymphomas," *Radiology,* **108:**675–680, 1973.

Glidewell, O., and J. F. Holland: "Clinical Trials of the ALGB in Acute Lymphocytic Leukemia of Childhood," *Proc Vth Int Symp Comparative Leukemia Res,* Padova, Italy (in press).

Holland, J., and E. Frei (eds.): *Cancer Medicine,* Lea & Febiger, Philadelphia, 1973.

Johnson, R. E.: "Total Body Irradiation (TBI) as Primary Therapy for Advanced Lymphosarcoma," *Cancer,* **35:**242–246, 1975.

Kaplan, H. S.: *Hodgkin's Disease,* Harvard, Cambridge, 1972.

Newall, J. and M. Freidman: "Reticulum Cell Sarcoma, Part III, Prognosis," *Radiology,* **97:**99, 1970.

Peckham, M. (ed.): "Symposium on Non-Hodgkin's Lymphomata," *Br J Cancer,* vol. 31, suppl. 2, H. L. Lewis, London, 1975.

Rappaport, H.: "Tumors of the Hematopoietic System," in *Atlas of Tumor Pathology,* Section III, Armed Forces Institute of Pathology, Washington, D. C., 1966.

Rubin, P. (ed.): *Clinical Oncology for Medical Students and Physicians: A Multidisciplinary Approach,* 4th ed., American Cancer Society, New York, 1974.

Schoenberg, D., A. C. Carr, D. Peretz, and A. H. Kutscher: *Psychosocial Aspects of Terminal Care,* Columbia, New York, 1972.

Smith, Dorothy, and Carol Germain: *Care of the Adult Patient,* Lippincott, New York, 1975.

Young, R. C., et al.: "Maintenance Chemotherapy for Advanced Hodgkin's Disease in Remission," *Lancet,* **1:**1339–1343, 1973.

Young, R. C., et al.: "Patterns of Relapse after Complete Remission in Hodgkin's Disease Treated with Nitrogen Mustard, Vincristine, Procarbazine and Prednisone Chemotherapy," *Proc Am Soc Clin Oncol,* 1975.

Zarafonetis, C. V. (ed.): *Proc Int Conf Leukemia-Lymphoma,* Lea & Febiger, Philadelphia, 1968.

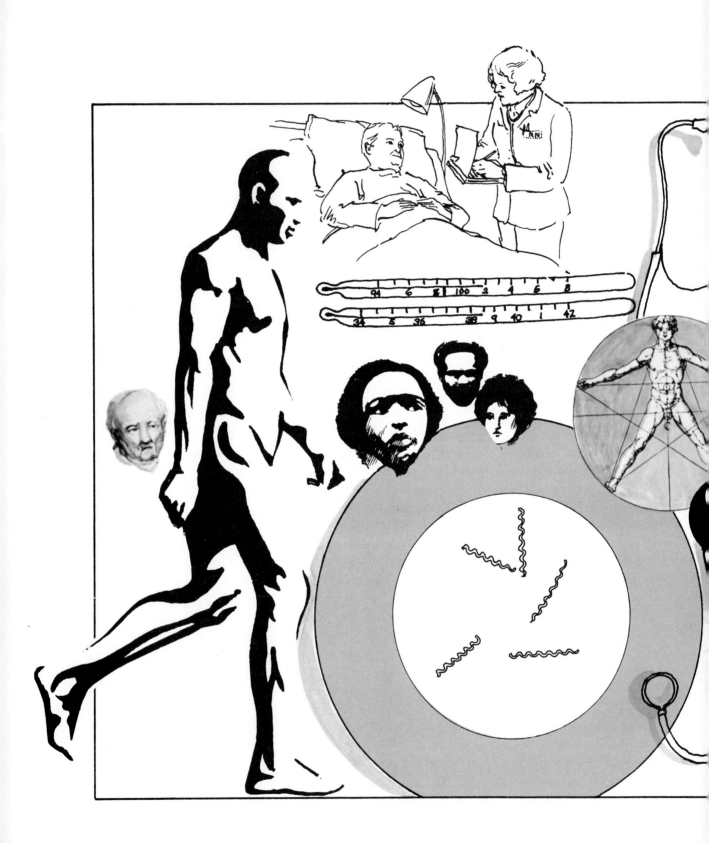

# PART 3
## INFLAMMATION AND IMMUNITY

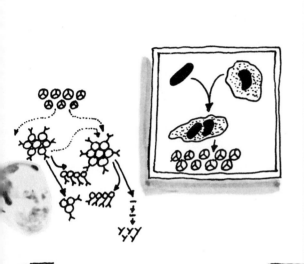

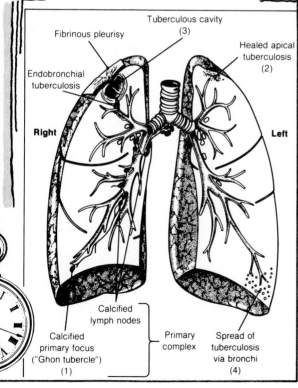

Tuberculous cavity (3)

Fibrinous pleurisy

Healed apical tuberculosis (2)

Endobronchial tuberculosis

**Right**

**Left**

Calcified lymph nodes

Calcified primary focus ("Ghon tubercle") (1)

Primary complex

Spread of tuberculosis via bronchi (4)

# 8

# THE CONCEPTS OF INFLAMMATION AND IMMUNITY*

Claire Ford Dunbar
Lora B. Roach

**M**icroorganisms, viruses, and the potential for bodily injury are part of everyone's environment. Without intrinsic protection, a person's interaction with these portions of the environment would result in an altered state of health. To preserve and protect the body against invasion by organisms and damage by injury, the immune system and the process of inflammation go into action.

Leukocytes and the reticuloendothelial system play vital roles in this protection of the body against injurious agents. This chapter therefore begins with a discussion of their structure and function. Following this discussion, the processes of inflammation and immunity, as well as physical assessment of the skin, are described. The emphasis in the physical assessment section is on inflammatory skin conditions and conditions of the skin that are part of an immune response.

## LEUKOCYTES

Leukocytes fall into two basic classifications, *granular* and *non-granular.* The division is based on the nuclear and cytoplasmic appearance of the various cellular components. Granular leukocytes (granulocytes) include *polymorphonuclear neutrophils, polymorphonuclear eosinophils,* and *polymorphonuclear basophils,* as shown in Table 8-1. The cell of origin for all granulocytes is the *myeloblast,* which is found in the bone marrow; the major function of granulocytes is phagocytosis.

Nongranular leukocytes include *lymphocytes* (large and small) and *monocytes.* Lymphocytes originate from lymphocytic stem cells in the bone marrow. However, before the lymphocyte is able to function, it must be processed in the lymphoid tissue. Lymphoid tissue includes the thymus, lymph nodes, spleen, tonsils, gut, and bone marrow. The majority of small lymphocytes, highly necessary for cellular immunity, are believed to be derived from processing in the thymus and are therefore referred to as *T cells* or *T lymphocytes.* Other lymphocytes are differentiated in an unknown lymphoid structure in man that is equivalent to the bursa of Fabricius in birds. These are known as *B cells* or *B lymphocytes* and are responsible for antibody production (humoral immunity).

Monocytes are produced in the bone marrow and have the monoblast as their cell of origin, as

* The inflammation and immunity section was written by Claire Ford Dunbar and the physical assessment section by Lora B. Roach.

shown in Table 8-1. They are believed to mature into macrophages as necessary for phagocytosis.

## Functional Characteristics

Leukocytes have several specialized properties that make them well suited for their role in inflammation and immunity. These specialized properties include *diapedesis, ameboid motion, chemotaxis,* and *phagocytosis.*

**Diapedesis** The peculiar ability of leukocytes to pass through the pores between cells, particularly the endothelial cells in blood vessels, is known as *diapedesis.* This process involves the passing through, little by little, of each individual leukocyte. Thus leukocytes, and particularly neutrophils, are able to squeeze between endothelial cells in the walls of the smallest vessels and get out into the tissues, where they move about by ameboid motion, as illustrated in Fig. 8-1.

**Ameboid motion** Granulocytes and, to a lesser extent, monocytes and large lymphocytes extend pseudopodia (footlike projections) and travel in a "fluid" manner known as *ameboid motion.* This movement occurs when a pseudopodium is extended by the forward part of the cell; the remainder of the cell then moves in the direction of the extended portion (Fig. 8-1). Frequently this movement by leukocytes within the tissues is in response to a chemotactic substance. The ameboid activity may be either *positive* (toward the substance) or *negative* (away from the substance).

**Chemotaxis** Chemical products within tissues either attract or repel leukocytes through a process known as *chemotaxis.* Substances resulting in positive (or attracting) chemotaxis include the products of inflammation, complement derivatives, and bacterial toxins. This process of attracting leukocytes is especially important in situations of inflammation; it enables these defensive cells to get to an area quickly to perform their protective function of phagocytosis (Fig. 8-1).

**Phagocytosis** The engulfing and subsequent destruction or inactivation of foreign substances by body cells is known as *phagocytosis* ("cell eating").

**TABLE 8-1**
CLASSIFICATION OF LEUKOCYTES

| Cell | Normal Blood Concentration | Description | Formation Site | Function |
|---|---|---|---|---|
| TOTAL LEUKOCYTES | 5000–9000/ml | | | |
| GRANULAR LEUKOCYTES | | | | |
| Polymorphonuclear neutrophils (PMN) | 62–65% of total leukocytes | Fine granules in cytoplasm; two- to three-lobed nucleus | Bone marrow (*myeloblast*) | Phagocytosis |
| Polymorphonuclear eosinophils | 2–4% of total | Large granules in cytoplasm; bilobed nucleus | Bone marrow (*myeloblast*) | Weak role in phagocytosis; increased concentration in the presence of foreign protein, perhaps a detoxifying function; increased in parasitic infection |
| Polymorphonuclear basophils | 0.2–0.5% of total | Large granules in cytoplasm; bilobed nucleus | Bone marrow (*myeloblast*) | Complete function unknown; resemble mast cells in the release of histamine and heparin; increased during inflammation |
| NONGRANULAR LEUKOCYTES | | | | |
| Lymphocytes | 25% of total | Nongranular cytoplasm; large globular nucleus | Bone marrow (lymphoblasts) go to thymus and bursal-equivalent lymphoid tissue to differentiate into thymic (T) and bursal (B) lymphocytes | T cells responsible for cellular immunity; B cells produce large lymphocytes and plasma cells which form the antibodies of humoral immunity |
| Monocytes | 5–7% of total | Nongranular cytoplasm; large, deeply indented nucleus | Bone marrow (monoblasts) | Phagocytosis; form tissue macrophages (histiocytes) that also participate in phagocytosis |

SOURCE: Adapted from Russell M. DeCoursey, *The Human Organism,* 4th ed., McGraw-Hill, New York, 1974, p. 329; and Maxwell Wintrobe, *Clinical Hematology,* Lea and Febiger, Philadelphia, 1974, pp. 228–229.

Neutrophils and macrophages participate most actively in phagocytosis, as both are rich in lysosomes, which contain potent digestive enzymes. The invading organism is surrounded by the phagocytic cell, forming a *phagocytized particle.* Lysosomes in the phagocytic cell fuse with the phagocytized particle, and the lysosomal enzymes proceed to digest the entire particle.

Immune phagocytosis occurs when antibodies (called *opsonins*) join with foreign particles and make them more susceptible to phagocytosis. Further detail on the process of phagocytosis is included in the discussions of inflammation and immunity.

## THE RETICULOENDOTHELIAL SYSTEM

Reticuloendothelial tissue is composed of cells with similar staining characteristics and similar functions. Its cells line blood vessels and lymph channels and are also found in other lymphoid tissue. The primary cell of this system is the nonmotile *tissue macrophage* (*histiocyte*). It appears to have two sites of origin within the body, emerging from unknown precursor cells within the connective tissue and from the blood monocytes. To form macrophages, monocytes enlarge and change their characteristics to become more phagocytic. Tissue macrophages are particularly helpful in surrounding and "walling off" invading organisms and foreign particles.

In the liver, local histiocytes referred to as *Kupffer cells* line the liver sinuses. Organisms that have passed through the gastrointestinal tract to the portal circulation are filtered by the Kupffer cells and phagocytized. In the alveoli, macrophages attack invading organisms that enter via the respiratory system. The histiocytes in the lymph nodes are a third local defense against bacteria. Destruction in the lymph node sinuses, like that in the liver and alveoli, prevents general dissemination throughout the body.

If organisms somehow manage to get through these barriers, macrophages in the bone marrow and spleen can still perform phagocytosis. These histiocytes have the further function of removing dead and abnormal cells from the blood. Additional defense is provided by macrophages that wander through the peritoneal and pleural spaces.

## INFLAMMATION

Inflammation is a protective mechanism exhibited by the tissues in response to an insult that may be

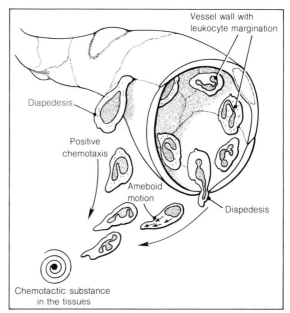

**FIGURE 8-1**

Leukocytic activity in response to the release of chemotactic substances to the tissues. (*Adapted from A. Guyton, Text of Medical Physiology, 5th ed., Saunders, Philadelphia, 1976, p. 69.*)

of various origins. The source may be thermal (hot or cold), chemical (drugs, poisons, foreign substances), or mechanical (trauma). The distinctive signs of inflammation are *redness, heat, swelling, pain,* and *loss of function.* These five so-called "cardinal signs" are due to the *chemical, vascular,* and *cellular* changes that occur as a result of the injury. These changes are described below in terms of localized injury or insult.

### Chemical Mediators

When tissue is injured, *histamine* is released by connective tissue *mast cells,* found adjacent to blood vessels. Histamine is the most important chemical mediator and is believed to be principally responsible for the *vasodilatation* and *increased capillary permeability* that occur. Other chemicals believed to have vital roles in this local tissue response include bradykinin, kallidin, slow-reacting substance A, and serotonin.

Histamine has a vasodilating effect when liberated locally and is a potent bronchial constrictor during systemic reactions (for example, in anaphylaxis). Much has yet to be discovered about the total chemical mediation of the inflammatory process; however, histamine's vascular effects have been fairly well documented.

## Vascular Changes

Initially, after localized injury, there may be a brief period of *vasoconstriction.* This is due to arteriolar contraction and may last for as much as 5 minutes.[1] The vasoconstriction is replaced by *dilatation* of the arterioles, occurring within 30 minutes of the localized injury.[2] The increased diameter of the vessels results in increased blood flow to the area and is responsible for the hyperemia, or *redness,* so characteristic of localized inflammation. This increase in circulation is also partially responsible for the *heat* felt when the inflamed tissue is touched. Increased permeability of the venules and capillaries occurs at the same time as hyperemia and results in the exudation of protein and fluid into the tissues.

Accelerated blood flow may continue for an extended period of time (as much as several hours) and is dependent on the severity of the insult. Gradually the rate of blood flow decreases, although the vessels remain dilated, causing stasis and stagnation. With the decrease in flow, leukocytes are seen to marginate along the walls of the vessels, as illustrated in Fig. 8-1. They adhere firmly to the vessels and are not dislodged easily. From here, leukocytes migrate out of the small vessels by diapedesis and move about within the tissue by ameboid motion.

The leukocytes are aided in diapedesis by the increase in capillary permeability, which permits large numbers of leukocytes to move into the area of injury. In addition to leukocytes, large amounts of protein, including fibrinogen, and some red blood cells pass into the tissues. As the osmotic pressure of the blood decreases, fluid leaves the blood and follows the protein molecules. The effect of the protein-fluid movement into the tissues is *extracellular edema.* It is this edema that is responsible for the characteristic *swelling* of local inflammation. The presence of *pain* in an inflamed area may also be due to the presence of edema, as pressure is greatly increased over sensory nerve endings. *Loss of function* is also largely attributable to the swelling, particularly over joints which are rendered immovable because of the edema and resultant pain. Within body organs, this localized inflammation may greatly interfere with the specialized function of the cells involved (for example, kidney, liver, or lung). Capillary permeability is *biphasic:* the initial phase rapidly follows the injury and rapidly subsides; the second phase occurs after a brief interval and persists for some time.

**Triple-response reaction** Vascular changes in inflammation are demonstrated by the triple-response reaction. Application of light pressure along an area of skin by a dull pointed instrument elicits a "white" reaction that is due to arteriolar vasoconstriction. However, when the same instrument is drawn across the skin with more pressure, the "triple response" is produced. The first stage of this response is the red reaction or vasodilatation that occurs as histamine is released from the injured tissue. The dull red mark made by the pointed object is soon surrounded by a bright red border or flare. This flare is the second phase of the triple response; it is believed to result from neurogenic arteriolar vasoconstriction. This natural response to mechanical injury is absent where skin is anesthetized or denervated. The third phase is marked by swelling that is localized along the line of pressure. This is called a *wheal,* and is the result of increased capillary permeability caused by the release of histamine and histamine-like substances.

The triple response demonstrates clearly, on a small scale, the redness, heat, swelling, and to some extent pain that are caused by the vascular changes in inflammation. The defensive function of the cellular changes could not take place without the vascular response.

## Cellular Activity

Fibrinogen, leukocytes, and histiocytes are responsible for most of the cellular activity that occurs in inflammation. Fibrinogen that has passed into the tissues quickly forms clots in the tissue spaces and local lymphatics, effectively walling off the inflamed area, thus preventing the generalized spread of any toxic substances. *Neutrophils* are the first cells to appear at the injured site. Next, tissue macrophages (histiocytes), already present in the inflamed area, migrate toward the organism or injury. Finally, large numbers of blood monocytes change and mature into macrophages and move into the tissues. These macrophages usually assume major phagocytic responsibility, consuming large amounts of bacteria, necrotic tissue, and other dead phagocytes. The quantity of cells traveling to an injured area varies with the specific tissue and the specific organism. With a large number of acute infections, neutrophil proliferation occurs, resulting in neutrophilia. In more chronic inflammations, neutrophils decrease and macrophages and lymphocytes become the primary defensive cells.

When acute infection is present, the *leukocytosis-promoting factor,* thought to be produced by inflamed tissue, can increase the number of neutrophils to as high as 25,000 per mm[3] of blood. Neutrophils, unlike monocytes, are stored in the bone marrow and are believed to be released in response to this factor. Production of additional neutrophils is secondarily stimulated by the same factor. The total number of leukocytes may rise to 15,000 or to even higher than 25,000 in severe systemic infections.

**Formation of pus**  When inflammation is due to bacteria rather than mechanical or thermal sources, the walling off of the inflamed area frequently results in *abscess* formation. An abscess is a cavity that is formed as phagocytosis takes place and damaged or necrotic tissue is consumed. The yellow or greenish fluid content of this abscess is referred to as *pus.*

*Suppuration,* or the formation of pus, occurs after phagocytic cells have performed their vital functions of engulfing and digesting bacteria and necrotic tissue. These phagocytic cells eventually die and, together with partially digested and undigested bacteria and necrotic tissue, form the cellular composition of pus. The enzymes liberated by the dead cells further act to digest the dead debris and account for the liquid consistency of *purulent exudate* (pus). The presence of undigested bacteria makes this exudate highly infectious.

The abscess may remain encapsulated, and the purulent contents may eventually be autolyzed and absorbed by surrounding tissues; it may rupture and drain into adjoining structures or to the body surface; it may remain encapsulated and quiescent; or it may form sinus tracts that drain continuously to the skin or other body organs. Healing of opened abscesses occurs by scar formation.

**Exudate**  The body liberates exudates, other than purulent, in response to bacterial and nonbacterial inflammation. The word "exudate" refers to the protein-containing fluid that collects within tissues or body cavities as a result of the pressure changes brought about by increased capillary permeability.

Exudate is said to be *mucoid* (sometimes called *catarrhal*) if it is produced by a mucous membrane. This clear, jellylike material may be readily identified in mild upper respiratory conditions such as the common cold.

*Serous* exudate is liberated from the cells lining body and joint cavities and blood vessels. This pale yellow or pinkish watery fluid is typified by the contents of a blister caused by a burn.

Chronic inflammation or severe injury to the tissues results in the passage of large amounts of fibrinogen into the inflamed area. The stringy, whitish-gray appearance of *fibrinous exudate* signals the deposition of fibrin as a result of severe capillary damage. Undebrided decubiti and surgical wounds are frequently covered with closely adhering fibrinous exudate that may or may not also be purulent. Fibrinous exudate may also be present in conditions such as pericarditis; if left untreated, scar tissue eventually forms, resulting in impaired cardiac function.

Normally only small numbers of red blood cells pass through the capillary membranes. However, with severe infection or injury to vascular integrity, large quantities of red blood cells may pass into the tissue spaces. This *hemorrhagic exudate* is evident when inflammatory necrosis or rupture of small blood vessels occurs in the skin, kidney, or endocardium as well as other body structures.

**Healing**  The goal of the inflammatory process is to return the damaged tissue to its normal structure and function. This is accomplished through the process of healing, or repair. Healing begins early in the inflammatory process; it is primarily achieved by the proliferation of connective tissue and the formation of a *fibrous scar;* specialized healing occurs by *regeneration* of the cells or tissues.

**S**car Formation  The formation of a scar involves the re-forming of blood vessels and the restoration of tissue integrity by *fibroblasts.* Soon after macrophages begin phagocytosis, new blood capillaries begin to form from the endothelium of blood vessels in the injured area. Though initially very fragile and highly permeable, these small vessels gradually develop and differentiate into arterioles, venules, and capillaries.

At nearly the same time as the formation of blood vessels, fibroblasts formed from nearby loose connective tissue enter the clotted exudate. After several days, when cellular debris has been removed, *collagen fibers* are laid down. These fibers arrange themselves in layers and at right angles, producing the consistently durable membrane of collagen known as a *scar.*

**H**ealing by First Intention  Healing by first intention is exemplified by the repair of a surgical incision or injury. The incised space that has been brought together by stitches is filled with some blood and serous exudate. Leukocytes and macrophages migrate to the area to remove this clotted material. New connective tissue begins to form early in the process. This is followed by capillary formation and the laying down of collagen fibers. The fine, early collagen fibers mature into coarser, tougher collagen. Two weeks after a surgical incision, collagen-replaced tissue (scar) should be approaching normal tissue in strength. The stitches from most uncomplicated surgical wounds are removed by the tenth postoperative day because the fibrous tissue is sufficiently durable.

Elastic fibers and sensory nerves eventually reform some time after the fibrous tissue. The scar, while initially very vascular, fades over time to become a paler version of the original skin color. It also appears to shrink in size and may eventually become just a fine line.

**Healing by Second Intention** The formation of granulation tissue is referred to as healing by second intention. It occurs when the edges of a wound or incision cannot be closely joined. Fibrinogen and cells contained in the exudate go to the surface of the wound; beneath this transparent layer, the wound appears red and granular. This granular tissue is highly vascular and bleeds easily; it continues to grow in area until the wound is filled with granulation tissue. Over time, the fibrous tissue formed by fibroblasts and found beneath the granulation layer strengthens, contracts, and closes the defect.

Because of the size of the scar formed by this type of healing, function of the body structure involved may be affected. The scar of second intention takes longer to acquire full strength as its fibers mature. It therefore takes longer to change color. The final contracture or shrinking of the scar may alter appearance or function.

Infected wounds, and gaping wounds that are quite deep, commonly heal by second intention. Infarcted areas of body organs also heal in this manner.

When colloid accumulation is excessive and prominent, the scar is referred to as a *keloid.* A second deviation in wound healing occurs when granulation tissue forms in excessive amounts that protrude from the wound. This is referred to as *exuberant granulation* or *proud flesh.*

**Regeneration** Various organs in the body are capable of reproducing, partially or completely, their own tissue. This regenerative ability preserves function through all but massive insults. Epithelial tissue, particularly mucous membrane and small blood vessels, regenerates quite well. Liver cells, including bile ducts, blood vessels, and connective tissue, appear to re-form completely. Other organs, such as the lung and kidney, reproduce some cells and tissues but not others. Bone, cartilage, and various glands also exhibit regenerative abilities.

## Systemic Inflammation

Systemic inflammation has been referred to several times in the preceding discussion of the inflammatory process. Some of these special effects of inflammation on the total organism warrant elaboration.

**Portals of entry** The skin is a very effective barrier to bacteria and viruses; the mucous membranes lining various organs of the body are less efficient. Consequently, despite local inflammatory reactions of vasodilatation, secretion of exudate, and all the other steps in the process, organisms sometimes enter the general circulation, frequently from entrance sites in the lung, bladder, intestine, or genital tract. Occasionally systemic inflammation results from massive infection of a wound.

Susceptibility of a person to generalized infection and poor wound healing is enhanced by poor nutrition (particularly ascorbic acid and protein deficiencies), decreased blood supply to the affected area, and concurrent stressors.

**Metabolic effects** The entire body responds to injury or infection by exhibiting the signs of inflammation on a larger or more general scale. There is a generalized stress response, with its release of adrenalin and sympathetic nervous system stimulation. The primary effects of this are manifested in an increased pulse rate and an acceleration of the metabolic rate. Adrenalin, along with corticosteroids, causes an increase in the blood glucose. Fats and proteins are mobilized to meet the increased metabolic needs. As toxic materials are liberated by damaged cells or microorganisms, they have a vasodilating effect, causing symptoms of shock to occur. Following these crisis periods, repair and recovery begin. This period of repair is marked by increased protein metabolism as the tissues strive to return to normal.

**Fever** The elevation of body temperature known as *fever* frequently accompanies infection. It is reflected by an increase in leukocytes and the erythrocyte sedimentation rate. Observable signs of its presence are chills, flushing, and diaphoresis; the pulse and blood pressure are usually elevated, and headache, confusion, and loss of appetite may be experienced. Fever may be caused by a hypersensitivity reaction or may be due to the direct action of pyrogens (bacterial or leukocytic) upon the anterior hypothalamus.

**Healing** Scar formation within localized areas of the body, as a result of systemic infections, may be helpful in restoring function or harmful in interfering with function. Specific inflammations are discussed further in Chap. 9.

## IMMUNITY

Resistance to invading organisms and foreign and tumor protein is referred to as *immunity.* Certain natural body processes, including the skin as a barrier, phagocytic cells, some chemical constituents in blood, and acid secretions of the gastrointestinal tract, function to protect from invading organisms or toxins. Not all protective responses to infectious organisms and foreign substances are innate, however; some are acquired. *Acquired immunity* is the focus of this section; it may be divided into two major types, *humoral* (thymus-independent) and *cell-mediated* (thymus-dependent).

*Immunocompetence* exists when the body is able to identify and inactivate or destroy foreign substances (antigens). The entire sequence of the immune response, from maturation of immunocompetent cells to antigen destruction, is illustrated in Fig. 8-2. Briefly, the sequence begins with processing of the foreign substance by the macrophages to form an identifiable antigen. This is followed by the activation of T lymphocytes to form *sensitized T cells* and the activation of B lymphocytes to form *antibodies.* Antibodies then join with antigen and inactivate it in several ways, and sensitized or reactive T lymphocytes react with antigen directly or through the release of chemical substances.

The special role of macrophages, the nature of antigen, humoral and cellular immunity, and vaccination are discussed in detail below.

### Special Role of Macrophages

Research indicates cooperation between humoral and cellular immunity. Part of this is related to the role of macrophages. As pointed out earlier, some macrophages are the enlarged product of monocytes that have matured in the lymphoid tissue. Also present in this tissue are the T and B lymphocytes. When invading organisms or foreign protein enter the lympoid tissue, they are first phagocytized by the macrophages. This process releases the antigenic material to the two groups of lymphocytes. T lymphocytes may then assist B lymphocytes in antibody formation against the antigen. It is this cooperative effort that helps make the total immune response so effective.

### Antigens

In general, the body exhibits *self-recognition* or *tolerance* for its own cells and structures; failure to do

this results in autoimmunity, as discussed in Chap. 10. Recognition and intolerance of foreign proteins and polysaccharides are vital to body defense; these foreign substances are of high molecular weight and are referred to an *antigens.* Commonly occurring sources of antigen for humans are bacteria, viruses, toxins, and foreign tissue. Antigens are capable of stimulating production of and reacting with specific antibodies or reactive lymphocytes. This characteristic of *specificity* makes particular antibodies or sensitized lymphocytes responsive to particular antigens. The immune response is produced against special areas referred to as *determinant groups,* located on the surface of the antigen. These localized areas direct the formation of the specific antibodies or small lymphocytes. Once formed, the antibodies or reactive lymphocytes, combine with the antigen only at these localized or active sites.

**Haptens** Low-molecular-weight substances that *combine* with known antigens (usually proteins) and are, therefore, capable of stimulating production of antibodies or sensitized lymphocytes are called *haptens.* When the body encounters the hapten a second time, the immune response is stimulated by this substance *alone.* Common haptens include certain drugs and chemicals, danders, and dust.

### Humoral Immunity

The production of circulating antibodies in response to an antigen is referred to as *humoral immunity.* Antibodies are derived from bursal (B) lymphocytes, as shown in Fig. 8-2.

When an antigen enters the lymphoid tissue, the B lymphocytes specific for that antigen enlarge and differentiate further into lymphoblasts, plasmablasts, and finally plasma cells. The mature plasma cells then divide to produce gamma globulin antibodies, or *immunoglobulins* (Ig). These antibodies pass from the lymphoid tissue into the lymph and finally into the blood, where they are circulated.

Some of the lymphoblasts formed do not differentiate into plasma cells but instead form new B lymphocytes called *memory cells.* These new B cells remain in a dormant state until activated by the original antigen. This is termed a *secondary response* and is longer and stronger than the *primary response.*

**Classes of immunoglobulin** Each immunoglobulin has a particular organization of amino acids composing its light and heavy polypeptide chains. Differences in the constant region of heavy

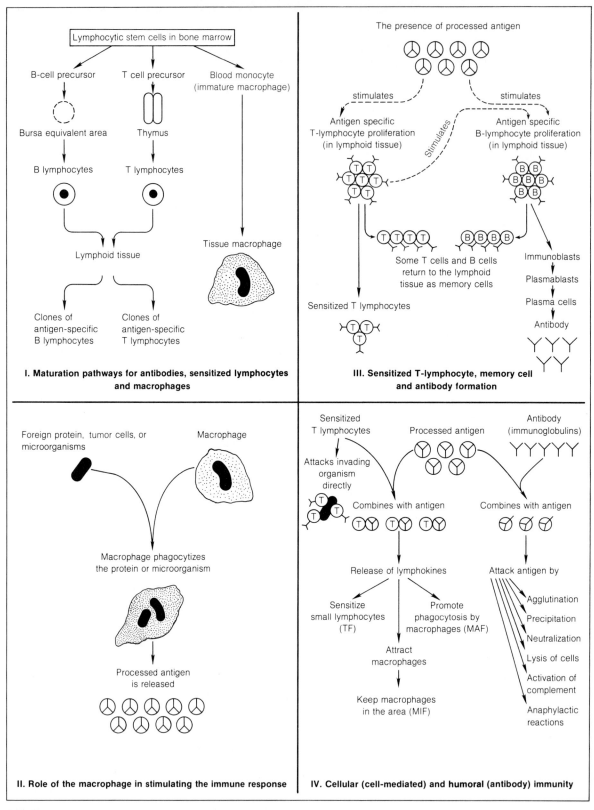

**I. Maturation pathways for antibodies, sensitized lymphocytes and macrophages**

**II. Role of the macrophage in stimulating the immune response**

**III. Sensitized T-lymphocyte, memory cell and antibody formation**

**IV. Cellular (cell-mediated) and humoral (antibody) immunity**

**FIGURE 8-2**

Immune response sequence. (*Adapted from Herman Eisen, Immunology, Harper and Row, Hagerstown, Md., 1974, p. 461; and John O. Nysather et al., "The Immune System: Its Development and Function," ATN, 76:10, Oct. 1976, pp. 1617–1618.*)

chains are the basis for the division of immunoglobulins into five classes, *IgM, IgG, IgA, IgD,* and *IgE.* These classes and their functions are summarized in Table 8-2. IgG is the most abundant antibody in human beings, followed by IgA, IgM, IgD, and IgE.

The *primary antibody response* is said to occur when B lymphocytes first encounter an antigen and begin producing antibody. In this response, *IgM* antibodies are produced within the first 48 to 72 hours after contact. A *secondary response* occurs when subsequent contact is made with the antigen. This response is stronger and longer than the primary response, and *IgG* is the major antibody present.

*IgE* attaches itself to the surface of cells and can remain attached for some time. This latter fact is important because of the role of IgE in atopic allergy. IgE (reaginic antibody) present in respiratory and intestinal mucosa is increased several times in atopic allergic reactions. Treatment in this situation is frequently by a process known as *desensitization* (hyposensitization), in which IgG (blocking antibody) is increased by administering progressively larger injections of the offending allergen (see Chap. 10).

**Methods of action**   Antigen-antibody reactions may be direct, may be mediated by complement, or may provoke an immediate hypersensitivity response (anaphylaxis), as illustrated in Fig. 8-2.

**D**irect Action   Antibodies directly inactivate antigens by lysis, precipitation, agglutination, and neutralization. *Lysis* occurs when antibodies act upon cell membranes to cause breakage and rupture of the cellular contents; *precipitation* involves the formation of insoluble antigen-antibody complexes which precipitate; *agglutination* is the clumping of antigen caused by some antibodies; *neutralization* occurs when antigens are rendered incapable of action because their active sites are directly affected by antibodies.

**C**omplement   A series of eleven proteins composing approximately 10 percent of the globulins in serum is known as *complement.*[3] These proteins react with (are *fixed* by) antigen-antibody complexes to enhance their effectiveness and mediate their action.

Complement proteins or particles, after reacting with the antigen-antibody complexes, exert their major actions on cell membrane. The effects of this action include lysis, anaphylatoxin production, chemotaxis, and enhancement of phagocytosis (opsonization).

*Lysis*   Complement proteins react with antigen-antibody (AgAb) complexes and can cause rupture of cells because of their effect on cell membranes. When they affect mast cells, histamine is released and the signs of inflammation develop. They may also affect red blood cells, bacteria, and even normal tissues.

*Anaphylatoxins*   Small polypeptide molecules derived from specific complement proteins in the serum have been identified as *anaphylatoxins.*

**TABLE 8-2**
CLASSIFICATION OF IMMUNOGLOBULINS

| Class | Quantity | Location | Function |
|---|---|---|---|
| IgG | About 75% of total immunoglobulins | Plasma and interstitial fluid | Produces antibodies against bacteria, viruses, and toxins; largely responsible for secondary immune response reactions; activates the complement system |
| IgA | About 15% of total | Large quantities in tears, saliva, milk, and other exocrine secretions, small quantities in serum | Functions in mucous membrane protection and defense of exposed body surfaces, particularly from infectious agents |
| IgM | About 10% of total | Serum | In combination with IgG, has specific antitoxin action; provides the "natural" antibodies that include the rheumatoid factor and the ABO isoantibodies; largely responsible for the primary immune response reaction; activates the complement system |
| IgD | Less than 1% of total | Serum | Unknown |
| IgE | Less than 1% of total | Serum and interstitial fluid; present also in exocrine secretions | Allergic reactions: atopy and anaphylaxis |

When these substances join with antigen-antibody complexes, they have a degranulating effect on mast cells, causing the release of histamine. The release of histamine causes increased capillary permeability and the other signs of inflammation discussed earlier.

*Chemotaxis* Certain complement fragments have been shown to attract granulocytes. This chemotactic effect is important in infection in order to move more phagocytic cells into the infected area.

*Opsonization* When a particular complement fragment joins with antigen-antibody complexes or antibody-sensitized cells, it causes their attachment to macrophages, granulocytes, and other cells. This makes them more susceptible to phagocytosis and is known as *opsonization.* Bacteria and viruses (antigens) that have already been joined by a specific antibody are destroyed more easily when attached by the complement fragment. This process is also referred to as *immune adherence.*

**A**naphylactic Reactions Certain antibodies, particularly IgE, may be quite harmful when they are present in increased numbers. (The resulting atopic conditions are discussed in Chap. 10.) Briefly, the reaction involved occurs because IgE attaches to cell membranes, including mast cells and basophils, which contain histamine; when these particular cells rupture, an inflammatory-type process results.

**Cellular Immunity**

T lymphocytes, which are processed in the thymus, are responsible for the production of the *small, sensitized lymphocytes* that furnish the body with *cellular* or *cell-mediated immunity* (Fig. 8-2). The presence of an antigen stimulates release of sensitized lymphocytes from lymphoid tissue into the lymph. From there, they travel into the body tissues to act upon foreign substances.

The "memory cells" for cellular immunity are formed in much the same manner as for humoral immunity. That is, some of the T lymphocytes divide into new T lymphocytes, instead of forming sensitized cells, and remain in the lymphoid tissue. A second introduction of antigen results in a longer and stronger secondary response.

Sensitized lymphocytes are capable of persisting in the tissues for months, perhaps even years, while humoral antibodies survive only hours or days. They have a wide variety of functions, including foreign-tissue (graft) rejection, delayed hyper-

sensitivity reactions, autoimmune responses, and preservation of immunologic tolerance. Additional functions include activation of macrophages in resistance to infection and action against insidious bacteria (tuberculosis, brucellosis) and many viruses. The protection against viruses may also provide some defense against related cancer cells: it has been found that some slow-growing tumors are heavily infiltrated with both lymphocytes and plasma cells.[4] The exact immune mechanisms of cancer-cell rejection are not fully known.

**Methods of action** Cell-mediated responses act by direct attack upon the antigen or by stimulation of mediator substances called *lymphokines* that enhance the action of sensitized lymphocytes, as shown in Fig. 8-2.

**D**irect Action The direct attack by sensitized cells is upon the cell membrane of the antigen, followed by the release of enzyme-like substances that destroy the invading cell. Sensitized T cells that react in this manner are referred to as T "killer" cells.

**M**ediators Once T cells have migrated to the antigen area they release a polypeptide substance known as *transfer factor*. This factor changes normal lymphocytes into reactive cells capable of enhancing the immune response.

A second substance, known as *macrophage-aggregating factor,* is released. This factor chemotaxically attracts more macrophages to the area of the sensitized lymphocytes. Other substances, known as *migration-inhibiting factor* and *macrophage-activating factor,* keep the large macrophages in the area and enhance their phagocytic action.

**Vaccination**

Vaccination to confer immunity is accomplished in one of three ways: (1) by injecting *dead* organisms that still retain their antigens but are not of sufficient virulence to cause disease, e.g., protection against diphtheria and whooping cough; (2) by injecting *attenuated* organisms, which are derived mutations that are incapable of producing illness, e.g., vaccination against smallpox and poliomyelitis; (3) by injecting *toxins* that have been specially processed without destroying the antigenic properties, e.g., immunization against botulism and tetanus.[5] Vaccination confers *active, acquired immunity* by stimulating the production of antibodies or sensitized lymphocytes. Immunity may also be conferred *passively* when an individual is given the antibodies or sensitized lymphocytes after their formation in another person or animal. An example of such a substance is tetanus antitoxin. The transfer of antibodies from mother to fetus via the placenta is another example of passive immunity.

## PHYSICAL ASSESSMENT OF INFLAMMATION AND IMMUNITY

Nursing assessment in terms of the immune response includes examination of the skin, mucous membranes, nails, and hair. Most of these structures are readily available for examination; however, the fact that integumental structures are so visible often results in their being overlooked. People tend to disregard or underestimate the value of things to which they have become accustomed. Other factors may also hamper accurate skin assessment; for example, people may deliberately conceal lesions or abnormalities with cosmetics, clothing, and jewelry or accidentally conceal them because of hair growth, collections of dust or grease, or heavy pigmentation of the skin.

Changes in color, texture, temperature, moisture, elasticity, and configuration of the integumental structures provide important clues to systemic and deep-tissue disorders of the immune response as well as to local and superficial ones. Significant information from skin assessment is obtained by making a thorough, purposeful examination, using the skills of inspection, mensuration, and palpation. During assessment, environmental factors affecting the skin should be controlled, when possible, to prevent inaccurate findings which could be misinterpreted. For example, the redness of excessive warmth and embarrassment can mimic or mask erythema, and the peripheral vasoconstriction from being chilled can mimic pallor.

### Inspection

*Inspection* requires the nurse to distinguish and accurately describe slightly differing shades of color, shapes, and sizes of tissues and lesions. *Mensuration* is an important adjunct to inspection and involves estimating sizes and shapes by inspection and palpation in addition to correctly using calibrated measuring tools. Mensuration is useful for assessing overall size and shape of tissue structures (e.g., an edematous leg, a distended abdomen) and the size, shape, and distribution of lesions. A small, pliable metal or plastic metric ruler and disposable metric tape measure are essential tools for mensuration.

Assessment of color requires a good light source, preferably non-glare daylight or a light that simulates daylight. If neither is available, a stand light with a bulb of at least 60 watts may be used. Fluorescent lighting is more commonly available and will serve well, except that subtle color changes may be masked.

**Skin color** The normal color of skin is determined by variables such as hereditary characteristics and the amount and distribution of exposure to sunlight. Within the influence of such variables, basic skin color is the result of three physiologic determinants: (1) superficial capillaries and venous plexuses that provide the red tones of oxyhemoglobin and the blue tones of reduced hemoglobin; (2) melanin that provides the shades of yellow, brown, and black; and (3) melanoid and carotene that provide additional tints of yellow. Light penetrates the superficial strata of the skin and is reflected back by the underlying pigment (hemoglobin, melanin, and carotene), giving the skin a normally translucent appearance. At approximately middle age the skin assumes a duller appearance, but with advancing age the epidermis becomes thinner and the skin regains a highly transparent quality.

The normal degree of *redness* in a person's skin reflects the state of the superficial capillaries. Some persons have a natural pallor because of the genetically determined quantity and depth of the capillaries (see Fig. 8-3). In natural pallor, the skin retains its healthy translucent appearance and the mucous membranes and nail beds are pink. A good example of natural pallor is skin that is continually protected by clothing (e.g., abdominal skin). Another genetic variant is the flushed appearance of persons with florid complexions. The redness is constant and conveys a healthy tone, as opposed to the bluish red of polycythemia vera or the edematous redness of inflammation.

The normal underlying red tones provide brown and black skin with its "healthy glow" or "living color."[6] The presence of the normal redness or glow is usually concealed by pigmentation, but its absence (pallor) becomes quite evident to the observant nurse.

Abnormal pallor and flushing of the skin reflect systemic or local disorders which produce changes in the quality and quantity of blood in the capillary bed of the skin. For example, acute blood loss causes peripheral vasoconstriction, resulting in white, waxy-looking, cool, moist skin. Chronic illnesses such as anemia and malignant disease re-

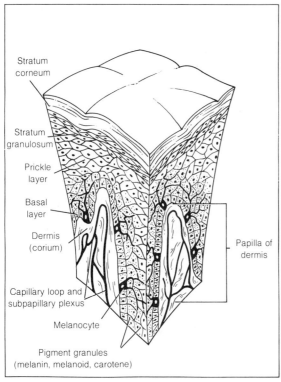

Stratum
corneum

Stratum
granulosum

Prickle
layer

Basal
layer

Dermis
(corium)

Papilla of
dermis

Capillary loop and
subpapillary plexus

Melanocyte

Pigment granules
(melanin, melanoid, carotene)

**FIGURE 8-3**

Cross section of the skin. The melanocytes, located among the
basal cells of the papilla, release granules of pigment which provide
the yellow, brown, and black skin tones; darkly pigmented skin
results from increased size and function of melanocytes. The blood
in the capillaries and subpapillary venous plexuses provide the
red and blue skin tones. The depth, number, and quality
(constriction, dilatation) of superficial vessels determine the degree
of normal redness. (*Redrawn by permission from Donald M.
Pillsbury, A Manual of Dermatology, Saunders, Philadelphia, 1971.*)

*Pallor* of the extremities may be an adaptation
to environmental factors rather than a pathologic
process. The person who is chilled by air conditioning or fearful and anxious about something will
often have pallor of the hands and feet. Smoking
will also cause significant peripheral vasoconstriction, resulting in pallor of the extremities.

*Cyanosis* occurs when the blood contains a
minimum of 5 g reduced hemoglobin per 100 ml
blood.[7] Failure to detect cyanosis is more often a
result of inattention than of difficulty in seeing it.
Usually the onset is gradual, and unless the nurse
regularly and deliberately inspects for a bluish tint,
the subtle changes go unnoticed. Many of the same
techniques are used to detect cyanosis as are used
for pallor, but palmar color change is more difficult
to recognize in the adult than the bluish color of the
lips, circumoral skin, cheeks, and earlobes of the
light-skinned person. Dark-skinned persons usually
have enough pigmentation to obscure cyanosis, so
the mucous membranes and nail beds are the best
areas for inspection.

*Methemoglobinemia* and *sulfhemoglobinemia*
may cause cyanosis with tones of violet and brown,
respectively. When cyanosis is severe, yet the person demonstrates no respiratory or cardiovascular
insufficiency, a careful history of drug and chemical
ingestion is imperative. Ingested substances which
may cause methemoglobinemia and sulfhemoglobinemia include sulfones, Bromo Seltzer, and
colored wax crayons (uncommon).[8] Percutaneous
absorption of aniline dye (e.g., shoe dye, marking
ink) is a less common cause.

*Abnormal flushing* may be a manifestation of a
wide variety of disorders, including systemic disease, fever, infection, and hypersensitivity reactions. Both systemic and psychologically induced
flushing occurs primarily in the skin of the "butter-
fly" area of the face (cheek to cheek across the
nose), neck, upper chest, and flexor surfaces of the
extremities.

Assessment of flushing should include observation of the shade, intensity, pattern, and distribution of the onset and evolution of the flush. Some
flushes are highly characteristic, such as the bright
pink or cherry-red flush of the lips, face, and upper
torso which usually accompanies carbon monoxide
poisoning. Others, including the flushing of embarrassment and of menopause, are quite similar and
require discerning observations for differentiation.
Flushing is difficult, but not impossible, to recognize in the black-skinned person. When flushing is
suspected (on the basis of subjective complaints),
the skin temperature of the flush area should be

sult in sallow skin (pale, sickly, yellowish color). The
brown-skinned person with pallor will appear yellowish brown, and the black-skinned person will
appear ashen gray; both color changes reflect the
loss of the normal underlying red tones (see Color
Plates 8-1 and 8-2).

Unless the palms are calloused and have heavy
deposits of carotene, they are excellent sites for
assessing the presence, and even the degree, of
pallor. To inspect someone's palms, have the person lie down with his or her hands at heart level,
because the blood flow to the hands will be greatest
in the supine position. Slightly hyperextend the person's fingers and look along the palm at a low
angle (20 to 30°) toward the fingers to assess the
color of the creases; compare with the color in a
person with normal hemoglobin and blood pressure.

compared with a different area of the body. Also, close inspection will often reveal a deeper "glow" to the skin in the flush area (see Color Plate 8-3).

When the skin or underlying structures are inflamed, the characteristic redness, heat, swelling, pain, and loss of function are present but to varying degrees, depending on the depth of the inflamed tissue and the magnitude of the inflammatory response. Problems of detection include (1) relatively inaccessible location of the inflamed tissues (e.g., pharynx, vagina), (2) material covering the inflamed area (e.g., cosmetics, hair, clothing, cast), and (3) heavy pigmentation concealing the signs.

A careful inspection of the less accessible areas will easily locate the bright redness of inflamed mucous membranes. Covering materials such as hair and clothing must be moved or removed to make possible a thorough examination; substances such as cosmetics, dirt, and grease must be removed in such a way as not to irritate the underlying skin surface, and the skin should be allowed to rest a few minutes before it is inspected.

Redness (erythema, flushing) alone does not imply inflammation, since any factor which causes peripheral vasodilatation will result in increased redness. For this reason, and because redness is difficult to see in the dark-skinned person, palpation is important when assessing the skin for inflammation. With light strokes of the fingertips, feel for "slick," tight skin suggesting edema, and with slightly firmer pressure, check for hardening of deep tissues or blood vessels. Compare the temperature of the reddened skin with that of nearby areas. The warmth of inflammation can also be palpated through a plaster cast. Normally the cast material is slightly cool, so any localized area of warmth on the cast, especially in conjunction with complaints of pain, is highly suggestive of an inflammatory process and should be investigated promptly.

Assessment of inflammation should always include observation for particular patterns, shapes, and locations of erythema and edema. Many disorders have characteristic patterns, such as the linear flare along the vein in phlebitis or the extensively diffuse, markedly hot, reddened, edematous appearance of cellulitis.

**Pigmentation** The yellow, brown, and black skin colors are provided primarily by the *melanocytes* (melanin-forming cells), which are located at the junction of the epidermis and dermis (Fig. 8-3). All persons have essentially the same number of melanocytes, but dark-skinned persons have in-creased secretion of melanin. The normal distribution of pigment varies in dark-skinned persons just as it does in light-skinned ones. Some have near-black skin, while others may have tan, freckled skin. Surfaces that are protected by clothing tend to be lighter than those exposed to the sun. One consistency is the absence of melanin deposits in the palms and soles of both light- and dark-skinned persons (except in the creases); however, when these surfaces are calloused, there may be heavy deposits of carotene and carotenoid. Because of the highly variable normal patterns, assessment of pigmentation should include a carefully obtained history of *change.*

Some changes, especially early ones, are very subtle and may not be recognized unless the nurse has an accurate mental picture of the person's normal or usual state. The importance of making and recording baseline observations cannot be over-emphasized, especially for persons with unusual patterns and increased amounts of pigmentation (hemoglobin as well as melanin and carotene).

The skin areas most likely to reflect systemic pigmentary disturbances include the face (particularly the circumoral area), backs of the hands, flexor surfaces of the wrists, genital area, axillae, areolae, and the midline of the abdomen.[9] Increased pigmentation in these areas may occur as a normal change in the pregnant woman (cloasma gravidarum). Also, surfaces of the aging skin that are exposed to sunlight normally have irregular patches of increased pigmentation ("liver spots," "age spots") and of depigmentation (vitiligo). The former are more noticeable in light-skinned persons, and the latter are particularly striking in dark-skinned persons.

Jaundice, the yellowish color of bile pigment (bilirubin) deposited in the skin and mucous membranes, may be difficult to distinguish from other causes of yellow color, including a fading suntan, excessive carotene, cholesterol, drugs (quinicrine), and industrial chemicals.[10] It is helpful to inspect the distribution pattern of the color for clues to the probable cause. A diffuse yellowish tint to the entire skin but not involving the sclera, mucous membranes, palms, and soles is probably the normal yellow coloration of melanin and carotene in persons of Oriental descent. Also, keep in mind that normally olive skin tone may appear quite yellowish under some types of artificial light. A fading suntan is often distinguishable by locating the untanned areas normally covered by a bathing suit or by the absence of yellow in the sclera and mucous membranes.

The yellow color of excess carotene is unevenly distributed and is most noticeable in the skin of the nose, forehead, palms, soles, elbows, and knees. Carotene gives the skin a canary-yellow or golden tone, whereas jaundice gives it a bronze color, sometimes with tones of orange or green. The distribution of color in jaundice includes all skin areas, the sclera, and the mucous membranes.

In addition to the sclera, examination of the palms and the lighter pigmented skin areas protected by clothing is helpful when observing for jaundice. A problem to be aware of is the influence of edema on skin color. The presence of edema increases the distance between the skin surface and the pigmented and vascular layers, thereby reducing the intensity of all color, including jaundice. If edema precedes jaundice, the serum bilirubin level must be much higher than the usual 2 to 3 mg/100 ml necessary to give the skin a yellow tone.

Jaundice is difficult to detect in darkly pigmented skin. If the palms are not heavily calloused and colored with carotene, they will show moderate to severe jaundice readily, but the earliest sign of jaundice is best observed in the sclera and mucous membranes. Scratch marks, denoting itching, may help determine the presence of jaundice, but itching has many causes and is present in only about one-fourth of those who have jaundice.[11]

**Nails** The fingernails, toenails, and nail beds provide many clues to a person's state of health. The normal nails have a high metabolic activity, so disorders which interfere with availability of oxygen and nutrients will cause changes such as ridges and transverse white lines (denoting severe malnourishment), brittleness (as in hypothyroidism), and angle and contour changes (accompanying clubbing).

Nails are composed of a modified keratin which is firm, flexible, smooth, and transparent. They cover highly vascular nail beds which provide their normal pink color (see Fig. 8-4). Although the nail-beds are usually free of pigment (melanin), some blacks will be found to have frecklelike deposits which obscure much of the vascular color and which must be carefully differentiated from abnormalities such as petechiae and ecchymoses.

Assessment of the nails includes inspection for variations (1) from the normally uniform pink *color* of the nail bed, (2) in the *shape* and *continuity* of the nails, (3) in the *angle* at the junction of the nail fold and the nail plate, and (4) in the *thickness* and *transparency* of the nails. Palpation is used to determine the presence of ridges, pits, and excess dryness (all abnormal) and to assess the qualities of flexibility and firmness.

The *capillary filling test* is used to evaluate both generalized and local vasomotor tone. The test is done with the subject's hand at his or her heart level. Apply pressure on the free edge of the nail, causing a blanching of the nail bed; upon release of the pressure, the color normally returns quickly (no longer than one second), and it appears to return from below the pallid spot as well as from the periphery. A slow return of color indicates a diminished quality of vasomotor function and is especially valuable in differentiating the pallor of an immobilized or slightly chilled extremity from the pallor caused by internal hemorrhage or a cardiovascular dysfunction (including a localized obstruction such as a tight arm cast). When the nail bed is naturally pale, the color may be increased with gentle pressure against the patient's finger pad during the test (Fig. 8-5).

The nail beds, when not pigmented, readily demonstrate cyanosis, but peripheral vasoconstriction caused by smoking, medications, or generalized chilling can displace cyanosis even though serious hypoxia is present. True cyanosis must be differentiated from "cold cyanosis," which is caused by an uncomfortably cold environment. Elevating (to about 15°) or lowering (to 30 to 90°) an extremity may intensify a slight cyanosis to make it more recognizable. The capillary filling test, when done on cyanotic nails or directly on cyanotic skin, shows a prolonged filling time, with the color returning slowly and moving inward from the periphery.

**Hair** Characteristics, patterns, and distribution of hair are genetically determined and sex-related. The downy (vellous) hair of the body and the terminal hair of the scalp, eyebrows, and eyelashes are all present at birth; the axillary, pubic, and coarse body and facial hair develop at puberty. The normal pattern for male pubic hair is a triangle with the base at the pubic bone and the apex at the umbilicus; normal for the woman is an inverted triangle with the base just above the pubic bone. Facial hair in the woman usually is indistinguishable from vellous hair, but some brunettes have a familial trait that results in dark, coarse hair resembling masculine facial hair.

The normal color, texture, and amount of hair (scalp, pubic, etc.) varies considerably according to genetic and age determinants and should be assessed with special emphasis on recent *change*. A thorough history of hair care should be obtained when disorders involving the scalp hair are present. For example, acute total alopecia (loss of hair) of the scalp may be the result of dye or bleach damage to the hair shafts rather than to disease, drug reaction, or other pathology; patchy alopecia may result from nervous behaviors such as twisting or pulling the hair or from prolonged use of tight curlers.

In addition to obtaining information about hair care and related behaviors, inspect the hair of the entire body for (1) recent unexplained *color* change, especially localized or patchy changes, and (2) increased or decreased *amount* of hair unrelated to the natural influences of age, balding patterns, etc. Examine the *texture* of the scalp hair by gently easing the finger and thumb along a lock of hair. Select the locks from hair least likely to be coated with hair spray. Determine how fine, coarse, pliable, or brittle the hair feels, especially noting inconsistencies from one area to another and between findings and the person's description of usual hair texture.

**M**ucous Membranes  Mucous membranes are highly transparent, which makes them especially valuable when assessing abnormalities in the content or function of superficial capillaries. For example, the erythema of inflammation and the cyanosis of reduced hemoglobin are both readily apparent in the lips and oral mucosa. Usually the normal mucous membranes have a clear pink color in both light- and dark-skinned persons, but exceptions will be encountered. For instance, full-blooded Negroes often have splotched or diffuse bluish pigmentation

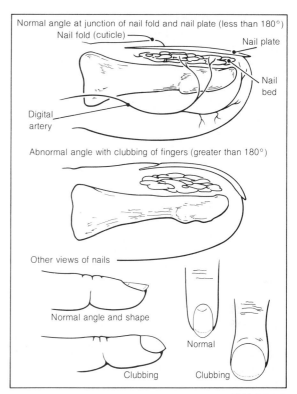

**FIGURE 8-4**
Cross section and contour of the nail.

**FIGURE 8-5**
The capillary filling test.

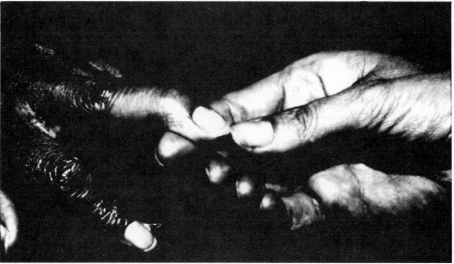

of the gums. In others, it is normal for the gum, buccal cavity, and borders of the tongue to have brown freckle-like deposits of pigment.[12] Early recognition of such normal variations is necessary in order to establish a base from which to assess color change.

The hard palate is an excellent site for detecting early jaundice and is less likely than the sclera to be yellow from other causes, such as carotene or drugs.

Other important signs of illness are frequently discovered during inspection of the mucous membranes; for example, Koplik spots of measles in the mouth, pigmentation of the lips and buccal mucosa in Addison's disease and the Peutz-Jeghers syndrome, a beefy red tongue in pernicious anemia, and the white membranous plaque of monilia (thrush) on the tongue or buccal mucosa. Certain lesions of the oronasal mucosa may signify similar lesions throughout the gastrointestinal or the respiratory tract. For example, monilia in debilitated persons may involve the respiratory passages and most of the gastrointestinal tract; the ulcerative lesions of the oronasal mucosa in agranulocytosis may extend through the entire digestive tract; angioneurotic edema of the lips or tongue may forewarn of extension to the epiglottis and larynx.

The genital mucosa is not readily accessible for inspection, and social taboos create additional restraints, but this area is a common site for infection and certainly should be included in an examination (see Chap. 4).

**Conjunctiva** The conjunctiva is the transparent mucous membrane lining the eyelids and sclera. Normally, the eyelid (palpebral) portion assumes the clear pink color of the oxygenated red blood cells below, and the scleral (bulbar) portion gives an opalescent character to the opaque white of the sclera. Although the conjunctiva is usually not pigmented, some blacks have frecklelike deposits of brown pigment in the portion of the sclera exposed by the palpebral fissure. An accurate history should help differentiate normal from pathologic pigmentation.

The conjunctiva is inspected by eversion of the lower lid as for administering eyedrops. The vascular color near the inner canthus may be normally lighter, so assessment for pallor and cyanosis should include inspection of the full length of the palpebral conjunctiva. Carotene-stained fatty deposits may be present near the periphery of the sclera, so inspecting the portion of the sclera revealed naturally by the palpebral fissure may provide a more accurate assessment for jaundice than

would looking beneath the lower lid. When there is a history of quinicrine ingestion, the central portion of the sclera is likely to be "falsely" colored yellow, so inspection of the peripheral sclera for jaundice is recommended.

Conjunctivitis, the nonspecific reaction of the conjunctiva to irritation and inflammation, may occur as *conjunctival* or *ciliary* injection (engorged blood vessels). Differentiation between the two is important, especially when the nurse must decide whether to recommend home care or referral to a physician for prompt therapy. Conjunctival injection is more prominent in the palpebral and the peripheral bulbar conjunctiva, becoming less pronounced near the limbus (outer edge of the cornea). Ciliary injection, which usually results from serious deep-seated eye disease (e.g., iritis, viral infection), is more intense at the limbus, becoming less pronounced near the periphery of the eye.

**Foreign Bodies** When inflammation of the skin is present, particularly following trauma, the possible presence of a foreign body such as a splinter of wood, glass, or metal must be considered. Special care is indicated during cleansing and examining the area to avoid advancing the object even deeper into the tissues. Small foreign objects are difficult to see, but the use of a magnifying lens with oblique lighting improves the chances of locating them. If a magnifying lens is not available, an otoscope (without the speculum) can be used.

**Swelling** Swelling of the skin denotes an abnormal condition such as edema, ascites, or subcutaneous emphysema; assessment is therefore directed toward collecting sufficient data to identify the cause. The swelling of generalized edema will be more pronounced in dependent tissues (feet and ankles of ambulatory patients; presacral and pretibial tissues of bedfast patients). To check for pitting edema, press a thumb firmly into the tissue over a bony surface for 5 to 10 seconds; a depression will remain when the thumb is lifted. In general, the deeper the depression and the slower the filling of the pit, the greater is the amount of edema. Tight, "slick" skin with subcutaneous induration (hardness) is characteristic of nonpitting edema. Unless inflammation accompanies edema, the skin usually feels slightly cooler than expected.

*Extensive edema* of the eyelids and periocular tissues may assume a blisterlike appearance. The skin of this area is so loose and thin that large amounts of fluid may collect, ballooning the skin outward.

*Subcutaneous emphysema,* resulting from air

leaking into the tissues, looks like edema, but application of pressure with the fingers produces crepitation (crackling sensation) and promptly differentiates between the two.

*Discolored swelling* may indicate an underlying hematoma or a contusion with edema. Examination of hemorrhagic lesions should always include an accurate and complete determination of color and size. A gradual increase in swelling suggests continued bleeding; color changes (from reddish purple to blue-black, to greenish brown, to yellow) provide guidelines for estimating the age of a lesion. The various colors of purpura may be masked by pigment in very dark skin, but usually the area is significantly darker than the surrounding skin, suggesting the presence of hemoglobin.

*Enlarged lymph nodes* are common causes of small, firm, swollen areas. A brief review of the lymphatic anatomy and a history of precipitating factors such as a sore throat, an insect sting, or a puncture wound will help differentiate enlarged nodes from other causes of nodules and tumors (see Chap. 4). A fairly common cause of nodules that should be considered is the fibroblastic response to a foreign body.

**L**esions  *Rashes* constitute a large proportion of the lesions affecting the skin, and the components of rashes include essentially every type of lesion (see Color Plates 8-4 through 8-10). Rashes accompany many allergic, infectious, and toxic states and may occur in a variety of forms and patterns. Assessment of rashes includes collecting information (by history and observation) about (1) the length of time between the beginning of the illness and the onset of the rash (prodromal period), (2) the site at which the rash first appeared, (3) the characteristics of the primary lesion(s), and (4) additional relevant information about symptoms of infection or allergy, history of drug ingestion, exposure to someone with a rash, etc. Direct observation of the rash is necessary to (1) identify the components, (2) differentiate the primary and secondary lesions, (3) determine the pattern of distribution and configuration, (4) determine the color and texture of the lesions and underlying tissues, and (5) identify the sequence (evolution) of the rash.

The components of rashes are classified as primary and secondary lesions (Fig. 8-6 and 8-7). A *primary* lesion is one that occurs early and is characteristic for the rash, as vesicles are characteristic of chickenpox. The primary-lesion category includes macules, papules, plaques, nodules, tumors, cysts, wheals, vesicles, bullae, and pustules.

*Secondary* lesions develop as modifications of primary ones or as an end result; for example, the crusts that form during chickenpox or the scars from smallpox. The category of secondary lesions includes crust, scale, fissure, excoriation, erosion, ulcer, striae, scar, and atrophy.

Identification and differentiation of lesions present a number of problems, some of which may be overcome by painstaking use of inspection, mensuration, and palpation skills. There is disagreement even among standard references concerning the size (and sometimes other characteristics) of various skin lesions, but the nurse can promote accurate diagnosis by recording exact measurements (metric) of height and diameter of individual lesions and patches of lesions.

Combinations of two or more components may be seen; for example, the maculopapular rash of measles and the common presence of petechiae with chickenpox vesicles in dark-skinned children.[13] Rashes are more difficult to assess in dark skins because the erythema is less conspicuous, but the papules, vesicles, and even petechiae may be detected by viewing the skin with diffuse oblique lighting. Palpation of the lesions will often differentiate the firm, solid papules from the softer and more yielding vesicles and the firm induration of wheals from the soft rebound of bullae.

*Distribution* includes the location and pattern of the rash. Many rashes assume characteristic distributions which are valuable to making a diagnosis. For example, drug-related rashes are often distributed primarily on the trunk and thighs in a diffuse pattern; vesicles of herpes zoster demonstrate a linear pattern following the segmental distribution of peripheral nerves; measles' rash begins behind the ears and along the hair line, spreading downward; and poison ivy rash tends to assume a linear pattern on exposed skin areas (hands, arms, face, legs). When describing and recording distribution of rashes, use accurate anatomic terms.

*Configuration,* the shape of single lesions or patches of lesions, is also characteristic for many rashes. For example, fungal lesions are usually annular in shape and the lesions of scabies are short, fine, tortuous "threads." Configuration is most accurately described with specialized terminology (discrete, confluent, punctate, circinate, gyrate, annular, serpiginous, linear, arcuate), but accurate descriptions are possible with carefully selected common terms (separate, merged, pointed, halo, scalloped, circular, snakelike, straight, arc-shaped).

Observation of *texture* includes the characteristics not only of the surface lesions but also of the underlying tissues and requires the use of palpa-

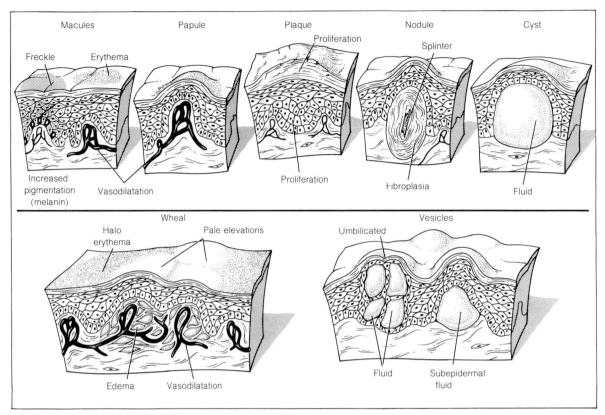

**FIGURE 8-6**
Primary lesions.

tion. *Color* is assessed in terms of the basic color (red, blue, etc), the shade or tint (pink, plum), and intensity (bright, dull, dark).

The *evolution* of a rash is the orderly change in the characteristics of the lesion from its onset to its final form; for example, the progression of urticaria from erythema to wheals to urticarial bullae, then gradual subsidence of the lesions, leaving no skin changes except perhaps excoriation from scratching.

*Primary lesions* A *macule* is a flat, circumscribed area of color which differs from the normal adjacent skin color (Fig. 8-6). Macules may be of any color, including the red of erythema, the brown tones of hyperpigmentation, and the variable colors of telangiectasia, petechiae, and ecchymoses; or depigmentation may cause absence of color. They may be of any size but are usually defined as being 1 mm to 1 cm in diameter. Examples include freckles, vitiligo, erythematous patches, measles, and petechiae.

A macular rash may be differentiated from sim-ple erythema by stretching the skin gently between the thumb and forefinger (as for administering an injection). This maneuver decreases the red tone of erythema but accentuates macules.[14] Hemorrhagic lesions (petechiae, ecchymoses) will also be accentuated by this maneuver. Another useful technique is to press a glass slide or piece of clear plastic firmly against the skin and inspect the color that remains. This technique is particularly helpful in differentiating a fresh purpuric lesion from erythema.[15]

A *papule* is a small, solid elevation of skin, usually less than 1 cm in diameter (Fig. 8-6). Papules assume a variety of colors (including natural skin tones) and shapes (pointed, flat-topped, rounded, etc.). Examples include verrucae, measles, varicella, secondary syphilis, and drug reaction. Assessment of papular lesions should include an accurate description of the size, color, contour, and texture of the lesion and of concomitant lesions or markings (erythema, excoriation, scales).

A *plaque* is a wide, firm expanse of skin elevation, more than 2 to 3 cm across and usually no higher or deeper than a papule (Fig. 8-6). Although some plaques are original lesions, most are clusters of papules, as in psoriasis and mycosis fungoides.

A *nodule* is a solid elevation of tissue that is larger than a papule and often involves deeper tissues (Fig. 8-6). Large nodules are generally referred to as *tumors*. Palpation will help determine the contour (round, oval), depth (dermis, subcutaneous), and size of a nodule. Examples of nodules include basal cell carcinoma, granuloma from foreign body reaction, and erythema nodosum. A *cyst* looks and feels much like a nodule or papule but may have a more compressible or elastic quality, because the content is often fluid or semifluid (Fig. 8-6). Cysts of the skin may be epidermal (keratinous) or intra-dermal (sebaceous).

*Wheals* (urticaria, hives) are localized, transient, edematous lesions characteristic of allergic reactions (Fig. 8-6). The elevation of skin is firm and may be rounded (resembling a blister) or flat-topped (forming a plaque), varying in size from tiny papules (4 mm) to huge plaques (12 cm). The raised area is whitish or pale pink, often with an erythematous halo. Unless the allergen is highly localized, e.g., a mosquito bite, wheals show a tendency to shift from one area to another within the space of a few hours and to increase and decrease in size with equal rapidity.

A *vesicle* is a small blister, containing serous or serosanguinous fluid. If the vesicle is larger than approximately 0.5 cm in diameter, it is referred to as a *bulla.* Vesicles and bullae may occur singly or in clusters and may originate in the epidermis (intra-epidermal) or at the epidermal-dermal junction (subepidermal) (Fig. 8-6). The walls of subepidermal vesicles are thicker and less tranparent than the intraepidermal ones and must be carefully differentiated from papules. Vesicles and bullae caused by viral infections may have a depressed center (umbilicated) instead of the usual smooth, round surface (Color Plate 8-9). Subepidermal vesicles in the dark-skinned person are difficult to distinguish from papules because the thick-walled vesicles have a dark coloration which further disguises the blisterlike quality. Vesicles are characteristic of many disorders, including varicella, variola, herpes simplex, herpes zoster, and contact dermatitis.

Vesicles may be identified by close inspection with sufficient light to detect the fluid content of the lesions. Side-lighting may help when the lesions are darkly pigmented by melanin or contain blood. Bullae are easily distinguished from wheals because of the obvious free fluid within the elevated skin of the bulla as opposed to the edema of a wheal. Gentle palpation may help differentiate between solid and fluid-filled elevations. Assessment of vesicles and bullae should include determination of size, color (contents), distribution, configuration, and concomitant lesions (petechiae, pustules, crusts).

*Pustules* are vesicles (or bullae) filled with purulent exudate, which may be sterile (e.g., iodine or bromide sensitivity, pustular psoriasis) or infectious (e.g., impetigo, acne vulgaris, varicella) and may be accompanied by erythema. The term "pustule" usually refers to small (less than 1 cm) superficial lesions; the deeper, larger lesions are called *abscesses, furuncles,* and *carbuncles.* Pustules vary in shape and color: they may be flat, round, conical, or umbilicated, and the color may be white, yellow, or greenish yellow, depending on the con-

**FIGURE 8-7**
Secondary lesions.

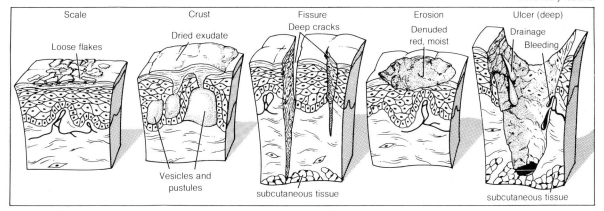

Scale — Loose flakes

Crust — Dried exudate — Vesicles and pustules

Fissure — Deep cracks — subcutaneous tissue

Erosion — Denuded red, moist

Ulcer (deep) — Drainage — Bleeding — subcutaneous tissue

tents. Pustules are assessed in the same manner as vesicles and bullae.

*Secondary lesions* *Scales* are flakes of abnormal stratum corneum (Fig. 8-7). They may assume a variety of characteristics, described as shiny, silvery, yellow, dull, fine, coarse, powdery, greasy, etc. Variations are seen even within a single disease entity. For example, the scale of psoriasis may be thin, silvery, and easily detached or coarse, adherent, and associated with an excessive accumulation of keratin. Assessment of scales includes identification of associated changes (e.g., erythema, plaque), in addition to the color and character of the scales.

*Crust* is dried exudate. Vesicles, bullae, and pustules rupture, releasing serous, serosanguinous, or purulent drainage which combines with tissue debris, soil, etc. and hardens into a crust or scab (Fig. 8-7). The color and nature of crusts are determined by the composition. The typical thick, soft, honey-colored crusts of impetigo are composed of vesicular and pustular fluid; green or blue-green crusts with a grapelike odor are typically composed of purulent exudate from *Pseudomonas* infection; brown, black, or dark-red crusts indicate the presence of blood, as seen in erythema multiforme. Assessment of crusts should include specific details of size, color, consistency, adherence, odor, and concomitant lesions.

*Fissures* are linear cracks in the skin which usually extend into the subcutaneous tissue (Fig. 8-7). They are often accompanied by pain and erythema and may result from such conditions as severe drying (chapping), *Candida* infection, allergy (chronic contact dermatitis), or riboflavin deficiency.

An *erosion* is loss of the epidermis, resulting in a superficial, reddened, weeping lesion (Fig. 8-7). Erosion accompanies many allergic and infectious rashes and lesions. An *ulcer* is an erosion into the dermis or deeper tissues (Fig. 8-7) and may result from a similar variety of causes. Assessment of fissures, erosions, and ulcers should include observations which will help to determine the cause. For instance, observe the location (especially in relation to pressure points), the appearance of the edges and base of the lesion (color, shape), the presence and type of drainage, and any associated lesions or changes.

*Scars* are the end result of healing by fibroustissue (collagen) replacement. Lesions which destroy portions of the stratum granulosum (Fig. 8-3) will result in scarring. Fresh scars, in both light- and dark-skinned persons, have a pink to purplish color because they are highly vascular under a thin covering of epidermis. As scars mature, they usually become white in light-skinned persons and heavily pigmented in dark-skinned persons. Hypertrophic scars (keloids) are more common in Negroes and may result from surgical incisions as well as from ulcers and other lesions. Atrophic scars leave firm, sometimes nodular, depressions in the skin. "Pitting" scars of this type are characteristic of acne. *Striae,* which are narrow, shiny stretch lines, may resemble scars, but they remain soft and thin whereas scars become firm and hard as they mature.

## Palpation

Palpation of the skin is the use of one's tactile sense to observe for abnormal changes in texture, configuration, temperature, elasticity, and moisture. Experience-based knowledge of these normal palpable qualities is especially helpful and can be developed through disciplined practice. The normal limits of all these qualities vary with such factors as age, sex, occupation, habits of skin care, and basic physiologic determinants.

**Texture** Texture is the "feel" of skin. Its *smoothness* depends on a combination of lubrication from the sebaceous glands and the absence of an excess collection of keratin (e.g., scale, callus). Thus skin normally protected from exposure and friction (especially areas covered by clothing) should feel smooth in comparison to the rougher texture of skin continually exposed to the drying, damaging rays of sunlight. Darkly pigmented skin that has been protected from the elements will have the same degree of smoothness and softness as lightly pigmented skin, The presence of lesions (papules, scale, plaque) will disrupt the normal smoothness of skin.

*Softness* is provided by fat cells underlying the base of the dermis and is influenced by the depth and character of the overlying keratin. The skin of obese persons, men as well as women, feels soft. Normal softness changes to hardness (induration) in the presence of nonpitting edema, plaque formations, and many other lesions.

The finger pads normally provide a fine discrimination of touch, so skin texture is palpated by using light stroking and "feeling" movements of the fingers.

**Configuration** Configuration of the normal skin pertains to the *symmetry* of its surface contours and characteristics. The underlying subcutaneous tissue, muscle, bone, and other structures determine the surface contours when there are no normal unilateral protrusions or depressions. Assessment of configuration includes inspection and palpation for asymmetry of contour and skin characteristics such as pigmentation, vascularity, texture, temperature, and moisture. Palpation for changes in configuration is accomplished in the same manner as for texture.

**Temperature** *Warmth* is determined primarily by the speed of blood flow through the cutaneous vascular structures (Fig. 8-3). Vasodilatation, with an increased amount and flow rate of blood, raises the skin temperature; vasoconstriction lowers the temperature. Edema, which increases the distance between the surface and the cutaneous vessels, will also lower the skin temperature.

The dorsal surfaces of the fingers are more sensitive to temperature differences than the palmar surfaces. A good way to palpate for temperature is to curve the fingers into a relaxed flexion and gently rest the middle phalanges on the skin to be tested (Fig. 8-8), then move them to another skin surface for comparison.[16]

**Elasticity** *Elasticity* is determined by the presence of elastic fibers in the subcutaneous tissues but is also influenced by turgor. With increasing age, the loss of elasticity causes the skin to wrinkle and assume a looseness which may be misinterpreted as poor turgor. *Turgor* (tissue tension) reflects the quantity of fluid within and between the cells of the skin (quality of hydration). The skin of the forehead, chest, abdomen, or anterior forearm is used for checking turgor and elasticity. Gently pinch the skin between the thumb and forefinger and lift upward slightly; a prompt return to the normal contour upon release denotes good hydration and elasticity.

**Moisture** *Moisture* on the skin is the result of sweat-gland secretion, which becomes palpable when increased function is stimulated by anxiety, excessive warmth, or increased activity. Moist palms, soles, and axillae are more indicative of psychic stimulation of perspiration, while generalized moisture more often accompanies warmth and activity.

The quality of *dryness* may be determined by any one or a combination of several factors. There may be decreased tissue hydration, decreased function of sebaceous and sweat glands, excessive removal of sebum from the skin, or increased depth of the stratum corneum. A "rough" dryness (chapping) is characteristic of excessive removal (or a deficient amount) of sebum. Tanning from exposure to sunlight is accompanied by increased dryness, but naturally dark skin has no greater tendency to dryness than light skin. Moisture and dryness are

**FIGURE 8-8**
Palpation for skin temperature.

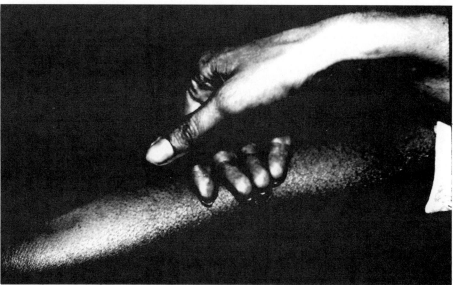

palpated by stroking the skin with the finger pads in the same manner as for texture.

## SUMMARY

Inflammation and immunity represent the body's defenses against invading organisms and foreign substances. The skin, as the protective barrier of the body, reflects the activities of these two defenses very accurately. Perceptive and detailed assessment of the skin is therefore vital. Nurses use primarily the assessment skill of observation, although palpation of the skin is also involved.

## REFERENCES

1   Lord Florey, *General Pathology,* 4th ed., Saunders, Philadelphia, 1970, p. 73.
2   Ibid.
3   Herman N. Eisen, *Immunology,* Harper & Row, Hagerstown, Md., 1974, p. 512.
4   Ibid., p. 621.
5   Arthur Guyton, *Textbook of Medical Physiology,* 5th ed., Saunders, Philadelphia, 1976, p. 85.
6   Lora B. Roach, "Color Changes in Dark Skins," *Nurs '72,* **2:**19–22, 1972, p. 21.
7   Ibid., p. 22.
8   William E. Clendenning and John T. Boyer, "The Skin and the Hematopoietic System," in T. B. Fitzpatrick et al. (eds.), *Dermatology in General Medicine,* McGraw-Hill, New York, 1971, p. 1321.
9   C. Philip Anderson, in Richard D. Judge and George D. Zuidema (eds.), *Physical Diagnosis: A Physiologic Approach to the Clinical Examination,* Little, Brown, Boston, 1963, p. 64.
10   Lora B. Roach, "Assessing Skin Changes: The Subtle and the Obvious," *Nurs '74,* **4:**64–67, March, 1974, p. 66.
11   Ibid.
12   Roach, "Color Changes in Dark Skins," p. 20.
13   R. T. D. Emond, *Color Atlas of Infectious Diseases,* Year Book, Chicago, 1974, p. 144.
14   Roach, "Assessing Skin Changes," p. 65.
15   Thomas B. Fitzpatrick and David P. Johnson, "Fundamentals of Dermatologic Diagnosis," in T. B. Fitzpatrick et al. (eds.), *Dermatology in General Medicine,* McGraw-Hill, New York, 1971, p. 16.
16   Roach, "Color Changes in Dark Skins," p. 21.

## BIBLIOGRAPHY

Allen, James H.: "Disorders of the Eyelids, Part 1," *Hosp Med,* **8:**30–48, August 1972; "Part 2," **8:**102–120, September 1972.

Briody, Bernard: *Microbiology and Infectious Disease,* McGraw-Hill, New York, 1974.
Brown, Marie Scott, and Mary M. Alexander: "Examining the Skin," *Nurs '73,* **3:**39–43, September 1973.
Caplan, Richard M., and Charles J. Hammer: "Skin Lesions: Identifying and Treating Common Fungal Infections," *Patient Care,* **7:**24–44, Oct. 1, 1973.
Caplan, Richard M., and Charles J. Hammer: "Skin Lesions: Watch for Common Fungal Infections," *Nurs Update,* **7:**3–8, February 1976.
Cirksena, William J., H. L. Albert, and James H. Knepshield: "Cutaneous Manifestations of Renal Disease," *Hosp Med,* **9:**61–74, September 1973.
Cooper, Max D., and Alexander R. Lawton: "The Development of the Immune System," *Sci Am,* November 1974, pp. 59–72.
DeCoursey, Russell M.: *The Human Organism,* 4th ed., McGraw-Hill, New York, 1974, pp. 327–333.
Derbes, Vincent J.: "Rashes: Recognition and Management," *Nurs '73,* **3:**44–49, March 1973.
Dharan, Murali: "Immunoglobulin Abnormalities," *Am J Nurs,* October 1976, pp. 1626–1628.
Haider, S.: "Infectious Diseases: Rashes," *Nurs Mirror,* **137**(S):1–8, Oct. 19, 1973.
Jacoway, John R. et al.: "Oral Cancer," *Hosp Med,* **8:**69–84, April 1972.
Jordan, William P., Jr., and William F. Schorr: "Finding the Cause of Contact Dermatitis," *Nurs Update,* **7:**3–9, April 1976.
Krall, Leo P. et al.: "Foot Lesions in Diabetes," *Hosp Med,* **9:**66–78, January 1973.
Krull, Edward A., Ira Mersack, and Dennis A. Weigand: "When the Problem Is Hair Loss," *Patient Care,* **7:**20–33, Mar. 1, 1973.
Mayer, Manfred M.: "The Complement System," *Sci Am,* November 1973, pp. 54–66.
Nysather, John O., Arnold E. Katy, and Janet L. Lenth: "The Immune System: Its Development and Function," *Am J Nurs,* October 1976, pp. 1614–1618.
Parrish, John A.: *Dermatology and Skin Care,* McGraw-Hill, New York, 1975.
Pillsbury, Donald M.: *A Manual of Dermatology,* Saunders, Philadelphia, 1971.
Rice, Alice K.: "Common Skin Infections in School Children," *Am J Nurs,* **73:**1905–1909, October 1973.
Robbins, Stanley, and Marcia Angell: *Basic Pathology,* 2d ed., Saunders, Philadelphia, 1976, pp. 31–67, 167–209.
Roberts, Sharon L.: "Skin Assessment for Color and Temperature," *Am J Nurs,* **75:**610–613, April 1975.

Robinson, Raymond C. V.: "Bacterial Infections of the Skin," *Hosp Med,* **8:**11–31, April 1972.

Samman, Peter D.: *The Nails in Disease,* Charles C Thomas, Springfield, Ill., 1972.

Sana, Josephine M., and Richard D. Judge: *Physical Appraisal Methods in Nursing Practice,* Little, Brown, Boston, 1975.

Schragger, Alan H.: "Common Skin Disorders and What to Do About Them," *Hosp Med,* **8:**79–103, May 1972.

Silverman, Mark E.: "Physical Signs in Infective Endocarditis," *Hosp Med,* **9:**94–104, January, 1973.

Smith, J. D., and John M. Knox: "Management of Precancer of the Skin," *Hosp Med,* **8:**40–60, February 1972.

Spiro, Joel M.: "Skin Clues to Neurologic Disease," *Consultant,* **15:**91–95, January 1975.

Tardy, M. Eugene, Jr., and Francis L. Lederer: "Visual Guide to the Diagnosis of Nasal Lesions," *Hosp Med,* **8:**8–33, October 1972.

Verbov, Julian: *Skin Diseases in the Elderly,* Lippincott, Philadelphia, 1974.

Weinstein, Gerald D., and Victor H. Witten: "Cancer of the Skin," *Hosp Med,* **8:**68–80, March 1972.

Wintrobe, Maxwell et al.: *Harrison's Principles of Internal Medicine,* 7th ed., McGraw-Hill, New York, 1974, pp. 342–346.

# 9

## DISRUPTIVE INFLAMMATORY RESPONSES*

Nina H. Williams

A delicate but peaceful interaction is ordinarily maintained between humans and their environment. Each of us is "infected" from birth with a wide variety of bacteria which are part of the natural microflora, but these organisms normally do not cause clinical disease. The body's defenses serve to limit the flora to areas where they are safely tolerated. Normal products of growing and dying cells are also removed by the body's defenses.

However, the balance between humans and their environment can be upset if an irritant is capable of breaching the body's natural protective barriers or if normal defense mechanisms are impaired. Clinical signs and symptoms result from the action of the irritant (e.g., virus destroying body cells), as well as from the host's reaction to the irritant (e.g., inflammation). Inflammation is the body's normal reaction to irritation, regardless of the nature of the initial irritant.

This chapter describes the inflammatory response in selected communicable diseases and disorders of the integumentary system. In the various examples, inflammation is induced by infection, infestation, trauma, chemical or physical agents, and antigen-antibody reactions.

### INFLAMMATORY RESPONSE IN COMMUNICABLE DISEASES

An understanding of the infectious process is necessary for the prevention and control of communicable diseases. The essential factors for the development of the infectious disease process are a *causative agent*, a *reservoir* for the causative agent, a *mode of escape* from the reservoir, a *mode of transmission* from the reservoir to the new host, a *mode of entry* into the new host, and a *susceptible host*.

The term *infection* indicates that a viable organism capable of causing disease is present within a person. What happens under such circumstances depends on the difference in magnitude between two opposing forces: those of infection and those of the host's resistance. When the infecting forces are sufficiently greater than the resisting forces, clinical manifestations of disease occur. Depending on the balance between the two forces, the disease

* The author acknowledges the assistance of William B. Taylor, M.D., Thomas F. Anderson, M.D., Marion Koch, R.N., Paul F. Durkee, M.D., Carol Barnett, R.N., Yvonne Backus, R.N. Marjorie Dutton, R.N., Jan Holloway, R.N., George H. Nolan, M.D., and Gloria Staiger, R.N., in reviewing the manuscript of this section.

may be so mild as to go unrecognized, so severe as to be fatal, or anywhere on a continuum between these two extremes. If the forces are equal a *carrier* state exists. No disease will occur if the resistive forces are sufficiently greater than the infecting forces.

*Bacteria* produce disease by either the invasion of tissues or the elaboration of toxins. Bacteria invade tissues which provide the appropriate pH, oxygen, temperature, and nutrients for growth and multiplication. Many microorganisms produce extracellular products which enhance the spread of the bacteria through the host's tissues. For example, when coagulase is secreted by an organism, it induces clotting which walls the organism off from the action of host defenses. Other factors produced by bacteria, such as collagenase, hyaluronidase, and streptokinase (fibrinolysin), dissolve host tissues to aid in the spread of the organisms. Some species of bacteria have a protective coat which prevents their ingestion by the host's phagocytes or enables them to survive it. The ability to kill phagocytes is associated with the organism's production of leukocidin, which destroys white blood cells. Thus, the bacteria are able to grow, multiply, and spread locally. Their presence in the host's tissues is irritating and evokes an inflammatory response. When the host defenses are insufficient to contain the invading microorganisms locally, the bacteria may travel along the lymphatics and reach the bloodstream. Widespread dissemination of infection leading to involvement of multiple organs can result.

When circumstances are unfavorable, some bacteria have the ability to change to a smaller, less active form, a *spore,* which resists drying, heat, and antiseptic agents. In more favorable situations, vegetative forms capable of invading human tissues grow from the spores. Other bacteria, in unfavorable circumstances, go through a series of changes known as *L forms* before reverting in better conditions to their original size and form.

Most of the harmful effects of bacteria can be attributed to chemical substances called *toxins;* these may be exotoxins or endotoxins. *Exotoxins* are proteins secreted by certain species of bacteria which are extremely toxic and specific in their action. Exotoxins act as antigens and can be neutralized by their homologous antibody (antitoxin). *Endotoxins,* by comparison, compose part of the bacterial cell wall and are released only upon disruption of the bacterial cell. Endotoxins are considerably less potent than exotoxins, and their actions are more varied and less specific. Among the many

effects of endotoxins are fever, diarrhea, hypotension, shock, transient leukopenia followed by leukocytosis, hyperglycemia, capillary hemorrhages, diffuse intravascular coagulation, and altered resistance to bacterial infections.

*Viruses* consist basically of a core of nucleic acid (RNA or DNA) surrounded by a protein coat. The protein coat is antigenic and specific for each type of virus. Thus, virus infections stimulate the production of antibodies which usually provide the host with immunity or resistance to reinfection with the same virus. Viruses are unable to function or multiply outside living cells.

Unlike bacteria, viruses damage host cells by direct invasion and not by the production of toxins. In many cases the infected cell is completely destroyed by the virus, and this destruction causes the signs of illness. Most viruses damage only specific kinds of cells, such as those in the liver or the mucous membrane of the nose and throat. In other instances viruses do not kill the host's cells but cause them to grow abnormally, as in the case of malignant cells. Viruses may also cause latent infection, remaining within the cell in a potentially active state but producing no obvious effect on the cell's functions.

Obviously, humans would be overcome by the forces of infection if they did not have effective means of resistance. There are anatomic barriers to invading organisms such as skin, nasal hairs, and the mucociliary blanket of the tracheobronchial tree. Cells of the reticuloendothelial system, polymorphonuclear leukocytes, and monocytes all have the ability to phagocytize microorganisms. Phagocytes engulf organisms and destroy them by means of enzymes. Cell-mediated and antibody-mediated immunity (see Chap. 8) develops against specific organisms. Viruses induce the production of a protein, *interferon.* When interferon is released by infected cells and taken up by other cells, the uninfected cells are rendered refractory to the viral infection.

The *inflammatory response* (see Chap. 8) constitutes the marshaling of all the nonspecific defense mechanisms. The increased blood and lymph flow which accompany inflammation serve to bring phagocytes to the scene and to flush away toxic bacterial products. Polymorphonuclear cells form the principal cellular response to bacterial invasion, while infiltration with lymphocytes and monocytes characterizes viral infection. Infiltration of inflamed areas with lymphocytes and plasma cells provides a mechanism for the development of immunity. The formation of fibrin aids in walling off the area of infection, and, finally, the local rise in temperature may be injurious to microorganisms.

## RHEUMATIC FEVER

Rheumatic fever is primarily a disease of children and young adults. It warrants detailed discussion in this section because of its suspected relationship to streptococcal infections. Rheumatic fever is an inflammatory process and is *not* infectious or communicable. However, the streptococcal sore throat thought to precede its occurrence *is* infectious and communicable. Many hospitalized adults live with the aftereffects of rheumatic fever, particularly the valvular damage referred to as rheumatic heart disease. For this reason, the nurse should be familiar with the total process and care of rheumatic fever.

### Pathophysiology

*Rheumatic fever* is an acute or chronic inflammatory process involving connective tissue throughout the body, especially the heart, joints, nervous system, and subcutaneous tissues. Most rheumatic fever patients have had a streptococcal infection within the preceding 2 to 4 months as demonstrated by antistreptococcal antibodies in the blood. In spite of this proof of association, no one knows how streptococci cause rheumatic fever. There is no evidence of streptococci on the heart valves or in the joints, causing direct bacterial invasion.

**Theories of causation** Although none have been proved unequivocally, there are at least five theories of causation. First, since only 1 to 3 percent of patients with untreated streptococcal infections develop rheumatic fever, it may be that susceptible individuals are *hypersensitive* to streptococci. Second, there is evidence that rheumatic fever may be the result of an *autoimmune* mechanism.[1] The streptococci may act as the original source of antigen, but immunologically similar tissue antigens that exist in the heart, blood vessels, and elsewhere can become the eventual target of the antibodies. Other theories of causation propose that there is *direct invasion* of the tissues by the unaltered streptococcus or by L forms; there is *direct toxic action* by substances produced by the streptococcus; or, lastly, there are *tissue changes* due to substances produced by the streptococcus, which predispose to eventual damage by an immunologic process.

**Major manifestations** The inflammatory process of rheumatic fever is manifested in many ways. Nonspecific reactions are fever, malaise, weakness, anorexia, abdominal pain, and weight loss. *Major manifestations* which may occur are carditis, polyarthritis, chorea, erythema marginatum, and subcutaneous nodules.

**C**arditis  The most serious of the manifestations of rheumatic fever is *carditis.* Rheumatic carditis develops in approximately 40 to 51 percent of initial attacks of rheumatic fever and involves any of the three layers of the heart (endocardium, myocardium, pericardium).[2] When the heart valves become involved in the inflammatory process, edema, ulceration, and erosion of valve flaps occur. *Valvular stenosis* results from fusion of valve leaflets which narrows the valve opening. Dilatation of valve rings, destruction of valve substance, or contraction of chordae tendineae produces regurgitation (blood leaks backward). The mitral valve is the site most frequently affected, particularly in females, followed by the aortic valve, which is damaged more often in males. The final consequence of both valvular stenosis and regurgitation is *congestive heart failure* due to an increased workload for the heart (see Chap. 27).

Inflammation of the myocardium may cause the heart muscle to become weak and flabby resulting in loss of contractile strength. Characteristic lesions called *Aschoff's bodies* may be seen in the myocardium. These appear as small nodules which consist of inflammatory cells and degenerating tissue. As the nodules age, they may become fibrotic and damage the arteries in the myocardium.

Rheumatic *pericarditis* results from a diffuse inflammatory reaction. Pericarditis may produce precordial pain, pericardial effusion, or a pericardial friction rub.

**P**olyarthritis  Red, hot, swollen joints which may be exquisitely tender characterize *polyarthritis.* It involves the large joints such as the knees, ankles, elbows, wrists, and hips most frequently. Characteristically, the joint pain is migratory, moving from one joint to another without causing permanent damage.

**C**horea  A neurologic manifestation of rheumatic fever which may develop as much as 6 months after the onset of the disease is *chorea.* In some cases it is the only clinical manifestation of rheumatic fever which occurs. The condition is characterized by involuntary muscle spasms and emotional lability.

Choreic movements are purposeless, nonrepetitive, spasmodic motions that may involve any voluntary muscle. The facial spasms give rise to bizarre grimacing and slurred speech. The hand movements make the patient clumsy and unable to perform tasks such as writing. The movements disappear during sleep. The emotional lability is characterized by irritability and by sudden outbursts of crying or aggression.

**E**rythema Marginatum A nonpruritic, flat, or slightly raised red rash that usually occurs on the trunk or extremities and accompanies rheumatic fever is *erythema marginatum.* The lesions extend and coalesce, forming larger lesions with an irregular outline. The rash is typically transitory, disappearing and then reappearing within a few hours.

**S**ubcutaneous Nodules   Firm, movable, nontender masses, less than 1 to 2 cm in size, are referred to as *subcutaneous nodules.* The scalp and the extensor surfaces of the hands and elbows are common locations. The nodules are more frequently seen in patients with severe rheumatic fever or carditis.

**Course and prognosis**   The course of rheumatic fever is highly variable. An acute attack may last a few weeks to a few months. Less than 1 to 2 percent of patients die during the initial attack; in these cases, death usually results from myocarditis.[3] Aside from carditis, each of the major manifestations of rheumatic fever subsides, leaving no residual effects. Although some individuals recover completely and never have another attack of rheumatic fever, one attack predisposes to subsequent recurrences. In recurrent attacks, the mortality rate increases to 2.3 to 3 percent.[4] The extent of cardiac damage increases with each subsequent attack. The long-term outcome of rheumatic fever depends primarily on the severity of cardiac involvement. Valvular heart disease remains the major cause of disability and death caused by rheumatic fever.

**First-Level Nursing Care**

Although the incidence of rheumatic fever is declining, it is still a major cause of death and disability in children and adolescents.[5] There still are approximately 100,000 new cases in the United States each year.[6] The initial attack of rheumatic fever occurs most frequently in school-age children between 6 and 15 years old, with a peak at about 8 years.[7] It is especially prevalent among poor, crowded, city dwellers who may be more prone to rheumatic fever because of malnutrition, greater exposure to streptococcal infections, little possibility of isolating streptococcal infections, and less money for medical care. Rheumatic fever occurs most frequently in temperate climates and during late winter and early spring when streptococcal infections are prevalent. It has a high familial incidence, but whether this is due to inheritance or environment is not known.

**Prevention**   Recognition of streptococcal pharyngitis remains vital to the prevention of rheumatic fever. Streptococci can cause an illness of varying severity in different individuals. Some infections will be so mild as to be unrecognized, while others cause severe manifestations. Symptoms include sudden onset of a sore throat, pain on swallowing, malaise, headache, and, in children, abdominal pain, nausea, and vomiting. On physical examination the throat is red with an exudate on the tonsils or tonsillar fossae; anterior cervical lymph nodes are enlarged and tender. A fever of 101 to 104°F is usually present, and the white blood cell count is greater than 12,000/mm³. A negative throat culture can exclude the diagnosis of streptococcal infection.

The optional treatment of streptococcal pharyngitis is a single dose of intramuscular long-acting benzathine penicillin G. An alternative is to administer penicillin or erythromycin orally over a 10-day period. The major disadvantage of oral treatment is that the patient may forget to take the medication or discontinue taking it once symptoms subside and never complete the full 10-day course of therapy. Penicillin must be present at effective tissue levels for at least 10 days to achieve eradication of the organism. From one-third to three-fourths of patients fail to complete oral antibiotic therapy.[8–11]

School-oriented programs, particularly in overcrowded schools in the large cities, provide an excellent opportunity for the school nurse or any trained personnel to examine children with pharyngitis and to make throat cultures. Mass culturing of schoolchildren has been undertaken in some communities. Teachers and parents should be informed about rheumatic fever and its prevention. Literature for the public is available from local chapters of the American Heart Association.

The limitations of primary preventive measures for rheumatic fever might be overcome if a safe, effective, and practical streptococcal vaccine were available. Because of the complexity of the problem, the streptococcal vaccine is still in the experimental stage.

## Second-Level Nursing Care

Because rheumatic fever manifests itself in many ways, the diagnosis is based on combinations of signs and symptons. Physicians still use as a guideline the criteria developed in 1944 by T. D. Jones and modified by the American Heart Association. The revised Jones Criteria list five major and five minor manifestations of rheumatic fever (see Table 9-1). The presence of two major manifestations or of one major and two minor manifestations indicates a high probability of rheumatic fever if there is also evidence of a preceding streptococcal infection.[12]

**Nursing assessment**  Evaluation of the patient should include a health history. Any streptococcal infection, previous incidence of rheumatic fever, or preexisting heart disease should be noted. In addition to the history, *physical assessment* of the individual for manifestations of rheumatic fever (see Pathophysiology) and a *psychosocial appraisal* are necessary to obtain information which may affect prognosis or determine the plan of care. It is helpful to know the patient's interests, hobbies, level in school, attitudes toward self, and relationships with family members. The physical characteristics of the home and the ability of the family to provide long-term care should be assessed.

**Diagnostic Tests**  There are no specific laboratory studies for diagnosing rheumatic fever. The *erythrocyte sedimentation rate* (ESR), *C-reactive protein test* (CRPA), and *white blood cell count* are all commonly elevated, indicating the presence of inflammation. Mild anemia may occur due to chronic inflammation. Ninety-five percent of rheumatic fever patients will have an increased titer of streptococcal antibodies which is evidence of a preceding streptococcal infection.[13] Tests for streptococcal antibodies include the *antistreptolysin O (ASO) titer,* the *antihyaluronidase (AH) titer,* and the *antistreptokinase (ASK or antifibrinolysin) titer.* Throat cultures may still be positive for group A beta-hemolytic streptococcus. An electrocardiogram frequently reveals a prolonged PR interval which is a common sign of acute rheumatic fever and does not necessarily indicate carditis.

**Nursing problems and intervention**  Major nursing problems include *fever, joint pain, chorea, malaise, loss of appetite,* and *potential cardiac involvement.* Interventions for these problems include drug therapy, rest, nutrition, and care of specific symptoms.

There is no specific cure for rheumatic fever, although there are supportive measures which can reduce the severity of the acute manifestations. Physicians differ on their recommendations for therapy. Generally, however, the degree of cardiac involvement is central in treatment decisions.

**Drug Therapy**  *Antibiotics* are given to destroy any remaining streptococci. The drug of choice is penicillin, although erythromycin can be used by those persons who are allergic to penicillin. The patient should be protected against exposure to persons with respiratory infections who could be harboring streptococci.

*Salicylates* (sodium salicylate or acetylsalicylic acid) and/or *corticosteroids* are prescribed to minimize the inflammatory process. The fever and arthritis improve dramatically with the use of salicylates. Although corticosteroids are very effective anti-inflammatory agents, they have serious side effects, and there is a tendency for the disease to flare up when the dose is reduced (rebound phenomenon). Some physicians prefer to use corticosteroids for the treatment of severe carditis or for patients whose signs and symptoms fail to improve with salicylates. Patients on steroids need to be prepared for potential side effects such as fat redistribution (the moon face, truncal obesity, and so forth), acne, hirsutism, gastric irritation, and increased susceptibility to infection. Patients should also be monitored for hyperglycemia, hypertension, and weight gain. Salicylates and steroids should be administered with milk, antacids, or meals to reduce gastric irritation. Unfortunately, neither steroids nor salicylates alter the duration of the rheumatic attack or prevent the damaging effects of rheumatic carditis.

**Painful Joints**  When the joints are painful, measures should be taken to protect the patient from unnecessary discomfort. When handling the af-

**TABLE 9-1**
REVISED JONES CRITERIA FOR GUIDANCE IN THE DIAGNOSIS OF RHEUMATIC FEVER

| Major Manifestations | Minor manifestations |
| --- | --- |
| Carditis<br>Polyarthritis<br>Chorea<br>Erythema marginatum<br>Subcutaneous nodules | History of previous rheumatic fever or evidence of preexisting rheumatic heart disease<br>Arthralgia<br>Fever<br>Abnormal erythrocyte sedimentation rate or C-reactive protein test<br>Electrocardiographic changes, mainly PR-interval prolongation |

fected extremity, care should be taken to minimize movement of the joint by supporting both above and below the joint. Because the arthritis is temporary and will cause no permanent deformity, the extremities can be supported in whatever position provides the most comfort. A cradle may be employed to keep the weight of the bed linens off the affected joints. Local applications of heat may afford the patient some relief.

Patients with rheumatic fever have traditionally been confined to bed for long periods of time. Because the value of prolonged bed rest has not been proved, some physicians feel it is unnecessary. A patient with painful arthritis, uncontrolled chorea, or severe congestive heart failure will usually be limited in activity. Because rheumatic fever is an inflammatory rather than an infectious process, isolation procedures are not necessary.

**C**horea  The patient with chorea is likely to be frustrated, embarrassed, and moody. It is important to reassure the patient and family members that the peculiar movements are due to a neurologic disorder, are temporary, and do not affect the intellect. Precautions against bruising and falling out of bed should be taken. Because choreiform movements disappear during sleep, sedatives may be ordered, and care should be organized to minimize interruptions.

**D**ecreased Appetite  Because of weakness and discomfort, the appetite may be decreased. Adequate nutrition should be encouraged by including food the patient likes, serving it attractively, and providing socialization during meals. A diet high in proteins and carbohydrates may be necessary to meet the increased demands for nutrients when fever and infection are present. Fluid intake should also be encouraged. In any febrile state, fluids are lost through perspiration and the high rate of protein metabolism.

**R**eferral  As with other long-term illnesses, the *education* of the patient and family members about the nature of rheumatic fever is imperative if they are to assume responsibility for treatment of the current attack and prevention of recurrences. The family may need guidance in the use of community resources. The Crippled Children's Commission and the American Heart Association may provide information and financial assistance.

Regardless of whether the patient is hospitalized, a community health nurse referral should be made. Through home visits the nurse can help the family plan home nursing care and follow up on the continuity of therapy.

### Third-Level Nursing Care

Patients with rheumatic fever are likely to be hospitalized for varying periods of time, ranging from a few weeks to a few months. In some cases, however, the patient is hospitalized only to establish the diagnosis and is then discharged with a home care plan.

**Nursing assessment**  Since cardiac complications have the most serious long-term implications for the patient, nurses need to teach patients and their families about the symptoms of carditis and congestive heart failure. Once the patient is hospitalized, the nurse needs to be equally observant for changes in the cardiac status.

**P**hysical Assessment  Inflammation of the heart valves results in *abnormal murmurs* heard on auscultation of the heart. A systolic murmur with a very high-pitched sound (called a *cooing-dove sound*), indicating mitral regurgitation, is typical. Enlargement of the left atrium and the left ventricle, with swelling of the valve leaflets and rings, produces a relative mitral stenosis heard as a middiastolic murmur (called the *Carey-Coombs murmur*).

Progressive damage to the heart may result in signs of congestive heart failure. The nurse should be alert for any *dyspnea, cough, fatigue, anorexia, abdominal pain, enlarged liver, gallop rhythm,* or *edema.*

**D**iagnostic Tests  In addition to the tests mentioned under First-Level Nursing Care, x-ray and electrocardiograph readings may be taken. Chest x-rays may reveal the left ventricular hypertrophy characteristic of congestive heart failure. Electrocardiographic tracings may show a lengthened PR interval; occasionally second-degree heart block is present.

**Nursing problems and intervention**  Nursing problems at this level include *joint pain, malaise, fever,* and the *cardiac symptoms.* Care for a rheumatic fever patient in the hospital is much the same as described under Second-Level Nursing Care. Additional therapy, specific to the cardiac involvement, may be added. This would include the routine drug, dietary, and fluid management of a patient with congestive heart failure (see Chap. 27). Administration of anti-inflammatory and antibiotic medications, and care of other symptoms, would be as previously described.

### Fourth-Level Nursing Care

Rehabilitation of the patient with rheumatic fever is facilitated by occupational therapy, schooling, and vocational preparation. Diversional activities are enjoyable, provide an acceptable outlet for releasing tensions, and help to develop talents and satisfactions. Maintaining contact with peers helps to keep the patient group-oriented rather than totally ego-centered. Continuation of schooling is essential, either through a hospital school or a visiting teacher. Prolonged interruptions in schooling are hard to make up and can delay the patient's recovery. The teacher needs to be kept informed about the patient's progress and whether there are any physical restrictions. Patients with rheumatic fever are not likely to be restricted in choice of occupation. However, heavy physical labor or employment under poor environmental conditions of dampness, crowding, or excessive exposure to infectious illness is not recommended.

Once limits on activity have been identified, the patient should be involved in plans for recovery and encouraged to be independent and active within the prescribed limits. Through education concerning rheumatic fever, patients and their families can form realistic expectations for the future with minimal psychologic effects from the threat of future rheumatic attacks or cardiac disability.

The long-term management of patients who recover from acute rheumatic fever will vary with the degree of cardiac involvement. Most patients will be relatively asymptomatic in childhood but may have progressive disability as adults. Valvular disease progresses over a period of years due to scar tissue formation. Patients with severe valvular stenosis or regurgitation resulting in congestive heart failure are candidates for open-heart surgery. The malfunctioning valves may be surgically repaired or replaced with prosthetic valves (see Chap. 27).

Every patient with rheumatic fever should be protected against subsequent streptococcal infections. Persons who have had a streptococcal infection within the last 3 months should be avoided. Rheumatic patients need to know the importance of seeing a physician for prompt antibiotic therapy should a sore throat occur. After an initial attack of rheumatic fever, the rate of recurrence of rheumatic fever following a streptococcal infection may reach 50 percent.[14] Patients should be told that it is important to avoid subsequent attacks of rheumatic fever

because the possibility of heart damage increases with each attack of rheumatic fever.

The most effective prophylactic regimen is a monthly injection of 1.2 million units benzathine penicillin which prevents streptococcal infections in 99 percent of patients treated.[15] Oral prophylaxis is slightly less effective possibly because patients do not take the drug as prescribed. The nurse's enthusiasm and encouragement are extremely important in motivating patients to continue taking prophylactic medication. Penicillin, sulfadiazine, or erythromycin given orally provides acceptable prophylaxis. Additional doses of prophylactic antibiotics must be given when patients with a history of rheumatic fever undergo surgical or dental procedures. This is because there is an increased risk of bacterial endocarditis when the heart valves are diseased.

The risk of recurrence of rheumatic fever is increased with the presence of rheumatic heart disease, with an increased number of preceding attacks of rheumatic fever, with a recent attack of rheumatic fever (within the previous 5 years), with exposure to streptococcal infections, and during childhood. When deciding whether prophylaxis should be discontinued, these factors are all considered. Most authorities recommend that antirheumatic prophylaxis be maintained for at least 5 years after the last acute attack and until the patient reaches the age of 25 years. When carditis is present, prophylaxis will probably be maintained for the rest of the patient's life.

## TUBERCULOSIS

Tuberculosis continues to be a health problem and is, therefore, of concern to the nurse, particularly the community health nurse. Patients with this disease often have concurrent health problems, and it behooves the nurse to be aware of the total patient being assessed.

### Pathophysiology

Tuberculosis is a destructive, infectious disease caused by the tubercle bacillus, *Mycobacterium tuberculosis*. Tubercle bacilli are nonmotile, acid-fast, and incapable of multiplication outside the body except under laboratory conditions. Tuberculosis is a chronic infection consistent with the slow rate of multiplication of tubercle bacilli (once every 14 to 24 hours). *Mycobacterium tuberculosis* is an obligate aerobe, which explains why the lungs are the most common site of infection. Tubercle bacilli are readily killed by burning, boiling for 5 minutes, autoclaving, or exposure to sunlight or ultraviolet irradiation.

In the United States tuberculosis infection is almost always acquired by inhaling tubercle bacilli in *droplet nuclei* produced when a person with active pulmonary tuberculosis speaks, laughs, coughs, or sneezes. *Large* droplets, visible to the naked eye, tend to settle too quickly to be inhaled or are caught on the mucociliary blanket of the tracheobronchial tree and cleared from the lungs without harm. Droplet nuclei are so small as to be invisible and may be deposited deeply in the respiratory bronchioles or alveoli, beyond the protective mucous blanket. There, the droplet nuclei may become implanted and establish an infection. Droplet nuclei can be carried by air currents, although they may remain viable for only a few hours. Out of doors the droplets undergo such great dilution that they create little hazard.

Although the tubercle bacilli can lie dormant in dark places outside the body, as in dust, they pose little threat of causing infection. Attached to dust or fomites, the tubercle bacilli are not likely to be inhaled or to be implanted in the alveoli or bronchioles.

**Primary tuberculosis**   The initial infection an individual experiences with tubercle bacilli is called *primary tuberculosis.* Since tubercle bacilli enter the body by inhalation, the majority of primary lesions are in the lower two-thirds of the lungs, where ventilation is greatest. Most frequently a single focus of infection develops (the *Ghon focus*), although multiple foci do occur (see Fig. 9-1).

When the tubercle bacilli invade the lungs, the body's defense mechanisms attempt to isolate and destroy the organisms. White blood cells and macrophages phagocytize bacilli, but the organisms continue to survive and multiply. Lymphocytes accumulate around the focus of infection. Eventually, fibroblasts appear in the periphery of the lesion, and a dense zone of scar tissue is laid down forming a capsule, or *tubercle,* which walls off the infected area.

Wandering white blood cells which engulf the tubercle bacilli carry some of them to regional (hilar) lymph nodes. This regional adenitis in the hilar lymph nodes, along with the inflammatory reaction at the site of infection, is referred to as the *primary complex.*

Three to ten weeks after the first infection, cellular immunity develops, marked by the appearance of T lymphocytes specifically sensitized to the tubercle bacilli or their proteins (*tuberculins*). It is this hypersensitivity which is detected by the tuberculin skin test and is usually successful in arresting the tuberculosis infection.

The central portions of the tubercles typically undergo a process of degeneration (*caseation*). The necrotic tissue in the lesion usually persists as a cheeselike mass called *caseous material.* The lesion heals by resolution, in which the caseous exudate is absorbed, or by fibrosis and calcification, in which calcium and lime deposits are deposited in the scar formation. Calcified lesions may be seen by x-ray for the rest of the person's life.

In the vast majority of cases primary infection is so well controlled by the body's defense system that it causes no apparent illness and heals without being diagnosed. Occasionally defenses fail and the patient develops *progressive primary tuberculosis.* In this situation the patient directly enters the stage of chronic tuberculosis.

The principal importance of primary tuberculosis is that during this stage tubercle bacilli are carried in the lymphatic system and bloodstream to other parts of the body where distant focal lesions are established. These metastatic foci most frequently occur in the apex of the lung (*Simon foci*) where the oxygen tension is high, but they may also develop in the kidney, ends of long bones, spine, brain, or elsewhere. This process is usually asymptomatic. Occasionally, such foci progress and produce destructive tuberculosis in a short period of time, but more commonly the body's defenses wall off the metastatic foci along with the primary infection.

**Latent (dormant) tuberculosis**   Even though the primary infection and metastatic foci heal, tubercle bacilli often remain alive, especially in the Simon foci in the upper lung lobes. While the tubercle bacilli usually remain dormant for the duration of the individual's life, they are still alive and may erupt into active tuberculosis at any time.

**Chronic (adult, postprimary, or reactivation) tuberculosis**   Most cases of tuberculosis among adults today are the result of reactivation of latent tubercle bacilli when the body's resistance is lowered for any reason. Various factors which may impair the body's defenses and increase the risk of latent infection developing into active tuberculosis include emotional stress, adolescence, pregnancy, old age, alcoholism, malnutrition, diabetes mellitus, silicosis, gastrectomy, prolonged treatment with corticosteroids, immunosuppressive therapy, and malignancies (especially malignancies of the reticuloendothelial system).

The most common site for chronic tuberculosis is in the Simon foci, although foci anywhere in the body can be the sites of late progression. The caseous material in the center of the lesion tends to soften and liquefy. If erosion into a bronchiole occurs, the highly infectious material drains into the tracheobronchial tree and is expectorated as *sputum*. Caseous material may also be aspirated to new areas of the lungs and give rise to new lesions. As the liquefied material drains out of the lesion, an air-filled sac or *cavity* is formed. Individuals with unusual resistance may live for many years with chronic pulmonary tuberculosis. *Pleural effusion* may occur due to the spread of caseous material into the pleural space, which in turn causes an inflammatory reaction. *Miliary tuberculosis* occurs when a necrotic focus erodes a blood vessel, suddenly spilling a large number of organisms into the bloodstream. This event overwhelms the body's defense mechanisms, seeding many organs simultaneously, and may be rapidly fatal without treatment. *Tuberculous meningitis* follows rupture of a caseous focus into the subarachnoid space and can also be rapidly fatal. Other forms of extrapulmonary tuberculosis include tuberculosis of kidney, bone, lymph nodes, reproductive organs, peritoneum, pericardium, adrenals, and larynx.

### First-Level Nursing Care

Although the morbidity and mortality rates for tuberculosis have fallen dramatically in the United States during the twentieth century, tuberculosis continues to be a serious public health problem. About 16 million persons (8 percent of the total population) are thought to have tuberculous infection.[16] While most of these infections are healed foci of latent tuberculosis, it is in this group that over 90 percent of new active cases of tuberculosis will arise.[17] Over 30,000 new cases of active tuberculosis are reported annually,[18,19] and over 250,000 total cases are under medical supervision in the United States.[20] Tuberculosis has dropped from the leading cause of death with over 200 deaths per 100,000 population in 1906[21] to 1.8 deaths per 100,000 in 1974.[22]

Tuberculosis is common among city dwellers where circumstances such as overcrowding, poor ventilation, and undernourishment favor the transmission of the disease. It is more common among nonwhite than white Americans probably because of both environmental conditions and immune response.[23,24] For unknown reasons, tuberculosis is

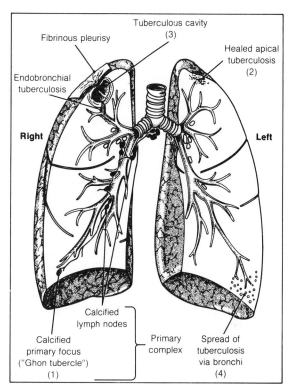

**FIGURE 9-1**

Pulmonary tuberculosis. Diagrammatic drawing of lungs shows progressive stages of pulmonary TB: (1) Healed and calcified complex of primary infection—primary focus and tributary lymph glands at base of right lung. (2) Healed lesion in left lung apex. (3) TB disease with cavity formation in right lung subapical region. (4) Disease spreads to opposite lower lobe through bronchial channels. (*Used by permission. Introduction to Lung Diseases, New York: American Lung Association, 1975, p. 35.*)

twice as common among males as females, especially those over 45 years of age.[25] Although tuberculosis is not inherited, children may develop the disease because of close contact with tuberculous parents.

**Prevention** Many factors are involved in the prevention of tuberculosis. Routine tuberculin testing of cattle and pasteurization of milk virtually eliminate the occurrence of bovine tuberculosis. Widespread public education about tuberculosis promotes early detection and prevents spread of the infection. Community action to improve economic conditions, nutrition, housing, sanitation, and health habits serves to reduce its incidence.

For those who have never been infected with tubercle bacilli, *bacillus Calmette-Guérin* (*BCG*) is available to induce immunity. BCG contains live, attenuated bovine tubercle bacilli incapable of producing active disease. Vaccination with BCG is about 80 percent effective in preventing tuberculous infection and almost 100 percent effective in keeping the infections that do occur from being fatal.[26] Although BCG is widely used in other countries, it is seldom used in the United States. Most authorities agree that the risk of tuberculosis among nonreactors in the United States is too small to justify using BCG vaccine. Because BCG changes the tuberculin skin test to a positive reaction, it interferes with the usefulness of tuberculin testing for case finding.

### Second-Level Nursing Care

Nursing care of patients with tuberculosis is administered primarily through clinic or outpatient services. Accurate assessment is essential to detect additional health problems that may contribute to the severity of the disease.

**Nursing assessment** Most patients with *primary tuberculosis* have no symptoms. Although infection may be discovered by a chest x-ray or physical examination, the primary method for discovering infection is usually the *tuberculin skin test.* When tuberculin, a protein fraction of tubercle bacilli, is injected intradermally into a person with tuberculous infection, latent or active, it causes a localized thickening of the skin over the next 24 to 72 hours because of the accumulation of sensitized T lymphocytes. The preferred method is to inject 0.1 ml of a solution containing 5 tuberculin units (TU) of purified protein derivative stabilized with Tween 80 (5 TU PPD-T or the Mantoux test) into the skin of the volar aspect of the forearm. If properly administered, a pale elevation resembling a mosquito bite is produced by the injection. The Mantoux test is read 48 to 72 hours later by observing and palpating the injection site for induration. An area of induration 10 mm or more in diameter is considered a positive reaction. Induration from 5 to 9 mm in diameter is classified as a doubtful reaction, and an induration less than 5 mm in diameter is a negative reaction. Other methods of tuberculin skin testing include jet gun injection and multiple puncture tests (e.g., Heaf, Sterneedle, Mono-Vacc, or tine).[27]

A positive reaction to the tuberculin skin test indicates that the individual has been infected with tubercle bacilli at some time in the past. The tubercle bacilli may be present as either latent or active

infection. In general, tuberculin reactivity persists throughout the individual's life, even after successful treatment of tuberculosis. Vaccination with BCG to induce immunity also produces a positive tuberculin reaction. A negative tuberculin reaction indicates that the individual has never been infected with tubercle bacilli.

Routine tuberculin testing should be performed on individuals who have a high risk of developing tuberculosis, such as the elderly, the poor, hospital employees, and the ill who have impaired body defenses. Persons with *positive tuberculin reactions* should have chest x-rays taken and should be examined for evidence of tuberculosis.

**Nursing problems and intervention** The major problem that must be dealt with when caring for patients with asymptomatic primary tuberculosis is *control of the infection.* This involves prophylactic drug therapy and identification of potentially infected persons.

When infection has occurred but there is no evidence of active tuberculosis, chemoprophylaxis is widely advocated. A single daily dose of 300 mg *isoniazid* (INH) taken orally for 1 year prevents latent infection from developing into active disease, as well as the possible subsequent spread of infection to other persons.

At the beginning of treatment with INH, the nurse should instruct the patient about the disease process, necessity of treatment, and importance of recognition and prompt reporting of signs and symptoms of toxicity (see Table 9-2). Patients should be helped to develop their own system of reminders to take the medication daily. Patients may also need information or assistance to obtain the medication. The nurse's enthusiasm and encouragement are extremely important in motivating patients to complete the full course of treatment.

Because administration of INH is not without risks, the American Thoracic Society has developed criteria for therapy to prevent tuberculosis.[28] In order of priority, chemoprophylaxis is recommended for: (1) household members and other close contacts of persons with recently diagnosed tuberculous disease; (2) positive tuberculin test reactors with chest x-ray findings consistent with tuberculosis; (3) newly infected persons; (4) positive reactors to tuberculin skin test with prolonged corticosteroid therapy, immunosuppressive therapy, hematologic and reticuloendothelial diseases, diabetes mellitus, silicosis, or gastrectomy; and (5) other positive skin test reactors, especially infants, adolescents, and the elderly.

**TABLE 9-2**
ANTITUBERCULOSIS MEDICATIONS

## PRIMARY MEDICATIONS

| Name | Usual Adult Daily Dosage and Route | Side Effects | Remarks |
|------|------|------|------|
| Isoniazid (INH) | 300 mg po (5–10 mg/kg po) | Toxicity: Peripheral neuritis (numbness, tingling, burning of feet or hands), anemia. Hypersensitivity: Hepatitis, nausea, vomiting, fever, rash. | For neuritis, pyridoxine 25–50 mg as prophylaxis, 50–100 mg as treatment. Serious side effects are rare. Mild and transient elevation of SGOT or SGPT may occur without cessation of INH. Discontinue drug with signs of hypersensitivity. Reduce dose in renal insufficiency. |
| Rifampin (RMP or RFN) | 600 mg po | Minimal; liver dysfunction, GI upset. | Extremely effective; PAS decreases its GI absorption. Warn patient it colors the urine orange. Monitor SGOT and SGPT. May alter serum levels of anticoagulants and interfere with birth control pills. |
| Ethambutol (EMB) | 25 mg/kg for 60 days, then 15 mg/kg po | Rare optic neuritis. | Optic neuritis reversible with discontinuation of drug. Ocular history and funduscopic examination advisable before use. Monitor visual acuity (Snellen chart) and red-green color discrimination. |
| Streptomycin (SM) | 0.75–1.0 g IM may be reduced to 2–3 times a week | Otic and vestibular toxicity, decreased hearing, vertigo, tinnitus, rare renal toxicity. Hypersensitivity: Fever, rash, malaise. | Frequently given with advanced disease. Monitor gross hearing (ticking of watch); if abnormal, take audiograms. Measure BUN and creatinine. Do not use with CM, KM, VM. Reduce dose in renal insufficiency. |
| Para-amino-salicylic acid (PAS) | 12–15 g po | GI irritation, Na load. Hypersensitivity: Rash, fever, malaise, hepatotoxicity. | Potentiates effects of INH. Give with meals or antacids. Avoid in patients with peptic ulcer or irritable bowel. |

## SECONDARY MEDICATIONS

| Name | Usual Adult Daily Dosage and Route | Side Effects | Remarks |
|------|------|------|------|
| Ethionamide (ETA) | 0.5–1.0 g po | GI irritation, hepatotoxicity. Hypersensitivity: Rash. | Temporarily stop with GI irritation or hepatotoxicity. Monitor SGOT and SGPT. |
| Pyrazinamide (PZA) | 1.5–3.0 g po | Hyperuricemia, hepatotoxicity, arthralgia. | Monitor uric acid, SGOT, and SGPT. Benemid or allopurinol to reduce serum uric acid. |
| Cycloserine (CS) | 0.5–1.0 g po | CNS toxicity: Psychosis, personality changes, convulsions, insomnia, irritability. Rash. | For CNS toxicity, pyridoxine 50–300 mg/day, sedatives, anticonvulsants. Avoid in patients with azotemia. Monitor serum drug levels if poor renal function. |
| Capreomycin (CAP or CM) | 1 g IM for 60–120 days then 1 g IM 2–3 times a wk | Nephrotoxicity, ototoxicity, hepatotoxicity, hypersensitivity. | Avoid with SM, KM, VM. Monitor gross hearing; if abnormal, take audiograms. Monitor BUN, creatinine, SGOT, and SGPT. |
| Viomycin (VM) | 1 g q 12 h for 2 doses twice a week IM | Similar to streptomycin but nephrotoxicity more common. | Monitor gross hearing; if abnormal, take audiograms. Monitor BUN, creatinine, urine. Do not use with SM, CM, KM. |
| Kanamycin (KM) | 0.5–1.0 g IM | Vestibular and auditory toxicity, nephrotoxicity. | Do not use with SM, VM, CM. Rarely used. |

SOURCE: Adapted with permission from John G. Weg, *Tuberculosis and Other Mycobacterial Diseases,* American Lung Association and its Medical Section, American Thoracic Society, 1976, p. 7.

### Third-Level Nursing Care

Hospitalization is usually recommended for new, active cases of tuberculosis. Hospital facilities are used to establish the diagnosis and detect other diseases that may be present. It is advisable that patients be under medical supervision while antituberculosis medications are started because of their possible adverse effects. Hospitalization prevents the spread of infection to friends and family while the patient is contagious. Hospitalization also provides an opportunity to help patients accept the diagnosis, to learn about tuberculosis and its treatment, and to plan for long-term outpatient care. Patients may need to be hospitalized for a couple of weeks to a few months.

**Nursing assessment** Because the onset of pulmonary tuberculosis is usually insidious, the disease may be well advanced by the time the patient seeks medical attention. The *health history* may reveal *fatigue, irritability, anorexia, weight loss, irregular menses, night sweats,* and *late afternoon low-grade fevers.* Chest symptoms include a *chronic cough* associated with the production of green or yellow sputum and *chest pain* of varying severity. *Hemoptysis* is unusual but prompts the patient to seek medical attention. Dyspnea does not occur until the lungs are extensively involved, unless there is a pleural effusion. In some patients the onset of pulmonary tuberculosis is relatively sudden, with *fever, chills, productive cough,* and *pleuritic pain.*

**P**hysical Assessment Physical findings may be unremarkable. While some persons with longstanding tuberculosis appear debilitated, most patients appear amazingly well. Rales may be heard on auscultation over the affected lung. Long-standing tuberculosis with extensive fibrosis may produce dullness on percussion, bronchial breath sounds, deviation of the trachea, and unequal lung expansion bilaterally. The nurse should be alert for any abnormal signs and symptoms which may be indicative of extrapulmonary tuberculosis.

**D**iagnostic Tests Routine diagnostic findings of pulmonary tuberculosis include a positive tuberculin skin test, abnormalities characteristic of tuberculosis visible on chest x-rays, and identification of *M. tuberculosis* from sputum cultures. Because tubercle bacilli reproduce slowly, a minimum of 3 weeks is usually necessary to obtain a positive culture report and 6 to 8 weeks is needed for a negative report. Stained smears of the sputum may

identify the organism more quickly, although culturing of *M. tuberculosis* is necessary to confirm the diagnosis. A series of at least three single, early morning sputum specimens should be collected from the patient. Heated aerosol treatments may help to induce sputum production in persons who have difficulty raising sputum spontaneously. When no sputum can be collected, gastric contents may be aspirated before breakfast, permitting the study of swallowed sputum.

On the evening prior to sputum collection the patient should receive the specimen container with instructions on how to obtain the sputum. Secretions tend to pool and collect in the lungs during sleep so that early morning coughing is likely to produce sputum. The use of antiseptic mouthwashes immediately prior to obtaining the specimen may affect the viability of the microorganisms and should be discouraged. The patient should be instructed to cough deeply in order to produce at least a teaspoonful of sputum from below the larynx. The opening and inside of the specimen container must be kept sterile. Patients should be instructed to inform the nurse as soon as the sputum specimen has been obtained so that it can be immediately delivered to the bacteriology laboratory.

**Nursing problems and interventions** *Chest symptoms* (pain, cough, etc.), *anorexia,* and *control of the infection* may be identified as the primary nursing problems in caring for a patient with active pulmonary tuberculosis.

*Chemotherapy* is the specific treatment for active tuberculosis regardless of the organ involved. If adequately treated, tuberculosis can be controlled in 95 percent of patients.[29] *Primary medications* listed in Table 9-2 are those which are most effective and most commonly used in the initial treatment of active tuberculosis. In the treatment of active disease at least two medications which affect the bacilli in different ways are prescribed concurrently to minimize the development of drug-resistant organisms. The choice of medications depends on the results of culture and sensitivity studies and the extent of the patient's disease. Because tubercle bacilli multiply slowly and many of the antituberculosis medications are bacteriostatic, therapy must be continued for at least 2 years to allow time for the body's defenses to contain all the organisms. Antituberculosis medications are more effective when administered in a single daily dose which obtains a single peak concentration of medication, rather than in divided doses throughout the day. Injectables are administered about one hour after oral medications so that the peak concentrations of the medications will occur simultaneously.

*Patient education* plays a highly significant role in successful chemotherapy. Patients need to understand that they are not cured of tuberculosis when their symptoms disappear and that failure to take their medications as prescribed will probably result in reactivation of the infection. Educational materials about tuberculosis for patient teaching are available from local branches of the American Lung Association (which was formerly called the National Tuberculosis and Respiratory Disease Association). Patients should be taught the names and doses of their medications and side effects which they should report to their physician. Patients are usually taught to take all oral antituberculosis medications before breakfast when intestinal absorption is rapid.

Chemotherapy renders the patient noninfectious within days to a few weeks, even before cultures for tubercle bacilli become negative. Patients and their families can be reassured that it is the unknown, undiagnosed person who creates a hazardous environment, not the diagnosed case. Although chemotherapy soon creates a chemical isolation, patients should be instructed about other ways to prevent the spread of infection. The responsibility of preventing the spread of infection lies with the patient, and nurses should help patients to understand this. Patients should be instructed to cover their nose and mouth with tissues when coughing or sneezing to prevent the spread of droplet nuclei; those unable to do this need to wear a mask. Patients should wear masks when visitors are in the room and when they leave the room for any reason until chemical isolation is produced. Open windows dilute the number of infectious particles in a room, thereby decreasing the possibility of inhalation by another person. Ultraviolet light in the room or air ducts decontaminates the environment. Since tuberculosis is not spread by fomites, only ordinary care is required for eating utensils, linens, personal articles, and so forth. The means of preventing the spread of infection, then, are chemotherapy, patient education, good ventilation, and ultraviolet irradiation.

Successful treatment of tuberculosis depends primarily on chemotherapy and patient education. A *well-balanced diet* is important for adequate recovery, but a special diet is unnecessary. The patient's weight and appetite should be monitored. Frequent oral hygiene and the absence of sputum containers in view during meals may help improve the appetite. Prolonged bed rest and climate control are of no value in the treatment of tuberculosis. Bed rest is prescribed only while the patient is clinically ill and weak. Therapeutic surgical intervention is rarely necessary since the advent of chemotherapy. Occasionally, resection of a diseased portion of a lung is necessary in patients with cavitary disease which is drug-resistant. Despite the fact that corticosteroids increase the chance of reactivation of latent tuberculosis, they may be life-saving when used in conjunction with antituberculosis medications for some patients who are very seriously ill, such as those with tuberculosis meningitis or pericarditis. Steroids are used to improve the patient's general clinical condition, to suppress inflammation, to reduce cerebral edema, and to hasten resorption of caseous exudate, pleural effusion, and pericardial fluid.

### Fourth-Level Nursing Care

Patients in the home should be supervised by community health nurses. It is important to ensure the continuity of chemotherapy, to monitor for side effects and toxicity of medications, and to provide continuing support and guidance for patients.

While a patient is receiving chemotherapy, sputum and chest x-ray examinations must be repeated at periodic intervals. Lifetime follow-up by annual x-ray examination is recommended for all persons treated for active tuberculosis.

Treatment failures which occur are usually due to neglect by the patient to take the prescribed medication but may also be due to inadequate initial chemotherapy, drug-resistant organisms, or discontinuation of therapy prior to complete healing. A study of reactivation of tuberculosis in New York City shows that reactivation tends to occur most often among persons at the lowest end of the socioeconomic scale, those who live alone, and alcoholics.[30]

When reactivation occurs, patients are generally treated with three or more medications which they have not received before. The *secondary antituberculosis medications* (see Table 9-2) are usually employed in conjunction with the primary medications for retreatment. Medications are given in maximum tolerated dosage, and side effects may occur, so it is advisable for initial therapy to be given in the hospital.

All cases of tuberculosis must be reported to the local health department. A careful investigation should be made to determine from whom the patient may have been infected and to whom the patient may have transmitted the infection. Examination of contacts, especially household members, should include a tuberculin skin test and chest x-ray.

Unfortunately, some persons still think of tuberculosis as a social stigma. Until the middle of the twentieth century, tuberculosis was a social disease that spread through communities. Persons with tuberculosis were separated from their families, lost their jobs, and were hospitalized for years in a sanatorium. Tuberculosis was feared as a major cause of death.

Although the whole outlook on tuberculosis has changed, many misconceptions still exist. Patients need a great deal of emotional support and understanding when they learn that they have tuberculosis. Education of patients and their families is extremely important. Chemotherapy for tuberculosis has little effect upon the leading of a normal life, and usually no restrictions are necessary. Tuberculosis is neither inherited nor passed on to the fetus during pregnancy. Patients can be encouraged to return to full activity soon after they are discharged from the hospital.

## SYPHILIS

Venereal disease (VD), particularly syphilis and gonorrhea, is still widely prevalent despite the existence of curative antibiotic therapy. A patient with a newly diagnosed case of syphilis usually requires only outpatient services, while patients in the late stages of the disease may require hospitalization.

### Pathophysiology

Syphilis (also known as lues or "bad blood") is a chronic infectious disease caused by the spirochete *Treponema pallidum.* Nearly all cases of syphilis are acquired by sexual contact with infectious lesions. *Treponema pallidum* enters the body through mucous membranes or breaks in the skin. Outside the human host, the organism is exquisitely fragile. The spirochete is destroyed within seconds by drying, heat, cold, soap and water, or disinfectants.

Untreated syphilis is characterized by four stages of disease: primary, secondary, latent, and late. Following an incubation period of anywhere from 10 days to 3 months, a *chancre* (see Color Plate 9-1), characteristic of *primary syphilis* appears where the treponeme entered the body. Portals of entry include the external genitalia, cervix, mouth, perianal area, and anal canal. Although a single sore is most common, mutliple chancres can occur.

A chancre is usually painless and indurated, with a serous exudate that is highly contagious. Regional lymph nodes may be enlarged. The chancre remains for 2 to 6 weeks and disappears without treatment, although the disease may persist.

The manifestations of *secondary syphilis* appear 2 weeks to 6 months after the healing of the chancre and are extremely variable. *Skin eruptions* commonly occur and may be macular, papular, pustular, or nodular lesions. Characteristically, the lesions are generalized, bilateral, and painless and appear on the palm of the hand and sole of the foot. *Mucous patches* which are slight erosions of the mucous membrane may occur in the mouth. *Condylomata lata* can occur in the genital region. These are raised, tabletopped, or mushroom shaped papules which are pale in color. Alopecia, generalized lymphadenopathy, and a flulike syndrome may also occur. All the moist skin and mucous membrane lesions of secondary syphilis are highly contagious. If not treated, the manifestations of secondary syphilis disappear after 2 to 6 weeks, and the patient enters the latent stage of syphilis.

During *latent syphilis* the untreated patient is without clinical manifestations of disease, although serologic tests for syphilis are positive. Latent syphilis is divided into two periods: *early latent,* asymptomatic syphilis of less than 4 years' duration, and *late latent,* asymptomatic syphilis of more than 4 years' duration. Approximately one-fourth of patients have recurrences of the mucocutaneous lesions of secondary syphilis during the early latent period.[31] Most patients with latent syphilis remain asymptomatic for the rest of their lives.

About one-fourth of patients with untreated latent syphilis develop clinically apparent *late (tertiary) syphilis.*[32] Symptoms occur many years after the primary infection. Complications which develop in late syphilis are frequently irreversible. The most common form of disease at this stage is the *gumma (late benign syphilis),* a granulomatous inflammatory lesion with an area of central necrosis. Gummas range in size from microscopic to several centimeters in diameter. Virtually any organ of the body may develop gummas. The most commonly involved site is the skin; other sites include bone, mucous membranes, upper respiratory tract, liver, and stomach. Gummas may heal spontaneously with scarring but are often chronic and destructive.

Other common forms of late syphilis are *cardiovascular syphilis* and *neurosyphilis.* Cardiovascular complications cause the majority of deaths in untreated syphilis. The most common forms of cardiovascular syphilis are aortitis, aortic regurgitation, and aneurysms of the thoracic aorta. Neurosyphilis can be asymptomatic, in which case the diagnosis is made by examining the cerebral spinal fluid which reacts positively to serologic tests for syphilis. Symptomatic neurosyphilis is characterized by cerebral infarcts (meningovascular neurosyphilis), widespread loss of nerve cells (*general paresis*), or degeneration of the dorsal roots of the spinal cord (*tabes dorsalis*). Manifestations of neurosyphilis include personality changes, psychosis, strokes, ataxia, paresthesias, and blindness.

The pathologic process is basically the same in the various stages of syphilis. *Treponema pallidum* shows a penchant for involving the blood vessels. It invades the perivascular lymphatics causing endothelial swelling, obliterative endarteritis, and infiltration by lymphocytes and plasma cells. After this, fibroblastic proliferation occurs, leading to fibrosis and healing. In cardiovascular syphilis, endarteritis obstructs the arteries supplying blood to the larger vessels, producing necrosis and destruction of tissue, particularly in the aorta. The lesions of neurosyphilis result from obliterative endarteritis of small arteries with subsequent death of nerve tissue.

*Treponema pallidum* is rarely demonstrated in gummatous lesions. Gummas are thought to be cellular hypersensitivity reactions to the treponemal infection, although this has not been proved.

A person with late syphilis will rarely infect others by sexual contact or blood donation. The one important exception is the pregnant syphilitic who may transmit syphilis to the fetus regardless of the duration of her disease. Congenital syphilis can result in multiple defects including abnormal teeth, decreased visual acuity, bone deformities, deafness, and cutaneous lesions with scarring.

### First-Level Nursing Care

The incidence of syphilis fell dramatically after the development of penicillin therapy in the 1940s, but has since risen. In 1974 there were 24,728 cases of primary and secondary syphilis reported in the United States and 84,164 reported cases of syphilis including all stages.[33] In 1973 syphilis was the third most common communicable disease reported in the United States.[34] The number of cases reported understates the actual problem because cases occur which are not diagnosed and many diagnosed cases are not reported to the health departments. The reported rate of primary and secondary syphilis is highest among the 15- to 39-year-old age group.[35] During the primary and secondary stages of syphilis there are twice as many males as females

reported with the disease.[36] This may be because the chancre occurs in less noticeable parts of the body in females so that the disease may go unnoticed. The reported incidence of syphilis is greater in urban than in rural areas.[37] These statistics may reflect differences in case finding, case reporting, and the availability of public clinics.

**Prevention** The inability to cultivate *T. pallidum* in vitro has hindered attempts to develop a vaccine for syphilis. Currently no vaccine is available.

Transmission of syphilis can occur by blood transfusions. All states require that blood donors have a serologic test for syphilis. If the test is positive, the blood can not be transfused into another person.

In the pregnant woman, spirochetes can cross the placenta, infecting the fetus. Untreated infection in the mother may result in abortion, stillbirth, prematurity, neonatal death, or congenital syphilis. Because penicillin crosses the placental barrier, treatment of the mother can cure the fetus. Most states require routine serologic testing for syphilis in pregnant women. Nurses can help make these laws effective by teaching patients the importance of early prenatal care and checking to see that routine serologies are performed. All female patients with venereal disease should be asked about pregnancy.

A premarital serologic test for syphilis before issuance of a marriage license is required in most parts of the country and is helpful in population screening. As with all venereal diseases, public education is essential in order to prevent complications. The reader is referred to Gonorrhea for further discussion of the prevention of venereal disease.

### Second-Level Nursing Care

Because the signs and symptoms can be absent or may go unnoticed, early syphilis may be detected by a history of exposure or a positive serologic test on routine screening. Serologic tests for syphilis are commonly performed on blood donors and hospitalized patients, and for premarital, prenatal, and preemployment examinations.

**Nursing assessment** Examination of the patient for manifestations of syphilis should be done with enough leisure so that the patient feels at ease and free to verbalize whatever problems are present. The manifestations of primary and secondary syphilis usually are not painful or incapacitating, and the patient's primary problem may be *anxiety* due to lack of understanding of the disease process. An explanation to the patient about the etiology, stages, treatment, and prevention of syphilis is important. It should be reassuring to patients with primary and secondary syphilis to know that the manifestations are temporary and the disease can be completely cured.

**Diagnostic tests**　Serologic tests for syphilis are based on antigen-antibody reactions. When *T. pallidum* invades a human host, it acts as an antigen and evokes the production of multiple antibodies of two basic types: nonspecific and specific. The nonspecific antibodies are called *reagins* and are present in other conditions besides syphilis. The specific *antitreponemal antibodies* are usually present only in those persons who have or have had syphilis.

*Nontreponemal* or *reagin tests* are used for routine syphilis screening. The *Venereal Disease Research Laboratory (VDRL)* flocculation test is the most widely used nontreponemal test. The VDRL test does not become positive until 1 to 4 weeks after the appearance of the chancre. The VDRL test may be falsely positive owing to the presence of reagins produced in response to other conditions such as viral infections, liver damage, atypical pneumonia, smallpox vaccination, pregnancy, lupus erythematosus, connective tissue disorders, leprosy, malaria, narcotic addiction, and aging. There are many other nontreponemal tests. Among the more commonly used tests are the *rapid plasma reagin (RPR)* agglutination test and the *Kolmer* complement-fixation test.

The *treponemal* tests are more specific for syphilis and clarify possible biologic false positive reactions obtained with nontreponemal tests. Two of the more common treponemal tests are the *fluorescent treponemal antibody absorption (FTA-ABS)* test and the *Treponema pallidum immobilization (TPI)* test. Once these tests become positive, they usually remain so, even after adequate therapy. If the patient has had syphilis before, this should be noted because it will cause the treponemal test to be positive.

Evaluation of the patient for syphilis should include dates and results of previous serologic tests for syphilis as well as remembered signs and symptoms. This information helps to establish the length of the current infection and how far back to determine contacts.

Serous exudate from the moist lesions of primary and secondary syphilis should be examined on a slide under a dark-field microscope for identification of *T. pallidum.* Cleansing or the use of topical medications is apt to destroy the surface treponemes making dark-field examination impossible. Patients should be cautioned to avoid home remedies prior to dark-field examination. The use of systemic antibiotics, such as tetracycline for acne, can also destroy surface treponemes and should be noted in the health history.

A *lumbar puncture* to procure a specimen of cerebrospinal fluid for examination is important in the evaluation of neurosyphilis. Significant tests performed on the spinal fluid include cell count, total protein, and VDRL. Frequently neurosyphilis can be detected in the absence of clinical manifestations, in which case the patient can be treated before symptomatic neurosyphilis occurs.

**Nursing problems and intervention**　*Control of infection* in the patient and any contacts is the major nursing problem. Interventions include drugs and case finding. The drug of choice for treating syphilis in all stages is *penicillin.* The Center for Disease Control recommends one dose of 2.4 million units benzathine penicillin intramuscularly, half in each buttock, for treatment of primary, secondary, or latent syphilis when the spinal fluid is normal.[38] An alternative treatment is 600,000 units aqueous procaine penicillin G (APPG) intramuscularly daily for 8 days. Treatment of syphilis in pregnant patients should be the same as for nonpregnant patients.

Before administering penicillin, the nurse should always ask if the patient has any known allergies, particularly to penicillin or other antibiotics. Following penicillin injections, patients should be observed for 30 minutes for hypersensitivity reactions. In a survey of 27,673 patients treated with penicillin, there were 11 cases of anaphylaxis and 183 reactions, of which urticaria was the most common hypersensitivity reaction.[39] Emergency supplies and equipment should be readily available (see Chap. 10 for discussion of anaphylaxis).

Patients who are allergic to penicillin can be given tetracycline hydrochloride 500 mg four times a day by mouth for 15 days or erythromycin in the same dosage. Tetracycline is not recommended for pregnant women because of its effects on unborn children.

A condition known as the *Jarisch-Herxheimer reaction,* consisting of fever, headache, malaise, and intensification of skin lesions, may develop a few hours after initiation of treatment for syphilis. This reaction is thought to result from the rapid release of endotoxin after the spirochetes are destroyed by antibiotics. Patients should be warned that these symptoms may occur. The symptoms subside after 24 hours and can be managed by bed rest and acetylsalicylic acid.

Case finding is extremely important at this level. Sensitive interviewing methods should be utilized to obtain the names of all sexual contacts of the patient. Referrals should be made to local community nursing agencies for follow-up care (see fourth level).

### Third-Level Nursing Care

Patients with severe forms of late syphilis may need to be hospitalized. The lesions of late syphilis may alter almost any bodily function, and nursing care appropriate to the specific problems is given.

**Nursing assessment** Neurosyphilis and cardiovascular syphilis cause the majority of problems in the late phase of this disease. Nursing assessment and care of these patients is oriented toward provision of comfort and halting the progression of the damage.

A health history will probably not reveal any of the symptoms of the earlier stages of syphilis. The primary infection usually will have occurred many years before and, most likely, was untreated or inadequately treated. Current symptoms described and exhibited by the patient will be characteristic of disrupted functioning of the nervous or cardiovascular system.

**N**eurosyphilis Involvement of the central nervous system may be asymptomatic or symptomatic. Asymptomatic neurosyphilis is diagnosed upon the basis of cerebrospinal fluid abnormalities. These may include a positive Wasserman or VDRL test. Left untreated, the chances of symptomatic neurosyphilis developing increase over time.

Symptomatic neurosyphilis may be manifested by personality changes, altered affect and judgment, diminished memory for recent events, and speech impairment. Physical assessment could reveal hyperactive reflexes, paresthesias, ataxia, alteration in temperature, pain, and position sense, as well as the Argyll Robertson pupil (reacts to accommodation but not light).

**C**ardiovascular Syphilis Involvement of the great vessels, particularly the aorta, is characteristic of cardiovascular syphilis. Signs of aortic regurgitation and cardiac insufficiency may develop; nursing intervention is appropriate to the disease's manifestations.

**Nursing problems and intervention** Cognitive, motor, and sensory impairment are nursing problems present in caring for a patient with neurosyphilis. Signs of cardiac insufficiency (fatigue, dyspnea, etc.) are the problems of cardiovascular syphilis. Intervention is symptomic and may include neurological and cardiac work-ups by the physician. Medication is the intervention of choice to halt the syphlitic organism.

Although permanent damage may be caused by gummas, cardiovascular syphilis, or neurosyphilis, antibiotic therapy may arrest the progression of the disease or result in clinical improvement. The recommended treatment of late benign syphilis, cardiovascular syphilis, and asymptomatic or symptomatic neurosyphilis is 7.2 million units benzathine penicillin G given in doses of 2.4 million units by intramuscular injection at weekly intervals.[40] An alternative treatment is APPG 9.0 million units total, given as 600,000 units by intramuscular injection daily for 15 days. Hospitalized patients may be given aqueous crystalline penicillin G intravenously. Patients who are allergic to penicillin can be given 500 mg erythromycin or tetracycline four times a day by mouth for 30 days.

### Fourth-Level Nursing Care

If treatment for syphilis is inadequate, relapses can occur, usually within the first 3 to 9 months. The response to treatment can be determined by following the VDRL titer 3, 6, and 12 months after treatment is initiated.[41] After 2 years nearly all patients adequately treated for early syphilis have a negative VDRL. Additional follow-up is recommended for patients with syphilis of more than 1 year's duration.[42] Retreatment is considered if manifestations of syphilis persist or recur, or the VDRL increases or fails to decrease. Patients need to understand the importance of having these tests performed.

All cases of syphilis must be reported to the local health department. As in gonorrhea an anonymous form of reporting is usually used, and an epidemiologic interviewer traces persons known to have been exposed to the lesions of syphilis. Patients are interviewed for the contacts dating over the duration of symptoms plus 3 months with primary syphilis, 6 months with secondary syphilis, and 12 months for latent syphilis. It is generally recommended that treatment of contacts be the same as for primary syphilis.

During the primary, secondary, and early latent stages, all lesions are believed to be contagious. In the care of a patient with untreated early syphilis, the use of gown and gloves is indicated for procedures requiring direct patient contact. Adequate penicillin therapy renders the patient noncontagious after 24 hours. Patients should be instructed to refrain from sexual activities for at least 24 hours after treatment is instituted.

A person who has had primary or secondary syphilis and has been adequately treated can become reinfected. For this reason, patients should be instructed to refrain from sexual contact with previous partners who have not received treatment. Reinfection is uncommon, though, in patients with latent or late syphilis, regardless of whether they receive adequate treatment.

In addition to experiencing problems associated with contracting a venereal disease (see Gonorrhea), the person with syphilis may be stigmatized. Syphilis is associated with promiscuity, crippling, blindness, and insanity. Because of culturally derived standards of behavior, the social worth of a person with syphilis may be judged less than it should be. This stigma may produce feelings of shame at being inferior and guilt for violating a moral code.[43] There is a natural desire on the part of syphilitics to keep knowledge of their diagnosis from others. Realizing the patient's desire for privacy, the nurse must be able to justify seeking information. Patients should be assisted with ways to manage information given to others. Nurses who treat syphilitic patients as worthwhile, thinking, feeling beings will behave in a helpful manner.

## GONORRHEA

Also known as "the clap" or "GC," gonorrhea is a submucous infection caused by *Neisseria gonorrheae.* Because of its prevalence, particularly among young people, a detailed description of the manifestations and nursing care of gonorrhea will be presented.

### Pathophysiology

*Neisseria gonorrhoeae* is a gram-negative diplococcus which is nonmotile and does not form spores. It is differentiated from other strains of *Neisseria* by its ability to ferment glucose. Although the gonococcus is an aerobe, most strains require an atmosphere of 3 to 5% carbon dioxide to initiate growth.

Gonorrhea is transmitted through direct sexual contact, whether it be oral, anal, or genital. Despite old wives' tales, there is almost no possibility of contraction of the infection from toilet seats, towels, or bed linens. *Neisseria gonorrhoeae* is unable to survive very long outside the warm, moist environment of the human body. It is readily killed by drying, sunlight, and ordinary disinfectants.

The gonococci penetrate mucous membranes in order to reach the submucous tissues in which they can survive. Capillary dilatation occurs with exudation of cellular elements and serum. Large numbers of leukocytes infiltrate the area and phagocytize gonococci. In the absence of specific treatment, the leukocyte infiltration is eventually replaced by fibroblasts which results in formation of a layer of fibrous tissue. The gonococci can also pass into the lymphatic system or bloodstream and spread to other parts of the body.

*Males* usually note symptoms 2 to 6 days following exposure to the gonococcus, although longer intervals are not uncommon. In perhaps 10 to 20 percent of males who become infected, symptoms never develop.[44] The disease begins as an irritation of the urethral meatus with a *clear mucous discharge.* Within a day or two the discharge becomes profuse, thick, and purulent. Its appearance is usually associated with a *painful* and *burning sensation* in the penis *during urination.* Inflammation in the tissues surrounding the urethra can make the *penis red, swollen, and tender to the touch.*

Before antibiotic treatment became available for gonorrhea, these symptoms persisted for an average of 2 months before disappearing. Today, most males readily seek treatment because the symptoms are so uncomfortable. Without treatment the gonococci may spread to neighboring structures. Unilateral epididymitis is the most common complication and is characterized by severe pain, tenderness, and swelling. Fibrous tissue formation can obliterate the lumen of the epididymis. Sterility can result from bilateral involvement. Other local complications which are now uncommon include inguinal lymphadenitis, prostatitis, periurethral abscess, seminal vesiculitis, cowperitis, and urethral stricture.

Gonorrhea in *females* is more likely to become chronic because of failure to secure treatment early and failure of health providers to offer screening cultures. As many as 80 percent of females with gonorrhea may be asymptomatic.[45] The clinical manifestations of gonorrhea in the female may include a *purulent, yellow discharge,* and a *red, swollen, tender vulva. Burning, frequency, and urgency of urination* are often present. The spread of discharge into the rectal area can cause anorectal discomfort and purulent drainage from the rectum. Acute inflammation of a Bartholin's gland is usually unilateral and results in redness, swelling, and purulent drainage. Occlusion of the duct with desquamated epithelial cells and leukocytes may result in a Bartholin's abscess.

In addition to the urethra and endocervix, other anatomic sites that can be directly infected by gonococci include the anal canal, pharynx, and conjunctiva. *Anorectal infections* frequently produce only mild symptoms or are asymptomatic. Signs and symptoms which may occur include anorectal burning or pruritis, purulent rectal discharge, bright-red rectal bleeding, and a feeling of fullness in the rectum with an urgent need to empty the bowel. *Pharyngeal infection* may be asymptomatic, or it may produce a sore throat with an exudate and enlarged, tender cervical lymph nodes. *Gonococcal conjunctivitis* in adults may result from touching the eyes with fingers contaminated with infectious genital secretions. An extremely purulent and destructive conjunctivitis is produced.

### First-Level Nursing Care

Gonorrhea is presently the most common reportable communicable disease in the United States. In 1975 the total number of reported cases of gonorrhea in the United States climbed to 1,032,303.[46] Because many cases of gonorrhea are not detected and many which are treated are not reported, the actual incidence of the disease is not known. In 1974 teen-agers composed nearly 29 percent of cases, while 87 percent were under the age of 30.[47] There were 11,510 reported cases of gonorrhea in children under the age of 14.[48] Large cities have rates of gonorrhea incidence five to ten times higher than smaller cities and towns.[49] Within the larger cities rates are as much as 10 times higher among low socioeconomic groups.[50] These differences may reflect a high rate of case finding and case reporting by public clinics where low socioeconomic groups in cities are usually treated.

Many factors may be influencing the spread of gonorrhea. As many as 80 percent of females with gonorrhea may be asymptomatic, thus providing a large pool of carriers.[51] Gonorrhea has a short incubation period which promotes its rapid spread. There are strains of gonococci that are becoming increasingly resistant to the large doses of antibiotics used to treat them, and these require ever-increasing doses for effective therapy. If follow-up tests are not done after treatment, these resistant strains may go unchecked for unwarranted periods of time.

**Prevention** Newborn infants whose mothers have untreated gonorrhea may acquire gonococcal *ophthalmia neonatorum* during the birth process. Infection to the infant is transmitted by direct contact between the baby's eyes and the infected tissues of the mother. Unlike syphilis, gonorrhea cannot spread from the bloodstream of the mother into the infant because the gonococcus cannot cross the placenta. Ophthalmia neonatorum is an acute conjunctivitis which can lead to corneal ulceration and subsequent blindness if not treated properly. The most effective means of prevention is the *instillation of 1% silver nitrate solution* into the eyes of infants at birth. In many areas of the country this prophylactic measure is required by law. The Center for Disease Control recommends examination of endocervical cultures of all pregnant women for gonococci as part of prenatal care.[52]

The common association of the venereal diseases with sexual promiscuity introduces an element lacking in other communicable diseases and seriously complicates prevention programs. *Education* about venereal disease as an illness of importance, that can be prevented, should be presented to the public. It is important that young people realize the danger of sterility, the need for notifying others who might have been infected, and the significance of preventive measures and prompt treatment.

Some preventive measures for venereal disease can be taken, and these should be taught to young people. *Cleansing* the genitals with warm water and soap before and after sexual intercourse can decrease the spread of venereal disease. Urinating before and immediately after intercourse may also help males cleanse the genitourinary tract of any invading organisms. The condom has been available for venereal disease prophylaxis for at least four centuries and is quite effective. A study by Arnold and Cogswell indicates that adolescents do take advantage of condoms when they are easily accessible and provided free of charge at local grocery stores, barber shops, pool halls, and restaurants.[53] Some of the intravaginal contraceptive preparations also seem to confer considerable protection against venereal disease.

State health departments are employing a variety of imaginative approaches to present factual information about venereal disease in a manner that will appeal to the public. Some of these activities include VD workshops, the use of radio and television programs, VD hot-lines, VD booths at regional fairs, VD literature in clinics and physicians' offices, VD teachers' guides, open houses in VD clinics, and courses for teachers on VD education.

McGrath and Laliberte surveyed basic knowledge of syphilis and gonorrhea held by junior and senior high school nurses in Massachusetts.[54] Because only 32 percent of the nurses were able to correctly answer at least 36 out of 40 questions, the investigators recommended that nurses increase their knowledge of venereal disease and available community resources. Many nurses are in a position to play a key role as a community contact, collaborating with and educating other health professionals about venereal disease, its treatment, and prevention.

Although no vaccine is currently available to prevent gonorrhea, research toward this end is taking place. Several small, controlled field trials with a gonococcus vaccine have been initiated, but its value in preventing gonorrhea has yet to be established.

### Second-Level Nursing Care

Patients who suspect that they have gonorrhea most frequently seek help in a community clinic or outpatient facility. Nurses are often responsible for the initial patient evaluation.

**Nursing assessment** The *health history* may reveal exposure to a person with gonorrhea, pain, difficulty voiding, or a purulent discharge. Patients should be examined for lesions, signs of inflammation, abnormal discharges, and pelvic lymphadenopathy.

**D**iagnostic Tests In males the diagnosis is most often made by identification of gram-negative diplococci on a smear of urethral discharge. Isolation of *N. gonorrhoeae* by culture is required when other sites are examined and when the diagnosis cannot be confirmed with a smear of the urethral discharge. In a female the endocervix is the most likely source to produce a positive culture. Because gonorrhea is frequently asymptomatic, case finding can be extended by obtaining cultures for gonorrhea during routine physical examinations.

In many situations proper management of culture specimens depends on nurses. Figure 9-2 describes proper techniques for obtaining, inoculating, and handling specimens. Thayer-Martin medium, which contains antibiotics to selectively inhibit most other organisms, is used to culture gonococci obtained from the endocervix, anal canal, and pharynx where large numbers of a variety of bacteria are normally present. After inoculation, the Thayer-Martin medium is placed in an atmosphere containing sufficient carbon dioxide to permit growth of the gonococci, such as a candle jar. Transgrow medium also suppresses contaminating organisms and is under 10% carbon dioxide atmosphere in bottles. Transgrow medium is recommended only when specimens cannot be delivered to the laboratory or incubator on the day they are taken.

A blood test for gonorrhea has recently been developed but is not yet in widespread use. Nurses should explain to patients that the blood study which is done for syphilis does *not* test for gonorrhea.

**Nursing problems and intervention** Major nursing problems for symptomatic gonorrhea include *the signs of the infectious process* (pain, discharge, etc.) and *control of its communicability.* Interventions include drug therapy and identification of patient contacts.

The preferred treatment for gonorrhea is still *penicillin,* despite increasing numbers of penicillin-resistant strains of gonococci. The recommended therapy is APPG 4.8 million units intramuscularly divided into at least two doses and injected at one visit into different sites, together with 1 g probenecid by mouth just before the injections.[55] Probenecid competes with penicillin for excretion by the kidney tubules, thus delaying its excretion from the body. Patients should be carefully observed for at least 30 minutes, for signs of sensitivity following administration of penicillin (see Syphilis).

An alternative therapy is to administer ampicillin 3.5 g orally together with probenecid. For patients who are allergic to penicillin, either tetracycline hydrochloride or spectinomycin hydrochloride can be used. However, ampicillin and spectinomycin are ineffective in pharyngeal gonococcal infection.

Patients need to understand that self-treatment with antibiotics taken for another problem is usually unsuccessful. The doses of antibiotics needed to treat gonorrhea are much greater than those used to combat other infections.

Most states have passed legislation permitting treatment of minors for venereal disease on the basis of their own consent. Adolescents are certainly more likely to obtain treatment if they realize parental notification is not necessary.

All cases of gonorrhea must be reported to the local health department. A trained epidemiologic interviewer is usually responsible for obtaining information from the patient about recent *sexual contacts.* In some areas nurses are responsible for epidemiologic interviewing. This type of interview requires considerable expertise, discretion, and sensitivity on the part of the investigator. Most states have an anonymous method for reporting cases of venereal disease to prevent identification of the patients. All the patient's sexual contacts within the last 30 days should receive the same treatment as those known to have gonorrhea.

Isolation of patients with gonorrhea is not necessary. Patients should be instructed not to engage in sexual activity for at least 24 hours after treatment. There is no evidence that an attack of gonorrhea produces immunity to subsequent infections. Patients should refrain from intercourse with untreated previous sexual partners to avoid reinfection.

The patient with venereal disease does not regard his or her complaint in the same light as any other infectious disease. Complex social, psychologic, or moral problems may be involved.

Patients with signs and symptoms may suspect their diagnosis and may be somewhat prepared for it. However, the diagnosis of gonorrhea may come as a particular shock to the asymptomatic patient who is diagnosed by a routine screening procedure. Patients in such cases are likely to be very upset and angry, especially if this is an indication that their sexual partner has been unfaithful. Disclosure of the diagnosis may be facilitated if the patient is told initially that a routine culture for gonorrhea is being done. Nurses should assist patients to explore ways to cope with their feelings and problems with their sexual partners.

Patients may have guilt feelings about contracting venereal disease or fear serious social repercussions from disclosure of their infection. Disclosure of sexual contacts may require that the patient admit to homosexuality, marital infidelity, promiscuity, prostitution, and so forth. Nurses need to examine their own attitudes about such situations and be prepared to approach each patient with understanding and an open mind. Patients with venereal disease may have many problems and fears and may be only too ready to discuss them if they sense a sympathetic attitude.

**Third-Level Nursing Care**

In females, extension of the gonococcal infection to the fallopian tubes is referred to as *acute salpingitis* (*pelvic inflammatory disease* or *PID*) and occurs in 10 to 15 percent of females with gonorrhea.[56] Infection can escape from the fallopian tubes into the pelvis resulting in pelvic *peritonitis.*

**Nursing assessment** The patient's history may include severe *abdominal pain, chills, fever, general malaise, nausea,* and *vomiting.* Physical assessment may reveal *swollen* and tender *inguinal lymph nodes* and a *purulent vaginal discharge.* Patients may experience an exquisite pain when the cervix is manipulated during the pelvic examination. Abnormal laboratory values commonly include an elevated erythrocyte sedimentation rate and leukocytosis. Partial or complete closure of the fallopian tubes can occur due to scar formation which may

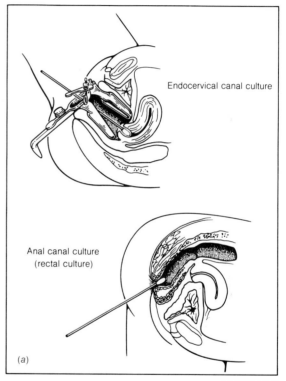

Endocervical canal culture

Anal canal culture (rectal culture)

(a)

**FIGURE 9-2**
Culture technique for the diagnosis of gonorrhea. (*From U.S. Dept. of Health, Education and Welfare, Public Health Service, Center for Disease Control. Used by permission of the publisher.*)
Women: (a) Endocervical Canal Culture
1. Moisten speculum with warm water; do not use any other lubricant.
2. Remove cervical mucus, preferably with a cotton ball held in ring forceps.
3. Insert sterile cotton-tipped swab into endocervical canal; move from side to side; allow 10 to 30 seconds for absorption of organisms to the swab.
Anal Canal Culture (rectal culture)
1. Insect sterile cotton-tipped swab approximately one inch into the anal canal. If the swab is inadvertently pushed into feces, use another swab to obtain specimen.
2. Move swab from side to side in the anal canal to sample crypts; allow 10 to 30 seconds for absorption of organisms to the swab.
(continued)

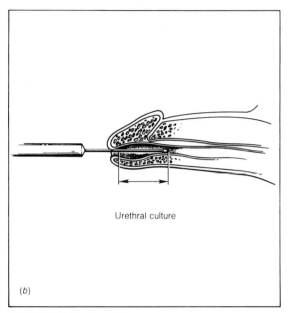

(b)

**FIGURE 9-2 (Continued)**
Men: (b) Urethral Culture.
1. Use sterile bacteriologic loop to obtain specimen from anterior urethra by gently scraping the mucosa. An alternative to the loop is a sterile synthetic swab (calgiswab) that is easily inserted into the urethra.
Anal Canal Culture.
1. These can be taken in the same manner as for women.

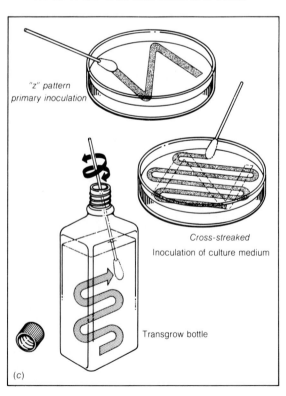

(c)

**FIGURE 9-2 (Continued)**
(c) Inoculation of culture medium.
1. Medium should be at room temperature prior to inoculation.
2. Do not place inoculated culture medium in the refrigerator or expose to extreme temperatures.
3. Thayer-Martin (TM) Plates
    A   Roll swab directly on TM medium in a large "Z" pattern; all surfaces of the swab should touch the medium.
    B   Cross-streak immediately with a sterile wire loop, preferably in the clinic. If not done previously, cross-streaking should be done in the laboratory.
    C   Place culture in a candle jar within 15 minutes; the medium side should be uppermost to prevent moisture from the lid falling on the culture. Be sure to relight the candle each time the candle jar is reopened.
    D   Begin incubation of plates the same day (but the sooner the better) at 35° to 36°C.
4. Transgrow bottles.
    A   Keep neck of bottle in upright position to prevent CO₂ loss.
    b   Remove cap of bottle only when ready to inoculate medium.
    C   Soak up all excess moisture in bottle with specimen swab and then roll swab from side to side across medium, starting at the bottom of the bottle.
    D   Tightly cap the bottle immediately to prevent loss of CO₂.
    E   When possible, incubate the Transgrow bottle in an upright position at 35°–36°C for 16–18 hours before sending to the laboratory and note this on accompanying request form. Resultant growth usually survives prolonged transport and is ready for identification upon arrival at the laboratory. (If an incubator is not available, store cultures at room temperature [25°C or above] for 16–18 hours before subjecting it to prolonged transport and extreme temperatures.)
    F   Package the incubated Transgrow culture and request form in a suitable container to prevent breakage and immediately transport to a central bacteriologic laboratory by postal service or other convenient means.
    G   At the lab, preincubated Transgrow bottles, will be examined immediately for *Neisseria gonorrhoeae;* other bottles are incubated at 35°–36°C for 24–28 hours and examined.

predispose to tubal pregnancy or result in sterility. Approximately 15 percent of females with one episode of gonococcal salpingitis become sterile.[57] Chronic pelvic inflammatory disease can lead to abnormal menstrual periods, pain with intercourse, low back pain, anemia, and periodic recurrence of the acute symptoms.

**Nursing problems and intervention**   *Signs of pelvic inflammation* (pain, purulent discharge) and *communicability* must be viewed as the most characteristic nursing problems encountered in caring for patients with acute salpingitis of gonococcal origin. Interventions include drug therapy, follow-up and prevention of complications.

Antibiotic therapy employed for uncomplicated gonorrhea may be prescribed for outpatients with gonococcal salpingitis. Hospitalization is considered under the following circumstances: when the diagnosis is uncertain, a pelvic abscess is suspected, the patient is pregnant, the patient fails to respond to outpatient therapy, or there is a history of noncompliance with treatment plans. Hospitalized patients may receive aqueous crystalline penicillin G 20 million units intravenously each day until clinical improvement occurs, followed by 500 mg ampicillin taken orally four times a day to complete 10 days of therapy.[58] Tetracycline hydrochloride may be given intravenously as an alternative treatment. If abscesses form, surgical drainage may be necessary.

The nurse should continually assess the character and amount of vaginal discharge. Placement of the patient in semi-Fowler's position promotes downward drainage. Patients should be instructed to practice careful handwashing and avoid touching their eyes with unclean hands to prevent gonococcal conjunctivitis. Application of heat, sitz baths, and analgesics may help to alleviate the discomfort.

Follow-up of patients with repeat pelvic examinations and cultures for *N. gonorrhoeae* is essential. Failure to examine and treat male sex partners is a major cause of recurrent gonococcal salpingitis.

*Disseminated gonococcal infection* results from the systemic spread of the organism via the bloodstream resulting in a variety of clinical manifestations including arthritis, tenosynovitis, skin eruptions, meningitis, endocarditis, pericarditis, toxic hepatitis, and, rarely, fulminant gonococcemia. A diagnosis of disseminated gonococcal infection is supported by the presence of *N. gonorrhoeae* on culture or on specific immunofluorescent stain of blood, synovial fluid, cerebrospinal fluid, or skin lesions. Patients with disseminated gonococcal infection should preferably be hospitalized and treated with high doses of intravenous aqueous crystalline penicillin G until clinical improvement occurs.

### Fourth-Level Nursing Care

Follow-up cultures should be obtained after completion of treatment to ensure eradication of the gonococci. If follow-up tests are not done, resistant strains of gonococci may go unchecked, allowing for the further spread of infection, development of complications, and transmission of the disease to others. The Center for Disease Control recommends spectinomycin intramuscularly to patients with gonorrhea that fails to respond to penicillin, ampicillin, or tetracycline.[59]

Patient education about the disease, its trans-

mission, and effects is imperative to prevent chronicity. Nurses have a key role in this prevention as they encounter patients in the clinic, hospital, or community. Case finding and reporting are also extremely important at this level (see second level).

## INFECTIOUS MONONUCLEOSIS

A familiar and rather common infectious disease, particularly in young people, is mononucleosis. Much is still to be learned about "mono," but what is known should be part of every nurse's store of knowledge.

### Pathophysiology

Infectious mononucleosis is an acute and self-limited illness, characterized by fever, sore throat, and lymphadenopathy. The outstanding pathologic feature of infectious mononucleosis is generalized involvement of lymph tissue. The lymph nodes and spleen become hyperplastic and produce excessive numbers of lymphocytes. The liver shows alterations associated with lymphatic proliferation in the portal tracts and sinusoids and hypertrophy of Kupffer cells.

The generalized, uncontrolled proliferation of one of the white blood cell series sometimes makes infectious mononucleosis similar to acute leukemia, but unlike leukemia the abnormal process of infectious mononucleosis is always self-limited and reversible. Patients who have suffered from infectious mononucleosis do not have a higher incidence of leukemia, lymphoma, or other malignant conditions subsequently.

Since 1968 evidence has been accumulating to demonstrate that infectious mononucleosis is caused by the *Epstein-Barr virus* (*EBV*), a herpes-like virus associated with Burkitt's lymphoma. Many studies show that only individuals without EBV antibodies contract infectious mononucleosis and the presence of EBV antibodies confers lifelong immunity.

Although the exact mode of transmission is unknown, most authorities agree that infectious mononucleosis is transmitted by the intimate oral exchange of saliva which can occur during kissing. The exact period of communicability is unknown, but EBV is present in throat washings from 1 week to many months after clinical illness.[60] Transmission by carriers seems likely, since the disease often occurs in the absence of contact with a known case. Infectious mononucleosis does not seem to be highly contagious, as roommates and family members of persons with the disease usually

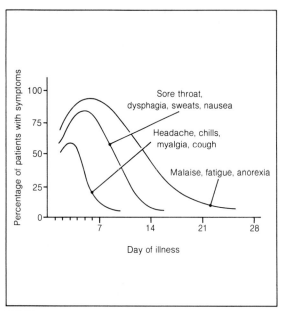

**FIGURE 9-3**
Usual frequency and duration of major symptoms in young adults with infectious mononucleosis. (*From S. C. Finch: "Clinical Symptoms and Signs of Infectious Mononucleosis," in Carter and Penman (eds.), 1969, p. 20. By permission of the publisher.*)

do not become ill. It may be that many persons have a mild or unrecognized case of mononucleosis as children and so acquire immunity.

Following an incubation period of 2 to 6 weeks, three stages of infectious mononucleosis can be identified: the prodromal period or onset, the stage of acute illness, and the convalescent period. During the *prodromal period* which lasts 3 to 5 days the patient has nonspecific symptoms such as fatigue, malaise, and anorexia. The *stage of acute illness* usually lasts from 7 to 20 days. Figures 9-3 and 9-4 show the usual frequency and duration of major signs and symptoms of infectious mononucleosis. During the *convalescent period* fatigue and weakness may persist. Usually 2 to 6 weeks, sometimes longer, are required for signs and symptoms to subside.

**First-Level Nursing Care**
Infectious mononucleosis occurs most frequently in young adults between the ages of 15 and 25. When infection occurs during childhood, it may be mild or asymptomatic and usually is not recognized as infectious mononucleosis. As the age of exposure and infection is delayed to young adult life, an increasing proportion of EBV infections cause clinical manifestations of infectious mononucleo-

sis. The incidence of infectious mononucleosis is greatest in high socioeconomic settings where sanitary standards delay infection until adolescence or young adulthood. Early fall and spring are periods of high incidence among college students. It is not presently possible to prevent the occurrence of infectious mononucleosis.

**Second-Level Nursing Care**
Mononucleosis has an onset that is similar to many "routine" viral and bacterial infections of the throat. It is important, therefore, that patients seek medical attention for common sore throats and that nurses be discriminating in their patient assessments.

**Nursing assessment** The typical and highly characteristic features of infectious mononucleosis in the young adult are *sore throat, fever,* and *cervical lymphadenopathy.* The sore throat may be accompanied by a grayish white exudative tonsillitis persisting for 7 to 10 days. The palate and uvula may appear covered with a gelatinous film. Tiny red circumscribed spots may be seen at the junction of the hard and soft palate (*palatal enanthem*) if a bright light is used for viewing the throat. Swallowing and eating may be quite difficult. Many patients claim the sore throat of infectious mononucleosis is the most severe they have ever experienced. Temperature elevations of 101 to 105°F may persist for 5 to 10 days. In some patients an intermittent fever pattern with morning remissions may persist for 2 weeks. Shaking chills and profuse sweats may accompany the fever. Lymph node enlargement is almost invariably present at some time. Most frequently the posterior cervical lymph nodes are bilaterally enlarged, firm, and nontender to touch. Generalized adenopathy may develop, and *splenomegaly* is common.

**Diagnostic Tests** Laboratory findings are typical and essential to a diagnosis of infectious mononucleosis. EBV antibodies are almost always present in titers of 1:80 to 1:320. Alterations in liver function tests are common. The white blood cell count is usually 12,000 to 20,000 per mm³ of which 60 percent are lymphocytes and monocytes. Atypical lymphocytes called *Downey cells* represent 10 to 20 percent of the lymphocyte population. The term *mononucleosis* came into use because these atypical white blood cells were originally thought to be monocytes. They combine the characteristics of both lymphocytes and monocytes.

Paul and Bunnell discovered that the serum of patients with infectious mononucleosis contains antibodies that clump (agglutinate) the red blood cells of sheep in concentrations far above normal. The antibody is called a *heterophil* since it reacts with more than one group or species. Usually normal persons have a heterophil titer (Paul-Bunnell test for agglutinins to sheep erythrocytes) of up to 1:28. The serum of patients with infectious mononucleosis characteristically contains a titer of 1:224 or higher.

**Nursing problems and intervention** *Severe sore throat, fatigue,* and *generalized discomfort* constitute the major nursing problems. As there is no specific treatment for infectious mononucleosis, therapy is symptomatic. *Bed rest* is recommended during the febrile period and for those who feel too weak to function. Activities should be coordinated to provide periods of uninterrupted rest for the patient. Isolation precautions are not necessary.

For relief of general discomfort and fever, an *analgesic* such as codeine or acetylsalicylic acid may be administered. Warm saline gargles and throat lozenges may help to relieve the sore throat. Semisolids, such as ice cream and gelatin dessert, and cold drinks should be encouraged.

*Antibiotics* are indicated only if the patient develops a concomitant bacterial infection, such as streptococcal pharyngitis. Throat cultures should always be obtained from patients with infectious mononucleosis. Ampicillin should be avoided because it is thought to precipitate rashes in mononucleosis patients.

### Third-Level Nursing Care

Hospitalization for uncomplicated infectious mononucleosis is usually not necessary. When home care is unavailable, though, students may be admitted to the school infirmary. The student hospitalized with infectious mononucleosis is usually concerned about prolonged hospitalization and its effects on grades and school activities. Flexibility in the hospital management and an understanding nurse can help to allay the patient's anxieties. Arrangements can often be made to allow the student to participate in selected activities. Hospitalization usually lasts 5 to 10 days.

Unusual clinical patterns and serious complications are rare. Splenomegaly may lead to *splenic rupture* which requires immediate surgical intervention to remove the spleen (see Chap. 23). The nurse should suspect splenic rupture if the patient complains of sudden abdominal pain and has signs of impending hypovolemic shock. Patients with

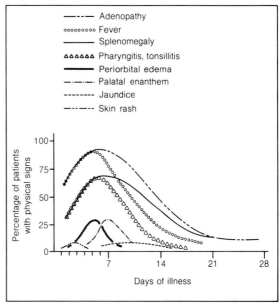

**FIGURE 9-4**
Usual frequency and duration of major signs in young adults with infectious mononucleosis. (*From S. C. Finch: "Clinical Symptoms and Signs of Infectious Mononucleosis," in Carter and Penman (eds.), 1969, p. 27. By permission of the publisher.*)

splenomegaly should be cautioned about straining at stool and abdominal trauma; abdominal palpation should be avoided.

In patients with severe exudative pharyngitis, acute *airway obstruction* may occur, which on rare occasions requires a tracheostomy. A short course of steroids may be administered to patients with severe pharyngitis. Steroids do not influence the course of the disease, but their anti-inflammatory effects usually reduce airway obstruction, lymphadenopathy, and splenomegaly.

Other uncommon complications include thrombocytopenic purpura, hemolytic anemia, pericarditis, liver failure, various neurologic manifestations, and death. The actual incidence of fatal complications is difficult to estimate but appears to be less than 1 per 3000 cases.[61] Between 1964 and 1973 an average of 21 deaths were reported each year in the United States due to infectious mononucleosis.[62]

### Fourth-Level Nursing Care

During the period of convalescence patients are encouraged to pace themselves and rest when they feel fatigued. An afternoon nap can be recommended. Prolonged bed rest produces deconditioning and is unnecessary. As long as splenomegaly is present, patients should avoid strenuous physical activity, contact sports, straining at stool, riding motorcycles or bicycles, and driving on bumpy roads. It is usually not necessary for students to drop out of school, particularly if they curtail extracurricular activities temporarily.

Patients should be cautioned that they may still transmit infectious mononucleosis to others during the convalescent period, although the exact period of communicability is unknown. Outbreaks of infectious mononucleosis are to be reported to the public health department. In most states it is not necessary to report individual cases.

Follow-up visits are important to evaluate splenomegaly and liver function. It is possible for exacerbation of signs and symptoms to occur during convalescence, although this is uncommon.

## MALARIA

Malaria is an infectious disease caused by protozoan parasites belonging to the genus *Plasmodium*. It is transmitted from person to person by the bites of infected female mosquitoes belonging only to the genus *Anopheles*. Malaria remains a major infectious disease problem in many parts of Africa, Asia, the Pacific, and Central and South America. Most cases of malaria that occur in the United States affect persons who travel to countries where the disease exists and who fail to take suppressive therapy.

Of the many species of *Plasmodia,* only four are responsible for malaria in humans: *P. vivax, P. ovale, P. malariae,* and *P. falciparum.* The clinical manifestations vary little among the species of plasmodia. Most deaths from malaria are in cases caused by *P. falciparum* in which the symptoms occur with great severity and complications are likely.

Once a human is bitten by an infected mosquito, parasites migrate to the liver and spleen. After an average period of 12 to 30 days, depending on the species of plasmodia, the parasites spill into the bloodstream where each invades a red blood cell. The parasite stays inside the red blood cell for 48 to 72 hours, feeding on the hemoglobin. The parasite divides into 10 to 20 small parasite segments which burst the red blood cell membrane and spill into the bloodstream. While the parasites are floating free in the bloodstream, the victim experiences a *malarial paroxysm* (attack). Some of the parasites are destroyed by the victim's immune mechanisms while others invade new red blood cells and the cycle is repeated. The malarial paroxysms occur at regular 48-hour intervals in per-

sons infected with *P. vivax* and *P. ovale.* Although *P. falciparum* has a cycle of 48 hours, parasites of all ages may be present at the same time resulting in continuous signs and symptoms rather than the typical, cyclical paroxysms. The cycle lasts 72 hours with *P. malariae.*

A malarial paroxysm is characterized by three stages: *chill, fever,* and profuse *diaphoresis.* The attack begins with malaise and a feeling of chilliness which suddenly develops into a severe shaking chill, usually lasting 10 to 60 minutes. Headache, nausea, vomiting, muscle aching, and diarrhea are frequent symptoms. The chills cause the body temperature to rise, reaching 103 to 107°F. The skin is hot, dry, and flushed; the headache intensifies; and the patient develops severe thirst and may become disoriented. This stage usually lasts 3 to 8 hours, until most of the parasites enter new red blood cells. Then, suddenly, there is a profuse diaphoresis that rapidly reduces the temperature to normal and leaves the patient feeling weak and exhausted. Between paroxysms, however, the patient may feel relatively well and may be able to engage in activities of daily living.

The diagnosis of malaria is based on the clinical picture and identification of plasmodia in a blood smear. Because the organisms are free in the bloodstream only during the chills and fever, blood smears should be taken during these first two stages of the paroxysm.

Left untreated, the paroxysms may become irregular and finally cease. The parasites persist in the liver, however, and relapses occur when they reinvade the bloodstream. Varying levels of immunity develop after repeated infections.

Patients with severe malaria can develop a variety of complications. Hypovolemia and sloughing red blood cells can interfere with circulation to almost any organ, causing such complications as gastrointestinal upset, respiratory insufficiency, renal failure, hemiplegia, convulsions, coma, and death. Blackwater fever is a disorder that occurs with *P. falciparum* infections in persons who have been treated with quinine. Clinically, the disease is characterized by chills, profuse vomiting, massive intravascular hemolysis, jaundice, hemoglobinuria, the passage of dark red to black urine, and acute renal failure. The overall mortality ranges from 20 to 50 percent. Chronic malaria can lead to anemia, debility, cachexia, hepatosplenomegaly, and increased susceptibility to infections, which is often the cause of death.

Acute malaria may be treated with a variety of drugs which are effective only when the parasite segments are free in the blood. The oldest drug known to be specific for malaria is *quinine sulfate*. However, a number of synthetic antimalarial agents are currently in use, including chloroquine, amodiaquine, pyrimethamine, and chlorguanide. Relapses of malaria can be prevented by the administration of primaquine which can eradicate those plasmodia residing in the liver. A strain of drug-resistant *P. falciparum* has developed which may be treated with a combination of quinine, pyrimethamine, and one of the sulfonamides or sulfones.

During paroxysms, the nurse is primarily concerned with keeping the patient comfortable, preventing dehydration, and reducing the possibility of transmitting the disease. The patient should be kept warm and given hot drinks during the chill stage. This probably does little to prevent the chill but provides comfort and psychologic support. Alcohol sponge baths, an ice cap to the head, and analgesics may be ordered during the febrile stage. Nourishing, cold drinks are encouraged during both febrile and diaphoretic stages. The patient's temperature must be closely monitored, and the nurse should be alert for early signs of complications. During the diaphoresis the linens and clothing should be kept dry and changed frequently.

Since malaria is a reportable disease, local public health authorities must be notified of the diagnosis. Isolation is not necessary, but care is essential in the handling and disposal of needles used for the patient, because contaminated needles can transmit the malaria-causing parasites. The patient should be advised never to give blood since the disease can also be transmitted through blood transfusions.

General preventive measures for malaria include identification of mosquito vectors, elimination of breeding places, destruction of larvae and mosquitoes with insecticides, and screening of homes. Although research is under way to produce a vaccine, there is no vaccine currently available for the prevention of malaria. Persons traveling to areas where malaria exists (endemic areas) should take personal precautions to wear protective clothing, make liberal use of insect repellants (see the section later in this chapter on mosquito bites), and avoid being outside during the night when mosquitoes are most likely to bite.

Although it is not possible to prevent infection, it is possible to suppress the symptoms of malaria. *Suppressive therapy* frequently consists of the oral administration of chloroquine and primaquine weekly while the person is in the endemic area and for 8 weeks after leaving the area. The nurse should explain to patients the necessity of taking all prescribed antimalarial medications in order to completely eradicate the parasites.

## INTEGUMENTARY SYSTEM'S RESPONSE TO INFLAMMATION

Inflammation is defined according to the presence of the cardinal signs of Celsus: redness, swelling, heat, and pain (see Chap. 8). On the basis of these manifestations skin diseases are classified as inflammatory or noninflammatory disorders.

## ACNE VULGARIS

Teen-aged persons and young adults are the target population of an unpleasant and uncomfortable condition known as *acne vulgaris*. Because of its tremendous implications for self-image and general health, the nurse needs to be aware of this problem and any nursing role in alleviating it.

### Pathophysiology

Acne vulgaris is a chronic condition involving the pilosebaceous unit of the skin. It is characterized by noninflammatory and inflammatory lesions located on the face, neck, and upper trunk.

*Noninflammatory acne* is essentially an obstructive disease in which accumulations of compacted keratin, sebum, and bacteria dilate the pilosebaceous ducts. The obstructive lesion is called a *comedo* and may be classified as open or closed. The *open comedo* (*blackhead*) is topped with dark material which probably is due to the compaction of keratinous material at the follicular orifice. In the open comedones the pilosebaceous ducts are open to the external environment, allowing the escape of sebum to the skin surface. The *closed comedo* (*whitehead*) does not have a visible opening, and the escape of sebum to the skin surface is prevented. Owing to its deep location in the skin, the closed comedo is more easily felt than visualized. If the skin is stretched, however, it appears as a small white or flesh-colored raised papule. Closed comedones are the main precursors of inflammatory acne lesions.

*Inflammatory acne* may result if a break occurs in the follicular wall and sebum leaks into the surrounding tissues. The free fatty acids in sebum are strong irritants, and it is hypothesized that they initiate the inflammatory acne lesions. In the dermis surrounding the disrupted follicle, there is a localized accumulation of inflammatory cells. Clinical manifestations of inflammatory acne include *pustules, papules, nodules,* and *cysts.* The inflammatory lesions of acne may cause extensive scarring.

The pathogenesis of acne vulgaris is complex and not fully understood. Some of the factors believed to contribute to the development of acne vulgaris are alterations in the pilosebaceous unit, hormonal stimulation, bacterial activity, and extrinsic influences.

Acne is confined to areas where the sebaceous glands are well developed and does not occur in the absence of actively functioning glands. Increased sebum production and hyperkeratinization of the *pilosebaceous unit* are associated with acne vulgaris. The increased keratinization encourages the formation of keratin plugs, leading to the development of comedones. It is possible that there may be changes in the quality of keratin or in the composition of sebum. There may also be an alteration in the pilosebaceous unit produced by faulty structure or function which increases the risk of plugging of the follicular opening or of rupture of the follicular wall with leakage of sebum into the surrounding tissues.

*Androgens* stimulate development of sebaceous glands and secretion of sebum in both males and females. Administration of androgen-dominant oral contraceptives and adrenocorticosteroids can cause acne vulgaris. Since acne patients usually have normal plasma levels of testosterone, researchers have developed the concept of "end-organ sensitivity." Two important discoveries in testosterone metabolism help to explain this concept.[63] First, dihydrotestosterone (DHT) is the cellularly active form of testosterone. Second, the skin is capable of converting testosterone to dihydrotestosterone. It has been shown that skin with acne produces 2 to 20 times more dihydrotestosterone than normal skin from corresponding areas.[64] It is not known whether acne results from increased sebum production secondary to the androgen stimulation or whether there are other androgen-mediated factors contributing to the acne formation.

Among the normal flora of the skin is *Propionibacterium (Corynebacterium) acnes* which is regularly found in acne lesions. *Propionibacterium acnes* produces an enzyme (a lipase) that converts the triglycerides of sebum to free fatty acids, which are believed to be the major inflammatory substances in sebum. It is also possible that *P. acnes* possesses other inflammatory or toxic substances that might contribute to the acne lesion.

*Extrinsic factors* which may influence the course of acne vulgaris include emotions, exposure to acnegenic substances, ingestion of acnegenic drugs, mechanical forces, and hot, humid climates. Exacerbations of acne may occur with stress such as examination times for students. A variety of substances which are common constituents of cosmetics may cause comedones. Any type of mechanical stress on the skin, such as supporting the head with hands, friction from hands or fingers, football helmets, and turtleneck sweaters, may aggravate acne vulgaris. The mechanical stress may rupture early comedones which are not yet observable, resulting in inflammatory lesions.

### First-Level Nursing Care

The prevalence of acne in any form among adolescents varies from less than 6 percent in some countries to 90 to 100 percent in the United States.[65] More research is needed to be able to explain the wide variations in acne incidence. Although acne can occur during middle adulthood, the ages of peak incidence are 14 to 17 in girls and 16 to 19 in boys.[66] Acne becomes more marked at puberty and adolescence perhaps because at that age certain endocrine glands of the body are at their peak activity, which influences the secretions of the sebaceous glands. The most severe forms of acne are found in about 3 percent of males and rather less frequently in females.[67] Although the mode of inheritance is unknown, acne vulgaris is thought to have a familial tendency.

**Prevention** Although it is not possible at this time to actually prevent acne, there is evidence that good health practices and early treatment help to control acne and minimize scarring. Young people should be taught in the preadolescent years about the natural course and care of acne. It should be emphasized that acne vulgaris is a condition that normally occurs in American adolescents and that it can be controlled but not prevented or cured.

### Second-Level Nursing Care

The school, community health, or clinic nurse may be the first to see a patient with acne. This initial assessment of the problem can result in effective medical follow-up of the patient.

**Nursing assessment** The nursing assessment should explore the *history* of the acne condition, previous treatment, its effectiveness, and possible causative factors, such as emotional stress, cosmetics, medications, or a familial tendency. The patient's face, neck, anterior chest, back, and upper arms are examined for the presence of *comedones, papules, pustules, nodules,* and *cysts.* The distribution, shape, surface characteristics, and color of the lesions are noted. An unusual distribution pattern may indicate that an external factor is traumatizing the skin. Crusts and scabs might indicate that the patient has been squeezing the acne lesions.

**Nursing problems and intervention** *Skin lesions* and *emotional side effects* are the outstanding nursing problems identified while caring for patients with acne vulgaris. Treatment of acne vulgaris is based on an understanding of the pathogenesis of the disease and geared to the specific lesions present. Many different treatment modalities are available which are aimed at different points in the disease process. A combination of treatment modalities is likely to be employed.

**T**reatment of Noninflammatory Acne  Mechanical removal of the open and closed comedones is an essential part of the management of acne. Open comedones may be expressed by the utilization of a *comedo extractor,* which basically consists of a loop or plate with a small central hole. The hole is placed directly over the blackhead and pressure is exerted against the skin. To express closed comedones, the physician first nicks the closed follicular orifice with a small needle or scalpel and then uses the comedo extractor.

A variety of therapeutic agents function by producing erythema and desquamation. They probably act in part by producing an increased rate of turnover of the horny layer lining the follicular duct, thus reducing the compaction necessary to produce the comedo and facilitating mechanical removal of comedones. *Peeling agents* include cleansing agents, astringents, topical acne preparations, cryotherapy, and ultraviolet light.

*Cleansing agents* include soaps and abrasive cleaners. Bacteriostatic soaps are not more helpful than plain soap. The frequency of washing is adjusted individually by the patient to produce mild drying of the skin.

*Astringents* contain mixtures of such materials as alcohol and acetone. They are used essentially in the same way as cleansing agents.

*Topical acne preparations* usually contain one or more of the following ingredients: sulfur, resorcinol, and salicylic acid. The over-the-counter acne preparations are effective for very mild forms of

acne. Benzoyl peroxide is more potent and comes as a gel or lotion. The patient should be instructed to apply the benzoyl peroxide sparingly at first, with the object of producing a little flaking and peeling, but not pain. The patient should understand that certain areas of the face, such as around the mouth, are more sensitive than others. More recently, topical vitamin A acid used once daily, or as tolerated, has been shown to be a very effective peeling agent. Vitamin A augments the action of chemical and physical agents so the patient should be instructed to avoid other local treatments unless specifically prescribed by the physician. Patients should not apply vitamin A while the skin is wet to minimize the stinging effects. Vitamin A increases susceptibility to sunburn, and so patients should be warned to avoid excessive exposure to sunlight. A sunscreen may be prescribed. Exacerbation may occur in the early weeks of treatment due to action on previously unseen comedones. Visible improvement should occur in 2 to 3 months.

Natural or artificial *ultraviolet light* may be used as a peeling agent. Many patients with acne vulgaris will improve during the summer months because of the ultraviolet light in the natural sunshine. Patients using ultraviolet lamps should be instructed to measure the distance to the lamp, to protect their eyes with goggles or sunglasses, and to set a timing device in case they fall asleep. The amount of ultraviolet light exposure recommended is that which will produce a mild erythema in 24 hours.

*Cryotherapy* produces erythema and desquamation similar to that produced by ultraviolet light. It is performed by the application of a slush made with sulfur, dry ice, and acetone or by brushing across the skin a piece of solid carbon dioxide that has been dipped in acetone.

**T**reatment of Inflammatory Acne  *Tetracycline* is the most widely used antibiotic in the treatment of inflammatory acne lesions, although other antibiotics are also effective. Tetracycline reduces the production of free fatty acids in the sebum. It is believed to do this by reducing the number of *P. acnes* or by inhibiting the synthesis of the lipase which converts triglycerides to free fatty acids. There is no proof, however, that the beneficial effect with tetracycline therapy results solely from a decrease in free fatty acids. Because the sebaceous glands appear to act as an excretory route for tetracycline, it is well concentrated in the sebum even when the patient is on doses as low as 250 mg/day. Tetracycline should not be given between the fourth fetal month and twelfth year of life in order to prevent discoloration of the teeth and enamel hypoplasia. Although side effects are uncommon, tetracycline may cause nausea, diarrhea, yeast vaginitis, photosensitivity, liver damage, and anaphylaxis. Degraded tetracycline can severely interfere with renal tubular function, and so patients should be warned not to use outdated medication. Absorption of tetracycline is enhanced if it is taken 1 hour before or 2 hours after eating a meal. Antacids, iron pills, milk, and other dairy products can bind with tetracycline and render it inactive. Recent work indicates that topical tetracycline also may be effective in treating inflammatory acne.

Intralesional injections of *corticosteroids* may prove helpful in the resolution of the more severe nodular and cystic lesions. This local effect of corticosteroids is contrary to their systemic effects where, in high dosage, they may produce acne. Systemic corticosteroids in low dosage may be used on a short-term basis for selected severe cases unresponsive to other modes of therapy.

*Estrogen-dominant oral contraceptives* can be valuable in the treatment of acne in some female patients because of the ability of estrogen to suppress sebum production. Acne may flare in the first few months of treatment, and it may be the fifth month of treatment before good results are seen. The benefits of therapy for acne should be weighed against the known hazards associated with oral contraceptives.

*Irradiation* is sometimes used for extremely severe acne. If sufficient dosages of x-rays are given, the sebaceous glands atrophy, resulting in clearing of the acne. However, after completion of treatment the sebaceous glands may regenerate, accompanied by recurrence of the acne. Since excessive x-rays may be carcinogenic, this treatment modality has been almost abandoned.

**G**eneral Considerations   The acne patient should be encouraged to eat a well-balanced diet and avoid excessive intake of any single item. Controlled studies have failed to demonstrate that acne flare-ups are caused by food substances.

Cosmetics, in general, need not be discouraged unless they are associated with the development of acne lesions. The use of water-base preparations and the avoidance of greasy, occlusive bases are recommended. All traces of makeup should be washed off before the patient goes to bed.

Manipulation of the lesions should be discouraged. This may best be accomplished by a simple explanation of the mechanism by which manipulation may introduce secondary bacterial infection or contribute to the rupture of follicular contents into the surrounding dermis, converting a previously noninflammatory lesion into a destructive inflammatory lesion and promoting scar formation. Mechanical irritation should be avoided. Unconscious habits such as touching the face or resting the head on the hands should be brought to the patient's attention so that they may be consciously avoided.

**Third-Level Nursing Care**
Despite the best methods of therapy available to date, it is not always possible to prevent the disfiguring scarring that results from the more serious inflammatory types of acne (see Color Plate 9-2). The *acne pit* is the most common disfiguring effect seen in acne. Pits range in size from less than a millimeter to 3 or 4 mm and are frequently seen on the cheeks. Larger pits appear as openings in the skin resembling holes made with an ice pick. In the more deeply seated acne lesions, follicular destruction results in scars that are irregular in outline and may be depressed, level with the skin, or elevated. While scars will often fill in over a period of 2 to 3 years, the final result is often unsatisfactory.

*Dermabrasion* (scraping, sandpapering, brushing, or planing of the skin) is the most common surgical treatment for acne scarring. The procedure involves the removal of the epidermis and some superficial dermis while preserving enough of the dermis to allow reepithelialization of the dermabraded area. Dermabrasion is not performed with the intent of curing acne but only of improving its scars. The object is to sand down the high points or elevations of the skin so that the low areas appear less deep. Most often dermabrasion is carried out with a motor-driven instrument which revolves at a high speed and has a cylinder of sandpaper or a wire brush attached to it. Anesthesia can be local for small dermabraded areas, but is more likely to be general when the entire face is treated.

Postoperatively serum from the wound forms a coagulum (crust) across the abraded surface. When no dressings are used, oozing may be noticed. The patient may experience the sensation of a recent sunburn. By the fifth day after treatment a thin epidermis regenerates, and the coagulum cracks and falls away during the following week. A generous layer of an ointment such as petroleum jelly or cocoa butter is applied daily to aid in removing the coagulum as well as lubricating the surface beneath. The dermabraded area usually remains erythematous for 4 or 5 weeks.

Pigment formation by the melanocytes in the basal layer of the epidermis begins about 4 weeks postoperatively. Patients need to be instructed to avoid excessive sun exposure and to use a good quality sunscreen for a period of 2 to 4 months following treatment in order to prevent hyperpigmentation from occurring.

Long-term results of dermabrasion may produce anything from no improvement or even worsening to very marked improvement benefiting the patient's appearance and psyche. Unfortunately, it is the rare case of acne scarring in which a superior result is achieved. Possible complications include prolonged erythema, milia, hyperpigmentation, and scarring. One procedure is usually not enough; frequently two or three dermabrasions will be necessary at intervals of 3 to 12 months.

The patient undergoing dermabrasion for acne scarring needs to understand the nature of the surgical procedure, the degree of improvement that can be expected, possible complications, and the postoperative course. An awareness of the various stages postoperatively should prevent unnecessary anxiety with the unsightly and slow recovery which is inevitable. Realistic expectations of the outcomes of dermabrasion can prevent patients from being angry and disappointed when dermabrasion does not improve their complexion and life-styles.

### Fourth-Level Nursing Care

Continued care and follow-up are essential in the control of acne vulgaris. Typically, the patient whose skin clears up dramatically with treatment is faithful to the therapeutic regime for a few months and then stops all care. In a few months to a year acne returns. A discussion of the waxing and waning chronic course of acne helps patients to realize the necessity of continuing treatment and prepares them for the longevity of the condition. Patients need continued reassurance, support, and understanding in order to continue treatment and cope with the slow progress and discouraging problems accompanying a chronic condition.

Patients need follow-up to ensure that they are carrying out treatment correctly and are achieving effective results. Instructions about treatment may have to be reviewed with patients, or a new treatment modality may be initiated. It is also important that the patient be monitored for untoward effects from medications.

The nurse needs to give emotional support to adolescents with acne since they are particularly sensitive about their body image at this time. Acne seldom hampers an outgoing, extroverted youngster, but it can be intolerable for a basically shy individual. Acne may disturb an adolescent's peer relationships and undermine self-confidence. The adolescent may use acne as an excuse to avoid anxiety-arousing relationships. An understanding and receptive attitude on the part of the nurse can help the adolescent through this difficult time.

The nurse can help the patient to keep a proper perspective of the total picture of acne by emphasizing how common acne is and encouraging patience since it takes months to see improvement after initiation of therapy. It may be necessary to refute public misconceptions relating acne with sexual intercourse, masturbation, uncleanliness, contagion, etc. It should be emphasized that the goal of treatment is not cure but rather control of acne, improving daily appearance, and minimizing scarring.

## DISTURBANCES DUE TO PARASITES AND INSECTS

The number of bites or lesions due to parasites or insects is very large. The major disturbances will be presented in *brief* form; they are scabies, pediculosis, flea bites, bedbug bites, chigger bites, mosquito lesions, and bee stings.

### Scabies

*Scabies* is a skin infection caused by a crab-shaped mite (*Acarus* or *Sarcoptes scabiei*). Both male and female parasites live upon the skin, but the female burrows into the superficial layer of the skin to deposit her eggs. The primary lesion, the burrow, is a gray-brown threadlike lesion a few millimeters in length which is usually difficult to see. The presence of the mite causes severe itching, especially at night, and inflammation which results in the formation of papules, vesicles, excoriations, and crusting (see Color Plate 9-3). The lesions are most commonly noted on the webs between the fingers but can also be found about the wrist, elbow, waist, axilla, popliteal spaces, buttocks, groin, genitalia, and areolae of the nipples. Transmission of scabies is by direct contact and to a limited extent from soiled sheets and undergarments freshly contaminated by infected persons.

The patient is bathed thoroughly with soap and water, and 1 percent gamma benzene hexachloride cream or lotion or 25 percent benzyl benzoate lotion is applied to the entire body at prescribed intervals. Treatment is irritating to the average skin and will not quickly relieve the pruritus. Patients should be made aware that they are likely to be uncomfortable for a week or more. Triamcinolone ointment may be prescribed for the pruritus.

## Pediculosis

*Pediculosis* is an infestation caused by lice and is readily transmissable to others by personal contact or by contact with articles that temporarily harbor them. Although any person may be accidentally infested, extensive lousiness is a sign of poor personal hygiene, chiefly lack of bathing. Lice can become a matter of major public health importance because they are vectors for typhus and relapsing fever.

Three types of lice are commonly encountered: the head louse (*Pediculus capitus*), the body louse (*P. corporis*), and the pubic louse (*Phthirus pubis*). Lice are oval and gray, about 2 to 4 mm long, and wingless with six legs. The females lay eggs called *nits* which are attached to hair or clothing by a sticky substance that hardens. Lice live on blood which they suck from the skin.

The primary symptom of any type of pediculosis is pruritus which is produced by the saliva of the louse. Itching leads to excoriations which can easily become secondarily infected. Dusky gray macules may be observed as the result of the insect's saliva acting on bilirubin, converting it to biliverdin.

Treatment is directed toward destruction and removal of nits and pediculi and toward cleansing and soothing of irritated skin. Gamma benzene hexachloride shampoo should be used to cleanse the scalp infested with lice. Nits can be removed manually or with a fine comb. The hair need not be cut. Combs and brushes are also disinfected with the shampoo.

*Pediculus corporis* lives in clothes and leaves them only to obtain blood from the skin (see Color Plate 9-4). Treatment of *P. corporis* includes sterilization of clothing by laundering followed by pressing with a hot iron. Seams of the clothing should be dusted with 1% gamma benzene hexachloride powder.

## Flea Bites

The *flea* (*Pulex irritans*) is a wingless insect which is attracted by moving objects and leaps to attain them. This often places it on an ankle or lower leg. It penetrates the skin and feeds on blood, producing a hemorrhagic spot surrounded by a pruritic wheal. Humans are attacked by dog or cat fleas only when these animals are absent. Flea disinfectant should be dusted on the pets and their living quarters.

## Bedbug Bites

Bedbugs (*Cimex lectularius* and *C. hemipterus*) are bloodsucking insects which live in cracks and crevices in the room and come out at night to obtain a blood meal. The bites are usually found in the morning grouped or arranged in a straight line on parts of the body that were not covered by bedclothes. Each lesion consists of a wheal, and vesicles may develop. The lesions may persist for 2 weeks. If itching is intense, it may be alleviated by the administration of oral antihistamines and topical corticosteroids. A professional fumigator should be consulted to rid the environment of bedbugs.

## Chigger Bites

Chiggers (*Trombicula, red bug, harvest mite*) are reddish mites found in grass and especially in blackberry bushes. The chigger attaches itself to the lower extremities, groin, axilla, or under the breasts, and punctures the skin to obtain blood. The presence of the mite causes a dermatitis which consists first of bright-red flecks which transform in a few hours into wheals. After 24 to 48 hours there are papules and nodules often with central puncta, and occasionally there are vesicles. Pruritus becomes quite intense. Although the chigger will leave the skin of its own accord, 25% benzyl benzoate emulsion or 1% gamma benzene hexachloride cream or lotion may be used to eliminate the organism. The pruritus may persist for some time, and so treatment is directed toward relief of itching. Oral antihistamines, topical corticosteroids, and clear fingernail polish applied to the chigger bites may produce relief of pruritus. Good mosquito repellents are also toxic to chiggers and can be used to prevent chigger infestations.

## Mosquito Bites

Mosquitoes (*Culicidae*) are capable of transmitting yellow fever, dengue fever, encephalitis, malaria, and filariasis. Lesions are produced by the mosquito's penetration of the skin and the droplets of mosquito saliva introduced prior to removing blood. The bite produces a small erythematous papule with or without a visible central punctum. The pruritus associated with the lesion may be relieved by topical corticosteroid ointment with 0.25% menthol and phenol.

Mosquito bites may be prevented by using commercial insect repellents which contain diethyltoluamide, ethyl hexanedoil, or dimethyl phthalate. For maximum efficacy, repellents should be applied liberally and frequently, such as every 2 hours.

After exposure to water and when exercising or sweating profusely, repellents should be reapplied. All exposed areas should be coated with repellent; nontreated areas only a few centimeters away from repellent may be bitten.

## Bee Stings

The *bee* or *wasp* sting results from a puncture of the skin by the insect's sharp stinging apparatus and injection of a chemically complex venom. Immediately after the sting an intense burning local pain occurs, followed some minutes later by edema, inflammation, and itching. The honeybee and some wasps leave part of the stinger and poison sacs in the wound to discharge more venom. The stinging apparatus should carefully be removed by scraping it off with a knife blade, the side of tweezers, or a fingernail. The sac or stinger should not be grasped since this forces remaining venom into the wound. Generally, bumblebees and most wasps do not leave the stinger.

Bee venom is acid, and ammonia or sodium bicarbonate should be applied after extraction of the stinger. Wasp venom is alkaline or neutral and should be treated with lemon juice or vinegar. An ice pack applied to the bite may help to reduce edema and pain. Administration of antihistamines may be of value.

An individual who is allergic to bee or wasp stings may have an immediate anaphylactic reaction or a delayed reaction following a sting (see Chap. 10). Persons known to be allergic to bee stings need to have an emergency kit available and someone able to administer emergency treatment when they are around bees. Treatment includes epinephrine, adrenocorticosteroids, antihistamines, and supportive care. A generalized reaction to a bee sting is an indication for desensitization which takes place over several years.

## HERPES SIMPLEX

Herpes simplex is an infectious disease caused by a virus, *herpesvirus hominis.* The disease usually occurs first in early childhood and is asymptomatic in 85 to 90 percent of patients. After the patient recovers from the primary infection, the herpes simplex virus probably remains latent throughout life. The disease, may be activated at any time, and recurrent attacks are common. The mechanism of reactivation is not fully understood, but trigger factors include trauma, fever, malaria, pneumonia, meningitis, physiologic stress, menses, and sunlight.

Two types of herpes virus are responsible for recurrent vesicular manifestations. Type I is responsible for *herpes labialis,* commonly called a *cold sore* or *fever blister.* The lesion most frequently occurs on the lips and around the mouth. It begins with a burning, tingling, and itching in the area, followed by multiple grouped tiny vesicles on an erythematous base. Crusting occurs after about 48 hours, and the lesion heals in 7 to 10 days. Type II herpes virus is responsible for *herpes progenitalis* in which herpetic lesions occur on the genitals. Healing may take 10 days to 6 weeks.

Herpes simplex is transmitted by direct contact such as kissing or intercourse. Pregnant women with genital herpetic infection can transmit the disease to the newborn during delivery unless preventive measures are taken.

A variety of therapeutic agents have been employed for the treatment of herpes simplex, although none of these has been proved to effectively shorten the duration of herpetic lesions. Treatment of herpes simplex is largely symptomatic and directed toward relieving discomfort and preventing secondary infection. When lesions are in the mouth, oral intake of food and fluids may be difficult. Rinsing the mouth with a topical anesthetic such as viscous Xylocaine may be helpful. The use of sitz baths, heat lamps, analgesics, or topical cornstarch may help alleviate discomfort associated with genital herpetic lesions. Herpes progenitalis presents a serious venereal disease problem because it is recurrent and there is presently no effective treatment.

## HERPES ZOSTER

Herpes zoster, commonly called *shingles,* is a painful infection of nerve structure believed to be caused by the same virus that causes chickenpox (varicella-zoster virus). Zoster is believed to result from activation of latent varicella-zoster virus that has been present in the patient since the time of the initial infection with the virus. The greatest incidence of herpes zoster occurs in adults over 40 years of age. Although it occurs in apparently well individuals, it is often seen in persons with chronic debilitating disease such as malignancies and in persons on immunosuppressive therapy.

The virus of herpes zoster causes an inflammation of the ganglions of the posterior nerve roots or the extramedullary cranial nerve ganglions. Skin manifestations occur along the course of the corresponding sensory nerve (see Color Plate 9-5). There are prodromal symptoms of pain, burning, or pruritus prior to the onset of other clinical signs. Subsequently, vesicles develop on a tender, erythematous skin following the distribution of the sensory nerve. During the acute stage of the illness, the patient may complain of fever, malaise, anorexia, and headache. The vesicles become pustular, break down, and form crusts. Brownish spots may remain after healing. The eruption is almost invariably unilateral. The site most frequently affected is the thorax. Another relatively common site is the fifth cranial nerve, causing pain in the eye and surrounding tissues. The acute painful stage of herpes zoster generally lasts 7 to 21 days before it gradually subsides and the pain disappears.

There is no specific therapy that will alter the course of herpes zoster. Nursing care is directed toward preventing secondary infection of the lesion and keeping the patient as comfortable as possible. Analgesics such as acetylsalicylic acid or narcotics may be ordered for pain relief. Systemic adrenocorticosteroids may be used to alleviate the inflammatory component of the disease.

While most patients have an uneventful recovery, some patients, especially the elderly, may develop a *postherpetic neuralgia* that causes pain which is unresponsive to treatment. Systemic corticosteroids given to treat herpes zoster have been shown to significantly reduce the incidence and duration of postherpetic neuralgia.

Zoster-immune globulin is available for passive immunization against herpes zoster. Because it is in short supply and not without risks, zoster-immune globulin is presently indicated only for patients in danger of developing severe, disseminated zoster.

## FUNGUS INFECTIONS (SUPERFICIAL MYCOSES, DERMATOPHYTOSES)

Superficial mycoses are highly communicable fungus infections involving the skin, hair, and nails. The microorganisms responsible for superficial mycoses are the fungi known as *dermatophytes*. *Microsporum, Epidermophyton,* and *Trichophyton* are three important genera of dermatophytes responsible for fungus infections.

The most common of the fungus diseases are those infections of the skin, hair, and nails generally referred to as *ringworm* or *tinea*. These diseases are classified as *tinea capitis* (ringworm of the scalp), *tinea barbae (*ringworm of the beard), *tinea corporis* (ringworm of the smooth skin or body), *tinea pedis* (ringworm of the feet or "athlete's

foot"), *tinea cruris* (ringworm of the groin), and *tinea unguium* (ringworm of the nails).

Ringworm is transmitted by both direct and indirect contact. The causative organism may be transmitted by combs, brushes, towels, or clothing. Opinions differ as to whether tinea pedis is contracted from areas about swimming pools and locker rooms. Household pets may be infected and at times serve as a source of fungus infection.

The fungi causing ringworm produce several types of lesions. In cases of *tinea capitis* the hairs become dry, dull, and lusterless and fall out easily, leaving a scaly denuded area. Inflammation of the scalp may be present as pustules or boggy, raised, suppurative lesions called *kerion. Tinea corporis* occurs on nonhairy smooth skin, forming a circular lesion that is slightly raised and erythematous about the periphery. The lesion may be vesicular, pustular, scaly, or crusted. *Tinea pedis* is characterized by cracking and scaling of the skin between the toes, with vesicular lesions that contain a thin watery fluid. The infection may spread to the soles of the feet and cause severe itching. Persons with fungus infections may develop skin eruptions on various parts of the body, especially the hands, which constitute an *allergic* reaction to the fungi or their antigenic products. These lesions do not contain fungi and are called *dermatophytids* ("id" lesions).

The diagnosis of fungus infections depends on clinical features, microscopic examination of hairs or scrapings from lesions, and cultures from the fungus. Fungus infections caused by *Microsporum* can be diagnosed by using a Wood light (filtered ultraviolet light). Hairs or lesions infected by *Microsporum* will fluoresce with a brilliant green light.

There is some variation in treatment depending on the site and extent of the fungus infection. *Griseofulvin,* a fungistatic antibiotic, is the treatment of choice for all forms of ringworm. The drug is administered orally, and absorption is enhanced if it is given with a fat-containing meal. Because griseofulvin is fungistatic rather than fungicidal, the hairs over the infected area may be clipped to prevent spread of the infection to other persons. Topical treatment may also be employed such as tolnaftate, miconazole, or benzoic and salicylic acid ointment (Whitfield's ointment). Acute tinea pedis with weeping lesions may be treated by foot soaks of potassium permanganate solution or Burrow's solution. Heat, perspiration, and physical activity tend to aggravate the pruritus of ringworm. In cases of tinea pedis, plenty of ventilation should be given the feet, such as by going barefoot or wearing sandals or lightweight socks. All treatment is continued until a complete cure has been achieved, because of the danger of recurrence.

## DISCOID LUPUS ERYTHEMATOSUS

*Discoid lupus erythematosus* is a chronic skin eruption which often leads to scarring and permanent disfigurement. The cause of discoid lupus erythematosus is unknown, although there is evidence that it may be an autoimmune disease. The areas most commonly affected are the face, scalp, neck, and external ears. It may start as a single lesion and gradually involve more and more areas. The lesions characteristically appear as erythematous, scaling macules, with atrophy at the center of the lesions giving them a discoid appearance (see Color Plate 9-6). After persisting for a variable length of time, the lesions usually heal with atrophy, scarring, pigmentary changes, and alopecia when the scalp is involved.

Discoid lupus erythematosus may be treated with topical fluorinated adrenocorticosteroids under an occlusive plastic dressing. Because exposure to sunlight may precipitate the appearance of new lesions and aggravate those already present, patients should be instructed to avoid sunlight and use a sunscreening agent. Although their mode of action is unknown at this time, some of the antimalarial drugs are used successfully in treating discoid lupus erythematosus. They are administered in doses considerably higher than those used in treating malaria and have numerous side effects. Chloroquine is one of the antimalarial drugs commonly used in treating discoid lupus erythematosus.

## PSORIASIS

*Psoriasis* is a chronic recurrent skin disease characterized by thick red plaques and papules covered by silvery white scales (see Color Plate 9-7). In the United States it is estimated that one or two people out of a hundred have psoriasis, making it one of the most common skin diseases in the country.[68] The onset of psoriasis is usually during early or middle adulthood, but it may occur at any age. Since there is a familial tendency, psoriasis is believed to be inherited.

While the actual cause of psoriasis is unknown, the disease is characterized by rapid proliferation of the cells in the epidermis. Normally, the epidermal cells develop, mature, and are replaced every 28 to 30 days. The epidermal cells of psoriatic lesions are reproduced every 3 to 4 days. The abnormal cells are not shed inconspicuously; they

accumulate, building up thick, red plaques, and shed large numbers of silvery-white scales.

In most patients psoriatic lesions are limited to a few on the elbows, knees, sacrum, or scalp. The lesions enlarge and may coalesce, forming extensive irregularly shaped patches. They are often arranged in remarkable symmetry. Pruritus is common; some patients have such extensive psoriasis that they are unable to work or must go to great lengths to do so. Psoriasis has a tendency to improve and then recur, even throughout life. Fingernails and toenails are frequently involved with pitting, ridging, discoloration, thickening, and separating of the nail plate. A form of arthritis occurs in about 10 to 15 percent of patients with psoriasis.

While the psoriatic lesions may develop spontaneously without an apparent cause, there are specific systemic and environmental factors which are known to influence the course of the disease. Psoriatic lesions often occur at the site of physical trauma, which may be the result of an allergic response, overexposure to ultraviolet light, or mechanical or chemical injury. The phenomenon in which lesions are induced by epidermal injury is known as the *Koebner reaction* or *isomorphic response.* Psoriasis can also be aggravated by systemic illness or emotional stress.

Although there presently is no cure for psoriasis, treatment temporarily clears most lesions. Therapy is directed at suppressing the rapid epidermal cell proliferation and reducing the products of the metabolic disorder: scaling, erythema, and pruritus. One of the most frequently used treatments is the combination of *topical coal tar* preparations and exposure to *ultraviolet light.* This is known as the *Goeckerman regime.* It is not clearly understood why the Goeckerman regime is effective in treating psoriasis. It has been thought that the ultraviolet light inhibits cell proliferation and the photosensitizing action of coal tar enhances the ultraviolet light effectiveness, but it is questionable that this is a complete and accurate explanation for the mode of action of this therapy.

*Adrenocorticosteroids* can be applied topically and occluded under a plastic wrap to promote drug penetration. A plastic tape with steroid impregnated into the adhesive can be used to treat small psoriatic lesions. The effectiveness of steroids is thought to be due to their anti-inflammatory property and their ability to inhibit cell division.

Psoriasis may also be treated with a combination of *anthralin paste* applied topically and exposure to ultraviolet light. Anthralin is an irritant and must be applied carefully to lesions.

A treatment developed more recently is the application of a *psoralen* compound followed by exposure to *long-wave ultraviolet light.* This is termed *photochemotherapy* because the therapeutic response requires the interaction of the light and the drug. Regression of psoriatic lesions is believed to be due to inhibition of DNA synthesis.

Cancer *chemotherapeutic agents* such as methotrexate are used for persons with extensive psoriasis that fails to respond to other forms of treatment. Methotrexate is an antimetabolite that is given to inhibit the rapidly proliferating epidermal cells. However, the drug is very toxic, especially to the liver. Because psoriasis is not life-threatening, the risks of systemic therapy with methotrexate and other antineoplastic agents are evaluated in relation to the severity of the disease.

Recent studies have demonstrated that in psoriatic lesions there is a mild deficiency of cyclic AMP, a messenger molecule that regulates many different cell functions. If this deficiency is the cause of rapid epidermal cell proliferation, agents can be used to elevate cyclic AMP levels and normalize the growth process in psoriatic skin.

Localized psoriasis can be controlled reasonably well on an outpatient basis, but generalized psoriasis is a major problem often requiring hospitalization. Some patients require occlusive dressings over the entire body. Day or night care centers may enable patients to receive treatment and still go to work or be with their families.

Although psoriasis is not a life-threatening illness, it can have devastating effects. Topical treatment can be messy, uncomfortable, time-consuming, and expensive, and can virtually preclude going about one's normal daily activities. People often mistakenly associate the skin lesions with uncleanliness or believe that the lesions are contagious. Consequently, they avoid the patient and fear personal contact with the psoriatic lesions. Persons with psoriasis tend to withdraw from business, social, and intimate contact.

The National Psoriasis Foundation founded in 1968 by Beverly W. Foster is making great efforts to aid patients in understanding their disease through publications and meetings throughout the country. Persons with psoriasis often benefit from sharing their feelings and experiences. The group therapy is of value in learning how to adjust to a chronic, disabling, and disfiguring condition.

**REFERENCES**

1   Zabriskie, J. B., K. C. Hsu, and B. C. Seegal: "Heart-Reactive Antibody Associated with Rheumatic Fever: Characterization and Diagnostic Significance," *Clin Exp Immunol,* **7:**147–159, August 1970.

2   Stollerman, Gene H.: *Rheumatic Fever and Streptococcal Infection,* Grune & Stratton, New York, 1975, pp. 90, 154, 224, 256.

3   *Ibid.*

4   *Ibid.*

5   Doyle, Eugenie F.: "Rheumatic Fever—A Continuing Problem," *Cardiovasc Nurs,* **10:**17–21, July–August 1974.

6   *Ibid.*

7   Stollerman: op. cit., pp. 90, 154, 224, 256.

8   Bergman, Abraham B., and Richard J. Werner: "Failure of Children To Receive Penicillin by Mouth," *N Eng J Med,* **268:**1334–1338, June 13, 1963.

9   Charney, Evan, et al.: "How Well Do Patients Take Oral Penicillin? A Collaborative Study in Private Practice," *Pediatrics,* **40:**188–195, August 1967.

10   Leistyna, Joseph A., and John C. Macauley: "Therapy of Streptococcal Infections," *Am J Dis Child,* **111:**22–26, January 1966.

11   Mohler, Daniel N., David G. Wallin, and Edward G. Dreyfus: "Studies in the Home Treatment of Streptococcal Disease. I. Failure of Patients to Take Penicillin by Mouth as Prescribed," *N Eng J Med,* **252:**1116–1118, June 30, 1955.

12   *Jones Criteria (revised) for Guidance in the Diagnosis of Rheumatic Fever,* American Heart Association, New York, 1967.

13   Wallach, Jacques: *Interpretation of Diagnostic Tests: A Handbook Synopsis of Laboratory Medicine,* Little, Brown, Boston, 1974, p. 148.

14   Johnson, Alvis: "Rheumatic Fever," *Nursing 74,* **3:**57–59, March 1974.

15   Stollerman: op. cit., pp. 90, 154, 224, 256.

16   *Introduction to Lung Diseases, USA,* American Lung Association, 1975, pp. 35, 41.

17   Sbarbaro, John A.: "Tuberculosis: The New Challenge to the Practicing Clinician," *Chest,* **68:**436–443, September 1975 (Suppl).

18   *Morbidity Mortality Annu Suppl, 1974,* **23:**2, 5, 12, 13, 14.

19   "Tuberculosis in 1975—United States," *Morbidity Mortality Weekly Rep,* **25:**75, March 6, 1976.

20   American Lung Association: op. cit., pp. 35, 41.

21   Stead, William W.: "Tuberculosis," in Maxwell M. Wintrobe et al. (eds.), *Harrison's Principles of Internal Medicine,* 7th ed., McGraw-Hill, New York, 1974, p. 859.

22   "Recommendation of the Public Health Service Advisory Committee on Immunization Practices," *Morbidity Mortality,* **24:**69, Feb. 22, 1975.

23   *Morbidity Mortality Ann Suppl, 1974,* pp. 2, 5, 12, 13, 14.

24   Stead, William W.: op. cit., p. 859.

25 *Morbidity Mortality Annu Suppl, 1974,* pp. 2, 5, 12, 13, 14.

26 Stead, William W.: *Fundamentals of Tuberculosis Today. For Students in the Health Professions,* Marquette University Press, Milwaukee, 1971, p. 6, 17, 22.

27 Committee on Diagnostic Skin Testing of the American Thoracic Society Scientific Assembly on Tuberculosis: *The Tuberculin Skin Test,* American Lung Association, New York, 1974.

28 American Thoracic Society. Official Statement: "Preventive Therapy of Tuberculosis Infection," *Am Rev Resp Dis,* **110:**371–374, September 1974.

29 Stead, William W.: *Fundamentals of Tuberculosis Today. For Students in the Health Professions,* pp. 6, 17, 22.

30 Edsall, John, J. Gary Collins, and John A. C. Gray: "The Reactivation of Tuberculosis in New York City in 1967," *Am Rev Resp Dis,* **102:**725–736, November 1970.

31 Clark, E. Gurney, and Niels Danbolt: "The Oslo Study of the Natural Course of Untreated Syphilis," *Med Clin North Am,* **48:**613–623, March 1964.

32 *Ibid.*

33 The 1975 Committee on the Joint Statement, William L. Fleming (chairman): *Today's VD Control Problem 1975,* American Social Health Association, New York, 1975, pp. 15, 16, 17, 53, 54.

34 *Ibid.*

35 *Ibid.*

36 *Ibid.*

37 *Ibid.*

38 "Syphilis—CDC Recommended Treatment Schedules, 1976," *Morbidity Mortality Weekly Rep,* **25:**101–102, 107–108, April 9, 1976.

39 Rudolph, Andrew H., and Eleanor V. Price: "Penicillin Reactions among Patients in Venereal Disease Clinics," *JAMA,* **223:**499–501, Jan. 29, 1973.

40 "Syphilis—CDC Recommended Treatment Schedules, 1976," pp. 101–102, 107–108.

41 *Ibid.*

42 *Ibid.*

43 Blackwell, Betty: "Stigma," *Behav Concepts Nurs Intervention,* coordinated by Carolyn E. Carlson, Lippincott, Philadelphia, 1970, p. 176.

44 Holmes, King K., and Harry N. Beaty: "Gonococcal Infections," in Maxwell M. Wintrobe et al. (eds.), *Harrison's Principles of Internal Medicine,* 7th ed., McGraw-Hill, New York, 1974, p. 789.

45 McInnes, Mary E.: *Essentials of Communicable Disease,* Mosby, St. Louis, 1975, p. 176.

46 "Cases of Specified Notifiable Diseases: United States," *Morbidity Mortality,* **24:**445, Jan. 3, 1976.

47 *Morbidity Mortality Annu Supp, 1974,* pp. 2, 5, 12, 13, 14.

48 *Ibid.*

49 Millar, J. D.: "The National VD Problem," *Epidemic Venereal Diseases,* Second International Venereal Disease Symposium, St. Louis: Pfizer Laboratories Division, Pfizer, Inc., and American Social Health Association, 1972, pp. 10–13.

50 *Ibid.*

51 McInnes: op. cit., p. 176.

52 Venereal Disease Control Advisory Committee: Gonorrhea—CDC Recommended Treatment Schedules, 1974, *Morbidity Mortality,* **23:**341–342, Oct. 5, 1974.

53 Arnold, Charles B., and Betty E. Cogswell: "A Condom Distribution Program for Adolescents: The Findings of a Feasibility Study," *Am J Public Health,* **61:**739–750, April 1971.

54 McGrath, Patricia, and Elizabeth B. Laliberte: "Level of Basic Venereal Disease Knowledge among Junior and Senior High School Nurses in Massachusetts," *Nurs Res,* **23:**31–37, January–February 1974.

55 Venereal Disease Control Advisory Committee, pp. 341–342.

56 Wiesner, Paul J.: "Clinical Complications of Gonorrhea," *Epidemic Venereal Diseases.* Second International Venereal Disease Symposium, St. Louis: Pfizer Laboratories Division, Pfizer, Inc. and American Social Health Association, 1972, pp. 22–26.

57 *Ibid.*

58 Venereal Disease Control Advisory Committee, pp. 341–342.

59 *Ibid.*

60 Miller, George, James C. Niederman, and Linda-Lea Andrews: "Prolonged Oropharyngeal Excretion of Epstein-Barr Virus after Infectious Mononucleosis," *N Engl J Med,* **288:**229–232, Feb. 1, 1973.

61 Penman, Hugh G.: "Fatal Infectious Mononucleosis: A Critical Review," *J Clin Pathol,* **23:**765–771, December 1970.

62 *Morbidity Mortality Annu Suppl, 1974,* pp. 2, 5, 12, 13, 14.

63 Price, Vera H.: "Testosterone Metabolism in the Skin," *Arch Dermatol,* **111:**1496–1502, November 1975.

64 Sansone, Gail, and Ronald M. Reisner: "Differential Rates of Conversion of Testosterone to Dihydrotestosterone in Acne and in Normal Human Skin—A Possible Pathogenic Factor in Acne," *J Invest Dermatol,* **56:**366–372, May 1971.

65 Frank, Samuel B.: *Acne Vulgaris,* Charles C Thomas, Springfield, Ill., 1971, p. 8.

66 Ebling, F. J., and A. Rook: "The Sebaceous Gland," in Arthur Rook, D. S. Wilkinson, and F. J. G. Ebling (eds.), *Textbook of Dermatology,* vol. II, Blackwell, Oxford, 1972, p. 1545.

67 *Ibid.*

68 Van Scott, Eugene J., and Eugene M. Farber: "Psoriasis," in Thomas B. Fitzpatrick et al. (eds.), *Dermatology in General Medicine,* McGraw-Hill, New York, 1971, p. 220.

## BIBLIOGRAPHY

Ad Hoc Committee Report: "Systemic Antibiotics for Treatment of Acne Vulgaris: Efficacy and Safety," *Arch Dermatol,* **111:**1630–1636, December 1975.

Anderson, Gaylord West, Margaret G. Arnstein, and Mary R. Lester: *Communicable Disease Control,* Macmillan, New York, 1962.

Carter, R. L., and H. G. Penman (eds.): *Infectious Mononucleosis,* Blackwell, Oxford, 1969.

Chessin, Lawrence, et al.: "Keeping Up with Infectious Mononucleosis," *Patient Care,* **6:**44–45, Oct. 15, 1972.

Curwen, William, et al.: "Office Dermatology Logical Lines to Acne Control," *Patient Care,* **9:**108–137, April 15, 1975.

Fisher, Louis B., and Howard I. Maibach: "Topical Antipsoriatic Agents and Epidermal Mitosis in Man," *Arch Dermatol,* **108:**374–377, September 1973.

Grabb, William C., and James W. Smith, eds: *Plastic Surgery: A Concise Guide to Clinical Practice,* Little, Brown, Boston, 1973.

Hoagland, Robert J.: *Infectious Mononucleosis,* Grune & Stratton, New York, 1967.

Imperato, Pascal J.: *The Treatment and Control of Infectious Disease in Man,* Charles C Thomas, Springfield, Ill., 1974.

Kligman, Albert M., and Otto H. Mills, Jr.: "Acne Cosmetica," *Arch Dermatol,* **106:**843–850, December 1972.

Lasagna, Louis: *The VD Epidemic,* Temple University Press, Philadelphia, 1975.

Locke, David M.: *Viruses: The Smallest Enemy,* Crown, New York, 1974.

Luckmann, Joan, and Karen C. Sorensen: *Medical-Surgical Nursing: A Psychophysiologic Approach,* Saunders, Philadelphia, 1974.

Maibach, Howard I., and William Akers: "Use of Insect Repellents for Maximum Efficacy," *Arch Dermatol,* **109:**32–35, January 1974.

March, Cyril H.: "Dermabrasion," *Am Fam Physician,* **1:**68–74, January 1970.

McDonald, Charles J.: "Chemotherapy of Psoriasis," *Int J Dermatol,* **14:**563–573, October 1975.

Mills, Jr., Otto H., and Albert Kligman: "Acne Mechanica," *Arch Dermatol,* **111:**481–483, April 1975.

Morton, Barbara M.: *VD A Guide for Nurses and Counselors,* Little, Brown, Boston, 1976.

Parrish, John A., et al.: "Photochemotherapy of Psoriasis with Oral Methoxsalen and Longwave Ultraviolet Light," *N Eng J Med,* **291:**1207–1211, Dec. 5, 1974.

Reisner, Ronald M.: "Acne Vulgaris," *Pediatr Clin North Am,* **20:**851–864, November 1973.

Stawiski, Marek A., et al.: "Papaverine: Its Effects on Cyclic AMP in Vitro and Psoriasis in Vivo," *J Invest Dermatol,* **64:**124–127, February 1975.

Stephenson, Carol: "Malaria: Coming Home with Mobile Americans," *RN,* **38:**53–54, June 1975.

*Syphilis, A Synopsis:* U.S. National Communicable Disease Center, Atlanta, Venereal Disease Program. Publication 1660, 1968.

Tanenbaum, Lewis, et al.: "Tar Phototoxicity and Phototherapy for Psoriasis," *Arch Dermatol,* **111:** 467–470, April 1975.

Top, Franklin H., and Paul F. Wehrle (eds.): *Communicable and Infectious Diseases,* Mosby, St. Louis, 1972.

Voss, Jack G.: "Acne Vulgaris and Free Fatty Acids: A Review and Criticism," *Arch Dermatol,* **109:** 894–898, June 1974.

Wintrobe, Maxwell M., et al.: *Clinical Hematology,* Lea & Febiger, Philadelphia, 1974.

# 10

# HYPERSENSITIVITY AND AUTOIMMUNITY*

Zane Robinson Wolf†
Andrea Thomson

**H**ypersensitivity or *allergic* states are said to exist when there is an increased or tissue-damaging reaction to an antigen by an individual. The term *allergen* is applied to an antigen which can cause allergic symptoms. Allergens may be of protein or haptenic origin and may exist in an individual's external or internal environment. Foreign proteins that may act as allergens include animal products (milk, egg white, danders), fish, insect parts, mold spores, and plant substances (pollen, dust, nuts, fruit). Haptenic allergens include chemicals found in common commercial products (detergents, cosmetics, drugs) and in many industrial processes. This chapter presents the current continuum classification of hypersensitivity responses with their clinical examples, followed by a discussion of *autoimmunity* and the most commonly occurring autoimmune disorders.

## HYPERSENSITIVITY

*Hypersensitivity reactions* are currently classified according to the mechanism of tissue destruction and the immunologic reactants involved, as illustrated in Table 10-1.[1] These reactions represent "tissue-damaging" immune responses. Normally, the body responds to the presence of antigen by mobilizing the humoral and cellular systems of immunity. This results in the production of antibodies or T lymphocytes to attack the foreign substance (see Chap. 5). Hypersensitivity responses are increased immune reactions to the presence of an antigen and may cause a variety of disruptive effects in the individual. It is important to note that differences in classification exist among the four types of hypersensitivity reactions; within each specific category, there may also be variations.

## TYPE I: IMMEDIATE HYPERSENSITIVITY

Type I represents the *classic immediate hypersensitivity* reactions which result from an antigen reacting with reaginic antibody (usually IgE class) that is fixed to the surface of tissue mast cells or basophils. Generally, these disorders are referred to as *anaphylactic responses* and include systemic anaphylaxis, cutaneous reactions, the atopic diseases (urticaria, allergic rhinitis, asthma), and drug reactions.

* The hypersensitivity section was written by Zane R. Wolf, and the autoimmunity section by Andrea Thomson.
† I would like to express my thanks to Bonnie Harris, R.N., Portsmouth, Va., for her kindness.

The mediators for the anaphylactic reactions are IgE (primarily), IgG, complement, and other pharmacological agents such as histamine, slow-reacting substance of anaphylaxis (SRS-A), prostaglandins, eosinophilic chemotactic factor of anaphylaxis (ECF-A), and kinins. These antibody-mediated (*humoral*) responses occur within minutes of allergen-exposure (usually within 15 to 20 minutes) in a sensitized individual.

Anaphylactic responses may be elicited only in a *sensitized* person. This means that the person has had an initial "sensitizing dose" of allergen with little or no reaction. Following a *latent period* of unspecified length, during which reexposure to the allergen caused little or no effect, the person experiences an allergic or hypersensitivity reaction upon exposure to yet another dose of the same allergen. This subsequent reexposure is termed the "shocking dose" and may actually contain only a very small quantity of allergen. This small amount is enough to produce a violent reaction in a sensitized individual.

### Systemic Anaphylaxis

A violent, generalized, immediate response to a specific allergen is termed *systemic anaphylaxis.* Drugs such as penicillin, foreign serums, stinging insect venom, contrast-media dyes, and allergen extracts used in hyposensitization treatment are the frequent causes of these life-threatening reactions.

**Pathophysiology** When a specific allergen enters the circulation, it can react in widespread areas of the body with IgE antibodies attached to basophils of the blood and to mast cells located immediately outside the small blood vessels. As a result of this reaction, histamine is released into the systemic circulation and causes peripheral vasodilation as well as increased permeability of the capillaries and marked loss of plasma from the circulating blood. Itching, urticaria, and smooth muscle contraction (especially bronchiolar constriction) are also the result of histamine. Slow-reacting substance of anaphylaxis is another mediator released from the cells causing spasm of the smooth muscles of the bronchioles. The additional release of bradykinin can increase vascular permeability and vasodilatation and contribute to vascular collapse.

Systemic anaphylactic responses in humans have the skin, lungs, mucous membrane, and vasculature as their major *target tissues.* Effects on these structures include hives, bronchiolar constriction, edema of the hypopharynx or larynx, hypotension, and, eventually, vascular collapse.

Left untreated, pulmonary involvement leads to obstruction as air is trapped in the lungs. Severe bronchiolar constriction and edema can result in the trapping of large quantities of air, thus decreasing the oxygen-carbon dioxide exchange, eventually resulting in hypoxia, hypotension, and death.

### Cutaneous Reactions

IgE antibodies are capable of sensitizing skin cells and are therefore referred to as *skin-sensitizing antibodies.* Their combination with skin cells causes an immediate cutaneous reaction in the presence of antigen. This cutaneous response is termed the *wheal and flare reaction.* It is characterized by a pale wheal surrounded by a red flare. The wheal is formed as edema fluid moves into the area exposed to the allergen; it is then surrounded by the red flare of hyperemia. Cutaneous reactions

**TABLE 10-1**
HYPERSENSITIVITY REACTIONS

| Type | Mediators | Reaction | Disorders |
|---|---|---|---|
| Type I: Immediate or anaphylactic | IgE, IgG, complement. Pharmacological agents: Histamine, SRS-A, prostaglandins, ECF-A, kinins | IgE causes release of mediator substances from basophils and mast cells. | Systemic anaphylaxis, cutaneous reactions, atopic disease. |
| Type II: Cytotoxic and cytolytic | IgG, IgM, complement | IgG and IgM react with antigen on target cell surfaces. Complement may be activated. Phagocytosis or lysis of target cell results. | Blood incompatibility reactions, some drug-induced hemolytic anemias, erythroblastosis fetalis. |
| Type III: Immune complex | IgG, IgM, IgE, complement, neutrophils, eosinophils, lysosomal enzymes | Antigen-antibody complexes activate complement and subsequently attract neutrophils. Lysosomal enzymes are released. | Arthus reaction, serum sickness, systemic lupus erythematosus, possibly some types of acute glomerulonephritis. |
| Type IV: Delayed (cell-mediated) hypersensitivity | T lymphocyte, macrophage, lymphokines | Sensitized T lymphocytes attach to antigen, release lymphokines, and are directly destructive. | Tuberculosis, contact dermatitis, transplantation rejection. |

are widely utilized as a means of allergen detection in allergic individuals.

## Atopic Diseases

Those persons who inherit the tendency for certain anaphylactic responses are termed *atopics,* and the responses are called *atopic diseases* (urticaria, allergic rhinitis, asthma). These diseases are produced by environmental allergens that include drugs, plant and animal products, and air pollutants. In general, the allergen comes in contact with the person by means of inhalation, ingestion, injection, or direct touching. Nasal mucosa, bronchi, or skin may show evidence of disease depending upon the route by which the allergen comes in contact with the body. Frequently, symptoms not associated with the portal of entry will occur; examples of this include hives and skin eruptions produced by allergen ingestion or inhalation, instead of direct contact.

Apparently it is the *tendency* to develop sensitivities to particular *allergens* that is inherited, rather than a specific sensitivity or a particular disease manifestation, such as asthma or allergic rhinitis. The reaction to a specific allergen also depends on the degree of exposure to that allergen; a severely atopic person will not experience ragweed hay fever in a location where pollen is absent.

The distinctive immunologic feature of atopy is the overproduction of atopic reagin-type antibodies to normally harmless antigens in the environment. This tendency to overproduce reaginic antibody, which belongs to the IgE class, is believed to be inherited by persons later termed atopic. Atopic individuals commonly have serum IgE levels two to six times higher than normal levels. The mechanism of action is the same as described previously; that is, IgE antibodies attach to cells throughout the body, particularly mast cells and basophils. Subsequent antigen-antibody reactions result in cellular rupture and the release of the mediator substances (histamine, SRS-A, etc.)

**Urticaria** The cutaneous reaction in atopic individuals is referred to as *urticaria* or *atopic dermatitis*. It may be manifest by the wheal and flare response, hives, vesicles, or blisters, as illustrated in Color Plates(s) 8-8, 8-9, and 8-10.

**P**athophysiology Urticaria results from antigen entering specific skin areas. Normally innocuous antigens produce localized anaphylactoid reactions in atopic persons. Histamine is released at the site causing vasodilatation and an immediate red flare; increased permeability of the capillaries then leads to wheal formation, occurring within a few minutes and lasting for minutes or hours. These transient wheals or "hives" vary in size from a few millimeters to huge coalescent lesions the size of a large plate. Histamine is also responsible for the pruritis and/or numbness that begins in the localized area. Subsequent wheals may occur elsewhere, particularly on points of pressure from clothing, belts, shoulder straps, or girdles. If urticaria is present on lips, mucous membranes, the periorbital area, or eyelids, there may be diffuse swelling around the affected region. Lesions of the lips, tongue, or buccal mucosa may be associated with laryngeal edema and airway obstruction. Gastrointestinal mucosa may be involved with associated cramps, nausea, and vomiting.

Common causes of urticaria include drugs (penicillin, aspirin, and codeine), foods (strawberries, shellfish, tomatoes, chocolate, and cheese), insect bites and stings, inhaled allergens, and intestinal parasites. Physical agents such as cold, sun, external heat, or heat due to cutaneous flushing and exercise may also cause urticaria. Diseases such as lupus erythematosus, acute rheumatic fever, serum hepatitis, and parasites also elicit a cutaneous reaction. Urticaria may be aggravated by high environmental temperatures and emotional stress. Individual urticaria lesions may disappear in 48 hours leaving no residual skin eruption, although new eruptions may continue to appear for indefinite periods.

*Angioedema* involves a pathophysiologic process that is similar to urticaria; however, it involves deeper skin layers and submucosa. It is frequently localized but may occur at multiple sites and in any area of the skin, upper respiratory tract, or gastrointestinal tract. Cutaneous lesions may burn, sting, itch, or cause no discomfort. Gastrointestinal involvement may be associated with dysphagia and colicky retrosternal pain. Angioedema of the larynx leads to hoarseness, stridor, and dyspnea; death due to asphyxiation is uncommon.

Both urticaria and angioedema are associated with dilatation and engorgement of the venules and capillaries. The role of antibody in urticaria and angioedema is demonstrated by a test involving passive transfer of the wheal and flare response from an affected individual to a normal recipient— *the Prausnitz-Küstner reaction.*

In this test, serum from an affected patient is placed in the skin of a normal recipient and after an appropriate interval the recipient is challenged (reinjected) at that site with the offending antigen.

Results show that the incidence of positive direct skin reaction, or passive transfer, is appreciable in circumstances where the affected patient's history clearly suggests an anaphylactic event. The responsible immunoglobulin is presumably an antibody of the IgE class.

**Allergic rhinitis**  IgE-mediated rhinitis (hay fever) is an antigen-induced, antibody-mediated, hypersensitivity reaction which occurs in the nose. The term *perennial allergic rhinitis* is used for continuous nasal disease, and *seasonal allergic rhinitis* for transient symptoms caused by exposure to seasonal aeroallergens.

The etiology of perennial allergic rhinitis may be difficult to discover. Seasonal occurrence of allergic rhinitis coincides with pollination of weeds, grasses, and trees. Allergic rhinitis due to local contamination of the patient's environment is diagnosed by carefully correlating the patient's symptoms with exposure to potential allergens at home, work, and play.

**P**athophysiology  The antigens (allergens) important in allergic rhinitis are airborne substances to which the atopic patient becomes sensitized. These aeroallergens are generally protein substances, such as the major allergen of ragweed pollen, which has been obtained in relatively pure form. Most other individual antigens important in allergic rhinitis have not yet been characterized, and some aeroallergens, such as mold spores, are recognized by correlation of their concentration in the air with the patient's symptoms and skin reactivity.

Pollens which cause allergic rhinitis are airborne in relatively high concentration and are produced by plants that disseminate their pollen by means of wind currents. The major types of pollen aeroallergens in the United States come from trees, grasses, and ragweed plants. The concentrations of pollen from these sources vary with the geographical area, and this is important both in the production of the patient's symptoms and in the establishment of the cause of the rhinitis. See Table 10-2.

Mold spores and house dust antigen are two other offending allergens of allergic rhinitis. Mold spores are derived from saprophytic fungi and are present in the air in significant concentration when suitable culture media, such as decaying vegetation in the fall and spring, combine with sufficient rainfall to provide adequate moisture. Barns, because of mold growing in hay or straw, and damp basements are places of high mold concentration.

House dust antigen composes a major source of general environmental allergen. It is derived from household environments and is not outdoor dust, such as road dust. House dust mites are thought to be a major antigenic component of house dust. Symptoms from house dust are generally perennial since the antigen is obviously present in a patient's environment throughout the year.

Animal dander can be a significant cause of allergic rhinitis. Animal antigens are derived from the epithelial surface or saliva of animals. Many household pets can be a source of animal dander which causes allergy.

Exposure to nonimmunologic stimuli may be followed by an increase in nasal symptoms. These nonimmunologic stimuli include tobacco smoke, perfumes, newspaper print, and alcohol; their presence in the patient's environment enhances the nasal response in IgE- or non-IgE-mediated rhinitis.[2]

IgE-mediated rhinitis results from the reaction of antigen with IgE antibody fixed to the surface of mast cells in nasal tissue and the resultant release of vasoactive mediators.[3] When pollen and mold spores land on nasal mucosa, their carbohydrate coat is digested by the lysozyme of respiratory mucus, releasing the cellular contents. The process of sensitization is poorly understood but leads to production of IgE or "reaginic" antibodies in lymphoid tissues lining the respiratory tract. When an allergen diffuses across the mucous membrane and makes contact with specific IgE antibody fixed to the surface of these cells, they are activated to secrete histamine and probably other mediators, such as SRS-A, into the surrounding tissues. This process probably accounts for the major manifestations of respiratory allergies. The sensitivity in hay fever is not confined to the mucous membranes but is general and exemplified by the ability of the entire skin to react.

The nature of the defect responsible for allergic rhinitis is unknown, but it is probably hereditary. The nasal mucosa of patients with allergic rhinitis also appears to be more susceptible to irritants than normal nasal mucosa. Studies indicate that persons with allergic rhinitis are also more susceptible than normal persons to infection by respiratory viruses.

Symptoms of allergic rhinitis include pruritis around the eyes, nose, throat, and mouth, especially the soft palate, nasal discharge, sneezing, lacrimation, and mucosal swelling with occlusion of the airway, making breathing and sleeping difficult. Patients may be listless, irritable, or depressed because of these symptoms. The severity of symptoms varies from day to day. Nasal mucosa pallor and edema are usually found. Nasal secretions are thin, clear, and sticky.

Swelling of turbinates and mucous membranes may result in obstruction of sinus ostia or the eustachian tube, thus occluding the nasal passages; infection of sinuses and the middle ear may be a problem. Infection of the sinuses or nose, in patients with allergic rhinitis, results in formation of nasal polyps. These polyps further obstruct nasal passages, increase symptoms, and exaggerate infection. The conjunctiva and the skin about the eyes, nose, and occasionally the mouth are reddened.

**Asthma** Asthma is classified as an allergic disease despite the fact that it is not always caused by hypersensitivity to an allergen. Hypersensitivity is found to be a predominant cause in only one-third of cases and a contributing factor in another third. Allergic rhinitis and urticaria sometimes precede development of asthma or may occur at the same time. The same inhaled pollens, molds, dusts, and danders are associated with both asthma and allergic rhinitis.

Asthma has been divided into extrinsic and intrinsic forms. *Extrinsic asthma* occurs when the allergy is due to substances originating extrinsic to the body. Patients with extrinsic asthma are atopic and typically have a past history of infantile eczema, allergic rhinitis, or gastrointestinal food intolerance. Symptoms usually start in childhood. There are immediate skin responses to extracts of several of the common allergens, and the results correspond to provoking factors described in the history. Occasionally extrinsic asthma occurs in association with a low atopic status where there was no disease in childhood. Asthma may be completely stopped in the latter group of patients when exposure to the offending allergen is stopped. *Intrinsic asthma* is not usually preceded by a history of atopy. Symptoms usually begin in adult life. Perennial nonallergic rhinitis and nasal polyps may be present. There is no relationship between wheezing and exposure to common allergens. This type of asthma often begins with an illness suggesting infection, and there may be apparent respiratory infection from time to time, but this is not the cause of the persisting symptoms.[4]

**P**athophysiology The onset of asthma frequently occurs at the height of severe seasonal allergic rhinitis or with viral infection. It may accompany pneumonitis, the inhalation of a gaseous irritant, or as an isolated event.

*Precipitating factors Exercise-induced* asthma usually follows exercise which is vigorous, steady, and prolonged for 5 to 10 minutes. Bronchoconstriction develops after the exercise stops.

Asthma attacks often follow *emotionally charged encounters* or stressful situations. In some patients these emotionally charged encounters seem to be the main reason for the episodes.

*Respiratory infections* are among the most common events provoking episodes of asthma, especially the more severe ones requiring hospitalization. Recent studies indicate that the infections which provoke asthma are due primarily to respiratory viruses. In adults, rhinoviruses and influenza viruses predominate.

*Viral infections* seem to usher in the asthmatic state. The first attack follows a respiratory infection closely. After the infection is over, chronic asthma may continue with episodes of increased bronchoconstriction occurring subsequent to infection by other viruses.

*Aspirin* and *aspirin-like drugs* may stimulate acute attacks of asthma in some patients, especially those in which inhalant allergy is not a prominent factor. Cold air, industrial dusts, irritant chemicals, perfumes, cosmetic sprays of various kinds, household deodorizing sprays, tobacco

**TABLE 10-2**
SELECTED AEROALLERGENS USED IN SKIN TESTS

1 Fescue: A winter grass which is sown in September and pollinates in June and July.

2 Southern Grass: Seven varieties: June, redtop, orchard, timothy, sweet varnel, Bermuda, and Johnson: in variance they pollenate from April to September (or grass specific to area in which patient lives).

3 Eastern trees: Nine varieties: maple, oak, beech, sycamore, elm, ash, willow, cottonwood, and walnut, pollenating from February to May (or trees specific to area in which patient lives).

4 A. P. dust: House dust.

5 Endo dust: Mattress dust.

6 Feathers: Contains duck, geese, and chicken.

7 Epidermals: Animal hair from cats, cattle, dogs, sheep, rabbit, horses, and goats.

8 Sorrell dock: A weed pollenating from May to June.

9 Smut: A mold found in the grass during the winter months.

10 Tobacco and tobacco smoke.

11 Pyrethrum: Found in hairspray and perfume.

12 Kapok: A stuffing material used in throw pillows and some furniture.

13 Karaya gum: A substance found in adhesives, dietic foods, and jelly beans.

14 Orris root: Found in cosmetics unless they are stated to be allergy free.

15 Newspaper.

16 English plantin: A weed pollenating from April through the summer.

17 Weed mix: Contains four weeds: pigweed, lamb quarters, yellow dock, and cockleburr.

18 Ragweed: A weed pollenating from August to October.

19 Several molds.

20 Mites.

smoke, cooking odors, paints, and petroleum solvents are only some of the irritants which provoke asthma. People with asthma are hyperirritable to these substances and respond to concentrations of irritants too low to affect normal persons. The stimulation of sensory nerve endings by these irritants in or beneath the bronchial epithelium causes reflex bronchoconstriction.

*Effects* When allergy to inhaled antigens is a cause of asthma, the mechanisms are probably the same as the mechanism described previously for IgE-mediated rhinitis. The allergic pathophysiology in asthma affects the mucosa of the lower respiratory tracts.

Paroxysms of *expiratory* dyspnea and wheezing, overinflation of the lungs, cough, and rhonchi are typical asthmatic symptoms. Early in the disease, wheezing and dyspnea occur in discrete attacks, separated by variable periods without subjective symptoms. With chronicity or recurrent bronchial infection, wheezing may become constant.

Other symptoms include tightness in the chest, dyspnea, audible wheezing, and a cough which may produce thick, mucoid sputum. As the asthma attack abates, the cough becomes more effective in bringing up sputum, thus relieving the symptoms. The sputum tends to be clear, scanty, and gelatinous, but it can be copious and frothy at times.

When asthma is chronic, the sputum following an attack may contain mucus plugs. Costal margin and intercostal aching may be present following a paroxysm, and a sense of warmth or irritation may be experienced substernally or at the suprasternal notch. During an attack of asthma the patient uses the accessory muscles of respiration, and the chest is held in a position of inspiration. Dyspnea is usually increased when the patient is in a recumbent position.

It is postulated that the basic defect in asthma may be found in one of the intricate chains of biochemical reactions, at the cell membrane, that are involved in the reciprocal control of the response of the cell. The cell membrane defect may involve many cells, including mast cells, sensory and motor neurons of the vagal reflex arc, and cells of smooth bronchial muscle and the mucus glands. In this view, the asthmatic attack results from a feedback amplification of the signal from the bronchial irritant receptor.[5]

**Allergic reactions to drugs** Allergic reactions to drugs or drug hypersensitivities are difficult to document since the symptom that the patient develops may be due not to the drug being taken, but to an unusual manifestation of a disease. When a drug hypersensitivity reaction is suspected, it is useful for the nurse to consider the following classification of terms:

**O**verdosage Symptoms are related to side effects that occur as a result of excessive intake or failure to metabolize or excrete a drug.

**I**ntolerance Symptoms are those of overdosage but occur in the presence of normal blood and tissue levels of the drug.

**I**diosyncrasy Symptoms are different from those of overdosage; a deviation from the usual response to a drug.

**S**ide Effects Pharmacological reactions to a drug which are undesirable, generally infrequent, and often unavoidable.

**S**econdary Effects Indirect but not inevitable consequences of the primary action of a drug.

**H**ypersensitivity Reactions to a drug which are unlike the normal action of a drug; involves an immunological mechanism.

Reactions to a drug not explained by the properties of the drug, but by the response of the patient to the drug, are termed *allergic*. An allergic reaction to a drug is associated with symptoms commonly seen in hypersensitivity states.

**P**athophysiology The drug causing a reaction acts as a *hapten* by combining with a protein within the body, thus stimulating the immune response. Drugs are among typical haptens initiating antigen-antibody reactions. A drug in such a combination either combines with an antibody or reacts with the cells of the sensitized person. The better the combination of the drug with the protein, the more severe may be the allergic reaction. In some instances it is thought that breakdown products of a specific drug may be the cause of a drug allergy. Selected manifestations of drug allergy and common drug allergens may be found listed in Table 10-3.

The immunologic basis of drug sensitivity may be deduced from the *cardinal features* of an allergic reaction. These features include sensitization by previous exposure, relatively marked specificity to a particular drug or drugs, and manifestations known to differ from the pharmacologic actions or toxic effects of the drug.

The route of administration influences the sensitization of a person to a drug. Drugs often sensitize when in contact with skin and mucous membranes. The oral route of administration induces the least sensitization, the parenteral route, the greatest sensitization.

Once allergy develops, very small amounts of a drug may initiate a drug reaction in extremely sensitive people. Allergic reactions to drugs appear to be less frequent in children than in adults, although severe allergic reactions to drugs may be observed even in very small infants. Aged people seem less prone to sensitization.

A patient who has experienced allergic symptoms in response to one drug may develop similar symptoms to another related drug. This cross-sensitization phenomenon may lead to a severe drug reaction if the relatedness of the drugs is not recognized. Cross-sensitizations occur between all the penicillins, between penicillin and cephalosporin derivations, between the phenothiazines, between neomycin and streptomycin, and between others.[6]

### First-Level Nursing Care

Persons with the potential for systemic anaphylaxis may be unaware of any sensitivity to drugs, serum, or stinging insect venom. Previous exposures to these allergens may have caused minimal symptoms such as local swelling to the insect bite or itching after penicillin therapy.

More than 20 percent of people in the United States are likely to experience an episode of urticaria and/or angioedema during their lives. Chronic urticaria, which occurs frequently or persistently for an extended time period, is more common in adults, especially women, than in children; the highest incidence occurs in people from 21 to 31 years of age. Urticaria and angioedema have been associated with allergic and nonallergic patients and have been produced as a result of transfusions and drug administration.

Allergic rhinitis, atopic dermatitis, and asthma are considered to be hereditary. When both parents have atopic disease, the allergy in their offspring is likely to be unusually severe. Children with a known tendency to atopic disease or with a family history should be protected from potential antigens to lessen the chance of sensitization. The introduction of potential allergens should be under medical supervision, since during infancy children may become sensitized to cow's milk, eggs, chocolate,

wheat, oranges, and fish and liver oils. The nurse in a well-baby clinic should counsel parents about these potential allergens.

Because of the hereditary nature of anaphylactic reactions, a pertinent family history is important for persons seeking medical attention for any reason. Detailed health histories prior to treatment for *any* disorder or eruption may uncover allergic or atopic problems, of which the patient may be unaware.

Careful questioning of the patient by the nurse concerning drug allergies is essential in preventing anaphylactic reactions. A few minutes spent in discussion of past drug therapy and possible side effects is most important in preventing further difficulty.

The nurse who administers serums or vaccines prepared from antigenically different animals, such as horse serum, should make sure a skin test is ordered and administered to the patient before giving the injection. Also, test doses of diagnostic dye media should always be given prior to radiographic procedures.

**TABLE 10-3**
MANIFESTATIONS OF DRUG ALLERGY
AND COMMON DRUG ALLERGENS

CUTANEOUS REACTIONS
Pruritis: common feature of many drug reactions
Urticaria: penicillin, aspirin
Exanthems: penicillins, barbiturates, phenazone, sulfonamides
Exfoliative dermatitis: heavy metals, barbiturates, sulfonamides
Bullae: iodides and bromides
Erythema multiforme: sulfonamides, barbiturates, phenazone
Lichenoid eruptions: gold salts, thiazides, mepracine, cloroquine
Fixed eruptions: phenolphthalein, phenazone, barbiturates, sulfonamides
Contact dermatitis: neomycin, streptomycin, penicillin, and others

PHOTOALLERGIC REACTIONS
Increasing abnormal sensitivity to light with eczematous, urticarial, papular, bullous, lichenoid skin reactions

SYSTEM REACTIONS
Fever: accompanies many drug reactions
Resembling anaphylactic shock: penicillin, local anesthetics serums, pollen
Bronchial asthma: aspirin, indomethacin, paracetomol, dextropropoxyphene, pentazocine
Serum sickness: penicillin
Vasculitis
Syndrome resembling lupus erythematosus: procainamide, isonicotinic acid, hydrazine, troxidone, promidone
Liver damage: certain testosterones, certain oral contraceptives, phenothiazines, chlorpropamide, phenylbutazone, hydrazine monoamine oxidase inhibitors, halothane, sulfonamides, methyldopa, diphenylhydantoin, para-aminosalicylic acid
Nephropathy: sulfonamides, bacitracin, capreomycin, amphotericin, troxidone, colistin methanesulfonate esciphonate, phenindione, penicillins, mercury compounds, gold salts, phenacetin
Blood dyscrasias: quinidine, chlorothiazide, quinine, antazoline, penicillin, phenacetin, para-aminosalicylic acid, sulfonamides, antithyroid drugs, hydantoins, gold salts, phenylbutazone, chlorpropamide

Since adverse reactions to drugs continue to increase as more therapeutic agents are prescribed, it is crucial that the nurse be involved in preventive assessment of the patient who takes both prescribed and over-the-counter drugs. Nurses in schools, industry, clinics, hospitals, and physician's offices should take the opportunity to teach patients about drugs. Descriptive leaflets on common drugs that are prescribed or taken without prescription may conserve the nurse's and patient's time. Using the leaflet as a guide, the nurse can assess the patient's knowledge of a drug and review the medication's action, as well as toxic and side effects. Correct route of administration, dosage, frequency of administration, and additional situational variables can be reviewed as necessary. The nurse should further assess the patient's ability to identify and report side and toxic effects. It may be difficult for a patient to call a nurse or a doctor for fear of annoying a busy health care practitioner with what, the patient believes, may be an insignificant problem or symptom. Patients should be encouraged to call and assured that any symptom is important to report.

An "allergic" individual with asthma, urticaria, or allergic rhinitis will more commonly experience an anaphylactic drug reaction. Individuals with inflammatory or necrotizing gastrointestinal lesions are more susceptible to drug reactions when medications are administered orally.

The nurse should encourage patients who have acquired a reaction to one drug to alert physicians and nurses of this reaction since an allergic reaction to one drug is frequently followed by allergic reactions to others. It is important that a patient with known drug allergies carry a list of these allergies in the form of a Medic-Alert bracelet or card in case of accident or hospitalization.

The patient who takes a number of drugs is more likely to experience an adverse drug reaction. This may be due to an additive effect, pharmacologic interactions, or incompatibilities. An increased frequency of drug reactions may occur in patients with renal or liver dysfunction. The nurse should counsel both of these groups of patients on the possibility of adverse drug reactions. The patient should be asked to describe the nature of any reaction, particularly excessive local swelling at injection sites or hives.

Before administering a prescribed drug, the nurse should determine if the patient has taken the medication previously and if there was a reaction. If so, the patient should be asked to describe the response. It is also important to find out about drug-use patterns and other patient allergies. If the patient seems confused or remembers the past allergic response to a drug incorrectly, the physician should be notified to protect the patient from a possibly severe allergic reaction. The patient should be advised that drug reactions usually occur within 7 to 10 days of taking the medication for the first time. If the patient is unaware of previous sensitization, a reaction can take place almost immediately at the time of a second administration of the drug. The nurse should have the patient remain in the clinic or office for 20 to 30 minutes after the injection of any agent, in the event that such an anaphylactic reaction occurs.

## Second-Level Nursing Care

Nursing assessment of patients with allergic conditions is particularly dependent upon an accurate health history and well-developed skills of observation. Interventions vary slightly with the allergic or atopic disease being treated but are based upon certain drugs and antiallergic programs of care.

**Nursing assessment** Nurses in community health clinic and outpatient screening situations may be the first professionals to evaluate the allergic patient. It is extremely important, therefore, that this initial evaluation reflect a highly detailed and accurate health history and physical assessment.

**H**ealth History The nurse should encourage the patient to describe in subjective terms what complaint is most annoying and any symptoms experienced. The persistence and onset of symptoms should be described, as well as the past health, including childhood feeding problems, eczema, and school-age diseases such as frequent colds or sinus problems. A work history will examine the environmental variables on the job, to determine if a relationship can be established between allergic symptoms and working conditions.

The nurse should then elicit data about the course of the allergic problem, including the onset of symptoms, whether symptoms are intermittent or continuous, how often the disease episodes occur, and how long the episodes last. The time when the patient has symptoms, in what place(s) the patient has difficulty, and what environmental variables cause allergic distress should also be noted. Seasonal changes and year-round symptons should be elicited, as well as the specific time of occurrence. Notes should be made of any variation on a weekly basis, since symptoms may decrease on a weekend when the patient is not in the work environment. The nurse can then question the patient about the onset and severity of symptoms during a 24-hour time period. Questions relative to environmental change aside from the work situation should also be asked. Do the allergic symptoms improve in a friend's house? Do they worsen when walking in fields, etc?

Environmental agents which stimulate or worsen allergic symptoms, such as house dust, mattress dust, animals, grasses, medications, and tobacco smoke, should all be explored. It may be necessary to request that the patient keep a diary, recording pertinent data about the allergic symptoms.

The seasonal variations of pollens and fungal spores, potential allergens in the patients' home, school, work, and hobby environments, exposure to animals, house dust, industrial dusts and fumes, and drugs (especially aspirin), as well as the relationship of irritant exposure to observable symptoms, should be investigated. At times the relationship of allergen exposure to symptoms may be difficult to determine, for example, the manifestations of asthma which occur several hours after exposure.

A detailed history should be collected by the nurse of all drugs taken during the previous few months, including dates the drugs were started and stopped. The patient needs to be reminded to recall over-the-counter drugs such as aspirin and laxatives. Foods and cosmetics should be investigated, since these substances may contain drugs. Family members may help to record the fullest, most accurate history.

The nurse may also document the family history of allergic disease on a "family tree" representation. Personal and social variables which may precipitate or aggravate allergy such as the use of cigarettes, liquor, and the association of nervous tension with allergic symptoms should be recorded.

Frequently, it is not possible to obtain this detailed history prior to administering care to an allergic patient. This situation occurs most often when the nurse encounters a patient experiencing *systemic anaphylaxis*. The nurse may see such a patient in any health care setting or in any aspect of daily life. Insect stings, foreign serum, and drugs most frequently initiate such severe reactions.

After an insect sting, drug dose, or foreign serum injection, the patient experiencing systemic anaphylaxis may describe feelings of apprehension and impending doom, feelings of warmth, wheezing, tightness or pain in the chest, lightheadedness,

itching, and shortness of breath. Such symptoms demand immediate, effective medical attention.

**P**hysical Assessment Allergic patients present with a variety of physical symptoms ranging from the hives of urticaria to the severe dyspnea of asthma. The allergic episode may be the patient's first attack or only one of many. It is essential that the nurse be aware of the possible existence of an anaphylactic reaction (type I) when encountering a patient with nasal congestion, clear, watery nasal discharge, sneezing, pruritis, hives, or expiratory dyspnea.

*Asthma* During an asthmatic attack, physical assessment should focus on the patient's oxygenation status. Transient cyanosis may be noted, and the pulse rate is increased. Auscultation of the chest may reveal the presence of rhonchi with *wheezing* being present on both inspiration and expiration. Observable *dyspnea* is most pronounced on *expiration.* Respirations may be quite rapid to the point of *hyperventilation* as the patient tries to overcome the feeling of obstruction. Sputum produced is usually clear and tenacious, although it may appear purulent in the presence of infection.

*Systemic Anaphylaxis* During systemic anaphylaxis, assessment will reveal several changes in oxygenation status. The patient will appear cyanotic with marked pallor. The pulse rate will be increased and the blood pressure decreased. Pulses may be difficult to palpate; capillary refill will be poor. The patient will be dyspneic, and respirations may be shallow and labored. Urticaria may be noted and should be described according to appearance and location. These changes usually are directly related to a preceding event such as a drug injection or insect sting.

**D**iagnostic Tests *Skin tests* with allergenic antigens or allergens are of value in detecting the specific allergen(s) responsible for the patient's symptoms. Exact correlation of the skin reactivity with environmental circumstances helps to identify the responsible allergen.

Skin tests are performed with crude aqueous extracts of pollen, dust, foods, animal dander, insects, and other substances.[7] A representative group of allergens is found in Table 10-2.

No method of standardization is very reliable since the extracts used are crude and the measurement of specific antigen has not been possible except for ragweed and a few grasses. Usually a small number of allergens are used to skin-test one patient. The more diffuse the patient history, the more tests are likely to be utilized.

Allergy extract preparations contain water-soluble antigens known to induce atopic reactions. Selection of the appropriate concentration for intracutaneous or intradermal skin testing is crucial, since the reaction may be misleading and dangerous if the concentration is too high.

The technique of skin testing is to inject an appropriate amount of antigen beneath the stratum corneum and barrier zone of the epidermis. The simplest method is to apply a drop of testing solution to a superficial scratch. This *scratch method* has a low level of sensitivity, because despite the fact that a concentrated solution is used, the method will detect only the stronger and more obvious reactions.[8]

Most allergy nurses will be involved in skin testing using the *intradermal* or *intracutaneous method.* This skin test is as much as 100 times more sensitive than the scratch method, but demands more care in administration if it is to be both reliable and safe for the patient. The nurse injects, under the patient's skin, approximately 0.02 ml of a solution which varies in strength (Figure 10-1). Sterile, disposable allergist syringes are preferable to tuberculin syringes for skin testing. Twenty-six-gauge, ½-inch nondetachable needles are available commercially in 1-cc syringe capacity. These needles have an intradermal bevel. If a larger volume is used, or if air gets into the skin, a nonspecific irritative reaction may be produced.

On the upper, outer arm of the patient the nurse numbers areas corresponding to the allergy extracts to be used (Fig. 10-2). Different dilutions (stronger and weaker concentrations) may be injected side by side and adjacent to each number on the arm. Ten to fifteen minutes later the diameter of the wheal reaction is measured with a millimeter ruler (Fig. 10-3). Reactions of 4 or 5 mm in diameter may be discounted, depending on the dilution used. Wheals from 7 to above 10 mm in diameter may be evaluated with more scrutiny as to the offending allergen, depending on the dilution used. Generally, when a very dilute solution shows a positive reaction, the allergen is more likely to be clinically significant. Both false positive and false negative skin tests may occur. The nurse can utilize the other upper arm for additional skin testing. Testing is best done on the arm so that a tourniquet can be applied at the first sign of an anaphylactic reaction.

Alarming systemic reactions to skin testing were relatively common before the extreme potency of certain antigens was appreciated; now the risk is low. The best way to avoid reactions is to restrict antigens for testing on the basis of the history; a patient who has a severe allergy to egg should not be tested for egg white sensitivity.[9]

Emergency trays should always be present when the nurse is skin-testing a patient. These trays contain an airway, Ambu bag, oxygen, tourniquet, intravenous fluids, and the following medications: Benadryl, sodium bicarbonate, epinephrine, and aminophylline.

Prior to the skin tests the patient should avoid taking medications which may inhibit skin reaction. These medications include antihistamines, especially hydroxyzine, and subcutaneous epinephrine and isoproterenol. Ephedrine, aminophylline, and corticosteroids are not currently thought to inhibit skin test reaction. Negative skin tests may indicate a lack of sensitizing antibodies, a weak antigen preparation, or the presence of medications which block the wheal and flare response.

Another laboratory test is the *serum IgE concentration.* This is normally low, with values of less than 1 $\mu$g/ml. This IgE level may be elevated in extrinsic asthma but remains normal in intrinsic asthma. IgE levels can also be elevated in persons with allergic rhinitis or eczema without asthma, in parasitic infestations, and in liver disease.

*Spirometry* may be used to evaluate the severity of airway obstruction during the various stages of asthma. It is a measure of the patient's vital capacity.

*Allergen inhalation tests* have been used extensively in research and, to some extent, in diagnosis. An aerosol of the allergen extract is used, delivered by a face mask, and inhaled through the mouth. One test extract is used each day, with solutions progressing from weaker to stronger. Laboratory studies, respiratory evaluation, and a history and physical examination of the patient are done prior to allergen inhalation tests.

A variety of deviations in blood studies occur when patients experience allergic reactions to drugs. These blood studies may reveal either nonspecific or specific abnormalities due to the pharmacologic actions of the drugs. Agranulocytosis, eosinophilia, lymphocytosis, and hemolytic anemia are some of the blood abnormalities. The nurse in the clinic or doctor's office should explain to the patient the necessity of drawing blood samples.

**Nursing problems and interventions** Major nursing problems for anaphylactic patients include the *allergic response* itself and the systemic ana-phylactic problems of *inadequate ventilation, vascular collapse,* and *anxiety.* Special problems of the *asthmatic patient* will be discussed separately.

**T**he Allergic Response   In an immunization clinic, outpatient facility, or emergency room, nurses must always be prepared for the possibility of a systemic anaphylactic reaction and have appropriate supplies on hand to counteract this response. Patients may not recall previous, slight drug reactions or may be unaware of sensitivities they possess. *Epinephrine* is the drug of choice in these situations and should be administered subcutaneously or intravenously, according to the physician's standing orders (usually 0.5 ml 1:1000 strength, every 5 to 10 minutes until symptoms subside).

Should the person be in a nonmedical environent when the reaction occurs, care would be supportive until the person can receive medical attention. If the allergy is to a stinging insect, the stinger should be scraped away cautiously with a fingernail, knife blade, or other available, sharp instrument. If the insect sting is located on an extremity, a tourniquet (belt, scarf, etc.) should be placed between the origin of the extremity and the sting. This proper application of the tourniquet slows the release of venom into the general circulation. If an intravenous medication is being administered, the nurse should stop it. A tourniquet may be applied above the IV injection site to slow absorption of the offending drug. A physician should be notified of the possible drug reaction. For stabilized, predictable allergic conditions that do not take the dramatic form of systemic anaphylaxis, *environmental control, hyposensitization,* and *medications* are the major therapeutic interventions.

*Environmental control*   The avoidance of offending allergens is the goal of environmental control. Avoidance of aeroallergens is difficult since these allergens are widely distributed. Measures to eradicate sources of allergenic pollen are unfeasible and ineffective. The dose of inhaled allergens can be reduced by sleeping with bedroom windows closed, air conditioning, riding in cars with closed windows, and avoiding trips to rural areas during known pollen seasons.

Some patients are able to escape offending pollen and spores by traveling to areas where these allergens are absent. These trips are expensive and inconvenient, and control of the patient's symptoms in the local community is more desirable.

A patient with severe IgE-mediated rhinitis due

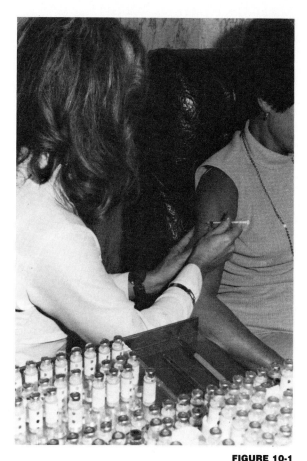

**FIGURE 10-1**
Allergy nurse injecting common aeroallergens into patient's upper arm. The wheal responses of the skin will be measured in 10 to 15 minutes.

to a single allergen such as cat dander will become asymptomatic if the cat is eliminated and the cat dander is removed by cleaning. Control of house dust concentration can be accomplished by encasing pillows and mattresses with plastic or airtight coverings, eliminating rugs and dust-collecting items in bedrooms, cleaning furnace filters, and maintaining adequate humidity. Air conditioning may improve symptoms by creating a constant flow of air and a cool environment, or aggravate them by circulating house dust and any mites or danders.

*Hyposensitization* Hyposensitization or *desensitization* is a process used in the treatment of atopic patients, particularly those suffering from pollen-induced allergic rhinitis (hay fever) or asthma. Progressively *increasing* concentrations of the offending allergen are given to the patient subcutaneously. The desired effect of these injections is an

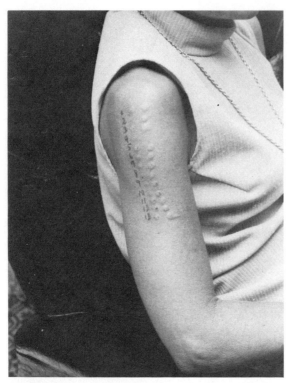

**FIGURE 10-2**
Intradermal or intracutaneous allergy test used to determine allergens to which a patient is sensitive. Note the wheals raised on the upper arm adjacent to numbers written in magic marker which correspond to allergens recorded on the patient's chart.

increase in plasma concentrations of IgG (*blocking*) antibody. IgG acts to prevent or reduce the contact of the allergen with IgE antibodies.

A program of elective desensitization is usually initiated 3 months prior to the specific allergen's season. Desensitization is usually prescribed for pollen, fungus, and dust allergies which can not be environmentally controlled.

The physician establishes a set of serial dilutions of the offending allergen. (If an "allergy nurse" mixes the extracts in preparation for hyposensitization treatment, following careful mixing protocols is important to ensure the greatest safety and effectiveness for the patient.) *Lower* dilutions begin the series of hyposensitization treatments. The patient is started on weekly or biweekly subcutaneous injections. The allergen dosage is gradually increased, as is the interval between injections. Accurate records must be kept. Generally, 20 to 25, but as many as 50 injections may be required to reach a maximum allergen dose. A maintenance dosage is then determined and may be continued, depending upon the time of year. Variations in therapy and reduction of dosage depend on the seasonal and perennial nature of the allergy and on patient symptoms.

Correct identification of the patient, the recorded history, and the extract are essential to avoid dangerous mistakes. The label of the allergenic extract should be read three times, before, during, and after filling the syringe. The hyposensitization injections are given subcutaneously; sites are rotated to avoid local hypersensitivity. It is essential to aspirate the needle to ensure that a blood vessel is avoided. Alcohol preparation of the skin is performed before the injection; after the injection an alcohol sponge is held in place to minimize seepage of allergen into small blood vessels.

The patient should wait in the clinic or office for at least 20 minutes after receiving treatment in the event an anaphylactic reaction occurs. The nurse should advise the patient to avoid strenuous exercise for an hour or more after receiving treatment to prevent a rapid rate of allergen absorption.

Local reactions, such as redness and swelling, appear commonly at the site of allergen injections. If these reactions are severe, the physician should evaluate the subsequent dose which the patient receives. Constitutional symptoms include increased nasal discharge, nasal stuffiness, pruritis of the nose and eyes, sneezing, wheezing, and conjunctival redness.[10] Systemic anaphylaxis may also occur, and emergency protocols should be followed by the nurse. In this event, a tracheostomy set must be available, and the physician summoned immediately. A syringe containing epinephrine should be nearby.

Throughout the course of hyposensitization therapy, the patient should be questioned by the nurse about exacerbation or improvement in symptoms. This should be documented in the patient's chart. Reevaluation of therapy by the physician may be necessary.

*Drug therapy* Concurrently during the course of hyposensitization therapy, the patient may develop symptoms of allergic rhinitis or urticaria. Symptomatic treatment involves the use of *antihistamines,* which control the sneezing and rhinorrhea of the allergic response and also may minimize the allergic conjunctivitis. They are thought to act as competitive inhibitors for histamines at receptor sites on reactive cells. The exact method of action is uncertain, and the antihistamines do not block all cellular activities of histamine. The nurse in the clinic or physician's office should advise the patient with seasonal allergies to take antihistamines during the pollen season. The patient with perennial rhinitis should take them continuously in order for them to act most effectively; prevention of symptoms occurs because the medications are taken prior to the release of histamine, thereby preventing its attachment to the cell receptor sites.

The nurse should also teach the patient about the side effects of these drugs which include both an excitatory effect and a depressing effect on the central nervous system. Dizziness, drowziness, dryness of the mouth and throat, disturbed coordination, and at times nausea and vomiting occur.

The sympathomimetic drugs (epinephrine, ephedrine, isoproterenol) with primarily alpha-receptor activity are effective vasoconstrictors of blood vessels of the mucosal surface. They have been used as topical agents in the nose for reduction of rhinitis from allergic and other causes.

*Topical corticosteroids,* such as dexamethasone nasal spray, are used transiently to control symptoms until the patient's nasal mucosa returns to a normal state; overuse should be discouraged. Oral adrenal corticosteroids have a dramatic effect in the control of IgE-mediated rhinitis. The exact mechanism for this therapeutic action is unknown. However, the long-term use of this therapy is not safe owing to the side effects and complications of corticosteroids. Oral corticosteroids may be used for 1 to 2 weeks during an increase in severity of symptoms at the height of the pollen season.

**Inadequate Ventilation**  Dyspnea, rapidly progressing to severe respiratory distress, is a most serious effect of systemic anaphylaxis. The administration of epinephrine should result in bronchiolar dilation and relief of this problem. Meanwhile, the nurse should support respiration by maintaining a patent airway, administering oxygen where possible, and resuscitation, when necessary. Occasionally, an emergency tracheostomy may be required to save the person's life. Most important of all interventions, after initial lifesaving care, is transport of the patient to a facility equipped to provide medical attention.

**Vascular Collapse**  The increased capillary permeability that occurs in systemic anaphylaxis can facilitate the loss of large amounts of fluid from the intravascular compartment. The eventual result of this loss is hypotension, shock, and circulatory collapse. Patients exhibit symptoms of hypovolemic shock and require appropriate intervention. Intravenous fluids (frequently 5% dextrose and water) should be started, if the patient is in a situation

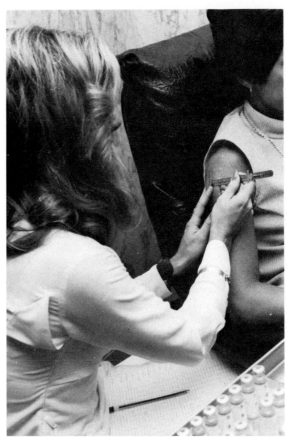

**FIGURE 10-3**
Allergy nurse measuring the diameter of the wheal 10 to 15 minutes after the intracutaneous injection of possible offending allergens. She is using a millimeter ruler.

where they are available. Otherwise, vital signs should be taken and close observations made, until the patient reaches a medical facility. (Refer to Chap. 28 for a complete discussion of shock.)

**Anxiety**  The inability to breathe, as well as generalized feelings of fear and disaster, cause great apprehension in the patient experiencing systemic anaphylaxis. Some feelings of anxiety may be relieved if the nurse approaches the situation in a calm, knowledgeable manner. Frequently, acting quickly while speaking quietly and calmly will provide the greatest comfort to an anxious patient.

The patient should be seen by a physician, even if emergency care is promptly effective. Hospitalization may be necessary to identify the causative agent(s). Teaching will be necessary, for the patient and the family, to prevent a recurrence. Patients should know of their own allergies and wear or carry identification to alert others.

Anxiety is also present in patients with allergic rhinitis and urticaria. These highly uncomfortable and chronically recurring diseases are not trivial to the suffering patient. Emotional support of the patient during the more symptomatic stages of allergic rhinitis is directed toward pointing out that the symptoms may become less acute with the change of season, better environmental controls, antihistamines, additional skin testing to identify altered sensitivities to offending allergens, and a modified program of hyposensitization.

The patient with urticaria should be advised to avoid causative drugs, foods, environmental conditions, and other agents. In the case of urticaria associated with other diseases, avoidance is impossible. Symptomatic treatment with cool temperatures and antihistamines may help the patient find comfort. Sedatives and tranquilizers may help the patient who is experiencing itching and the fear that the urticaria and angioedema are more serious than they actually are. Listening to the fears of the patient and reassuring the patient about the cause of the urticaria, if known at the time, may bring relief from stress.

**A**sthma  Approximately 4 percent of the United States' population is suffering from asthma, and 7 percent have had it at some time. In the adult, continuous respiratory symptoms sometimes suggest chronic bronchitis or emphysema, and the possibility of asthma may not be considered at first.

The differentiation of chronic bronchitis and emphysema from bronchial asthma generally presents a difficult problem. Patients with atopic asthma frequently have a personal or family history of allergic disease, or an onset of symptoms in infancy or childhood. Dyspnea which occurs between attacks of wheezing is suggestive of emphysema or chronic bronchitis.

After diagnosis, the patient may receive symptomatic treatment to control or prevent asthmatic attacks. The selection of the pharmacologic agent depends on the duration, severity, and precipitating factors causing the asthma. The drugs most commonly used in acute or chronic asthma are the sympathomimetic agents *epinephrine, ephedrine,* and *isoproterenol;* all are bronchodilators. The bronchodilators relax the smooth muscle of the bronchi through direct stimulating action on the beta-adrenergic receptors of the autonomic nervous system, thus relieving bronchoconstriction. The patient should be counseled by the nurse to avoid overuse of these aerosols. Overuse is associated with loss of effectiveness and a rebound effect of increased bronchospasm that follows the initial bronchial dilatation. In addition, the nurse should be aware that overuse of these agents has been linked to myocardial necrosis and an increase in deaths due to asthma.

Methylxanthines are effective bronchodilators and may be used either alone or when an additive effect is desired. Aminophylline is commonly used and may be administered orally, intravenously, or rectally. Expectorants may be used to increase the volume of bronchial secretions; these include glyceryl guaiacolate, ammonium chloride, potassium chloride, and water.

The patient also may receive adrenal corticosteroids; the chief action of these steroids in asthma is thought to be suppression of inflammation and stabilization of the cell membranes and lysosomes. The nurse should instruct the patient to maintain the dose of the steroid without abruptly stopping the drug. The patient must also be warned that the side effects of steroid therapy may occur.

Antibiotics may be used in the treatment of concurrent or preexisting bacterial infections of the respiratory tract. Infections can induce or complicate the asthmatic attack.

The patient should be counseled to take the medications as prescribed, report any untoward side effects to the physician, correctly and safely use the nebulizer, drink sufficient fluid to liquefy respiratory secretions (at least 3000 ml in 24 hours), administer epinephrine subcutaneously if wheezing is not relieved by the nebulizer, go to the emergency room if wheezing persists, avoid the offending allergen(s) in the environment, and notify the physician if symptoms of respiratory infection are present. This knowledge and these skills should be taught by the nurse according to the patient's individual needs. Because the amount of medical and nursing information may be quite overwhelming to the patient, the nurse must assess the patient's ability to learn this treatment regimen and must reinforce areas when necessary.

Asthma restricts the activity of the patient and disrupts family and social life. The cost and stress of emergency room visits and hospitalization can be financially and emotionally draining to the patient and the family. Nurses should be cognizant of these factors and refer patients to appropriate social service agencies for help.

### Third-Level Nursing Care

The patient experiencing systemic anaphylaxis in the hospital setting exhibits the same symptoms and receives the same initial intervention as the patient in a clinic setting. Should the symptoms not be relieved with epinephrine, additional measures are necessary.

Patients may also be hospitalized with severe allergic rhinitis, urticaria, or asthma. Care for allergic rhinitis and urticaria is basically the same as that described for level two. Asthma, however, involves more complex and intensive care.

**Nursing assessment** The nurse in the hospital setting should elicit exact information about allergies and record it on nursing history forms. The name of allergens and the symptoms manifest must be noted in several places, including the front of the patient's chart, the medication and nursing-care plan Kardexes, and on the patient's bed. As soon as the patient is able, a detailed health history, as outlined in Second-Level Nursing Care, should be obtained.

Physical assessment of a patient experiencing an unrelieved episode of systemic anaphylaxis usually reveals the following effects: asthmatic wheezing, cyanosis, severe pruritis, urticaria of the face and upper chest, apprehension, tightness or pain in the chest, cough, and circulatory failure as indicated by pallor, lightheadedness, imperceptible pulse, and dropping blood pressure. The patient's state of hydration, cardiac status, and respiratory embarrassment are assessed initially and carefully monitored thereafter.

If these effects are not quickly treated, death will follow rapidly. Intervention is directed toward relief of *bronchospasm* and subsequent management of respiratory distress as well as removal of the cause of the allergic response.

If an attack of *asthma* is severe, breath sounds and wheezing may become very faint owing to the bronchial plugging that is interfering with alveolar ventilation. Should the attack be prolonged and unresponsive to therapy, it is referred to as *status asthmaticus.* The patient appears greatly fatigued from the labor of breathing and often finds the most comfortable position to be sitting upright or leaning slightly forward. Talking and eating are very difficult for the patient because of the energy required and their interference with breathing. Skin turgor and mucous membranes should be checked frequently for early signs of dehydration.

The effort of respiration causes the patient to use accessory muscles to aid each breath. This may be observed in the supraclavicular, intercostal, and subcostal areas of the chest. Should status asthmaticus remain unresponsive, breath sounds may become absent (*silent chest*) and cardiac arrest ensue.

**Diagnostic Tests** Routine blood and urine studies are made, and samples are collected to test serum electrolytes, blood gases, and arterial pH. The $p_{CO_2}$ is elevated, the $p_{O_2}$ decreased, and the plasma bicarbonate decreased, indicating acidosis. The patient needs continuous contact with a nurse at this time not only for support through the studies, but especially to allay the fear of being alone and suffocating.

Pulmonary scans may be done to evaluate pulmonary blood flow. Chest x-rays may reveal unexpanded lung portions and areas with poor ventilation.

Following the crisis period, allergy testing will need to be done in the hospital setting, if the causative agent is unknown. Appropriate care must be taken during the testing to prevent a severe anaphylactic response.

**Nursing problems and interventions** Major nursing problems for acutely ill allergic patients are the severe *bronchospasm* and potential *vascular collapse* of systemic anaphylaxis, and *status asthmaticus.*

*Bronchospasm* may be treated with intravenous aminophylline or hydrocortisone in addition to epinephrine. Respiration can be aided with the administration of oxygen, insertion of an airway, and intermittent positive pressure breathing. Constant monitoring of vital signs is necessary. On the basis of these findings and central venous pressure readings, additional fluids and/or plasma expanders may be ordered for the patient. Albumin may be prescribed to pull fluid back into the vascular compartment and prevent *vascular collapse.*

**Status Asthmaticus** If asthma progresses so that the patient is critically ill, hospitalization is essential. Usually the patient receives epinephrine for treatment of the acute attack. Failure to respond to this therapy may cause the patient to progress to *status asthmaticus.*

Common causes of status asthmaticus include respiratory infection, discontinuation of therapy (especially corticosteroids), misuse of nebulized sympathomimetic drugs, and massive exposure to allergen(s).

Several principles of treatment aim to bring the patient out of this life-threatening situation and alter the cycle of factors which maintain the asthma. *Rest* is essential, since the patient in status asthmaticus is fatigued. The effort of breathing is great. The nurse and physician should reassure the patient by their presence and competence. Sedation is administered cautiously to foster rest. It is essential that the patient cough up any secretions in order to avoid mucous plugs in small-diameter airways.

The *fluid needs* of the patient are great, since fluid loss occurs through diaphoresis and exhaled water vapor. Intravenous hydration is often initiated in the emergency room. Small sips of fluids may increase the patient's comfort; they may not be advisable in the severely dyspneic patient. Oral fluids should be warm or at room temperature since cold fluids may cause a reflex bronchospasm, thus increasing the severity of the attack. The diet should be liquid or semisolid, with feedings small and spaced, so that a large quantity of food does not increase the patient's dyspnea. Supplemental electrolytes are added as necessary to intravenous fluids.

The mucus may become thick and gluelike during an asthmatic attack, making it difficult for the patient to expectorate the sputum. The subsequent formation of mucous plugs may cause distal atelectasis and pneumonitis. *Iodides* appear to exert an expectorant effect. Potassium iodides and syrup of hydriodic acid are the most commonly used oral preparations. Robitussin, Quibron, Verequad, and Asbron are used also. Since coughing may cause a prolonged asthma attack, it is best that the nurse maintain oral and intravenous fluid intake to assist the patient to be rid of these secretions.

Frequently, patients with status asthmaticus fail to respond to *epinephrine;* in this case, *aminophylline* given intravenously or rectally is used to relieve the severity of the attack. The medication is "piggybacked" and run from ½ to 2 hours. Side effects, including tachycardia, nausea, vomiting, and diarrhea, are not uncommon with aminophylline administration. Their occurrence should be observed for carefully and reported to the physician. Should side effects to aminophylline be unusually severe, the drug may be discontinued and replaced with another bronchodilator.

*Sodium bicarbonate* or *sodium lactate* may be given to treat metabolic or respiratory acidosis. These drugs also appear to help epinephrine exert a better pharmacologic effect. Arterial pH, $p_{CO_2}$ and $p_{O_2}$ values are measured to guide the use of these alkalinizing agents. The agents are given intravenously and must be judiciously prescribed according to the patient's serum sodium levels.

Control of respiratory infection is warranted through the use of broad-spectrum *antibiotics.* This therapy is initiated after the nurse obtains sputum speciments for culture and sensitivity.

The use of *corticosteroids* is evaluated for the patient in status asthmaticus, and these drugs are usually given in large doses, especially if the patient has been maintained on them prior to this severe episode. Reduction in dosage is determined by the patient's clinical state.

*Oxygen* is given by nasal catheter or Venturi mask to maintain arterial oxygen tension between 60 and 100 mmHg. The oxygen should be humidified and given at room temperature. Cold oxygen may cause increased bronchospasm. A mechanical respirator may be used to ensure continued alveolar ventilation. It is important that the nurse support the patient and the family emotionally, since the severity of the asthmatic attack and the use of oxygen therapy may imply an ominous prognosis.

Bennett or Bird *intermittent positive pressure breathing* (IPPB) machines may be used to nebulize bronchodilator solutions for therapeutic purposes. Oxygen therapists and nurses assist the patient to obtain the best pharmacologic effects. Isoproterenol in the usual 1:200 concentration is diluted in warm saline and added to the nebulizer. Intermittent positive pressure breathing treatment is given regularly three times a day before meals, since the patient breathes more easily on an empty stomach.

*Postural drainage,* if ordered, should be carried out immediately after IPPB treatment to remove respiratory secretions. The patient needs both psychological and physical support from the nurse and respiratory therapist at this time because of the possible hazards of throat irritation, cough, bronchospasm, and copious and thickened secretions.

An *ultrasonic aerosol generator* may be used to reduce the viscosity of bronchial secretions. The physician closely evaluates the patient at this time and may find it necessary to *lavage* the bronchial tree using a catheter and warmed normal saline.

*Bronchoscopy* may be necessary to assist secretion removal and lessen the patient's dyspnea. A special indication for bronchoscopy exists when the asthmatic patient develops a "silent chest," that is, when wheezing stops and breath sounds are absent on auscultation. Removal of retained secretions may restore the patient's ability to ventilate adequately.

The moribund asthmatic patient appears on the verge of death in spite of the use of therapy. Exhaustion, hypoxia, hypercapnia, heart failure, and circulatory collapse may contribute to this state. Samples are drawn frequently for arterial blood gases and evaluated to assess respiratory or metabolic acidosis. Drug intoxication from overtreatment must also be considered. Endotracheal intubation or inflated-cuff tracheostomy tubes with automatic ventilation are used during apnea or when the patient's inspiratory efforts are too weak to cycle the machine. Adequate humidification is essential. Sterile tracheostomy technique should be maintained by the nurse. Curarelike drugs may be used to paralyze muscles and thus assist mechanical ventilation.

It is crucial that the nurse caring for the patient in status asthmaticus maintain *psychosocial support* of both patient and family. Verbal reassurances, explanations of therapies used, and nonverbal communications such as touch and time spent with the patient are supportive. Care of this critically ill patient and the family should be sensitive and comforting.

Asthma which appears first in middle or later adulthood is frequently related to respiratory infection or to unknown causes and carries a less favorable prognosis than asthma with onset in early adulthood. The aspirin-sensitive group of asthmatic patients do most poorly; their attacks are prolonged, intractable, and inexplicable in onset.

Treatment for asthma is highly individualized regarding medications, inhalations, physiotherapy, and teaching. Most deaths and complications could possibly be prevented if the patient and family were taught to follow prescribed medical and nursing regimes at home.[11] Respiratory disorders are anxiety-provoking for the patient because they threaten the ability to breathe comfortably. The nurse in the outpatient clinic, community health agency or hospital should recognize this and establish a climate of trust with the patient in order to help allay this anxiety and foster a cooperative, participating, health-directed interaction.[12]

### Fourth-Level Nursing Care

Prevention and follow-up care of allergic patients are largely dependent upon the offending allergen and the specific allergic state. The recovery period may be protracted with patients having status asthmaticus, whereas allergic rhinitis and urticaria may appear to clear completely following each episode.

**Status asthmaticus** Following the resolution of status asthmaticus, the nurse should continue to assess hydration status and kidney function through daily weights, urinary output, and indices of edema. Oxygen exchange is evaluated as the patient is weaned from the respirator. Postural drainage and chest physical therapy are maintained, as are bron-

chodilating medications and IPPB treatments. The amount, color, and viscosity of the sputum should be evaluated and recorded. Activity levels progress according to the patient's tolerance. The patient can ambulate while receiving oxygen treatment.

The teaching plan for home care is initiated so that the patient is knowledgeable about drugs, including names, times of administration, actions, and undesirable side effects. In addition, the use of the nebulizer and proper cleaning of this equipment, factors to be avoided which may precipitate an asthmatic attack, subcutaneous administration of epinephrine when nebulizer therapy fails to stop the wheezing, the benefits and risks of steroid therapy, symptoms of infection, and the necessity of return clinic or office appointments should be reviewed by the nurse.

Disodium cromoglycate (DSCG) has recently been used in the treatment of asthma and may be ordered for the patient's home use. It causes inhibition of the antigen-induced release of mediators from mast cells by a yet unknown mechanism. This medication is used as a powder and inhaled from a capsule placed in an inhaler. The inhalation of DSCG prior to inhalation of an allergen prevents the asthmatic response. The patient should be taught that using more than 20 mg four times a day probably does not improve therapeutic value and that the drug is ineffective when used after exposure to the allergen. However, beginning treatment as early as possible is reasonable to avoid delay in achieving a therapeutic effect. Patients with extrinsic asthma who are steroid-dependent can be weaned from steroids after the initiation of DSCG therapy.

The patient should review with the nurse the environmental controls necessary to minimize or eliminate the offending allergen from the environment. Hyposensitization therapy may be continued to reduce bronchial reactivity. Allergen hyposensitization may be of little value if continued over 2 years; in some instances the patient's asthma is aggravated with each injection. The nurse performing hyposensitization treatment should assess the patient's symptoms with each visit to the clinic or physician's office.

During the convalescence of the patient, it is helpful to involve a family member in all aspects of care in order to assist the patient when the illness becomes more severe and to provide emotional support.

**Systemic anaphylaxis** The nurse should counsel the patient in the prevention of further episodes of systemic anaphylaxis. Prevention of systemic anaphylaxis is accomplished by avoiding situations where stinging insects are in large numbers, spraying areas with insect repellants, avoiding insect-attracting substances (perfumes, aftershave lotions, bright colors), wearing long, tightly closed shirt sleeves and pant legs when in rural settings, and carrying prescribed medications for immediate treatment should a reaction to an allergen occur. In clinics, community health nursing agencies, emergency rooms, and patient care units, protocols should be established for nurses to initiate treatment for systemic anaphylaxis until the physician can arrive on the scene.

Kits which contain epinephrine, other drugs, and a tourniquet are available for the patient. The physician should explain and the nurse should reinforce the individual's treatment regimen. The nurse should instruct the patient and the family in subcutaneous self-injection technique and in tourniquet application, when necessary.

If the patient is recovering from an anaphylactic reaction to a drug, it is imperative that both the patient and family be taught the importance of recalling the name of the drug that caused the reaction and the symptoms of the allergic reaction which were experienced. The nurse can give the patient the address of the Medic-Alert bracelet manufacturer, to stress the crucial nature of drug allergy.

The physician will frequently prescribe a different drug for the patient who experiences a reaction since suitable alternatives are often available with similar pharmacologic benefits. Occasionally, adrenal steroids have been used to suppress the symptoms of hypersensitivity while the patient receives a drug which triggers allergic reactions. Desensitization has also been used to minimize the chances of allergic reaction. This involves the administration of progressively larger doses of the drug. Desensitization is considered dangerous, however, since patients have experienced fatal anaphylactic reactions when receiving systemic doses of the offending drugs.

**General considerations** Environmental control, medications, and hyposensitization treatment will continue over a long period of time for patients with allergic disease. The course of these disorders may last for the patient's lifetime. The nurse should offer the patient hope and encouragement that therapeutics may be developed in the future to minimize the symptoms of allergic disease. Meanwhile, it is vital to identify and stress the strengths within the patient's life, so that discouragement does not replace active, useful living.

## TYPE II: CYTOTOXIC AND CYTOLYTIC REACTIONS

Allergens can cause cellular destruction by lysis (*cytolysis*) or by direct destruction without lysis (*cytotoxicity.*) A group of cells that are particularly susceptible to cytotoxic and cytolytic reactions are the formed blood elements (erthrocytes, platelets, and leukocytes). Cellular membrane components (such as blood group antigens) and haptens (for example, drugs like chloramphenicol) are the antigens responsible for type II responses. IgG, IgM, and complement serve as mediators for these reactions which can take hours or days to become clinically manifest.

*Blood incompatibility reactions* will be discussed as an example of type II responses. Other conditions of this type include hemolytic disease of the newborn as well as drug-induced hemolytic anemias, leukopenias, and thrombocytopenias.

### Blood Incompatibility Reactions

Blood incompatibility reactions occur when blood group antigens (A, B, or D), present in the membranes of *donor* red blood cells, encounter antigen-specific antibodies (anti-A, anti-B, or anti-D) in the *recipient's* blood. The donor is the person giving the blood and the recipient receives the blood.

**Pathophysiology** Blood types or groups are named for the antigen (A or B) present in the erythrocyte membrane. These antigens are referred to as *agglutinogens* or *alloantigens* (substances compatible in some members of a species but not others). Human blood types may be A, B, AB, or O. Blood group A has the A agglutinogen, B has the B agglutinogen, AB has both A and B agglutinogens in each red blood cell, and O has neither A nor B. (See Table 10-4.)

Each individual also possesses certain antibodies that are called *agglutinins* or *alloantibodies.* Anti-A agglutinins are present in persons of the B blood group, and anti-B agglutinins are present in group A persons; group AB persons have *neither* and group O persons have *both* anti-A and anti-B agglutinins. (See Table 10-4.)

**A**BO Incompatibility The most common cause of intravascular hemolysis of red blood cells is ABO incompatibility. When bloods are mismatched so that anti-A or anti-B agglutinins are mixed with red blood cells containing A or B agglutinogens, respectively, the red blood cells agglutinate as the agglutinin antibodies attach themselves to the red blood cells. These agglutinins are either bivalent

(IgG type) or polyvalent (IgM types); therefore a single agglutinin can attach to two different red blood cells at the same time. This causes the cells to adhere to one another.

The red blood cells then clump, and the resulting clumps plug small blood vessels throughout the systemic circulation. In a few hours to a few days, phagocytic white blood cells and the reticuloendothelial system destroy the agglutinated cells. *Intravascularly,* this destruction takes place because of complement-mediated lysis. *Extravascularly,* the opsonized cells (those having attached antibodies) are destroyed by the reticuloendothelial cells in the spleen, liver, and lungs.

Lysis of red blood cells causes hemoglobin to be released into the plasma (hemoglobinemia) and the urine (hemoglobinuria). Filtering out the hemoglobin in the kidneys may result in tubular damage and, eventually, acute renal failure.

**Rh Incompatibility** The major cause of extravascular transfusion reactions is Rh incompatibility. These reactions occur when a person who is Rh-negative, and possesses anti-Rh antibodies, receives blood from an Rh-positive donor.

The Rh blood group system contains more than 30 antigens and antibodies. Two separate terminologies identify the antigens in the Rh group: one is the Fisher-Race terminology, and the other is the Weiner terminology. The most common Rh antigen is the D (Fisher-Race terminology) or $Rh_0$ (Weiner terminology) factor. Eighty-five percent of persons possess the D ($Rh_0$) antigen on their red blood cells, react with anti-D serum, and are therefore referred to as *Rh-positive* (Rh+). The other 15 percent of persons do *not* possess the D ($Rh_0$) antigen on their red blood cells and are referred to as *Rh-negative* (Rh−). Rh− persons form anti-D antibodies when transfused with Rh+ blood. A second transfusion of Rh+ blood will cause these sensitized Rh− persons

to have a severe hemolytic reaction. (See Table 10-5.)

## Other Transfusion Reactions

Various allergic responses and certain nonimmune complications compose the other forms of transfusion reactions. *Allergic reactions* may be characterized by urticaria, swelling of lymph nodes, sore throat, joint pains, fever, and eosinophilia; angioedema and asthma have also been noted. These reactions may occur days after transfusion and may result from the transfer of reagins to which the recipient is sensitive. *Febrile reactions* are characterized by chills and fever that occur an hour or more after the transfusion; toxic substances in blood tubing and bacterial protein are among the offending agents. *Circulatory overload* can occur when large volumes of blood are given or small amounts are infused rapidly, especially in patients with heart disease. Symptoms develop between 1 and 24 hours after transfusions, and death may result from pulmonary edema. *Miscellaneous effects* of transfusions include hyperkalemia, hypocalcemia, syphilis, malaria, hepatitis, bleeding diathesis, and air embolism. While these other reactions are included for completeness, the focus of the four levels of nursing care is specific for *allergic* and *incompatibility* reactions.

## First-Level Nursing Care

Blood transfusions are most frequently utilized when blood volume is decreased, as in hemorrhagic shock. Anemic, thrombocytopenic, surgical, hypovolemic, and hemophilic patients, as well as those requiring exchange transfusions, may receive whole blood, packed red blood cells, and other blood components to improve physiologic status. The patient receiving whole blood transfusions or packed red blood cells *must* be carefully observed

**TABLE 10-4**
ABO BLOOD GROUP NAMES AND COMPATIBILITIES*

| Blood Group or Type | Red Blood Cell Agglutinogen(s) | Serum Agglutinin(s) | Compatible Donor Blood Groups or Types | Incompatible Donor Blood Groups or Types |
|---|---|---|---|---|
| A | A | Anti-B | A and O | B and AB |
| B | B | Anti-A | B and O | A and AB |
| AB | A and B | Neither (universal recipient) | A, B, AB, and O | None |
| O | Neither (universal donor) | Anti-A and Anti-B | O | A, B, and AB |

* ABO blood groups are named for the antigen (agglutinogen) found in the red blood cells. Compatibility is based on the antibodies (agglutinins) present in the serum.

by the nurse and physician. Patients who have received several transfusions are more likely to experience transfusion reactions than patients receiving their first transfusion.

**Prevention**  Even in the most hurried situations, prevention of transfusion reactions should be possible. Prevention begins with a thorough evaluation of the potential donor. Persons donating blood should be free of colds, allergies, hepatitis, syphilis, and chronic disease. Vital signs should be taken, and findings must reveal an afebrile, normotensive person. Most agencies that receive blood from donors also have minimum weight requirements. Satisfactory donor health must be established before the blood is taken.

It is essential that donor blood and recipient blood go through the process of *typing* and *cross matching*. *Typing* establishes the blood group of both the donor and the recipient, thereby identifying the presence of antigens A, B, and D (Rh$_0$). *Cross matching* is a procedure for determining if clumping of red blood cells will take place in serum from the other person's blood. Major cross matching occurs when the donor's red blood cells are mixed with the recipient's serum. Minor cross matching occurs when the recipient's red blood cells are combined with the donor's serum. Both combinations are incubated for 15 minutes and observed for clumping.

Further prevention of blood transfusion reaction can be accomplished through careful collection and labeling of blood. The label should contain the blood type, the full name of the patient, the hospital number and/or bottle number, and the name of the physician. Detailed labeling of the blood to be transfused also includes the date the blood was collected, the name of the donor, and the names of the place where the blood was collected and the hospital or clinic where the blood is to be transfused.

The nurse should participate in checking blood labels with the physician prior to administration,

especially in the hurried atmosphere of emergency situations when many successive blood transfusions are necessary for life support.

The intravenous tubing must be flushed with *isotonic saline* solution before and after blood is administered. Nonphysiological solutions cause hemolysis of red blood cells in the intravenous (IV) line.

Blood should be administered at room temperature. If there is any question about the labeling of the blood or the amount of time it has been unrefrigerated, it should *not* be given.

The nurse should observe all patients receiving blood transfusion for 15 minutes following the beginning of the transfusion and at prescribed intervals throughout the transfusion. The patient should be encouraged to call in the event unusual feelings or symptoms occur.

### Second-Level Nursing Care

Blood transfusions normally take place within the hospital setting. Patients receiving blood in an emergency room situation have probably experienced severe blood loss.

**Nursing assessment**  Observation and accurate assessment of the patient are vital to prevent a severe transfusion reaction. In order to do this, the nurse should have observed the preventative measures listed under First-Level Nursing Care and completed an individual health history and physical assessment.

Health History  When possible, a complete health history should be obtained from the patient. It is especially important to elicit information about any previous transfusions.

Patients experiencing an *incompatibility* reaction often describe feelings of restlessness and anxiety, generalized tingling sensations, pain in the back and thighs, nausea, and vomiting. If the reaction is an allergic response, the patient may complain of itching, shortness of breath, and light-headedness.

Physical Assessment  An individual experiencing a transfusion reaction usually has an elevated temperature, pulse, and respiratory rate. The blood pressure, particularly in allergic responses, may be decreased. Hives may be present in allergic reactions, often appearing on the back and extremities. Jaundice, dyspnea, oliguria, and hematuria may be observable in severe reactions.

Far-advanced reactions may cause the patient

**TABLE 10-5**
Rh INCOMPATIBILITY WITH ANTIGEN D (Rh$_0$)*

| Rh Type | D or Rh$_0$ Antigen on Red Blood Cells‡ | Anti-D or Anti Rh$_0$ Antibodies in the Serum‡ | Percentage of Persons |
|---|---|---|---|
| Rh+ | + | 0 | 85 |
| Rh− | 0 | +† | 15 |

* Fisher-Race terminology uses D, Weiner terminology uses Rh$_0$.
‡ + = present, 0 = not present.
† Antibody formation occurs after sensitization to Rh+ blood.

to be severely dyspneic and hypotensive. Intervention must be rapid to prevent renal failure, vascular collapse, and death.

**Diagnostic Tests** Laboratory tests utilized in a suspected case of transfusion reaction include examination of the blood and urine of the patient for hemoglobinemia, bilirubinemia, and urinary pigments. A serologic review of recipient and donor blood is also done and includes reexamination of a pretransfusion sample of the patient's blood, the tube of blood that was cross matched for the recipient, and the blood that was transfused.

**Nursing problems** Major nursing problems with cytolytic transfusion reactions include *chills and fever, pain in the back and thighs, oliguria, hypotension,* and *anxiety.* Allergic transfusion reactions have similar symptoms with the additional problems of *dyspnea* and *urticaria.*

**Interventions** Nursing interventions are directed toward stopping the infusion and combating any incompatibility effects already present. In an emergency room situation, care is instituted to stabilize the patient before transfer to a hospital unit.

The first and most important action is to *discontinue the infusion of blood* and *notify the physician.* Care should be taken to maintain a patent intravenous line. Therefore, the IV line should be flushed with isotonic saline and kept patent with an appropriate IV solution, usually 5% dextrose in water or a saline preparation, as ordered.

The blood should be saved and returned to the laboratory for examination. It may be reexamined for type and cross match as well as culture and sensitivity.

Emergency care to combat respiratory and hypotensive symptoms should be instituted. Because reactions typically occur in an inpatient situation, details of this care can be found under Third-Level Nursing Care.

**Third-Level Nursing Care**
Because of the specific nature of transfusion reactions, the effects on the patient are the same as those detailed in the health history and physical assessment described under Second-Level Nursing Care.

**Nursing problems and interventions** Discontinuing the blood infusion should be the first action taken in any suspected reaction. The importance of this intervention cannot be overemphasized. Fol-

lowing this, care is directed toward the effects of the reaction, whether due to incompatibility or allergy.

**Dyspnea and Wheezing** Care for respiratory difficulties may include oxygen administration, epinephrine (bronchodilator) and, at times corticosteroids (anti-inflammatory effect). Patients should be placed in a position which facilitates breathing, usually with the head of the bed elevated. This may be contraindicated if the patient is also hypotensive. Judgments must be individually made under the physician's supervision.

**Hypotension** Symptoms of shock are secondary to the reaction's effect upon the vasculature. The administration of epinephrine should result not only in the relief of dyspnea but in peripheral vasoconstriction and an increased blood pressure. Fluids administered intravenously, including dextrose preparations, saline solutions, plasma expanders, and blood, will often be necessary to achieve and maintain an adequate blood pressure. Vital signs should be monitored frequently. Vasopressor drugs may be necessary to combat severe hypotension. (Total discussion of hypotension is found in Chap. 28.)

**Urticaria** To lessen the urticaria in mild reactions, antihistamines, such as Benadryl, may be ordered intramuscularly or by mouth. Severe reactions may necessitate the use of epinephrine and corticosteroids.

**Oliguria and Hematuria** Urinary output is extremely important as a measure of renal function. The insertion of an indwelling catheter may be indicated to achieve maximum accuracy. Intake and output readings should be taken with the vital signs, until both are stabilized. Urine specimens should be tested for the presence of blood as an indication of hemolysis. If oliguria is marked, osmotic diuretics and intravenous fluids may be prescribed to promote diuresis.

**Severe Anxiety** Patient apprehension may be aggravated by the presence of chills, fever, and pain. Antipyretics may be ordered to lower the elevated temperature. Severe anxiety may warrant the use of sedation; frequently antihistamines have a sedative side effect and will serve this purpose.

**Circulatory Overload** While not a cytolytic or cytotoxic reaction, circulatory overload must be mentioned to complete the list of problems associated with transfusion reactions. (The reader is referred to Chap. 24 for a thorough discussion of congestive heart failure and circulatory overload.) Circulatory overload occurs when the blood or packed cells are administered too rapidly for the individual's cardiovascular system to respond to the additional volume. Respiratory congestion, dyspnea, frothy pink-tinged sputum, peripheral and pulmonary edema, tachycardia, and other signs of heart failure signal this complication.

### Fourth-Level Nursing Care

The nurse should advise the patient who has experienced a transfusion reaction to relate this information to nurses and physicians if the reality of future whole blood or packed red blood cell administration occurs. Measures to maintain a positive state of health should be taught to the patient who has a chronic disorder which requires periodic transfusion. Avoidance of blood transfusion is the most effective preventive measure to eliminate the allergic response. The patient should be advised to keep a mental or written record of this and any other transfusion reactions. It is also important to teach patients their blood group and Rh types so they, too, can be observant and knowledgeable during any future transfusions.

### TYPE III: IMMUNE COMPLEX HYPERSENSITIVITY RESPONSES

Immune complex responses or diseases have as their causative agent the *antigen-antibody complexes* or *microprecipitates* that are formed in the circulation or interstitial fluids when an allergen encounters a specific antibody. Diseases are produced when these complexes situate in tissues and interact there with the humoral and cellular mediators of immunologic inflammation. These mediators include IgG, IgM, IgE, complement, neutrophils, eosinophils, and lysosomal enzymes. Immune complex reactions may occur within minutes or may take days.

Most pathogenic complexes are destroyed by reticuloendothelial phagocytes. However, some escape and tend to localize and accumulate in the filtering structures of the body, such as glomeruli, blood vessels, and lymphoid tissue.

The Arthus reaction and serum sickness will be discussed as examples of type III responses. However, many human diseases such as systemic lupus erythematosus, rheumatoid arthritis, and glomeru-

lonephritis are suspected of having immune-complex hypersensitivity origins. In these diseases the antigen has yet to be definitively identified.

### The Arthus Reaction

The Arthus reaction is the cutaneous form of the immune-complex reaction and is named for the French physiologist who originally described it. Originally, it was elicited by injecting horse serum, subcutaneously, into rabbits. The injections were given on a weekly basis and caused no observable response at first. However, after several weeks, a localized area of inflammation was observed at each injection site. Arthus reactions occur when sensitized individuals, having a high level of precipitating antibody (IgG class), are reinjected with the antigen. The Arthus reaction is an example of a focal area of immune-complex tissue injury.

**Pathophysiology**  It has been found that Arthus reactions may affect structures other than the skin, such as the pericardial sac, blood vessels, lung, glomeruli, and joint spaces.

Arthus lesions are characterized by a destructive inflammation of small blood vessels known as *vasculitis*. The process leading to vasculitis begins when antigen-antibody complexes (microprecipitates) are deposited in the tissues. Complement is fixed by the complexes, neutrophils are attracted to the area, lysosomal enzymes are released by the cells causing tissue damage, and the resultant increased permeability permits the immune complexes to lodge in vessel walls, causing inflammation and necrosis.

Thrombi form within the small vessels, and blood flow is slowed. The affected area becomes edematous and has all the signs of classic inflammation. Eventual resolution of the reaction occurs when the immune complexes are phagocytized.

### Serum Sickness

The *serum sickness syndrome* is closely related to the Arthus reaction and may even be its disseminated form. It was first described by von Pirquet and Schick in persons who had received a single large dosage of an antiserum prepared in horses or rabbits. The syndrome was apparent 7 to 14 days after the injection. Today, antiserums prepared in animals are less frequently used. Nurses may encounter them in the form of horse antiserums to human lymphocytes, and tetanus and rabies antiserums. However, serum sickness can be caused by other antigens and haptens, especially drugs.

**Pathophysiology** Unlike the Arthus reaction, serum sickness occurs in the presence of antigen excess. It may be "one shot" (acute), chronic, or accelerated.

Classic "one-shot" serum sickness occurs after a *single* large dose of an antigen, such as an antitoxin produced in a horse, or a drug. The reaction is usually self-limited and clears within several days.

Seven to fourteen days after antigen exposure, as immune complexes are formed, the characteristic serum sickness symptoms are exhibited. These include fever, lymphadenopathy, urticaria, and painful joints. The syndrome may also include glomerulonephritis, arthritis, vasculitis, myocarditis, endocarditis, and neuritis.

The immune complexes become quite large and very susceptible to phagocytosis. This results in their efficient removal from the body and elimination of the disease, generally without serious effect.

**C**hronic Serum Sickness.   Chronic serum sickness occurs as a result of repeated exposure to an antigen. The continuous antigen exposure maintains the presence of immune complexes in the circulation and may cause damage to the kidney, heart, joints, and blood vessels. This form of serum sickness may involve many organs of the body, affecting cardiac, renal, and musculoskeletal function.

**A**ccelerated Serum Sickness   If the patient has received the same type of foreign serum previously, an accelerated reaction may occur after 1 to 5 days. Local itching, swelling, and redness at the injection site are some of the symptoms which may begin the serum sickness reaction 24 to 48 hours before the onset of systemic symptoms.

### First-Level Nursing Care

Prevention of serum sickness involves the active immunization of the population with tetanus and diphtheria toxoids. This eliminates the need for foreign or heterologous serum administration. Patients whose occupation puts them at risk to tetanus following injury, and those who are especially sensitive to horse dander and horse serum, should be cautioned by the nurse in the clinic, community health nursing agency, and allergist's office to maintain active tetanus immunization. Booster injections of tetanus toxoid are sufficient to protect an adequately immunized person following injury, to the extent that no tetanus antitoxin is necessary. There appears to be an adequate rise in tetanus

antitoxin titers, following toxoid booster injections, lasting more than 10 years following primary immunization.

### Second-Level Nursing Care

Serum sickness has an insidious nature and, therefore, requires careful assessment and evaluation. Its symptoms may seem nonspecific at first or be very typical.

**Nursing Assessment** The patient's *health history* should be taken with emphasis on any foreign antiserum or large drug dosages in the preceding 1 to 3 weeks. The nurse should determine the specific onset of symptoms in relationship to the time of foreign substance exposure.

Patients will often describe itching and a rash as their initial symptoms. They may also have joint pain, headache, nausea, and vomiting.

*Physical assessment* may reveal lymphadenopathy, beginning in the regional nodes near the site of the injection. Swollen joints may indicate the presence of effusion. Measurement of vital signs will usually reveal an elevated temperature. Cardiac involvement may be indicated by arrhythmias that are detectable on auscultation. Neurological assessment may reveal weakness and sensory losses.

Serum sickness may range in severity from transient urticaria to life-threatening laryngeal edema. Complete recovery usually occurs over time, although vascular inflammatory changes may cause death.

**D**iagnostic Tests   If the history does not suggest horse serum allergy, intracutaneous tests may be started to document hypersensitivity. It is very important to establish the responsible antigen or hapten.

Several laboratory study deviations are present if serum sickness is diagnosed. The total white blood count may be low, normal, or slightly elevated. Eosinophilia may occur late in the disease, and atypical lymphocytes may be evident. The sedimentation rate is slightly elevated. Urine studies may reveal protein, casts, and erythrocytes. If the heart is involved, electrocardiograph tracings may show transient conduction abnormalities.

**Nursing problems and intervention** Nursing interventions in serum sickness involve symptomatic relief of problems rather than definitive cure. *Urticaria* commonly occurs, and drug therapy is the primary intervention for relief of the rash and itching. Small doses of epinephrine, antihistamines, and corticosteroids are the drugs of choice. Local antipruritic lotions may be applied. If there is *joint involvement,* salicylate preparations including aspirin may be prescribed for pain and inflammation. Other care is symptomatic depending upon the severity of the symptoms.

Generalized *weakness* may be present because of neurological involvement and the inflammatory process. Patients should be told that it may take some time for normal strength and energy levels to return. Activity recommendations should include gradual resumption of previously assumed activites.

### Third-Level Nursing Care

Patients are usually hospitalized for severe episodes of "one-shot" serum sickness that require intensive therapy. The other indication for hospitalization is the life-threatening accelerated serum sickness response.

**Nursing Assessment**  Health history and physical assessment processes are similar to those discussed under Second-Level Nursing Care. Patients requiring hospitalization will, however, seem much weaker, generally more uncomfortable, and anxious. They may have respiratory distress and edema that are causing visible discomfort. Cardiac and neurological symptoms may be intensified.

**Nursing Problems and Interventions**  With severe serum sickness, care will focus on the *urticaria, joint symptoms,* and *fever.* Corticosteroids and adrenocorticotropic hormone (ACTH) are often used. *Respiratory problems* may also be severe. Emergency equipment to support respiration should be available. Detailed care is similar to that described earlier for systemic anaphylaxis.

### Fourth-Level Nursing Care

The nurse and physician should discuss with the patient the nature of the hypersensitivity reaction to the foreign serum. The patient should never be given it again. As with all allergic responses Medic-Alert tags or identification cards should be used to alert emergency health care workers to the patient's severe reactions in the event of foreign serum injection or penetrating wounds. Adequate active immunization for tetanus should be stressed as being crucial to eliminating the necessity of taking equine serum antitoxin. Human tetanus antitoxin (TAT) gives higher blood levels of antitoxin and less risk of serum reactions.[13]

If it is essential that a person sensitive to horse serum receive equine serum sometime in the future, dilutions of 1:100 in initial doses of 0.005 ml may be prescribed. The dose is doubled every 30 minutes until a therapeutic dose or a drug reaction is reached. Recovery from an episode of serum sickness may take some time but is usually complete.

## TYPE IV: DELAYED HYPERSENSITIVITY RESPONSE

*Delayed hypersensitivity reactions* involve the combination of an antigen with a sensitized T lymphocyte. In these tissue-damaging reactions, the effects of delayed hypersensitivity are produced either by means of released *lymphokines* (products secreted by lymphocytes) or by direct T-lymphocyte-mediated cell destruction (see Chap. 8).

These reactions may take hours or days to occur from the time of antigen exposure. Tuberculosis skin tests, contact dermatitis, and transplant graft rejection are the major examples of delayed hypersensitivity reactions. However, these responses may also have a role in autoimmune diseases and processes caused by microorganisms.

The classic example of a delayed (*cell-mediated*) hypersensitivity response is the effect of a *tuberculin skin test* in a person who has already been sensitized to the tubercle bacillus. This sensitization will have occurred at the time of a previous tuberculous infection. After an *intracutaneous* injection of tuberculin, a firm, raised area of *induration* and *erythema* appears at the site. The reaction begins in 8 to 12 hours and reaches a peak in about 2 days. Severe reactions may involve extended induration and even necrosis. Cells found to be present in the area are T lymphocytes and macrophages.

Allergic contact dermatitis and renal transplant rejection will be discussed in total, including related nursing care. Renal transplants are discussed because of the frequency of their occurrence. However, the transplant of *any vascular organ* may be endangered by the same rejection process.

### Allergic Contact Dermatitis

*Allergic contact dermatitis* or allergic contact eczema is the result of a specific, delayed, cell-mediated allergic reaction to antigen applied to the skin of a sensitized patient. Its appearance may vary with the specific antigen involved.

**Pathophysiology**  Contact dermatitis is caused by a variety of agents, ranging from complex substances present in plants such as poison ivy to simple chemicals or elements including paraphenyl-enediamine (found in dyes) and nickel. The offending agent of contact dermatitis acts as a hapten by combining with dermal protein as it penetrates the skin. The hapten-dermal protein combination performs as an antigen. Lymphocytes within the skin exposed to the antigen become altered, so that they recognize the antigen. These lymphocytes then travel to local lymph glands and proliferate, forming a clone of sensitized lymphocytes. The reaction of these sensitized lymphocytes with the skin containing the antigen result in the release of pharmacological agents which stimulate eczematous changes in the skin.[14]

The initial sensitization of the skin may develop over a period of years, although patients may become allergic after a few weeks of close contact with a new environmental agent. After sensitization, reexposure is followed by lesions appearing 18 or more hours later or perhaps in a shorter time period.

In the *acute phase* of allergic contact dermatitis, papules and vesicles predominate on the skin along with erythema, edema, and bullae. In the *subacute phase,* vesicular changes are less evident and may be interspersed with crusting, scaling, and early thickening and lichenification with minor or no papulovesicular features. These lesions are described in Chap. 8. Pruritis and discomfort of the affected skin may be severe.

The clinical course is characterized by exacerbations following exposure to the allergen and remissions following elimination of exposure. Contact dermatitis may be present at the same time as other skin disease such as fungus infection or stasis dermatitis.

**First-Level Nursing Care** Since literally thousands of materials in the environment can cause allergic contact dermatitis, it is difficult for community health, industrial, and campus health clinic nurses to stress avoidance of contact irritants.

Genetic factors, local concentration of antigen, duration of exposure, local variations in skin permeability, and development of immune tolerance are some of the important factors determining whether a person develops sensitization to a contact agent. The elderly are less susceptible to sensitization than the middle-aged. Sensitization to more than one agent occurs in approximately 20 percent of patients with contact dermatitis. This may be due to genetic predisposition or because contact dermatitis lowers the threshold of sensitization by other agents. Cross sensitivity between

closely related antigens may make a patient susceptible to more than one agent.

**P**revention   The nurse should be involved in teaching people in home and work situations to be cautious of exposure to the common sources of contacts found in Table 10-6. In addition to Table 10-6, lists of common contact agents are available for artists, commercial painters, carpenters, laborers, bakers, cleaners, dyers, furriers, photographers, leatherworkers and shoemakers, mechanics, metal workers, health care workers, and people in contact with domesticated and wild plants.

The community health nurse may investigate industrial settings and prepare health teaching programs to decrease the incidence of contact dermatitis in specific occupational groups of workers. Routine inspection of factories with particular attention to production methods tends to limit the exposure of the worker to potent allergens.

The nurse who seeks to prevent contact dermatitis may be involved in encouraging a factory to replace existing contact allergens with alternative chemicals. Frequently, industrial processes may not be easily changed, and so the nurse may counsel workers to reduce skin contact through the use of special equipment, protective clothing, and en-

**TABLE 10-6**
AGENTS CAUSING CONTACT DERMATITIS

*Rhus* (poison) plants:
Poison ivy, oak, sumac

Nickel:
Nickel-plated earrings
Metallic push-button telephones

Paraphenylenediamine (PPDA):
Hair dye

Formaldehyde and formaldehyde-releasing makeup preservatives

Benzocaine:
Anesthetic liquids, sprays, creams, ointments

Chromates:
Cement
Coolants
Chrome-tanned shoes

Ammoniated mercury:
Thiomerosal
Preservatives in lubricants

Ethylenediamine hydrochloride:
Mycolog cream

Neomycin:
Neomycin ointment on stasis ulcers and chronic otitis media

Mercaptobenzothiazole:
Rubber compounds
Insecticides
Parasiticides
Antipruritics used in veterinary medicine

SOURCE: Alexander A. Fisher: *Fifty Years with Contact Dermatitis,* vol. 19, Curtis, Philadelphia, 1977, pp. 18–32.

vironmental cleanliness. Potential sensitizers should be removed from the skin with soap and warm running water. If washing facilities are convenient to workers, they will wash frequently. Detergents and waterless cleansers may also be used.

Nurses who perform preemployment history and physical examinations may advise a person with known previous contact dermatitis to seek a less-threatening work environment. Educational measures to prevent contact dermatitis should be begun by nurses to prevent or minimize the exposure of the housewife, gardener, painter, or factory worker to contact allergens.

**Second-Level Nursing Care** An allergy nurse or a community health nurse will frequently be involved in identifying the most likely causative agents of contact dermatitis.

**N**ursing Assessment A form listing common offenders is useful when taking the *history* of a patient with contact dermatitis. The list may remind the patient of a substance which had seemed unimportant. Individuals frequently describe a rash and severe itching as their only symptoms. *Physical assessment* often reveals that the distribution of lesions is on the exposed surfaces of the face, neck, dorsal surfaces of the hands and feet, and the lateral aspects of the forearms and legs. The eyelids, sides of the neck, and genitalia are also frequent sites of eruption. If the contact agent is within the clothing of the patient, the distribution of lesions may be unusual, with the palms, soles, and areas well covered by hair being free of lesions.

*Patch test* The allergy nurse participates in *patch testing* a patient after an episode of contact dermatitis. Patch testing is the standard method of detecting contact sensitivity. Three methods are used to select suspected contact irritants for subsequent patch testing:

1  A history of the distribution of lesions on the patient's skin will indicate offenders such as jewelry, watch bands, shoes, and belts.

2  A history of the time and place of symptoms indicates the cause of the dermatitis. Seasonal, weekend, and vacation skin changes may coincide with contact dermatitis. A change in job or moving also may provide a clue, as may something in the patient's work situation, household objects, indoor and outdoor plants, clothing, cosmetics, hobbies, and skin ointments. The patient's thoughts about possible contact

irritants should be considered carefully. The patient may be asked to recall all activities for the previous 48 hours. A community health nurse or allergy office nurse may survey a patient's home or place of work when the contact irritant is elusive.

3  Contact substances known to be potent sensitizers should be investigated. (see Table 10-6.)

The patch test is given to determine the causative agent or agents of allergic contact dermatitis. *Patch testing* reproduces a small area of contact dermatitis by applying the suspected agent to unbroken skin. A positive test is determined when a delayed skin response occurs in 24 to 48 hours and is like the gross appearance of the primary lesion of the allergic contact dermatitis.

During patch testing, specific precautions are considered:

1  The proper concentration of test material must be used with adequate dilutions prepared prior to patch testing. A chemical burn could occur with high concentrations, and a positive patch reaction could be interpreted incorrectly.

2  When the patient is experiencing a severe contact dermatitis eruption, patch testing should be delayed. False-positive reactions could occur, as could an exacerbation of the primary skin lesions.

3  Highly sensitive patients should be advised to lift up the corner of the patch if itching or burning is experienced. If redness is present, the patch should be removed and the area washed with soap and water before the 48-hour period has elapsed.

4  A patient receiving ACTH or corticosteroids should not be patch tested, since these drugs may suppress delayed hypersensitivity reactions.

5  Materials for patch testing are selected according to the history and distribution of lesions, since patch testing may induce sensitization.

If a large number of tests are applied at one time, patch tests are placed on the dorsal surface of the back (see Fig. 10-4). The skin of the upper arms may be used if the number of tests is small. If the hands, feet, or face have erupted with the lesions of contact dermatitis, the patch test is done as close to these areas as possible. The face is avoided in patch testing.

For patch testing on the back, the nurse places the patient in a prone position, washes the area with alcohol, and allows it to dry. The tests are placed in rows on the skin, the distance between patches being 2 to 3 inches. Liquid contact offenders are applied directly to the skin with a dropper. Solid materials are placed on a small area of the skin and moistened. Oil-soluble articles are placed on the skin and touched with mineral or olive oil. A square of gauze 1 by 1 cm is placed on each area, and a 2 by 2 cm square of typewriter paper is placed over the gauze to protect the test area from the adhesive.

Adhesive tape, such as Micropore tape, is applied over the paper to hold the patch in place. The patches are numbered, and the materials applied to the skin are identified on the chart with the appropriate numbers. The nurse may perform the patch test or assist the physician. The nurse should instruct the patient to avoid bathing the area for 48 hours, to have someone renumber the areas if the numbers rub off, and to inspect any area which itches, burns, or appears red. These areas should be washed with soap and water.

The patient should return to the office in 48 hours. The patches will be removed, then read after 10 to 15 minutes so that the effect of mechanical irritation is decreased. Reaction to the adhesive tape should be noted. A positive patch test reaction may persist for several days. If the patient is allergic to adhesive tape, a binder bandage may be used to hold the patches in place. The center of the patch of skin is read with the following interpretations:

+      (1+) mild erythema
++     (2+) severe erythema, smooth skin
+++    (3+) erythema and papules
++++   (4+) erythema, papules, and vesicles

After the patch tests have been read, the skin should be washed with ether, soap and water, or alcohol, depending on the solubilities of the substances tested. Patients are frequently seen 24 hours after the initial reading of the patch test (72 hours after application of the test) in order to identify delayed positive results.

**N**ursing Problems and Intervention  The major nursing problems with contact dermatitis are the *rash* and *pruritis*. Interventions include avoidance of the allergen, drug therapy, wet dressings, and antipruritic lotions, creams, and ointments.

After the offending contact agents have been identified through patch testing, the nurse gives the patient a list of sources of these agents. By comparing this list with substances in the home and work environment, the patient will be able to *avoid* or *minimize exposure* to the causative agent of the

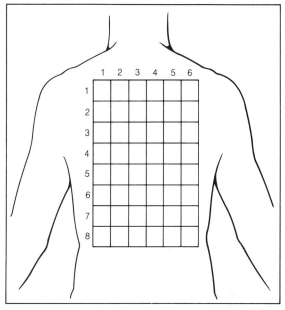

**FIGURE 10-4**
Diagram of the back of a patient indicating patch test divisions and numbering method used to determine contact irritants causing allergic contact dermatitis.

allergic contact dermatitis. In addition, washing with soap and water may assist in removing the hapten from the skin of the patient to prevent or minimize eczematous eruption. The patient should be instructed to avoid woolen clothing and starched collars and cuffs which will irritate the skin.

The nurse should discuss with the patient the action, side effects, and toxic effects of the antihistaminics (Phenergan, Benadryl, Chlor-Trimeton) and other antipruritic drugs, such as Temaril and Periactin, which the physician may order to relieve the pruritis. In addition, the nurse should advise the patient that a cool environmental temperature will reduce itching, and that keeping fingernails short will lessen the possibility of self-inflicted excoriation and superimposed infection to the susceptible skin surface. Distraction by reading or watching television could help decrease the discomfort of the itching. Tepid colloidal baths with Aveeno, or cornstarch and soda bicarbonate, may also decrease itching.

Wet dressings can be applied when the skin lesions are weeping. The nurse should tell the patient to protect the bed or furniture at home from the moisture, as well as to apply the ordered solution in the correct concentration. The patient can use a bulb syringe to add more solution to the dressings as they dry. The dressings should be applied loosely and removed periodically to avoid macerating the skin and to allow the patient to inspect it.

Topical corticosteroid creams, lotions, or ointments may be ordered to decrease the inflammatory response of the skin to the contact irritant. The patient may apply the cream, lotion, or ointment to the affected skin as the lesions progress from moist to dry. Occlusive plastic dressings may be used. The nurse should demonstrate the application of topical corticosteroid medications to the skin, cautioning the patient to avoid using excessive amounts due to the danger of systemic absorption. Calamine or neocalamine lotion may also be used.

**Third-level nursing care**   In acute, severe allergic contact dermatitis, such as severe poison ivy dermatitis, the patient will be hospitalized. While the nursing assessment and problems are similar to those discussed in Second-Level Nursing Care, the lesions may be open and weeping. Care must be meticulous and is frequently time-consuming.

**Intervention**   The discomfort of a severe allergic contact dermatitis can be lessened by systemic administration of corticosteroids. When the source is known and further exposure to the agent can be prevented, a 5- to 10-day course of treatment with systemic corticosteroids is indicated for severe, vesicular contact dermatitis. Therapeutic action of the steroids is probably due to suppression of the inflammatory response to cellular injury. Intravenous and oral preparations of corticosteroids may be administered. The nurse should observe the patient for toxic effects of short-term steroid therapy including peptic ulceration, psychoses, susceptibility to infection, and hypercoagulability of the blood.

In the acute phase of the dermatitis, compresses may be applied, on 1 hour and off 1 hour, throughout a 24-hour time period. The nurse should keep the ordered solutions cool and remove surface debris with sterile forceps between dressing changes. The patient and the family should be assured that the dermatitis is not a communicable disease and the patient cautioned against scratching the lesions. Protection against infections and adequate hydration are important nursing considerations. Safety precautions should be taken when the patient gets into and out of slippery colloidal baths.

**Fourth-level nursing care**   Rehabilitation of the patient with contact dermatitis involves identification and avoidance of the contact irritant. If the der-

matitis is not severe, the patient may possibly miss little or no work by being careful to avoid the contact agent through use of cotton-lined rubber gloves or special equipment such as long-handled brushes for household tasks.

After a severe eruption of contact dermatitis, recovery may be slow. Social service personnel should be notified of the financial, psychological, and social problems present or anticipated because of a serious vesicular skin eruption. It may be necessary for the patient to change jobs at an economic loss. Housewives, farmers, and dentists may not be able to change their occupations. Teaching avoidance and minimization of exposure to the contact irritant is essential.

Chronic contact dermatitis develops from exposure to chemical insults and contact with the allergen. Few patients can afford to avoid normal activities such as dishwashing and gardening. However, nurses should instruct patients to avoid these activities for months and perhaps even years if possible, despite the fact that the skin looks normal. The community health nurse may wish to inspect the factory or home to determine if preventive measures are being maintained and to reinforce previous teaching.

## Renal Transplant Rejection

*Renal homograft rejection,* the gradual tissue destruction which follows the grafting of a kidney from one person to a genetically different individual of the same species, is an example of a delayed hypersensitivity reaction (cellular). Other vascularized organ transplants (heart, liver, etc.) experience similar changes.

The immune responses which occur following kidney transplantation cause death of all cells in the transplanted kidney unless specific therapy is used to lessen the impact of the immune reaction. When tissue typing obtains the best possible match between donor and recipient, graft rejection is minimized by greater similarity of antigenic structure.

**Pathophysiology**   Three different types of renal transplant rejection have been identified. These episodes differ in time of occurrence and also in the pathophysiologic mechanisms that appear to be involved. Survival of a transplanted kidney depends on the patient's ability to pass through the rejection episodes which will occur.

**Acute Intermediate Rejection**   When an unsensitized patient is allografted (receives a kidney from an individual of the same species), a series of pathophysiologic events follows which can affect graft survival. *Acute intermediate rejection* usually occurs after the first week and within 4 months of grafting. In cadaveric transplants this danger lasts up to approximately 2 years. The acute (cellular) rejection pattern is mediated by the small thymus—derived lymphocytes, which recognize the transplant antigens as foreign as they pass through the transplanted kidney. The antigens are picked up by the lymphocytes, which then become sensitized. The sensitized cells then destroy graft cells on contact, without the need for complement or other serum factors. Round cells, probably small lymphocytes, migrate between the endothelial cells and infiltrate around the small vessels of the transplanted kidney. These round cells may reach large numbers within 24 hours. The number of infiltrating cells continues to increase during the first 48 hours after transplantation. Additional cells resembling small lymphocytes accumulate, as do macrophages. The cells which resemble small lymphocytes produce immunoglobulins by the third day. Therefore, *both* humoral (antibody) and cellular (small lymphocytes) immunities appear to be operating during acute kidney transplant rejection.

Sensitized lymphoid cells (small lymphocytes) release mediators of inflammation and cell damage upon recognition of the foreign tissue. These cytotoxic factors directly injure the membranes of adjacent cells. The lymphoid cells divide and further amplify the rejection process. Phagocytic macrophages are present, as are agents which enhance vascular permeability.

During this time complement is fixed, producing eventual cellular damage to the kidney. Capillary permeability increases, causing interstitial edema. Lymphoid cells continue to accumulate, as do plasma cells and polymorphonuclear leukocytes. These further alter the cellular structure of the kidney. By the tenth day, the small vessels have become plugged with fibrin and platelets, decreasing vascular perfusion and limiting the function of the allografted kidney. Either complete destruction of the graft or return to normal function with or without evidence of permanent damage can occur. The longer the interval between transplantation and acute rejection, the less likely it is that rejection will occur and the more likely that damage will be reversible.

**H**yperacute Rejection   Hyperacute (acute humoral) rejection occurs within the first 48 hours (often within a few minutes) after transplantation and is a dramatic event. After the donor kidney is in place in the recipient, the clamps are taken off the blood vessels, and the kidney fills normally with blood and becomes pink. In a short time, however, it becomes soft, blue, and mottled. The blood flow decreases and ultimately the entire kidney is progressively destroyed by vascular changes and ischemia. Humoral antibodies to donor antigens are implicated; preexisting antigenic exposure through a previous transplant, blood transfusion, pregnancy, or bacterial antigens may have stimulated antibody formation.

**C**hronic (late) Rejection   Late, or chronic, rejection is a rejection pattern seen in patients who have experienced long periods of immunosuppressive therapy. Extensive and progressive proliferation is produced in the glomerular capillaries and the endothelium of blood vessels, with progressive narrowing and eventual occlusion of the lumen. Serum antibody appears to be implicated. The patient commonly develops a nephrotic syndrome. The rejection progresses slowly over a period of years until the kidney is destroyed. The symptoms of late rejection will appear within 2 years of the transplant; these symptoms include proteinuria, hypertension, and depressed renal function. Final failure of the transplanted kidney may take 5 years. Late rejection, like hyperacute rejection, is primarily a humoral phenomenon and, once fully developed, is not reversible.

**E**ffects of Rejection   Initial oliguria and anuria due to tubular necrosis frequently occur immediately after cadaveric renal transplantation. These symptoms combined with temperature elevation (when the temperature has been normal), enlargement of the kidney with tenderness, proteinuria, and hypertension signal the necessity to consider renal transplant rejection.

The diagnosis of rejection is difficult in the early postoperative period, because the patient could be oliguric from tubular necrosis. Observation of the transplant recipient is crucial during the first few postoperative days, since acute rejection may be suppressed with adequate treatment.

**First-level nursing care**   Staff nurses and clinical specialists in dialysis units are involved in the preparation of the candidate for renal transplantation. These "candidates" are chronic renal failure patients who are dependent upon hemodialysis for survival. The kidney transplant offers the patient the hope of a dialysis-free existence; the reality of this existence may be more difficult than the patient anticipated.

**P**revention of Rejection Prevention of kidney transplant rejection is a desirable goal for the chronic dialysis patient; however, absolute freedom from rejection episodes is not likely. In the preoperative period the nurse should be available as a listener, encouraging the patient to ventilate feelings and ask questions about the chances of, and treatment for, rejection episodes.

While awaiting transplant surgery, the nurse prepares the patient for the surgical experience and the events that follow. Structured preoperative teaching plans have been used to minimize the stress of surgery for the candidate. The maintenance of high-level psychosocial and physiologic wellness is difficult for the chronic renal failure patient. The nurse should advise the patient to adhere to the rigors of fluid, diet, and medication regimens in order to stay within the narrow parameters of physiologic control.

The physiologic suitability of a kidney from cadaveric or living related donors is considered carefully. It is desirable to obtain a graft which is the most genetically compatible since the reaction of the host to the graft will be minimized. When donor and recipient are siblings, or when a parent is the donor, there is greater statistical chance of antigenic similarity between donor and recipient than when a cadaver or unrelated donor is used. It is expected that the immune system of the patient will attempt to reject the transplanted kidney unless the donor is an identical twin.

*Laboratory tests* Methods of *histocompatibility matching* have been developed to identify antigenic similarities between donor and recipient prior to transplantation. Histocompatibility matching ensures that relatively compatible donor and recipient pairs are selected. This matching process may decrease the need for large doses of immunosuppressive drugs and may increase the possibility of a successful outcome, with maintenance of the transplanted kidney for as long as possible. Leukocyte typing and mixed lymphocyte culture are the most promising methods used currently.

In *leukocyte typing,* the leukocytes of the patient and a group of standard antiserums are used to characterize many or all of the strong human leukocyte locus A (HL-A) histocompatibility antigens on the human leukocyte membrane. This is done for both donor and recipient, the two patterns being compared to determine to what extent the donor is compatible with the recipient.

*Mixed lymphocyte culture* (MLC) is another method of detecting degrees of histocompatibility between donor and recipient. The lymphocytes of the donor and recipient are mixed in tissue culture. When significant antigenic differences exist between the two, the response will be transformation into blasts, DNA synthesis, and mitosis. The MLC does not differentiate between subtle differences in incompatibility.

Kidney transplantation is not performed across the ABO red blood cell antigen carrier. It is important that the blood types of donor and recipient be compatible.

Another relevant laboratory test is the *cytotoxic antibody test* which is measured by performing a direct cross match between the donor's lymphocytes and the recipient's serum much in the manner of HL-A typing.

The nurse should explain the histocompatibility matching tests to the patient and the family. In the event a living related donor is anticipated, it is possible that the family may place undue pressure on the successful match. If so, it is possible for a member of the transplant team to tell the family that the match was not appropriate and that a cadaveric kidney should be considered. This allows the family member who is unwilling and fearful to evade the donor situation while remaining in good family standing.

*Immunosuppression* In addition to preoperative histocompatibility tests, there are other methods to decrease antigen-antibody reactions *after* kidney transplantation.

*Pharmacologic agents* are the most commonly used immunosuppressive agents which minimize and prevent rejection episodes. These drugs are listed in Table 10-7. Azathioprine (Imuran), corticosteroids (usually prednisone), and antilymphocyte globulin (ALG) are the most commonly used drugs. Azathioprine is usually started 2 to 10 days before surgery, and corticosteroids are generally administered immediately before the transplantation. ALG is most often given, IM or IV, 5 to 7 days prior to surgery and for 2 to 3 weeks after.

*Thoracic duct fistulas* have been used, selectively, to deplete the body of lymphocytes. The duct is cannulated a week or more before surgery and drained of 3 to 7 liters of lymph per day. With a thoracic duct fistula, rejecting crises do not appear as soon, either with or without azathioprine and glucocorticoid medication.

*Patient counseling* Nurses in transplant and hemodialysis units are involved in the preventive aspects of rejection. If the patient chooses to know, the statistics of rejection should be made available by the physician. The patient may be aware of the possibility of rejection, having discerned this fact from other dialysis patients. Shifts in family dynamics often occur when renal transplantation is anticipated. Emotional reactions flow between family, donor, and recipient. Representative emotional reactions between donor, recipient, and family are seen in Fig. 10-5. Recipients of either a cadaveric kidney or one from a living, related donor have, in most instances, experienced economic pressures and disturbances in social roles prior to the transplant event. These disturbances and pressures are shared by the family unit. The nurse should support the transplant candidate and the family through the pressures of the pretransplant period.

**Second-level nursing care**  After recovery from the renal transplantation, the patient returns home on medications which must be taken to suppress rejection. Kidney transplant centers may have nurse clinical specialists who teach patients according to their specific learning needs about the medications which they are taking. These nurses may be "on call" to the transplant patient for questions and discussion of any problems or symptoms experienced.

**N**ursing Assessment  Rejection reactions generally occur during hospitalization, and their appearance and detailed care will be discussed under Third-Level Nursing Care. However, late reactions may occur gradually, over a long period of time.

The patient's *health history* may reveal a decrease in urine volume, some weight gain, and malaise. *Physical assessment* may reveal a slightly elevated body temperature and an elevated blood pressure. There may be some tenderness on palpation of the graft area. (All these findings may not be present in every patient.)

*Laboratory studies* are directed toward measurement of renal function. The nurse should be familiar with the findings. Blood urea nitrogen and serum creatinine levels may be elevated, creatinine clearance decreased, and proteinuria present.

**N**ursing Problems and Intervention  Major nursing problems for the patient experiencing late transplant rejection are *oliguria, fever, graft site tenderness,* and *hypertension.*

Intervention in the clinic or outpatient situation is limited to immediate care and referral to an appropriate facility for further care. The patient should be advised, by the physician, of any pertinent find-

ings. These findings should be reinforced by the nurse.

**Third-level nursing care**  Nursing care in this level is directed toward patients experiencing hyperacute and acute rejection reactions, as well as those entering the hospital with late (chronic) reactions.

**N**ursing Assessment  Early assessment of transplant rejection is essential if the process is to be halted or reversed. The time of occurrence of a reaction may be within minutes of the surgery or days to years later. The first rejection occurrence is most often seen within 2 weeks after surgery.

The patient's rejection signs and symptoms will vary somewhat from the hyperacute and acute types to the more chronic type. Physical assessment of the patient experiencing hyperacute and acute reactions will show an *increased body tem-*

**TABLE 10-7**
COMMONLY USED IMMUNOSUPPRESSIVE DRUGS

AZATHIOPRINE (Imuran), an antipurine
Acts to suppress antibody synthesis to the antigenic substance of the kidney and prevents rejection. Oral route usually; intravenous route available. Toxicity includes bone marrow depression with profound leukemia contributing to morbidity and mortality from infections; also hepatitis. May be given the day before transplantation; always administered when patient has his or her kidney intact.

PREDNISONE, a corticosteroid
Acts to inhibit development of cellular and humoral immunity by causing T lymphocytes to disappear from circulation; depression of antibody formation; anti-inflammatory effects by inhibition of granulocytes as they enter areas of inflammation. Oral route for prednisone; intravenous route for methylprednisolone. Toxicity includes cushingoid changes, peptic ulceration, thrombophlebitis, psychoses, hyperglycemia, myopathy, osteoporosis, hypokalemia, acidosis, impaired wound healing, and, with larger doses, aseptic necrosis of femoral heads and/or tibial plateaus. May be started 1 week prior to transplant.

CYCLOPHOSPHAMIDE, an alkylating agent
Acts to cause inhibition of delayed hypersensitivity by direct action on the immune system; has significant anti-inflammatory action. Oral route. Toxicity and side effects include sterile hemorrhagic cystitis, thrombocytopenia, alopecia, transverse nail ridging, skin hyperpigmentation, myelosuppression. May be given in place of Imuran with liver function problems.

ANTILYMPHOCYTIC GLOBULIN (ALG)
Produced by injecting lymphocytes into horses, goats, rabbits, and other animals. Lymphocyte source is from human lymph nodes, spleen, thoracic duct, thymus, and human cells in tissue culture. ALG production has varied in its standardization, thus each batch can vary in potency. It is postulated that it acts when given intravenously by absorbing and coating the outside of the lymphocytes. Complement is fixed by the antibody, and these cells are susceptible to phagocytosis by the reticuloendothelial system. There is a fall in peripheral lymphocytes. Suppresses cell-mediated immune reactions. Intramuscular route. Toxicity includes thrombocytopenia, inflammatory reactions at site of intramuscular injections, fever, hypotension, allergic and anaphylactic symptoms. May be given prior to transplantation and 30 days afterward.

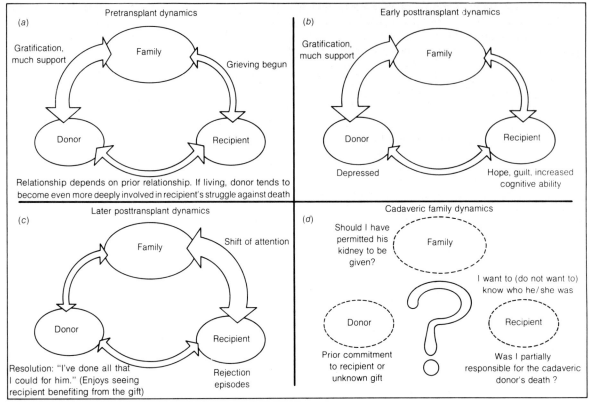

**FIGURE 10-5**
Schematic drawing which represents possible donor, recipient, and family dynamics during the
kidney transplant experience. Thick lines represent increased interactions; thin lines indicate
less dynamic interactions.

perature, *weight gain* (due to sodium retention),
*reduced urine volume, swelling over the graft side,
tenderness upon touching the graft site, irritability,
and restlessness.* Signs of the chronic rejection
response are detailed under Second-Level Nursing
Care.

Laboratory studies are performed, as indicated
under Second-Level Nursing Care, to aid the physician in diagnosing rejection reactions. Renal arteriography may be used to identify any vascular
changes.

**N**ursing Problems and Intervention   Major nursing
problems include *weight gain* and *oliguria,* as well
as *swelling and tenderness* at the graft site. These
are indicative of renal failure and a rejection reaction. Intervention is directed toward suppression of
the hypersensitivity reaction, where possible, or
surgical removal and hemodialysis, when suppression is ineffective. The physician will prescribe
therapy according to whether rejection is hyperacute, acute, or chronic.

*Hyperacute rejections,* due to preformed circulating antibodies, have no satisfactory treatment.
The transplanted kidney must be removed. Besides
the physical postoperative care, the patient and
family frequently experience disappointment and
depression. If the donor is a living relative, the guilt
at having "wasted" a family member's kidney may
be almost intolerable. The nurse should stress the
willingness with which the donor gave the kidney
and offer the hope of transplantation in the future
and hemodialysis in the present. The donor also
may reflect depression that the "gift" was in vain
and should be supported by the nurse.

*Acute rejection* is treated by increased dosages
of prednisone given orally (up to 300 mg daily) or
methylprednisolone given intravenously (1 to 3 g
daily or on alternate days). The high dose of glucocorticoids is maintained until renal function has improved, usually occurring in a week to 10 days. Dosages are gradually tapered to maintenance levels.
Azathioprine is maintained at the same dose or
reduced according to decreased glomerular filtra-

tion rates. ALG dosage is unmodified, and radiation to the kidney is commonly used as an antirejection measure. Radiation is used since lymphocytes are killed by small doses of radiation and since radiation is anti-inflammatory. Whole-body radiation was used formerly but has been abandoned, as has extracorporeal radiation to blood and lymph. Local radiation to the allografted kidney is used immediately after transplantation and during an acute rejection episode. The nurse caring for the patient in an acute rejection episode should support the patient and family with explanations of therapy during this crisis situation.

Host resistance is decreased by the drug and radiation therapy, increasing the patient's susceptibility to infection. Reverse or protective isolation may be required to exclude the patient from external infection. Occasionally, sterile environments are available, and the patient can receive this added protection.

*Chronic rejection* is very difficult to treat. Glucocorticoid doses are increased in the same manner as for acute rejection, with the gradual decrease in dosage lasting over a longer time period. Azathioprine, cyclophosphamide, and ALG doses may be left the same.

A chronic rejection episode is an irreversible event. Eventual graft removal and a return to maintenance hemodialysis will be necessary. Prednisone should be decreased to allow for adrenal recovery. Azathioprine may be discontinued abruptly.

Patients will need continuous nursing support whether they return to hemodialysis or go home with an, as yet, unrejected kidney. A detailed discussion of the care of patients receiving hemodialysis may be found in Chap. 14.

*Weight gain* and *oliguria* are treated as in chronic renal failure. This therapy includes fluid and sodium restriction, low-protein diet, and dialysis. A detailed discussion of this care may be found in Chap. 14.

**Fourth-level nursing care** After recovering from the acute phase of *acute* rejection, the patient returns home to begin careful monitoring of kidney function through urine output, blood pressure, and weight recordings, and taking any prescribed immunosuppressive agents and antacids. Once the acute rejection episode is past, the patient should be encouraged by the nurse to be hopeful about the future of the transplanted kidney and to be careful about taking the exact amount of prescribed medications.

The patient should be taught the symptoms of rejection and cautioned to notify the transplant unit if any occur. In addition, the patient is advised to be wary of infections because of decreased bodily resistance secondary to corticosteroids and cytotoxic agents. Because of changes in normal local defenses, the inflammatory process, and the cellular and humoral immune system, urinary tract infections due to the postoperative presence of a retention catheter, pneumonia, wound infection, and skin infections may occur following transplant surgery. Bacteria and opportunistic fungi are the greatest offending microorganisms. Mycobacterial, viral, and protozoal infections also occur. The nurse should encourage the patient and family to notify the transplant unit should any symptoms of infection occur. Direct contact with persons having a cold, a virus, or any other infection should be avoided.

In addition, the patient should be counseled to always take the Imuran (azathioprine) and prednisone in the ordered dosage. The dosage of these medications may be varied according to laboratory studies, and so the patient and family must be able to identify the correct drug and change the dosage as the physician alters the prescribed amount.

Family dynamics must also be assessed since the patient is now enjoying greater cognitive ability and a sense of well-being. Prior to transplantation the family structure may have shifted to accommodate the patient's illness. Social role functions of the patient on hemodialysis are partially or totally abdicated due to uremia. The transplant recipient may return to the family structure and assume previous role functions. This may disturb the family members who enjoyed having to meet dependency needs of a uremic patient. Further, sexual desire may increase in the transplant recipient, disturbing family stability. The transplant recipient also may experience overwhelming gratitude to a living related donor or guilt in the death of the cadaveric donor.

The euphoria of the immediate posttransplant period is replaced by the reality of drugs, rejection episodes, and change of appearance due to steroid medications. Patients may feel guilty that their bodies rejected the kidney.

The nurse in transplant units and clinics must be available to listen to the hopes, guilts, and stresses of the transplant patient and the family. The focus should be on the patient's ability to cope successfully with stress by pointing out positive coping strategies in the past.

The nurse should be aware that the patient has faced death previously and may contemplate kidney rejection as being equivalent to death. Hope can be offered by reminding the patient of drugs available to suppress rejection and of the reality of hemodialysis. If a transplant patient group exists in the area, the nurse may refer the patient so that mutual experiences can be shared.

Social service agencies can be utilized to assist with economic problems as can psychologists or psychiatrists who are members of the multidisciplinary transplant team. It is possible that the transplant recipient may be able to seek employment again through vocational rehabilitation agencies.

## AUTOIMMUNE RESPONSE

One of the more perplexing problems in medicine and immunology concerns the immunologic differentiation of "self" and "nonself." Major questions relating to this phenomenon are: How do the defense mechanisms of the body know when to attack (foreign protein) and when to tolerate self (body protein)? Why do people develop pathologic immune responses to their own tissue antigens? To date there is no simple or unified answer to this enigma. Current research has led to theories which may help to explain the development of autoimmunity and suggest new approaches in the treatment of patients who have an autoimmune disease. It is the intent of this section on the autoimmune response to define what the concept of autoimmunity means, to identify the nursing problems that arise owing to autoimmune diseases, and to identify what nurses can do to support these patients.

### Definition

The phenomenon of *autoimmunity* (autosensitization or autoallergic reaction) is thought to arise from the concept that an organism can react immunologically against itself. Basically it is believed to be a pathological process in which either *cellular* (lymphocytes) or *humoral* (antibodies) substances are produced against the body's own tissues. Apparently a breakdown occurs in the processes by which the body ensures that immune responses are directed against only foreign material; that is, the host loses the specific immune ability to recognize the body's own proteins (immunologic tolerance). A person, in a sense, develops a delayed or immediate hypersensitivity to the body's own cells or tissues which causes damage and even death. As a rule, the damage is concentrated in one organ or in one type of tissue.

### Theories of Causation

Over the years many theories have been proposed to explain the mechanisms and causes of autoimmune disease. It appears that the subject of autoimmunity is still vague in nature, and one can see that it is filled with many possibilities, probabilities, and some guesswork. Therefore, to eliminate confusion, only the most current and/or well-known theories will be summarized.

**Genetic theory** The genetic theory states that the predisposition to develop an autoimmune disease may be partially determined by genetic or hereditary factors. It is known, for example, that autoimmune conditions occur most often in families of affected individuals and that females are more frequently affected than males. Exactly how these genetic influences operate is still unclear.

**"Forbidden" clone theory** This theory contends that during embryonic development, a large number of *clones* (cells that are able to transmit "immunologic" memory to their descendants concerning specific antigens) of potential antibody-forming cells develop, each with a different immunologic pattern. Each antibody-produced clone has a corresponding *antigenic determinant* which is not present in the body or does not freely circulate in the body. These cells are, therefore, preadapted to react with the determinant (antigen). If a mutation occurs in lymphoid cells or if there is an activation of a "forbidden" clone of cells due to injury, disease, or a change in the body's metabolism, these cells will react with the body's own proteins and cause an autoimmune response.

**Tissue injury theory** The tissue injury theory states that an autoimmune response occurs after there is injury to the body's tissue such as with a myocardial infarction, general tissue damage after an automobile accident, or burn. The injury apparently alters the body's tissues to the point that the body can not recognize its own protein. Because of this loss of the ability to identify "self," an autoimmune response occurs to this supposed foreign tissue.

**Heterophil antigen** The heterophil theory suggests that autoimmunity occasionally develops because of the close resemblance of the body's own proteins (heterophilic antigen) to foreign antigens that enter the body. For instance, a certain strain of beta-hemolytic streptococcus releases a toxin that has an antigen structure similar to that of the heart muscle, heart valves, and synovial membrane. This antigen causes the immune system to develop autoimmunity against these tissues and is thought to produce rheumatic heart disease.

**Hapten theory** The hapten theory contends that a hapten enters the body and combines with body protein. The hapten itself is not antigenic to the body, but when it combines with body protein, it then can potentiate an autoimmune response. When this occurs, the body protein begins to act as a foreign antigen because of the way it was modified after it combined with the hapten. Conjugation of cell proteins with a hapten, such as a drug or industrial chemical, causes such autoimmune responses.

**Altered immune mechanism theory** The altered immune mechanism theory states that autoimmune diseases are related to and/or caused by alterations of the immune apparatus. This basic defect in one's capacity to generate certain immune responses is present prior to the onset of the autoimmune disease. As a consequence, it appears experimentally that animals are unable to recognize and suppress autoreactive lymphocytes. Therefore, "forbidden" clones of these autoreactive cells proliferate and create havoc with the body's own tissues.

In summary, there is no single explanation which can account for autoimmune diseases. Therefore, they must be viewed as the end result of an interaction involving several of these factors.

**Classification**

Currently classification of autoimmune disorders has been attempted in several ways. Categorization may be by: (1) Organ system, (2) operative immune mechanisms (humoral versus cellular), or (3) accessibility or nonaccessibility of antigenic determinants. Because there is much disagreement and confusion over the best way to categorize autoimmune disease, drawing up a list of these diseases is difficult, if not impossible. Therefore, Robbins and others offer, with great caution, lists of *probable and possible autoimmune diseases*[15] (Table 10-8).

**TABLE 10-8**
SOME AUTOIMMUNE DISORDERS IN MAN

| Organ or tissue | Disease | Antigen |
| --- | --- | --- |
| Thyroid | Hashimoto's thyroiditis (hypothyroidism) | Thyroglobulin Thyroid cell surface and cytoplasm |
| | Thyrotoxicosis (hyperthyroidism) | Thyroid cell surface |
| Gastric mucosa | Pernicious anemia (vitamin $B_{12}$ deficiency) | Intrinsic factor (I) Parietal cells |
| Adrenals | Addison's disease (adrenal insufficiency) | Adrenal cell |
| Skin | Pemphigus vulgaris Pemphigoid | Epidermal cells Basement membrane between epidermis-dermis |
| Eye | Sympathetic ophthalmia | Uvea |
| Kidney glomeruli plus lung | Goodpasture's syndrome | Basement membrane |
| Red blood cells | Autoimmune hemolytic anemia | Red blood cell surface |
| Platelets | Idiopathic thrombocytopenic purpura | Platelet surface |
| Skeletal and heart muscle | Myasthenia gravis | Muscle cells and thymus "myoid" cells |
| Brain | ? Multiple sclerosis | Brain tissue |
| Spermatozoa | Male infertility (rarely) | Spermatozoa |
| Liver (biliary tract) | Primary biliary cirrhosis | Mitochondria (mainly) |
| Salivary and lacrimal glands | Sjögren's disease | Many: secretory ducts, mitochondria, nuclei, IgG |
| Synovial membranes, etc. | Rheumatoid arthritis | Fc domain of IgG |
| | Systemic lupus erythematosus (SLE) | Many: DNA, DNA-protein, cardiolipin, IgG, microsomes, etc. |

SOURCE: Adapted with permission from I. Roitt: *Essential Immunology*, Blackwell, Oxford, 1971.

Probable autoimmune diseases:

1  Autoimmune hemolytic anemia

2  Hashimoto's chronic thyroiditis

3  Systemic lupus erythematosus

4  Rheumatoid arthritis

5  Lupoid hepatitis

6  Myasthenia gravis

7  Glomerulonephritic (nephotoxic) disease

8  Sjögren's syndrome

9  Autoimmune encephalomyelitis

10  Autoimmune thrombocytopenia purpura

Possible autoimmune diseases:

1  Polyarteritis nodosa

2  Systemic sclerosis (scleroderma)

3  Polymyositis-dermatomyositis

4  Autoimmune adrenalitis

5  Autoimmune orchitis

6  Pernicious anemia

The remainder of this chapter will discuss rheumatoid arthritis, lupus erythematosus, myasthenia gravis, polyarteritis nodosa, Sjögren's syndrome, polymyositis-dermatomyositis, scleroderma, and Hashimoto's thyroiditis as representative diseases with suspected autoimmune origins.

## RHEUMATOID ARTHRITIS

Rheumatoid arthritis is a chronic systemic disease characterized by nonsuppurative inflammatory changes in the body's connective tissues. It has a particular affinity for articular and periarticular structures of *diarthrodial joints* (those which possess a cavity and are freely moving). Knowledge of the diarthrodial joint and its synovial structure is essential to an understanding of the inflammatory changes of exudation and proliferation in joints, tendon sheaths, and bursae (see Chap. 31).

The bones in this type of joint are united by a joint capsule and by ligaments and tendons. The joint capsule consists of a dense fibrous connective tissue which merges with adjacent ligaments, tendons, periosteum, and fascia. The inner aspect of the joint capsule is lined by the synovial membrane that consists of layers of flat cells which cover the inner surfaces of the joint capsule and part of the articular cartilage. It is this vascular connective tissue that produces synovial fluid. The large capillary surface of the synovial membrane allows for formation of a dialysate of plasma which serves the needs of the cartilage. The important component of this fluid is a mucopolysaccharide called *hyaluronic acid* which supplies the viscosity needed for joint lubrication. This lubrication minimizes friction in the joints. The synovial fluid also provides oxygen and nutrients for the articular cartilage which covers the articular (joint) surfaces of the bones. This is an important function because adult articular cartilage lacks nerves and blood vessels.

### Theories of Causation

The etiology of rheumatoid arthritis in unknown. Investigation as to causation is being explored primarily in relation to autoimmune, infectious, hereditary, environmental, and psychosomatic factors.

**Autoimmune factors**  Impressive evidence supports the importance of an immunologic mechanism in the pathogenesis of rheumatoid arthritis. Evidence to support this theory was the discovery of the rheumatoid factor (RF) in the serum of patients with rheumatoid arthritis. This factor has an affinity for denatured gamma globulin probably in the patient's synovial membrane. It was this discovery that led to the classification of rheumatoid arthritis as an autoimmune disease.

**Infectious factors**  The inflammatory nature of rheumatoid arthritis implied an infectious process. However, overwhelming negative results of bacteriologic studies suggest that rheumatoid arthritis is probably not due to a bacterium. Attention is now focused on viruses because there are several viral infections that produce transient arthritis even though no virus has been found in the synovium.

**Hereditary factors**  It was noted by clinicians that rheumatoid arthritis seemed to occur most often within the same families, raising the question of heredity as a contributing factor. Several studies of twins support the possibility that rheumatoid arthritis occurs twice as often in people who are blood relatives and therefore are genetically predisposed or susceptible to this disease. These statistics suggest a hereditary influence, but no clear-cut genetic pattern has been identified.

**Environmental factors** Other researchers favor an environmentally based theory because of the following findings: (1) The onset for a large number of people has occurred in the spring of the year, and (2) many people have increased symptomatology when the humidity increases and the barometric pressure decreases.

**Psychosomatic factors** The literature abounds with research relating to the personalities and psychological mechanisms of patients with rheumatoid arthritis. There is little support for the theory that certain "personality types" relate to the cause of this disease, but the course of rheumatoid arthritis appears to be influenced by emotional factors.

### Pathophysiology

Rheumatoid arthritis usually starts insidiously. It generally begins with an inflammatory reaction in the joints.

**Joint manifestations** The inflammatory process of rheumatoid arthritis occurs especially in the synovial membrane and in the immediately subjacent joint capsule (Fig. 10-6). This *synovitis* is manifested by warm, red, swollen joints resulting from distention of tissue by the accumulation of edema fluid and inflammatory cells. This, in turn, produces much pain due to the pressure on sensory nerve endings. Consequently, the patient's mobility of the joint becomes quite limited. At this early stage the cartilage is likely to be quite normal. Often before the appearance of overt swelling, vague stiffness called "morning stiffness" will occur, as well as poorly localized aching. This stiffness is probably due to the overdistention of a normally slack joint capsule with fluid, coupled with inactivity during the hours of sleep. At the same time, people often demonstrate numerous constitutional symptoms which are probably due to the systemic inflammatory reaction. These include fever, loss of appetite, weight loss, fatigue, and generalized weakness.

In this inflammatory process, the synovium becomes infiltrated with a cellular material (chiefly lymphocytes and plasma cells) along with considerable edema, vascular congestion, and fibrinous exudate. Because of the inflammatory process there often is an increase in the amount and turbidity of synovial fluid.

Besides synovitis, *tenosynovitis* (inflammation of the tendon sheath) is common and most frequently affects the extensor and flexor tendons of the wrists (Fig. 10-7). This inflammation, in addition to causing pain, often presses on the nerves and

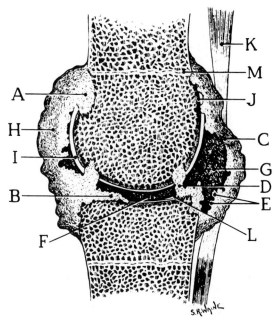

SYNOVIAL MEMBRANE

A - Invasion of Subchondral Bone
B - Erosion of Articular Cartilage (Pannus)
C - Fibrotic Area
D - Fibrous Adhesions
E - Multiple Villi

JOINT SPACE

F - Narrowed
G - Loculated Effusion

H - Laxity of Thickened Capsule and Ligaments
I - Articular Cartilage
J - Subchondral Bone
K - Muscle
L - Fibrocartilage
M - Old Epiphyseal Plate

**FIGURE 10-6**
Some changes in a synovial joint in rheumatoid arthritis. Compare with a normal synovial joint illustrated in Chap. 31. (*Reprinted with permission from Hamerman, D., Sandson, J., and Schubert M., "Biochemical Events In Joint Disease," Journal of Chronic Disease,* **16:**1963, p. 837.)

causes the development of the *carpal tunnel syndrome* (median nerve neuropathy).

If the inflammatory process becomes chronic, a secondary phenomena of *joint effusion* occurs. This represents the spilling into the joint space of the more mobile elements of the inflammatory exudate in the synovial membrane and joint capsule—mainly the exuded fluid and motile inflammatory cells. These effusions cause swollen boggy joints (Fig. 10-7). Knee effusions may be complicated by the development of popliteal (Baker's) cysts that often extend into the calf. The cysts are connected to the joint space and originate as a herniation directly from the joint, or via a bursa in the popliteal space.

As the inflammation continues, the synovial membrane begins to thicken and become shaggy and forms fingerlike projections called *villi* (hypertrophic villous synovitis). In addition, *subcutaneous nodules* or *granulomas* (aggregates of lymphocytes and plasma cells) form in these villi and in other connective tissue. The joint capsule also becomes markedly thickened by dense connective tissue. Granulation tissue gradually begins to form a *pannus* (scar tissue) which extends over the surface of the cartilage and then burrows into the subchondral bone. The basic pathologic process of rheumatoid synovitis is this development of chronic granulation tissue which erodes the adjacent cartilage, tendons, and in some cases subchondral bones and replaces it with a pannus. Atrophy of the subchondral and juxtarticular bones contributes to alterations in the shape of the joint and in the orientation of the opposing bones.

The exact events in the *pathogenesis* of rheumatoid joint inflammation are not clearly defined, but it seems that this process has an important immunologic component. It has been proposed that the antibodies produced by lymphocytes and plasma cells of the synovial membrane combine with antigens in the synovial membrane or with antigens in the synovial fluid. The antigen-antibody complexes that are formed may then fix and activate complement which causes the generation of numerous chemotactic substances. The polymorphonuclear leukocytes then ingest the complexes, form vacuoles, release lysosomal enzymes, and finally cause the cell to die. The enzymes released are believed to injure the articular cartilage and enhance pannus formation. The amount of damage done to the cartilage is a major factor in determining the degree of articular disability. If the bone becomes badly denuded of its cartilage and then atrophies, fibrous adhesions may form between the panni on the opposing joint surfaces. If these adhesions are extensive enough to obliterate most of or all the joint space, *fibrous ankylosis* occurs. *Bony ankylosis* (firm union) between bony surfaces occurs when there is complete obliteration not only of the joint space but of the joint itself. This interferes with motion of the joint and may cause total immobility.

In rheumatoid arthritis the connective tissue in periarticular structures and other connective tissues may also become chronically inflamed. This process weakens the tendons, ligaments, and other supporting structures of the joint resulting in in-

**FIGURE 10-7**
Hands of a 45-year-old man with rheumatoid arthritis of 2 years' duration. Note swelling of metacarpophalangeal (MCP) and proximal interphalangeal (PIP) joints and of the extensor sheath on the dorsum of the hands (tenosynovitis). (*Reprinted with permission from Rodman, G., et al., Primer on Rheumatic Diseases, 7th ed., JAMA, **224**:5, April 30, 1973.*

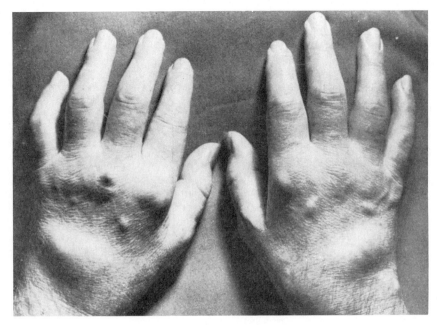

stability and/or partial dislocation (*subluxation*) of the joint (Fig. 10-8). This happens because joint stability is largely a function of ligaments that control motion of the joint. Subluxation also may occur if a joint loses vertical height owing to the wasting of cartilage or if subchondral bone collapses. Then, the ligaments become too long to provide adequate tension.

*Atrophy* of muscles commonly occurs owing to disuse and the generalized inflammatory effect on connective tissue in muscles (systemic myositis). This combined with the numerous other inflammatory effects on the articular and periarticular structures contributes to anatomical deformities, as well as to the loss of function of joints and peripheral structures.

**Systemic manifestations** As has been pointed out, rheumatoid arthritis is mainly a disease of joints, but major systemic manifestations may occur. Usually the extraarticular lesions are of minor significance, but when they do occur they may cause serious problems in terms of a patient's prognosis. The Arthritis Foundation divides the extraarticular manifestations into four categories: rheumatoid granulomas, major organ involvement, systemic complications, and the effects of vasculitis.

**R**heumatoid Granulomas As noted earlier, subcutaneous nodules occur most commonly over pressure areas and tendon sheaths. They have

also been encountered almost anywhere connective tissue is inflamed.

**O**rgan Involvement Generally, the specific symptomatology within the *cardiopulmonary system* depends greatly on the degree, location, and chronicity of the inflammation. Pathology of the heart is due to generalized inflammation or localized nodules. The cardiac manifestations are numerous, but very few cause significant functional impairment of the heart.

The *pleuropulmonary lesions* of rheumatoid arthritis are chronic, diverse, and generally non-life-threatening. They include chronic effusions, nodular pulmonary disease due to rheumatoid nodules, diffuse interstitial fibrosis, and Caplan's syndrome (rheumatoid pneumoconiosis).

*Ocular manifestations* have occurred primarily in the sclera, iris, and ciliary body due to generalized inflammation and localized subcutaneous nodules. Major complications of scleritis occur causing uveitis, cataracts, secondary glaucoma, and perforation.

*Neuropathy* is usually caused by local or generalized inflammation and sometimes by localized rheumatoid nodules. Diffuse neuropathy is the most common neuromuscular manifestation of rheumatoid arthritis. Most patients complain of numbness or burning pain and have decreased reflexes. Generally there are only minor motor and sensory changes with minimal residual problems. However, some persons develop rapid, generalized

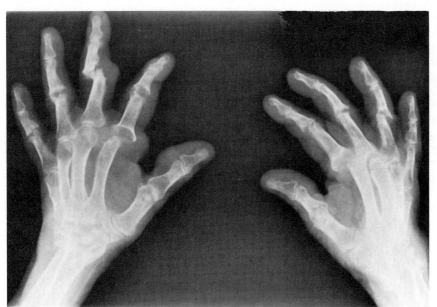

**FIGURE 10-8**
Both hands of a patient with advanced rheumatoid arthritis demonstrate marked and symmetrical destructive changes of the carpal, metacarpal-phalangeal and proximal interphalangeal joints bilaterally. Ulnar deviation of the phalanges, subluxations, loss of the ulnar styloid process, and characteristic sparing of the distal interphalangeal joints from this process are also evident.

neuromuscular involvement which leads to severe sensorimotor neuropathy with paralysis. Their prognosis for life is poor.

**S**ystemic Complications  Chronic active rheumatoid arthritis usually is associated with a moderate decrease in hemoglobin, but the level is rarely low enough to cause symptoms per se. The pathogenesis is obscure, but there is general agreement that the degree of *anemia* is related to the amount of inflammation or to an iron deficiency usually caused by chronic blood loss from aspirin gastritis.

Generalized *osteoporosis* is not uncommon (Fig. 10-9). The causes are probably multiple: (1) Excessive, generalized protein catabolism and poor nutrition, (2) loss of physical vigor and activity as the joint disease progresses, (3) in older people, the loss of the anabolic effects of androgens and estrogens, (4) the release of substances, such as prostaglandins, by the inflamed synovium that have been identified as calcium-releasing factors for bone, and (5) the inflammatory process, itself, within the joint. It is important to note that the degenerative process is aggravated by some medications such as corticosteroids. Most of the fractures that occur due to degenerative changes involve the collapse of the porotic dorsal and lumbar vertebrae which cause severe pain and disability.

A third systemic complication is known as *Felty's syndrome.* It occurs in persons with chronic rheumatoid arthritis and is characterized by *splenomegaly* and *leukopenia.* The splenomegaly is believed to be due to antinuclear antibodies (ANA) which have a particular affinity for leukocytes. Other features commonly associated with this syndrome are rheumatoid nodules, lymphadenopathy, chronic leg ulcers, peripheral neuropathy, anemia, thrombocytopenia, and Sjögren's syndrome. The dangerous aspect of this syndrome is a depression primarily of polymorphonuclear leukocytes, causing simple infections to become life-threatening.

People with chronic rheumatoid arthritis have the tendency to deposit amyloid (well-defined connective tissue components) in many tissues, perhaps because of prolonged inflammation or repeated immune stimulation. The clinical manifestations are varied and depend entirely upon the area of the body involved. The kidneys are particularly susceptible to *amyloidosis.*

**V**asculitis  In *rheumatoid vasculitis,* inflammatory changes occur in venules, arterioles, and arteries. Some patients develop digital arteritis which is limited to the fingers and may cause only focal ischemic lesions. However, total occlusion of the digital artery may occur causing frank gangrene of the entire digit.

*Raynaud's phenomenon* precedes or accompanies rheumatoid arthritis in about 10 percent of patients. Spasms of digital arteries cause blanching and numbness and even gangrene of fingers.

### Remissions and Exacerbations

Generally, the course of rheumatoid arthritis varies greatly and is characterized by remissions and exacerbations. At the onset predicting the course the disease will follow is almost impossible. In general, it follows one of two courses—*episodic* or *sustained.* In some cases rheumatoid arthritis may be very mild with its effects confined to a few joints causing little or no impairment of function. Three-fourths of all persons who have these early problems, for less than a year, will improve, and 15 to 20 percent may show complete remission.[16] However, it is more common for patients to have continuous chronic inflammation which leads to synovial hypertrophy, pannus formation, and cartilage destruction.

Factors associated with a poor prognosis, in respect to joint function, include: (1) Persistent disease for greater than a year, (2) onset before 30 years of age, (3) sustained disease, (4) presence of subcutaneous nodules, and (5) high titers of RF.[17]

It is important to note, however, that in observations extending over 10 to 15 years, 50 to 70 percent of the patients studied remained capable of full-time employment and after 15 to 20 years, only 10 percent were completely incapacitated.[18]

In a very small number of patients the disease pursues a rapidly progressive and systemically directed course which generally causes major joint destruction and frequently diffuse systemic vasculitis. It is then called *malignant rheumatic disease* or more commonly *vasculitis* (necrotizing inflammation of vessel walls).

### First-Level Nursing Care

On the basis of current evidence relating to the etiology of rheumatoid arthritis, prevention is not yet possible. Nurses should, however, be aware of some of the significant epidemiological factors related to this condition. Of the 3.6 million people with this disease, there seems to be a predilection for females (3:1) and a peak of onset between 20 and 50 years of age.[19] It is relatively rare in children and young adults. It does show an increasing prevalence with advancing age, beginning in middle life.

## Second-Level Nursing Care

It is important to detect rheumatoid arthritis at an early stage to give the patient a better chance for a more comfortable life. Patients are frequently diagnosed for the first time on an outpatient basis.

**Nursing assessment**   Rheumatoid arthritis may be insidious or acute in onset and may be manifest by mild or severe symptoms (Fig. 10-10). Patients will frequently seek medical attention when discomfort in the joints is interfering with normal functioning.

**H**ealth History   Usually the patient will describe an insidious process that started with fatigue, weight loss, morning stiffness, weakness, and vague muscle and joint pains. A loss of appetite may accompany the weight loss. A low-grade fever, hot and cold sensations, and excessive sweating are other initial symptoms. Finally, joint involvement will have increased in severity, the joints of the hands and feet being most frequently involved early in the disease. The patient will describe pain, swelling, and stiffness in these joints.

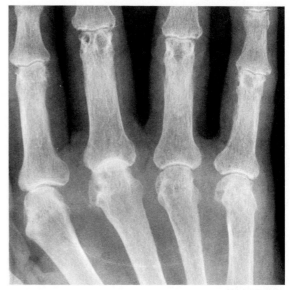

**FIGURE 10-9**
Magnified view of a patient's metacarpal-phalangeal and proximal interphalangeal joints of one hand demonstrating periarticular osteoporosis, joint space narrowing, and marginal erosions at synovial attachments. These changes are characteristic of rheumatoid arthritis.

**FIGURE 10-10**
Common clinical features of rheumatoid arthritis.

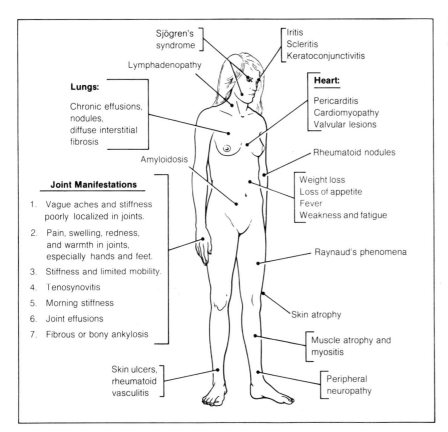

A minority of patients will have an acute onset of the disease in which there are very painful, swollen joints. These patients describe intense discomfort that is very debilitating.

**P**hysical Assessment  In assessing the patient for early signs of disease, an accurate record of vital signs, weight, and dietary history must be made. This will establish the degree of *fever,* if any, present due to the systemic inflammatory process, as well as the patient's nutritional status as measured by body weight. The nurse should have the patient identify the degree and location of any *pain* as well as the time when *fatigue* occurs. *Vasomotor instability* may be evaluated by observation for excessive body sweating and by the patient's subjective description of hot and cold sensations.

In adults, the joint symptoms originate in the hands (especially the metatarsophalangeal joints) and are generally bilaterally symmetric. Rheumatoid arthritis also affects large peripheral joints such as the knees, ankles, wrists, and elbows and other diarthrodial joints including the jaw (temporomandibular), intervertebral facetal joints, and the cricoarytenoid joints of the larynx. Painful swelling, especially in the wrist, commonly occurs and is due to tenosynovitis (Fig. 10-7). Patients often complain of paresthesias and pain in the first three fingers of the hand, which are often worse at night. The nurse should note whether there is any sensory loss in the median nerve distribution, weakness in abduction and opposition of the thumb, atrophy of the ulnar muscle, or tender swelling on the volar aspect of the wrist. Sometimes nerve conduction time across the wrist is prolonged and should, therefore, be evaluated with an electromyogram.

In assessing the patient, the nurse must observe which joints are involved and evaluate the pain, swelling, stiffness, range of motion, synovial thickening, and deformities. The *pain* generally is more evident on motion but also is present at rest. The *swelling* commonly is fusiform in appearance and presents a spindle-shaped appearance with thickening of the periarticular structures (soft-tissue swelling), especially around the proximal interphalangeal joints (Fig. 10-7). The *range of motion* is most accurately evaluated with a goniometer by a physical therapist, but may be observed grossly by the nurse. While observing for *inflammatory changes* in the periarticular areas, the nurse should look for subcutaneous nodules over pressure areas such as over the olecranon and along the shaft of the ulna. In addition it is important to

look for any unusual muscle atrophy or weakness with a grip test and a muscle test. The grip strength is usually decreased because of myositis, disuse, or pain in joints. The nurse should note the duration of *morning stiffness,* because it is a useful indirect measure of the activity of the rheumatic inflammatory process. If the patient has morning stiffness for longer than an hour, it is a sign that there is much inflammation in the involved joints.

An assessment of the patient's personality and emotional reaction to the disease is very important. Because of the chronic and debilitating nature of this process, depression and discouragement are common. Facial expression, body posture, and verbal affect give vital clues as to the patient's reaction to the disease.

**D**iagnostic Tests  (See Table 10-9). The nurse should tell the patient that several blood samples will be needed. If the patient has active, acute, or chronic rheumatoid arthritis, the erythrocyte sedimentation rate and C-reactive protein are usually elevated, often a mild anemia (normocytic hypochromic) is present, and there is a moderate hypergammaglobulinemia. The white blood cell and platelet counts are generally normal. The RF sometimes is present in early disease, but the presence of lupus erythematosus (LE) cells and ANA is uncommon.

If one joint in particular is inflamed, a *synovial fluid* analysis may be done. After explaining the test to the patient, the nurse should clean the surface of the skin over the joint with alcohol followed by a hexachlorophene scrub. Then the skin is painted with tincture of iodine and allowed to dry for at least 2 minutes before joint injection can be done. None of the synovial fluid findings is specific to rheumatoid arthritis, but three are particularly helpful in the diagnosis because they reflect varying degrees of inflammation within the joint: (1) A low synovial fluid complement, (2) the presence of RF in synovial fluid, and (3) the presence of RA cells. If after all these tests a reasonable question still exists about the diagnosis, a *synovial biopsy* can be done. If the pathology report indicates cell hyperplasia of the lining, edema of the synovial membrane, hyperemia, and infiltration of polymorphonuclear leukocytes, plasma cells, lymphocytes, and giant cells, then rheumatoid arthritis is much more likely. Early in the disease *x-rays* of the inflamed joints demonstrate only effusions and soft-tissue swelling. Rarely will definite bone changes be noted. It also is important to obtain chest x-rays and an EKG for the

**TABLE 10-9**
COMMON DIAGNOSTIC FINDINGS IN RHEUMATOID ARTHRITIS AND SLE

| Diagnostic Tests | Rheumatoid Arthritis | Systemic Lupus Erythematosus |
|---|---|---|
| HEMATOLOGY<br>Erythrocytes (RBC)<br>Normal: ♂ 4.8–5.5 million/mm³<br>♀ 4.4–5.0 million/mm³ | Anemia is common and proportionate to disease activity | Hemolytic anemia<br>Neutropenia |
| Leukocytes (WBC)<br>Normal: 5000–10,000/mm³ | Normal or slight leukocytosis | Mild leukopenia |
| Thrombocyte (platelet) count<br>Normal: 200,000–500,000/mm³ | Normal | Thrombocytopenia |
| Erythrocyte sedimentation rate (ESR)<br>Normal: 0–20 mm/h | Moderate to severe elevation | Moderate to severe elevation (85%) |
| SEROLOGY<br>Serum complement<br>Normal: 140–160 | Normal or somewhat elevated | Low |
| Serum protein or gammaglobulin<br>Normal: 1.3–3.2 g/100 mg serum | Moderate hypergammaglobulinemia | Hyperglobulinemia (50%) |
| Rheumatoid factor (RF)<br>Normal: negative | Positive (80%) | Positive (10–30%) |
| Antinuclear antibodies (ANA)<br>Normal: negative | Positive (25–60%) | Positive (95–100%) |
| Lupus erythematosus cell (LE cell)<br>Normal: not present | Present (10–25%) | Present (80%) |
| Anti-DNA<br>Normal: not present | Negative | Present |
| C-reactive protein<br>Normal: not present | Positive (90%) | Positive (30%) |
| Wasserman<br>Normal: negative | Negative | False positive |
| Coombs<br>Normal: negative | Negative | Rarely positive |
| URINE<br>Urinalysis<br>Normal: negative | Negative | Proteinuria, hematuria, and sometimes cells and casts |
| SYNOVIAL FLUID<br>Synovial fluid<br>Normal: negative | Purulent<br>Low viscosity<br>Decreased complement<br>RF present<br>Increased WBC | Noninflammatory<br>Decreased complement<br>ANA present |
| BIOPSIES<br>Synovial biopsy<br>Normal: negative | Nonspecific chronic synovitis | Rarely done |
| Skin biopsy<br>Normal: negative | Negative (rarely done) | Nonspecific chronic inflammation |
| X-RAYS<br>Normal: negative | Musculoskeletal<br>  Periarticular osteoporosis<br>  Loss of joint space<br>  Bone destruction<br>Cardiopulmonary<br>  Nodules<br>  Caplan's syndrome<br>  Pleurisy<br>  Honeycomb lung | Musculoskeletal<br>  Rarely bone destruction<br>Cardiopulmonary<br>  Pleural effusions<br>  Atelectasis<br>  Cardiomegaly |

present and future evaluation of possible visceral complications.

**Nursing problems and interventions** Because most problems resulting from rheumatoid arthritis are related to the degree of inflammation, the primary objective of nursing care is to reduce the inflammatory process. At this early stage of illness, *fatigue, weight loss, fever, vasomotor instability, joint symptoms,* and the disease's *chronicity* are all problems requiring knowledgeable, skilled nursing intervention. All these problems may be treated with a combination of *drug therapy, systemic rest,* and a *well-balanced diet* (Fig. 10-11). Specific intervention for joint symptoms and the emotional effects of chronicity will be discussed separately.

The initial drug of choice is *acetylsalicylic acid (aspirin).* Salicylates in doses of 5 to 6 g in divided doses after each meal and before bedtime are prescribed to reduce the pain, inflammation, and fever. It is important that the patient realize that a medication to cure this disease does not yet exist. The nurse must stress that to maintain the anti-inflammatory effect of salicylates, the aspirin must be

taken regularly in order to sustain a blood level between 18 and 25 mg percent.

Besides informing patients of the reasons for taking this medication, the nurse must teach them the common side effects that may occur—tinnitus, loss of auditory acuity, and gastric distress. The patient should take salicylates along with milk, food, antacids, or a large amount of water. The patient should be taught that tinnitus usually indicates high therapeutic blood levels. If tinnitus occurs, the dosage is usually decreased by one tablet every 2 or 3 days until it stops. The patient should also be made aware of the numerous preparations of aspirin that are available: plain, soluble, enteric coated, with buffer added or as a suppository. The plain tablet will be by far the least expensive form, but the enteric-coated form may be necessary because of gastrointestinal distress. Often it is not as well absorbed, so blood salicylate levels need to be checked more frequently (Table 10-10).

*Systemic rest* (total body) is helpful when a person's disease is active because rheumatoid arthritis is a systemic disease. The degree of rest depends on the type and severity of the manifestations at the

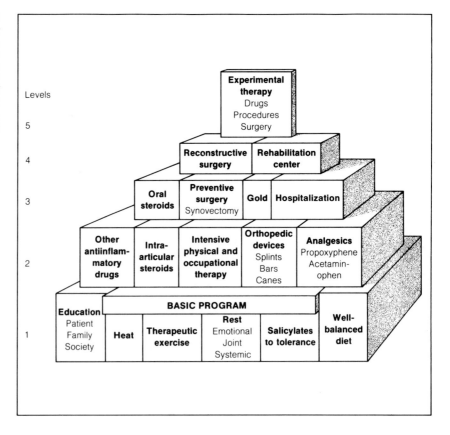

**FIGURE 10-11**
Pyramidal treatment program for rheumatoid arthritis. The measures in levels 2 to 5 are added to the basic program to meet specific therapeutic challenges. (*Adapted with permission from Smyth, C. J., "Therapy of Rheumatoid Arthritis—A Pyramidal Plan," Postgraduate Medicine,* **51:**6, 1972, p. 5.)

| Drug | Recommended Dosage and Frequency | Effect | Side Effects | Nurse should advise patient |
|------|----------------------------------|--------|--------------|------------------------------|
| Acetylsalicylic acid (aspirin) | 600–1200 mg po 4 times daily | Analgesic Anti-inflammatory Antipyretic | GI disturbance and bleeding, allergic reaction, tinnitus, platelet dysfunction, purpura, salicylism. | To take medication 30 min before exercise or physical therapy to lessen pain. To take medication regularly to maintain blood level of 18–25 mg%. To take medication with food, antacids, or milk. To use time-release forms at night if experiencing unusual morning stiffness. That buffered or enteric-coated tablets are available if plain aspirin is not tolerated. That ringing in ears generally means dosage is too high. The prothrombin time must be done every few months because aspirin prolongs prothrombin time. To store medication in sealed container. That urine may be green-brown. |
| Indomethacin (Indocin) | 25–50 mg po 2–3 times daily | Anti-inflammatory (nonsteroid) Analgesic Antipyretic | Nausea and vomiting, anorexia, epigastric distress, headaches, dizziness, vertigo, nervousness irritability, drowsiness, tinnitus, blurred vision, urticaria, leukopenia. | To take after meals or with antacids or milk. That if clinical relief is not obtained within 6–8 weeks, medication is generally discontinued. To store medication in light-resistant container. |
| Phenylbutazone (Butazolidin) or oxyphenbutazone (Tandearil) | 100 mg po 1–2 times daily for long-term use | Anti-inflammatory (nonsteroid) Analgesic | Nausea and vomiting, epigastric distress, reactivation and precipitation of peptic ulcer, aplastic anemia, agranulocytosis, leukopenia, thrombocytopenia with occasional purpura, cutaneous eruptions, stomatitis, edema, blurred vision, corneal deposits, headache, vertigo. | To take medication after meals or with milk. To discontinue medication immediately if cutaneous, hematologic, GI, or CV side effects appear. To carefully watch for signs of fluid retention—low-salt diet may be necessary. That this medication generally is prescribed with anticoagulant therapy. That if benefits of medication are not seen within 1 week, medication will be discontinued. That periodic CBCs are essential. To have ophthalmological exams every 6 months. |
| Gold salts | Gradually build to 50 mg IM weekly until ESR drops. Maintenance dosage: 50 mg every 3–5 weeks. | Anti-inflammatory | Dermatitis (ranges from erythema to exfoliative dermatitis), lesions of mucous membrane, metallic taste in mouth, thrombocytopenia, agranulocytosis, leukopenia and aplastic anemia, renal disorders (when taking Myochrysine ranging from proteinuria to nephrotic syndrome) nitritoid-type reactions (flushing, fainting, dizziness and sweating most common). | That frequent urinalysis is required. That medication may take several months to work. That if toxic side effects occur, medication will be discontinued until problems are resolved. Nurse should always give deep IM in upper gluteal quadrant and shake medication vigorously before giving IM. |
| Hydroxychloroquine sulfate (Plaquenil) or chloroquine (Aralen) | 200 mg po 2 times daily initially Maintenance dose: 200 mg po once daily | Anti-inflammatory | Skin eruption, unsteadiness, difficulties with visual accommodation, mild nausea and indigestion, leukopenia, peripheral neuropathy, dark pleomorphic skin lesions, corneal infiltrations, permanent retinopathy. | That medication may require several months to take effect. That ophthalmological evaluation is mandatory every 3 months. To wear sunglasses if exposed to bright light for an extended period of time. To store medication in light-resistant container. |
| Prednisone or its equivalent | Use the least amount that will control the rheumatoid inflammation. 10 mg po taken every morning is the upper limit except for acute flare-up | Anti-inflammatory | Serious disorders of any of the major systems. The majority of side effects are in fact manifestations of the hyperadrenal state (Cushing's syndrome): hirsutism, acne, moon face, abnormal fat deposit, purple striae, obesity with increased appetite, hyperglycemia with glucosuria, edema, hypertension, congestive heart failure, emotional disturbance. Also negative nitrogen balance, osteoarthritis, decreased wound healing, GI distress, premature cataracts occur. | To take oral preparation after meals. That routine checks of vital signs, weight, lab studies are vital. To never stop or change the dosage of the medication without medical advice. To store medication in light-resistant container. |
| Ibuprofen (Motrin) | 300–400 mg po 3–4 times daily | Anti-inflammatory (nonsteroid) Analgesic; antipyretic | GI distress, skin rashes, dizziness, amyblyopia, decreased prothrombin time. | That CBCs plus prothrombin times should be checked regularly. |

time. In mild disease, generally 2 to 4 hours spread out over the day is suggested. The nurse should stress the importance of a firm mattress and necessary supportive devices (small pillows under the neck or between the knees) in order to help the patient maintain normal posture and to prevent flexion deformities which are so common in this disease. Often patients complain that they feel worse after resting because they experience stiffness upon rising. An explanation by the nurse of what is causing the temporary stiffness helps to allay the patient's fears that the rest harms rather than helps.

Finally, the nurse must stress the importance of a *well-balanced diet.* There is no specific food known to be contraindicated, and generally there is no need to use supplemental vitamins. If a patient is overweight, a weight reduction diet is necessary. By losing weight the patient will lessen the strain on weight-bearing joints.

**Joint Disturbances**   The nurse's primary objective in providing care for involved joints is to reduce the pain, stiffness, and inflammation, to preserve function, and to prevent any deformities. Often the treatment program consists of increasing the dose of aspirin or trying a different nonsteroidal anti-inflammatory or antimalarial agent, plus prescribing analgesics, intraarticular injections of corticosteroids, physiotherapy, and systemic and articular rest (Fig. 10-10).

As pointed out earlier the dosage of salicylates varies with their effectiveness in relieving the pain and inflammation. Sometimes patients are unable to tolerate high doses of aspirin or it is not effective enough, so nonsteroidal anti-inflammatory agents such as phenylbutazone (Butazolidin), indomethacin (Indocin), and ibuprofen (Motrin) may be prescribed (Table 10-10).

*Phenylbutazone* (Butazolidin) and *oxyphenbutazone* (Tandearil) have anti-inflammatory and analgesic effects. The reason they are not used regularly for rheumatoid arthritis is because they frequently produce serious toxic effects. These include peptic ulcer, dermatitis, stomatitis, sodium and water retention, and hematologic side effects of anemia, leukopenia, and thrombocytopenia. Because of these toxic effects, it is necessary for the patient to have weekly blood counts for the first few months. Once the patient is stabilized, only monthly checks are necessary. Besides informing the patient of these potential problems, the nurse should advise the patient to cease taking the medication and see the physician if any of these problems

begin to develop. Generally, these drugs are not recommended for long-term use because of the frequency of the side effects and the lack of sustained benefits.

*Indomethacin* (Indocin) is a nonsteroidal anti-inflammatory agent that produces anti-inflammatory, analgesic, and antipyretic effects. Although it is not as toxic as Butazolidin, it still causes numerous side effects. These include headache, nausea and vomiting, anorexia, peptic ulcer, abdominal pain, diarrhea, depressions, mental confusion, and psychosis. The patient should be advised of these potential problems and be warned against driving and doing hazardous activities while taking this medication. Generally this drug is not recommended for long-term use because of the frequency of the side effects and the lack of sustained benefits. It appears that Indocin is used most frequently at bedtime to help relieve morning stiffness.

*Ibuprofen* (*Motrin*) is a relatively new nonsteroidal drug that produces an anti-inflammatory and analgesic effect. It is given to people who cannot tolerate aspirin. The most frequent adverse reaction is gastrointestinal including abdominal distress, pain and cramps, indigestion, epigastric pain, bloating, nausea and vomiting, ulceration, skin rashes, dizziness, amblyopia, and decreased prothrombin time. Besides teaching the patient to watch for these adverse reactions, it is important for the nurse to make sure blood counts and prothrombin times are checked periodically.

More commonly, a *pure analgesic* drug such as acetaminophen (Tylenol) or propoxyphene hydrochloride (Darvon) is given along with aspirin. It is important for the nurse to explain that these medications cannot be substituted for aspirin because they do not relieve the inflammation.

If patients continue to have persistent constitutional signs and symptoms and arthritic complaints after being on salicylates for several months, *antimalarials* may be prescribed. *Hydroxychloroquine sulfate* (*Plaquenil*) 200 mg/day or *chloroquine* (*Aralen*) 200 mg/day appear to produce an anti-inflammatory effect, but the benefit is seldom evident in less than 3 months and the maximum improvement often requires many months. The incidence of side effects is directly related to the dosage. Their most serious side effect is a tendency to produce irreversible retinopathy and retinal pigmentary changes which can cause blindness. Should any such symptomatology occur, the medication should be discontinued immediately. The initial and less serious side effects include malaise, headache, nausea, vomiting, and skin rash. If either of these drugs is used, it is very important for the patient to have an ophthalmological evaluation at least every 3 to 6 months and to wear sunglasses if prolonged exposure to light is anticipated.

Sometimes *intraarticular injections of long-acting corticosteroids* are used to relieve the pain for patients with acute inflammation of a single joint or a few joints. This is a nonspecific local technique aimed only at local suppression of inflammation within the joints. The knees, ankles, shoulder, elbows, wrists, and joints of the hands are most accessible for these injections. It is wise for the nurse to be aware that this procedure may introduce an infection. Therefore the site of the injection should be prepared appropriately. The nurse should advise the patient to look for any signs of infection and to rest the joint for a few hours after the injection. A number of long-acting synthetic steroids are available for use. The total dose depends on the size of the joints. The duration of the effect is generally 1 to 2 weeks in active joints and may even be as long as several months. Injections may be repeated every 2 to 3 weeks for several times and then every 6 to 8 weeks. If relief of pain and inflammation after the injection lasts less than a week, repetition of the procedure is not advisable. Often a synovectomy is considered at this point.

In addition to medications, *physiotherapy* is prescribed to provide physical agents to relieve pain and morning stiffness, to relax muscle spasms in order to help prevent deformities, to strengthen weakened muscles and improve function, and to shorten the period of disability from the disease. Several general types of physical therapy are used for patients with rheumatoid arthritis (Fig. 10-11). They include *heat, cold, massage, rest,* and *exercise.*

*Heat* may be applied locally or systemically and be dry or moist. The primary reasons for local applications of heat are to relax muscles, improve local blood flow, mobilize edema, and enhance analgesia. Heat is applied systemically to promote muscle relaxation and analgesia and to increase metabolism, pulmonary ventilation, and oxygen consumption. Many arguments remain regarding what effect these treatments have and which are most beneficial. In general, one finds that simple forms of heat, such as hot packs, hot tub baths, and hot paraffin baths, are used most often to relieve pain and relax muscles. Because of these effects, heat is frequently applied before the patient does any exercise.

*Cold* is also used but to a lesser degree because of the lack of evidence to support a therapeutic effect. Patients often state that cold does

decrease pain locally, especially during acute flare-ups.

A gentle stroking *massage* is sometimes used to induce muscle relaxation. Although deep massage increases the peripheral blood flow, it should not be used because it causes muscle contractions and pain. Massage should not be done directly to an actively inflamed joint but rather around surrounding muscles.

*Therapeutic exercise* is currently an important type of physiotherapy to preserve or improve range of motion in inflamed joints, to prevent muscle atrophy and increase muscle bulk, to maintain a useful pattern of joint motion, and to achieve maximum function of the upper and lower extremities. A patient's exercise program is generally prescribed on the basis of a physical examination and muscle and joint tests done by a physical therapist, occupational therapist, and physiatrist.

The nurse's responsibilities in regard to physical therapy are numerous. First, one should note what the purpose of the program is—muscle strengthening, relaxation, reeducation, or maintenance of range of motion and coordination. Specific exercises should then be prescribed. Often, the nurse can teach the patient about the more basic maintenance exercises that can be done at home. Obviously, in order to do this, the nurse must understand the principles behind the exercises, their purpose, and how to do them.

The nurse must know the importance of maintaining normal range of motion in all joints and keeping muscle strength at its maximum, while minimizing stress on the joint surfaces. This is necessary because muscle strength around involved joints will relieve stress on cartilage, protect normal joint function, and ensure the preservation of range of motion. The basic types of exercise are passive, isometric, isotonic, and resistive.

*Passive* exercises are implemented when the physical therapist or nurse moves the part while the patient relaxes. The objectives of this type of exercise are to prevent joint adhesions and shortening of muscles, and to mobilize edema while maintaining normal range of motion. They are initially used several times a day to aid the bedfast patient who is acutely ill and has severely inflamed joints.

*Isometric* (static or "muscle setting") exercises are done when the patient exercises muscles without moving the joint. These exercises often are used by patients with swollen and painfully inflamed joints or severely damaged joints, to preserve muscle strength. This type of exercise is accomplished by tightening muscles without moving the joint, holding them tense for a count of 6, then relaxing then for a count of 10. This cycle is generally repeated several times during the day until the patient can progress to active joint exercises.

*Isotonic* exercises are those in which motions are performed by the patient without assistance or resistance. They help to maintain or improve muscle strength and joint range of motion.

*Resistive* exercises are active exercises accomplished by the patient with additional resistance, either manual or mechanical. The major objective of any resistive exercise is the development of strength. The nurse should be aware that resistive exercises are performed primarily in non-weight-bearing positions to avoid additional trauma to the joint. Generally any of the active exercises should be performed initially three to five times on four different occasions daily. As the patient progresses, the number of repetitions will be increased to 10 or 20.

The nurse should keep in mind several precautions while supervising any of these exercises. Patients should not be encouraged to do exercises to the point of unusual pain or to do them quickly. Pain should not last longer than one-half hour after exercise; if it does, it is a sign that the exercise may be too strenuous. Often, advising the patient to take pain medications before they do their exercises is helpful. Exercises should be performed slowly because rapid motions fatigue muscles quickly, and a sudden jerk may cause damage to the joints. The nurse should stress the following facts about the patient's exercise program. A balance between exercise and rest in order to prevent unnecessary physical and emotional fatigue is imperative, for overactivity often causes unnecessary fatigue and pain. In addition, patients should do their exercises regularly (two to four times per day), at home, as a preventive measure. Frequently, written instructions serve as a reminder to the patient of how and when to do exercises and how to prepare the necessary equipment, as with a paraffin bath.

Besides supervising some of these exercises, the nurse can continually assess the patient's ability to ambulate and transfer, the type of gait used, and the posture assumed when lying down, sitting, and walking. It is not uncommon for patients to complain of much stiffness when they first stand up. The nurse should suggest that before standing up the patient limber up both knees by flexing and extending them. Posture is also very important since faulty alignment in sitting and standing favors fatigue,

strains, articular irritation, and deformities, while hindering proper functioning of the thoracic and abdominal organs.

In addition to systemic rest, research has shown that *localized rest* of an inflamed joint is helpful (Fig. 10-11). This generally is done with bed rest or with orthopedic supports or splints. The splint not only provides rest for the inflamed joint, but relieves spasms and pain and, over time, prevents deformities or reduces those already present. The nurse should advise the patient to remove all supports every day so that range of motion exercises can be done. It is important for the nurse to know that the splints are initially made by the occupational therapist to fit the shape of the extremity, with or without deformities. This is necessary because forceful extension of joints will only aggravate flexor muscle spasms and pain. Over time, the pain, muscle spasms, and flexion deformities generally decrease. Therefore, every 1 or 2 weeks the splints are reshaped to fit the joint again. Patients should be advised to wear the splints as much as possible, especially at night when involuntary flexion occurs and when the patient moves around and easily bumps the joints.

**C**hronicity   Knowledge of the progression of this disease and fear of its chronicity often cause patients to become *anxious* and *afraid* before and after being diagnosed with rheumatoid arthritis. The nurse must remember that no matter what the degree of disease activity is, individuals will need a great deal of reassurance, honesty, emotional support, and education. Nurses must work to motivate the patient and to prevent unnecessary worry and depression. Being totally honest with the patient in lay terms about the nature of the disease, its treatment, limitations, and prognosis often helps to develop a trust relationship. Ideally, this will help to inspire confidence and permit the patient to relax. Often it is a good idea to get the patient involved with outside interests or activities, so that total concentration is not upon the illness. Referring the patient to a recreational therapist may be necessary and desirable.

**Third-Level Nursing Care**

It is important to regularly follow patients with rheumatoid arthritis in order to promptly identify and treat acute exacerbations or complications. Nursing assessments and interventions are vitally important in the prevention and treatment of any deformities and complications.

**Nursing assessment**  At times, the conservative treatment program does not control the inflammatory process, and a severe exacerbation or a major complication occurs. At this point, the patient must be hospitalized for the purpose of continued evaluation with diagnostic tests as described earlier.

**H**ealth History  Many of the symptoms that patients experience at this point in time are the same problems that occurred earlier in the disease process (see Second-Level Nursing Care), except many have become chronic problems or are more severe. They generally are due to the continued inflammatory process of rheumatoid arthritis.

**P**hysical Assessment  To assess these problems, the nurse must follow the patient's vital signs, weight, and laboratory studies while regularly evaluating the degree of morning stiffness, weakness, and fatigue.

Total physical assessment of involved joints is particularly important. The redness, swelling, and pain that may not have been as apparent early in the disease are prominent now. The covering skin often appears purplish red instead of brightly erythematous. The joint is warm to touch and painful to move. Surrounding muscles exhibit weakness and atrophy from disuse. Range of motion and normal function are severely limited. Muscle extension over affected joints is especially reduced.

Actual joint deformity may be present in the form of flexion contractures, particularly of the fingers, knees, and hips. Two common deformities of the fingers are referred to as "boutonnière" and "swan neck" deformities (Fig. 10-12). Ulnar deviation may be observed as the patient's fingers devi-

**FIGURE 10-12**
The two common deformities seen in rheumatoid arthritis of the fingers are the boutonnière deformity and the swan neck deformity. The *boutonnière lesion* is produced by a synovitis of the proximal interphalangeal joint with stretching of the central tendon slip and the lateral bands. The *swan neck lesion* is the result of contracture of the lateral bands with hyperextension of the proximal joint and flexion of the distal phalanx. (*Reprinted with permission from Physical Therapy, Journal of the American Physical Therapy Association, vol. 44, no. 8.*)

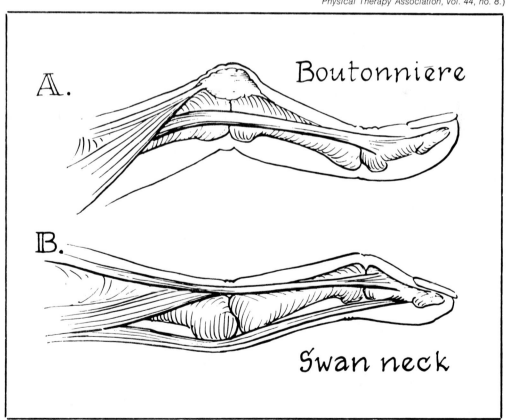

ate, at the metacarpal-phalangeal joints, inward and laterally toward the ulnar side of the wrist. Subluxation, or partial dislocation, of joints may be present (Fig. 10-8). Torn ligaments and tendons may also have occurred, contributing to joint instability, malfunction, and fatigability.

Continued synovitis with synovial membrane proliferation and joint effusion may result in palpable, swollen "boggy" joints. If the inflammatory process is not controlled, fibrous or bony ankylosis results. These affected joints are detectable by partial or total inability to flex or extend a particular joint.

Detailed descriptions of the patient's ability to do self-care, to ambulate or transport, and to tolerate activity should be made *before* a plan of intervention is determined.

**D**iagnostic Tests   Laboratory tests often will show a consistently increased titer of RF in the serum, a depressed synovial fluid complement, and a marked hypergammaglobulinemia. A patient might also demonstrate continued anemia, leukocytosis, increased sedimentation rate, elevated temperature, and increased heart rate. Synovial biopsies commonly reveal new villous growth covered with lymphoid nodules and plasma cells. Particular attention is paid to the x-rays, for they often show erosions in the subchondral bone and articular cartilage as well as deformities of the joints (Table 10-9, Figs. 10-8, 10-9, and 10-12).

**Nursing problems and interventions**   Weight loss, anemia, chronic fatigue, fever, and morning stiffness continue to be debilitating problems for the patient. As the disease progresses, however, the *joint inflammation* and the *systemic complications* become the predominant focus of nursing and medical interventions.

The continuing objective of therapy is to reduce the inflammatory process. Interventions include *medications* (particularly gold and corticosteroids), a *high caloric diet, total bed rest, heat, physical therapy, occupational therapy, traction, surgery* and, finally, *immunosuppressive agents* (Fig. 10-11).

**J**oint Inflammation   Any diarthrodial joint may be affected by rheumatoid arthritis. Symptoms are highly dependent on the joint involved. Depending on the actual joint affected, interventions may vary somewhat, for example, in the application of heat. Ambulation or transport assistance will also differ between a patient with hip involvement and a pa-

tient with cervical spine involvement. Nursing interventions must vary accordingly and be highly individual to the patient.

*Drug therapy*   Frequently *gold* therapy is instituted for the patient whose disease is uncontrolled within a few months by a conservative treatment program (Table 10-10). Gold salts remain the mainstay in long-range control of rheumatic inflammation in early rheumatoid arthritis because they are generally safer than oral steroids. Although it is unclear how the drug acts, it does appear to decrease inflammation. The nurse should always thoroughly shake the medication before giving a deep intramuscular injection, in order to prevent local irritation. The patient generally is given a "test" injection of 10 mg to check for an allergic reaction. If there are no untoward local or systemic effects, 25 mg will be given 1 week later. Thereafter, 50 mg/week is administered until a total dose of 1 g has been given or until side effects occur. If the patient shows no definite improvement within 12 weeks, the injections are stopped. If there is improvement, the injections are reduced to a maintenance dose of 50 mg every 3 to 5 weeks.

Side effects may occur such as photosensitivity and damage to mucous membranes, skin, kidneys, and bone marrow. The most frequent problems are a skin rash that itches and scales slightly and a metallic taste in one's mouth. Frequently mouth ulcers occur later. If gold treatment is continued at this point, severe exfoliative dermatitis may occur. It is very important for the nurse to check for any of these problems before giving the patient another injection. If gold is continued when proteinuria occurs, the patient runs the risk of a full-blown nephrotic syndrome with possible permanent kidney damage. The most effective agent for treatment of any of these toxic side effects is corticosteroids.

If the patient does not respond to gold, *corticosteroids* are prescribed (Table 10-10). Corticotropin and synthetic adrenal corticosteroid hormones (ACTH) are the most potent of all anti-inflammatory agents in the treatment of rheumatoid arthritis. We now are aware of the many serious side effects of these drugs when used over a long period of time. Therefore, use for rheumatoid arthritis is reserved for patients who are unable to function in activities of daily living because of continuous pain and inflammation despite treatment with other medications such as aspirin and gold. Corticosteroids also may be used when patients have an acute onset of rheumatoid arthritis with marked systemic manifestations. Corticosteroids should be given in addition to, and not as a substitute for, aspirin because they do not prevent the progression of joint destruction. The primary objective in giving these drugs is to lessen the symptoms of the disease. Unfortunately, while most patients initially respond rapidly to steroids, suppression of the disease does not continue, and progressively higher doses are often required. The well-known side effects of these higher dosages do not justify long-term administration (refer to Chap. 5).

The suggested initial dose is between 5 and 15 mg and is to be taken once every day in the morning. This dose should be maintained 4 to 6 weeks and then slowly tapered to the lowest possible dose per day. Serious side effects appear to rise sharply in patients who take greater than 10 mg per day for a long period of time.

The nurse should stress to the patient how important are regular physical examinations and routine laboratory tests. The patient's vital signs and weight should be followed, and any significant changes in the urinalysis, blood sugar, blood count, serum electrolytes, and chest x-rays noted. Should any of these patients require surgery, they are routinely given additional amounts of corticosteroids to avoid the risk of postoperative adrenal insufficiency. It is important for these patients to carry a card that states they are receiving steroid therapy.

*Diet therapy* Besides providing the additional medications of gold or corticosteroids, the nurse provides other supportive measures. Sometimes a *high caloric diet* with high protein is recommended if a patient's weight significantly decreases. Giving iron supplements generally is not helpful for the anemia, because it is related to the disease activity and recedes as the disease is brought under control with anti-inflammatory medications. If a patient develops anemia secondary to chronic blood loss, then iron is prescribed. It often becomes necessary for the patient to increase the number of hours of rest each day to lessen the fatigue and to give the total body a chance to rest physically and emotionally.

*Bed rest* In severe disease, *total bed rest* may be necessary until one sees objective and subjective improvement. There are many arguments against complete and total bed rest because of the numerous effects of prolonged immobility. Once improvement occurs and stabilizes for about two weeks, this rest schedule may be liberalized, depending on the situation. Should the patient be required to

spend many hours in bed, it becomes crucial for the nurse to pay close attention to prevention of any complications due to immobility itself. The equipment used to facilitate bed rest includes a firm mattress for maintenance of good posture and items such as foot boards, splints, and sandbags to help the patient maintain proper body alignment. All these efforts are directed toward prevention of flexion deformities. Proper positioning with supportive devices plus repositioning the patient every 2 hours is essential. It is wise to place the patient in a supine position, with supportive devices like trochanter rolls, much of the time with joints extended. Because in most diarthrodial joints the flexor group of muscles is stronger, patients will have a greater tendency to want to flex their extremities. Some supportive equipment can be deleterious if used improperly. For example, a big pillow under the patient's head or knees only encourages flexion deformities. When the patient begins to feel better and gets up more often, it is important to teach the value of gradually increasing exercise along with properly supporting any weakened joints with canes, splints, and metatarsal bars.

*Heat* Hubbard tank therapy and/or warm moist compresses are also used to facilitate muscle relaxation and relief of pain. It must be remembered, however, that if joints are red and swollen, applying heat locally may only aggravate them. This seems to be a very individualized response and needs close evaluation. Heat application may also be in the form of dry heat (heating pads), ultrasound, or diathermy. Paraffin baths for painful fingers and hands may be advised and the technique taught to the patient, as necessary. Warm tub baths and showers, where physically possible, are often the simplest way of achieving increased comfort and mobility from warmth.

*Physical therapy* Active exercises may be contraindicated when joints are acutely inflamed, but passive range of motion should be provided to prevent contractures, mobilize edema, maintain muscle strength, and lessen the severity of the generalized stiffness. Once improvement occurs, the patient should be encouraged to perform active exercise three or four times per day while increasing overall activity. This exercise should help the patient to lessen the generalized body stiffness and weakness due to myositis and disuse.

The physical therapist will continue to evaluate joints and muscles in greater detail. Assistive devices that the patient might need such as canes, crutches, or braces will be suggested. The nurse should remind the patient not to aggravate any flexion deformities or weaknesses in the joints. When the patient does get up, providing supportive devices such as splints and braces will lessen the chance of a problem. A close evaluation of the patient's gait will provide information about the needs that the patient might have for properly supportive shoes.

It is quite common for Plastizote inserts and metatarsal bars and pads to be put into shoes. The inserts relieve the flattened arches, and the bars decrease the pressure on painful metatarsal heads. Roomy shoes or properly fitted orthopedic shoes are helpful for painful, arthritic feet. Besides relieving pain, such devices help to provide balance. It is important for the nurse to advise the patient to wear good supportive shoes with a snug fit at the heel and a good leather sole.

*Occupation therapy*  Occupational therapists make detailed assessments of the patient's upper extremities in particular and then teach preventive exercises and provide any necessary assistive equipment for activities of daily living. Such assistive devices as raised toilet seats and chairs, grab bars, and zippered clothes all help the patient to maintain independence. Catalogs of such equipment are available to the patient and nurse through the Arthritis Foundation.

The occupational therapist can teach the patient work simplification and preservation techniques that can lessen the rate of joint destruction and prevent the occurrence of deformity. Besides teaching the patient to do appropriate exercises to maintain muscle strength and range of motion, the occupational therapist stresses the importance of conserving energy, respecting pain, and avoiding deforming postures and forces.

*Traction*  Skeletal traction may be used to relieve symptoms such as pain, to improve function, and to correct deformities and prevent progression of the disease. Skeletal traction is used mainly in the lower extremities to correct flexion deformities of the hips and knees and subluxation of the knees. If this works, one can expect to see results within 1 or 2 weeks. At that point a plaster cast is applied for 2 to 4 weeks while physical therapy exercises are begun. (See Chap. 40 for a discussion of traction.)

*Surgical intervention*  If medical measures such as casts and splints, traction, or corrective exercise fail to correct deformities, then one of the following

may be considered: synovectomy, manipulation of the joint, or surgery of juxtaarticular connective tissue, joints, or bones.

The ultimate selection of the appropriate procedure depends upon many things such as the stage of the patient's disease, age, motivation, the joint involved, and the type of deformity. It is important for the nurse to be aware of the patient's overall condition including weight and general physical well-being. Although active disease is no longer seen as a deterrent to surgery, being aware of the most recent results of diagnostic tests is still important. Besides the patient's current physical assessment, the nurse must be aware of the patient's current medical treatment program. It is important to note whether a person is taking steroids because of the predisposition to suppurative infections after surgery. However, this is not a contraindication to surgery. If a patient is taking these medications, a more gradual rehabilitation program is established. Once a total assessment has been made of the patient, the orthopedic surgeon decides which procedure needs to be done.

A *synovectomy* may be performed in order to prevent further destruction of bone and cartilage. In a synovectomy part or all of the synovial membrane of the joint is removed to prevent recurrent inflammation. The rationale for this procedure is based on the current research which suggests that the basic pathophysiology responsible for joint destruction occurs in the synovial membrane. Therefore any procedure which removes this tissue helps prevent further joint damage. It is important that the nurse explain the objectives of the surgery and what can be expected postoperatively. Synovectomies are regarded as palliative procedures, because apparently it is impossible to remove all the synovium, allowing the disease to recur. Research has shown that the regenerated synovium, for unknown reasons, appears to cause lesions that are milder and therefore less destructive. Also, the immediate results, especially 1 to 3 years after synovectomies, indicate that there is definite pain relief and improvement in weight bearing and in the ability to use the joints. Postoperatively, most patients experience localized pain and edema around the surgical site, but usually a few days after surgery the pain decreases, and the patient begins to do range-of-motion and active exercises.

*Manipulation* is the forceful stretching of a quiescent rheumatic joint done under general anesthesia for relief of adhesions within and around the joint, and for contractures in the muscle and fascia. After the manipulation, the joint is placed in a plaster cast until the soreness subsides. At this point physical therapy and exercises are begun. If the deformity is resistant to these measures, then reconstructive surgery is considered.

Newly devised surgical techniques and improved biomaterials have expanded the range and success of *reconstructive surgery.* In such surgery the inflamed or diseased tissues (synovium, joint capsule, or cartilage) are removed, and the joint is reconstructed. The objective is to provide relief of pain and restoration of alignment, motion, and power. Pain, generally, is the major indication for all reconstructive surgery in arthritis, although motion, strength, and joint control are also important facets. Reconstructive surgeries to be discussed here include tendon transfers, osteotomy, arthroplasties, and arthrodesis.

The objective of *tendon transfers* is to help prevent progressive deformity due to muscle spasms. These deformities, essentially, are increased by the pull of normal muscles in an abnormal direction. This muscle pull can be redirected surgically so that it corrects the deformity. Tendon transfers commonly are done to correct ulnar drifts (Fig. 10-8).

An *osteotomy* (cutting of a bone) is used in chronic rheumatoid arthritis mainly after a joint becomes ankylosed in a faulty position for function. Basically the objective of this surgical procedure is to realign bones and, therefore, correct the deformity and relieve the pain. Generally, the osteotomy is fixed by internal measures such as wire, screws and plates, bone grafts, and fixation material. The postoperative nursing care is similar to the treatment of a fracture at a comparable site, because, in essence, an osteotomy is a controlled fracture (see Chap. 40).

An *arthroplasty* attempts to recreate a joint as nearly like the original as possible (with or without replacement of joint parts). The objective is to maintain or improve the motion of a joint and relieve unremitting pain. Numerous arthroplastic procedures involving implantation of new joints and silicone rubber implants have been used for many joints (Fig. 10-13), including the shoulder, elbow, wrist, hand, fingers, hip, knee, ankles and foot. The many types of surgical procedures and prostheses in use are constantly being improved and modified as experience with them increases. Essentially these operations form a new joint when ankylosis is present or when the articular surfaces have been badly damaged. The primary indication for an arthroplasty is unremitting pain. In addition, mobility is improved, as well as appearance, espe-

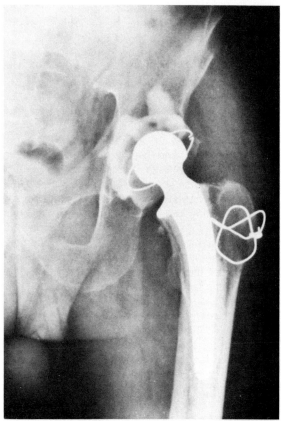

**FIGURE 10-13**
A total hip prosthesis in place two months after hip replacement.

cially in the joints of the hand. Preoperatively the nurse should explain the operative procedure and its goals and instruct the patient about movement after surgery and the exercises that will be necessary. It is very important to tell the patient that a surgically constructed joint will not equal a normal joint. However, if the exercise program is faithfully followed, motion in the joint and strength in the muscles will be developed, and function should closely approximate that of a normal joint.

Preoperatively, a patient with a *total hip arthroplasty* should be instructed in how to move and turn postoperatively. This includes hip-hiking, buttock elevation, recumbent urination and defecation, and use of the trapeze. The correct way to turn a patient after surgery is very important in order to prevent dislocation of the operated hip. The leg on the patient's operated side must be abducted at all times, and so an abduction pillow should always be placed between the patient's knees. Turning should be done by at least two nurses. One should stand on the nonoperated side of the patient, reach across the patient, grasp the shoulder and buttock, and gently roll the patient onto the nonoperative side while the other nurse supports the leg on the operated side during the turn. Then three pillows should be placed behind and three in front of the legs. The importance of coughing and deep-breathing exercises to prevent hypostatic pneumonia, as well as isometric quadricep and gluteal exercises and ankle pumps should be stressed.

Postoperatively, an air mattress, thigh-length elastic stockings, and heel protectors should be used to offset the effects of immobility. For the first few days the nurse should evaluate the nerve function and the circulatory status of the operative extremity. Routine dressing changes and observations for any signs of infection, skin breakdown, or urinary retention should be done. When positioning the patient in bed, it is important to place sandbags against the medial aspect of the upper, unaffected limb and against the chest wall on the unaffected side to remind the patient to lie flat. Placing the abductor pillow between the legs is also necessary. At this time, the nurse should stress the importance of exercise and use of the unaffected extremity to maintain muscle strength. Reminding the patient to keep the operated leg abducted and toes pointed upward to avoid dislocation is also important.

The first day after surgery the patient should begin active foot and ankle motions and gentle flexion and extension of the knees. The surgeon will assist the patient in slow and limited flexion of the hip. On the fourth postoperative day the patient should begin muscle-setting exercises, e.g., quadricep-setting and gluteal-setting, and may stand beside the bed with full weight bearing while the legs are abducted. On the seventh day, walking is allowed with the use of crutches or a walker. During the second week the patient, while supine, should begin roller-skating exercises to abduct the hip joint and strengthen abductor muscles. The patient also may lie prone every day to stretch the flexors and provide extension of the hip. The hip of the unoperated leg should be held to prevent compensatory adduction. Any unusual fatigue or muscle soreness should be noted. The nurse must continually work with the patient to prevent adduction and external rotation of the hip at all times. The importance of these exercises to maintain hip motion and to build muscle strength can not be overstressed. During the third week the patient may sit in a high chair and walk with crutches, walker, or cane. The nurse should give written instructions to all patients upon discharge delineating their exercises and

activity limitations. They should be advised to avoid all extremes of flexion, adduction, and internal rotation in order to prevent hip dislocation and not to sleep on the operative side for 2 months after returning home. In addition, the patient will need to use two crutches for walking, with no increase in weight bearing on the operative leg for 6 weeks. At that time another x-ray of the operated hip will be taken, and the patient's weight bearing and range of activities are increased depending on the radiological findings.

*Knee arthroplasties,* while less common, may be done to partially (hemiarthroplasty) or totally replace the knee joint. The primary indication for this procedure is unremitting pain due to joint destruction. Preoperatively the patient should be instructed about movement and exercises after surgery. The surgical procedure generally takes 1 to 2 hours. Postoperatively it is important for the nurse to regularly evaluate the patient's nerve function and circulatory status, and especially observe for any signs of infection, a major complication. Early mobilization with weight bearing in the postoperative period is the rule. The patient should be advised to use a cane to facilitate balance during this activity. Generally patients spend 2 weeks in the hospital doing the necessary exercises to increase muscle strength and joint range of motion before they are discharged.

The new procedure of *silicone rubber arthroplasty* is now used to help make hands functional again. It is designed for use in the metacarpophalangeal or proximal interphalangeal joints. A primary indication for this surgery is unremitting pain, unstable joint, x-ray evidence of major joint destruction, irreducible ulnar drift, or contracted intrinsic musculature. Preoperatively, the patient should be taught active hand and finger exercises and familiarized with the dynamic splinting that will be used for several weeks after surgery. Postoperatively, the hand should be continuously elevated to control swelling and increase patient comfort. A plaster slab and soft vinyl compression dressing should be used to immobilize the hand and reduce the pain and swelling. For the first 24 hours an hourly neurovascular check should be done to note the degree of swelling, capillary filling, sensation, temperature, pulses, and effect of motion on the operated side. The original dressing is removed 3 days after surgery, and a guided splinting program is started. During the first few days the nurse should frequently check for unusual swelling and finger positioning in order to assess the need for readjustment of the splint. The patient may begin at this time to actively flex, extend, abduct, and adduct the fingers within a reasonable limit of fatigue and pain. Gradually more vigorous exercises are added that facilitate maximum active flexion and extension. Upon discharge, the nurse should assess the patient's understanding of the need to continue doing the exercises and taking medications that control the disease process plus using the dynamic splints for several more weeks at home.

An *arthrodesis* is the operative fusion of a joint in the best position for function. The objective is to relieve pain in badly damaged joints, but unfortunately it also eliminates motion of that joint. It is performed occasionally in chronic arthritis. Generally, it is beneficial in joints when stability is important and where other joints may compensate for the loss of function. This procedure is considered only with severe destruction of a joint and when previous surgery, e.g., synovectomies, joint debridement, osteotomies, and arthroplasties, have failed. Basic nursing concerns, postoperatively, include checking for any circulatory or nerve impairment due to the cast and for any signs of bleeding or infection. Elevating the limb for 3 to 5 days after surgery often decreases the swelling and, thus, lessens the pain. The patient must be advised that the joint will generally be immobilized in a cast for 2 to 3 months and that weight bearing will not be permitted during that time.

*Experimental drug therapy* Despite treatment, local and systemic aspects of the disease may persist and cause a threat to survival or, at least, severe crippling. It is at this time that cytotoxic or immunosuppressive agents may be tried (Fig. 10-11).

**S**ystemic Manifestations Patients with seropositive rheumatoid arthritis often develop *rheumatoid nodules* over pressure areas such as the olecranon and in various other connective tissues throughout the body. These nodules may cause pain locally and sometimes ulceration. They are usually obvious from physical examination or on x-ray. Medical treatment is unsatisfactory. Excision may be necessary, depending on the location, but frequently they recur.

Specialized tissues throughout the body may become involved in the inflammatory process. The *sclera* may be inflamed (scleritis) causing redness and pain. Treatment is not satisfactory. Topical steroids may reduce some of the acute inflammation and prevent some of the necrosis. Inflammation of the lacrimal and salivary glands (Sjögren's

syndrome) may occur, producing dryness of the eyes with lack of tears and dryness of the mouth (see the Sjögren's Syndrome section).

*Pulmonary manifestations* are generally asymptomatic, but occasionally patients demonstrate dyspnea on exertion and a cough with scanty sputum. This is most common in rheumatoid pneumoconiosis (Caplan's syndrome) and diffuse interstitial fibrosis ("rheumatoid lung"). Besides a physical examination, chest x-rays or sometimes biopsies help to secure a diagnosis. Treatment is supportive with anti-inflammatory agents and exercises that encourage full expansion of the lungs.

*Cardiac manifestations* of rheumatoid arthritis generally are asymptomatic, but patients may demonstrate arrhythmias, pericardial tamponade, or rheumatoid nodules in the pericardium. A chest x-ray and EKG are of assistance in diagnosing these problems. Corticosteroid therapy has been successful in resolving these life-threatening problems.

Some patients experience numbness of their feet, hyperesthesia and burning pain due to *nerve compression syndromes,* and mild chronic sensory polyneuropathy. A neurological examination plus conduction tests help to identify the cause of these problems. Corticosteroids have been successful in relieving some of the symptoms.

The problems of *splenomegaly* and *leukopenia* (*Felty's syndrome*) occur in a small percentage of patients with rheumatoid arthritis. X-rays of the abdomen and blood tests help diagnose this syndrome. A major nursing concern is that these patients are very susceptible to infection when the neutrophilic leukocytes decrease. Corticosteroids sometimes help to reverse these complications. If the patient experiences recurrent infections and severe anemia or bleeding, a splenectomy may be done to help improve the white blood cell count.

Generalized *rheumatoid vasculitis* (arteritis) is very rare but frequently fatal in patients with rheumatoid arthritis. People may develop subacute lesions of small blood vessels of the muscles, heart, nerves, and other tissues or may develop a fulminant widespread necrotizing arteritis of medium and large vessels. In the less severe form, problems that occur include skin lesions, chronic leg ulcers, bleeding due to erosions of the mucosa of the gastrointestinal tract, and peripheral neuropathy. The clinical picture of the more advanced vasculitis (malignant rheumatoid arthritis) is characterized by the problems of polyneuropathies, skin infarction and ulceration, digital gangrene and visceral ischemia, and often high fevers. Laboratory tests often demonstrate an elevated RF, white blood cell count, and erythrocyte sedimentation rate. The dosage of steroids is generally raised to between 30 and 60 mg/day for an undetermined time. If this is not successful, penicillamine may be tried (Fig. 10-11). This drug has been used with some success in relieving symptoms and lowering the RF in rheumatoid arthritis, especially rheumatoid arthritis associated with vasculitis. The prognosis of life in these patients is poor. Death often occurs due to thrombosis, bleeding, infection, malnutrition, and/or congestive heart failure.

### Fourth-Level Nursing Care

Helping to identify a patient's *rehabilitation potential* is a great challenge for the nurse who works with the patient with rheumatoid arthritis. The nurse should assess the patient's physical and emotional state by assisting in functional, vocational, and psychosocial assessment.

The most common persistent nursing problems that occur during the patient's convalescence are exacerbations, chronic fatigue, weakness, pain, stiffness, physical disability, and numerous psychosocial difficulties in accepting and adjusting to this chronic disease.

The threat of an occurrence of an exacerbation is an ever-present problem for people with rheumatoid arthritis. A nurse who is assessing the patient's rehabilitation potential must be aware of some of the factors that may be related to these exacerbations which include: acute and chronic infections, weather changes, and physical and emotional stress. Therefore the nurse should screen all patients carefully for any signs of infection so that it can be treated early. The nurse also should assess what type of climate aggravates their arthritis and advise them to avoid exposure to it if at all possible. Finally, incidents and behaviors that may possibly cause stress for patients should be identified along with strategies that will lessen their effect.

**Functional assessment** Muscle power, stability and range of motion of joints, degree of pain, and ability to perform activities of daily living must be evaluated. Muscle weakness is an important observation because weakness in rheumatoid joints makes the joints unable to provide adequate stability. This can predispose them to more unnecessary trauma. In a *functional assessment* of a patient the nurse along with occupational and physical therapists will assess the following: (1) Ability to manage self-care (bed management, dressing, washing, and eating), (2) ambulation (ability to stand, walk, and manage steps), (3) ability to use transport (getting in and out of a car, driving a vehicle, and using public transportation), and (4) activity tolerance.

If possible, a home evaluation should be done to assess the physical layout of the house. The nurse should note in particular: (1) The basic layout of the home, for example, where steps are located, (2) facilities that are available for the patient's personal care such as safety bars and raised toilet seats, (3) types and height of furniture and work areas, and (4) general safety features such as sturdy railings. This often is a good time for the nurse to review with the patient the routine activities performed in a normal week. Listing all the activities in chart form often helps the nurse to advise specifically which portions of the schedule might be modified to achieve adequate rest while getting the tasks, hobbies, and exercises done. This also is an opportune time for the nurse to support some of the basic principles that the occupational therapist has taught the patient about work simplification and joint protection.

**Vocational assessment** The effects of rheumatoid arthritis are reflected not only physically but also socially, economically, psychologically, financially, vocationally, and avocationally. Therefore a *vocational* (work) evaluation should be done by the nurse with the assistance of vocational counselors and social workers. Features of rheumatoid arthritis which can be occupational hazards include the presence of: (1) Morning stiffness, (2) increased fatigue and decreased activity tolerance, (3) active inflammation of numerous joints for long periods of time causing pain and limitation of movement, and (4) joint deformity, instability, and limitation along with muscle wasting and weakness. It is a good practice to go with the patient to the job situation to make a more thorough evaluation.

**Psychosocial assessment** A *psychosocial* evaluation should be done by the nurse, with the assistance of family members and other allied health professionals, because of the effect this health problem has on one's psychological and social well-being. Here the nurse should identify the patient's understanding of and attitude toward the disease as well as any emotional response. A person's "psychological economy" is a major force in determining success or failure in the attainment of one's rehabilitation goals. All too often people suffer constant pain and failure and become hopeless and depressed, and eventually fall prey to total

dependence and quackery. Since success in rehabilitation is dependent on active participation by
the patient, motivation is necessary if rehabilitation
goals are to be achieved. At times, psychological
testing may be a wise course to follow in order to
facilitate a complete assessment. Also included in a
psychosocial evaluation would be a patient's economic status, work history, supportive persons and
marital stability, motivation level, problem-solving
mechanisms, coping abilities for life situations in
general, ego strength, and self-image, to mention
just a few. This type of assessment will help the
nurse develop better insight into the personality
and life experiences of the patient, thus facilitating
better assessments and more individualized therapy
and teaching.

All the data collected regarding the patient's
prognosis, functional capacity and potential, and
economic situation will help the rehabilitation team
establish the patient's *rehabilitation potential.* Once
this is established, necessary treatment programs
can begin. The overall objective of all treatment is a
patient's functional independence and protection
of joints against further damage. The treatment program may include: (1) medications, (2) surgery,
(3) physical and occupational therapy, (4) psychological assistance, and (5) vocational evaluation
and retraining.

When thinking about the overall rehabilitation
program, the nurse should not lose sight of the ultimate objective of any rehabilitation program which
is to return the patient to an acceptable place in
society where function is within limits, but to the
maximum of individual capacity. This not only calls
for good nursing assessment and intervention, but
appropriate identification of agencies and people
to use in making referrals and providing care for the
patient. Often a community health nurse is in a
good position to identify these needs on the basis
of assessment of the patient in the home situation.

Including the patient's family in the overall
rehabilitation program and helping them make
necessary adjustment to the patient's needs are
crucial. It also is important for the nurse to make
the patient and the family aware of the community
resources for the arthritis patient such as the Arthritis Foundation, social security benefits, and other
miscellaneous services assisting with housing, general health care, finances, travel, and transportation. The Arthritis Foundation is especially helpful
as it provides free patient-education booklets and
information about treatment centers, group physical therapy programs, and home living assistance
programs.

## SYSTEMIC LUPUS ERYTHEMATOSUS

Systemic lupus erythematosus (SLE) is an uncommon chronic inflammatory disease of connective
tissues. Its varied clinical manifestations are associated with lesions of connective tissue in the vascular system, the dermis, and the serous and synovial membranes. The disease varies greatly in severity but generally runs a long and chronic course
with occasional exacerbations.

### Theories of Causation

The etiology of SLE is unknown. Investigation as to
causation is being explored primarily in relation to
autoimmune, genetic, and viral factors.

**Autoimmune**  The autoimmune theory suggests
that a delayed hypersensitivity (allergic) reaction
may be responsible. The patient appears to develop
antibodies against several bodily tissues. The antibodies produced include anti-DNA, anti-RNA, ANA,
LE cells, and antibodies against red blood cells and
clotting factors. Because of the numerous antibodies against self-constituents and because cell-
mediated mechanisms may be involved, many
people draw the conclusion that the primary defect
in SLE is the immune system's inability to recognize
"self." There is clear evidence that ANA are responsible for two important features in SLE: the production of LE cells and hematoxylin bodies which are
believed to be the cause of lupus nephritis. Whether
immune complexes initiate SLE is not clear today,
but obviously the fixation of complement by antigen-antibody complexes causes the inflammatory
process of SLE. (See the discussion of type III immune complex hypersensitivity responses earlier in
this chapter.)

**Genetic**  A genetic influence in SLE has been
theorized. There is a tendency for the disease to
occur in particular families and in identical twins;
the immediate relatives of patients with SLE often
demonstrate elevated gamma globulins and ANA
without symptoms. SLE also occurs in more than
one generation. Experimentally it was found that
inbred mice developed manifestations of autoimmune SLE.

**Viral**  The viral theory suggests that viruses may
be the pathogenic agents in SLE. Experimentally
an autoimmune nephritis similar to SLE was virus-
induced. Some investigators suggest that a viral
agent is important because of increased titers of
antibodies that occur against several viruses—

measles and parainfluenza. Also, inclusions in a patient's connective tissue have been found resembling paramyxovirus.

## Pathophysiology

There is no characteristic pattern of clinical features at the onset of SLE. A single organ may be involved, or many systems may be affected simultaneously. It should be pointed out, before the pathology of SLE is described, that even if a patient is dying in an acute stage, only a few histological lesions may be present. This is, however, not the rule.

The changes in the connective tissue due to the inflammatory process include a variety of lesions. Some are nonspecific while others are relatively characteristic. The *fibrinoid degeneration* (fibrinous exudate consisting of nuclear protein, fibrin and mucopolysaccharides, complement components plus immune complexes) of connective tissue that occurs is a nonspecific change which often is widely distributed in numerous connective tissues. The more specific and characteristic pathological changes in SLE are: (1) *Vasculitis* in arterioles and small arteries, (2) *granulomatous growths* on heart valves producing verrucous (nonbacterial) endocarditis, (3) fibrosis of the spleen ("onion-skin" lesions), (4) thickening of the basement membrane of glomerular capillaries ("wire-loop" lesions), and (5) "hematoxylin bodies" (lesions involving cellular necrosis and nuclear alteration). Besides fibrinoid deposits, the lesions in SLE often contain autoantibodies, polymorphonuclear infiltrate, gamma globulin, and complement.

The degree of inflammation and eventual fibrotic changes in connective tissues are crucial in determining the severity of the symptoms in different organs and blood vessels (Table 10-11). Pathologic changes of the *skin* are common (80 percent) and cause atrophy of the epidermis and plugging of the hair follicles and gland orifices.[20]

Sixty percent of patients have *nonspecific glomerulonephritis* as evidenced by a thickened basement membrane of the glomeruli, necrotic glomerular capillaries, and thrombosis.[21] There are four major histologic findings in the *kidney:* (1) Acute fibrinoid necrosis of arterioles and small arteries, (2) focal proliferative lupus nephritis (glomerulitis), (3) membranous lupus nephritis, and (4) diffuse proliferative lupus nephritis. Focal nephritis is characterized by a few lesions in some of the glomeruli; progressive renal disease and death from renal insufficiency are very unlikely at this point. There is severe basement membrane

thickening of glomerular capillaries in membranous lupus nephritis which often causes profuse proteinuria and a nephrotic syndrome that may or may not cause serious problems. In diffuse proliferative lupus nephritis the basement membrane plus the glomeruli is involved which often causes arterial hypertension and eventual renal failure.

In the *central nervous system* there may be widespread vasculitis of small cerebral blood vessels causing local edema, atrophic endothelial cells, and an inflammatory infiltrate. The neurological manifestations of SLE vary greatly depending on the degree of inflammation and vasculitis. Ninety percent of patients have *musculoskeletal* symptoms due to a nonspecific swelling along with inflammatory infiltrate of the synovium.[22] Generalized inflammation of the connective tissue of the *heart* along with vasculitis occurs in 50 percent of SLE patients and causes myocarditis and pericarditis. Inflammation of the *pleura* and *pulmonary system* causes pleuritis and pneumonitis.

Necrosis and cellular proliferation of *lymph nodes* and enlargement of the *spleen* and *liver* occur owing to the inflammatory process. Hematological abnormalities such as anemia, leukopenia, and mild thrombocytopenia purpura occur because of the generalized inflammatory state of the connective tissues and to autoantibodies against *blood-forming cells*. Finally, *gastrointestinal* manifestations are common due to vasculitis of the bowel along with mucosal ulceration.

**Types of SLE** There is no characteristic pattern of SLE. Often the onset is insidious and reveals a puzzling combination of clinical symptomatology involving many systems. The course is extremely variable and unpredictable. Generally SLE is divided into two types: *acute* SLE which is rather severe in nature and *subacute* which accounts for the majority of the cases and is much milder in nature. SLE no longer poses its formerly serious threat to survival, as long as certain organs are not badly damaged like the heart, central nervous system, or kidney, and as long as the onset is not in childhood. Because renal problems are treated more vigorously, renal failure no longer is the major cause of death. Cerebral lupus and secondary infections cause most of the deaths. The present therapy and prognosis of patients with SLE is still far from satisfactory; greater than 50 percent of patients with renal and neurological involvement die within 10 years of onset.[23]

**TABLE 10-11**
INFLAMMATORY CHANGES DUE TO SLE

| Body Structure | Pathological and Histological Changes | Clinical Manifestations |
|---|---|---|
| Skin | Plugging of hair follicles and gland orifices<br>Degeneration of basal cell layer<br>Edema of cutis | "Butterfly" rash on bridge of nose and malar regions<br>Patchy erythematous rashes on face, neck, and extremities<br>Ulcers of skin<br>Altered pigmentation<br>Alopecia<br>Thickening of skin<br>Purpura<br>Urticaria<br>Atrophy<br>Scars<br>Pain and itching |
| Kidney | Thickened basement membrane of glomeruli ("wire-loop" lesion)<br>Necrosis of glomerular capillaries | Hematuria<br>Proteinuria<br>Headaches, nausea and vomiting, anorexia<br>Arterial hypertension<br>Nonspecific glomerulonephritis<br>Nephrotic syndrome<br>Renal failure |
| Central nervous system | Inflammation of small cerebral vessels<br>Vasculitis | Mental disturbances<br>Convulsions<br>Chorea, ptosis, diplopia<br>Hemiparesis, motor aphasia<br>Cerebrovascular accident |
| Musculoskeletal system | Thick layer of fibrinlike material covering thickened synovial membrane<br>Minimal erosion of articular cartilage | Polyarthralgias<br>Morning stiffness<br>Myalgias<br>Polyarthritis<br>Tenosynovitis<br>Mild deformities<br>Atrophy of muscles |
| Cardiovascular system | Generalized inflammation of connective tissue myocardium, pericardium, and major blood vessels | Pericarditis<br>Precordial pain and sinus tachycardia<br>Diffuse myocarditis leading to congestive heart failure<br>Raynaud's phenomenon |
| Respiratory system | Generalized inflammation of the connective tissue in the pleura and pulmonary system | Dyspnea, shortness of breath, chest pain<br>Pneumonitis<br>Pleurisy<br>Atelectasis (basilar) |
| Eye | Localized vasculitis of retina<br>Inflamed nerve endings | Hemorrhages and cytoid body in retina |
| Liver, spleen, and lymph nodes | Periarterial fibrosis of spleen ("onion-skin" lesion)<br>Necrosis and cellular proliferation of lymph nodes | Hepatomegaly<br>Splenomegaly<br>Lymph node enlargement |
| Blood | Autoantibodies present against blood-forming cells | Fatigue, easy bruising and bleeding, petechiae<br>Anemia<br>Leukopenia<br>Thrombocytopenia purpura |
| Gastrointestinal system | Vasculitis of intestinal wall and mucosal inflammation | Anorexia, nausea, and vomiting<br>Diarrhea and constipation<br>Abdominal pain<br>Dysphagia<br>Peritonitis<br>Mucosal ulceration of mouth, pharynx, and vagina |

### First-Level Nursing Care

Because the cause of SLE is unknown, prevention is not possible at this time. Nurses should, however, be aware of some of the significant epidemiological factors related to SLE. It is an uncommon disturbance that is predominantly found in females (7:1) of the child-bearing age group—about half those affected develop signs of SLE between 15 and 25 years of age.[24] There is no peak age of onset for males. It occurs more frequently in black Americans and Asians than in Caucasians, and it is rare in Africans. It is most common in sunny countries.

### Second-Level Nursing Care

It is vital to detect SLE at an early stage to give the patient a chance for a more favorable prognosis. Because the initial diagnosis may take place in an outpatient setting, nurses may have a vital role in the patient's assessment.

**Nursing assessment** The clinical picture of SLE at onset is highly variable. Early in SLE major clinical features generally reflect involvement of one or more of the following systems: *musculoskeletal, cutaneous, nervous, renal, gastrointestinal, cardiovascular,* or *pulmonary* (Table 10-11). The body structure initially affected often remains the predominant one throughout the disease.

Health History The patient frequently describes an insidious process that starts with numerous *constitutional symptoms* including chills, a low-grade fever (especially in the afternoon), generalized aching, weakness and fatigue, malaise, loss of appetite, and decreased weight. These are due to the on-going systemic inflammation. Women may note that their *menstrual periods* are irregular or have stopped. This is usually related to the anemia of SLE.

Often, patients will notice painful erythematous or scaly rashes on their face, neck, or extremities which may be induced by exposure to the sun. Some patients are particularly sensitive to cold, and after exposure to the cold, the skin on their hands and feet shows several distinct color changes. Alopecia and hyperpigmentation are also frequent initial problems. Some patients note that they seem to bruise easily or have pinpoint bleeding into the skin. Finally painful ulceration of the mouth, pharynx, and vagina may occur early in the disease.

Other initial symptoms may be due to inflammation of the pleura, pericardium, and myocardium. These include shortness of breath, dyspnea,

rapid heart beat, precordial pain, and pedal edema. The nurse should note any dyspnea or edema and have the patient describe the degree and location of any pain.

Weakness, painful joints (arthralgia) and muscles (myalgia), and stiffness are the most frequent initial problems. These are a result of inflammation of the synovial membrane and muscles. The patient should be asked to describe the character and location of the pain in the joints and muscles, and how long and to what degree they feel stiff during the day.

When the gastrointestinal tract is involved, the patient may experience a variety of symptoms. Pain in the abdomen, anorexia, nausea and vomiting, and diarrhea or constipation are frequent complaints.

Patients will often describe headaches, anorexia, or nausea and vomiting, particularly if the kidneys are initially involved in the disease. The severity of these symptoms should be noted.

Sometimes patients may state that they seem quite forgetful. Transient states of depression or psychosis, paranoia, hyperirritability and anxiety may also be experienced. All these symptoms are due to involvement of the central nervous system.

Physical Assessment Assessing the patient with SLE is a continuous challenge for a nurse because of the numerous problems that can occur due to inflammation throughout the body structures (Table 10-11).

While assessing the patient for *dermal involvement,* the nurse should note any atrophy or scars as well as the location, size, and character of any lesions or rashes. Hair loss, including a description of where and what quantity, should be noted. The texture and pigmentation of the skin may be altered also, and these changes should be recorded.

Generalized inflammation of the pericardium and myocardium, as well as vasculitis, is responsible for the *cardiopulmonary findings* of SLE. Auscultation may reveal sinus tachycardia; murmurs, arrhythmias, or friction rubs. Inflammation of the pleura (pleuritis) and pulmonary system may cause observable dyspnea and shortness of breath. In assessing these problems, the nurse should note the patient's respiratory rate and what may aggravate breathing.

Inflammation of the synovial membranes and muscles is the cause of the *musculoskeletal disturbances* found so frequently in SLE patients. Joints may appear red and swollen, particularly in the hands, feet, and large joints. Mobility may be decreased, and the joint may be painful when touched; muscle atrophy and weakness may contribute to these findings. Notation should be made of the location and degree of any swelling, tenderness, atrophy, or loss of function.

*Gastrointestinal symptoms* are primarily subjective and described in the health history. However, the abdominal examination may reveal enlargement of the liver and/or spleen. The reasons for this enlargement are not completely understood.

Inflammatory lesions of the glomeruli are responsible for the *renal findings* in SLE patients. Massive hematuria may be present with severe kidney involvement. Other effects are largely subjective or detectable by laboratory tests.

Changes due to inflammation of small cerebral blood vessels may include observable *anxiety, depression,* or *hyperirritability.* Body postures, facial expressions, rate of speaking as well as the nature of verbal responses should be noted. These observations may provide clues to the patient's emotional and psychological state.

Hemolysis due to the presence of antibodies against red blood cells and blood-clotting factors is the primary cause of the anemia and thrombocytopenia purpura commonly found in patients with SLE. These conditions may be observable as pallor, bruises, bleeding, or petechiae in the skin or mucous membranes. The severity and location of any of these findings should be noted.

**D**iagnostic Tests  The diagnosis of SLE rests heavily on laboratory tests (Table 10-9). The patient should be informed that several blood and urine samples will be needed. Serologically, one commonly finds an elevated erythrocyte sedimentation rate, mild anemia, moderate leukopenia, changes in electrolytes, thrombocytopenia, hypergammaglobulinemia, and decreased complement as well as a false positive test for syphilis. ANA, LE cells, and anti-DNA antibodies are generally present, as well as an occasionally positive RF test. The ANA is the best screening test, unless the patient is on massive steroids, because essentially all patients with SLE are positive, even in inactive disease. Also, antibodies against DNA are highly specific for SLE. The total serum complement is one of the best ways to follow the course of SLE. Urea clearance and 24-, 12-, and 3-hour urinalyses are collected to evaluate general renal function and the presence of abnormal proteins, red and white blood cells, and casts. Proteinuria is the best indicator of disease activity in the kidney. A skin biopsy may be done if there is skin involvement. If one joint is particularly inflamed, a synovial fluid analysis may be performed. An EKG is often ordered to confirm an arrhythmia. Chest x-rays are taken to observe for any significant enlargement of the heart. Sputum specimens and chest x-rays help to identify the cause and degree of respiratory involvement.

**Nursing problems and interventions**  *Dermal lesions, cardiopulmonary dysfunction, joint inflammation, gastrointestinal upset, renal dysfunction, bruising or bleeding* as well as *anxiety* and other central nervous system symptoms constitute the major nursing problems in caring for a patient with SLE. Interventions are in terms of general therapies and specific care of problems.

**G**eneral Therapies  If the diagnosis of SLE is confirmed, medical treatment is prescribed to control the inflammation, to prevent the main causes of death or "toxic" manifestations, and to avoid potentially exacerbating situations. Because no specific *medication* is available to cure the disease, the type and intensity of treatment are based upon the severity of the illness and the organ systems that are involved. Since there is a high rate of spontaneous clinical remission of SLE, many patients with mild complaints may require little or no medication. If the disease is not active or if patients are experiencing only a moderate exacerbation, salicylates may reduce most of the common problems such as fever and joint pain.

At this time, the nurse commonly gives between 3.6 and 7.2 g *aspirin* every day to relieve the inflammation. *Acetaminophen (Tylenol)* does not have an anti-inflammatory effect, but it is used for patients who can not tolerate aspirin for the purpose of controlling any fever. If salicylates are not effective enough, sometimes Indocin and phenylbutazone may be tried before low dosages of steroids are begun. *Indocin,* a nonsteroidal anti-inflammatory drug, may be used to control arthritis and fever and sometimes acute pericarditis. Another nonsteroidal anti-inflammatory agent, *phenylbutazone,* is given in a few limited cases when aspirin has failed to relieve these mild symptoms, or if the patient can not tolerate prednisone. If the mild symptoms are not relieved with salicylates or a nonsteroidal anti-inflammatory agent plus rest, *antimalarial* compounds may be added to the medical regime. These medications often exert a beneficial effect on some of the cutaneous lesions, and sometimes they relieve symptoms of the systemic disease. However, these drugs are used less often now because of their uncertain value and because of serious retinal damage that often occurs with prolonged use. It is important for the nurse to advise any patient who is taking an antimalarial compound to avoid excessive exposure to the sun and to use them sparingly because of the frequency of adverse reactions.

*Rest* is very important in the active phase of SLE. The nurse should advise patients not to keep irregular hours and not to become fatigued. Instead, they should gradually increase their activity over the months as these problems gradually decrease. It is best for patients to rest when they feel tired and to get a full night's sleep.

Rarely is a special *diet* necessary without major system involvement. A well-balanced diet is adequate to support the patient's overall health.

**D**ermal Lesions   If the type of lesion is not clearly identified after physical examination a skin biopsy may be done. The nurse should teach the patient to apply topical corticosteroid cream as ordered, usually in small amounts every 2 hours to the erythematous lesions and rashes. This reduces inflammation and therefore the pain. Generally high doses of aspirin and low doses of prednisone control the other skin and mucosal manifestations. If the mucous membranes are ulcerated, the patient may be advised to est bland foods or only drink liquids until substantial healing has begun. Patients should gradually increase their exposure to the sun in order to assess sensitivity to it. The wisest guideline a nurse can provide is to encourage the use of common sense. Patients should not intentionally overexpose themselves to the sun and should avoid the use of sunlamps. Often sunscreens, sunglasses, and protective clothing will lessen the occurrence of skin eruptions, especially if the patient is taking antimalarials.

Some patients take *antimalarials* for the skin manifestations until they disappear. The initial dose of antimalarials such as chloroquine or Plaquenil is 500 to 750 mg/day until a remission occurs. It is then decreased to 250 mg or less and maintained at that dosage for no longer than a year because of dangerous side effects (refer to Rheumatoid Arthritis section.)

**J**oint Inflammation   In addition to taking substantial doses of salicylates for the musculoskeletal problems, the patient may be advised to exercise regularly by walking, swimming, and bicycling. This helps keep joints mobile and lessens dysfunction. Patients may perform these activities any time as long as the exercises do not produce fatigue or pain. They also should maintain their daily activities at a constant rate, gradually adding more activities over time.

**G**astrointestinal Upset   It is important for the nurse to tell the patient that gastrointestinal problems are generally controlled with aspirin and low dosages of prednisone. Symptomatic relief may be offered through the use of antiemetics, laxatives, and bland diets.

**Third-Level Nursing Care**

It is vital to follow patients with SLE regularly in order to promptly identify and treat any acute exacerbation or life-threatening complication that may arise. At times it may be necessary to hospitalize these patients owing to poor control with a conservative treatment program. This may also be necessary during a severe exacerbation or involvement of a major system of the body.

**Nursing assessment**   The *health history* that the patient describes will vary with the acuteness of the disease process and the anatomic distribution of lesions. Symptoms are generally due to the continued inflammatory process of SLE. Many of the problems that occurred earlier in the disease process have become more severe (Table 10-11).

**P**hysical Assessment   To assess these problems, the nurse must follow the patient's vital signs, intake and output, weight, and laboratory studies while regularly evaluating each major system of the body with a thorough physical assessment.

*Cardiopulmonary findings* may be increased in severity. Arrhythmias, dyspnea, and orthopnea are present if acute pericarditis develops. These symptoms are detectable by a rapid and irregular pulse and difficult, irregular respirations. Dyspnea may be intensified with any exertion. The patient appears to be very uncomfortable and in distress as a result of the dyspnea as well as the intense precordial pain. Close monitoring of vital signs and the patient's general physical status are vital ongoing assessments in this situation. Shortness of breath and dyspnea may also be present if pleurisy or pneumonitis occurs as a result of inflammation or secondary lung infections. (Refer to Chap. 22 for details of lung assessment.)

Vascular involvement of the *bowel* resulting in infarctions and hemorrhage may cause bloody diarrhea, severe abdominal pain and distention, and a paralytic ileus. The patient's abdomen may be tender on palpation. Bowel sounds vary with the degree of involvement, possibly being accelerated with diarrhea or decreased with an ileus.

*Renal* problems arise owing to membranous lupus nephritis or diffuse proliferative lupus nephritis. The patient's blood pressure and temperature are elevated. Edema may be palpable in dependent areas of the body, particularly the feet and legs. The patient's weight should be taken and followed closely for any sign of further fluid retention.

There are many complications due to severe inflammation and vasculitis in the *central nervous system.* The patient may have observable ptosis (drooping of the eyelids) and may describe diplopia. Diplopia may be assessed further by an ophthalmological examination with prisms. Nystagmus may also be present and should be defined as vertical or horizontal. The patient may have difficulty walking or tolerating the weight of bedclothing because of peripheral neuropathy. Areas of the body affected by this condition should be noted. Severe, progressive neurological involvement may cause the patient to have seizures increasing to the point of status epilepticus. (Detailed discussion of assessment of the seizure patient is found in Chap. 33). The state of consciousness must be closely evaluated as coma may occur. Vital signs and the neurological examination must be assessed frequently to detect subtle changes in the person's condition.

Involvement of superficial blood vessels may result in vascular spasms. This condition is known as *Raynaud's phenomenon* and is discussed in detail in Chap. 29. In the patient with SLE, Raynaud's phenomenon may be observable as ulcerative, sensitive and eventually gangrenous digits. Palpation or examination may be very difficult because of the pain.

Hematological problems may increase in severity owing to autoantibodies that destroy red blood cells and platelets. If hemolytic anemia occurs, the patient should be observed for malaise, shaking chills, and fever. The urine should be observed and tested for hematuria, and any apparent discomfort noted, particularly pain in the back and abdomen.

Bruising and petechiae must be observed for and noted. Stools and gastric secretions should be tested for blood. Nosebleeds and other frank bleeding must be recorded according to severity and location. These findings may be indicative of the acute onset of idiopathic thrombocytopenic purpura.

**D**iagnostic Tests The diagnostic findings of a patient with severe SLE are quite variable, and depend on the severity of the presenting problems (Table 10-9). One may find a significantly elevated BUN, ESR, and gammaglobulinemia, severe anemia, leukopenia, and thrombocytopenia plus marked depression of serum complement levels. The findings from the *urinalysis* may include a decrease in urine volume, decreased specific gravity, marked proteinuria, leukocyturia, hematuria, and increased numbers of casts. A renal biopsy often reveals thickening of the basement membrane of the glomerular capillaries plus an inflammatory infiltrate, fibrin, and circulating immune complexes. *X-rays* of the chest may show pleural effusions, atelectasis, cardiac enlargement, or pericardial effusions. Often a low vital capacity and reduced diffusing capacity are detected with *spirometry* and *arterial blood gases.* The *cerebrospinal fluid* of patients with central nervous system involvement frequently has increased protein, mild lymphocytosis, and an abnormally low complement level. Often EMI scans of the brain, angiography, or a myelogram may be done to identify the location and degree of damage in the central nervous system.

**Nursing problems and interventions** Nursing problems are the same as described under Second-Level Nursing Care; however, the severity is increased enough to require hospitalization. *Cardiopulmonary insufficiency, fluid and electrolyte disturbance* due to severe gastrointestinal involvement, *edema, hypertension,* and other signs of renal failure, *bleeding* and other hematological problems, as well as severe *pain* and discomfort from peripheral blood-vessel involvement, are some of the nursing problems encountered in caring for a patient with advanced SLE.

**G**eneral Therapies When the patient develops severe problems due to the continuing inflammatory process, high dosages of steroids and immunosuppressives are prescribed plus adequate nutrition, increased rest, physical therapy, and sometimes surgery (e.g., splenectomies for thrombocytopenia purpura). The primary objective of these measures is to control the inflammation.

*Corticosteroids* have been and remain the mainstay in treatment. High dosages of corticosteroids are, however, reserved for acute generalized exacerbations of SLE or for serious involvement of vital organ systems. Often, initial daily dosages of 60 mg prednisone or more may be needed. Generally, if there is not significant improvement within

48 hours, the dosage will be increased to the amount required to control life-threatening problems. When there is significant objective improvement of the disease, the dosage is slowly reduced to the lowest possible amount. Patient-education about this medication is particularly crucial at this time, because of the dosages that are prescribed. Patients should be informed that steroids are a life-saving measure and that close supervision is imperative. It is advisable for the patient to carry an identification card at all times stating the name of the medication being taken.

The patient should be informed about the potential toxic effects that may occur. Some of the most severe include suppression of the immune system, diabetes mellitus, irritation of peptic ulcers, avascular necrosis of the hips, and secondary infections. Nurses must be aware that people on steroids have suppressed adrenal glands, and are often incapable of responding to stress due to surgery or an accident. Therefore, it is necessary to monitor these patients very carefully when such stressors are present. Since one of the major causes of death in patients with SLE is secondary infection, the nurse should be on the alert for any signs of infection. The nurse also should regularly check the results of routine laboratory tests including urinalyses, 2-hour postprandial blood sugars, complete blood count, serum electrolytes, and chest x-rays.

The second major group of medications used in advanced therapy is *immunosuppressants*. These agents include both alkylating compounds and antimetabolites. Immunosuppressants are used on an experimental basis because of the uncertainty of their action and numerous toxic effects. Therefore, their use is reserved for patients who do not experience significant improvement with prednisone and who have serious side effects or life-threatening situations.

Another important general nursing measure is the provision of appropriate *psychological* and *emotional support* for the patient and the family. This is vital because of the seriousness of the disease.

**C**ardiopulmonary Insufficiency   Chest x-rays often reveal cardiomegaly and pericardial effusions. A pericardial paracentesis may need to be done by the physician to relieve the acute problems. In addition, the nurse may give high doses of corticosteroids or immunosuppressives, as ordered, plus diuretics, digitalis, and morphine (for the pain). The patient may be placed on total bed rest and on a low-sodium diet with restricted fluids.

**R**aynaud's Phenomena   The pain and discomfort of this condition may be lessened by providing warmth and protection for the digits. Patients should also be advised that the elimination of smoking may relieve symptoms (see Chap. 29 for a detailed discussion).

**R**enal Involvement   Diuretics, antihypertensives, total bed rest, and a low-sodium and low-protein diet may be prescribed for renal involvement. If acute renal failure occurs, the patient may develop tremors, nausea, vomiting, convulsions, and signs of cerebral irritation. There may be a rapid decrease in urine volume or oliguria, and the blood urea nitrogen becomes very high. Massive doses of corticosteroids plus immunosuppressives, antihypertensives, and diuretics would be given. Renal dialysis may also be indicated at this point. Anticonvulsants will be used to control any seizures. A thorough discussion of renal failure may be found in Chap. 14.

### Fourth-Level Nursing Care

Once the acute problems have stabilized, the nurse must work with the rehabilitation team to identify a patient's *rehabilitation potential*. The nurse should assess the patient's physical and emotional state and contribute to the overall functional, vocational, and psychosocial assessment. The most common and persistent nursing problems that occur during a patient's convalescence are *exacerbations, continued muscle weakness, pain, fatigability, numerous physical disabilities,* and *psychosocial difficulties* in adjusting to this disease.

The possible occurrence of an exacerbation is an ever-present problem for people with SLE. The nurse who assesses the patient's rehabilitation potential must be aware of the numerous factors that may be related to exacerbations. These include exposure to the sun, an abrupt change in steroid dosage, physical and emotional stress, pregnancy, fatigue, infection, and numerous drugs. Therefore, the nurse must advise patients that excessive exposure to the sun can cause skin lesions and sometimes more acute systemic problems. If patients are taking corticosteroids, they should be informed that eliminating, increasing, or decreasing the dosage of the medication without supervision may cause an exacerbation. The nurse should help the patient identify activities that may cause unnecessary stress and then plan a strategy to lessen their potential effect. The patient should be informed that pregnancy may aggravate SLE, especially if major organs are involved in the disease. The working, resting, and living habits of patients should also be assessed in order to help the patient identify particular habits that may be unnecessarily stressful. Because infections may cause a exacerbation, patients should avoid exposure to infection and seek treatment immediately if one develops. Finally, patients need to be informed about the numerous drugs that have apparently aggravated SLE. These include sulfa derivatives, any drugs that the patient is known to be allergic to, penicillin (only during remission), hydantoin (Dilantin), mazantoin, diphenylhydantoin, oral contraceptives, Apresoline, hydralazine, procainamide, isoniazid, and foreign proteins like tetanus toxoid. These drugs should be taken only on the advice of a physician.

The *functional evaluation* is done to identify the patient's overall strength, tolerance to activity, degree of pain, and ability to perform activities of daily living. Assessing the patient's everyday activities is necessary in order to advise the patient how to best conserve energy and time. If the patient has permanent problems or disabilities due to the residual involvement of a major organ system like the cardiovascular or musculoskeletal systems, a physiatrist, occupational therapist, and physical therapist can provide more specific data for the functional assessment.

Major areas of concern in a *vocational assessment* are the patient's tolerance of the pace and type of activities on the job or in the work situation. It also is important to note any special physical limitation, such as a cardiac arrhythmia, that might limit the ability to work.

Because SLE affects a patient's psychological and social well-being, a *psychosocial assessment* is an important evaluation to be done by the nurse. One would want to evaluate the patient's and the family's understanding of and attitude toward SLE as well as their emotional response and ability to adjust to it. All too often patients become so frightened of the disease and its prognosis that they become overly dependent on their family and physician. Sometimes major psychological problems develop. If this is noted, the patient should be referred to a psychiatrist and neurologist to identify the cause—it may be the disease process itself or the patient's psychological response to it. Numerous social variables (as outlined in the Rheumatoid Arthritis section) must also be examined in a psychosocial evaluation.

Once these data are collected, a rehabilitation potential is established and the treatment program is begun. The nurse must be aware of the far-reaching effects of SLE on the patient. These involve pain, disability, work loss, disruption of family life, depression, financial costs, chronic illness, and

possible adverse reactions to the treatment program. Therefore the nurse must be understanding of the patient's feelings, fears, and anxieties and render support as needed. The nurse should not frighten patients by telling them to avoid all sunlight, to rest all the time, or to never become pregnant. All too often fears are aroused by overly protective professionals and family members. Often, available literature is frightening or so vague it causes patients to worry. Most patients with SLE can complete an education, marry and have children, and hold a job, as long as the disease process is controlled and major systems do not suffer permanent damage.

Once SLE is no longer active, the patient should be encouraged to continue to work or study part time, and then full time. Good judgment must be used in regard to avoiding fatigue, anxiety, and other factors that precipitate an exacerbation. Control of the disease process is the key in determining the patient's rehabilitation progress. When the patient first returns from the hospital, it is a good idea to provide a referral to a community health nurse for continued follow-up. When the patient becomes strong enough to return to work, the community health nurse may refer the patient to a vocational counselor for evaluation. Finally, the nurse must be aware of community resources, such as the Arthritis Foundation, which exist to provide various types of support for the patient and the family.

## MYASTHENIA GRAVIS

*Myasthenia gravis* is a health problem of presumed autoimmune origin with possible involvement of all striated muscles, but especially those innervated by the bulbar nuclei, e.g., voluntary muscles subserving ocular movement, facial expression, mastication, deglutination, and respiration. Muscles of the neck, trunk, and limbs are often affected.

### Pathophysiology

There are two common types of myasthenia: *ocular* and *generalized*. Only the extrinsic ocular and levator palpebrae muscles are involved in *ocular myasthenia*. This involvement causes drooping of the eyelids (ptosis) and double vision (diplopia).

*Generalized myasthenia* can involve the facial, pharyngeal, laryngeal, respiratory, and ocular muscles as well as the skeletal muscles of the trunk and limbs. This peripheral neuromuscular disorder generally has an insidious onset and is characterized by severe weakness and fatigability of various voluntary muscles. The manifestations are most likely due to some myoneural conduction block. Knowledge of how the myoneural junction functions is essential for an understanding of the clinical manifestations of myasthenia, its treatment, and the appropriate nursing care.

The *myoneural junction* is the connection between the end of a myelinated nerve fiber and a skeletal muscle fiber (Fig. 10-14). When a nerve impulse reaches this junction, the end plate secretes acetylcholine which increases the permeability of the plasma membrane of the muscle. This allows sodium leakage to the inside of the muscle fiber, which alters the membrane potential beneath the end plate. If the end plate potential becomes great enough, it will cause an action potential to move along the muscle fiber and cause the muscle to contract. Shortly after acetylcholine has stimulated the muscle fiber, it is destroyed by cholinesterase. This enables the plasma membrane of the muscle to repolarize and become ready to be stimulated by the next nerve impulse. This natural substance is necessary so that acetylcholine does not remain in contact with the muscle membrane indefinitely and therefore transmits a continuous succession of impulses. Myasthenia gravis occurs as a result of blockage of the conduction of these impulses at the myoneural junction.

**Theories of causation** The etiology of myasthenia gravis is unknown. Investigation as to the causation is being explored primarily in relation to autoimmune and genetic factors.

**A**utoimmune  As with all autoimmune reactions, the trigger event remains an enigma. Much data support the importance of an immunologic mechanism in the pathology of myasthenia gravis. They include the following findings: (1) Autoantibodies are present against voluntary muscle and thymic cells, as well as numerous other antibodies including ANA, RF, and antibodies against the thyroid gland and gastric mucosa. (2) There is a high incidence of thymic hyperplasia and an increase in the number of "germinal centers" within the thymus. (3) Thymectomies often produce remissions. (4) Lymphocytes formed in the thymus are responsible for producing antibodies that react against skeletal muscle. (5) Myasthenia frequently occurs in patients who demonstrate other possible autoimmune diseases like rheumatoid arthritis and SLE. The role the antibodies play in the pathology of this disorder is uncertain.

There also is evidence that contradicts the autoimmune hypothesis. The autoantibodies do not localize at the myoneural junction, and not all patients demonstrate autoantibodies. Therefore, many researchers now feel that the thymus gland may release a nonimmune humoral substance, because of the fact that many people improve after thymectomies.

**G**enetic  Some research supports a *genetic* predisposition to develop myasthenia. The family incidence is higher than chance, and these individuals appear to have some constitutional predisposition to abnormal immune reactivity, as demonstrated by the presence of various autoantibodies.

**Changes**  Pathophysiologic changes in myasthenia gravis are limited to voluntary muscles and the thymus. Only a few histologic lesions are found in skeletal muscles, nerves, and the thymus of patients with myasthenia gravis. Frequently, skeletal muscle appears normal except for collections of lymphocytes ("lymphorrhages") around blood vessels or isolated atrophic and necrotic muscle fibers. Sometimes degeneration of the muscle fibers occurs along with a more extensive inflammatory cellular response.

Normally the thymus undergoes atrophy in adult life, but in patients with myasthenia gravis there can be numerous changes. Patients over 30 years of age may develop thymomas (10 to 15 percent) or demonstrate lymphocytic proliferation in the form of "germinal centers" in the thymus medulla (70 percent).[25]

The basic problem appears to be a defect in the transmission of the nerve impulse at the myoneural junction. The most consistent abnormalities are widening and simplification of synaptic clefts and gross thickening of the capillary basement membrane. Because of this defect, a characteristic myasthenic reaction occurs; i.e., when a voluntary muscle is stimulated at intervals of seconds by a faradic current, the muscle contractions become progressively weaker and soon cease, but they generally return after a short rest. This reaction accounts for the primary symptoms of myasthenia.

Generally myasthenia runs a chronic progressive course with occasional spontaneous remissions, but there can be great variability. The prognosis is quite unpredictable. The mortality rate is 15 times that of the general population.[26] Death commonly occurs in patients with generalized myasthenia during the first 2 years after diagnosis due to respiratory paralysis or an infection of the respiratory system. If myasthenia is present for many years, it generally runs a more benign course.

If a patient has just thymic hyperplasia, there may be a more intermittent course, but patients with thymic tumors tend to have a progressive course, especially those with malignant tumors.[27]

## First-Level Nursing Care

As the cause of myasthenia gravis is unknown, prevention of the disease is not yet possible. Nurses should, however, be aware of some of the significant epidemiological factors related to myasthenia. It is a rare disease (33 per million) which occurs three times more frequently in females than in males.[28] The onset of the disease may occur at any age, but the peak age of onset for patients with thymic hyperplasia is 15 to 40 years of age. When symptoms begin after 50 years of age, a thymic tumor is usually present, and there is no sex preponderance.[29]

## Second-Level Nursing Care

Early in myasthenia gravis major clinical features usually reflect involvement of ocular muscles or a more generalized involvement of voluntary muscles.

**Nursing assessment**  Myasthenia gravis may be insidious or acute in onset and may be manifested by mild or severe symptoms. Patients often seek medical attention initially because of fluctuating muscle weakness.

Health History  In most cases the diagnosis of myasthenia is suggested by the history and physical examination. The patient usually describes an insidious process of weakness and rapid exhaustion that occurs first in very active muscles like the extraocular muscles of the face, tongue, and upper extremities. The patient may notice *ptosis* of the eyelids with *inability to close the lids, diplopia* (frequently induced by reading or embarrassment), and the *inability to smile normally. Difficult chewing, swallowing* (dysphagia), *speaking* (dysarthria), and *breathing* are other initial symptoms. Finally patients often state that their arms feel so weak that they cannot raise them; they may be unable to climb stairs or get up from a chair. There is a tendency for the *weakness* to fluctuate during brief periods such as in the course of a single day or over longer periods. Generally, the muscle weakness is greatest at the end of the day or after exercise and is partially relieved by rest. The sensation of generalized "stiffness" is quite common, as are *paresthesias* (numbness and tingling) of the hands,

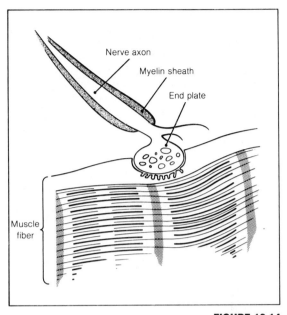

**FIGURE 10-14**
Schematic illustration of a normal myoneural junction.

thighs, and face. Rarely do patients complain of pain and discomfort in muscles.

Physical Assessment  In assessing the patient for early signs of myasthenia gravis, the nurse identifies symptoms that occur owing to ocular and generalized muscle involvement.

Ocular manifestations of myasthenia are often the initial symptoms and are present in a majority of patients. Observation may reveal unilateral or bilateral *ptosis*. The patient may be *unable to close the eyelids* against resistance or open them widely when asked to do so. Both of these findings are due to weakness of the levator palpebrae muscles and are frequently induced by bright lights, by looking fixedly at an object above eye level, or by an emotional disturbance.

The patient should also be assessed for the presence of *diplopia,* as this condition is indicative of unequal weakness of the extrinsic ocular muscles. This may be done via an ophthalmological examination with prisms.

Evaluation of facial pharyngeal and laryngeal muscle involvement is essential. Facial nerve involvement will cause the patient's facial appearance to be expressionless. When asked to smile, the person's lips move unnaturally to form a "snarl" (Fig. 10-15). There may also be an inability to whistle or purse the lips. Observation of the patient's ability to chew, swallow, and speak gives information as to

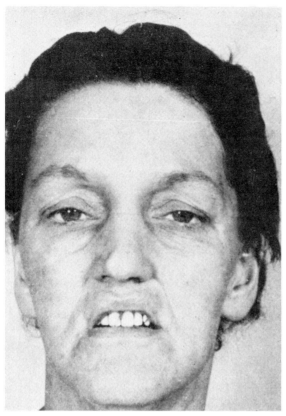

**FIGURE 10-15**
Patients with myasthenia gravis may demonstrate a characteristic facial "snarl" when they attempt to smile due to weakness of facial muscles. (*Reprinted with permission from Walton, John N., (ed.), Disorders of Voluntary Muscles, Churchill Livingstone, Edinburgh and London, 1974.*)

pharyngeal and laryngeal muscle weakness. There may be a preference for soft foods because chewing is impaired, and food intake may be decreased because choking accompanies attempts to swallow. The patient's weight should be taken to determine any changes. Having the person count out loud as far as possible in one breath will help in evaluating the degree of dysarthria (difficulty in speaking). The speech has an unusual sound, a nasal quality, and becomes progressively unintelligible as the person continues to speak. The quantity of speech completed should be noted, as this is usually diminished by weakness.

Strength in the upper extremities may be assessed by having the patient raise both arms. The effort required and the length of time the position is held should be noted.

It is critically important that the patient be assessed for respiratory muscle involvement. The fre-

quency and character of the respirations should be noted as well as any changes in the vital capacity, as measured by a spirometer. The character of the cough, the ability to clear the throat, and the nature of any dyspnea should be described and noted.

**D**iagnostic Tests   If the diagnosis of myasthenia is suspected, it can be confirmed by the response to a short-acting anticholinesterase compound *edrophonium (Tensilon)*. This drug is preferred when cranial muscles are being tested because the response is prompt and dramatic. First, the nurse should evaluate a patient's baseline strength. Then the physician injects 2 mg intravenously, followed in 30 seconds by an additional 8 mg if the first injection does not produce an increase in strength. The nurse should always have intravenous atropine available as an antidote. If the test is positive, i.e., there is increased muscle strength, the symptoms are said to be due to myasthenia gravis.

To provide more evidence, an *electromyogram* (EMG) may be done. A characteristic decline in the amplitude of the evoked muscle action potential is seen in affected muscle, but the response may be normal in ocular myasthenia. Also, *electrical stimulation* may be useful to demonstrate fatigability of the affected muscles (positive Jolly reaction). No other laboratory test provides such clear diagnostic evidence. Standard *roentgenograms of the chest* are done to identify the presence of thymomas. Thyroid function should be tested, also. Serum protein electrophoresis, an LE cell preparation, a latex fixation test for RF and ANA, and tests for muscle antibodies and lymphocyte sensitivity are run to evaluate any significant immunologic response.

If laboratory tests and the patient's history suggest that the patient may have myasthenia gravis, there are several measures besides those mentioned earlier that can be used to assess muscle weakness. They include bilateral hand squeezes or devices such as a dynamometer or ergogram, as well as a fatigue test. This test requires that the patient hold both arms outstretched for at least 1 minute. If the arms sag or tremble, then the shoulder girdle is quite weak.

**Nursing problems and intervention**   Specific nursing problems include *ptosis, dysphagia, dysarthria, dyspnea,* and *facial muscle weakness.* Interventions include medication and symptomatic care.

**D**rug Therapy *Anticholinesterase* drugs are the backbone of treatment for the numerous problems due to myasthenia. They increase the response of the muscles to nerve impulses and improve muscle strength by inhibiting cholinesterases. Drugs currently being used include neostigmine bromide (Prostigmin), ambenonium chloride (Mytelase), and pyridostigmine bromide (Mestinon). Most patients prefer *Mestinon* because they feel there is less diarrhea and abdominal cramping and its effect lasts longer (3 to 8 hours). Often a time-release spansule is provided for patients at bedtime so that they do not awaken with unusual weakness. *Mytelase* acts over 4 to 5 hours and is most toxic but produces maximum strength. *Prostigmin* acts over 3 to 4 hours. The dosages of any of these medications are highly variable, for some patients have no symptoms with neostigmine 60 mg three times a day, and others take dosages five times that amount and still need an injection of neostigmine 1 to 1.5 mg shortly before meals. The dosage is gradually increased until optimal effect has been achieved. Generally the dosage is kept at the lowest amount possible in order to prevent a "cholinergic crisis." It is not uncommon for patients who take anticholinesterase medications to experience side effects.

The most common nursing problems that arise owing to this medication include *anorexia, nausea, diarrhea,* and *abdominal cramps.* Atropine sulfate often is given as necessary, or along with the regular dosage of anticholinesterase to control these symptoms. *Gastric distress* frequently occurs because these medications are very irritating to the intestinal mucosa. Therefore, the nurse should encourage the patient to take the medication with milk, soda crackers, ice cream, or antacids in order to lessen these problems. The nurse must assess the amount and frequency of diarrhea and listen to the bowel sounds to evaluate the degree of peristalsis. It is important to control this problem in order to maintain a patient's personal hygiene, skin integrity, and proper electrolyte balance.

In addition to anticholinesterases, patients are given *ephedrine sulfate* 25 mg three times a day to increase the tone of skeletal muscles. *Potassium chloride* is also given because the effect of cholinergic drugs is believed to be potentiated when a patient has adequate serum levels of potassium.

The nurse should inform the patient about several matters in regard to these medications. The patient should clearly understand that the medications do not cure myasthenia and that they generally must be taken for the rest of one's life. It also is important to teach the patient the side effects of the medications and what they may indicate—a myasthenic or cholinergic crisis, or an exacerbation. In order to do this the patient must be made aware of

when the drug effect peaks and falls off. It is also important to point out that anticholinesterases are often poorly absorbed by the gastrointestinal tract, and an extra dosage may have to be ordered at times. It must be stressed how important it is to take medications *on time* and not to alter the dosage without appropriate training and medical supervision.

**M**uscle Weakness *Diplopia* responds poorly to medication, and so the nurse should cover one eye with a patch or make sure that one lens is frosted. Ptosis also responds poorly to medications, and eyelid crutches may be used. If the patient is unable to close the eyelids, methylcellulose should be used to lubricate the conjunctiva and prevent corneal damage.

Because of *dysphagia,* scheduling the patient's anticholinesterase medications 20 to 30 minutes before eating may be wise so that full advantage can be taken of the effect of the medication. Grinding up the medication may also be helpful. Perhaps smaller, more frequent semisolid or fluid meals that are high in potassium may be needed. Above all, the patient should not be rushed, for this only causes fatigue unnecessarily.

To lessen the problem of *dysarthria,* the nurse should help the family to establish clear and simple means of communicating verbally and nonverbally with the patient. Because involvement of the respiratory muscles causes part of this problem, it is important that emergency respiratory equipment be available at all times. The nurse should teach the patient's family how to use this equipment at home and should advise the patient to wear an identification bracelet with the medical diagnosis on it. Encouraging the patient to speak in shorter sentences is important in order to prevent unnecessary fatigue.

*Breathing* is made difficult by the respiratory muscle involvement. The primary nursing objective is to ensure that the patient gets adequate ventilation with the least amount of energy expenditure. After teaching the patient why this problem occurs, the nurse should help the patient to plan physical activities so that unnecessary dyspnea is minimized. Encouraging breathing and diaphragmatic exercises helps the patient to maintain strength in the respiratory muscles. Sometimes advising the patient to sleep with several pillows under the head may facilitate easier breathing. Patients with myasthenia should be advised to particularly avoid exposure to people with upper respiratory infections, because of their increased susceptibility. Sedatives of any type should not be given to a patient who is having difficulty breathing. The nurse should continually assess the severity of the weakness and the ways exercise and rest affect it. This can be done with a fatigue test and by using bilateral hand squeezes or devices to evaluate muscle strength.

The primary nursing objective is to help maintain the patient's present muscle strength as well as to prevent muscle atrophy and calcium depletion due to disuse. The nurse must educate the patient and the family about the activities that appear to cause the muscle weakness and then help the patient to plan each day differently to avoid fatigue. This would include emphasizing how important a good night's sleep is, perhaps a nap during the day, and reasonable pacing of activities that may cause fatigue. The patient should be encouraged to do regular active and active-resistive exercises every day as an important preventive measure. The nurse may do a home evaluation to help the patient decide what is the most efficient way to organize the living situation in order to prevent unnecessary waste of energy.

### Third-Level Nursing Care

If a conservative treatment program does not control the disease process or major complications occur, hospitalization may become necessary. Difficulties experienced earlier in the disease process are often more severe at this time.

**Nursing assessment**  During an acute exacerbation, the patient often relates a *health history* similar to that in Second-Level Nursing Care, but with symptoms that have increased in severity. This is often true of generalized muscle weakness and respiratory muscle involvement.

*Physical assessment* may reveal a severely malnourished person because of progressive dysphagia and regurgitation of food and fluids. The patient's weight should be taken and compared with previous records. Skin turgor and moistness of mucous membranes should be assessed for any sign of dehydration.

Severe involvement of the lingual, facial, palatal, laryngeal, and respiratory muscles may result in a distinct nasal twang, indistinct speech, and often an inability to speak (aphonia). This may be assessed by having the patient count or answer simple questions.

The most critical evaluation, at this time, is the patient's respiratory status. The degree of dyspnea should be noted and whether it is present at rest. If the patient is completely unable to breathe independently, emergency intervention is imperative.

The degree of weakness of the muscles of the trunk and limbs should be assessed. This may be done by asking the patient to hold the head up and to move different areas of the body. Patients with severe involvement cannot hold their heads up and frequently cannot move any of their muscles.

The patient may appear frightened and anxious. The nurse should remember that the person is generally very alert mentally and therefore aware of what is happening. Thorough explanations of all examinations should be given.

**D**iagnostic Tests  When a patient is hospitalized for any of these severe problems, the Tensilon test may be repeated to assess the cause of the problems. As time passes, the Tensilon test may be readministered in order to assess any significant change in the state of the disease and to regulate the dosage of anticholinesterases. Additional diagnostic tests that are used depend on the particular problems that a patient is experiencing. For example, a patient's arterial blood gases and vital capacity will be monitored regularly if the patient is having difficulty breathing. Fluoroscopy may be used to evaluate the patient's ability to swallow.

**Nursing problems and interventions**  *Malnutrition, aphonia, severe respiratory impairment, generalized weakness,* and *emotional stress* are among the nursing problems commonly identified in caring for a patient with myasthenia gravis.

**G**eneral Therapies  If a patient needs to be hospitalized for uncontrolled muscle weakness or a severe exacerbation, the dosage of the anticholinesterase medication may be increased and given intramuscularly or intravenously.

If the dosage of the anticholinesterase is increased, the nurse must be alert for any signs of a "cholinergic crisis." Signs of this crisis include *severe diarrhea, nausea* and *vomiting, hypersalivation* and *lacrimation, pallor, miosis,* and *hypotension.* Although *bradycardia* is uncommon with oral medications, it may occur and lead to a cardiac arrest. In the most severe cases of crisis, *confusion* and *coma* occur due to blockage of the cerebral synapses. Continually monitoring a patient's vital signs, arterial blood gases, and intake and output are important nursing actions in assessing the severity of the problems. The most valuable indication of the severity of side effects is the size of the pupil;

it should never be allowed to contract to less than 2 mm diameter in normal room light. All anticholinesterase medications are usually withdrawn, and the patient is given atropine sulfate 2 mg intravenously every hour until signs of atropine toxicity develop. A cuffed endotracheal tube may be passed, and artificial ventilation and suctioning should be provided if cholinergic paralysis occurs. If these problems are prolonged, a tracheostomy may be needed. When the crisis has passed, the anticholinesterases are given again but generally at about half the precrisis dosage.

If the patient is not controlled within a few days by a higher dosage of anticholinesterases, the physician may consider a thymectomy, to reduce the body's immune response. When a *thymectomy* is done, the result is unpredictable, for it may be immediate, delayed, or not occur at all. Generally, the improvement is gradual and the maximum benefit is seen at about the third year after surgery. This surgery tends to produce a much lower mortality and greater chance of complete remission or substantial improvement when the person is a female, has had the disease less than 5 years, or does not have a thymoma. After 7 years from the onset, there is less chance of improvement, but it still may occur. It is still not possible to clearly select patients who will benefit from the operation.

The other types of medications that can be tried at this point include ACTH, cortisone and its derivatives, and immunosuppressive agents. ACTH has been used because of its effect in shrinking thymic and lymphatic tissue for patients who do not respond well or are resistant to cholinergic medications. Initial deterioration is common, and so it must be given in the proper setting. Now, because of our ability to support ventilatory status, repeated courses of larger doses of ACTH have been used with considerable benefit. Generally 100 units ACTH is given every day for 10 days. Remissions induced by ACTH often last 3 to 6 months, but then a repeated course is necessary. Cortisone and its derivative are less effective than ACTH and have the same dangers, but they are used in patients who are unresponsive to cholinergic medications. Generally, patients are started on 60 mg and then slowly tapered to 5 to 15 mg every other day. Many people still question whether it is advisable to treat patients with a chronic disease with steroids because they often are weak and debilitated. Several *immunosuppressive* agents (methotrexate, azathioprine, and cyclophosphamide) have been used when steroids were ineffective, but many feel that there is no clear indication that they are better than steroids.

**Malnutrition** To treat malnutrition, intravenous feedings and nasogastric tube feedings may be ordered. Nasogastric feedings should contain no more than 200 ml at a time, to prevent overfilling the stomach. Care should be taken to make sure tube feedings are being absorbed. Failure to aspirate the stomach contents prior to each tube feeding might result in vomiting and aspiration by the patient. Suction equipment should always be next to the patient's bed.

**Severe Respiratory Impairment** Sometimes a rocking bed that utilizes gravity in order to externally aid respiration may be used for *dyspneic* patients. If severe weakness occurs, placing a mask over the patient's mouth and nose may be necessary so that the weak respirations can trigger the IPPB machine. If there is temporary paralysis of the respiratory muscles, a positive pressure machine is used. Perhaps a *tracheostomy* may be indicated in order to prevent an obstruction and to facilitate the removal of secretions by suctioning. When the patient is on a respirator, the dosage of anticholinesterases should be greatly decreased in order to decrease the pulmonary secretions and gastrointestinal side effects. Once the crisis is passed, the normal dosage of medication is resumed. Other important nursing measures include regular postural drainage, sterile suctioning when needed, and frequent turning of the patient. Often prophylactic antibiotics are given to try to prevent respiratory infections. It is important for nurses to remember that a number of antibiotics, including streptomycin, dihydrostreptomycin, gentamycin, kanamycin, neomycin, and polymyxin A and B, have a depressant effect on the myoneural junction. Therefore, these drugs must be used with great caution.

**Generalized Weakness** During this critical time, the patient should receive the highest level of nursing care. The patient should be placed in a highback chair to support weak neck muscles when sitting. When there is severe generalized muscle involvement, the nurse must provide all physical care and assure the patient that someone will be within reach at all times. Patients frequently will have *stress incontinence* because of the inability to control their external sphincters. Appropriate nursing measures should be provided to ensure cleanliness in order to prevent skin breakdown and to prevent unnecessary embarrassment of the patient.

**Fourth-Level Nursing Care**

Helping to identify a patient's *rehabilitation potential* is a continuous and challenging process for the nurse who works with patients with myasthenia gravis. This consists of assessing the patient's physical and emotional state by assisting in a functional, vocational, and psychosocial assessment.

The most common and persistent nursing problems that occur during the patient's convalescence are *exacerbations, chronic muscle weakness* and *fatigue,* numerous psychosocial *difficulties in accepting* and *adjusting* to this disease, and continuous *fear* of the unknown as to whether the disease will remain controlled. The possibility of the occurrence of an exacerbation is an ever-present problem for people with myasthenia gravis. A nurse who is assessing the patient's rehabilitation potential must be aware of the factors that may be related to these exacerbations which include physical and emotional stress, pregnancy, infections, and numerous drugs. Therefore, the nurse should work with the patient to identify the activities or events that seem to cause physical or emotional stress and then help to modify this activity in order to eliminate the stressor.

The effects of pregnancy are variable, but often an exacerbation may occur at or soon after delivery. The nurse must make careful and frequent assessments of the status of the patient's myasthenia before, during, and after the delivery plus have emergency equipment available at all times.

Infections often cause worsening of the symptoms of myasthenia, so it is important for the nurse to advise the patient to avoid unnecessary exposure to people with upper respiratory infections because of the respiratory muscle involvement in myasthenia gravis. Adequate sleep plus regular, nutritious meals also help patients to maintain their resistance to infections. If a patient does get an infection, antibiotics like neomycin and streptomycin are prescribed, with caution, because of the blocking effect they may have on the myoneural junction. There are many other medications that tend to affect patients with myasthenia gravis. It is best to avoid the use of curare, quinine, quinidine, chloroform, morphine, and ether because of their depressant effects. Other medications that have been suspected in effecting a worsening of myasthenia include ACTH, corticosteroids, thyroid compound, sedatives, and other respiratory depressants. Finally, the use of enemas has precipitated fatal myasthenia crises, perhaps because of the potassium depletion.

**Functional assessment**  The degree of muscle weakness and fatigue must be evaluated. Therefore a functional evaluation should be done to identify the activities that appear to cause any increased muscle weakness and fatigue. It must be remembered that although permanent disabilities are rare, there will be some physical limitation in the patient's strength and tolerance to exercise. This is because the anticholinesterase medications generally relieve only 80 percent of the problems due to myasthenia gravis. With this information in mind, the nurse should work with the patient to modify everyday activities, to conserve energy and time, so that they do not cause unnecessary weakness and fatigue.

**Vocational assessment**  When a patient's disease is stabilized to the point that everyday activities do not cause unusual weakness and fatigue, a vocational assessment should be done. A nurse may help in this assessment, when possible, by going with a vocational counselor and the patient to the former place of employment to ascertain the physical and emotional requirements and potential stressors of the job. The circumstances of the job must allow the patient to sit down and rest when necessary, and the job must not be unusually stressful physically.

**Psychosocial assessment**  A psychosocial assessment is an important evaluation because all too often, even with proper medical management, rehabilitation problems revolve around the psychosocial difficulties of the patient and the family. It is important for the nurse to evaluate the patient's and family's understanding of and attitude toward myasthenia, as well as their emotional response and ability to adjust to it. Should any unusual fears or problems occur relating to the patient's adjustment to the disease, it may be necessary for a psychologist to provide a psychological evaluation.

After these data are collected, the nurse can work with the rehabilitation team to establish the patient's rehabilitation potential. The ultimate objective is to help patients with myasthenia to learn how to live as nearly normal a life as possible. It is best for these people to do as much as they physically are able to do without overdoing unnecessarily. The rehabilitation program that helps the patient to achieve this goal includes appropriate patient education about the disease, medication, safe activity level, and measures to prevent exacerbations.

Once the patient's disease is controlled, it is wise to urge continuance of the former life-style, job, and other activities, with suggested modifications to prevent muscle weakness and fatigue.

When a patient returns home, the nurse can provide a referral to a community health nurse for continuous follow-up. The patient's progress and adjustment to this health problem can then be better evaluated. In addition, the nurse should inform the patient about the Myasthenia Gravis Foundation and other community organizations which provide various types of support for patients with this disease.

## OTHER AUTOIMMUNE DISEASES

It is not possible within the limits of this section to cover all the diseases that have suspected autoimmune origins. Therefore, only a few more representative diseases will be described.

### Polyarteritis Nodosa

Polyarteritis nodosa is an uncommon collagen vascular disease that produces inflammation and necrosis in the walls of small and medium-sized arteries. No single etiologic agent or pathogenic mechanism has been identified. Some research has indicated that because there is a deposition of immune complexes of foreign antigens and antibodies in areas of fibrinoid necrosis of blood vessels, it may be an autoimmune disease.

*Pathological findings* commonly include segmental necrosis, fibrinoid degeneration and inflammation of the media and adventia of small and medium-sized arteries, along with infiltration by polymorphonuclear leukocytes. The usual renal lesion is glomerulitis with focal fibrinoid changes and marked proliferation of Bowman's capsule. The involved vessels often have depositions of immune reactants like immunoglobulin and complement as well as fibrin and albumin. This pathology commonly results in thrombosis and obstruction to blood flow. Generally, the healing process results in fibrosis and thickening of the artery with resulting circulatory impairment of the affected tissues. Sometimes only a portion of the circumference of an artery may be affected leading to localized dilatation and rupture.

Although it occurs primarily in middle life, it may occur at any age, with an incidence about three times as great in females as in males. Whether it is acute or chronic, the disease often is fatal within 5 years after the onset owing to failure of the heart, kidneys, or other vital organs.

The clinical symptoms are determined primarily by the location and severity of the arteritis and by the extent of the secondary circulatory impairment. The most common sites of involvement are the kidneys (80 percent), heart (70 percent), liver (65 percent), and gastrointestinal tract (50 percent), as well as the lungs, muscles, skin, pancreas, peripheral nerves, brain, and testes.[20] The most common *nursing problems* are *low-grade fever, malaise, weakness,* and *weight loss.* Others include severe pain in the abdomen or loins, diffuse muscle aches and pain, arthralgias, arthritis, bloody diarrhea, hypertension due to renal disease, cardiac failure, peripheral neuritis, bronchial asthma or pneumonia, purpuric skin rashes, and infarction of the liver and testes. Besides observing for these clinical manifestations, it is important for the nurse to note any significant changes in laboratory findings. Eosinophilia, leukocytosis, and thrombocytosis sometimes are observed. Proteinuria and microscopic hematuria are common urinary abnormalities. Sometimes a patient's serum gamma globulins are elevated along with a positive RF and an elevated sedimentation rate. A definite diagnosis depends on a biopsy of the skin, subcutaneous tissues, or muscles from the site of an acute reaction where autoantibodies against vascular wall antigens are found.

Nursing care consists of symptomatic and supportive measures of the major systems that are involved. *Analgesics* and high dosages of *corticosteroids* usually are given initially to control the inflammatory process and pain. The steroids are often tapered to a maintenance dose, but they are only partially effective for long-term therapy. *Salicylates* are given to control the fever. A balanced diet with adequate caloric intake is necessary in order to maintain the patient's weight. Advising patients to rest, especially when their disease is active, is important.

### Sjögren's Syndrome

Sjögren's syndrome is a rare benign chronic disorder of the connective tissues that occurs primarily in females between 40 and 65 years of age. The disease appears insidiously, and generally is characterized by dryness of the eyes with lack of tears (keratoconjunctivitis sicca), dryness of the mouth (zerostomia), and enlargement of the salivary and lacrimal glands. In addition, a collagen-vascular disease such as rheumatoid arthritis, SLE, or progressive systemic sclerosis commonly is present. In the fully developed syndrome, nasal, pharyngeal, vaginal, and vulvar dryness also occur as well as generalized dryness of the skin.

Sjögren's syndrome is believed to be an autoimmune disease because of the presence of autoantibodies against the lacrimal and salivary glands as well as numerous other autoantibodies. The concept of a slow viral infection as a causative factor is also considered.

The classic lesion in Sjögren's syndrome is a lymphocytic and plasma cell infiltrate of salivary, lacrimal, and other exocrine glands in the respiratory and gastrointestinal tract and vagina. The gradual atrophy and destruction of these glands are believed to be associated with this massive infiltration of their parenchyma.

Major *nursing problems* that occur are due to the dysfunction of the salivary and lacrimal glands. They include a *burning* and *scratchy sensation* in the patient's eyes due to lack of tears, *photophobia,* a *dry mouth,* and *difficulty in swallowing* and *speaking* due to nasal and pharyngeal dryness. The diagnosis of Sjögren's syndrome is confirmed by many tests. Ocular staining detects keratoconjunctivitis sicca, and the Schirmer test measures the amount of tear secretions. In evaluating the salivary glands, one measures the amount and type of salivary flow and does sialography to visualize radiologically the salivary duct system. In addition, common hematological findings include an elevated ESR, anemia, leukopenia, and eosinophilia. The immunological abnormalities detected in the serum include diffuse elevation of gamma globulin, normal or elevated complement, a positive RF, and the presence of ANA and other autoantibodies.

*Nursing care* consists of treating the disease manifestations locally, because systemic therapy with medication is ineffective. The most effective therapy for dry eyes is the application of artificial tears as often as necessary in order to prevent corneal ulcers. Advising patients to wear glasses to protect their eyes from foreign bodies is also important to prevent unnecessary trauma and possible infection. Treatment of the zerostomia must include keeping the mouth well lubricated by frequently drinking a lot of fluids, by sucking on hard candy, and by avoiding any medication that would decrease salivary secretions. Immaculate oral and dental care must be emphasized, because dental caries and loss of restorations are frequent problems for these patients. It is important to continually observe for the occurrence of any localized infection so that it is treated promptly. If the dryness involves the upper respiratory tract, the nurse must be alert for signs of inflammation because superimposed infections commonly occur.

### Polymyositis and Dermatomysositis

Polymyositis and dermatomyositis are uncommon chronic diffuse inflammatory diseases of striated muscle which generally occur insidiously. They cause muscle weakness and atrophy principally in the limb girdles, neck, and pharynx. Dermatomyositis frequently is accompanied by a prominent skin rash.

No single *etiological agent* has been identified. Some feel that this problem has an autoimmune basis because there are numerous similarities between this disease and other connective tissue disorders having more substantial evidence for an autoimmune origin. Several infectious agents have been suspected, but the myxovirus is of greatest interest currently because of the identification of inclusions similar to this virus in the affected muscle fibers.

The characteristic *pathological* lesions in the muscles include degeneration of the muscle fibers along with an infiltrate of chronic inflammatory cells. Edema, hyperkeratosis, and atrophy occur in the dermis along with an inflammatory infiltrate.

These disorders may occur at any age, and females are affected twice as often as males. Prognosis for children and young adults is quite good. However, the overall survival for adults, who are 50 years of age and older at diagnosis, is 53 percent.[31] This is probably due to the fact that malignant neoplasms are found in a higher proportion of these patients.

The clinical symptoms are determined by the location of the muscle and other connective tissues involved. The most common *nursing problems* include *weakness* and *pain* in the proximal muscles which may eventually limit the patient's ability to walk, use the arms, speak, and swallow. *Skin rashes* may occur on the face, neck, hands, knees, and ankles. They may, with time, cause *stiffness* and *contractures* particularly in a patient's fingers because of skin atrophy, fibrosis, and calcification. Some pain and stiffness occur due to mild polyarthritis and polyarthralgias, but rarely does joint destruction occur. Sometimes the viscera are involved resulting in colicky abdominal pain and constipation. Essentially, all patients experience different degrees of constitutional symptoms and some weight loss.

In order to help facilitate a complete assessment, the nurse must be aware of some of the common diagnostic tests that should be performed. The diagnosis is most often confirmed by muscle biopsy and electromyographic findings. The activity of the disease is followed by detecting the levels of enzymes released by the affected muscle tissue in the serum. Screening for tumors is important because of the unusually high incidence of malignancy.

Nursing care consists of symptomatic and supportive measures. Providing *corticosteroids, immunosuppressive* or *cytotoxic* agents as ordered, to control the acute or chronic inflammatory process, helps to sustain improvement in patients with straight-forward polymyositis or dermatomyositis. However, some children and adults with a coexisting malignancy or Sjögren's syndrome will often respond poorly or only temporarily. Long-continued maintenance dosages of prednisone often are necessary. Early detection and removal of malignancies often can be followed by remarkable improvement in the muscle symptoms. *Analgesics* should be given for the pain. Encouraging patients to get adequate rest while still doing regular active exercise is important in sustaining muscle strength and in preventing permanent musculoskeletal disability. Helping patients to maintain their weight and a good nutritional status plus preventing constipation are also important nursing considerations.

## Systemic Sclerosis (Scleroderma)

Scleroderma is an uncommon generalized connective tissue disease which is characterized by fibrotic thickening (sclerosis) and inflammatory changes throughout many organs of the body, especially the skin. It is most common between 30 and 50 years of age and is twice as common in females as it is in males.[32]

No single *etiologic agent* for scleroderma has been identified. It may be due to a derangement in the metabolism of connective tissue or to a defect in the immune system. However, a great deal of evidence supports the view that it is an immunologic disorder because of the presence of numerous autoantibodies, elevated gamma globulins, and serum complement, and because it overlaps and resembles other possible autoimmune diseases such as rheumatoid arthritis.

The characteristic *pathological lesions* in the connective tissue include inflammation and fibrotic and degenerative changes along with vascular lesions. The most prominent changes occur in the skin, musculoskeletal system, esophagus, and intestinal tract. In addition, lesions often occur in the heart, lung, kidneys, and peripheral nerves.

The course of the disease is steadily progressive and leads to cardiac failure, hypertensive renal disease, pulmonary complications, or intestinal malabsorption and cachexia. These occur in 50 percent of patients within 2 or 3 years after diagnosis.[33]

The clinical symptoms are determined by the location and severity of the organ system involved. The most common initial *nursing problems* are *pain* in the fingers, wrists, knees, or ankles and *swelling, stiffness,* and a *reddish discoloration* in the

terminal digits. These symptoms occur owing to Raynaud's phenomenon (90 percent), to inflammatory changes in the skin, and to polyarthritis.[34] Myositis often causes generalized *muscle weakness. Dysphagia* and *esophageal reflux* occur because of ulcers and/or aperistalsis of the esophagus. Less frequently pulmonary alveolar thickening occurs and causes dyspnea and cough. If the kidneys are involved early, highly malignant hypertension occurs. As the disease progresses, many other major nursing problems may occur which include flexion contractures, pulmonary and malignant hypertension, right- or left-sided heart failure, renal failure, severe ulceration, and aperistalsis of the gastrointestinal tract which causes marked malabsorption and cachexia. Besides observing for these clinical manifestations, the nurse must be aware of any significant laboratory findings. Frequently these patients demonstrate anemia early in the disease, and if there is renal involvement, proteinuria and microscopic hematuria occur. Significant immunological findings include a positive RF and LE cell reaction, an elevated gamma globulin, the presence of ANA, and occasionally a false positive test for syphilis.

At this point in time no treatment has been found that significantly affects the inflammatory and fibrotic changes in this disease. *Corticosteroids* and *antihypertensives* have had only a limited effect. However, patients who have had *nephrectomies* and *renal transplants* have done well. It is important for the nurse to note any signs of an infection, so that it can be treated early and aggressively with antibiotics. Regular monitoring of a patient's vital signs, respiratory capacity, urinary output, and significant changes in the gastrointestinal tract are important nursing actions. Encouraging patients to actively exercise is important in order to maintain muscle strength, although even extensive physical therapy does not totally prevent contractures. Advising patients to protect their extremities from extreme cold also is important. Because of numerous gastrointestinal problems, it is best to have patients eat small frequent meals with the head of the bed elevated and to then follow the meal with an antacid.

## Hashimoto's Chronic Thyroiditis

Hashimoto's disease is a common form of chronic thyroiditis characterized by enlargement of the thyroid gland. Hypothyroidism consequently occurs because of the destruction of the secretory cells of the thyroid gland and the presence of autoantibodies against the thyroid gland and thyroglobulin.

The presence of numerous autoantibodies

against thyroid tissue has caused investigators to feel that it may be an autoimmune disease, but experimental research has not confirmed this. A genetic predisposition is also considered because of a higher incidence of the disease or presence of thyroid autoantibodies in a patient's family members.

*Pathological* findings commonly include a diffuse infiltration of the thyroid gland by lymphocytes and plasma cells with eventual fibrotic changes and a decrease in the size of thyroid secretory cells. The larger size of the gland is due to the increase in the lymphocytes and plasma cells which virtually alter the character of the thyroid gland so much that it begins to resemble lymphoid tissues.

This disease occurs 30 times as often in females, as compared with males, and there is a strong peak incidence in females about the time of menopause. The course is generally chronic, and approximately one-third of the patients develop hypothyroidism and myxedema.[35]

The major *nursing problem* occurring early in the disease is the marked *enlargement of the thyroid gland.* With time it may cause pressure locally and produce *dysphagia* and possible *respiratory distress.* Problems due to hypothyroidism such as *lethargy* or *apathy* develop slowly over time. Besides being aware of these potential problems, the nurse must be aware of the laboratory tests which help to confirm a diagnosis. Thyroid autoantibodies are present, and decreased thyroid activity occurs, although false positive antibody tests are relatively common. Therefore, the diagnosis should be confirmed by a needle biopsy of the enlarged thyroid gland.

Nursing measures are directed toward decreasing the size of the thyroid gland and preventing hypothyroidism. Therefore, replacement therapy with *thyroxine* 0.2 to 0.3 mg/day or *desiccated thyroid* 120 to 200 mg/day is provided to correct or avoid the hypothyroidism. *Corticosteroids* frequently reduce the size of the thyroid gland and sometimes decrease the titers of thyroid autoantibodies. Rarely is radiation therapy necessary to reduce the size. A *partial thyroidectomy* is done as a last resort because of the risk of the occurrence of myxedema.

## REFERENCES

1 Patterson, Roy, C. R. Zeiss, and John F. Kelly: "Classification of Hypersensitivity Reactions," *N Engl J Med,* **295:**277–279, Jan. 29, 1976.

2 Solomon, William R.: "Hay Fever, Allergic Rhinitis, and Bronchial Asthma," in John M. Sheldon, Robert G. Lovell, and Kenneth P. Matthews (eds.), *A Manual of Clinical Allergy,* 2d ed., Saunders, Philadelphia, 1967, pp. 78–97.

3 Patterson, Roy: "Rhinitis," *Med Clin North Am,* **58:**43–54, January 1974.

4 Hargreave, Frederick E., and Jerry Dolovich: "Immunology of Pulmonary Disease," in Geoffrey Taylor (ed.), *Immunology in Medical Practice,* Saunders, Philadelphia, 1975.

5 Reed, Charles E.: "The Pathogenesis of Asthma," *Med Clin North Am,* **58:**55–61, January 1974.

6 Ackroyd, J. F.: "Drug Hypersensitivity," in *Immunology in Medical Practice,* pp. 317–366.

7 Wintrobe, Maxwell M., et al.: *Harrison's Principles of Internal Medicine,* 7th ed., McGraw-Hill, New York, 1974, pp. 368–375.

8 Slavin, Raymond G.: "Skin Tests in the Diagnosis of Allergies of the Immediate Type," *Med Clin North Am,* **58:**65–69, January 1974.

9 Samter, Talmage, Rose, Sherman, and Vaughn, *Immunological Diseases,* 2d ed., Little, Brown, Boston, 1971, p. 816.

10 Sheldon, John M., Robert G. Lovell, and Kenneth P. Matthews: "Specific Therapy: Avoidance and Hyposensitization," *A Manual of Clinical Allergy,* Saunders, Philadelphia, 1967, p. 102.

11 Moody, Linda E.: "Nursing Care of Patients with Asthma," *Nurs Clin North Am,* **9:**195–207, March 1974.

12 Hargreaves, Anne G.: "Emotional Problems of Patients with Respiratory Disease," *Nurs Clin North Am,* **3:**479–487, September 1968.

13 Sheldon et al., op. cit., pp. 456–483.

14 Greaves, Malcolm W.: "Immunology of Skin Diseases," in *Immunology in Medical Practice,* pp. 293–316.

15 Robbins, Stanley L.: *Pathological Basis of Disease,* Saunders, Philadelphia, 1974, pp. 1466–1470.

16 Rodman, Gerald P. (ed.): "Primer on the Rheumatic Diseases, 7th ed., *JAMA,* **224:**25–38 (Suppl), April 30, 1973.

17 *Ibid.*

18 *Ibid.*

19 Huskisson, E. C., and Dudley Hart: *Joint Disease: All the Arthropathies,* Williams & Wilkins, Baltimore, 1973, pp. 109–110.

20 *Ibid.*

21 *Ibid.*

22 *Ibid.*

23 Rodman, Gerald P. (ed.): op. cit., pp. 39–49.

24 *Ibid.*

25 Simpson, John A.: "Myasthenia Gravis and Myas-

thenic Syndromes," in *Disorders of Voluntary Muscles,* 3d ed., Churchill-Livingstone, London, 1974, pp. 653–692.

26  Beeson, Paul B., and Walsh McDermott (eds.): *The Textbook of Medicine,* 14th ed., Saunders, Philadelphia, 1975, pp. 802–805.

27  *Ibid.*

28  *Ibid.*

29  Flacke, Werrer: "Treatment of Myasthenia Gravis," *N Engl J Med,* **288:**27–31, Jan. 4, 1973.

30  Rodman, Gerald P., (ed.): op. cit., pp. 60–64.

31  Whitake, J. N., and W. K. Engle: "Vascular Deposits of Immunoglobulin and Complement in Inflammatory Myopathy," *N Engl J Med,* **286:**333–338, 1972.

32  Rodman, G. P.: "Progressive Systemic Sclerosis (Scleroderma)," in Joseph L. Hollander and Daniel J. McCarty (eds.), *Arthritis and Allied Conditions.* 8th ed., Lea & Febiger, Philadelphia, 1972, pp. 962–1005.

33  Beeson, Paul B., and Walsh McDermott (eds.): *The Textbook of Medicine,* 14th ed., Saunders, Philadelphia, 1975, pp. 124–128.

34  Rodman, Gerald P. (ed.): "Primer on the Rheumatic Diseases," pp. 60–64.

35  Volpé, Robert, et al.: "The Pathogenesis of Grave's Disease and Hashimoto's Thyroiditis," *Clin Endocrinol,* **3:**239–261, 1974.

## BIBLIOGRAPHY

Barnes, C. G., et al.: "Felty's Syndrome: A Clinical Pathological Survey of 21 Patients and Their Response to Treatment," *Ann Rheum Dis,* **30:**359–374, 1971.

Bartholomew, Lee E., et al.: "Management of Rheumatoid Arthritis," *Am Fam Physician,* **13:**116–125, 1976.

Bayles, Theodore B.: "Salicylate Therapy for Rheumatoid Arthritis," in Joseph L. Hollander and Daniel J. McCarty (eds.), *Arthritis and Allied Conditions,* Lea & Febiger, Philadelphia, 1972, pp. 448–454.

Beaumont, Estelle: "Ravages of Rheumatoid Arthritis—Rehabilitation of Both Body and Spirit," *Nursing '75,* **5:**44–49, June 1975.

Beland, Irene L.: *Clinical Nursing, Pathophysiological and Psychosocial Approaches,* 2d ed., Macmillan, New York, 1970, pp. 781–786.

Belzer, Folkert, and Oscar Salvatierra: "Renal Transplantation, Organ Procurement, Preservation, and Surgical Management," in Barry M. Brenner and Floyd C. Rector (eds.), *The Kidney,* Saunders, Philadelphia, 1976, pp. 1796–1816.

Bergman, R. A., R. J. Johns, and A. K. Afilfi: "Ultra-

structural Alterations in Muscles from Patients with Myasthenia Gravis and Eaton-Lambert Syndrome," *Ann NY Acad Sci,* **183:**88, 1971.

Bilka, Paul J., et al.: "Rheumatoid Arthritis Therapy: Three-step Therapy for Rheumatoid Arthritis," *Patient Care,* **8:**21–27, May 15, 1974.

Bitter, T., et al.: "Immunosuppression in Systemic Lupus Erythematosus," in *Rheumatology–an Annual Review,* vol. 5, New York: Karger, 1974.

Bluestone, Rodney M. B.: "Systemic Lupus Erythematosus and other Connective Tissue Disorders," *Postgrad Med,* **58:**28–35, October 1975.

Bluhm, Gilbert B.: "The Treatment of Rheumatoid Arthritis with Gold," *Semin Arthritis Rheum,* **5:** 147–166, November 1975.

Bohan, A., et al.: "Polymyositis and Dermatomyositis," *N Engl J Med,* **292:**403–407, Feb. 20, 1975.

Bowden, Susan A.: "New Surgery for Arthritic Hands," *Nursing '76,* **6:**46–48, August 1976.

Brunner, Carolyn M., and John S. Davis IV: "Immune Mechanisms in the Pathogenesis of Systemic Lupus Erythematosus," *Bull Rheum Dis,* **26:**854–861, 1975–1976.

Burnet, Sir MacFarlane: *Auto-immunity and Auto-immune Disease,* Davis, Philadelphia, 1972.

Calabro, John J.: "Long-term Reappraisal of Indomethacin," *Drug Ther,* **5:**46–60, February 1975.

Craven, Ruth F.: "Anaphylactic Shock," *Am J Nurs,* **72:**718–721, April 1972.

Dameschek, W., and S. O. Schwartz: "The Presence of Hemolysins in Acute Hemolytic Anemia," *N Engl J Med,* **218:**75, 1938.

Dubois, Edmund L.: *Lupus Erythematosus: A Review of the Current Status of Discoid and Systemic Lupus Erythematosus and Their Varieties,* 2d ed., University of Southern California Press, Los Angeles, 1974.

Ehrlich, George E. (ed.): *Total Management of the Arthritic Patient,* Lippincott, Philadelphia, 1973.

Ehrlich, Paul: "On Immunity and Specific References to Cell Life," *Proc R Soc Lond,* **66:**424–448.

Eisen, H. N.: *Immunology—An Introduction to Molecular and Cellular Principles of Immune Response,* Harper & Row, New York, 1974.

Falconer, Mary W., et al.: *The Drug, The Nurse, The Patient,* 5th ed., Saunders, Philadelphia, 1974.

Fassbender, H. G.: *Pathology of Rheumatic Diseases,* Springer-Verlag, New York, 1975.

Felty, A. R.: "Chronic Arthritis in the Adult, Associated with Splenomegaly and Leucopenia. A Report of 5 Unusual Cases of an Unusual Clinical Syndrome," *Bull Johns Hopkins Hosp,* **35:**16–20, 1924.

Fink, Jordan N., and Abe J. Sosman: "Therapy of

Bronchial Asthma," *Med Clin North Am,* 801–808, May, 1973.

Fried, J. F., et al.: "Estimating Prognosis of Systemic Lupus Erythematosus," *Am J Med,* **57:**561–565, 1974.

Good, Robert A., and David W. Fischer (eds.): *Immunobiology,* Sinauer Associates, Stamford, Conn., 1967.

Guyton, Arthur C.: *Textbook of Medical Physiology,* 5th ed., Saunders, Philadelphia, 1976, p. 86.

Harris, Jules (ed.): "Symposium on Clinical Immunology," *Med Clin North Am,* **56,** March 1972.

Harvey, A. M., et al.: "Systemic Lupus Erythematosus: Review of Literature and Clinical Analysis of 138 Cases," *Medicine,* **33:**291, 1954.

Hollander, Joseph L., and Daniel J. McCarty (eds.): *Arthritis and Allied Conditions,* Lea & Febiger, Philadelphia, 1972.

Holt, Peter J.: *Current Topics in Connective Tissue Disease,* Churchill Livingstone, New York, 1975.

Jennings, Kate R.: "The Cheerful Operation—Total Hip Replacement," *Nursing '76,* **6:**32–37, July 1976.

Kemph, John P., Eric A. Bermann, and Henry P. Coppolillo: "Kidney Transplant and Shifts in Family Dynamics," *Am J Psychiatry,* **125:**1485–1490, May 1969.

Kinder, R. R., et al.: Systemic Scleroderma: A Review of Organ Systems, *Int J Dermatol,* **13:**382–395, November–December 1974.

Kintzel, Kay C.: *Advanced Concepts in Clinical Nursing,* Lippincott, Philadelphia, 1971.

Langstaff, S. R.: "Rheumatoid Arthritis Treated with Penacillamine," *Nurs Times,* **71:**918–920, June 12, 1975.

Larson, Carroll B., and Marjorie Gould: *Orthopedic Nursing,* 8th ed., Mosby, St. Louis, 1974.

Lewis-Faning, E.: "Report on an Inquiry into the Aetiological factors Associated with Rheumatoid Arthritis," *An Rheum Dis,* vol. 9, Suppl 94, 1950.

Lister, Joann: "Nursing Intervention in Anaphylactic Shock," *Am J Nurs,* **72:**720–721.

Matthews, W. B.: "Myasthenia Gravis," *Nurs Times,* **71:**1807–1812, Nov. 13, 1975.

Milgram, F., and E. Witebsky: "Auto-Antibodies and Auto-Immune Disease," *JAMA,* **181:**706–716, 1962.

Mills, J. A., et al.: "Value of Bedrest in Patients with Rheumatoid Arthritis," *N Engl J Med,* **284:**453–458, 1971.

Mitchell, N., and Shepard, N.: "The Effects of Synovectomy on Synovium and Cartilage in Early Rheumatoid Arthritis," *Clin Orthop,* **89:**178–196, 1972.

Najarian, J., et al.: "Renal Transplantation: Criteria for Evaluation and Selection of Patients and Immunological Aspects of Transplantation," in Barry M. Brenner and Floyd C. Rector (eds.), *The Kidney,* vol. II, Saunders, Philadelphia, 1976, pp. 1745–1792.

O'dell, A. J.: "Hot Packs for Morning Stiffness," *Am J Nurs,* **75:**986–987, June 1975.

Rabin, B. S., and A. Winkelstein: "Theories of Autoimmunity," *Bull Rheum Dis,* **26:**842–847, 1975–1976 series.

Rodman, G. P.: "Progressive Systemic Sclerosis (Scleroderma)," in Joseph L. Hollander and Daniel D. McCarty (eds.), *Arthritis and Allied Conditions,* 8th ed., Lea & Febiger, Philadelphia, 1972, pp. 962–1008.

———: "Primer on the Rheumatic Diseases," 7th ed., *JAMA,* vol. 224, no. 5 (Suppl), April 30, 1973.

Ropes, M. W., et al.: "1957 Revision of Diagnostic Criteria for Rheumatoid Arthritis," *Bull Rheum Dis,* **9:**175–176, 1958.

Rusk, Howard A.: *Rehabilitation Medicine,* 3d ed., Mosby, Saint Louis, 1971.

Samter, Talmage, Rose, Sherman, Vaughan: *Immunological Diseases,* 2d ed., Little, Brown, Boston, 1971, pp. 906–915.

Sell, Steward: *Immunology, Immunopathology and Immunity,* 2d ed., Harper & Row, New York, 1975.

Shean, Martin A.: *Sjögren's Syndrome,* Vol. II in *Major Problems in Internal Medicine,* Saunders, Philadelphia, 1971.

Sheldon, John M., Robert G. Lovell, and Kenneth P. Matthews (eds.): "Status Asthmaticus and Aids for Respiratory Allergy," in *A Manual of Clinical Allergy,* 2d ed., Saunders, Philadelphia, 1967, pp. 161–175.

Shoemaker, Rebecca A.: "Total Knee Replacement," *Nurs Clin North Am,* **8:**117–125, March 1973.

Shulman, Lawrence E., and Harvey, A. McGehee: "Systemic Lupus Erythematosus," in Joseph L. Hollander and Daniel J. McCarty (eds.), *Arthritis and Allied Conditions,* Lea & Febiger, Philadelphia, 1972, pp. 893–917.

Simpson, John A.: "Myasthenia Gravis: A New Hypothesis," *Scot Med J,* **5:**419, 1960.

———: "Myasthenia Gravis and Myasthenia Syndromes," in *Disorders of Voluntary Muscles,* 3d ed., Churchill Livingston, London, 1974.

Stewart, William D., Julius L. Danto, and Stuart Maddin: *Synopsis of Dermatology,* 2d ed., Mosby, St. Louis, 1970.

Stiller, C. R., A. S. Russell, and J. B. Dossetor: "Autoimmunity: Present Concepts," *Ann Intern Med,* **82:**405–410, 1975.

Strauss, A. J. L., et al.: "Immunofluorescence Demonstration of a Muscle Binding, Complement Fixing Serum Globulin Fraction in Myasthenia Gravis," *Proc Soc Exp Biol Med,* **105:**184, 1960.

Swezey, Robert L.: "Essentials of Physical Management and Rehabilitation in Arthritis," *Semin Arthritis Rheum,* **3:**349–368, Summer 1974.

Thier, Samuel O., Lee W. Henderson, and Richard K. Root: "Renal Transplantation, Medical Management of Transplant Recipient," in B. M. Brenner and F. C. Rector (eds.), *The Kidney,* Saunders, Philadelphia, 1976, pp. 1819–1860.

Turk, D. C., and I. C. Porter: *A Short Textbook of Medical Microbiology,* Year Book, Chicago, 1973.

Veits, H. R.: "Myasthenia Gravis," *N Engl J Med,* **251:** 97–141, 1954.

Vignos, Paul J.: "Psycho-social Problems in Management of Chronic Arthritis," in George Ehrlick (ed.), *Total Management of the Arthritic Patient,* Lippincott, Philadelphia, 1972, pp. 111–128.

Walton, John N. (ed.): *Disorders of Voluntary Muscle* 3d ed., Churchill Livingstone, London, 1974, pp. 653–692.

Ziff, J.: "Viruses and Connective Tissue Disease," *Ann Intern Med,* **75:**951–958, 1971.

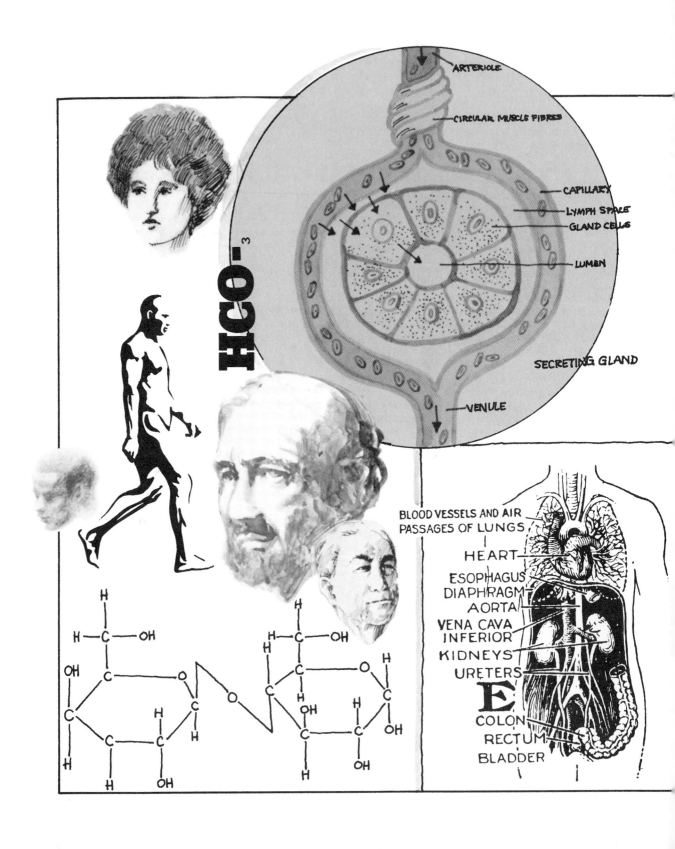

HCO₃⁻

ARTERIOLE

CIRCULAR MUSCLE FIBRES

CAPILLARY

LYMPH SPACE

GLAND CELLS

LUMEN

SECRETING GLAND

VENULE

BLOOD VESSELS AND AIR
PASSAGES OF LUNGS

HEART

ESOPHAGUS

DIAPHRAGM

AORTA

VENA CAVA
INFERIOR

KIDNEYS

URETERS

COLON

RECTUM

BLADDER

# PART 4

## FLUID AND ELECTROLYTE DYNAMICS

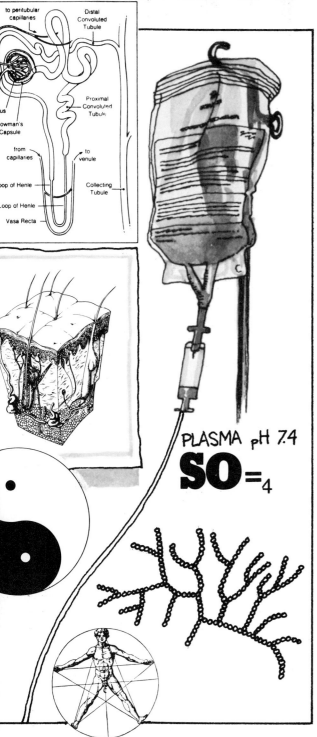

to peritubular capillaries

Distal Convoluted Tubule

Proximal Convoluted Tubule

Bowman's Capsule

from capillaries

to venule

Loop of Henle

Loop of Henle

Collecting Tubule

Vasa Recta

PLASMA pH 7.4

SO=4

# 11

# THE CONCEPTS OF FLUID AND ELECTROLYTE DYNAMICS*

Mary Marmoll Jirovec
JoEllen Wilbur Nolan

**W**ater is vital to life. Life first originated in water, which sustained it by bringing all necessary substances to the organism while carrying away all wastes. The water within the human body functions in much the same way. By living out of water, however, the body must maintain the composition of its fluids independently of its environment. Because it is in constant interaction with its environment, water and various substances are constantly passing into and out of the body. These exchanges must be equalized for fluid and electrolyte balance to occur.

## FLUID AND ELECTROLYTE BALANCE

Water is the universal solvent, and body fluids consist of water and dissolved substances which provide an internal environment in which the vital chemical and physical reactions occur and through which substances can be carried to and from the cells. Changes in body fluids affect all the bodily processes, and, because of this, an elaborate system has evolved to maintain balance. Water distribution, electrolytes, the movement of fluid and electrolytes, acid-base balance, the role of the kidney, hormonal control, and the role of the skin in fluid and electrolyte balance will be discussed.

### Water Distribution

The adult body is approximately 50 to 70 percent water, a percentage that varies with a number of factors. Fat contains little water so that people who are overweight have a lower percentage of body water. Women have less body water than men because of a higher proportion of fat. As a person ages, body water decreases so that the elderly can be expected to hold less body water than a younger person. In fact, 75 to 80 percent of an infant's weight is water.

Water found in the body is generally in the *extracellular fluid* (ECF) and the *intracellular fluid* (ICF). The intracellular fluid is found within the cells and comprises 75 percent of the total body water. The other 25 percent is extracellular, or outside the cells. The extracellular fluid can be further divided into *intravascular, interstitial,* and *transcellular fluids,* as well as the water found in connective tissue and bone. Intravascular fluid is plasma found within the circulatory system, while the interstitial

* The Fluid and Electrolyte Balance section was written by Mary Marmoll Jirovec, and the Physical Assessment of Fluid and Electrolyte Dynamics by JoEllen Wilbur Nolan.

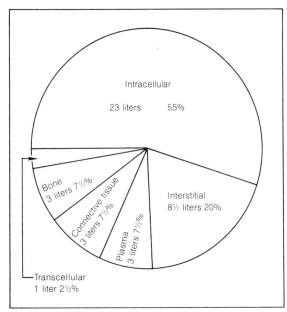

**FIGURE 11-1**
Fluid distribution in the body.

fluid is found between the cells. Transcellular fluids are similar to interstitial fluid in that they are found outside of cells, but are a product of secretion and diffusion from the cells and are generally found in special locations such as cerebrospinal fluid or intraocular fluid. Saliva, pancreatic juices, bile, intestinal juices, thyroid secretions, and semen are all examples of transcellular fluids. Figure 11-1 illustrates the percentages of the various body fluids.

### Electrolytes

Electrolytes are substances that break down into positively and negatively charged particles when placed in water. These charged particles are called ions. Ions with a positive charge are called *cations* and ions with a negative charge are *anions.* Ions in solution, then, have a valence or charge and combine according to that valence with oppositely charged ions. Sodium ion, $Na^+$, carries one positive charge and can combine with a chloride ion, $Cl^-$, which carries one negative charge, to form sodium chloride, $NaCl$. Calcium ion, $Ca^{2+}$, carries two positive charges and therefore can combine with two chloride ions to form calcium chloride, $CaCl_2$.

Electrolytes are active chemicals, and they are constantly breaking down and combining in water. This chemical combining power is expressed in *milliequivalents* (meq), and one milliequivalent is equal to the combining power of one milligram of

hydrogen. The combining power of the other electrolytes is measured against this standard. *Tonicity* refers to the concentration of a substance dissolved in water. As the concentration of a *solute* (the substance dissolved in water) increases, so the tonicity increases. A fluid is considered *isotonic* if it is the same concentration as the body fluids; 0.9% NaCl is an isotonic solution. When a solution has a solute concentration greater than the body fluids, it is considered *hypertonic.* A solution with a solute concentration less than the body fluids is a *hypotonic* solution.

The body fluids vary according to the composition of electrolytes found within them. The cations found within the body are sodium ($Na^+$), potassium ($K^+$), calcium ($Ca^{2+}$), and magnesium ($Mg^{2+}$). The anions are chloride ($Cl^-$), bicarbonate ($HCO_3^-$), phosphate ($PO_4^{3-}$), sulfate ($SO_4^{2-}$), and various organic acids such as proteinate and carbonic and lactic acids. All of the body's cations and anions are found in all fluid compartments, but the relative amounts of each vary greatly. Potassium, magnesium, and phosphate are the principle electrolytes of the intracellular fluid, while sodium, calcium, and chloride are primarily found in the extracellular fluid. Plasma differs from interstitial fluid only in that it contains large amounts of proteinate. Table 11-1 summarizes the electrolyte composition of the intracellular interstitial and intravascular fluids.

**Functions of electrolytes** In general, electrolytes have three major functions in the body. They play a vital role in water distribution by determining the *osmotic pressure* of the various fluids. Electrolytes are also necessary for *transmission of impulses.* Nerve cells carry impulses, muscle cells move, and gland cells secrete as a result of a change in their electrochemical state. This change involves the movement of sodium and potassium ions. As stated earlier, sodium is found primarily outside cells and potassium inside. A chemical stimulus such as acetylcholine or a mechanical stimulus such as a pin prick causes the $Na^+$ ions to enter the cells and the $K^+$ ions to leave. This movement of positively charged ions is the electrochemical change that results in impulse transmission, muscle movement, or secretion. Electrolytes also play a vital role in *acid-base balance,* functions which will be discussed more fully in the sections on movement of fluid and electrolytes and acid-base balance later in this chapter.

The specific functions of the various electrolytes are primarily related to their location. Because *sodium* is the primary extracellular cation, it functions to maintain the tonicity of the ECF and, therefore, the movement of water between the fluid compartments. Sodium affects neuromuscular and myocardial impulse transmission. *Potassium* is the primary intracellular cation functioning to maintain the tonicity of the ICF. Its effects on impulse transmission are especially evident in skeletal muscle and the myocardium.

While sodium and potassium play a vital role in the genesis of electrical changes within the body, calcium also performs a variety of functions. *Calcium* controls cell membrane permeability by lining the pores of the cell. This is especially evident in skeletal muscle. As calcium increases, permeability decreases. With less calcium there is an increased permeability with excessive ion diffusion resulting in nerve impulses and muscle contraction. Calcium appears to have an opposite effect on heart muscle, stimulating depolarization and contraction. Calcium also influences cell adhesion and helps to maintain intracellular connections. It is needed for the release of acetylcholine, the secretion of several glands, the formation of bone, and blood coagulation. *Magnesium* participates in the metabolic activities of the cells by taking part in the activation of a variety of enzyme systems. It also exhibits an inhibitory effect on skeletal muscle similar to that of calcium.

*Phosphate* is unique in function because the addition of phosphate to molecular structure makes replication, an essential feature of life, possible. Phosphate, then, is necessary for growth. It is also necessary to maintain adequate adenosine triphosphate (ATP) levels and, thus, energy levels. The best known function of phosphate is in bone metabolism.

## Movement of Fluid and Electrolytes

The fluid and electrolytes of the body are in perpetual motion. There is a constant exchange between the body's internal and external environments as well as between the various compartments within the body. In health these exchanges are balanced.

Water can be gained from the external environment in a variety of ways. The most obvious is ingestion of water and the water fraction of foods. Water is also gained from the oxidation of foodstuffs and body tissues. In less normal circumstances, water can be gained by tube feedings, parenteral fluids, or rectal feedings. The average 24-hour intake consists of 1300 ml oral fluids, 1000 ml fluid from foods, and 300 ml water from oxidation, totaling 2600 ml.

The ways in which water can be lost to the external environment are even more diverse. The most obvious of these is the production of urine. Water is also lost through evaporation with expired air, through gastrointestinal discharges, and through unconscious sweating. This type of sweating, as well as the water lost through the lungs, is called *insensible water loss.* The minimum amount of urine necessary to excrete urea in a 24-hour period is 600 ml. This minimum urine output and the water lost through the lungs, gastrointestinal tract, and insensible sweating is *obligatory* and is lost regardless of intake. It totals about 1500 ml/day.

**TABLE 11-1**
ELECTROLYTE COMPOSITION OF BODY FLUIDS

| Electro-lytes | Intra-cellular, meq/liter | Inter-stitial, meq/liter | Plasma, meq/liter | Measured as | Normal Range |
|---|---|---|---|---|---|
| $Na^+$ | 10 | 146 | 142 | Serum sodium | 136–145 |
| $K^+$ | 141 | 4 | 5 | Serum potassium | 3.5–5.5 |
| $Ca^{2+}$ | 1 | 2.5 | 5 | Total calcium | 4.5–5.5 |
| $Mg^{2+}$ | 40 | 1.5 | 3 | Serum magnesium | 1.5–3.0 |
| $HCO_3^-$ | 10 | 30 | 27 | $CO_2$ content<br>$CO_2$ combining power | 24–33<br>24–35 |
| $Cl^-$ | 4 | 115 | 103 | Sodium chloride | 98–106 |
| $PO_4^{3-}$ | 140 | 2 | 2 | Phosphorus | 1.2–3.0 |
| $SO_4^{2-}$ | 10 | 1 | 1 | Sulfur | 0.3–1.5 |
| Organic acids | — | 5 | 6 | Lactic acid<br>Total organic acid | 0.9–1.9<br>2–10 |
| Protein | 40 | 1 | 16 | Proteinate | 14.6–19.4 |

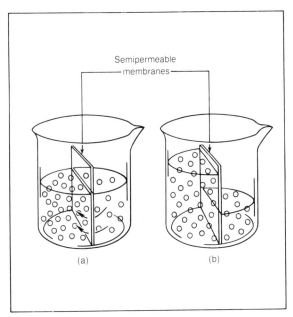

**FIGURE 11-2**

Osmosis. In (a) a concentration gradient exists between the two sides of the semipermeable membrane causing the movement of water to the more concentrated side as shown in (b).

The average 24-hour output consists of 1500 ml urine, 200 ml in stool, 300 ml through the lungs, and 600 ml in insensible sweating, equaling the 2600 ml taken in. Normally this exchange of water between the internal and external environments is equal and balance is maintained.

This balance is most often disrupted when output is either inadequate or excessive. Excessive water can be lost to the environment through profuse perspiration, vomiting, diarrhea, gastrointestinal suctioning, intestinal fistulas, ostomies, burns, wound or ulcer exudates, breast milk, hemorrhage, draining fistulas, mouth breathing, or various centeses. These abnormal losses must be compensated for by increased intake for balance to be maintained.

**Basic principles of movement** Fluid and electrolyte balance is dependent not only upon exchanges between the internal and external environment but upon exchanges between the intravascular, interstitial, and intracellular fluids. These exchanges are dependent upon osmosis, diffusion, active transport, filtration, pinocytosis, flow, hydrostatic pressure, and colloid osmotic pressure.

*Osmosis* is the movement of water across a semipermeable membrane from an area of lesser solute concentration to an area of greater solute concentration. A semipermeable membrane is one that will allow water to pass through but not some of the dissolved substances in the water. In this way a concentration gradient is created between the two sides of the membrane causing water to move to the more concentrated side (Fig. 11-2).

*Osmotic pressure* is the drawing power of a particular solution for water. If the solution consists of nonprotein substances, then it exerts *crystalloid osmotic pressure*. If the substances are protein, then the result is *colloid osmotic pressure* (oncotic pressure). The drawing power of albumin, which cannot pass through the capillary wall, holds water in the vessels and therefore accounts for the colloid osmotic pressure of plasma.

*Diffusion* is the movement of substances from an area of greater concentration to an area of lesser concentration (Fig. 11-3). Osmosis then is the diffusion of water through a semipermeable membrane. Because ions and molecules move randomly, they continue to bounce off each other until the concentrations within a given area are equalized.

In the body three types of diffusion occur. Substances can diffuse through *pores in the cell membranes.* This is dependent upon the size of the molecule in relation to the pore and the electrical charge of the molecule. The pores of cell membranes are lined with positively charged ions, especially calcium, and positively charged proteins so that other cations are repelled. Substances that are able to diffuse through the pores more easily are water, urea, hydrated $Cl^-$, hydrated $K^+$, and hydrated $Na^+$. The lactate ion, glycerol, and ribose diffuse less easily while sugars such as galactose, glucose, sucrose, and lactose are not able to pass through the pores.

A second way diffusion occurs in the body involves *fat-soluble substances* which dissolve into the fatty part of the cell membrane, pass through, and diffuse out. Examples of substances that diffuse in this manner are alcohol and oxygen. *Facilitated diffusion* involves a substance insoluble to the cell membrane. The substance combines with a carrier to become fat-soluble, and then dissolves into the cell membrane and passes through. Once through, the substance breaks away, freeing the carrier to return to the outside surface and repeat the process. Glucose enters cells through facilitated diffusion. The rate of facilitated diffusion is dependent upon the concentration gradient between the two sides, the amount of carrier available, and the rate of chemical reaction between the substance and the carrier.

Diffusion occurs when there is a *concentration*

gradient between two areas, with substances going from areas of greater concentration to less concentrated areas. It also can occur as a result of an electrical gradient, with ions moving toward opposite charges until the charge is balanced. Lastly, diffusion can occur as a result of a pressure gradient, with the increase in pressure on one side causing movement to the other side. Diffusion must be considered in terms of net movement, as it occurs in both directions. Net diffusion is determined by gradients.

Substances cannot diffuse against a concentration gradient. When it is necessary to move substances in this way the body utilizes what is called active transport. Active transport is similar to facilitated diffusion, except that it occurs against a concentration gradient and therefore requires energy. Several substances are actively transported, examples of which are $I^-$ by the glandular cells of the thyroid; $Na^+$, $Ca^{2+}$, $I^-$, and $HCO_3^-$ by the intestinal epithelial cells; $H^+$, $Ca^{2+}$, $Na^+$, and $K^+$ by the tubular epithelial cells of the kidneys; and amino acids by all cells. Sugars generally move by facilitated diffusion except where the concentration gradient requires active transport, as in the intestinal lumens and renal tubules. There is also an active transport system in muscle cells to supply them with glucose and amino acids during activity.

Active transport involves a carrier system which is specific for certain ions. The most famous of these is the so-called sodium pump. Cells contain high concentrations of protein anions which tend to pull the cation sodium, and therefore water, by osmosis into the cells. If this were allowed to happen indefinitely, the cells would eventually swell and burst. To counteract this tendency there is a carrier system that actively transports sodium out of the cells. After the carrier releases $Na^+$ at the outer surface it picks up $K^+$ and carries it into the cell. For every 3 $Na^+$ transported out 2 $K^+$ are carried in. The $Na^+$ builts up a positive charge outside the cells causing $Cl^-$ to diffuse out and the resultant NaCl pulls out water by osmosis. In this way, the osmotic pressure inside the cell is balanced by pressure outside, and the cell doesn't swell. $Ca^{2+}$ and $Mg^{2+}$ are actively transported by all cells in a similar manner.

Filtration is the movement of water and dissolved substances through a permeable membrane from an area of greater to an area of lesser pressure. The pressure differences are caused by hydrostatic pressure, which is the pressure exerted by a column of fluid on the sides of the container as a result of the weight of the fluid. The higher the column of fluid, the greater the hydrostatic pressure

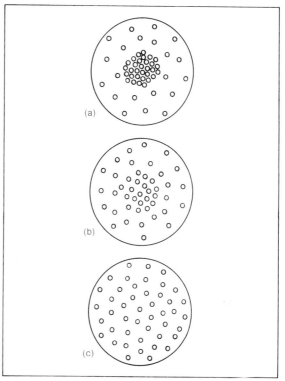

**FIGURE 11-3**

Diffusion. As molecules randomly move they bounce off each other and the unequal concentrations in (a) become progressively more equal (b) until fully equalized (c).

toward the bottom of the column. In the body, the heart supplies the pressure needed to maintain the hydrostatic pressure in the blood vessels. In filtration, movement occurs only in one direction, while diffusion is random with movement in both directions.

More recently described, and less well understood, are two phenomena that also contribute to the movement of fluid and substances within the body. The first of these is flow, which is the movement of fluid with solutes through pores rather rapidly. The pore size determines which solutes pass. Pinocytosis is the ability of the cell membrane to completely engulf a droplet of fluid and transfer the entire droplet to the inside of the cell.

**Capillary fluid dynamics** The movement of fluid in and out of the capillaries is dependent upon the pushing power of hydrostatic pressure and the pulling power of colloid osmotic pressure. At the arterial end of the capillaries, the capillary hydrostatic pressure (CHP) equals 25 mmHg, while the interstitial hydrostatic pressure (IHP) is −7 mmHg.

The interstitial colloid osmotic pressure (ICOP) equals 4.5 mmHg. The negative IHP and the ICOP along with the CHP move fluid out of the capillaries. This pressure totals 36.5 mmHg and is countered by the capillary colloid osmotic pressure (CCOP), 28 mmHg, holding fluid into the capillaries. The resultant pressure gradient of 8.5 mmHg causes a net movement of water and solute out of the capillaries.

At the venous end of the capillaries the opposite occurs because of a change in the CHP, which decreases to 9 mmHg. Thus combining CHP with the negative IHP and the ICOP gives a total pressure of 20.5 mmHg for outward movement. Meanwhile, the CCOP remains at 28 mmHg, resulting in a net pressure gradient of 7.5 mmHg which causes fluid to move back into the capillaries. At the arterial end, 8.5 mmHg moves fluid out, while 7.5 mmHg moves nine-tenths of that fluid back into the capillaries at the venous end (Fig. 11-4). The other one-tenth is picked up by the lymphatics, which drain this excess fluid and also pick up any large molecules such as proteins which may have leaked into the interstitial fluid. The lymphatic capillaries are suitable to this task as they are permeable to anything that will fit their lumens. In effect, then, much of the lymphatic fluid is interstitial fluid.

The movement of fluid and solutes in and out of the capillaries occurs as a result of the pressure gradient through diffusion, pinocytosis, and flow. Sodium, chloride, glucose, water, urea, sucrose, and to a lesser extent myoglobin and hemoglobin, all diffuse through the pores of the capillary membrane. Fat-soluble substances such as oxygen, carbon dioxide, anesthetic gases, and alcohol dissolve into the capillary membranes and pass through. The rate of their passage is much quicker than the rate for substances that must fit through the capillary membrane pores. Large molecules such as plasma proteins, glycoproteins, and polysaccharides pass between the blood and interstitial fluid through pinocytosis or by flow through slits between the capillary epithelial cells.

## Acid-Base Balance

There are several types of compounds in the body: oxides such as carbon dioxide, salts such as sodium chloride, acids such as hydrochloric acid, and bases such as sodium hydroxide. Of special interest

**FIGURE 11-4**

Pressure dynamics in capillary bed. Capillary hydrostatic pressure (CHP), interstitial hydrostatic pressure (IHP), and interstitial colloid osmotic pressure (ICOP) move fluid out of the capillaries while capillary colloid osmotic pressure (CCOP) moves fluid into the capillaries.

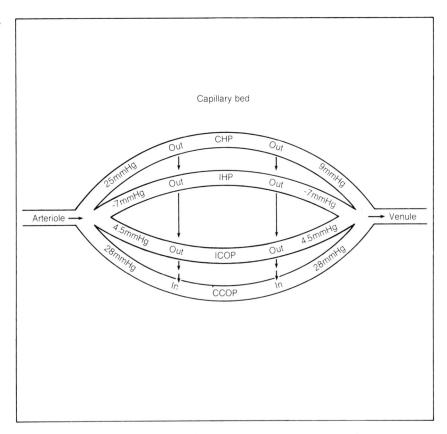

in the body are acids and bases. Water ($H_2O$) is a neutral substance containing an equal number of hydrogen ions ($H^+$) and hydroxyl ions ($OH^-$). An acid is a substance that when placed in water can dissociate and increase the $H^+$ concentration; acids are $H^+$ donors. When placed in water a base increases the $OH^-$ concentration and therefore neutralizes the $H^+$ ions; bases are $H^+$ acceptors. A strong acid readily gives up its $H^+$, while a weak acid dissociates less readily. Similarly, a strong base readily attracts the $H^+$ ion, while a weak base does so to a lesser degree.

The acid-base balance in the body is important because $H^+$ ions are produced throughout the body. For instance, glucose is metabolized to lactate and $H^+$. The reaction continues with the addition of oxygen so that carbon dioxide and water are formed and neutrality is maintained.

$$\text{Glucose} \rightarrow 2\ \text{lactate}^- + 2H^+ + 3O_2 \rightarrow 6CO_2 + 6H_2O$$

Similarly, the end products of fat metabolism combine with oxygen to form carbon dioxide and water. The end products of protein metabolism form the neutral substances of carbon dioxide, water, and urea.

If metabolism were limited to these reactions, there would be no acid-base problem in the body. Most amino acids, however, contain sulfur which oxidizes to sulfate with the production of $H^+$. Sulfate cannot be broken down further in the body and must be excreted as such.

$$\text{Methionine} + O_2 \rightarrow \text{urea} + CO_2 + H_2O + SO_4^- + 2H^+$$

The metabolism of phosphoproteins also produces $H^+$. Acid-base balance can again become significant when carbohydrates or fats are incompletely oxidized, as when the oxygen supply is inadequate.

Acid-base balance in the body refers to the hydrogen ion concentration in the body. Slight changes in this concentration cause marked alterations in the body's chemical reactions, decelerating some and accelerating others. The symbol used to express the hydrogen ion concentration is pH. A decrease in the pH denotes an increase in $H^+$ concentration and, therefore, *acidity*. An increase in the pH reflects a decrease in the $H^+$ concentration, or *alkalinity*. The normal pH of the body ranges from 7.35 to 7.45 with 7.0 and 7.8 being the limits compatible with life.

Three systems have evolved to control the $H^+$ concentration and, therefore, the pH of the body. These are the buffer systems, respiration, and the kidneys. The *buffer systems* are the most immediate and can neutralize excess acid or base within seconds. *Respiratory changes* can alter acidity or alkalinity in 1 to 3 minutes, while it takes the *kidneys* several hours to alter the pH.

**Buffer systems** Buffer systems are paired substances consisting of an acid and a base which act together to neutralize either acids or bases as they are added to the system containing the buffer. The way in which buffer systems are able to maintain acid-base balance is expressed in the Henderson-Hasselbalch equation

$$pH = pK + \log \frac{\text{acid}}{\text{base}}$$

where $pK$ is the midpoint within the range of acidity to alkalinity that a particular buffer system is effective. Each buffer system has its own $pK$. A simplified explanation of the equation, then, states that the pH or $H^+$ concentration of a particular fluid is determined by the range within which the buffer system is effective and the ratio of acid to base present in the system.

Probably the most important buffer system in the body is the bicarbonate buffer system. While the substances in this system are not powerful acids or bases, their concentrations can be regulated by the body. The system consists of sodium bicarbonate ($NaHCO_3$) and carbonic acid ($H_2CO_3$). According to the Henderson-Hasselbalch equation, in order to maintain the pH at the normal 7.4 the ratio of bicarbonate to carbonic acid must be 20:1. This ratio can be maintained because the kidneys are able to increase or decrease bicarbonate while respiration can increase or decrease the carbonic acid.

The bicarbonate buffer system is expressed in the following equation:

$$H^+ + HCO_3^- \rightleftharpoons H_2CO_3 \rightleftharpoons CO_2 + H_2O$$

The bicarbonate ($HCO_3^-$) can pick up an acid ($H^+$) and form carbonic acid ($H_2CO_3$); 99.9 percent of carbonic acid becomes carbon dioxide and water. All of these reactions are termed *reversible* because they can occur in both directions. The bicarbonate concentration is controlled by the kidneys and the carbonic acid concentration by the lungs. The following equation shows that adding hydrochloric acid (HCl) to sodium bicarbonate ($NaHCO_3$) yields carbonic acid ($H_2CO_3$) and sodium chloride (NaCl), a neutral salt. The carbonic acid then becomes carbon dioxide and water.

$$HCl + NaHCO_3 \rightarrow H_2CO_3 + NaCl$$
$$\Updownarrow$$
$$CO_2 + H_2O$$

$CO_2$ is exhaled during respiration.

When a base such as sodium hydroxide (NaOH) is added to the bicarbonate buffer system, sodium bicarbonate and water are formed.

$$NaOH + H_2CO_3 \rightarrow NaHCO_3 + H_2O$$

Excess $NaHCO_3$ can be eliminated by the kidneys. This same pattern of reactions exists for the buffer systems of the other salts of bicarbonate such as calcium bicarbonate, potassium bicarbonate, and magnesium bicarbonate. The primary intracellular bicarbonate buffer systems are those of potassium and magnesium.

The phosphate buffer system is one-sixth the concentration of the bicarbonate buffer system and consists of $NaH_2PO_4$, a weak acid, and $Na_2HPO_4$, a weak base. When a strong acid is added, a weak acid is formed and the pH remains relatively stable.

$$HCl + Na_2HPO_4 \rightarrow NaH_2PO_4 + NaCl$$

When a strong base is added, a weak base is formed to maintain the pH.

$$NaOH + NaH_2PO_4 \rightarrow Na_2HPO_4 + H_2O$$

The most plentiful buffer system in the body is the protein buffer system which accounts for three-quarters of all buffering. To a large extent it occurs inside the cells. It is able to buffer because some proteins have free acid radicals and others have free base radicals. Therefore, they are able to release acids or bases as needed to regulate the pH.

**Respiratory control**   Over 99 percent of the carbonic acid in the body dissociates into carbon dioxide and water. Therefore, by increasing or decreasing respirations, $CO_2$ can be conserved or lost and the carbonic acid concentration affected. As respirations increase, more $CO_2$ is lost and the carbonic acid concentration is decreased, causing an increase in pH and alkalinity, called *alkalosis*. As respirations are decreased, less $CO_2$ is lost and the carbonic acid concentration increases, causing a decrease in pH and an increase in acidity, called *acidosis*. The pH of the blood stimulates the respiratory center so that respirations are increased in acidosis and decreased in alkalosis.

**Kidney control**   The kidneys function to maintain acid-base balance in two ways. They regulate bicarbonate concentration by excreting the excess or reabsorbing what is needed; they also excrete excess $H^+$. Figure 11-5 illustrates the mechanisms through which the kidneys are able to do this. In order to reabsorb sodium bicarbonate from the tubules and excrete the hydrogen ion, the tubule epithelial cells combine carbon dioxide and water under the influence of carbonic anhydrase (an enzyme) to form carbonic acid. The carbonic acid then dissociates into bicarbonate ion and hydrogen ion. The hydrogen ion is secreted into the tubule in exchange for the sodium ion that dissociates from the sodium bicarbonate in the tubule. The hydrogen ion then combines with the bicarbonate ion to form carbonic acid. This becomes water, which is excreted, and carbon dioxide, which enters the tubular epithelial cells to be reused to form carbonic acid. The sodium ion that was reabsorbed from the tubule is secreted into the extracellular fluid where it combines with the bicarbonate ion that the epithelial cell has secreted to form sodium bicarbonate. The end result of all this is that an hydrogen ion is lost and the sodium bicarbonate has been conserved.

As the pH decreases and the hydrogen ion concentration begins to exceed the available bicarbonate, the excess hydrogen combines with a phosphate buffer or ammonia and is excreted. As the pH increases, the amount of bicarbonate in the tubules exceeds the available hydrogen ions so the excess bicarbonate is lost in the urine. The kidney is able to regulate acid-base balance by either excreting excess base or excreting acid and conserving base.

### The Role of the Kidney in Fluid and Electrolyte Balance

"It is no exaggeration to say that the composition of the body fluids is determined not by what the mouth takes in but by what the kidneys keep: they are the master chemists of our internal environment."[1]

**Anatomy**   The body contains two kidneys, one on each side of the vertebral column in the posterior part of the abdomen and outside the peritoneal cavity. The kidney is a bean-shaped organ that weighs approximately 170 g. Each kidney is composed of approximately 1 million nephrons each functioning independently as a unit. The outer layers of the kidney are called the *cortex* and the inner part the *medulla*.

The *nephron* is the functional unit of the kidney. It is composed of a vascular network called the *glomerulus* and *tubules* (Fig. 11-6). The vascular glomerulus is surrounded by *Bowman's capsule* which opens into the *proximal convoluted tubule.* The proximal tubule drains into a thin, hairpin tubule called the *loop of Henle.* This is followed by the *distal convoluted tubule* which finally drains into the *collecting tubule.*

Nephrons in the kidney differ only in the length of their loop of Henle. *Cortical nephrons* have short loops and are found in the renal cortex. *Juxtamedullary nephrons* originate in the cortex but have long loops of Henle which extend down into the renal medulla. The importance of this will become clear when the countercurrent mechanism is discussed.

Normally, the blood supply to an organ consists of arteries to and veins from the organ. In the kidney, however, the blood supply is unique. The renal artery emerges from the aorta and carries blood a short distance to the *afferent arteriole* (Fig. 11-6). The blood then passes through the capillary network of the glomerulus and into the *efferent arteriole.* From there it either enters the *peritubular capillaries* or flows through long vessels that follow the loop of Henle of the juxtamedullary nephrons into and out of the renal medulla. These long ves-

sels are called *vasa recta.* Both the peritubular capillaries and the vasa recta flow into venules which empty into the renal vein and finally the inferior vena cava.

**Physiology**   The kidneys function to remove the end products of metabolism from the body and to control the concentrations of practically all substances in the body fluids. They accomplish this task by filtering approximately one-fifth of the plasma through the glomerulus and into Bowman's capsule and then reabsorbing wanted substances while eliminating unwanted substances through the urine.

**G**lomerular Filtration   Glomerular filtration is the passage of plasma through the vascular glomerulus into Bowman's capsule. It occurs as a result of a pressure gradient between the glomerulus and Bowman's capsule. As in the capillary beds, the pressure gradient is determined by a combination of hydrostatic pressure and colloid osmotic pressure. The glomerular capillary hydrostatic pressure is 70 mmHg and tends to push plasma out of the

**FIGURE 11-5**
Kidney regulation of acid-base balance.

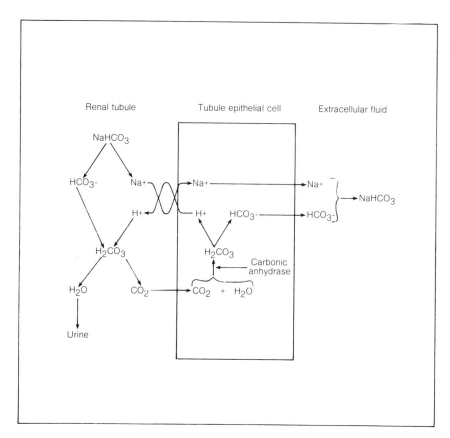

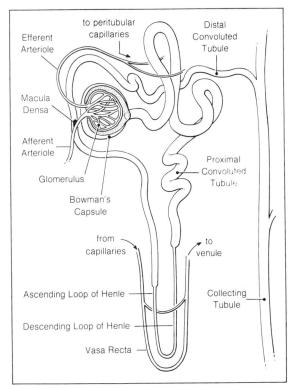

**FIGURE 11-6**
Structure of renal nephron.

capillaries. This pressure is countered by the glomerular capillary colloid osmotic pressure, 32 mmHg, and the hydrostatic pressure in Bowman's capsule, 14 mmHg.

The resultant 24 mmHg gradient is the filtration pressure and causes a net movement of 19 percent of the renal plasma flow to move into Bowman's capsule. This amount of filtrate is called the *filtration fraction*. The glomerular filtrate is basically plasma minus the protein. Some hemoglobin and albumin leaks into the filtrate but not in significant amounts.

Kidney function is dependent upon adequate amounts of plasma being filtered into Bowman's capsule, which in turn is dependent upon the maintenance of glomerular capillary hydrostatic pressure. This is accomplished through an internal mechanism that regulates the afferent and efferent arterioles. As renal blood flow and, therefore, filtration decrease, efferent constriction exceeds afferent constriction, thus increasing pressure. The increased pressure, then, increases filtration. If efferent constriction is severe, as happens in prolonged hypotension, the blood flow through the glomerulus becomes sluggish. As the plasma stays in the glomerulus longer, large amounts of fluid are lost

to the capsule and the colloid osmotic pressure in the capillaries rises. The fluid then is pulled back into the capillaries and net filtration decreases.

In circumstances when blood flow to the kidney increases, as happens with hypertension, the afferent arteriole constricts and the efferent arteriole dilates to decrease the pressure in the glomerular capillaries. Through these mechanisms the kidneys are able to maintain normal glomerular filtration under a wide range of vascular pressures. Renal blood flow will remain constant if aortic pressure does not drop below 80 mmHg or rise above 250 mmHg. Outside of these parameters renal blood flow and, therefore, glomerular filtration fall or rise respectively.

The mechanism through which the kidneys are able to accomplish this *autoregulation* is not well understood. Studies have demonstrated a close spatial relationship between a portion of the distal tubule and a point between the afferent and efferent arterioles known as the *juxtaglomerular apparatus*.[2] Experimental evidence indicates that the macula densa cells of the juxtaglomerular apparatus may be stimulated by the concentration of NaCl in the tubules or vascular stretch receptors in the glomerulus to alter afferent and efferent arteriole constriction.[3,4]

The glomerular filtration rate can also be altered by *sympathetic stimulation*. In mild sympathetic stimulation there is equal constriction of the afferent and efferent arterioles so that blood is shunted elsewhere but the filtration rate is not changed. As sympathetic tone increases, afferent constriction is initially greater than efferent with a resultant decrease in glomerular filtration. With prolonged sympathetic stimulation, the efferent constriction exceeds the afferent constriction, increasing glomerular pressure and the filtration rate.

**T**ubular Reabsorption and Secretion    As the glomerular filtrate passes through the tubules, many changes occur. Almost 99 percent of the water is reabsorbed, other substances reabsorbed partially or entirely, and still others actively secreted into the fluid. The peritubular capillary system is highly permeable. In the glomerulus, large quantities of fluid but not albumin are filtered out of the blood so that what remains is highly concentrated. The peritubular capillaries also empty into a venule so that hydrostatic pressure in them is decreased. The result is an increased peritubular capillary colloid osmotic pressure and a low hydrostatic pressure pulling fluid from the renal tubules through highly permeable membranes into the peritubular capillaries.

Much of this movement occurs by passive diffusion; but the kidneys control the movement by actively absorbing certain substances and secreting others. Because active transport both into and out of the tubules requires a carrier, the amount of carrier dictates the amount of a particular substance that can be reabsorbed or secreted. This amount is known as the *renal threshold*. If more of a particular substance is filtered into the tubules than can be reabsorbed, the excess is lost in the urine. Renal thresholds exist for glucose, phosphate, sulfate, amino acids, vitamin C, urate, plasma protein, hemoglobin, lactate, and acetoacetate.

*Tubular transport of electrolytes* One of the most important transport systems in the kidney is the *active reabsorption of sodium* occurring throughout the tubular system. As sodium is reabsorbed into the peritubular fluid, an electrical gradient develops with positive sodium ions outside the tubules and negativity inside. As a result of this, anions, especially chloride, diffuse out of the tubules. The sodium chloride outside the tubules increases the concentration of the peritubular fluid, exerting an osmotic pressure which pulls water out of the tubules. Other electrolytes such as calcium, magnesium, potassium, phosphate, and urate ions are reabsorbed from the tubules in a similar manner.

Because the tubules are only slightly permeable to *bicarbonate,* a more elaborate system has developed to conserve it. The mechanisms of bicarbonate conservation were discussed in the section on acid-base balance. Basically, the bicarbonate ion combines with hydrogen to form carbonic acid which dissociates into carbon dioxide and water. The carbon dioxide then diffuses into the epithelial cell where it is used to form a new bicarbonate ion.

As the tubules actively reabsorb these electrolytes, they are also actively secreting others. *Potassium* is secreted into the urine in the distal and collecting tubules. The proximal as well as the distal and collecting tubules also secrete *hydrogen ions.* Most of the electrolytes, especially sodium, chloride, and bicarbonate, are excreted in the urine in concentrations similar to their concentrations in the extracellular fluid. Potassium is an exception to this and is excreted in quantities greater than its concentration in extracellular fluid.

*Tubular transport of metabolic end products* One of the most important functions of the kidney is removal from the body of the end products of metabolism. The tubules accomplish this through a process of *selective reabsorption and secretion.* Metabolic end products are filtered into the glomerular filtrate. As water is reabsorbed from the tubules the concentrations of the end products increase in proportion to their ability to permeate the tubular epithelial cells.

The permeability of the epithelial cells to urea is much less than their permeability to water; therefore, only about 40 percent of the urea filtered into the tubules is reabsorbed. About 85 percent of the urate ion, sulfates, phosphates, and nitrates are reabsorbed. Nevertheless, large quantities of these are still lost in the urine. No creatinine is reabsorbed by the tubules and, in fact, still more is secreted into the tubules. Inulin is neither reabsorbed nor secreted, so that whatever is filtered through the glomerulus is lost in the urine. Para-aminohippuric acid (PAH) is secreted by the proximal tubules and not reabsorbed.

Ammonia is secreted by the distal tubular cells in proportion to the urine acidity. As the pH of the urine falls and the $H^+$ concentration increases, ammonia is secreted into the tubules to combine with the $H^+$ and form ammonium chloride, which is then excreted.

*Tubular transport of nutritionally important substances* The kidneys must conserve glucose, amino acids, and proteins in order to prevent debilitation. They accomplish this by reabsorbing all of the glucose and amino acids in the proximal tubules. As mentioned earlier, however, the kidneys have a threshold for this reabsorption. Therefore, if abnormally large amounts of these substances are filtered through the glomerulus, the excess will be lost.

Small amounts of albumin leak into the glomerular filtrate but are too large to be reabsorbed. Research indicates that the proximal tubular epithelial cells are able to conserve the filtered albumin.[5] By taking the albumin into the cell through pinocytosis, 90 percent of the leaked albumin is conserved. The epithelial cells then digest the albumin to form polypeptides and amino acids. These either remain in the cell or are returned to the circulation. In this way only trace amounts of albumin are lost in the urine. Because of the renal threshold for albumin, increased amounts leaked into the filtrate are lost in the urine.

*Countercurrent mechanism* The discussion to this point has examined the movement of a variety of substances in and out of the tubules. The mechanism whereby the urine is able to become more concentrated than the peritubular fluid is called the *countercurrent mechanism.* The mechanism is dependent on the length of the loop of Henle, and the longer the loop, the greater the concentrating power.

The purpose of the countercurrent mechanism is to increase the concentration of the medullary interstitial fluid. The collecting tubules pass through the medulla on their way to the renal pelvis. By passing through a highly concentrated area, water diffuses out of the tubule and the urine becomes more concentrated. The amount of water movement is controlled by the varying permeability of the collecting tubules.

Large quantities of sodium and, therefore, chloride are reabsorbed throughout the tubules. In the loop of Henle, however, this reabsorption greatly increases the concentration of the interstitial fluid (Fig. 11-7). The descending loop is highly permeable to sodium and chloride so that both diffuse into the tubule as water diffuses out. In the ascending loop the sodium and chloride are actively transported out of the tubules. Because the ascending loop is impermeable to water, sodium chloride is able to leave the tubule while water is not. A cycle is created whereby sodium chloride is absorbed by the descending loop and given up by the ascending loop. As more and more new sodium enters from the glomerular filtrate, the concentration in the medullary interstitial fluid builds up.

The special structure of the vasa recta prevents the excess sodium chloride from being removed by the blood. The vasa recta flows in the opposite direction of the loop of Henle so that as it descends it passes the ascending loop and picks up sodium chloride that is being transported out of the tubules. As the vasa recta ascends it passes the descending loop and gives up its sodium chloride to the lower concentration within the loop.

As the filtrate descends the loop of Henle, it becomes increasingly more concentrated. As it ascends the loop it becomes increasingly dilute until its concentration is actually less than that of the glomerular filtrate. From here its concentration is mediated by the antidiuretic hormone (ADH), which controls the size of the pores of the epithelial cells in the distal and collecting tubules. As ADH decreases, the pores become smaller, water cannot pass and is, therefore, not reabsorbed, resulting in a dilute urine. As the concentration of ADH increases, the pores enlarge and water passes easily. In the distal tubules the concentrations of the tubular and peritubular fluids are equal. As the collecting tubule passes through the medulla, the highly concentrated medulla pulls water out and the urine becomes concentrated.

## Hormonal Influences on Fluid and Electrolyte Balance

The regulation of the fluid volume in the body is mediated by the antidiuretic hormone and aldosterone. Their functioning ability in turn is greatly affected by the glomerular filtration rate. Small changes in this rate greatly affect the water and sodium presented to the tubules. Once presented, ADH governs water conservation and aldosterone controls sodium.

**The antidiuretic hormone**   The antidiuretic hormone (Vasopressin) controls the permeability of the walls of the collecting tubule as it passes through the hypertonic medullary interstitial fluid. As ADH increases the tubule becomes more permeable to water, which then diffuses into the interstitial fluid and is conserved. As ADH decreases, the tubule becomes less permeable to water, so that water is unable to diffuse out of the tubule and is lost to the urine.

Many factors have been shown to affect ADH secretion. Osmoreceptors in the internal carotid artery stimulate the hypothalamus. The neurosecretory cells of the hypothalamus then secrete ADH, which is transported along axons to nerve endings in the posterior pituitary gland. There the ADH is stored until it is needed.

The posterior pituitary releases ADH in response to a variety of conditions. These many stimuli seem to be mediated through the *hypothalamoneurohypophyseal complex.* ADH secretion is very much affected by changes in the body fluids. Increases in tonicity and dehydration, both with and without changes in tonicity, stimulate its release. Changes in blood volume stimulate volume receptors in veins in the thorax and baroreceptors in the arteries so that decreases in volume or pressure increase ADH production. Likewise, increases will decrease production.

The relationship between blood volume and ADH has many implications. Persons experiencing positive pressure breathing decrease their intrathoracic blood volume and, therefore, increase ADH. With negative pressure breathing the opposite occurs and water is lost to the urine. Persons standing or sitting for prolonged periods of time decrease intrathoracic pressure and water is conserved. Likewise, the night reclining position increases the pressure and diuresis occurs. This is especially relevant for persons with difficulties of salt retention, because they have a greater antidiuretic effect when upright.

Both emotional and physical stress such as surgery, trauma, pain, fear, infection, or vigorous exercise will stimulate ADH secretion. Warmth has been shown to increase ADH while cold decreases its production. Anesthetics, morphine, Demerol, barbiturates, acetylcholine, ferritin (a substance released from ischemic liver), and nicotine all increase antidiuretic hormone. The only effective inhibitor of ADH is ethyl alcohol. This effect, however, is limited and short-lived. Hypercalcemia blocks the action of ADH.

The thirst center in the hypothalamus lies in close proximity to the center for ADH, so that some of the stimuli that increase ADH production cause a conscious desire for water. Once activated, the stimuli for thirst are inhibited by the act of drinking and fullness in the gastrointestinal tract. In this way the ingested water is given time to be absorbed by the body before more is taken in.

In doses larger than is required for antidiuresis, ADH has a vasopressor effect. Research has shown different sensitivities of vascular beds to the pressor effects of ADH. The muscles have the greatest sensitivity, with the mesentary vascular bed next, and the kidneys showing the least response to vasoconstriction by ADH.[6]

**Aldosterone** Aldosterone is a mineral cortocoid secreted by the adrenal cortex. Its primary function is to regulate sodium concentration. All of the mineral corticoids, as well as the glucocorticoids and sex steroids, have a role in sodium concentration but to a very small degree. Aldosterone, in fact, accounts for 95 percent of the mineral corticoid activity and is 50 times as potent as the others.

Aldosterone secretion can be stimulated by a decrease in sodium concentration in the extracellular fluid, increases in extracellular potassium, decreases in blood volume and cardiac output, or both physical or emotional stress. It acts by increasing the reabsorption of sodium from the tubules, which in turn develop a negativity in comparison to the peritubular fluid, and potassium diffuses into the urine. Aldosterone, then, causes sodium retention and potassium loss.

*Renin,* a hormone released from the kidneys, plays a role in aldosterone secretion. Decreases in renal blood flow and renal arterial pressure stimulate volume receptors in the afferent arterioles. This causes renin to be released from the juxtaglomerular cells. Renin activates angiotensin which stimulates aldosterone secretion. The distal tubules then conserve sodium and lose potassium in response to aldosterone secretion.

**Fluid and electrolyte effects of other hormones** There are several other hormones that

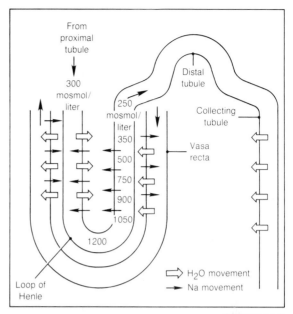

**FIGURE 11-7**
Countercurrent schema for concentrating urine.

have an effect on fluid and electrolyte balance, *parathyroid hormone* (PTH) being the one which has the greatest effect. It directly affects the gastric mucosa to increase calcium absorption and increases the rate of calcium reabsorption from the renal tubules. There is an inverse relationship between its effects on calcium and phosphate; as PTH increases calcium reabsorption, it increases phosphate excretion. With decreases in PTH less calcium is reabsorbed and more phosphate is retained. PTH also increases bone absorption so that both calcium and phosphate are mobilized. The calcium then is conserved and the excess phosphate lost in the urine. Research has shown that PTH depresses bicarbonate reabsorption, but the exact mechanism and extent of this action is not known.[7]

There appears to be a second parathyroid hormone which decreases the concentrations of calcium in the extracellular fluid. The hormone is called *calcitonin* and much research is needed before its action will be fully understood. The thyroid secretes a calcitonin called *thyrocalcitonin* which decreases the extracellular calcium concentration. *Thyroid hormone,* itself, tends to increase bone absorption.

*Growth hormone* increases bone formation, calcium excretion, and sodium and potassium retention, while it decreases the excretion of phosphorus. The *adrenal steroids* have been shown to decrease bone absorption and absorption of calcium from the intestine and increase calcium and phosphorus excretion in the tubules. They also have a mild mineralocorticoid effect. The effects of the *sex steroids* on calcium are not fully established, but they seem to increase bone formation and inhibit bone absorption. The kidney itself secretes a hormone, *prostaglandin,* which exerts a local diuretic effect.

## Micturition

After urine passes through the collecting tubules, it flows into the renal pelvis where it accumulates. As urine in the pelvis increases, pressure rises and peristaltic contractions that begin at the pelvis spread down the ureter forcing urine toward the bladder. The ureters are small, smooth muscular tubes that contain both sympathetic and parasympathetic fibers and are innervated with many pain fibers. Any blockage in the ureters results in intense peristaltic waves and excruciating pain. The pain impulses also cause sympathetic stimulation which leads to renal vasoconstriction and a decrease in urine production.

After passing through the ureters, the urine collects in the bladder, which functions to both store the urine and eliminate it from the body. As urine accumulates, the bladder relaxes to prevent pressure from building and urine from backing up into the ureters. When the tension on the walls of the bladder reaches a certain threshold, the micturition reflex is stimulated. Parasympathetic fibers stimulate the detrusor muscle of the bladder to contract and the internal sphincter relaxes. The external sphincter is voluntarily relaxed and the urine passes through the urethra and out of the body. Micturition, then, is the final step in ridding the body of unwanted fluid, electrolytes, and substances.

## The Role of the Skin in Fluid and Electrolyte Balance

The human body is enclosed in a specialized envelope—the skin—which acts as a barrier between the body and its external environment. It both protects the body from its environment and keeps it in constant communication with the environment.

Figure 11-8 illustrates the normal structure of the skin. It is composed of two main layers, the *dermis* and the *epidermis.* Proceeding from the innermost to the outermost layer, the dermis consists of the *stratum reticularis* and the *stratum papillaris.* The reticular layer is composed primarily of elastic and collagenous fibers. The papillary layer lies under the epidermis and consists of papillae which carry capillaries, nerve fibers, and sensory end organs to the epidermis. The dermis contains the glands, hair follicles, vessels, lymph, and nerves.

The epidermis is composed of epithelial cells that form, move to the surface, and slough off by passing through four or five layers. In the *stratum germinativum* the cells multiply by mitosis. They then move through the *stratum spinosum* to the *stratum granulosum* where they die. In the palms and soles they then go through the *stratum lucidum* before becoming part of the *stratum corneum.* The stratum corneum is the outer layer of all skin and is made up of dead cells composed of keratin, a water-repellent protein.

The skin performs many vital functions not the least of which is maintaining fluid and electrolyte balance. It has certain waterproof qualities that are instrumental in preventing fluid loss. The surface of the skin, however, does contain some water which is being continually lost to the air through evaporation. The lost water is replaced by diffusion of water from the deeper layers of the skin (Table 11-2). This water loss through evaporation is the insensible loss mentioned earlier in the chapter and is a function of the environmental temperature.

The skin also assists with temperature regulation primarily through the functioning of the *eccrine sweat glands.* These sweat glands are composed of a secretory coil and a duct that comes almost to the surface of the skin. The coil produces an isotonic ultrafiltrate of plasma which the duct then selectively reabsorbs in a manner similar to the way the renal tubules function. Aldosterone controls the concentration of sweat in the same way it effects urine. The sweat produced is a hypotonic solution of primarily sodium, chloride, and potassium with very little glucose. The body rids itself of excess heat through sweating. To a small degree the sweat glands also function as excretory organs.

The skin functions to protect the body from a variety of threats, preventing microorganisms, excess water, and most chemicals from entering the body. It protects against excess sunlight by the production of melanin pigment. Melanocytes lie just below the dermis and distribute melanin to the stratum germinativum as needed.

Lastly, the skin protects against mechanical injury. Almost every skin surface has been shown to have a basic geometrical design that allows the relatively inelastic stratum corneum to accommodate deformities and manipulation without cracking.[8] The reticular layer of the dermis has the combined characteristics of a viscous fluid and an elastic solid which further allows the skin to withstand deformities. Fluid surrounds the fibers in the skin so that upon deformation, the fluid is easily displaced and the fibers move closer together.

The skin contains many sensory end organs and, itself, serves as one of the most important sense organs. The role of the skin in perception is discussed fully in Chap. 31.

The skin contains two other glands whose functions are not readily apparent. The *apocrine gland* is a type of sweat gland that produces a substance that causes a characteristic odor when acted upon by bacteria. This odor, which is unique to each individual, appears to be the only function of these glands. The *sebaceous glands* secrete a lipid substance whose function is not clear. It may serve as an emollient for the stratum corneum, it may have bacteriostatic and fungistatic effects, and it may be related to odor.

## PHYSICAL ASSESSMENT OF FLUID AND ELECTROLYTE DYNAMICS

Physical assessment of fluid and electrolyte dynamics can be invaluable in evaluating a patient's fluid status. A careful history can point the investigator toward a specific imbalance, but cannot by itself fully evaluate the patient's status. Laboratory tests can identify specific deficits or excesses but, alone, give little information regarding the magnitude of the imbalance. Data from the history, laboratory tests, and physical examination must be collected and integrated in order to formulate an accurate impression of the patient's state of hydration.

The following section will discuss inspection, palpation, percussion, and auscultation in the assessment of body hydration. In each section appropriate assessments will be reviewed and specific findings related to fluid loss and fluid retention discussed.

### Baseline Measurements

Before beginning any physical examination, it is helpful to take some baseline measurements. Much can be told about body hydration from the patient's weight and vital signs. The patient's weight should be compared to previous weight records, a comparison which is helpful in estimating the volume of fluid changes. Fluid losses result in weight losses, while fluid excesses result in weight gains.

The patient's temperature, pulse, respirations, and blood pressure can supply valuable information when assessing fluid and electrolyte balance. The vital signs of a well-hydrated patient will not

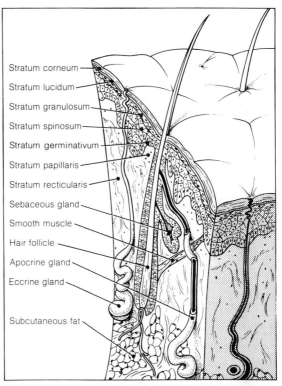

**FIGURE 11-8**
Normal skin and appendages.

change. If hypertonic dehydration is present, there will be an increase in temperature resulting from inadequate amounts of water for removal of the heat of metabolism. If hypotonic dehydration is present, the temperature may be subnormal because of reduced energy output. With severe loss of fluid volume, the pulse becomes rapid and weak. As shock ensues, respiration will increase while the blood pressure falls.

When fluid excess is present, the pulse may be slightly increased and bounding in character. The blood pressure, also, may be increased. The temperature generally remains unchanged. One of the

**TABLE 11-2**
WATER CONTENT OF SKIN

| Skin Layer | Water Content, % |
| --- | --- |
| Stratum corneum | 2 |
| Stratum granulosum | 10 |
| Stratum papillaris | 71 |
| Stratum reticularis | 61 |
| Subcutaneous fat | 30 |

best indicators of fluid excess is the respiratory rate, as the patient often experiences an increase in respirations and may be short of breath. An evaluation of difficulty breathing upon exertion should also be made.

### Inspection

The first step in every physical examination is inspection. Assessment of the patient's fluid and electrolyte status should include evaluation of the patient's general hydration and intake and output. A systematic approach to inspection of the patient should be used so that important clues to the patient's general hydration are not overlooked.

**General hydration**   The overall *appearance and behavior* of the patient should be assessed. The well-hydrated patient will be conscious, alert, and able to respond to questions with speed and accuracy. In severe dehydration the blood volume is significantly decreased, and the patient will often display visible signs of anxiety, agitation, exhaustion, or fear. When the fluid loss is complicated by metabolic acidosis, cerebral disturbances, delirium, and coma may be present. The patient with fluid excess generally will not experience behavioral changes, although the patient will often be extremely apprehensive if the excess fluid is interfering with respirations.

The *posture* of the well-hydrated patient will be unaffected. The patient who is slumped and weak may be presenting signs of excessive fluid and/or electrolyte loss. One can elicit much information from the posture of an overhydrated patient. If the fluid excess is presenting too great a demand on the heart, the patient will be more comfortable in a sitting as opposed to a recumbent position.

The patient's *face and body* should be generally observed. The skin should appear smooth, firm, and normally colored. The face and eyes should have a bright, alert appearance. When fluid loss is present, the patient's skin often appears shrunken and wrinkled and has a pallor or grayish discoloration. This color change is difficult to assess in dark-skinned patients and is best observed in the nailbeds. The patient with severe fluid loss will appear emaciated.

The appearance of the face and body of the patient with fluid excess will be dependent on the location of the fluid. Early fluid retention will often not cause noticeable changes in appearance. As retention increases, however, the fluid will begin to collect and the patient should be observed for signs of edema. The skin over an edematous area often appears red and glistening. Fluid will often collect in dependent locations; the eyelids, extremities, flanks, and abdomen should be observed for fluid accumulation. Fluid in the peritoneal cavity is called *ascites* and will be evidenced by a distended abdomen and bulging of the flanks with the umbilicus appearing flat or protuberant.

Once the patient's face and body have been assessed generally, specific attention should be focused on the *oral cavity.* The condition of the tongue and mucous membranes of the mouth are valuable indicators of the state of hydration. Normally they will appear moist. Fluid loss results in decreased salivary flow causing the mucous membranes and tongue to become dry. One of the most reliable signs of dehydration is a dry tongue with longitudinal furrows. There will not be any noticeable changes in the mucous membranes in fluid excess.

Progressing in a systematic order the *jugular veins of the neck* should then be inspected. The appearance of the jugular veins often reflect circulating blood volume. With fluid loss there will be decreased filling of the veins when the patient is in the recumbent position. There is distention of the jugular veins in the erect position when the extracellular fluid volume is increased.

**Intake and output**   Many questions concerning hydration are answered by carefully evaluating the patient's intake and output. When assessing the patient's *intake,* all avenues of possible fluid intake should be considered. Intake is more inclusive than just the patient's oral fluids. Solid food may be 70 percent water and metabolism of carbohydrate, protein, and fat yields water from oxidation. Other avenues of intake include parenteral fluids, gavage feedings, and all irrigations, e.g., nasogastric and Foley catheter irrigations.

*Output* should also be considered in terms of all possible avenues. In addition to normal sensible and insensible fluid loss, the patient may have abnormal losses of fluid resulting from prolonged vomiting, diarrhea, excessive diuresis, copious sweating, wound, burn or fistula drainage, or bleeding. Also to be considered as avenues for fluid loss are all forms of suctioning and drainage tubes including gastric suctioning, tracheostomy suctioning, T-tube and Penrose drainage, colostomies, and enterostomies. Fluid losses should be evaluated in terms of the amount and type of fluid. Usually the losses involve water and electrolytes, and a disturbance in electrolyte balance and acid-base equilibrium can be a frequent complication.

Inspection of urine concentration is especially valuable in evaluating fluid status. This includes assessment of the *color* of the urine and the *specific gravity*. The normal color of urine varies from dark amber to pale yellow. Urine that is dark indicates a strong concentration in that the kidney is maximally conserving water, as in dehydration. The kidneys conserve water by excreting small volumes of highly concentrated urine that is rich in nitrogenous wastes and with little solute excretion. When urine is a pale yellow it indicates a reduced concentration that can occur with excessive water intake and overhydration, as well as by starvation and a low protein diet. Urinary concentration is lowered when urinary solutes are increased.

Specific gravity varies from 1.001 to 1.040, reflecting the body's need to conserve water. The normal range is 1.010 to 1.030. A low specific gravity in the presence of excessive water elimination is indicative of excessive water intake or is seen in conditions such as diabetes insipidus and uncontrolled diabetes mellitus. When urine specific gravity is low in the absence of diuresis it suggests an inability of the nephron to conserve water properly and kidney failure. The maximum urinary specific gravity that can be attained by the kidney is 1.040. In dehydration the urine is strongly concentrated with a specific gravity greater than 1.030. A high specific gravity in the absence of glucose or protein suggests good renal function and an antidiuretic response.

Assessment of urine output necessarily includes *inspection of the bladder.* The distended bladder may extend to the level of the umbilicus. A bulge may be observed in the midline of the abdomen. If this is noted the nurse should have the patient void and inspect again.

In considering intake and output many questions will be answered and problems resolved by setting up a *fluid data sheet.* Records should be kept on a 24-hour basis. Under intake the date, time, and patient's weight should be recorded. Then the type of intake should be noted including oral liquids, food, parenteral fluids, and amount of solutions used in irrigating tubes, if not subtracted from the output of the tube. Under output the nurse should record insensible losses, urine, diarrhea, vomitus, sweat, blood, and any drainage from tubes. The total intake and losses should be estimated and the net differences calculated.

## Palpation

Palpation is used to confirm the findings of the inspection. Inspection and palpation are inseparable and the nurse should continue to observe while palpating.

**Skin** The skin is a large depot for body fluid and electrolytes and much can be learned about body hydration with careful palpation. The skin should be palpated for temperature, turgor, texture, and the presence of edema. Normally, the skin will feel warm. In contrast, the skin of the patient with fluid loss is often cool and moist, resulting from the vasoconstriction and sympathetic stimulation associated with hypovolemia. The skin of the mildly dehydrated patient will be warm, but will feel dry. In overhydration the skin over edematous areas is often cool to the touch.

*Skin turgor* refers to the skin's elasticity or its ability to return to its normal position after being stretched. The technique for determining skin turgor is to lift a fold of skin over the sternum with the thumb and index finger and then release the skin (Fig. 11-9). Normally the skin will return rapidly to place. If the fold persists for a time after pinching, there is decreased turgor associated with dehydration. Dehydration is also suspected if the skin is loose, wrinkled, and lax in areas not previously subjected to chronic sun damage.

In assessing skin for the *presence of edema* it should be palpated carefully to determine the texture. Texture refers to the quality of the skin surface. The skin may feel tough and hard when distended by fluid. The technique for determining the degree of edema is to apply firm pressure with the thumb against a bony surface (the subcutaneous aspect of the tibia, fibula, or sacrum). When the thumb is withdrawn note if indentation persists. Persistence of indentation indicates fluid is present and is referred to as *pitting edema*. The depth of indentation is measured in millimeters. In evaluating the amount of fluid retention, it should be remembered that up to 10 lb of fluid can accumulate before it is detectable as pitting edema.

**Eyeballs** If a patient's eyes appear to be sunken, it is a sign that dehydration is present. The eyes should then be palpated to obtain confirming evidence. To determine intraocular pressure ask the patient to look downward and place the tips of both index fingers on the upper lid. Apply pressure on the sclera but not the cornea. Two fingers should be used because one cannot distinguish globe indentation from displacement of the eye into orbital fat. As one finger rests on the globe, the other should be advanced to indent the eyeball. The fingers should alternate several times. The rebound of

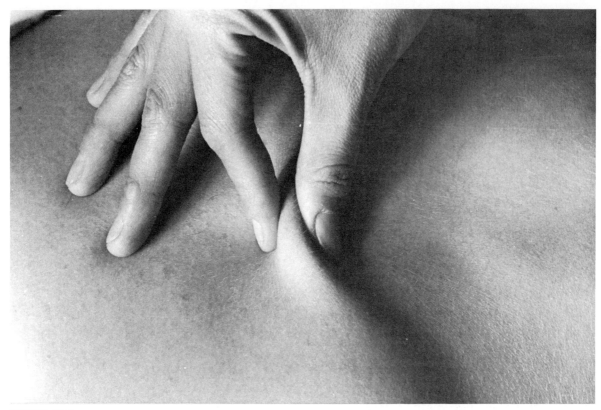

**FIGURE 11-9**
Technique for determining skin turgor. A fold of skin over the sternum
is lifted with the thumb and index finger and then released.

the depressed sclera against the withdrawing finger is the best detector of normal intraocular tension. In dehydration, intraocular fluid will be lost,
decreasing tension. The eyeball will feel spongy
and soft. A hard consistency of the eyeball is indicative of increased intraocular tension as in glaucoma.

**Abdomen**   It must be remembered that palpation
of the abdomen occurs only after auscultation and
percussion. Careful palpation of the abdomen can
detect signs of fluid in the peritoneal cavity and distention of the bladder.

The nurse can assess for ascites by determining the presence of a *fluid wave* (Fig. 11-10). To determine the presence of a fluid wave the patient
should be supine. Either the patient or an assistant
should place the ulnar edge of one hand lightly
against the middle of the abdomen. This limits
transmission of the wave through the tissues of the
abdominal wall. The nurse should place one hand
on the patient's left flank while tapping the patient's
right flank with the other hand. The wave of fluid to

the left side will be felt. Transmission of the fluid
wave is not immediate. There may be a false positive test if the patient is obese or if the patient has
an ovarian cyst with encapsulated fluid. The fluid
wave cannot be obtained if the volume of ascites is
only moderate and abdominal distention is slight.
Sometimes it is helpful to perform the test during
the expiratory phase of a cough.

Palpation of the abdomen is often difficult with
massive ascites. *Ballottement* of fluid may be the
only way to palpate the liver and spleen or a suspected mass. The technique involves lightly thrusting the fingers into the abdomen. This tends to displace the fluid, causing the mass to bound upward
producing a tapping against the palpating fingers.

The abdominal examination necessarily includes palpation for a *distended bladder.* It is sometimes difficult to palpate the bladder and is often
better determined by percussion. It is palpated in
the suprapubic region. Palpate again after the patient has voided. In palpating the bladder the nurse
should note its size, shape, tenderness, pulsations,
mobility, and consistency.

## Percussion

Percussion is the tapping of the structures of the body to produce a sound by which the density of the underlying tissue may be assessed. Careful percussion of the chest and abdomen can identify the presence of underlying fluid. When fluid replaces air containing lung or occupies the pleural space, dullness replaces the normal resonance. The percussion note will be dull to flat depending on the degree of effusion. It will be flat (absolute dullness) when there is a large amount of fluid and very little air present in the underlying tissue. To further identify fluid in the underlying lung, the level of diaphragmatic dullness should be percussed bilaterally during quiet respiration. Pleural effusion usually results in dullness in the lowermost part of the thorax.

To percuss the abdomen for the presence or absence of fluid in the peritoneal cavity, the maneuvers of shifting dullness and puddle examination should be used. *Shifting dullness* is based on the principle that fluid will seek the lowest level (Fig. 11-11). Therefore, when the patient is supine, fluid goes to the sides and back producing a dull percussion note laterally. To perform the maneuver the patient should be supine and the nurse should percuss the level of dullness laterally and mark it with a body pencil. A tympanitic note will be percussed in the midline because the fluid will have fallen to the back. The patient should then be turned to one side for a few minutes and the level of dullness percussed and marked. A new level of dullness closer to the midline indicates the probability of fluid, as the fluid will have gravitated to the dependent flank and the level of dullness will move toward the midline. The percussion note will be tympanitic on the nondependent side. The maneuver should be repeated on the other side. Percussion of shifting dullness will not detect much less than 500 ml of free fluid in the abdominal cavity, and with the obese patient it is difficult to perform.

The *puddle exam* detects as little as 120 ml of free fluid in the abdominal cavity (Fig. 11-12). The patient should be prone for 5 minutes and then rise to the knee chest position. Free fluid in the peritoneal cavity will run to the most dependent area, the periumbilical region. If a dull percussion note is heard in this area it indicates fluid. The puddle exam is not affected by obesity.

The abdomen should be percussed in the suprapubic region to detect a *distended bladder.* If the bladder is distended, there will be dull percussion notes in this region.

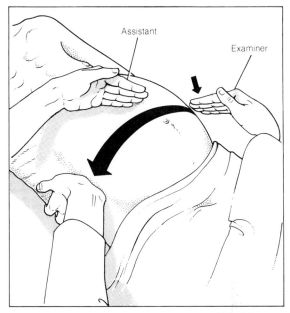

**FIGURE 11-10**

Fluid wave. The nurse taps the right flank and palpates the resultant fluid wave on the left flank. The assistant's hand limits transmission of the wave through the abdominal wall.

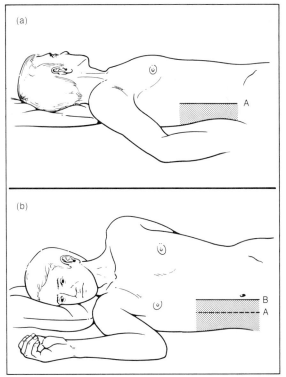

**FIGURE 11-11**

Shifting dullness. (*a*) With the patient supine, each flank is percussed and the level of dullness noted. (*b*) When the patient is turned to the side, the area of dullness percussed will change (shift).

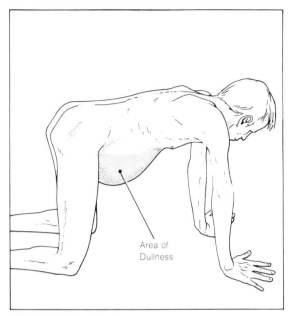

**FIGURE 11-12**
Puddle exam. Dullness is percussed in the periumbilical region when the patient is in the knee chest position.

## Auscultation

Auscultation of the chest and abdomen can further help to identify the presence of underlying fluid. Fluid accumulation will cause decreased sounds where sounds should be heard.

Normal vesicular *breath sounds* are soft, low pitched, and heard mainly during inspiration. Breath sounds will be decreased or absent when fluid separates the air passages from the stethoscope, as with pleural effusion. When effusion is moderate, breath sounds may be heard underlying the effusion. Even when breath sounds are inaudible through the stethoscope, auscultation with the ear directly over the chest may reveal faint bronchial breathing.

To evaluate *voice sounds* have the patient speak in a normal voice and auscultate the chest. The patient should repeat his words in an exaggerated whisper. When there is fluid between the lung and chest wall there is decreased voice intensity.

Auscultation of the abdomen should follow inspection because abdominal sounds will be altered by percussion and palpation. Bowel sounds are generally not diminished by fluid in the peritoneal cavity. *Succussion splash,* a maneuver used to determine the presence of increased air and fluid in the stomach, produces a sound when the patient is rocked from side to side. The nurse should place the stethoscope over the epigastrium and shake the patient. A characteristic slushing and gurgling sound is heard if fluid is present.

## REFERENCES

1   Homer W. Smith, *From Fish to Philosopher: The Story of Our Internal Environment,* CIBA Pharmaceutical Products, Summit, New Jersey, 1959, p. 4.
2   J. Schnermann, "Regulation of Single Nephron Filtration Rate by Feedback," *Clin Nephrol,* **3**(3):75–81, 1975.
3   Ibid.
4   M. R. Per Omvik and F. Kiil, "Renal Autoregulation: Evidence for the Transmural Pressure Hypothesis," *Am J Physiol,* **228**:1840–47, June 1975.
5   J. E. Bourdeau and F. A. Carone, "Protein Handling by the Renal Tubule," *Nephron,* **13**(1):22–34, 1974.
6   P. G. Schmid, F. M. Abboud, M. G. Wendling, E. S. Ramberg, A. L. Mark, D. D. Heistad, and J. W. Eckstein, "Regional Vascular Effects of Vasopressin: Plasma Levels and Circulatory Responses," *Am J Physiol,* **227**:998–1004, November 1974.
7   M. L. Karlinsky, D. S. Sager, N. A. Kurtzman, and V. K. G. Dillay, "Effect of Parathormone and Cyclic Adenosine Monophosphate on Renal Bicarbonate Reabsorption," *Am J Physiol,* **227**:1226–31, December 1974.
8   F. A. Schellander and J. T. Headington, "The Stratum Corneum—Some Structural and Functional Correlates," *Br J Dermatol,* **91**:507–515, November 1974.

## BIBLIOGRAPHY

### Fluid and Electrolyte Balance

Anthony, C. P., and N. J. Kolthoff: *Textbook of Anatomy and Physiology,* Mosby, St. Louis, 1971.
Berman, L. B.: "Practical Nephrology: Urine Isn't Everything," *JAMA,* **231**:978, March 3, 1975.
Bland, John H.: *Clinical Metabolism of Body Water and Electrolytes,* Saunders, Philadelphia, 1963.
Burgess, A.: *Nurse's Guide to Fluid and Electrolyte Balance,* 2d ed., McGraw-Hill, New York, 1978.
Cadnapaphornchai, P., J. L. Boykin, T. Berl, K. M. McDonald, and R. W. Schrier: "Mechanism of Effect of Nicotine on Renal Water Excretion," *Am J Physiol,* **227**:1216–1220, November 1974.
Champion, R. H.: "Sweat Glands," in R. H. Champion et al. (eds.), *An Introduction to the Biology of the Skin,* Davis, Philadelphia, 1970.
Erslev, A. J.: "Renal Biogenesis of Erythropoietin," *Am J Med,* **58**:25–30, January 1975.

Gardner, W. D., and W. A. Osburn: *Structure of the Human Body,* Saunders, Philadelphia, 1973.

Gibson, T., and R. M. Kenedi: "The Structural Components of the Dermis and Their Mechanical Characteristics," in W. Montagna et al. (eds.), *Advances in Biology of Skin,* vol. X: *The Dermis,* Appleton-Century-Crofts, New York, 1970, pp. 19–38.

Gillman, T.: "The Dermis," in R. H. Champion et al. (eds.), *An Introduction to the Biology of the Skin,* Davis, Philadelphia, 1970, pp. 76–113.

Goldberger, E.: *A Primer of Water, Electrolytes, and Acid-Base Syndromes,* Lea and Febiger, Philadelphia, 1970.

Guyton, A. C.: *Textbook of Medical Physiology,* Saunders, Philadelphia, 1966.

Langley, L. L.: *Review of Physiology,* McGraw-Hill, New York, 1971.

Maxwell, M. H., and C. R. Kleeman: *Clinical Disorders of Fluid and Electrolyte Metabolism,* 2d ed., McGraw-Hill, New York, 1972.

Metheny, N. M., and W. D. Snively, Jr., *Nurse's Handbook of Fluid Balance,* Lippincott, Philadelphia, 1974.

Montagna, W., and P. F. Parakkal: *The Structure and Function of the Skin,* Academic, New York, 1974.

Needleman, P., G. R. Marshall, and E. M. Johnson: "Determinants and Modification of Adrenergic and Vascular Resistance in the Kidney," *Am J Physiol,* **227:**665–666, September 1974.

Norman, J. N., J. R. Shearer, A. J. Napper, I. M. Robertson, and G. Smith: "Action of Oxygen on the Renal Circulation," *Am J Physiol,* **227:**740–744, September 1974.

Schrier, R. W., and T. Berl: "Nonosmolar Factors Affecting Renal Water Excretion, Part I," *N Engl J Med,* **292:**81–88, January 9, 1975.

Schrier, R. W., and T. Berl: "Nonosmolar Factors Affecting Renal Water Excretion, Part II," *N Engl J Med,* **292:**141–145, January 16, 1975.

Sharer, J.: "Reviewing Acid-Base Balance," *Am J Nurs,* **75:**980–983, June, 1975.

Snively, W. D.: *Body Fluid Disturbances,* Grune and Stratton, New York, 1962.

Statland, H.: *Fluid and Electrolytes in Practice,* Lippincott, Philadelphia, 1954.

Weisberg, H. F.: *Water, Electrolytes, and Acid-Base Balance,* Williams and Williams, Baltimore, 1962.

Zins, G. R.: Renal Prostaglandins, *Am J Med,* **58:**14–24, January 1975.

## Physical Assessment

Bates, Barbara: *A Guide to Physical Examination,* Lippincott, Philadelphia, 1974.

Beeson, Paul B., and Walter McDermott: *Textbook of Medicine,* Saunders, Philadelphia, 1975.

DeGowin, Elmer L. and Richard L. DeGowin: *Bedside Diagnostic Examination,* Macmillan, New York, 1969.

Hughes, James G.: "Common Fluid and Electrolyte Problems in Pediatrics," *Synopsis of Pediatrics,* 4th ed., Mosby, St. Louis, 1975, pp. 139–156.

Judge, Richard D., and George D. Zuidema: *Methods of Clinical Examination: A Physiologic Approach,* Little, Brown, Boston, 1974.

Metheny, Norma Milligan, and W. D. Snively: *Nurse's Handbook of Fluid Balance,* Lippincott, Philadelphia, 1974.

Prior, John A., and Jack S. Silberstein: *Physical Diagnosis,* Mosby, St. Louis, 1973.

Selkurt, Ewald E.: "Body Water and Electrolyte Composition and Their Regulation," *Basic Physiology for the Health Sciences,* Little, Brown, Boston, 1975, pp. 487–501.

Welt, Louis G.: "Disorders of Fluids and Electrolytes," in M. M. Wintrobe et al. (eds.), *Harrison's Principles of Internal Medicine,* 7th ed., McGraw-Hill, New York, 1974, pp. 1343–1356.

# 12

# FLUID AND ELECTROLYTE IMBALANCES

Diane Chapell Hagen
Deena B. Hollingsworth

**W**ater and electrolytes are constantly being gained from and lost to the environment. These exchanges must be accomplished within a narrow margin for balance to be maintained. Any deviation will result in imbalance. A thorough comprehension of the concept of fluid and electrolyte dynamics is essential to an understanding of the imbalances. This chapter will draw heavily upon the information presented in Chap. 11. The reader is encouraged to review the concept of fluid and electrolyte dynamics in order to understand the imbalances of sodium/water, potassium, calcium, and magnesium, and acid-base dynamics that will be explored.

## PATHOPHYSIOLOGY OF FLUID AND ELECTROLYTE IMBALANCES

The pathophysiological changes associated with fluid and electrolyte imbalances exhibit widespread effects throughout the body. The specific changes, their causes, and their effects on the individual will be explored for each imbalance. Levels of nursing care during imbalance will then be examined in general, followed by specific therapies for each imbalance.

In order to understand fluid and electrolyte imbalances, one should have an understanding of the normal functions of the electrolytes and the normal regulators of fluid and electrolyte balance. The *regulators* include intake, output, acid-base balance, hormonal influences, and cellular integrity. The reader may find a review of these areas (in Chap. 11) helpful prior to proceeding to the discussion of the various imbalances. The imbalances will be explored according to defects in the regulators and the causes of the defects that result in imbalance.

### Water and Sodium Imbalances

Because water and sodium imbalances usually occur in unison, it is difficult to examine one without including the other. The two are interdependent in their roles in maintaining the tonicity of the body fluids. *Tonicity* refers to the concentration of a substance dissolved in water. *Isotonic* fluids are of the same concentration as body fluids. A *hypertonic* solution has a solute concentration greater than that of body fluids, while fluids with concentrations less than that of body fluids are *hypotonic*. Table 12-1 summarizes the types of fluid changes in the body and their effects on the tonicity of the extracellular fluid (ECF) compartment. Water and sodium imbalances will be examined according to hypotonicity and hypertonicity of body fluids and fluid depletion or excess.

**Isotonic depletion** As illustrated in Table 12-1, when isotonic fluids are lost, the ECF becomes depleted. Any patient who loses large amounts of fluid with electrolytes is susceptible to *isotonic ECF depletion.* The most common cause of fluid depletion is gastrointestinal loss such as vomiting or diarrhea. Other possible causes include hemorrhage, nasogastric suctioning, and repeated enemas.

Weight loss is the most sensitive indicator of this and is accompanied by weakness and lethargy. Interstitial depletion will be manifested in poor tissue turgor, dry skin, and dry, sticky mucous membranes. Intravascular hypovolemia will be reflected in a lowered blood pressure, increased pulse, and oliguria. Severe ECF depletion results in shock, which is discussed in Chap. 28.

**Isotonic excess** *Isotonic ECF excess* results when isotonic fluids are gained (Table 12-1). It causes increases in the interstitial fluid compartment, intravascular fluid compartment, or both. It can result from an excessive intake of electrolyte solutions, as when intravenous normal saline is infused too rapidly, in excessive amounts, or in the presence of compromised renal function. Likewise, a situation where there is inefficient excretion of fluid and electrolytes, as in patients with congestive heart failure, renal failure, increased aldosterone, cerebral damage, or cortisone therapy, can

lead to an isotonic ECF excess. Increases in the interstitial fluid often result in edema or in the accumulation of fluid in body compartments. Increases in intravascular fluid result in circulatory overload. A more thorough discussion of the dynamics of ECF excess and related nursing care is found in Chap. 14 in relation to renal failure and in Chap. 24 in relation to pump failure.

**Hypotonic syndrome** *Hypotonic syndrome* is characterized by hyponatremia or a low serum sodium. It results from a loss of sodium in excess of water (hypertonic loss) or a gain of water in excess of sodium (hypotonic gain—see Table 12-1). An understanding of hypotonic syndrome is dependent upon knowledge of the normal regulators of sodium and water balance—intake, output, aldosterone, and the antidiuretic hormone (ADH). Table 12-2 summarizes the causes of ECF hypotonicity in relation to these regulators. The various causes result in either net losses of sodium or net gains of water.

In hypotonic syndrome, the cell is bathed in a solution that is less concentrated than the fluid inside the cell. The resultant change in the osmotic gradient causes water to be drawn into the cell, making it swell and become bloated. This disrupts cellular function and results in a variety of nonspecific effects on the patient which are manifested as confusion, lethargy, headache, anorexia, nausea, vomiting, abdominal cramps, diarrhea, and generalized weakness. If the ECF volume is increased, edema may be present.

**Hypertonic syndrome** Hypertonic syndrome is characterized by hypernatremia or an elevated serum sodium level. It results from a loss of water in excess of sodium (hypotonic loss) or a gain of sodium in excess of water (hypertonic gain—Table 12-1). As in hypotonic syndrome, an understanding of hypertonic syndrome is dependent upon knowledge of the normal regulators of sodium and water balance. Table 12-3 summarizes the causes of ECF hypertonicity in relation to these regulators. The end result is either a net loss of water or a net gain of sodium.

In a hypertonic syndrome, the cell is surrounded by a solution that is more concentrated than the fluid inside the cell. The increase in ECF osmotic pressure pulls water out of the cells, causing them to become dehydrated or shrink (*crenation*). Cellular function is disrupted, causing a variety of nonspecific effects on the patient. If conscious, the patient will experience extreme thirst.

**TABLE 12-1**
RELATIONSHIP BETWEEN NET GAINS AND LOSSES OF WATER AND SODIUM (HYPOTONIC AND HYPERTONIC FLUIDS) AND TONICITY OF EXTRACELLULAR FLUID

| Fluid Changes | ECF Volume | Serum Sodium Concentration | Consequence |
| --- | --- | --- | --- |
| Hypotonic loss | Decreased | Increased | Hypertonic syndrome |
| Isotonic loss | Decreased | Unchanged | Isotonic fluid depletion |
| Hypertonic loss | Decreased | Decreased | Hypotonic syndrome |
| Hypotonic gain | Increased | Decreased | Hypotonic syndrome |
| Isotonic gain | Increased | Unchanged | Isotonic fluid excess |
| Hypertonic gain | Increased | Increased | Hypertonic syndrome |

**TABLE 12-2**
SUMMARY OF THE NORMAL REGULATORS OF SODIUM AND WATER BALANCE
AND DEFECTS IN THE REGULATORS THAT RESULT IN HYPOTONIC SYNDROME

| Normal Regulators | Regulator Defects | Causes of Defects | $Na^+/H_2O$ Changes | Changes in ECF Volume | Result |
|---|---|---|---|---|---|
| Intake | Inadequate $Na^+$ ingestion | Prolonged low-$Na^+$ diets | $Na^+$ gain< $H_2O$ gain | May be decreased | Hypotonic syndrome |
| | Excessive $H_2O$ intake | Infusion of electrolyte-free solutions Inhaling large amounts of fresh $H_2O$ (near drownings) Replacing electrolyte losses with $H_2O$ | $H_2O$ gain> $Na^+$ gain | Increased | Hypotonic syndrome |
| Output | Excessive loss of $Na^+$ with water | Nasogastric tube irrigation with plain water Tissue losses through cellular destruction (wasting diseases and burns) Renal losses through inability to conserve $Na^+$ or diuresis | $Na^+$ loss> $H_2O$ loss | Decreased | Hypotonic syndrome |
| Aldosterone | Inadequate aldosterone effect | Adrenal cortical insufficiency | $Na^+$ loss> $H_2O$ loss | Decreased | Hypotonic syndrome |
| ADH | Excessive ADH effect | Inappropriate ADH syndrome | $H_2O$ gain> $Na^+$ gain | Increased | Hypotonic syndrome |

The patient may also be confused, stuporous, or, in extreme cases, comatose. The skin and mucous membranes will be dry and may appear erythematous. Tissue turgor, however, remains fairly normal unless ECF volume is greatly decreased. Hyperpnea, hypotension, and tachycardia may also develop if ECF is depleted. The patient's temperature may be elevated secondary to dehydration. Unless there is a simultaneous osmotic diuresis, oliguria will be present.

**TABLE 12-3**
SUMMARY OF THE NORMAL REGULATORS OF SODIUM AND WATER BALANCE
AND DEFECTS IN THE REGULATORS THAT RESULT IN HYPERTONIC SYNDROME

| Normal Regulators | Regulator Defects | Causes of Defects | $Na^+/H_2O$ Changes | Changes in ECF Volume | Result |
|---|---|---|---|---|---|
| Intake | Excessive $Na^+$ intake | Ingestion of large amounts of salt without water Inhaling large amounts of salt water (near drownings) High solute loads, i.e., tube feedings without adequate water | $Na^+$ gain> $H_2O$ gain | Increased | Hypertonicity |
| | Inadequate $H_2O$ ingestion | Failure to drink | $H_2O$ gain< $Na^+$ gain | Decreased | Hypertonicity |
| Output | Excessive $H_2O$ loss | Excessive sweating (hypotonic solution) Osmotic diuresis as a result of mannitol, hypertonic glucose, or ketoacidosis Chronic renal failure | $H_2O$ loss> $Na^+$ loss | Decreased | Hypertonicity |
| Aldosterone | Excessive aldosterone effect | Primary aldosteronism Cushing's syndrome | $Na^+$ gain> $H_2O$ gain | Increased | Hypertonicity |
| ADH | Inadequate ADH effect | Diabetes insipidus Posthypophysectomy with excessive water loss | $H_2O$ loss> $Na^+$ loss | Decreased | Hypertonicity |

## Hypokalemia

*Hypokalemia* may be defined as a low serum potassium, generally less than 3.5 meq/liter. If one has an understanding of the normal regulators of potassium, deduction of the factors leading to hypokalemia naturally follows. The causes of hypokalemia in relation to these regulators are presented in Table 12-4.

When the normal functions of potassium are known, the nurse can predict those problems which might be associated with a decreased serum potassium. In hypokalemia there is not enough potassium to maintain normal function. This is especially evident in impulse conduction of skeletal and cardiac muscle. Potassium is a myocardial depressant and stabilizes the normal polarized cardiac cell. Thus a low serum potassium may lead to increased *myocardial irritability* or instability which may precipitate an automatic firing of cells and cardiac arrhythmias. A weak or irregular pulse is common. Sensitivity to digitalis is also increased.

Nerve conduction in both smooth and skeletal muscle is disturbed. *Anorexia* and *nausea* may progress to vomiting. Intestinal motility may be decreased, leading to prolonged emptying of the stomach, failure to pass stools or gas, abdominal distention, and, in severe imbalance, *paralytic ileus.* Neuromuscular weakness, often accompanied by muscle cramps, is common but usually not evident until the hypokalemia is more severe (serum $K^+$ less than 2.5 meq/liter). The weakness is most prominent in the legs; however, with profound hypokalemia, the respiratory muscles become involved and the patient may suffer a respiratory arrest.[1] Postural hypotension manifest by dizziness and a tendency to faint is also common.

## Hyperkalemia

Excess potassium is termed *hyperkalemia* and is indicative of an elevated serum potassium level, greater than 5.5 meq/liter. In order to understand the dynamics of potassium excess, the approach used in assessing the hypokalemic state should be employed. The causes of hyperkalemia are presented in Table 12-5. If normal function is known, the nurse can predict abnormal function or expected problems. In review, potassium is a myocardial depressant and stabilizes the polarized cardiac cell; therefore, it plays a major part in cardiac irritability (stability). An elevated potassium level has an increased depressant effect which disrupts the normal electrical potential of the cardiac cell and may lead to arrhythmias or sudden cardiac standstill. The effects of hypokalemia and hyperkalemia on the neuromuscular system are similar; nerve conduction of skeletal muscle is disrupted, leading to flaccidity, weakness, and cramping.

**TABLE 12-4**
SUMMARY OF THE NORMAL REGULATORS OF POTASSIUM BALANCE
AND DEFECTS IN THE REGULATORS THAT RESULT IN HYPOKALEMIA

| Normal Regulators | Regulator Defects | Causes of Defects | Result |
|---|---|---|---|
| Intake | Inadequate intake of potassium | Decreased intake of $K^+$<br>Change in diet, i.e., fasting, anorexia, NPO status<br>Poorly executed weight reduction plans<br>Prolonged parenteral fluid therapy with potassium-poor fluids | Hypokalemia |
| Output | Abnormal $K^+$ loss via kidney | Excessive diuresis, especially with $K^+$-wasting diuretics<br>Tubular wastage of $K^+$ in some chronic renal diseases | Hypokalemia |
| | Abnormal $K^+$ loss via GI tract | Diarrhea<br>Nasogastric suction or irrigation<br>Vomiting | Hypokalemia |
| Acid-base balance | $K^+$ shifts into cell in exchange for $Na^+$ and $H^+$ | Alkalosis | Hypokalemia |
| Hormonal influences | Excessive aldosterone effect leads to increased excretion of $K^+$ and increased absorption of $Na^+$ | Increased secretion of aldosterone<br>Cushing's disease<br>Treatment with steroid medications | Hypokalemia |
| Cellular integrity | Leakage of intracellular $K^+$ | Tissue damage: surgery, trauma, burns<br>Wound drainage | Hypokalemia |

**TABLE 12-5**
SUMMARY OF THE NORMAL REGULATORS OF POTASSIUM BALANCE
AND DEFECTS IN THE REGULATORS THAT RESULT IN HYPERKALEMIA

| Normal Regulators | Regulator Defects | Causes of Defects | Result |
|---|---|---|---|
| Intake | High $K^+$ intake | Increased dietary intake (in presence of impaired renal function)<br>Rapid infusion of highly concentrated potassium salts<br>Failure to discontinue KCl supplements when need has ceased | Hyperkalemia |
| Output | Inability to excrete potassium via normal route | Acute or chronic renal failure | Hyperkalemia |
| Acid-base balance | Acidosis causes $K^+$ to move out of cell in exchange for $H^+$ | Severe respiratory or metabolic acidosis | Hyperkalemia |
| Hormonal influences | Decreased aldosterone leads to increased serum $K^+$ (aldosterone causes $Na^+$ and $H_2O$ reabsorption and $K^+$ excretion) | Adrenal cortical insufficiency<br>Aldosterone inhibitors (i.e., Aldactone) | Hyperkalemia |
| Cellular integrity | Release of intracellular potassium | Rapid massive use of protein (major infections, crush injuries, burns)<br>Presence of devitalized tissue (e.g., burns)<br>Extravascular blood (e.g., hemorrhage into a body cavity) | Hyperkalemia |

## Hypocalcemia

With knowledge of the normal regulators of calcium balance, deduction of the factors which lead to hypocalcemia or decreased serum calcium (less than 4.5 meq/liter) can be made. Table 12-6 summarizes the causes of hypocalcemia according to the normal regulators. Poor calcium intake is among the leading causes of hypocalcemia. Milk or milk products are the best dietary source of calcium, and without sufficient amounts, an adequate intake of calcium is difficult if not impossible to achieve. Reasons for little or no milk in the diet are numerous and may include personal dislikes, milk intolerance or allergy, and various economic factors. One can experience an increased calcium loss through the kidneys or a decrease in the absorption of calcium from the gastrointestinal tract because of diarrhea or a metabolic problem. Calcium is more readily absorbed in an acid medium; therefore, significant gastrointestinal alkalinity will impair absorption.

**TABLE 12-6**
SUMMARY OF THE NORMAL REGULATORS OF CALCIUM BALANCE
AND DEFECTS IN THE REGULATORS THAT CAN RESULT IN HYPOCALCEMIA

| Normal Regulators | Regulator Defects | Causes of Defects | Result |
|---|---|---|---|
| Intake | Inadequate intake of $Ca^{2+}$ in diet | Intolerance to milk protein<br>Allergies<br>Poor economic status<br>Old age<br>Alcoholism | Hypocalcemia |
| Output | Increased $Ca^{2+}$ loss via kidney | Chronic renal insufficiency | Hypocalcemia |
| | Decreased $Ca^{2+}$ absorption via GI tract | Diarrhea<br>Malabsorption syndrome<br>Inadequate vitamin D | Hypocalcemia |
| Parathyroid gland | Decreased parathyroid hormone (PTH) | Hypoparathyroidism:<br>Spontaneous or secondary to thyroidectomy<br>Postoperative complication of removal of parathyroid adenoma | Hypocalcemia |
| Acid-base balance | Poor ionization of $Ca^{2+}$ in alkalotic medium. Shift of ionized $Ca^{2+}$ to bound $Ca^{2+}$ | Metabolic alkalosis | Hypocalcemia |

Disturbances in acid-base balance may also cause hypocalcemia. It is important to remember that only about 50 percent of the serum calcium is ionized and, therefore, physiologically effective. The rest is bound, generally to proteins. Calcium is more readily ionized in an acidotic medium and less so in an alkalotic medium. Therefore, hypocalcemia may be hidden during acidosis and aggravated by alkalosis.

Finally, the parathyroid gland plays an important part in the secretion of parathyroid hormone (PTH). A decreased PTH will have the greatest effect on the hypocalcemic state. It decreases available calcium by decreasing bone absorption and increasing calcium excretion and phosphate absorption by the kidney. It also decreases the absorption of calcium from the gastrointestinal tract.

The primary effects of the decreased calcium are manifested in skeletal and heart muscle. As the serum concentration of calcium falls below normal (generally less than 4.8 meq/liter), the nervous system becomes increasingly excitable with symptoms manifested peripherally. The nerve fibers become highly excitable and discharge spontaneously, giving rise to paresthesias and spasm of skeletal and smooth muscle. The resultant symptom complex is *tetany.* Other tetanic contractures involving the extremities and the larynx are common. The spasm may occur spontaneously or be induced by ischemia (positive Trousseau's sign) and is most readily seen in the forearm and hand. Laryngeal involvement may produce stridor or suggest asthma, while severe laryngospasm may lead to asphyxia and respiratory arrest. Epileptiform seizures can occur, generally taking the form of grand mal seizures; however, Jacksonian seizures have also been docu-

mented.[2] Perception will also be affected with varying degrees of numbness and paresthesias. The myocardium is affected similarly, leading to decreased contractility and arrhythmia.

There may be emotional disturbances including irritability, emotional lability, depression, memory lapse, confusion, delusions, and hallucinations. Psychoses and psychoneuroses become strong indications for a serum calcium determination.

## Hypercalcemia

The factors that lead to an elevated serum calcium or hypercalcemia (greater than 5.2 meq/liter) can also be deduced from knowledge of its normal regulators. Table 12-7 summarizes the causes of hypercalcemia according to these regulators.

Although excessive intake of calcium alone is not a causal factor, it must be taken into consideration. More common is the excessive use of milk and absorbable alkali compounds or the *milk-alkali syndrome* associated with the treatment of peptic ulcer disease.

Bone plays an important role in calcium regulation. The bone requires weight-bearing stress to facilitate *osteoblastic* or building-up activity. Those patients who are immobilized for long periods of time suffer from increased *osteoclastic* (breaking down) activity, and calcium is mobilized from their bones. Increased intake of vitamin D facilitates reabsorption of calcium from the bone and enhances absorption from the intestinal tract. Bone destruction associated with metastatic neoplasms can also be responsible for elevated serum levels of calcium.

From an earlier discussion, the reader should recall that ionized calcium is the only physiologically effective form and that ionization takes place

**TABLE 12-7**
SUMMARY OF THE NORMAL REGULATORS OF CALCIUM BALANCE
AND DEFECTS IN THE REGULATORS THAT CAN RESULT IN HYPERCALCEMIA

| Normal Regulators | Regulator Defects | Causes of Defects | Result |
|---|---|---|---|
| Intake | Excessive calcium intake | Excessive intake—not primary causal factor<br>Excessive intake of milk and absorbable alkali | Hypercalcemia |
| | Increased GI absorption | Increased intake of vitamin D | |
| Bone | Increased calcium release from bone | Prolonged immobilization<br>Metastatic disease of the bone<br>Increased PTH | Hypercalcemia |
| Acid-base balance | Increase of ionized calcium available; shift of bound $Ca^{2+}$ to ionized $Ca^{2+}$ | Acidosis | Hypercalcemia |
| Parathyroid activity | Excessive PTH effect | Hyperparathyroidism with increased secretion of PTH | Hypercalcemia |

more readily in an acid medium. It follows then that patients suffering from acidosis will have an increase in ionized calcium and therefore become susceptible to hypercalcemia.

Parathyroid hormone, secreted by the parathyroid gland, plays an important part in calcium balance. An increase in PTH leads to increased absorption of calcium from bone and the gastrointestinal tract. It also decreases excretion of calcium by the kidney in exchange for phosphate. Overstimulation of bone by the parathyroid causes increased osteoclastic activity (absorption of calcium from the bone and release into the serum) and may lead to bone destruction, pain, and osteoporosis. In the kidney, high concentrations of calcium in the urine may cause salts to precipitate, forming renal calculi.

The primary effects of increased serum levels of calcium are seen in skeletal muscle, the heart, and the gastrointestinal tract. Calcium plays an important role in allowing sodium to enter the cell, enhancing depolarization. When there is an excess of calcium, this "gate" is blocked, leading to decreased permeability which produces a sedative or depressive effect on the central and peripheral nervous systems. The patient may tire easily, and complain of lethargy, weakness, hypotonia, depressed or absent tendon reflexes, or headache.

In the heart, calcium acts as a stimulant, increasing myocardial contractility. This action is closely related to that of potassium and is manifest as cardiac arrhythmias. As arrhythmias increase, cardiac output falls, affecting the blood pressure.

Anorexia, nausea, and vomiting with resultant weight loss are the most common gastrointestinal manifestations of hypercalcemia. Peptic ulcers may develop. Many patients complain of constipation because of dehydration and smooth muscle hypo-tonia. Abdominal bloating, pain, and diminished bowel activity may be evidenced.

It is also important to note that a high incidence of psychiatric disturbances has been associated with hypercalcemia. Emotional changes such as disturbances in affect and drive, depression, and apathy are manifestations of lesser degrees of hypercalcemia, while severe cases may present as acute psychoses in the form of delirium, disorientation, confusion, hallucinations, and paranoia.[3]

### Hypomagnesemia

Hypomagnesemia is a low serum level of magnesium (less than 1.5 meq/liter). Approximately 50 percent of the magnesium in the blood is normally bound to protein, and so total serum magnesium levels may not accurately reflect the level of ionized magnesium available. If the normal regulators of magnesium balance are known, those factors which lead to hypomagnesemia naturally follow. Table 12-8 summarizes the causes of hypomagnesemia according to these regulators. Hypomagnesemia rarely occurs alone. It most often is seen in conjunction with other electrolyte deficits. Since magnesium acts as a depressant, the early effects are similar to those seen in early hypocalcemia, with increased neuromuscular irritability being the most evident.

### Hypermagnesemia

As in hypomagnesemia, with the normal regulators of magnesium balance in mind, identification of the factors leading to an elevated serum magnesium (greater than 3.0 meq/liter) follows naturally. A brief summary of the causes of hypermagnesemia is found in Table 12-9. Since magnesium normally depresses or stabilizes central nervous system,

**TABLE 12-8**
SUMMARY OF THE NORMAL REGULATORS OF MAGNESIUM BALANCE
AND DEFECTS IN THE REGULATORS THAT CAN RESULT IN HYPOMAGNESEMIA

| Normal Regulators | Regulator Defects | Causes of Defects | Result |
|---|---|---|---|
| Intake | Decreased amount of $Mg^{2+}$ available through ingestion | Chronic alcoholism with poor nutritional patterns<br>Fasting or severely restricted diets<br>Prolonged IV intake with $Mg^{2+}$ free solution in presence of poor nutrition<br>Failure to absorb $Mg^{2+}$ | Hypomagnesemia |
| Renal function | Increased loss of $Mg^{2+}$ | Renal tubular damage<br>Postdiuretic electrolyte imbalance<br>Hemodialysis | Hypomagnesemia |
| Gastro-intestinal tract | Decreased absorption of $Mg^{2+}$ | Severe acute or chronic diarrhea or steatorrhea | Hypomagnesemia |

peripheral neuromuscular, and cardiac impulse transmission, increased magnesium results in profound depression of these areas and may be manifested as muscle weakness, flaccidity, decreased deep tendon reflexes, and central nervous system depression. The cardiac depression is manifested by a decrease in cardiac output with a fall in blood pressure and a compensatory tachycardia. This may be further antagonized by the vasodilatation which accompanies excess magnesium in the periphery. The central nervous system and neuromuscular depressions caused by hypercalcemia can be further antagonized by excess magnesium.

## FIRST-LEVEL NURSING CARE

Because the causes are well known, fluid and electrolyte imbalances are *avoidable.* Preventive nursing care focuses on identifying patients in all settings who could potentially develop imbalances and instituting appropriate measures to counteract the problem before it materializes.

Of primary importance is careful monitoring of both intake and output. All possible avenues of fluid movement into and out of the body should be considered. Nurses must be aware of the amount of fluid as well as the type being lost or gained. In a sense, a mental yardstick needs to be developed which can assist the nurse in measuring the potential losses and excesses.

*Oral intake* is an obvious route of fluid gain. The type of fluids taken in, however, is of prime importance. A patient may be taking nothing by mouth and at the same time be allowed ice chips. Over time this can represent a significant gain of hypotonic fluid. The fluid equivalents of different amounts of ice chips should be tabulated and used consistently. Patients on restricted diets or those fasting for testing procedures are also prone to fluid and electrolyte imbalance.

Nurses should become more conscientious label-readers. The composition of liquid diets should be examined. Some solutions for tube feedings are extremely high in sodium and can represent a significant solute load unless adequate water supplementation is made.

Individuals who for various reasons are unable or not motivated to eat a nutritionally balanced diet are also susceptible to fluid and electrolyte imbalances. Adolescents who go on fad diets are in this group. The elderly, the poor, the debilitated, and patients who are psychotic or confused often eat inadequate diets. The elderly, especially, are prone to imbalance because of poor gastrointestinal absorption and their liberal use of antacids and laxatives. These tend to decrease intestinal acidity, further impairing electrolyte absorption. Alcoholism and food intolerances can contribute to poor nutrition and subsequent susceptibility to imbalances.

Patients receiving intravenous (IV) fluids are especially prone to the development of imbalances. The intravenous solutions used and supplements added should be closely monitored. The amount and type of fluids to be given need to be clearly stated. What is meant by a "keep-open" IV must be well defined and monitored. Patients receiving intravenous fluids for over a week are especially vulnerable and should be watched closely.

Other avenues of fluid intake that should be monitored include nasogastric tube irrigations, catheter irrigations, tracheostomy instillations, and enemas. The types and amounts of fluids used should be considered when assessing overall fluid balance.

*Fluid loss* from the body can occur in several ways, and all must be appreciated so that adequate replacement can occur. Urinary output is the most obvious and should be carefully monitored when indicated.

A less obvious but no less important route of fluid loss is through perspiration. Sweat is a hypotonic solution. During excessive sweating, large amounts of water may be lost in excess of sodium. Athletes are especially prone to this. Replacement

**TABLE 12-9**
SUMMARY OF THE NORMAL REGULATORS OF MAGNESIUM BALANCE
AND DEFECTS IN THE REGULATORS THAT CAN RESULT IN HYPERMAGNESEMIA

| Normal Regulators | Regulator Defects | Causes of Defects | Result |
|---|---|---|---|
| Intake | Increase of $Mg^{2+}$ intake with compensated renal function | Chronic ingestion of magnesium-containing antacids<br>Use of magnesium salts as cathartics<br>Acute administration of magnesium salts | Hypermagnesemia |
| Output | Inability to excrete magnesium | Renal insufficiency | Hypermagnesemia |

with fluids that contain electrolytes qualitatively similar to the fluid that is lost is an important preventive measure. Tap water will not replace lost electrolytes, and commercial beverages which contain glucose, potassium, chloride, and sodium as well as water should be encouraged. Gatorade thirst quencher is an excellent example. Cola beverages, fruit juices, and broths are also beneficial.

Fluid and electrolytes can also be lost from the gastrointestinal tract. Patients with vomiting or diarrhea can potentially develop multiple imbalances. Nasogastric tubes attached to suction are a constant source of fluid and electrolyte loss. Irrigating a nasogastric tube with a hypotonic solution can "wash out" electrolytes. Plain water should never be used, and isotonic saline should be routinely included in the irrigating setup to avoid imbalances. Any retention of irrigating fluid should be noted so that the intake and output can be calculated accurately.

The amount and type of fluid from any tube must be considered when planning for the patient's fluid and electrolyte balance. This can include fluids from Foley catheters, T tubes, gastrostomy tubes, intestinal tubes, Hemovacs, tracheal suctioning, oral suctioning, and wound drains. If losses are replaced, imbalance can be prevented.

Patients with certain *pathologic conditions* are prone to fluid and electrolyte problems. Patients with renal disease are particularly at risk. Those who could potentially develop renal disturbances such as the patient in shock or who has suffered massive trauma must especially be monitored. Cardiac patients, because of the hemodynamic changes that occur, are also prone to imbalance. Those with hormonal disturbances that affect fluid and electrolyte balance such as aldosteronism or Cushing's syndrome are considered at risk. Skeletomuscular disturbances, especially those requiring prolonged bed rest, can result in calcium imbalance. If the nurse is aware of which individuals are particularly susceptible to the development of fluid and electrolyte imbalance, careful and regular assessments can be made and measures instituted so that imbalances do not occur.

Several medications interfere with the normal regulators of fluid and electrolyte balance. These include diuretics and steroids, which may alter water, sodium, and/or potassium balance; electrolyte supplements, which can lead to electrolyte excess; magnesium-containing antacids; antacids in general which decrease gastrointestinal acidity, resulting in impaired calcium absorption; and magnesium sulfate, used for the hyperreflexia asso-

ciated with preeclampsia. Nurses should be especially aware of patients taking any of these drugs.

**Prevention**

Fluid and electrolyte imbalances can be readily prevented. All patients, especially those prone to the development of imbalance, should be carefully monitored regarding their fluid and electrolyte status. If noted early, loses can be easily replaced. Fluids similar to those lost should be encouraged. For more acutely ill patients, slushes can be made from electrolyte-rich fluids. For some patients electrolyte supplements may be indicated. Adequate nutritional intake should be restored. Diets should be planned within the appropriate economic and sociocultural parameters of food selection and availability. If necessary, assistance with shopping and meal planning should be offered. For the poor, referrals should be made to obtain economic assistance.

Besides replacing losses as they occur, excesses in fluid and electrolyte intake should be countered to prevent imbalance. This may be accomplished by simply restricting the intake of water or the electrolyte that is in excess or by the use of diuretics. Whatever the potential imbalance, the nurse is in a unique position to prevent its occurrence.

## SECOND-LEVEL NURSING CARE

Mild degrees of fluid and electrolyte imbalance are frequently seen in a community setting. The nurse can be instrumental in detecting imbalances early and intervening to prevent severe disruptions from developing. While any patient can develop an imbalance, the patients identified in first-level nursing care should be especially monitored.

### Nursing Assessment

In all settings, patients should be carefully assessed to detect early fluid and electrolyte imbalances. Because the initial effects on the patient are often vague and nonspecific, careful attention should be given all aspects of the nursing assessment.

**Health history** A careful and thorough *health history* can contribute valuable information to the nurse's data base. All avenues of fluid losses and gains should be explored with the patient. The patient should be asked about fluid intake in the recent past. Any changes in the color or amount of urine must be examined. Abnormal losses associated with vomiting, diarrhea, or excessive sweating are especially significant.

The patient's previous history including medications currently being taken should be particularly noted and special attention given to conditions or drugs that alter fluid and electrolyte balance. Patients with peptic ulcers, for instance, may be drinking excessive amounts of milk which can alter calcium balance.

Vague complaints that may be indicative of imbalance, especially sodium and potassium disruptions, should be explored. Malaise, weakness, and lethargy are common complaints. Gastrointestinal difficulties such as anorexia, nausea, constipation, diarrhea, or abdominal cramping may also be noted. The patient should be questioned about neurological complaints such as a numbness of the fingers or a tingling or burning sensation in the extremities and around the lips which are indicative of hypocalcemia. Leg pain reflective of osteoporosis and pain associated with renal colic and/or constipation may be indicative of calcium excess.

**Physical assessment**  In the *initial* phases of fluid and electrolyte imbalances, the findings during *physical assessment* are often not remarkable. Water losses may be elicited by testing tissue turgor (Chap. 11) and evaluating mucous membranes. The patient's weight may also be a sensitive indicator of fluid gains or losses. At this point vital signs are usually normal, as are the chest and abdominal examinations. A neurological examination may reveal changes associated with calcium imbalance. These will be discussed in detail in Third-Level Nursing Care.

**Diagnostic tests**  The most useful diagnostic tool for identifying fluid and electrolyte imbalances early is determination of *serum electrolytes*. While the values are reflective of the level of the electrolytes in the plasma and not the whole body, they are useful indicators of electrolyte balance. Depending on the individual patient situation, they are often elevated or depressed in varying combinations. Sodium and potassium losses, for instance, are often associated with chloride losses. Magnesium losses seldom occur alone and may be found in conjunction with calcium losses.

While the serum electrolytes are sensitive indicators of electrolyte balance, the *hematocrit* will reflect water balance. The hematocrit is expressed as the percentage of red blood cells in relation to the total blood volume. Increases in the hematocrit reflect fluid losses, while decreases may indicate fluid excess. The *urine Sulkowitch test* may be used to provide an index of urinary calcium excretion.

**Nursing Problems and Interventions**

When patients have mild fluid and/or electrolyte imbalances, the disruption can often be reversed with prompt care. The initial nursing problem is the *imbalance*. Restricting excesses and supplementing deficits will generally reverse this. Nursing care focuses on diet teaching. The specific foods that must be encouraged or avoided are discussed under the specific therapies in Third-Level Nursing Care. Dietary intake may also need to be supplemented with electrolyte preparations. The medications being taken should be reviewed. Often, dosages, especially of diuretics, will need to be adjusted.

While the imbalance is being corrected, the patient must often cope with problems of *weakness, nausea, diarrhea,* or *constipation.* Rest should be encouraged. The patient's normal daily activities should be evaluated for opportunities to increase rest periods and decrease exertion. Nausea and diarrhea should be treated symptomatically until they subside. Patients suffering from constipation should be encouraged to drink 2000 to 3000 ml fluid daily and to increase dietary bulk as tolerated.

## THIRD-LEVEL NURSING CARE

Severe fluid and electrolyte imbalances are most often seen in the hospital. Often the imbalance is masked by the more severe effects of the underlying pathologic process. Acute illness is often associated with losses of fluid and electrolytes. The elderly living alone or in poorly run nursing homes may also develop severe imbalances before care is instituted.

### Nursing Assessment

All patients in the hospital should be monitored for fluid and electrolyte imbalances. Many factors in addition to the illness itself make patients susceptible to imbalance. These include fluid restrictions in preparation for tests or procedures, medication regimes, and intravenous fluids.

**Health history**  The *health history* related in severe imbalance will be similar to that discussed in Second-Level Nursing Care. Often, however, the patient is too ill to relate the history. The family or significant others should be questioned when possible. If the patient has been at home, the family may describe a bedridden patient often suffering from nausea, vomiting, or diarrhea. Nursing home personnel should be questioned when patients arrive from long-term care facilities. If the patient develops an acute imbalance while hospitalized, the nurse's notes and intake and output record should be utilized to identify precipitating factors.

**Physical assessment** With severe fluid and electrolyte imbalance, *physical assessment* will reveal several effects on the patient. Cerebral functioning should be evaluated. Depending on the imbalance, varying degrees of confusion, irritability, and/or psychoses may be evident. The abdominal examination may also reveal changes. Distention may be noted, pain elicited, and/or bowel sounds diminished. Vital signs also often evidence imbalance. The blood pressure and pulse should be carefully evaluated. With some imbalances heart sounds will evidence arrhythmia. During the chest examination, breath sounds are usually normal.

A complete neurological examination should be done. Muscle strength and perception should be tested bilaterally. Varying degrees of muscle weakness and paralysis are common with several imbalances. Deep tendon reflexes should be tested. Evidence that they are diminished or absent may indicate a severe imbalance.

Hypocalcemia is associated with muscle spasms and tetany. The presence of Chvostek's and Trousseau's signs are especially indicative of hypocalcemia. To test for Chvostek's sign, tap the VIIth cranial nerve (facial nerve) where it passes over the angle of the jaw (in front of the ear) lightly. Twitching of the facial muscles on the same side is a positive finding. Trousseau's sign can be elicited by placing a tourniquet or inflating a blood pressure cuff on the upper arm just above the patient's systolic blood pressure point and leaving it for 3 minutes, causing ischemia of the peripheral nerves and increasing excitability. The resultant carpal spasm with contraction of the thumb and fingers and an inability to open the hand is considered a positive Trousseau's sign (see Fig. 12-1).

**Diagnostic tests** As with second-level nursing assessment, the serum electrolytes and hematocrit are the most sensitive indicators of fluid and electrolyte imbalances. With more severe imbalance, the *urine specific gravity* provides a simple method of evaluating renal function. Mildly elevated *fasting blood sugars* may also be seen in patients with hypokalemia.

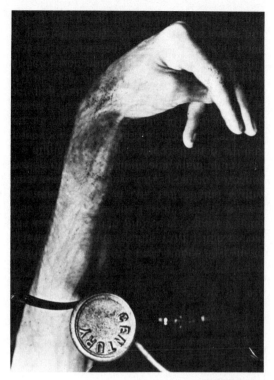

**FIGURE 12-1**

Trousseau's sign in a patient with hypoparathyroidism. (*From Maxwell and Kleeman, 1972. By permission of the publisher.*)

Because potassium and calcium imbalances can affect myocardial functioning, an *electrocardiogram* (*EKG*) may also be used. When the serum potassium falls below 3.0 meq/liter, the EKG may evidence a flattened T wave and prolongation of the QT interval (see Fig. 12-2). With excess calcium levels the EKG may reflect a shortened ST segment.

The EKG changes associated with hyperkalemia are also illustrated in Fig. 12-2. Initially there is a high peaking of the T waves (especially in the chest leads) associated with a normal or decreased QT interval, which differentiates it from other disorders manifested by elevated T waves. With a progressive rise in serum potassium, prolongation of the PR interval occurs, followed by disappearance of the P wave and finally prolongation of the QRS complex. At extremely high levels (greater than 9 or 10 meq/liter), the QRS complex becomes wide and smooth, joining with the T wave to give the appearance of a continuous sine wave. This is manifest as ventricular flutter progressing to ventricular fibrillation or standstill.

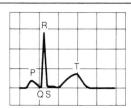

**Normal tracing (serum potassium 4-5.5 meq/liter)**: PR interval = 0.16 second; QRS interval = 0.06 second; QT interval = 0.4 second (normal for an assumed heart rate of 60).

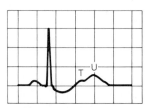

**Hypokalemia (serum potassium ± 3.5 meg/liter)**: PR interval = 0.2 second; QRS interval = 0.06 second; ST segment depression. A prominent U wave is now present immediately following the T wave. The actual QT interval remains 0.4 second. If the U wave is erroneously considered a part of the T, a falsely prolonged QT interval of 0.6 second will be measured.

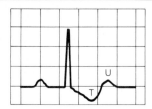

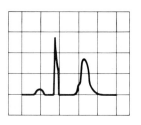

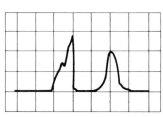

**Hypokalemia (serum potassium ± 2.5 meq/liter)**: The PR interval is lengthened to 0.32 second; the ST segment is depressed; the T wave is inverted; a prominent U wave is seen. The true QT interval remains normal.

**Hyperkalemia (serum potassium ±7 meq/liter)**: The PR and QRS intervals are within normal limits. Very tall, slender, peaked T waves are now present.

**Hyperkalemia (serum potassium ±8.5 meq/liter)**: There is no evidence of atrial activity; the QRS complex is broad and slurred, and the QRS interval has widened to 0.2 second. The T waves remain tall and slender. Further elevation of the serum potassium will result in ventricular tachycardia and ventricular fibrillation.

**FIGURE 12-2**
Correlation of serum potassium level and the EKG. (Assuming serum calcium is normal.) The diagrammed complexes are left ventricular epicardial leads. (*Reproduced, with permission, from M. U. Goldman: Principles of Clinical Electrocardiography, 9th ed., Lange, Los Altos, Calif., 1976.*)

### Nursing Problems and Interventions

The problems associated with fluid and electrolyte imbalance often affect myocardial functioning, muscle strength, and perception. *Arrhythmias* are common, especially with potassium and calcium imbalances. Cardiac monitoring is frequently indicated. Until the imbalance is corrected, vital signs should be monitored carefully along with EKG tracings.

Some degree of *muscle weakness* or *paralysis* may also be a problem. Care must be symptomatic until the imbalance is reversed. If paralysis is present, the patient will be susceptible to the hazards of immobility. Patients with *diminished perception* must be protected from injury. The skin, especially, should be examined for evidence of breakdown. Special care must be provided for patients with *muscle spasms* associated with tetany. This is discussed under the specific therapy for hypocalcemia. If *confusion* is a problem, safety must be provided. Side rails, restraints as necessary, and close observations become nursing obligations. When severe nausea and vomiting accompany the imbalance, *dehydration* may develop. The vomiting is often dealt with symptomatically, while adequate fluid replacement is paramount.

The most obvious nursing problem associated with fluid and electrolyte changes is the *imbalance* itself. Intervention will depend on the underlying cause. In general, deficits must be supplemented and excesses eliminated or restricted. This often involves *intravenous therapy*.

**Parenteral administration** Intravenous "setups" usually consist of three major components (Fig. 12-3).

Component 1    Container of solution and any prescribed additives

Component 2    IV administration set (may include auxillary fluid chamber)

Component 3    The IV line and the IV site

The *container of solution* is one of the most vital parts of intravenous infusions. The solution not only holds fluids and electrolytes but often nutrients and medications. It is given intravenously and, therefore, will have an immediate impact. Because of this, the type, amount, and sterility of the fluid are extremely important.

Intravenous orders should always be evaluated against the nurse's perception of the patient's fluid and electrolyte needs. The intake and output, weight record, information in the nursing notes obtained during report or rounds and from laboratory tests, as well as the nurse's own observations, should be examined in relation to intravenous infusions. Any discrepancies should be clarified with the physician before the infusion is administered.

Once the amount and type of solution have been determined, it may be the nurse's responsibility to prepare it. This should be done maintaining the strictest of sterile conditions. If sterility is broken, bacteria will be introduced directly into the bloodstream.

As important as the type of fluid is the amount. Overly rapid administration of fluid intravenously can result in overexpansion of the blood volume with increased workload on the heart and kidneys. The potential for the development of congestive heart failure and pulmonary edema exists when patients with compromised cardiac or renal status are "overdosed" with fluids. For this reason, small-volume bottles should be used for elderly patients or those with small body masses.

The *administration set* plays an important part in the amount of fluid the patient receives. It can deliver 10, 12, or 15 drops per milliliter (macrodrip) or 60 drops per milliliter (microdrip). The macrodrip set should be used if rapid administration of fluid is needed or when the administration rate is faster than 100 ml/hour. The microdrip set should be used when the fluid volume needs to be smaller or more finely controlled. These situations include patients with compromised renal or cardiac status, patients on "keep-open" rates, and patients who require an intravenous route for the administration of medication only.

Some sets may have an *auxiliary fluid chamber.* This is an optional component and may be a tubular chamber calibrated in milliliters with a volume of 100 to 150 ml. It may also consist of five plastic nodular chambers each of which contains 10 ml. This type of auxiliary chamber may be clamped off at any level so that 10 to 40 ml can be delivered at any one time. Auxiliary chambers are especially useful when delivering fluids to children or people

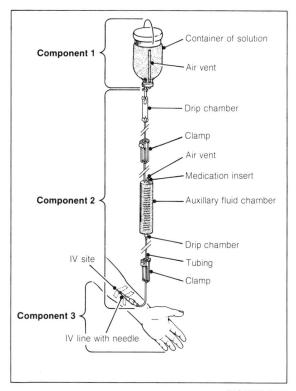

**FIGURE 12-3**
Components of an intravenous "setup."

with small body masses or blood volumes, elderly people, people with compromised renal or cardiac status, patients needing only small amounts of fluid over a period of time, and patients receiving intravenous medications that require dilution.

The *intravenous line* and *intravenous site* make up the final component. Either a pliable catheter or needle-like line may be used. Increased stability and longevity may be achieved by the use of a long intravenous catheter.

When an IV catheter is in place for more than 48 hours, there is an increased risk of sepsis and thrombophlebitis. The nurse should evaluate the site often for redness, tenderness, edema, pain, or warmth. The site should be cleaned and the dressing changed daily.

**Specific therapies**  While the fluid and electrolyte imbalances have many similarities, specific imbalances must be countered with electrolyte-specific interventions for balance to be maintained. These therapies will now be examined in relation to each imbalance.

**H**ypotonic Syndrome The nursing management of hypotonicity is dependent upon the underlying cause and the associated fluid imbalance. When hypotonicity is due to *water gain* in excess of a sodium gain, the aim is to correct the basic flaw by withholding water and decreasing the dilutional tendency. If it is a product of *sodium loss* in excess of water loss, the problem would likely be solved with infusions of isotonic saline. In some situations hypertonic saline may be infused, although indications for this are rare. If the pathologic process is severely complicated by hyponatremia, if it is necessary to correct the concentration of sodium rapidly, or if it is necessary to restrict the volume of fluid taken in, hypertonic saline may be of use. When it is used, the nurse must be alert to overcorrection of the serum sodium leading to hypernatremia and the development of an increased ECF volume.

**H**ypertonic Syndrome Care of the patient with hypertonic syndrome always involves hypotonic fluid replacement. This may be accomplished with oral or rectal tap water, intravenous administration of an electrolyte-free solution such as 5% dextrose in water, or intravenous administration of hypotonic electrolyte solutions such as 0.45% sodium chloride.

**H**ypokalemia Potassium loss can often be replaced with oral potassium supplementation. The first approach to this problem would include a diet with a higher potassium content. Traditionally high sources of $K^+$ include bananas, oranges, potatoes, carrots, and celery. Table 12-10 lists the potassium content of various foods and fluids. The nurse can utilize this information to plan with the patient a well-balanced but varied diet.

**TABLE 12-10**
RELATIVE POTASSIUM CONTENT OF CERTAIN FOODS AND LIQUIDS

| HIGH $K^+$ | LOW $K^+$ |
| --- | --- |
| Milk | Ginger ale |
| Coca-Cola | Pepsi-Cola |
| Coffee | Seven-Up |
| Tea | Kool-Ade soft drink mix |
| Potatoes | Beef |
| Jell-O gelatin dessert | Chicken |
| Peanut butter | Cottage and cheddar cheeses |
| Nuts | Dietetic gelatin |
| Chocolate | Margarine |
| Oranges | Enriched white bread |
| Tomatoes | |
| Bananas | |
| Carrots | |
| Celery | |

It may be necessary for the patient to be placed on one of the oral potassium supplements. These often contain chloride and allow for the chloride losses that are often associated with potassium losses. Chloride as well as potassium is essential to repair deficits and avoid the complications of hypochloremia or metabolic alkalosis. Potassium supplements are bound to bicarbonates, citrates, or gluconates, and nurses should be cognizant of the preparation being used.

Potassium supplements are extremely unpalatable and should be made as acceptable as possible. Dissolving or diluting the preparation in fruit or vegetable juice may help disguise the taste and provide additional potassium. Tomato juice is often used. Giving an undiluted preparation can also cause severe gastric irritation and nausea. Chilling the preparation after it is mixed will increase palatability. Again, allowing the patient to participate is important. If the preparation is offensive and unacceptable, the patient is not likely to continue taking it at home. Patients should be cautioned to follow instructions carefully, such as dissolving tablet supplements, and be told why this is important. They should be aware of the relationship between the $K^+$ supplement and their other medications as well. If they fail to understand these relationships, they may fail to take their supplement but continue to take the medication which necessitated $K^+$ replacement. Periodic review of medication dosages and schedules is advisable; it may be helpful to have patients bring medications with them to their appointments so that these can be validated.

It may be necessary for the hypokalemic patient to be treated with *intravenous infusions of potassium chloride* (KCl), which can give rise to several nursing problems. KCl is very irritating to the vascular intima; therefore, a concentration of less than 80 meq/liter of solution is recommended, and under no circumstances should KCl be given undiluted or by direct IV "push."[4] In selecting an IV site, the nurse should look for a large vessel to facilitate further dilution of the KCl. Protection against and observation for infiltration become important as potassium chloride may cause tissue necrosis and sloughing. The nurse should therefore check those patients with KCl additives more often for the characteristic signs of redness, irritation, and pain. Nursing responsibility to guard against vein and tissue damage due to careless administration of KCl cannot be overemphasized.

Generally the rate of administration should not exceed 20 to 25 meq/(liter)(hour) in the average-sized adult; however, in certain emergency situations such as digitalis toxicity with lethal cardiac arrhythmias or muscular paralysis, the rate may be increased. It is important to remember that $K^+$ is a cardiac depressant and large doses may exert a toxic effect on the heart. It can enhance the degree of conduction block or cause coronary artery spasm. For this reason, high concentrations of KCl should not be administered rapidly into a central venous pressure line because of its direct route of access to the myocardium. Renal function should be monitored since the primary route of exit for $K^+$ is the kidneys. The infusion should be continued with caution if urinary output falls below 50 ml/ hour.

**H**yperkalemia Intervention during hyperkalemia should be directed at decreasing potassium intake and increasing potassium loss. It should be obvious that modifying the dietary potassium intake is a primary means of decreasing the potassium load. Nurses share the responsibility for teaching and coordinating their patients' dietary plans with other members of the health care team. If the hyperkalemia is the result of renal failure, this dietary restriction will be a long-term plan. The nurse should help the patient become familiar with foods high and low in potassium. (Refer to Table 12-10.) The patient and the family should be assisted in varying the diet with the "allowed" foods in order to avoid the monotony which often leads to "cheating" and intake of excluded foods. An understanding of the relationship between the dietary problem and restrictions is vital to the cooperation of these patients and their families.

Dangerously high serum potassium levels require more aggressive intervention. They are usually lowered with a three-part approach. First, *diuretics* may be prescribed by the physician when normal renal excretion of potassium has not successfully lowered the serum level. Diuretics work by many principles, but in the final analysis they increase potassium excretion as they increase output of water and sodium chloride through the kidney.

The next step involves the use of *cation-exchange resins.* These are generally sodium-containing resins such as sodium polystyrene sulfonate or Kayexalate, administered orally or rectally. They exchange sodium ions for potassium ions through the gastrointestinal mucosa and are then excreted. They are often given in conjunction with sorbitol to avoid fecal impaction. Kayexalate is extremely unpalatable; therefore, the nurse should experiment to find a palatable vehicle. The mixture needs to be diluted to avoid a thick, stiff preparation which is difficult to swallow. Chilling the mixture may also make ingestion somewhat easier.

When giving Kayexalate rectally, one should use a large-lumen Foley catheter (with a large-volume inflation balloon) as the rectal tube. After insertion of the tube, the bag should be inflated to aid in retention of the enema. The solution should be instilled slowly and the catheter clamped for 30 to 45 minutes. At the end of the time, the clamp is released and the enema is expelled. It is often necessary to repeat the procedure at frequent intervals until the serum potassium falls to a safer level.

Finally, correction of severe hyperkalemia may also be achieved by *dialysis.* Both peritoneal dialysis and hemodialysis remove potassium; although the latter is more efficient, the former is easier to use. It is important to note that both procedures are considered as last measures and generally are utilized only in life-threatening situations. The reader is referred to Chap. 14 for a more complete discussion of these dialysis methods and related nursing care.

Another serious problem associated with hyperkalemia is *cardiac depression.* When cardiac function is seriously threatened, the critical nature of the situation warrants shifting the potassium back into the intracellular fluid where it is less apt to be harmful. Calcium gluconate is often used as a temporary measure to counteract the depressant effect of hyperkalemia on the myocardium. Nursing considerations which accompany the administration of calcium include the maintenance of a long, stable intravenous line and monitoring the electrocardiogram. The calcium should be diluted and given by direct intravenous push or added to an intravenous solution for infusion. It should be administered slowly to prevent overloading with high concentrations.

*Metabolic acidosis* is often associated with severe hyperkalemia. It results in the movement of hydrogen ions into the cell, thus forcing potassium ions into the extracellular fluid. This shift compounds the high levels of potassium that already exist. To correct the acidosis, sodium bicarbonate is given intravenously. This increases the serum pH, drawing hydrogen ions out of the cells and thus allowing potassium to reenter. Potassium reentry may be further facilitated by the administration of hypertonic glucose in conjunction with insulin.

**H**ypocalcemia With mild hypocalcemia, a dietary intake high in calcium is indicated. If an oral calcium salt is necessary, long-term care should focus on a teaching plan. Calcium gluconate is a less concentrated solution than calcium chloride and, therefore, not as irritating to the gastrointestinal tract. Calcium is best absorbed in an acidic medium. Taking the supplement with orange juice will maximize its absorption. If gastrointestinal upset is a problem, patients can take the calcium with meals but should avoid drinking milk or other alkaline products.

For more severe imbalance, *calcium replacement* is the treatment of choice. Calcium may be administered orally or parenterally as calcium gluconate or calcium chloride. It is important to remember that the effect of calcium is transitory and an additional dose may be necessary. Caution should be exercised when giving calcium to digitalized patients since calcium and digitalis act on the same portion of the cardiac cycle and both are cardiac stimulants. Intravenous infusion of calcium carries many nursing responsibilities. Calcium may cause vessel irritation and should, therefore, be administered through a long, stable intravenous line. Care should be taken to avoid infiltration, especially when using calcium chloride, as the tissue may become necrotic and slough off. Infusions should be administered at a slow rate to avoid high serum concentrations and the associated cardiac depression. It is also suggested that the patient be monitored closely for changes in the cardiac rhythm, rate, and blood pressure.

*Tetany* often develops with hypocalcemia and can be very distressing and exhausting for the patient from both a physical and emotional standpoint. The nurse should be aware of those factors which exacerbate tetany and limit or control them as much as possible. The patient should be kept quiet and free from stress since the associated hyperventilation can precipitate tetany by creating an alkalotic state. The symptoms of tetany are more pronounced when there is pressure on a motor nerve as when patients cross their legs or rest an arm over a chair. The observant nurse can teach patients the pitfalls associated with such activity. If *seizures* develop, the patient should be protected from injury (see Chap. 33). With *laryngospasm,* preservation of a patent airway becomes paramount.

**H**ypercalcemia  Elevated *serum calcium* levels can best be treated by restricting the calcium intake, specifically by limiting the dietary allowance of dairy products. Severe hypercalcemia is a medical emergency and most often results from acute parathyroid intoxication, vitamin D intoxication, or

malignant neoplasms of the bone. *Dehydration* associated with the severe nausea and vomiting that often accompany hypercalcemia can develop. Adequate fluid replacement, maintaining a stable intravenous line, encouraging fluids (up to 4000 ml/day), and keeping an accurate intake and output record are important interventions.

Prevention of *renal calculi* is an important part of nursing management. Increasing fluid intake to 3000 to 4000 ml/day, maintaining an acid urine, and preventing urinary tract infections will aid with this (see Chap. 14). The increased fluid will dilute the calcium concentration and decrease the chance of stone formation. Calcium salts precipitate more readily in an alkaline solution; therefore, keeping the urine at a lower pH will lessen precipitation. Acid-ash food products such as cranberry or prune juice should be encouraged.[5]

*Surgical intervention*  Hyperparathyroidism may necessitate a *parathyroidectomy.* Preoperative care is directed toward preventing dangerously high serum calcium levels and the associated problems discussed in the previous section.

The postoperative period presents new problems which are the reverse of those seen preoperatively. Mild tetany is not uncommon, due to the normal drop in serum calcium following the surgery. These patients need close monitoring for more severe forms of tetany, especially laryngospasm. The nurse should check regularly for signs of increased muscle irritability as evidenced by positive Chvostek's and Trousseau's signs. If tetany becomes severe, intravenous use of calcium gluconate will relieve the symptoms.

Large quantities of calcium salts may be required postoperatively, especially in those patients with previous bone disease. Removal of the parathyroids reduces bone resorption. The "hungry-bones" syndrome characterized by hypocalcemia and severe tetany can develop. These patients should be encouraged to eat a high-calcium diet and ambulate as early as possible in order to aid in the recalcification process.[6]

The patient who has had a parathyroidectomy often needs long-term follow-up. Serum calcium levels should be monitored as secondary hypocalcemia may occur. Acute pancreatitis may also occur, and patients should be advised to seek medical attention if they suffer from abdominal discomfort.[7]

**H**ypomagnesemia  The resolution of hypomagnesemia may be achieved (if only temporarily) by replacement with magnesium, in the form of magnesium sulfate, for example. However, the underlying cause of the deficit will have to be resolved if balance is to be maintained. The amount and route of administration for magnesium salts are dependent on the degree of depletion and its cause. Symptomatic deficiencies are usually treated parenterally. When giving parenteral magnesium salts, the nurse should monitor the cardiac rhythm and the patient's reflexes to detect the depressive effects of magnesium. The presence of deep tendon reflexes diminishes the likelihood that respiratory depression and paralysis associated with excess magnesium will develop. However, it is advisable to have a self-inflating breathing bag, airways, and oxygen readily available in case a respiratory emergency should occur. Calcium preparations are often given to counteract the potential danger to myocardial functioning that magnesium intoxication secondary to rapid infusions poses.

Once normal magnesium levels have been achieved in the acute setting, long-term maintenance of normal levels becomes the nursing objective. This may be accomplished by long-term supplementation with oral magnesium, but more important is the modification of the underlying problem, specifically to decrease losses and increase intake. Examples would include recommending that the patient avoid alcohol or counseling for a more balanced diet.

**H**ypermagnesemia   Elevation in the serum magnesium level is a serious problem which requires thorough nursing care. Hypermagnesemia mimics hypercalcemia, and nursing approaches are similar. Urinary and serum magnesium levels and the deep tendon reflexes should be monitored. As stated earlier, a decrease or disappearance of these reflexes may indicate toxicity or excessive depression by the magnesium and *respiratory paralysis* can potentially develop. The nurse should monitor respiratory status by checking tidal volume and utilizing auscultation of the chest. Respiratory support equipment should be readily available.

Toxic effects on the heart are generally preceded by respiratory depression; however, the nurse should monitor the cardiac rhythm for evidence of depression such as *heart blocks* (see Chap. 26). Increased levels of magnesium mimic the effect of hyperkalemia on the myocardium and are evidenced as flushing, diaphoresis, and hypotension. The nurse should have a preparation of *calcium salts* readily available to antagonize these cardiac depressant effects. It is important to note

that while magnesium and calcium both depress skeletal muscle, magnesium depresses the myocardium and calcium stimulates it. Calcium, therefore, can be used as an antagonist to the myocardial effects of magnesium.

## FOURTH-LEVEL NURSING CARE

Rehabilitation of the patient who has developed a severe fluid and/or electrolyte imbalance focuses on preventing its reoccurrence. Much of the preventive interventions examined in First-Level Nursing Care are applicable to preventing reoccurrence of an imbalance. Follow-up care is especially important. The patient should be evaluated regularly, and nursing assessment should include routine serum electrolyte levels.

Patients with fluid and electrolyte imbalances need to be taught what constitutes abnormal losses and should be encouraged to contact their nurse or physician if losses occur. The importance, proper use, and significance of taking medications and/or supplements should be emphasized. Patient understanding of diet restrictions and medications should be periodically reevaluated. Consider, for example, the therapeutic triad of a digitalis preparation, a diuretic, and a potassium supplement which is commonly associated with recurrent hypokalemia. Patients admitted to the hospital with digitalis intolerance or toxicity and hypokalemia probably represent a population who were not prepared to manage their therapeutic regime. Thus, any patients who have such an admitting diagnosis or who are receiving this drug repertoire should be engaged in a practical teaching exercise. This teaching is appropriate prior to discharge from an acute setting and again in the community.

The teaching of patients being treated with this therapeutic triad should begin with a discussion of the correct dosages and times of administration. This information should be reviewed repeatedly, and the patient should be able to state when the pills are to be taken in reference to daily activities. A brief, simple discussion of the interrelationships of the triad is helpful to the patients' understanding the importance of taking medications as prescribed. The importance of taking KCl in full doses and ways to prepare it should be discussed. Teaching the patient how to take a radial pulse and what to do if it is less than 60 may avoid further problems. Avenues of action should be discussed. What does the patient do if he or she develops gastrointestinal problems and cannot take one or more of the medications? Digitalis toxicity may develop in the presence of a decrease in serum $K^+$. The patient should be made aware of signs and symptoms such as visual disturbances, anorexia, an increase or decrease in the pulse, palpitations, or "fast heart beat," any of which may signal digitalis toxicity, and the patient should be encouraged to seek help if these occur. Many dangerous cardiac arrhythmias are associated with digitalis toxicity and may prove lethal if untreated. Printed material to which the patient can periodically refer after discharge is always helpful.

## OTHER DISRUPTIONS IN FLUID AND ELECTROLYTE BALANCE

Fluid and electrolyte balance can be disrupted when the normal locations of fluid and electrolytes within the body are altered. Any disturbance in the normal regulators of fluid and electrolyte balance, especially the hormonal regulators—the antidiuretic hormone and aldosterone—can also result in imbalance. These internal shifts of fluid and hormonal disturbances will be briefly examined.

### Internal Shifts of Fluid

Earlier in this chapter changes in tonicity and how they effect movement of fluid between intercellular and extracellular compartments were explored.

*Fluid shifts between the two extracellular compartments—the intravascular fluid (IVF) and the interstitial fluid (ISF)—will now be examined.*

An understanding of fluid dynamics of the ECF is dependent upon an understanding of the normal regulators of fluid exchanges between the interstitial fluid and the intravascular fluid. These regulators include factors which foster movement of fluid from the intravascular fluid compartment to the interstitial fluid compartment such as capillary hydrostatic pressure (CHP), interstitial hydrostatic pressure (IHP), and interstitial colloid osmotic pressure (ICOP), and those which foster movement from the interstitial fluid compartment to the intravascular fluid compartment such as capillary colloid osmotic pressure (CCOP) and lymphatic drainage. These pressure differences are mediated by the capillary permeability. A thorough discussion of capillary fluid dynamics can be found in Chap. 11.

With a clear understanding of normal fluid dynamics between the IVF and ISF, the causes of imbalance can be deduced. Table 12-11 summarizes the causes of extracellular fluid shifts according to the normal fluid exchanges within the ECF compartment.

**Fluid shift into the interstitial space**   When a shift of fluid from the intravascular compartment to

**TABLE 12-11**
SUMMARY OF THE NORMAL REGULATORS OF ECF DYNAMICS AND DEFECTS IN THE REGULATORS THAT CAN RESULT IN FLUID SHIFTS

| Normal Regulators | Regulator Defects | Causes of Defects | Direction of Shift |
|---|---|---|---|
| Capillary hydrostatic pressure (CHP) | Increased CHP | CHF with decrease venous return leads to pooling of blood<br>Allergic response with histamine release, arteriolar dilatation, and increased blood flow | IVF→ISF |
| Capillary colloid osmotic pressure (CCOP) | Decreased plasma protein with decreased intravascular colloid osmotic pressure | Liver disease with decreased synthesis of plasma proteins<br>Dietary protein deficiency<br>Increased loss of protein via kidney<br>Leakage of protein from burned skin | IVF→ISF |
| | Increased plasma protein with increased intravascular colloid osmotic pressure | Excessive infusion of colloidal solutions, i.e., Dextran, albumin, plasma | IVF←ISF |
| Interstitial colloid osmotic pressure (ICOP) | Increased capillary permeability leads to leakage of proteins into ISF and increasing ICOP | Burns (early)<br>Allergies<br>Radiation therapy | IVF→ISF |
| | Decreased capillary permeability with decreased ICOP | Second stage of burns<br>Mobilization of edema fluid | IVF←ISF |
| | Decreased return of proteins and fluid to IVF via lymphatics leads to increased ICOP | Removal of lymphatic glands with mastectomy<br>Obstruction of lymphatics with cancer | IVF→ISF |

the interstitial compartment occurs, there is a net loss of circulating blood volume which may compromise the cardiovascular system. Blood pressure may be decreased with a compensatory tachycardia and vasoconstriction. Oliguria due to decreased renal perfusion develops.

*Edema,* or an increase in the interstitial fluid volume, may also occur as the exchange of fluid between the two compartments is disrupted. It may be generalized or localized, subtle or grossly evident. Fluid distribution is influenced by gravity; therefore, fluid may pool in dependent areas such as the lower extremities or the sacrum. This type of edema is known as *dependent edema.*

Edema also occurs in other body cavities. It is known as "third spacing" and may manifest itself as a collection of fluid in the abdomen (*ascites*), in the pleural cavity (*hydrothorax*), or the pericardial sac (*pericardial effusion*). The term *anasarca* refers to massive and generalized edema. Physical manifestations of edema may not develop until there is a large increase in the ISF volume. Nursing care in relation to problems of fluid shifts into the interstitial fluid compartment is explored in detail in relation to burns (Chap. 13), renal failure (Chap. 14), hepatic dysfunction (Chap. 19), and pump failure (Chap. 24).

### Fluid shift into the intravascular space

When a shift of fluid into the intravascular compartment occurs, there is an expansion of the intravascular volume (plasma volume). This can increase the workload on the heart and kidneys, and in severe cases circulatory overload can occur. Nursing care in relation to circulatory overload is discussed in Chap. 13 in relation to the fluid dynamics associated with burns and in Chap. 24 in relation to the patient with pump failure.

### Diabetes Insipidus

*Diabetes insipidus* is a clinical problem which illustrates well the fluid and electrolyte imbalances that have been discussed. Essentially, it results from a defect in the chain of events which normally lead to the secretion of the antidiuretic hormone (ADH) from the neurohypophysis. It may occur as a result of a lesion or injury to the hypothalamus or hypophysis. Surgical hypophysectomy for treatment of metastatic carcinoma of the breast may also lead to the development of diabetes insipidus.

Normally, ADH promotes water reabsorption from the distal and collecting tubules. Decreases in ADH may lead to excessive water loss (10 to 30

liters/day). Patients with such water loss have a decrease in blood volume with concentration of the extracellular fluid. They may exhibit a fall in blood pressure and severe thirst secondary to polyuria. Their urine is characteristically pale and dilute (specific gravity less than 1.010) with a decreased osmolarity.

It is important to replace these fluid losses either by mouth or intravenously. To facilitate this, the nurse should keep a meticulous intake and output record. Serum electrolytes, especially potassium, as well as the urine electrolytes and osmolarity should be monitored. Specific intervention might include offering the patient electrolyte-rich solutions in addition to plain water and checking urine output and specific gravity on an hourly basis. A flowsheet at the bedside will facilitate coordination of therapy with patient responses and foster communication. It should provide a continuous record of the date, time, vital signs, intake (both by mouth and intravenously), urine volume and specific gravity, and laboratory data including serum and urine electrolytes, osmolarity, and hematocrit. A section for notations regarding thirst, fatigue, alertness, and clinical signs of dehydration or electrolyte depletion is helpful. During the acute phase of diuresis, intravenous intake may be titrated hourly according to urine output and specific gravity.

In some instances, synthetic ADH (Pitressin) is given to compensate for the lack of intrinsic ADH. Some preparations are injectable, while others are nasal insufflations. With the latter, chronic rhinopharyngitis and gastritis often develop. Allergic reactions may also occur. The therapeutic effect of Pitressin is evaluated according to changes in urine volume and specific gravity. It is advisable to administer Pitressin to coincide with polyuria in order to prevent marked fluctuations in body water content and fluid compartment shifts. It is also important to time its administration so that the patient's nighttime rest will not be disrupted by frequent urination. The normal actions of ADH may create some side effects such as pallor due to vasoconstriction and intestinal cramping. Pitressin can cause coronary artery constriction and should be administered with caution to patients with a history of coronary artery insufficiency.

### Primary Aldosteronism

In general, *aldosteronism* is a syndrome associated with hypersecretion of aldosterone. In primary aldosteronism the stimulus for the excessive aldosterone comes from the adrenal gland and results primarily from aldosterone-producing adrenal adenomas (*Conn's disease*).

Aldosterone normally acts on the renal tubules to control reabsorption of sodium and thus the concentration of sodium in the body fluids. Sodium reabsorption is accompanied by water reabsorption and increased secretion of potassium. Knowing this, the nurse can anticipate those problems which logically accompany an excess of aldosterone.

An overproduction of aldosterone may be treated by surgical correction of the underlying cause or with antagonists such as Aldactone. Until the problem is corrected, however, the nurse must deal with the problems which arise from an excess of aldosterone. *Hypernatremia* occurs from the increased reabsorption of sodium and with it comes *hypertension*. One would expect edema naturally to follow frank hypernatremia, but the intense polydipsia and secondary polyuria will cause the sodium to be "washed out" via the kidneys, thus decreasing the accumulation of edema fluid. Secondary to the polyuria is a loss of potassium which may lead to *hypokalemia,* fatigue, and muscle weakness. These patients are often placed on sodium-restricted diets and oral potassium supplements, which have been discussed earlier. The nursing responsibilities include careful monitoring of vital signs, potassium replacement, intake and output, and urine specific gravity. The nurse should ensure an adequate intake of the appropriate amount and type of fluid and always evaluate for signs of possible edema and fluid overload.

## ACID-BASE IMBALANCES

Acid-base imbalances occur when the normal ratio of acids to bases in the body is disrupted. *Acidosis* is a state of either increased acid or decreased base and reflects a high hydrogen ion ($H^+$) concentration in relation to base. It is characterized by a low blood pH. *Alkalosis* is a state of either increased base or decreased acid. It reflects a low $H^+$ concentration in relation to base and a high blood pH. The normal pH of arterial blood is 7.35 to 7.45. Thus a pH less than 7.35 indicates acidosis, while a pH greater than 7.45 indicates alkalosis.

There are four major classifications of acid-base imbalances—respiratory acidosis, metabolic acidosis, respiratory alkalosis, and metabolic alkalosis. The pathophysiology of these will be discussed, followed by nursing care relevant to all acid-base imbalances and specific therapies for each.

### Pathophysiology

Whenever the balance between acids and bases is disturbed, the body uses its resources to compensate for the imbalance. The most immediate compensatory mechanism is the *buffer systems* which immediately neutralize the excess. The *lungs* provide the second compensatory mechanism and are able to rid the body of excess acid by excreting more $CO_2$. Indirectly, the lungs can regulate base by retaining $CO_2$ and thus increasing acidity. The third compensatory mechanism is that of the *kidneys.* They are directly involved in the regulation of acids and bases by excreting acid ($H^+$) and retaining base ($HCO_3^-$) in conditions of acidity or excreting excess base in conditions of alkalinity.

**Respiratory acidosis**  An acidotic state resulting from a malfunction of the respiratory system is known as respiratory acidosis. It is caused by retention of carbon dioxide ($CO_2$) which increases carbonic acid producing a fall in the pH. Carbon dioxide is retained when respirations are slow, shallow, or ineffectual (hypoventilation). Any condition which leads to hypoventilation can cause $CO_2$ retention and respiratory acidosis. Such conditions include:

Airway obstruction

Upper abdominal incisions with "splinting"

Pneumonia, atelectasis

Medications (anesthesia, narcotics, barbiturates, tranquilizers)

Inadequate ventilation with mechanical ventilators

Pulmonary emphysema with alveolar destruction

The retention of $CO_2$ is usually accompanied by hypoxia. Individuals who retain large amounts of $CO_2$ will frequently develop somnolence, decreased attention span, or fixity of purpose which is related to the anesthetic effects of carbon dioxide. Flushing and decreased blood pressure may occur as a result of carbon dioxide's ability to cause vasodilatation. Other symptoms exhibited by these patients such as restlessness, tachycardia, and cardiac arrhythmias can be attributed to the associated hypoxia.

**Metabolic acidosis**  A fall in blood pH as a result of either too much acid or too little base results in metabolic acidosis. It occurs when the kidneys are unable to compensate for an increase in acidity. Table 12-12 summarizes the causes of metabolic acidosis according to factors that regulate acid-base balance.

When metabolic acidosis develops, the body attempts to compensate with both respiratory and metabolic changes that work to decrease acid and/or increase base. The lungs may excrete $CO_2$ as a means of decreasing excess acid while the kidneys eliminate $H^+$ and conserve bicarbonate.

Metabolic acidosis is most commonly seen in acute settings as the result of diabetic ketoacidosis or acute impairment of oxygenation as happens during a cardiac arrest. A healthy person during strenuous exercise develops a metabolic acidosis. The condition, however, is self-limiting because the hypoxia forces the person to rest, which allows the body to oxygenate the tissues, eliminating the lactic acid buildup.

The effects of metabolic acidosis on the patient are variable and depend on the underlying cause. For purposes of discussion the focus here will be on the acidosis that results from inadequate tissue perfusion. In the presence of inadequate perfusion, the cell is deprived of the oxygen needed for normal aerobic metabolism. Anaerobic metabolism with its accumulation of lactic acid results and is referred to as *lactic acidosis.*

The *neuromuscular, gastrointestinal,* and *respiratory* systems are most often affected. Early, the patient may complain of a headache and lethargy. As the acidosis worsens, lethargy progresses to drowsiness and, if untreated, to stupor, coma, and death. Anorexia and nausea progressing to vomiting and diarrhea are common. The lungs exhibit a powerful compensatory effort in the presence of metabolic acidosis by attempting to excrete acid in the form of carbon dioxide. This is seen as rapid, deep respiration (*Kussmaul respirations*).

As the pH drops, the acidotic condition can exert harmful effects on the *cardiovascular* system. An acidotic condition will impair the mechanical ability of the heart to contract and may result in a drop in cardiac output with an associated fall in blood pressure. Drugs which normally stimulate myocardial contractility, electrical conduction in the heart, or blood pressure may not be as effective in the presence of acidosis. Hyperkalemia is common as potassium moves out of the cells in exchange for $H^+$ in an attempt to decrease the extracellular acid.

**Respiratory alkalosis** Decreased levels of carbon dioxide (hypocapnia) lead to respiratory alkalosis. An increased rate and depth of respiration can result in a loss of $CO_2$ and contribute to the development of respiratory alkalosis.

Essentially, any condition which causes *hyperventilation* (deep, rapid respiration) can lead to the development of respiratory alkalosis. These conditions include anxiety, fear, pain, or fever. Aspirin intoxication initially stimulates the respiratory center leading to hypocapnia. An injury or lesion in the central nervous system may have the same effect. Mechanical ventilation can also produce hyperventilation and resultant respiratory alkalosis. It has been observed that a mild degree of respiratory alkalosis occurs in a large percentage of postoperative patients.[8]

Severe respiratory alkalosis can produce vasoconstriction which may reduce cerebral circulation. Additionally, the alkalotic state may decrease the ionization of calcium, causing it to be more easily bound to protein. This shift of calcium from the

**TABLE 12-12**
SUMMARY OF THE METABOLIC REGULATORS OF ACID BALANCE AND DEFECTS IN THE REGULATORS THAT RESULT IN METABOLIC ACIDOSIS

| Normal Regulators | Regulator Defects | Causes of Defects | Result |
|---|---|---|---|
| Production of acid | Increased production of acid | Ketoacidosis with increased fat metabolism<br>Cellular anoxia with lactic acid buildup | Metabolic acidosis |
| Intake of acid | Increased intake of acid | Acidifying salts, i.e., calcium chloride, ammonium chloride | Metabolic acidosis |
| Acid excretion | Decreased excretion of acid | Renal dysfunction as result of decreased renal blood flow, hypovolemia, or renal disease | Metabolic acidosis |
| Loss of base | Increased loss of base ($HCO_3^-$) in excess of chlorides | Dehydration<br>Carbonic anhydrase inhibitors (Diamox) | Metabolic acidosis |

free, ionized compartment to the bound state will *lower serum calcium.* All these effects are manifest as complaints of headache, numbness and tingling of the hands and around the mouth, and, in very severe cases, tetany or related tetanic equivalents.

The main compensatory mechanisms are chemical and chemical-cellular buffering. Initially in response to the decreased carbon dioxide, hydrogen ions shift out of the cell in exchange for potassium which enters the cell. This exchange may result in a lowered serum potassium and *hypokalemia.* If the alkalosis continues, the kidneys compensate by reducing tubular losses of acid and increasing bicarbonate excretion. Respiratory alkalosis is usually short-lived, and renal compensation does not have time to develop.

**Metabolic alkalosis** Metabolic or renal dysfunction that elevates the blood pH in the absence of compensation or when compensation is incomplete causes metabolic alkalosis. It involves either an increase in base or a decrease in acid and can follow an increased loss of body acid, excessive alkali administration, or hypokalemia. Body acids may be lost from vomiting, diarrhea, or nasogastric suction. Chloride depletion resulting from gastric losses of hydrochloric acid or diuretics complicates the alkalosis by stimulating retention of bicarbonate by the kidney. Large amounts of alkali taken by mouth, such as sodium bicarbonate for indigestion, can lead to increased serum bicarbonate levels. This is especially likely in the presence of compromised renal function.

The mechanism by which hypokalemia causes metabolic alkalosis is under question. When serum potassium falls, hydrogen is exchanged for intracellular potassium. As the hydrogen moves into the cells, an excess of bicarbonate occurs, leading to metabolic alkalosis. Recent studies, however, have shown the potassium depletion associated with metabolic alkalosis to be a consequence of accelerated sodium-cation exchange in which potassium as well as hydrogen is secreted in response to the demand for cation excretion and in the presence of an anion deficiency (chloride).[9] The use of potassium supplements that do not contain chlorides is inappropriate as they fail to correct the original deficit.

Metabolic alkalosis affects primarily the *neural, gastrointestinal,* and *respiratory* systems, although the alkalotic patient is also susceptible to atrial tachycardia. Neurological effects include twitching and tremors. If *hypocalcemia* develops as calcium becomes bound to protein, tetany can progress to convulsions and coma. Nausea and vomiting are often present, and diarrhea may be evident. As the alkalosis becomes severe, hypoventilation develops.

Compensation for metabolic alkalosis is both renal and respiratory and consists of lowering the levels of base or increasing the levels of acid. The lungs can contribute acid in the form of carbon dioxide by diminishing ventilation, which raises the level of $CO_2$. Oxygen demand will limit the compensatory hypoventilation. The renal system initially compensates by excreting base and conserving acid (H ions); however, this is limited by the available $CO_2$ that results from hypoventilation. $CO_2$ facilitates acid secretion by the renal tubules (see Chap. 11).

**First-Level Nursing Care**

In order to prevent acid-base imbalances, patients who are at risk to their development should be identified in all health care settings. With an understanding of the normal avenues through which acids and bases are gained and lost, those patients susceptible to abnormal losses or gains can be identified.

*Respiratory acidosis* involves excessive gains in carbon dioxide ($CO_2$). Any patient prone to hypoventilation and, thus, excessive $CO_2$ retention can develop respiratory acidosis. This would include postoperative patients, those who have taken respiratory depressants, patients with muscle weaknesses such as those with neuromuscular disruption, the elderly, and obese persons. Patients with respiratory disturbances that disrupt the normal $CO_2/O_2$ exchange are also susceptible to respiratory acidosis. To prevent its development, the nurse should offer ventilatory assistance. This may range from teaching the patient to take deep breaths to placing a patient on a mechanical respirator (see Chap. 30).

*Metabolic acidosis* is characterized by an excessive buildup of metabolic acids in the body. These can include hydrogen ions, lactic acid, or ketone bodies. Patients who can potentially develop an excess of one or more of these acids include those with compromised renal function, those with inadequate tissue perfusion that results in hypoxia, and those with diabetes mellitus. Preventing metabolic acidosis involves managing the underlying disturbance properly.

*Respiratory alkalosis* involves an excessive loss of carbon dioxide. It results from hyperventilation, and patients with acute anxiety, fearful, in pain, or with fever should be watched and cautioned against hyperventilation. Patients with aspirin intoxication must also be considered at risk.

*Metabolic alkalosis* is characterized by an excessive loss of metabolic acids or excessive gain in metabolic base. The latter neutralizes the acids, resulting in an overall decrease in acidity. Patients with gastrointestinal disturbances are most susceptible to this condition. The losses associated with vomiting and diarrhea should be minimized and replacement therapy instituted for metabolic alkalosis to be prevented. Patients with gastrointestinal ulcers who take antacids regularly should be taught the correct type and usage of these medications.

### Second-Level Nursing Care

For acid-base imbalances to be identified and corrected early, a thorough nursing assessment is paramount. Patients at risk to the development of imbalance should be especially monitored in the community.

**Nursing assessment** The changes associated with early acid-base imbalances are vague and non-specific. The most valuable tool in assessing patients is the *health history*. Patients should be carefully questioned about avenues of acid-base loss or gain. Losses may include hyperventilation, vomiting, and diarrhea. Gains may be reflected in hypoventilation or respiratory disruption, oral intake, or other disturbances such as renal failure, diabetes mellitus, and cardiac problems. Medications the patient is taking should be elicited and any past illnesses noted. Patients with early acid-base imbalance may complain of vague neurological and gastrointestinal symptoms. These may include headache, restlessness, lethargy, drowsiness, nausea, and/or vomiting.

During the *physical assessment* the findings in early imbalance will not be remarkable. The patient's vital signs should be taken, although changes are not often evident until the imbalance is more severe. Throughout the nursing assessment the overall mental state of the patient should be evaluated. The skin should be observed as respiratory acidosis is often accompanied by flushing. The respiratory rate is often noted to be decreased in respiratory acidosis and increased during respiratory alkalosis. As a compensatory mechanism it may be increased in metabolic acidosis and decreased in metabolic alkalosis.

The most accurate *diagnostic tests* associated with acid-base imbalances are the blood gases and pH determination. These require a sample of arterial blood and are most frequently done in a hospital setting. They will, therefore, be discussed under Third-Level Nursing Care. In a community health setting, the *serum electrolytes* may reflect acid-base imbalance. Potassium and chloride losses, because of their association with metabolic alkalosis, are especially useful. The serum calcium may be lowered during alkalosis.

**Nursing problems and interventions** The primary nursing problem in early acid-base disturbance is the imbalance itself. If identified early, measures can be instituted to correct it.

Mild *respiratory acidosis* is most often seen in patients with chronic obstructive lung disease. These patients should be taught to manage their condition in order to prevent decompensated respiratory acidosis. Sputum should normally be thin and clear and patients should be alert to any change in color and thickness. Provided there are no cardiac or renal contraindications, large amounts of fluid should be encouraged to keep the secretions thin and mobile. A high-humidity environment is helpful in easing expectoration of secretions. The family can be taught postural drainage and percussion and vibration techniques to aid in the mobilization and expectoration of the patient's secretions (see Chap. 30 for a more complete discussion).

It is especially important to alert the patient to situations which can lead to acute carbon dioxide retention. These include respiratory infections, stress, and exposure to allergens with resultant bronchospasm. A change in environment or medication regime may also lead to an acute problem. Both patients and their families should be cognizant that these situations are potentially dangerous, and help should be sought. There should be a consistent health worker to whom the patient may refer when questions or problems arise.

Chronic *metabolic acidosis* is most often seen in patients with chronic renal failure. Adequate long-term nursing care in the community is the best approach to preventing severe imbalance (see Chap. 14).

Nurses working in ambulatory care settings may occasionally have contact with patients who hyperventilate and develop *respiratory alkalosis*. This most frequently occurs in emergencies and severely anxious, stressful, or painful situations. It is important that the nurse recognizes this early and intervenes appropriately. Rebreathing of carbon dioxide with a closed paper bag is helpful in assisting patients to control their respirations by focusing on a direct activity and replenishing lost carbon dioxide. If the hyperventilation is associated with apprehension or anxiety, the patient should be guided in recognizing the source so that future episodes can be minimized.

Early signs of *metabolic alkalosis* are nonspecific. In the community, those patients with complaints of continuous vomiting and diarrhea should become suspect. It becomes important for the nurse to teach the patient how to replace lost potassium in the diet and to seek medical attention if the symptoms persist.

### Third-Level Nursing Care

When acid-base imbalances become severe, hospitalization is required. Most often patients who develop severe imbalances have already been hospitalized for other acute conditions that have contributed to the acidosis or alkalosis.

**Nursing assessment**  Severe acid-base imbalances are often difficult to assess because changes are overshadowed by the underlying pathology. The *health history* will be similar to that discussed under Second-Level Nursing Care. With acutely ill, hospitalized patients, special attention should be given to artificial losses and gains. These would include drainage from tubes, irrigating solutions, intravenous infusions, and fluid instillations. The types and amounts of intravenous fluids being used

should especially be noted and all medications reviewed.

During the *physical assessment* several changes will become evident. Table 12-13 summarizes the physical assessment findings relating to acid-base imbalances. Assessment should focus on perception, coordination, gastrointestinal status, respiratory status, and cardiac functioning. At the onset the skin should be assessed for color changes.

Because of the many nonspecific effects of acid-base imbalances, *diagnostic tests* are most useful in identifying the imbalance. The most important of these are tests of the *arterial blood gases.* Arterial blood is needed for the blood gas determination. Generally the femoral, brachial, or radial artery is used to obtain the sample. It is important to assess the status of the radial site for hematoma or adequacy of pulses before using it for arterial puncture. Allen's test for collateral circulation should be done prior to a radial puncture. This is accomplished by occluding the ulnar and radial arteries at the wrist. After the hand is blanched, release the pressure over the ulnar artery. The palm should regain its color indicating adequate collateral circulation. After the puncture has been done, digital pressure should be applied to the site for a full 5 minutes (longer if the patient is anticoagulated). The specimen should be handled with

**TABLE 12-13**
PHYSICAL ASSESSMENT FINDINGS DURING ACID-BASE IMBALANCES

| | Physical Assessment Findings | | | |
| | Acidosis | | Alkalosis | |
| | Respiratory | Metabolic | Respiratory | Metabolic |
|---|---|---|---|---|
| PERCEPTION AND COORDINATION | Somnolence Decreased attention span Fixidity of purpose Restlessness | Headache Lethargy Drowsiness Stupor | Headache Numbness and tingling Tetany Convulsions Hyperreflexia | Twitching and tremors Tetany Convulsions |
| GASTROINTESTINAL STATUS | | Anorexia Nausea Vomiting Diarrhea | | Nausea Vomiting Diarrhea |
| RESPIRATORY STATUS | Hypoventilation Hypoxia | Compensatory hyperventilation (Kussmaul respirations) | Hyperventilation | Compensatory hypoventilation |
| CARDIAC STATUS | Lowered blood pressure Tachycardia Arrhythmia | Lowered blood pressure | | |
| GENERAL | Flushed skin | | | |

care and the syringe sealed adequately after excess air is ejected before it is sent to the laboratory.

The normal values for arterial blood gases are:

| | |
|---|---|
| pH | 7.35 to 7.45 |
| $p_{CO_2}$ | 35 to 45 mmHg |
| $HCO_3^-$ | 22 to 26 mmHg |
| $p_{O_2}$ | 80 to 110 mmHg |
| $O_2$ saturation | 95 percent or more |

While the $p_{O_2}$ and $O_2$ saturation values are important in evaluation of the oxygenation status of the body, they are not essential for understanding acid-base imbalances. Thus, for the purposes of this discussion the pH, $p_{CO_2}$, and $HCO_3^-$ values will be considered.

Arterial blood gas values should be examined using the following format. First, the pH should be considered. This is the prime indicator of either acidosis or alkalosis. A decreased pH indicates the former and an increased pH the latter. Secondly, the respiratory parameter, the $p_{CO_2}$, should be examined. An increase will indicate respiratory acidosis while a decrease respiratory alkalosis. Thirdly, the $HCO_3^-$ which is the metabolic parameter should be evaluated. A decrease indicates metabolic acidosis, while an increase shows a metabolic alkalosis.

Table 12-14 summarizes sample arterial blood gas findings and their appropriate interpretation. It should be noted that Example 2 represents classic values associated with respiratory arrest.

**Nursing problems and interventions**  With severe acid-base imbalances, nursing intervention must focus on the problem of the imbalance itself and associated difficulties the patient may be having. Nursing care must be planned to treat the underlying condition, support compensatory mechanisms, and neutralize excesses.

Acute carbon dioxide retention and its resultant *respiratory acidosis* require aggressive care. The goals of nursing and medical interventions are to lower the carbon dioxide level, correct the underlying hypoxia, and elevate $p_{O_2}$ levels to those which are more normal for that patient. Finally, the underlying problem must be corrected or stabilized by treating factors which altered the physiology. This aim is accomplished by aggressive bronchial hygiene which may include suctioning, humidification, postural drainage, percussion, and vibration. In more severe cases intubation and ventilatory assistance may be necessary. A more thorough discussion of the care related to chronic obstructive lung diseases may be found in Chap. 30.

Nursing intervention in *metabolic acidosis* is related to the underlying cause. Lactic acidosis associated with inadequate tissue perfusion and poor oxygenation requires care directed toward improving the oxygenation status and circulatory function and reversing fluid and electrolyte disorders. Attempting to elevate the blood pH is a common denominator in all situations of metabolic acidosis.

The drug used most often to reinforce a low reserve of bicarbonate, combating acidosis and hyperkalemia, is intravenous sodium bicarbonate. Nursing responsibilities when giving sodium bicarbonate include the use of a long, stable intravenous line and administering the drug slowly, as rapid excessive administration may lead to overalkalinization which is difficult to correct. The exception occurs with cardiac arrest situations where an intravenous "push" is acceptable. Nurses should exercise caution as sodium bicarbonate is a hypertonic sodium solution which may provide an excessive sodium load and provoke overexpansion of the

**TABLE 12-14**
ARTERIAL BLOOD GAS DETERMINATIONS

| | pH | Interpretation | $p_{CO_2}$ | Interpretation | $HCO_3^-$ | Interpretation | Primary Imbalance |
|---|---|---|---|---|---|---|---|
| EXAMPLE 1 | 7.52 | Increased: Alkalosis | 30 | Decreased: Respiratory alkalosis | 24 | Normal | Respiratory alkalosis |
| EXAMPLE 2 | 7.20 | Decreased: Acidosis | 60 | Increased: Respiratory acidosis | 18 | Decreased: Metabolic acidosis | Respiratory and metabolic acidosis |
| EXAMPLE 3 | 7.50 | Increased: Alkalosis | 48 | Slightly increased | 30 | Increased: Metabolic alkalosis | Metabolic alkalosis with respiratory compensation |

intravascular compartment, circulatory overload, and pulmonary edema. For this reason they should monitor vital signs including urine output and cardiac rhythm. Sodium bicarbonate should be titrated according to arterial blood gases.

Nursing intervention in acute *respiratory alkalosis* is directed toward the underlying cause of the disorder. In the presence of good cardiac, respiratory, and renal function, most patients will resolve this problem without intervention. Care generally involves adjusting the respiratory and/or emotional support for the patient.

Management of *metabolic alkalosis* is a reflection of the cause. Alkalosis which is the result of potassium and chloride loss responds to the administration of potassium chloride supplements. Isotonic saline may also be required. The nurse must always keep in mind the nature of the lost fluids when considering appropriate replacements. Certainly sodium, potassium chloride, and water replacements must all be considered. Vital signs should be monitored to detect hypotension and tachycardia which suggest hypokalemia. The respiratory rate will decrease if compensation is occurring. An accurate intake and output record is necessary to plan for replacement of lost fluid and electrolytes.

With both respiratory and metabolic alkalosis, *hypocalcemia* can become a problem. Patients should be regularly assessed for indications of neural irritability. Usually, as the alkalosis is resolved, the serum calcium returns to normal levels.

### Fourth-Level Nursing Care

When caring for patients who have experienced acute acid-base imbalances, the nurse should remember that patient education and close follow-up are critical in forestalling recurrence. The nurse can draw upon the discussion under Second-Level Nursing Care for tips that will aid in patient and family teaching. Readmission for acute imbalances signals that the patient may not have been adequately prepared, and a practical teaching exercise should be instituted.

### REFERENCES

1  Maxwell, M. H., and C. R. Kleeman, *Clinical Disorders of Fluid and Electrolyte Metabolism*, McGraw-Hill, New York, 1972, p. 635.
2  McGann, Marlene R., "Secondary Hyperaldosteronism," *Am J Nurs*, **76:**634, April 1976.
3  Maxwell and Kleeman, *op. cit.*, p. 405.
4  *Ibid.*, p. 414.
5  Tripp, Alice, "Hyper and Hypocalcemia," *Am J Nurs*, **76:**1142, July 1976.
6  Luckman, Joan, and K. C. Sorenson, *Medical-Surgical Nursing: A Psychophysiologic Approach*, Saunders, Philadelphia, 1974, p. 1364.
7  Maxwell and Kleeman, *op. cit.*, p. 437.
8  Lyons, A., and R. Moore, "Post-traumatic Alkalosis: Incidence and Pathophysiology of Alkalosis in Surgery," *Surgery*, **60:**93, July 1966.
9  Maxwell and Kleeman, *op. cit.*, p. 332.

### BIBLIOGRAPHY

Bay, W. H., et al.: "Hypernatremia and Hyponatremia: Disorders of Tonicity," *Geriatrics*, **76:**53–64, August 1976.

Beland, Irene L., and Joyce Y. Passos: *Clinical Nursing: Pathophysiological and Psychosocial Approaches*, 3d ed., Macmillan, New York, 1975.

Betson, C.: "Blood Gases," *Am J Nurs*, **68:**1010, May 1968.

Burrell, Zeb L., and Lenette O. Burrell: *Intensive Care Nursing*, Mosby, St. Louis, 1969.

Davenport, H. W.: *The ABC's of Acid-Base Chemistry*, 5th ed., University of Chicago Press, 1969.

Dutcher, I.E., and H. C. Hardenburg: "Water and Electrolyte Imbalances," in L. E. Meltzer, F. Abdellah, and J. R. Kitchell (eds.), *Concepts and Practices of Intensive Care for Nurse Specialists*, Charles Press, Philadelphia, 1969.

Ganong, W. F.: *Review of Medical Physiology*, Lange, Los Altos, Calif., 1973.

Goodhart, Robert S., and Maurice E. Shils: *Modern Nutrition in Health and Disease*, 5th ed., Lea & Febiger, Philadelphia, 1973.

Goodman, Louis S., and Alfred Gilman: *The Pharmacological Basis of Therapeutics*, 5th ed., Macmillan, New York, 1975.

Guyton, A. C.: *Textbook of Medical Physiology*, 5th ed., Saunders, Philadelphia, 1976.

Harrison, T. R., et al.: *Principles of Internal Medicine*, 7th ed., McGraw-Hill, New York, 1974.

Hudak, Carolyn M., Barbara M. Gallo, and Thelma Lohr: *Critical Care Nursing*, Lippincott, Philadelphia, 1973.

Kee, Joyce L.: "Fluid Imbalances in Elderly Patients," *Nursing '73*, **3:**40–42, April 1973.

Kubo, Winefred, et al.: "Fluid and Electrolyte Problems of Tube Fed Patients," *Am J Nurs*, **76:**912–916, June 1976.

Kurdi, William J.: "Refining Your I.V. Therapy Technique," *Nursing '75*, **75:**41–47, November 1975.

Lee, Carla A., Violet R. Stroot, and Ann C. Schaper: "What To Do When Acid Base Problems Hang in the Balance," *Nursing '75,* **75:**32–37, August, 1975.

Luckman, Joan, and Karen C. Sorenson: *Medical-Surgical Nursing: A Psychophysiologic Approach,* Saunders, Philadelphia, 1974.

Lyons, A., and R. Moore: "Post-traumatic Alkalosis: Incidence and Pathophysiology of Alkalosis in Surgery," *Surgery,* **60:**93, July 1966.

McGann, Marlene R.: "Secondary Hyperaldosteronism," *Am J Nurs,* **76:**634–637, April 1976.

Max M.: "Acute Hypercalcemic Crisis," *Heart Lung,* **76:**624–626, July-August 1976.

Maxwell, M. H., and C. R. Kleeman: *Clinical Disorders of Fluid and Electrolyte Metabolism,* 2d ed., McGraw-Hill, New York, 1972.

Potassium Imbalances: Programmed Instruction, *Am J Nurs,* **67:**343, February 1967.

Reed, Gretchen M., and Vincent F. Sheppard: *Regulation of Fluid and Electrolyte Balance: A Programmed Instruction in Physiology for Nurses,* Saunders, Philadelphia, 1971.

Shapiro, B. A.: *Clinical Applications of Blood Gases,* Year Book, Chicago, 1973.

Tripp, Alice: "Hyper and Hypocalcemia," *Am J Nurs,* **76:**1142–1145, July 1976.

Vinsant, M. O., M. I. Spence, and D. C. Hagen: *A Commonsense Approach to Coronary Care: A Program,* 2d ed., Mosby, St. Louis, 1975.

Weldy, Norma Jean: *Body Fluid and Electrolytes: A Programmed Presentation,* 2d ed., Mosby, St. Louis, 1976.

# 13

# THE SKIN AND FLUID AND ELECTROLYTE IMBALANCES

Valerie C. Stillyards

The skin is the largest organ of the human system. It provides the body with a protective barrier against many hazards in the external environment, including invasion of bacteria, chemicals, or excess water. It provides protection from mechanical injury and prevents the loss of body fluids. In addition, the skin contains multiple nerve endings which relay valuable information regarding the external environment to the central nervous system. The skin also has an important cosmetic function, as changes in the appearance of the skin can significantly alter a person's self-image and affect interpersonal relationships.

## BURNS

Anything that destroys the skin's integrity will affect its functions. Burns cause widespread destruction and significantly alter the skin's ability to mediate between the person and the external environment. The extent of the impairment will be relative to the depth of the burn injury and the surface area of skin involved.

### Pathophysiology

Burn injuries are usually described according to the depth of the injury. Common terminology includes *first-, second-,* and *third-degree,* or *partial-* and *full-thickness* burns. First- and second-degree burns are partial-thickness burns, while a third-degree burn is a full-thickness injury. In a first-degree burn only the epidermis is damaged. A common example is a sunburn, and the skin is typically red and dry. Second-degree burns involve both the epidermis and some of the dermis. Sufficient epithelial cells remain to produce new epidermis. A second-degree burn has a pink-red appearance and is characterized by either moisture or blisters (see Color Plate 13-1). Nerve endings remain, causing the injury to be painful. Partial-thickness burns can potentially heal spontaneously in the absence of infection.

In a third-degree or full-thickness burn both the epidermis and dermis are destroyed. There may also be destruction of subcutaneous tissue, muscle, and even bone, if the heat source was intense or if there was a prolonged exposure to heat. The full-thickness injury is characterized by a dry, leathery appearance and is usually white, gray, or charred in color (see Color Plate 13-2). Nerve endings as well as specialized structures such as hair follicles and sweat glands are destroyed. Because both the epidermis and dermis are destroyed, regeneration of skin is not possible. Grafting is necessary to close the wound.

**Local changes**  Thermal injury damages the skin cells and underlying tissues. The extent of the damage will depend upon the severity of the injury. Besides the cellular destruction, capillary dynamics are altered. The capillaries dilate and increase in permeability resulting in a loss of fluid and electrolytes as well as plasma proteins into the local tissue. These losses result in what is typically referred to as *burn edema*. Besides the changes in capillary permeability, the heat often thromboses blood vessels in the vicinity of the burn, decreasing circulation to the area.

**Systemic changes**  These local changes result in many systemic changes which have profound effects on the patient. The severity of the systemic changes will depend upon the extent of burn injury.

**F**luid and Electrolyte Changes  With the skin destroyed, the body is no longer able to minimize water loss to the environment and *insensible water loss* is greatly increased. The amount of water evaporation from the burn wound will be determined by the temperature and humidity of the environment. As much as 3 to 5 liters of fluid per square meter of burn may be lost in 24 hours.

The local burn injury also causes *fluid shifts*. As the capillaries dilate and increase in permeability, fluid is lost from the vessels. To compensate for this loss, fluids from undamaged tissues are pulled into the circulation. Eventually, as the burn wound becomes edematous and the body becomes dehydrated, hypovolemia develops (see Chap. 27). Fluid losses associated with burn edema continue for 24 to 48 hours, with the peak loss occurring in about 6 to 8 hours after the injury. The wound edema continues until the third or fourth postburn day when it becomes *mobilized* and is reabsorbed into the circulation. Reabsorption of the edema fluid is generally complete 7 to 8 days after the injury.

During the initial fluid shifts in the early postburn period, *sodium* is lost into the edema fluid. With remobilization, however, sodium returns to the vascular space, increasing its concentration in the serum. *Potassium,* primarily an intracellular cation, is lost from the damaged cells of the burn wound, resulting in an initial increase in serum potassium. This excess is excreted by the kidneys, and hypokalemia often develops during the second postburn week.

Severe burn injuries also result in *acid-base imbalances.* The hypovolemia from fluid losses, vessel thromboses, and sluggish microcirculation result in a decrease in tissue perfusion. Hypoxia develops and cells revert to anaerobic metabolism. The buildup of lactic acid leads to metabolic acidosis. At the same time the anxiety and pain associated with a burn often cause the patient to hyperventilate. Too much $CO_2$ is blown off and respiratory alkalosis develops.

Generally, unless severe shock develops causing renal ischemia, the *kidneys* continue to function and try to compensate for the widespread fluid and electrolyte changes. The losses of water and sodium from the intravascular space result in increased production of aldosterone and the antidiuretic hormone (ADH). Aldosterone causes the kidney to conserve sodium while ADH conserves water. The result is a scant amount of concentrated urine.

**C**hanges in Oxygenation  Fluid losses affect the patient's oxygenation status. There is an overall *hypovolemia* that decreases cardiac output, and the body compensates with vasoconstriction of peripheral vessels. The fluid losses also increase the blood viscosity which leads to "sludging" in the microcirculation. The sluggish microcirculation and vasoconstriction result in inadequate tissue perfusion and cellular hypoxia.

This cellular hypoxia is complicated by the local thromboses associated with the injury and the *destruction of red blood cells* (RBC). At the time of the burn injury, red blood cells are hemolyzed by the heat. This causes an immediate decrease in circulating RBC which is masked by the hemoconcentration. Some RBC are partially damaged at the time of injury. These damaged cells have a shorter survival rate and delayed hemolysis occurs several days and sometimes weeks after the injury. Severe anemia often develops when the burn fluid is mobilized from the wound. The hemoglobin liberated from the destroyed corpuscles is eliminated in the urine. *Hemoglobinuria* usually indicates a deep injury and is often seen in patients who have sustained an electrical burn.

Oxygenation status can also be complicated by *respiratory difficulties.* The respiratory tract can be damaged as a result of inhalation of the products of combustion, causing swelling and irritation of tissues. If the injury is severe, tracheal edema can develop. The injury as well as the immobilization and hypoxia associated with severe burns make the lungs susceptible to bacterial invasion from the environment or from the burn wounds themselves.

Metabolic Changes Energy requirements are greatly increased following thermal injury. As water is lost through evaporation, body heat is lost and must be replenished for the body to maintain normal temperature. Each liter of fluid evaporated is associated with a loss of 576 kilocalories of heat. The body begins to mobilize its energy stores to meet the demand. Glucose and fat stores are quickly used up forcing the body to begin to breakdown protein. The protein catabolism is increased further by the increase in adrenocorticosteroid hormones that are secreted in response to the physical stress. Protein is lost not only through catabolism but as a direct result of thermal destruction and from the burn exudate. Negative nitrogen balance quickly develops and the patient rapidly loses weight.

Patients with severe burns often develop *stress ulcers*. These patients have been found to have normal or decreased amounts of gastric HCl. The ulcer appears to develop as a result of decreased ability of the mucosa to protect itself from the acid and may be related to congestion in the mucosal capillaries. The term *Curling's ulcer* refers to the ulcers associated with burns originally described by Curling in 1842.[1] *Gastric dilatation* and *adynamic ileus* frequently occur in patients who have sustained severe thermal injury. They are usually transient, lasting 24 hours or less.

Inflammatory Changes The thermal injury itself causes a massive inflammation. The resultant wound exudate is an ideal medium for bacteria growth, while at the same time, the systemic changes limit the body's ability to fight infection. Infection is a common complication in thermal injury and most frequently occurs in the wound itself, the lungs, and the venous cutdown site. It worsens all the problems the patient is already coping with and can convert partial-thickness to full-thickness burns. Most burn deaths are a result of some type of sepsis.

Changes in Perception and Coordination Because the skin contains sensory end organs, destruction of skin results in various perceptual changes. In partial-thickness burns the sense organs are not destroyed and the patient often experiences severe *pain* over the site of injury. In full-thickness burns the nerve endings are destroyed, with *loss of sensation* in the area. Patients with full-thickness burns often have areas of partial-thickness injury which are painful.

Changes in coordination are not an immediate

problem in thermal injury. As full-thickness wounds heal, however, integrity is restored by stretching the surrounding skin to cover the exposed subcutaneous tissue. If surrounding skin is not sufficient to cover a wound, it will remain an open, granulating area, or be covered by thin epithelium which is an insufficient barrier against the external environment. The stretching of skin over an area is called *contraction* and often results in a functional deformity as the stretched skin limits range of motion and impairs coordination.

**Causes** Burns are thermal injuries and result from contact with a heat source. The more extensive the contact with the heat, the greater the damage. Some of the many sources of heat include the sun, fires, explosions, boiling liquids, hot metal, chemicals, and electricity. First-degree burns usually result from ultraviolet exposure (sunburn) or from a very short flash. A second-degree burn often results from a short flash or scalds from spilled liquids. Immersion scalds, flames (especially those involving clothing), chemical contact, and electrical injury usually result in third-degree burns.

### First-level Nursing Care

In the United States, 12,000 lives are lost annually as a result of fire. It has been estimated that another 300,000 Americans survive burn injuries; 50,000 of these people require hospitalization varying from 6 weeks to 2 years. The United States, the richest and most technologically advanced nation in the world, leads all the major industrialized countries in per capita deaths and property loss from fire.[2]

The nurse can be instrumental in preventing burn injury. Teaching patients about the safety hazards that can cause burn injuries should become a routine aspect of patient care. Patients should also be taught how to cope with fire once it has started.

The community health nurse is in an especially advantageous position to prevent thermal injuries. Home assessments should include evaluation of safety hazards, and the patient should be helped to minimize dangers. Parents should be encouraged to discuss these dangers with their children and to plan avenues of escape if fire occurs. Children should be taught how to get out of the house and where to go. A planned meeting place will minimize the chance that someone will enter the burning building in search of others. At regular intervals, the school nurse should conduct fire safety education programs; including the parent-teacher association in such a program would insure reinforcement of the safety principles at home. Children should be taught how to properly use equipment that can potentially cause burn injury. Nurses in all settings can contribute to the prevention of burn injury by being aware of areas of higher incidence and common accidents and dangers that result in injury. Burns in children are often the result of a battering. If child abuse is suspected, a complete psychosocial and environmental assessment should be made.

Although burns occur in all areas of the country, a greater number occur in the southern states. This increase has been attributed to the common use of *open fires* for heating and cooking and to the use of temporary forms of heating such as *open space heaters.* The risk of burn injury is also greater in the predominantly nonwhite ghetto areas of larger cities where crowded conditions and substandard housing prevail. Outdoor grills are also a source of burn injury. The misuse of starter fluid often results in an unexpected flash.

Although people are burned in industrial and transportation accidents, the majority of burn injuries occur in the home. *Flammable liquids* and *flammable clothing* are involved in many of these injuries. Numerous sources of ignition are cited: *kitchen ranges, open space heaters, gas water heaters, outdoor fires,* and *smoking materials.* The misuse of *gasoline* for cleaning tools, paint brushes, etc., is an extremely dangerous practice. The gasoline vapor can easily be ignited by the pilot light of a gas heater often located in the garage. The storage of large amounts of gasoline should be discouraged; 1 gallon of gasoline has the explosive force of 30 sticks of dynamite.

Many people, especially children, are scalded with *hot liquids.* Small children may pull saucepans of hot food or water onto themselves, or, left unsupervised in the bathtub, may turn on the *hot water faucet.*

*Matches, cigarette lighters,* and *lighter fluid* are associated with a large number of burn injuries each year, particularly in the young and the elderly. Children under 10 years of age are often burned as a result of playing with matches. An elderly person may not be able physically to light a match safely or to extinguish a clothing fire if one starts. Some injuries are caused by a person smoking while under the influence of alcohol or drugs. The use of firecrackers on the 4th of July is always associated with thermal accidents. *Electricity* from power lines, unprotected wall sockets, and defective wiring is another common cause of burn injury. Excessive *exposure to the sun* can result in varying degrees of burns. Fair-skinned individuals are especially vulnerable to sunburn.

**Prevention of burns**   There are numerous safety hazards which, if corrected, could prevent thermal injury. Some of the more common measures will be discussed here.

Patients should be taught how to properly use open space heaters. They should be adequately guarded and vented. Venting is needed to prevent the buildup of carbon monoxide, which may cause asphyxiation. A sand or dirt box should be kept near the outdoor grill so that a fire that begins to get out of hand can be immediately extinguished. People should also be taught to check the wind before starting a fire so the fire can be located properly. The use of an asbestos or wire screen in front of the fireplace will decrease the chance of a fire starting.

Building codes may also help in the prevention of burn injuries as these codes regulate the type of materials used for a building, and to some extent, its design and location. Codes vary from area to area and, unfortunately, many local governments do not at this time have building codes. A building code may, for example, specify that a gas water heater be located at least 24 inches from the ground. This is to prevent gasoline vapors, which are heavy and stay close to the ground, from being ignited by the pilot light. Nurses should be aware of local codes and become advocates for stricter enforcement. Any suspicion of a gas leak should be reported immediately.

Scalds may be prevented by improved design of hot liquid containers and range tops and thermostat control of bath water temperature. Parents should be taught to turn pan handles inward and out of a child's reach. Young children should not be left unsupervised or in the care of older siblings who are not of an age to take this kind of responsibility.

Electrical injuries may be prevented by the use of safety caps on electrical outlets, the replacement of frayed wiring, and the correct ampere fuse. Often 30-ampere fuses are used where a 15-ampere fuse ought to be located. Patients should be taught the dangers of electrical overload, and the use of extension cords and multiple outlets should be discouraged.

Emphasis is now being placed on the use of flame resistant fabrics for clothing and some household furnishings, such as mattresses, carpets and rugs. Two federal laws have been passed which enable the federal government to set flammability standards and to inform the public about the hazards associated with flammable fabrics. The Flammable Fabrics Act was originally passed in 1953 to regulate the manufacture of highly flammable clothing, such as brushed rayon sweaters. This act was amended in 1967 to permit regulation of a wider range of clothing and interior furnishings.

The Consumer Product Safety Act passed in 1972 created the Consumer Product Safety Commission, with broad jurisdiction over product safety, and transferred responsibilities under the Flammable Fabrics Act to the Commission. Several federal standards have been passed to implement the Flammable Fabrics Act. A standard effective on May 1, 1975 involved children's sleepwear. This includes any garment size 7 to 14 worn primarily for sleeping or activities relating to sleeping, such as nightgowns, pajamas, and robes. Diapers and underwear are excluded. This standard also states that flame-resistant sleepwear must bear a permanent label providing instructions for proper care to protect the garments from agents or treatments known to cause significant deterioration of the flame resistance.

It should be pointed out, however, that flame-resistant does not mean flameproof. Flame-resistant fabric will burn, but it is able to resist flames more effectively than ordinary fabrics.

Some manufacturers have voluntarily started to use resistant fabrics for other clothing, including clothes for adults. The public should be educated to look for labels stating that the material is flame-resistant when buying clothes.

### Second-level Nursing Care

Burn injury can occur anywhere, and burn patients can be found in any of a variety of community settings. Nursing care at the time of injury focuses on the initial assessment, emergency intervention, prevention of further injury, and care of the initial nursing problems.

**Nursing assessment**   During the initial assessment a brief *history* of how the injury occurred should be obtained. This may give valuable information regarding the probable depth of injury. The nurse should also determine if the patient has any past history of illnesses or allergies which may be significant. Assessment of the burn should focus on the location, area involved, and probable depth of injury.

Maintenance of a patent airway is always the first priority in an emergency situation. The location of the burn can give clues as to difficulties in this area. Any burn involving the face, neck, or upper chest can cause respiratory damage. If the patient was burned in a standing position, the likelihood of inhaling the products of combustion is increased.

The approximate area of body surface involved should also be quickly assessed. Depth of injury can be approximated by knowing how the injury occurred and by the appearance of the burn wound. Partial-thickness burns appear pink-red and are moist, while a full-thickness burn is generally dry and may have a charred appearance (see Color Plates 13-1 and 13-2).

**Emergency intervention**   The first step in emergency intervention is to put out the fire. The patient should be moved away from the fire and the flames smothered with a rug or any other available heavy material, or by having the person roll over on the ground. If necessary, dirt or sand can be used to smother the flames. The next steps involve the regular first aid procedures of establishing a patent airway and applying pressure to points of external hemorrhage, if the burn injury is associated with other trauma. The application of towels soaked in ice water will stop the effect of heat on the tissues and may bring some pain relief.

Injuries caused by chemicals should be immediately washed with copious amounts of water to remove the chemical. With chemical burns of the eye, repeated eyewashes should be given. If a large area of the body is involved, clothing should be removed and the chemical may be washed away by having the person stand under a shower. Ointments, creams, and home remedies should not be applied to the burns, and oral fluids should not be given.

With nonchemical burns, it is not necessary to remove the patients clothing except for constricting clothes and shoes. If the hands are burned, rings should be removed before edema forms. Wound contamination should be avoided. A clean sheet serves as a suitable temporary covering.

After the initial emergency care, the patient should be *transported* to an appropriate facility. All burn wounds involving more than a superficial injury require the attention of a physician. A second-degree burn of less than 15 percent and a third-degree injury of less than 2 percent of the body surface may be considered minor burns and treated on an outpatient basis. A second-degree burn of less than 30 percent or a third-degree burn of less than 10 percent may be classified as a moderate injury, and the patient should be taken to an adequately equipped and staffed community hospital. More extensive burns, those involving the face, hands, or feet, those associated with respiratory tract injuries, and electrical burns are considered critical. These patients will require specialized care in a general hospital or burn facility. In the case of an extensive burn injury, the hospital emergency room should be notified, if at all possible, in order to have the hospital personnel ready to receive the patient.

A critically burned patient requiring transfer to a larger hospital may be safely moved during the first 48 hours following the injury. Resuscitative intravenous fluids should be started and an indwelling Foley catheter inserted for accurate measurement of urine. Oxygen therapy, if required, should be instituted. A nurse or a physician may be needed to accompany the patient during the transportation period.

**Nursing problems and interventions**  During the initial period following a burn injury, the systemic changes are not sufficiently widespread to cause significant problems. Most patients will remain in a relatively stable condition for 1 hour or more following the accident. However, the barrier functions of the skin have been lost and *possible wound contamination* can occur at the accident site. Contamination often results from rolling on the ground to extinguish the fire, from the hands of people administering first aid, or from exposure of the wounds to the air. A clean sheet provides a suitable temporary dressing and should be placed over the wound as soon as possible.

Most burn patients experience *pain.* Partial-thickness burns are painful because nerve endings are intact, while patients with full-thickness burns usually have areas of partial-thickness injury which are painful. Until the patient reaches a facility where pain medication is available, the application of cold will result in pain relief. Once available, narcotics are generally used to relieve pain, and small amounts are given by the intravenous route only. Intramuscular administration is avoided because absorption will be poor during the period of decreased circulation. Once circulation is restored, the narcotics will be absorbed and an overdose can result.

*Anxiety and listlessness* are commonly seen in patients following a burn injury. The patient as well as family and friends will need to be reassured. The nurse should remain calm and try to control hysteria. Often giving a person something to do such as calling an ambulance or getting a sheet is helpful. The nurse should stay near the patient, explaining the surrounding activity and offering support. Fear is common. If others were injured in the accident, the stress of losing a family member often increases the patient's anxiety.

**Third-level Nursing Care**

As soon as the patient arrives at an acute care setting, a more complete history and physical examination should be done and proper care instituted.

**Nursing assessment**  An accurate *health history* can help to determine the severity of the injury. How, when, and where the injury occurred should be determined. Symptoms related to the burn as well as other injuries should be explored. Other health problems, past illnesses, allergies, and the most recent tetanus immunization should also be determined. Social and family history is another important consideration. A burn injury not only involves the patient but the immediate family unit, and this information will be important to consider when planning the patient's rehabilitation. With this information as background a careful *physical examination* of the burn wound should be made.

**E**valuation of the Burn Wound  To determine the severity of a burn injury, the depth of the wound and size of the area involved are evaluated. The depth of injury can be determined by careful observation of the wound itself. The appearance of partial and full thickness burns is illustrated in Color Plates 13-1 and 13-2. A partial-thickness injury is pink-red with moisture or blisters. A full-thickness burn usually has a dry, leathery, white or gray charred appearance. Third-degree burns are also present if the burn area is anesthetic and hairs can be pulled out easily without pain.

*Rule of nines*  The size of a burn is expressed as a percentage of total body area. To calculate this percentage, diagrams are used and burned areas are shaded. The most frequently used method of calculation is called the *rule of nines* (Fig. 13-1). The head and each upper extremity are given the value of 9 percent of the body surface. Each lower extremity is given a value of 18 percent of the body surface. The anterior and posterior trunk are each rated at 18 percent and the perineum is valued at 1 percent, to make a total of 100 percent. Although this method is fairly simple, as it does not require the use of calculation tables, it is somewhat inaccurate. This inaccuracy is particularly true when a burn on a child is to be calculated, as there is no allowance for differences in the proportion of head and lower extremities in children as compared to adults.

A more accurate method of estimating the surface area of a burn injury is that developed by Lund and Browder, adapted from tables formulated by Berkow in 1924. This method takes into consideration changes in surface areas of various body parts that occur during different stages from infancy through childhood. The area of the head makes up a large proportion of the total skin area of infants as compared to adults, while the lower extremities in infants account for a smaller surface area than in adults. Again, a diagram is used and the burned areas are shaded. In this method the areas affected by growth are given different values depending upon the age of the patient (Fig. 13-1).

Evaluation of Systemic Changes  About 1 hour after the burn injury, the patient will begin to demonstrate the widespread systemic changes. The body's ability to cope with the changes will be manifested in the physical examination. To assess *fluid and electrolyte status,* the turgor of normal skin and mucous membranes should be evaluated.

As dehydration develops, tissue turgor becomes poor, mucous membranes dry, and the patient will complain of thirst. The eyeballs will feel soft on palpation and edema over the burn area may be visible. In third-degree burns the dry, leathery surface called the *eschar* often prevents swelling, masking the fluid losses under the wound surface. Urine output will be scant and appear dark amber in color.

Measurement of vital signs will give information regarding *oxygenation status.* The pulse will be increased and may be thready while the blood pressure may be decreased. Respirations, also, may increase as a result of hypoxia and anxiety. If respiratory damage has occurred, rales may be heard during the chest exam. In the absence of cardiac difficulties, heart sounds will be normal. If shock is developing, unburned skin will appear pale and will feel cool and clammy. The nailbeds and lips will be dusky or cyanotic, and capillary refill will be poor.

The remainder of the physical exam will not be remarkable during the initial assessment. As soon after injury as possible the patient should be weighed so that this baseline weight can be used to evaluate fluid and metabolic status. During the

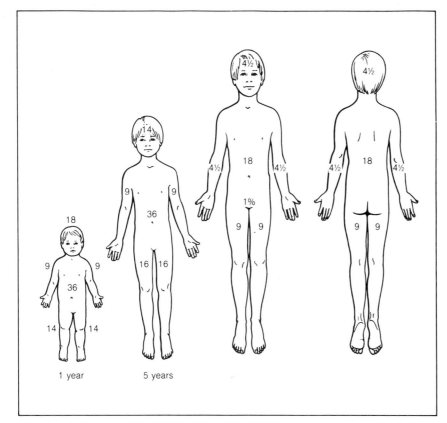

**FIGURE 13-1**
Rule of nines with modification for children and infants.

acute phase of a burn careful physical assessment should be done on a regular basis. Changes in the patient's condition can occur rapidly and careful nursing assessments can help to modify or institute interventions. During the initial assessment, for instance, bowel sounds are usually present. If adynamic ileus develops, however, they may diminish or disappear.

*Laboratory tests*   Several laboratory tests are helpful in evaluating the patient's condition. *Serum electrolytes* give valuable information regarding fluid and electrolyte imbalance. Initially the serum sodium is often decreased while potassium is increased. The increased *hematocrit* also reflects fluid losses. The *red blood cell count* will be indicative of the extent of corpuscle destruction as will the presence of *hemoglobinuria.* The *serum protein electrophoresis* will reflect the protein losses into the wound edema. The serum and urine osmolality will also aid in determining the patient's fluid and electrolyte requirements.

**Nursing problems and interventions**   The patient with a thermal injury will present a variety of extremely challenging nursing problems. A thorough understanding of the dynamics involved will aid the nurse to adequately care for the patient.

**F**luid and Electrolyte Imbalances   In the early postburn period, *fluid and electrolyte losses* are significant and, if allowed to continue without intervention, will result in hypovolemic shock. To evaluate the extent of the losses, the patient should be closely monitored. Accurate intake and output should be recorded on an hourly basis, and note should be made of the type of fluid and route of intake or output. Urine output should be especially monitored to insure maintenance of kidney function. The insertion of an indwelling Foley catheter will be required in most cases to obtain accurate urine collection and measurement. A suitable urine output is usually considered to be approximately 1 ml/kg body wt/hour. This means that a satisfactory urine output for an adult patient would be 50 to 70 ml/hour, whereas for an infant the amount would be considerably less, usually in the range of 10 ml/hour. The urine specific gravity should also be measured and recorded hourly. In most cases, the aim of fluid therapy is to maintain a urine specific gravity of 1.010 to 1.025. Body weights aid in the determination of fluid requirements and should be measured on a daily basis. It is often most con-

venient to do this after the patient has been in the tub. A rapid increase in body weight usually is indicative of an excess of fluids.

Patients with a burn injury of less than 20 percent of the total body surface may not require intravenous fluid therapy. However, in the elderly or the very young patient, fluid replacement may be necessary. Fluid therapy formulas have been developed to serve as a guideline in determining the amount of fluid the patient is to receive. These formulas act only as a guide because the depth of the injury cannot be measured and the formulas do not encompass the age of the patient nor any past medical history.

The first to be developed was the *Evans formula* (see Table 13-1). In it, the amount of fluid to be replaced is calculated by considering both the size of the wound and the weight of the patient. The total estimated amount of colloids and crystalloids (electrolytes) is given during the first 24 hours. One-half of this amount is given during the next 24 hours, with an appropriate amount of dextrose and water to cover insensible water loss. To avoid overhydration in extensive burns of over half the body, the requirements in these patients should be estimated as though only 50 percent of the body surface had been burned.

The *Brooke formula* is a modification of the Evans formula. Table 13-2 illustrates the estimation of fluid requirements using the Brooke formula.

More recently developed, the *Parkland formula* is based on the premise that plasma volume expansion is dependent on the rate of intravenous infusion and not the type of fluid infused (see Table 13-3). It uses only an electrolyte solution during the first 24 hours postburn. Dextrose and water are used during the second 24 hours to meet fluid requirements. Colloid is given only if urine output is not maintained with the dextrose and water.

If these formulas are not used, the physician may elect to administer Ringer's lactate at a rate sufficient to maintain a urinary output of an appropriate quantity and specific gravity, i.e., in infants, 10 to 20 ml/hour; in adults, 50 to 70 ml/hour with a specific gravity of 1.010 to 1.025. In addition, a piggyback infusion of albumin, prepared as a 5 percent solution in Ringer's lactate, is administered at a slow, constant rate to maintain the patient's serum albumin level above 2 g/100 ml, the minimum level. The constant, slow infusion of albumin will maintain serum albumin levels during the period of capillary permeability following the burn injury. This plan of fluid resuscitation was designed by physicians at the Shriners Burns Institute, Galveston, to aid physicians who are not familiar with treating children who have been seriously burned.

In the early postburn period, if fluid loss to the burn edema is severe and intravenous fluid therapy inadequate, *hypovolemic shock* may develop (see Chap. 27). The nurse should carefully monitor the patient's vital signs and hourly urinary output for any significant changes. Decreased urine output, increased pulse rate, and restlessness are early signs which, if noted, will allow necessary changes in treatment to be made before shock develops.

On the third or fourth postburn day the edema fluid begins to be reabsorbed. If excess fluids are given, *circulatory overload* can develop (see Chap. 24). The patient needs to be watched closely for increases in blood pressure, pulse, respirations, or urine output. Problems seldom arise if intravenous fluids are adjusted appropriately and kidney function is adequate.

*Renal failure* is seldom a problem, even with severe burns, if the hemodynamic changes are treated adequately. While the hemoglobinuria that results from the red blood cell destruction can predispose to renal damage, acute renal failure associated with burns is usually a result of ischemia.

Most burned patients complain of thirst in the early stages of treatment. This complaint is usually inappropriate and may not indicate that intravenous fluid therapy is insufficient. If given a choice, the patient may drink large amounts of salt-poor fluid, such as tap water, resulting in *water intoxication*. It is characterized by weakness, confusion, disorientation, vomiting, and, finally, convulsions. Prevention is the most effective treatment. The nurse should ensure that the patient's oral fluid intake is limited to the amounts ordered by the physician. If water intoxication develops, it is treated with diuretics and fluid restrictions.

**M**etabolic Problems  An almost universal problem that develops after a severe burn injury is a *negative nitrogen balance.* As tissue is destroyed, its protein content is lost. Nitrogen is also lost in the burn exudate. At the same time, the stress response initiated by the trauma mobilizes other body proteins to meet the energy requirements. High urinary nitrogen levels are usually found 2 to 3 days postburn and may continue until grafting is almost complete. These, coupled with the increase in metabolic rate, result in a nitrogen deficit which contributes to the general debilitation of the patient. If

not corrected, wound healing will be delayed and the patient will be more susceptible to infection.

Nutrition is a vital part of the care of the burned patient. While the burn wounds are open, extensive *calorie loss* occurs through evaporation. This can result in a rapid loss of body weight. The increase in caloric requirements is coupled with an increase in protein requirements. Following a severe burn injury, daily protein requirements may be increased to as much as 2 to 4 times the normal.

A daily diet providing between 50 and 80 calories/kg body wt and 2 to 3 g protein/kg body wt is needed for an adult burn patient. In addition, multi-

**TABLE 13-1**
EVANS FORMULA FOR FLUID RESUSCITATION THERAPY

| | |
|---|---|
| First 24 hours | |
| Colloids (blood, dextran, plasma) | 1 ml/kg body wt/% burn |
| Crystalloids (physiologic saline) | 1 ml/kg body wt/% burn |
| Second 24 hours | |
| One-half the amount of colloid and crystalloids given during first 24 hours | |
| Water (5% glucose in water) dependent upon the age and size of the patient to replace insensible water loss | |

**TABLE 13-2**
BROOKE FORMULA FOR FLUID RESUSCITATION THERAPY*

| | |
|---|---|
| First 24 hours | |
| Colloid (plasma, dextran)† | 0.5 ml/kg body wt/% burn |
| Electrolyte (Ringer's lactate) | 1.5 ml/kg body wt/% burn |
| Dextrose/water‡ | 2000 ml |
| Second 24 hours | |
| One-half the amount calculated for colloid and electrolyte during the first 24 hours, but the same amount of electrolyte-free water (2000 ml dextrose/water) | |

* For calculating fluids, 50% burn is upper limit in adults, 30% in children.
† Unless concomitant injuries demand it, blood is not given until hematocrit level has fallen and need is demonstrated.
‡ This requirement is relatively greater in children, being 160 ml/kg up to 2 years of age, 100 ml/kg at 2 to 5 years, and 80 ml/kg at 6 to 8 years.
SOURCE: S. I. Schwartz et al. (eds.), *Principles of Surgery*, 2d ed., McGraw-Hill, New York, 1974.

**TABLE 13-3**
PARKLAND FORMULA

| | |
|---|---|
| First 24 hours | |
| Colloid | None |
| Electrolyte (Ringer's lactate) | 4 ml/kg body wt/% burn |
| Dextrose/water | None |
| Second 24 hours | |
| No further electrolyte is administered. Hydration and urine flow are maintained by dextrose/water, and colloid is administered only if it is required to maintain urine output. | |

SOURCE: S. I. Schwartz et al. (eds.), *Principles of Surgery*, 2d ed., McGraw-Hill, New York, 1974.

vitamins and ascorbic acid are given to aid in tissue healing, and, for some patients, supplemental iron is also given. The patient should be served high protein, high calorie meals. If unable to tolerate regular-size meals, initially, small meals served at more frequent intervals should be offered. Cooperation between the patient, nurse, and dietician will ensure that the patient's food likes and dislikes are considered. In addition to regular meals, supplemental feedings should be given. These are often commercially prepared high-protein liquids, although homogenized cow's milk can be an excellent supplement. Some patients may develop diarrhea as a result of the osmolarity of the high-protein supplements and may tolerate cow's milk better.

Extremely sick patients may need to be fed through a nasogastric tube. Tube feedings are usually a blenderized high-protein diet mixed with a commercial protein supplement. Care should be taken before each feeding to check for any residual gastric contents and bowel sounds. The patient should be watched carefully to prevent aspiration of the gastric contents during the procedure. An adequate water intake is also necessary for patients receiving tube feedings. This is usually given at the end of the feeding to clear the feeding tube.

In order to monitor the patient's nutritional intake, a calorie count chart listing the patient's food and fluid intake may be used. Both the calorie and protein intake can then be calculated and adjustments made as necessary.

As a result of the loss of areas of the skin, the body's ability to maintain a constant temperature is compromised and the patient experiences *heat loss.* To prevent chilling, the thermostat in the patient's room is set at 75°F and additional heat from radiant heat lamps and warming blankets may be necessary. Procedures requiring patient exposure should be performed as quickly as possible. In addition, only the area of the body undergoing wound care should be exposed. The high thermostat settings and the use of additional sources of heat are often uncomfortable for visitors and personnel. The reasons for the environmental manipulation should be explained to visitors and instructions on appropriate dress given. Uniforms should be worn that maximize comfort.

Patients of all ages and with both minor and major burn injuries may develop *Curling's ulcer.* With a major burn injury, this can be a serious complication. The use of milk and antacids has been found to reduce its incidence. Some physicians prefer that the patient drink milk on an hourly basis, while others prefer a regimen alternating milk and antacid. The development of an ulcer is usually evidenced by gastrointestinal hemorrhage and is initially treated conservatively. Should conservative therapy be unsuccessful, surgical management is then considered. See Chap. 17 for a thorough discussion of gastrointestinal ulcers.

*Gastric dilatation* and *paralytic ileus* may also occur following a burn injury. Acute gastric dilatation is often seen immediately following the injury, as a result of stress. The condition can occur, however, at a later time during treatment, probably as a result of fear, pain, and decreased motor activity. The reason for the development of a paralytic ileus is not clear; in some instances it is associated with septicemia. When caring for a burned patient, the nurse should routinely listen for bowel sounds and observe the patient's abdomen for signs of distention. Abdominal distention, nausea, vomiting, pain, absence of bowel sounds and movements should be noted and oral intake stopped until the patient is evaluated by a physician. With both gastric dilatation and paralytic ileus decompression of the stomach is done using a nasogastric tube. For the patient with ileus, no food or fluids are given orally until bowel sounds return. With gastric dilatation, the tube is removed after 48 hours if fluids are tolerated.

**P**roblems in Oxygenation   Oxygenation status can be affected by pulmonary difficulties. *Pulmonary edema* may be seen early during burn therapy (see Chap. 24). Pulmonary burns are rare but damage can result from inhalation of the products of combustion which results in edema. It can also result from an overload of intravenous fluids. Fluid requirements in the elderly and the very young may be overestimated. Pulmonary edema is characterized by dyspnea, a productive cough with frothy and, sometimes, blood-tinged secretions, and a rapid increase in pulse rate. The patient may become agitated due to hypoxia.

When pulmonary edema develops, immediate treatment is necessary. The head of the bed should be elevated and intravenous fluids, especially saline solutions, should be slowed to a rate that will keep the intravenous line open. Oxygen is often administered and *intermittent positive pressure breathing treatments* with bronchodilators or antifoaming agents may be used. Digitalis is administered in a fully digitalizing dose, and the physician may order the administration of a diuretic, such as furosemide. If the extremities are not burned, rotating tourniquets may be employed.

Pulmonary problems can also develop later as

a result of hypostatic or infectious *pneumonia* or from *atelectasis*. These later complications are best treated prophylactically by encouraging the patient to cough and deep breath, by frequent position changes, and by early ambulation. If a pulmonary infection does develop, in addition to the use of antibiotics, supportive respiratory therapy, such as humidified air, oxygen, or intermittent positive pressure breathing with bronchodilators, may be necessary. In severe cases, the use of an endotracheal or tracheostomy tube may become necessary. A tracheostomy is generally avoided if at all possible, particularly if it has to be performed through burned skin, as this allows drainage from the burned area to enter the pulmonary tree via the tracheostomy. Extremely careful aseptic technique is required for both the endotracheal and tracheostomy tube to prevent further pulmonary infection.

One of the more serious problems affecting oxygenation status is the development of *shock* and the several nursing problems that result from it. Initially, it can occur if fluid losses are not met with adequate intravenous replacement therapy. After the early fluid changes have been resolved, shock can develop from a septicemia arising from infection of the burn wound. A complete discussion of the patient in shock can be found in Chap. 28.

Up to 40 percent of the *total red blood cell mass* can be hemolyzed as a result of thermal injury. Initially, the hematocrit will not reflect this destruction because of the fluid losses. Blood replacement is not undertaken until the hematocrit begins to manifest red blood cell loss. Multiple transfusions may then be given according to need.

**C**hanges in Inflammation and Immunity  The thermal injury itself results in a massive inflammation of the wound area. The burned surface, deprived of the normal protection of skin, is an attractive site for infection. At the same time immunosuppression generally results from severe burns. If infection becomes extensive, septicemia can develop. This is a major cause of death in burned patients.

The nurse plays a vital role not only in preventing infection, but in recognizing developing septicemia early. Patients normally experience a drop in temperature after burn wounds are exposed. Excessive use of heat lamps or heating pads can cause temperature elevations. These episodes of hypo- or hyperthermia should be avoided. Any that occur and are not related to these circumstances may be indicative of sepsis. Other early indicators are changes in the patient's sensorium, especially lethargy, increased respiratory rate, lowered blood pressure, and abdominal distension. Changes in the appearance of the burn wound such as a pale, unhealing appearance, foul-smelling drainage, or darkened areas are indicative of bacterial invasion.

Infection of a burn wound can be minimized if the wound is adequately cleansed and early closure provided. The important aspects of wound care include methods of treatment, tubbing and debridement, surgical debridement, topical chemotherapy, isolation precautions, and surgical coverage.

*Methods of wound care*  Three methods have been developed for treating burn wounds. The first of these is the *open or exposure method* and involves leaving the wounds completely exposed to the atmosphere. This method is generally used for minor burns, areas difficult to dress, or newly grafted sites. The wounds require careful cleansing to prevent bacterial growth and the patient needs strict isolation. Often when being treated by the exposure method, patients complain of feeling cold. A tentlike arrangement of sheets is used to cover the patient, and heat lamps aid in maintaining normal body temperature.

When using the *semiopen method* of wound care, wounds are covered with a layer of sterile, fine mesh gauze impregnated with a topical antibacterial agent. The patient is bathed daily or more often if wounds are grossly contaminated, and new dressings are applied under strict sterile technique. In addition, extremely soiled dressings are changed as needed throughout the day. This method of wound care is suitable for even severe burns.

Using the *occlusive method* of treatment, wounds are covered with many layers of gauze dressing which are left intact often for periods up to 10 days. Exudate is kept in contact with the wound surface causing it to be a warm, moist medium for the proliferation of bacteria. For this reason, and the added disadvantage that the wound cannot be inspected daily, the occlusive treatment has fallen into disuse.

*Tubbing and debridement*  For healing to occur, necrotic tissue on the wound must be removed. The easiest method for cleansing the wound is to bathe the patient in either a bath tub or a Hubbard tank. The latter is a specially designed tub fitted with motors to agitate the water. The agitation aids in cleansing the wounds. Various substances that aid in cleansing may be added to the bath water; the more commonly used agents are detergent, prepodyne whirlpool concentrate, and sodium hypochlorite 1:120.

The bath water should be at body temperature. The patient's outer dressings should be loosened and the patient lowered into the water. The dressings will float off in the water. The patient generally stays in the water for 15 to 20 minutes, during which time limb exercises may be performed under the supervision of a physical therapist. Many patients are able to move their joints more freely when immersed in water. The patient should not be left unattended during the tubbing procedure. At the end of the soaking period the bathing solution is drained and the wounds rinsed with tap water. The patient is moved to a stretcher for debridement.

*Debridement* is the removal of eschar, the leathery covering of dead tissue that forms following a full-thickness burn. Loose pieces of tissue are removed by using a forceps and curved scissors. Sterile technique should be employed throughout this procedure. To prevent bleeding, only loose eschar should be removed. The procedure should be performed as gently as possible to prevent further tissue damage and to minimize discomfort.

During the debridement procedure, the wounds should be carefully examined for evidence of sub-eschar abscesses, decreases in granulation, color changes, or necrotic areas indicative of bacterial invasion. Evidence of these should be reported to the physician immediately.

*Enzyme debridement agents* are commercially prepared concentrations of enzymes which, when applied to the burn wound, hasten dissolution of the eschar. The use of these agents is still relatively controversial and further research is needed before their effectiveness can be determined.

*Escharectomy* Surgical excision of eschar is often performed to remove the dead tissue and allow for early closure of the wound. Circumferential full-thickness burns of an extremity or the trunk may also require surgical intervention because the obligatory wound edema that forms under the inelastic band can cause pressure severe enough to compromise circulation to the part or decrease chest expansion.

The procedure is usually performed within 48 hours of the injury. The patient is anesthetized and the dead tissue gradually excised down to viable tissue. This is called a *tangential excision.* In the case of a very deep burn, the eschar and the subcutaneous tissue are removed down to the underlying fascia. After escharectomy skin grafts or a biological dressing are applied. If the patient is extensively burned, sections of the burned area will be excised at one time, thus lessening the amount of stress for the patient. A waiting period of 2 to 3 days is allowed between procedures. Blood replacement is necessary during the procedure and careful monitoring of the patient in the postoperative period is required. Escharectomy is advantageous in that it decreases the chances of burn wound sepsis and shortens the hospitalization time.

*Topical chemotherapy* Because infection develops so readily and can convert a partial-thickness burn into a full-thickness injury, topical agents are used for their antibacterial effects. *Mafenide 1%* (*Sulfamylon*) is available as a white ointment which may be applied directly to the burn wound or impregnated into a fine mesh gauze dressing. It is applied at least once or twice daily. It has the disadvantage of causing pain on application. It is also a carbonic-anhydrase inhibitor and thus interferes with the kidney's ability to secrete hydrogen ions. Metabolic acidosis is a common complication and is compensated for by an increase in the respiratory rate. When mafenide 1% is used, blood gas and pH determinations are necessary to monitor the patient's condition.

*Silver sulfadiazine* also is available as a white ointment and is applied either on a fine mesh gauze dressing or directly to the wound. It causes no pain or burning on application and is not a carbonic-anhydrase inhibitor. There are no apparent electrolyte imbalances associated with its use. It does not, however, penetrate eschar as deeply as does mafenide.

*Silver nitrate* has been used for many years in burn therapy and is still used by some physicians. It is used in a hypotonic solution (0.5 to 1%) and is applied to the wound on thick layers of gauze dressing. The gauze needs to be constantly saturated to be effective, which may involve a great deal of nursing time. There are several disadvantages associated with its use. Because it is hypotonic, it draws sodium, potassium, calcium, and chloride out of the tissues. Sodium, chloride, and potassium supplements will be needed during its use. Calcium supplements are seldom needed because the unbound serum calcium usually remains unchanged. Silver nitrate also causes black discoloration of any surface, and institutions using it generally resort to using dark colored linens and decor.

*Isolation procedures* In an effort to minimize the chance of bacterial contamination, isolation procedures are routinely employed. The patient's external and internal environments are potential reservoirs of infection. *Escherichia coli* are organisms normally found in the gastrointestinal tract which can contaminate the burn wound. Antimicrobial drugs are sometimes used to prevent this; however, good aseptic technique and personal hygiene are important in controlling autocontamination.

Isolation procedures that protect the patient from contaminants in the external environment are designed relative to the location of the burn center in the hospital and consistent with the philosophy of the medical and nursing personnel. Procedures are formulated not only to protect the burned patient from other patients, personnel, and visitors but to protect the rest of the patients in the hospital from burned patients. Burn wards vary in their use of isolation procedures and the requirements range from having personnel and visitors change into scrub clothes, cap, mask, and overshoes upon entering the unit to a completely "open ward" policy.

Strict sterile technique is necessary when performing wound care and careful handwashing before and after each patient contact is extremely important in the prevention of cross-contamination. Supplies and equipment should be assigned to each individual patient and not used from patient to patient. Housekeeping techniques, including the handling of soiled linen and trash, also play an important role in controlling infection.

*Wound coverage*   Wound coverage is extremely important in decreasing the chances of infection. Temporary coverage can be achieved through the use of "biological dressings." These may be skin from another person, a *homograft,* or from an animal, a *xenograft* or *heterograft.* Homografts usually involve cadaver skin. Occasionally, skin may be taken from a living donor. Because the supply of homografts is limited, xenografts are commonly used. They are most frequently obtained from pigs, *porcine xenograft,* and are available in individually packaged squares and in square-foot rolls.

Biological dressings are applied following the bathing procedure. Sterile technique is used during the application and, as the procedure is not painful, no anesthesia is required. The xenograft is laid onto the wounds and the gauze backing material is peeled away. It may be held in place with a tubular mesh dressing. Exudate which collects beneath the porcine skin is expressed by rolling the xenograft with cotton-tipped applicators and blotting the exudate with gauze at the edges of the graft. The exudate is cultured and if there is evidence of inflammation, the xenograft is removed, the patient bathed, and more xenograft applied. If no inflam-

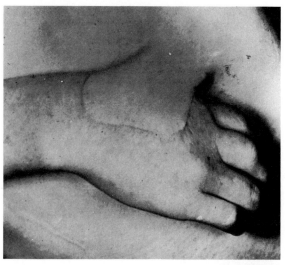

**FIGURE 13-2**
Abdominal pedicle flap applied to dorsum of hand. Scar on hand has been turned back to resurface the raw side of pedicle and a portion of the donor site. Flap will be separated from the abdominal wall in 18 days. (*From S. I. Schwartz et al. (eds.), Principles of Surgery, 2d ed., McGraw-Hill, New York, 1974, by permission.*)

mation is present, the xenograft is left in place for periods of time up to 5 days.

Xenografts are used to prepare granulation beds to receive autografts and to prevent loss of body fluids. In addition, it has been found that this early coverage of the wound helps alleviate pain and therefore allows for earlier rehabilitation. Xenografts may be used in addition to grafts of the patient's own skin when a large surface area of the body is burned and sufficient donor sites are not available to cover all the wounds during one procedure.

Research is being done on the use of immunosuppressants to delay rejection of homografts in patients with extensive burns.[3,4] These grafts provide wound closure until the patient's own donor sites heal and more skin can be taken.

*Autografts* are grafts of the patient's own skin. They can be *free grafts* in that they are completely separated from the donor site or *pedicle grafts* which remain attached to the donor site in order to maintain a vascular connection as depicted in Fig. 13-2. Pedicle grafts are used when more tissue than skin has been destroyed and other tissue such as fat, tendon, muscle, or nerve is being replaced along with the skin. After the graft has established a blood supply at the recipient site, the pedicle is separated from the donor site.

Free grafts can vary in thickness. In full-thickness grafts both the epidermis and dermis are

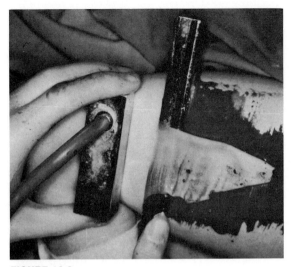

**FIGURE 13-3**
Removal of thick split-thickness graft with a free-hand knife. The largest possible grafts can be taken by this method. (*From S. I. Schwartz et al. (eds.), Principles of Surgery, 2d ed., McGraw-Hill, New York, 1974, by permission.*)

transferred. Full-thickness grafts are usually small because the donor site will have to be sutured closed or covered with a split-thickness graft. Split-thickness grafts are most commonly used and involve the transfer of the epidermis and part of the dermis.

Autografting is an operative procedure usually performed under general anesthesia. The donor sites are shaved and prepared in the operating room. The thighs and buttocks are primary choices as donor sites because they are accessible, they are composed of fairly firm tissue, and skin traction may be readily applied. When areas such as the back or scalp are used, infiltration of the subcutaneous tissue is necessary to provide a smooth surface for skin removal. If it is necessary to use the scalp as a donor site, the patient should be forewarned that the skin graft is only partial thickness, and, therefore, will not result in baldness or hair being transferred to other parts of the body. Skin from the abdomen is often used to graft the face and hands because the pigment is the nearest match for those areas. In the case of the extensive burn injury, the same donor site may be used several times. If skin is taken at a depth of 0.005 to 0.010 inch and the area kept infection-free, healing will take place in 10 to 14 days and the donor site may be reused.

The granulation bed, the recipient site, is prepared by removing exuberant granulation tissue either by scraping with a knife or scrubbing the area with a brush or coarse gauze. Bleeding is controlled by the applications of warm saline soaks.

A dermatone is most often used to remove donor skin although a knife may be used (see Fig. 13-3). Those commonly used are the Brown, Reese, and Padgett dermatomes. The Brown dermatome, an air-driven instrument, is often used for large, split thickness grafts. Once the skin is removed, it is spread, dermal side up, onto fine mesh roller gauze and kept moist with neomycin solution. When the necessary amount of skin has been obtained, application of the graft to the burn wound is performed. The strips of skin are placed dermal side down onto the granulation bed. There should be as little space as possible between the grafts without overlapping of the skin. Use of the full strip of skin in this fashion is called *"sheet grafting"* (see Fig. 13-4).

Several techniques have been developed to expand the skin graft to cover a larger area. The *postage stamp* technique was an early technique in which the skin graft was cut into small pieces and applied to the granulation bed in such a way that there were spaces between the grafts. A more recent method called *"mesh"* or *"split"* grafts involves the use of an instrument which meshes the skin and allows it to be stretched (see Fig. 13-5).

Occasionally, an excess of skin is taken. If this occurs, it may be wrapped in vaseline gauze and stored in neomycin solution at a temperature of 23°F (−5°C) for a period up to 2 weeks. This bank skin can then be used if some loss of the skin graft occurs.

When several grafting procedures are required to cover extensive burn wounds, areas such as the face, hands, and arms are usually grafted first, followed by the anterior trunk and legs. Once these grafts have taken, the posterior aspects requiring autografts are covered.

Following the grafting procedure, much care is required to ensure a graft take and healing of the donor sites. Donor sites are dressed with dressing materials such as glycerine gauze or scarlet red gauze depending upon the preference of the surgeon. Sometimes they are left without dressings. Heat lamps are used to dry the donor sites. As healing takes place, the gauze becomes loosened at the edges and may be trimmed away.

Autografts may be covered initially with dressings, usually consisting of neomycin gauze next to the graft, a bulky gauze dressing, and then an elastic bandage. These are usually left in place for 3 days and then either changed or removed entirely. This type of dressing is especially useful over a mesh graft, as a light pressure dressing will often help the graft to adhere.

Many surgeons prefer to leave the graft open, in which case frequent, meticulous care is needed to ensure adhesion. When a graft has "taken," by the third to fifth day it assumes a pink appearance which reflects the development of vascular connections. The grafts are rolled with cotton-tipped applicators to remove the exudate that forms underneath. The exudate is expressed to the edges of the graft and then blotted with gauze. If exudate is allowed to collect beneath the graft it will prevent adherence and provide a media for bacteria growth. Frequently, during the first 24 hours following surgery, this procedure needs to be performed every 15 minutes. Some shrinking of the grafts does occur, leaving small raw areas between the grafts. These areas are dressed with gauze impregnated with nitrofurazone, scarlet red (an aniline dye), or one of the topical antibacterial agents used in the earlier stage of burn care.

*Immunization*  Bacteria such as *Clostridium tetani* are present in the soil and the intestines of humans and animals. In wounds such as burns, where dead tissue is present, tetanus can develop. The patient's immunization record should be evaluated and if active immunization against tetanus has not occurred, protection must be given. Most often hyperimmune human antitetanus γ-globulin will be given and will provide protection for at least 6 weeks.

Studies have also shown that actively immunizing patients with a polyvalent vaccine against *Pseudomonas aeruginosa* decreases these life-threatening infections and may prove to be an effective adjunct to treating burned patients.[5]

**P**erceptual Problems  The most striking perceptual change following burn injury is related to pain. Full-thickness burns are anesthetic; however, they are often surrounded by areas of partial-thickness injury which can be excruciatingly painful. The amount of pain is generally inversely proportional to the depth of injury. Narcotics are usually required for pain relief in the first few days following the burn accident. As mentioned earlier, these should be given intravenously. Due to the possibility of addiction and the possible contribution of narcotics to problems such as anorexia and gastrointestinal disturbances, their continued use is not recommended. Short-acting barbiturates or tranquilizers such as diazepam may be used, particularly prior to bathing and dressing procedures.

After the first few days, pain is most often associated with dressing changes. The use of "white noise" and distractions to decrease pain is discussed in greater detail in Chap. 39. Anxiety often contributes to the pain a patient may experience. This may be greatly relieved by nursing measures, and the relationship between the patient and staff is extremely important in this respect. Emotional support to the patient, in addition to performing proce-

**FIGURE 13-4**
Autografts using sheet grafting.

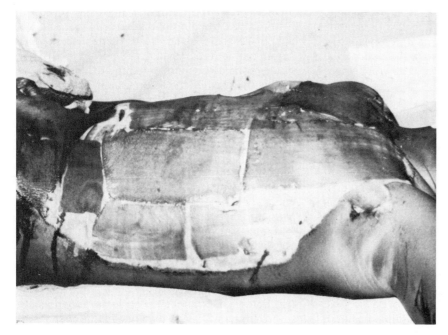

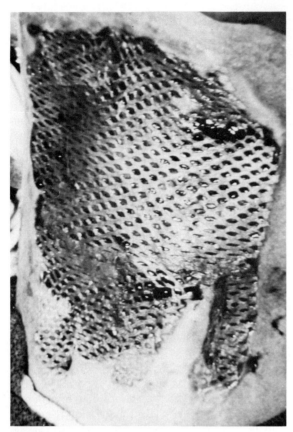

**FIGURE 13-5**
Autograft using mesh or split graft.

dures in a gentle and efficient manner, will result in the patient gaining confidence in the personnel. Often, with reassurance and a careful explanation of the procedure to be performed, the patient will be able to tolerate procedures such as wound care without the use of analgesics.

**Coordination Problems** Coordination is not affected initially but can be greatly impaired when healing occurs as the result of contracture formation. *Joint contractures* and the development of hypertrophic scars and keloid bodies cause not only physical limitations but often distressing cosmetic deformities (see Fig. 13-6). Contractures occur when scar tissue forms over a joint area. The more common areas affected are the neck, axilla, and elbow.

Careful and meticulous nursing care can do much to prevent contracture formation. In the acute phase of burn injury, positioning is vitally important. Most patients, if allowed to do so, will place themselves in the most comfortable position, usually the fetal position, which predisposes to joint contractures. The patient should be positioned with joints in a neutral position. The knees and elbows should be extended and the shoulders abducted. Extension splints may be used for the upper and lower extremities. Hand splints made of isoprene are often helpful in maintaining extension of the interphalangeal joints and optimal wrist, metacarpophalangeal, and thumb position. The neck can be positioned with an isoprene neck conformer to prevent flexion. Passive exercises are used as tolerated.

As soon as the patient's condition allows, the joints should be actively mobilized. Active range of motion exercises can be done while the patient is confined to bed or during the tubbing procedure in the hydrotherapy tank. Many patients find exercising while in water easier and less discomforting. Dynamic splinting may be used between exercise periods to maximize joint movement. Early ambulation is encouraged not only to prevent contracture deformities but to promote a feeling of independence. Patients who have burns of the legs should have their legs wrapped with elastic bandages when ambulating to prevent venous stasis. Walkers and parallel bars may also be used when the patient first begins to walk.

To prevent contracture formation following grafting procedures or when healing has occurred but full maturation of the scar tissue has not been reached, *skeletal traction* is often used. Hypertrophy of the scar tissue occurs in some patients following healing of a partial thickness burn or in the area of a grafted full-thickness injury. Application of pressure using elastic bandages or elasticized garments can be used to prevent this. Hypertrophy generally occurs 6 months to 1 year following the injury when the scar tissue is immature and has a fairly bright pink appearance. Once the scar tissue has matured and becomes a lighter color, the application of pressure is not effective in reducing the hypertrophy.

Whatever the method or methods employed to minimize contractures, close coordination between the nurse and the physical therapist should be maintained. The physical therapist often fits the patient for the various braces and splints and aids in exercising and ambulation. The nurse and the physical therapist should develop an exercise program and conferences should be held on a regular basis to evaluate the patient's progress.

**Psychological Changes** Patients experiencing severe burns will evidence a variety of changes of which the nurse should be aware.[6] During the *acute stage* the physical injury along with the anxiety and stress surrounding the accident often results in an altered mental state. These changes can range from mild confusion to delirium. This should be considered an acute organic brain syndrome and its symptoms are often decreased with the use of tranquilizers.

During the *intermediate stage* of the burn, the patient's psychological reactions are often associated with pain. Dependency needs increase, the patient becomes discouraged, and cooperation often decreases. The pain can be decreased with the use of sedatives and narcotics. Frank uncooperativeness during painful procedures, however, can be difficult to handle, and desirable behavior should be positively reinforced. Rationalization can

also be employed, explaining the reasons for various procedures or regimes. Using other patients as models and developing an esprit de corps may help in maximizing the patient's cooperation.

The nurse-patient relationship is of prime importance, particularly as the patient must receive a great deal of emotional support from the nursing staff during the hospitalization period. In addition to the fears associated with death, disfigurement, invalidism, and pain following a burn accident, the patient must cope with a strange environment, a strange group of people, and confusing procedures. During the initial contact with the patient, the nurse may be able to alleviate some of these extra fears by giving the patient some orientation to the surroundings and explanations of the procedures in understandable terms.

**FIGURE 13-6**
(*a*) Severe contracture produced by full thickness skin loss in burn wound of neck and face. Note ectropion of lower lip. (*b*) Release of contracture in same patient shown in (*a*). Contracture was released by excising scar tissue and resurfacing the defect with several split-thickness skin grafts. Note absence of wrinkling of graft and restoration of cervical profile. Facial scars ultimately will be excised and resurfaced. (*From S. I. Schwartz et al. (eds.), Principles of Surgery, 2d ed., McGraw-Hill, New York, 1974, by permission.*)

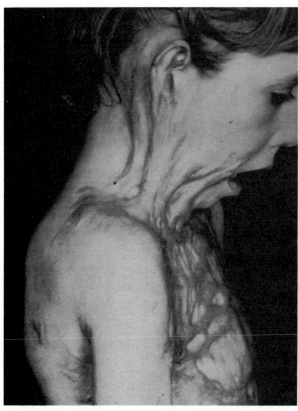

A

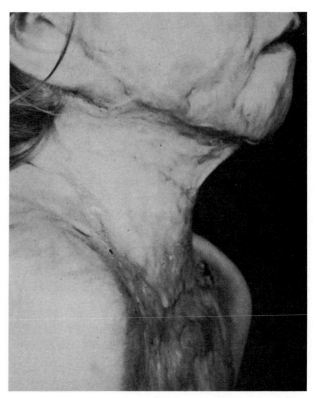

B

It is important that all members of the burn care team use a consistent approach for each patient, and this should be discussed at regular care-plan meetings. Inconsistencies may place the patient in a position to manipulate the nursing staff. An effective method is to establish a form of contract with the patient wherein careful explanations and guidelines as to what is expected of the patient are given before each procedure. Requests from the patient should be considered and the contract should be made as mutually acceptable as possible.

When performing procedures, the nurse should realize that the manner in which the procedure is carried out will influence the nurse-patient relationship. Procedures should be performed competently and so as to cause as little discomfort as possible. Patients should be encouraged to participate in their own care as much as possible.

**Fourth-level Nursing Care**

The burned patient has experienced extensive physical and psychological problems which will require long-term nursing care. In preparation for discharge, a careful assessment should be made of the patient's physical or psychological limitations, if any, as well as the family strengths and weaknesses, social and economic background, and community resources to which the patient will be returning. In the case of a patient without a family network, arrangements may have to be made for a public health nurse to provide follow-up care. For a child, communication between the school and the hospital personnel is important to prepare for the child's return to the classroom.

The patient or a family member must be fully instructed in *care of the wounds* and the *care and application of any braces or splints* which are to be used. This instruction should be given over a period of days prior to discharge, starting with a demonstration of the techniques involved and ending with the patient or family member giving a return demonstration of these procedures. In addition, the patient should be given written instructions for these techniques and for any exercise program to be performed at home. Also, any limitations of physical activity should be carefully listed. It is helpful to the patient to be given a telephone number to call if questions or difficulties arise upon returning home. This provides an important "lifeline" for some patients when they are newly discharged.

In addition to physical preparation, *psychological preparation* for discharge must be taken into consideration. It is often helpful for a patient to have a pass from the hospital several times before the final discharge. This will give the patient an opportunity to meet people outside the "safe" burn ward environment.

During the recuperative stage of a burn, the patient experiences many problems that must be resolved.[7] These often involve anxiety over separating from the hospital and staff, changes in body image, concerns about social acceptance, vocational and financial worries, and mobilizing the courage to overcome deficits. Patients often tend to withdraw, regress, and become depressed. They have experienced a significant change in body image. This is especially so if the patient is young or if the head or neck are burned. Initially this will cause anxiety which will be followed by grief and mourning. Self-esteem is often lowered. The nurse should encourage patients to discuss the change in body image. It is important to explore how the patient views the change, and regular sessions with a psychiatric nurse practitioner may be helpful. Individual and/or group psychotherapy may be indicated on a long-term basis. *Burn Recovery* is a group of former burn patients organized to help in adjusting to these problems.

*Follow-up* care is extremely important after burn injury. Most often the patient returns in 2 to 6 weeks. At this time both physical and psychological conditions should be evaluated. Physical therapy may need to be continued on a long-term basis.

The physical evaluation should be done by the physician, physical therapist, and nurse. The patient's understanding of wound care and the use of braces and splints should be evaluated. Wounds should be examined for any breakdown of skin grafts or evidence of contractures. Braces and splints should be adjusted or remade if necessary. The patient should also be interviewed privately, away from the clinic, by the social worker, psychiatric nurse, and/or psychologist to evaluate the patient's psychological adjustment following the burn injury. Further outpatient visits should be scheduled on an individual basis dependent upon the patient's physical and psychological needs.

Following a burn injury many patients require some reconstructive surgery for either functional or cosmetic deformities (see Fig. 13-7). This surgery is usually delayed until 6 months or even 1 year following the acute injury to allow the scar tissue to mature and the patients overall condition to improve. Functional deformities are usually corrected prior to cosmetic deformities, although sometimes simultaneous reconstruction is performed. The reconstructive surgery must obviously be individualized. Some patients may require very little surgery, whereas a patient who has survived a major burn injury may be faced with many surgical procedures. The long-term care of a burned patient must focus on physical rehabilitation, psychosocial counseling, vocational training, and family support.

## REFERENCES

1  T. B. Curling, "On Acute Ulceration of the Duodenum in Cases of Burns," *Med. Chir. Trans. London,* **25:**260, 1842.

2  *America Burning,* Report on the National Commission on Fire Prevention and Control, 1973.

3  D. Hughes, E. A. Caspary, and H. M. Wisniewski, "Letter: Immunosuppression by Linoleic Acid," *The Lancet,* **2**(7933):501–502, September 13, 1975.

4  John F. Burke, J. W. May Jr., N. Albright, W. C. Quinby, P. S. Russell, "Temporary Skin Transplantation and Immunosuppression for Extensive Burns," *N Engl J Med,* **290:**269–271, January 31, 1974.

5  J. W. Alexander and M. W. Fisher, "Immunization Against Pseudomonas in Infection After Thermal Injury," *J Infect Dis,* **130:**supplement:S152–158, November 1974.

6  J. A. Jorgensen and J. J. Brophy, "Psychiatric Treatment Modalities in Burn Patients," in J. H. Masserman (ed.), *Curr Psychiat Ther,* vol. 15, Grune and Stratton, New York, 1975.

7  Ibid.

## BIBLIOGRAPHY

Artz, C. P. and T. A. Moncrief: *The Treatment of Burns,* Saunders, Philadelphia, 1969.

Feller, I., and J. C. Archambeault: *Nursing of the Burned Patient,* Institute for Burn Medicine, Ann Arbor, 1973.

Jacoby, Florence Greenhouse: *Nursing Care of the Patient with Burns,* Mosby, St. Louis, 1972.

Jelenko, C., III: "Studies in Burns: Water Loss from the Body Surface," *Ann Surg,* **165:**83, January 1967.

Krizek, T. J., J. E. Hoopes, and R. W. Steenburg: "Management of Burns, Cold, and Electrical Injuries," in W. F. Ballinger, B. Rutherford, and G. D. Zuidema (eds.), *The Management of Trauma,* Saunders, Philadelphia, 1968.

Larson, Duane, S. Abston, and A. Goldman: "The Burned Child," *Tex Med,* **67:**58–67, April 1971.

Lunan, H. N.: "Topical Treatment of the Burn Patient," *Am J Hosp Pharm,* **32:**599–605, June 1975.

Manafo, William W.: *The Treatment of Burns: Principles and Practice,* Grenn, St. Louis, 1971.

Moncrief, J. A., and A. D. Mason: Evaporative Water Loss in Burned Patients, *J Trauma,* **4:**180, March 1964.

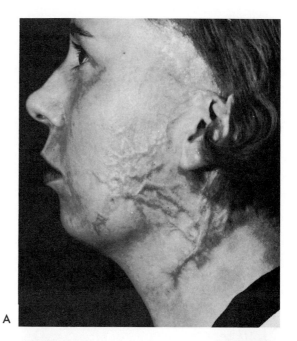

A

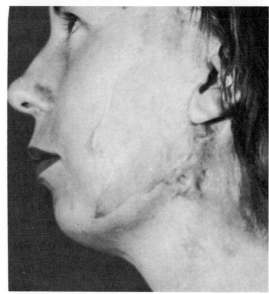

B

**FIGURE 13-7**

(*a*) Hypertrophic scar produced by deep second degree burn. Although a significant amount of full thickness skin has not been lost, overproduction of collagen has produced an unsightly scar. (*b*) Patient shown in (*a*) following excision of facial portion of scar and application of a thick split-thickness skin graft. Cervical portion of scar will be resurfaced later. A single graft covering facial and cervical areas would obliterate submandibular groove. Note that scar at junction of graft and skin is most prominent near angle of mouth where motion and tension are unavoidable. Although different in texture, height and thickness from normal skin, the graft provides a smooth surface over which cosmetics can be applied more effectively than over previous scar. (*From S. I. Schwartz et al. (eds.), Principles of Surgery, 2d ed., McGraw-Hill, 1974, by permission.*)

Polk, Hiram C., and H. Harlan Stone (eds.): *Contemporary Burn Management,* Little, Brown, Boston, 1971.

Schwartz, S. I., R. C. Lillehei, G. I. Shires, F. C. Spencer, E. H. Storer: *Principles of Surgery,* 2d ed., McGraw-Hill, New York, 1974.

"Transplantation and Burns," *Lancet,* **1**(7914):1017–1018, May 3, 1975.

Willis, B., D. L. Larson, and S. Abston: "Positioning and Splinting The Burned Patient," *Heart and Lung—The Journal of Critical Care,* **2**:696–700, September–October 1973.

# 14

# THE KIDNEY AND FLUID AND ELECTROLYTE IMBALANCES

Marcia Moeller Grant

As humans interact with the external environment, the kidneys play a vital role in maintaining fluid and electrolyte balance. Nurses are involved daily with the prevention, recognition, and care of patients with fluid and electrolyte imbalances resulting from changes in kidney functioning. No patient is immune.

Renal disease respects no one; it is found in newborns, the young, and the elderly. It is seen in both sexes, in all socioeconomic groups, and in every geographic area of the world. There are diseases affecting the kidneys which are more prevalent in some areas than in others; there are some diseases which affect one sex more than another, but no one is free from the threat of renal disease.[1]

While the primary role of the kidney is the regulation of fluid and electrolyte balance, additional life-preserving functions include the excretion of metabolic waste products and the secretion of endocrine substances involved with the regulation of blood pressure, renal blood flow, and maturation of red blood cells. The expansion of knowledge of the mechanisms by which these functions are carried out, along with the clarification of the pathophysiology of renal disease, and the success of the artificial kidney and renal transplantation, have led to the development of many nursing roles in caring for renal patients. Nurses are responsible for the prevention, recognition, and assessment of early renal disease, the care of the hospitalized patient with established renal disease, the education and management of the dialysis patient, and rehabilitation of the patient with chronic renal failure. Both the critical care and long-term education of patients with renal failure requires in-depth education for specialty nursing roles. Nonetheless, the appropriate daily care of patients in all settings requires that nurses be prepared in fundamental knowledge of the kidney disorders and resulting fluid and electrolyte imbalances.

## RENAL FAILURE

Renal failure results in a reduction of renal function with associated accumulation of nitrogenous wastes. It occurs in an adult when urine output is less than 400 ml in 24 hours (*oliguria*), or less than 50 ml in 24 hours (*anuria*). *Azotemia* refers to the accumulation of nitrogenous wastes reflected in the elevation of blood urea nitrogen (BUN) and creatinine. Azotemia may begin even before urinary output decreases, and may progress to *uremia,* a toxic syndrome caused by the accumulation of nitrogenous wastes and excess substances in the body and characterized by marked deterioration in renal tissue, water and electrolyte imbalances, hypertension, nausea, vomiting, headache, and, eventually, convulsions and coma. Azotemia, while serious, is not life-threatening; uremia is fatal if untreated.

Acute renal failure differs from chronic renal failure in the time of onset and the physical, psychological, and sociological aspects of care. *Acute renal failure* may be reversible with successful treatment, resulting in no residual dysfunction. However, it is a very serious disturbance, and continues to have mortality rates which vary from 25 to 70 percent, depending upon the initiating cause.[2] *Chronic renal failure* has a gradual onset accompanied by irreversible damage to tissue. It imposes major changes on the patient's life-style in terms of the physical aspects of care, the decrease in activity and strength, the financial burdens, and the psychological stress apparent in both the patient and the family. Interrelationships between acute and chronic renal failure occur, since an episode of acute renal failure may lead to the establishment of chronic renal disease, and patients with chronic renal disease may experience periods of acute failure. Acute and chronic renal failure will each be explored in depth. Specific renal conditions, such as glomerulonephritis, renal calculi, pyelonephritis, and nephrosis among others, will then be reviewed.

**Acute Renal Failure**

Acute renal failure is a broadly applied term that includes a wide variety of conditions. The causes of acute renal failure can be categorized as prerenal, postrenal, and intrarenal, according to their pathogenesis. *Prerenal failure* is caused by factors outside the kidney which decrease renal blood flow by either vasoconstriction or a reduction in blood pressure, and, therefore, reduce glomerular perfu-

sion. This reduction can be caused by local interference with blood supply as is seen in renal artery obstruction by a thrombus or an embolus, or by hypovolemia associated with hemorrhage, burns, cardiac insufficiency, and septic shock. Prolonged or excessive prerenal failure can result in intrarenal disease.

*Postrenal failure* is caused by obstructions to the flow of urine into the bladder or the urethra. These obstructions include calculi, tumors, and trauma with resulting blockage of ureteral and/or urethral drainage. As the flow is blocked, urine backs up into the renal pelvis and parenchyma. Anuria, rather than oliguria, is generally present.

*Intrarenal failure* occurs most frequently and is caused by damage to the renal tissue itself, resulting in malfunctioning of the nephrons. The variety of etiologic factors include *primary renal diseases,* such as acute glomerulonephritis and acute pyelonephritis, *systemic diseases,* such as disseminated lupus erythematosus and polyarteritis nodosa, and a variety of conditions which lead to a condition commonly known as *acute tubular necrosis* (ATN). ATN can follow major surgery, crush lesions, major trauma, incompatible blood transfusions, and septicemia. The causes of acute renal failure are summarized in Table 14-1.

**Pathophysiology** Acute renal failure results in specific pathophysiological changes and their clinical manifestations. Differences, however, occur between prerenal, postrenal, and intrarenal failure. In prerenal and postrenal failure, the pathophysiology is related to the initiating cause, while a variety of pathologies result in intrarenal failure. A discussion of all of these pathologies is not within the scope of this chapter. The pathophysiology associated with glomerulonephritis and pyelonephritis are discussed later in the chapter. The present discussion will be limited to those changes found in ATN, the most common cause of acute intrarenal failure. Regardless of the underlying pathophysiological changes, however, the effects on the patient and nursing care are applicable to all types of acute renal failure.

The specific pathophysiological changes that occur in ATN vary with the cause. During *renal ischemia,* the tubular cells are damaged from lack of oxygen and slough off, plugging the tubules. As a consequence of *transfusion reactions,* specifically those in which red blood cells are lysed, hemoglobin molecules accumulate in the renal tubules causing blackage, thus preventing adequate renal functioning. *Nephrotoxic substances* cause ATN by

**TABLE 14-1**
CAUSES OF ACUTE RENAL FAILURE

| Prerenal | Intrarenal | Postrenal |
|---|---|---|
| Renal artery obstruction | Acute tubular necrosis | Calculi |
| Embolus | Glomerulonephritis | Trauma |
| Thrombus | Incompatible blood | Tumors |
| Hypovolemia | transfusions | |
| Burns | Lupus erythematosus | |
| Cardiac insufficiency | Polyarteritis nodosa | |
| Hemorrhage | Pyelonephritis | |
| Septic shock | Septicemia | |

obstructing the intrarenal structures with crystals. Substances that can be toxic to the kidneys are many and include uricosuric drugs, cytotoxic drugs, sulfonamides, many antimicrobials, organic iodinated x-ray contrast media, some organic solvents, inorganic mercurials, massive doses of salicylates, and paraldehyde. On rare occasions, ATN develops spontaneously with no apparent etiological factor involved.

**E**ffects on the Patient   As tubular cells are damaged, many changes in renal functioning occur. These changes are most often reflected in a *decrease in urine output.* The patient usually has a drop in urine output to 50 to 150 ml in a 24-hour period. Occasionally, acute renal failure may occur without oliguria, and the initial sign is a rise in the blood urea nitrogen.

Investigations into the cause of this decrease in renal functioning have suggested two mechanisms by which oliguria develops.[3] In the first, the production and drainage of urine is physically obstructed by sloughed cells, debris, or casts in the tubules. In the second mechanism, depicted in Fig. 14-1, the tubular damage results in a failure by the proximal tubule to conserve sodium. As sodium is lost in the urine, the renin-angiotensin system is activated. An increase in renin activates angiotensin, causing renal arterial vasoconstriction. The result is an increase in renal glomerular arteriolar resistance, a decrease in total renal blood flow with cortical ischemia, and a decrease in glomerular filtration. Urine production is therefore diminished.

The most profound effects of renal failure are manifested in *changes in fluid and electrolyte balance.* The changes follow a definite course which can be described in three phases. First is the *oliguric phase* which consists of that period of time during which the urinary output is below 400 ml in 24 hours. This phase usually lasts from 8 to 14 days. The longer it lasts, the poorer is the patient's prognosis. A relatively early sign of the oliguric phase is *hyponatremia,* which results from the inability of the tubules to conserve sodium. More sodium than water is lost and a hypotonic syndrome results, characterized by excess body water. Besides water retention by the kidneys, excess water results from endogenous water production from oxidation and an initial excess intake by the patient.

The oliguric phase is also characterized by a retention of certain substances. *Hyperkalemia* develops as the obligatory potassium loss from the kidneys decreases. Moderate *hypermagnesemia* develops, but does not produce severe effects on

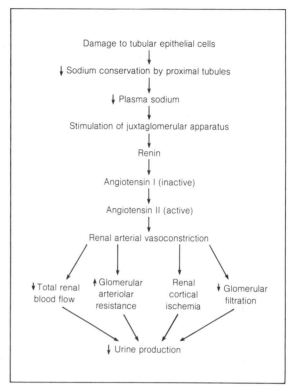

**FIGURE 14-1**
Pathophysiological changes associated with oliguria in acute tubular necrosis.

the patient. The kidneys are also unable to excrete hydrogen ions. *Metabolic acidosis* results from inadequate elimination of acids in the urine, an increase in ketonic acids as body fats are mobilized to combat the catabolism, exhaustion of the bicarbonate buffer ion, inadequate reabsorption of bicarbonate by the kidney, and the inability of the kidneys to acidify phosphate salts. A thorough discussion of the effects these fluid, electrolyte, and acid-base changes have on the patient can be found in Chap. 12, and the reader is encouraged to review that chapter for a better understanding of renal failure.

Besides these fluid and electrolyte changes, the *metabolic end products* (nitrogenous wastes) are retained. These include urea, creatinine, and uric acid, the end products of protein metabolism. As the plasma levels of these substances rise, changes in oxygenation, metabolism, the immune response, perception, and coordination result.

Following oliguria, the patient enters the *diuretic phase,* during which the kidney begins to recover and urine production increases. In the early period, however, while urinary output is above 400 ml in 24 hours, the urine may be hypotonic and the BUN will continue to rise or remain high for several days. In the late diuretic phase, the BUN begins to fall until it reaches a normal level. Elimination of magnesium, potassium, and acids also returns to normal, and fluid and electrolyte balance returns.

The final phase is the *recovery phase,* which begins when the BUN stabilizes at normal. During the recovery phase, the anemia, which will be discussed later, improves, but signs and symptoms may continue for 4 to 5 months before normal activities can be resumed.

The effects of renal failure on *oxygenation* are widespread. The excess body fluid during the oliguric phase can lead to circulatory overload. As renal failure progresses, anemia resulting from decreased erythropoietin production by the kidney develops in the second week. The hypervolemia and anemia lead to an increase in cardiac output and blood pressure, and in severe cases, to left ventricular failure. Bleeding disorders are not uncommon, and are usually related to a decrease in platelets. Lastly, the accumulation of nitrogenous wastes in the blood can produce pericarditis and pleuritis, compromising both circulation and respiration.

*Metabolic changes* related to the accumulation of urea and creatinine in the blood are the apparent causes of gastrointestinal disorders. Anorexia is very common in renal failure, and nausea, vomiting, diarrhea, and hiccups also occur. Gastrointestinal ulcers may complicate matters further.

*Changes in the immune system response* also occur. As renal failure develops, patients exhibit a decreased resistance to infection. In fact, infection is a frequent cause of death in these patients. Wound healing is decreased, and the frequency of pneumonia and cystitis is increased.

*The changes in perception and coordination* are related to the accumulation of urea and creatinine in the blood. As they accumulate in the blood, they interfere with the central nervous system and peripheral nerves. The patient may become confused, anxious, irritable, agitated, and may have bad dreams or hallucinate. As toxic substances increase, the patient may progress from muscle twitching (asterixis) to seizures and, finally, coma.

**First-level nursing care** Prevention of acute renal failure in the community setting involves the careful monitoring of high-risk patients with diseases in which renal failure is a potential complication. Patients with diabetes mellitus, hypertension,

and lupus erythematosus, for example, need to be followed carefully and regularly so that control of disease progression can be minimized and complications can be prevented. Nurses in clinics and physician's offices need to teach and encourage patients to carry out treatments related to their disease and to be alert for changes that may indicate progression of the pathology and possible complications.

The industrial nurse is able to prevent renal problems in several ways. Employees with chronic diseases should be encouraged to maintain prescribed treatment and to report changes that may indicate beginning complications. Referral to the physician for prompt treatment may result in the prevention of tissue damage. For example, prompt treatment of the diabetic patient who has influenza may bring about rapid adjustment of metabolic complications which could compromise functioning renal tissue. The industrial nurse can prevent renal failure associated with severe trauma or chemical intoxication through the establishment and management of accident prevention programs. As recently as November 1974, 15 of 41 people employed at a drug company in Tennessee were treated for acute renal failure associated with carbon tetrachloride poisoning.[4]

In the hospital setting, prevention of acute renal failure is accomplished by careful monitoring of the fluid and electrolyte status of trauma patients, by the prompt recognition and treatment of patients with hypovolemia, and careful follow-up on surgical patients with high-risk chronic diseases. With swift intervention when fluid and electrolyte changes occur, the prevention of renal complications is possible. Table 14-2 summarizes populations at risk and interventions that can prevent acute renal failure.

**Second-level nursing care** Acute renal failure is less often seen in a community setting because its pathogenesis often involves an acute condition that will have required hospitalization—hypovolemia, shock, and conditions necessitating transfusions. An alert nurse working in a community setting, however, can be instrumental in the early identification of renal failure associated with nephrotoxic substances so that the patient can be referred for appropriate care.

**Nursing Assessment** An accurate and detailed nursing assessment will ensure a general data base upon which the patient can be evaluated. Patients may seek help because they notice changes in their urine output. During the *health history,* the patient may relate a decrease in urination or note that urine output does not increase with increased fluid intake. The patient should be carefully questioned about any drugs taken in the recent past. Recent diagnostic tests, especially those involving contrast media, should be explored. Lastly, the patient's employment should be discussed, and any chemicals the patient may have been exposed to should be noted.

*Physical assessment* of the patient first developing renal failure will not be remarkable. Depending on the patient's intake, some fluid retention may be elicited early. Dependent locations should be palpated for edema. At this early stage, a general inspection will not reveal noticeable changes. Breath sounds and heart sounds will be normal in the absence of concomitant disease. The heartbeat may be increased and bounding, and peripheral pulses, also, may be bounding. The abdominal examination will be essentially normal, although pain at the costal-vertebral margin may be indicative of active kidney infection. The neurological evaluation will also be unchanged.

*Diagnostic tests* Perhaps invaluable in early identification of renal failure are the diagnostic tests which provide information on subtle changes that are difficult to elicit through the health history and physical assessment. The routine *urinalysis* gives a number of measurements related to the integrity of functioning renal tissue. The *urine specific gravity* is a measurement of urine concentration. The normal range for specific gravity, 1.010 to 1.025, fluctuates daily as the fluid intake is increased and decreased, thus reflecting the ability of the kidney to produce either concentrated or dilute urine. In most renal diseases, the concentrating ability of the kidneys is decreased and a small urine output of fixed specific gravity is produced. During acute renal failure, the nurse is often responsible for the collection and testing of hourly urine specimens for specific gravity. The specimen should be fresh, the cylinder and urinometer should be clean and checked against distilled water for accuracy, and the nurse should carefully read the scale at eye level. Accuracy in carrying out the test is essential.

Other abnormal substances found on urinalysis may indicate changes compatible with acute renal

**TABLE 14-2**
PREVENTION OF ACUTE RENAL FAILURE

| Clinical Setting | Predisposing Factors | Preventive Measures |
|---|---|---|
| *Diagnostic radiology* | | |
| Cholecystographic examination | Advanced age, nephrosclerosis, jaundice, repeat examinations with double dose | Avoidance of dehydration, proper spacing of procedures |
| Renal angiography | Nephrosclerosis and hypertension, renal insufficiency | Limitation of amount of contrast material |
| *Surgical procedures* | | |
| Aortic surgical treatment | Cross clamping of aorta, cholesterol emboli | Correction of hypovolemia, measures prior to, |
| Open-heart surgical treatment | Excess hemodialysis with extracorporeal circulation, hypovolemia from surgical trauma and blood loss | during, and after surgical treatment with maintenance of adequate urine output, careful typing and cross matching of transfusions |
| Biliary surgical treatment | Obstructive jaundice, poor hepatic function | |
| *Pregnancy* | | |
| Abortions | Infections, hypovolemia, and nephrotoxic abortifacients | Adequate antibiotics, early radical hysterectomy |
| Toxemia | Disseminated intravascular coagulation | Heparinization |
| Pre- and postpartum hemorrhage | Abruptio placentae, placenta previa | Early recognition of hemorrhage and adequate transfusion of blood |
| *Pigment release* | | |
| Transfusion reactions | Renal ischemia: anesthesia, surgical treatment, dehydration, hypovolemia | Careful major and minor cross matching, early diagnosis of reaction |
| Intravascular hemolysis | Paroxysmal cold hemaglobinuria, glucose-6-phosphate dehydrogenase deficiency | Early diagnosis and recognition |
| Myoglobinuria | Predisposing muscle disorder, excessive exertion with poor physical condition, tissue trauma | |
| *Proteinuric states* | | |
| Nephrotic syndrome | Dehydration, hypotension | Adequate hydration and prevention of hypovolemia and adequate urine volume |
| Multiple myeloma | Dehydration with use of radiographic contrast media | |
| Dysproteinemias | | |
| Low-molecular-weight dextran | Nephrosclerosis | |

SOURCE: M. H. Maxwell and C. R. Kleeman, *Clinical Disorders of Fluid and Electrolyte Metabolism,* McGraw-Hill, New York, 1972.

failure. *Protein,* not found normally, is present when albumin is lost through deteriorating nephrons. The presence of *white blood cells* and *bacteria* may result from a urinary tract infection involving renal tissue. During renal failure associated with blood transfusions, drug toxicities, and crush injuries, *red blood cells* are present. Since accuracy in identifying these substances is increased when fresh urine specimens are examined, a major responsibility of the nurse is the prompt collection and delivery of specimens.

The most common blood test used to identify early renal failure is the *blood urea nitrogen.* The BUN is the major nitrogenous waste produced during metabolism. It rises steadily during acute renal failure, and then falls gradually as renal functioning returns to normal. Since the BUN may be elevated by other factors, for example, increased protein intake, dehydration, and fever, other measurements are done to substantiate the presence of renal failure. The serum *creatinine,* a normal end product of metabolism, rises rapidly during renal failure and is less influenced by nonrenal factors. *Uric acid,* an end product of purine metabolism, increases as renal damage occurs. Electrolyte levels also change during renal failure and are monitored frequently to detect early imbalances. Serum *sodium* levels fall initially as the sodium conservation mechanisms of the kidney are lost. *Calcium* levels are decreased as a result of the increases in serum *phosphorus.* Decreased renal elimination leads to increases in *sulfate, phosphate, potassium,* and *magnesium.* Among these, potassium elevation is the most serious and can result in cardiac abnormalities. *Serum glucose, lipids,* and *cholesterol* levels rise as urinary elimination deteriorates. Since these blood tests involve a simple blood sample from the patient, nursing responsibilities include the prompt reporting of abnormal test results to the physician so that early treatment may be initiated.

**N**ursing Problems and Interventions  Whenever acute renal failure is suspected, the patient should be immediately referred for medical evaluation and appropriate care. Acute renal failure is a serious condition which will require immediate hospitalization. At this stage of the disturbance, nursing problems are not dealt with in the community.

**Third-level nursing care**  In the hospital the patient with acute renal failure will require intense and effective nursing care. A thorough nursing assessment should be done, problems identified, and nursing care planned that will minimize damage during the acute phase.

**N**ursing Assessment  The *health history* during third-level nursing care will be similar to that in second level. The hospitalized patient, however, may reveal significant information in relation to the cause of the failure. This may include a previous history of hypovolemia, shock, trauma, antibiotic therapy, infection, renal calculi, or systemic disease.

When acute renal failure is well established, *physical assessment* reveals significant changes. General inspection of the patient will generally show fluid overload, as evidenced by distention of the neck veins, edema, puffy eyelids, and weight gain. The skin will be pale or slightly yellow because of the accumulation of urochrome in the tissue. Urochrome is derived from urobilin and is the substance that gives urine its characteristic color. Bruises may be present if the platelets are diminished. Vital signs may reveal on elevated blood pressure, an increased and bounding pulse, and some shortness of breath. Breath sounds may include moist rales, and if fluid overload is severe, frothy sputum may be present.

When metabolic acidosis develops, Kussmaul breathing begins as the patient tries to compensate by eliminating carbon dioxide (see Chap. 12). The presence of excessive serum potassium may depress cardiac activity and produce sinus bradycardia and, eventually, sinus arrest. The abdominal examination will be generally normal.

The neurological examination often shows various degrees of disturbance depending on the extent of specific imbalances. If hyponatremia is present, mental confusion may result. When hyperkalemia is present and severe, the patient may become confused and anxious and exhibit muscular weakness and paralysis. With metabolic acidosis, anorexia and weakness may occur, and if untreated, the patient may become apathetic, with decreased consciousness and eventual coma. In hypocalcemia, muscle twitching occurs. A positive Chvostek's sign may be elicited even when other indications of calcium deficiency are not apparent (see Chap. 12). As hypocalcemia increases, tetany and convulsions may occur. The patient in acute renal failure may develop any of a variety of electrolyte imbalances. Complete nursing assessment in relation to these imbalances is discussed in Chap. 12.

*Diagnostic tests*  While physical assessment demonstrates a wide range of changes, diagnostic tests remain invaluable in adequately evaluating the patient's renal function. When renal failure is well established, the laboratory tests discussed in second-level nursing care will reveal a more severe degree of failure. Renal function tests may also be used to adequately assess the patient and to determine the amount of renal damage present following the acute period.

The *glomerular filtration rate* (GFR) measures renal functioning by identifying the rate at which known substances are filtered by the glomeruli and eliminated in the urine. The methods used are tests of clearance, referring to the volume of plasma that is completely "cleared" of a substance in a given unit of time. *Clearance tests* involve the injection of a specified amount of a substance, such as inulin, urea, or mannitol, that is eliminated by the normal kidney at a known rate. Samples of both serum and urine are collected at intervals and examined for their content of the injected substance. The degree of change from normal is identified, and the GFR is then calculated. In acute renal failure, damage to the kidneys is indicated by a decrease in clearance rates and decreased GFR. Nursing responsibilities for patients undergoing clearance tests include explaining the procedure to the patient and collecting the timed urine and blood specimens. Accurate labeling of each specimen is of prime importance in carrying out the tests, and is often the responsibility of the nurse who collects the specimens and sends them to the laboratory.

*Renal blood flow* can be evaluated by aortography, which involves the injection of a radiopaque dye into the aorta followed by a series of kidney x-rays. Visualization of kidney circulation can reveal obstructive prerenal failure from cysts, tumors, and renal artery thrombosis. During and following the examination, the patient should be observed for allergic responses, especially if the dye used contains iodine. The site of injection should be checked for local redness or swelling, since the dye can leak into the surrounding tissues and cause local inflammation.

The *phenolsulfonphthalein test,* commonly called the PSP test, is used to determine the rate and amount of blood flow to the kidneys, the integrity of tubular functioning, and the patency of the urinary tract. Injection of a specified amount of the PSP dye is followed by the collection of urine specimens precisely at 15, 30, 60, and 120 minutes after dye injection. The specimens are then analyzed for the presence of dye. Nursing responsibilities include explaining to the patient the nature of the procedure and the importance of adequate water ingestion before the dye is injected. This ingestion of water is necessary so that enough urine will be produced to provide specimens at precisely the times needed.

An additional diagnostic test used in acute renal failure is the *electrocardiogram* (ECG), which reflects the electrical activity of the heart. During acute renal failure, as serum potassium levels rise, specific EKG changes include a prolonged PR interval, initially, tall and peaked T waves, a prolonged QRS segment, and, eventually cardiac arrest. Patients in impending renal failure should have cardiac monitors so that rising potassium levels can be detected and treated early. The nurse should report pertinent abnormalities swiftly so that prevention and prompt treatment of electrolyte abnormalities can take place.

**N**ursing Problems and Interventions   Both nursing assessment and diagnostic test results will reveal a variety of nursing problems in the hospitalized patient with acute renal failure. Fluid and electrolyte problems are profound and successful nursing interventions may be life-saving.

*Fluid excess* occurs rapidly from the inability of the kidneys to produce urine and can lead to edema and congestive heart failure if untreated. Fluid restriction is used to decrease the intake of fluid and may be limited to 500 ml/day. Stimulation of urinary output may be carried out by injection of 25% mannitol, which acts as an osmotic diuretic stimulating the formation of large amounts of urine if any functioning renal tubules are present. Given soon after the onset of oliguria, this diuresis may be effective in "unplugging" the renal tubules and reversing renal failure. Because fluid excess can occur rapidly, continuous evaluation is needed for replacement and restriction of fluids. Accurate intake and output records provide an excellent means of recognizing the onset of fluid volume overload. To increase the accuracy of the information on these records the nurse should

1   Clearly identify patients on intake and output at the bedside, in the nurses' station, and in the utility room

2   Post charts of the capacity in milliliters of common containers within view of charting areas

3   Involve the patient in recording intake and output

4   Calculate for the appropriate inclusion or exclusion of ice in iced drinks, depending on patient consumption

5   Include fluid loss from all body sources by noting stool number and consistency, respiratory secretions, and perspiration

The life of the patient in acute renal failure is so dependent on the regulation of fluid and electrolyte balance that the accuracy of the intake and output records cannot be overemphasized. As urinary output is being evaluated, the specific gravity should be checked every hour or as frequently as possible depending on available specimens. Daily body weights can reveal even small gains in fluid balance, since rapid changes in body weight reflect changes in body fluid rather than changes in muscle and fatty tissue. The patient should be weighed at the same time each day with the same clothing and using the same scale.

Careful monitoring of changes in vital signs and an increase in central venous pressure can be used to detect early evidence of circulatory overload. Increases in pulse rate and venous pressure, shortness of breath, distention of neck veins, and a rising blood pressure need to be reported quickly. Although rare, pulmonary edema may occur with extreme shortness of breath, necessitating emergency treatment (see Chap. 24). Fluid restrictions will be ordered by the physician, with the distribution of the specific amounts determined by the nurse. Both intravenous and oral medications, as well as the patient's fluid desires throughout the day, should be taken into consideration when distributing the ordered fluid intake. Because of potential damage, care must be taken to avoid the use of diuretics in patients with renal impairment. By careful evaluation and management of the patient, complications of fluid excess can be detected and prevented by the nurse.

*Hyponatremia* in the patient with acute renal failure is associated with failure of the kidney to conserve sodium, as well as the dilution of body sodium by fluid excess. Correction of low serum sodium is managed generally by restriction of fluid intake. Sodium replacement is usually avoided because it promotes additional water retention and can precipitate congestive heart failure. The patient should be watched for additional losses of sodium through vomiting, diarrhea, or increases in urine output. As sodium levels drop below normal, further losses can precipitate signs of sodium deficit. Indications of severe hyponatremia, such as apathy, apprehension, anorexia, or abdominal cramps, should be reported. Serum sodium levels should be monitored daily and abnormalities reported.

The most serious of the electrolyte imbalances that occurs with acute renal failure is *hyperkalemia.* The smaller the urine output, the greater is the danger of potassium excess. The nurse should watch the patient carefully for signs of increased restlessness, anxiety, muscular weakness, and flaccid paralysis. The patient needs cardiac monitoring and should be watched for decreases in pulse rate and sinus bradycardia. Reflections of hyperkalemia include an initial prolonged PR interval, tall and peaked T waves, a prolonged QRS, and finally cardiac standstill. The nurse must be alert to these changes and ready to report them promptly and initiate cardiopulmonary resuscitation should standstill occur. To prevent potentially lethal cardiac changes, potassium intake should be carefully controlled by potassium-free intravenous solutions, medications that do not contain potassium, and dietary restriction. Potassium-rich foods, such as meats, legumes, milk, fresh fruits, fruit juices, coffee, and tea are often eliminated.

If hyperkalemia is severe, potassium output may be improved by the administration of ion-exchange resins. These pick up potassium ions in exchange for sodium ions in the gastrointestinal tract, thus improving both hyperkalemia and hyponatremia. During administration of this medication, the nurse should assess the patient for symptoms of increasing sodium levels and fluid retention, and report any positive findings. Short-term and rapid correction of dangerously rising potassium levels may be accomplished by several methods: (1) the administration of concentrated glucose with insulin to drive serum potassium into the cells, (2) the use of calcium to counteract the effects of potassium on the heart, and (3) the administration of sodium bicarbonate to increase the plasma pH, which in turn causes potassium to move into the cells. Long-range correction of potassium excess is accomplished either by peritoneal dialysis or hemodialysis. The complex care of patients undergoing dialysis is elaborated below. Hyperkalemia presents a life-threatening situation for the patient in acute renal failure, and the continuous monitoring of the patient for signs and symptoms requires carefully planned nursing care. This may be best accomplished in an intensive-care environment where the equipment for monitoring and treating the patient is readily available.

*Metabolic acidosis,* which occurs because of the failure of the kidney to excrete metabolically produced acids, may be first detected by the nurse while checking the patient's vital signs. Increased depth and rate of respiration will occur as the lung attempts to compensate for the increased metabolic acids by eliminating more carbon dioxide. This compensatory mechanism may partially correct the patient's pH. Additional signs and symptoms of metabolic acidosis include weakness, anorexia, apathy, and eventual coma; therefore, nursing care includes watching for changes in consciousness and physical strength. Patients whose status is changing rapidly need to be protected from any accidental injury.

A less common electrolyte imbalance is *hypocalcemia,* which generally occurs with *hyperphosphatemia.* Excess phosphorus is normally excreted by the kidneys, but as they fail, phosphorus accumulates. The increase of serum phosphorus decreases the serum calcium because of the reciprocal relationship between these electrolytes. Despite the calcium deficit, the patient in acute renal failure may not show signs of tetany because the metabolic acidosis present increases the ionization of available calcium. However, if the acidosis is corrected with alkaline fluids, calcium ions will be decreased and muscle twitching, tetany, and convulsions can occur. The nurse can detect early signs of calcium deficit by checking serum calcium levels and watching for neuromuscular irritability. Chvostek's sign involves tapping the facial nerve just anterior to the external auditory meatus. Contraction of the facial muscle is a positive sign which indicates hypocalcemia and impending tetany and should be reported promptly. Lowered serum calcium also increases the effects of hyperkalemia on the heart muscle, and can increase cardiac arrhythmias. As the calcium deficit is treated with calcium gluconate by the oral or intravenous route, the patient should be closely observed. Desired results may become apparent immediately through improvement in the electrocardiogram.

The mechanisms for oxygenating the body tissues is compromised in acute renal failure for several reasons. Fluid excess may lead to *hypertension* which can result in a cerebrovascular accident if untreated. The patient's blood pressure should be monitored regularly, and increases higher than previous readings reported. Treatment with fluid restriction, dialysis, and drugs is used to prevent complications. *Respiratory congestion* occurs as the fluid overload accumulates in the pulmonary vessels, interfering with the passage of oxygen from the lungs into the bloodstream. Until the fluid overload is corrected, oxygen is administered, and turning, coughing, and deep breathing become more vigorous to reduce the chances of pneumonia. A chest X-ray is often done to evaluate respiratory status.

Without the hormone erythropoietin from the kidney, fewer red blood cells and platelets are produced, and the patient becomes *anemic.* Decreased red blood cells diminish the oxygen delivered to cells, and if the anemia is severe enough, oxygen and transfusions may be required. Packed cells are often used to avoid adding to fluid overload. The nurse should administer the blood slowly over approximately 4 hours (or as specified), watching for signs and symptoms of blood reactions and fluid overload. *Bleeding problems* are associated with a decrease in platelet production as well as decreased serum calcium levels. Without platelets there is excessive bleeding from injuries, and if levels are low enough, spontaneous bleeding in the gastrointestinal tract and in subcutaneous tissue may occur. If the patient has acute renal failure precipitated by massive surgery or trauma, disseminated intravascular coagulation (DIC) may result (see Chap. 28). The nurse needs to carefully inspect the patient's skin for any bruises and monitor the urine and stool for visable and occult blood. Both should be routinely tested with a disposable hemastick. Bleeding after intramuscular injections is common and indicates the need for using small gauge needles and applying direct pressure after injections. Blood needed for laboratory tests should be obtained using as small a needle as possible and with minimal vein trauma. Careful observation and gentle handling of patients will decrease tissue oxygenation problems.

Patients with acute renal failure may develop *infections* which can be fatal. Pneumonia, as mentioned earlier, is not uncommon. Wound infections may also develop and may be prevented by scrupulous aseptic technique and daily inspection. Since cystitis commonly occurs, catheterization of the patient should be avoided. However, accurate urine measurement is essential and may require catheterization. Maintaining a closed drainage system with daily catheter care should be implemented to assist in minimizing the development of urinary tract infections. Treatment of infections is accomplished through the cautious use of antibiotics, as the accumulation of these toxic substances in the bloodstream will cause further damage to renal tissue and must be avoided.

Metabolic changes occurring during acute renal failure are associated with *catabolism* from the inflammatory process and urinary protein losses from the deteriorating renal tissue. As proteins are metabolized, a persistent *azotemia* develops. To counteract these changes, protein, calories, and electrolytes are carefully regulated. Protein intake is restricted to that amount needed to meet daily requirements and yet prevent further accumulation of nitrogenous wastes. The amount of protein allowed depends on the amount of renal failure, the activity of the patient, the presence of healing wounds, and the basal protein needs. Restriction may vary from 10 to 40 g/day and on occasion may be eliminated altogether. The provision of adequate calories is necessary to prevent the use of body protein and fat for energy.

Dietary restrictions may result in limited choices of food for the patient, and coupled with the patient's *nausea, vomiting, anorexia,* and *gastrointestinal bleeding,* present a difficult challenge to the nurse. Initiation of a diet history is needed to identify the patient's food likes and dislikes. Preparation of an appropriate environment at mealtimes can include removing unnecessary equipment from the patient's room and allowing family members to be present and assist the patient. Helping the patient at mealtime is a high priority in planning care.

Small frequent meals may produce adequate intake despite the presence of nausea. Exceptions to the elimination of potassium-containing foods may be considered as food intake drops. For example, milk shakes may be allowed even though they are high in potassium, if they are the only source of potassium for the patient. Consultation with the dietitian is invaluable in planning the patient's meals. Evaluation of the patient's metabolic problems involves checking the patient's daily weight, recording dietary intake, checking the patient's skin for breakdown, and watching laboratory results for acidosis, nitrogenous wastes, and electrolyte levels.

Toxic levels of accumulating urea and creatinine can cause *drowsiness* and *agitation* and lead to further *neuromuscular irritability.* The patient may become confused, anxious, and complain of nightmares. Uremic symptoms occur, as demonstrated by muscular twitching, hallucinations, and convulsions. In order to prevent these symptoms, the nurse needs to observe the patient regularly and report changes that indicate an increase in neuromuscular irritability. If drowsiness and anxiety increase, the nurse may request additional laboratory measurements to follow the increase in BUN. A fairly early indication of irritability is the "restless leg symptom,"[5] wherein the patient continues to move both legs and is unable to lie still. Transfer to the intensive care unit is needed when increasing neuromuscular irritability points to the need for continuous surveillance. If seizures become imminent, the patient's bed should be padded with extra pillows and the nurse should prepare for the administration of diazepam.

Changes in the skin are associated with the accumulation of urea, creatinine, and uric acid. Paleness occurs from anemia and a yellowish tinge from the deposition of urochrome is apparent. The skin color differs from jaundice in that it does not occur in the sclera and because it stains the washcloth when the skin is washed. These skin changes cause severe *pruritus* and *skin breakdown.* Itching may be relieved by vinegar and water or by topical lotions. Benadryl may be ordered by the physician. Daily hygiene is essential and may be needed even more frequently, depending on the condition of the patient's skin and the presence of an elevated temperature which increases perspiration. Careful inspection, a plan for regular turning, and protecting body prominences with soft fabric are essential nursing interventions.

As the patient's physical needs are being met, *psychosocial aspects* of care should not be overlooked. The onset of acute renal failure is a frightening experience for both the patient and family. Frequent explanations and reassurances should be offered, and involving the family in patient care will foster support systems for all involved. The patient should be encouraged to verbalize feelings and anxieties throughout the illness.

**D**ialysis   An effective treatment used to reverse the symptoms of acute renal failure is dialysis. Through this process removal of excess potassium, urea, uric acid, creatinine, and body water can be readily accomplished. Dialysis is a physical procedure which involves the differential *diffusion* of substances across a semipermeable membrane which separates two fluid compartments containing substances of different concentrations.[6] A pressure gradient is produced, resulting in the diffusion of substances to the less concentrated compartment. This diffusion continues until equilibration is achieved (see Fig. 14-2).

Osmosis and filtration may also occur during dialysis. *Osmosis* is the movement of solvent or fluid across a semipermeable membrane, and during dialysis it permits either drainage of excess body fluids or administration of needed body fluid supplements. The direction of flow will depend on the patient's fluid and electrolyte status and the contents of the dialysate. *Filtration* is the movement of both fluid (solvent) and dissolved substances (solute) across a semipermeable membrane under force. If hydrostatic pressure is increased on one side of the membrane used for dialysis, fluid and dissolved substances are driven into the opposite compartment.

Two methods of dialysis are available—peritoneal dialysis and hemodialysis. Peritoneal dialysis is most frequently used in acute renal failure and will be discussed here. Hemodialysis involves the use of the artificial kidney and is generally used when chronic dialysis is required. It will be discussed in the section on chronic renal failure.

*Peritoneal dialysis* In *peritoneal,* or intracorporeal, *dialysis,* a dialysate solution is introduced into the peritoneal cavity where it remains for a period of time before being drained out. The peritoneal lining itself acts as a semipermeable membrane, allowing substances in high concentration to move out of the bloodstream and into the dialysate solution in the peritoneal cavity. Because it involves a safe technique, rapidly learned by personnel and available to almost all hospital situations, peritoneal dialysis is used frequently for acute renal failure.

The dialysate solution used during peritoneal dialysis contains sodium, potassium, chloride, calcium, magnesium, lactate, and glucose in amounts needed to produce an osmolality above that of body tissues. This increased tonicity promotes the loss of excessive body water. Commercially prepared dialysate solutions generally come in 1.5, 4.25, and 7% glucose solutions, and are selected for use depend-

ing on the patient's total body water balance. Higher concentrations are used to promote loss of excess body water and lower concentrations to prevent loss of body water.

The patient is frequently uncomfortable from the toxic effects of renal failure and may welcome the institution of dialysis. The nurse should explain the procedure to the patient in order to decrease unwarranted fears and establish patient cooperation. Baseline information will include body temperature, vital signs, blood electrolyte levels, weight, and cardiac monitoring. After the consent form is signed, the patient should empty the bladder. A sedative will then be administered. Following local anesthesia, the physician introduces the trochar and inserts the multiple-holed catheter into the pelvic gutter (Fig. 14-3). A purse-string suture and dressings are used to secure and pad the catheter as it leaves the abdomen. The catheter is connected by tubing to the dialysate containers and the collecting containers (Fig. 14-3). By use of clamps on the lines to and from the abdominal catheter, the direction of fluid flow can be maintained.

**FIGURE 14-2**
Dialysis process.

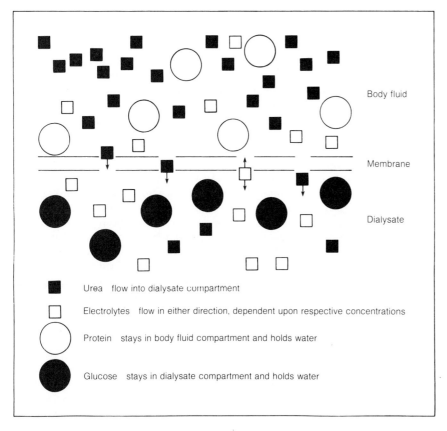

Urea   flow into dialysate compartment

Electrolytes   flow in either direction, dependent upon respective concentrations

Protein   stays in body fluid compartment and holds water

Glucose   stays in dialysate compartment and holds water

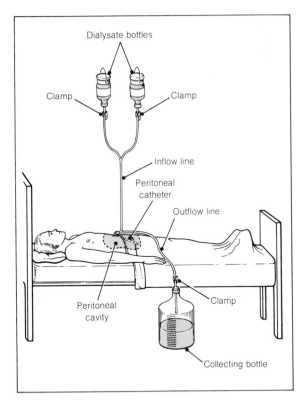

**FIGURE 14-3**
Set-up for peritoneal dialysis.

The nurse should administer the dialysate fluid at body temperature, which allows for the most efficient exchange of substances and limits peritoneal discomfort. The dialyzing solution should be allowed to run in over a period of 10 to 15 minutes. The tubing is then clamped and the solution allowed to remain in the abdominal cavity for 30 to 60 minutes. The indwelling period must be prescribed by the physician according to individual patient needs. The fluid is then allowed to drain out of the abdominal cavity. The amount of fluid to be drained out is also determined by the physician, and should be carefully monitored by the nurse. Often only 200 ml in excess of the dialysis fluid is removed with each cycle, since additional amounts can cause hypovolemia. Drainage may continue over a period of 20 minutes. It is often helpful to change the patient's position in order to foster drainage. When drainage is completed, the next cycle of dialysate fluid is begun. Dialysis exchanges continue for 36 to 48 hours, depending on the individual patient situation. Longer periods are not used because of the danger of introducing infection.

*Nursing responsibilities* during peritoneal dialysis involve monitoring and evaluating the patient's responses. Vital signs should be checked every 15 minutes for the first hour and then hourly to determine whether excessive fluid loss or fluid overload is occurring. At the start of each indwelling and drainage period, the patient's tubing should be checked for kinks and the catheter checked for position and leakage.

Precise *dialysis records* are a major nursing responsibility, and should identify the amount of fluid administered, the amount drained on each cycle, and a calculation of the patient's fluid balance. The physician's order must state whether drainage should equal the amount instilled or be a specified amount below and/or above that amount. The overall limits for accumulated excesses and deficits should also be stated, and the physician notified of exceptions. Table 14-3 gives an example of an intake and output record used for peritoneal dialysis fluid balance calculations.

The drainage fluid may be pink tinged initially as a result of bleeding associated with catheter insertion. After the first few exchanges, however, it should be clear and straw colored. If bleeding persists or becomes visible, it should be reported. Heparin may be administered in the first few bottles to prevent clotting and clogging of the catheter.

Nursing care should be administered during the drainage periods, as patients are often more comfortable during these periods and able to move about more. Eating is easier during drainage periods and the patient's daily weight should be taken at the end of a drainage period. Regular skin care, oral hygiene, position changes, and coughing and deep breathing to prevent pulmonary complications are part of the needed routine care.

To minimize *infections,* sterile techniques should be used when caring for the patient's abdominal catheter. Evaluation of nursing procedures should be instituted to prevent any other contamination. For example, if the bottles of dialysate are warmed in a water bath, they should be dried before hanging to prevent contaminated fluid from the outside of the bottle from running down the tube and into the peritoneal catheter opening.[7] The patient should be placed in a chair and ambulated as equipment permits.

The head of the bed may be elevated to minimize pressure on the diaphragm and allow for adequate lung expansion, thus preventing atelectasis and pneumonia. Prolonged and unrelieved pressure on the diaphragm can lead to respiratory arrest. *Abdominal discomfort* and *fullness* are the most frequent patient complaints and are minimized by warming the fluid and decreasing the rate of administration. Abdominal pain accompanied by abdominal tenderness, an elevated temperature, or cloudiness of the drainage fluid must be reported immediately, as each may indicate a developing peritonitis. Treatment must be prompt and usually consists of the administration of antibiotics into the peritoneal cavity through the dialysis catheter.

Fluid imbalances can occur during dialysis, and include *fluid overload* and *dehydration.* The patient should be observed for the occurrence of either complication. Positive findings, especially if confirmed by trends in the fluid balance record, should be reported promptly. Rapid loss of body fluids into the peritoneal cavity and then out of the body can lead to a drop in fluid volume, blood pressure, and eventually shock. Signs of *hypernatremia* and *hyperglycemia* (from the glucose in the dialysate solution) can occur, and can be detected and treated early through careful monitoring of the patient and reporting of abnormal electrolyte and glucose laboratory determinations.

In addition to the information on the dialysis record, charting should include the total number of exchanges, any added medications, and vital signs, weight, catheter site and dressing condition, and the presence of abdominal and respiratory symptoms. Patient observations should continue hourly following dialysis until a stable condition is apparent. The nurse caring for the patient undergoing peritoneal dialysis will be busy keeping the patient comfortable and well informed, and maintaining the system of dialysis exchanges, observations, and records. A recent development, a peritoneal dialysis machine, may assist the nurse in caring for this patient by automatically starting and stopping the administration and drainage times in the cycle. The results of peritoneal dialysis will be rewarding as the patient's fluid and electrolyte imbalances are corrected and progress to recovery becomes evident.

**D**iuretic Phase   As the patient responds to treatment and nursing care, and renal function begins to return, the diuretic phase begins. During this phase, which generally lasts 1 week, nursing care should focus on carefully monitoring the patient for indications of dehydration, sodium losses, and potassium losses. The recovering kidney is unable to selectively retain and secrete various substances. If the patient is given free access to water and sodium and is sufficiently recovered to be alert and able to swallow fluids independently, sodium and water regulation will generally occur through appropriate thirst signals and improving renal functioning. The nurse should be aware that potassium losses may be significant and often require replacement.

**Fourth-level nursing care**   For the recovery phase, the patient is often discharged from the hospital. It is extremely important in this phase to provide a long enough period of time for the recovery of renal tissue. At first, regulation of fluid and electrolyte balance may still be difficult, and frequent laboratory tests will be necessary to detect and prevent imbalances from occurring. The convalescent phase often lasts from 4 to 5 months. The nursing care needed includes support of medical follow-up, nursing support, and the prevention of complications and recurrences.

Medical follow-up includes regular evaluation of returning kidney functioning and regulation. The patient has few overt symptoms at this time and often needs *nursing support* and encouragement to continue seemingly unneeded medical care. Encouragement to keep medical appointments may be necessary. Referral to a home care nursing agency should be made. Follow-up should focus on dietary instruction with application to the home situation, monitoring of the blood pressure and other signs indicative of complications, and the need to plan for physical rest and emotional support for the patient and family.

*Preventing the recurrence* of acute renal failure is related to the initial cause of the failure, whether prerenal, postrenal, or intrarenal. Prevention of infections is necessary for all patients who have had an episode of acute renal failure. This

**TABLE 14-3**
PERITONEAL DIALYSIS RECORD

| Exchange Number | Time Infused | | Time Drained | | Volume | | Balance (+ or −) | Cumulative Balance | Dialysate | Comments |
|---|---|---|---|---|---|---|---|---|---|---|
| | Start | Stop | Start | Stop | In | Out | | | | |
| 1 | 9:00 | 9:10 | 9:40 | 10:00 | 2000 | 1800 | −200 | −200 | | |
| 2 | 10:00 | 10:10 | 10:40 | 11:00 | 2000 | 2200 | +200 | 0 | | |
| 3 | 11:00 | 11:10 | 11:40 | 12:00 | 2000 | 2100 | +100 | +100 | | |

may mean that the patient needs to stay away from crowds where exposure to pathogenic organisms would be high. Daily weight records should be kept so that the patient is able to evaluate whether or not fluids are being retained. If a special diet is prescribed, the preparation of the necessary foods should be clarified. The patient should be aware of signs and symptoms that are indicative of fluid or electrolyte imbalances and should be reported to a physician. Since it may be 4 to 5 months before the patient can return to work, financial difficulties may arise for the patient's family, and referral to the social service personnel would be appropriate.

### Chronic Renal Failure

Chronic renal failure is a progressively debilitating health problem resulting in irreversible damage to the parenchyma of the kidney. Because the onset is slow, the adaptive ability of kidney tissue forestalls symptoms of renal failure until 80 to 90 percent of the renal tissue is irreversibly damaged.[8] The *causes* of chronic renal failure have been classified into several groupings, and one such classification can be found in Table 14-4. The causes include both diseases which are primarily renal in nature, such as glomerulonephritis and nephrosclerosis, and those which originate elsewhere, such as diabetes mellitus and lupus erythematosus. Chronic renal failure is becoming a more prevalent problem as improvements in care result in earlier diagnosis. These improvements also make possible the maintenance of renal function and the successful substitution of diseased kidneys by chronic dialysis and kidney transplantation. Approximately 60,000 to 100,000 people die each year in the United States from primary chronic renal disease, and, of these patients, 6,000 to 20,000 are likely to be eligible for dialysis and transplantation.[9] Expansion of

**TABLE 14-4**
CAUSES OF CHRONIC RENAL FAILURE

| GLOMERULAR DISEASE | INTERSTITIAL NEPHRITIS |
|---|---|
| Glomerulonephritis, acute and chronic | Chronic hypercalcemia |
| Lupus erythematosus (systemic) | Chronic analgesic ingestion |
| Polyarteritis nordosa | Antibiotics, diuretics, and other drugs |
| Diabetes mellitus | Heavy metal poisoning |
| | Gout |
| VASCULAR DISEASE | |
| Hypertension | HEREDITARY DISEASE |
| Renal artery stenosis | Polycystic kidney disease |
| Nephrosclerosis | Familial amyloidosis |
| | Medullary cystic disease |
| INFECTIONS | |
| Pyelonephritis | OBSTRUCTIVE DISEASE |
| Tuberculosis | Calculi |
| | Tumors |

facilities and personnel to care for these patients is already beginning.

**Pathophysiology**  Changes in renal functioning are similar to those occurring in acute renal failure. A set of four stages is used to describe the gradual changes: diminished renal reserve, renal insufficiency, renal failure, and uremia. In *diminished renal reserve,* approximately 50 percent of the nephrons are destroyed or nonfunctional. Azotemia is not yet present, and the excretory and regulatory functions of the kidney are maintained. *Renal insufficiency* occurs when the patient begins to have nocturia associated with the loss of renal concentrating ability. Along with this loss, the patient experiences mild azotemia and may develop a mild anemia from decreased erythropoietin release. Stress on patients with renal insufficiency may precipitate the next stage, *renal failure.* This is a more serious stage, and electrolyte problems include a marked azotemia, acidosis, hyperphosphatemia, and hypocalcemia. Fluid problems include a decline in urine flow with a resultant water retention. Anemia is present all of the time. The fourth and final stage is the *uremic stage,* also referred to as end stage renal disease, during which the accumulation of nitrogenous wastes, urea, uric acid, and creatinine reaches levels dangerous to survival. Major water and electrolyte imbalances occur and threaten the patient's life. Without treatment the patient rapidly develops the additional complications of hypertension, gastrointestinal hemorrhage, central nervous system disorders evidenced by muscular twitching, tingling, and convulsions, and finally death.

**E**ffects on the Patient  *Fluid and electrolyte imbalances* are usually not evident until the third stage, renal failure, is present. Then imbalances are associated with changes in the regulation of body water, electrolytes, and body pH. *Water balance* is compromised in patients with chronic renal failure because, while the thirst mechanism and secretion of the antidiuretic hormone (ADH) is normal, the renal tissue fails to respond normally to ADH, and decreased urine concentration results. The urine osmolality parallels the osmolality of serum and does not change during periods of water ingestion or water deprivation. This causes the patient to be susceptible to both fluid deficit and fluid excess.

*Fluid deficit* can occur during abnormal decreases in the ingestion of water or excessive water losses. For example, an episode of nausea, vomiting, and diarrhea can cause rapid dehydration from the inability of the kidney to conserve needed body water. If the patient is well enough to walk around and respond to thirst, the ingestion of adequate water by mouth may compensate for the fluid loss.

*Fluid excess* occurs from excessive water intake. As functioning renal tissue is gradually lost, less and less urine is produced, even to the point of anuria. Ingestion of water may continue from habit rather than need, and produce overhydration. During hospitalization, patients may become overhydrated through attempts by personnel to provide adequate water. Fluid excess causes pump failure when the heart is no longer able to handle the excess fluid load. Water intoxication occurs when water is ingested without sodium and is not excreted by the kidneys. The serum sodium is diluted by the excess water, causing a drop in the serum sodium level. Overhydration is more common as the patient reaches end-stage renal disease.

In chronic renal failure, patients are prone to *sodium imbalances.* Since sodium conservation occurs primarily in the renal medulla, deterioration of this area produces excessive sodium loss and *hyponatremia* which lead to decreased extracellular fluid. As the circulating blood volume decreases, the glomerular filtration rate decreases and renal function is further compromised. Sodium excesses (*hypernatremia*) can occur in patients with end-stage renal disease when urine volume drops to very low levels. Then, even a restricted salt intake can produce retention of sodium and water with edema and pump failure.

The potassium imbalance most frequently encountered in chronic renal failure is potassium retention or *hyperkalemia.* Potassium levels rise rapidly as oliguria and anuria develop. Dangerous levels can occur rapidly when an increased metabolic rate releases more potassium.

Imbalances of calcium and phosphorus are related to the reciprocal relationship between these electrolytes (calcium is decreased when phosphorus is increased and vice versa). This relationship is affected by parathormone, which regulates the serum calcium levels. As the glomerular filtration rate decreases, the serum phosphorus level rises, producing *hyperphosphatemia.* This, in return, stimulates the secretion of parathormone. Normally, this would increase serum calcium levels. However, parathormone is ineffective in chronic renal failure and *hypocalcemia* results. Recently, it was demonstrated that the kidney produces an active metabolite of vitamin D, which is necessary for parathormone activity. Patients with chronic

renal failure have such low levels of active vitamin D that parathormone activity is ineffective.[10] It has also been found that bone is resistant to the action of parathormone in patients with chronic renal disease.[11] Therefore, these patients are apt to have hyperphosphatemia and hypocalcemia. The degree of hypocalcemia is rarely low enough to produce tetany, but may drop to those levels during the administration of alkali to treat acidosis.

A mild *hypermagnesemia* can occur when urine output is low and a normal magnesium intake continues. It may also be precipitated when magnesium-containing laxatives and antacids are administered.

The acid-base imbalance commonly found in the patient with chronic renal failure is *metabolic acidosis.* It occurs gradually and is dependent on the loss of a major proportion of nephrons. In the early stages functioning nephrons compensate for damaged nephrons and produce an increase in hydrogen ion excretion. As failure becomes more widespread, acid excretion is decreased, and metabolic acidosis occurs. The degree of acidosis is generally mild and the pH is rarely below 7.35. However, the acidosis can increase rapidly with an increase in production of body acids, as during fever or an increased intake of acid-producing foods.

The *accumulation of uremic toxins*—urea, uric acid, and creatinine—increases gradually throughout the first and second stages of chronic renal failure. In the third stage, the levels become toxic and may produce fatal neurological complications. Skin changes result from the deposition of urochrome pigments, and combined with anemia, produce a pale yellow skin tone. A crust of uric crystals, referred to as *uremic frost,* can accumulate on the skin. Pruritus is common and difficult to relieve, producing damage to the skin and resulting in infections because of uncontrolled scratching by the patient.

*Metabolic changes* in chronic renal failure occur primarily in the third and fourth stages and are a result of uremic toxins and gastrointestinal bleeding. The gastrointestinal tract is irritable and inflamed, resulting in *nausea, vomiting,* and *diarrhea,* which further complicate the fluid and electrolyte imbalances. *Gastrointestinal bleeding* is not uncommon. The rising accumulation of ammonia in the body produces the characteristic taste and odor in the patient's mouth. *Stomatitis* and *parotitis* occur, and an associated *pancreatitis* may further impair digestion.

*Changes in oxygenation* occur during the third and fourth stages. *Hypertension* is associated with increased extracellular fluid volume resulting from the inability of the kidneys to excrete excess fluid, as well as an increase in renin, which is produced by the damaged kidney. Renin stimulates aldosterone secretion with resulting salt and water retention. The accumulation of extracellular fluid volume can cause *pericarditis, cardiac tamponade, pleuritis,* and *congestive heart failure. Anemia* is caused by a decrease in the production of erythropoietin by the kidney. Patients also encounter *bleeding problems* as a result of a defect in platelet production by bone marrow. While the numbers of platelets produced may be normal, their effectiveness is decreased. Changes in blood coagulation occur and result in subcutaneous hemorrhage. There is a potential for profuse hemorrhage from any wound as the severity of uremia increases. Patients with untreated chronic renal failure often die of massive gastrointestinal hemorrhage.

*Changes in immunity* result in an increased occurrence of infections. Patients often experience delayed hypersensitivity to antigens and a prolonged survival of skin allografts.[12]

*Changes in perception and coordination* are caused by the accumulation of nephrotoxins. Initially the symptoms are mild and include irritability, emotional lability, insomnia, and a decrease in concentrating ability. As nephrotoxins accumulate, symptoms become more severe and include increased deep tendon reflexes, stupor, coma, convulsions, and eventual death. Peripheral neuropathy includes disturbances reflected in *numbness* and *paresthesias.* Changes in motor innervation to the extremities, such as foot drop, can also occur and can eventually result in quadriplegia. The central nervous system manifestations and the sensory neuropathy can be reversed, but the motor neuropathy is generally permanent.

**First-level nursing care** Prevention of chronic renal failure in the community setting involves the provision of adequate health care for patients with diseases that can cause renal damage—diabetes mellitus, lupus erythematosus, and acute rheumatic fever. Because various chemicals and medications can also lead to gradual and progressive kidney damage, nurses in all settings should become familiar with them (Table 14-5). Nurses in industrial settings should focus on safety programs needed for nephrotoxic chemicals, and nurses in office and clinic settings need to implement adequate health histories of drug therapy so that potential renal toxicity becomes evident. Patient instruction for prescribed medications should include informa-

tion about needed fluid intake with certain antibiotics and the dangers of saving a few pills to treat the next infection or other family members. The nurse's preventive role includes genetic counseling for parents with hereditary renal diseases. Families with such risks who participate in genetic counseling will need support and assistance during this difficult decision-making process. The risks should be explained and the nurse should act as a prime supporter.

Patients with frequent *urinary tract infections* are also at risk to the development of chronic renal failure from repeated kidney infections. The flow of urine makes the spread of an infection from the urinary tract to the kidney a real danger. *Cystitis,* infection of the bladder, is the most common of these infections and occurs more often in females; it is especially prevalent after sexual intercourse. Cystitis in males is often associated with prostatic hypertrophy and urinary retention.

Urinary tract infections often result from contamination from the large intestine. Prevention of these infections should focus on teaching proper perineal hygiene. Women especially, because of a short urethra and the proximity of the meatus to the anus, should be taught to always clean themselves by wiping from the front to the back. In this way, organisms from the anus will not be drawn to the meatus or vagina. A clean tissue should be used with each wipe. Cotton underwear will also help to absorb rectal secretions and prevent their sliding into the area of the meatus.

When urinary tract infection does develop, prompt treatment is imperative to prevent its spread to the kidney. The patient will often experience burning, especially on urination, frequency, urgency and low back pain. Fluids should be taken liberally and antibiotics are often utilized. Sitz baths may also be helpful in soothing the discomfort. If systemic manifestations such as fever, malaise, muscle aches, nausea, and/or vomiting develop, the possibility of kidney infection should immediately be explored. For patients with repeated urinary tract infections, an intravenous pyelogram is often done to assess renal damage.

**Second-level nursing care** Even though early indications of chronic renal failure are subtle and nonspecific, referral and prompt treatment are invaluable in minimizing destruction of renal tissue and may, indeed, reverse pathological changes.

**N**ursing Assessment A careful and detailed *health history* may reveal the need for more definitive evaluation of the patient. Gradually increasing fatigue and evidence of mild nocturia may be present. All changes in urination should be noted. Careful questioning may reveal a history of chronic exposure to nephrotoxic substances, urinary tract infections, or pyelonephritis. The most revealing aspects of the history may be the presence of other chronic diseases that can lead to renal failure. The *physical assessment* will reveal few, if any, symptoms. A mild weight gain and slight hypertension may be present. The chest, abdominal, and neurological examinations will be essentially normal.

*Diagnostic tests* may provide the earliest evidence of chronic renal failure and are of great importance in the community setting. A slight rise in the serum creatinine level may be present. A routine urinalysis can reveal the presence of albumin or red blood cells. One of the ways that has been suggested for early detection of renal failure is the establishment of community diagnostic centers where susceptible individuals can be tested for bacteriuria, hematuria, albuminuria, and renal calculi.[13]

**N**ursing Problems and Interventions  With positive identification of any of these signs, chronic renal failure may be suspected. At this point nursing problems are not dealt with on an outpatient basis, and the patient is usually referred to an acute care setting for a complete diagnostic work-up and early treatment.

**Third-level nursing care**  Because extensive renal damage may occur before difficulties arise, patients in the hospital with chronic renal failure may have variable symptoms. The stage of illness present may range from renal insufficiency to renal failure to uremia, or the patient may be in a stable form of end-stage renal disease on a chronic dialysis program.

**N**ursing Assessment  A careful *health history* of the hospitalized patient may reveal the same information as that indicated under second-level nursing care. Additional changes precipitating hospitalization may include a recent decrease or cessation of urine output and evidence of fluid retention. More dramatic events such as disorientation and convulsions may have occurred in the previously untreated patient who is first seen when uremia is well established. A careful history of other chronic diseases and exposure to industrial chemicals should be elicited.

The *physical assessment* may reveal few findings if the patient has renal insufficiency, while a striking picture may be evidenced if uremia is established. The more toxic patient will be irritable, thin but edematous, with pale yellow itchy skin. Bruises will be present. Hypertension will vary from mild to severe, and moist rales, dyspnea, and frothy sputum will occur with fluid volume excess. Evidence of retinal changes consistent with chronic hypertension may be present. The abdominal examination may reveal fluid retention, and the patient may complain of nausea and vomiting. The extremities will be edematous as the severity of fluid retention increases. The neurological examination will vary according to the toxicity of the patient and the presence of electrolyte imbalances. Muscular twitching may progress to tetany and convulsions. Slight confusion may progress to frightening hallucinations and complete disorientation.

*Diagnostic tests*  The severity of renal failure will be revealed by the results of the diagnostic tests. Serum values found in acute renal failure will be present and include elevated BUN, creatinine, and uric acid levels, as well as elevations in potassium, sodium, and magnesium. Azotemia will be marked when uremic symptoms are present. Metabolic acidosis may be revealed in blood gas analysis with a slightly lowered blood pH and a lowered carbon dioxide level. Urinalysis will reveal protein losses and may contain red blood cells and bacteria as well. Anemia will be apparent in a lowered red blood cell count. Clearance tests will show a steady decrease in glomerular filtration rate as the number of damaged nephrons increases. The *phenolsulfonphthalein test* will also reflect diminished renal function.

The *renogram* involves the intravenous injection of a radioactive substance followed by a recording of the uptake and excretion of the sub-

**TABLE 14-5**
NEPHROTOXIC CHEMICALS AND MEDICATIONS

| METALS | ANTIBIOTICS |
|---|---|
| Mercury | Penicillin |
| Arsenic | Neomycin |
| Gold | Kanamycin |
| Lead | Amphotericin |
| Copper | |
| Uranium | OTHER MEDICATIONS |
| Cadmium | Sulfonamides |
| | Salicylates |
| POISONS | Furosemide |
| Carbon tetrachloride | Thiazides |
| Methyl alcohol | Phenindione |
| Phenols | Diphenylhydantoin |
| Ethylene glycol | |

stance as it is eliminated through the kidney. Areas of ischemia and partial or complete obstruction are revealed. The radioactive material used is in tracer doses, so that no special precautions are necessary for the protection of either the patient or the nursing personnel. Patients should be prepared to be placed in both prone and upright positions. They may be asked to void at the end of the procedure for the determination of average urinary flow rates and bladder residual testing.

A *renal biopsy* is used to determine the extent of pathological change present. Contraindications include the presence of only one functioning kidney, bleeding disorders, kidney tumors or cysts that could be disseminated during the biopsy, uncooperative patients, and pregnancy. The procedure is carried out under local anesthesia in the radiology department, with the position of the biopsy needle confirmed by radiopaque dyes and fluoroscopy. Following biopsy a small dressing is placed over the wound.

Postbiopsy nursing care should focus on watching for bleeding, a common complication. Microscopic hematuria may be seen in 50 percent or more of these patients, and gross hematuria may be present in 5 percent or less. The patient's vital signs should be monitored every 15 minutes for the first 1½ hours, every 30 minutes for the next 2½ hours, every hour for 6 hours, and then every 4 hours. Urine specimens, collected for approximately 24 hours, are examined on the unit for gross hematuria. The patient's hematocrit is checked several times following the procedure. Patients should remain on bed rest for 24 hours and be watched for flank pain, a drop in the blood pressure, extreme weakness, light-headedness, fainting, a flushed feeling, perspiration, and/or a rapid pulse.

Treatment for bleeding involves bed rest and, on rare occasions, surgical intervention. At discharge, the nurse should instruct the patient to avoid strenuous activity such as heavy lifting, contact sports, horseback riding, or any activity that can cause jolting to the kidney area for at least 2 weeks. The signs and symptoms of bleeding should be explained and patients should be instructed to report their occurrence to the physician immediately. While hazards are few, they can be prevented when detected early by close nursing observation and proper instruction.

The *intravenous pyelogram* (IVP) is probably the most commonly ordered test when renal pathology is suspected. The procedure involves the injection of a radiopaque dye intravenously followed by a series of x-rays of the kidneys, pelvis, ureters, and bladder. Preparation of the patient for IVP is primarily a nursing function. Visualization of the contrast material as it moves through the kidneys, ureters, bladder, and urethra is possible only if the colon is clear of gas and feces. Preparation begins the night before the procedure and involves the administration of a cathartic, enemas, or both. Fluids and food are omitted for 12 to 15 hours prior to the test to keep the bowel clear, as well as to increase the concentration of the dye in the urine by mild dehydration of the patient. Because of the debilitating effects of this preparation, caution should be used when preparing older patients, the young, and persons with already existing disease that may further effect fluid and electrolyte balance. Complications are rare, but include an allergic response to the radiopaque dye. The nurse should observe the patient for itching, hives, wheezing, or respiratory distress indicative of such a reaction and have the necessary equipment and medications easily available in case of anaphylactic shock. The frequent x-rays following injection of the dye may require the patient to remain on the x-ray table for a rather long period of time. Padding the table with a soft bath blanket can ease discomfort. Following completion of the procedure, the nurse should observe the patient for allergic manifestations and provide fluids and foods as soon as permitted to prevent fluid and electrolyte imbalances.

The *24-hour urine volume* is used to determine whether the kidneys are producing the 500 ml minimal urine volume required for the daily excretion of nitrogenous wastes. Urine volumes below this level indicate a serious decrease in the amount of functioning renal tissue. The specimen may also be analyzed for electrolyte contents to determine what electrolyte losses are occurring. Monitoring such losses can be used to determine the daily electrolyte intake required to keep the patient in electrolyte balance. The nurse's responsibility includes the accurate collection and labeling of specimens, instruction of the patient to ensure cooperation in the collection of the specimens, and prompt transportation of the specimen to the laboratory for analysis.

**N**ursing Problems and Interventions   The results of the nursing assessment and the diagnostic tests of the patient with chronic renal failure will present a wide range of nursing problems. As more damage occurs to nephrons, the problems become life-threatening for the patient. Early nursing intervention can interrupt fatal processes and may reverse pathological changes. Because the problems are so similar to those occurring with acute renal failure, the reader is encouraged to review that section.

*Fluid excess* develops gradually and predictably as renal functions are decreased. Intake and output records should be precise and include all sources of fluid intake and loss. All dependent areas, ankles, and coccyx should be palpated for evidence of fluid retention, and the patient's weight should be recorded daily. Fluids will most likely be restricted, requiring careful communication among personnel and patient for accuracy. If fluid excess becomes acute, congestive heart failure and pulmonary edema may result. Patients should be observed carefully for signs of increasing pulse rate, chest congestion, dyspnea, and a bounding heart rate. Frequent observation of the patient during the night can reveal congestion resulting from reabsorption of fluid from the extremities.

*Diuretics* are used to decrease fluid retention. Patients are frequently started on minor diuretics, such as chlorothiazide, and then progress to the more powerful diuretics such as ethacrynic acid and furosemide. Patients should be watched for hyponatremia and hypokalemia associated with rapid fluid loss. They should be informed of the action, dose, and side effects of the specific medications being used, as well as the signs and symptoms of side or toxic effects that should be reported. A frequent adverse effect of diuretics is damage to the renal tubules. Their use, therefore, needs to be accompanied by regular and thorough monitoring of the patient's progress. Overhydration leading to potential heart failure may be treated by the initiation of dialysis.

Disorders of sodium balance are not as common, but *hyponatremia* may occur with a salt-wasting disease such as pyelonephritis. A record of sodium intake and the analysis of sodium output are generally used to identify the patient's needs. Careful dietary instruction is needed to ensure accurate intake. *Hyperkalemia* is much more common and can cause great difficulties, and patients should be watched for signs of irritability, nausea, and heart block. An ECG monitor should be attached to the very ill patient so that hyperkalemia can be identified early. Serial electrolytes should be run regularly and the physician informed of abnormalities. Potassium intake is drastically reduced, making dietary adjustments and instruction essential. If the potassium levels rise severely, the administration of cation exchange resins (see Chap. 12) and/or the initiation of dialysis may be necessary.

*Hyperphosphatemia* and *hypocalcemia* occur as renal impairment prevents excretion of phosphate. Antacids are administered to produce the exchange of phosphate and calcium in the large intestine, and administration of high doses of vitamin D may be used to improve the gastrointestinal absorption of calcium. The nurse should carefully monitor the patient's serum levels and report abnormalities. If calcium deficiency continues, the nurse should observe the patient for sore, painful feet, muscle weakness, spontaneous fractures, and joint pain. Mild pain medication may provide relief from bone pain.

As the number of functioning tubules diminishes, excretion of acid decreases, and *metabolic acidosis* results. Administration of sodium bicarbonate and sodium citrate are generally very effective in correcting the problem. During treatment, the patient should be watched for signs of tetany, as hypocalcemia can result as the pH rises. The nurse should be ready to administer calcium, if needed.

Dietary restriction of protein is used to prevent the accumulation of nitrogenous wastes and resulting *azotemia*. The nurse is responsible for instructing the patient and family about these restrictions. Protein is restricted in total amount and in amino acid content. Eggs and milk are generally used because they contain all essential amino acids. Animal meat, fish, and fowl are restricted because of their sulfur-containing, nonessential amino acids. Protein restriction is lifted when dialysis is initiated, since waste products are cleared by the machine.

The management of *hypertension* is accomplished by the reduction of fluid volume and the administration of antihypertensive medications. Patients should be taught the actions and side effects of these medications and methods for self-administration at home. Many of the antihypertensive medications cause orthostatic hypotension and patients may experience dizziness or falling when changing from a lying to a sitting position or from a sitting to a standing position. These difficulties can be minimized if the patient is instructed to hesitate a few minutes after changing position and before moving on to a new activity or position. See Chap. 28 for a more thorough discussion of caring for the patient with hypertension.

*Anemia* generally has a slow onset through the early stages of chronic renal failure. Frequently the anemia comes about so gradually that the patient is unaware of a problem and only experiences fatigue on occasion. Folic acid and ferrous sulfate are administered and some patients may need blood transfusions. Such patients should be watched closely for signs and symptoms of hyperkalemia following the administration of blood. *Gastrointestinal bleeding* is not uncommon, and patients should be observed for hematemesis, occult blood in the stool, and bloody diarrhea. Antacids are used to decrease gastrointestinal irritability.

The patient's skin needs special care to prevent *skin breakdown.* Deposition of urochrome gives a yellowish tinge to the skin and rubs off during bathing. As the uremia increases, uric crystals form on the skin and careful and frequent skin care is needed. Pruritus may become severe. Lotions and soothing ointments may be used to increase patient comfort. Decreased platelets produces bruising of the skin, and the patient may begin to hemorrhage. Inspection and care of the skin is a high priority in planning nursing care.

Symptoms of *neurological involvement* begin when azotemia becomes severe. The patient initially has muscular twitching, numbness, tingling, and seizures. As neurological symptoms increase in severity, it is important to revise the nursing care plan to include adequate safety measures for the patient. Increasing muscular activity indicates that seizures may begin, and the establishment of seizure precautions is appropriate. The nurse should have anticonvulsant medications available for administration. The occurrence of decreased attention and beginning confusion indicate the need for increased surveillance of the patient to prevent falls and injuries. Hiccups may occur, and are sometimes treated with sedatives. Neurological symptoms may be reversed when dialysis is begun.

Finally, *infections* must be prevented or detected early. Any infectious process increases the work of the kidney and may increase the progression of renal damage. Patient instruction concerning prevention of infection is a major nursing priority. Patients should be taught to avoid large crowds of people, especially when epidemic type infections such as influenza and upper respiratory infections are prevalent. Good hygiene practices should be encouraged, as well as immunizations recommended by the physician. Some patients may be taking preventive antibiotic therapy and will need instruction on the methods of administration, recording, and side effects that should be reported. Early detection of infectious disease involves teaching the patient the early signs and symptoms of respiratory and urinary tract infections and the need to report such signs to the physician for prompt treatment.

Patients being treated for chronic renal failure will also be undergoing treatment for the underlying cause of the progressive renal damage. For example, the patient's diabetes mellitus or lupus erythematosus will be treated along with the problems of beginning renal failure. Nursing care for these specific problems is discussed in Chaps. 20 and 10, respectively.

*Hemodialysis* In *hemodialysis,* or extracorporeal dialysis, blood leaves the body and circulates through a machine where dialysis occurs. The blood is then pumped back into the body. Hemodialysis requires specialized equipment and personnel, and is instituted when long-term dialysis is planned or when very rapid removal of toxic substances is needed to save the patient's life. It is used for patients with intoxication from dialyzable drugs such as alcohols, aspirin, some antibiotics, and barbiturates.

Hemodialysis is used for patients with chronic renal failure whose medications and diet are no longer sufficient in treating complications and for patients in the third and fourth stages of chronic renal failure. There are presently more than 20,000 patients in the United States at this end-stage renal disease point where dialysis is mandatory for survival, and it is estimated that this number will increase to 50,000 to 60,000 by 1986.[14] Although peritoneal dialysis is used for some of these patients, the overwhelming majority are treated with hemodialysis because of its advantages in long-term treatment. A comparison of peritoneal dialysis and hemodialysis is found in Table 14-6. Peritoneal dialysis is used for patients who cannot tolerate the systemic heparinization needed for hemodialysis, whose cardiovascular status is incompatible with rapid changes in body fluids, or for whom access to the bloodstream is no longer possible. Nursing care while the patient is undergoing hemodialysis involves additional education and experience in a highly specialized area. However, basic information on the procedure and complications will assist nurses in caring for patients before and after each session. The reader is encouraged to explore additional sources of information for further preparation in hemodialysis nursing.

During hemodialysis, blood leaves the body through a cannula or needle and circulates through a dialysis machine in which the diffusion of materials occurs across a semipermeable membrane within the machine. Blood then returns to the body via tubing connected to another cannula or needle. Electrolytes, nonelectrolytes, and water move out of the blood dependent upon the substances found in the dialysate. One treatment involves approximately 4 to 8 hours and is repeated 2 to 3 times a week.

There are two procedures used to permit access to the bloodstream during hemodialysis: the external shunt and the internal fistula. The *external shunt,* pictured in Fig. 14-4, is composed of two cannulas, one placed in a vein and one in an artery. During the dialysis procedure the arterial cannula is connected to the tubing that goes to the dialysis machine, and the tubing that exists from the dialysis machine is connected to the venous cannula. Between dialysis treatments, a small connecting tubing of soft, pliable, clot-resistant material such as high-grade Silastic is used to join the arterial and venous cannulas. Shunts can be used within 48 hours of formation and last 4 to 9 months or longer.

The major problems associated with external shunts include clotting, infection, and awkwardness for the patient. Since the connecting tubing is outside the body, special dressings are used to protect the area. Although it is an infrequent occurrence, the connecting tubing can come apart and lead to exsanguination. As a result, most patients with external shunts should carry a set of bulldog clamps with them at all times and should be instructed in their use.

The *internal fistula* (Fig. 14-5), the newer of the two procedures, is a surgically created fistula between an adjoining artery and vein. Within a few weeks or months of the surgical connection, the arterialized vein dilates from the increased blood flow and becomes very prominent. Fistulas can be established in the forearms or the legs. During dialysis, needles are inserted into the fistula, one to allow blood to flow to the dialysis machine and the other to return blood to the patient. The obvious disadvantage of the fistula is that it requires venipunctures with large bore needles to provide adequate blood flow for each hemodialysis treatment. The advantages of a fistula are great in that the

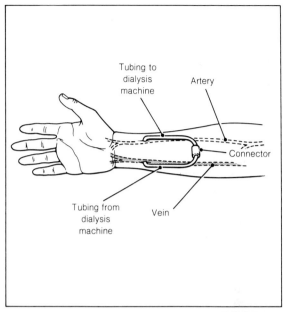

**FIGURE 14-4**
External shunt for hemodialysis.

problems of clotting and infection are virtually eliminated, the patient has free use of the limb, and hemorrhage is nonexistent. A summary of the comparison of the external shunt and the internal fistula is presented in Table 14-7.

The psychological preparation of the patient for hemodialysis begins a considerable period of time before treatment is begun. The establishment of the blood access route can be used to initiate a dialogue with the patient about feelings regarding chronic hemodialysis. Establishment of a relationship with the patient and allowing the patient to feel comfortable in expressing any feelings about the illness are important steps in providing emotional support.

Physiological assessment of the patient is also needed. Baseline information should include the patient's weight, temperature, blood pressure,

**TABLE 14-6**
COMPARISON OF HEMODIALYSIS AND PERITONEAL DIALYSIS

|  | Hemodialysis | Peritoneal Dialysis |
|---|---|---|
| Personnel preparation | Specialized educational programs | Skilled, on-the-job training |
| Length of treatment | 4–8 hours | 24–48 hours |
| Equipment | Special machines | Routine hospital materials |
| Site | Blood vessels in the extremities | Abdomen |
| Exchange membrane | Dialysis machine | Peritoneal lining |
| Complications | Dysequilibrium syndrome, fluid and electrolyte imbalances, exsanguination | Peritonitis, protein loss |

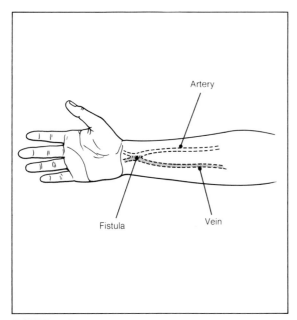

**FIGURE 14-5**
Internal fistula for hemodialysis.

pulse, fluid and food status, and clotting time. The assessment will continue at intervals throughout dialysis so that complications can be detected and treated promptly.

Prior to connecting the patient to the dialysis machine, heparinization is done to keep the blood anticoagulated within the hemodialysis machine. During and after hemodialysis the patient's clotting time is determined, and observations for additional signs of potential bleeding are monitored closely.

A number of complications can occur during hemodialysis in addition to bleeding problems. The major fluid and electrolyte imbalance that may occur is called the *dysequilibrium syndrome* and occurs in patients with severe azotemia who exhibit agitation, restlessness, twitching, jerking,

confusion, and eventually grand mal seizures toward the end or immediately after dialysis. The faster the exchange of nephrotoxic substances, the more common the syndrome, hence it is seen most frequently with highly efficient dialysis machines. The syndrome is thought to be related to large and rapid changes in water, pH, and osmolality between the serum and cerebrospinal fluid.[15] Changes in the ratio of urea found within the serum and the cerebrospinal fluid, plus the relative alkalosis that occurs during hemodialysis, are responsible for the symptoms. Prevention of this complication includes shorter periods of initial dialysis for patients with severe azotemia.

Additional fluid and electrolyte imbalances that may occur during hemodialysis include fluid overload, hypertension, hypotension from excess fluid loss, electrolyte imbalances, and cerebral manifestations. Monitoring the patient's vital signs and electrolyte levels during hemodialysis is done to prevent these complications.

Several problems in oxygenation can occur while patients are on hemodialysis. If pericarditis is present, *cardiac tamponade* may occur from the heparinization during hemodialysis. *Cardiac arrhythmias* occur occasionally and are related to either underlying heart disease or the lowering of serum potassium in the patient on digitalis products. An *air embolus* can occur from an air leak into the blood tubing and the symptoms produced include chest pain, cough, cyanosis, and cardiac arrest. Immediate notification of the physician and initiation of life-saving techniques are required.

The two most serious problems that can occur while a patient is on hemodialysis is the delivery of an *incorrect dialysis solution* and *exsanguination* from disconnection of the blood tubing or cannula, or blood loss into the machine. Both of these complications can be prevented by following safety techniques in preparing the dialysate bath and ob-

**TABLE 14-7**
COMPARISON OF EXTERNAL SHUNT AND INTERNAL FISTULA

| Characteristics | External Shunt | Internal Fistula |
|---|---|---|
| Appearance | Tubing entering vessels from outside of body | No skin openings, large dilated vessel visible |
| Activity | Restricted use of cannulated extremity | Nonrestricted |
| Average length of use | 4–9 months and longer | 2 years and longer |
| Complications | Clotting, infection, limited extremity use, exsanguination | None |
| Daily care | Inspection and sterile dressing change | None |
| Effects on dialysis treatment | Painless tubing connection, free extremity movement | Venipuncture required, limited extremity movement |

serving the patient frequently during the procedure. Most patients rapidly develop a pattern of reaction to the hemodialysis treatment and are able to tell if something is wrong by feelings of restlessness and discomfort. Reports of such feelings should be followed by a thorough check of the entire set-up and functioning of the machine.

*Renal transplant* As knowledge of the antigen-antibody response has expanded, the success of *renal transplant* for the treatment of end-stage renal failure has increased. Of 389 renal transplants performed from 1951 to 1972, 47.6 percent of the patients have functioning graft kidneys and 18.2 percent are being maintained on maintenance dialysis because of graft failure.[16] Within this group there have been 62 successful pregnancies. Transplantation as the therapy of choice for patients with end-stage renal failure is preferred by most patients and recommended by most physicians.

The procedure for transplantation begins with the selection of the recipient who is free from irreversible systemic disease and the selection of a suitable donor. Grafts from closely related living donors have a much higher success rate than grafts from cadavers. This fact often produces strain within the family as a potential donor may be fearful of giving a kidney and the resulting guilt may be a problem (see Chap. 10). Preparation includes tissue typing to determine the degree of immunological difference between donor and recipient.

Preoperatively, the recipient may have a bilateral nephrectomy if infection or hypertension present problems. The kidney is removed from the donor and placed in the iliac fossa of the recipient. The renal vessels are anastomosed and the ureter omplanted into the bladder. Postoperatively, the patient receives routine postoperative care, dialysis if needed, and immunosuppressive therapy to reduce rejection.

The *nursing problems* for the preoperative renal transplant patient include providing emotional support for the patient and family, reinforcing the patient's knowledge about the procedure, and explaining the drainage tubes and medications to be expected postoperatively. Following surgery the patient should be observed for signs of hemorrhage and the development of pneumonia. Fluid and electrolyte imbalances should be prevented and urinary output reestablished. Urine production may begin within a few hours or not for several days or weeks. Immunosuppressive therapy demands that patients be carefully observed for leukopenia, infections, hypotension, and decreased wound healing.

The most serious complication following renal transplantation is rejection, which may occur within the first week or as long as 1 to 2 years following surgery. The usual symptoms of rejection include fever, a swollen tender kidney, and indications of renal failure such as hypertension, decreased urine volume, and weight gain. Acute reversible rejection is treated with increased immunosuppressant therapy. Long-term chronic rejection is insidious and present treatment is not available to reverse the process. Transplant rejection is discussed in detail in Chap. 10.

**Fourth-level nursing care** Patients on chronic hemodialysis programs are usually found in either low-cost care facilities where patients come in for treatment or in the home where family members assist with the dialysis procedure. Nursing personnel are responsible for much of the needed care and support for the patient's rehabilitation to be effective. Physical assessment and monitoring for complications both in fluid and electrolyte imbalances, oxygenation problems, and metabolic changes are necessary. Patients should be taught shunt care, which involves the daily observation of the shunt for adequate blood flow and clotting, and of the skin for beginning signs of infection. Each of these complications needs to be reported for follow-up care at the dialysis center. Patients should be taught the details of dialysis care, family involvement in care, and dietary restrictions of protein, fluid, and electrolytes.

*Hypertension* continues to be a problem, and changes in pressure should be monitored regularly by the patient and the nurse. While most of this hypertension is a result of fluid overload and will respond to decreased volume, approximately 20 percent is caused by high levels of circulating renin. Treatment may necessitate the removal of the kidneys, thus increasing the patient's anemia and calcium deficiencies. Regular laboratory testing is done to check for anemia and electrolyte deficiencies, which are treated with folic acid, ferrous sulfate, occasional blood transfusions, and electrolyte supplement.

The *stresses* of dialysis are real and have been grouped by Wright as follows: actual or threatened losses, such as loss of kidney functioning; injury or threat of injury, such as opening of a cannula and resulting hemorrhage; and frustration in drives or instinctive needs, such as imposed dietary restrictions.[17] These stresses also include economic pressures from loss of income and increased expenses, an increase in dependency, and a decrease in sexual functioning. The usual emotional responses to these stresses include anxiety, depression, denial, and depersonalization. Denial often is especially strong and is frequently manifested in dietary indiscretions. The patient will usually utilize previously established coping strategies.

The nurse working with the patient can assist the patient and family in dealing with these stresses by clarifying information and teaching patients about dialysis, dietary management, and medications. It is appropriate to reward patients with honest praise as much as possible. The establishment of a working relationship among the nurse, patient, and family over a period of time can do much to maintain communication.[18] Often patients and their families will benefit from group and/or individual counseling.

The economic pressures for the patient with chronic renal failure have been changing rapidly in the last few years. In April 1974, the so-called "kidney amendment" was passed by the federal government and allowed for federal financing of care for all citizens with end-stage renal disease. Two therapies in particular were reimbursable—kidney dialysis and transplant. Since the cost of dialysis can range anywhere from $6,000 to $30,000 per year, the provision of these funds by the federal government has made treatment for end-stage renal disease possible for every citizen, not just a select few, as previously. The pattern of care for patients with end-stage renal disease on dialysis is changing from isolated areas to the development of a nationwide network of kidney centers organized to assure that each patient will have access to the system and coordinated care.

Hemodialysis can often be coordinated with the patient's occupational schedule and a program can be developed with work time planned around dialysis treatments. Employers need to be impressed with the potential contributions that can still be made by dialysis patients. With kidney centers established throughout the country, travel can often be planned and arrangements made for the patient to receive treatments from another center.

## GLOMERULONEPHRITIS

*Acute glomerulonephritis* is a diffuse inflammation of the glomeruli of both kidneys, nonsuppurative in nature. It affects children and adults and is the cause for renal failure in the greatest percentage of patients in dialysis and transplant programs. The prognosis is quite good. Complete cure is generally found in 80 to 85 percent of children and slightly less in adults; death in the acute stage occurs in about 2 to 5 percent, death in 3 to 18 months after onset occurs in another 4 percent, and the remaining patients progress to chronic glomerulonephritis.[19]

Acute glomerulonephritis is generally preceded by a streptococcal infection of the upper respiratory tract which occurs 10 to 14 days before the onset of symptoms. Then the abrupt onset of edema, hypertension, and abnormal urinalysis occurs. The patient demonstrates hematuria and proteinuria, mild to moderate elevations in blood pressure, and fluid retention in dependent areas. The treatment is nonspecific and related to the presenting symptoms. The fluid and electrolyte imbalances are treated with sodium and water restriction. Sometimes diuretics are administered. The hypertension usually responds to the decrease in body fluids from the sodium restriction, but may on occasion be treated with antihypertensive medications. Bed rest and sedation are used to decrease the metabolic rate and, in general, decrease the stress on the kidney tissue. In the occasional patient in whom renal failure occurs, dialysis is initiated.

*Chronic glomerulonephritis* involves bilateral renal tissue damage and related renal insufficiency, and differs from acute glomerulonephritis in both onset and clinical course. The patient is unaware of any precipitating symptoms and rarely has any physical disability when the diagnosis is made. The discovery of the disease usually occurs when a routine physical examination reveals mild proteinuria and moderate hypertension. Once the diagnosis is established, the patient may have good health for 10 to 30 years. Eventually renal insufficiency becomes apparent, and episodes of proteinuria and azotemia increase in severity. The treatment of chronic glomerulonephritis is symptomatic during the long onset and early years. Hypertension is usually treated with antihypertensive medications, and edema by salt and water restriction. Some patients are given penicillin to prevent additional streptococcal infections. In renal insufficiency, conservative management of symptoms occurs. When uremia becomes apparent, dialysis may be initiated. Nursing care parallels that described above under acute and chronic renal failure.

## RENAL CALCULI

Stones can be found at every level of the urinary tract, from the renal pelvis to the bladder. These concretions are formed within the body and are called *calculi* or lithiasis. They are a part of the history of medicine, having been identified in Egyptian mummies and treated during Hippocrates' time. Their occurrence is still prominent, affecting approximately 1 of every 1000 patients hospitalized in the United States.[20] No age group is excluded, but the majority of patients are between the ages of 20 and 55.

### Pathophysiology

The etiology of stone formation is not known. The occurrence in hot climates is associated with an increased insensible fluid loss combined with inadequate fluid intake, which results in concentrated urine and precipitation of urinary salts. Infections of the urinary tract are associated with stone formation, especially if the infecting organism is a urea-splitting organism such as *Escherichia coli, Staphlococcus,* or *Streptococcus.* Any patient who has urinary stasis is prone to urinary tract calculi formation from precipitation of urinary salts. A small organic matrix begins to gather layers as precipitation occurs. Most calculi, about 85 percent, are composed primarily of calcium. The remaining 15 percent are usually uric acid stones with only a few composed of cystine, glycine, and calcium oxalate.

Calculi can be found in the kidney pelvis and may be multiple, ranging from gravel to many small stones to a large stone obstructing the entire renal pelvis (a *staghorn calculus*). Smaller stones formed in the renal pelvis may pass down the ureter, lodging and obstructing the ureter or going through to the urinary bladder. Formation of stones can also occur in the urinary bladder and either remain there or pass through the urethra and out during urination.

**Effects on the patient** The clinical manifestations of urinary tract calculi depend on the location, size, and movement of the stones. In some instances no symptoms are present and the diagnosis is made when an x-ray reveals radiopaque calculi. If the stone moves down the ureter, the diameter of the stone can fill the inside of the ureteral passageway, causing irritation, inflammation, and obstruction. *Hematuria* is evident, and severe pain, called *renal colic,* occurs as the peristaltic movements in the ureter move the obstruction along. If infection accompanies the calculus, pyuria, burning on urination, and frequency may be present.

### First-level Nursing Care

Prevention of calculi outside the hospital involves health education for community groups with emphasis on adequate daily fluid intake. Discussion of this aspect of preventive health is especially important for persons anticipating moving to or visiting hot climates and for those on regular exercise programs. Insensible fluid loss can increase enormously depending on exercise and environmental temperature. Since people vary considerably in their estimation of adequate fluid intake, an approach that seems to work is to emphasize the need for adequate urinary output, especially following periods of exercise and during the night when urine tends to be concentrated. The nurse who cares for homebound and frequently bedridden patients with other chronic diseases needs to plan for adequate intake and adequate urinary output to prevent the formation of stones. Since stasis of urine in either the kidney pelvis or the bladder can lead to the precipitation of stone forming salts, patients should be turned frequently. Figure 14-6 compares urinary stasis in the renal pelvis during the upright and prone positions, illustrating the need to get patients up in the sitting position as soon as possible, and to turn patients on bed rest every 2 to 4 hours.

Any patient with a high concentration of calcium in the urine is prone to renal calculi. This includes patients with hyperparathyroidism, excessive milk, alkali, or vitamin D ingestion, and bone pathologies. Immobility increases bone reabsorption making paralyzed patients susceptible from the calcium mobilization and from urinary stasis. Patients with gout are prone to uric acid stones.

Patients who have a family history of stone formation or have already had a stone, are at risk to the development of calculi and need preventive instructions. They should be taught to maintain urinary output and be observant for the passage of sandy urine and stones. If the initial stone has been collected and analyzed, a change in the pH of the urine or the dietary intake of the predominant salt can be used to create an environment where reoccurrence of calculi is less likely. The more common approaches to changing the urine pH are an acid ash diet to increase the acidity of the urine when the calculi are composed of calcium, and an alkaline ash diet to increase the alkalinity of the urine for uric acid stones. Cranberry juice is especially effective in acidifying the urine, and, in addition, seems to have a bacteriostatic effect. Hospitalized patients with increased risk of calculi formation include patients on bed rest or whose fluid intake has been decreased. Schedules for turning and ambulating patients are necessary to decrease this complicating occurrence.

### Second-level Nursing Care

Early identification of patients with urinary calculi can be done in the community setting during the *health history.* The nurse should inquire about the occurrence of recent travel in warm climates, infections of the urinary tract, and periods of time during which bed rest was increased. During *physical assessment* the patient will reveal tenderness over the kidneys and flank pain. These signs and symptoms should be followed up with further *diagnostic testing.* Helpful in revealing renal calculi is the urinalysis, with evidence of increased sediment, concentration, and actual stones being posi-

tive findings. The nurse is responsible for collection of these specimens and reporting positive findings to the physician. An x-ray of the abdomen may confirm the location of a stone and indicate whether surgical removal of the stone is necessary.

If the pain the patient experiences is not incapacitating, and the patient is not dehydrated, *nursing problems and interventions* may be handled with the patient at home. The care for such a patient would be similar to that discussed under third-level nursing care. The community-based nurse, however, must focus on instructing the patient and family to manage the condition until the stone is eliminated.

### Third-level Nursing Care

The patient hospitalized for treatment of existing calculi will need thorough nursing care. The *nursing assessment* should begin with the health history, which will reveal hematuria, pyuria, urinary retention, and colicky pain. The pain will vary depending on the location of calculi and subside in minutes or persist for hours. If the stone is located in the renal pelvis or high in the ureter, renal colic

**FIGURE 14-6**
Urinary stasis.

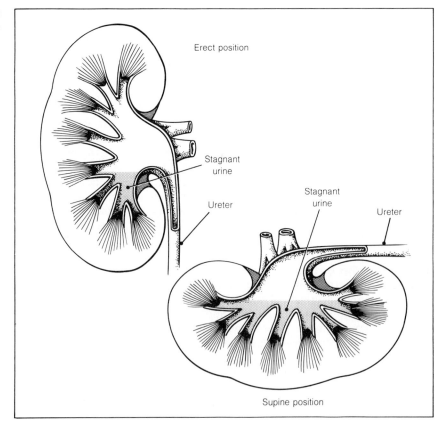

results, with pain primarily in the flank area of the affected side. Pain in the flank is often associated with a low back syndrome and patients should be questioned about this. If the stone is located in the lower ureter, the pain generally radiates across the side of the abdomen and into the genital area on the affected side. Physical assessment will reveal an acutely ill patient who is sweating, nauseated, vomiting, and pale. The abdominal examination will reveal tenderness over the kidney, and the pulse may be weak and rapid. To distinguish renal colic from low back pain, the flank area should be bluntly percussed with a closed fist. Any resultant pain may be indicative of renal pathology. Other findings during the physical assessment will be negative.

Patients with suspected urinary calculi will have diagnostic tests to pinpoint the location of the calculi. X-ray of the kidneys, ureters, and bladder will reveal stones with calcium as the predominant material. Serum analysis may show elevated calcium, phosphorus, or alkaline phosphorus levels which correlate to the composition of the stone. During *cystoscopy* a lighted tube is passed through the urethra and into the bladder under anesthesia. Bladder stones may be located and sometimes removed, or ureteral catheters passed to the kidney to locate stones, relieve an obstructed renal pelvis and promote healing of affected tissues. Following this procedure, patients should be observed for hematuria and the passage of any urinary calculi.

**Nursing problems and interventions** The *pain* of a moving urinary calculi is excruciating and needs prompt nursing interventions. Analgesics and antispasmotics may be ordered, and should be given liberally during acute episodes of pain. Moist heat and hot water bottles may be used over the flank area to increase the patient's comfort. The patient with colic is generally very restless and should be instructed to ask for assistance in getting out of bed. Patients should be checked routinely to avoid falls or other accidents.

If obstruction of one or both ureters occurs, a *decrease in urine* will result. *Hydronephrosis,* the collection of urine in the renal pelvis, may complicate matters, and is treated with antibiotic therapy and the establishment of urinary drainage. Occasionally acute renal failure will occur. Since *nausea* and *vomiting* generally are present, the patient frequently becomes dehydrated and additional fluids are given parenterally. *Dehydration* can lead to further precipitation of urinary calculi, and should be avoided when possible. Nursing care should include the establishment of accurate and inclusive intake and output records and the maintenance of the patient's hydration in the face of both increased losses and decreased intake from gastrointestinal symptoms. In all patients with potential calculi, a method for straining the urine is essential. Using gauze to strain the urine will prevent loss of uric acid stones which tend to crumble. If *infection* is present, antibiotics are administered. The nurse should be alert to the occurrence of side effects from antibiotics and ensure an adequate intake of fluids for the potent antibiotics that may cause damage to renal tissue. *Paralytic ileus* associated with reflex activity from the pain of colic may occur and be treated by a nasogastric tube to provide for release of gas from the small bowel (see Chap. 18).

**S**urgical Treatment of Calculi   Almost 90 percent of the stones formed in the urinary tract pass through the tract and out of the body into the urine spontaneously. For the other 10 percent surgical removal is needed. If the stone is within the kidney, a *nephrolithotomy* is performed and the kidney opened to remove the stone. If the stones are located in the ureter, a *ureterolithotomy* is performed. If the stones are in the bladder, a *cystotomy* is performed, and the stones removed through the abdominal wall. An alternate to the cystotomy is the process of removing the stones from the bladder via the transurethral route, called a *litholapaxy.* In this procedure, a stone crusher is passed transurethrally, and the stone is crushed while inside the bladder, making spontaneous passage easier.

*Preoperative nursing care*   Preoperative preparation for the surgical intervention of urinary calculi includes the treatment of dehydration and electrolyte losses. Observation for these imbalances is an important nursing intervention. Psychological preparation of the patient should include an explanation of the results expected from the surgical procedure. If removal of a kidney is necessary, discussion of this loss with the patient is essential. Many patients do not know that normal functioning is possible with one kidney. Techniques for deep breathing and coughing should be taught preoperatively to ensure the patient's cooperation in the early and often painful post-operative period.

*Postoperative nursing care*   The nursing care of the patient postoperatively involves specific interventions to prevent problems. Because of the location of the incision directly below the diaphragm and across the side and flank area, deep breathing and coughing are very difficult and painful for the patient. Postoperative *atelectasis* and *pneumonia* are not uncommon, and indicate the need for a regular and vigorous plan for turning, deep breathing, and coughing. Because of the amount of *pain* experienced by the average patient with a flank incision, the nurse may expect to administer the pain medication every four hours for 24 to 48 hours after surgery. Pain medication should be administered at an appropriate time interval prior to assisting the patient with deep breathing and coughing. Patients frequently complain of muscular aches and pain other than in the incisional area. These discomforts are generally caused by the position during the surgical procedure, since the patient may be strapped on one side with the flank or waist area jacknifed upward to provide visualization of the kidney. Massage and moist heat, if allowed, will ease this discomfort.

Another usual problem in the postoperative period is the *maintenance of urinary drainage.* Depending on the surgical approach and the location of the calculi, several urinary drainage tubes may be present. Catheters may be placed in the renal pelvis, the ureters, and the urethra. If placed through the renal cortex and medulla and then into the pelvis, the tube is called a *nephrostomy* catheter and exits from a stab wound near the incisional area. A *pyelostomy* tube can be placed in the same fashion, using a similar approach through the flank but going directly into the pelvis and avoiding the renal cortex and medulla. Either tube allows direct drainage of urine from the kidney when the ureter has been obstructed preoperatively. When an incision is made into the ureter, a *ureterostomy* tube may be inserted to splint the area postoperatively and provide for adequate drainage of urine through the ureter. The ureterostomy tube is also placed through a flank incision, or stab wound, and thus exits from the abdominal wall. A *ureteral catheter* is inserted up the ureter via the bladder, using a cystoscope. The catheters used for ureteral catheterization are considerably smaller than those for kidney and bladder drainage. Catheters are inserted into the urinary bladder via two methods. A *cystostomy* tube can be inserted directly through the abdominal wall. The bladder can also be catheterized via the urethra by use of a *urethral catheter,* the only catheter inserted by a nurse. All other catheters are inserted by the physician.

Important aspects for the nurse to be aware of in dealing with the patient's catheters are to know the kind, size, location, and expected drainage from each. Catheters should never be clamped unless specifically ordered. On occasion, both ureteral catheter(s) and a urethral catheter may be placed via the urethra. Each catheter may drain urine and should be individually marked as to the drainage site and attached to separate drainage bottles or bags so that identification of the amounts of urine collected from each catheter is available. Charting should include the individual amounts drained from each.

Catheters may also be irrigated, if ordered. The location of the catheter should be taken into account when identifying the amount of solution to use for irrigation. The capacity of the renal pelvis is only 4 to 6 ml of fluid, and even less for children, so that only very small amounts of fluid are used to irrigate nephrostomy and pyelostomy tubes. Ureteral catheters are generally not irrigated. The urinary bladder can be irrigated via a urethral catheter with from 75 to 100 ml of fluid without causing any distress for the patient. Irrigations should be carried out using sterile technique, gentle instillation, and gravity drainage.

Patients generally have *drains* that allow for urine and serous drainage directly through the incision. This causes considerable drainage on the dressing covering the surgical wound, requiring frequent inspection, reinforcement, and changing of the surgical dressing. Montgomery straps are commonly used because dressings may have to be changed more than once on each shift. Because of the variety of drains and catheters possible for these patients, it is imperative that the nurse administering postoperative care know exactly the kind, number, and location of each tube or drain. Drainage can be either bloody urine, serous drainage, or clear urine. The amount and color of the drainage should be noted when the patient enters and leaves the recovery room postoperatively and is transferred back to the surgical unit. Expectations of the color and amount of drainage should be clarified with the surgeon so that identification of postoperative bleeding and obstructive complications is prompt.

*Hemorrhage* is a complication primarily of renal calculi surgery involving the parenchyma of the kidney. The nurse should be on the alert for increased pulse rate, falling blood pressure, restlessness, and pallor. Drainage tubes and dressings should be inspected regularly for signs of bleeding and compared to previous observations for changes in color and amounts. If hemorrhage is suspected or obvious, the physician must be notified immediately. If the drainage from catheters is very bloody, observations for clotting and resulting obstruction of the drainage tubes should be made at least once a shift. The physician should be notified and an irrigating set should be available if obstruction occurs. Dehydration and electrolyte imbalances from preoperative renal damage may occur. Observation for *renal shutdown* is imperative for all patients undergoing major surgery involving kidney tissue. Careful intake and output records which include the amount, color, and source of urinary drainage are imperative.

Decreased intestinal peristalsis may occur because of either renal colic or severe pain. The need for analgesia, turning, and getting the patient up as soon as possible are all good approaches to preventing the gastrointestinal complications of nausea, vomiting, and gaseous distention. On occasion patients may have to have a nasogastric tube inserted so that gaseous distention of the bowel may be relieved.

### Fourth-level Nursing Care

Patients with urinary calculi need follow-up care after discharge from the hospital. If patients are discharged with urinary drainage tubes in place, instruction on daily dressing changes, provision for adequate rest periods, and follow-up medical care is necessary. Examination of the urine continues at 3- or 4-month intervals, so that future stone formation may be identified earlier. Health teaching should emphasize the need for adequate urinary output to prevent stasis. Special dietary instruction may be necessary, depending on the analysis of the calculi. Patients may be on low calcium diets in which milk and milk products are restricted, or they may be on alkaline ash or acid ash diets. The adaptations necessary to implement these diets in the home situation are the major priorities for the nurse. An alkaline ash diet consists primarily of milk, fruits, and vegetables with only small amounts of protein. Acid ash foods include meat, whole grains, eggs, cheese, cranberries, prunes, and plums.

Following an incision in the flank area, patients need to be instructed to avoid straining or lifting heavy objects for at least 1 year. The nurse should encourage the patient to keep appointments with the physician so that urinary sediment can be analyzed, and the follow-up care needed to prevent and detect recurrence completed.

### PYELONEPHRITIS

Pyelonephritis is an infectious disease of the kidneys, generally divided into acute and chronic phases. *Acute pyelonephritis* may be caused by organisms ascending from the lower urinary tract or

descending to the kidney via the bloodstream. Predisposing factors include anomalies of the kidney, pregnancy, calculi, diabetes, neurogenic bladder, and introduction of instruments or a catheter into the bladder. Usual clinical manifestations include a rapid onset of fever, nausea, vomiting, and flank pain. Laboratory findings reveal both bacteria and white cells in the urine, and leukocytosis. If most of the renal tubules are involved, the kidney loses its ability to concentrate urine, and both water and electrolytes are rapidly lost. Treatment involves the administration of antibiotics based on the culture and sensitivity of organisms identified in the urine. Many patients with acute pyelonephritis are diagnosed and treated in physicians' offices. The nurse is responsible for explaining the medication therapy and instructing the patient in maintaining a high fluid intake and monitoring intake, output, and signs of fluid and electrolyte imbalances. If damage to the kidney parenchyma occurs, renal shutdown and resulting failure may result, requiring dialysis to save the patient's life. Nursing responsibilities in these situations have been described earlier. Following clearing of the initial symptoms, follow-up care is needed for medication administration and urine checks.

*Chronic pyelonephritis* occurs when repeated bacterial infectious processes have resulted in scarring of the renal parenchyma, with damage to tubules, vessels, and glomeruli. Its onset is more subtle, and symptoms of an acute infectious process are seldom present. Patients complain of chronic fatigue and lassitude and eventually develop hypertension. A careful history may reveal unexplained fevers in the past or diagnosed acute pyelonephritis. Urinary obstruction frequently accompanies chronic pyelonephritis. Glomerular filtration rate is decreased, as well as the ability to concentrate urine. Renal failure may eventually occur and dialysis must be instituted. Nursing care for patients undergoing dialysis has been described earlier in this chapter.

### POLYCYSTIC DISEASE OF THE KIDNEYS

Polycystic disease of the kidneys is a familial problem which comes in two forms, one affecting adults and the other affecting infants and children. It is characterized by the replacement of renal parenchyma by multiple tightly packed cysts. The adult form is a regular autosomal dominant heredity disorder, while the childhood form is an autosomal recessive disorder. This is an important distinction because it points to the likelihood of preventing transmission of the disease through genetic counseling of potential parents with a family history. The nurse may be actively involved with making arrangements for patients to receive genetic counseling, explaining to them what genetic counseling is all about, and listening and supporting them as they make their decisions about the process.

The adult form of the disease is a slowly progressive disease, initially asymptomatic and eventually characterized by hematuria, mild hypertension, and flank pain. Accompanying urinary tract infections are common. Uremia develops gradually. Fluid and electrolyte imbalances include severe salt wasting because of the involvement of the renal medulla. Oral sodium supplements are necessary to compensate for sodium losses. If end-stage renal disease occurs, dialysis and kidney transplant may be initiated. Nursing care associated with this treatment has been described earlier.

## HYDRONEPHROSIS

*Hydronephrosis* is the dilation of the kidney pelvis caused by the obstruction of urinary flow out of the kidney. The obstruction may be a calculi, a tumor, or infectious scarring. Hydronephrosis is not a disease itself, but rather a complication of obstructive disease. Treatment is aimed at relief of the obstruction and differs according to the cause.

## NEPHROTIC SYNDROME

The nephrotic syndrome is characterized by massive proteinuria, edema, hypoproteinemia, lipidemia, and lipiduria. It has many causes, including glomerulonephritis, diabetes mellitus, lupus erythematosus, sickle cell anemia, nephrotoxins, allergies, infections, and pregnancy. It develops when the glomerulus is injured in any way. The permeability of the glomerular capillary membrane increases and protein is lost in the urine. All forms of nephrosis present with massive proteinuria. As albumin is lost, the plasma colloid osmotic pressure decreases and fluids and electrolytes are lost into the interstitial spaces. This is seen clinically as edema. Treatment includes the administration of high doses of corticosteroids, which results in a sustained remission of the disease in most adults. Careful skin care and frequent positioning and inspection are of high priority in planning care for the patient. The decrease in plasma proteins increases the patient's susceptibility to infections. Thus the protection from infectious sources is appropriate. The patient's diet may be restricted in both protein

and sodium. On rare occasions, an abdominal paracentesis may be done for massive edema.

## NEPHROSCLEROSIS

*Nephrosclerosis* is defined as a hypertensive vascular disease which involves the renal vasculature. The disease has several forms, which may be characterized as a general arteriosclerosis, an arteriolar (benign) nephrosclerosis, and an accelerated form of hypertensive disease, generally called malignant hypertension. As the blood supply to renal tissue is decreased, renal damage occurs. Most patients die from problems other than renal failure, namely stroke and heart disease. The few patients who demonstrate massive renal involvement have symptoms similar to those of chronic glomerulonephritis, and nursing care has been elaborated in that section.

## TUBERCULOSIS OF THE KIDNEY

Spread of pulmonary tuberculosis to the kidneys is the most common site for the occurrence of a secondary localized tuberculosis infection. The high oxygen tension of the renal arterial blood supports the survival of the tubercle bacillus for long periods of time. The patient generally presents with signs of hematuria, pyuria, and the presence of the tubercle bacillus in the urine. Frequently pain, urinary frequency, and dysuria are present. Successful treatment is accomplished with chemotherapy, including streptomycin, para-aminosalicylic acid, and isoniazid. Nursing approaches that are appropriate include the identification of high-risk patients among those patients known to have tuberculosis. A careful follow-up on any urinary tract symptoms is necessary in order to detect the tuberculosis spread early. Nursing care includes instructing the patient and family in protective care and ensuring that medications are taken.

## NEPHROPTOSIS

Nephroptosis is a condition which occurs when the fat pad that normally holds the kidney in place is absent, and the kidney sags into the pelvic cavity. Symptoms are produced by obstruction of the ureters which accompanies the sagging movement of the kidney, and include acute pain, nausea, vomiting, and on occasion, chills and fever. The acute attack is referred to as *Dietl's crisis.* Treatment involves the surgical procedure, *nephropexy,* wherein the kidney is sutured into its normal anatomical location. Nursing care during the acute attack involves positioning the patient in a supine position with a pillow placed under the hips so that the tension on the kidney and ureter is minimized. Problems associated with the pre- and postoperative care of the patient undergoing nephropexy are similar to those discussed above under the surgical treatment of renal calculi.

## REFERENCES

1   E. L. Becker, "Foreword," in F. H. Netter, *The CIBA Collection of Medical Illustrations,* vol. 6; *A Compilation of Paintings on the Kidneys, Ureters, and Urinary Bladder,* CIBA, Summit, New Jersey, 1973, p. vii.
2   R. W. Schrier and J. D. Conger, "Acute Renal Failure: Pathogenesis, Diagnosis, and Management," in R. W. Schrier (ed.), *Renal and Electrolyte Disorders,* Little, Brown, Boston, 1976, p. 289.
3   P. Freedman and E. C. Smith, "Acute Renal Failure," *Heart and Lung,* **4:**873–878, November–December 1975.
4   *Morbidity and Mortality Weekly Report,* U.S. Department of Health, Education, and Welfare, Public Health Service, **24**(7):59–60, February 15, 1975.
5   A. C. Alfrey, "Chronic Renal Failure: Manifestations and Pathogenesis," in R. W. Schrier (ed.), *Renal and Electrolyte Disorders,* Little, Brown, Boston, 1976, p. 333.
6   R. C. Pabico, "Dialysis in Chronic Renal Failure," in G. L. Hansen (ed.), *Caring for Patients with Chronic Renal Disease,* University of Rochester, Rochester, 1972, p. 40.
7   J. D. Harrington and E. R. Brener, *Patient Care in Renal Failure,* Saunders, Philadelphia, 1973, pp. 86–102.
8   R. B. Freeman, "Pathophysiology and Conservative Management of Chronic Renal Disease," in G. L. Hansen (ed.), *Caring for Patients with Chronic Renal Disease,* University of Rochester, Rochester, 1972, p. 16.
9   R. B. Freeman, "Introduction of the Problem of Chronic Renal Disease," in G. L. Hansen (ed.), *Caring for Patients with Chronic Renal Disease,* University of Rochester, Rochester, 1972, p. 1.
10   A. C. Alfrey, "Chronic Renal failure: Manifestations and Pathogenesis," in R. W. Schrier (ed.), *Renal and Electrolyte Disorders,* Little, Brown, Boston, 1976, p. 331.
11   S. G. Massry, J. W. Coburn, D. B. N. Lee, J. Fowsey, and C. R. Cleeman, "Skeletal Resistance to Parathyroid Hormone in Renal Failure: Studies in 105 Human Subjects," *Ann Intern Med,* **78:**357–364, March 1973.
12   Alfrey, A. C. "Chronic Renal Failure: Manifestations and Pathogenesis," in R. W. Schrier (ed.), Little, Brown, Boston, 1976, p. 338.
13   D. Zschoche (ed.), "Concepts in Hemodialysis," *Critical Care Update!,* **3:**26–27, March 1976.
14   D. B. McLaughlin and F. L. Shapiro, "Regional Kidney Disease Network Offers Efficient Care, Operation," *Hospitals,* **50:**89–92, January 1, 1976.
15   C. F. Gutch and M. H. Stoner, *Review of Hemodialysis for Nurses and Dialysis Personnel,* Mosby, St. Louis, 1975, pp. 143–144.
16   Advisory Committee to the Renal Transplant Registry, "The Eleventh Report of the Human Renal Transplant Registry," *JAMA,* **226:**1197–1204, December 3, 1973.
17   R. G. Wright, P. Sand, and G. Livingston, "Psychological Stress During Hemodialysis for Chronic Renal Failure," *Ann Intern Med,* **64:**611–621, March 1966.
18   P. M. MacElveen, "Cooperative Triad in Home Dialysis: Care and Patient Outcomes," in M. V. Batey (ed.), *Communicating Nursing Research,* vol. 5, Western Interstate Commission for Higher Education, Boulder, Colo., 1972, pp. 134–147.
19   F. H. Netter (ed.), *The CIBA Collection of Medical Illustrations,* vol. 6, *A Compilation of Paintings on the Kidneys, Ureters, and Urinary Bladder,* CIBA, Summit, New Jersey, 1973, p. 131.
20   M. B. Strauss and L. G. Welt (eds.), *The Kidney,* Little, Brown, Boston, 1971, p. 973.

## BIBLIOGRAPHY

Abram, H. S.: "Survival by Machine: The Psychological Stress of Chronic Hemodialysis," *Psychiatry Med,* **1**(1):37–51, 1970.
Berne, T. V. and B. H. Barbour: "Hemodialysis for Postoperative Acute Renal Insufficiency," *RN,* **35**(3): ICU5–ICU11, March 1972.
Blagg, C. R., R. O. Hickman, J. W. Eschbach, and B. H. Scribner: "Home Hemodialysis: Six Years' Experience," *N Engl J Med,* **283**(21):1126–1131, November 19, 1970.
Cummings, J. W.: "Hemodialysis—Feelings, Facts, Fantasies," *Am J Nurs,* **70**(1):70–79, January 1970.
DiPalma, J. R.: "Preventing Drug Toxicity in Renal Failure," *RN,* **38**(6):65–69, June 1975.
Dolan, P. O., and H. L. Greene: "Renal Failure and Peritoneal Dialysis," *Nurs '75,* **5**(7):41–49, July 1975.
Downing, S. R.: Nursing Support in Early Renal Failure," *Am J Nurs,* **69**(6):1212–1216, June 1969.

Fennell, S. E.: "Percutaneous Renal Biopsy," *Am J Nurs,* **75**:1292–1294, August 1975.

Horoshak, I: "A Special Kind of Kidney Patient," *RN* **38**(1):55–59, October 1975.

Kintzel, J. E. and E. M. Cameron: "The Insulted Kidney: Medical and Nursing Intervention for Patients Undergoing Dialysis or Renal Homotransplantation," in K. C. Kintzel (ed.), *Advanced Concepts in Clinical Nursing,* Lippincott, Philadelphia, 1971, pp. 277–291.

Metheny, N. M. and W. D. Snively: *Nurses' Handbook of Fluid Balance,* 2d ed., Lippincott, Philadelphia, 1974.

Nassen, A.: "Arteriovenous Shunt Implantation: An Adolescent's Perception and Response," *Am J Nurs,* **70**(10):2171–2176, October 1970.

O'Neill, Mary I.: "Home Dialysis: A Most Encompassing Nursing Situation," *ANA Clinical Sessions, 1972,* Appleton-Century-Crofts, New York, 1972, pp. 141–148.

O'Neill, Mary (ed.): "Symposium on Care of the Patient with Renal Disease," *Nurs Clin N Am,* **10**:411–516, September 1975.

Read, M. and M. Mallison "External Arteriovenous Shunts," *Am J Nurs,* **72**(1):81–85, January 1972.

Santopietro, M.: "Meeting the Emotional Needs of Hemodialysis Patients and Their Spouses," *Am J Nurs,* **75**(4):629–632, April 1975.

Schlotter, L.: "Hemodialysis: What Do You Teach the Dialysis Patient," *Am J Nurs,* **70**(1):83, January 1970.

Stroat, V. R., C. A. Lee, and C. A. Schoper: *Fluids and Electrolytes: A Practical Approach,* Davis, Philadelphia, 1974.

Visel, J. M.: "Clinical Aspects of Renal Biopsy," *Heart and Lung,* **4**:900–902, November–December 1975.

Williams, S. R: *Nutrition and Diet Therapy,* Mosby, St. Louis, 1969.

Wolf, Z. R.: "What Patients Awaiting Kidney Transplant Want To Know," *Am J Nurs,* **76:**92–94, January 1976.

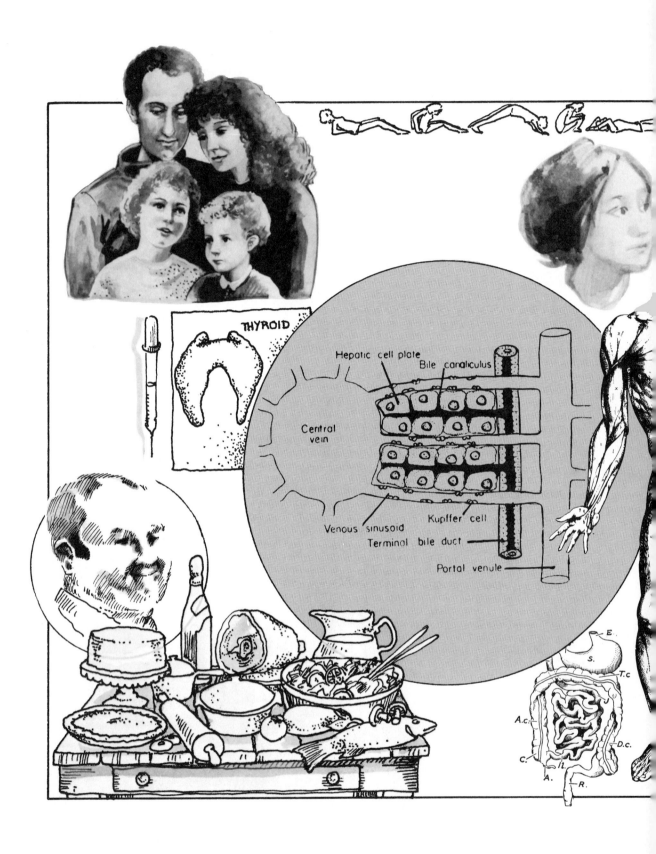

THYROID

Hepatic cell plate
Bile canaliculus
Central vein
Venous sinusoid
Kupffer cell
Terminal bile duct
Portal venule

E.
S.
T.c
A.c
D.c
C.
I.
A.
R.

# PART 5
## METABOLISM

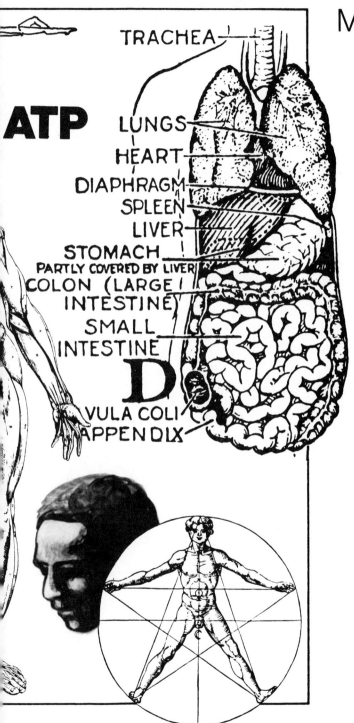

**ATP**

TRACHEA

LUNGS

HEART

DIAPHRAGM

SPLEEN

LIVER

STOMACH
PARTLY COVERED BY LIVER

COLON (LARGE
INTESTINE)

SMALL
INTESTINE

**D**

VULA COLI

APPENDIX

# 15
# THE CONCEPT OF METABOLISM*

Mary Marmoll Jirovec
Anne Fero Chestnut

**M**etabolism involves change. Defined literally, it encompasses all the material changes in a cell. Changes in matter correspond to changes in energy, and energy is at the core of metabolism. When metabolism is defined from a broad perspective, it includes all the bodily processes that contribute to changing the chemical energy contained in food to mechanical energy, heat, or cellular chemical energy.

## ENERGY EXCHANGES

Because energy can be neither created nor destroyed but is changed from one form to another, the body's energy requirements must be obtained from its external environment. This interaction between man and environment is one of the most dramatic exchanges. Chemical energy contained in food is removed from the environment and taken into the body through *ingestion.* The food is then mechanically and chemically broken down by *digestion.* Once broken down, the nutrients are taken into the body from the gastrointestinal tract during *absorption.* Indigestible foodstuffs are then returned to the environment by *elimination.* During carbohydrate, fat, and protein metabolism, the absorbed food is changed in various ways in order to liberate for immediate use or store the chemical energy it contains. *Hepatic influences* play an integral role in changing carbohydrates, fats, and proteins. Lastly, the various metabolic processes are controlled by *hormonal influences.*

## METABOLISM

Energy may be defined as the capacity to do work. The purpose of all the body's metabolic processes is to obtain energy. Metabolism allows muscles to contract, nerves to conduct, cellular components such as proteins, fatty acids, cholesterol, phospholipids, hormones, hemoglobin, enzymes, genes, and antibodies to be synthesized, glands to secrete, and substances to be actively transported across membranes. The body obtains its energy by changing the potential energy contained in the chemical bonds of food to kinetic or moving energy such as muscle contraction or to potential energy contained in chemical bonds within the body. When energy is transferred from one form of potential energy to another, some kinetic energy

* The section on metabolism was written by Mary Marmoll Jirovec and the section on physical assessment by Anne Fero Chestnut.

will be lost. The term *entropy* refers to the amount of energy lost. In the body this occurs by loss of heat. Therefore, energy changes within the body can be measured by heat. The greater the temperature, the greater the changes in energy.

Energy is liberated from food by oxidation. When foods are burned outside the body, the energy is lost as heat. Inside the body this energy is coupled with enzymes and energy transfer systems to create potential energy for use in the body. During this oxidation and coupling, entropy occurs and energy is lost to the environment as heat. External work also increases entropy and decreases the energy content of the body. The more work done, the greater will be the energy needs.

In man the primary chemical bond used to store energy is adenosine triphosphate (ATP). This compound has three phosphates attached by high-energy bonds. If one of the phosphates is removed, the compound becomes adenosine diphosphate (ADP) and energy is released. If another phosphate is removed, the compound becomes adenosine monophosphate (AMP) and again energy is released for use by the body. ATP, then, is the "energy currency" of the body. As food is oxidized, the energy is used to form the high-energy phosphate bonds.

$$\text{AMP} \xrightarrow{\text{energy}} \text{ADP} \xrightarrow{\text{energy}} \text{ATP}$$

As the body needs energy, the phosphate radicals are given up.

$$\text{ATP} \xrightarrow{\text{energy}} \text{ADP} \xrightarrow{\text{energy}} \text{AMP}$$

ATP is the primary energy-rich bond found in the body. Other chemicals are present which also contain high-energy bonds and thus are sources of energy for the cell. These include acetyl coenzyme A, glycerophosphate, glucose-6-phosphate, creatine phosphate, and many more.

The rate of energy exchange within the body is expressed as the *metabolic rate*. Several factors influence an individual's metabolic rate. There are sex differences, with women generally having a lower rate than men. This rate decreases even more with menopause. Metabolic rate is also decreased during menstruation. It tends to decrease with age and increase during periods of growth as during the last trimester of pregnancy. The metabolic rate varies with the seasons, decreasing in warm weather and increasing in cold. Cultural differences have also been observed. Australians, Chinese,

Indians, and Syrians were found to have lower rates than other Caucasians living in the same area, while American Indians in the area had higher metabolic rates.[1] Manual labor increases the rate. It is increased with increased protein ingestion and decreased with lowered intake of protein. Drugs can influence the metabolic rate; epinephrine, caffeine, camphor, atropine, and nicotine (from smoking) increase it, while morphine, barbiturates, and chloral hydrate decrease it.

## Ingestion

*Ingestion* or the intake of food is the necessary first step in normal metabolism. *Hunger* is the awareness of the need to ingest food. It is usually accompanied by hunger pains, increased salivation, and food-searching behavior. While hunger is an awareness of a need, *appetite* is a desire to ingest food. Hunger is influenced by physiological changes, while appetite can be influenced by a multiplicity of factors. Appetite often persists when hunger is appeased. *Satiety* is the lack of desire to eat after food ingestion.

Hunger and satiety are under nervous system control. The *feeding center* is located in the ventrolateral nuclei of the hypothalamus and is most likely stimulated by the blood glucose level and/or possible receptors in the gastrointestinal tract that determine the calorie content of food. The *satiety center* is located in the ventromedial nuclei and, when stimulated, inhibits the feeding center. The satiety center may be stimulated by increases in blood glucose and stomach distention.

If eating were solely controlled by these physiological mechanisms, imbalances between food intake and energy output would not exist. Ingestion, however, can be influenced by sensory stimulation in relation to the sight and smell of food or auditory reminders of food, cultural factors, affluence, boredom, increases in energy requirements, and drugs such as the barbiturates. Ingestion is generally inhibited by stomach distention, dehydration, increases in blood glucose, increases in the temperature of the hypothalamus, and drugs such as amphetamines.

Once food is taken into the mouth, it must be swallowed for ingestion to be complete. This is accomplished by holding the bolus of food between the upper surface of the tongue and the roof of the mouth. The soft palate rises to close off the nasopharynx. The larynx moves under the epiglottis to prevent entry into the trachea. The tongue, then, propels the bolus back and into the esophagus.

## Digestion

*Digestion* encompasses all the processes that change food into a form that can be absorbed into the body. It begins in the mouth, continues in the stomach, and is completed in the small intestine. It is dependent on the ability of the gastrointestinal tract to both move food through the tract and secrete substances to break it down. Table 15-1 summarizes the secretions into the gastrointestinal tract and their functions.

**Mouth**   Digestion begins in the mouth where food is mechanically broken down by chewing and mixed with saliva. In general, saliva is a hypotonic solution containing sodium, calcium, bicarbonate,

**TABLE 15-1**
GASTROINTESTINAL TRACT SECRETIONS

| Location | Secreting Structures | Secretion | Action |
|---|---|---|---|
| Mouth | Parotid glands<br>Sublingual and submandibular glands | Ptyalin<br>Mucus | Starch digestion<br>Lubrication<br>Dissolve food to activate taste buds<br>Bactericidal effect |
| Esophagus | Epithelial cells | Mucus | Lubrication<br>Protection<br>Neutralization of acids and bases |
| Cardiac portion of stomach | Cardiac glands | Mucus<br><br>Electrolytes | Protection<br>Lubrication<br>Buffering action |
| Fundus and body of stomach | Mucus neck cells<br>Parietal cells<br><br>Chief cells | Mucus<br>Hydrochloric acid<br>Intrinsic factor<br>Pepsinogens | Protection<br>Protein digestion<br>Vitamin $B_{12}$ absorption<br>Protein digestion |
| Pyloric portion of stomach | Pyloric glands | Mucus<br>Electrolytes | Protection<br>Buffer acid |
| First few centimeters of duodenum | Brunner's glands | Alkaline mucus | Neutralize acid<br>Protection |
| Small intestine | Goblet cells<br><br>Epithelial cells of crypts of Lieberkühn<br><br><br>Inside epithelial cells of crypts of Lieberkühn | Mucus<br><br>Isotonic fluid<br><br>Enterokinase<br>Amylase<br>Peptidases<br>Maltase<br>Sucrose<br>Lactose<br>Isomaltose<br>Intestinal lipase | Lubrication<br>Protection<br>Lubrication<br>Absorption<br>Activates trypsin<br>Carbohydrate digestion<br>Protein digestion<br>Disaccharides to monosaccharides<br><br><br><br>Neutral fats to glycerol and fatty acids |
| Pancreas | Acini and ducts leading from acini | Isotonic fluid high in $NaHCO_3$ and KCl<br>Pancreatic amylase<br>Pancreatic lipase<br><br>Proteolytic enzymes (trypsin, chymotrypsins, carbopolypeptides, ribonuclease, deoxyribonuclease) | Lubrication<br>Buffer acids<br>Starch to disaccharides<br>Fats to fatty acids, glycerides, and glycerol<br>Proteins to amino acids |
| Gallbladder | Hepatic cells of the liver | Isotonic fluid<br>Bile salts<br><br><br><br><br>Bile lipids<br>Bile protein<br>Bilirubin<br>Alkaline phosphatase | Solution<br>Emulsify fats<br>Aid in absorption of fatty acids, monoglycerides, and fat soluble vitamins (A, D, E, and K)<br>Facilitate lipase action<br>By-product of bile salt formation<br>Result from leakage<br>Waste product<br>No specific function in digestion |

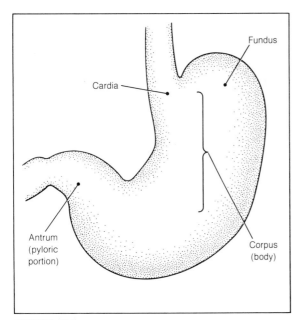

**FIGURE 15-1**
Anatomical divisions of the stomach.

potassium, mucus, and amylase (ptyalin). It begins starch digestion as well as lubricating, dissolving, and serving a bacteriocidal function (Table 15-1). Secretion of saliva is stimulated by nervous reflexes. The sight, smell, thought, or taste of food can increase or decrease secretion. Oral tactile stimulation or chewing movements also increase salivation.

**Esophagus** The bolus of food from the mouth is propelled into the esophagus which runs from the pharynx to the stomach. The esophagus functions to carry the food to the stomach. It accomplishes this movement by peristaltic waves. These are waves of contraction that are generally preceded by active relaxation. They can occur in both directions, but generally stimulation at the beginning of the esophagus causes forward movement to the stomach. Mucus, which is secreted throughout the gastrointestinal tract, is the only secretion of the esophagus. It contains mucin, water, and inorganic salts and functions to lubricate the esophagus, protect the mucosa from esophageal contents, and neutralize acids and bases. The last segment of the esophagus is the cardiac sphincter which prevents the gastric contents from reentering the esophagus.

**Stomach** The stomach serves as a reservoir to hold the food and slowly feed it into the intestine. Anatomically the stomach can be divided into four areas: the cardiac, fundus, body, and pyloric portions which are depicted in Fig. 15-1. Each contains specialized cells which secrete fluids that aid in digesting the food while in the stomach. The stomach is capable of both mixing and peristaltic movements so that the food can be both mixed with gastric secretions and propelled into the intestine.

Table 15-1 summarizes the various types of gastric secretions and their functions. The major secretions of the stomach are mucus, pepsinogen, and hydrochloric acid (HCl). Small amounts of gastric lipase and gastric amylase can also be found in gastric juice, but their digestive functions are not significant.

The parietal cells produce HCl by actively secreting hydrogen and chloride ions into the stomach while bicarbonate ($HCO_3^-$) is returned to the plasma. The $HCO_3^-$ is eliminated in the urine in order to maintain acid-base balance and accounts for the postprandial alkaline tide seen in the urine. The chief cells secrete pepsinogen which is a precursor of pepsin. In an acid pH of 6 or less, pepsinogen converts to pepsin, which in turn causes more pepsinogen to become pepsin. The cardiac glands, mucous neck cells, and pyloric glands all secrete mucus which forms a film over the gastric epithelial cells to protect them against the action of pepsin and HCl. The mucus further protects the stomach lining by buffering the strong acid as it comes in contact with it.

There are three phases of gastric secretion which come under nervous and hormonal control. In the *cephalic phase* the sight, smell, touch, or taste of food cause parasympathetic stimulation and an increase in gastric secretions. In the *gastric phase* bulk in the stomach results in vagal stimulation which increases secretion and motility. Food in the stomach also stimulates epithelial "gastrin" cells in the gastric mucosa to secrete gastrin which is absorbed into the circulation. Gastrin increases gastric motility and secretion of acid. It also moderately stimulates pepsin and intrinsic factor production. In the *intestinal phase* of gastric secretion bulk in the small intestine stimulates the enterogastric reflex which decreases secretion. At the same time fat in the small intestine causes the release of enterogastrone into the circulation which decreases gastric activity. Histamine released from damaged cells also stimulates acid production, as does an increased serum calcium level. Ethanol acts as a local gastric irritant and at the same time stimulates gastrin secretion. Caffeine increases acid production, probably by the same mechanism.[2]

**Small intestine** In the small intestine digestion of all ingested foods is completed. This is accomplished with secretions from the intestine itself, pancreas, and liver and with both mixing and peristaltic movements. Table 15-1 summarizes the secretions found in the small intestine. The secretions function to break down carbohydrates to monosaccharides, fats to glycerol and fatty acids, and proteins to amino acids so that they can be assimilated into the body.

The *secretions of the small intestine* itself are primarily under nervous system control. Locally, direct mechanical or chemical stimulation, as when there is food in the intestine, will increase intestinal secretions. Parasympathetic stimulation increases motility and secretion, while sympathetic stimulation decreases them. Several reflexes affect motility and secretion in the small intestine; these are summarized in Table 15-2. In most cases distention or irritation of certain tissues will result in a decrease in intestinal motility and secretions. There is also a hormone produced by the small intestine, *duocrinin,* which may have a stimulatory effect on intestinal secretions. Recent studies have suggested that pancreatic enzymes as well stimulate the intestinal epithelial cells to release enzymes[3]

Control of *pancreatic secretions* is both neural and hormonal. During the cephalic phase of digestion parasympathetic stimulation increases pancreatic secretions. Locally, food in the intestines initiates local reflexes which result in increased secretion. Two hormones secreted by the mucosa of the duodenum affect pancreatic secretion. As gastric contents enter the duodenum, *secretin* and *pancreozymin* are released. Secretin stimulates the production of alkaline fluids from the pancreas, while pancreozymin increases secretion of an enzyme-rich fluid.

*Bile secretion* occurs continually in the liver. After it is secreted, it either is stored in the gallbladder or empties directly into the intestine. Peristalsis causes periodic relaxing of the sphincter of Oddi so that bile not stored in the gallbladder periodically spurts into the intestine. The bile in the gallbladder is released into the intestine when the gallbladder contracts. During the cephalic phase of gastric secretion, parasympathetic stimulation causes mild contraction. The primary mechanism for gallbladder contraction is related to a hormone— *cholecystokinin.* Fat in the intestine causes the intestinal mucosa to secrete this hormone. It is absorbed into the blood and stimulates the gallbladder to contract. At the same time the sphincter of Oddi is relaxed.

## Absorption

Once food has been adequately broken down, *absorption* occurs—primarily in the small intestine. The stomach absorbs water while the large intestine absorbs water and electrolytes. Some monosaccharides and amino acids could be absorbed in the large intestine but normally do not reach it.

The absorbing surface of the small intestine is increased sevenfold by the presence of *villi*—small fingerlike projections. Villi are most numerous in the duodenum and begin to disappear in the terminal ileum. Food is absorbed best in the proximal small intestine. Most absorption of fats, protein, and glucose is complete halfway down the jejunum. Only 10 percent of the ingested protein will be found in the distal ileum.

*Carbohydrates* are ingested as polysaccharides, disaccharides, and monosaccharides. Polysaccharides are absorbed only in minute quantities while some dissaccharides are absorbed and

**TABLE 15-2**
REFLEXES AFFECTING INTESTINAL ACTIVITY

| Reflexes | Stimulant | Effect on intestinal activity |
|---|---|---|
| Gastroenteric | Gastric distention | Increased |
| Intestinal-intestinal | Overdistention or irritation in one part of intestine | Increased in affected part and decreased in other parts |
| Peritoneal-intestinal | Distention or irritation of peritoneum | Decreased |
| Renointestinal | Distention or irritation of kidney | Decreased |
| Vesicointestinal | Distention or irritation of bladder | Decreased |
| Somatointestinal | Distention or irritation of abdominal skin | Decreased |

hydrolyzed internally. Most are broken down to monosaccharides and absorbed as glucose, fructose, and galactose. This absorption occurs by passive diffusion and active transport.

Ingested *fats* are emulsified and hydrolyzed by bile and lipases to glycerol, fatty acids, and mono-glycerides, diglycerides, and triglycerides. Glycerol is absorbed into the portal circulation. The fatty acids and glycerides are absorbed by the intestinal epithelium probably through pinocytosis, synthesized into fats, and carried away by the lymph. Fats travel in the lymph in droplets called *chylomicrons.* The fats are emptied into a vein from the thoracic lymph duct.

*Proteins* are broken down into amino acids and absorbed into the bloodstream. When large quantities of amino acids are present, some will enter the lymph. The exact nature of the transport system that allows amino acids to be absorbed is not known, but it does occur against a concentration gradient.

The greatest amount of *iron* is absorbed in the duodenum as soluble ferrous iron. Iron is usually ingested as the insoluble ferric form and needs to be converted to ferrous. This occurs at a low pH as when ascorbic acid has been ingested. When the acidity is decreased, as happens after ingestion of milk or antacids, the ferric iron forms insoluble iron salts and is not absorbed. *Calcium* is absorbed in both the stomach and duodenum and also needs an acid pH to prevent it from forming insoluble calcium salts. Dietary proteins and vitamin D facilitate calcium absorption.

There are several intestinal secretions which are reabsorbed. The large quantities of water and electrolytes are all readily reabsorbed. The enzymes which are proteins and the fats, cholesterol, and protein from desquamated epithelial cells are digested and absorbed. Ninety-five percent of the bile acids are reabsorbed in the lower part of the small intestine. Bilirubin is changed to urobilinogen by the action of bacteria, and some of this is reabsorbed. The mucus that is secreted undergoes spontaneous liquefaction.

## Elimination

After food is digested and all usable substances absorbed, the indigestible material needs to be removed to maintain the patency of the gastrointestinal tract. The large intestine primarily functions in this capacity. Before expelling its contents, it extracts any useful substances from the feces. Most often these are water and electrolytes.

The only digestion that occurs in the large intestine results from bacterial action.

To aid in elimination, the large intestine secretes mucus which protects the epithelial lining and causes the feces to adhere. When irritating or toxic substances are present in the large intestine, it secretes water and electrolytes to dilute the contents and move them rapidly through to the external environment. Tactile stimulation of the intestinal mucosa and parasympathetic stimulation also increase these secretions.

Flatus is a normal constituent of the gastrointestinal tract which is eliminated through the large intestine. It originates from swallowed air, the action of bacteria on food, and the diffusion of gases from the blood.

*Defecation* is the expelling of the contents of the large intestine into the environment. It is caused by a wave of contraction that begins about midway along the transverse colon. The rectum is passive and receives the feces. As they accumulate in the rectum, peristaltic waves of the descending colon are initiated. The interior sphincter relaxes and the external sphincter is voluntarily relaxed, resulting in a bowel movement. Defecation is often initiated by reflexes. In the *duodenocolic reflex,* filling of the duodenum causes mass movements in the colon. Similarly, filling of the stomach results in mass movements (*gastrocolic reflex*).

## Carbohydrate Metabolism

Carbohydrates are absorbed primarily as glucose, although some fructose and galactose are also absorbed. The latter two are converted to glucose by the liver. Several things can happen to glucose after absorption. It can be broken down and used for energy—*glycolysis.* It can be stored primarily in the liver and skeletal muscle as glycogen—*glycogenesis.* Or it can be synthesized into fat for storage—*lipogenesis.*

Glucose can enter the body by injection, from gastrointestinal absorption, and through internal secretion. During internal secretion the liver and skeletal muscle convert glycogen back to glucose—*glycogenolysis.* The liver also can make glucose from fats and proteins—*gluconeogenesis.* It does this by deaminizing amino acids or using fats and converting them to glucose.

Glucose is either stored for later use or used immediately. It is taken up by cells through a process of facilitated diffusion. The process which liberates energy from glucose is outlined in Fig. 15-2. Once inside the cell it is immediately combined with a phosphate radical to hold it in the cell. If not stored as glycogen, it will be broken down for energy. This breakdown (glycolysis) splits the glucose into two molecules of pyruvic acid through 10 successive steps that produce four hydrogen ions, heat, and two ATP molecules. Pyruvic acid becomes two molecules of acetyl co-enzyme A (CoA), liberating two carbon dioxide molecules and four hydrogen ions.

Acetyl CoA then enters the Krebs cycle (tri-carboxylic acid cycle). In the cycle it combines with oxaloacetic acid to form citric acid. In successive steps of the cycle several molecules of water are added, carbon dioxide and hydrogen ions released, and one molecule of ATP formed. The last reaction forms oxaloacetic acid, and the cycle begins anew with another molecule of acetyl CoA. The hydrogen ions released during the cycle are oxidized to form water, and during this process 30 ATP molecules are formed.

This schema of glucose breakdown encompasses 95 percent of the glycolysis in the body. A second route, the phosphogluconate pathway, can be followed by glucose; it is less well understood but accounts for up to 30 percent of the glycolysis that occurs in the liver.

Oxygen is needed to remove the end products of glycolysis. In the absence of oxygen, pyruvic acid will build up. If this occurs, glycolysis will cease and with it the energy supply. To prevent the buildup of pyruvic acid when oxygen is not available, the body converts to anaerobic metabolism. Pyruvic acid is changed to lactic acid and allowed to diffuse out of the cell, thus clearing it of the end products of glycolysis. When oxygen again becomes available, the reaction is reversed and lactic acid is converted back to pyruvic acid. The heart especially is able to convert lactic acid to pyruvic acid and thus use it for energy.

## Fat Metabolism

The major types of lipids in the body are the glycerides (e.g., triglyceride composed of fatty acids and glycerol), phospholipids, and cholesterol. As much as two-thirds to three-fourths of the energy needed by cells can come from fats. This is accomplished primarily through the use of triglycerides for energy.

Triglyceride is broken down into glycerol and fatty acids. Glycerol can be used by the cells in the Krebs cycle for energy. Fatty acids are picked up by the liver and through successive steps that release many ATP molecules converted to acetyl

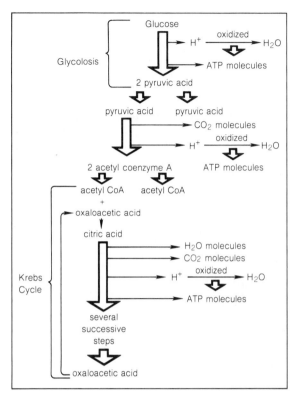

**FIGURE 15-2**
Aerobic carbohydrate metabolism.

CoA. Two acetyl CoA molecules quickly combine to form acetoacetic acid which diffuses into the blood and goes to the cell, where it again becomes two acetyl CoA molecules which enter the Krebs cycle. Acetoacetic acid is a ketone body and in abundance can form acetone, which is volatile and is expired through the lungs.

Fats not used for energy can be stored in adipose tissue or synthesized into other lipids in the liver. Adipose tissue is composed of triglycerides (fatty acids and glycerol) and is synthesized from fatty acids in the bloodstream and glucose. Adipose tissue is constantly exchanging fatty acids with the blood. When energy is needed, adipose tissue releases fatty acids and glycerol into the circulation. The liver not only degrades triglycerides and fatty acids for use as energy but synthesizes glucose from fats (gluconeogenesis) and synthesizes other lipids from triglycerides.

The primary lipids formed by the liver are phospholipid and cholesterol. When ingested, cholesterol causes only a slight increase in the cholesterol level as the liver will compensate by synthesizing less. Ingestion of saturated fats, however, results in an increased synthesis of cholesterol, increasing its level in the body. Conversely, ingestion of unsaturated fats will tend to decrease the cholesterol concentration.

Cholesterol serves several functions. About 80 percent of it is used to form cholic acid which forms the bile salts necessary for fat digestion. It also helps to form hormones (especially the adrenal cortical steroids and the sex hormones) and the water-resistant quality of the corneum of the skin. Cholesterol as well as the phospholipids are necessary to the physical integrity of cells by forming the insoluble cell membrane.

The liver cells synthesize 90 percent of the phospholipids. They are transported in the blood as lipoproteins. Ninety-five percent of all blood lipids are in the form of lipoproteins which are synthesized in the liver. Phospholipids serve several functions in the body. They help transport fatty acids through the intestinal mucosa into the lymph; they insulate nerve fibers; they are used in phosphate tissue reactions; they act as carriers in active transport; they form thromboplastin; and they form some of the structural elements of the body.

### Protein Metabolism

Protein composes about three-fourths of the body's solids. It is obtained from the diet as amino acids. There are 21 different kinds of amino acids. Eleven of them can be synthesized by the body and are called *nonessential* amino acids. The other 10 cannot be synthesized by the body or are synthesized in very small quantities and are, therefore, *essential* to the diet. Amino acids absorbed from the gastrointestinal tract and formed by the body are used to synthesize the various proteins of the body. This process is called *anabolism* and is the building up of body protein. *Catabolism* is the opposite of this or the breakdown of body proteins. The body proteins include fibrous proteins, globular proteins, enzymes, genes, oxygen transporting protein, muscle protein, hormones, and various substances such as creatinine glycocholic acid (bile acid), and histamine.

The plasma concentration of amino acids is fairly constant. As amino acids are absorbed from the intestines, they very rapidly move into cells by active transport, where they are conjugated into cellular protein for storage (anabolism). As the concentration of plasma amino acids decreases, the process is reversed (catabolism). Any tissue that needs amino acids uses them from the common

blood supply, and other tissues replenish what has been used.

Individual cells are able to store only a certain amount of excess protein. The liver, kidney, and intestinal mucosa have the greatest capacity for this. The liver also uses amino acids to synthesize plasma proteins; gamma globulins are synthesized in reticuloendothelial cells and the lymph. Amino acids not synthesized into body proteins are used for energy or stored as fat. The liver makes this possible by deaminizing amino acids and using the deaminized compounds to synthesize glucose (gluconeogenesis) or fats (lipogenesis). The ammonia that results from deaminization is made into urea which is eliminated in the urine. Figure 15-3 summarizes protein metabolism. A certain amount of protein is degraded by the liver every day; it equals about 30 g and is considered *obligatory protein degradation*.

### Hepatic Influences on Metabolism

The liver plays an integral role in metabolism. It is a large, vascular, complex organ located in the upper right quadrant of the abdomen. Its functional unit is the lobule, and the liver contains 50,000 to 100,000 lobules. Figure 15-4 illustrates the normal structure of the liver lobule. It is formed around a central vein which empties into the hepatic vein. The hepatic plates radiating from the central vein are composed of two layers of hepatic cells. The bile canaliculi between the cells drain into the terminal bile duct. The portal vein from the mesentary flows into the portal venules which feed into the venous sinusoids between the plates. The venous sinusoids drain into the central vein. The sinusoids are lined with epithelial and Kupffer cells.

Bile circulation from the liver begins in the bile canaliculi. These drain into the terminal bile duct which flows first into the right or left hepatic ducts and then into the common hepatic duct. This is joined by the cystic duct from the gallbladder to form the common bile duct. The common bile duct terminates in the ampulla of Vater, where it is joined by the pancreatic duct and enters the intestine through the sphincter of Oddi.

The blood circulation to the liver summarized in Fig. 15-5 has a unique feature which allows blood from the mesentery rich with the products of absorption to pass through the liver before going to the rest of the body. This is accomplished by the portal vein, which flows from the intestines into the liver. Blood flows from the two branches of the portal vein through portal tracts to the sinusoids. The hepatic artery carries oxygenated blood to the liver, and the sinusoids contain a mixture of arterial blood and portal vein blood. The hepatic vein carries this blood to the vena cava.

The widespread functions of the liver are outlined in Fig. 15-6. First, the liver plays a variety of roles in maintaining normal *metabolism.* As blood glucose increases, two-thirds of the extra glucose will be immediately stored in the liver as glycogen (glycogenesis). As blood glucose falls, glycogenolysis immediately occurs. If this does not meet the need, the liver makes glucose from amino acids and glycerol (gluconeogenesis). The liver also converts galactose and fructose absorbed from the intestine to glucose. It makes fats from other fats, as well as glucose and amino acids (lipogenesis). When glucose is not available for energy, it oxidizes fatty acids, releasing ketone bodies into the blood for energy.

The liver synthesizes amino acids and converts one type into another. Besides synthesizing amino acids, it synthesizes cholesterol, phospholipids, and lipoprotein from fats, glucose, and amino acids

and plasma proteins from amino acids. The liver converts carotene to vitamin A and stores vitamins A, D, and E. The last of the liver's metabolic functions involves digestion as the liver produces bile salts that are essential to fat breakdown.

The liver *detoxifies* several substances listed in Fig. 15-6. In general it does this by converting lipid-soluble substances to substances less lipid-soluble or water-soluble so that they can be eliminated in the urine. The Kupffer cells lining the sinusoids are highly phagocytic and absorb and digest over 99 percent of any bacteria in the portal circulation as well as foreign colloids, tumor cells, endotoxins, and particulate antigens. Since portal blood comes from the intestines, it always contains some colon bacilli, making this filtration system extremely valuable. The liver converts the ammonia from deaminization of amino acids and the large quantities of ammonia absorbed from the intestine to urea, which is excreted in the urine. This is one of the most vital functions of the liver. Lastly, it removes bilirubin, an end product of red blood cell breakdown, from the blood and makes it water soluble by conjugating it so that it can be eliminated in the bile.

**FIGURE 15-3**
Protein metabolism. (*Adapted from Jirovec,* 1974.)

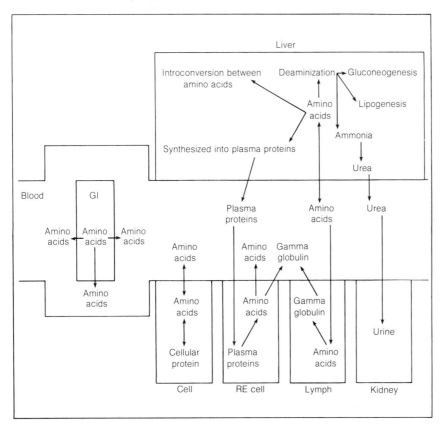

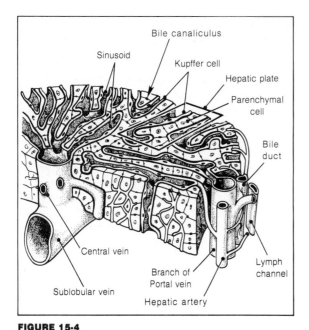

**FIGURE 15-4**
Schematic view of liver lobule.

The final area of liver function involves *oxygenation status*. The liver is a storehouse of iron, a necessary component of red blood cell formation. It also stores vitamin $B_{12}$ which aids in the normal maturation of red blood cells. Up to a liter of blood is also stored. The liver participates in the normal clotting sequence by storing vitamin K and synthesizing several clotting factors.

## Hormonal Influences on Metabolism

Hormones, secreted principally by the endocrine system, have widespread effects on metabolic functions. They accomplish these effects by controlling the rates of reactions, transport of substances, growth, and secretion of substances throughout the body. A *hormone* can be defined as a chemical substance that is secreted by specialized cells and carried by the blood to other areas of the body where it exerts its effect. Hormones that have a specific local action, like the previously discussed gastrointestinal hormones, are termed *local* hormones. This section will discuss the *general* hormones, which are secreted by endocrine glands and whose metabolic effects are widespread.

**FIGURE 15-5**
Graphic summary of the hepatic blood flow. (*Original drawing courtesy of Irene B. Alyn.*)

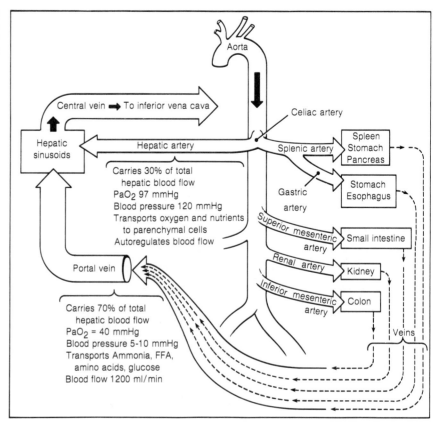

**FIGURE 15-6**
Functions of the liver. (*Adapted from Jirovec, 1974.*)

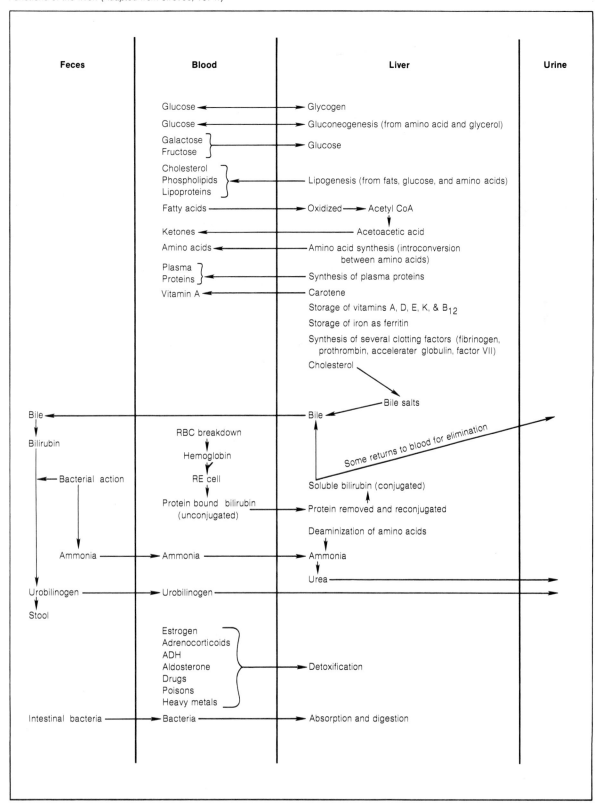

The general hormones in the human are summarized in Table 15-3. Many of the hormones play a principle role in fluid and electrolyte balance and are discussed in detail in Chap. 11. Another group of hormones affects cellular growth and proliferation in relation to reproduction. This section will discuss the hormones whose actions are principally metabolic in nature. They include some of the anterior pituitary hormones, the glucocorticoids, thyroxine and triiodothyronine, and the pancreatic hormones. The metabolic effects of the sex hormones will also be discussed.

**Anterior pituitary hormones** The anterior pituitary (adenohypophysis) is sometimes called the master gland of the body because it functions principally to control secretion in other glands. It is governed by the hypothalamus. All the stimuli of the nervous system pass through the hypothalamus, supplying it with the necessary information to mediate adenohypophyseal secretion. The hypothalamus stimulates the adenohypophysis by secreting certain neurosecretory substances that travel along minute blood vessels called hypo-thalamic-hypophyseal portal vessels. These substances are called *releasing factors.* There are specific releasing factors for the various adeno-hypophyseal hormones. Thyrotropin-releasing factor (TRF) stimulates secretion of the thyroid-stimulating hormone (TSH), and luteinizing-releasing factor (LRF) increases production of both luteinizing hormone (LH) and follicle-stimulating hormone (FSH). There is also a somatotropin-releasing inhibiting factor which inhibits the secretion of the growth hormone (GH).[4] Cortico-tropin-releasing factor (CRF) stimulates adrenocor-ticotropin (ACTH) secretion but has not yet been isolated.[5] There are probably many other releasing and inhibiting factors still to be discovered.

TSH and ACTH both have effects throughout the body. Their effects, however, are secondary in that they are mediated through another hormone. TSH increases the growth of thyroid tissue and secretion of the thyroid hormones. ACTH increases secretion of the adrenocortical hormones. Both work on a feedback mechanism. As the level of the target hormone increases, secretion of the adeno-hypophyseal hormone decreases.

**TABLE 15-3**
SUMMARY OF GENERAL HORMONES, THEIR SITES OF ACTION, AND PRINCIPAL EFFECTS IN THE BODY

| Gland | Hormone | Site of Action | Principal Effect |
|---|---|---|---|
| Anterior pituitary (adenohypophysis) | Growth hormone (GH, STH) | Body as a whole | Growth |
| | Adrenocorticotropin (ACTH) | Adrenal cortex | Secretion of steroids |
| | Thyroid-stimulating hormone (TSH) | Thyroid | Production of thyroid hormones |
| | Follicle-stimulating hormone (FSH) | Ovarian follicle | Growth and estrogen production |
| | Luteinizing hormone (LH) | Ovarian follicle | Corpus luteum formation and estrogen production |
| | Luteotropic hormone (LTH) | Corpus luteum | Progesterone secretion |
| Pituitary intermediate lobe | Melanocyte-stimulating hormone (MSH) | Skin | Deposition of pigment |
| Posterior pituitary (neurohypophysis) | Antidiuretic hormone (vasopressin, ADH) | Renal tubule | Water reabsorption |
| | Oxytocin | Uterus | Contractility and mammary milk ejection |
| Adrenal cortex | Glucocorticoids (cortisol) | Most cells | Changes in carbohydrate, fat, and protein metabolism |
| | Mineralocorticoids (aldosterone) | Renal tubules | Sodium retention |
| | Androgenic hormones | Throughout body | Male sex characteristics and anabolism |
| Adrenal medulla | Epinephrine and norepinephrine | Nerves | Sympathetic response |
| Thyroid | Thyroxine and triiodothyronine | Most cells | Increased metabolic rate |
| | Thyrocalcitonin | Bone | Decreased bone activity and decreased calcium |
| Pancreas | Insulin | Most cells | Glucose transport into cells |
| | Glucagon | Liver, muscle, and fat | Increased blood glucose level |
| Ovary | Estrogen | Reproductive tissue | Cellular proliferation of sexual organs and tissues related to reproduction |
| | Progesterone | Uterus | Secretory changes in the endometrium |
| Testis | Testosterone | Throughout body | Male sex characteristics and anabolism |
| Parathyroid | Parathormone | Bone | Increased bone absorption and serum calcium |

Normally, the level of thyroid hormones is maintained through this feedback mechanism. External factors, however, can affect TSH secretion. Both exposure to cold and emotional reactions that stimulate the sympathetic nervous system will increase TSH release. ACTH secretion is controlled by the hypothalamus through various stresses. Any kind of stress, both physical and emotional, will cause an increase in ACTH production.

The adenohypophyseal hormones appear to have an inverse relation to each other. For instance, as secretion of TSH increases, secretion of ACTH decreases. Because of this relation, in the absence of adrenal cortical secretion, ACTH secretion will increase antagonizing FSH and LH secretion and causing atrophy of the gonads. When ACTH secretion is decreased, MSH (see Table 15-3) activity will increase.

The *growth hormone (GH)* has a direct effect on the body's metabolism. It increases the size and quantity of body cells by increasing protein synthesis in all cells. It also tends to decrease carbohydrate use. The exact reason for this effect is not well understood, but GH causes an increase in blood glucose that is refractory to the effects of insulin. Lastly, GH increases fat mobilization and its use for energy. The anterior pituitary secretes an exophthalmos-producing substance and also lipolytic factors which increase fat breakdown.

**Adrenocorticoids** The adrenal cortex secretes over 30 hormones which include mineralocorticoids, glucocorticoids, androgens, estrogens, and progesterone. Of these, aldosterone accounts for 95 percent of mineralocorticoid secretion, and cortisol accounts for 95 percent of glucocorticoid secretion; these are the principal secretions of the adrenal cortex. Aldosterone is discussed in Chap. 11. The effects of cortisol will be discussed here.

The metabolic effects of cortisol are widespread and function to make glucose available for immediate use in an emergency. Cortisol secretion will be increased in periods of stress. It affects *glucose metabolism* by increasing gluconeogenesis and glycogenolysis in the liver. To a mild degree it also decreases glucose utilization in the periphery. The result of these changes is an increase in the blood glucose level. Cortisol affects *protein metabolism* by increasing the transport of amino acids into the liver while decreasing their transport into extrahepatic cells. Protein stores in these cells are decreased and amino acids from them are mobilized. The liver uses the increased amino acids to increase deaminization in order to provide more glucose through gluconeogenesis, to synthesize protein, and to form plasma proteins.

*Fat metabolism* is affected by mobilization of fatty acids from adipose, making them available for energy. Fat stores, however, tend to be increased and often are abnormally distributed because the increase in blood glucose stimulates insulin secretion. Because of the decrease in peripheral glucose use, the insulin facilitates glucose uptake by adipose tissue. In large amounts cortisol also has an *anti-inflammatory effect.* The exact mechanism of this is not well understood, but it is thought to suppress cell-mediated immunity and is accompanied by a decrease in eosinophils and lymphocytes.

**Thyroid hormones** The thyroid gland is located below the larynx on either side and anterior to the trachea. It functions to accumulate iodine and combine it with tyrosine to form thyroid hormones. The iodine needed to form thyroid hormones is obtained from the diet which should contain 1 mg iodine a week. Two-thirds of this will be lost in the urine, while the other third is actively transported into the thyroid (iodine pump).

The principal thyroid hormones are thyroxine ($T_4$) and triiodothyronine ($T_3$). They differ only in their strength and duration of action. $T_3$ tends to be of greater potency, have a shorter half-life, circulate less tightly bound to protein, and be more widely distributed in tissues when compared with $T_4$. Evidence indicates that $T_3$ may be the metabolically active thyroid hormone with $T_4$ being deiodinized to $T_3$ before being used.[6]

The exact mechanism through which $T_3$ and $T_4$ exert their effect is not known but may be related to an increase in available enzymes. They cause an increase in enzymatic reactions, increasing the metabolic rate of most tissues. The brain, retina, spleen, testes, and lungs are not affected by this. The increase in metabolic rate causes increases in both anabolism and catabolism. The growth rate is increased, but at the same time negative nitrogen balance develops when the supply of fats and carbohydrates is exhausted.

The thyroid hormones increase glucose absorption from the gastrointestinal tract and increase glucose use by the cells. This glucose excess can increase fat formation, but the accelerated metabolic rate quickly uses up the glucose. Fatty acids and amino acids must be mobilized to meet the need. They decrease serum and liver lipids, but the exact mechanism involved is not known. Vitamins are an essential part of cellular enzymatic reactions, and the increased reactions increase the vitamin needs. Thiamine and vitamin $B_{12}$ are especially related to this, with the other B vitamins and ascorbic acid needed to a lesser degree. Small amounts of the thyroid hormones are also needed by the liver to convert carotene to vitamin A. $T_3$ and $T_4$ increase the activity of the other endocrines, increase bone absorption, and excite the mental processes.

**Pancreatic hormones** The pancreas, which plays a vital role in digestion, also secretes two endocrine hormones which are essential to normal carbohydrate metabolism—*insulin* and *glucagon.* Insulin is secreted by beta cells and glucagon by alpha cells of the islets of Langerhans. These are located throughout the pancreas but are most numerous in the tail. Their actions are diametrically opposed so that they work in conjunction to maintain the glucose concentration of the blood.

**Insulin** Glucose enters cells through a process of facilitated diffusion, and insulin is the facilitator that makes this possible. Insulin will increase glucose transport through cell membranes. The brain, intestinal mucosa, and renal tubular epithelial cells are the only cells that do not need insulin to take up and use glucose. The skeletal muscle and adipose tissue are especially dependent on it. With increased glucose uptake, there is a decrease in blood glucose concentration. Glucose not used for energy is readily stored as glycogen.

The effects of insulin on the liver are not completely understood. Initially, as insulin decreases blood glucose, the liver will break down glycogen. After a while, however, as more glucose enters the liver, glycogenesis occurs. Because certain products of glucose metabolism are used to form fat, decreases in insulin which will be accompanied by decreases in glucose metabolism lessen fat formation. At the same time fatty acids are mobilized to meet the energy requirements not being met in an insulin-deficient state. As insulin increases, fat formation also increases when adequate quantities of glucose are available. Insulin also blocks the breakdown of triglycerides to fatty acids. Very small amounts have this antilipolytic effect.

Because insulin promotes the use of glucose, indirectly it spares protein. To a moderate degree insulin also has an anabolic effect by enhancing amino acid transport through the cell membrane. Insulin, then, affects growth, and without it growth hormone has no effect. Lastly, insulin increases the transport of phosphate and potassium into cells.

Insulin has widespread effects on carbohydrate as well as protein and fat metabolism. Its concentration is inversely related to the blood glucose level. As insulin increases, blood glucose decreases. With no insulin glucose transport into cells is one-fourth of normal, and the blood glucose level will increase. The blood glucose level mediates insulin secretion; as it increases, secretion increases, decreasing the glucose level and, therefore, decreasing insulin secretion.

**Glucagon** Functioning in ways opposite to insulin is glucagon. Table 15-4 compares the effects of insulin and glucagon. While insulin decreases the blood glucose, glucagon increases it. It does this by increasing the breakdown of glycogen from liver and skeletal muscle. It also enhances gluconeogenesis by the liver. If fats are not available, amino acids will be used for this, and catabolism will occur. Glucagon also promotes fat mobilization making glycerol and fatty acids available for use. Lastly, it has a positive inotropic effect on the heart.

Glucagon secretion is stimulated by a low blood glucose level. Because insulin causes this, insulin secretion will cause glucagon to be released. Because glucagon increases the blood glucose, its secretion will stimulate insulin production. It is thought that these two hormones work together to maintain a normal glucose concentration in the blood. This function is vital because glucose is the only nutrient that can be used by the brain, retina, and germinal epithelium. Without it, these structures starve and cannot function.

**Sex hormones** The sex hormones play a variety of roles in maintaining the gonads and reproduction. They also have a few metabolic effects which are significant. *Testosterone* enhances protein anabolism in general, resulting in larger muscles. Secondary to this, it increases the metabolic rate. *Estrogen* also increases the total body protein but to a lesser degree than testosterone. Its anabolic effects tend to concentrate more in the sexual organs. Like testosterone, it increases the metabolic rate but, again, to a lesser degree. Lastly, estrogen tends to increase the formation of subcutaneous fat especially in the breasts, buttocks, and thighs. *Progesterone* has a mild catabolic effect which is not significant except in pregnancy, when amino acids are mobilized.

## PHYSICAL ASSESSMENT OF METABOLISM

Metabolism is an all-encompassing physiological phenomenon affecting each organ, tissue, and cell of the body. Thus, the methods by which metabolism is assessed are highly significant and complex. They range from the general perspective of overall nutrition, including body build, stature, and the distribution of fat deposits, to the specific assessment of organs, physical structures, and their surrounding environment. The total gastrointestinal system from the mouth to the anus is included. The logical way to proceed in metabolic assessment is to begin with the general appearance of the client's nutritional state and thoroughly assess the gastrointestinal tract beginning with the oral cavity and progressing through the abdomen to the anus and rectum.

### General Nutritional State

The effect of nutrition upon the body is a very well-known and important factor in human growth and development. Adequate nutritional status will be reflected throughout the body. Similarly, poor nutritional status will be manifested in a variety of observable changes. A well-nourished person will generally appear alert and responsive with good coloring. The hair will appear shiny and lustrous and facial skin smooth and moist. Eyes will be bright and lips moist, and the neck glands will not be enlarged. On examination of the oral cavity, the tongue will be healthy with no lesions, gums pink and firm, and the teeth clean and white. The patient's weight will be normal, the posture good and abdomen flat. Muscles will be well developed and firm, and the patient will be attentive and relaxed. The patient will give a history of a good appetite, regular bowel movements, restful sleeping habits, and an overall feeling of vitality. A poorly nourished patient will exhibit changes in all or some of these areas. Chapter 16 discusses the changes associated with poor nutrition.

**Body build**  It is generally accepted knowledge that there are wide variations in normal body build. As you observe the person for the first time, it is important to notice the general body build. There are three common human body types which are generally considered as normal.

The *asthenic,* or ectomorph, is one common body type. An individual with such a body build is slender and may look underweight. This person is characterized by a delicate bone structure and slight muscular development of the extremities. Other features may include narrow shoulders, a decreased anteroposterior chest diameter, and long arms and legs.

A second type is the *sthenic,* or mesomorph. This category includes the athletic or muscular person, with large bone structure, increased muscle mass in the extremities (as well as in the neck and pectorals), and broad shoulders.

A third type is the *pykinic,* or endomorph. This individual appears to have a large amount of body fat. Such a person appears soft and well-rounded, but might have either a small or a large bone structure. The abdomen and breasts may protrude and appear flabby, and the arms and legs may be short and stubby in comparison with individuals of the other body types.

Because it is known that the naked eye can be deceived, some examiners feel that in addition to the observation of body types, it is helpful to determine skeletal proportion in order to correctly evaluate the level of growth and development in an individual. Such measures of skeletal proportion in normal adults are the span and the skeletal segments. The *span* is the length from outstretched fingertip to outstretched fingertip, which should equal the height from head to toe. There are upper and lower *skeletal segments.* The upper skeletal segment is measured from the top of the skull to the top of the symphysis pubis. This measurement should equal the lower skeletal segment, which is the distance from the top of the symphysis pubis to the heel.

The complete assessment of body build includes the determination of height and weight and a comparison with prepared charts of averages which are based on sex and bone structure. It is important to note the dress of the individual and the time of day when the measures of height and weight are taken. Extra pounds may be added after a meal, and height and weight may both be affected if shoes are worn.

**Fat distribution**  Another body characteristic which is connected with nutrition is that of fat and muscle distribution. This determination requires more than a simple assessment of fatness or thinness. Normally, women tend to have more fat cells

**TABLE 15-4**
EFFECTS OF INSULIN AND GLUCAGON

| Insulin | Glucagon |
| --- | --- |
| Decreases blood glucose | Increases blood glucose |
| Increases glucagon secretion | Increases insulin secretion |
| Glycogenesis | Glycogenolysis |
| Decreases gluconeogenesis | Increases gluconeogenesis |
| Lipogenesis | Lipolysis |
| Mild anabolism | Slight catabolism |
| Increases phosphate and potassium transport | Inotropic effect on heart |

than men and their center of gravity is along an imaginary line through their hips. Men have more muscle mass than women, and their center of gravity is through their shoulders. This is obviously a generalization, as the examiner may encounter an extremely muscular woman or an extremely soft and flabby man.

In discussing weight, one describes the condition of being overweight as *obesity* and the condition of being underweight as *cachexia.* There are two common types of obesity. The most prevalent is *exogenous obesity.* It is caused by overeating, or increasing the caloric intake while not increasing the caloric expenditure. With this type of obesity the fat distribution is generalized and is deposited over most areas of the body: the face, the trunk, and the extremities. A method commonly used to assess this type of obesity is for the examiner to pick up skin between thumb and forefinger to estimate the amount of subcutaneous fat. The second type of obesity is called *endogenous* and is caused by endocrine or other systemic diseases. The fat distribution is more apt to be localized in certain areas. For example, with Cushing's disease the fat is located around the face and trunk or girdle area. This person may have normally slender legs.

Obesity should not be confused with edema, which is a collection of water, usually found in dependent areas such as the ankles and the sacrum. Edematous areas will pit or depress with pressure and be slow to return to the normal state. This is not the case with obesity.

Cachexia can be easily detected by observation and is usually quite a startling sight. The person will appear to have sunken eyeballs. The face will have a gaunt look due to loss of tissue around the cheeks and temples. There will be a hollow look about the supraclavicular area and the axilla. The ribs will be prominent. A person who is obese and suffers a substantial weight loss may not exhibit signs of cachexia. In such a case, some of the first observations of the loss of body fat would be loose, flabby folds of skin. The loss of body fat in young persons may be observed as numerous wrinkles.

In general, when evaluating a person's weight, it is important to observe the rate of change from his or her normal weight. It is necessary to note whether this change is associated with illness or trauma. The body build and distribution of body fat observed by the examiner make up the general evaluation of nutritional state. Beginning with the observations of nutritional state, the examiner can proceed to a more detailed assessment of metabolism.

## Oral Cavity

A careful examination of the oral cavity is important when assessing the nutritional status and the overall metabolism of an individual. It is the place where nutrition begins, and it is one of the most accessible areas for examination. The various structures in the oral cavity can give clues to local diseases such as gingivitis (inflammation of the gums) and neoplasms, as well as systemic diseases such as anemia and hypothyroidism.

**Mucous membranes** The mucous membranes of the mouth should first be examined for color. They are normally coral to pale pink, with patchy pigmentation being normal for the black population. A bright-red color may indicate inflammation caused by infection or ulcers. Localized white patches beneath the surface of the membranes indicate ischemia. When the pallor is generalized, it could be a sign of anemia. Patches of white that appear to be clinging to the surface of the membranes may be a sign of *Monilia* (thrush). General cyanosis is indicative of systemic hypoxia. Brown membranes may indicate Addison's disease or other metabolic disturbances.

The membranes should also be examined for the presence of nodules, irritations, sores, or masses, and the salivary glands should be inspected for blockages. The surface of the mucosa is normally flexible with a rich supply of blood vessels. The presence of ulcers may be the result of trauma or viral diseases. Swelling most often results from inflammation, reactive hyperplasia, cysts, congenital deformities, or neoplasms.[7]

With the exception of the lips, the membranes are kept moist by salivary gland secretions. In observing the salivary glands, the examiner may notice an abnormal increase in salivation. This condition is called *ptyalism* and can be caused by mucosal irritation, drugs, or toxic levels of heavy metals.

**Lips** The lips are normally a pinkish red in color and are susceptible to swelling and bleeding with trauma and inflammation. The insides of the lips are lubricated by salivary fluids. During the examination, the color of the lips should be observed. Again, pallor may indicate anemia, while cyanosis is often caused by oxygen deficit.

Congenital problems and surgical scars should also be noted. Sores or lesions may be present. One of the most common lesions of the lips is that caused by the herpes simplex virus. This infection is often called a *cold sore* or fever blister, and consists of a vesicle, progressing to a scab, and disappearing in 10 to 14 days. It may return at intervals, especially during periods of stress. Swelling and nodules may suggest infection or neoplasms. The latter is usually manifest as a thickened plaque, a warty growth, or a crust that does not heal. It is most commonly found on the lower lip. The *chancre* of primary syphilis may appear on the lips and look somewhat like a neoplasm except that it is usually found on the upper lip. *Cheilosis* is a fissuring or cracking of the lips at the corners of the mouth and is a rather common problem. It is often caused by too much saliva escaping from the mouth. This is frequently the case with people who have poorly fitting dentures. Rarely, cheilosis may be caused by a riboflavin (vitamin $B_2$) deficiency.

Finally, the examiner should check the symmetry of the oral cavity and the performance of its motor and sensory functions. If one corner of the mouth droops and the person is drooling, there may be a problem with the facial nerve. Numbness of the lips may be due to nerve damage or may be the effect of anesthesia.

**Gingivae**  The normal gums are pale red to bright pink in color and are firm to the touch. Reddened, swollen, or spongy gums may be indicative of gingivitis, abscesses, dental calculus, bleeding disorders, or scurvy. They may also be a side effect of Dilantin (diphenylhydantoin) therapy or even pregnancy.

The normal gingivae are attached to the teeth and should have sharp margins around each tooth. Gingival tissue fills in the interdental spaces with shallow crevices of no more than 1 to 2 mm in depth. In cases of gingivitis or pyorrhea, these crevices may extend beyond this depth. The gum margins may recede, exposing more of the teeth. In advanced stages, the teeth may become loose and eventually fall out. A recession of the gums may be normal with increasing age. In younger people it may be a sign of pyorrhea, but it could also merely be the result of incorrect brushing.

Bleeding gums may be normal after intensive manipulation. However, since this condition may also be a sign of scurvy or a bleeding disorder, its presence should be cause for further evaluation.

**Teeth**  The teeth are used to prepare food for digestion and are vital to overall metabolism. The examiner should check the number of teeth and if any are missing determine the reason. Then the color should be noticed. The average adult has 32 white-enameled teeth. Dark enamel may be caused by such severe conditions as trauma or abscess. They may also be the result of caffeine or nicotine stains.

Irregularly shaped tooth crowns may be caused by congenital hypoplasia or dental caries. Notched or barrel-shaped teeth (Hutchinson's teeth) may indicate the presence of congenital syphilis.

During palpation of the teeth increased mobility may be found. This may be a sign of primary or metastatic malignancy if the hypermobility is localized. More commonly, it is the result of peridontal disease.

A tooth may be percussed if there is a possibility of an abscess at its roots. If there is an abscess of the tissue at the root of the tooth (periapical), the person will feel pain when the tooth (or teeth) involved is tapped. This maneuver is helpful in localizing the affected area as well as differentiating true dental pain from that pain which may be referred from other areas (such as the heart).

Dental caries (cavities) are the most common of the dental diseases. They may be severe, resulting in peridontal problems and tooth loss, or they may be a minor condition affecting one or more teeth. Tooth decay can be significant, yet hidden from view. Frequent dental x-rays should be a part of each person's annual health examination.

**Tongue**  The tongue is necessary for chewing and swallowing as well as for tasting. These three functions are important for digestion as well as nutrition. The healthy tongue is approximately the color of the normal mucosa (coral to pale pink). A tongue with white, prominent papillae surrounded by a deep-red color may be the "strawberry tongue" of scarlet fever. As with the mucous membranes, white patches may suggest *Monilia*.

The top of the tongue (dorsum) is covered by papillae, giving it a moderately rough coat. If the dorsum of the tongue appears shiny and smooth, a niacin deficiency or pernicious anemia may be suspected. A heavily coated tongue may indicate a decreased food intake, since the brushing effect of the food as it is chewed helps to cleanse the tongue. The reason for the decrease in oral intake should be determined. In rare cases, heavy dark fur may appear on the posterior dorsal surface. This is usually due to elongated papillae, and it may be caused by a fungus infection secondary to the administration of antibiotics. A "geographic tongue" is the result of different formations of papillae and is considered benign except in some childhood cases when a connection with allergies has been noted.[8] The undersurface (ventral) is smooth with large veins.

With the elderly person, these veins may become varicosed and quite prominent.

The examiner should note the overall size of the tongue. An enlarged tongue may indicate myxedema (hypothyroidism) or neoplasms. Asymmetrical tongue enlargement is more indicative of hemangioma or lymphangioma.

The tongue should protrude in a straight line. Deviation to either side would indicate impairment of the hypoglossal nerve. The examiner should check to see if there is severe restriction of movement due to an abnormally shortened frenulum.

Finally, the examiner should inspect the sides, the ventral and dorsal surfaces, as well as the floor of the mouth under the tongue, looking for nodules, indurations, or white spots. Any of these would suggest the presence of a malignancy. The area under the tongue seems to be the common location for malignancies in the oral cavity.

There are serious problems such as neoplasms which are not found on the surface and cannot be detected simply by looking. Palpation should be carefully undertaken with each examination. The examiner's finger should be protected by a glove or a finger cot, and precautions should be taken against biting by uncooperative patients. All areas of the tongue should be palpated as well as the floor of the mouth. Special attention should be given to this latter area.

**Swallowing** The ability to swallow is a result of the coordination of many structures and systems. Abnormalities should not be overlooked as many nutritional deficiencies can be caused by painful or difficult swallowing. *Dysphagia* (difficulty in swallowing) must be differentiated from a sore throat. When a client volunteers information which points to true dysphagia, it should always be taken seriously and an appropriate examination completed. If the impairment in the ability to swallow is restricted to solids, the problem is likely to be mechanical, e.g., an obstruction. A neurological problem is suspected if there is trouble swallowing liquids, as this act demands a more sophisticated motor control. With any suspected throat pathology that impairs the ability to swallow, the problem of choking and aspiration must be explored.

### Abdomen

For the physical examination, the abdomen is usually marked into quarters. A vertical line is drawn from the xiphoid process to the symphysis pubis and a horizontal line is drawn through the umbili-

cus to each side. Another method less commonly used marks the abdomen into nine areas. To determine a true clinical picture, it is important to know the underlying organs and structures in relation to these areas. See Fig. 15-7. The structures found in each quadrant are listed in Table 15-5.

Positioning of the patient throughout the abdominal examination is very important. If the abdominal muscles are not relaxed, they may make a complete assessment of the area impossible. The person being examined should be supine with the head elevated on one or two pillows, arms at the sides, and knees slightly raised. The person should be uncovered from the nipples to the symphysis pubis. Every effort should be made to relax the client. This includes a calm, relaxed manner on the part of the examiner. For the extremely apprehensive person, deep breathing and much verbal reassurance might be necessary. Inspection and auscultation of the abdomen should precede percussion and palpation as the latter two may alter normal organ functions and influence assessment results.

**Inspection** There are several components to consider during inspection of the abdomen. They include the skin, vasculature, abdominal architecture, umbilicus, and movement.

**S**kin The skin should be examined for abnormal color such as pallor. Pale coloring may indicate anemia. Jaundice, if present, may suggest liver disease. Darkened or splotchy areas (hyperpigmentation) may be present in cases of Addison's disease. There may be scars due to injury or surgery. Observed rashes may result from allergies or infections. There may also be signs of strain which indicate stretching followed by a weight loss, as in pregnancy (striae).

Next, examine the hair distribution. There may be an overabundance or, in some cases, there may even be a complete absence of hair. The normal hair pattern in the female pubic area is that of a triangle, while the male has an inverted triangle. Abnormalities in the hair pattern could mean a hormonal imbalance.

**V**asculature Discolorations and marks due to vascular conditions should be noted. The abdominal veins are rarely noticeable on the healthy abdomen. If they are seen, the blood in them flows away from the umbilicus. With obstruction of the hepatic portal circulatory system the umbilical blood vessels,

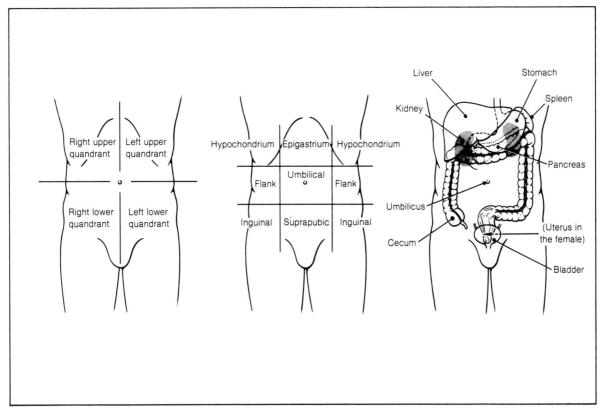

**FIGURE 15-7**
Divisions of the abdomen and abdominal organs.

closed since birth, are reopened. The flow of blood through these vessels will be toward the umbilicus. The direction of blood flow can be determined by stripping the veins with the fingers (see Palpation below). These umbilical vessels cause a pattern known as *caput medusae,* or "snake hair."

**A**bdominal Architecture   The human abdomen is basically symmetrical. First, observe this symmetry. Bumps or bulges which are symmetrical may indicate such things as a full bladder or pregnancy. An assymetrical bulge could be caused by a hernia. Notice the shape of the abdomen as the person lies on his or her back. The abdomen may be flat, which is normal with people of average build. A rounded abdomen may be caused by obesity or abnormal distention. Causes of abdominal distention are often listed as the five F's—flatus, feces, fetus, fluid, and fat. Enlarged organs as well as tumors can also cause distention. The distention may be generalized or localized. If localized, note the location and the structures lying underneath. The assessment of

distention will be discussed further in Auscultation, Percussion, and Palpation below.

The person may have a *scaphoid* abdomen, which is concave with the skin apparently falling away. This may be normal with the thin individual.

**TABLE 15-5**
STRUCTURES OF THE ABDOMEN
ACCORDING TO QUADRANT

| RIGHT UPPER QUADRANT (RUQ) | LEFT UPPER QUADRANT (LUQ) |
|---|---|
| Liver | Stomach |
| Gallbladder | Spleen |
| Pancreas (head) | Pancreas (body and tail) |
| Right kidney | Left kidney |
| Duodenum | Splenic flexure of colon |
| Hepatic flexure of colon | |
| RIGHT LOWER QUADRANT (RLQ) | LEFT LOWER QUADRANT (LLQ) |
| Cecum | Sigmoid colon |
| Appendix | Descending colon |
| Right kidney (lower pole) | Left kidney (lower pole) |
| Right ovary and fallopian tube (female) | Left ovary and fallopian tube (female) |
| Right spermatic cord (male) | Left spermatic cord (male) |

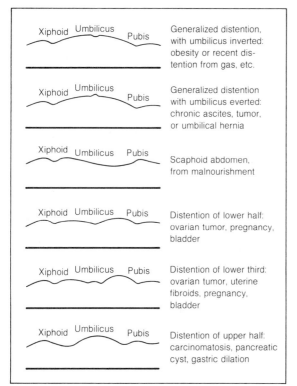

Xiphoid  Umbilicus  Pubis — Generalized distention, with umbilicus inverted: obesity or recent distention from gas, etc.

Xiphoid  Umbilicus  Pubis — Generalized distention with umbilicus everted: chronic ascites, tumor, or umbilical hernia

Xiphoid  Umbilicus  Pubis — Scaphoid abdomen, from malnourishment

Xiphoid  Umbilicus  Pubis — Distention of lower half: ovarian tumor, pregnancy, bladder

Xiphoid  Umbilicus  Pubis — Distention of lower third: ovarian tumor, uterine fibroids, pregnancy, bladder

Xiphoid  Umbilicus  Pubis — Distention of upper half: carcinomatosis, pancreatic cyst, gastric dilation

**FIGURE 15-8**
Abdominal profiles. Careful inspection of the profile of the abdomen from the side may give the first clue to abnormality, directing attention to a specific region and prompting a search for further signs. (*From DeGowin and DeGowin, Bedside Diagnostic Examination, 1976. By permission of the publisher.*)

However, it may also be caused by emaciation due to poor nutrition or malignancy. Figure 15-8 depicts various abdominal profiles and possible causes.

**U**mbilicus  The normal umbilicus is somewhat recessed. If it is flat or bulging, abnormal distention may be the cause. The umbilicus will protrude due to free fluid in the abdominal cavity (*ascites*). It may be inverted in cases of obesity. The umbilicus is normally located slightly below the midline. It is not normally in the exact center of the abdomen as one might expect. If the umbilicus is found to be above the midline, a mass in the lower abdomen, most commonly a pregnancy, is indicated.

**M**ovement  Several important movements of the abdomen are observed during inspection. The first is *respiratory movement.* The normal abdomen protrudes slightly with inspiration due to the descent of the diaphragm. It recedes with expiration. The second movement which may be observed is *peristal-*

*sis.* In the healthy individual, of normal weight, peristalsis is not usually seen. However, it may be observed on the abdomen of a thin person. Visible peristaltic waves occur with bowel obstruction. The location and the direction of these observable peristaltic waves should be noted.

The third type of movement which may be observed is a *pulsation.* Cardiac pulses are frequently seen in the epigastric area of thin people. This pulsation can be seen as a slight bulge. Abnormal pulsations transmitted to the abdomen may originate in the heart with tricuspid insufficiency. In the aorta they may be caused by an aneurysm. In the liver they may be the result of congestion. Masses near major vessels may also give rise to increased abdominal pulsations.

**Auscultation**  The next step in the physical examination of the abdomen is auscultation. As mentioned earlier, this precedes percussion and palpation. Ausculatory findings are often altered by the manipulation of the abdomen and underlying organs. The examiner should listen for at least 3 to 5 minutes with the diaphragm of the stethoscope held lightly over each section or quadrant of the abdomen.

There are three major types of abdominal sounds: bowel sounds, vascular sounds, and friction rubs. It is important to be able to assess these sounds and describe them according to frequency, quality, and location.

Normal *bowel sounds* are caused by air mixing with fluid during peristalsis. They may vary according to the amount of food which has been eaten. They are described by frequency, intensity, and pitch. Frequency shows the speed of the waves of contraction. The intensity describes the strength of the peristaltic waves, and pitch reflects the amount of tension in the intestinal wall. The location of the waves will aid the examiner in determining the structures or organs involved. These sounds are thought to originate primarily from the small intestine and are high pitched and gurgling. The sounds from the colon are lower pitched and have a rumbling quality.

A sound resembling a rush of fluid from one side of the stomach to the other is referred to as a *succussion splash.* This sound may be heard normally if the examiner places the stethoscope over the stomach of an individual who has recently drunk a large amount of fluid and, with a hand on either side of the patient's upper abdomen, rocks the patient from side to side.

High-pitched, tinkling sounds are caused by intestinal fluid and air under pressure in a dilated bowel. Rushes of high-pitched sounds with abdominal cramps may be present. Both of the above sounds suggest early intestinal obstruction.

Normally, bowel sounds occur at a rate of 5 to 35 per minute. Again, this varies in relation to oral intake. An increase in bowel sounds may be present immediately after the client has taken something by mouth, especially large amounts of fluids. An increase may also be heard during a bout of diarrhea and during early intestinal obstruction. A decrease in sounds is an indication of paralytic ileus, peritonitis, or progressive bowel obstruction.

With partial bowel obstruction there are high-pitched, frequent, and very intense sounds from the peristaltic waves. The portion of the bowel above the obstruction increases pressure and creates a strong enough contraction to force the intestinal contents through the smaller obstructed lumen. There seems to be no regular rhythm to these contractions. There may or may not be cramps with the peristaltic waves.

Often after this intense peristaltic activity there is a decrease in bowel sounds while tired muscles try to rest and recover their ability to work again. As the bowel obstruction progresses, there may be an increase of tinkling sounds. These are caused by many small gas bubbles in the obstructed intestinal juices rising to the surface and breaking. The bowel sounds become higher pitched and less intense as the bowel becomes "tired." Eventually, in late or complete obstruction, there will be silence. The examiner should be careful to listen for several minutes before assessing an absence of bowel sounds, since this is a rather serious observation.

The second general type of sound heard during auscultation of the abdomen is the *vascular sound.* Arterial bruits (murmurs) and venous hums are both included in this category. Abdominal *bruits,* vascular sounds described fully in Chap. 22, may be heard in the young healthy person, although these should still be carefully evaluated. A bruit which is considered to be of possible pathological importance is that heard during the examination of the older client or one who may be prone to arterial changes (e.g., the diabetic, the hypertensive). In this situation, the bruit is heard with a light pressure over the area with the diaphragm of the stethoscope. The sound is still audible in the same location as the client is moved to different positions. Such sounds are usually caused by turbulent blood flow in either a dilated or constricted blood vessel. Bruits can be caused by congenital or arteriosclerotic narrowing. They may also be the result of inflammation, tumors, or other masses pressing on blood vessels.

It is important for the examiner to make sure that the abdominal bruit heard is not a cardiac murmur transmitted to the abdominal area. Differentiation can easily be made by palpating the carotid artery while listening to the abdomen with the stethoscope. If the sound heard with the stethoscope is slightly later than the carotid pulse, it can be assumed to be a true abdominal bruit, since there is a significant circulatory lag. If the pulse and bruit are felt and heard simultaneously, the sound is probably that of a heart murmur. The examiner must concentrate, as the murmur or bruit may be very faint.

A *venous hum* is a rare occurrence. If present, it is heard over the epigastric and umbilical areas. It is a low-pitched, continuous sound which is softer than a bruit. The hum is caused by collateral circulation or anastamoses of the portal and systemic venous circulation.

The third sound heard with the stethoscope is the *friction rub.* It is also quite rare and is characterized by a soft, grating sound which varies with respiratory movements. It indicates an inflammation of the surface of an organ such as the liver or spleen. This inflammation can be due to a tumor of the liver or infarction of the spleen.

**Percussion**   The normal or abnormal presence of air or fluid in the abdomen is noted by percussion. When the patient is recumbent, the air present in the gastrointestinal system will rise to the surface. This gives the normal percussion sound of tympany. Tympany is normally found over the air bubble in the stomach and over any air present in the bowel. Free air in the abdomen will also cause this sound. The percussion note will vary with the content of the gut. An increase in fluid under the percussing finger will sound dull or flat.

Different characteristics of the flat or dull percussion sound may also be noted. If the flatness is localized, it could mean a fluid-filled tumor. However, if the flatness moves when the individual changes position, it could indicate free fluid in the abdominal cavity (ascites).

Other abnormal conditions which cause a significant change in the note are intestinal obstruction and paralytic ileus. Both of these cause an increase in air in the gut and result in a tympanic note.

The abdominal organs and underlying masses cause distinct sounds when percussed. Thus, percussion is important in the assessment of abnormal masses and organ enlargement. Organs usually percussed are the stomach, liver, spleen, and occasionally the kidneys, although the latter can be percussed only with some difficulty.

It is important to percuss both borders of the liver to determine if it is enlarged or is merely a normal liver which is displaced downward. The lower border of the liver is percussed by starting at the midclavicular line (MCL) below the umbilicus in an area of resonance and percussing until a flat or dull sound is heard. To find the upper border, percuss from the resonant note heard in the lungs in the midclavicular line downward until dullness is heard. Measure the distance between the two borders. A liver is considered normal-size if it measures 6 to 12 cm in length.

Dull sounds from the spleen may be found in the left anterior axillary line (AAL) between the ninth and eleventh intercostal spaces. Ask the person to take a deep breath and percuss the eleventh intercostal space. If the note changes from tympany to dullness during inspiration, it is a positive sign of splenic enlargement.[9] Dullness above the ninth intercostal space is suggestive of an enlarged spleen, an enlarged kidney, or consolidation of the left lung.

**Palpation** Palpation is used to verify assessments done by the previous methods, add new information, and identify muscle development and tone. It may also indicate painful or tender areas. Palpate each quadrant and slowly increase the pressure. It may be helpful to have the person breathe in and out with the mouth open to relax the abdominal muscles. If the person is extremely ticklish, the examiner may choose to disregard the problem or use the person's hand to begin the palpation.

Before palpation of some of the more important organs and masses is discussed, several important basic elements in assessment must be reviewed. One is the method of differentiating the superficial tenderness of the abdominal wall from the visceral tenderness which is deep in the peritoneal cavity. The person being examined is asked to tense the abdominal muscles by lifting the legs and head at the same time. If discomfort is still felt, it is considered to be in the more superficial muscles. During this maneuver, if attempts to elicit pain or discomfort are unsuccessful, the cause may be considered deeper, i.e., under the abdominal musculature.

Rigidity of the abdominal musculature is an important finding during the abdominal examination. It may be voluntary or involuntary. The first occurs with fear and nervousness. The latter indicates peritoneal irritation or lesions.

The presence of abdominal pain or tenderness during the examination is also important to note. The characteristics of this subjective symptom need to be carefully assessed. The examiner should determine whether the discomfort is superficial, in the wall of the abdominal muscle, or deep in the viscera, as described above. Next, the discomfort or tenderness should be localized as much as possible to aid in the differential diagnosis. For example, pain in the right lower quadrant in a line two-thirds of the way from the umbilicus to the iliac crest is likely to be appendicitis, whereas pain in the right upper quadrant may indicate the presence of liver disease. Abdominal pain may be diffuse and radiating and is often difficult to locate specifically.

*Rebound tenderness* is elicited by pressing into the abdomen with the palpating fingers and quickly releasing the pressure. Increased pain with the release of pressure indicates peritoneal inflammation. It is necessary to make sure the finding of rebound tenderness is not due to an increase in palpating pressure just before the release. If this were true, the increase in discomfort could not be called rebound tenderness.

It should be remembered that both the area of the epigastrium and the abdominal aorta may be normally sensitive or tender with deep palpation. Pain in these areas does not necessarily mean that disease is present.

During palpation for organs and masses, findings need to be described with respect to size, location, consistency, pulsality, tenderness, and mobility. Smoothness, irregularity, and the presence of nodules are also important descriptions.

**Liver** The technique most often used on the liver is bimanual palpation (see Fig. 15-9). The palpating fingers are placed below the percussed lower border of the liver, and they are pointed toward the right costal margin. As the person exhales, the fingers are advanced deeper and upward, until the lower edge of the liver "flips" over the fingertips. With a normal liver this is usually all that is possible to feel. Some normal livers are not possible to palpate. A normal liver edge is usually found not more than 1 to 2 cm below the costal margin. This distance may be increased by a congenitally displaced liver or an overexpanded lung. The maximum limit for a normal liver is considered to be 5 cm below the costal margin.

As the examiner becomes proficient in feeling the edge of the liver, a description of this edge is necessary. When palpable, the normal liver has a regular, firm edge with a smooth surface. A dull edge usually indicates a large amount of swelling, while neoplasms feel irregular with nodules. Continual or deep palpation of the liver edge may cause slight discomfort in the healthy individual. If the liver is not palpable, the tenderness may be assessed by striking the upper and lower quadrants on each side and comparing the sensations. Increased discomfort in the right upper quadrant may indicate liver disease.

**G**allbladder    The gallbladder is located in the right upper quadrant and is normally not palpable. A technique for palpation of this organ consists of hooking the thumb of the left hand around the right costal margin with the fingers resting on the right rib cage. During inspiration, an enlarged, tender gallbladder will be caught between the thumb and the ribs, causing patients to stop breathing in mid-inspiration and "catch their breath" (referred to as *Murphy's sign*). With a jaundiced person, the right upper quadrant should be palpated for a small mass attached to the liver, which moves with respiration. Locating this would indicate an enlarged gallbladder.

**S**pleen    Palpation of the spleen is bimanual and is done in the left upper quadrant over to the mid-axillary line. The normal spleen is not palpable; it usually must be enlarged two to three times before it can be felt. If the examiner is right-handed, the left hand is placed under the lower left rib cage. The right hand is pressed underneath the ribs. The person is asked to take a deep breath. The spleen moves downward with inspiration and, if enlarged, will hit the palpating fingers of the right hand. If an enlarged spleen is suspected and not felt, the person may be rolled to a right decubitis position. This position will bring the spleen close to the anterior surface of the abdomen where it may be palpable. A greatly enlarged spleen may be palpated in the lower left quadrant. If the spleen is palpable, the number of centimeters from the costal margin should be noted.

**K**idney    As with the spleen and the liver, bimanual palpation is used for the kidneys. Each kidney may be palpated in the costavertebral angles or the flanks. With a thin person, the lower part of the right kidney may be occasionally palpated. However, normally the left kidney is very rarely palpable. Because it is placed higher in the left upper quadrant, if it is successfully palpated this would

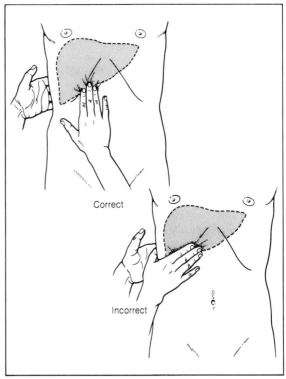

**FIGURE 15-9**
Bimanual technique for palpation of the liver.

usually indicate an increase in size. The consistency, size, and tenderness of both kidneys should be noted in the examination. An enlargement may indicate polycystic disease, hydronephrosis, or neoplasms.

One method used to check for kidney tenderness is to strike the costavertebral angles posteriorly with the ulnar surface of the hand. This is called the *Murphy punch*. Tenderness found by this test is indicative of inflammation or infection.

**O**ther Organs    During the abdominal examination other organs may also be palpated. An enlarged urinary bladder which is filled with urine may be palpable in the suprapubic area. It should be palpated after the person voids. The cecum may be palpable in the right lower quadrant. It feels like a soft, air-filled mass and is easily manipulated. The sigmoid colon may be felt in the left lower quadrant as a movable, tender, sausage-shaped mass.

**V**ascular Structures    The abdominal aorta is usually felt in the epigastrium slightly to the left of the midline. It is necessary to palpate it in order to ascertain its lateral dimensions. In thin, elderly people, or those with anterior curvature of the spine, the aorta will be palpated as soft and pulsatile from midepigastrium to the pelvic area. In a younger individual or one with a normal spine, palpating the aorta is often difficult; when palpable, it is normally tender. Careful distinctions should be made between a normal aorta and an aortic aneurysm. An enlarged, pulsatile mass with lateral pulsation is indicative of an aneurysm. Often the aneurysm is felt in the midportion of the abdomen and causes pain. If there is a leak from the aneurysm, the blood often collects posterior to the peritoneum and causes increasing back pain.

The palpation of abnormal veins and arteries seen during inspection should be undertaken next. These vessels should be stripped as depicted in Fig. 15-10 to determine the direction of blood flow. The significance of this is discussed earlier in Inspection.

### Anus and Rectum

Assessment of metabolic status necessarily includes an examination of the anus and rectum.

Maintenance of gastrointestinal elimination is vital to normal metabolism. An efficient examiner may find important information concerning the patient's state of health and the presence of serious pathology.

**Inspection**  The buttocks should be gently spread and the anus and perineal area examined. These areas often show signs of irritation, sweating, and itching. The skin may be thickened. The anal area is often the site of fissures, external hemorrhoids, and remnants of resolved hemorrhoids (skin tags). Hemorrhoids containing blood clots (thrombosed) may be purple or dark red in color. The examiner may ask the person to bear down (Valsalva maneuver). This may cause cracks or fissures to appear at the anus. A perirectal abscess will show as a bulge. Other swellings, bumps, or lesions should be noted. Occasionally, as the person bears down, a rectal prolapse will extend through the anal orifice. Two to three centimeters posterior to the rectum, at the tip of the coccyx, is the pilonidal area. There may be a dimple, sinus, or inflamed pilonidal cyst in this area.

**FIGURE 15-10**
Methods for stripping a blood vessel. (*a*) Exert pressure on vessel with both fingers together. (*b*) Maintain pressure and separate fingers to strip vessel of blood. (*c*) Release one finger and observe time for blood to fill. (*d*) Repeat procedure releasing the other finger. Compare the filling times. The direction of the faster filling is the direction of blood flow.

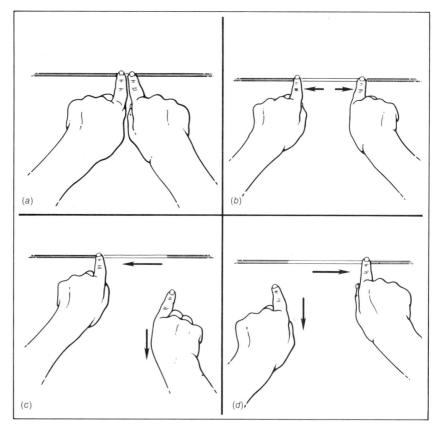

**Palpation** The technique of palpation of the anus and the rectum consists of positioning the client, gently inserting the palpating finger, and positioning the finger in important areas. All possible surfaces of the anus and rectum should be examined. The person being examined may be somewhat nervous. Although the finger is much smaller than feces which normally pass through the anal orifice, having a rectal examination may be psychologically uncomfortable. Such nervousness may cause tenderness and increased resistance in the anal orifice. Adequate explanation of the procedure should precede the examination. The person should be told that as the finger is inserted into the anal canal, the feeling may be similar to having a bowel movement.

The gloved examining finger should be well lubricated and the fleshy part placed against the anal opening. As the sphincter relaxes, the finger is inserted gently and the person is allowed to relax before the examination is begun. At the beginning, or any time during the examination, the examiner may ask the person to bear down. This not only facilitates insertion of the palpating finger, but also may bring within reach lesions which are high in the rectum. The anal sphincter is evaluated for muscle tone and tenderness. Increased tone may be caused by nervousness, tension, a scar which causes a narrowing of the opening, or an irritating lesion. An abnormally relaxed anal sphincter may be secondary to childbirth, surgery, trauma, or neurological disease. Tenderness of the sphincter may be due to hemorrhoids or an anal fissure.

Internal hemorrhoids cannot ordinarily be felt unless they are thrombosed. Such hemorrhoids are described as *hard cords* and may be very painful. Any abnormalities noted during inspection should be palpated. After the palpation of the anal canal is completed, the finger is inserted deeper and the right lateral, left lateral, and posterior walls of the rectum are palpated. The examiner feels for polyps, masses, nodules, or any other abnormalities. The anterior rectal wall is then palpated. In the male, the prostate gland will be felt as a firm, heart-shaped mass with two lobes which may normally be tender. With the female, the cervix can normally be palpated. It will feel like a small, rounded mass on the anterior wall and should not be confused with an abnormal finding. Cancer of the abdominal organs often metastasizes to the anterior peritoneum of the rectum. In the male, these lesions may be felt as hard nodules just above the prostate. In the female, they are felt in the cul-de-sac (pouch of Douglas), which is a space between the rectum and vagina.

Malignancies are often felt as irregular, hard nodules or ulcerative masses. Polyps are felt as masses easily pushed about with the finger. None of the above should be confused with the prostate gland or the cervix.

Naturally, the most common mass in the rectum is the feces, which feel firm, soft, and not attached to the walls of the rectum. An impacted stool may be hard and lumpy, but it will also be freely movable and unattached.

## SUMMARY

Metabolism encompasses a multiplicity of bodily processes that contribute to supplying the body with energy. A clear understanding of these physiological processes and the assessment skills that can be employed to evaluate an individual's metabolic status are essential to nursing care.

## REFERENCES

1  Zollner, N., and S. Estren (eds.), *Thannhauser's Textbook of Metabolism and Metabolic Disorders,* vol. I, Grune & Stratton, New York, 1962, p. 31.
2  Konturek, S. J., "Gastric Secretion," in E. D. Jacobson and L. L. Shanbour (eds.), *Physiology Series One, Volume 4, Gastrointestinal Physiology,* University Park Press, Baltimore, 1974, p. 245.
3  Alpers, D. H., and F. J. Tedesco, "The Possible Role of Pancreatic Proteases in the Turnover of Intestinal Brush Border Proteins," *Biochim Biophys Acta,* **401:**28–40, August 5, 1975.
4  Peterson, R. E., and R. Guillemin, "The Hormones of the Hypothalamus," *Am J Med,* **57:**591–600, October 1974.
5  Kaplan, S. A., "Hypothalamic Releasing Substances and Inhibitors," *Am J Dis Child,* **128:**451–452, October 1974.
6  Martin, J. B., "Regulation of the Pituitary-Thyroid Axis," in S. M. McCann (ed.), *Physiology Series One Vol. 5, Endocrine Physiology,* University Park Press, Baltimore, 1974.
7  Judge, Richard D., and George Zuidema (eds.), *Methods of Clinical Examination: A Physiologic Approach,* 3d ed., Little, Brown, Boston, 1974, p. 83.
8  Bates, Barbara, *A Guide to Physical Diagnosis,* Lippincott, Philadelphia, 1974, p. 70.
9  Burnside, John, *Adams' Physical Diagnosis,* 15th ed., Williams & Wilkins, Baltimore, 1974, p. 169.

## BIBLIOGRAPHY

### Metabolism

Ball, E. G.: *Energy Metabolism,* Addison-Wesley, Reading, Mass., 1973.

Brown, J. H. U., and S. B. Barker: *Basic Endocrinology,* Davis, Philadelphia, 1966.

Brunner, H., et al.: "Gastric Emptying and Secretion of Bile Acids, Cholesterol, and Pancreatic Enzymes during Digestion," *Mayo Clin Proc,* **49:**851–860, November 1974.

Carlson, L. D., and A. C. L. Hsieh: *Control of Energy Exchange,* Macmillan, London, 1970.

Francis, M. G., and M. H. Peaslee: "Effects of Social Stress on Pituitary Melanocyte-Stimulating Hormone Activity in Male Mice," *Neuroendocrinology,* **16:**1–7, 1974.

Gorbman, A., and H. A. Bern: *A Textbook of Comparative Endocrinology,* Wiley, New York, 1962.

Gray, G. M.: "Carbohydrate Digestion and Absorption: Role of the Small Intestine," *N Engl J Med,* **292:** 1225–1230, June 5, 1975.

Guyton, A. C.: *Textbook of Medical Physiology,* Saunders, Philadelphia, 1976.

Hargreaves, T.: *The Liver and Bile Metabolism,* Appleton-Century-Crofts, New York, 1968.

Jirovec, M.: *Metabolism,* Boston University Print Shop, 1974.

Johnson, L. R.: "Gastrointestinal Hormones," in E. D. Jacobson and L. L. Shanbour (eds.), *Physiology Series One,* vol. 4, *Gastrointestinal Physiology,* University Park Press, Baltimore, 1974.

Langley, L. L.: *Review of Physiology,* McGraw-Hill, New York, 1971.

Levitan, R., and D. E. Wilson: "Absorption of Water Soluble Substances," in E. D. Jacobson and L. L. Shanbour (eds.), *Physiology Series One, Vol. 4, Gastrointestinal Physiology,* University Park Press, Baltimore, 1974.

Magee, D. F.: *Gastrointestinal Physiology,* Charles C Thomas, Springfield, Ill., 1962.

Marks, V.: "Effect of Drugs on Carbohydrate Metabolism," *Nutr Soc Proc,* **33:**209–214, December 1974.

Miller, A. T.: *Energy Metabolism,* Davis, Philadelphia, 1968.

Tepperman, J.: *Metabolic and Endocrine Physiology,* Year Book, Chicago, 1973.

Truswell, A. S.: "Drugs and Lipid Metabolism," *Nutr Soc Proc,* **33:**215–224, December 1974.

Unger, R. I.: "The Pancreas as a Regulator of Metabolism," in S. M. McCann (ed.), *Physiology Series One,* vol. 5, *Endocrine Physiology,* University Park Press, Baltimore, 1974.

Weiss, J.: "Etiology and Management of Intestinal Gas," *Curr Ther Res,* **16:**909–920, September 1974.

### Physical Assessment

Bates, Barbara: *A Guide To Physical Diagnosis,* J. P. Lippincott, Philadelphia, 1974.

Beneson, Abram S.: *Control of Communicable Diseases in Man,* 12th American Public Health Association, Washington, 1975.

Brown, Marie Scott, and Mary Alexander: "Physical Examination: Part 10, Mouth and Throat," *Nursing '74,* 57–61, August 1974.

DeGowin, Elmer, and Richard DeGowin: *Bedside Diagnostic Examination,* 3d ed., Macmillan, New York, 1976.

Ganong, William F.: *Review of Medical Physiology,* 6th ed., Lange, Los Altos, Calif., 1973.

Govoni, Laura: *Drugs and Nursing Implications,* 2d ed., Appleton-Century-Crofts, New York, 1971.

Hochstein, Elliot, and Albert L. Rubin: *Physical Diagnosis,* McGraw-Hill, New York, 1964.

Kraft, Jacob: "The Acute Abdomen," *Emergency Med,* **5**(2):145–151, February, 1973.

Mitchell, Pamela H.: *Concepts Basic to Nursing,* McGraw-Hill, New York, 1973.

"Patient Assessment: Examination of the Abdomen," *Am J Nurs,* **74:**9:1679–1702, September 1974.

Prior, John A., and Jack Silberstein: *Physical Diagnosis,* 4th ed., Mosby, St. Louis, 1973.

Stern, Thomas: *Clinical Examination,* Year Book, Chicago, 1964.

Willacker, Jean: "Bowel Sounds," *Am J Nurs,* **73:**12: 2100–2101, December 1973.

Williams, Sue Rodwell: *Essentials of Nutrition and Diet Therapy,* Mosby, St. Louis, 1974.

Wintrobe, Maxwell M., et al. (eds.): *Harrison's Principles of Internal Medicine,* 7th ed., McGraw-Hill, New York, 1974.

# 16
# DISTURBANCES IN INGESTION

Barbara Braden

Ingestion is one of the human being's most basic interactions with the environment. This interaction involves taking food substances from the environment into the body for use in metabolic processes. Ingestion is the necessary first step in normal metabolism. Any disturbance in this first step of metabolism will lead to disturbances in subsequent metabolic processes. Disturbances of ingestion range from too little to too much intake of certain food substances. Ensuing metabolic disturbances can vary from abrupt to insidious in onset, severe to mild in symptomatology, and acute to chronic in consequent problems.

## MALNUTRITION

Malnutrition is a state of impaired functional ability or development caused by an inadequate intake of essential nutrients or calories to provide for long-term needs.

Despite the fact that the United States is among the most affluent countries in the world, malnutrition exists in many segments of its population. The Ten State Nutrition Survey, the largest nutrition survey ever conducted in the United States, had delineated the major nutritional problems and the populations in which malnutrition most frequently occurs. In brief, this survey indicates that low-income populations are the most likely to be malnourished and that iron-deficiency anemia and obesity are the prevalent nutritional problems.[1] If present trends toward rising food costs, high unemployment, and an increasingly aged population continue, the incidence of malnutrition will increase and become more serious.

Malnutrition can result in or result from physical illness. Whatever the cause, malnutrition constitutes a deviation from high-level wellness and deserves the attention of the nurse and other health-care professionals. The nurse needs a repertoire of assessment skills and nursing interventions to deal effectively with malnutrition and associated problems.

### Pathophysiology

The amount and quality of food consumed by a person is influenced by a number of factors, psychological, sociocultural, economic, and physical. In most instances these factors work together to influence the maintenance of a varied and nutritionally adequate diet. However, on occasion these same factors will have a negative effect on food intake.

For instance, a feeling of psychological well-being will usually foster a healthy appetite, while depression may cause loss of appetite. Cognizance of both positive and negative aspects of the factors influencing intake will assist the nurse in assessing real and potential problems of malnutrition as well as in planning effective nursing interventions.

**Psychological causes of malnutrition** The psychological influence on food intake includes choosing foods which one associates with security, comfort, and sociability, feelings of masculinity and femininity, and perceptions of one's body image or health status.

In recent years, *food faddism* has been documented as a growing cause of malnutrition. Examples of these food fads are the macrobiotic diet, vegetarian diet, organic food diets, and others. The macrobiotic diet is among the most dangerous, while certain properly selected vegetarian diets can be nutritionally adequate. The appeal of these diets appears to be psychological. The advocates of fad diets may be searching for spiritual peace, protesting against the "establishment," or reacting to fear of real or perceived health problems. Whatever the basis, the consequences of such diets can be severe malnutrition and lack of medical treatment for serious illnesses.

Another increasing psychosocial problem frequently associated with malnutrition is *chemical dependency*. Theories vary on the psychological cause of chemical dependency. Chemical dependency leads to malnutrition when the addict begins to substitute the abused chemical for food. This is especially common in alcoholic dependency. Deficiency diseases such as pellagra and beriberi are rarely seen in the United States except in alcoholics.

The problem of malnutrition as a result of *social isolation* and disintegration of the family is becoming more evident. Eating is linked with sociability and social occasions. This psychological relationship probably stems from pleasant memories of eating with family and friends at home and in other happy circumstances. When the social element is removed from the eating situation, food preparation time diminishes, food selection is primarily based on convenience, and loss of appetite commonly occurs. Chronic social isolation accompanied by poor nutrition is typical of the situation experienced by many aged persons. However, similar circumstances are arising in the modern family. Family mealtimes may give way to snacks eaten on the run in the busy family. Even when adequate time is available for meal preparation, eating schedules staggered to fit various family members' needs may leave some members eating alone. The food habits and nutritional status of children probably suffer most in this situation.

*Anorexia nervosa* is the least common but most dramatic example of malnutrition with a psychological etiology. It is characterized by self-imposed starvation accompanied by extreme weight loss. This disease, seen predominantly in adolescent females, is generally thought to stem from a faulty perception of body image. Since some patients literally starve themselves to death, the initial treatment goal may be to correct the malnutrition. Though traditional treatment is psychotherapeutic, recent theories of physiologic etiology have prompted experimental treatment with levodopa.

**Sociocultural and economic causes of malnutrition** According to the findings of the Ten State Nutrition Survey, "income is a major determinant of nutritional status, [but] other factors such as social, cultural and geographic differences also have an effect on the level of nutriture of a population group."[2]

It is not surprising that *income* has the greatest impact on nutritional status when one considers the components of food procurement. First, one must be able to reach a food source. This is difficult when money is not available for transportation or purchase of housing close to the marketplace. Second, one must have money to buy the food and the nutritional knowledge to select the proper foods. Poverty not only limits buying power but may also affect the amount of education attained: a relationship has been found between the number of years of school completed by the person usually responsible for buying and preparing food and the nutritional status of children.[3] Third, once food is obtained, proper storage and preparation facilities are necessary. Housing which provides these facilities is not always attainable by the poor.

Though malnutrition is more common and more severe among the poor, affluence does not guarantee nutritional health. Snack foods, sweets, and other sources of "empty calories" may replace more nutritious foods in the diets of the affluent. Consequently nutritional deficiencies are possible and dental caries are probable.

Various *ethnic groups* are found to have a higher incidence of malnutrition than others, even in comparison with groups of similar income range. "Evidence of malnutrition [is] found most commonly among blacks, less commonly among Spanish-Americans, and least among white persons.''[4] The primary exception to this is vitamin A deficiency, which appears to be most common among low-income Spanish-Americans.

The exact nature of the cultural traditions within ethnic groups that contribute to malnutrition is difficult to uncover. It has been observed that Mexican-American women residing in the Southwest traditionally eat only what is left after their husband and children finish and that Indians living with large extended families share meager supplies with the group. Traditional Chinese dietary beliefs can cause nutritive problems, especially during pregnancy and lactation, because of the general exclusion of milk from the diet, the belief that iron will ''harden the bones and contribute to a difficult delivery,'' and the avoidance of fruits and vegetables in the first postpartum month.

With the exception of limits imposed by poverty, cultural patterns of eating that would consistently lead to malnutrition are not readily discerned among blacks and Appalachian whites. However, extreme poverty forces priority setting among such essentials as food, clothing, and shelter, and if shelter or clothing take priority over food, nutritional deficiencies can result.

**Physical causes of malnutrition** Physical illness can lead to malnutrition in various ways. Some illnesses cause an increase in metabolic need which exceeds the quantity or quality of metabolic fuel a person is able to ingest. Such illnesses include those accompanied by prolonged fever, body burns, extensive trauma, hyperthyroidism, and cancer. The symptoms occurring with illness, the stress of hospitalization, or side effects of treatment can also cause a disturbance of ingestion. Anorexia is a commonly occurring disturbance of ingestion resulting from these factors.

*Anorexia,* defined as loss of appetite, occurs in illnesses of every sort. It is a common side effect of drug therapy and occasionally signals drug toxicity. The desire to eat may also be diminished with the psychological stress of hospitalization and by unpleasant sights or odors. When nausea accompanies anorexia, any motivation to eat is extinguished. *Nausea,* like anorexia, may arise from visceral discomfort, chemical products of illness and therapy, or psychological distress. A third disturbance to be differentiated from anorexia and nausea is sitophobia. *Sitophobia,* ''the fear of eating because of subsequent or associated discomfort,'' may be seen in patients with regional enteritis or after gastric resection. Not adequately appreciated is the presence of sitophobia in patients in the late stages of chronic obstructive pulmonary disease (COPD). The increase in both mucus production and the work of breathing that accompanies ingestion of food causes the patient with COPD to become dyspneic and short of breath. The memory of this discomfort and the physical inability to tolerate the concomitant disturbance in oxygenation discourages the patient from eating. Severe malnutrition can result.

Other physical disturbances of ingestion include inability to self-feed, inability to chew, and inability to swallow. *Inability to self-feed* may occur in patients with extreme weakness or neuromuscular problems affecting the upper extremities. One should also be aware of self-feeding problems in patients who have perceptual disturbances (disorientation, sightlessness, diplopia) or are confined to bed in positions which hinder feeding. Feeding assistance may allow adequate nutrition, but this will not always be true.

*Inability to chew* occurs with dental problems, ankylosis of the jaw, facial injuries requiring jaw wiring, and dysarthria sometimes associated with hemiplegia. Persons who are edentulous (without teeth) and those who have poorly fitted dentures, loose teeth, or painful caries and peridontal disease often limit their food intake to soft foods. Though mechanically soft diets can be nutritionally adequate, diets followed by these people frequently are not sound. Persons with problems in jaw articulation, especially those whose jaws are wired shut to repair facial injuries, must rely primarily on liquid nourishment. Balanced liquid diets are commercially available, but those who care for themselves at home may use more convenient but nutritionally deficient liquids.

*Inability to swallow* (dysphagia) can cause severe malnutrition. This problem may be seen in neuromuscular disorders affecting the muscles of swallowing or with structural defects in the throat and esophagus. Neuromuscular problems which commonly affect swallowing are myasthenia gravis, dermatomyositis, amyotrophic lateral sclerosis, and hemiplegia. As a result of these diseases, the muscles of swallowing are unable to effectively propel food into the esophagus.

*Structural defects* which are obstructive in nature include cancer of the throat and esophagus and esophageal burns. Esophageal burns from ingestion of caustic substances such as lye or drain cleaners usually result in scar tissue and stricture formation. Strictures or tumors may cause partial or complete obstruction of the esophagus; passage of food through the esophagus into the stomach is at best difficult and sometimes impossible. Esophageal atresia is a congenital anomaly in which the esophagus ends in a blind pouch before reaching the stomach. These conditions can easily lead to severe malnutrition.

An *esophageal-tracheal fistula* is an abnormal tubular opening which allows communication between the esophagus and the trachea. These fistulas may be congenital but may also be induced by, for example, pressure necrosis and trauma from tracheal intubation. Whatever the cause, esophageal-tracheal fistulas allow food to enter the lungs, making food ingestion a life-threatening situation.

*Achalasia* is a condition which begins as a motor disorder and results in a structural defect. In this condition, diminished or absent esophageal peristalsis in combination with incomplete relaxation of the cardiac sphincter results in dilatation of the distal portion of the esophagus. Achalasia rarely produces sufficient obstruction or symptomatology to induce anything more than mild malnutrition.

**Cellular changes and effects on the patient**
The basic pathophysiologic processes of malnutrition are set forth in the following passage from Gifft, Washbon, and Harrison:[5]

Nutritional deficiency may be primary in origin (due to lack of sufficient quantities of the nutrient in the diet) or secondary to any one of many conditions which may interfere with absorption or utilization of the nutrient or which may elevate the need for the nutrient. The speed with which a deficiency syndrome develops and the degree to which it is manifest depends on the relative severity of the dietary inadequacy, the extent of body stores of the nutrient, and the capacity of the body to adapt successfully to lower intakes of the particular nutrient. Although the speed of progress may vary greatly, deficiency disease develops according to the following general pattern:

1. Exhaustion of nutrient reserves

2. Tissue depletion

3. Biochemical lesion (metabolic pathways do not proceed normally)

4. Clinical lesions (physiological signs and symptoms observable by physical examination)

This pattern holds whether the diet is deficient in one nutrient or in several. Deficiencies in only one nutrient are not rare, but biochemical or clinical lesions indicative of one deficiency raise the possibility of others and should prompt further investigation.

Broadly speaking, the essential nutrients are carbohydrates, proteins, fats, minerals, vitamins, and water. Deficiency states involving vitamins and selected minerals are outlined in Table 16-1. The pathophysiology of malnutrition that occurs with inadequate intake of carbohydrates, fats, and proteins is discussed below.

Carbohydrates are the body's usual source of energy. As the dietary intake of carbohydrate falls, other sources of energy—proteins and fats—must be utilized. This is especially serious because proteins used for energy are not available for anabolic processes. In other words, carbohydrates have a protein-sparing effect, and the two must be taken in simultaneously to achieve the optimal anabolic use of protein.

If proteins and fats are also deficient in the diet, body stores will be burned for energy. After glycogen stores in the liver are depleted, fat is mobilized from adipose tissue. Oxidation of large amounts of fat for energy will result in the accumulation of acidic byproducts known as *ketone bodies*. When fat stores are exhausted, the body will use the protein in its tissues for energy, producing nitrogen wastes. This process initially results in loss of weight and finally in a wasted, emaciated appearance as the patient develops a negative nitrogen balance. By this time the patient is usually apathetic and susceptible to infections and has a variety of skin and hair changes due to protein, fat, and vitamin deficiencies. Figure 16-1 summarizes the physical changes associated with malnutrition. If malnutrition goes untreated and is severe, coma and death can eventually occur.

**First-level Nursing care**
Malnutrition develops over a long period of time. Short-term disturbances of ingestion are not likely to deplete the body stores of a healthy person. Likewise, if a long-term disturbance of ingestion is detected early in its course, malnutrition may be preventable. This is especially true of a disturbance of ingestion with a physical cause, since people with physical illnesses are more likely to seek help from health professionals. Keen observation, careful questioning, and knowledge of the problems that put people at risk of developing malnutrition will assist the nurse in assessing and identifying preventable problems.

**Nursing assessment of physical factors**  Anorexia may be suspected when patients complain of loss of appetite. These complaints may be expressed in a number of ways: ''Nothing tastes good anymore''; ''I just can't eat''; ''I'm off my feed.'' The

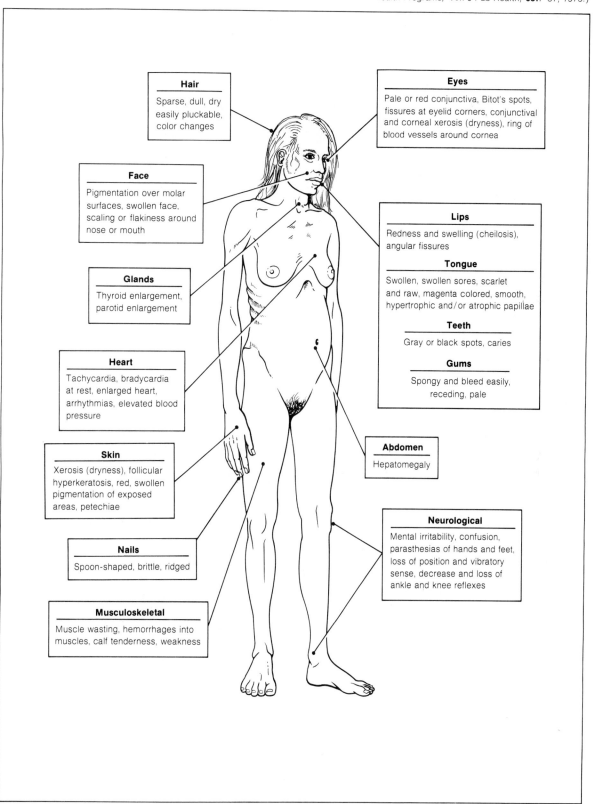

**Hair**
Sparse, dull, dry easily pluckable, color changes

**Eyes**
Pale or red conjunctiva, Bitot's spots, fissures at eyelid corners, conjunctival and corneal xerosis (dryness), ring of blood vessels around cornea

**Face**
Pigmentation over molar surfaces, swollen face, scaling or flakiness around nose or mouth

**Lips**
Redness and swelling (cheilosis), angular fissures

**Tongue**
Swollen, swollen sores, scarlet and raw, magenta colored, smooth, hypertrophic and/or atrophic papillae

**Glands**
Thyroid enlargement, parotid enlargement

**Teeth**
Gray or black spots, caries

**Gums**
Spongy and bleed easily, receding, pale

**Heart**
Tachycardia, bradycardia at rest, enlarged heart, arrhythmias, elevated blood pressure

**Abdomen**
Hepatomegaly

**Skin**
Xerosis (dryness), follicular hyperkeratosis, red, swollen pigmentation of exposed areas, petechiae

**Neurological**
Mental irritability, confusion, parasthesias of hands and feet, loss of position and vibratory sense, decrease and loss of ankle and knee reflexes

**Nails**
Spoon-shaped, brittle, ridged

**Musculoskeletal**
Muscle wasting, hemorrhages into muscles, calf tenderness, weakness

**TABLE 16-1**
SUMMARY OF NUTRITIONAL DEFICIENCIES OF VITAMINS AND SELECTED MINERALS

| | Pathogenesis | Clinical Findings | Diagnosis | Treatment | Rich Food Sources* |
|---|---|---|---|---|---|
| VITAMIN A Hypovitaminosis | Long-term inadequate dietary intake; malabsorption, as in sprue or pancreatitis; reduction of serum transport in kwashiorkor. | Mild or early signs: dry skin, night blindness, follicular hyperkeratosis; severe or late signs: xerophthalmia, atrophy, skin keratinization, keratomalacia, Bitot's spots. | Serum vitamin A below 20 μg/100 ml indicates low stores, less than 10 μg/100 ml indicates deficiency | 15,000 to 25,000 IU of vitamin A once or twice daily, given in conjunction with bile salts, or intramuscularly if absorption is impaired | Liver, kidney, milk fat, fortified margarine, egg yolk, yellow and dark-green leafy vegetables, apricots, cantaloupe, peaches |
| Hypervitaminosis | Ingestion by an adult of 100,000 to 200,000 IU a day for several years; long-term excessive intake of vitamin A preparations can cause its occurrence in children | Anorexia, weight loss, hair loss, hyperostosis, hypercalcemia, hepatomegaly, splenomegaly, anemia, skin rash, CNS manifestations | Serum vitamin A above 400 μg/100 ml | Withdraw vitamin or its source | |
| VITAMIN D Hypovitaminosis | Inadequate dietary intake, lack of sunlight, absorption defect such as sprue or pancreatitis, chronic renal disease | Active rickets in children; epiphyseal enlargement; beading of ribs, craniotabes; osteomalacia in adults | Increased serum phosphatase —to 20 Bodansky units in rickets; serum phosphorus and urinary calcium usually fall; product of serum calcium times phosphorus is less than 35 mg/100 ml | 2,500 USP units daily for 1 month, plus adequate intake of calcium and phosphorus | Vitamin D milk, irradiated foods; some in milk fat, liver, egg yolk, salmon, tuna fish, sardines |
| Hypervitaminosis | Prolonged ingestion of 5,000 to 150,000 USP units daily | Hypercalcemia, renal damage, metastatic calcification | Serum calcium over 11.5 mg/100 ml | Withdraw source of vitamin; use corticosteroids or sodium phytate to reverse hypercalcinuria. | |
| VITAMIN B₁ (thiamine) Hypovitaminosis | Inadequate dietary intake: increased need during thyrotoxicosis or with a high carbohydrate intake; chronic alcoholism; reliance on polished white rice as a staple food | Anorexia, symmetrical footdrop, ataxia, loss of ankle and knee jerks, muscle tenderness, burning feet, paresthesias; later or more severe symptoms (beriberi) include edema, polyneuritis, paralyses, cardiac insufficiencies manifested by tachycardia, dyspnea | Daily thiamine excretion in the urine of less than 50 μg; reduced erythrocyte transketolase activity | Thiamine hydrochloride, 20 to 50 mg orally, IV, or IM, in divided daily doses for 2 weeks, then 10 mg/day orally | Pork, liver, organs, meats, legumes, whole-grain and enriched cereals and breads, wheat germ, potatoes (synthesized in intestinal tract) |
| VITAMIN B₂ (riboflavin) Hypovitaminosis | Insufficient dietary intake; low consumption of milk and milk products can contribute to deficiency | Early or mild stages: oral pallor, scaly and greasy skin in nasolabial folds, ears, and eyelids, conjunctivitis, weight loss, weakness, photophobia —symptoms vary greatly and often occur along with thiamine and niacin deficiency; late or severe symptoms: cheilosis, fissures of nares, magenta tongue, moderate edema, anemia, corneal vascularization, scrotal dermatitis | Urinary riboflavin excretion of less than 50 μg/day | Riboflavin, 40 to 50 mg/day, IV, IM, or orally until all symptoms have cleared | Milk and dairy foods, organ meats, green leafy vegetables, enriched cereals and breads, eggs |
| VITAMIN B₆ (pyridoxine) Hypovitaminosis | Dietary deficiency severe enough to cause clinical signs is rare but occurs in infants; look for deficiency in malab- | Anemia, usually normoblastic but sometimes megaloblastic; hemoglobin can drop to less than 4 g/100 ml; convulsions | Use tryptophan load test: give 10 g of d-l tryptophan; patient who excretes more than 50 mg of xanthurenic acid per day in | B₆, 10 to 50 mg/day IV or IM, plus other B complex factors; pyridoxine can relieve nervous symptoms and weakness of | Pork, glandular meats, cereal bran and germ, milk, egg yolk, oatmeal, legumes |

| | | | | | |
|---|---|---|---|---|---|
| | sorption syndromes, increased renal clearance, or persons taking oral contraceptives, isonicotinic acid hydrazide, hydralazine, or D-penicillamine | can occur in deficient infants | the urine is deficient in pyridoxine | pellagra when niacin fails and can cure glossitis and cheilosis when riboflavin fails | Liver, kidney, milk and dairy foods, meat, eggs |
| VITAMIN B$_{12}$ (cyanocobalamin) Hypovitaminosis | Restricted intake of animal products, as in pure vegetarianism; most common cause is lack of intrinsic factor and consequent malabsorption of the vitamin (pernicious anemia) | Dietary deficiency: megaloblastic anemia; glossitis, achlorhydria, jaundice, paresthesias, subacute combined degeneration of the cord; nausea, nutritional amblyopia, dorsal-funiculi and pyramidal-tract syndromes | Serum B$_{12}$ less than 120 pg/ml; mean corpuscular volume greater than 100; Schilling test for pernicious anemia: urine excretion of radio-cobalt-labeled B$_{12}$ less than 2% per day unless intrinsic factor also given | For dietary deficiency, give 15 to 25 $\mu$g/day orally; for pernicious anemia, give loading dose of 200–500 $\mu$g IM, follow with 50 to 100 $\mu$g IM 3 times a week for 2 weeks, then 50 to 100 $\mu$g IM each month (Note: Folic acid will improve the anemia and glossitis temporarily, but not the neurologic degeneration) | |
| FOLIC ACID (folacin) Hypovitaminosis | Decreased absorption, as in sprue; low dietary intake, especially if aggravated by pregnancy; increased requirement in hemolytic disorders such as thalassemia and sickle cell disease; use of oral contraceptives can increase requirements; anticonvulsants can interfere with absorption of folate; therapy with methotrexate, pyrimethamine, or triamterene can block folic acid metabolism | Megaloblastic anemia, malabsorption. Increased risk of spontaneous abortion, abruptio placentae, fetal abnormalities | Serum folacin less than 3 ng/ml, red blood cell folacin less than 140 ng/ml; mean corpuscular volume greater than 100; increased urine excretion of formiminoglutamic acid after a 15-g dose of L-histidine | 5.0 mg folic acid orally, twice daily. | Green leafy vegetables, organ meats (liver), lean beef, wheat, eggs, fish, dry beans, lentils, cowpeas, asparagus, broccoli, collards, yeast (synthesized in intestines) |
| NIACIN (nicotinic acid) Hypovitaminosis | Low niacin and tryptophan intake, since niacin can be synthesized from tryptophan in protein; maize diets can cause niacin deficiency when niacin and its precursor tryptophan are low; niacin largely unavailable for absorption unless food is prepared with alkali; deficiency can occur with malignant carcinoid tumors and Hartnup disease and during treatment with isonicotinic acid hydrazide | Pellagra: early or mild symptoms include soreness of skin and tongue, burning and pruritus on back of hands, late symptoms include roughening of skin exposed to light or friction, with cracking and black crusts caused by hemorrhages; diarrhea, scarlet-red tongue, depression, rigidity | Urinary excretion of nicotinamide less than 0.2 mg in 6 h or less than 0.5 mg/g of urinary creatinine | Nicotinamide (niacinamide) 50 to 500 mg/day, IV, IM, or orally (niacin in similar doses causes vasodilation), along with therapeutic doses of thiamine, riboflavin, and pyridoxine | Fish, liver, meat, poultry, many grains, eggs, peanuts, milk, legumes, enriched grains |
| VITAMIN C (ascorbic acid) Hypovitaminosis | Inadequate intake of green vegetables or citrus fruits; poor preparation of food, including overcooking, prolonged exposure to air, addition of alkali | Early or mild signs: edema, spongy or bleeding gums, porosity of dentine, hyperkeratotic hair follicles; late or severe symptoms: muscle changes, swelling of joints, bleeding tendency, anemia, loosening of teeth, poor wound healing; costochondral beading in children | Leukocyte-platelet ascorbic acid of less than 0.2 mg/100 ml, plasma ascorbic acid less than 0.2 mg/100 indicates recent low intake; x-ray studies of long bones reveal rarefaction | Sodium ascorbate injection, 100 to 500 mg IM, or ascorbic acid, 100 to 500 mg orally, each day for as long as deficiency lasts | Puerto Rican cherry, citrus fruits, tomatoes, melons, peppers, greens, raw cabbage, guava, strawberries, pineapple, potatoes |

**TABLE 16-1**
SUMMARY OF NUTRITIONAL DEFICIENCIES OF VITAMINS AND SELECTED MINERALS (Continued)

| | Pathogenesis | Clinical Findings | Diagnosis | Treatment | Rich Food Sources* |
|---|---|---|---|---|---|
| IRON Deficiency | Low intake, especially if combined with pregnancy; low iron stores at birth, prematurity, the low iron content of milk, and rapid growth contribute to iron deficiency in children; blood loss can cause iron deficiency in children or adults | Iron-deficiency anemia (microcytic, hypochromic); fatigue, pallor of mucous membranes, koilonychia, atrophy of the lingual papillae | Mean corpuscular hemoglobin concentration less than 32%, serum iron below 50 $\mu g$/100 ml, iron-binding capacity above 450 $\mu g$/100 ml; reduced or absent stainable iron reserves in bone marrow | 200 mg of ferrous sulfate, gluconate, or fumarate orally each day; iron dextran, IM or IV when quick response is critical | Liver, meat, egg yolk, legumes, whole or enriched grains, dark green vegetables, dark molasses, shrimp, oysters |
| IODINE Deficiency | Poor iodine content of local soils and produce can contribute to low intake; reduced uptake of iodine after ingestion of goitrogens | Hyperplasia of thyroid (goiter), cretinism, deaf-mutism, stunted growth | 24-h excretion of urinary iodine less than 20 to 25 $\mu g$/g of creatinine | Iodized salt; saturated solution of potassium iodide or Lugol's solution, 2 drops in water 3 times daily | Iodized table salt, seafoods, water and vegetables in nongoitrous regions |
| IODINE Excess | Iodine intake from cough medicine | Goiter | 24-h urinary excretion over 400 $\mu g$ | Withdraw iodine source | |
| PROTEIN Deficiency | Intake of low-level or poor-quality protein; weaning children onto protein-poor foods causes kwashiorkor in low socioeconomic groups; deficiency aggravated by infections, diarrhea, parasitic infestations | Kwashiorkor in children, causing growth failure, edema, apathy, skin changes, sparse or depigmented hair, enlarged and fatty liver, muscle wasting; blood changes include anemia, hypoalbuminemia, hyperglobulinemia, low levels of urea, potassium, cholesterol, alkaline phosphatase, amylase, lipase; in adults, weight loss, hypoalbuminemia, hair loss, fatigue, anemia, muscle wasting | Serum albumin less than 3.0 g/100 ml; ratio of nonessential to essential amino acids in serum raised to more than 2.0 | Requires knowledgeable and experienced personnel: gradually increase dietary protein to 3–4 g per kg of body weight per day and give protein of high biologic value, such as milk; replace fluid and electrolyte deficiencies with oral or parenteral therapy; give vitamin supplements; prescribe antibiotics when indicated | Protein foods (meat, fish, poultry, eggs, milk, cheese, legumes, nuts) |
| PROTEIN AND CALORIE Deficiency | Deficient intake of all nutrients, including calories and protein; marasmus in children always complicated by infections or parasites | Marasmus in children, characterized by weight loss, emaciation without edema, apathy, skin changes, gastroenteritis, anemia, vitamin deficiencies; in adults, weight loss, muscle wasting, fatigue | Same as for kwashiorkor; total serum protein levels may not drop | Same as for kwashiorkor | |

* Rich food sources from M. V. Krause and M. A. Hunscher: *Food, Nutrition, and Diet Therapy*, Saunders, Philadelphia, 1972.

preceding statements or the observation by the nurse that the patient is not eating well should be followed up by careful questioning. It is important to differentiate anorexia from nausea and sitophobia. Inquiring whether nausea or any type of discomfort is associated with eating will help in making this distinction. Finding out whether any type of food appeals to the patient may uncover a simple dislike for the food served or cultural preferences which influence eating. This information will also help the nurse in planning interventions. Determining when the patient began experiencing anorexia will assist the nurse to place the problem in perspective with previous events (e.g., initiation of medications and therapies, course of illness) and to assess the seriousness of the problem. In addition, the nurse should be alert to contributing factors such as anxiety, depression, unpleasant environmental sights or odors, or the possible inability of the patient to smell or taste.

Identification of nausea as a problem is fairly simple, since most patients have experienced this unpleasant sensation before, are able to recognize it when it recurs, and will readily admit to having it if questioned properly. Alternate means of asking the patient about nausea might be "Are you sick to your stomach?" or "Do you feel as if you could vomit?" Information should be elicited concerning how long the nausea has lasted, whether it is constant or intermittent, what aggravates or relieves it, whether it is accompanied by vomiting, and, if so, the characteristics of the vomitus. As in assessment of the anorectic patient, a review of events preceding the nausea and of contributory emotional, physical, and environmental factors may be helpful.

Inability to self-feed is relatively easy to assess. Cursory observation of the patient's upper-extremity strength and coordination will yield most of the information necessary to identify this problem. If some doubt still exists, the patient should be evaluated while eating. Apparent fatigue while feeding should be noted, as well as the amount and type of food the patient is able to propel from the plate to the mouth. One must not overlook the patient whose perceptual state may be interfering with self-feeding and adequate intake.

To assess the patient's ability to chew, the mouth should be examined. Presence or absence of dentures, denture fit, multiple caries, loose teeth, and signs of peridontal disease should be noted. Patients should be asked what foods, if any, they are able to chew, as many make amazing adaptations to their problem. Again, the nurse can learn much by direct observation of the patient at meal-times. The exception to this, of course, is the patient with facial injuries or jaw wiring. In such cases the inability to chew is a foregone conclusion and assessment will be limited to the ability to take liquids.

Inability to swallow can result from several physical problems. Diagnoses mentioned earlier in association with the inability to swallow will provide clues. If suspicion exists, the nurse should ask the patient whether swallowing is difficult. If the patient is unable to provide this information because of disorientation or aphasia, the gag reflex should be checked before feeding by stimulating the back of the throat with a tongue blade. Persistent choking, sputtering, or regurgitation of food after feeding is indicative of a swallowing problem. Complaints which suggest swallowing problems related to pathology in the lower esophagus are heartburn and substernal fullness or pain following meals. The nurse may also notice a fetid odor on the breath in patients retaining food in the lower esophagus.

**Nursing assessment of psychological and socioeconomic factors** In our society, the highest-risk person is the one who is poor. Assessment of the presence or degree of poverty is not an easy task. Poverty-level income guidelines change from year to year, and the ability of a person or family to stretch the income to meet basic needs is dependent on many factors. Furthermore, clues to economic status are generally subjective in nature and may be difficult to discern, especially in depersonalizing settings such as a hospital. However, some demographic data, such as occupation of the head of the household, level of education, and size of the household may be available or obtainable by questioning. If the nurse is familiar with the poverty "pockets" in the geographic or urban area where the patient resides, tentative assumptions may be made on that basis. The nurse should also be alert to the high incidence of poverty among elderly and nonwhite segments of the population. In patients who appear to be of low socioeconomic status, discreet questions regarding nutritional practices, food consumed in the last 24 hours, and problems in food procurement are in order. An even more extensive assessment should be made of pregnant women, especially pregnant adolescents and frequently pregnant women, in low socioeconomic groups. Lastly, the nurse should never assume that obese patients are ingesting an adequate diet. While the diet of obese patients may be high in calories, it may be low in specific nutrients.

The elderly deserve special attention, since psychological and physical factors may be present in combination with poverty. Physical and psychological problems should be assessed first. Disoriented or deviant behavior or affect should be noted, since these may be symptoms of vitamin B complex or vitamin C deficiencies.[6] Data concerning nutritional practices, general eating patterns, opportunities for socialization, and problems of food procurement should be collected. The following quotation suggests some appropriate lines of questioning and empathy for problems encountered by the elderly:

Perhaps the most unfortunate of all are those elderly individuals living in slum housing, afraid to leave their rooms because of street crime, having inadequate cooking facilities and refrigeration, who are completely dependent for food on neighbors, who may or may not serve them regularly. These are the elderly—racked by poverty, friendlessness and despair.[7]

Two groups of high-risk persons, the chemically dependent and the food faddists, are difficult to identify when they present themselves for treatment of other problems. These groups are represented in nearly every age group and at every income level. In assessing food faddism as a potential cause of malnutrition, it is necessary to examine the motivation for following the diet. If the motivation is to treat illness, even obesity, the potential for danger exists—danger not only of developing malnutrition but also of delaying treatment of serious illness. If the nurse discovers that a patient is treating an illness with dietary measures, assessment should shift immediately to the illness. Food fads or food cults adopted for spiritual, psychological, or ecological reasons may be very sound, but further investigation is warranted. The nurse should conduct the interview with an accepting attitude so as to assure the patient's cooperation and a receptive disposition toward nutritional education.

Probably the most common food cult at this time is vegetarianism. The first information to be elicited from a vegetarian is the extent of dietary limitation. Some vegetarians may exclude only red meat from their diets; others may exclude all meat but include milk, eggs and other dairy products (ovo-lacto-vegetarians); and pure vegetarians will exclude all animal products. Comprehensive assessment of the adequacy of these diets may necessitate a one-week record of dietary intake to be evaluated by a dietitian. A skillfully planned ovo-lacto-vegetarian diet is likely to be quite adequate, but only careful evaluation will reveal the skill of the planner. The pure vegetarian diet requires more skill in planning for adequacy and even then is almost certain to be deficient in vitamin $B_{12}$. It should be kept in mind that vegetarian diets are high in folic acid and this may mask early signs of vitamin $B_{12}$ deficiency and delay diagnosis until the deficiency is severe enough to cause irreversible neurologic damage.

**Prevention of malnutrition** Basically, prevention of malnutrition involves instituting measures which alleviate or compensate for the problem identified as creating the potential for malnutrition. For instance, the problem of loose dentures accompanied by an inability to chew may be alleviated by obtaining new dentures, while a patient's inability to chew due to facial injuries may be compensated by providing a nutritionally complete liquid diet. Depending on the nature of the problem involved, the nurse may institute preventive measures independently or in collaboration with other health care professionals. Naturally, a dietitian will be an integral part of the nurse's resource base when nutrition is a problem. The nurse and the dietitian should work together to provide for consistency and reinforcement in diet teaching. A social worker will be invaluable for assisting the poverty-stricken patient in maximum utilization of welfare and nutrition programs. Other problems may require referral to a physician or a dentist. The nurse should also be familiar with community resources to assist with problems of the elderly and of chemical dependency. Occasionally, a nutrition book written for lay consumption can be recommended to a patient. The nurse must be extremely cautious in such recommendations, ensuring first that the book offers sound nutritional advice and second that the patient is able to utilize this type of written teaching tool.

**Second-level Nursing Care**

It is often believed that malnutrition occurs only in underdeveloped, overpopulated countries. In reality, however, various forms and degrees are found throughout the industrialized world. As seen earlier, it is most common in low-income groups, but affluence does not guarantee wisdom in food choice. Nor is any socioeconomic group free of the physical or psychological problems that lead to malnutrition. Therefore the nurse should be alert to the possibility of malnutrition in all communities and with all patients.

**Nursing assessment** Nursing assessment of malnutrition includes a dietary history, physical assessment, and diagnostic tests.

**D**ietary History One of the most useful tools in assessing early malnutrition is an accurate and complete dietary history. An effective way to begin a dietary history is to assist the patient in recalling all food intake the day preceding the interview. This dietary history should cover a 24-hour period, so that early morning, late evening, and nighttime intakes are included. In addition to eliciting information on food eaten at mealtimes, it is necessary to inquire about liquids, snacks, and use of nutritional or vitamin supplements. The 24-hour intake should be evaluated to determine the frequency of use of the four basic food groups. If any food group seems deficient in the diet, the nurse should explore the possibility that this food group is chronically omitted. The nurse should also ascertain whether the 24-hour history is representative of the patient's usual eating habits. If it is not, information on the usual eating habits should be gathered.

Besides evaluating the patient's diet according to the four basic food groups, the nurse should appraise the diet for the presence and amount of "empty calories"—candy, potato chips, soft drinks, alcoholic beverages, and the like which contribute little or nothing other than calories to the diet and may actually be replacing more nutritious foods. Along these same lines, the nurse should attempt to find out whether tobacco, coffee, or drugs such as amphetamines or cocaine are being used, as these substances tend to suppress the appetite.

Once the quantity and quality of the patient's daily food intake has been established, the nurse needs to determine the usual eating patterns. Does the patient skip meals? Are small, frequent meals taken, or three larger meals? While skipping meals is not a nutritionally sound practice, eating small, frequent meals can be wholesome provided that the four basic food groups are appropriately represented. Does the patient eat alone or with family or friends, and is the emotional atmosphere at mealtime pleasant or distressful? Although eating alone frequently leads to inadequate intake, an unpleasant emotional atmosphere at group meals can be even more limiting.

If the patient's diet seems to be inadequate, the nurse should explore the possible basis for this. The discussion concerning food habits may reveal the patient's general level of knowledge. If it has not, asking the patient to identify what he or she would consider an ideal meal plan can be helpful. In this way one may ascertain whether poor food choice is due to nutritional ignorance and identify specific areas of teaching need. Cultural and socioeconomic influences on food choice and eating patterns should also be evaluated. If socioeconomic level appears to be a problem, the nurse should assess consequent problems with food procurement as listed earlier in this chapter. If the patient is part of a family unit, the number of persons in the family should be determined along with the general level of income.

Lastly, emotional or physical problems which may create a disturbance of ingestion should be assessed. These assessments are covered in detail in the section on First-level Nursing Care.

**P**hysical Assessment In early malnutrition, the patient will not present with striking symptomatology. Initially, the body compensates for the nutritional lack by mobilizing its own stores. Physical findings at this point are usually nonspecific. When physical findings are viewed in combination with one another and with the dietary history, however, a pattern may emerge which can alert the nurse to the possibility of malnutrition.

Initial assessment of *height, weight, and vital signs* may reveal some abnormalities. If the patient is under the norm for height, malnutrition may have been a problem during childhood but is not necessarily a present problem. The patient's weight should be evaluated by using charts which correlate height and body build with ideal weight. A patient who is malnourished will frequently fall significantly below this norm for weight. Heart rate, respiratory rate, and blood pressure may be slightly increased in early malnutrition, primarily as a result of anemia.

Fatigue, lethargy, and pallor may be evident in the *general appearance and activity* of the malnourished patient. Pallor should be assessed more fully by checking the nail beds and mucous membranes of the mouth and eyes for paleness. The patient should be questioned concerning exercise tolerance and general level of energy to validate the impression of fatigue. In children this lack of energy may be more apparent, since lethargic behavior and lack of curiosity is so uncharacteristic of a healthy child.

The *mouth* should be checked thoroughly. The tongue should be inspected first and any redness, abnormal texture, or complaints of soreness should arouse suspicion of nutritional deficiency. Dental caries and signs of periodontal disease (recessed, reddened gums that bleed easily) should be noted.

These problems, if painful, can cause a person to limit intake. The presence of rampant caries may indicate a diet which is high in carbohydrates, especially in the form of between-meal sweets. Periodontal disease, though primarily caused by dental plaque, may be due secondarily to deficiencies of protein, vitamin C, vitamin A, and iron.

Early signs of vitamin deficiencies may show up in the *skin*. Dry skin, follicular hyperkeratosis, and soreness of the skin are some indicators. Follicular hyperkerotosis can best be detected by feeling the skin for roughness caused by keratotic plugs projecting from the hair follicles. More localized symptoms include burning and pruritus on the back of the hands and greasy scales in the nasolabial folds and on the eyelids. Other early signs of vitamin deficiencies involve the *eye*. The conjunctiva should be assessed for pallor or redness. Night blindness or photophobia should also arouse suspicion of certain vitamin deficiencies.

**D**iagnostic Tests  Simple diagnostic studies for screening are appropriate at this level of assessment. Hemoglobin and hematocrit readings may reveal anemia, which can result from a variety of deficiencies. A tape test of the urine may show the presence of ketones and a low pH if food intake is very low. If a high level of glucose is present in the urine in association with ketones and a low pH, starvation is likely to be occurring as a result of a lack of insulin. If clinical signs, dietary history, and simple laboratory studies strongly suggest malnutrition, a 24-hour urine specimen and blood may be collected for more sophisticated laboratory assessment (see Table 16-1).

**Nursing problems and interventions**  When nutritional deficiencies are discovered early, vitamin supplementation and diet therapy will usually alleviate the problem. The nurse, in collaboration with the physician and the dietitian, may be able to identify specific nutritional inadequacies by evaluating the assessment data. The assessment data may also help the nurse to identify food-procurement constraints such as low income or poor food-preparation facilities, which affect the patient's ability to obtain adequate nutrition. In planning diet teaching, the nurse should take into consideration the specific deficiencies identified, the constraints operating in the patient's situation, and the patient's general level of nutritional knowledge. Food suggestions should be discussed with the patient to determine which foods are acceptable and which are not. The final food plan should contain foods rich in the deficient nutrient (see Table 16-1) which are acceptable and procurable for the individual patient.

Though a well-rounded diet is an inexpensive and adequate source of vitamin intake for a healthy person, in certain instances vitamin supplements may be necessary, as when an actual deficiency state has developed. In the very early stages of malnutrition, oral vitamin supplements will often suffice. The patient should be cautioned to take only the prescribed dose, since fat-soluble vitamins can accumulate in the body to the point of toxicity.

The nurse should become familiar with community resources which assist the poor, the elderly, and the chemically-dependent in obtaining food and nutritional supplements. The social worker and the dietitian may be helpful in providing additional information and referral services.

### Third-level Nursing Care

Ideally, malnutrition should be diagnosed early in its course and the patient treated in the community. In industrialized societies, however, with severe poverty, isolation, lack of health care, extreme ignorance or faddism, untreated illness, or chemical dependence, a patient may develop severe malnutrition and require hospital care. Table 16-1 summarizes specific nutritional deficiencies and differentiates, when possible, early signs of deficiency from late signs. Often a patient who is severely malnourished will manifest several deficiencies simultaneously (see Fig. 16-1).

**Nursing assessment**  The general appearance of the severely malnourished patient will depend on the type of dietary restriction that caused the malnutrition. For instance, the alcoholic may eat very little food but take in sufficient calories to maintain body weight. The semistarved patient, however, will exhibit a marked loss of subcutaneous fat and muscle wasting, resulting in an emaciated, sunken appearance. Brown pigmentation may be present over the cheeks and under the eyes, and parotid enlargement may be noticeable. The patient will be weak and inactive and may exhibit bradycardia at rest as the body adapts to the diminished supply of energy.

The specific findings on physical examination are depicted in Figs. 16-1 through 16-4. It is easily seen that severe malnutrition can affect almost every part of the body. Only the ear examination and breath sounds will be essentially normal. Even so, breath sounds should be checked in the acutely ill patient to detect incidental problems. Also, in severe thiamine deficiency, congestive heart failure with pulmonary congestion may result in diffuse rales throughout the lungs.

Knowledge of certain special techniques and terminology will help the nurse in eliciting the physical signs of malnutrition. For instance, a severely malnourished patient may have xerosis of the skin, conjunctiva, cornea, and mucous membranes of the mouth. Xerosis refers to a dry, crinkled appearance. It may show up in the conjunctiva and cornea as a dull, dried appearance. Mucous membranes which are xerotic lose their shininess and translucency.

In assessing the hair, color changes are best observed by combing the hair upward and observing for a line of color change. This change usually occurs in persons with black hair, and the change is to a lighter color. In testing the hair for pluckability, the nurse should gently pull on three or four strands of hair without warning the patient. The hair may be pulled out effortlessly and without pain or reaction from the patient.

In examining the tongue, a tongue blade should be used to explore all areas. If the tongue appears to be abnormally smooth, it should be scraped with a tongue blade and reevaluated. If all or part of the tongue remains smooth after scraping, the proportion remaining smooth should be estimated and recorded. The patient with a reddened, swollen tongue should be asked about any pain associated with eating.

Musculoskeletal weakness can be tested by having the patient attempt to rise from a squatting position. Muscle tenderness is best evaluated by pressing firmly, but not squeezing, the belly of the muscle.

**Nursing problems and interventions**  The patient with severe malnutrition will present a variety of problems to the nurse. The usual patient is emaciated and weak and may have a gait disturbance. The general condition of skin, mouth, and tongue is poor and may be complicated by open lesions, which cause considerable discomfort when the mouth and tongue are involved. The patient may be irritable or even confused and combative. Frequently a bleeding tendency is also present.

Because the patient is *weak* and has a limited amount of energy, the nurse must plan to conserve the patient's energy for the most important tasks of the day. Often this will mean maintaining the patient on bed rest and conserving energy for diagnostic tests, feeding, turning in bed, and short periods of ambulation. Bed rest for the emaciated patient with *poor skin integrity* presents many prob-

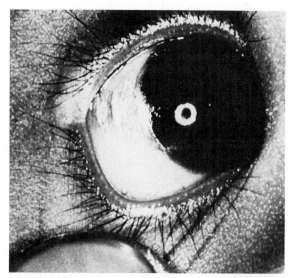

**FIGURE 16-2**
Bitot's spots associated with vitamin A deficiency.

lems of skin care. The skin should be cleansed with plain water or a soothing, medicated preparation if ordered by the physician. Thorough rinsing and gentle drying should follow. If open lesions are present in certain areas, these areas should be avoided when applying lotion. If lesions are generalized, any lotion used should be prescribed by the physician. Gentle massage should be applied to bony prominences, and the patient should be repositioned as frequently as every 30 minutes. Bed rest can also cause respiratory and vascular complications, so the patient should be assisted in coughing, deep breathing, and ambulating. The nurse should be cognizant of the patient's safety when ambulating and should observe and record any *disturbance in gait*.

Because of the *poor condition of the mouth,* good oral hygiene must be provided. The nurse should start with a soft-bristle toothbrush and mild toothpaste. If bleeding, trauma to the gums, and discomfort are induced by brushing, a gentler means of oral hygiene should be tried. A mild mouthwash can be used, or an anesthetizing agent such as lidocaine viscous mouthwash may be ordered by the physician. A cotton-tipped applicator dipped in hydrogen peroxide may be used to gently remove dried blood. The patient's lips may be lubricated very lightly with glycerine, provided open sores are not present.

Patience and empathy are necessary when the patient is *irritable.* If *confusion* or *combativeness* is a problem, safety measures must be taken to pre-

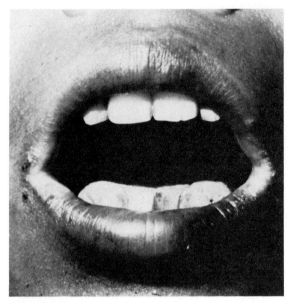

**FIGURE 16-3**
Angular fissures and cheilosis of the lips associated with deficiency in vitamin B complex (especially riboflavin).

vent the patient from being injured. For the patient with a bleeding tendency and poor skin integrity, a vest restraint and padded side rails will usually provide adequate safety and minimize skin trauma. Wrist or ankle restraints should be used only when absolutely necessary and then should be well padded and applied loosely. Environmental stress, especially noise, should be reduced, while orienting factors should be maximized.

Some interventions for the patient with a *bleeding tendency* have already been mentioned. In addition to these, the nurse should use small-gauge needles when giving injections and apply gentle pressure for several minutes to the injection site. If the patient is to be shaved, an electric razor should be used to avoid nicks.

In addition to treating the patient symptomatically, the nurse must remember that the primary problem is malnutrition and that the underlying cause may be a disturbance of ingestion. Identification of the underlying disturbance will assist the nurse in planning nutritional interventions. Occasionally the underlying disturbance precludes oral intake of table foods. In these instances gavage, elemental feedings, or hyperalimentation may be necessary to provide adequate nutrition.

**Gavage**   The term *gavage* refers to the process of feeding a patient through a tube in the stomach. Most commonly this is a nasogastric tube or a gastrostomy tube. If the patient cannot take food orally, gavage is the most advantageous alternative for providing nutrition, because (1) it maintains an active digestive process and (2) it provides more calories and more nutrients than the 5% dextrose solutions given by the peripheral intravenous route. The feeding given through a tube is a liquid with a balanced nutrient composition. Although it is pos-

**FIGURE 16-4**
Swollen, spongy, bleeding gums associated with vitamin C deficiency.

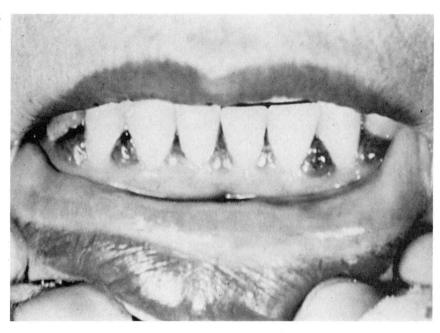

sible to blenderize common foods for use in tube feeding, commercial preparations are available and frequently used (see Fig. 16-5).

The most common complications associated with gavage are diarrhea and dehydration. These can be largely avoided by proper administration techniques. The nurse should remember the following principles when administering tube feedings:

1. Keep the feedings refrigerated to prevent bacterial growth.

2. Pour one feeding from the refrigerated supply, return the remaining supply to the refrigerator, and allow the single feeding to come to room temperature (approximately 1 hour).

3. Assess the location of the tube to verify its placement in the stomach prior to the feeding.

4. Flush the tubing with water *before* and *after* feedings to clear the tubing. Consult with the physician on the amount of fluid intake to be provided in addition to the feedings.

5. Give the feeding slowly by gravity drip (see Fig. 16-5).

6. Maintain accurate intake and output records for evaluation of fluid status.

Diarrhea is to be expected for the first few days after initiation of tube feedings. To minimize this, the feedings may begin small and be gradually increased. If diarrhea persists, give the feedings more slowly, with more water, and be certain they are at room temperature. The dietitian and the physician should be notified of persistent diarrhea so that alleviating measures may be employed.

**FIGURE 16-5**
Principles of tube feeding.

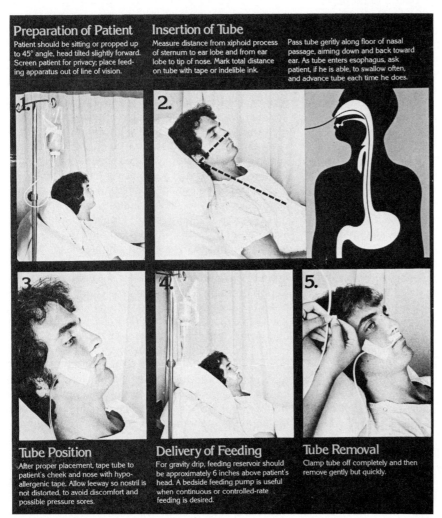

### Preparation of Patient
Patient should be sitting or propped up to 45° angle, head tilted slightly forward. Screen patient for privacy; place feeding apparatus out of line of vision.

### Insertion of Tube
Measure distance from xiphoid process of sternum to ear lobe and from ear lobe to tip of nose. Mark total distance on tube with tape or indelible ink.

Pass tube gently along floor of nasal passage, aiming down and back toward ear. As tube enters esophagus, ask patient, if he is able, to swallow often, and advance tube each time he does.

### Tube Position
After proper placement, tape tube to patient's cheek and nose with hypoallergenic tape. Allow leeway so nostril is not distorted, to avoid discomfort and possible pressure sores.

### Delivery of Feeding
For gravity drip, feeding reservoir should be approximately 6 inches above patient's head. A bedside feeding pump is useful when continuous or controlled-rate feeding is desired.

### Tube Removal
Clamp tube off completely and then remove gently but quickly.

**Elemental feedings** Elemental feedings are commercially prepared liquid feedings containing nutrients in simple chemical form which require little or no digestive breakdown before absorption. Elemental feedings are sometimes referred to as "predigested" feedings. These feedings are used when the patient has a disturbance of digestion with or without a concomitant disturbance of ingestion. Elemental feedings may be taken orally or as a tube feeding. Whichever route is used, the feeding must be taken slowly over a 1-hour time period. Otherwise, administration of this feeding via a tube is carried out under the same principles as other gavage feedings.

If elemental feedings are to be taken orally, interventions must be planned to overcome the unpleasant taste and smell of the preparations. The feeding should be served cold or as a slush in a cup with a plastic lid over it. The patient should be instructed to sip the feeding through a straw and to place the straw as far back in the mouth as possible. A basin of ice should be provided to keep the feeding cold over the hour required to drink it. Because this process can occupy much of the day, the patient may become discouraged. The nurse should give the patient frequent support and progress reports.

**Hyperalimentation** In some cases oral feedings or tube feedings will not suffice in meeting nutritional needs, and parenteral hyperalimentation may be necessary. The patient with a disturbance of ingestion or digestion combined with excessive catabolism is the usual candidate for parenteral hyperalimentation. One liter of hyperalimentation solution can provide 70 to 80 g of protein in the form of crystalline amino acids, 1000 to 2000 calories in a 20 to 50% dextrose solution, electrolytes, and vitamins. The high osmolarity of this solution, while one of its life-saving properties, can also cause some serious problems. To administer this solution in a peripheral vein would cause inflammation and thrombosis, so it is given via subclavian catheter. Up to a point, the body adapts to the infusion of a hyperosmolar solution by secreting more insulin. If the infusion rate is suddenly decreased, hypoglycemia can develop rapidly because of the extra insulin available. On the other hand, overly rapid infusion can pull body fluids into the intravascular space, causing cellular dehydration, potassium depletion, and possibly circulatory overload. When the patient's nutritional needs dictate a rapid infusion rate, extra insulin must be supplied parenterally.

Despite the complications associated with parenteral hyperalimentation, it is often the only way to save the patient from severe malnutrition. The subclavian catheter is literally a lifeline, and it is the nurse's responsibility to maintain the patency of the catheter and prevent possible complications. The patency of the catheter can be compromised by mechanical factors such as kinking or occlusion with blood clots. The catheter and IV tubing should be checked for kinks, and proper tube positioning should be meticulously attended to, especially during dressing changes. Blood clots may form in the lumen of the catheter if they are not constantly flushed away by the continuous drip of solution or if blood is allowed in the catheter beyond the tip. To prevent this, constant infusion rates must be maintained and the IV tube never allowed to run dry. Precautions should be taken to prevent blood from being withdrawn or administered through the line. Finally, swelling of the neck or face should be observed for as a sign of infiltration.

*Preventing complications* is largely a matter of preventing infections and maintaining the proper infusion rate. To prevent infections, stringent aseptic technique is used during insertion of the catheter and dressing changes. The physician performs the subclavian catheterization, and the nurse assists in maintaining aseptic technique by closely monitoring and immediately informing the physician of any contamination. The nurse will be responsible for dressing changes and must be equally careful at that time. The dressing procedure is carried out with the patient positioned flat in bed. Procedures concerning skin preparation may vary from one hospital to another but should include a skin scrub and antibiotic ointment applied to the catheter insertion site. The nurse should use this opportunity to check the insertion site and catheter tubing. The IV tubing and filter should be changed during dressing changes, and the change should be carried out under strict sterile technique. Surgical masks should be worn. If the dressing remains dry and intact, it is changed every 48 hours. The dressing should be made occlusive with adhesive tape or plastic surgical drape, and neither the patient nor the nurse should tamper with it between dressing changes. Should the dressing somehow become wet or disrupted, it should be changed immediately. Medications generally are not added or piggybacked with hyperalimentation solution because of the possibility of precipitation in the tubing. In addition to these preventive measures, vital signs should be taken every 4 hours and the physician notified of any temperature elevation or any other unusual change in vital signs.

To maintain the infusion rate properly, an infusion pump with an alarm system is often used; without a pump the drip rate should be checked at least every half hour. If the flow rate falls behind, the patient should be checked for signs of hypoglycemia. Whatever deficit is incurred should be spread over the remainder of the 24-hour infusion period. The recalculated drip rate should not constitute an increase of more than 10 percent over the originally ordered rate, and the physician should be notified of any change. The nurse should *never* attempt to "catch up" rapidly, as excessive infusion over a short period of time is very dangerous. If this should happen accidentally, the nurse should (1) slow the drip, (2) observe the patient for signs such as nausea, headache, and increased lassitude, (3) test the urine for glycosuria, and (4) notify the physician.

The nurse must also carry out certain *monitoring procedures.* The patient's urine should be tested every 6 hours to detect glycosuria. This test may be performed on fractional urine samples or second-voided specimens, according to the physician's preference. Positive results should be reported to the physician, who determines the flow rate and dosage of parenteral insulin accordingly.

A careful record of intake and output and of daily weight should be kept. After an initial fluid weight gain, the well-regulated patient should gain about ¼ lb/day. Excessive gains may precede fluid overload, while losses may indicate dehydration. Electrolyte studies are also made frequently, and the nurse should be especially cognizant of disturbances in potassium and calcium levels.

At intervals, fat emulsions may be given in peripheral veins to supply essential fatty acids not present in hyperalimentation solution. It is important to check these solutions before administration for any oiling out of the emulsion. These solutions should never be given through a filter, nor should they be mixed with other solutions or have additives mixed in. They should be started at a rate of 1 ml/minute for the first 15 to 30 minutes; if no adverse reactions occur, the rate can be increased to 125 ml/hour.

### Fourth-level Nursing Care

In most cases, rehabilitation of severe malnutrition begins in the hospital with gradual reestablishment of food intake and normal exercise tolerance. The diet teaching should be started in the hospital and continued in the community. It is important to involve the family in the teaching, but the nurse should concentrate on the person who assumes responsibility for meal planning and preparation. Again, the social worker should be involved if food procurement and full utilization of community so-cial services are a problem. These patients will require follow-up in the home. Periodic visits should be made to assess the adequacy of the diet and the physical status of the patient. Diet teaching should be reinforced during each visit. The nurse should carefully assess and record any remaining physical signs of malnutrition and be alert to lessening or worsening of these signs in subsequent visits. Most physical signs of malnutrition are reversible, and careful rehabilitation of these patients should result in a return to high-level wellness.

### ORAL RECONSTRUCTION

Oral reconstruction is considered separately because it results in a profound disturbance of ingestion and poses unusual nursing problems in both the acute and the rehabilitative phases. Oral reconstruction is usually undertaken to resect cancerous lesions, although facial trauma may sometimes require reconstructive surgery. Frequently the resection of cancerous lesions in the oral cavity will necessitate a radical procedure. Because almost every structure in the oral cavity participates in the act of swallowing, radical resections of any oral structure will affect the patient's ability to swallow to some extent.

*Total glossectomy* is among the most disabling of the oral reconstructive procedures and requires skillful care. Not only is the tongue removed, but certain muscles of the pharynx are affected. In the immediate postoperative phase, the priority nursing problem is provision of an adequate airway. Glossectomy patients will have a tracheostomy and will require frequent suctioning because of aspiration of saliva. The patient should be positioned on either side to allow for drainage of saliva into a kidney basin. Gauze wicks may also be used to divert saliva. After the first few postoperative days, less care need be taken to divert saliva, but frequent suctioning should continue to remove any aspirated saliva. As the patient relearns swallowing in an attempt to handle salivary flow, the nurse will notice a decrease in the amount of saliva suctioned from the tracheostomy.

Nutritional needs up to this point are usually met by tube feedings via a nasogastric, cervical pharyngostomy, or gastrostomy tube. Hyperalimentation may be necessary in some instances. Once the patient begins to effectively swallow saliva and healing is satisfactory, swallowing retraining can begin. Soft foods such as custard, jello, and purees are used more successfully than liquids, which tend to be aspirated. The patient should never be left during feeding times, as suctioning may be necessary and emotional support is imperative. After taking liquids, the patient may need to throw the head back to facilitate rapid movement past the larynx. Some aspiration may still occur, but the patient should try to complete the swallowing process and then clear the larynx with a small cough. Swallowing retraining may take several months, and the patient may need to continue tube feedings for nutritional supplementation after dismissal.

Oral reconstruction for cancer may involve skin grafting in the oral cavity and radical neck dissection. The nurse should observe for bleeding from all sites, including donor sites for grafts. Although early hemorrhage is easily managed, late hemorrhage, from 8 to 20 days postoperatively, can be life-threatening. The appearance of even small amounts of bright red blood should alert the nurse to the possibility of impending major vascular hemorrhage. The physician should be notified and anticipatory measures carried out as directed. In the event of major hemorrhage, direct pressure should be applied to the bleeding vessel while emergency surgical treatment is rapidly mobilized.

Oral hygiene is very important in preventing infection. Because the surgical sites in the mouth may be complex and delicate grafts may be present, the surgeon will sometimes perform any oral hygiene measures in the first few postoperative days. If the nurse is to provide oral hygiene to these patients, a prescription should be obtained for any mouth preparation used, suture lines should be carefully avoided, and steps should be taken to prevent aspiration.

Patients who have had a total glossectomy will be unable to communicate and will suffer from severe disturbances in body image. They will need much emotional support before and after the surgery. Postoperative communication, which may involve the use of a slate, paper and pencil, or predetermined signals, should be planned with the patient in the preoperative period. Whenever possible, questions asked in the postoperative period should be answerable by "yes" or "no" signals. It is also important to teach the family how to communicate with the patient and to provide them with emotional support. Because of the drastic change in body image, psychological care given by the nurse can be a crucial factor in the patient's adjustment and rehabilitation from this disabling and disfiguring surgery.

## OBESITY

More than one-third of middle-aged Americans are overweight, and the incidence of obesity appears to

be increasing. A relationship between obesity and affluence has often been assumed to explain the high incidence of this problem in Western societies. However, recent studies performed on large numbers of obese subjects in all age groups have proved this assumption to be false. In fact, a strong inverse relationship between obesity and socioeconomic status has been demonstrated.[8] One study found that by age 6, obesity was nine times more prevalent in lower-class girls than in those of upper class.[9] No clear explanation for this phenomenon, combined with the rise in obesity in affluent Western societies, is available. It is clear, however, that excess weight exacts a physical, psychological, and sociological toll of its victims and constitutes a major health problem in the United States today.

### Pathophysiology

When caloric intake exceeds the body's caloric need for energy expenditure, the body stores the excess calories, primarily as fat. If this imbalance continues on a long-term basis, the proportion of body fat relative to lean body mass becomes abnormally high. This excess in body fat occurs in different patterns at the cellular level, depending on the developmental period at which the fat stores are first laid down. These patterns are described in relation to adipocytes (fat cells) as hyperplastic-hypertrophic and hypertrophic. The *hyperplastic-hypertrophic pattern* results from an excessive caloric intake during critical phases of adipocyte proliferation. The pattern is characterized by an excess number of adipocytes containing an excess amount of fat. The *hypertrophic pattern* results from excessive caloric intake after the body's adipocyte count is stable. It is characterized by a normal number of adipocytes containing an excess amount of fat.

Irrespective of cellular patterns, obesity can also be classified as mild, moderate, or severe according to the degree to which body weight exceeds height-weight norms. The mild obesity category comprises persons who are 10 to 20 percent overweight; the moderate obesity category includes those who are 20 to 50 percent overweight; and the severe obesity category contains those who are 50 percent or more overweight.

**Causes of obesity**  The causes of obesity may be exogenous or endogenous. Exogenous obesity results from a disturbance in a person's interaction with the external environment. Endogenous obesity results from a disturbance in a person's internal environment. Exogenous obesity is by far the more common. The basic disturbance is, as previously mentioned, the ingestion of more calories than necessary to meet energy needs. Psychological, sociocultural, economic, and physical factors may influence this excessive ingestion.

**P**sychological Factors   Much research has been done over the years on the psychological factors related to obesity. At one time it was thought that certain personality disorders led to overeating. Current thought is that most of the psychological characteristics identified earlier as the causes of obesity are actually the results of obesity. One example is the tendency in severely obese persons toward social isolation. This tendency may be construed as the cause of obesity: people eat themselves into social unattractiveness for the purpose of repelling social contact. Others view it as a result of obesity, observing that the social interaction of obese persons increases when their weight decreases.

Psychological conditioning, however, can have a great effect on eating habits. This conditioning frequently begins early in life in instances where food is used as a reward or an appeasement. The anxious mother may respond to a crying baby by feeding it, thus establishing an association between relief of stress and eating. Conditioning may also dictate the types of food eaten. Cookies, candy, ice cream, and cake may be held out as rewards for good behavior, while raw fruits and vegetables or the promise of pleasant physical activities would be healthier. Conditioning continues to operate in the adult when such activities as watching television, going to movies, reading the paper, and attending social functions become associated with eating high-calorie snack foods or beverages.

**S**ociocultural Factors   Some sociocultural factors blend with conditioning factors as a cause for obesity. Traditional social celebrations such as weddings, graduations, housewarmings, and holidays are incomplete without an abundance of food and drink. This association is so ingrained that well-meaning friends of successful dieters often insist on celebrating their success with food! Other sociocultural factors blend with physical factors in causing obesity. The American diet is high in fat, which provides more calories per gram than protein or carbohydrates. At the same time, a high-fat diet may interfere with a person's physiologic mechanisms for "recognizing" the amount of food necessary for maintaining normal weight.

Strictly sociocultural factors which have a strong relationship with obesity are social mobility, number of generations in the United States, and ethnic and religious affiliations.[10] Obesity has been found more prevalent in socially downward mobile subjects and in first-generation and second-generation immigrants to the United States. Although not all ethnic groups were represented in the study and the small number of subjects made tests of statistical significance difficult, it appeared that among lower-class subjects, Czech and Hungarian backgrounds had the strongest ethnic influence on obesity. By religious affiliation, the greatest prevalence of obesity was found among Jews, followed in order by Roman Catholics, Baptists, Methodists, Lutherans, and Episcopalians. The causative factors of obesity which operate in these groups remain unclear.

**E**conomic Factors   Studies in this country and other Western societies demonstrate a strong inverse relationship between obesity and social class. This finding is most pronounced among American women. Recent research on Navaho Indians, comparing the Navahoes acculturated to surrounding white culture with traditional Navahoes, strongly suggests that Western sociocultural factors account for the inverse relationship.[11] In other words, it appears the Western social factors, perhaps fashion or fad, may exert control over the weight of the affluent while little affecting the poor. It is possible that social factors explain the increasing thinness of American women and the increasing obesity in American men over the last twenty years. However, the actual social determinants of obesity remain to be studied.

**P**hysical Factors   Though there is strong suspicion that a biochemical or metabolic cause for *exogenous obesity* exists, conclusive evidence for this has not been found. Certain physical factors are known to influence body weight; for instance, genetic factors have a strong influence on the development of obesity. Children with no obese parentage have a 7 percent incidence of obesity; those with one obese parent, 40 percent incidence; and those with two obese parents, 80 percent incidence. Studies on twins raised in separate environments and on adopted children show that the genetic influence is much stronger than the environmental influence on the control of body weight.

One physical factor is overfeeding during critical periods of adipocyte proliferation. These critical periods occur in late gestational life, early infancy, and adolescence. As mentioned earlier, excess caloric intake at these times results in an increase in the total number of body fat cells. This seems to explain the fact that four-fifths of fat babies become fat adults.

Physical inactivity, especially as seen in a convenience-oriented society, may not be accompanied by a decrease in caloric intake. This causes an imbalance between caloric intake and energy expenditure, with fat storage resulting. Business executives, the elderly, and physically disabled persons are prone to obesity for this reason.

*Endogenous obesity* results from various disturbances of metabolism. The incidence of endogenous obesity is small, and the disturbances do not ordinarily result in massive obesity. Hypothyroidism, with its accompanying decrease in basal metabolic rate, is a common cause of endogenous obesity. The increased cortisol secretion in Cushing's syndrome causes weight gain with deposition of adipose tissue in certain areas. Patients with Cushing's syndrome have a characteristic moon face, "buffalo hump," and truncal obesity as a result. Hyperinsulinism caused by hypersecreting islet-cell tumors can cause increased food intake and increased food storage. Generally, however, the weight gain as a result of hyperinsulinism is small.

**Effects of obesity** The *psychological effects* of obesity vary greatly and appear to be related to the degree of obesity and the age of onset. A person who has been moderately to severely obese from childhood may have a pronounced disturbance in body image and low self-esteem. This results from the generally punitive attitudes of our society toward obese persons. On a daily basis, the obese person is faced with the contempt of a society which equates obesity with lack of self-control and slovenliness. Because of this attitude, job promotions, job opportunities, and acceptance into schools and clubs may be denied obese persons. Store clerks may delay assistance to obese persons. The obese person may hold these same attitudes and frequently develop self-contempt and a low self-esteem.

Social interactions can become a source of humiliation and result in a withdrawal from social settings. If, because of early conditioning, a person associates food with comfort or relief of stress, then overindulgence in food will follow these unsatisfying social interactions. After many unsuccessful attempts at dieting, the obese person may seek help only to find that health professionals hold the same contempt for and punitive attitude toward obesity as society at large. With the background of strong conditioning and low self-esteem, it is small wonder that the obese person can rarely endure the long-term dieting necessary to lose large amounts of weight.

Obesity also has profound *physical effects.* Excess weight is associated with a high mortality rate. The leading causes of mortality are hypertension, gallbladder disease, and diabetes mellitus. The mechanism by which obesity contributes to these pathologies varies. Hypertension and gallbladder disease appear to be related to increased body fat. With the increase in body fat and the concomitant increase in cholesterol turnover and cholesterol in the bile, gallstones may be formed. Increased stores of fat also require more blood to be circulated, thus increasing cardiac output, stroke volume, and blood pressure. Eventually the heart will enlarge. Hyperlipidemia may develop and, along with hypertension, increase the risk of vascular disease.

The effects of obesity on endocrine disease are usually dependent on the duration rather than the magnitude of obesity. Pancreatic function is altered over a period of time. As the obese person gains weight, the body's adipocytes fill with fat and become very large. The larger the cells become, the less responsive they are to insulin. As less glucose is utilized, hyperglycemia develops and leads to hypersecretion of the islet cells. The patient's glucose tolerance is impaired, and plasma insulin levels may be elevated in the fasting state and after glucose administration. Finally, prolonged hypersecretion of the islet cells can cause pancreatic exhaustion. For this reason, adult-onset diabetes mellitus is often precipitated by obesity. In the person whose pancreas has a genetically impaired secretory capacity, weight gain alone can bring about diabetes. In this same person, weight loss may control the diabetes. Other endocrine functions are also affected by obesity. Abnormal menstrual cycles and amenorrhea may result. The release of growth hormone is impaired. The secretion of adrenal steroids is increased, along with the excretion of 17-hydroxycorticosteroids in the urine.

Obesity also has an effect on pulmonary function because chest wall fat restricts chest movement. It can increase the work of breathing to a far greater extent than congestive heart failure. Postanesthesia atelectasis is common because of hypoventilation. An occasional severely obese patient will develop *Pickwickian syndrome.* This syndrome is characterized by hypoventilation, somnolence, polycythemia, and cyanosis. During sleep, respirations may be periodic and cyanosis pronounced. The carbon dioxide tension of arterial blood is increased, and the oxygen tension may be decreased. Loss of weight will cure the disease, but ventilatory support may be necessary in extreme cases.

Other complications of obesity are impaired

venous return from the lower extremities, impaired wound healing, osteoarthritis of the lower spine and weight-bearing joints, and skin problems aggravated by excessive moisture and friction. The reasons for the two latter complications are obvious. Poor venous return from the lower extremities is the result of fat-laden muscles which are inefficient venous pumps. Thus dependent edema, thrombophlebitis, and varicosities can be problems. Wound dehiscence is a common complication in the postsurgical obese patient, because sutures tend to break through friable fatty tissue. In addition, large fat cells impinge on capillary blood flow so that subcutaneous wound layers are poorly perfused and healing is slow.

### First-level Nursing Care

Once obesity is established, it is very difficult to control. Prevention of obesity is nearly as difficult as control because of the long-term nature of preventive measures when a genetic predisposition is present. However, the pains taken in prevention can circumvent a lifetime of physical and emotional misery.

The first step in prevention is the identification of commonly affected groups. The poor, those persons in or past their middle years, and children with one or more obese parents are frequently affected. Children of all socioeconomic groups are the prime targets of prevention, because they tend to become obese adults. Childhood obesity is the product of overnutrition during phases of adipocyte proliferation, so the nurse should focus on pregnant women, mothers of small infants, and adolescents.

Prevention of obesity primarily consists of early counseling. Pregnant women should receive good diet counseling throughout the prenatal period. Although pregnancy is not a time for stringent caloric restriction, these women should be counseled against dietary excesses. This will prevent the gaining of an excessive amount of weight and may protect the offspring from future obesity. It should be noted that women who are frequently pregnant tend to become accustomed to a larger food intake and easily become obese.

Diet counseling should continue after the baby is born to assure adequate nutrition to both mother and child. However, to avoid adverse conditioning, the mother should be advised against feeding the baby every time it cries. The mother of a fat baby should be given extra attention in diet teaching. A dietitian or a pediatrician can help the nurse in modifying the infant's diet.

Adverse conditioning of children may take place when parents force children to "clean up their plate." Mothers who complain that their young children are not eating well should be assisted in evaluating and planning for adequate family diets. However, it is important to caution these women that children should not be forced to eat past their feeling of satiety at mealtimes. As long as the child eats food from all four basic groups and is not allowed to consume many "empty calories" between meals, the diet consumed voluntarily should be adequate. Rewards for good behavior should not revolve around food, and between-meal snacks are best limited to raw fruits and vegetables.

Counseling adolescents is somewhat more difficult. Though many are body-conscious enough to attempt weight maintenance, food may become an issue in their struggle for independence. It is extremely important to involve adolescents in diet planning and to make allowances for their preferences. Group teaching is especially effective with adolescents.

In counseling patients eating on a low income, the nurse should stress the less expensive sources of protein. Fish and poultry are especially good suggestions because of their low fat content. Older patients are best advised of these sources of protein and of the benefits of fruits and vegetables in the diet. All patients should be encouraged to get adequate exercise.

### Second-level Nursing Care

During the *nursing assessment* of early or mild obesity, the nurse should consult height-weight charts. If the patient's weight is 10 to 20 percent higher than the norm, mild obesity may be a problem. However, the nurse should critically examine the patient's general body build and muscularity before concluding that the patient is obese. Moderate obesity can be detected on sight or by examination for folds of fat. The moderately obese person is 20 to 50 percent overweight. If the patient has a problem with obesity, a physician should determine whether the obesity is endogenous or exogenous before treatment is instituted.

The nurse may wish to obtain a 24-hour dietary recall from the patient. Techniques for eliciting and evaluating a 24-hour recall are discussed in the section on malnutrition. If the patient is more than mildly obese and is willing to pursue a long-term weight reduction program, it is helpful to ask for a one-week food diary. Patients who keep such diaries should record precisely what they eat, how much, at what time of day, where they were, whom they were with, and how they felt. This assists both the patient and the nurse to fully evaluate eating habits and faulty patterns. The amount and type of daily exercise should also be determined, as inactivity may be contributing to the obesity.

**Diet teaching** A good diet program has four planned components: (1) a well-balanced, calorie-deficit diet plan, (2) a plan for modifying faulty eating habits, (3) a plan for increased exercise, and (4) a plan for positive reinforcement of results.

A diet plan utilizing an exchange list will usually have better results than simple calorie counting. Calorie counting allows the patient to substitute rich foods for more nutritious fare or to skip meals as compensation for planned overindulgence. An exchange diet has a three-meal framework and provides for all basic food groups. The patient should be strongly encouraged to eat all three meals and to measure and weigh all foods as specified. If this is done faithfully, over the course of the diet, the patient will develop concrete concepts of normal food portions and meal patterns. It also provides a framework more adaptable to eating outside the home. A list of low-calorie vegetables should be included in the exchange lists to be eaten as snacks. Alcoholic beverages should be eliminated because they add "empty calories" to the diet and stimulate appetite while reducing inhibitions. The nurse should never assume that one teaching session is sufficient and should reassess and reinforce teaching on every patient visit.

Faulty eating patterns should be assessed and steps taken to correct these patterns. The tendency of obese persons to eat only in the evenings should be immediately corrected. All food should be consumed slowly and while sitting at a table. No other activities, such as watching television or reading the paper, should be paired with eating. If extra calories are being consumed at identifiable times, such as while cooking or clearing the table, measures should be planned which assist the patient in changing this habit.

An exercise program should be planned which gradually increases the patient's activity level. Activities such as walking, bicycling, and swimming are appropriate. The patient should be encouraged to omit "short cuts" such as elevators and to use opportunitites in a normal day to increase the activity level. Calisthenics, while helping to tone muscles, expends few calories and may give the patient a false feeling of accomplishment.

Because obese patients have used food as a positive reinforcement for many years, food deprivation can lead to depression and anxiety. A plan for positive reinforcement should be instituted. A simple plan is to require weekly weigh-ins. This affords the nurse an opportunity to deal with problems as they arise and to give the patient support. The patient should be led to expect a maximum weekly weight loss of ½ to 1 kg (1 to 2 lb). Praise and support should be given for any weight loss, and gains should be handled with sympathy and optimism for future success. These patients have a battered ego, and to lower their self-esteem further by a punitive or disapproving attitude will lead to certain failure. Patients should also be encouraged to frequently reward their own good behavior with shopping trips, movies, and other pleasant activities. In situations where weight loss will require long-term dieting, referral to groups such as TOPS (Take Off Pounds Sensibly) or Weight Watchers should be considered, as group reinforcement and support can be invaluable.

**Drug therapy** Anorexigenic agents are sometimes used to assist the obese patient in appetite control. Most of these drugs are amphetamines and have undesirable side effects such as central nervous system stimulation and addiction. Some new compounds have reduced these side effects while retaining the anorectic properties, most notably fenfluramine. Weight loss should be attempted without drugs because of the previously mentioned side effects and because the patient does not acquire the sense of dietary self-control necessary to maintain weight loss. In some cases, however, the side effects of drug therapy may be preferable to the side effects of obesity.

**Psychological counseling** Some patients may require psychological counseling to achieve success in weight control. Counseling is usually aimed at increasing the patient's awareness of external cues which stimulate eating and assisting the patient to develop coping mechanisms to deal with anxiety and frustration. Behavior modification groups led by skilled therapists may provide this in conjunction with other benefits to ease the patient's struggle to lose weight.

Although some patients experience depression during the dieting process, many will begin to have more satisfying personal relationships as their self-esteem improves. In the event that emotional problems become apparent in a dieting patient, the nurse should refer the patient to professional counseling immediately.

### Third-level Nursing Care

Most obese patients are treated in ambulatory settings; massively obese patients, however, may require hospitalization. Reasons for hospitalization vary. Usually the patient is admitted for a complete physical examination in preparation for a treatment prescription. If radical medical or surgical treatments are attempted, hospitalization is mandatory. Occasionally the patient is admitted for developing complications such as heart failure or Pickwickian syndrome.

**Nursing assessment** The nurse should evaluate the need for a *dietary history* when the patient is admitted. If complications are developing or the patient is admitted for a prolonged fast, the dietary history is not necessary, but it is helpful in the case of the patient admitted for a diagnostic workup preceding dietary treatment. General information concerning the age of onset and general progression of obesity should be elicited first. The patient should be asked about previous successes and failures in dieting. These questions should be asked in a sensitive manner. For example, the nurse should ask the patient what types of diets have been attempted and which were most successful. Questions such as "Have you ever tried dieting?" demonstrate lack of sensitivity and ignorance of the usual dieting patterns of the obese. The patient should also be asked about any emotional effects of previous diets, especially depression. Evaluation of food intake and the circumstances surrounding food intake can be undertaken or may be postponed until the general course of treatment is decided.

The nurse should keep in mind that childhood obesity is the hyperplastic-hypertrophic type. The increased number of adipocytes seem to create their own "metabolic demand" and make weight loss difficult to sustain. This knowledge should temper the nurse's attitude toward such patients and their many dietary failures. Anticipation of this should not prompt pessimism but should help the nurse to handle the frustrations associated with treatment failure.

**P**hysical Assessment The nurse should measure the height and weight of the patient on a balance scale, noting the time of day and the amount of clothing worn. If the patient's weight is more than 50 percent above the norm on height-weight charts, obesity is severe. General body conformation abnormalities should be noted—e.g., pendulous abdominal aprons—and skin folds should be checked for excoriation or skin lesions. The blood pressure and pulse should be taken, though they may be difficult to palpate. Hypertension and mild tachycardia

may be present. Tachycardia will be more pronounced after exercise.

Heart sounds will be distant but should be normal if there is no cardiac involvement. The nurse should note the point on the chest where heart sounds are best heard, as they may be a clue to cardiac enlargement. If heart failure is present, a gallop rhythm may be heard. Breath sounds will be distant and may be diminished in the bases due to hypoventilation. Rales may be heard if the hypoventilation is beginning to cause atelectasis. Chest-wall excursion may also be limited because of the restrictive effect of excessive overlying fat. The eye and ear examinations, as well as the neurological examination, should be normal.

**D**iagnostic Tests A fasting blood sugar, glucose tolerance test, ketonuria-glycosuria test, serum cholesterol, and electrocardiogram are usually taken. The outcome of the first three is important. Findings on these tests will differ according to the duration of the obese state, but their primary purpose is to detect diabetes mellitus resulting from insulin antagonism or pancreatic exhaustion. Serum cholesterol may or may not be elevated; elevation would indicate a possible predisposition to atherosclerosis. An electrocardiogram is taken to evaluate the patient's general cardiac status. Further electrocardiography may be done with exercise stress. The oxygen consumption of the respiratory muscles, the oxygen uptake of the excess adipose tissue, and hypoventilation may all contribute to hypoxia during exercise, which may cause arrhythmias detectable only on stress testing.

**Nursing problems and interventions** Personal hygiene and skin problems can be troublesome for the massively obese patient. *Perineal hygiene* is a particular problem when a pendulous abdomen, massive thighs, and heavy skin folds produce moisture, trap secretions, and obscure the area. The nurse should assist the patient in perineal care as much as possible, being careful to wash in all skin folds. If a whirlpool both is available in the hospital, the patient should be bathed in it at least twice a week. All skin folds should be cleansed thoroughly and a powder applied to absorb moisture and reduce friction. If *skin excoriation* is present in the folds, cotton wadding should be tucked inside to absorb the excess moisture. If the skin fold can be pulled up and secured with tape, the excoriated skin can be exposed to air several times a day.

The patient will also have general *problems with movement.* The nurse should evaluate the need for an oversize bed and obtain one if the patient cannot move about adequately. The bed should be kept in a position at which the patient's feet can just touch the floor, as higher or lower positions will create safety hazards. The patient should be out of bed and ambulatory as much as possible to avoid the hazards of immobility, especially thrombophlebitis, thromboembolism, and hypostatic pneumonia. When the patient is ambulating, the nurse should be alert to shortness of breath and complaints of dyspnea on exertion. The pulse rate should be taken before and immediately after ambulation until the nurse has ascertained the amount of exercise the patient can tolerate. If the patient is on bed rest, leg exercise, turning, coughing and deep breathing are in order.

**Severe dietary intervention** In severely obese patients, a fast may be used to hasten weight loss. Several studies have reported fewer undesirable emotional effects with fasting than with deficit diets. Complete fasting, while inducing ketosis accompanied by anorexia, also may deplete body protein. For this reason many physicians prefer a modified fast which maintains the nitrogen balance. With the modified fast, the patient is fed 1 to 1.5 g of protein per kilogram of weight. Fluids are taken liberally, and limited amounts of leafy vegetables are added for bulk. Vitamin supplements are necessary adjuncts to any fast. These patients must be monitored closely, and those with a tendency to hyperlipidemia should have serum cholesterol levels taken frequently.

The nurse should observe these patients for signs of orthostatic hypotension, dizziness, or fainting around the third to fourth day. The body will usually adapt to the low intake after a week. The nurse should also observe the patient for any signs of depression, anxiety, or agitation.

**Surgical intervention** In some severely or morbidly obese patients, surgical intervention may be the treatment of choice. *Jejunoileal shunts* are the most successful and most common type of surgical intervention. These procedures are associated with many complications, however, and are still considered by most physicians to be in the experimental category. Strict criteria are therefore applied to potential surgical patients. The patient's weight must be 100 to 150 percent of normal. Massive obesity must have been a problem for at least 5 years, and attempts at conservative treatment must have failed. Complications such as diabetes mellitus, hypertension, osteoarthritis, or hyperlipidemia

must be present, but diseases such as coronary insufficiency, liver disease, and serious or correctible endocrine disease must not. The patient should be under 50 and emotionally stable, must understand the risks and complications, and must be willing and able to cooperate with the postoperative treatment and examinations.

Jejunoileal shunts are surgically constructed to divert food from large areas of digestive and absorptive surface in the jejunum and ileum, thus creating a surgically induced malabsorption. The most common surgical procedure (see Fig. 16-6) involves resection of most of the 6 meters (20 feet) of the ileum and jejunum, with an end-to-end anastomosis of the remaining 40 cm ($\approx$15 inches) of the proximal jejunum and 10 to 20 cm ($\approx$4 to 8 inches) of the distal ileum. The resected portion of intestine is closed at one end, while the other end is attached to either the transverse or sigmoid colon for drainage. The desired result of this surgery is weight loss, which usually brings the weight to within 23 kg ($\approx$50 lb) of the patient's ideal weight. After 2 years the patient's weight reaches plateau, as the remaining intestine adapts by adding more absorptive surface. Other desirable side effects of the surgery are a fall in serum cholesterol, blood pressure reduction, and improvement in the glucose tolerance curve.

Complications can arise in the immediate postoperative phase and at a later date. *Common complications* in the immediate postoperative period are wound infection and dehiscence, pneumonia, atelectasis, and pulmonary embolism. Later, persistent and severe diarrhea can lead to acute electrolyte imbalances with losses of potassium, magnesium, and calcium. Hypocalcemia may especially be a problem; it is discussed in detail in Chap. 12. Mild hepatic dysfunction is common, and on rare occasions cirrhosis may develop. Vitamins, especially $B_{12}$, can be depleted and must be supplemented. Renal calculi of the calcium oxalate type may occur, though the mechanism for this is unknown. Rarely does any complication other than cirrhosis require surgical reconnection.

Nursing responsibilities in the *preoperative period* are to prepare the patient for the postoperative course and to assure informed consent. These patients may have more pain postoperatively than most patients because of extensive surgical trauma. Careful teaching of postoperative procedures such as turning, leg exercises, deep breathing, and coughing will help in obtaining the patient's later cooperation. The physician is responsible for informing the patient of the effects and risks of the surgery, but the nurse should collaborate with the physician in reinforcement of this teaching.

In the *postoperative period,* the nurse must give special care to prevent complications. Close attention to the wound and to patient complaints will help in detecting early signs of wound infection and dehiscence. The nurse should frequently encourage the patient to take very deep breaths, pausing several seconds at maximum inspiration. Coughing is necessary only when sputum is raised to the upper airways, and then the nurse should splint the entire abdomen during the cough. The patient must turn and move in bed and may need liberal parenteral analgesics to do so; in addition, an oversized bed and extra assistance will facilitate this.

Once oral intake resumes, diarrhea will begin. For the first few weeks, watery stools may occur 15 to 20 times daily. Fluid restrictions and medications may be ordered to decrease the frequency of diarrhea. The nurse may need to help patients with perineal care and should apply powder or soothing preparations if rectal excoriation is developing. Diarrhea will persist 3 to 5 times daily throughout the first year and possibly into the second year. Because diarrhea is a symptom of the malabsorption purposely induced to cause weight loss, this symptom is controlled only if severe fluid and electrolyte disturbances are a problem.

In giving postoperative care and in discharge teaching, the nurse should remember that oral medications will not be well absorbed. The need for parenteral analgesia may therefore continue into the second postoperative week. Female patients should be informed that birth-control pills may not be adequately absorbed and an alternative means of contraception is necessary. Pregnancy is not advised for 2 years postoperatively, as there is risk of in utero fetal malnutrition during this period. Discharge teaching should also include instruction on a low-fat diet, supplemented with foods rich in potassium, and any electrolyte or vitamin supplements indicated. Alcoholic intake is forbidden, as it can contribute to liver complications. The nurse should emphasize the absolute necessity of following prescribed regimes and keeping all appointments with the physician to prevent complications.

### Fourth-level Nursing Care

Rehabilitation of the obese patient begins in the treatment phase. Many of the principles discussed in diet teaching under Second-level Nursing Care apply after weight is lost. This requires long-term contact and individualized care. In discussing indi-

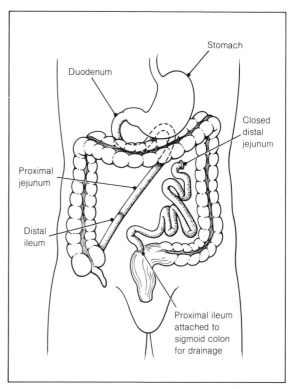

**FIGURE 16-6**
Jejunoileal shunt.

vidual problems, the nurse should assist the patient to develop good problem-solving techniques. Most patients need special assistance in generating low-calorie alternatives to eating and drinking in social situations.

Rehabilitation does not end when patients achieve their ideal weight. Normal caloric intake must be reinstituted gradually as the body adapts to the decreased energy supply during dieting. Weight gains during this period warrant an immediate reduction in caloric intake. The patient's weight should stabilize within 2 to 3 months. Because of the difficulty in changing ingrained habits, and possibly because of a "metabolic demand" in patients obese since childhood, the weight lost is frequently regained. The patient will need continued support if weight loss is to be maintained. The group support available through behavior modification groups and organizations such as TOPS and Weight Watchers can be a valuable adjunct for weight maintenance.

The nurse must be patient, understanding, and encouraging when advocating weight reduction, assisting in weight loss, and monitoring weight maintenance. The fact that lost weight is frequently regained should not discourage the nurse or the patient in these endeavors. It is important to remember that the increase in the quality of life and health can make even temporary weight loss worthwhile.

## REFERENCES

1   *Ten State Nutrition Survey, 1968–1970,* U.S. Department of Health, Education and Welfare Publication HSM 72-8134, 1972.

2   Ibid., p. 9.

3   Ibid., p. 10.

4   Ibid., p. 9.

5   Helen H. Gifft, Marjorie B. Washbon, and Gail G. Harrison, *Nutrition, Behavior and Change,* Prentice-Hall, Englewood Cliffs, N.J., 1972, p. 213.

6   M. L. Mitra, "Confusional States in Relation to Vitamin Deficiency in the Elderly," *J Am Geriatr Soc,* **19**(4):536–545, June, 1971.

7   George Christakis, "Nutritional Assessment in Health Programs," *Am J Public Health,* **63**:1–37, November Supplement, 1973.

8   Illonna J. Rimm and Alfred A. Rimm, "Association between Socioeconomic Status and Obesity in 59,556 Women," *Prev Med,* **3**:543–473, December, 1974.

9   Albert Stunkard, Eugene O'Aquili, Sonja Fox, and Ross D. L. Fillion, "Influence of Social Class on Obesity and Thinness in Children," *JAMA,* **221**(6):579–584, Aug. 7, 1972.

10   P. B. Goldblatt, M. E. Moore, and A. J. Stunkard, "Social Factors in Obesity," *JAMA,* **192**:1039–1044, 1965, as reported in A. J. Stunkard, "Presidential Address, 1974: From Explanation to Action in Psychosomatic Medicine: The Case of Obesity," *Psychosom Med,* **37**(3):195–236, May-June, 1975.

11   J. L. Garb, J. R. Garb, and A. J. Stunkard, "The Influence of Social Factors on Obesity and Thinness in Navaho Children," as reported in A. J. Stunkard, Presidential Address, 1974: From Explanation to Action in Psychosomatic Medicine: The Case of Obesity," *Psychosom Med,* **37**(3):195–236, May–June, 1975.

## BIBLIOGRAPHY

Bray, G. A.: "The Overweight Patient," *Adv Intern Med,* **21**:267–308, 1976.

Chang, Betty: "Some Dietary Beliefs in Chinese Folk Culture," *J Am Diet Assoc,* **65**:436–438, October 1974.

Crisp, A. H., and B. McGuiness: "Jolly Fat: Relation between Obesity and Psychoneurosis in General Population," *Br J Med,* **1**:7–9, Jan. 3, 1976.

Gormican, Annette, and Eileen Liddy: "Nasogastric Tube Feedings," *Nurs Digest,* 59–62, January 1974.

Grant, JoAnn Nallinger: "Patient Care in Parenteral Hyperalimentation," *Nurs Clin North Am,* **8**(1):165–182, March 1973.

Hallberg, D., L. Backman, and S. Espmark: "Surgical Treatment of Obesity," *Prog Surg,* **14**:46–83, 1975.

Heydman, Abby Hitchcock: "Intestinal Bypass for Obesity," *Am J Nurs,* **74**(6):1102–1104, June 1974.

Howard, Lyn: "Obesity: A Feasible Approach to a Formidable Problem," *Am Family Practitioner,* **12**(3):153–163, September 1975.

Jeffers, Camille: "Hunger, Hustlin' and Homemaking," *J Home Econ,* **61**(10):14–20, December 1969.

Johanson, A. J., and N. J. Knorr: "Treatment of Anorexia Nervosa by Levodopa," *Lancet,* **2**:591, Sept. 7, 1974.

Margen, Sheldon, and Lindsey H. Allen: "What to Look for in the Nutritional Examination," *Consultant,* 43–52, March 1976.

Mawson, A. R.: "Anorexia Nervosa and the Regulation of Intake: A Review," *Psychol Med,* **4**:289–308, August, 1974.

Meyers, Eugene N.: "Rehabilitation of the Oral Cavity after Resection for Cancer," in John Conley and John T. Dickinson (eds.), *Plastic and Reconstructive Surgery of the Face and Neck,* vol. 2, *Rehabilitative Surgery,* Grune & Stratton, New York, 1972, pp. 213–217.

Nizel, A. E.: "Nutrition and Oral Problems," *World Rev Nutr Diet,* **16**:226–252, 1973.

Raper, Nancy R., and Mary M. Hill: "Vegetarian Diets," *Nutri Rev,* **32**(Suppl. 1): 29–33, July, 1974.

Read, M.S.: "Malnutrition, Hunger, and Behavior," *Journal of the American Diabetes Association,* **63**:379, October 1973.

Rosillo, Ronald H., Mary J. Wetty, and William P. Graham: "The Patient with Maxillofacial Cancer. II. Psychologic Aspects," *Nurs Clin North Am,* **8**(1):153–158, March 1973.

Rynearson, E. H.: "Americans Love Hogwash," *Nutr Rev,* **32**(Suppl. 1): 1–14, July 1974.

Stunkard, A. J.: "Presidential Address, 1974: From Explanation to Action in Psychosomatic Medicine: The Case of Obesity," *Psychosom Med,* **37**(3):195–236, May–June 1975.

Stunkard, A. J., and John Rush, "Dieting and Depression Reexamined," *Ann Intern Med,* **81**(4):526–533, October 1974.

Todhunter, E. Neige: "Food Habits, Food Faddism and Nutrition," *World Rev Nutri Diet,* **16:**286–317, 1973.

Tolstrup, Kay: "The Treatment of Anorexia Nervosa in Childhood and Adolescence," *J Child Psychol Psychiatry,* **16:**75–78, January 1975.

*Ten State Nutrition Survey, 1968–1970.*

Welty, Mary J., William P. Graham, and Ronald H.

Rosillo: "The Patient with Maxillofacial Cancer, I." *Surg Treatment Nurs Care,* **8**(1):137–151, March 1973.

Wettengel, Paul J. (ed.): "Intralipid," *Pharm Newsletter* (Creighton Memorial St. Joseph Hospital, Omaha, Neb.), **3**(2):1–5, March 1976.

Wintrobe, Maxwell M. et al.: *Harrison's Principles of Internal Medicine,* McGraw-Hill, New York, 1974.

# 17
# DISTURBANCES IN DIGESTION

Nancy Guardino Safer

**E**ach person must interact with the environment in order to maintain a dynamic equilibrium for the preservation and promotion of a healthy society. This equilibrium is frequently challenged during a person's life span, and the result may be a deviation from the state of health.

One of the major threats to the health of Americans today is gastrointestinal disease, which can take credit for a multibillion-dollar economic loss yearly, often disabling people during the most productive period of their lives. Digestive disease is the primary reason for hospitalization in this country and also one of the major causes of death.

If nurses are to be truly committed to health and the quality of life, they must be prepared to offer in-depth assessment, intervention, and rehabilitation to the person who is suffering a disturbance in digestion. Their skillful counseling and health teaching, early detection, and referral may help prevent disability from the wide spectrum of digestive problems affecting such large numbers of our population.

## DISTURBANCES OF GASTRIC DIGESTION

Many of the altered physiologic mechanisms which result in disturbances of gastric digestion produce similar clinical pictures. The nurse plays a vital role, through observation, assessment, and intervention, in accurate definition of problems and development of an appropriate therapeutic approach.

### Peptic Ulcer

Peptic ulcer is a sharply defined break in tissue which may involve the mucosa, submucosa, and muscular layers of the digestive tract exposed to acid. Although peptic ulcer occurs throughout the world, studies attempting to correlate it specifically with diet, geography, climate, culture, or class have not been successful in establishing any definite patterns.

Chronic ulcerations in the stomach and those in the duodenum have many similarities in clinical manifestations, course, and complications. However, they also display many differences, and it is currently a matter of controversy whether they can both be considered to represent the same disease process (see Table 17-1). While gastric ulcers are more common in the older age groups of both sexes, duodenal ulcers seem to be found more frequently in men during young adulthood and middle age. The duodenal ulcer is most often related to stress and life-style, leading to stereotyping of the "ulcer personality" as a competitive, successful, nervous, compulsive executive in a position demanding high-powered decision making and affording little opportunity for relaxation.

**Pathophysiology** As mentioned previously, peptic ulcers occur in areas of the digestive tract where acid is found, that is, the lower esophagus, stomach, and duodenum. They may also occur in the jejunum after gastroenterostomy. Ulceration does not occur in the actual membrane which secretes acid but is found in adjacent mucous membranes which are not normally accustomed to acid conditions. It is important to remember, at this point, that normal gastric secretions are capable of digesting any tissue and that the digestive tract mucosa is usually protected from autodigestion by its mucous coating and by dilution and neutralization of the acid by food, saliva, and duodenal fluids. The development of ulceration, then, can be viewed as due to an imbalance between the digesting power of acid secretions and the ability of the mucosa to resist this digestive action. The mucosal resistance can be decreased by factors such as inadequate blood supply, inadequate regeneration of epithelial tissue, and an inadequate quantity of mucus.

Persons with *duodenal ulcer* usually secrete more acid than normal persons and have an increased parietal cell (acid-secreting cell) mass. Faulty removal of acid in the duodenum is also implicated. Even without the normal stimuli for acid secretion, the hypersecretion associated with duodenal ulcers continues and occurs at unusual times, such as between meals and overnight. Persons with duodenal ulcer secrete 3 to 20 times more acid than normal persons overnight or during fasting. This is thought to be the result of vagal stimulation. The output of pepsin is also increased in

duodenal ulcer, and this increases the digestive capacity of the secretions.

On the other hand, persons with *gastric ulcer* secrete normal to low amounts of acid, a consistent finding that has not as yet been completely explained. This was formerly thought to be simply a hyposecretion of gastric acid, but recent thinking leans toward the belief that hyposecretion is not in operation here and that, instead, excessive acid may be lost through back-diffusion of the acid into the gastric mucosa which has become abnormally permeable to acid. This increased permeability may be a result of the action of bile and pancreatic juice, which refluxes into the stomach when there is incompetence of the pyloric sphincter mechanism.

Most peptic ulcers are small in size—duodenal ulcers average about 1 cm and gastric ulcers 1 to 2.5 cm. Gastric ulcers usually occur on or near the lesser curvature of the stomach, while duodenal ulcers are commonly found in the first 2 cm distal to the pylorus.

Hypertrophy of the mucosa is common in duodenal ulcer, whereas atrophy is usually found in gastric ulceration. It is thought that this gastric atrophy may predispose to carcinoma, but it is important to remember that *most* gastric ulcers are benign.

*Healing* of peptic ulcers proceeds from the botton upward; as the healing process advances, a layer of epithelium grows over the area where tissue has been eroded. If the ulceration was very small and superficial, complete healing may take place, with the mucosa appearing normal, but in the healing of large ulcers, the new mucosa is thinner and the damaged muscle is replaced by fibrous tissue.

**P**redisposing Factors and Causes Many predisposing factors and causes of peptic ulcer have been set forth. Some have been proved to have a definite relationship to the disease process, while others remain controversial, needing further study. *Emotional and psychogenic factors* have long been implicated as etiologic agents in the pathogenesis of peptic ulcer. As mentioned previously, this relationship seems more apparent with duodenal ulcers. The exact causal relationship is not clear but may involve a mechanism of increased gastric secretion from vagal stimulation. Long-term vagal stimulation may result in hyperplasia and hypertrophy and, eventually, an increase in parietal cell mass.

*Drug-induced* injury to the gastric mucosa has been a recognized cause of ulceration. Aspirin, probably one of the most misused drugs in our

**TABLE 17-1**
SOME DIFFERENTIATIONS BETWEEN GASTRIC AND DUODENAL ULCERATIONS

| Factor | Duodenal | Gastric |
| --- | --- | --- |
| Age | Young adulthood | Older age and middle age |
| Sex | Mainly male | Both male and female |
| Emotional stress | Yes | No |
| Acid secretion | Increased | Normal to low |
| Nocturnal pain | Yes | No |
| Usual location | First 2 cm distal to pylorus | On or near lesser curvature |
| Appearance of mucosa | Hypertrophied | Atrophied |

modern society, is often singled out. Aspirin can penetrate the gastric mucosa and enter the cells. It also may affect the production of gastric mucus and allow acid diffusion back into the gastric mucosa. This back-diffusion then produces vasodilatation, the release of histamine, and possible submucosal hemorrhage. When considering how widely aspirin is used and in such staggering quantities, it is nevertheless amazing to discover that it has been estimated that the 20 to 30 billion tablets of aspirin consumed in the United States within the period of 1 year lead to a loss of 10 billion ml of blood. This loss is about twice as much as the total amount used for blood transfusions during the same period of time.[1]

Ulcerations often develop in persons who are receiving long-term steroid therapy. It has been suggested that steroids may suppress cell-mediated immunity causing abnormality of the mucosal structure, or may affect the type and amount of mucus produced thus altering the resistance of the mucosal barrier. It is important to remember that the symptoms of peptic ulcer may be masked by steroid therapy and, therefore, patients should receive antacids prophylactically and have stools routinely examined for the presence of occult blood. Other drugs such as Reserpine which can increase gastric acidity should be used very cautiously in persons with a history of peptic ulcer. Besides these drugs, alcohol and caffeine are also often implicated in the pathogenesis of peptic ulcer although definitive relationships have not been established. Caffeine stimulates gastric acid secretion and alcohol is thought to alter the mucosal barrier permitting back-diffusion of acid.

*Genetic factors* have also been considered among the causes of peptic ulceration. However, there is still no clearcut evidence linking heredity with the disease process. Some have tended to lean toward a genetic explanation of causation after finding a very frequent incidence of peptic ulcer in some families, frequent development of ulcerations among siblings of people with diagnosed ulcers, and, at times, ulcers in twins. People with blood type O seem to develop duodenal ulcers much more frequently than persons in the other blood groups. On the other hand, findings indicate a high percentage of males develop peptic ulcer disease in comparison to females, and the actual occurrence is only about 15 percent of the population. The answer to causation may eventually be found in a combination of genetic and environmental factors.

There have been some theories linking *cigarette smoking* with duodenal ulcer but the mechanism is not clear and it is difficult to document a cause and effect relationship. A significant increase in duodenal reflux back into the stomach has been found after smoking both in people with and without duodenal ulcers.

Gastric ulceration and bleeding as consequences of *severe systemic stress* are now being recognized. Some are classified specifically, such as *Curling's ulcer* which occurs after severe burns and *Cushing's ulcer* which is commonly found after central nervous system damage. However, all may be considered acute stress ulcerations and may occur as a sequel to a variety of severe systemic problems such as sepsis, trauma (including surgery), burns, central nervous system damage, hyperparathyroidism, jaundice, respiratory failure, and uremia. These ulcers are usually multiple, small erosions most commonly found in the body and near the fundus of the stomach. A decreased blood flow and ischemia seem to be prime factors in the pathology of stress ulcers. Systemic illnesses may disrupt the protective gastric mucosal barrier, with resulting ulcerations from back-diffusion of small amounts of acid. These erosions are painless, often occurring without warning, and so are difficult to detect early. It has recently been documented that a high incidence of gastrointestinal bleeding in patients with cancer is most likely due to stress ulcerations.

Several possible causes of peptic ulcer and the pathophysiologic changes which occur during the disease process have been discussed; it is important now to look at the effect these changes have on a person. The major effect of this altered physiology on the patient is *pain.* This pain will often set up a vicious cycle which will eventually prompt the person to seek medical attention: the greater the distress from pain, the greater the disturbance of the stomach and increase in gastric acid secretion and, completing the cycle, the greater the pain. Some patients will also suffer from *vomiting,* especially following bouts of severe pain, but this cannot be considered a typical finding in peptic ulcer. The vomiting may be preceded by nausea, and pain relief is often experienced after vomiting. Infrequently, patients may experience nausea and vomiting in the absence of pain. Vomiting, when present, is usually the result of pyloric obstruction. Eventually the time comes when the persistent pain and distress is affecting every aspect of the person's life.

**First-level nursing care** Peptic ulcer is all too often diagnosed and treated only after a major complication has occurred, such as massive bleeding, or the pain has finally become intolerable and the person is forced to seek medical advice. In view of this it is a prime responsibility of the nurse to thoughtfully identify problems which can lead to peptic ulcers and to be active in communicating methods of prevention to the population being served. Many possible predisposing factors have been previously mentioned. In the light of these, an accurate patient and family history is an invaluable tool for the nurse. Many potential ulcer-related problems may be identified, such as incidence of peptic ulcer within the family, patterns of drug ingestion—especially drugs known to cause gastric irritation—and other habits, such as smoking and alcohol consumption. An extremely important part of the history is a detailed assessment of the patient's life-style. For example, questions concerning occupation, feelings about work, and use of leisure time can all give valuable information about the patient's daily life. It is important to try to determine at this time what methods of dealing with stress are usually used and whether the person sees these stress responses as effective ones.

After identification of potential problems, prevention of peptic ulcer becomes the major goal of nursing care. At this point, teaching and counseling are the most effective tools the nurse can utilize. The patient must be assisted to identify stressful situations that provoke anxiety. Alternative ways of dealing with such situations should be explored. The effects of various drugs and of cigarettes should be emphasized. The nurse cannot dictate a change in habits or life-style patterns, but accurate, objective information will give patients a basis for making their own decisions about life-style and initiating some changes. After getting to know the person and setting up a therapeutic relationship, the nurse can often recommend some type of relaxation technique such as exercise, yoga, or transcendental meditation. Many people have found such techniques useful in alleviating the tension and anxiety so prevalent in our complex society. If the teaching and counseling by the nurse do not seem to be helping the patient, psychotherapy —individual, group, or family—may be beneficial.

**Second-level nursing care**  When peptic ulcer occurs, the major role of the nurse involves early case finding and appropriate referral, as well as active intervention. In uncomplicated cases of ulceration, hospitalization is often not necessary and the patient is frequently treated successfully in the community.

**N**ursing Assessment  Early detection and case finding are greatly aided by an accurate *health his-*

*tory.* When evaluating a patient who may have a peptic ulcer, the primary feature of the health history is the description of pain. Patients most often describe the character of the pain as burning, gnawing, aching, or cramplike. The degree of pain should be documented—whether it is mild, moderate, severe, or, in some cases, absent. The pain is usually localized in the epigastrium but may also be felt in the back at the level of T8 to T10, as shown in Fig. 17-1. The pain is usually cyclical, demonstrating chronicity and periodicity. Symptoms may last for only a few days or weeks but often are chronic, lasting for many years. The pain is also periodic, appearing for a few weeks, subsiding for a significant amount of time (months or years), and then recurring.

During the health history it is important to determine the relationship of the pain to food consumption. The discomfort may sometimes be relieved by the ingestion of food, but a typical pattern of pain for gastric ulcer is the occurrence of pain about 60 to 90 minutes after a meal and for duodenal ulcer 2 to 4 hours after eating. Patients with duodenal ulcer are likely to be awakened by pain overnight unless they eat very late in the evening. These patients tend to continue to secrete large amounts of gastric acid overnight. The influence of possible acid secretion during REM sleep has been implicated. Since the stomach is empty of food, these secretions are not buffered and enter the duodenum at a low pH. It is also important at this time to inquire whether the patient has discovered ways to relieve the pain. For example, does taking an antacid or eating something alleviate the distress? If the patient has also been troubled by vomiting, the nurse should elicit a description of such episodes, determining whether they are preceded by nausea; what, if any, is their relationship to the pain; and, if related, whether they help relieve the pain.

The *physical examination* of a patient with uncomplicated peptic ulcer usually does not yield much significant data. Appearance of the patient, vital signs, and chest, heart, and neurologic examinations are usually within normal limits. One finding may be an area of localized tenderness in the epigastrium over the ulcer site. Otherwise the physical examination is usually unremarkable, making an accurate health history very important.

*Diagnostic tests*  Several diagnostic tests may be used to confirm the presence of a peptic ulcer. A *barium swallow* is often one of the early procedures performed. A definitive finding in the case of peptic ulcer is the visualization of a sharply defined crater.

The patient is given a substance containing barium which is radiopaque. Barium collects in the ulcer, making it visible on x-ray. The procedure itself, as well as the use of a laxative or an enema following the study to avoid constipation or impaction from the barium, should be explained to the patient. Unfortunately, a barium study is not always a reliable indication of ulcer disease; often superficial ulcerations do not retain enough barium to be visualized.

Recent years have seen the rapid development of *gastrointestinal endoscopy.* The procedure involves the use of a long, flexible, lighted fiberscope which is passed through the mouth into the stomach and allows direct visualization of the gastric mucosa. Endoscopy is often used after x-ray studies to provide further information on the appearance of the crater, the ulcer margins, and the adjacent wall. Specimens for cytology studies can also be obtained during the procedure.

A local anesthetic may be applied to the pharynx to facilitate insertion of the tube. To empty the stomach, the patient should be instructed to take nothing by mouth for several hours preceding the test. After completion of the test, the nurse should determine that the gag reflex has returned before the patient takes anything orally. Although complications of this procedure are rare, perforation of the esophagus or the stomach has occurred in 1 to 2 percent of examinations. Swelling of tissues of the throat can also occur. The nurse should therefore observe for bleeding, fever, abdominal pain, dysphagia, and dyspnea.

Another diagnostic test commonly performed when peptic ulcer is suspected is *gastric analysis.* The gastric contents are removed by aspiration through a nasogastric tube and the gastric secretions analyzed for acidity. The patient is required to fast for about 8 hours prior to the test. A basal analysis is done in the morning, after an overnight fast, to determine acidity when there has been no stimulation. A stimulated analysis may be performed using a substance such as histamine to stimulate the gastric-secretion response. In both analyses, acid outputs are significantly higher in patients with duodenal ulcer than in those with gastric ulcer or in normal persons.

Throughout all diagnostic testing the major role of the nurse should be one of support to the patient, offering explanations and understanding. The procedures may be uncomfortable and frightening, but much of the anxiety can be alleviated by a sensitive nurse.

**N**ursing Intervention  The goals of intervention for the patient diagnosed as having a peptic ulcer are

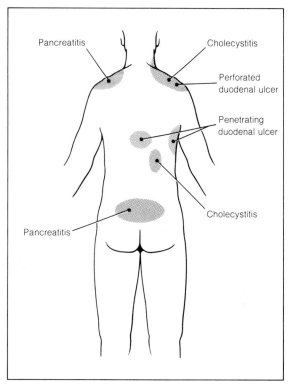

**FIGURE 17-1**
Common sites of referred abdominal pain (posterior view) due to peptic ulcer, pancreatitis, and cholecystitis. (*Adapted from A. H. Robins, GI Series, Physical Examination of the Abdomen, Part 5, A. H. Robins Co., Richmond, Va., 1972.*)

relief of pain, healing of the ulceration, and prevention of complications and recurrences. In the absence of complications, the outlook for patients is very favorable with therapy consisting mainly of diet, medication, and counseling.

*Diet therapy*  Traditional bland diets used in the therapy of peptic ulcer have been extremely rigid and restrictive. The therapeutic value of such a severe regimen has never been justified, and the imposition of unnecessary restrictions may take its toll in increased tension and anxiety. It is now therefore advocated that the diet be as liberal as possible. It should be remembered that ulceration is a rather long-term disruption. The patient who is placed on a severely restricted diet will probably follow it until symptomatic relief is obtained, then go off the diet and suffer tension and guilt feelings which may cause more harm than the restricted foods. Bland diets or the Sippy diet (frequent, small intake, alternating milk and an antacid) are still sometimes used in the acute stage when severe pain may be present.

*Caffeine* has long been known to stimulate gastric acid secretion. Even with the current liberalization of ulcer diets, therefore, most physicians still recommend the restriction of regular coffee and advise the patient to drink decaffeinated coffee. It is also usual practice to restrict not only coffee but all other beverages containing caffeine, such as tea and cola drinks. However, a recent study examined the effects of caffeine alone, regular coffee, and decaffeinated coffee on acid secretion.[2] The surprising finding was that the effects of caffeine alone were minimal compared to the powerful acid stimulation of regular coffee and decaffeinated coffee. The findings suggest that there may be a substance in coffee (regular or decaffeinated) which is capable of independently stimulating acid secretion. Patients with peptic ulcer are also advised to stop *smoking* and to restrict their intake of *alcohol*. Again, these restrictions are difficult to justify, but until more definitive studies are made, caffeine, cigarettes, and alcohol will remain on the restricted list.

In spite of the controversy over specific restrictions, the most important dietary aspect of treatment is *eating frequently*. Large variations in gastric acidity can be avoided by neutralization with small, frequent meals that give symptomatic relief of ulcer pain. Most patients have identified the foods that cause them distress and will eliminate those foods from their diet. These should be the only specific restrictions, thus allowing the diet to be individualized.

One of the most vital aspects in successful diet therapy for peptic ulcer is the counseling of the patient and family. It is important to stress the positive aspects of diet rather than the restrictions. The key point is advising small, frequent meals, explaining that there is more acid present when the stomach is empty and that keeping small amounts of food in the stomach will help neutralize this acid. The patient should have a clear understanding that *how* one eats is much more important than *what* one eats. Regular patterns for eating that include having meals at the same time every day, with regular snacks in between, should be established. Meals should be eaten in a relaxed, unhurried environment. If the patient has been experiencing nocturnal pain, it can be advised that an alarm be set for an hour before the usual time of the pain and a light snack be eaten at that time. If the patient has been advised to give up smoking but has not done so, there should certainly be a warning against smoking on an empty stomach. Although there is no clear-cut evidence that smoking retards ulcer therapy, there is documentation that smoking on an empty stomach often produces pain and epigastric distress in patients with ulcers. All in all, an ulcer diet should not prove to be an extreme hardship for the patient. The patient should be taught to choose a nutritionally sound diet from a wide variety of foods, avoiding those found to cause discomfort. Often only extremely spicy foods need to be avoided; otherwise, the patient is able to enjoy a normal diet.

*Drug therapy* Medication is the second therapeutic approach and is aimed at the symptomatic control of ulcer distress until healing can take place. Probably the most commonly used medications in ulcer treatment are the *antacids*. Although they have no direct effect on ulcer healing, they achieve relief of the pain associated with acidity. In addition to neutralizing the acid content, antacid therapy inactivates pepsin, which can also damage the mucosa.

The two major classifications of antacids are systemic and nonsystemic. The *systemic antacids* are absorbable, and although their main action may be local, the absorption can produce systemic effects. When such an alkaline substance is taken in relatively high doses over an extended period of time, a severe disruption of the patient's acid-base balance may result. Alkalosis is a major problem in the milk-alkali syndrome, which may occur when a patient takes large doses of a systemic antacid together with large amounts of milk over a prolonged period of time. Manifestations of this syndrome include nausea, hypercalcemia, and renal insufficiency with azotemia. The systemic antacids are the most rapid-acting in terms of neutralizing acid, but their potential systemic side effects make them unsuitable for the treatment of peptic ulcer, since rather long-term antacid therapy is usually advised.

In the second group are the *nonsystemic antacids*, which form insoluble compounds in the intestine and thus are not absorbed. Their action is almost completely local, and they therefore do not have such a serious effect on the acid-base balance. These antacids are much more suitable for chronic or long-term use. Taken orally, in liquid form, most antacid preparations begin to act within 5 minutes, with effects lasting about an hour. Many patients prefer to take antacids in chewable-tablet form because they find them more palatable. These preparations are less effective than the liquid suspensions because they provide less surface area for interaction with the hydrochloric acid, but they may be convenient in temporary situations, as when a person is away from home for the day.

The nonsystemic antacids are not without their side effects. Depending on the preparation, the most common of these effects is either diarrhea or constipation. Preparations containing magnesium (e.g., milk of magnesia, Maalox) may often cause diarrhea and should be given cautiously to people with fluid and electrolyte imbalances or malabsorption syndromes. Antacids containing magnesium are contraindicated for anyone with renal failure, since the magnesium may be retained and the patient may develop a toxicity manifested by lethargy, coma, and respiratory and circulatory collapse. Other commonly used nonsystemic antacids contain aluminum (e.g., Amphojel, Gelusil) and may cause constipation. Often by alternating the use of two antacids, the patient can be assisted in maintaining normal bowel patterns. Since it takes, on the average, about 6 weeks for complete healing of a peptic ulcer, the patient is usually maintained on antacid therapy for at least this amount of time.

Besides antacids, *anticholinergic drugs* such as propantheline bromide (Pro-Banthine) have long been used in the management of peptic ulcer. When given in large doses, these drugs reduce gastric acid secretion and so help to alleviate pain. For some time there has been controversy over the use of anticholinergics in the treatment of ulcers, because, in order to effectively reduce gastric secretions, the drugs must be given in large doses. Toxic side effects include extreme dryness of the mouth, nausea and vomiting, decreased visual acuity, and difficulty in urinating. The present controversy centers on whether the benefits of the drugs justify risking these side effects. Because of the possible ocular and urinary tract problems, anticholinergics are contraindicated for patients with glaucoma or prostatic hypertrophy.

*Sedation* is often used for the patient with a peptic ulcer. Sedatives may not have a direct action on gastric secretions but will promote relaxation and sleep. There is also some thought that sedation may in some way contribute to decreasing the amount of nocturnal acid secretion in duodenal ulcer. In relation to episodes of nocturnal pain, the use of a *synthetic hydrogen receptor antagonist,* Cimetidine, is currently under investigation. This drug seems to inhibit acid output with minimal side effects. It is a long-acting antagonist, and because of its duration of action, it is hoped that it will be effective in inhibiting overnight gastric secretions. More clinical trials are needed, however, to fully assess its therapeutic potential in duodenal ulcer.

*Teaching and counseling*   The third major nursing intervention for patients with peptic ulcer is teaching and counseling, which are key factors in preventing complications and recurrences. The patient and the family need to understand the basic disease process in order to understand and accept the rationale for therapy. Dietary counseling has been discussed previously. Besides understanding what medications are to be taken and the reason for their use, the patient should also be instructed to avoid medications, especially nonprescription drugs such as aspirin, which may irritate the gastric mucosa. If the patient has some other condition, such as arthritis, which may necessitate the use of a gastric irritating drug, antacid therapy may have to be continued indefinitely. The patient should also be instructed to avoid excessive sporadic physical activity, since recurrences of ulceration have been associated with physical fatigue. This is a good opportunity for the nurse to encourage consistent, moderate daily exercise as an adjunct to health.

The patient and family will need specific counseling not only in regard to diet and medications but also in recognizing and reducing some of the stress which may be inherent in their life-style. The patient should be encouraged to ask questions about anxieties: conflicts and stresses should be identified, and approaches to problem solving should be decided on. Through this process the patient will often be able to identify a pattern of stressors and find healthier ways of coping with them. If the patient seems to be exhibiting or identifying severe emotional problems, psychotherapy may be the appropriate intervention. Whatever steps are taken, the most important thing the nurse can do is *listen:* what is the patient saying about himself or herself and his or her life?

**Third-level nursing care**   With adherence to the medical regimen, ulcers usually heal within 6 to 8 weeks. However, occasionally an ulcer does not respond to medical care and complications may follow, the most common being pyloric obstruction, perforation, and hemorrhage. These complications are acute and require the assistance of a hospital setting.

The assessment skills of the nurse are of vital importance when complications interrupt the course of peptic ulcer. Many subtle clinical changes may signal potentially life-threatening situations. Because of the amount of time spent in direct contact with the patient, the nurse is usually the health-team member in the best position to observe and assess these changes.

When the threat of possible complications exists, the interviewing and communication skills of the nurse are also fundamental to providing quality care. Throughout the course of any complication, these skills can be utilized to decrease the patient's stress by offering consistent explanations and support. Surgical treatment of complications is frequently carried out on an emergency basis, and the support of the nurse is invaluable, since there may be little time to prepare the patient for the surgical procedure. Acceptance will come more easily and with less anxiety if the patient has already established a trusting relationship with the nurse.

**Pyloric Obstruction**  Pyloric obstruction may be a complication of either duodenal or gastric ulcers which are located near the pylorus. Some degree of stenosis (narrowing of the lumen) occurs frequently in peptic ulcer but is usually not severe enough to produce clinical symptoms. Obstruction develops when inflammation and edema around an ulcer cause the lumen to narrow to the point where passage of food into the small intestine is disrupted. The luminal narrowing, which decreases gastric

emptying, results in gastric dilatation. The increased bulk in the stomach increases peristalsis, and these changes are manifested clinically by vomiting of sour-smelling, undigested food, loss of appetite, weight loss, distention after a meal, and classic ulcer pain. Physical assessment of the patient may reveal a distended abdomen, visible peristaltic movement, and a succussion splash due to the presence of fluid and air.

During the initial 36- to 48-hour period, the patient will probably be treated with continuous gastric suction through a *nasogastric tube.* The tube is passed through the nares, pharynx, and esophagus to the stomach and is then connected to a suction machine to facilitate removal of air and fluid contents from the stomach, as shown in Flg. 17-2. The pressure of the suction can vary according to the machine used, and the suction created may be continuous or intermittent. Since continuous suction may cause adherence of the tube to the mucosal lining and disrupt the flow of gastric contents, intermittent suction is commonly used.

The insertion of a nasogastric tube may be a frightening and uncomfortable experience for the

**FIGURE 17-2**
Placement of nasogastric tube.

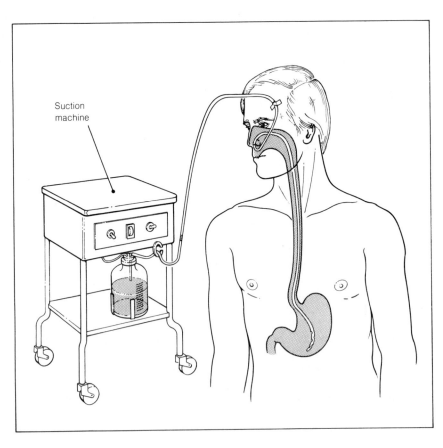

Suction machine

patient. A thorough explanation should therefore be given before any part of the procedure is undertaken. Hyperextension of the neck while the patient is in a sitting position facilitates passage of the tube. It is helpful for the patient to swallow to promote downward movement of the tube, and it may be more comfortable to do so while taking small amounts of water. When passage is completed, the proper positioning of the tube in the stomach should be determined. It is easy to pass the tube into the lungs, which can have disastrous consequences if not detected. A small amount of fluid can be aspirated through the tube to be sure that it is in the stomach and that gastric contents are returning. A second way to verify proper placement of the tube is to push air through the nasogastric tube while listening over the stomach with a stethoscope. The air can be heard entering the stomach if the tube is in place. After proper placement of the tube has been verified, it may be taped to the nose, being careful to avoid any undue pressure.

A major nursing responsibility after a nasogastric tube is inserted is to maintain functioning of the suction apparatus and patency of the tube. To facilitate this, irrigation at regular times with a specific solution is sometimes ordered. The nurse should always check the placement of the tube in the stomach before instilling fluids. Frequent changes of position and frequent observation of the entire system will help prevent loss of patency. If the nurse observes distention, nausea, vomiting or if the patient complains of feeling full, there is usually a disturbance in the patency of the system.

The tubing should be arranged and secured so that the patient can move freely. Since the tube is uncomfortable and irritating, good mouth and nose hygiene with lubrication is especially important. The nurse should carefully observe the drainage resulting from the suction, noting appearance, amount, and color. Since large amounts of fluid may be lost, an accurate intake and output record is essential.

During the time the tube is in place the patient does not receive any oral intake. The suctioning of gastric contents can contribute to fluid and electrolyte disturbances, so there is usually intravenous replacement of nutrients, fluids, and electrolytes. After about 48 hours the patient is given several small liquid feedings. If these are tolerated, the suction will be discontinued and the tube removed. At times the obstruction may subside on its own or resolve with the outlined medical therapy. However, as the edema subsides, the narrowing may be severe enough to require surgery. The most common

operative procedures used are vagotomy with antral resection, selective vagotomy, and partial gastrectomy with pyloroplasty. A later section on Gastric Surgery gives a more complete discussion.

**P**erforation   Perforation is the most serious complication of peptic ulcer and the most common cause of death, occurring in 1 to 2 percent of all ulcers. Ulcer perforation seems to occur most commonly during the day (especially late afternoon) and after a meal. It may also occur following trauma to the abdomen, coughing, vomiting, extreme emotional tension, straining at defecation, or any type of strenuous exercise. Duodenal ulcers perforate most frequently. They may perforate into the peritoneal cavity, causing a generalized peritonitis, into the pancreas, or into the lesser peritoneal sac, causing a localized peritonitis. The rapid escape of gastric and intestinal contents results in chemical irritation.

The most striking *clinical manifestation* is severe upper abdominal pain of sudden onset. The pain becomes increasingly severe and persistent and may be referred to the shoulders because of irritation of the diaphragm and phrenic nerves (Fig. 17-1). Nausea and vomiting are common if the perforation has occurred soon after a meal. Paralytic ileus develops, fluid is lost into the peritoneal cavity and the gastrointestinal tract, and the consequent hypovolemia may be manifested by signs of shock. The patient is often in an extreme state of anxiety and may be experiencing respiratory difficulty. As significant amounts of fluid escape into the peritoneal cavity, circulating volume decreases and respiratory demands increase.

On *physical assessment* the patient is often found to have a tender, rigid, boardlike abdomen and decreased peristaltic sounds, owing to the paralytic ileus. Within about 12 hours bacterial peritonitis develops with elevated temperature, further signs of shock, and malaise. At this point the condition urgently indicates surgery. The most common surgical procedure is simple closure of the perforation with a patch of omentum. Other more definitive procedures frequently used are vagotomy and pyloroplasty or vagotomy and antrectomy.

**H**emorrhage   Hemorrhage, another serious complication of peptic ulcer, results from penetration of the ulcer into an artery, vein, or capillary or from bleeding from highly vascular granulation tissue at the ulcer base. Twenty-five percent of duodenal ulcers hemorrhage at some time during the course of the disease, and bleeding is even more common and more severe in gastric ulcers. The risk of bleeding also increases with age. Hematemesis or melena may be the first *clinical manifestation* and may quickly progress to signs of shock as blood loss continues. There is often a sharp reduction in ulcer pain because of the buffering effect of alkaline blood on the gastric acid. Diagnosis is usually made by inserting a nasogastric tube to determine the bleeding site. X-ray, endoscopy, and arteriography may also be done. At times, a string test may help identify the bleeding site: the patient swallows a cotton tape with radiopaque markings, and fluorescein is injected intravenously; when the tape is removed after a few minutes, areas of fluorescence indicate areas of bleeding.

Immediate *interventions* include transfusing blood to alleviate shock. Gastric lavage through the nasogastric tube with iced saline may be used to produce vasoconstriction and control bleeding. The patient is placed on total bed rest with the foot of the bed elevated, and vital signs are taken frequently. Gastric suction is maintained, and the patient is usually sedated. When active bleeding has stopped, hourly antacids may be administered through the nasogastric tube. Intravenous fluids are given to maintain urinary output. The nasogastric tube usually remains in place for 48 hours, and the nurse should be especially observant for any signs of renewed bleeding. There has been some recent use of intra-arterial infusions of vasoconstrictor drugs, such as Pitressin and epinephrine, to control bleeding once the active site of hemorrhage has been determined. Infusion of these drugs results in the formation of a clot at the bleeding point and thus reduces hemorrhage. This mode of treatment may prove especially valuable for patients who are poor surgical risks, since if the bleeding cannot be controlled with medical treatment in a short time, surgery is the next line of treatment. Surgery will be necessary when a patient continues to bleed for more than 24 hours or when there are any signs of renewed bleeding. The surgical procedures commonly used are a partial gastric resection or a vagotomy and pyloroplasty.

Not only does the risk of hemorrhage increase with age, but also the mortality from gastrointestinal bleeding. In persons under 50 years of age, the mortality is about 1 percent; after the age of 50, mortality increases sharply to 5 to 15 percent.

**Gastric Surgery** When peptic ulcers do not respond to the medical therapeutic regimen or when severe complications occur, surgical treatment may be required. Several different operations are used in the treatment of peptic ulcer, but the goal of all surgical procedures is the same: to reduce acid. This may be accomplished by interference with either the vagus nerve or gastrin, the two primary stimuli for acid secretion. Acid may also be reduced by decreasing the number of parietal cells. Although all the operations reduce acidity, none are totally effective for all patients.

When a *subtotal gastrectomy* is performed, about 70 to 80 percent of the stomach is removed and an anastomosis made to either the duodenum (Billroth I) or the jejunum (Billroth II), as shown in Figs. 17-3 and 17-4. This reduces the parietal cell mass and so reduces acid secretion. It also diverts acid from the ulcer area.

Another common procedure is complete *truncal vagotomy,* in which branches of the vagus nerve innervating the stomach are divided. This reduces acid secretion by eliminating the neural stimulus. Decreasing the vagus tone also decreases stomach motility, causing it to empty more slowly, so a *pyloroplasty* (enlarging of the pyloric sphincter) may be done with a vagotomy to aid in gastric emptying.

Selective *parietal cell vagotomy* is a procedure which has gained favor in recent years. The vagal supply to the body and fundus of the stomach is removed, but supply to the antral and pyloric regions is preserved. Therefore only the acid-secreting cells of the stomach are affected by denervation, and the function of the pyloric and antral portions remains, allowing normal emptying of the stomach.

Whatever type of surgery is to be performed, the patient should be as fully prepared as possible by the nurse. If the surgery is elective and planned, there will be time and opportunity for extensive teaching and explanation. If the surgery is done on an emergency basis, adequate teaching will be difficult. However, the patient may be helped immensely by the nurse who recognizes the frightening nature of the situation. Recognition of the patient's anxiety and offers of support will add to the patient's comfort. To avoid unpleasant surprises, all patients should be told preoperatively that they will awaken with a nasogastric tube in place and will be receiving intravenous fluids.

Along with the observations and interventions common to all surgical patients, the nurse must be especially observant of the drainage from the nasogastric tube postoperatively, noting color, amount, and odor. The drainage may be initially bright red but should change to dark red within about 12 hours and back to normal greenish yellow within 36 hours. Besides the possible complications of any surgical procedure, such as shock, infection, hemorrhage, respiratory problems, and thromboses, the nurse should also be aware of complications unique to a gastrointestinal procedure. These may include gastric dilatation, obstruction, hemorrhage, and suture-line leakage resulting in abscess formation or peritonitis.

The nasogastric tube is kept in place and the patient receives nothing by mouth for several days. After this time, with the nasogastric tube still in place, the patient may be given small amounts of clear fluid by mouth. About an hour later the gastric contents are aspirated to see how much of the fluid remains. When fluids are being tolerated well, the nasogastric tube is removed and the patient's diet gradually progresses to regular, frequent, small feedings.

**Fourth-level nursing care**   The patient who has undergone gastric surgery will require long-term care and follow-up. The patient is susceptible to several chronic complications, which the nurse plays a vital role in minimizing. *Anemia* can result from decreased absorption of vitamin $B_{12}$ due to reduced production of intrinsic factor. This anemia can be treated by administration of vitamin $B_{12}$. *Reflux gastritis* frequently occurs if the pyloric sphincter was removed during the surgical procedure. If the resulting pain, nausea, vomiting, and weight loss cannot be medically controlled by diet and antispasmodics, corrective surgery may become necessary. Another complication may be the development of *marginal ulcers* near the area of anastomosis after gastric resection. The finding of such ulcerations may also necessitate further surgery.

**D**umping Syndrome   Following gastric resection, a disturbing, uncomfortable metabolic problem occurs in about 50 percent of patients. It is known as the *dumping syndrome* and is caused by a number of events, beginning with rapid emptying of gastric contents—"dumping." Food and fluid are moved quickly into the small intestine and cause distention. This hypertonic intestinal content then draws extracellular fluid from the plasma, thus decreasing the circulating blood volume and producing vasoconstriction. The patient's discomfort begins about 5 to 30 minutes after a meal and usually is described as a feeling of fullness and nausea. The reduced blood volume may be clinically manifested by sweating, pallor, a feeling of warmth, headache, palpitations, and vertigo. The extremely rapid removal of gastric contents also causes a quick elevation of blood glucose. In an

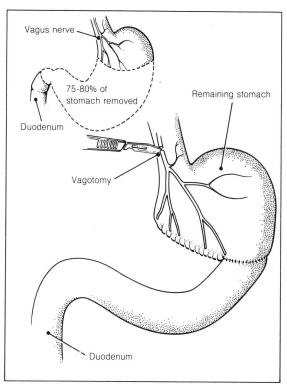

**FIGURE 17-3**
Billroth I resection.

attempt to compensate for this, there is an oversecretion of insulin, resulting in hypoglycemia 2 to 3 hours after a meal. At this time the patient may experience weakness, sweating, anxiety, and tremors.

The dumping syndrome can be caused by all foods but seems to be more severe following ingestion of foods high in glucose, especially if they are taken with liquids. Surgical correction of this problem is rarely needed, but if it does become necessary a piece of jejunum is usually sutured between the stomach and duodenum. For most patients the symptoms will subside in about 6 to 12 months. The nurse can help the patient control this syndrome through diet teaching, follow-up, and counseling.

The patient and family should be taught to select a high-protein, high-fat, low-carbohydrate diet and to set up a pattern of small, frequent feedings rather than three large meals a day. Fluids should not be taken during or immediately following meals, and a large amount of sugar should not be eaten at one time. The patient should be instructed to eat in a semirecumbent position and to lie down after meals to help delay gastric emptying and reduce small-bowel distention. Sedatives and

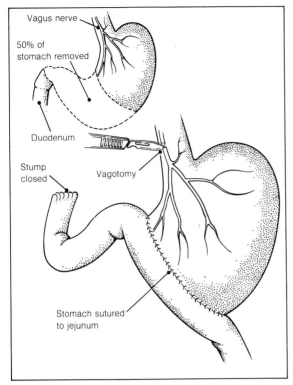

**FIGURE 17-4**
Billroth II resection.

antispasmodics are sometimes prescribed to increase the length of time contents remain in the stomach.

**L**ong-term Follow-up   The importance of follow-up care, such as x-rays every 3 to 6 months, needs to be stressed to the patient and family. It is important for them to understand that convalescence may be slow and that continued health supervision is needed. This slow recovery is often extremely difficult for the anxious, aggressive, tense person who seems to be susceptible to ulcer disease.

As in other phases of peptic ulcer, the nurse must take the time to know the family in order to counsel them and offer support in adjusting routines of home, work, and sleep, including avoidance of anything the patient finds irritating to the gastric mucosa, such as salicylates, fatigue, and stressful situations.

Throughout all levels of nursing care during the course of a peptic ulcer, restoration and maintenance of health must be foremost in the nurse's mind. Even though peptic ulcer is often a puzzling problem, the prognosis for the patient is usually very good.

## Indigestion

Indigestion (dyspepsia) is a gastrointestinal disturbance manifested by a feeling of fullness, epigastric distress, acid reflux, heartburn, and flatulence. It may have a functional or organic basis. The organic form is usually found in conjunction with diseases of the gastrointestinal tract. The functional type is far more common and is often associated with inadequate diet patterns or emotional distress. Persons with the functional form of indigestion need to be taught the basics of good nutrition, the importance of relaxed, regular eating habits, and avoidance of or alternative methods of dealing with tension and anxiety.

## Nausea and Vomiting

*Nausea* is a subjective, uncomfortable sensation in the epigastrium and back of the throat during which one feels like vomiting. The feeling is accompanied by a decrease in gastric contractions and spasms of the duodenum. It commonly occurs with gastric or pancreatic disease, pyloric or intestinal obstruction, and severe pain of any kind.

*Vomiting* is a powerful ejection of gastric contents through the mouth and may or may not be preceded by nausea. Just prior to vomiting, the stomach and gastroesophageal sphincters are relaxed. The glottis is closed and the larynx and soft palate are elevated. Then the diaphragm descends forcefully and the abdominal-wall muscles contract, thus squeezing the relaxed stomach and expelling its contents. This series of events may be initiated by stimulation of the chemoreceptor trigger zone or the vomiting center in the medulla by some type of neural, chemical, humoral, or emotional stimulus. The most effective short-term symptomatic treatment is administration of a phenothiazine drug such as prochlorperazine (Compazine), which may act on the chemoreceptor trigger zone or the vomiting center to achieve an antiemetic effect. Although drugs may give symptomatic relief, the underlying cause of the nausea and vomiting must be determined and treated.

The nurse should observe the vomitus for color, amount, consistency, and any unusual appearance. It is important to assess what factors seem to stimulate vomiting and attempt to control them. Vomiting is an extremely unpleasant experience, and frequent mouth care should be offered to the patient. The patient must also be carefully observed for signs of fluid and electrolyte imbalance due to the vomiting. When losses are primarily from the stomach, hydrogen and chloride, especially, are lost and alkalosis can develop. Electrolyte imbalance is less of a problem when the source of the vomitus is the small intestine. With all vomiting, however, fluid is lost from the body and dehydration can develop. Toleration of food and fluids must be carefully assessed, and it is often helpful to give an antiemetic drug before meals.

### Gastritis

Gastritis is an inflammation of the gastric mucosa which may be found in either an acute or a chronic form. The *acute* inflammation is often due to an irritating drug or chemical such as aspirin, alcohol, spices, or food contaminated with *Staphylococcus.* It may be manifested clinically by malaise, bouts of nausea and vomiting, epigastric pain similar to that of peptic ulcer, and hematemesis. Diagnosis is usually made on the basis of the history and gastroscopy. The disturbance is often self-limiting if the irritant is removed. Supportive therapy includes a reduced oral intake, administration of parenteral solutions to maintain fluid and electrolyte balance if necessary, antiemetic drugs, and antacids.

The *chronic* form of gastritis features recurrent inflammation and a progressive atrophy of the stomach wall and lining. It may be caused by chronic duodenal reflux, nutritional deficiencies, stasis of gastric contents, certain endocrine problems, or autoimmune mechanisms. It is believed by some that this type of gastritis may have an association with gastric carcinoma. Clinical signs may be completely absent or may include indigestion, vomiting, and ulcerlike epigastric pain which is not relieved by antacids. Treatment is primarily symptomatic and includes such measures as small, frequent feedings and the avoidance of known gastric irritants.

### Gastroenteritis

Gastroenteritis is an acute irritation of the stomach and small bowel, often caused by viruses or bacteria. Clinical symptoms frequently include severe abdominal cramping, vomiting, and diarrhea. The disturbance usually has a short course of only a few days and does not carry much risk of complications except for the very young or very old. Persons who should be watched carefully are those who have been ill or debilitated and may suffer a rapid shift of fluids and electrolytes. Treatment usually consists of resting in bed and taking in large amounts of fluids for several days.

### Gastric Cancer

As mentioned earlier, gastric carcinoma is often considered to be one of the complications of peptic ulcer (especially gastric ulceration), but this complication is extremely rare. It is usually found that the ulceration occurs after the carcinoma rather than before it. Since it is often difficult to distinguish a benign peptic ulcer from an ulcerating carcinoma, however, any chronic gastric ulcer which is at all questionable will usually be treated surgically.

Although the incidence of gastric cancer has been declining in the United States during recent years, there is still substantial mortality. It occurs frequently in Japan, and in Iceland it is responsible for 35 to 45 percent of cancer deaths in males. Attempts have been made to link these geographic predispositions to dietary customs, since a large amount of smoked meat and fish is consumed in those countries. There is no clear evidence at this time, but exposure to dietary carcinogens may play a part in the etiology of gastric cancer. Other carcinogenic agents which have been implicated include talc (rice is treated with talc in Japan), coal, phenol, reheated fats, and peat.

Gastric carcinoma is found mainly in males, in persons over 65, and among persons of the lower socioeconomic groups. In the United States, nonwhites have a higher incidence of gastric carcinoma than whites.

The earliest metastasis of gastric cancer is usually to the lymph nodes and then into other abdominal organs via the lymph and portal drainage from the stomach. Unfortunately early symptoms are usually vague and medical assistance is not sought. There is often slight epigastric distress which at times can mimic the pain of peptic ulcer. If such pain does not respond to routine ulcer therapy within 4 to 6 weeks, a diagnosis of gastric cancer has to be considered. The patient may or may not exhibit loss of appetite and weight loss. The finding of epigastric masses is usually an ominous, late sign indicating metastases to other abdominal areas.

*Early detection,* then, seems to be the key factor in control of gastric carcinoma. This is difficult because of the insidious onset and the lack of definitive clinical manifestations. However, a high-risk population can be defined, including those exposed to possible carcinogenic agents, patients with pernicious anemia and accompanying gastric changes, those with chronic gastritis, and those with hiatal hernia and frequent reflux of acid gastric juices.

Surgery is the only hope for cure of gastric carcinomas. A subtotal or total gastric resection may be done. The cure rate, based on 5-year survivals, is still extremely low because the problem is not usually diagnosed until the late stages. Chemotherapy and radiation therapy are also used for gastric carcinoma, but their effect is one of controlling symptoms rather than curing the disease. Recent therapy, especially for cancers which cannot be completely removed at the time of gastrectomy, involves giving a single, massive dose of electron-beam therapy at the time of the surgical procedure. It is still too early to evaluate the effectiveness of this approach.

### Zollinger-Ellison Syndrome

The Zollinger-Ellison syndrome consists of three basic problems: a non–beta cell tumor in the pancreas (gastrinoma), extreme hypersecretion of gastric acid, and peptic ulceration. The tumors release excessive amounts of gastrin, producing excessive secretion of gastric acid and eventually resulting in peptic ulceration. About 60 percent of the pancreatic tumors are malignant, and the disorder has a much higher incidence in men. Although the syndrome may be found in all age groups, it is much more common during the third to fifth decades.

The major clinical manifestations of the Zollinger-Ellison syndrome are diarrhea, steatorrhea (large amounts of unabsorbed fat in the stools), and ulcer pain. The large amounts of gastric acid that lead to ulceration and pain, on entering the intestines inactivate lipase and precipitate the bile salts, decreasing fat digestion and resulting in steatorrhea. Gastrin also decreases salt and water absorption, leading to diarrhea.

The treatment of choice for this disorder is removal of the organ primarily affected—the stomach. Because of the extremely high incidence of multiple lesions, simple removal of the tumor will not suffice. Survival rates are good after total gastrectomy (55 percent 5-year survival). Even though metastases are common, the tumors grow slowly and the prognosis after surgery is good. In several instances spontaneous regression of metastases has been noted after total gastrectomy.

### Hiatus Hernia

Hiatus hernia refers to the protrusion of part of the stomach into the chest cavity through a gap in the diaphragm. If the protrusion occurs intermittently, it is termed *sliding hernia.* The stomach is forced into the thoracic cavity when the subject is in a recumbent position but reenters the abdominal cavity on return to an upright position. Hiatus hernia occurs most often in obese middle-aged females. It is often found that the esophagus is shorter than normal, a condition that may be due to a congenital defect or, more commonly, to scarring after trauma and inflammation.

Most of the clinical symptoms are caused by a reflux of acid gastric secretions into the esophagus, setting up an inflammatory process. This gives rise to substernal heartburn and epigastric pain occurring soon after meals. The discomfort usually becomes worse upon lying down, bending forward, or any kind of exertion. The pain may be associated with a feeling of fullness, belching, nausea and vomiting and usually disappears within 1 hour after meals. The discomfort may sometimes mimic that of peptic ulcer. At other times the pain may radiate to the back, jaws, shoulders, and arms, much like the pain of angina pectoris.

Treatment includes use of antacids and a bland diet of small, frequent feedings. These measures are taken to prevent distention from large volumes of food and to reduce and control the acidity of gastric secretions. The obese patient should receive specific nutritional counseling and a reducing diet. The nurse should explain to the patient the nature of the disorder and advise against frequent bending forward, tight clothing, and the like. If the patient complains of distress at night, the head of the bed should be elevated. If the discomfort becomes extreme, surgical repair may be carried out.

## DISTURBANCES OF INTESTINAL DIGESTION

Disorders of intestinal digestion, like those of gastric origin, require accurate history taking, careful observation, in-depth assessment, intelligent intervention, and sensitive counseling by the nurse. Because of the close interrelationships of structure and function in the gastrointestinal system, the nurse's observations will greatly assist in recognizing disorders and initiating a beneficial therapeutic regimen for the patient.

### Cholecystitis

*Cholecystitis* is an inflammation of the gallbladder. It may be acute or chronic and is often associated with the presence of calculi or gallstones—*cholelithiasis.*

**Pathophysiology** Although the exact mechanism for the initiation of the inflammatory process is not known, it is thought that it may originate from obstruction of the cystic duct either by a stone or by a bacterial invasion. The presence of calculi is the more common precipitating factor. As a result of the inflammation, the gallbladder wall becomes thickened and edematous and the diameter of the cystic-duct lumen increases in size. If the inflammation and edema spread to the common duct, the temporary obstruction of bile elimination will result in jaundice. Long-term jaundice is usually caused by stones obstructing the common duct. If the cystic duct is completely occluded, the gallbladder will become distended with inflammatory exudate and bile. Following the acute attack, the surface mucosa heals, scarring the gallbladder wall. Depending on the amount of tissue involved, future gallbladder function may or may not be affected. If the inflammation becomes chronic, there is an increased thickening of the gallbladder wall and dilatation of the cystic duct lumen, allowing potential passage of calculi into the common duct.

Gallbladder disease has traditionally been associated with "fat, fertile, fortyish females." These four descriptive terms have been seriously questioned in recent years. Gallbladder disease does occur slightly more often in women than in men, but one study found no evidence supporting increased incidence during the forties.[3] Higher incidence of the disease was correlated with higher parity only in younger age groups. Obesity, however, had a consistent positive correlation and seems to be the factor with the strongest relation to gallbladder disease.

As previously indicated, cholecystitis may also be caused by a bacterial invasion without calculi. The bacteria usually reach the gallbladder through the bile, blood, or lymphatics. Chemical, enzymatic, and allergic factors are also being implicated in the etiology of cholecystitis. For instance, it is thought that enzymatic activity after reflux of pancreatic secretions into the gallbladder may initiate an inflammatory process.

Gallstones (cholelithiasis), the major cause of cholecystitis, are estimated to be present in about 16 million Americans. They are thought to occur in persons who may have stagnation of bile in the gallbladder, such as pregnant women, those with some type of organic obstruction to bile flow, and those who are immobilized for prolonged periods. It is believed that gallstones may also be due to abnormal composition of the bile or inflammation of the gallbladder and ducts. The exact causative role of each of these factors has not been determined. The majority of persons with gallstones remain asymptomatic ("silent" gallstones). Chemically, the stones are composed of one or more substances normally found in the bile which have precipitated. These substances include cholesterol, calcium bilirubinate, and calcium carbonate.

Besides the predisposing factors already mentioned, patients with diabetes mellitus have a higher incidence of gallstone formation (30 percent as compared to 12 percent in the general population) and suffer more complications from gallbladder disease. This predisposition is found only in juvenile, insulin-dependent diabetics and does not apply to those with adult onset of the disease.

The possible role of diet in the etiology of gallbladder disease is also being examined. Studies on groups of Japanese people living in Japan, in Hawaii, on the West Coast of the United States, and in central areas of the United States reveal that as people moved closer to the central United States and therefore had diets much higher in animal fats, the likelihood of cholelithiasis increased. The role of genetic factors in gallstone formation has also been questioned, since there is a much higher incidence of gallstone formation in the American Indian than in other Americans.

The effect of gallbladder disease on the patient may range from no visible effects through mild discomfort to extreme pain and debilitation. The common problems affecting patients with biliary disease result from a disturbance of gallbladder function. Decreased digestion of fats is manifested clinically by loss of appetite, nausea and vomiting, weight loss, distention, and flatulence. The inflammation and presence of calculi result in varying degrees of pain. The reduction of bile elimination by obstruction causes a back-up and accumulation of bilirubin in the blood, leading to jaundice.

**First-level nursing care** Since gallbladder disease is a rather common problem in the United States, the nurse should be aware of groups of persons who may be predisposed to its development and work toward early detection of problems.

The nurse needs to recognize predisposition in ethnic groups such as Italians, Jews, and Chinese. The obese and those with sedentary life-styles also have a higher incidence of gallbladder disease. Pregnancy seems to be implicated in the formation of cholesterol stones, and hemolytic anemias are often associated with stones containing bilirubin compounds. As mentioned earlier, insulin-dependent diabetics are also in the high-risk group. Because there is no concrete knowlege of causes, prevention is difficult. The above-mentioned groups can be advised to follow a low-fat diet, but this has been proved beneficial only for the obese.

**Second-level nursing care** The patient with chronic gallbladder disease often experiences only mild to moderate symptoms and with appropriate care can remain in the community.

**N**ursing Assessment The *health history* usually reveals that the patient is experiencing a distaste for or intolerance of fatty foods and complains of vague episodes of epigastric distress. Sometimes the distress is described as a recurring type of pain, often accompanied by nausea and vomiting. The patient is frequently able to relate these episodes to large meals.

The *physical examination* often reveals some right-upper-quadrant tenderness on palpation, and a mass may sometimes be felt. At times, actual calculi can be felt by careful bimanual palpation. If gallstones have passed through the dilated cystic duct and are obstructing the common bile duct, jaundice will be present. The nurse should especially observe the skin, mucous membranes (especially in the mouth), sclerae, and inner aspects of the forearms for evidence of jaundice. The patient should be examined for indications of jaundice in natural light when possible, since artificial lighting may distort the findings. Other aspects of the physical examination are essentially normal in uncomplicated chronic gallbladder disease.

*Oral cholecystography,* which permits visualization of the gallbladder with the assistance of radiopaque substances, is the most commonly used method of diagnosing cholecystitis. The radiopaque substances routinely used include iopanoic acid (Telepaque), sodium ipodate (Oragrafin), and sodium tyropanoate (Bilopaque). These materials are given by mouth and, after reaching the gallbladder, are reabsorbed more slowly than the bile, so that they eventually accumulate to a high enough concentration to cast an opaque shadow on an x-ray film. Visualization is best 10 to 15 hours after ingestion of the dye, therefore the radiopaque material (usually six tablets) is administered after dinner the evening before. The gallbladders of about 25 percent of people cannot be visualized after this first dosage of the contrast dye. Nausea, vomiting, or any process interfering with absorption may be responsible for this. Repetition of the dose of radiopaque material the next evening allows visualization about 92 percent of the time. If the second test fails, bile excretion is impaired and biliary disease is confirmed.

Because of the problem of nonvisualization on the first test, some authorities recommend a change in the preparation routine. Instead of giving six tab-

lets of dye the night before the examination, it is suggested that the patient receive twelve tablets beginning 2 days before the actual test (that is, six tablets each day). This modified preparation results in a higher percentage of visualization during the first examination. Since nausea, vomiting, and diarrhea are common side effects when these contrast materials are ingested, the nurse must be aware that these events prior to the testing could disrupt absorption and alter test findings. Besides oral cholecystography, *ultrasonic scanning* can also aid in diagnosis. This is especially useful in the detection of very small calculi.

**N**ursing Problems and Interventions Patients with chronic cholecystitis often do not feel very ill and may seek assistance only when the *epigastric distress or pain* becomes very frequent and annoying. Antispasmodics may be given to decrease smooth-muscle spasms. Patients often complain of increased discomfort after meals or report a specific *intolerance to fatty foods*. They are, therefore, often placed on a low-fat diet so that stimulation of gallbladder contraction will be decreased. Unless the patient suffers from a specific intolerance to fats, however, the restriction is not always reasonable. Since the gallbladder responds to most foods, protein, fat, and carbohydrate will all produce a release of cholecystokinin and thus stimulate the gallbladder. On the other hand, a low-fat diet should always be advised for the obese patient. The diet in most cases should be geared to what the patient can tolerate. The patient should be taught to select a nutritionally sound diet, avoiding those foods which cause discomfort. Many people find that not only fats but fibrous foods such as cabbage, onions, melons, and berries may cause distress. If fat is to be restricted, the patient will need guidance in selecting lean meats and preparing them by roasting, broiling, baking, or stewing instead of frying. The patient who is having a problem with intolerance to fats may also be given oral replacement of bile salts. This replacement therapy will assist in emulsifying fats and may stimulate some output of bile. Other than a mild cathartic action, bile-salt replacement has little adverse effect on the gastrointestinal tract.

Although it is not usual, chronic cholecystitis may at times be accompanied by *infection*. With this as a possibility, antibiotics are often used for patients who are diabetic or those over the age of 60. Ampicillin or a cephalosporin are commonly used because they reach high concentrations in the bile.

**E**xperimental Treatment   In order to avoid eventual surgical procedures, especially in people with minimal distress, dissolution of gallstones by the administration of chemical agents is being studied. Chenodeoxycholic acid is one such agent currently being investigated. This substance has an effect on bile by replenishing bile acids and by decreasing cholesterol synthesis and secretion in the liver. It is thought to dissolve cholesterol stones by restoring the balance between bile acid and biliary lipids. Although the drug is not yet generally available, during experimental work it has been administered to over 600 patients and has been found to totally or partially dissolve calculi in about 70 percent of them.[4] Dissolution of calculi occurs over a period of 6 to 30 months. Questions are being raised, however, concerning the safety of this treatment, since an increase in liver enzymes and some histologic changes have been found on liver biopsy. The changes seem to be transient but will have to be carefully studied before chenodeoxycholic acid can be considered a truly viable alternative to surgery. Another criticism of this form of therapy is that it does not eliminate important stone-forming factors. When calculi are present, the gallbladder wall is thickened and there is poor contraction. Even if the gallstones are dissolved, the changes are not reversible, and the gallbladder will probably form new calculi.

**Third-level nursing care**   Patients with chronic cholecystitis, usually including cholelithiasis, can develop an acute inflammation which will require hospitalization. Most often the cystic duct dilates, allowing passage of stones from the gallbladder into the common duct, where they impact and obstruct the flow of bile. An acute inflammation results from the obstruction and consequent infection. If untreated, the end of this progressive course is usually perforation of the gallbladder, with either local or diffuse peritonitis. It is extremely rare for the inflammation to subside without treatment.

**N**ursing Assessment   An important focus of the nursing assessment is the intense right-upper-quadrant pain the patient usually experiences. This pain is often referred to as biliary colic and results from dilatation and muscular contraction over a stone lodged in the bile duct. The pain usually begins a few hours after a heavy meal, is abrupt in onset, and often radiates to the right shoulder (Fig. 17-1). Extremely intense pain is often accompanied by nausea, vomiting, and diaphoresis. The nurse will frequently find abdominal rigidity on palpation,

and a mass may be felt in the right upper quadrant. Palpation will also elicit upper abdominal tenderness, which is increased on inspiration. At times the pain is accompanied by fever and chills, which indicate the presence of infection. This often occurs when a gallbladder with a large stone becomes fused with the duodenum or transverse colon, setting up a communication channel for infection of the gallbladder and biliary ducts with enteric organisms.

The nurse should also carefully assess the patient for jaundice, clay-colored stools, and dark urine, all of which occur within 24 hours of the onset of common-bile-duct obstruction. While gathering data from the patient's health history, the nurse should especially note whether the patient has previously suffered similar episodes of abdominal pain. If so, the nurse should ascertain whether the patient had biliary calculi visualized on previous cholecystography and what was done to relieve the pain. Since the pain frequently mimics that of an acute myocardial infarction, other problems need careful assessment.

When a patient is suffering from acute obstructive gallbladder disease, *intravenous cholangiography* is often done in lieu of oral cholecystography. It is used because of the time factor involved in acute disease since it can be performed in 1 to 2 hours, yielding more immediate diagnostic information. It may also be used when there is concomitant liver disease, pancreatitis, or peritonitis, all of which would decrease concentration of the oral contrast material in the gallbladder and make visualization inadequate. It is important for the nurse to know that mild reactions to the dye injected (usually meglumine iodipamide) include a feeling of warmth, nausea, cough, and urticaria. Nursing care should include careful observation for more severe allergic reactions. Since most contrast mediums contain iodine, the nurse should determine whether the patient has a history of reactions to *any* dye which may have been used in previous testing.

In addition to intravenous cholangiography, *percutaneous cholangiography* may be performed, which can localize the site and extent of bile-duct obstruction from any cause, including calculi, strictures, and inflammation, as illustrated in Fig. 17-5. A long, spinal-type needle is inserted through the liver and the dye is injected directly into the biliary ducts. Ductal filling is then observed by fluoroscopy and the obstructive site determined. The patient must be observed carefully for bleeding from the site, pain, and infection. Recently *endoscopic retrograde cholangiopancreatography* (ERCP) has also been used as a diagnostic measure. The procedure consists of cannulating the bile ducts through a flexible fiberscope and directly visualizing obstructive sites.

In addition to x-ray studies that visualize the gallbladder and ductal system, certain blood, urine, and stool laboratory tests are significant. With acute obstructive cholecystitis the patient will usually have a moderately elevated *leukocyte count* (12,000 to 20,000). The *serum and urine bilirubin* levels will be elevated. The nurse should remember to collect urine specimens for bilirubin in dark containers, since light alters bilirubin composition. A decreased amount of *urobilinogen in the feces* is also a common finding in biliary obstruction. The nurse should therefore observe for clay-colored stools and record all changes in color of urine and feces. *Serum amylase* levels are commonly elevated in acute cholecystitis, but this is a rather nonspecific finding, since amylase has many sources.

**N**ursing Problems and Interventions  The patient with acute cholecystitis usually feels extremely ill, and the major nursing problem is control of the *colicky abdominal pain.* Pain control is, of course, important for the patient's comfort, but extreme

**FIGURE 17-5**
Contrast studies of the biliary tract.
*A.* Cholelithiasis. Multiple radiopaque stones in a gallbladder with impaired concentrating ability.
*B.* Cholelithiasis. Nonopaque stones of varying sizes shown as negative shadows outlined by concentrated eye.
*C.* Cholelithiasis. Numerous small stones grouped in a layer near the bottom of the ballbladder.
*D.* Percutaneous transhepatic cholangiogram. The needle has punctured a dilated bile duct. Contrast medium shows marked distention of bile ducts. (*From M. M. Wintrobe et al. (eds.), Harrison's Principles of Internal Medicine, 7th ed., McGraw-Hill, New York, 1974, p. 1561.*)

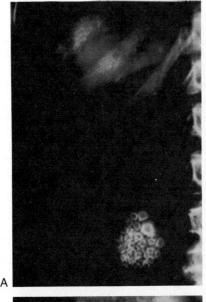

A

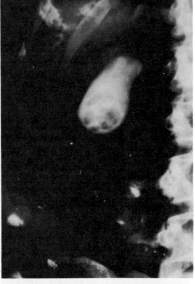

B

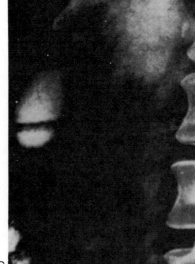

C

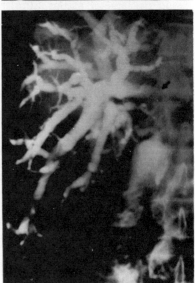

D

pain may also impair respiration, and when there is abdominal guarding and little movement, the patient is subject to the many hazards of immobility. The patient with this type of severe pain is given nothing by mouth, and a nasogastric tube is passed. With a nasogastric tube in place, acid is kept out of the duodenum, the release of cholecystokinin is prevented, and therefore stimulation of gallbladder contractions is decreased. Anticholinergic drugs are often administered to decrease secretions and muscle spasm. Narcotic analgesics may be ordered to control the pain. Since morphine tends to increase contraction of the sphincter of Oddi, it is usually avoided, and meperidine (Demerol), which is less likely to cause contractions, is often the drug of choice for pain relief. To combat inflammation and infection, antibiotics may also be ordered. Drugs which tend to concentrate in the bile, such as ampicillin, tetracycline, and the cephalosporins are frequently used.

Another common nursing problem occurring in the patient with acute cholecystitis is *jaundice*. Obstructive jaundice is often accompanied by intense *itching of the skin (pruritus)* from the high concentration of bile salts in the blood. The itching is difficult to relieve and does not respond well to local applications of lotions or to antihistamines. It may sometimes be relieved by the administration of cholestyramine resin, which binds bile salts and therefore decreases their accumulation in the blood. However, the resin is a bulky powder which must be mixed with a liquid for administration, and most patients find both the taste and the consistency disagreeable. Mixing the powder in a fruit juice may help to make it more palatable. The nurse must be especially careful to prevent skin breakdown in the jaundiced patient. Because of the intense itching, many patients will scratch in their sleep. Nails should be kept short and clean, and protective mitts can be worn overnight.

*Nausea with vomiting* is another commonly identified nursing problem in these patients. Again, giving nothing by mouth and inserting a nasogastric tube will help control this clinical problem by removing stomach contents and decreasing stimulation of the gallbladder. Antiemetics may also be administered to the patient in an attempt to control the nausea and vomiting. The phenothiazines (Thorazine, Compazine, Phenergan) are the most potent and most commonly used antiemetic drugs. They act on the chemoreceptor trigger zone, decreasing stimulation of the vomiting center. Besides phenothiazines, central nervous system depressants such as sedatives and barbiturates will de-

press the vomiting center. It is important for the nurse to remember that sedatives used in conjunction with phenothiazines will have a potentiated effect. Anithistamines such as diphenhydramine (Benadryl) are sometimes used as antiemetics, but their major effectiveness seems to be in the control of motion sickness, since they act mainly upon the vestibular apparatus. Anticholinergic agents are also used at times to reduce gastric-acid secretion, which may contribute to nausea and vomiting. Drowsiness is the most common side effect produced by antiemetic drugs. The nurse must take this into consideration in maintaining a safe environment for the patient. The presence of any stimuli for vomiting must be assessed and an attempt made to prevent the patient's interaction with them. It is often helpful to administer antiemetic medication before meals or scheduled activities.

Placement of a nasogastric tube or severe nausea and vomiting may quickly lead to *fluid and electrolyte imbalance* in the patient with acute cholecystitis. The nurse must be especially careful to maintain an accurate intake and output record, since a large amount of fluid may be lost through nasogastric suctioning and emesis. The laboratory electrolyte values should be monitored closely during this time. Since the patient is losing large amounts of fluid and is receiving nothing by mouth, intravenous replacement of fluid and electrolytes (especially potassium) will be ordered. The usual amount infused averages 3 to 4 liters/day, but if there is a large gastric output through the tube, additional fluids may be ordered. Besides intake and output, an accurate daily weight is helpful in assessing fluid balance. To be of value the weight must be taken at the same time every day, on the same scale, with the patient wearing the same amount of clothing. If done accurately and monitored carefully, intake and output and daily weights can give valuable information for ongoing assessment of the patient's fluid and electrolyte status. Imbalances can be detected and corrected early, before they become severe.

*Adequate nutrition* also becomes a nursing problem with these patients. When the common bile duct is obstructed, there is an inadequate amount of bile to facilitate digestion and absorption of the fat-soluble vitamins, and a vitamin deficiency is a commonly resulting clinical problem. Besides fluid and electrolyte replacement, therefore, the patient must also receive vitamin supplements.

The nurse should be especially aware that a deficiency of vitamin K can lead to *bleeding tendencies* in the patient. Therefore a primary aspect of nursing care is protecting the patient from any injury which might result in bleeding. If blood samples are drawn or injections must be given, a small-gauge needle should be used and pressure applied to the puncture site. The site should be observed carefully to make sure further bleeding does not occur. Laboratory results pertinent to coagulation must be followed carefully at this time. The prothrombin time will indicate the relative impairment of prothrombin and fibrinogen activity in the coagulation process due to the deficiency of vitamin K. An acceptable level for the patient's prothrombin time is about twice the control value. If the prothrombin time becomes prolonged, vitamin K may be administered. The nurse must carefully watch for signs of gastrointestinal hemorrhage, bleeding from any trauma, and epistaxis. All urine, feces, and nasogastric drainage should be tested for the presence of blood.

Throughout all phases of intervention, the nurse must be aware of the *possibility of complications* arising from acute cholecystitis with obstruction. Complications may include peritonitis due to perforation of the gallbladder, pancreatitis, biliary fistula, and liver abscess. If the gallbladder perforates, a stone may travel into the duodenum or jejunum, where it becomes entrapped and produces an acute intestinal obstruction. Calculi may perforate into the stomach and eventually be vomited by the patient. Stones passing into the large bowel may be eliminated in the feces. The nurse should keep in mind that the older the patient and the longer the duration of gallbladder disease, the more common and the more frequent are the risks of complications from acute cholecystitis.

*Surgical intervention*    If conservative medical therapy does not result in a significant reduction of symptoms within 24 to 36 hours, surgical intervention becomes the treatment of choice. It should be noted that surgery is also the only reliable treatment for chronic cholelithiasis, although conservative therapy may be carried out for a long time, often many years.

The usual surgical procedure is a *cholecystectomy* (removal of the gallbladder) accompanied by a *choledochotomy* (exploration and drainage of the common bile duct). *Cholecystostomy* (removal of calculi from the gallbladder) may be performed on an emergency basis if the patient is assessed as a poor surgical risk. It is only a temporary measure, however, and by no means the procedure of choice, since the organ itself is left, with the likelihood that calculi will form again in a few months. Whenever possible, surgeons prefer to wait until the acute symptoms of cholecystitis, especially the fever, chills, and pain, have subsided before performing a cholecystectomy. Patients are often placed on a temporary regime of cephalosporin drugs both pre- and postoperatively to decrease the incidence of serious infections.

During a cholecystectomy the gallbladder is removed and the cystic duct sutured. Bile will then travel directly into the common bile duct and the duodenum. Drains are usually placed during gallbladder surgery to determine whether there is any leakage of bile or blood. If there is no drainage after about 5 days, the drains are removed. When the common bile duct has been explored and calculi removed by choledochotomy, a *T tube* may be placed in the duct (Fig. 17-6). This tube maintains patency of the duct immediately after surgery and allows for drainage of bile. The tube is usually left in place from 7 to 10 days, and a cholangiogram is then done to demonstrate the patency of the duct before the tube is removed.

After a cholecystectomy and choledochotomy, the patient will have a nasogastric tube in place to prevent distention and vomiting. Nutritional requirements will be initially met with intravenous fluids, but as bowel sounds begin to return, usually within 48 hours, oral intake will begin and the diet will be gradually increased. Prevention of pulmonary complications by frequent turning, coughing, and deep breathing is important during the first postoperative days. Fowler's position and analgesia will ease pain and facilitate movement. Ambulation should begin as soon as possible to relieve the distention due to flatus and prevent respiratory complications.

The patency of the T tube is extremely important, and any kinking or obstruction to the flow should be avoided. The drainage should be observed and accurately measured. For the first few days it averages about 300 to 500 ml and then begins to decrease. It may contain blood the first few hours and then changes to the green-brown color of bile. If excessive amounts of drainage are noted and continue over several days, there is the probability of ductal obstruction, necessitating reexploration. After several days the tube may be clamped while the patient eats to retain the bile and assist in fat digestion. During this postoperative period, the nurse should be carefully observing the patient's stools, watching for the return to brown color which indicates bile is once again entering the duodenum. If excessive drainage from the T tube continues, the bile is sometimes returned to the patient either through the nasogastric tube or in oral feedings.

The site at which the T tube is brought out through the skin must receive special attention. Since bile is extremely irritating to the skin, it is important to keep the dressing clean and dry. A protective agent such as karaya gum may help prevent skin breakdown in the area around the tube. The nurse must be careful to maintain a free drainage system and prevent any tension on the tubing which can lead to dislodgement. The diet will be gradually increased after removal of the nasogastric tube, but low fat content is usually advised for several months, according to individual tolerance.

Although gallbladder surgery is associated with a low mortality rate, complications may occur and the nurse must be aware of their possibility. Peritonitis may result from the seepage of bile into the peritoneal cavity and be manifested by severe pain, fever, and chills. Jaundice, continuing clay-colored stools, and excessive T tube drainage may indicate obstruction of the bile duct. This may be due to a retained stone, edema, or the presence of a biliary fistula. A subhepatic abscess may sometimes occur, necessitating surgical drainage.

**Fourth-level nursing care** The prognosis after gallbladder surgery is extremely good. When counseling a patient postoperatively, therefore, it is not necessary for the nurse to advise many restrictions or drastic changes in life-style. The patient should try to avoid excessive fatigue and should not lift heavy objects for about 4 weeks to avoid disruption of the abdominal incision. Driving a car, climbing stairs, and sexual intercourse are permissible whenever the patient feels ready. A common fear of patients is that such activity will pull their healing wound apart, and they need to be reassured that these activities will not cause enough stress to disrupt the abdominal incision. There are usually no specific dietary restrictions imposed, because bile is still being produced. However, due to the absence of the gallbladder, it is being released continuously, so many patients may find it more comfortable to avoid large, fatty meals. Even though the patient has had the gallbladder removed surgically, it is possible that the liver may still produce lithogenic bile, hence recurrent stones may develop in some people. For this reason, and especially when working with older people who have a higher complication rate, it is important for the nurse to stress the importance of follow-up health care.

### Pancreatitis

Inflammation of the pancreas actually encompasses a wide spectrum of disorders ranging from acute pancreatitis, a serious, severely incapacitating illness, to chronic pancreatitis, a series of recurring episodes of inflammation and pain which may eventually lead to pancreatic insufficiency.

**Pathophysiology** The pathophysiologic changes which occur during *acute pancreatitis* can be directly related to the liberation of proteolytic enzymes which are normally secreted by the pancreas. Although the pathogenesis is still not entirely clear, the normal mechanism of pancreatic secretion is disturbed and the enzymes are secreted into the pancreatic tissue itself rather than into the duodenum. As a result of this abnormal enzyme release, there is actual autodigestion of the gland, setting up an acute inflammatory process. Although all pancreatic enzymes are released, it is trypsin which directly causes the chemical irritation and serious destruction of tissue.

In the first few days the pancreas becomes edematous, with vascular engorgement in response to the irritation. Most edema occurs in the head of the pancreas. In some cases there may be a spontaneous reduction of the edema without further pathologic changes. In other instances, however, the process goes on as the gland continues to enlarge, obstructing the pancreatic duct, increasing vascular engorgement, and resulting in ischemia. Areas of necrosis then appear, encircled by infiltrates of leukocytes. Within a short time there is necrosis of arteries, producing hemorrhage—most commonly into the pancreas and retroperitoneal tissue—and

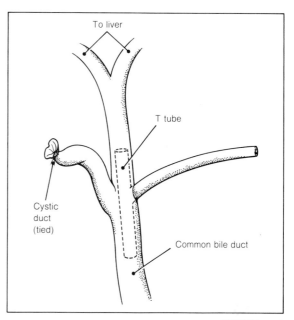

**FIGURE 17-6**

T tube inserted in common bile duct after cholecystectomy.

the veins may become thrombosed. Bacteria then tend to invade the necrotic tissue, and the necrosis and hemorrhage proceed to suppuration. This process may affect only certain localized areas of the gland or may invade the entire pancreas. The actual amount of tissue destruction and resulting clinical manifestations depend on the quality of blood supply to the tissue, the amount of obstruction reducing the flow of pancreatic juice, and the effect of the pancreatic juice itself on the glandular tissue. Although the inflammation may become chronic, the inflammation and edema usually subside after about a week and the necrotic areas are replaced by growth of fibrous tissue.

*Chronic pancreatitis* may be the end result of recurring bouts of inflammation. The repeated cycles of edema, necrosis, and hemorrhage gradually destroy increasing amounts of glandular tissue, which is replaced with fibrotic areas. The pancreas becomes increasingly hard and nodular. There is ever-increasing calcification of glandular tissue and pancreatic ducts, leading to a loss of acinar and islet tissue. This diffuse destruction of tissue ultimately leads to pancreatic insufficiency and many metabolic problems, including diabetes mellitus.

Whether the process is acute or chronic, the exact pathogenesis of pancreatitis has not as yet been determined (see Table 17-2). Obstruction of pancreatic ducts, increased secretion of pancreatic juices, vascular ischemia, and trauma have all been factors implicated in the etiology. Alcohol has been recognized as a causative factor in both acute and chronic pancreatitis, but the mechanism is not known. In recent years elevated triglyceride levels associated with alcohol consumption have been

implicated. It has been found that many alcoholics with acute pancreatitis have abnormal serum lipids and that between one-third and two-thirds of patients with pancreatitis also have a drinking problem.

Gallbladder disease has also been documented as a causative factor in the etiology of pancreatitis, both acute and chronic, perhaps when a biliary calculus becomes lodged in the ampulla of Vater. The resulting reflux of bile into the pancreatic duct may well begin the inflammatory process.

These two factors—alcoholism and biliary-tract disease—are believed to be responsible for most cases of pancreatitis. However, other factors such as trauma, infection, metabolic-nutritional disturbances, and drug reactions are thought to have possible roles. The possible role of an autoimmune mechanism is also being studied. Specific antibodies to pancreatic tissue have been found, but whether they are the cause of the inflammation or the result of the necrosis is not yet clear.

Chronic pancreatitis has long been recognized as a possible sequel to hyperparathyroidism. There is also a form of chronic pancreatitis linked to a hereditary metabolic disorder transmitted as a dominant, autosomal gene. In comparison with the more common form of chronic pancreatitis, this hereditary form begins in early childhood and is rarely associated with alcoholism or gallbladder disease.

Since pancreatitis is really a wide range of disorders, its effects on the patient can also cover a wide spectrum of severity. Some patients may present with extreme, incapacitating symptoms, while others may be relatively free of clinical problems. The usual presenting problems which occur in varying degrees of severity include pain, nausea, vomiting, fever, and abdominal tenderness.

**First-level nursing care** The nurse must utilize knowledge and skills to assess actual and potential problems which may lead to pancreatitis. Besides assessing the predisposing factors, the nurse must assume a role in the prevention of pancreatitis. Through teaching and counseling, early diagnosis and treatment of gallstones can be encouraged. Counseling of the alcoholic is more difficult, but the nurse should help the patient identify the existence of problems and select methods of coping with these issues. The potential effects of alcohol on the pancreas can be shared with the patient in a nonjudgmental manner. Although the decision to discontinue the use of alcohol must come from the patient, support can be offered during the decision-

**TABLE 17-2**
COMMONLY IMPLICATED ETIOLOGIC FACTORS
IN THE DEVELOPMENT OF PANCREATITIS

| Acute | Chronic |
|---|---|
| Alcohol | Alcohol |
| Biliary disease | Biliary disease |
| Trauma | Hyperparathyroidism |
| Infection | Hereditary metabolic disorder |
| Drug reactions (salicylates, glucocorticoids, immuno-suppressants) | |
| Metabolic—nutritional disturbances (pregnancy, ketoacidosis, uremia) | |
| Autoimmune mechanism | |

making process as well as information regarding community and health resources which may be of further help (see Chap. 19).

**Second-level nursing care** *Chronic pancreatitis* is a long-term disease and is frequently detected on an outpatient basis. The *health history* usually reveals a vague discomfort and feeling of fullness in the epigastrium. The patient may report a good appetite in the presence of weight loss. This weight loss and the appearance of frequent frothy, foul-smelling stools results from the disturbance in digestion and absorption of fats. As replacement by fibrous tissue becomes more extensive, invading and destroying larger areas of acinar and islet tissue, there are further metabolic disturbances contributing to weight loss, steatorrhea, and azotorrhea (increased levels of nitrogen in the feces). When islet-cell destruction is great enough, the patient will report symptoms of diabetes mellitus. During the history taking the nurse should carefully assess the presence of contributing disorders, especially alcoholism. The *physical assessment* at this time is essentially normal except for the weight loss and some possible tenderness in the epigastrium during palpation. Laboratory data will show an elevation of the pancreatic enzymes amylase and lipase in the serum. There may also be hyperglycemia and glycosuria due to the destruction of islet tissue. X-ray studies commonly reveal calcification of the pancreas.

**N**ursing Problems and Interventions   Proper care and counseling of both patient and family in the community can result in minimal disruption of the patient's life-style. Critical to the prognosis is the patient's willingness and ability to cooperate with the therapeutic regime. Chronic pancreatitis is often characterized by remissions and exacerbations. As the disease progresses, larger areas of the gland are destroyed and larger numbers of cells not functioning, with a resultant decrease in acute symptoms.

The nursing problem of *pain* or epigastric discomfort may often be dealt with conservatively. The patient should be counseled to change position or apply warm packs to the abdomen. Antacids are sometimes used to neutralize acid and thus decrease stimulation of the pancreas. If the patient does not obtain relief from these measures, pain medication may be ordered. Because of the chronic nature of the disease, narcotics should be given cautiously and only as a last resort. Nonnarcotic oral analgesics are safest and easiest for home use.

Morphine causes spasms of the sphincter of Oddi and should not be used.

*Inadequate nutrition* is another nursing problem commonly identified during chronic pancreatitis. Diet teaching should focus on frequent feedings of a bland, low-fat, high-carbohydrate, and high-protein diet. Supplemental fat-soluble vitamins may also be indicated. Irritating, stimulating foods are eliminated to decrease pancreatic secretions and reduce the workload of the damaged gland. The nurse should advise the patient and family to avoid large, heavy meals and rich foods in order to keep pancreatic secretions at a low level. The patient and family can also be instructed to inspect stools for foul odor, frothiness, and floating and to report these indications of steatorrhea. Pancreatic extracts (pancreatin, Viokase, Cotazym) may be administered to the patient to augment deficient amounts of pancreatic enzymes and help to control the progression of pancreatic insufficiency. The tablets are usually enteric-coated to prevent destruction by gastric pepsin and are taken with each meal.

Since chronic pancreatitis usually follows a recurring pattern, an important nursing problem is control and possible prevention of *exacerbations* in the attempt to avoid further pancreatic damage. The patient should be taught the importance of avoiding alcohol, caffeine, overeating, and any other factors which may increase pancreatic secretion.

*Hyperglycemia* is another problem requiring instruction of the patient. Depending on the severity of islet-tissue destruction, the patient may require insulin or oral hypoglycemic drugs. The patient should be counseled to report polydipsia, polyphagia, polyuria, weight loss, weakness, or dizziness. With hyperglycemia, diet instruction will need to be modified to include calorie restriction. A more thorough discussion of nursing care related to hyperglycemia can be found in Chap. 20.

Since, in many instances, chronic pancreatitis can result in total pancreatic insufficiency, hospitalization and transplantation of the pancreas or of islet cells is currently being studied. At this time only one pancreas transplanted to a human being has remained functional for 1 year.[5] However, transplants have been successful in rats, with both exocrine and endocrine functions being maintained.

**Third-level nursing care** *Acute pancreatitis* can result from an exacerbation of the chronic form of the disease, with symptoms progressively increasing in severity, or, more commonly, can be of sudden onset, totally incapacitating the patient and making immediate hospitalization necessary.

**N**ursing Assessment   Most of the systemic effects seen in acute pancreatitis are thought to result from the absorption of pancreatic enzymes and by-products of pancreatic digestion by the blood. The nursing assessment usually begins with an evaluation of *pain,* since the patient most often presents complaining of severe midepigastric pain of abrupt onset. The pain may radiate to the lumbar and dorsal areas of the back (Fig. 17-1), and the patient often reports sudden onset occurring after a large meal or heavy alcohol intake. The pain remains severe and constant and is often more intense in a supine position than when sitting or lying on the side. At times the pain may radiate over the entire abdomen, to the flanks, or to the substernal area, at which point it must be differentiated from the pain of angina or myocardial infarction.

Vomiting is almost always present at this time. It usually occurs in the absence of nausea and commonly continues even after the stomach has been emptied. The patient reports that the vomiting is frequent and forceful. The vomitus usually appears watery and may contain some bile. Instead of relieving the pain, vomiting seems to increase it, since it increases pressure in the pancreatic ducts, causing further obstruction to pancreatic secretions. The patient may also have a low-grade fever.

Overall inspection of the patient may reveal the presence of *jaundice,* which occurs in about 25 percent of patients with acute pancreatitis. The jaundice primarily results from the obstruction of the terminal common bile duct by pancreatic edema. Jaundice will first become noticeable about 24 to 36 hours after complete obstruction. During inspection the nurse may also observe ecchymotic, mottled areas on the skin of the flanks (Grey Turner's spots), thought to be caused by the presence of pancreatic enzymes in the skin. There may also be discoloration of the abdominal wall as the result of vascular damage by trypsin. These *skin manifestations* are usually seen in very severe cases.

During the *abdominal examination,* the nurse will find abdominal tenderness, muscle rigidity, and guarding. Peritonitis occurs as the result of pancreatic juices leaking into the retroperitoneal space. There may be paralytic ileus with abdominal distention from the toxins which have entered the peritoneal cavity. Peristalsis is usually diminished, and eventually bowel sounds may disappear as paralytic ileus develops. The abdominal examination may also reveal ascites. It is thought that bradykinin and kallikrein are released from the injured pancreas. Their vasodilating effects on the mesenteric vessels result in a loss of plasma colloids into the peritoneum and tissues. The colloids in the peritoneum lead to an osmotic pressure gradient that pulls fluid into the cavity. This free fluid often averages more than 3 liters in severe cases.

Signs of *shock* may be outstanding during assessment. The massive loss of fluid and plasma from the circulation results in a severely depleted circulating blood volume and hypovolemic shock. The nurse may find restlessness and apprehension, pallor, cyanosis, tachycardia, cold and clammy skin, hypotension, diaphoresis, a rapid, feeble pulse, and respiratory difficulties. Neurogenic shock may also be implicated in the symptomatology: since the pancreas lies near the celiac plexus nerves, if these nerves become involved they can affect the circulation.

Laboratory *diagnostic tests* usually focus on serum levels of amylase and lipase, since these pancreatic enzymes are released into the bloodstream early in the disease process. The serum amylase is elevated within a few hours and peaks in the first 24 to 48 hours. The maximum normal value is 200 Somogyi units/100 ml of blood. Many consider a value of more than 300 units to be diagnostic of pancreatitis; others feel that only a value of more than 1000 units is definitely diagnostic of acute pancreatitis. Amylase levels usually return to normal after 2 to 10 days. The serum-lipase level elevates later, reaching a peak in about 72 hours. It also returns to normal levels more slowly than amylase. There may also be elevation of blood-sugar levels due to islet-cell damage.

**N**ursing Problems and Interventions   Probably the most immediate nursing problem during an attack of acute pancreatitis is the relief and control of *pain.* A strong narcotic analgesic is needed to relieve this severe pain, but morphine is avoided because of its tendency to constrict the sphincter of Oddi. The nurse must attempt to control the pain before it becomes unbearably severe. Positioning will sometimes help the patient rest after the administration of pain medication. The patient with acute pancreatitis can often rest more comfortably on one side with the knees and back flexed. Since the patient may be receiving prolonged pain medication, the nurse must consistently evaluate its effectiveness in relieving pain and controlling discomfort. The danger of narcotic addiction must also be recognized.

*Shock,* as a nursing problem, is also of prime

importance when caring for a patient with acute pancreatitis. Vital signs should be checked hourly or at more frequent intervals if unstable. A central-venous-pressure catheter or Swan-Ganz catheter is usually inserted in order to monitor hemodynamics. If the pressure falls below 5 cm of water, blood, plasma, albumin, or dextran may be administered to expand the circulating volume. Large amounts of saline may also be given by infusion to replace fluid lost to the tissues. It is extremely important to monitor the fluid intake and urinary output and accurately record them, noting volume and appearance of the urine. During this period of shock, steroid drugs are sometimes used to decrease inflammation and enhance blood flow. However, since steroids have been implicated as possible etiologic factors in pancreatitis, they should be used with care.

The *pancreatic secretions* themselves present another nursing problem during an acute attack of pancreatitis. Oral intake of food is eliminated and a nasogastric tube is inserted and connected to suction in order to decrease stimulation by gastric acid. Anticholinergic drugs are often given to inhibit pancreatic secretions; however, the value of this is being questioned, since the doses of these drugs usually given may not be large enough to produce this effect. Increasing the dosage does not provide an ideal solution, since large doses may result in tachycardia, urinary retention, and increased severity of the intestinal ileus which is commonly present in pancreatitis. Trasylol, an enzyme inhibitor, may be given intravenously to neutralize trypsin.

*Adequate nutrition* also becomes a problem when pancreatic secretions are reduced. There has been recent interest in an enteric-coated pancreatic digestive enzyme* that will have very predictable enzyme activity in the small bowel. The active component is protected from gastric acidity but begins to act within 12 minutes in the alkaline environment of the intestine. The drug breaks up into small beads and mixes with the food, so that enzymes are available as long as food is being passed into the intestine and allow almost total digestion of carbohydrates, fats, and proteins. Vitamin replacement may also be indicated to improve nutrition.

Since necrosis of the pancreas sets up ideal conditions for bacterial invasion, the prevention of *infection* becomes a nursing problem. Broad-spectrum antibiotics such as penicillin, tetracycline, and

cephalothin are usually administered in an attempt to ward off secondary infection. The nurse must also be aware of the possibility of pulmonary infection. Severe pain and immobilization can contribute to pulmonary problems. Ascites may cause shortness of breath by exerting pressure on the diaphragm. Positioning, turning, coughing, and deep breathing as well as the use of intermittent positive-pressure breathing may reduce the risk of respiratory problems.

*Fluid and electrolyte imbalance* frequently occurs with acute pancreatitis. The nasogastric suction and elimination of oral intake make it necessary to replace fluids and electrolytes intravenously. To evaluate fluid and electrolyte balance, the nurse must maintain an accurate intake and output record, observe carefully for signs of electrolyte depletion or elevation, monitor vital signs, and observe changes in the skin and mucous membranes.

The patient usually recovers on this medical regimen, but the mortality rate is about 15 percent. Surgery is rarely performed and is not considered the treatment of choice. No operation has been found to give consistently good results. A drainage procedure such as the Roux-EN-Y involves opening an obstructed duct and anastomosing it to the jejunum. A more aggressive approach may involve partial or near-total pancreatectomy.

**Fourth-level nursing care** To reach the goal of rehabilitation of the patient and prevention of recurrent attacks of pancreatitis, the nurse must utilize teaching as a basic, vital tool. The patient and family must be helped to understand what the disease is in order to accept the therapeutic regimen. Patients are usually advised to follow a low-fat diet of small, frequent meals in order to keep pancreatic secretion to a minimum. Patients should also be cautioned to avoid alcohol and beverages containing caffeine, since they stimulate secretions. The nurse should stress that adherence to the prescribed diet is one of the major factors in preventing recurrence. Instruction on checking stools is also important. The patient should check for a foul smell, frothiness, and floating and report any of these observations. The nurse should also encourage the patient to maintain regular medical follow-up care to assist in preventing recurrence of the disease.

**Pancreatic Tumors**

Carcinoma of the pancreas rarely occurs before the age of 40, and the highest incidence is found in the

---

* Experimental product by Johnson and Johnson, New Brunswick, N.J.

sixth and seventh decades, primarily in males. The disease follows a rapid, fatal course. Most patients with carcinoma of the pancreas die within a year after the first appearance of symptoms, and about one-half the deaths occur within 3 months. Metastasis occurs first in the regional lymph nodes and the liver. Further spread may involve the lungs, intestines, adrenals, and bone.

Surgery is sometimes performed in the hope of treating pancreatic cancer but does not seem to improve the extremely poor prognosis. Radiation and chemotherapy are commonly employed as palliative measures which may reduce symptoms temporarily. The goal of nursing care also is support and control of symptoms. Relief of pain, psychological support, and stimulation of appetite are the major nursing problems.

### Pancreatic Cysts

The most common cystic lesion found in the pancreas is the pseudocyst, which is a collection of enzyme fluid, necrotic tissue, and blood encapsulated by connective tissue and adhering to the upper abdominal viscera or the lesser omental sac. Pancreatic pseudocysts usually occur as a late complication of acute pancreatitis or recurrent chronic pancreatitis. They may also occur following trauma to the abdomen. These lesions arise in any part of the pancreas and can rupture into nearby organs—most often the colon and stomach. Secondary infection, with hemorrhage into the pseudocyst, may occur and is a poor prognostic sign.

The clinical manifestations of a pseudocyst are very similar to those of pancreatitis. There is a constant aching, dull pain in the upper abdomen which may radiate to the back. The pain is often accompanied by anorexia, weight loss, and low-grade fever. Jaundice may be present in those patients who have a pseudocyst in the head of the pancreas.

Some pseudocysts, usually the smaller ones, may resolve spontaneously. In other cases it becomes necessary to treat the underlying causes of pancreatic disease, such as alcoholism or gallbladder disease. Surgery is sometimes done, anastomosing the pseudocyst to the nearest part of the upper gastrointestinal tract in order to provide drainage of the cyst.

### Malabsorption Syndrome

Malabsorption syndrome is a group of disorders characterized by faulty intestinal absorption of water and nutrients, especially fats. The most common clinical manifestation of malabsorption is steatorrhea (fatty stools). Two malabsorption syndromes, adult celiac disease and tropical sprue, will be briefly explored.

**Adult celiac disease** Adult celiac disease, also known as nontropical sprue and idiopathic steatorrhea, is thought to be a genetically controlled enzymatic or metabolic defect resulting in an intolerance for gluten. The basic hereditary defect seems to be lack of an intestinal enzyme responsible for hydrolyzing a peptide contained in dietary gluten. The villi of the small intestine become shortened or distorted, offering less available surface area for absorption of nutrients. Although the defect is hereditary, patients do not usually become symptomatic until the third to sixth decade. The most common presenting complaint is that of frequent, loose, foul-smelling, greasy stools (steatorrhea). This decreased fat absorption contributes to other clinical manifestations. The excessive loss of fat lessens caloric supply of the body, with resulting weight loss and malnutrition. Along with fats there is also decreased absorption of the fat-soluble vitamins and clinical symptoms of their deficiency, for example, bleeding tendencies from decreased vitamin K and hypocalcemia due to vitamin D deficiency (see Chap. 16).

There is also impairment of protein and carbohydrate absorption, contributing to weight loss and muscle wasting. Severely reduced absorption of protein leads to a loss of nitrogen in the stools (azotorrhea). Malabsorption of protein can also lead to edema and decreased resistance to infections.

Since the only effective treatment for adult celiac disease is the elimination of gluten from the diet, the major role of the nurse is helping the patient and family understand the disease and the dietary restrictions. A gluten-free diet eliminates all cereal grains except rice and corn. Soy flours may be used. Besides avoiding the specific grains, patients must be advised to read all package labels, since cereal grains or flour may be added to many products.

If the patient adheres to a gluten-free diet, the outlook is optimistic. Within several weeks there is a decrease in steatorrhea and a concomitant weight gain. After a few months there may be partial regeneration of the intestinal villi.

**Tropical sprue** Tropical sprue is another example of a malabsorption problem. Its highest incidence occurs in people living in parts of the Far East, India, and the Caribbean. It is generally thought that both nutritional deficiencies and bacterial invasion of the small bowel may be causative factors in its development. Although it is similar to adult celiac disease in its pathology and clinical manifestations, a reduction in size or number of intestinal villi is less commonly found and the pathologic changes are less severe. A gluten-free diet is totally ineffective in tropical sprue, but the pathology is reversible with folic acid therapy. The first clinical problems the patient may notice are fatigue and bulky, frothy stools. Usually within a period of a few weeks, a marked loss of weight is noted. Finally there is diarrhea and depletion of iron stores, leading to anemia.

The usual therapy involves administration of a broad-spectrum antibiotic such as tetracycline, in conjunction with daily administration of folic acid. This regimen quickly reduces diarrhea, stimulates appetite, and results in weight gain. After total remission of the disease, the patient is often maintained on a daily dosage of folic acid.

## REFERENCES

1   F. J. Ingelfinger, "The Side Effects of Aspirin," *N Engl J Med*, **290**:1196–1197, May 23, 1974.
2   Sidney Cohen and Glenn H. Booth, Jr., "Gastric Acid Secretion and Lower Esophageal Sphincter Pressure in Response to Coffee and Caffeine," *N Engl J Med*, **293**:897–899, Oct. 30, 1975.
3   Ronald A. Bernstein et al., "Relationship of Gallbladder Disease to Parity, Obesity, and Age," *Health Serv Rep*, **88**:925–936, December 1973.
4   Halpert, Bela, "Gallbladder and Biliary Ducts," W. A. D. Anderson (ed.), *Pathology*, Mosby, St. Louis, 1971, pp. 1261–1270.
5   Claude E. Welch, "Abdominal Surgery, Pt. III," *N Engl J Med*, **293**:957–964, Nov. 6, 1975.

## BIBLIOGRAPHY

AMA Council on Drugs: *AMA Drug Evaluations*, American Medical Association, Chicago, 1971.

Athanasoulis, Christos A.: "Infusion of Vasopressin," *Emergency Med*, **7**:39–46, April 1975.

Bates, M.: "Hiatus Hernia," *Nurs Mirror*, **141**:50–55, Sept. 4, 1975.

Bernstein, Ronald A., et al.: "Relationship of Gallbladder Disease to Parity, Obesity, and Age," *Health Serv Rep*, **88**:925–936, December 1973.

Bigelow, J.: "Roundtable: Gallbladder Disease," *Patient Care*, **9**:30–106, Aug. 1, 1975.

Blackburn, George L., et al.: "New Approaches to the Management of Severe Acute Pancreatitis," *Am J Surg*, **131**:114–124, January 1976.

Brodie, David A.: "Stress Ulcer," *Emergency Med*, **7**:35–37, April 1975.

Buchan, D. J.: "Mind-Body Relationships in Gastrointestinal Disease," *Can Nurse*, **67**:35–37, March 1971.

Burhenne, H. Joachim, and William G. Obata: "Single Visit Oral Cholecystography," *N Engl J Med*, **292**:627–628, Mar. 20, 1975.

Cameron, John L., et al.: "A Pathogenesis for Alcoholic Pancreatitis," *Surgery*, **77**:754–763, June 1975.

"Case Records of the Massachusetts General Hospital: Case 1-1976," *N Engl J Med*, **294**:37–42, Jan. 1, 1976.

Clark, M. L.: "Medical Treatment of Peptic Ulcer," *Nurs Mirror*, **139**:48–50, Sept. 6, 1974.

Clearfield, Harris R.: "Stanching the Hemorrhage," *Emergency Med*, **7**:49–52, April 1975.

Cohen, Sidney, and Glenn H. Booth, Jr.: "Gastric Acid Secretion and Lower Esophageal Sphincter Pressure in Response to Coffee and Caffeine," *N Engl J Med*, **293**:897–899, Oct. 30, 1975.

Colcher, H.: "Current Concepts: Gastrointestinal Endoscopy," *N Engl J Med*, **293**:1129–1131, Nov. 27, 1975.

Comer, Steven J., et al.: "Pancreatic Abscess," *Am J Surg*, **129**:426–431, April 1975.

Coyne, Martin J. et al.: "Treatment of Gallstones with Chenodeoxycholic Acid and Phenobarbital," *N Engl J Med*, **292**:604–607, Mar. 20, 1975.

De Risi, Lucy L.: "Starving in the Midst of Plenty: Adult Celiac Disease," *Am J Nurs*, **70**:1048–1053, May 1970.

Dinoso, Vicente P., Jr.: "Hot Pancreas, Hot Belly: Medical Management," *Emergency Med*, **7**:186–187, April 1975.

French, Ruth M.: *Guide to Diagnostic Procedures*, McGraw-Hill, New York, 1975.

Gambill, Earl E.: "Diagnosing Pancreatitis," *Emergency Med*, **7**:179–185, April 1975.

Given, Barbara A., and Sandra J. Simmons: *Gastroenterology in Clinical Nursing*, Mosby, St. Louis, 1975.

Griffin, George E., and Claude H. Organ: "The Natural History of the Perforated Duodenal Ulcer Treated by Suture Plication," *Ann Surg*, **183**:382–385, April 1976.

Grossman, Morton I., et al.: "Peptic Ulcer," in Paul Beeson and Walsh McDermott (eds.), *Cecil-Loeb Textbook of Medicine*, Saunders, Philadelphia, 1975, pp. 1198–1217.

Henry, Lyle G., and Robert E. Condon: "Ablative Surgery for Necrotizing Pancreatitis," *Am J Surg*, **131**:125–128, January 1976.

Herrington, J. Lynwood, John L. Sawyers, and William

A. Whitehead: "Surgical Management of Reflux Gastritis," *Ann Surg,* **180:**526–537, October 1974.

Horn, Robert C.: "Alimentary Tract," in W. A. D. Anderson (ed.), *Pathology,* Mosby, St. Louis, 1971, pp. 1129–1131.

Ingelfinger, F. J.: "The Side Effects of Aspirin," *N Engl J Med,* **290:**1196–1197, May 23, 1974.

Johnston, Ivan D. A.: "Duodenal Ulcers," *Nurs Mirror,* **136:**24–26, May 11, 1973.

Kowlessar, O. Dhodanard: "Diseases of the Pancreas" in Paul Beeson and Walsh McDermott (eds.), *Cecil-Loeb Textbook of Medicine,* Saunders, Philadelphia, 1975, pp. 1243–1252.

Lacy, Paul E., and John M. Kissane: "Pancreas and Diabetes Mellitus," in W. A. D. Anderson (ed.), *Pathology,* Mosby, St. Louis, 1971, pp. 1280–1285.

Lamb, Carolyn (ed.): "When Complications Upset Ulcer Therapy," *Patient Care,* **7:**65–100, Oct. 15, 1973.

Langman, M. J. S.: "Duodenal Ulcers," *Nurs Mirror,* **136:**38–39, May 4, 1973.

Lindenauer, S. Martin, and Thomas L. Dent: "Management of the Recurrent Ulcer," *Arch Surg,* **110:**531–536, May 1975.

Longstreth, G. F. et al.: "Cimetidine Suppression of Nocturnal Gastric Secretion in Active Duodenal Ulcer," *N Engl J Med,* **294:**801–804, Apr. 8, 1976.

Richardson, Charles T., and John H. Walsh: "The Value of a Histamine $H_2$-Receptor Antagonist in the Management of Patients With the Zollinger-Ellison Syndrome," *N Engl J Med,* **294:**133–135, Jan. 15, 1976.

Robinson, Corinne H.: *Normal and Therapeutic Nutrition,* Macmillan, New York, 1972.

Rubin, Phillip: "Cancer of the Gastrointestinal Tract," *JAMA,* **228:**883–896, May 13, 1974.

Sawyers, John L. et al.: "Acute Perforated Duodenal Ulcer: An Evaluation of Surgical Management," *Arch Surg,* **110:**527–530, May, 1975.

Schwartz, Seymour et al.: *Principles of Surgery,* McGraw-Hill, New York, 1974.

Simmons, Sandra, and Barbara Given: "Acute Pancreatitis," *Am J Nurs,* **71:**934–939, May 1971.

Skillman, John J.: "Pathogenesis of Peptic Ulcer: A Selective Review," *Surgery,* **76:**515–523, September 1974.

Sodeman, William A., and William A. Sodeman, Jr.: *Pathologic Physiology: Mechanisms of Disease,* Saunders, Philadelphia, 1974.

Sleisenger, Marvin H.: "Diseases of Malabsorption," in Paul Beeson and Walsh McDermott (eds.), *Cecil-Loeb Textbook of Medicine,* Saunders, Philadelphia, 1975, pp. 1217–1243.

Spenney, Jerry G.: "GI Hemorrhage," *Emergency Med,* **5:**107–113, July 1973.

Sun, David C. H.: "Duodenal Ulcer: Treat the Crisis, Avoid the Recurrence," *Consultant,* **14:**27–28, February 1974.

Tauxe, Robert V., Lucius F. Wright, and Basil I. Hirschowitz: "Marginal Ulcer in Achlorhydric Patients," *Ann Surg,* **181:**455–457, April 1975.

Thompson, James C. et al.: "The Effects on Gastrin and Gastric Secretion of Fine Current Operations for Duodenal Ulcer," *Ann Surg,* **183:**599–608, May 1976.

Trapnell, J. E.: "Acute Pancreatitis," *Nurs Mirror,* **139:**52–54, Dec. 19, 1974.

Van Heerden, Jonathan A., and William H. ReMine: "Pseudocysts of the Pancreas," *Arch Surg,* **110:**500–505, May 1975.

Walsh, John H., and Morton I. Grossman: "Gastrin, Pt. I," *N Engl J Med,* **292:**1324–1334, June 19, 1975.

Walsh, John H., and Morton I. Grossman: "Gastrin, Pt. II," *N Engl J Med,* **292:**1377–1384, June 26, 1975.

Way, Laurence W.: "Diseases of the Gallbladder and Bile Ducts," in Paul Beeson and Walsh McDermott (eds.), *Cecil-Loeb Textbook of Medicine,* Saunders, Philadelphia, 1975, pp. 1308–1319.

Welch, Claude E.: "Abdominal Surgery, Pt. I," *N Engl J Med,* **293:**858–863, Oct. 23, 1975.

Welch, Claude E.: "Abdominal Surgery, Pt. III," *N Engl J Med,* **293:**957–964, Nov. 6, 1975.

Wolferth, Charles C.: "The Operation Nobody Wants," *Emergency Med,* **7:**193–196, April 1975.

Yajko, R. Douglas, Lawrence W. Norton, and Ben Eiseman: "Current Management of Upper Gastrointestinal Bleeding," *Ann Surg,* **181:**474–480, April 1975.

# 18

# Disturbances in Elimination

Carol E. Hartman

The human gastrointestinal tract receives substances from and returns waste products to the external environment. Physical, psychosocial, and economic changes in the environment can alter gastrointestinal activity. This is frequently reflected in disturbances in *intestinal elimination*.

Disturbances in elimination are manifested in many ways. A common example is "traveler's diarrhea" which frequently occurs when people physically change environments. A more refined diet has led to increases in diverticular problems. Diarrhea and constipation are common consequences of psychosocial stresses. Social customs governing elimination can also lead to disturbances. As the pace in daily activities increases, the urge to eliminate is inhibited for convenience. Forsaking the primitive squatting posture for defecation has also led to problems. The mistaken belief that one must have a bowel movement every day to be healthy results in large expenditures for laxatives and elimination aids. The economic impact of man's elimination is considerable. Inflammatory bowel disease, intestinal obstructions, diverticular disease, and hemorrhoids are among the more common disturbances in elimination discussed in this chapter.

## INFLAMMATORY BOWEL DISEASE

Inflammatory bowel disease is a broad concept that includes ulcerative colitis, Crohn's disease, appendicitis, diverticulitis, and infectious diarrheas. A common elimination disturbance caused by inflammatory bowel disease is diarrhea, a very liquid or frequent stool. The nature and duration of the diarrhea will depend on the particular inflammatory disorder.

### Ulcerative Colitis

The best known of the chronic inflammatory bowel disturbances is ulcerative colitis, which involves inflammation and ulceration of the large bowel. Its exact cause is not clear, but several theories of causation have been proposed. Initially, ulcerative colitis was thought to result from some *infectious agent*. The possibilities of an *allergic reaction* to milk protein or of *autonomic stimulation* of blood vessels supplying the intestine were also suggested. Visceral responses to psychological and emotional stresses led to the *psychosomatic theory* of causation, which became popular in the 1950s. There may also be a *genetic predisposition* for developing ulcerative colitis. Currently, the role of *altered immunologic mechanisms* as a cause is receiving attention.[1] Lymphocytes from patients with ulcerative colitis have cytotoxic effects on intestinal epithelial cells. The presence of antibodies to human colon tissue may indicate an autoimmune phenomenon or may be a secondary effect of tissue breakdown. In the final analysis a combination of factors may enter into the etiology of ulcerative colitis.

Ulcerative colitis can occur at any age. Its peak occurrence, however, is between the ages of 15 and 25, with another small peak between 30 and 40 years of age. The incidence is higher in Jews than in non-Jews. Both sexes are affected, but it is more common in females than in males. Often there is a family history of chronic inflammatory bowel disease. Ulcerative colitis is frequently associated with *traumatic emotional experiences* involving real, threatened, or symbolic losses: one study found that major losses occurred within 4 months of diagnosis,[2] suggesting an interactive response between mind and body.

**Pathophysiology** The inflammation associated with ulcerative colitis first involves the mucosa and then the submucosa and usually begins in the distal colon, spreading proximally. The colonic mucosa becomes engorged and very friable, causing it to bleed easily. Multiple, irregular, superficial ulcerations and crypt abscesses develop, and mucus secretion increases. Bloody discharges and pus are common. As the inflammation progresses, areas of bowel may slough. Some of these ulcerated areas heal with normal mucosa, while others are replaced with scar tissue.

Ulcerative colitis is characterized by remissions and exacerbations. During remission the colon appears normal but microscopic examination reveals small, latent abscesses. During exacerbations the inflammation may remain localized or progressively involve more and more of the large bowel. Repeated episodes leave the colon scarred, with thickened walls, a narrowed diameter, and shortened length.

**Metabolic Changes** The most widespread effects of chronic inflammation in the colon are manifested in metabolic changes. Normal elimination through the large bowel is interrupted, and *diarrhea* results. The stools increase in frequency, with 20 or more bowel movements a day during the acute stage of the inflammation. The stool becomes loose and often contains blood and mucus. In-

continence is often a problem. With extensive loss of bowel mucosa and inflammation of the submucosa, an acute dilatation, *toxic megacolon,* can occur.

Patients with ulcerative colitis often experience *loss of appetite* and ingest inadequate amounts of both water and food. Ingestion stimulates bowel motility and increases diarrhea. The patient may therefore fear eating and avoid food and fluids. In order to compensate for the inadequate intake of nutrients, the body mobilizes its own energy stores, and *catabolism* occurs. Weight loss results, and in severe cases *metabolic acidosis* can develop (see Chap. 12). As the protein stores are depleted, negative nitrogen balance ensues.

**Fluid and Electrolyte Imbalances** Changes in fluid and electrolyte dynamics are a direct result of the losses associated with diarrhea. *Dehydration* occurs, its severity depending on the amount of loss in relation to the intake of fluids and electrolytes. With severe diarrhea, potassium and sodium can become depleted.

**Changes in Perception** Perceptual changes are manifested in various degrees of discomfort. Pain is usually felt as *lower abdominal cramping.* Since multiple nerve endings are stimulated by the increased peristalsis, the pain is often diffuse and difficult to localize. In addition, cramping activity in the sacral area is frequently accompanied by urgency of defecation. The defecation itself is often painful and does not relieve the cramping, because the initial stimuli from the peristaltic activity has not been relieved. Another perceptual change is *blurred vision,* the result of eye manifestations found in some patients with ulcerative colitis.

**Changes in Oxygenation** Oxygenation status is compromised by *anemia.* This results from chronic loss of blood in the stool and is accompanied by iron deficiency. Decreased synthesis of vitamin K results in lowered prothrombin levels, increasing *blood loss.* Decreased synthesis of vitamin $B_{12}$, iron deficiency, and the effect of a chronic inflammation on the bone marrow result in *impaired maturation of red blood cells.* As the colon involvement becomes widespread, over half the patients have significant anemia and iron deficiency. Further local impairment of oxygenation may result from *thromboembolic phenomena* as the blood becomes more viscous from increased numbers of platelets and white blood cells and from dehydration.

Changes in Cellular Growth   In children and adolescents, normal cellular growth can be retarded and sexual development delayed. With any age group, long-standing ulcerative colitis can lead to abnormal cellular growth. *Malignant changes* are not uncommon. The intestinal epithelium proliferates, leading to polyps, which can progress to cancer. Studies have shown that the average time for a polyp in the large bowel to progress to cancer is 10 to 15 years.[3] The risk of malignant changes becomes greater with each decade of disease as well as with extensive colonic involvement. Universal disease, that involving the entire colon, carries the highest risk for developing cancer. The ulcerations may heal with no defects in the bowel mucosa. In many instances, however, portions of the mucosa and the underlying layers of bowel are replaced with scar tissue. As the scar tissue contracts, the colon narrows and shortens. Strictures of the colon may develop, leading to partial or total obstruction.

Changes in Immunity   Patients with ulcerative colitis often manifest widespread changes in their immune system response. Inflammations involving the *joints* or the *liver* often parallel the activity in the colon. Ten to twenty percent of patients with ulcerative colitis experience some kind of joint involvement. As the colitis improves, the peripheral joint pains subside. It is thought that small immune complexes in the serum of patients with inflammatory bowel disease may be important in the pathogenesis of these extracolonic manifestations. Other inflammations found in patients with ulcerative colitis do not seem to correlate with activity in the colon. These include *uveitis,* inflammation of the iris, ciliary body and choroid; *conjunctivitis,* inflammation of the conjunctiva; and *skin lesions* such as erythema nodosum and pyoderma gangrenosum. *Erythema nodosum* is characterized by tender, red raised nodules in the extensor surfaces of arms and legs. In *pyoderma gangrenosum,* purulent cutaneous ulcerations are the characteristic lesions (see Color Plate 18-1). It is thought that a defect in the cellular immune system may account for some of these manifestations.[4]

**First-level nursing care**   With lack of knowledge about the cause of ulcerative colitis and the conditions which lead to its development, little can be done to identify high-risk groups and prevent occurrence. The nurse who works with mothers and children may be able to identify situations in which the parents could be assisted to help the child express feelings of anger and aggression in a direct but socially acceptable way. The child would thus build a repertoire of useful coping mechanisms for life stresses. Perhaps the need for expression in somatic symptoms would then be unnecessary. The nurse in a school setting may be in a position to do similar counseling with children and teachers. Similarly, persons of all ages should be helped to explore coping mechanisms that allow feelings to be turned outward rather than inward.

**Second-level nursing care**   Patients with ulcerative colitis are often diagnosed and treated initially on an outpatient basis. If the care and treatment is successful, hospitalization may never be necessary. The patient will initially be seen in any of a variety of community settings, and the *nursing assessment* should include a health history, physical assessment, and diagnostic tests.

Health History   Any disturbance in elimination should be carefully explored in the health history. When the patient uses the term *diarrhea,* the nurse should inquire about the character and frequency of stools and collect details on the amount, color, and character of the stools as well as time of day, relation to meals, and any associated discomfort. Patients with ulcerative colitis usually complain of diarrhea occurring both day and night as often as 5 or 6 times in a 24-hour period. The diarrhea is often described as being unrelieved by home remedies. The stools are described as soft or loose and watery, frequently streaked with blood and mucus. Patients are often distressed by severe abdominal cramping, unrelieved after bowel movements, and sometimes by soiling because of the urgency of defecation. The cramping frequently becomes more severe after eating or with activity, but it also wakes them. Many patients with ulcerative colitis complain of decreased appetite, weight loss, and fatigue, and a number mention stiffness and joint pains as well.

When a patient complains of diarrhea, additional information should be obtained in order to determine the cause. Asking the following questions elicits useful information: Do contacts (family, friends, coworkers) have a similar problem? Has there been foreign travel? Are there emotional stresses? Have there been disruptions in relationships or significant losses? Are other diseases present? Is there exposure to heavy metals in work or leisure activities? What is the intake of food and fluids? Has appetite been affected? Is there nausea or vomiting? Has the weight changed? Is the patient taking any medications, especially laxatives, antibiotics, or steroids? Are there allergies?

The health history should also focus on the patient's *psychosocial and emotional status.* A history of significant changes in the past year can give the nurse some idea of the amount of stress the person is undergoing and what the usual coping mechanisms are. Patients with ulcerative colitis frequently are anxious to please and to conform. Neatness, orderliness, and punctuality are common traits. Often there are outward appearances of energy, ambition, and efficiency which cover exaggerated feelings of inferiority. There is often low tolerance for frustration and a lack of well-directed expressions of anger. Anger accompanied by a sense of helplessness and despair or a loss or a disrupted relationship often precedes an attack of ulcerative colitis. The person is usually quite perceptive of hostility and tends to brood and withdraw. Mothers of patients with ulcerative colitis have been described as controlling and domineering.

The effects of ulcerative colitis are not confined to the colon. The abdominal cramping and the frequency and urgency of diarrhea interfere with many activities. The patient with ulcerative colitis may restrict social activities and relationships with others. During exacerbations, keeping up with job responsibilities may be difficult.

**P**hysical Assessment  Physical assessment of the patient with ulcerative colitis often reveals a variety of signs and symptoms. Exploration of the *metabolic changes* focuses on weight and abdominal and rectal examinations. Inspection of the abdomen often reveals a flat or concave shape with visible peristalsis. Bowel sounds are generally increased. On palpation the abdomen is often tender. In chronic ulcerative colitis, the sigmoid colon is often palpable and feels firm and pipelike. On rectal examination, one usually finds an empty rectum and a tight sphincter. Tenderness is often referred to the sacral area. Irritations around the anus are common. The patient's weight should be noted and compared with previous weight records if available. Patients with ulcerative colitis usually show a progressive weight loss, reflecting the catabolism that occurs. Inspection may reveal a generalized loss of muscle mass. A low-grade fever is often found.

*Oxygenation status* should be carefully assessed to evaluate the degree of anemia present.

Ulcerative colitis patients with anemia usually appear pale—best seen in the nail beds and conjunctivae. Capillary refill is usually brisk. Fingers and toes may feel cool to the touch. If the anemia is severe, the nurse may note an increased pulse and dyspnea on exertion. Bruises, indicating an increased bleeding tendency, may be found. Unequal calf size and a positive Homan's sign indicate the presence of thrombophlebitis, which develops in many patients with ulcerative colitis. The chest examination is usually normal.

The diarrhea associated with ulcerative colitis compromises the patient's *fluid and electrolyte status.* With mild dehydration one sees dry mucous membranes and weight loss of about 4 percent of the body weight. Urine appears concentrated, and its specific gravity ranges from 1.020 to 1.025. The patient experiences mild thirst. In moderate dehydration there is severe thirst, a dry skin as well as dry mouth, poor skin turgor, and a scant amount of more concentrated urine. About 6 percent of the body weight is lost. Depletion of potassium frequently is exhibited by weakness, flabby muscle tone, decreased or absent deep tendon reflexes, and cardiac arrhythmias.

The widespread changes in the *immune system* manifested in some patients with ulcerative colitis may be found throughout the body. General observation may reveal the presence of skin lesions. Round, raised, tender, red nodules, usually found on the extensor surfaces of the arms and legs, and purulent cutaneous ulcerations are characteristic skin findings in patients with ulcerative colitis. Jaundice points to liver involvement. On examination of the mouth one often finds ulcerations. Assessment of the musculoskeletal system may reveal tender, warm, swollen joints, bony deformity, and limitation of motion. Usually a few joints are involved, and the pattern of involvement is symmetrical. Limitation of motion in the back, particularly around the sacroiliac joint, is also found in some patients. On gross eye examination one may find reddened conjunctivae, sluggish pupillary responses to light, small pupil size, and blurred vision. Visual fields and extraocular movements are usually not involved.

The changes in *cellular growth* in the young patient are assessed by comparing the patient's height and weight with established norms. The youth with ulcerative colitis is often smaller than average. The development of secondary sex characteristics and the onset of menarche are often delayed, and the menstrual cycle may be irregular.

**D**iagnostic Tests A variety of laboratory tests aid the nurse in assessing the patient with ulcerative colitis. *Stool specimens* are examined for blood, mucus, and organisms. A *complete blood count* helps establish the existence of anemia and leukocytosis. *Hematocrit* and *hemoglobin* readings are usually sufficient to evaluate the patient's blood loss during treatment. *Serum electrolytes* may reflect losses from diarrhea and inadequate replacement. Metabolic catabolism is often reflected in *decreased serum protein* levels.

A *barium enema* is frequently used to diagnose ulcerative colitis and to follow the patient's response to treatment. This is a radiologic examination of the colon and involves the instillation of barium, a radiopaque substance, through the rectum. Because patients frequently have difficulty retaining the barium during the examination, a rectal tube with an inflatable balloon is often used. The progress of the barium is followed on a fluoroscopy screen. After x-rays are taken, the patient is allowed to expel the solution and additional films are taken.

Preparation for a barium enema includes preparing the patient for what to expect and cleansing the colon. A clean colon is essential for adequate results. The specific preparation varies according to the protocol of the radiologist performing the test but often involves a clear-liquid diet, a cathartic at noon and again at 4 P.M. the day prior to the test, increased fluids and, on the day of the examination, cleansing enemas. One study recommends that at least 240 ml of fluid be taken every hour for 8 to 10 hours.[5] The use of cathartics and cleansing enemas may be too rigorous for the patient with ulcerative colitis, and the nurse should inquire whether a modification of the usual protocol is indicated. Irritation from these measures can result in significant bleeding.

Another radiologic examination, an *upper gastrointestinal (GI) series with small bowel followthrough,* may also be done. In preparation for this, the patient takes nothing by mouth for 6 to 8 hours prior to the examination. Barium is then given by mouth, and a series of x-rays are taken as the barium progresses through the gastrointestinal tract. The total examination usually takes several hours, and the patient is not allowed food or fluids until it is completed. After any barium study, it is important that the patient expel the barium. Increasing fluids is usually effective, but a mild laxative may be needed to prevent impaction with hardened barium.

A *sigmoidoscopy* is often done to visualize the rectum and sigmoid colon directly and evaluate the extent of disease. Biopsies can also be obtained. The procedure involves the insertion of a sigmoidoscope (a rigid, straight instrument fitted with a light and lens) through the anus into the rectum and sigmoid colon. As with the barium enema, preparation for the examination focuses on cleansing the colon and instructing the patient. The procedure should be explained and the patient warned that some discomfort and cramping may occur. For adequate visualization the bowel mucosa needs to be free of stool. Methods of bowel cleansing vary but usually involve some combination of increased fluids and cathartics the preceding day and tap-water or saline enemas on the day of the examination. A light diet is usually advised the evening before and the morning of the examination.

During the examination the nurse should help the patient assume the proper position. The knee-chest position is most commonly used, although a left lateral position is adequate. Draping the patient to avoid unnecessary exposure and embarrassment is a prime responsibility of the nurse. Caution should be exercised in case the patient becomes dizzy. The nurse should also observe the general condition of the patient and give explanations and encouragement as the sigmoidoscopy is performed.

Another examination that may be done on an ambulatory basis is a *colonoscopy.* It involves direct visualization of the entire colon through the use of a flexible fiberscope (see Fig. 18-1). During a colonoscopy the physician is able to take biopsies and photograph areas of the bowel. Polyps may be removed through the scope, thus eliminating an abdominal approach for benign lesions. The length of time the procedure takes depends on the location of the lesions. Diverticular disease, discussed later in the chapter, makes passage of the scope more difficult. Thorough cleansing of the bowel is needed for an adequate examination. In preparation for colonoscopy the patient is often given clear liquids for two or three days prior to the procedure, a laxative the day before, and nothing by mouth the day of the procedure. Cleansing enemas with tap water or sodium bicarbonate solution are given at least 3 hours before, or even the evening before, the examination.

The patient needs a thorough explanation of the procedure. There may be discomfort and cramping when air is introduced and when the

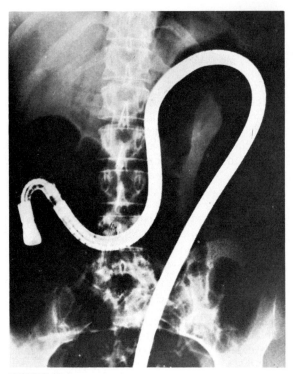

**FIGURE 18-1**
Plain film of the abdomen showing flexible fibercolonoscope introduced into the right colon. (*From S. I. Schwartz et al. (eds.), Principles of Surgery, 2d ed., McGraw-Hill, New York, 1974, by permission.*)

colonoscope is being advanced around the flexures. Premedication, usually some combination of meperidine and diazepam, is given to relax the patient.

At the start of the procedure the patient should be placed in a left lateral decubitus position. As the scope is inserted, resistance may occur at bends in the colon and the patient may be moved to a supine position to aid in insertion. During the procedure the nurse should attend to the patient's physical and mental comfort. If there is undue discomfort, additional medication may be given. Talking with the patient, giving explanations of what is being done, and sometimes letting the patient watch part of the procedure through a teaching attachment are effective in reducing anxiety and gaining cooperation.[6] Perforation and bleeding can occur with colonoscopy, and the nurse should be alert to these.

**N**ursing Problems and Interventions  The nurse can help the patient with ulcerative colitis cope with many problems. Probably one of the most distressing of these is the *diarrhea.* This can be controlled somewhat with medication and diet modifications. There is no indication that any special diet is able to prolong remissions, but some diet modifications may decrease discomfort. Cooked foods are often tolerated better than raw fruits and vegetables. When new foods are added to the diet, it is wise to add one at a time so that tolerance to each one can be judged. It is usually suggested that hot, spicy foods be omitted. If there is a history of milk intolerance, milk can be left out of the diet. Some patients find that they can take small amounts of milk products even though milk itself causes bloating, flatulence, and diarrhea.

The nurse should help the patient understand the chronic nature of the disease and that medications used in ulcerative colitis are taken on a long-term basis. The medications help control but do not cure the disease. *Salicylazosulfapyridine* (Azulfidine) is an antiinfective agent that is effective in reducing inflammation and improving symptoms. It is initially given in dosages of 3 to 4 g/day and then decreased to 2 g/day for 6 to 12 months. It is important that the patient maintain an adequate fluid intake and urinary output to prevent crystalluria, which could damage the kidneys.

*Corticosteroids* are useful in suppressing symptoms of ulcerative colitis. During an acute exacerbation, oral prednisone, 40 to 60 mg/day, is given in divided doses. The dose is gradually reduced according to the clinical response until 20 mg every day or every other day is effective. Treatment continues over several months in a dose of 10 to 15 mg every other day. Steroids may also be administered through a retention enema. This route controls the local inflammation of the colon and can be used over a longer period of time than oral therapy with fewer systemic complications. The nurse instructs on preparation and administration of the enema solution. A discussion of nursing care associated with steroid therapy can be found in Chap. 21.

Since some studies of ulcerative colitis indicate a problem with the immunologic system, *immunosuppressive agents* such as azathioprine (Imuran) and 6-mercaptopurine have been used for therapy. Results on disease activity in the colon thus far are not impressive. In some cases there was no healing, and in others, increased ulcer formation was found.[7]

The patient with ulcerative colitis is apt to develop *dehydration,* and it is important that an adequate intake to replace losses from diarrhea be maintained. Bland fluids may be tolerated and at the same time supply nutrients as well as fluid. If there is an increase in perspiration or in diarrhea, the patient should increase the fluid intake accordingly.

Over a period of time the patient often experiences some degree of *weight loss.* The nurse should instruct the patient about a well-balanced, nutritious diet and help plan for increased intake of calories, protein, and vitamins. Sometimes adequate intake may be achieved with small but more frequent feedings. Weights should be measured regularly, and realistic goals for weight gain should be established with the patient. Vitamin, calorie, and protein supplements may be necessary if the patient has difficulty maintaining the desired weight.

The patient with ulcerative colitis who has *anemia* is advised to plan for rest periods and to increase dietary intake of iron. The nurse should identify foods rich in iron for the patient. If iron losses are greater than can be replaced in the diet, supplemental iron may be needed. Oral iron supplements are better absorbed with orange juice or other sources of ascorbic acid. Taking them with foods such as milk can inhibit absorption. The patient should be advised that the stool will be black when taking iron. Checking the stool regularly for occult blood is necessary to detect blood loss. Some patients do not tolerate oral iron supplements, and the hematocrit and hemoglobin determinations indicate insufficient blood response. For these patients an intramuscular dextrose-iron complex may be used. To prevent leakage and staining of the skin, the preparation should be administered deeply, using the "Z track" technique.

There may be *perianal excoriations* from loose stool. The nurse should advise the patient to use soft tissue and cleanse well after each bowel movement. Sitting in a warm tub of water, drying thoroughly, and applying cornstarch lightly is also soothing.

Patients with ulcerative colitis often must cope with many *emotional problems.* There may be problems handling life stresses, particularly those involving losses. Unmet dependency needs and conflicts with conformity are commonly identified. Acknowledging feelings of anger may be difficult for the patient with ulcerative colitis. The patient may become discouraged and fearful of exacerbations of the disease.

The nurse needs to establish a good working relationship with the patient. Acceptance of patients with openness and honesty in the relationship is crucial, since these patients are perceptive of hostility in others and easily hurt. Listening to patients express feelings about their life and relationships is often helpful. Encouragement and reinforcement for successful coping is useful. The nurse should provide information and allow time for the patient to express feelings. Consistency in the relationship is important. If changes can be anticipated, the patient may be better able to cope if there has been an opportunity to talk through the coming event and its effects.

The nurse can also become a too-important support for the patient, who may find this unbearable. Unkept appointments may be a clue that the patient is feeling vulnerable. Discussing the situation and providing an opening for the patient to express feelings is useful. Acceptance of the patient's feelings is important. The nurse's withdrawal without an explanation or some exploration with the patient does not meet the patient's needs and often aggravates the situation.

Repeated sigmoidoscopic examinations are necessary to follow the activity of the disease and to detect proliferative changes, which often become malignant. Frequently the patient views these intrusive procedures as intentional trauma. The nurse should be aware of this possibility and, again, offer the patient an opportunity to express feelings.

Hospitalization for acute exacerbations may disrupt the patient's coping mechanisms, and sometimes the necessity of surgery is hard to accept. Preparation for hospitalization, explanations of the alterations in elimination which follow an ileostomy, and exploration of the meaning for the patient is often best accomplished by someone who has known the patient over a period of time.

Patients with ulcerative colitis should be assisted with any *socioeconomic problems.* Ulcerative colitis is found in persons from all socioeconomic levels, and each patient's needs are different. Sometimes housing and living conditions are inadequate because of limited economic resources. The expense of medication is frequently a concern. There are apt to be problems with family relationships. Stresses at work may also be aggravating the ulcerative colitis. The nurse can offer information about community resources the patient may find helpful. Frequently the patient exhibits a low tolerance for frustration, but each successful event helps build confidence. Referral to a social worker is often beneficial both for the patient and the family.

**Third-level nursing care** Hospitalization and intensive medical care is required for severe exacerbations of ulcerative colitis. Failure of medical therapy to control the patient's symptoms or the development of complications makes the ulcerative colitis patient a candidate for surgical intervention.

Nursing Assessment During an acute attack of ulcerative colitis, the findings on nursing assessment will be similar to those found in a less acute stage but more severe. The patient often has severe diarrhea, with 20 or more stools a day, and the stool contains more blood, mucus, and pus than feces. The patient complains of severe abdominal cramping, urgency of defecation, and often fecal incontinence. The patient may appear very thin, with little muscle mass and little padding over bony prominences. Fatigue and weakness are common. During the abdominal examination peristalsis is often visible and extreme tenderness is found. Bowel sounds are increased, reflecting a hyperactive bowel.

If blood loss has been severe, the pulse may begin to increase and the blood pressure decrease. Postural blood pressure readings are an excellent assessment technique to indicate the development of hypovolemia. After the patient sits up, a decrease in the systolic pressure of more than 10 mmHg and a concurrent increase in the pulse rate indicates a volume problem.

Hypovolemia also results from fluid losses associated with the diarrhea. As dehydration develops, the blood pressure falls further. Tissue turgor becomes poor, the mucous membranes become sticky, and the patient complains of severe thirst. Urine output decreases and becomes concentrated. The patient's temperature is often elevated. With progressive dehydration, the patient may become quite lethargic. Daily weights are important, as the amount of weight loss reflects the severity of dehydration.

With severe diarrhea, electrolytes as well as fluid are lost and the patient often develops hypokalemia, a low serum potassium. This electrolyte deficiency is exhibited by weakness, flaccid muscles, decreased or absent deep tendon reflexes, and cardiac arrhythmias.

Nursing Problems and Interventions During an acute exacerbation of ulcerative colitis, the patient is extremely ill and presents many challenging problems for the nurse. The most immediate of these is the development of *hypovolemia.* Restoration of volume with intravenous fluids is urgent to maintain perfusion of vital organs and requires careful monitoring of the patient's response. The frequency of monitoring may be hourly but is determined by the severity of the volume deficit and the response to fluid replacement. Central venous pressure, as well as the usual vital signs, is often measured. Measuring urine output and determining specific gravity are useful in evaluating the effect of therapy. After some of the volume has been replenished, the hematocrit reading may reveal a severe *anemia,* requiring blood transfusions. As soon as adequate urinary output is established, potassium salts are included in the intravenous fluids to treat the *hypokalemia,* which contributes to decreased bowel tone and, if not corrected, can play a part in precipitating toxic megacolon.

The control of *persistent diarrhea* presents other challenges to the nurse. In order to decrease the motility of the intestinal tract and in turn the abdominal cramping and frequency of rectal discharges, the patient is often given nothing by mouth. This, along with the dehydration, makes frequent mouth care important.

*Opium derivatives* will also decrease intestinal motility and may be used initially to control diarrhea. Because of their addicting potential, opiates are not advised for long term use. Diphenoxylate (Lomotil), a synthetic derivative of meperidine with small amounts of atropine, slows peristalsis and is often preferred. Anticholinergic drugs, although not very effective in controlling the spasms and diarrhea in ulcerative colitis, may be used. However, they are often contraindicated because of their systemic effects. Dilatation of the colon and bowel obstruction can be precipitated by indiscriminate use of antidiarrheal medications. An order for medication after each loose stool clearly calls for judgment on the part of the nurse. The total 24-hour dose of diphenoxylate should not exceed 20 mg. The amount is decreased as the diarrhea subsides.

*Intravenous corticosteroids* may be used to decrease inflammation and thereby help control the diarrhea. These drugs are particularly important if the patient received oral corticosteroids previously. Intravenous *antibiotics* may also be necessary to prevent or treat generalized sepsis in an acute exacerbation of ulcerative colitis. Occasionally antibiotics may prolong or increase the diarrhea, and the nurse must be aware of the patient's response to treatment.

If there is *urgency* to defecate the patient may want the security of a bedpan nearby. It should be clean and covered and easy for the patient to reach. A padded bedpan may be more comfortable and may also help prevent trauma to the coccyx and ischial areas. A bedside commode is often preferred by patients.

Frequent loose stools contribute to *perianal irritation* and skin breakdown. If urgency is so great that the patient loses sphincter control, maintaining skin integrity becomes more difficult. Cleansing well after each bowel movement is necessary to remove the irritants. After thorough drying, a light application of cornstarch is soothing. Control of *odors* requires careful attention. Prompt emptying and thorough cleansing of bedpans are essential. Soiled linen should be removed from the patient's area. Ventilation and the use of mechanical deodorizers are generally more satisfactory than deodorizers that attempt to mask an odor by superimposing another.

*Debilitation* is commonly seen with chronic inflammation and persistent diarrhea. Because the patient is in a poor nutritional state, skin breakdown may develop readily; therefore frequent changes of position are necessary. Foam mattresses, alternating pressure pads, or water beds are useful adjuncts to a regular turning schedule. When the patient's intake does not compensate for the protein losses, negative nitrogen balance often results. Intravenous fluids can replace volume but do not provide adequate protein and calories. To overcome this deficit, hyperalimentation is often used to provide bowel rest and improve nutrition. (Hyperalimentation is discussed in Chap. 16.) The inflammatory process in the bowel often decreases with the use of hyperalimentation.[8] In any event, the improved nutrition makes the patient a better risk for surgery, if it is needed.

Since activity promotes anabolism, the patient should be encouraged to ambulate while receiving hyperalimentation, if the physical condition is otherwise stable. Therapy with hyperalimentation is gradually decreased after the patient is able to resume oral intake. Supplemental feeding of elemental formulas may also be used to increase nutritional intake. However, the patient often finds these unpalatable and difficult to take (see Chap. 16).

The patient's activity needs to be balanced with adequate rest. Because diarrhea frequently disturbs rest, it is especially important that nursing-care activities be planned and organized to allow the patient some uninterrupted rest periods. If the person with ulcerative colitis requires complete bed rest, the nurse also attends to those measures that

prevent other hazards of *immobility*. Dorsal and plantar flexion and active leg exercises are important to maintain vascular tone and to prevent venous stasis. For this purpose antiembolic stockings are often worn. Changing position, deep breathing, and coughing improve circulation and promote lung expansion. Monitoring breath sounds aids the nurse in detecting potential pulmonary complications arising from immobility and excessive fluid replacement.

Frequently the problems in care of the patient with ulcerative colitis arise not so much from the physical care required as from the *emotional and psychological* requirements. Many believe that initially the ulcerative colitis patient benefits from being totally dependent in care during an acute exacerbation. This seems to meet some of the emotional needs and allows energy expenditure for tissue maintenance and repair. The nursing plan should be deliberate, with provisions for gradually increasing the patient's independent participation in care.

The behavior exhibited by the ulcerative colitis patient often drives the nursing staff away. It helps if the nurse tries to understand the reasons for the behavior and plans approaches to work with the patient. The nurse can help meet security and dependency needs by planned attention. An effective relationship may be established which will allow anger to be acknowledged and expressed directly. At the same time realistic limits should be set.

Patients with ulcerative colitis usually benefit from consistency in care. In view of the sensitivity to rejection by others, changes of assignments and days off can be interpreted as desertion by the nursing staff. It is important to inform patients of plans in advance and make sure they know who is responsible for care.

Family interpersonal relationships should also be evaluated. The problem stimulus is often intertwined in family dynamics. Family therapy or individual therapy may be beneficial.

Patients with ulcerative colitis may develop several *complications*. Common ones are toxic megacolon, perforation, stricture formation, and malignant changes. When complications develop, the nurse is guided by the care standards for the particular complications. Although the sequence of events associated with toxic megacolon and perforation differs, both result in adynamic intestinal obstruction, peritonitis, and often generalized sepsis. Stricture formation and malignant changes can lead to mechanical intestinal obstruction. Intestinal obstructions are discussed later in this chapter; perforation is discussed in Chap. 17.

*Surgical intervention* Debilitating diarrhea with cramping, toxic megacolon, obstructions, and the increased risk of cancer in persons with long-standing ulcerative colitis are indications for a *proctocolectomy and ileostomy.* An ileostomy allows the ileum to open to the external environment. The surgical procedure brings the terminal ileum through the abdominal wall, creating an opening for intestinal elimination. The remainder of the colon and rectum is removed (see Fig. 18-2*b*). Since the newly created opening does not have sphincter control and the contents of the ileum are liquid, it is necessary for the patient to wear an appliance to catch the drainage. While an ileostomy can be temporary, when done for ulcerative colitis it is generally a *permanent* alteration of the route for elimination.

Recently, an ileostomy modification which involves the creation of an *intra-abdominal pouch* and an artificial sphincter has been developed[9] (Fig. 18-2*e*). Proponents of this procedure say that the complexity and time of care are reduced. As the capacity of the pouch increases the patient is able to empty it three or four times a day by inserting a catheter. Problems of obtaining a good-fitting appliance and of maintaining skin integrity are reduced.[10] On the other hand, some find catheterizing the pouch inconvenient. The surgical procedure itself is not without risk, since operating time is longer than with an ileostomy. If complications such as perforation, fistula, or obstruction develop and require reoperation, as much as 45 cm of the small intestine may be lost.[11]

When bowel surgery will bypass the usual route for elimination, it is helpful to have the patient express concerns and ask questions regarding the management of the ostomy preoperatively. In a nonemergency situation there can be fittings of various appliances, and the site of the ostomy can be planned for the individual body contours in advance of the surgery. If available, an enterostomal therapist may be a helpful resource. Since bowel function is usually very private, there is limited knowledge of ostomies by the general public. It takes time for the patient to adjust to the altered body image. Volunteers from an ostomy club can be useful visitors. In most communities, the American Cancer Society maintains a list of suitable visitors who have ostomies.

*Preoperative bowel preparation* usually includes a low-residue or clear liquid diet, cathartics, and cleansing enemas. Sometimes oral antibiotics which are not readily absorbed from the gastrointestinal tract are given to reduce the number of intestinal organisms. However, it is impossible to "sterilize" the bowel, and preoperative oral antibiotics are not used routinely by all surgeons. The patient who has had corticosteroid therapy for treatment of colitis will need extra steroids preoperatively and in the immediate postoperative period.

*Following surgery* the patient will have the newly created stoma, an abdominal incision, and a perineal incision. The relationship between an ileostomy stoma and the abdominal incision is shown in color plate 18-2. In the operating room the stoma is fitted with a drainage bag and the primary abdominal incision is carefully protected from stomal discharges. An oiled-silk or plasticized skin drape

**FIGURE 18-2**
Surgical interventions of the bowel which alter elimination.

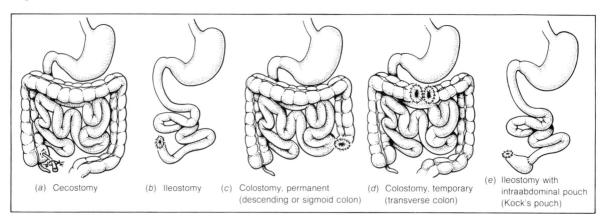

(*a*) Cecostomy   (*b*) Ileostomy   (*c*) Colostomy, permanent (descending or sigmoid colon)   (*d*) Colostomy, temporary (transverse colon)   (*e*) Ileostomy with intraabdominal pouch (Kock's pouch)

makes an effective barrier. The perineal incision may be packed and left open rather than being sutured. The patient will have a nasogastric tube connected to intermittent suction to remove gastric secretions and swallowed air until the bowel regains normal motility. Nothing will be given by mouth, and fluids will be administered intravenously. An indwelling urinary catheter may be used for several days.

*Relief of pain* is necessary so that the patient will move, breathe deeply, and cough. These activities are important to maintain good pulmonary function and decrease the risk of atelectasis and pneumonia, which are early complications of general anesthesia and abdominal surgery. Complications from blood loss also arise early. The nurse should check the dressings for evidence of external bleeding and monitor blood pressure and pulse to detect internal hemorrhage. Laboratory values such as the hematocrit and hemoglobin will provide further information regarding internal bleeding.

Postoperatively the patient has potential for *fluid and electrolyte imbalances* for several reasons. Initially one is concerned with the amount of blood lost during the operation. Then external or internal hemorrhage in the immediate postoperative period becomes a possibility. Neuroendocrine responses initiated by the trauma of surgery result in sodium and water retention. In one or two days diuresis with losses of water and potassium occurs. The removal of gastric secretions through the nasogastric tube results in the loss of large amounts of fluid and electrolytes that are usually reabsorbed. As the ileostomy begins to function there is increased loss of sodium as well as water, since the colon, which normally conserves water and sodium, has been removed. The patient may also have serosanguineous drainage from the perineal wound, and this protein loss may further decrease the effective circulating volume. If hyperalimentation was being given prior to surgery, this therapy will probably be continued until the patient is able to take adequate nutrition and fluids orally.

Accurate assessment of intake and output is essential. Records of output include the source of drainage, so that appropriate replacement of fluid and electrolytes can be planned. Serum electrolytes will be followed closely in the immediate postoperative period. Nursing observations should include levels of consciousness, mental alertness, and muscle tone, as well as the indicators of dehydration or fluid overload.

Cleanliness and freedom from odor contribute to the patient's sense of well-being. A good tight seal on the drainage bags and good ventilation decrease odor problems. Disposal of used equipment should be in closed containers outside the patient's immediate unit.

Protection of the skin from the ileostomy drainage should begin at once. The ileostomy drainage contains secretions rich in digestive enzymes. It takes only a short time for exposed skin to become red, painful, and excoriated. The stoma and surrounding skin should be washed with mild soap and water, rinsed well, and dried thoroughly. The stoma lacks nerve endings for pain, so it can be touched gently for cleansing. The skin can be protected with karaya powder or rings and plain tincture of benzoin. Stomahesive (Squibb) and Reliaseal (Davol) are examples of products which are satisfactory for skin protection. Stomahesive can be placed on oozing skin. As shown in color plates 18-3 and 18-4, the skin protector and appliance are fitted close to the stoma so that the skin is not exposed to irritating materials. To further protect the skin, adhesives should not be removed more often than necessary. If the bag can be opened on the end, the drainage is emptied without removing the adhesive each time. With some of the permanent appliances the adhesive need not be removed more often than every week. The amount of time between changes of the appliance varies with the individual. An adhesive remover may be applied with an eyedropper or soft gauze to facilitate removal but should be washed off thoroughly.

Even after explanation before surgery, the patient often is unable to comprehend what the ileostomy will be like. It may be difficult for the patient to look at the incision and stoma, especially if its existence is being denied. It is not uncommon for the patient to name or depersonalize the stoma as a means of coping. It takes time to incorporate this change into one's body image.

Patients are often repulsed by the drainage and the alterations in elimination. The nurse can acknowledge these feelings and yet proceed in a matter of fact way to care for the stoma, skin, and equipment. Telling the patient what is being done sets the stage for the patient's active participation later. As with all teaching-learning, the pace and sequence depend on the learner and on learner readiness.

The groundwork for the rehabilitation of the patient with an ileostomy may begin in second-level nursing care. Specific measures related to the care of the ostomy are begun in third-level nursing care. Further aspects of rehabilitation are discussed in fourth-level nursing care.

**Fourth-level nursing care**  Many patients seek minimal information and frequently change the subject when nurses begin discussing how to care for and live with an ostomy. The patient should know the essentials of care before being discharged, but may not have had time to accept the ostomy during hospitalization. Much energy is directed toward recovering from the surgery. However, the nurse should cover information related to care of the skin, changing the appliance, obtaining supplies and equipment, and control of odor. Resources for help after hospitalization should be addressed. There may be questions about food, clothing, and activities. Going home for visits during hospitalization to help the patient anticipate what the needs might be and to provide for a smoother transition from hospital to home has been suggested.[12] Discharge planning should include referral to the community health nurse for follow-up of nursing problems. At the very least the patient should have a name and number to call as questions arise.

Before going home the patient should have the equipment needed for care of the ileostomy and know where to obtain additional supplies. Since the stoma may become smaller, disposable equipment may be used temporarily. When healing has taken place and the stoma has attained a stable size, a permanent appliance can be fitted. Once the patient has gained weight, it may be necessary to have the appliance refitted as body contours change. Weight loss or weight gain necessitates checking the appliance for proper fit.

Essential qualities of the permanent appliance are good fit and ease of application and cleansing. Once these are determined, cost, durability, and aesthetics are considered in the selection. It is helpful if the patient can see displays of available equipment and then select the type that best meets individual requirements (see Fig. 18-3).

At first the drainage from the ileostomy is liquid. As the body adjusts to the alteration, some water reabsorption takes place in the ileum. Eventually the stool may have a soft consistency. Some recommend bismuth subgallate by mouth to reduce odors and to thicken discharge. Changing the appliance is best done when the ileostomy is quiescent—normally early in the morning, in the evening, or between meals. The time, of course, should be at the individual's convenience. With an ileostomy, odors are not usually a problem if the appliance fits well. The appliance should be cleaned thoroughly. Soaking in a dilute solution of vinegar (1 or 2 tablespoons in a quart of water), drying well, and airing between uses are recommended.

Usually there are no *dietary restrictions* following an ileostomy. The patient should be encouraged to experiment with new foods and discover which foods to avoid. Only one new food should be tried at a time, so that any intolerance can be pin-

**FIGURE 18-3**
Variety of appliances used for the collection of fecal and urinary excretions. (*Photo courtesy of United Surgical Corporation.*)

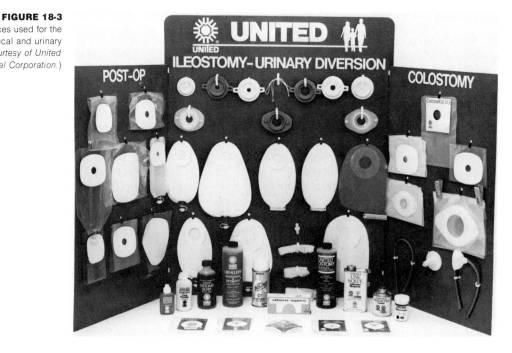

pointed. Generally, the patient should avoid foods which previously had laxative effects or caused gas. A well-balanced diet is desirable. The person with an ileostomy is chronically depleted of salt and water and does not tolerate sodium losses. The patient should be taught to increase salt and water intake when there is increased perspiration or gastrointestinal upsets.

*Skin problems* sometimes develop because the patient is allergic to the appliance material or because perspiration under the appliance provides a good environment for fungal growth. Mycostatin powders are recommended by some. Trying different equipment may also solve the problem.

Obstruction of an ileostomy is rarely a problem. However, if the stoma is very small or contracted, it may be necessary to dilate it regularly so that the little finger is easily inserted. Decreasing foods which are high in indigestible material may also help.

After convalescence, there is no medical reason why the person with an ileostomy cannot carry on normal work and social activities, but sometimes encouragement to resume activity that involves other people is needed. Swimming is not a problem if the appliance fits properly. As patients learn to manage their ostomies, travel can be planned without difficulties.

Intercourse for a woman may be painful until the perineum heals. Sometimes perineal nerve damage interferes with sexual activity in the male, but usually satisfying sexual activity is possible. However, there may be some feelings on the part of both the patient and the sexual partner to be resolved. The patient must adjust to a significant change in body image, and self-esteem is often diminished. It is important to consider past sexual adjustments. The nurse can provide an opening for discussion of these concerns. Women with ileostomies have become pregnant and successfully borne children. Articles authored by ileostomates attest to successful rehabilitation in all spheres of life.

The United Ostomy Association publishes helpful materials for patients. It also sponsors conferences and local ostomy groups in which people share solutions to problems in managing and living with an ostomy. Local branches of the American Cancer Society furnish some of these publications to patients and professionals.

Although one is encouraged to pursue individual interests, sometimes fellow members in an ostomy club pave the way for acceptance of the body change and provide an opportunity to begin talking about the change. In addition, sharing experiences covering a broad range of topics, e.g., equipment, travel, and sexual adjustments, is helpful in total rehabilitation.

### Crohn's Disease

Crohn's disease, sometimes called regional enteritis or transmural colitis, is another chronic inflammatory disease of the bowel. As with ulcerative colitis, the cause is unknown and there are spontaneous remissions and exacerbations. Crohn's disease has been thought to be a disease of the small intestine particularly affecting the terminal ileum. The disease process may involve the whole bowel, however, and have systemic manifestations as well.[13]

In contrast to the contiguous spread in ulcerative colitis, the inflammatory process in Crohn's disease is scattered and clearly demarcated from portions of normal bowel. These "skip" lesions are described as *cobblestone markings*. Fistula tracts from the colon or small bowel to bladder, vagina, and skin often develop. Scarring may narrow the lumen. Acute inflammation in the terminal ileum is sometimes confused with acute appendicitis. The effects of Crohn's disease are similar to those of ulcerative colitis. Surgical intervention is not advised. If it is attempted, as much of the bowel as possible is retained. Following surgery, the recurrence rate of Crohn's disease is high.

### Appendicitis

Appendicitis, an acute inflammation of the vermiform appendix of the cecum, is a common surgical problem in people under 40. Obstruction of the appendiceal lumen from fecaliths, foreign bodies, tumors, or twisting initiates inflammation. Complications of acute appendicitis are perforation, abscess formation, and generalized peritonitis.

Appendicitis occurs in all age groups, but in the young and in the elderly, early signs may be missed. The onset is usually characterized by vomiting and periumbilical pain, which later localizes in the right lower quadrant. The pain is aggravated by movement, bowel sounds are decreased, and constipation is usual. There is tenderness on abdominal and rectal exams. The white blood count is elevated to between 10,000 and 20,000/mm$^3$, and the temperature is usually elevated.

Laxatives and enemas are *avoided* when there is abdominal pain, as stimulation of the bowel can precipitate perforation. Food and fluid should be withheld. Pain medication should not be given until the diagnosis has been confirmed, so that symptoms will not be masked. Positioning in semi-Fowler's position with knees flexed may provide some comfort.

The treatment for appendicitis is an appendectomy, and recovery is usually uneventful. As soon as bowel sounds return, the diet can be advanced rapidly. Ambulation is begun the day of surgery. If the appendix ruptures, however, peritonitis ensues and recovery is delayed. The patient then requires antibiotics, intravenous fluids, and often nasogastric intubation. Perforation into the peritoneum is discussed in greater detail in Chap. 17.

### Infectious Diarrheas

Many *acute* inflammations of the bowel are caused from food or water contaminated with organisms or their toxins and are referred to as *bacterial gastroenteritis* or *enterocolitis.* They are characterized by acute diarrhea lasting a few hours or days. Occasionally chronic diarrhea results.

Thorough handwashing before food preparation and eating, cleanliness in food preparation, proper refrigeration, and adequate cooking of meats, poultry, and egg products are preventive measures which cannot be overstressed. Using boiled water in areas of questionable sanitation is also useful. Fecal contamination of food or water supplies accounts for outbreaks of gastroenteritis with *Salmonella, Shigella,* pathogenic strains of *E. coli,* and *V. cholerae.* Improper cleansing of fiberscopes has been incriminated in transferring *Salmonella.*[14]

Fluid and electrolyte replacement is necessary with prolonged diarrheas. Intestinal absorbants and drugs to decrease motility may give symptomatic relief but should be used judiciously. Antibiotics are often not used unless there is evidence of systemic involvement, as their use can lead to resistant strains of organisms and in some cases prolong the time organisms are found in the stool.

The onset of *amebic diarrhea* is usually more gradual than that of bacterial gastroenteritis. Cysts and motile amebae can be found in warm, fresh stools or in specimens fixed with a special preservative. Treatment is with amebicides, some of which are effective in the lumen while others work in the tissues. Follow-up requires six successive stool specimens. Reexamination of stools is frequently indicated in 3 months.

*Worm infestations* may be a factor in persistent diarrheas. History and laboratory findings are especially enlightening. Since many worms gain entry in man by penetrating the skin of the feet and legs, wearing shoes in unsanitary areas and avoiding snail-infested waters in some parts of the world are preventive measures.

An important roundworm infection in the United States is *trichinosis.* The larvae are ingested in infected pork and mature in the stomach and duodenum. After mating, the female worms burrow into the mucosa of the small intestine, giving rise to gastrointestinal symptoms about 4 days after the infected meat is eaten. Larvae migrate in the bloodstream and encyst in striated muscles. Systemic disruptions range from mild to fatal, depending on the number of larvae and the tissues invaded. Larval invasion is characterized by myositis, fever, prostration, periorbital edema, and at times myocarditis and encephalitis. Infected meat cannot be detected by inspection, so all pork and pork products should be thoroughly cooked before eating. Cooking kills Trichinella, but smoking and pickling do not. Utensils for preparing pork should be thoroughly cleaned before being used for other food.

## INTESTINAL OBSTRUCTIONS

Elimination from the gastrointestinal tract can be interrupted by an obstruction anywhere along the bowel. The obstruction can be partial, allowing small amounts of intestinal contents to pass through the bowel, or complete, stopping passage of all intestinal contents.

### Pathophysiology

The pathophysiologic changes that occur in intestinal obstruction are illustrated in Fig. 18-4. Obstruction of the intestinal lumen causes an accumulation of fluid and gas proximal to the site of the obstruction, distending the bowel. The distention increases intestinal secretions and decreases absorption, resulting in a further buildup of fluids. During the first few hours after the lumen is blocked, peristalsis increases in an attempt to push contents past the obstruction. With increasing distention, venous return is diminished so that fluid from the capillaries is lost to the lumen, peritoneal cavity, and bowel wall. The edematous bowel wall becomes permeable, and bacteria and fluid within the lumen enter the peritoneal cavity, causing peritonitis. The pressure eventually compromises the arterial blood supply and necrosis of the bowel wall develops. The increased peristalsis and the accumulation of fluid and gas result in elevated intraluminal pressures. The small intestine can accommodate pressures up to 120 mmHg, but the colon has lower pressure limits.[15] The last stage of intestinal obstruction, if high pressures are unrelieved, is the bursting of the intestine and the spilling of its contents into the peritoneum. In response to this foreign material, the peritoneum becomes inflamed and secretes fluid faster than it can be reabsorbed, resulting in ascites, an accumulation of fluid in the peritoneal cavity.

**Causes** Intestinal obstructions arise from a variety of causes, some of which are illustrated in Fig. 18-5. The causes, generally, are considered mechanical, nervous, or vascular in origin. *Mechanical obstructions* are physical blockages of the intestinal lumen either from within or from outside the bowel. Hernias, neoplasms, adhesions, foreign bodies, intussusception, and volvulus cause mechanical obstruction. An intestinal obstruction of *nervous origin* results when the impulses to the bowel for propulsive movements are absent, diminished, or uncoordinated. This is called *adynamic ileus.* An obstruction can also develop when the bowel becomes damaged by *impaired blood supply,* as happens in occlusion of mesenteric vessels.

**H**ernias Hernias account for about 1 percent of the intestinal obstructions (Fig. 18-5b). They can be defined as protrusions of the contents of the peritoneal cavity through incompetent openings or weaknesses in the abdominal wall. Serosal lined sacs are formed and may contain fat, omentum, and portions of bowel. Some hernias are pronounced only with straining and subside when the person lies down. Others are noticeable at all times but can be manipulated to return the hernia contents to the peritoneal cavity. These hernias are considered *reducible.* At the other end of the spectrum are *incarcerated* hernias, in which segments of viscera are caught and cannot be reduced, and *strangulated* hernias, in which the blood supply to the hernia contents is cut off. Hernias can potentially obstruct the intestines. This most commonly occurs in the small intestine, because the colon is relatively fixed retroperitoneally.

   *Inguinal hernias* are the most common and are found more in men than in women. They form in defects of the posterior inguinal floor and can be direct or indirect. *Indirect inguinal hernias* arise where the cord structures enter the inguinal canal and are sometimes felt in the scrotum. *Direct inguinal hernias* arise in defects of the inferior medial area of the inguinal floor. Other common

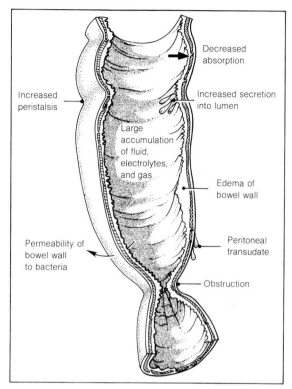

**FIGURE 18-4**
Pathophysiology of intestinal obstruction and peritonitis. (*Adapted from Nadrowski, 1974.*)

sites for hernias are in the *femoral* and *umbilical* areas and at *surgical incisions.*

**A**dhesions Mechanical obstruction of the bowel can also develop from *contraction of scar tissue.* Repeated ulcerations of the bowel may be repaired with scar tissue, and as this tissue contracts, strictures are apt to develop. Strictures may also develop at sites of surgical anastomosis. Bands of scar tissue, called adhesions (Fig. 18-5a), develop outside the bowel. The adhesions may entrap portions of the bowel, causing obstruction. Obstruction from adhesions can develop months after abdominal surgery, intra-abdominal chemotherapy, or radiation.

**N**eoplasms Elimination can also be interrupted when the intestinal lumen is blocked by a *tumor* (Fig. 18-5c). *Polyps* and *cancer* are the most common neoplasms causing obstruction. In familial polyposis, a Mendelian autosomal dominant trait, hundreds to thousands of polyps may develop with no symptoms for years. If these polyps are untreated, cancers with multiple primary sites arise and obstruction often results.

Cancer of the rectum and colon is the most common type of intestinal neoplasm. It was predicted that 101,000 Americans would develop colorectal cancer during 1977.[16] Persons at greater risk for developing colon cancers include those with ulcerative colitis of more than ten years' duration, those with gastrointestinal polyposis, and members of families with a history of colorectal cancers and polyps. These cancers tend to occur slightly more often in women than in men.

A great number of colon and rectal cancers evolve from a polyp. The average time for malignant changes to develop is 10 to 15 years, after which, in 1 to 2 years, they encircle the lumen, causing an obstruction. They generally spread by direct extension and by metastasis to the regional lymph nodes, liver, lungs and bone.

**Intussusception** Intussusception is the telescoping of one portion of the bowel into another, forming an obstruction (Fig. 18-5f). In children this happens spontaneously, whereas in adults often a polyp gets caught in the fecal stream, beginning the telescoping of the bowel. In children this mechanical obstruction may be relieved with a barium enema, but in adults, surgical correction is necessary.

**Volvulus** Another example of mechanical obstruction is *volvulus,* the twisting of the bowel upon itself (Fig. 18-5d). Volvulus more commonly involves the small intestine, although redundant loops of sigmoid may also twist around the mesentery, giving symptoms of obstruction. Factors associated with volvulus formation are a high-residue diet, chronic constipation, habitual abuse of laxatives and enemas, and previous abdominal operations. As with intussusception, a barium enema may correct the obstruction in children, but in adults, surgical intervention is needed.

**Foreign Bodies** Any foreign body ingested or formed within the body is a potential cause of intestinal obstruction. Dry, impacted stool often causes symptoms of obstruction. Impacted barium from inadequate elimination after barium studies

**FIGURE 18-5**
Some causes of intestinal obstruction.

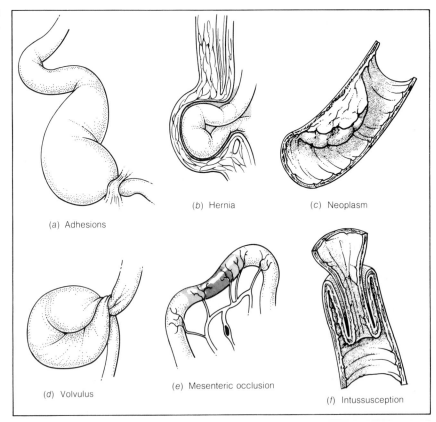

(a) Adhesions

(b) Hernia

(c) Neoplasm

(d) Volvulus

(e) Mesenteric occlusion

(f) Intussusception

is not uncommon. Foreign bodies such as fruit pits and gallstones have also obstructed the bowel. Many patients who develop obstruction from foreign materials have a lumen already narrowed from strictures or cancers. *Phytobezoars*—masses composed of vegetable matter usually found in the stomach—have caused obstructions in persons who have previously had extensive gastric surgery. A variety of foods from citrus pulp to grape leaves have been found in obstructions. More rarely, and usually in patients with psychiatric problems, balls of hair called *trichobezoars* are found. Large round-worms can also cause intestinal obstructions.

**A**dynamic Ileus  The bowel can be considered obstructed if a portion of it no longer produces pro-pulsive movements to advance the intestinal con-tents. This is the case in *adynamic ileus,* also re-ferred to as *paralytic ileus.* Impulses that stimulate propulsive movements are absent, diminished, or uncoordinated. Adynamic ileus may occur after general anesthesia, after abdominal surgery, with electrolyte imbalances (especially hypokalemia), with peritoneal irritation, after trauma, during acute infections, or as a consequence of metabolic im-balance. *Toxic megacolon,* an acute dilatation of the colon seen with massive bowel destruction in ulcerative colitis and Crohn's disease, is a form of ileus. Drugs used to decrease intestinal motility can also precipitate an ileus in an already disturbed bowel.

When the arterial blood supply to a portion of the intestine is interrupted, that segment initially goes into spasm and then relaxes, resulting in an adynamic ileus. If the circulation is not restored, infarction occurs and the bowel becomes nec-rotic.[17] *Mesenteric ischemia* arises from occlu-sions with emboli or with narrowing of vessels in extensive atherosclerosis or from vasoconstriction of the splanchnic vessels in response to a fall in cardiac output (Fig. 18-5e). The elderly, extremely ill patient is particularly susceptible to intestinal ob-structions of vascular origin, but many patients in severe shock also develop multiple intestinal infarctions.

**Effects on the patient**  As the bowel becomes obstructed, the immediate effect is *distention.* The distention at first is localized, but if the obstruction persists in the lower portion of the bowel, the dis-tention soon becomes generalized. In mechanical obstruction, the increase in peristalsis proximal to the obstruction is manifested in *increased bowel sounds* and *severe, colicky abdominal pain* that

coincides with the peristaltic contractions. If the small intestine becomes distended, the pain is usu-ally referred to the periumbilical area. Pain from large-intestine distention is referred to the sacral area. With an adynamic ileus, the bowel sounds are diminished or absent and the abdominal pain is constant. With a partial obstruction, diarrheal stools are common, but with complete obstruction, after the bowel distal to the obstruction is empty, the patient is unable to pass any stool or flatus.

Intestinal obstructions result in many *fluid and electrolyte changes.* Fluids and electrolytes are lost to the intestinal lumen as secretion increases while absorption decreases. Further fluids and electro-lytes are lost to the peritoneal cavity as capillary permeability increases, allowing serum to leak into the peritoneum. As obstruction persists, the bowel wall becomes permeable and bloody luminal fluid escapes into the peritoneum. In response to this irritant, the peritoneum itself becomes inflamed, producing more fluid than can be absorbed. These losses are manifested in *dehydration* and *ascites.*

*Vomiting* further compromises fluid and elec-trolyte balance. The nature of the vomitus depends on the location of the obstruction. When the ob-struction is high in the small intestine, the patient soon vomits large amounts of gastric and intes-tinal secretions. This vomitus is often bile-stained. If the obstruction occurs in the ileum or colon, vomiting occurs later and the vomitus often con-tains fecal material. With intestinal obstructions, more bicarbonate than acid is usually lost in the vomitus, and *metabolic acidosis* results. To com-pensate for the acidosis, the respirations increase in an attempt to blow off excess $CO_2$ (acid). The ascites and distention, however, impinge on res-pirations, disturbing this compensatory mech-anism. When the obstruction occurs near the distal end of the large intestine, vomiting usually does not occur. Distention is more pronounced than with small-bowel obstruction, and the patient experi-ences an intense feeling of constipation.

*Impaired oxygenation* of the bowel mucosa and bowel wall is significant in the development of necrosis and perforation in intestinal obstruction. Fever and leukocytosis are systemic manifestations of the tissue necrosis, peritonitis, and sepsis. Gen-eralized abdominal distention interferes with res-piratory ventilation, thereby decreasing the oxygen available for all cellular functions.

*Metabolic changes* in intestinal obstruction re-sult from decreased absorption from a distended bowel and from food and fluid restrictions. The life-threatening complications of complete intestinal obstructions usually develop rapidly, however, and overshadow catabolic changes.

### First-level Nursing Care

First-level nursing care is aimed at prevention and early identification of conditions which can lead to obstructions. The nurse involved with well-child care and with school, camp, and preemployment physical examinations is in a position to detect hernias early. The three commonly described hernias are ventral, inguinal, and femoral. Ventral hernias occur in the abdominal wall and are frequently seen in the umbilicus or at operative sites. They are usually readily seen on inspection and will recede with pressure, allowing the nurse to feel the opening.

An inguinal hernia occurs through an opening in the inguinal canal. To assess the inguinal canal in a male, the nurse should indent the scrotum on each side with the little finger until the inguinal ring is felt. The ring may be dilated if the examiner's fingertip can enter. The patient should also be asked to cough or bear down so that the ring can be reassessed. If a hernia is present, a mass will be felt. Inguinal hernias in the female are usually tender and bulging.

The femoral canal may be evaluated by placing the right index finger on the right femoral artery. The middle finger will be on the femoral vein and the ring finger on the canal. It is normally not palpable. A hernia can be felt as a soft mass.

Any lump in the groin area should be investigated. The subject should be referred for medical evaluation and elective surgical repair before complications develop. If surgery is not feasible, as may be the case with extremely obese, elderly, or debilitated patients or with some cardiac patients, certain precautions that minimize the possibility of incarceration and strangulation should be emphasized. These include applying firm pressure over the hernia before coughing or straining, investigating and treating chronic coughs, not flying in an unpressurized airplane without a truss or a pressure dressing if the hernia is large, and avoiding heavy lifting.

To avoid obstruction from foreign bodies, the state of the teeth should be assessed and the importance of adequate chewing emphasized. This is especially important in persons with previous gastrointestinal surgery. Simple instruction in chewing food thoroughly may be adequate. If not, repair of the teeth or well-fitting dentures may be necessary to ensure proper chewing. Hard, indigestible seeds and fruit pits should be avoided.

Popcorn and nuts, if not well chewed, can also precipitate obstruction, especially if other conditions have narrowed the lumen. The very young and the elderly usually manage food better if the pits and seeds are removed before serving.

Since cancer is a major cause of obstruction, public education regarding the early warning signs of cancer is appropriate. The early warning signs published by the American Cancer Society are a useful adjunct to patient education. A thorough discussion of early detection of cancer can be found in Chap. 5.

First-level nursing care to prevent obstruction also includes work with family members of the person with a diagnosis of familial polyposis. The family should be informed of risk to future offspring, and the importance of follow-up on a regular basis for all family members should be emphasized.

*Constipation* is the passage of hard, dry stools with difficulty or unusual delay in defecation and is a common complaint. In the hectic pace of contemporary society, people inhibit the urge to defecate, feces are retained longer in the colon, and more water is absorbed, making the stools harder and more difficult to pass. Constipation can be a manifestation of local disease in the colon and rectum or of depression and general metabolic disorders. Many drugs have constipating effects. More commonly, however, complaints of constipation relate to the idea that a bowel movement every day is essential for health and to the abuse of laxatives, cathartics, and enemas.

If no bowel pathology is present and a person is concerned about improved bowel function, some simple suggestions may help. These include moderate exercise, a balanced diet including some roughage, fluid intake of at least 2000 ml every day, and establishing a regular time to respond to the urge to defecate. Some people find taking one or two glasses of fluid before breakfast, eating a good breakfast, and allowing some toilet time after breakfast are effective. The addition of three tablespoons of bran to the daily diet adds bulk and decreases the transit time of wastes through the intestine.

Laxatives and cathartics should not be used regularly in spite of the advertisements that bombard us. Their chronic use can damage the myoneural plexuses and the bowel mucosa and lead to electrolyte loss. A vicious cycle is established.

Persons who are immobilized, who are not aware of the need to defecate, or who are dependent on others to get them to the toilet are candidates for fecal impactions. If a person is not competent or not able to take care of elimination needs, the family or caretakers should make note of defecations. The nurse can be helpful in working with the family or caretakers. Increasing fluid intake, eating foods that help maintain a soft stool, and providing time for defecation may prevent an impaction. A stool softener may be helpful. Medications should be used judiciously, as dependency often occurs. Patients should be taught to avoid the chronic intake of laxatives. Contracting the abdominal muscles is something an immobilized patient can do to try to retain muscle tone. The nurse should also review other prescriptions which may be contributing to constipation and discuss plans with the physician to see whether modification may be possible.

### Second-level Nursing Care

The most common nonacute intestinal obstruction results from fecal impactions. They are commonly seen in elderly persons at home or in nursing homes.

When giving a *health history,* the patient, family, or caretaker is often unable to remember the last bowel movement. Rather, diarrhea or incontinence is often complained of because small amounts of liquid stool ooze around an impaction. The patient may also complain of a feeling of constipation, bloating, and anorexia. Knowledge of the amount and type of intake is useful in the assessment.

The *physical examination* focuses on the abdomen and rectum. Inspection and percussion of the abdomen may reveal distention. Bowel sounds are usually normal. Masses of fecal matter are often palpable. Hard feces may also be felt during the rectal examination.

Once the presence of a fecal impaction is established, *nursing interventions* should be instituted before the obstruction becomes acute. If fecal material is felt during the rectal examination, in many instances, it can be broken up and removed manually. An oil retention enema helps to soften any remaining stool, which can then be evacuated with a cleansing enema. The measures to prevent future impactions discussed in first-level nursing care should be taught. If these measures prove inadequate, a stool softener may be helpful.

### Third-level Nursing Care

Most intestinal obstructions other than those from fecal impactions are acute conditions requiring hospitalization. If a patient is thought to have an obstruction, immediate referral should be made for a thorough evaluation.

**Nursing assessment**   A careful *health history* of the patient with an obstruction may give many clues about the site involved and the underlying cause. The patient should be questioned about any previous illness, with special attention to a history of cancer, polyps, chronic constipation, and chronic inflammations such as diverticulitis or ulcerative colitis. Previous abdominal operations should also be noted.

Early symptoms the patient experienced should be explored. Obstructions in the small bowel usually begin with nausea and vomiting, with distention appearing later. Conversely, large-bowel obstructions begin with distention. A decrease in the diameter of the stool and small amounts of liquid stool are also early signs of beginning large-intestine obstruction. Vomiting is a later development. The patient should be questioned about the duration of the vomiting and the nature of the vomitus. In small-bowel obstructions it consists of gastric and intestinal juices and is bile-tinged. Fecal matter, however, often appears in the vomitus associated with obstruction in the large bowel.

**P**hysical Assessment   During physical examination, special attention should be given to the abdominal and rectal examinations. The abdomen will appear distended, and if the obstruction is fairly recent, peristalsis may be visible. Incarcerated hernias or volvulus may be apparent. With mechanical obstruction, bowel sounds are generally increased, while they are decreased or absent in adynamic ileus. During percussion, the abdomen will sound tympanic and ascites may be evident. The patient's abdomen will be tender. In large-bowel obstructions fecal matter is often palpable. An obstruction in the rectum may be felt during the rectal examination.

Because large volumes of fluid are being lost in intestinal obstructions, it is important to assess fluid and electrolyte status. The amount of fluid lost to the peritoneal cavity can be estimated during the abdominal examination, using the criteria of shifting dullness, the fluid wave, and the puddle technique (see Chap. 11). The amount lost through vomiting should also be determined. Depending on the degree of dehydration, the patient will experience mild to extreme thirst and may have sticky mucous membranes and poor tissue turgor. The patient's urine is likely to be scant and dark amber in color and have an increased specific gravity, reflecting the kidney's effort to conserve water. As dehydration becomes severe, hypovolemia will develop. The patient should be closely observed for increases in pulse or respiration and decreases in blood pressure, since a patient with intestinal obstruction is a prime candidate for shock. If the intestinal obstruction involves a strangulated or infarcted bowel that has necrosed, fever may be present.

**D**iagnostic Tests   When intestinal obstruction is suspected, certain diagnostic tests may be used. An x-ray of the abdomen often reveals increased fluid and gas levels in an obstructed bowel. Other tests usually done include sigmoidoscopy, colonoscopy, and sometimes a barium enema. Barium is not given orally if obstruction is suspected, as it will not be possible to eliminate it. These tests are discussed in more detail in the section on inflammatory bowel disease. If acute mesenteric ischemia is suspected, angiography may be done to locate occlusions and areas of low perfusion. Laboratory tests usually reflect the dehydration and inflammation. The hematocrit reading is often increased and the white blood count elevated.

**Nursing problems and interventions**   The most pressing problem is the *abdominal distention.* Pressure within the bowel must be relieved before the patient's condition can be stabilized. This is most frequently accomplished through decompression. For high obstruction, a nasogastric tube connected to intermittent suction is inserted. This aids in preventing fluid and gas accumulation. More frequently, however, a long, weighted tube, illustrated in Fig. 18-6, is inserted nasogastrically and gradually advanced to the site of obstruction. Early in the insertion process the position of the tube is assessed to ensure that it has not entered the lungs. Intermittent suction through this tube then removes accumulated fluid and gas. Positioning the patient on the right side aids in passage of the tube through the pylorus, and Fowler's position or walking then helps to advance it through the intestine. Once the tube reaches the jejunum, the physician may order the tube advanced periodically. The tube is lubricated well and advanced the distance ordered as the patient swallows. The use of viscous Xylocaine along with a water-soluble jelly for lubricating the tube relieves some of the nasal discomfort. Extra tubing should be coiled loosely so that the weight of the tube does not interfere with its movement through the bowel. The position of the tube is checked regularly with x-ray or fluoroscopy.

The patient's progress during decompression should be evaluated regularly. Careful assessment of the abdomen will aid in this. It is often helpful to measure abdominal girth at regular intervals. The drainage should be measured accurately so that adequate intravenous fluid and electrolyte replacements can be planned. Intravenous fluid administration requires careful monitoring, since rapid replacement of fluid can further increase the fluid accumulation in the bowel lumen. If the obstruction is in the large bowel, the patient may be allowed a liquid diet, which will be absorbed before it gets to the site of obstruction.

As with any nasogastric tube, *mouth care* is very important. If the patient is too weak or uncomfortable to carry this out independently, assistance from the nurse adds to the patient comfort. Mouthwash diluted with water and ice is refreshing if used to supplement regular cleansing procedures. A water-soluble jelly or mouth cream keeps lips soft and comfortable. Lozenges may soothe the throat.

*Maintaining patency* of the tube is important if decompression is to be successful. Irrigation of the tube with normal saline may be ordered. It is difficult, however, to recover the irrigating fluid immediately, and the amount used should be recorded so that an accurate output can be calculated.

To remove the decompression tube, one should pull it gradually; too-rapid removal could damage the bowel. Since the tube is being pulled against peristalsis, the patient may experience some nausea. As the tube is withdrawn, the weighted portion can be brought out through the mouth and the mercury or weight removed. Swift disposal of the tube and thorough mouth care is imperative after removal, since there is often fecal material and odor on the tube.

In *adynamic ileus,* decompression and replacement of potassium levels may promote the return of bowel function. Mild activity and changing of position may help to eliminate flatus and thereby decrease distention. Recent authors have described various positions such as a headstand that aid in relieving flatus.[18] These positions for relief of flatulence have not been widely tested, but in selected patients various positions could be tried. More traditional measures to relieve distention in adynamic ileus include the insertion of a rectal tube for 20 to 30 minutes, flushes in which a mild enema solution is alternately administered and siphoned off, and medications such as neostigmine and prostigmine, which stimulate peristalsis. Narcotic analgesic medications delay the return of bowel function.

Another urgent problem arising from unrelieved obstruction and inadequate restoration of circulating volume is the development of *hypovolemia* and shock. Care of the patient in shock is discussed in detail in Chap. 28.

Patients with intestinal obstructions often demonstrate other *fluid and electrolyte imbalances.* Intake and output needs to be recorded accurately. Daily weights are also helpful in assessing hydration. Generally, the patient's only intake will be intravenous fluids. Special attention should be given to ensure that the patient's parenteral fluid replacement is adequate. Serum electrolytes should be assessed regularly to aid in planning for replacement fluids.

**S**urgical Intervention   Most mechanical obstructions require surgical intervention. The specific procedure will depend on the cause. With strangulated hernias, the hernia is repaired and necrotic bowel removed. Neoplasms are generally removed. With mesenteric infarction, an embolectomy and vascular reconstruction may be done. Likewise, adhesions, intussusception, and volvulus all require various surgical repairs. Some common operations associated with bowel obstruction are discussed below.

*Hernia repairs*   Reducible hernias may be repaired under local or general anesthesia by returning the abdominal contents to the peritoneal cavity and closing the defect in the abdominal wall. If the hernia is strangulated, immediate surgical intervention is necessary. The trapped bowel is freed, any gangrenous portion is resected, the remaining bowel is anastomosed, and the defect in the abdominal wall is closed. The care of the patient following a strangulated hernia operation is similar to that required after a bowel resection.

After repair of an inguinal hernia the male patient may experience painful scrotal swelling. Ice bags and a scrotal support may be helpful. The scrotum may be elevated with a rolled towel or a soft sling while the patient is in bed. Urinary retention and abdominal distention are to be reported promptly so that measures can be taken to prevent strain on the repair. Early ambulation, standing to void, and using the toilet for defecation are clearly indicated in the postoperative period.[19] After hernia repairs, many patients are fearful of bursting the incision. They are often afraid to ambulate and need to be encouraged to stand straight. The gas pains that patients experience usually subside quickly once a regular diet and bowel movements resume. The hernia patient should be taught to place a hand firmly over the incision when cough-

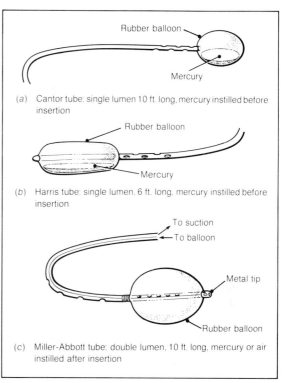

(*a*)   Cantor tube: single lumen 10 ft. long, mercury instilled before insertion

(*b*)   Harris tube: single lumen, 6 ft. long, mercury instilled before insertion

(*c*)   Miller-Abbott tube: double lumen, 10 ft. long, mercury or air instilled after insertion

**FIGURE 18-6**
Tubes used for intestinal decompression.

ing. Conditions which predispose to recurrences of hernias are incisional infections, obesity, repeated episodes of coughing, straining at stool, and heavy lifting. After simple hernia repair, patients are usually able to return to sedentary work in 1 week and to more strenuous work in 4 to 6 weeks.

*Surgical decompression*   If the patient is too ill for extensive surgery to repair an obstruction, a surgical decompression may be done. This is a palliative procedure that involves the insertion of a cecostomy tube through an opening in the bowel near the cecum (Fig. 18-2*a*). The cecostomy tube is then used to drain the intestine either by gravity or with intermittent suction. The drainage is thick and foul-smelling. To maintain patency of the tube and ensure drainage, frequent irrigation with normal saline is needed. Drainage around the cecostomy tube necessitates thorough cleansing of the skin and frequent dressing changes.

*Bowel resection*   If the patient's condition warrants, a more definitive approach to the obstruction is made. The diseased portion of the bowel may be removed and the healthy segments anastomosed. Because the bowel is to be entered, an attempt is made to rid the bowel of all fecal material. If the patient is allowed oral intake, a low-residue diet is often given for several days and clear liquids are given the day before surgery. Cleansing enemas are used. Poorly absorbed oral antibiotics (neomycin) or sulfonamides (succinylsulfathiazole) may be administered for several days before surgery to reduce the number of bacteria in the colon. Some physicians think, however, that the complications from these drugs are greater than the benefits and therefore do not use them.

*Postoperatively,* the patient will have a nasogastric tube to remove fluid and air and thus prevent tension on the suture line. The nurse should observe for hemorrhage and carry out all the measures for preventing cardiovascular and respiratory complications following general surgery. Parenteral fluids are given until the tube is removed and bowel sounds return. When clear liquids are ordered, they are offered in small amounts at frequent intervals. If clear liquids are tolerated, the diet progresses to full liquids and then to a soft diet.

*Temporary colostomy* A temporary colostomy may be used if there is a possibility that the lower bowel will heal and can be reanastomosed, retaining rectal sphincter control. Although this procedure may be used to relieve bowel obstructions, it is often an attempt to rest the distal portion of the intestine and is more commonly used, following trauma to the abdomen or severe diverticulitis, in an effort to decrease drainage through fistulae and allow healing to occur. A temporary colostomy involves bringing a loop of bowel to the exterior and creating two openings (Fig. 18-2d). The proximal opening drains fecal material. The distal opening connects to the distal bowel and rectum, which are left in place. Occasionally the openings in the loop of bowel are not made until the abdominal incision has had a chance to heal. The loop of bowel is then opened with cautery. Although this procedure is not painful, the odor of burned flesh is disagreeable. Following surgery there may be discharges of mucus, blood, and sloughed tissue through the rectum.

If the distal bowel is inflamed and infection is suspected, instillations of antibiotic solutions may be ordered. The solution is instilled into the distal opening and expelled per rectum. Irrigations of the proximal opening may be undertaken to establish regular elimination. The degree of success with irrigation depends on the portion of bowel used for the colostomy as well as the patient's motivation.

Because the colostomy will be temporary, some patients prefer to wear a bag to collect the drainage rather than undertake irrigation. The length of time a temporary colostomy is kept varies, but 3 to 6 months is not uncommon before reanastomosis is done.

*Permanent colostomy* A permanent colostomy is most often done for colorectal cancer when the lesion is too close to the rectal sphincter to allow adequate resection of the tumor and still retain sphincter function. A permanent colostomy may also be necessary following extensive trauma to the bowel which results in large, gangrenous areas of colon that cannot be resected. Depending on the site of the pathology, a colostomy may be performed anywhere along the large intestine. The colon is opened and brought out through the abdominal wall (see Color Plate 18-5). This becomes the terminal end of the bowel, and the distal bowel and rectum are removed (Fig. 18-2c). For effective management of drainage and skin protection, the stoma should be situated away from bony prominences and abdominal folds, as illustrated in the color plates. Drains and packing are common in the perineal wound whether or not it is sutured, and there is often copious serosanguineous drainage. Frequent perineal care is essential. When the patient can be out of bed, sitz baths are given. Most patients find these soothing, and the perineal drainage decreases.

The preoperative and postoperative care of a patient with a colostomy is similar to that for a patient with an ileostomy, discussed earlier in this chapter. Table 18-1 gives a comparison of an ileostomy and a colostomy.

The primary difference between an ileostomy and a colostomy is the nature of the discharge. With time and training, colostomies of the descending colon generally discharge formed stool. The degree of stool formation will depend on the location of the colostomy. Stool will become more formed as the colostomy site comes closer to the rectum.

Colostomies can usually be trained to evacuate at regular intervals. This can be accomplished with suppositories, finger dilation, or irrigations. Some knowledge of the patient's bowel pattern prior to the surgical intervention, the daily activities and responsibilities, and the availability of bathroom facilities is useful in establishing with the patient the frequency and the best time for evacuation. All too frequently evacuation in the hospital is done at the nurse's convenience! Once home, that patient is required to readjust the schedule. Once the time has been determined, the training method should be employed regularly. Irrigating the colostomy is a common method. In the hospital, irrigations should be performed using the same equipment that the patient will use at home. When the patient can sit comfortably, the bathroom is the best place for the irrigation. The usual irrigating equipment consists of a container for solution, soft tubing or flexible cone, lubricant, a stoma guard, and an irrigating sleeve to facilitate discharge of solution into the toilet. Some patients substitute a large bulb syringe and a soft catheter for the solution container and tubing. Tap water at body temperature is the usual solution. Although some recommend cool water, most patients experience severe cramping with this. One usually tries for an adequate evacuation with the least amount of solution possible. Initially about 500 ml is used. The patient should be cautioned not to exceed 2 liters of solution. With large amounts of irrigating solution, the risk of depleting electrolytes increases.

The container of fluid should be hung no more than 18 inches above the stoma; the patient's shoulder level is a good guide. With the patient seated comfortably on or in front of the toilet, the irrigating sleeve should be directed into the toilet. The tubing should be lubricated well with water-soluble jelly and air cleared from the tubing. Then, with the solution flowing slowly, the tubing is inserted gently about 6 inches into the stoma. Because the bowel can be perforated, force should not be used to insert the tube. If resistance is met, it may be necessary to wait a short time before advancing the tube. Rotating the tubing slightly sometimes make insertion easier. Since there is no sphincter, some of the solution will return as it is being given. After the bulk of the irrigating solution and stool is expelled, the sleeve may be rinsed and rolled up and the end clamped. Other activities can then be carried out, allowing time for additional drainage before final cleansing of the skin and stoma. Control of drainage is not usually established in the short time of hospitalization, so a drainage bag is used between irrigations. After several weeks, control of the colostomy may be so well established that irrigations may no longer be necessary and the patient may need to wear only a soft dressing or tissue between evacuations. Whether or not the patient will be irrigating the colostomy regularly, it is advisable that some instruction be given in case problems of expelling stool occur at home and necessitate an irrigation.

*Diet* is one of the most effective methods of ensuring regular evacuations. Problems of diarrhea, constipation, and flatus encountered by the colostomy patient are frequently related to diet. If diarrhea is a problem, avoiding high-residue foods will decrease bowel stimulation. The patient should maintain an adequate fluid intake to prevent dehydration. If constipation develops, the residue in the diet should be increased. Flatus can be controlled to some extent by avoiding gas-forming foods.

The patient will be adjusting postoperatively to a significant change in body image. Grieving for the loss of normal body functioning is common. Patients should be encouraged to talk about their feelings and their thoughts about the colostomy. Often a spouse will need support in adjusting to the change. Elimination is a private function, and involving others in it is often a source of embarrassment.

### Fourth-level Nursing Care

Patients with colostomies should be referred to a community health nurse for follow-up physical and psychosocial care. Many communities have "ostomy specialists," nurses specially trained in all aspects of caring for ostomy patients. Usually the ostomy nurse will work with the patient in the hospital and follow through in the community.

Before beginning a teaching plan, it is extremely important to assess the patient's acceptance of the colostomy. The degree of acceptance will reflect the patient's readiness to learn. The patient should be encouraged to verbalize concerns. Often misconceptions about future difficulties cause undue anxiety. Discussing the patient's reactions with the family is often helpful.

The teaching plan should focus on care of the colostomy and on diet. In general, the measures in fourth-level care discussed under ileostomy apply to the colostomy patient. The ileostomate has liquid

**TABLE 18-1**
COMPARISON OF ILEOSTOMY AND
DESCENDING OR SIGMOID COLOSTOMY

|  | Ileostomy | Colostomy |
| --- | --- | --- |
| Stool consistency | Liquid | Soft, formed |
| Appliance needed | Yes | Not always |
| Evacuation regularity | No | Often achieved |
| Irrigations/Suppositories | No | Usually |
| Diet | Well-balanced | Well-balanced, omit gas-forming foods |
| Fluid requirement | Increased | No change |
| Body-image changes | Yes | Yes |
| Activity limitations | No | No |
| Stoma location | Right abdomen | Usually left abdomen |

drainage and must use an appliance for drainage. Diet is not effective in controlling stool. The colostomate, on the other hand, will have more formed stools, and control of evacuation may be achieved with irrigation and diet, so that appliances are often not needed. As with the ileostomy patient, it should be possible for the person with a colostomy to return to work and to participate fully in social and recreational activities. Initially, however, the patient's life may center around the stoma and its care. An inordinate amount of time may be spent in irrigations. The person with a colostomy may avoid social contacts and withdraw because of sensitivity about odors. Often the patient is not aware that anything more than the control achieved in the hospital is possible. The nurse who is aware of some of the common problems faced by these patients can ask questions to open communication with the patient and help in finding solutions. The goal is to have the patient manage the colostomy with a minimum of time and effort so that it does not become a major focus of life. Patients should be encouraged to resume their normal activities. All sporting and social activities can be enjoyed. It usually takes time for the patient to become comfortable with the colostomy care before full activities are resumed.

The regularity of evacuations and the patient's ability to care for the colostomy should be reevaluated on a regular basis. At the same time the condition of the stoma and surrounding skin should be assessed. Strictures around the stoma and prolapse of the stoma are possible complications and may require surgical revision. The patient is often taught to dilate the stoma manually at regular intervals to prevent stricture formation.

Any difficulties with diarrhea or constipation should be explored. With each of these problems, the diet should be evaluated and problem foods identified. The patient should be advised that only water safe for drinking is safe for irrigation. Ostomy clubs are helpful in assisting the patient to adjust to the drastic change in body image. Often the family as well as the patient needs support in making the adjustment.

## DIVERTICULAR DISEASE

Diverticular disease, on the increase in the Western world over the past 70 years, has been called the most common abnormality of the Western colon. Thirty-five percent of persons over 40 years and 45 percent of those over 60 years have diverticular disease. The condition in black Americans was rare before World War II but is now more common. An increase of diverticular disease is predicted for other countries now developing economically and adopting the highly refined diet of the Western world.

*Diverticuli* are acquired herniations of colon mucosa through weak areas of the colon musculature. These weak areas correspond to spaces between the longitudinal muscles in the colon. The acquisition of diverticuli is related to segmentation and increased intraluminal pressure in the colon. If segmentation is complete and contents are not propelled forward, the increased pressure contributes to the herniation of the colon mucosa.[20] Maintaining soft, easily passed stools reduces the intraluminal pressure in the colon segments. Drugs such as morphine sulfate and prostigmine increase intraluminal pressures and are best avoided. Feces may be trapped in the herniations. Stools may be small, hard, and constipated.

To prevent diverticuli, general health education related to diet and prevention of constipation is needed. Including vegetable and cereal fibers in the diet and relying less on highly refined foods offer some promise of preventing diverticular disease.[21] Increasing bulk in the stool also helps retain water to make a softer stool.

The presence of a number of diverticuli is called *diverticulosis.* When the outpouchings become irritated, inflamed, and tender, the condition is referred to as *diverticulitis.* Small perforations, pericolic abscesses, and fistulas are common in diverticulitis. The patient with diverticulitis usually experiences pain in the left lower quadrant. Diarrhea frequently occurs, and pus, mucus, and blood may appear in the stools. Nursing care is similar to that discussed under Ulcerative Colitis. If elevations in temperature and white blood count accompany the abdominal pain and stool changes, the treatment includes a clear liquid diet and antibiotics. If the condition is more severe and there are suspicions of perforation and peritonitis, the patient is given nothing by mouth. Antibiotics, fluids, and electrolyte replacements are given intravenously. In patients in whom there is perforation, a temporary colostomy may be performed to divert the fecal stream and to allow healing of the distal colon. If the diverticuli are confined to a well-defined portion of the bowel, a bowel resection may be done.

With repeated episodes of acute inflammation, scars and adhesions may develop and lead to intestinal obstruction, which also requires surgical intervention. A more thorough discussion of these operations is found under Intestinal Obstructions.

# HEMORRHOIDS

Hemorrhoids are varicosities of the hemorrhoidal plexus which drains the rectum and anal canal. Predisposing factors for hemorrhoids are weakness of hemorrhoidal-vein walls, straining at stool, and increased venous stasis, as in prolonged standing and in pregnancy. Portal hypertension often leads to hemorrhoids. Symptoms range from mild discomfort to severe pruritus and pain. Rectal bleeding is common.

Conservative treatment of hemorrhoids includes preventing constipation, increasing soft bulk, and using stool softeners or mineral oil. Cleansing with soft tissue and sitz baths after bowel movements may give relief from minor discomfort. Hemorrhoids protruding through the anal sphincter can be replaced with a lubricated finger to reduce discomfort and prevent strangulation.

Single hemorrhoids above the anorectal junction can be treated by injection, rubber-band ligation, or cryosurgery on an ambulatory basis. After these procedures, medication and sitz baths help relieve pain. A brown, serous anal discharge, especially after cryosurgery, may require the wearing of absorbent dressings for 2 to 3 weeks.[22] Severe hemorrhoids with recurrent prolapse, strangulation, or infection are best treated with *hemorrhoidectomy,* the surgical excision of hemorrhoids.

After hemorrhoidectomy, common problems are pain, hemorrhage, and urinary retention. Ice packs initially may provide comfort. Analgesics are often needed for the first 24 to 48 hours and again after the first bowel movement. Sitz baths are started 1 to 2 days after surgery for comfort and cleanliness and are usually continued after bowel movements for 1 to 2 weeks after the patient goes home. The nurse should check for rectal bleeding and teach the patient what signs to watch for.

Urinary retention can be prevented by fluid restriction following anorectal surgery. In one study, the need for postoperative catheterization was reduced by limiting fluids to 250 ml and giving no coffee or tea until the first spontaneous voiding or catheterization.[23] With this fluid restriction, bladder capacity is not reached for 18 to 24 hours and, unless there is significant distention, the patient may safely go without voiding for as long as 36 hours postoperatively. Reassuring the patient of the ability to void and getting the patient out of bed also facilitate voiding.

Review of measures to prevent constipation should be included postoperatively. Mineral oil, stool softeners, and bulk laxatives may all be used after rectal surgery for a short time. Heeding the urge for a bowel movement is important, as hard, constipated stool is more difficult to pass and may cause bleeding as well as pain.

## REFERENCES

1   R. Wright, "Immunological Aspects of GI Disease," *Proc R Soc Med,* **67:**574–580, June 1974.

2   I. Hislop, "Onset Setting in Inflammatory Bowel Disease," *Med J Aust,* **1**(25):981–984, June 22, 1974.

3   Basil Morson, "The Polyp-Cancer Sequence in the Large Bowel," *Proc R Soc Med,* **67:**451–457, June 1974.

4   R. Wright, *op. cit.*

5   R. Miller, "The Clean Colon," *Gastroenterol,* **70:**289–290, February 1976.

6   Christine Curtis, "Colonoscopy: The Nurse's Role," *Am J Nurs,* **75:**430–432, March 1975.

7   B. Korelitz and S. Sommers, "Responses to Drug Therapy in Ulcerative Colitis Evaluation by Rectal Biopsy and Histopathological Changes," *Am J Gastroenterol,* **64**(5):365–370, November 1975.

8   S. C. Truelove and D. P. Jewell, "Intensive Intravenous Regimen for Severe Attacks of Ulcerative Colitis," *Lancet,* **1**(866):1067–70, June 1, 1974.

9   Nils G. Kock, "Ileostomy without External Appliance," *Ann Surg,* **173:**545–550, April 1971.

10   O. H. Bearhs and M. H. Adson, "Ileal Pouch with Ileostomy Rather Than Ileostomy Alone," *Am J Surg,* **125:**154–158, February 1973.

11   G. Bruce Thow (moderator), "Symposium: Present Status of the Continent Ileostomy," *Dis Colon Rectum,* **19**(3):189–212, April 1976.

12   Bettie S. Jackson, "Colostomates: The Mosaic of Stress and Implied Care," *Aust Nurs J,* **4:**24–27, May 1975.

13   F. W. Nugent, "Crohn's Colitis Comes of Age," *Am J Gastroenterol,* **63:**471–475, June 1975.

14   H. Chmel and D. Armstrong, *"Salmonella Oslo,"* *Am J Med* **60:**203–208, February 1976.

15   Leon F. Nadrowski, "Pathophysiology and Current Treatment of Intestinal Obstruction," *Rev Surg,* **31**(6):381–407, November-December, 1974.

16   *1977 Cancer Facts and Figures,* American Cancer Society, New York, 1976.

17   Si-Chun Ming and J. McNiff, "Acute Ischemic Changes in Intestinal Muscularis," *Am J Pathol,* **82:** 315–326, February 1976.

18   A. K. Blackwell and W. Blackwell, "Relieving Gas Pains," *Am J Nurs,* **75:**66–67, January 1975.

19   Theodore Jones, "A Comparative Study of Inguinal Herniorrhaphy," *Am Surg,* **41:**20–27, January 1975.

20  N. S. Painter, "Diverticular Disease of the Colon: The Effect of the High Fiber Diet," *R Soc Health J,* **4:**194–198, 1975.

21  D. Burkitt, in Allen Ginsberg (ed.), "The Fiber Controversy: Denis P. Burkitt vs. Albert I. Mendeloff," *Digestive Dis,* **21:**103–112, 1976.

22  J. C. Goligher, "Cryosurgery for Hemorrhoids," *Dis Colon Rectum,* **19**(3):213–218, April 1976.

23  H. Randolph Bailey and James A. Ferguson, "Prevention of Urinary Retention by Fluid Restriction Following Anorectal Operations," *Dis Colon Rectum,* **19**(3):250–252, April 1976.

## BIBLIOGRAPHY

Aston S. J., and H. I. Machlfeder: "Intussusception in the Adult," *Am Surg,* **41**(9): 576–580, September 1975.

Basler, R., and H. Dubin: "Ulcerative Colitis and the Skin," *Arch Dermatol,* **112:**531–534, April 1976.

Bates, Barbara: *A Guide to Physical Examination,* Lippincott, Philadelphia, 1974, pp. 158–178, 179–187, 205–242.

Beck, William S.: *Human Design,* Harcourt Brace Jovanovich, New York, 1971.

Beeson, Paul B., and Walsh McDermott (eds.): *Textbook of Medicine,* Saunders, Philadelphia, 1975.

Beland, Irene L., and Joyce Y. Passos: *Clinical Nursing: Pathophysiological and Psychosocial Approaches,* Macmillan, New York, 1975.

Best, W. R., J. Becktel, J. Singleton, and F. Kern: "Development of a Crohn's Disease Activity Index," *Gastroenterology,* **70:**439–444, March 1976.

Boley, S., S. Sprayregen, J. Vieth, and S. Siegelman: "An Aggressive Roentgenologic and Surgical Approach to Acute Mesenteric Ischemia," in Lloyd Nyhus (ed.), *Surgery Annual 1973,* Appleton-Century-Crofts, New York, 1973, pp. 355–378.

Bonfils, S. and M. de M'Uzan: "Irritable Bowel Syndrome vs. Ulcerative Colitis: Psychofunctional Disturbance vs. Psychosomatic Disease?" *J Psychosom Res,* **18:**291–296, August 1974.

Brocklehurst, J. C.: "Management of Anal Incontinence," *Clin Gastroenterol,* **4:**479–487, September 1975.

Buhac, I., and J. Balint: "Diarrhea and Constipation," *Am Family Physician,* **12:**149–159, November 1975.

Campbell, A. C., J. M. Skinner, P. Hersey, P. Roberts-Thomson, I. C. MacLennan, and S. C. Truelove: "Immunosuppression in the Treatment of Inflammatory Bowel Disease. I. Changes in Lymphoid Sub-populations in the Blood and Rectal Mucosa Following Cessation of Treatment with Azathioprine," *Clin Exp Immunol,* **16**(4):521–533, April 1974.

DeLuca, Joanne C.: "The Ulcerative Colitis Personality," *Nurs Clin North Am,* **5:**23–24, March 1970.

Dericks, Virginia C.: "The Psychological Hurdles of New Ostomates: Helping Them Up and Over," *Nurs '74,* **4:**52–55, October 1974.

Dilawari, J., J. Lennard-Jones, A. MacKay, J. Ritchie, and H. Sturzaker: "Estimation of Carcinoembryonic Antigen in Ulcerative Colitis with Special Reference to Malignant Change," *Gut,* **16:**255–260, April 1975.

Durham, Nancy: "Look Out for Complications of Abdominal Surgery," *Nurs '75,* **5**(2): 24–31, February 1975.

Engel, George: "Studies of Ulcerative Colitis. III. The Nature of the Psychological Processes," *Am J Med,* **19:**231–256, August 1955.

Engel, George: "A Life Setting Conducive to Illness: The Giving-up—Given-up Complex," *Ann Intern Med,* **69:**293–300, August 1968.

Erbe, Richard W.: "Inherited Gastrointestinal-Polyposis Syndromes," *New Engl J Med,* **294:**1101–1104, May 13, 1976.

Falchuk, K., and K. Isselbacher: "Circulating Antibodies to Bovine Albumin in Ulcerative Colitis and Crohn's Disease," *Gastroenterology,* **70:**5–8, January 1976.

Farman, J., J. Twersky, and S. Fierst: "Ulcerative Colitis Associated with Hypertrophic Osteoarthropathy," *Digestive Dis,* **21:**130–135, February 1976.

Gallagher, Ann M.: "Body Image Changes in the Patient with a Colostomy," *Nurs Clin North Am,* **7:**669–676, December 1972.

Gilat, T., J. Ribak, Y. Benaroya, Z. Zemishlany, and I. Weissman: "Ulcerative Colitis in the Jewish Population of Tel-Aviv Jafo I. Epidemiology," *Gastroenterology,* **66:**335–342, March 1974.

Gilat, T., P. Lilos, Z. Zemishlany, J. Ribak, and Y. Benaroya: "Ulcerative Colitis in the Jewish Population of Tel-Aviv. Yafo III. Clinical Course," *Gastroenterology,* **70:**14–19, January 1976.

Gorbach, S., B. Kean, D. G. Evans, D. J. Evans, and D. Bessudo: "Traveler's Diarrhea and Toxigenic *Escherichia coli,*" *N Engl J Med,* **292:**933–936, May 1, 1975.

Greenstein, A. J., D. B. Sachar, B. S. Pasternack, and H. D. Janowitz: "Reoperation and Recurrence in Crohn's Colitis and Ileocolitis," *N Engl J Med,* **293:**685–690, Oct. 2, 1975.

Hoberman, Laqrence J., E. Eigenbrodt, W. Kilman, L. Hughes, R. Norgaard, and J. Fordtran: "Colitis Associated with Oral Clindamycin Therapy," *Digestive Dis,* **21:**1–17, January 1976.

Hill, M.: "The Role of Colon Anaerobes in the Metabolism of Bile Acids and Steroids, and its Relation to Colon Cancer," *Cancer,* **36**(6 Suppl): 2387–2400, December 1975.

Hill, M., and B. Drasar: "The Normal Colonic Bacterial Flora," *Gut,* **16**:318–323, April 1975.

Hornick, R. B.: "Acute Bacterial Diarrheas," *Adv Intern Med,* **21**:349–361, 1975.

Howard, Phillip: "Let's Simplify and Clarify the Anatomy and Surgery of Groin Hernias," *Am J Surg,* **128**:65–70, July 1974.

Jackson, Bettie S.: "Colostomates' Reactions to Hospitalization and Colostomy Surgery," *Nurs Clin North Am,* **11**(3):417–425, September 1976.

Jensen, Vicki: "Better Techniques for Bagging Stomas. Part III: Ileostomies," *Nurs '74,* **4**:60–63, September 1974.

Lennard-Jones, J., J. Misiewicz, J. Parrish, J. Ritchie, E. Swarbrick, and C. Williams: "Prospective Study of Outpatients with Extensive Colitis," *Lancet,* **1**(866):1065–1067, June 1, 1974.

Lennard-Jones, J., J. Ritchie, W. Hilder, and C. Spicer: "Assessment of Severity in Colitis: A Preliminary Study," *Gut,* **16**:579–584, August 1975.

Lennenberg, Edith, and Alan N. Mendelssohn: *Colostomies: A Guide,* United Ostomy Association, Los Angeles, 1971.

Localio, S. A.: "Curative Surgery of Midrectal Cancer with Preservation of the Sphincters," in L. Nyhus (ed.), *Surgery Annual 1974,* Appleton-Century-Crofts, New York, 1974, pp. 213–245.

Luckmann, Joan, and Karen C. Sorenson: *Medical-Surgical Nursing, a Psychophysiological Approach,* Saunders, Philadelphia, 1974.

Madden, J. L., and S. Kandaloft: "Electrocoagulation in the Treatment of Cancer of the Rectum," in L. Nyhus (ed.) *Surgery Annual 1974,* Appleton-Century-Crofts, New York, 1974, pp. 195–212.

Marston, A., R. Kieny, E. Szilagyi, and G. Taylor: "Intestinal Ischemia," *Arch Surg,* **111**:107–112, February 1976.

Mendeloff, A., in T. Almy (moderator): "Panel I: Prevalence and Significance of Digestive Disease," *Gastroenterology,* **68**:1351–1371, May 1975.

Meuwissen, S., S. Katolina, D. Pape, D. Agenant, H. Oushoorn, and G. Tytgat: "Crohn's Disease of the Colon," *Digestive Dis,* **21**:81–88, February 1976.

O'Connell, T., B. Kadell, and B. Tompkins: "Ischemia of the Colon," *Surg Gynecol Obstet,* **142**(3):337–342, March 1976.

Painter, N. S., and D. Burkitt: "Diverticular Disease of the Colon, A 20th Century Problem," in A. Smith (ed.), *Clin Gastroenterol,* **4**:3–21, January 1975.

Price, J. E., S. Michel, and L. Morgenstern: "Fruit Pit Obstruction," *Arch Surg,* **111**:773–775, July 1976.

Rodkey, G. V., and C. E. Welch: "Colonic Diverticular Disease with Surgical Treatment: A Study of 338 Cases," *Surg Clin North Am,* **54**:655–674, June 1974.

Rush, Alice: "Cancer and the Ostomy Patient," *Nurs Clin North Am,* **11**(3):405–415 September 1976.

Shafer, Kathleen, Janet Sawyer, Audrey McCluskey, Edna Beck, and Wilma Phipps: *Medical-Surgical Nursing,* Mosby, St. Louis, 1975.

Sharpton, B., and R. Cheek: "Volvulus of Sigmoid Colon," *Amer Surg,* **42**:436–440, June, 1976.

Sherlock, Paul: "Etiology of Gastrointestinal Cancer: Heredity vs. Environment," *Digestive Dis,* **21**:68–70, January 1976.

Sleisinger, Marvin H., and John S. Fordtran: *Gastrointestinal Disease,* Saunders, Philadelphia, 1973.

Silverstein, Fred, and Cyrus Rubin: "The New Look into the Gastrointestinal Tract," in H. F. Dowling (ed.), *Disease-A-Month,* Year Book, Chicago, February 1976.

Spiller, G. A., and R. Amen "Dietary Fiber in Human Nutrition," *Crit Rev Food Sci Nutr,* **7**:39–70, November 1975.

Taylor, I., H. Duthie: "Bran Tablets and Diverticular Disease," *Br Med J,* **1**:988–990, April 24, 1976.

Tedesco, Francis J.: "Clindamycin-associated Colitis," *Digestive Dis,* **21**:26–32, January 1976.

Thayer, W.: "Are the Inflammatory Bowel Diseases Immune Complex Diseases?" *Gastroenterology,* **70**:136–137, January 1976.

Watt, Rosemary C.: "Ostomies: Why, How and Where: An Overview," *Nurs Clin North Am,* **11**(3):393–404, September 1976.

Watson, Pamela, Robin Wood, Nancy Wechsler, and Linda Christensen: "Comprehensive Care of the Ileostomy Patient," *Nurs Clin North Am,* **11**(3):427–444, September 1976.

Weinstein, M., and M. Roberts: "Recurrent Inguinal Hernia: Followup Study of 100 Postoperative Patients," *Am J Surg,* **129**:564–569, May 1975.

Weissman, J., G. Craun, D. Lawrence, R. Pollard, M. Saslaw, and E. Gangarosa: "An Epidemic of Gastroenteritis Traced to a Contaminated Public Water Supply," *Am J Epidemiol,* **103**:391–398, April 1976.

Welch, Claude E.: "Abdominal Surgery: First of Three Parts," *N Engl J Med,* **293**:858–863, Oct. 23, 1975; "Second of Three Parts," **293**:908–912, Oct. 30, 1975.

Wentworth, Arlene, and Barbara Cox: "Nursing the Patient with a Continent Ileostomy," *Am J Nurs,* **76**(9):1424–1428, September 1976.

Yahle, Margaret-Ellen: "An Ostomy Information Clinic: A Community Resource," *Nurs Clin North Am,* **11**(3):457–467, September 1976.

# 19

# DISTURBANCES IN HEPATIC FUNCTION

Irene B. Alyn

The liver functions in a multiplicity of roles as human beings interact with the environment. It plays an integral part in maintaining a ready energy supply for cellular use and in storing and converting energy from the environment. It detoxifies a wide variety of substances and prepares many of them for elimination into the external environment. In several ways the liver also participates in meeting the oxygenation requirements of the body. This discussion will focus on the many internal and external factors that can result in disturbances in hepatic function. The reader is encouraged to review the normal structure and functions of the liver described in Chap. 15 before beginning this section.

## PATHOPHYSIOLOGICAL CHANGES IN LIVER DAMAGE

There are a variety of injurious agents that can damage the liver. Dysfunction, therefore, has been classified in several ways. Parenchymal damage can result from inflammation, cirrhosis, infiltrations, space-occupying lesions, or functional disorders.[1] Inflammation of the liver is called *hepatitis* and most often results from viral infection, although it can be of toxic or drug-induced origin. When damage occurs from alcohol ingestion, severe inflammation with necrosis, or biliary disease, *cirrhosis* can develop. The liver can be *infiltrated* by glycogen, fat, amyloid, lymphoma, and granuloma. *Space-occupying lesions* include not only tumors but abscesses and cysts.

Regardless of the cause of hepatic dysfunction, the resultant effects on the patient are similar. Differences lie in the extent and duration of liver damage. In general, the pathophysiological alterations which occur include changes in cellular growth and proliferation, decreased immunocompetence, fluid and electrolyte imbalances, metabolic disruptions, inadequate oxygenation of cells, and distortions of perception and coordination. Table 19-1 summarizes the pathophysiological changes associated with liver disease.

### Changes in Cellular Growth and Proliferation

Liver cells have a unique ability to regenerate. This process takes about 2 to 4 weeks. Functional capacity is maintained in the absence of approximately 75 percent of the total liver mass. Because of this, damage may occur without noticeable effects on the patient. Within the limits of the liver's regenerative capacity, damage can be followed by complete

**TABLE 19-1**
SUMMARY OF PATHOPHYSIOLOGICAL CHANGES IN LIVER DAMAGE

| Changes | Mechanism | Effects |
|---|---|---|
| Variations in cellular proliferation | Decreased estrogen detoxification results in increased estrogenic action | Decreased axillary hair<br>Decreased pubic hair<br>Pectoral alopecia<br>Testicular atrophy<br>Gynecomastia<br>Decreased libido<br>Impotence<br>Palmar erythema<br>Spider angiomas |
| Decreased immunocompetence | Decreased efficiency of Kupffer cells and splenic congestion | Increased blood bacteria<br>Increased susceptibility to infection |
| Fluid and electrolyte imbalance | Decreased synthesis of albumin results in decreased plasma colloid osmotic pressure | Edema<br>Ascites<br>Pleural effusion |
| | Scar tissue blocking liver microvasculature results in increased portal hydrostatic pressure | Increased ascites |
| | Decreased detoxification of ADH and aldosterone | Sodium and water retention<br>Potassium loss |
| Metabolic imbalances | Decreased glycogenesis, glycogenolysis, gluconeogenesis, and oxidation of fatty acids | Weight loss<br>Lassitude<br>Fatigue<br>Varying blood glucose levels (related to ingestion) |
| | Decreased lipogenesis | Decreased serum cholesterol |
| | Decreased amino acid breakdown and synthesis results in increased blood amino acids | Aminoaciduria and negative nitrogen balance<br>Fetor hepaticus |
| | Decreased bile production results in decreased fat digestion | Intolerance to fatty foods<br>Anorexia<br>Nausea<br>Vomiting<br>Flatulence<br>Diarrhea or constipation |
| | Decreased absorption of fat-soluble vitamins and decreased vitamin storage | Vitamin deficiencies |
| Changes in oxygenation | Decreased storage of vitamin $B_{12}$ results in RBC fragility | Anemia<br>Increased cardiac output |
| | Decreased storage of iron | Cardiomegaly<br>Clubbing of the fingers |
| | Decreased synthesis of fibrinogen, prothrombin, and factors V, VII, and X with decreased storage of vitamin K | Bleeding tendency<br>Increased prothrombin time<br>Ecchymoses<br>Purpura |
| | Scar tissue blocking liver microvasculature results in increased portal hydrostatic pressure | Esophageal varices with possible rupture and hemorrhage<br>Splenomegaly<br>Dilated periumbilical veins<br>Hemorrhoids |
| | Decreased conjugation of bilirubin | Jaundice<br>Mahogany-colored urine<br>Clay-colored stools<br>Pruritus |
| Changes in perception and coordination | Increased blood ammonia level results in interference with normal brain metabolism | Altered mental state<br>Asterixis |
| | Decreased detoxification of drugs | Increased susceptibility to sedatives, hypnotics, etc. |

resolution. If it is extensive, however, the liver can fail, or regeneration can be irregular with fibrous tissue replacement and disruption of liver lobules.

Some hormones contribute to cellular growth and proliferation. Estrogen, which the liver detoxifies, promotes the growth and development of the secondary female sex characteristics. In liver dysfunction, detoxification is decreased, resulting in an increased estrogenic action. These are losses of axillary, pubic, and general body hair (*pectoral alopecia*). The skin softens, and in males the testicles atrophy and *gynecomastia* develops. There is a decrease in libido, and impotence is often a problem. *Palmar erythema* develops, and the *spider angiomas* (spider nevi) (see Color Plate 19-1) associated with hepatic disease are also thought to be a result of the increase in estrogen levels, although the exact mechanism for their development is not understood.

## Decreased Immunocompetence

The reticuloendothelial system (RES) is composed of cells that line many of the vascular and lymph channels and are capable of phagocytizing or forming immune bodies against bacteria, viruses, and foreign agents. The major functioning of the RES is accomplished by lymphocytes, reticulum cells of the spleen, Kupffer cells of the liver, and reticulum cells of bone marrow. Since the liver has both sessile (Kupffer cells) and mobile (lymphocytes) macrophages of the RES and one-fourth of the lymph is produced in the liver, pathophysiology of the liver profoundly influences the competence of the immune system. Disruption of hepatic lobules may cause portal hypertension and splenic congestion, further altering the body's host defense system. The reader is referred to Chap. 8 for further discussion of the immune response.

The liver also plays a vital role in phagocytizing bacteria in the blood. Many colon bacilli are present in the portal circulation, and the Kupffer cells remove 99 percent of these from the blood as it passes through the liver. During liver damage, the efficiency of this purifying system is lessened, increasing the blood bacteria level. The lack of blood flow through the sinusoids and destruction of parenchymal and Kupffer cells make the patient prone to infection.

## Fluid and Electrolyte Imbalance

Liver pathology can lead to profound changes in fluid and electrolyte balance. The liver is the only organ that synthesizes albumin, the plasma protein responsible for maintaining colloid osmotic pressure in the vasculature. With decreased albumin, the plasma colloid osmotic pressure is decreased, allowing fluid to escape to the interstitial fluid spaces. This is noticeable as edema in dependent locations such as the ankles, in the abdomen as ascites, and in the lungs as pleural effusion. The ascites will be further increased if scar tissue formation blocks the liver microvasculature, increasing the pressure in the portal vein. The increase in portal hydrostatic pressure in the presence of decreased colloid osmotic pressure enhances fluid losses into the peritoneal cavity.

The liver also functions to detoxify the antidiuretic hormone (ADH) and aldosterone. The actions of both of these are increased during liver dysfunction, increasing water and sodium retention and potassium loss. The excess fluid conserved by the kidneys is lost to the edema fluid, however, and the intravascular dehydration remains.

## Metabolic Imbalances

The metabolic role of the liver is, perhaps, its major function. The liver has an integral part in carbohydrate, fat, protein, and vitamin metabolism and in fat digestion. In liver disease there is a decrease in glycogenesis, glycogenolysis, gluconeogenesis, lipogenesis, oxidation of fatty acids, and amino acid breakdown and synthesis. This generally results in weight loss, lassitude, and fatigue. The body's ability to maintain normal blood glucose levels and cellular nutrition is less efficient. This deficit of glucose results in degradation of fat and protein to provide energy for the body. With chronic cirrhosis of the liver, hyperglycemia and decreased glucose tolerance are often evident. Decreased lipogenesis affects the fatty component of cell membranes, phospholipids, and steroid hormones and is manifested in lowered serum cholesterol levels. The impaired amino acid metabolism and the mobilization of amino acids for gluconeogenesis increase the blood amino acid level, resulting in aminoaciduria (loss of amino acids in the urine). A negative nitrogen balance ensues. The sweet odor on the breath (*fetor hepaticus*) of patients in liver failure is due to the inability of the liver to adequately metabolize the amino acid methionine.

These metabolic processes in the liver become a major source of heat in the body. However, in the presence of liver pathology, the body's ability to maintain normal temperature is curtailed. The liver's ability to synthesize phosphocreatine used in the formation of ATP is also impaired. The adrenocorticosteroids are detoxified by the liver, but as this detoxification decreases in liver pathology, the increased serum hormone levels decrease production of the steroids, and normal levels are generally maintained by a feedback mechanism.

Because the liver stores several vitamins and converts carotene to vitamin A, liver disease is often accompanied by *vitamin deficiencies.* Glossitis may be present as a result of deficiencies in vitamin B complex. Iron and protein deficiencies may contribute to this condition. Peripheral neuropathy resulting from insufficient vitamin $B_6$ and nicotinic acid is common. A more complete examination of the vitamin deficiencies and their manifestations may be found in Chap. 16. Vitamin deficiencies are complicated further by a decreased absorption of the fat-soluble vitamins (A, D, E, and K). The bile salts formed by the liver are necessary for normal fat breakdown in the intestines. With liver damage normal bile formation is compromised, affecting the digestion and absorption of fats. The patient often experiences an intolerance to fatty foods, anorexia, nausea, vomiting, flatulence, and diarrhea or constipation.

### Changes in Oxygenation Status

The liver functions in several ways to maintain the circulating blood volume and an adequate number of red blood cells. Normally the liver stores approximately 500 ml blood (about 10 percent of the total blood volume); with increased right atrial pressure, up to a liter can be stored. When blood is lost, vasopressor substances are released by the liver, and blood which is normally stored is placed into the circulation. Vitamin $B_{12}$ and iron which are stored in the liver are deficient in liver pathology. Red blood cells do not mature properly and become fragile. Adequate iron is not available to produce hemoglobin, and *anemia* is a common consequence. This can be complicated further by alcohol ingestion which has a direct inhibitory effect on erythropoiesis.[2] Anemia results in increased cardiac output, as well as cardiomegaly and clubbing of the fingers.

Disruption of the normal clotting mechanisms also occurs. Vitamin K, necessary for the formation of several clotting factors, is absorbed less readily because of inadequate bile and stored in the liver to a lesser degree. At the same time synthesis by the liver of fibrinogen, prothrombin, and factors V, VII, and X are decreased resulting in a bleeding tendency. As the prothrombin time increases, *ecchymoses* are often evident and *purpura* may be noticeable.

When healing occurs in a cirrhotic or severely damaged liver, scar tissue forms and blocks the microvasculature. This blockage increases the circulatory pressure which is communicated to the portal vein. *Portal hypertension* develops. Collateral circulation opens to relieve the pressure increases, and blood begins to bypass the liver (Fig. 19-1). As the portal pressure continues to rise, the collaterals become overdistended. The result is esophageal varices, splenomegaly, dilated periumbilical veins, and hemorrhoids. The esophageal varices are the most severe complication and can rupture, resulting in hemorrhage.

Another liver function disrupted in the presence of pathology is related to, but does not directly affect, oxygenation. There is a decrease in the liver's ability to pick up unconjugated bilirubin, an end product of the breakdown of red blood cells, and conjugate it via the action of glucuronyl transferase so that it is water soluble and can be eliminated in the bile. As less bilirubin is removed, it becomes concentrated in the serum and is deposited in the tissues. This is visible as *jaundice,* a characteristic yellowing of the skin. Jaundice can occur in four different ways and is not always a result of liver damage.

1 When erythrocyte breakdown is accelerated, as happens in hemolytic states, the demand on the hepatic cells is greater than their ability to conjugate the bilirubin supplied them. There is an increase in unconjugated bilirubin.

2 In liver pathology, such as cirrhosis and hepatitis, the transport mechanisms for bilirubin within the liver are interrupted and there is an increase in unconjugated bilirubin.

3 In the newborn physiological jaundice develops because of a deficiency in glucuronyl transferase, the enzyme that conjugates bilirubin. Unconjugated bilirubin is increased.

4 Obstruction of the bile canaliculi by fibrous regeneration, tumor growth, or obstruction of the bile ducts by stones interferes with bile excretion which backs up into the general circulation. There is an increase in conjugated bilirubin.

Jaundice is usually accompanied by dark, mahogany-colored urine as bilirubin is excreted through the kidneys and light, clay-colored stools as urobilinogen disappears from the feces. *Urobilinogen,* formed by the action of bacteria on bilirubin in the intestines, is either excreted in the feces or reabsorbed and recirculated through the liver and bile ducts. A small amount is excreted in the kidneys. When the bile ducts are completely obstructed, no bilirubin reaches the intestine to form urobilinogen. Therefore, no urobilinogen is excreted in the urine. An abnormal concentration of urobilinogen is found in the urine only in parenchymal cell damage.

Jaundice is usually accompanied by severe itching (pruritis). The absence of bile in the feces, when bile flow is not obstructed, is usually concurrent with the absence of pruritus, suggesting that it is due to some substance excreted in the bile. Further, pruritus disappears when liver cells fail, indicating that whatever is responsible for itching in the jaundiced individual is manufactured by the liver.[3]

## Changes in Perception and Coordination

Abnormalities in perception and coordination develop as the liver's ability to convert ammonia to urea for excretion in the urine is compromised. Ammonia interferes with normal brain metabolism. Some ammonia results from the deaminization of amino acids, but the bulk of the blood ammonia is absorbed from the intestines. When liver function is impaired, urea is not formed and ammonia builds up in the blood. If portal hypertension is present, portal systemic shunts develop. The ammonia-rich blood absorbed from the intestines flows along collateral veins, bypassing the liver and further increasing the ammonia level. If bleeding occurs in the gastrointestinal tract, even more ammonia will be formed by bacterial action on the blood. The end result of high ammonia concentrations in the blood is an altered mental state and a flapping tremor of the hands (*asterixis*). As the ammonia level increases in the serum, the patient progresses from a state of lethargy to personality changes, which include combativeness, noisiness, and abusive behavior, and finally to coma. This final state is referred to as *hepatic coma.*

Liver pathology also interferes with the detoxification of drugs, poisons, and heavy metals. There is an increased intolerance for sedatives and hypnotics, which include morphine, barbiturates (except phenobarbitol and barbitol), Librium, and paraldehyde.

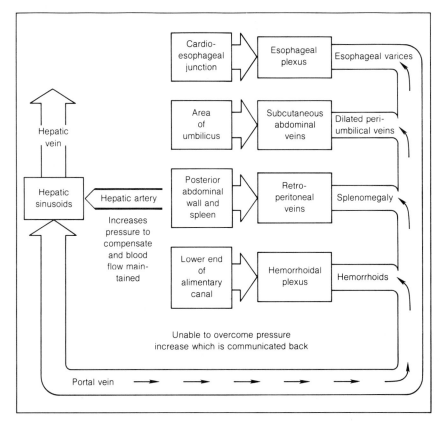

**FIGURE 19-1**

Graphic summary of hepatic blood flow in portal hypertension.

# HEPATIC CIRRHOSIS

*Hepatic cirrhosis* is a term used to describe a chronic process involving disruption of the normal configuration of hepatic lobules leading to parenchymal cell death and regeneration with scarring. Regenerated hepatic cells are nodular cells and distort the shape of the liver, compress intrahepatic venous and lymphatic radicles, and thereby cause obstruction to blood and lymph flow through the liver. If the obstruction is great enough, portal hypertension results.

Pathologists have outlined three morphological classifications of cirrhosis of the liver:

Micronodular: Also called portal, associated with continued alcohol intake

Macronodular: Previously referred to as postnecrotic (posthepatitis) cirrhosis

Mixed micronodular-macronodular: Variable mixture of liver cell death and regeneration with concomitant deposition of fat, iron, and fibrous tissue

*Causes* of hepatic cirrhosis are numerous, but it occurs most frequently in alcoholics. In addition to alcohol, other major factors to consider in the etiology of hepatic cirrhosis are viral hepatitis, chronic cholestasis, Wilson's disease, hemochromatosis, hepatic venous obstruction, fibrocystic disease, hepatotoxins, galactosemia, and glycogen storage disease. The focus of this discussion is alcohol-induced hepatic cirrhosis (alcoholic cirrhosis, Laennec's portal cirrhosis).

*Alcoholic cirrhosis* is characterized by fatty infiltration, destruction of parenchymal cells, and disruption of normal lobular architecture by alcoholic hyalin and fibrous tissue. These changes have been attributed to the toxicity of ethyl alcohol, malnutrition, and immunological reactivity.[4] Each of these three factors alone or in combination contributes to the cirrhotic process in the alcoholic. The magnitude of the hepatic cellular failure and portal hypertension will depend on the amount, type, and duration of alcohol intake. As cirrhosis progresses, more and more of the liver's functions are increasingly disturbed, and the patient with severe cirrhosis will evidence all the pathophysiological changes described in the previous section.

## First-Level Nursing Care

Widespread damage can be done to the liver by excessive alcohol consumption. Preventing alcoholic cirrhosis is contingent upon preventing alcohol abuse. *Alcoholism is a disease.* The National Institute of Mental Health defines it as a chronic disease, or disorder of behavior, which is characterized by repeated alcohol consumption in excess of that dictated by customary dietary use or social norms. As a disease, alcoholism interferes with the individual's health, interpersonal relations, and economic functioning.

The most immediate effect of alcohol is on the brain. It acts much like a narcotic, depressing cerebral function. The effects of alcohol on the various parts of the brain are listed below. The part whose normal functioning is disturbed by the smallest concentration of alcohol in the blood is listed first.

*Frontal lobes:* Feeling of well-being, false confidence, weakening of will power

*Parietal lobe:* Distorted sensation, loss of technical skill, inability to write, speech disturbances

*Cerebellum:* Disturbance in equilibrium and coordination

*Occipital lobes:* Loss of distance perception, double vision, loss of color perception

*Thalamus and medulla:* Depression of respiration and other autonomic nervous system functions; subnormal temperature, stupor, shock, death

While the focus of this discussion is care of the alcoholic in order to prevent liver cirrhosis, alcoholism causes widespread pathology throughout the body. These changes are summarized in Table 19-2. Perhaps the greatest threat to an alcoholic patient's health is the combination of drinking and driving. As many as 50 percent of all traffic fatalities can be linked to alcohol consumption.

Besides affecting health, drinking can have serious *effects on interpersonal relations.* A typical pattern in the process of the development of alcoholism is that, as the alcohol intake is less well controlled, the person tends to "drop out" of some or most interpersonal interactions. All too frequently family and friends allow this disengagement to occur to be momentarily "rid of the problem." Forced interaction, of course, is an excuse to resume drinking.

After years of drinking, psychological changes occur in the alcohol-dependent person. Alcoholics alibi for and defend their drinking of alcohol, they hide the quantity and frequency of their drinking from themselves and others, and, finally, they spend most of their time thinking about or engaging in drinking. They usually become irritable and may not conform socially in interpersonal interactions.

Finally, alcoholism interferes with the individual's *economic functioning.* As the need to drink increases both before and during working hours, judgment and performance suffer. Even the most tolerant and empathetic employer will reach a limit. Jobs are frequently lost, putting a further strain on both the alcoholic and the family.

Alcoholism affects all age groups. It is found in both males and females and can affect people from virtually any ethnic or cultural background. Its incidence was thought to be extremely rare in persons under twenty; however, the occurrence of teen-age alcoholism is increasing at an alarming rate.

Before care of the alcohol-dependent person can be effective, self-recognition by the alcoholic that a problem exists is essential. This often does not readily occur because psychological and physiological manifestations of chronic alcoholism include distortion of the ability to objectively perceive and critique one's own behavior and its impact on others.

In order to care for alcohol-dependent patients, nurses must identify and try to understand their own *attitudes* toward alcoholic patients. These attitudes can have a profound influence on nursing care. Nurses must look into themselves in an effort to understand their negative or ambivalent feelings. Once identified, these feelings can be accepted. The heightened self-awareness will help to control and temper hostilities.

Even before the alcoholic patient has sought help, nurses are frequently in a position to counsel and support *families.* The nurse should counsel the family to talk with the patient when sober and point out their reactions to the drinking. The family should impress upon the patient their love and concern, and they should help in efforts to decrease or stop alcohol intake. Few alcoholics seek help early unless pressure is exerted by the employer, family, or friends; however, demeaning nagging is of little value. Threats should be made only if the family is prepared to carry them out. It is critical to the maintenance of the family not to let the events of one member's drinking become the focus of all interactions within the home. Family members should be counseled not to alibi for the patient if work or social engagements are missed.

Once the alcoholic has sought help, nursing care should focus on helping the patient to condition coping mechanisms, offering psychological support, and coordinating resources. The patient needs to learn to tolerate stresses previously handled with alcohol consumption. With the patient's help, the nurse should identify activities, interactions, and/or events that tend to precede alcohol intake. Situations that are most stressful should be avoided initially. This may be especially difficult in social situations where not drinking is considered odd and unacceptable. Business people, especially, are often "expected" to have a cocktail. The nurse should explore with the patient methods for handling pressures from friends and acquaintances. It is often easiest to politely answer, "No, thank you, I'm an alcoholic." A firm "no, thank you" or ordering a soft drink may also deter persistent friends. Behaviors and situations that enabled the patient to remain sober in the past should be reinforced.

Failures to remain sober should be handled sympathetically and nonjudgmentally. The incident should be maximized and the reasons for the relapse explored with the patient and family in an attempt to prevent its recurrence.

**TABLE 19-2**
EFFECTS OF ALCOHOLISM ON VARIOUS ORGAN SYSTEMS

| Site | Result |
| --- | --- |
| Brain | Acute: Blackouts or amnesias<br>Chronic: Chronic brain syndromes—<br>Korsakoff's syndrome/psychosis<br>and Wernicke's syndrome<br>Personality changes |
| Nervous system | Acute: Peripheral polyneuropathy<br>Temporary nerve palsies<br>Chronic: Peripheral polyneuropathy with<br>muscle wasting |
| Musculature | Acute: Alcoholic myopathy<br>Chronic: Chronic myopathy—severe<br>muscle wasting |
| Heart | Alcoholic cardiomyopathy |
| Liver | Alcoholic hepatitis<br>Cirrhosis<br>Liver failure |
| Pancreas | Acute: Pancreatitis—permanent damage<br>unlikely with treatment<br>Chronic: Pancreatitis—permanent,<br>progressive damage |
| Hematologic system | Iron-deficiency anemia<br>Bone marrow depression<br>Thrombocytopenia |
| Lungs | Decreased vital capacity<br>Respiratory infections<br>Tuberculosis |
| Reproductive system | Male: Temporary or permanent impotence<br>Female: Potential birth defects |

SOURCE: Pamela K. Burkhalter: *Nursing Care of the Alcoholic and Drug Abuser,* McGraw-Hill, New York, 1975.

If the patient is to be successful, family therapy may be necessary. This is especially true regarding the husband, wife, and/or teenage alcoholic. The core of the problem of alcoholism is often intertwined in family relations. Family therapy allows all members to search out and uncover the problem.

The patient and family should be made aware of community resources that may be beneficial. Participation in group psychotherapy, Alcoholics Anonymous, Alanon for family members, health facilities, or support from clergy or friends may be suggested. Because of the increased prevalence in teen-age alcoholism, prevention programs are being started in many high schools. Nurses can play a significant role in helping communities recognize this problem and in initiating programs to prevent its spread.

**Second-Level Nursing Care**
Assessment by the nurse of the effects of chronic alcohol ingestion is a challenge. Because of the liver's regenerative capacity, when alcoholic cirrhosis is first developing, often referred to as *alcoholic hepatitis,* the pathological changes will not be widely manifested. Initially, the effects on the patient will be as much a result of the direct effects of alcohol as they will be from liver damage.

**Nursing assessment** After the initial assessment has led the practitioner to think that inflammation or destruction of liver cells is occurring, a careful, detailed *health history* should be sought. It usually reveals a recent episode of heavy drinking and complaints of anorexia, nausea, and fatigue. Since certain alcoholic beverages are more toxic than others (bourbon is more toxic than vodka), the type of alcohol ingested ought to be elicited. The patient should be questioned about any known weight loss. A change in the way clothes fit is a good indication. Changes in bowel habits and the color of urine and stools should be elicited.

Upon *physical assessment* the patient may demonstrate a variety of changes. A general inspection should be made with special attention given skin color and secondary sex characteristics. When jaundice first appears, it is best observed in the sclera. The classic image of an alcoholic is often presented—flushed face, bloodshot eyes, decreased visual acuity, and spider angiomas of the upper extremities, chest, back, and face. The patient may have a fever. The abdominal examination will reveal hepatomegaly and some abdominal tenderness. The skin will feel dry and the mucous membranes may reveal various vitamin deficiencies. In the early stages of alcoholic cirrhosis the chest examination may be normal. Neurological evaluation often reveals intellectual deterioration and decreased sensation in the periphery.

**D**iagnostic Tests When alcoholic cirrhosis is suspected, the diagnosis can be confirmed by a variety of liver function tests. These studies are summarized in Table 19-3. *Dye clearance studies* involve the injection of substances, Bromsulphalein (BSP) or indocyanine green, which, after injection into the body, are picked up by the liver and excreted. The amount of the substance remaining in the blood after a certain period of time reflects current liver functioning.

There are also several biochemical studies which reflect liver function. The *total serum bilirubin* indicates the liver's ability to conjugate and excrete bilirubin and will be slightly increased with hepatic damage. *Direct serum bilirubin* measures conjugated bilirubin and is not increased in alcoholic cirrhosis unless biliary obstruction is a problem. *Serum alkaline phosphatase* which is excreted in the bile will also be slightly increased. The *serum proteins,* especially albumin, which are manufactured by the liver will be slightly decreased at this early stage of cirrhosis.

Thousands of enzymes are necessary for the many chemical reactions carried out by the liver. With tissue injury, these *enzymes* [transaminases such as serum glutamic oxaloacetic transaminase (SGOT) and serum glutamic pyruvic transaminase (SGPT)] are released into the bloodstream, increasing their concentrations. *Prothrombin time* will be prolonged as cirrhosis develops. *Serum cholesterol* is also decreased as lipogenesis in the liver is impaired.

The immunocompetence of the liver has recently been evaluated by *injection of PHA* (a purified hyalin). With hepatic damage the injection of PHA results in decreased responsiveness of lymphocytes[5] to the substance and can help differentiate alcoholic hepatitis from cholecystitis or cholelithiasis.

**Nursing problems and interventions** When alcoholic cirrhosis first develops, the prognosis for cure is excellent. The major problem affecting that prognosis is the patient's *drinking.* If drinking can be controlled, the liver may heal and the patient's health return. The patient should be encouraged to stop drinking and told the prognosis with and without alcohol. The nurse should coordinate the care, talk with the alcoholic, encourage sobriety, and try to meet as many dependent and physical needs as are warranted. At this time, the alcoholic is preoccupied with personal misery, does not answer questions directly, and may appear constantly vigilant—startling easily and being unusually alert.

*Fatigue* is also a problem, and the patient should be encouraged to get adequate rest and sleep. The patient's work and activity patterns should be reviewed and plans made to provide rest periods. It is often helpful to include the family in this planning.

For liver regeneration to occur, *adequate nutrition* is essential. Fever and jaundice often recede as nutrition improves. The diet is very important because alcohol has a direct toxic effect on the liver and because malnutrition contributes to hepatic cellular pathology. Dietary teaching should focus on eating a high-carbohydrate, high-calorie, high-protein diet. Protein supplements in liquid or solid form may be given. Vitamin and mineral supplements, especially folic acid, vitamin $B_6$, thiamine, iron, and potassium, are often used. The patient must recognize the necessity for sobriety. However, if this is not feasible, the nurse should encourage eating when the blood is free of alcohol and advise selectivity in the type of alcoholic beverage ingested.

### Third-Level Nursing Care

When large amounts of alcohol are consumed over an extended period of time, severe alcoholic cirrhosis develops with widespread hepatocellular failure and portal hypertension. The patient is acutely ill and will require hospitalization.

**Nursing assessment** The patient's *health history* usually includes a history of alcohol intake, weight loss, anorexia, jaundice, swelling of legs and abdomen, fatigue, abdominal pain, hemorrhage from the mouth or vomiting of blood, diarrhea, and impotence. Depending on the severity of ammonia intoxication, the patient's mental state may be altered.

Upon *physical assessment* the nurse will observe many of the physical changes associated with hepatic failure (spider nevi, palmar erythema, peripheral edema, purpuric lesions, gynecomastia, pectoral, pubic, and axillary alopecia, and jaundice). During the abdominal examination ascites will be evident and can be confirmed by testing for shifting dullness, the puddle examination, and fluid wave. These maneuvers are discussed in Chap. 11. The liver and spleen will be enlarged, and the superficial veins of the abdomen may be dilated (caput

medusae). The patient may also complain of abdominal tenderness.

During the chest examination there may be dullness and decreased breath sounds over areas of pleural effusion. If hypovolemia and cardiomyopathy are severe, heart sounds may evidence failure. Neurological evaluation may reveal asterixis. The patient should be asked to outstretch both arms and hands while the nurse observes for flapping tremor. Sensation in the periphery should also be evaluated.

**D**iagnostic Tests The dye clearance studies and biochemical studies discussed in Second-Level Nursing Care will reveal an increased degree of liver damage. The SGOT, SGPT, LDH, serum alkaline phosphatase, serum bilirubin, and prothrombin times will be increased. The serum albumin, manufactured in the liver, will be decreased, while the serum globulins are increased. Proteinuria may be present if the kidneys are functional; otherwise, oliguria may occur.

A *photoscan* (scintiscan) may also be done to obtain an outline of the size and configuration of the liver. This information is useful both for the establishment of a diagnosis and as a guide for *liver biopsy.* The biopsy is performed to show not only the presence of cirrhosis but to confirm the extent of hepatic cellular damage. The liver may be so fibrous that aspiration biopsy is difficult to perform and produces only a few hepatic cells.

Prior to liver biopsy the patient's prothrombin time should be determined, vitamin K administered, and the patient should void. The biopsy is accomplished by asking the patient to take a deep breath and hold it while the physician inserts a needle intercostally into the liver and aspirates the hepatic cells. The needle is quickly removed and the patient instructed to breathe, remain still, and stay in bed. A sealer such as collodion may be applied after the cannula is removed.

Asceptic technique should be maintained throughout the procedure. Because of the vascularity of the liver, bleeding is a danger. Vital signs should be carefully monitored following the procedure, and the patient should be kept supine or on the right side. The right-side position causes the abdominal contents to fall against the liver, affording a certain amount of pressure to decrease bleeding.

*Peritoneoscopy* may be used to identify the type of cirrhosis present. To evaluate the extent of the circulatory changes associated with portal hypertension, *radiography* may be used. Some of the studies include hepatoportography, celiac arteriography, and splenoportography.

*Esophagoscopy* or *esophagogastroscopy* is used to directly visualize the esophageal varices and gastric mucosa. *Wedged hepatic vein pressure* and *portal vein pressure* may also be taken. An *electroencephalogram* will reveal the encephalopathy that results from ammonia intoxication.

**Nursing problems and interventions** Identification of nursing problems in alcoholic cirrhosis is overwhelming initially, but when each problem is related to the underlying pathological change, the reason for the problem and a plan of intervention are easier to outline.

Correction of the patient's *weight loss* and *malnutrition* are of prime importance if any healing of

**TABLE 19-3**
TESTS OF LIVER FUNCTION

| Test | Normal | Comment |
|---|---|---|
| 1 Blood clotting and blood cell count | | |
| Prothrombin time | 12–15 s | Prothrombin time most important test in assessing liver pathology. In liver disease, blood takes longer to clot owing to decreased ability of the liver to synthesize the protein prothrombin. Also, there is decreased absorption of vitamin K which is essential for prothrombin synthesis. Failure of the liver to return the prothrombin time to normal in presence of vitamin K indicates clinically significant liver cell damage. The degree of liver impairment can fairly accurately be estimated by the degree of prothrombin abnormality. |
| Hematocrit | 35–45% | |
| WBC | 5000–10,000 cells/mm$^3$ | Normal early in cirrhosis and hepatitis. Leukopenia with enlarged, overactive spleen. Leukopenia accompanies fever in hepatitis. |
| 2 Clearance studies | | |
| Indocyanine green (ICG) | Less than 5% remain- | Procedure: Patient fasts for 12 h before |
| Bromsulphalein (BSP) | ing in serum 45 min after injection of 5 mg/ kg body weight | test. Dose is reduced if clinical symptoms already present. Dye retained in liver cell damage. |
| 3 Serum enzyme studies | | |
| SGPT | 5–35 units/ml | Damage to liver cells causes release of |
| SGOT | 5–40 units/ml | these enzymes into blood, but the in- |
| LDH | 400 units/ml (varies with method used) | creased levels in the serum do not directly correlate with the amount of liver impairment. Elevations occur in other diseases. Blood withdrawn from vein. |
| Alkaline phosphatase | 2–5 Bodansky units (varies with method) | Synthesized in liver, bone, and kidney and excreted in the biliary tract. A measure of biliary obstruction |
| Gamma glutamyl transpeptidase | | Enzyme found in biliary tract and not in cardiac or skeletal muscle. Elevated in hepatitis. More sensitive in detecting hepatic disease than alkaline phosphatase. |
| 4 Special tests | | |
| Hepatitis B surface antigen (HBsAg) | | HBsAg is normally absent from the serum and, if present, is diagnostic for viral hepatitis, type B. Tests for HBsAg include counterelectrophoresis and radioimmunoassay. Not found in serum of patients with type A viral hepatitis. |
| Liver scan | | Through the injection of a radioactive substance, the therapist can visualize the size and shape of the liver. Serves as a guide for liver biopsy. |
| Liver biopsy | | Used to determine microscopic, cellular pathology of liver cells. |

the liver cells is to occur. The diet should be one that is high in both carbohydrates and calories. The protein content should be moderate and will be mediated by the degree of ammonia intoxication. The patient should be encouraged to eat, offered frequent snacks, and provided with an environment that is conducive to eating. Liquid protein supplements (Sustagen) may be needed initially until the patient can progress to a nutritious diet. Supplemental vitamin therapy is usually given intravenously. The patient will experience *fatigue,* and energy should be conserved with adequate rest.

If the patient is having difficulty with *nausea* or *vomiting,* frequent oral hygiene should be emphasized. Movement should be minimized. The air in the patient's room should be fresh, clean, and de-

| | Test | Normal | Comment |
|---|---|---|---|
| | Hepatic hemodynamic studies (in patients with suspected cirrhosis) | | Splenoportogram is used to determine the adequacy of portal blood flow. Diminished in cirrhosis. Endoscopy to view esophageal varices. Measurement of portal vein pressure. |
| 5 | Metabolic studies | | |
| *a* | Protein metabolism | | |
| | Serum albumin | 3.5–5.5 gm/100 ml | Serum proteins are synthesized by the liver. Serum albumin is markedly decreased in liver cellular damage. Gamma globulin is usually elevated in liver disease and markedly elevated in chronic active liver disease |
| | Plasma fibrinogen | 0.2–0.4 gm/100 ml | |
| | Serum globulin | 2.5–3.5 gm/100 ml | |
| | Total protein | 6–8 gm/100 ml | |
| | Serum protein electrophoresis: | | |
| | Albumin | 50–65 % of total | |
| | Alpha$_1$ globulin | 4–7.5 % | |
| | Alpha$_2$ globulin | 7–12 % | |
| | Beta globulin | 10–16 % | |
| | Gamma globulin | 10–20 % | |
| | Ammonia | 30–70 $\mu$g/100 ml | In liver disease, less ammonia is converted to urea, and thus the serum ammonia concentration increases. |
| *b* | Carbohydrate metabolism | | |
| | Galactose or glucose tolerance tests | Removed from blood in 1–2 h | Injected intravenously, and serial samples are drawn from the vein. If serum galactose remains elevated after 75 min, liver function is impaired. If serum glucose remains elevated after 1–2 h, the liver cells are damaged or utilization of glucose by body tissues is impaired. |
| *c* | Fat metabolism | | |
| | Serum cholesterol | 150–250 mg/100 ml | Blood drawn after low-cholesterol diet. Cholesterol esters 70% of total cholesterol. Lipids decreased in liver parenchymal cell damage, elevated in biliary duct obstruction. |
| | Serum phospholipids | 125–300 mg/100 ml | |
| | Triglycerides | 30–135 mg/100 ml | |
| *d* | Bilirubin metabolism | | |
| | Serum bilirubin | | Venous blood drawn. Bilirubin is a product of RBC hemoglobin breakdown, and elevation may cause jaundice. Total bilirubin measures both direct and indirect bilirubin. Direct bilirubin elevated with obstructed biliary ducts or impaired excretion of conjugated bilirubin. Indirect bilirubin elevated with accelerated erythrocyte hemolysis, absence of glucuronyl transferase, and/or damaged liver cells. |
| | Direct (conjugated, soluble) | 0.2 mg/100 ml | |
| | Indirect (not conjugated, not water soluble) | 0.8 mg/100 ml | |
| | Total bilirubin | 1.0 mg/100 ml | |
| | Urine bilirubin | None | A measure of conjugated bilirubin. If bilirubin present in urine, shaking the specimen results in a yellow tint in the foam. Urinary and fecal urobilinogen decreases with bile duct obstruction. Antibiotics reduce the urobilinogen levels. Fecal urobilinogen seldom measured. |
| | Urobilinogen | | |
| | Urine | 0–4 mg/24 h | |
| | Feces | 40–280 mg/24 h | |

odorized. Antiemetics (e.g., Tigan) are often given orally, parenterally, or, most frequently, by suppository. The cirrhotic patient is frequently *anemic.* To improve this problem, vitamin $B_{12}$ and iron preparations are usually given to supplement the diet.

*Ascites* is another problem requiring intervention by the nurse. Patience is the key to successful management of the cirrhotic patient with ascites because resolution of the problem requires weeks to months. Intervention is governed by the severity of the ascites. If retention of fluid in the peritoneal cavity is great enough to interfere with respiration and eating, or to cause an umbilical hernia, paracentesis may be performed and 1000 to 2000 ml fluid removed. Because the fluid is rich in serum proteins, the depleting effect its removal has on body proteins must be recognized. It is unusual for the physician to drain more than 1000 ml.

*Paracentesis* is a minor surgical procedure done at the bedside. The procedure should be fully explained. The patient should be instructed to void, and vital signs should be taken. With the patient positioned in a chair or in high Fowler's position, the abdomen is draped and prepared with antiseptic solution. The site of insertion is then anesthetized and a trocar with an obturator is inserted. The obturator is removed and tubing attached to the trocar which remains in the peritoneal cavity. The prescribed amount of fluid is then drained into a container by gravity. Finally, the trocar is removed and a dressing applied. The patient's vital signs should be taken until stable, and the patient's condition and response to the procedure noted. The amount and description of fluid removed should be recorded, and specimens sent to the laboratory. Because ascites usually returns, paracentesis provides only temporary relief and may have to be repeated over time.

Control of the problem of *edema* is concomitant with controlling ascites. Knowledge of why the edema and ascites have developed directs the nurse to magnify efforts to maintain the prescribed diet, restrict fluid intake, and record more accurately the urine output and urinalysis data. Sodium should be restricted to 200 to 500 mg/day, fluid to 1000 to 1500 ml/day, and spironolactone (Aldactone) administered by the nurse. Daily urinalysis to determine the sodium ($Na^+$) and potassium ($K^+$) concentrations should be done as a guide for diuretic therapy. The dose of spironolactone is increased until the urinary $Na^+:K^+$ ratio is greater than 1. Diuresis which occurs at this point in the therapy is usually sufficient to begin resolution of the ascites. The nurse should keep a flowsheet to record intake and output, electrolytes, and daily weight. Hyponatremia, hypokalemia, dehydration, and renal failure are complications of vigorous diuretic therapy. The nurse should encourage the patient to rest which promotes diuresis and to eat only the diet prescribed. The sodium content of the medications being administered should be calculated in the total sodium intake of the patient.

Patients with advanced hepatic cirrhosis are also susceptible to *infection.* All possible infection sites should be cleansed regularly and watched closely. Cutdown sites, central venous catheter sites, and subclavian sites for hyperalimentation should be handled aseptically and an antibiotic ointment applied. Turning, coughing, and deep breathing should be encouraged and the patient's temperature monitored. Antibiotic therapy should be instituted when indicated.

Because of the bilirubin buildup in tissues, *jaundice* and *pruritus* are problems. Controlling pruritus requires ingenious nursing intervention. The drug cholestyramine (Cuemid) may be administered to supplement the following nursing actions:

1   Establish that the etiology of the pruritus is bilirubin deposits in the skin and not drug allergy or electrolyte imbalance.

2   Tissue anoxia increases pruritus, and so the nurse should encourage adequate rest, balanced diet, high fluid intake, iron supplements, and good room ventilation (without causing drafts). These nursing interventions are also important because vasodilatation resulting from fever, hypoxemia, and/or increased blood volume can cause pruritus.

3   Since perspiration contributes to itching, clothing should allow evaporation. Anxiety needs to be controlled and exertion avoided. Bed sheets should be changed frequently.

4   Emotional stress promotes pruritus and prolongs the symptoms; therefore, enjoyable distractions and a degree of emotional tranquility are desirable.

5   Dry skin tends to be itchy, especially if it is alkaline. Have the patient avoid frequent bathing, hot baths, alkaline soap, and irritating clothing which tend to increase pruritus and, therefore, scratching. Whirlpool bath (vibration) and pressure on the skin (not scratching with the nails) may help to relieve the itching. Bland emollient creams may be applied to the skin.

6   Avoid an itch-scratch-itch cycle if possible by keeping the patient's nails short, preventing sweating

(especially at night), and providing diversion and reassurance. Although not yet supported by nursing research, a theory holds that pruritus possibly is worse during late evening and night because temperature and vasodilatation are greatest during those times.

Patients with hepatic damage are more *susceptible to certain drugs.* The nurse should be selective when administering medications and give only those drugs known to have little or no hepatotoxic effects. The therapeutic value of a drug should be weighed against the risk of further liver damage. Because of the increased sensitivity, narcotics, sedatives, and hypnotics should be used with extreme caution. Smaller doses will be needed because of the cumulative and potentially fatal effect these drugs will have.

*Changes in body image* are often experienced by patients with cirrhosis. Gross ascites can cause significant alterations in self-perception. The male alcoholic, especially, must adjust not only to ascites but to enlarged breasts, hair loss, soft skin, atrophied testicles, and impotence. These changes can be extremely depreciating to the patient's self-esteem and masculine image. The changes should be faced honestly by the nurse, and the likelihood of their resolution explained to the patient.

**H**epatic Coma   One of the most difficult problems encountered is that of *ammonia intoxication.* The increased serum ammonia interferes with brain metabolism, altering the mental state. The patient should be monitored closely for changes in mental status. Any confusion, disorientation, changes in handwriting, speech, and mood, or asterixis should be noted. The importance of individualized patient care by one nurse is especially important in recognizing subtle changes.

In an effort to decrease the blood ammonia level, potassium, which is necessary for cerebral metabolism of ammonia, is given. Ammonia is formed in the intestines by the action of bacteria on protein. To decrease intestinal protein, its intake is limited. Tap water enemas may be given to remove protein-rich blood that may result from bleeding esophageal varices. Antibiotics that are absorbed poorly and, therefore, become concentrated in the intestines are given to decrease intestinal bacteria. Neomycin is most commonly used and may be given orally or instilled by enema. Since ammonia is formed during muscle contraction, rest is important. The blood ammonia level is also decreased by lactalose which, when degraded in the large bowel,

decreases the pH of the stool, preventing formation of ammonia and promoting ammonia ion excretion. Hemodialysis and exchange blood transfusion may also be used to temporarily decrease the serum ammonia.

Since the protective reflexes, such as coughing and blinking, are lost during hepatic coma, all the problems associated with a *loss of consciousness* need to be evaluated. These include monitoring vital signs and preventing hypoxia. The nurse should be cognizant of eye and mouth care to prevent drying and ulceration. The patient with impending hepatic coma has difficulty ambulating and is unsteady. As coma progresses, protection from falling and seizure precautions should be provided.

Flowsheets to record patient progress, intake and output, and electrolyte and neurological status are helpful. The prognosis is generally poor if hepatic coma lasts for over 24 hours. *Skin breakdown* in a patient who is malnourished, immobile, jaundiced, and edematous can occur in less than 24 hours. Careful attention to skin care, passive exercises, and turning of the patient are indicated. To keep the skin dry, bed sheets should be changed frequently and a Foley catheter inserted. The nurse should ensure proper alignment of the patient's extremities and support an ascitic abdomen to keep it free from pressure.

As precoma progresses to coma and postcoma, the nurse cannot be certain when the patient can and cannot hear. The ability to hear should be assumed, and the patient should be addressed directly. The family should be instructed about this, the need for turning, and the prognosis.

In some cases hemoperfusion, artificial liver support, and extracorporeal assist have been attempted to detoxify the blood and to afford regeneration of hepatocytes. To date, safe, practical models useful on humans have not been found. Liver transplantation has had variable results.

**E**sophageal Varices   As the liver becomes increasingly cirrhotic, the microvasculature is further interrupted and portal hypertension increases. The collateral circulation that subsequently develops flows along vessels that are weaker than normal vessels. As the pressure in the collaterals increases, they become overdistended. Esophageal varices and hemorrhoids result.

The most common problem associated with esophageal varices is *bleeding.* Varices tend to bleed as the pressure increases. Normal portal vein pressure is 6 mmHg or less but may increase to

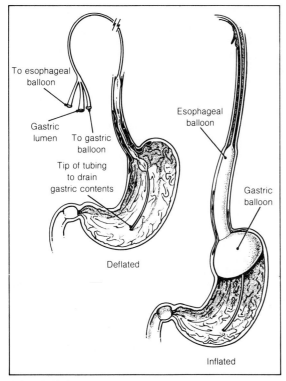

**FIGURE 19-2**
Diagram of properly placed Sengstaken-Blakemore tube.

20 mmHg in hepatic cirrhosis. Bleeding can also result if infection is present or if rough foods constantly rub the area. If bleeding occurs, an endoscopy is often performed to determine whether the bleeding is from varices or a result of erosive gastritis or peptic ulcer.

Nursing care of a patient with esophageal varices initially focuses on careful monitoring to detect bleeding. Regular and careful assessment of the patient's status should be instituted, and any indication of bleeding reported immediately. The earliest indications will include restlessness, pallor, tachycardia, and a cooling of the skin. These will be followed by hypotension. It is especially important to identify bleeding early because the liver is very susceptible to cell damage from ischemia and because the patient already has a diminished ability to sustain stress.

If hemorrhage occurs, the site of bleeding is often confirmed by esophagoscopy. Depending on the patient's condition and on the severity of the bleeding, treatment may include any one of the following: (1) gastric lavage with ice-cold saline continuously until returns are clear, (2) administration of alpha- and/or beta-adrenergics, (3) administra-

tion of fresh blood or plasma, and/or (4) insertion by an endoscopist of a Sengstaken-Blakemore tube.

During the acute stage of the bleeding the patient will require close monitoring; vital signs should be taken frequently. Hepatic coma becomes a real danger because of the high protein load present when blood is digested. If the prothrombin time is significantly prolonged, vitamin K may be administered.

The *Sengstaken-Blakemore tube* is commonly used to control hemorrhage. It is a three-lumen tube composed of a catheter that goes into the stomach for suctioning, a lumen that ends in a gastric balloon, and one that ends in an esophageal balloon. It functions to stop bleeding by applying pressure to the esophageal varices.

As depicted in Fig. 19-2, the Sengstaken-Blakemore tube is inserted by an expert who ensures its proper placement and functioning. The pharynx is anesthetized, and the patient intubated to prevent aspiration during insertion. Before insertion, the stomach and esophageal balloons are checked for leaks. The tube is then passed into the stomach. The gastric balloon is inflated first with Hypaque (200 ml) and double-clamped securely. Pressure is exerted on the tube to pull the gastric balloon against the cardioesophageal junction. The correct position of the balloon is assured by x-ray. The esophageal balloon is then inflated to 20 (or up to 40) mmHg pressure and double-clamped. Continuous pressure, less than 1 kg, is exerted on the tube to keep the gastric balloon against the cardioesophageal junction.

Use of the Sengstaken-Blakemore tube, while invaluable in arresting hemorrhage, carries many dangers. Because of the possibility of gastric and esophageal erosion, the balloons should be deflated in 24 hours. The esophageal balloon should be deflated first to prevent dislodgement and airway obstruction. If after 48 hours no additional bleeding occurs, the tube is removed. Once removed, it should be cut and destroyed to prevent reuse. While in place the tube should be monitored closely. In the event it dislodges and obstructs the airway, scissors, kept at the bedside, should be used to cut the tube, thus deflating the balloons.

*Surgical intervention*  If bleeding from esophageal varices continues after medical management, the patient may be considered for surgery. Although a poor surgical risk, subsequent bleeding episodes with esophageal varices are associated with a higher mortality rate than surgery.[6] *Portosystemic shunts* are generally employed to divert the blood flow from the high-pressure portal venous system to the low-pressure systemic veins and, in doing so, relieve the pressure in the esophageal varices. Figure 19-3 illustrates the major portosystemic shunts. One of the difficulties with portosystemic shunts is the encephalopathy that results from the blood ammonia level. Depending on the procedure used, all or part of the portal venous blood flow is diverted away from the liver, and the ammonia absorbed from the intestinal tract begins to accumulate in the blood and, thus, interferes with cerebral functioning.

A procedure recommended by some is a *distal splenorenal shunt*.[7] This procedure, depicted in Fig. 19-4, drains blood from the esophageal varices and spleen. It relieves the distention in these areas while hepatic blood flow is essentially unchanged. Collateral veins to the esophageal plexus are ligated and the splenic vein is ligated with its distal end sutured to the side of the renal vein. Postoperatively, nursing care of these patients is similar to that of any patient having undergone a shunting procedure. Because these patients are generally poor surgical risks, care should especially focus on preventing complications following surgery. Bleeding is often a problem, and the patients' vital signs and prothrombin time should be monitored. These patients also need to be watched closely for developing encephalopathy.

**D**elirium Tremors   Alcoholic patients often experience withdrawal symptoms when alcohol ingestion is stopped. This frequently occurs 3 to 4 days after hospitalization and is usually short-lived. The symptoms that develop are called *delirium tremors* and are characterized by profound confusion, illusions, delusions, vivid hallucinations, tremors, agitation, sleeplessness, and increased autonomic activity. The exact mechanism for the development of delirium tremors is not well understood. They usually last 3 days or less and are followed by a deep sleep. The patient awakes with no memory of the experience.

Nursing care during delirium tremors focuses on safety of the patient and nurse. The patient is confused and often becomes violent, requiring restraint. Restraints should be applied properly and checked frequently. Side rails should be kept up, and the patient protected from falling or self-injury. Two people should be present when the restraints are removed. During the tremors the patient will be bedridden, and so care should also focus on the hazards of immobility. Because of liver damage, sedatives and hypnotics should be used

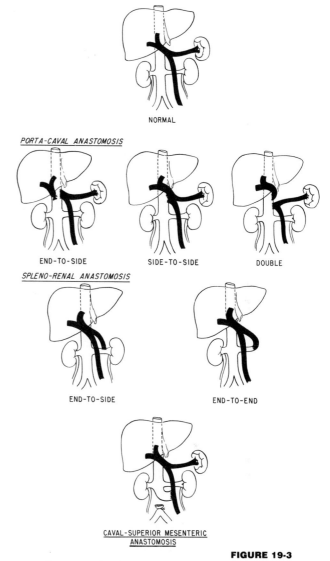

**FIGURE 19-3**
Diagrammatic representation of major portosystemic shunts. (*From S. I. Schwartz et al. (eds.): Principles of Surgery, McGraw-Hill, New York, 1974. By permission of the publishers.*)

cautiously. A variety of drugs have been used to control the withdrawal symptoms. Currently, the most popular medication is *chlordiazapoxide* (Librium). It has proved to be effective, is long-acting, and has a wide margin of safety. Other drugs that may be used with varying adverse and/or toxic effects are the barbiturates, phenothiazines, haloperidol, paraldehyde, and hydroxyzine.

### Fourth-Level Nursing Care

The prognosis of the person with alcoholic cirrhosis is good if sobriety can be maintained. A *low-*

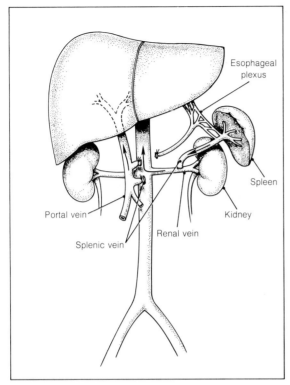

**FIGURE 19-4**
Distal splenorenal shunt. Arrows indicate blood flow through anastomosis.

*salt, nutritious diet* is also essential. Since alcohol (7 calories/g) is a major source of calories, the person who has relinquished alcohol intake requires help from the nurse in planning and eating a well-balanced diet to replace with food the calories once imbibed through drinking alcohol. Written diet instructions discussed with the patient and family or friends are useful. Frequent follow-up visits by a community health nurse are essential.

The *activity level* of the person recovering from alcoholic cirrhosis is governed by the symptoms. Because hepatic blood flow diminishes with moderate exercise, rest periods are advised initially and adjusted by the patient at home according to the level of fatigue. The patient may return to work but should be advised to avoid straining such as lifting heavy objects if portal hypertension and esophageal varices are a problem.

The patient and those with whom he or she lives should be taught to recognize symptoms of *encephalopathy.* When symptoms occur, measures to decrease the blood ammonia level should be taught. These include increased potassium intake and avoidance of hepatotoxic drugs. The patient

should be cautioned against driving when any signs of encephalopathy are present and about the dangers of over-the-counter drugs. A list of foods high in potassium and drugs to be avoided should be given for home use.

If ascites and peripheral neuropathy are significant problems for the alcoholic cirrhotic patient, special advisement by the nurse on *sexual difficulties* (fatigue, decrease of libido, impotence, physical awkwardness due to ascites) may help make any adjustment less ominous for the patient and spouse. *Peripheral neuropathy* is not readily reversible. The patient should be taught to measure bath water temperature, use heating pads and hot water bottles cautiously, and smoke with care. Because stress decreases hepatic blood flow, any reduction of stress at home, at work, or in the community is therapeutic.

Follow-up care is extremely important for the patient with alcoholic cirrhosis. Community support systems such as Alcoholics Anonymous should be made available. Hepatic cirrhosis results in many complex nursing problems which should be assessed on a regular basis by a community-based nurse. Understanding of the therapeutic regime should be periodically reevaluated, and gaps or misunderstandings corrected. Community-based nursing care should continue for years and should focus on supporting the patient in efforts to overcome alcoholism and liver disease.

## VIRAL HEPATITIS

*Hepatitis,* inflammation of the liver, is a major uncontrolled public health problem for several reasons: the causative agents have not been identified, there are no specific therapeutic drugs for its treatment, its incidence has increased in relation to illicit drug use, and it is communicable prior to the appearance of observable clinical symptoms. To further intensify the problem, it is easily disseminated to others and usually results in an extended period of convalesence with concomitant loss of time from school or work.

Two main types of viral hepatitis have been identified, type A and type B. They are caused by different viruses, have different incubation periods, and have different modes of transmission. However, both manifest similar symptoms and pathological changes within the hepatic tissue.

Recently, a type of viral hepatitis that is neither type A nor type B has been discovered; it is sometimes referred to as type C. Little information is available about type C viral hepatitis except that it occurs in patients who have had multiple (at least 15 units) blood transfusions.

## Pathophysiology

Viral hepatitis results in inflammation of the hepatic cells, hyperplasia of the Kupffer cells, bile stasis, and necrosis. The severity of the inflammation varies. It can be so mild that the patient is unaware of the problem or so severe as to cause death. Hepatitis affects the patient in three stages—the prodromal or initial stage (preicteric stage), the icteric or jaundiced stage, and the recovery period.

During the *prodromal period,* which lasts from 1 to 3 weeks, the patient experiences vague gastrointestinal and general body symptoms. Fatigue, malaise, lassitude, weight loss, and anorexia are common. Many patients develop an aversion to food and cigarettes. Less commonly nausea, vomiting, diarrhea, arthralgias, and flulike symptoms occur. The liver becomes enlarged and tender, and intermittent pruritus may develop. One to four days before the icteric stage, the urine darkens from bilirubin and the stool lightens as less bilirubin is conjugated and excreted.

The *icteric stage* is characterized by the appearance of jaundice which peaks in 1 to 2 weeks and persists for 6 to 8 weeks. During the icteric stage the acuteness of the inflammation is subsiding. The gastrointestinal symptoms begin to disappear, and after 1 to 2 weeks of jaundice, the liver decreases in size and becomes less tender. During the icteric stage the postcervical lymph nodes and spleen are enlarged. The final stage is that of *recovery* and lasts 3 to 4 months. The patient generally feels well but fatigues easily.

## Type A Viral Hepatitis

The Center for Disease Control reported 2746 deaths in 1971 directly attributable to type A viral hepatitis. Currently there are about 50,000 known cases of type A viral hepatitis each year in the United States. The actual incidence is probably much higher because not all persons who contracted type A hepatitis were diagnosed and their illness reported.

Type A viral hepatitis, previously called *infectious hepatitis (IH), epidemic hepatitis,* and *short-incubation hepatitis,* is caused by a filterable virus which has not been isolated—a fact which makes early detection and vaccine development extremely difficult.

The chief mode of transmission of type A virus is from infected feces directly to the mouth or indirectly to the mouth through contaminated water, shellfish, or food. Parenteral transmission of type A virus is also possible through transfusion of whole blood, blood serum, or plasma from infected persons. Once the type A virus gains entry into the body, the incubation period is 15 to 50 days before mild symptoms ensue.

**First-level nursing care**  The nurse should be aware that young, low-income persons living in crowded facilities with minimal sanitation standards are most vulnerable to being infected with type A viral hepatitis. Individuals less than 25 years of age more frequently contract this disease than adults over 25 years of age possibly because adults already have been exposed to type A viruses and are therefore immune. Aged adults also seem to be susceptible to type A viral hepatitis. Recognition of the candidate for type A viral hepatitis aids the nurse in assessing clients and in taking appropriate precautions to prevent spread of the disease.

Prevention of type A viral hepatitis is dependent upon education of the public. Nurses can assess the health needs of communities and strengthen their knowledge of and motivation to practice safe sanitation. General rules that should be included in a health education program to prevent type A viral hepatitis are:

1   Avoid direct contact with stool, blood, or other body secretions (saliva, semen) of known or probable carriers of type A virus. Wear gloves and avoid sexual contact with these individuals.

2   Wash your hands thoroughly and frequently.

3   Avoid puncture of the skin with needles or lancets which were in contact with an infected person. Throw away syringes, needles, and pins that were used on or by an individual with type A hepatitis. Autoclaving is the only safe way to destroy the type A virus.

4   Do not drink water or eat shellfish that potentially are polluted with type A virus.

5   Recognize high-risk persons and seasons (fall and winter) and take extra precautions.

6   Obtain an injection of human immune serum globulin (ISG), 0.02 to 0.05 ml/kg body weight (usually about 5 ml is administered), if exposed in close contact to a person thought to have type A hepatitis.

7   Provide individual toothbrushes, eating utensils, and thermometers for family or institutional group members.

**Second-level nursing care** During the *prodromal phase,* which lasts from 1 to 3 weeks, the patient is infectious. Because of the nonspecific physical changes experienced during this phase, frequently the individual does not seek health care and may not be diagnosed.

**N**ursing Assessment  Obtaining an accurate *health history* is valuable in the prodromal phase because the diagnosis of type A viral hepatitis cannot be made by a simple laboratory test but is based upon history, physical examination, and laboratory data. Exposure to icteric persons, experience with blood transfusions or injections, participation in camping or disaster conditions such as flooding, a tornado, or chemical contamination of waterways, and recent complaints of gastrointestinal upset, fatigue, and weight loss are suggestive of this disease. Aver-

sion to food or smoking should especially be noted, and the patient should be asked about any urine and stool color changes.

The *physical assessment* in this stage is not remarkable. The patient may have a fever, less than 39°C, and during the abdominal examination the liver will be found to be enlarged and tender. The remainder of the physical examination will be normal.

*Diagnostic tests* During the prodromal phase, diagnostic tests can be very helpful in identifying the problem. Table 19-4 summarizes the laboratory data. (The relevance of the various tests is summarized in Table 19-3.) At this stage BSP will be retained and *liver biopsy* will show diffuse inflammation of both portal and central areas of the liver lobule. A more thorough discussion of these diag-

**TABLE 19-4**
COMPARISON OF TYPE A AND TYPE B VIRAL HEPATITIS

|  |  | Type A (infectious) | Type B (serum) |
|---|---|---|---|
| 1 | Epidemiology | | |
|  | Incubation | 15–50 days | 50–150 days |
|  | Season | Fall, winter | Any season |
|  | Age | Children, young adults, aged | Any age |
|  | Source of infection | Feces, clams, oysters, blood | Blood, feces |
| 2 | Laboratory data | | |
| a | Blood | | |
|  | SGPT, SGOT | High in prodromal phase | High in prodromal phase |
|  |  | Rapid drop in icteric phase | Remains elevated for months |
|  |  | Elevated 10 to 15 times normal | Elevated 10 to 15 times normal |
|  | Lactic dehydrogenase (LDH), isocitric dehydrogenase (ICD) | Elevated 5 to 10 times normal | Elevated 5 to 10 times normal |
|  | Alkaline phosphates | Elevated | Elevated |
|  | Aldolase | Elevated 10 times normal | Elevated 10 times normal |
|  | Gamma glutamyl transaminase (GGT) | Elevated | Elevated |
|  | 5-Nucleotidase | Slightly elevated | Slightly elevated |
|  | Albumin | Decreased | Decreased |
|  | IgM | Elevated | Elevated |
|  | Bilirubin | Elevated in icteric and early convalescence | Elevated in icteric phase |
|  |  |  | Elevated in icteric and convalescence |
|  | Leukopenia | With onset of fever | With onset of fever |
|  | HBsAg | Negative | Positive |
| b | Urine | | |
|  | Urobilinogen | Normal early, increased in convalescence | Normal or increased |
|  | Bilirubin | Increased early | Increased |
| c | Feces | | |
|  | Urobilinogen | Decreased | Decreased |
|  | Bilirubin | Decreased | Decreased |
|  | Virus | Viral particles 2 weeks before jaundice | Virus suspected |
| 3 | Immunity | | |
|  | Immunity | Lifetime immunity posthepatitis | Immune posthepatitis |
|  |  | Immune only to type A | Immune to type B |
|  | Prophylaxis | ISG useful | ISG not useful unless a high titer of HBcAb established |

nostic tests may be found in Hepatic Cirrhosis above.

**N**ursing Problems and Interventions The patient with type A viral hepatitis may often be cared for at home. Because the most acute stage is often passed when the diagnosis is confirmed, the physician may decide against hospitalization. The decision is based on the severity of the patient's illness and the feasibility of home care. Often the patient is hospitalized for a short time to confirm the diagnosis and then returned to the community.

The primary nursing problem during the prodromal period is *preventing dissemination of the disease.* These infected persons are nonjaundiced, mobile individuals who do not feel acutely ill and may or may not adhere consistently to safe sanitation practices. They are, therefore, a major source of spread of type A virus. The feasibility of caring for the patient at home should be assessed. Ideally, a community health nurse should evaluate this in a home visit. If it is determined that the patient feels well enough to be at home and the family is able to institute safe procedures, a plan should be drawn up that includes teaching the patient and family:

1   Safe hand-washing techniques

2   Simple isolation procedures

3   Use of disposable dishes, cups, and silverware

4   Nonuse of communal items (tooth brushes, wash clothes)

5   Proper disposal of garbage

6   Handling of linens, underwear, etc., by separate washing

7   Separate toilet and bath facilities

8   Avoidance of close contact with the patient (abstinence from sexual contact)

9   Avoidance by patient of alcohol and *all* drugs except those prescribed

The patient and family members may require help in acknowledging the need for these preventive practices when the individual does not appear critically ill and registers only a few mild complaints. Talking with them to interpret the reasons for the isolation procedures and restrictions is especially important. The family should also be counseled not to avoid or fear the patient and to continue interactions with him or her. Surveillance of these patients until they are noninfective is crucial. Home

care should include periodic evaluation of the isolation procedures. Breaks in procedure should be explained by the nurse, and correct practice retaught.

Human ISG, administered to all individuals who have been exposed to persons with type A viral hepatitis, is protective if injected during the incubation period. The adult dose of immune serum globulin is usually a single intramuscular injection of approximately 5 ml (0.02 to 0.05 ml/kg body weight). ISG stimulates antibody production and provides immunity for 6 to 8 weeks.

Because the patient experiences varying degrees of *anorexia* and *fatigue,* these are also nursing problems in the preicteric phase. The patient should be encouraged to eat a high-caloric, balanced diet. Small, frequent meals are often more palatable to the patient. While strict bed rest is not warranted, the patient should be encouraged to avoid strenuous physical exercise and to regularly rest in bed or in a chair.

**Third-level nursing care** Patients with type A viral hepatitis are most often hospitalized if they are acutely ill; having difficulty with vomiting and, therefore, fluid and electrolyte imbalance; or unable to be cared for at home. Often hospitalization finds the patient past the prodromal phase of illness and into the icteric phase.

**N**ursing Assessment The *health history* will have the same focus as that taken in the prodromal phase. During the icteric phase, however, the patient will relate definite urine and stool color changes and may complain of pruritus. The most striking finding on *physical assessment* will be the appearance of jaundice—most noticeable in the sclera. Jaundice usually precipitates within 1 week after the onset of prodromal symptoms; however, some persons with type A viral hepatitis do not become jaundiced throughout their entire illness. The abdominal examination will find the liver decreasing in size 1 to 2 weeks after jaundice appears. The tenderness will also subside. Because the spleen becomes enlarged, it will be palpable. Palpation of lymph nodes will reveal postcervical node enlargement. Laboratory tests are summarized in Table 19-4.

**N**ursing Problems and Interventions The patient with type A viral hepatitis is considered infectious from about 3 weeks before jaundice appears to 3 weeks after. *Preventing dissemination of the infection* remains a nursing problem during hospitalization. Isolation techniques should be employed, and the staff and visitors instructed in the rationale and proper procedures. Precautions should be taken with needles, food tray, linens, stool, urine, and any body secretions.

During this time the patient may become *irritable* or *depressed*. *Anxiety* regarding the jaundice and *resentment* of the isolation precautions may become evident. Isolation is usually continued with the aim of preventing viral spread, minimizing contacts, and promoting rest. The patient, however, may become restless and disoriented if isolation is extreme. The nurse should recruit the help of the patient's family and/or friends in providing sufficient diversional activities to prevent boredom and promote rest. Staff should be cautioned not to avoid the patient and to schedule regular interaction.

Adequate nutritional intake may be a problem at this stage owing to *anorexia*. The nurse should be careful to not allow the patient to receive contradictory messages about the importance of food. While nutritious intake of food and fluids is essential for hepatic cell regeneration, serving food on paper plates and trays is also indicated. A soggy paper plate in the context of prolonged confinement is no stimulus to eat for a person who is already anorectic and even may be viewed by the patient as a rejection of individual value. A diet high in carbohydrate and protein served as tolerated by the patient is indicated unless the hepatitis is severe and danger of coma exists. Food and fluids available on demand may contribute to adequate nutrition.

An adequate fluid intake, as much as 3 liters/day, is important in preventing complications which may arise from markedly decreased activity and/or bed rest. If *vomiting* is a problem, intravenous fluids may be indicated.

During the icteric phase the patient must also cope with *jaundice*. Reassurance from the nurse that it is transient is helpful. Family members and friends should be prepared for their visit with the patient. They should be informed that the patient has jaundice which will recede and they may mention to the patient that they notice the color change. Jaundice is often accompanied by *pruritus*. Nursing intervention in relation to this itching is discussed in Hepatic Cirrhosis above.

Throughout the course of hepatitis, *stress* should be minimized. It results in a prolongation of the amount of time the patient experiences symptoms.[8] The nurse should assess, with the patient's help, factors which are most stress-producing and attempt to resolve the precipitating causes. Including the family in minimizing stress is often valuable.

**Fourth-level nursing care**   The role of the nurse in fourth-level nursing care of the patient with type A viral hepatitis is to minimize residual damage to the hepatic cells. The nursing interventions employed during second- and third-level nursing greatly influence the success of nursing care during this phase of the patient's illness.

The patient tends to feel better during this phase. A sense of well-being returns, as does appetite, while jaundice, liver tenderness, and abdominal pain disappear. The patient experiences less fatigue and may need reminding of the need to pace activities. Young patients especially may find a more restful pace difficult to follow. For those living away from home, peer pressure to join in group activities and a fast-paced life-style are often persuasive deterrents to the nurse's instructions. Regular follow-up care will be needed to reemphasize the importance of rest and sleep for eventual complete recovery. Since school is usually missed, especially during hospitalization, arrangements to minimize the backup of school work should be made early in the illness. This is often a source of great concern for the patient.

The nurse should teach patients that although they usually have a lifetime immunity to type A viral hepatitis, resistance to infection will be lowered for several weeks or longer. Alcohol should be avoided for up to 6 months, and the patient should not donate blood in the future. The patient, family, and/or friends may require help in understanding the mode of transmission of viral hepatitis and in correcting any sources of contamination in the home or at work.

Complete recovery is possible within 4 months with continued care following the acute phase of the disease. Follow-up care of the patient should focus on an adequate diet and proper rest. The patient should return for checkups until the laboratory findings and physical examination are normal. The SGPT, SGOT, and LDH may remain abnormal for months. Cholesterol, WBC, bilirubin, and prothrombin time should return to normal as hepatic cell function is restored.

## Type B Viral Hepatitis

Type B viral hepatitis (serum hepatitis) occurs less frequently and has a higher mortality rate than type A. The type B virus is transmitted when the blood of an infected human comes in contact with the blood or mucous membrane of another person. Spread of the virus, then, is through blood transfusion, skin prick or cut, kissing, or sexual intercourse. Professional personnel are especially vulnerable to the disease during surgery, vaginal deliveries, hemodialysis, or parenteral therapy for a person with type B viral hepatitis. Only 0.0005 ml blood from the type B–infected person transmitted to another individual's blood or mucous membrane is required to spread the infection. Even piercing of ears, acupuncture, or tatooing with contaminated instruments can cause type B viral hepatitis. It can also be transmitted from the gastrointestinal tract via urine, menstrual secretions, saliva, semen, or feces.

The incidence of posttransfusion hepatitis has been reduced since the isolation of the type B virus. The factor isolated, originally called Australian antigen,[9] is the hepatitis B surface antigen (HBsAg). The complete virion probably consists of a core antibody (HBcAb) and the surface antigen (HBsAg). HBsAg can be identified in the blood of carriers of type B virus.

The incubation period of type B viral hepatitis is 50 to 150 days; thus, this type is sometimes called *long-incubation hepatitis.* The pathophysiological changes and effects on the patient are identical to those of type A viral hepatitis. The only difference between the two is the morality rate and the presence of circulating HBsAg in patients with type B.

**First-level nursing care** Type B viral hepatitis is found worldwide and occurs in all seasons. There is no one type of individual or special age that is predisposed to the illness. Drug addicts are a high-risk group for contact of type B viral hepatitis because of their use of communal needles.

The spread of the disease can be minimized by:

1 Identification of carriers of type B virus through blood screening for HBsAg

2 Use of disposable equipment (syringes, needles, intravenous bottles, and infusion packs)

3 Sterilization by autoclaving of instruments, utensils, and other nondisposable objects used in patient care

4 Donation of one's own blood prior to elective surgery

5 Wearing of gloves when indicated to avoid direct contact with the patient's blood, secretions, or feces

6 Recognition that the feces are contaminated and taking precautions not to spread the virus

7 Avoidance of unnecessary transfusion (no one-unit transfusions) and commercially obtained blood or plasma

8 Testing of blood for HBsAg during pregnancy, hemodialysis, and prior to surgery and taking precautions to prevent the spread of the virus

Administration of ISG to prevent type B viral hepatitis is of questionable value and may be dangerous. Injections of ISG to patients with high titers of HBsAg were reported to prevent hepatitis for 6 months.[10] On the other hand, injection of ISG could allow development of a "subclinical" case of type B viral hepatitis. The individual then may have only mild symptoms without jaundice and, therefore, never be diagnosed. In this condition the person is a carrier who is unknowingly disseminating the virus through blood, feces, or secretions. Before immunization for type B virus is attempted, the antibody potency should be established.

**Second-level nursing care** Type B viral hepatitis follows a course similar to type A. The onset, however, is insidious, while type A has an abrupt onset. Type B differs from type A in the degree of sickness and number of concomitant illnesses. It is thought that the high mortality rate associated with type B may be due to the fact that most patients who are given blood transfusions are already quite ill. On the other hand, it is not definite that lowered host resistance, rather than a higher virulence of the type B virus, causes the high mortality rate. Table 19-4 compares type A and B viral hepatitis.

**N**ursing Assessment The *health history* will be similar to that in type A but should include direct questioning regarding blood transfusions, drug addiction, recent surgery or cuts, ear piercing, acupuncture, or tatooing. The findings on *physical assessment* will mimic those of type A but may include findings of concomitant problems such as urticarial rash, arthralgia, pharyngitis, and bruising. The *laboratory tests* are summarized in Table 19-4. The presence of HBsAg in the serum distinguishes type B from type A viral hepatitis.

Patients with type B viral hepatitis are generally more acutely ill and require hospitalization. The community nurse has a role in being aware of patients at risk for developing the infection and in early identification of its appearance. If hepatitis is suspected, the patient should be immediately referred for confirmation and treatment.

**Third-level nursing care** The *nursing assessment* in the icteric phase of type B is similar to that of type A. After the rapid onset of jaundice, the arthralgia, pharyngitis, fever, and rash recede. Unlike type A, however, malaise generally continues, and the patient feels quite miserable.

The *nursing problems and interventions* are also the same as those for type A, and the reader should review that section. Besides the problems of anorexia, nausea, vomiting, fatigue, emotional reactions, jaundice, and pruritus, bleeding may be a problem. Easy bruising can be a serious sign necessitating serial prothrombin times and vitamin K administration.

Because of the persistent malaise, a special effort by the nurse to ensure rest is indicated. The patient often feels better in the morning than in the evening, and activities and rest periods should be planned accordingly. The nutritional plan often includes vitamin supplements, especially vitamin B. The patient with type B viral hepatitis often has other major chronic diseases which require attention.

Isolation precautions similar to those used with type A should be instituted. Parenteral precautions are especially important, and needles, syringes, intravenous bottles, and infusion packs (lines of tubing) should be disposed of in a safe way. Needles may be broken off at the hub, placed in a container, and destroyed. Plastic syringes collected in a flammable container are rendered unusable when burned. Nursing personnel who are responsible for safe disposal of contaminated equipment should conclude these functions regularly so that large collections of contagion do not accumulate in the patient area.

The nurse will also have an opportunity to interpret to nursing service and hospital administrators the need for increased expense involved in the care of the patient with type B viral hepatitis. Private rooms, disposable equipment, special handling of nondisposable items, and individualized care of patients are expensive in the context of care for one patient. On the other hand, if dissemination of the virus to nursing and medical personnel and to other patients or family members occurs, consideration of the additional cost of treating these individuals helps put in context the escalated cost of caring for one hospitalized patient with viral hepatitis. Although it is difficult to estimate, the "cost" to the family and to the employer due to loss of interaction with or work produced by the diseased individuals should be projected to explain the need for taking precautions to prevent the spread of viral hepatitis.

The nurse, in conjunction with the nurse epidemiologist or infection control committee, should collect data to show that the techniques used to prevent viral spread are effective. Since major accountability for care of patients with viral hepatitis rests with nurses, they are responsible for seeking new methods of care, including prevention of the disease.

**Fourth-level nursing care** Fourth-level nursing care of the patient with type B viral hepatitis is centered around providing complete recovery from the illness, encouraging follow-up care, and health teaching. Rehabilitation of the patient cannot be achieved without the cooperation of the patient.

During the lengthy convalescent phase, ranging from 6 weeks to 6 months, the patient may eat any food which will ensure a well-balanced diet. The nurse should assess the patient's knowledge of nutrition and provide any dietary information needed by the patient. Sometimes larger meals are tolerated in the morning. Within the limit of fatigue, daily exercise can be undertaken.

Follow-up care on an outpatient basis usually includes weekly visits for 3 weeks, then monthly visits for the next 3 months until symptoms are negative. Follow-up should include laboratory data, especially on enzymes. Enzyme studies should be repeated 6 weeks after they first return to normal.

The nurse should tell the patient who has had type B viral hepatitis not to dine in restaurants until the enzymes are near normal levels. The patient may need to be reminded not to donate blood and to avoid new and intimate contacts (kissing, intercourse) until the HBsAg assay is negative on two subsequent analyses. Patients need help and encouragment, if they are going to be able to prevent spreading the disease and avoid becoming depressed or hyperattentive to possible complications or symptoms of posthepatitis syndrome. *Posthepatitis syndrome* is a constellation of vague symptoms that include weakness and malaise. They may last for 6 to 12 months. Nursing care focuses on reassuring the patient, who can become very discouraged.

The nurse can help the patient evaluate when it is safe to resume work. This will depend on the type of job held by the patient, the amount of physical labor required of the employee, and the opportunity for part-time employment. Persons who are food handlers or work with chemicals which are potentially hepatotoxic will need special counseling regarding employment changes.

Immunity to type B viral hepatitis is lifelong once the disease has been contracted. It is necessary to know that immunity is for specific subtypes (x, a, d, y) of type B and not for the type A virus.

## CANCER OF THE LIVER

Primary carcinoma of the liver frequently follows cirrhosis of the liver and is usually lethal within several months. The patient may or may not report pain, jaundice, and ascites. Metastatic carcinoma of the liver and primary carcinoma of the liver are difficult to differentiate. Metastatic carcinoma is reported to occur 25 times more frequently than primary carcinoma of the liver.

The most outstanding features of carcinoma of the liver are the extreme weakness experienced by the patient, the huge size to which the liver develops (from a normal of 1 to 5 or 10 kg), and the alarming rapidity of the downward clinical course. Patients usually experience a continual ache in the epigastrium or back and do not complain of extreme pain. Anorexia is profound and weight loss rapid. During the terminal stage, hemorrhage is common and hepatic coma often develops.

Photoscan shows diagnostic malconfiguration of the liver. Hepatic functions are all abnormal. Malignant cells may be found in bloody ascitic fluid, anemia and leukocytosis are marked, and fever may be present.

The medical treatment is palliative with special attention to restoring liver function. Surgical intervention by resection is sometimes possible if the tumor is localized.

Nursing interventions are directed toward ensuring patient comfort. Needs are anticipated and meaningful interaction with the patient is essential. The intervention requires sensitivity to the fear, anxiety, anger, and guilt felt by the patient; tolerance of regression; and special expressions of love and encouragement. The nurse can learn much about the value of life through interactions with the patient and family.

## TRAUMA TO THE LIVER

The extent of hepatic trauma depends upon the offending agent, the area traumatized, and the force of the penetration or impact. There are two main types of liver trauma: penetrating wounds and blunt injuries. Blunt injuries to the liver are the most serious and may result in fracture of the liver capsule and parenchyma. Even if the liver capsule is intact, extensive parenchymal cell damage may have occurred due to trauma. Secondary complications include hematoma, hemobilia (hemorrhage into the biliary passages), and intraperitoneal hemorrhage.

The treatment of hepatic trauma includes clini-cal assessment of the injured patient, aggressive treatment of shock, and early transfer to the operating room. In surgery the wound is debrided, hemorrhage controlled, and drainage of the hepatic wound provided. Postoperatively antibiotics are administered, and drainage from the wound is cultured. Intravenous fluids are ordered as needed to correct hypoalbuminemia, hypoglycemia, and vitamin K deficiency. Platelets or fresh whole blood is transfused cautiously to correct thrombocytopenia.

Complications of the trauma, surgery, and/or treatment may include infection, hemorrhage, biliary fistulas and hemobilia, stress ulcer of the gastric mucosa, pulmonary embolism and renal failure.

Interventions by the nurse are primarily those of good preoperative and postoperative care. The nurse working in an emergency room or trauma unit needs broad knowledge and the ability to respond accurately under stress and in a setting of confusion.

Trauma or accidental injury occurs in a vehicle-oriented society and one in which the crime rate is high. It is the leading cause of death in young adults. Advances in health sciences have resulted in the technical abilities to save the life of the person with major hepatic trauma. However, emergent and advanced technology is primarily available only in urban areas, and at times, the health team is so involved with machines that the need of the person to talk about and react to the trauma is thwarted as the patient is transported from one group of personnel to another. Owing to the requirement for emergency treatment, the patient frequently endures these stresses without family or friends. Nurses can be helpful in remedying this situation.

## REFERENCES

1   M. M. Wintrobe et al. (eds.), *Harrison's Principles of Internal Medicine,* 7th ed., McGraw-Hill, New York, 1974, p. 1512.

2   J. Carbone, L. Brandborg, and S. Silverman, "Gastrointestinal Tract and Liver," in M. Krup and M. Chatton (eds.), *Current Medical Diagnosis and Treatment,* Los Altos, Calif., Lange, 1976, pp. 372–374.

3   S. Sherlock, *Diseases of the Liver and Biliary System,* 5th ed., Blackwell Scientific Publications, Oxford, 1975, p. 267.

4   C. Leevy, C. Tamburro, and R. Zetterman, "Liver Disease of the Alcoholic," *Med Clin North Am,* **59**:4: 909–918, July 1975.

5   *Ibid.*

6    S. I. Schwartz et al., *Principles of Surgery,* 2d ed., McGraw-Hill, New York, 1974, p. 1201.

7    R. A. Malt, "Portasystemic Venous Shunts," *N Engl J Med,* **295:**1:24–29, July 1, 1976, and **295:**2:80–86, July 8, 1976.

8    K. Baranowski, H. Green II, and J. T. Lamont, "Viral Hepatitis: How To Reduce Its Threat to the Patient and Others (Including You)," *Nursing '76,* **6:**31–38, May 1976.

9    B. Blumberg, H. Alter, and S. Visnick, "A "New" Antigen in Leukemia Sera," *JAMA,* **191:**541, February 15, 1965.

10    M. Conrad, "Endemic Viral Hepatitis in U.S. Soldiers: Causative Factors and the Effect of Prophylactic Gammaglobulin," *Can Med Assoc J,* **106:**Suppl:456–460, February 26, 1972.

## BIBLIOGRAPHY

Alter, H. J., et al.: "Health-care Workers Position for Hepatitis B Surface Antigen: Are Their Contacts at Risk?" *N Engl J Med,* **292:**9:454–447, February 27, 1975.

Anderson, W., and T. Scotti: *Synopsis of Pathology,* 9th ed., Mosby, St. Louis, 1976.

Beland, I.: *Clinical Nursing: Pathophysiological and Psychosocial Approaches,* 3d ed., Macmillan, New York, 1975.

Bergerson, B.: *Pharmacology in Nursing,* 13th ed., Mosby, St. Louis, 1976.

Bogoch, A. (ed.): *Gastroenterology,* McGraw-Hill, New York, 1973.

Brunner, L. S., and D. A. Suddarth: *Lippincott Manual of Nursing Practice,* Lippincott, Philadelphia, 1974.

———— and ————: *Textbook of Medical-Surgical Nursing,* 3d ed., Lippincott, Philadelphia, 1975.

Burkhalter, P. K.: *Nursing Care of the Alcoholic and Drug Abuser,* McGraw-Hill, New York, 1975.

Carey, L. C. (ed.): "Surgery of the Liver, Spleen, and Pancreas," *Surg Clin North Am,* **55**(2):461–473, April 1975.

Conn, H., R. Rakel, and T. Johnson: *Family Practice,* Saunders, Philadelphia, 1973.

*Control of Communicable Diseases in Man,* 11th ed., American Public Health Association, New York, 1970.

Dane, D. S., C. Cameron, and M. Briggs: "Virus-like Particles in Serum of Patients with Australia-Antigen-Associated Hepatitis," *Lancet,* **1:**695–698, April 4, 1970.

Dordal, E.: "Fluid Accumulation in Liver Disease," *Mod Treat,* **9:**33, February 1972.

Editorial: "Is Halothane Hepatitis an Imaginary Disease?" *Med World News,* **15:**14–16, January 11, 1974.

Frohlich, E. D. (ed.): *Pathophysiology: Altered Regulatory Mechanisms in Disease,* 2d ed., Lippincott, Philadelphia, 1976.

Fung, W., et al.: "Differentiation between Acute Alcoholic Hepatitis and Acute Infectious (viral) Hepatitis," *Am J Gastroenterol,* **59:**221, March 1973.

Gabuzda, George J.: "Cirrhotic Ascites: An Etiologic Approach to Management," *Hosp Prac,* **8:**67–74, August 1973.

Garibalde, R., B. Hanson, and M. Gregg: "Import of Illicit Drug-Associated Hepatitis on Viral Hepatitis Morbidity Reports in the United States," *J Infect Dis,* **126:**288, September 1972.

Gillies, D., and Alyn, I.: "How Well Do You Understand Cirrhosis?" *Nursing '75,* **5:**38–43, January 1975.

———— and ————: *Patient Assessment and Management by the Nurse Practitioner,* Saunders, Philadelphia, 1976.

Givens, B. A., and S. J. Simmons: *Gastroenterology in Clinical Nursing,* 2d ed., Mosby, St. Louis, 1975.

Guyton, A.: *Medical Physiology,* 5th ed., Saunders, Philadelphia, 1976.

Krugman, S.: "Hepatitis: Current Status of Etiology and Prevention," *Hosp Prac,* **10:**39–46, November 1975.

———— and J. Giles: "Viral Hepatitis, New Light on an Old Disease," *JAMA,* **212:**1019, May 11, 1970.

Lieber, C. S.: "Liver Adaptation and Injury in Alcoholism," *N Engl J Med,* **288:**356–362, Feb. 15, 1973.

Luckman, J., and K. Sorensen: *Medical-Surgical Nursing: A Psychophysiological Approach,* Saunders, Philadelphia, 1974.

Mallory, F.B.: "Cirrhosis of the Liver. Five Different Types of Lesions from Which It May Arise," *Bull Johns Hopkins Hosp.,* **22:**69–75, 1911.

McDermott, W. V., Jr.: *Surgery of the Liver and Portal Circulation,* Lea & Febiger, Philadelphia, 1974.

Mandell, J.: "Psychogenic Retention of Water," *Am Heart J,* **65:**572–574, April 1963.

Mazzur, S.: "Menstrual Blood as a Vehicle of Australia-Antigen Transmission," *Lancet,* **1:**749, April 7, 1973.

Moidel, H., E. Giblin, and B. Wagner (eds.): *Nursing Care of the Patient with Medical-Surgical Disorders,* 2d ed., McGraw-Hill, New York, 1976.

Pitcher, J. L.: "Safety and Effectiveness of the Modified Sengstaken-Blakemore Tube: A Prospective Study," *Gastroenterology,* **61:**291–298, September 1971.

Robbins, S., and M. Angell: *Basic Pathology,* 2d ed., Saunders, Philadelphia, 1976.

Rothschild, M., et al.: "Alcohol-Induced Depression of Albumin Synthesis: Reversal by Tryptophan," *J Clin Invest,* **50:**1812–1818, September 1971.

————, M. Oratz, and S. Schrieber: "Regulation of Albumin Metabolism," *Annu Rev Med,* **26:**91–104, 1975.

Rosen, R. A., and R. Morecki: "Correlation Conferences in Radiology and Pathology—Ascites and Fever," *NY State J Med,* **74:**1020–1023, June 1974.

Rubin, E., and C. S. Lieber: "Fatty Liver, Alcoholic Hepatitis and Cirrhosis Produced by Alcohol in Primates," *N Engl J Med,* **290:**128, January 17, 1974.

Saba, T. M.: "Physiology and Physiopathology of the Reticuloendothelial System," *Arch Intern Med,* **26:**1031–1052, December 1970.

Saunders, S. J., and J. Terblanche: *Liver,* Proceedings of an International Liver Conference with Special Reference to Africa, University of Cape Town Medical School, Pitman Medical, New York, 1973.

Schaffner, F.: "Electronmicroscopy of Virus, Alcohol and Drug Induced Hepatitides," in S. Saunders and J. Terblanche (eds.), *Liver,* Pitman Medical, London, 1973, pp. 46–47.

Schiff, L. (ed.): *Diseases of the Liver,* 4th ed., Lippincott, Philadelphia, 1975.

Schmid, R.: "Bilirubin Metabolism in Man," *N Engl J Med,* **287:**14:703–709, October 5, 1972.

Seixas, F., K. Williams, and S. Eggleston (eds.): "Medical Consequences of Alcoholism," Part II, *Ann NY Acad Sci,* **252:**10–234, April 25, 1975.

Shafer, K., et al.: *Medical-Surgical Nursing,* Mosby, St. Louis, 1975.

Shear, L.: "Ascites: Pathogenesis and Treatment," *Postgrad Med,* **53:**1–3:165–170, January 1973.

Smith, D., and C. Germain: *Care of the Adult Patient,* 4th ed., Lippincott, Philadelphia, 1975.

Storlie, F.: *Patient Teaching in Critical Care,* Appleton-Century-Crofts, New York, 1975.

Tamburro, C., and C. Leevy: *Acute Viral Hepatitis in Conn H. Current Therapy,* Saunders, Philadelphia, 1974, pp. 356–359.

Victor, M., and R. Adams: "Alcohol," in M. Wintrobe et al (eds.), *Harrison's Principles of Internal Medicine,* 7th ed., McGraw-Hill, New York, 1974, pp. 671–681.

Villarejos, V., et al.: "Role of Saliva, Urine and Feces in the Transmission of Type B Hepatitis," *N Engl J Med,* **291:**1375–1378, December 26, 1974.

Wakim, K. G.: "Basic and Clinical Physiology of the Liver: Normal and Abnormal," *Anes Analg,* **44:**634–710 (Suppl) September-October, 1965.

Williams, R., and M. Murray-Jyon (eds.): *Artificial Liver Support,* Pitman, New York, 1975.

Witte, M., and C. Witte: "Progress in Liver Disease: Physiological Factors Involved in the Causation of Cirrhotic Ascites," *Gastroenterology,* **61:**742, November 1971.

# 20
# DISTURBANCES IN GLUCOSE METABOLISM

Delores Schumann

The metabolism of glucose is a dynamic component of the body's internal environment. It is a vital mechanism that must keep pace with changing conditions in both the internal and external environments. Both excesses and deficiencies in glucose create specific clinical entities. This chapter examines the common disturbances of glucose metabolism, considers the impact upon the health of those affected, and discusses the function of the nurse in preventing and managing these conditions and in restoring susceptible populations to an optimal health state.

## DIABETES MELLITUS

The most common disturbance of carbohydrate metabolism is *diabetes mellitus.* It is characterized by a disorder in the metabolism of insulin and of carbohydrate, fat, and protein. It also involves a defect in the structure and function of blood vessels. Diabetes is an abbreviated term for diabetes mellitus and will be used throughout this chapter. Since the beginning of the century, mortality associated with diabetes has increased significantly. Today this problem ranks fifth among death-causing disease in the United States. Some authorities suggest that its proper place is third, as the deaths of diabetic patients are often caused by complications of diabetes, and, therefore, the cause of death is not listed as diabetes mellitus. More alarming is that the incidence of diabetes has increased by more than 50 percent since 1965.

### Pathophysiology

The exact mechanisms involved in the development of diabetes remain unclear. It can arise when the production of insulin is inadequate or when glucose is in excess. Researchers investigating diabetes in juveniles have reported a possible *autoimmune mechanism.*[1] The immune system of juvenile diabetics was found to produce antibodies that killed pancreatic cells. As beta cells are destroyed, less insulin is produced. What triggers the autoimmune mechanism is not known. One theory implicates a *viral infection* at an early age.[2] As the child fights off the infection, an immune defect causes production of antibodies against both the virus and the child's own beta cells.

The *genetic* implications in the development of diabetes have long been recognized, but there is little agreement about the nature of the genetic mechanisms involved. Diabetes was once considered to be transmitted as a Mendelian single autosomal recessive trait. Now the hypothesis that a single genetic trait can bring about impaired metabolism and lead to a vascular defect is seriously questioned. More favored is a multifactorial or polygenic hypothesis in which genes at several loci act together to bring about this condition. One genetic trait may give rise to the metabolic derangement of insulin deficiency while another causes the premature vascular disease. Although these traits are independent of one another, they coexist.

Underproduction of insulin can also follow damage or *destruction of the pancreatic islet cells.* This can be caused by pancreatectomy, pancreatitis, pancreatic neoplasms, cystic fibrosis of the pancreas, pancreatic infections, or cytotoxic drugs. A hereditary condition called *hemochromatosis* also reduces pancreatic function by depositing iron pigments in pancreatic cells.

Work by Unger and associates[3] suggests that a bihormonal abnormality may cause diabetes mellitus. A relative or absolute excess of glucagon and a relative or absolute deficiency of insulin may be the etiological cofactors. This has been supported by observations of hyperglucagonemia whenever hyperglycemia is found. Another possible etiological mechanism may involve proinsulin, the precursor of insulin. It may be that conversion of proinsulin to insulin is abnormal in some diabetics.

Excessive blood glucose levels can also precipitate diabetes. Hyperglycemia over time exhausts the beta cells and "wears them out." Persons with a genetic predisposition to the development of diabetes are especially vulnerable to this. It partly accounts for the recent increase in the incidence of diabetes. In an affluent society, increased consumption of carbohydrates accompanied by decreased exercise all contribute to higher blood glucose levels. When food supplies have been low, as in the European countries during World War II, the incidence of diabetes declined.

*Overweight* persons are especially susceptible to diabetes. Enlarged fat cells are less responsive to insulin, and glucose uptake by them is lessened. This decrease in the use of insulin by fat cells combines with excessive carbohydrate ingestion to increase the blood glucose level. To compensate, overweight persons must hypersecrete insulin to sustain normal glucose metabolism. The risk of diabetes is reported to be greater in subjects with central adiposity of the trunk as contrasted to equally fat persons who have more of their total body fat in the subcutaneous depots of their extremities.[4]

Judged by the commonly used diagnostic tests for diabetes, carbohydrate intolerance increases with *aging.* Although no age group is spared, 80 percent of the diabetic population is more than 40 years old. If the plasma glucose values of 60 to 100 mg/deciliter (dl) (100 ml) are considered normal for the population as a whole, persons over the age of 40 will have a higher incidence of elevated blood glucose levels than younger persons. When glucose tolerance tests are done, the abnormality is more marked at the end of the first hour of the test than by the close of the second hour. There are two schools of opinion with respect to aging and glucose intolerance: one considers the decline in glucose tolerance as a pathologic process, while another views it as an adaptive decline and expectation of aging in the general population. It is important to remember that once persons reach the age of 40 they may have higher blood glucose values when the current criteria for normal are applied. Whether or not this is true diabetes remains a researchable issue.

There are several factors which have a *diabetogenic effect.* That is, they cause hyperglycemia and, in susceptible individuals, can precipitate frank diabetes. *Pregnancy,* for instance, has such an effect. The variety of hormones elaborated by the placenta and the increased maternal levels of cortisol during gestation diminish the effectiveness of insulin. The placenta also degrades maternal insulin. Women who have limited ability to secrete insulin may be unable to augment the output sufficiently to overcome the elevation in blood glucose.

Some medications can induce hyperglycemia. *Glucocorticoids* do this by stimulating gluconeogenesis. The *estrogen* component of birth control pills also induces a resistance to the hypoglycemic effects of insulin. In some persons *oral thiazides* have a diabetogenic effect. The exact mechanism for this is not known, but potassium has been shown to have a corrective effect.

*Physiological or psychological stress,* with its resultant increases in epinephrine, norepinephrine, and glucocorticoid secretion, leads to increases in the blood glucose level. Stressors can include a loss, severe trauma, myocardial infarction, infection, or cancer. In susceptible individuals some type of stress often precipitates the development of diabetes. The onset of diabetes in persons following an acute stress such as a myocardial infarction may be transient, reflective of the increase in blood glucose that results from the stress response mechanism. After the acute episode, the diabetes may disappear, or only diet control may be necessary.

Many *endocrine disorders* are associated with increases in blood glucose levels. Excesses in growth hormone (as in acromegaly) and hypersecretion of the adrenal cortex (as in Cushing's syndrome) cause hyperglycemia. Overactivity of the thyroid gland most likely increases the blood glucose level by potentiating the effects of the catecholamines.

Whatever the provoking circumstance, the functioning beta cells attempt to secrete insulin in sufficient quantities to decrease the blood glucose and maintain normal levels. Eventually the strain upon the islet cells outstrips their ability to produce insulin. Beta cell exhaustion follows and initiates a chain of events that distorts the normal metabolic processes.

**Metabolic changes**  Inadequate amounts of insulin prevent glucose from entering the cells, and it becomes concentrated in the blood. The abnormally high blood glucose level is called *hyperglycemia*. Glucose normally filters from the blood into the urine in the glomerulus and is reabsorbed by the renal tubules. As the blood glucose rises, the amount filtered through the glomerulus increases and the renal threshold for glucose reabsorption is exceeded. Glucose is then in the urine (*glucosuria*). Renal thresholds vary with individuals. Most frequently, glucosuria can be expected when the blood glucose reaches 180 mg/dl.

While the blood is rich in glucose, the body cells, unable to obtain glucose because the insulin transport system is inadequate, become energy-depleted. Proteins and fats are mobilized (*proteolysis* and *lipolysis*) to supply energy. The low levels of circulating insulin cannot exert their usual antilipolytic effects, and fatty acids are mobilized from adipose tissue. The liver converts the fatty acids to ketones for use by the cells as energy. Because the cells are being deprived of glucose, the liver also increases gluconeogenesis and glycogenolysis in an effort to supply the necessary glucose. In the absence of insulin, this only drives the blood glucose levels higher.

As fat and protein stores are mobilized and utilized for energy, *weight loss* occurs. At the same time the patient is continually hungry and eats excessively (*polyphagia*), while deriving no benefit from the increase in food intake. The ingested carbohydrates and proteins are converted to glucose, which is not able to enter the cells. Cells that depend on insulin for glucose transport are starved and their functions disrupted.

The increase in plasma lipids associated with diabetes can result in distinctive yellow lesions of the skin called *xanthomas*. Xanthomas are associated with high lipid levels and are not limited to

diabetes. With hypercholesterolemia, *xanthelasma palpebrarum* can develop. These are soft, slightly raised yellow plaques which develop on and around the eyelids (see Color Plate 20-1). *Papular xanthoma* (xanthoma diabeticorum, eruptive xanthoma) result from increases in the plasma triglyceride levels. They are characterized by a sudden onset and are usually found over the buttocks, elbows, or back of the thighs. These papules are yellow with a red periphery.

**Fluid and electrolyte imbalances**  Several changes in fluid and electrolyte dynamics are associated with diabetes. As hyperglycemia increases, the blood becomes hypertonic and pulls water from the intracellular fluid space. This results in cellular dehydration. Dehydration is worsened as the glucosuria results in an osmotic diuresis and large quantities of water are lost with the glucose in the urine. This increases both the frequency of urination and quantity of urine (*polyuria*). The patient becomes excessively thirsty and drinks large amounts of fluid (*polydipsia*).

In a more intense diabetic state, *nephropathy*, pathologic changes in the kidney, can occur over a period of time. It usually is caused by a variety of structural changes. These changes include atherosclerosis of muscular arteries and alterations in the small blood vessels of the kidney. The basement membrane of the renal capillaries becomes progressively thickened and folded. Glycoprotein is also deposited in the capillaries. The thick basement membrane is permeable to large molecules, and albumin is lost in the urine (*proteinuria*). These changes are referred to as *glomerulosclerosis*. If urinary tract infection is present, the increased permeability of the basement membrane will allow white blood cells and casts to be excreted as well.

As glomerulosclerosis continues, about 15 years after insulin therapy is started, a nephrotic syndrome (*Kimmelstiel-Wilson's syndrome*) can develop. With the loss of protein in the urine, hypoalbuminemia develops, intravascular colloid osmotic pressure decreases, and fluid is lost to the interstitial fluid space. This results in edema of the eyes, face, and lower extremities. Hypertension develops as kidney function decreases, and uremia can occur. As the renal impairment becomes severe, glucosuria decreases. The kidney also degrades insulin less effectively. The diabetic state itself falsely appears to improve, and the usual insulin dose becomes more effective.

**Changes in immunity and inflammation**  Several factors contribute to the diabetic patient's susceptibility to infection. Glucose concentration is increased not only in the blood and urine, but in the tissues. The skin especially becomes a reservoir for glucose, which leaves the skin in diabetic patients more slowly than nondiabetics. This provides an excellent medium for bacterial and fungal growth. At the same time if diabetes is poorly controlled and ketoacidosis develops, host resistance is altered. There is a delay in the mobilization of granulocytes to the site of the lesion and an apparent leukocyte defect[5] in which the phagocytic function of the leukocytes is impaired. Cutaneous infections, especially fungal, are frequent and often occur in moist skin folds. Boils and furuncles can develop, and minor cuts in the skin become easily infected. In women vulvovaginitis is common. Because of the glucose content in the urine, bladder infections can develop.

**Changes in oxygenation** Oxygenation is affected by a variety of vascular changes that affect tissue perfusion. These include large-vessel and microvasculature lesions. Diabetic patients are more likely to develop *arteriosclerosis* and *atherosclerosis*. Arteriosclerosis frequently affects the lower extremities, and arterial occlusion of the tibial and popliteal arteries is most frequent.

Besides the large vessel arteriosclerosis, *microvascular abnormalities* occur. The basement membrane of virtually every capillary bed becomes thickened. Prime targets for microvascular changes are the kidney, retina, and the skeletal muscle. Thickening of the basement membrane of the capillaries is so distinctive with diabetes mellitus that it may be noted before other signs and symptoms develop.

The incidence of the vascular changes associated with diabetes increases as the duration of diabetes increases and is not related to adherence to the therapeutic regime. Over time *coronary artery disease* results from the atherosclerosis. *Hypertension* develops from the microvascular abnormalities, arteriosclerosis, atherosclerosis, and renal damage. Involvement of the cerebral vasculature can lead to *cerebrovascular accidents*.

The vascular disease can also result in skin lesions. *Necrobiosis lipoidica diabeticorum* (NLD) is a lesion that develops in the pretibial area. The skin becomes ulcerated and necrotic. As healing occurs, the lesion is covered with a thin cutaneous layer and becomes reddish yellow in color (see Color Plate 20-2). These occur most frequently in insulin-dependent women.

*Diabetic dermopathy* (shin spots, atrophic pre-tibial macule) also evolves from the microvascular pathology and results from small hemorrhages. Initially this condition takes the form of small, well-defined, dull-red inflammations. The borders slope upward to a slightly depressed center. After many months healing occurs with thin atrophied scars and diffuse brown pigmentation. These occur most frequently on the anterior and lateral aspects of the legs.

Perhaps the most destructive skin lesion is that associated with arteriosclerosis. As arterial circulation is obstructed, the skin becomes smooth and shiny and begins to atrophy. The muscles to the affected limb also atrophy. The distal end of the extremity becomes mottled and reddish blue when dependent. If elevated, it shows a waxy pallor. If pallor is present when the extremity is dependent, the obstruction is more severe. As the obstruction develops, *gangrene* and *ulceration* result (Fig. 20-1). Gangrene is discussed in greater detail in Chap. 29.

**Changes in perception and coordination** Diabetes is associated with multiple neuropathies which impair perception and coordination. Dysfunction of the cerebrum, spinal cord, and/or peripheral nerves can occur. The etiology of these neuropathies is not well understood. A relationship to vascular changes or a thickening of the basement membranes of the Schwann cells has been suggested. The neuropathies can be bilateral or unilateral. They vary in their degree of perceptual impairment and paralysis. They can occur in mild or severe diabetes and in diabetes of long or more recent duration. They may develop slowly or be abrupt in onset.

*Peripheral neuropathy* occurs most frequently in the lower extremities and is characterized by pain and parethesias. The pain becomes worse at night and is relieved by walking. It has been described as a burning, a dead feeling of the feet, or a sensation of walking on pillows. The mere touch of bed clothes on the feet may be intolerable.

Neuropathic changes cause distortions of the muscle and bony structure of the foot (*Charcot's joints*). Toes become cocked up, and the metatarsal heads are exposed. Changes in the toe position require adjustments in walking so that the metatarsal heads are not subjected to pressure. Swelling slowly develops. The joints shorten and the foot widens, the longitudinal arch flattens, and the foot assumes a rocker-bottom appearance. An abnormal gait results. The foot is painless, making ambulation possible. *Neuropathic ulcers* are

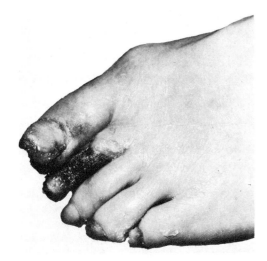
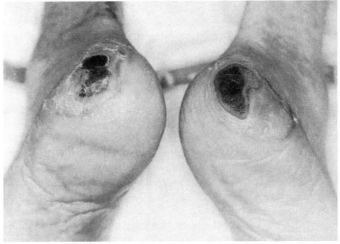

**FIGURE 20-1**

(A) Gangrene of several toes of an adult onset diabetic woman with arteriosclerosis obliterans. Treated with successful transmetatarsal amputation. (B) Bilateral heel gangrene in an insulin dependent diabetic with juvenile onset. The lesion was due to pressure on the heels, had excellent arterial supply, and was successfully managed by local excision. (*Photographs courtesy of Henry Haimovici, M.D.*)

painless, circular lesions with a punched-out appearance that often develop at pressure points on the foot.

*Upper-extremity neuropathy* is usually less severe. When the hands are affected, numbness and atrophy of the muscles of the interosseous spaces develop. Atrophy between the thumb and first finger is most common. Painless burns on the hands from smoking or preparing foods hint of the severity of sensory impairment.

*Visceral neuropathies* also develop and involve the autonomic nerves supplying the gastrointestinal tract. Gastric emptying is delayed, and absorption becomes irregular and unpredictable. In the small intestine malabsorption and diarrhea can occur. Vesical dysfunction can develop and is characterized by bladder paralysis and urinary retention.

If the pelvic autonomic nervous system is affected, several *sexual difficulties* can occur. Retrograde ejaculation may develop. That is, while orgasm is achieved, normal ejaculation does not occur. Because the bladder neck is incompetent, the seminal fluid flows back into the bladder rather than being thrust outward. For the male diabetic impotence is the most difficult of the sexual problems. It usually develops slowly. Normal sexual interest is maintained, but there is a slow onset of erectile dysfunction. Erection cannot be achieved at intercourse, nor with masturbation. The disorder is believed to be due to impaired transfer of the nervous impulse that leads to penile artery dilatation, thus hindering engorgement of the corpora cavernosa and spongiosum. If plasma testosterone and the prostate are normal, the prognosis is poor. Androgen therapy is ineffective. Diabetic women often complain of orgasmic difficulty. This develops gradually during the first years after the onset of diabetes.

A multitude of changes found in the eye are associated with diabetes. *Disturbances in visual perception* are not uncommon in diabetic patients. Blindness occurs 25 times more frequently in diabetics as compared with nondiabetic patients. This discussion will focus on the more common changes that alter visual perception.

*Ocular motor paralyses* occur with neuropathy of the IIIrd, IVth, and VIth cranial nerves. They can result in headache, eye pain, double vision, and/or ptosis. They are generally self-limiting and subside spontaneously. *Glaucoma* occurs more frequently in diabetic patients and most likely results from the microvasculature changes which block the flow of fluids out of the eye, thus increasing intraocular pressure. *Cataracts* develop at an earlier age in diabetic patients and result from the accumulation of fructose and sorbitol in the lens. Glaucoma and cataracts are discussed in greater detail in Chap. 38.

*Diabetic retinopathy* is the most destructive of the visual changes associated with diabetes. It usually appears about 10 years after the diagnosis of diabetes mellitus is made. *Noninfiltrative retinopathy* is characterized by dilatation of the retinal veins. The veins become torturous, and microaneurysms develop. These are often accompanied by small hemorrhages and retinal exudates. Usually, the changes associated with noninfiltrative retinopathy do not alter vision. Occasionally, if hemorrhage occurs in the area of the fovea, a scotoma (an area of blindness) may result.

The greatest loss of vision is associated with *proliferative retinopathy*. Ten percent of patients with diabetes for 10 years or more develop this type of retinopathy. It involves the changes associated with noninfiltrative retinopathy in addition to the formation of new vessels and fibrous tissue proliferation. The mechanism responsible for the development of new vessels is not clear; they may appear before other changes are noted. The new vessels that are formed are weak and hemorrhage easily. They also may attach to the vitreous. Normally, the vitreous draws away from the retina with age. In proliferative retinopathy this process often results in tearing of new vessels, vitreous hemorrhage, or retinal detachment if fibrous proliferation has resulted in strong vitreoretinal attachments.

**Stages of diabetes mellitus** Persons with a genetic predisposition for diabetes are believed to progress to a true clinical case in four stages. The first stage is called *prediabetes*. The patient is asymptomatic and blood tests are normal. However, basement membranes may be thickened, and subclinical abnormal glucose metabolism may exist. The second stage is termed *suspected* or *subclinical diabetes*. The person remains asymptomatic and blood tests are normal. Under stress, however, these tests become abnormal.

During the third stage of *chemical* or *latent diabetes*, the patient may experience a reactive hypoglycemia after meals. Insulin release has become sluggish and occurs only as the blood glucose reaches a very high level as when virtually all the glucose has been absorbed from the intestinal tract. This insulin spurt drops the blood glucose level, quickly stimulating a sympathetic response. The patient perspires and experiences nervousness, tremors, and palpitations associated with the release of epinephrine. During this third stage hyperglycemia is found with postprandial blood glucose determinations and glucose tolerance tests. The final stage is *overt* or *clinical diabetes*. The characteristic changes and effects are present, and blood glucose tests are abnormal.

## First-Level Nursing Care

Prevention of diabetes mellitus should focus on the population in general and persons predisposed to its development in particular. In all health settings nurses should make their patients weight conscious. The dangers of developing diabetes as well as the other complications of obesity should be impressed upon all patients, and the interactive nature between weight gains and diabetes stressed. A more thorough discussion of weight control can be found in Chap. 16.

Nurses should also identify patients at risk to the development of prediabetes. Reliable indicators for the prediabetic patient include the presence of diabetes in close relatives, obesity, neurological or vascular changes in the eye or kidney that resemble those seen in diabetes, and abnormal obstetrical histories. Special attention should be given to mothers of large babies, as infants born to diabetic women are often 20 to 25 percent heavier than average.

Women are at greater risk to developing diabetes than men. This is primarily related to their degree of adiposity. Ethnic and racial factors also help to identify risk patients. After age 45 non-Caucasian women in the United States have an incidence about twice that of whites. Pima Indians in south-central Arizona show an overall prevalence of 50 percent diabetes among those 35 years and older. This is 10 times higher than for the same age group in the United States and Western Europe. Other Indian tribes have similarly high rates. The occurrence of diabetes in the Pimas points to the obesity among persons 40 years and older and the aggregation of diabetes in families. Equally striking is the fact that diabetes is rare in the Athanbaskan and Alaskan Eskimos. Persons of certain Jewish background were once considered prone to diabetes. This view is no longer held; obesity was found to be a major factor in the population studied.

Early identification of subclinical diabetes allows health teaching to occur that can postpone, perhaps indefinitely, the development of diabetes. Nurses functioning in a primary health care setting have a unique opportunity to screen patients. Programs that evaluate large numbers of people can be planned and implemented. This can be done in collaboration with schools, with industry, or as a part of special community occasions such as fairs. An evaluation program may be set up as a separate event (Diabetes Detection Week) so that the population of an entire town can participate.

The Dextrostix method may be used for mass

screening. Capillary blood is applied to a paper test strip. The strip is then rinsed with water after exactly 60 seconds and the color intensity evaluated. The technique eliminates the need for venipuncture and requires only a prick to obtain capillary blood from the fingertip or earlobe.

Urine tests for glucosuria may be used but are not satisfactory as the *only* diabetic screening test. Some persons, particularly the elderly, have high renal thresholds for glucose, and glucose will not be found in the urine even when the blood level is high.

If prediabetes is suspected, the 2-hour postprandial blood glucose test should be used. A blood specimen is drawn 2 hours after ingestion of a meal with 75 to 100 g carbohydrate. At the end of 2 hours a blood glucose of 100 mg/dl is suspicious, while a level in excess of 120 mg/dl is indicative of diabetes. Anyone with a level that is suspicious or higher is referred for additional tests to establish the diagnosis.

Patients suspected of being prediabetic should have their blood glucose levels checked regularly. They should be especially monitored during periods of stress, such as a severe illness, infection, or trauma.

All patients who are at risk to developing diabetes should be counseled about proper diet, weight control, regular exercise, and avoidance of diabetogenic drugs. They should be encouraged to avoid foods that contain refined sugar. Corticosteroids, birth control pills containing estrogen, and thiazides should be avoided if possible.

Nurses may also be called upon to provide genetic counseling for families with a history of diabetes. Prediction is difficult because if both parents have diabetes, only about 50 percent of their children are found to be prediabetic.[6] Precise counseling is not possible until the exact mode of the inheritance is known. Known statistics offer some guidelines. If both parents have had diabetes since childhood or if an identical twin is diabetic, there is a 100 percent genetic susceptibility to diabetes. If one parent and one sibling have diabetes or one parent and an aunt or uncle on the opposite side have it, the chance of being susceptible to its development is 50 percent. If one sibling is affected, there is a 25 percent chance; if just one parent or both grandparents on one side are diabetic, the chances of being susceptible drop to 20 percent.[7]

### Second-Level Nursing Care

In a community setting the nurse often encounters a patient with latent diabetes or one who has a mild degree of overt diabetes. Diabetes often develops later in life, and this type has been called *adult-onset diabetes.* These patients often have some endogenous insulin secretion which makes them resistant to the development of ketoacidosis. Diabetics who do not require exogenous insulin replacement are considered *insulin-independent diabetics.* The Commission on Diabetes has recommended that diabetic persons be classified as insulin-dependent or insulin-independent, drawing attention to the differences in management. This replaces the formerly used terminology of adult-onset and juvenile-onset or ketosis-prone.

**Nursing assessment** A thorough health history, physical assessment, and laboratory analysis of blood and urine are vital to the management of the insulin-independent client. Because exogenous insulin is not required, neither the disease nor its complications are likely to be extensive.

The most pertinent feature of the *health history* is the reactive hypoglycemia. Patients often relate feelings of nervousness, irritability, and tremors, and perspire 3 to 5 hours after a meal. This is an early phenomenon and is often the presenting complaint. As the diabetes progresses, this disappears. In insulin-independent diabetes, symptoms develop slowly, and patients often will not experience any changes. Other patients may complain of some or all of the classic symptoms—polyuria, polydipsia, polyphagia, and weight loss. Patients may find that they fatigue more easily.

A complete *physical assessment* should be done to evaluate the existence of any of the common complications associated with diabetes. A thorough discussion of the findings on physical assessment may be found in Third-Level Nursing Care. The complications in insulin-independent diabetes are generally less frequent and less severe.

**D**iagnostic Tests  Because the pathophysiological changes and their effects on insulin-independent diabetics are often not easily identified by the history and physical examination, laboratory tests are invaluable in establishing the diagnosis. *Urinalysis* should include glucose, albumin, organisms, white blood cells, and casts. The presence of glucose in the urine is not diagnostic of diabetes but serves as a guide during management. The presence of albumin may serve as an index to glomerulosclerosis. Organisms, white blood cells, and casts may indicate infection.

Laboratory tests that confirm the diagnosis of diabetes are the fasting blood glucose, the 2-hour postprandial blood glucose, and the glucose tolerance test. Several preparatory measures are common to these tests. Food is omitted for at least 8 hours prior to the test but not longer than 16 hours before to eliminate starvation effects. Water is permitted, but coffee, tea, and cigarettes are not allowed because they stimulate metabolism. Venous blood is used for the analysis; capillary blood is unsatisfactory because its glucose content is variable and it may be mixed with lymph.

The *fasting blood glucose level* of a normal person is 60 to 100 mg/dl blood by the true blood glucose method. In diabetes this is elevated above normal limits. Both the postprandial blood glucose and the glucose tolerance test require that a glucose load be given as a challenge to the body's metabolism. Glucose is mixed into a solution, or a liquid commercial product is used. The solution must be ingested over a 5-minute interval. The excessive sweetness of the solution may induce nausea and vomiting. Chilling the solution or flavoring it with lemon juice enhances its palatability. If the patient is markedly nauseated or vomits, the test is invalid and must be rescheduled.

The *postprandial blood glucose* is determined by giving the patient a glucose load orally and evaluating the serum glucose level 2 hours after ingestion. The expectation is that the glucose level returns to normal 2 hours following ingestion of the glucose challenge. If the patient shows a slower descent to normal, a glucose tolerance test is done to confirm the diagnosis.

Because of the diagnostic importance of the *oral glucose tolerance test* (OGTT), nurses must take the initiative to guarantee its accuracy. A high-carbohydrate diet should be consumed for 3 days prior to the test. Authorities differ in the recommended amount of carbohydrate, but the usual range is 150 to 300 g/day. Patients should be provided with written instructions about the dietary requirements and a suitable meal and snack plan to ensure the required intake.

Drugs that influence glucose tolerance must be discontinued 3 days prior to the test. Estrogen-progestin contraceptives, steroids, diuretics, salicylates, and diphenylhydantoin influence glucose metabolism and should be omitted when possible. Since many drugs affect glucose metabolism, it may be desirable to eliminate all medications during the preparation time.

Glucose tolerance tests should be scheduled for ambulatory patients only. Illness, endocrine problems, or any stressful emotional or physical event invalidates the test because the multiple hormones released under these circumstances influence blood glucose levels. The test should be done in the morning as glucose tolerance is known to decrease later in the day.

Procedurally, a fasting blood glucose and a urine specimen are collected before the test as controls. After ingestion of the glucose load, specimens of blood and urine are collected at 1-, 2-, and 3-hour intervals and evaluated for their glucose content. Glucose levels are elevated in diabetes. Specimens may be collected at additional times and the test extended for the fourth and fifth hours in some institutions.

An alternative method for determining glucose tolerance is by completing an *intravenous glucose tolerance test* (IVTT). The intravenous method is less desirable because it does not simulate the normal route for acquiring glucose. The results are similar to the OGTT.

The *intravenous tolbutamide response test* may also be used to confirm suspected diabetes mellitus. The tolbutamide stimulates endogenous insulin secretion and therefore is indicative of pancreatic function. The patient should be instructed to fast the night before the test. In the morning a baseline fasting blood glucose is taken. Tolbutamide is then given, and blood samples taken after 20 and 30 minutes. The *oral tolbutamide response test* follows a similar procedure. With both tests, the blood glucose of diabetic patients decreases more slowly than in nondiabetic persons. After the test the patient should be given orange juice or a glucose preparation and instructed to eat breakfast.

Since elevated *plasma lipids* are associated with a high incidence of atherosclerosis, serum cholesterol and serum triglycerides are measured. If the lipids are elevated, a *lipoprotein typing (profile)* will identify the specific abnormality. Type IV abnormality, with a high triglyceride level and a cholesterol level that is elevated to a lesser extent, is common in diabetes. A type II abnormality in which there is primarily an elevation in blood cholesterol may also be found in some diabetics. See Chap. 29 for a more detailed discussion of lipoprotein typing.

**Nursing problems and interventions**  The primary problem of the insulin-independent diabetic patient is in *maintaining the blood glucose levels* within normal limits. This can be accomplished by focusing on an activity plan, a diet plan, urine testing, and oral hypoglycemics.

**A**ctivity Plan    Regular, moderate physical activity is extremely advantageous to the insulin-independent client. Exercise increases the release of epinephrine which inhibits insulin production. At the same time, it enhances glucose uptake by the cells independently of available insulin. Exercise also improves the condition of the blood vessels and the muscle power of the heart.

Patients should be taught to develop an exercise regime appropriate to their life-style. Patients often misinterpret an activity plan to mean strenuous exercise or an organized sport. Activities do not need to be exhausting, expensive, or time-consuming. Substitution of walking for driving the car for short distances, climbing stairs rather than riding elevators, gardening, or washing the car are suitable ways to expend energy. It is not uncommon for the insulin-independent person to have been physically active but to have become increasingly sedentary with progressing years. When stressing an activity plan, consider the age, interests, and general physical condition of the patient and severity of the diabetes. The most important aspect of the plan is regularity. Significant decreases in activity will result in elevated blood glucose levels.

**D**iet Plan    The dietary plan remains the foundation in managing the diabetic client. The goal is to plan a diet that is consistent with the insulin resources of the patient. The principles of dietary treatment are similar for the insulin-independent and insulin-dependent client. Planning a program to achieve ideal body weight is a primary goal. A characteristic of the insulin-independent client is obesity. Diabetologists are emphasizing that clients should be given a trial period on a weight-reducing program before any other therapy is added. Normalizing weight often restores carbohydrate tolerance toward normal.

The *diet prescription* is written on the basis of the patient's ideal body weight (IBW) in kilograms. Basal caloric needs can be estimated by multiplying the ideal weight by a caloric multiplication factor. Table 20-1 illustrates the caloric multiplication factors for persons of varying weights. Persons of normal weight who engage in moderate activity need 35 calories/kg IBW daily. If they are sedentary but of normal weight, only 30 calories/kg IBW is prescribed. If the client engages in heavy activity, the diet prescription is based on 40 calories/kg IBW.

After determination of the optimum calories, the carbohydrate, fat, and protein allotments are distributed accordingly. The American Diabetic Association advocates that 45 percent or more of the calories be in the form of carbohydrates. The recent emphasis on liberalized carbohydrate intake is aimed at preventing the atherosclerosis associated with diabetes. Allowance for this amount of carbohydrate automatically decreases the fat and cholesterol in the diet. Current recommendations are that 14 percent of the calories should be derived from protein. The remaining total calories should be derived from fat. Saturated fats and cholesterol may also be restricted. The physician may use the results of the patient's lipoprotein typing to determine specific dietary restrictions.

The liberalized carbohydrate intake does not mean that the diabetic is free to eat carbohydrate at random. Concentrated carbohydrates are restricted. The nutritional value of fruits and vegetables with their ready supply of vitamins and minerals should be emphasized.

*Regulation of dietary intake*    Authorities differ as to the best therapeutic approach to the diet. Some advocate *chemical regulation* in which all foods are weighed on a food scale. This degree of calculation or precision is usually unnecessary, but the Joslin Clinic in Boston, Massachusetts, finds it valuable in helping patients learn about food measurement and sizes. At the other extreme are the liberal physicians who believe that careful regulation will not postpone the onset of vascular problems. Hence, they permit clients an unmeasured or "free" diet that eliminates only sugar or foods high in sugar. This is called *clinical regulation.*

The majority of physicians support and select the *exchange method of regulation,* a system based on standard household measures. In the exchange system foods are divided into six types (exchange lists), and foods from within each list can be substituted (exchanged) for one another because they have the same food value. The composition of the food exchanges can be found in Table 20-2. Table 20-3 illustrates the exchange lists. If the client is

**TABLE 20-1**
DIABETIC DIET CALCULATION (CALORIES PER KILOGRAM IDEAL BODY WEIGHT PER DAY)

|  | Sedentary | Moderate Activity | Marked Activity |
|---|---|---|---|
| Overweight | 20–25 | 30 | 35 |
| Normal | 30 | 35 | 40 |
| Underweight | 35 | 40 | 45–50 |

**TABLE 20-2**
COMPOSITION OF FOODS IN THE EXCHANGE LISTS

| List | Type of Exchange | Carbo-hydrate, grams | Protein, grams | Fat, grams | Calories |
|------|------------------|----------------------|----------------|------------|----------|
| | | | | Composition | |
| I | Milk | 12 | 8 | Trace | 80 |
| II | Vegetable | 5 | 2 | | 25 |
| III | Fruit | 10 | | | 40 |
| IV | Bread | 15 | 2 | | 70 |
| V | Meat | | 7 | 3 | 55 |
| VI | Fat | | | 5 | 45 |

allowed one bread exchange, a slice of bread, one-half bagel, one-half cup cooked cereal, or a small, white potato may be selected. The diet prescription is given the patient in terms of exchanges. The dietitian or nurse then plans with the patient the distribution of the exchanges for a 24-hour period. The patient's life-style and normal eating patterns must be considered. A typical lunch from an 1800-calorie diet might include two meat exchanges, two bread exchanges, one vegetable exchange, one fruit exchange, and one milk exchange.

**TABLE 20-3**
DIABETIC EXCHANGE LISTS FOR MEAL PLANNING (USED WITH PERMISSION OF AMERICAN DIABETIC ASSOCIATION)

LIST 1   MILK EXCHANGES (INCLUDES NONFAT, LOW-FAT, AND WHOLE MILK)

This list shows the kinds and amounts of milk or milk products to use for one Milk Exchange.

NONFAT FORTIFIED MILK

| | |
|---|---|
| Skim or nonfat milk | 1 cup |
| Powdered (nonfat dry, before adding liquid) | ⅓ cup |
| Canned, evaporated skim milk | ½ cup |
| Buttermilk made from skim milk | 1 cup |
| Yogurt made from skim milk (plain, unflavored) | 1 cup |

LOW-FAT FORTIFIED MILK

| | |
|---|---|
| 1% fat-fortified milk | 1 cup |
| (omit ½ Fat exchange) | |
| 2% fat-fortified milk | 1 cup |
| (omit 1 Fat Exchange) | |
| Yogurt made from 2% fortified milk (plain, unflavored) | 1 cup |
| (omit 1 Fat Exchange) | |

WHOLE MILK (OMIT 2 FAT EXCHANGES)

| | |
|---|---|
| Whole milk | 1 cup |
| Canned, evaporated whole milk | ½ cup |
| Buttermilk made from whole milk | 1 cup |
| Yogurt made from whole milk (plain, unflavored) | 1 cup |

LIST 2   VEGETABLE EXCHANGES

This list shows the kinds of vegetables to use for one Vegetable Exchange. One Exchange is ½ cup.

Asparagus
Bean sprouts
Beets
Broccoli
Brussels sprouts
Cabbage
Carrots
Cauliflower
Celery
Cucumbers
Eggplant
Green pepper
Greens:
  Beet
  Chards
  Collards
  Dandelion
  Kale

Greens:
  Mustard
  Spinach
  Turnip
Mushrooms
Okra
Onions
Rhubarb
Rutabaga
Sauerkraut
String beans, green or yellow
Summer squash
Tomatoes
Tomato juice
Turnips
Vegetable juice cocktail
Zucchini

The following raw vegetables may be used as desired:
Chicory
Chinese cabbage
Endive
Escarole

Lettuce
Parsley
Radishes
Watercress

Starchy vegetables are found in the Bread Exchange List.

The foods eaten by the diabetic need not be "different" or costly. Purchase of special foods is unnecessary. Foods that are not permitted are the concentrated carbohydrates—table sugar, candy, honey, molasses, Karo syrup, jams and jellies, pies, cakes, cookies, pastries, regular soft drinks, and candy-coated gum. Canned foods that have been packed in syrup can be drained and rinsed to remove the excess syrup. The foods should be those selected and prepared for other family members. "Dietetic" foods are generally costly, often contain forms of sugar, and do not contribute any special nutritive substances. Nonnutritive sweeteners can be used in coffee, tea, or other beverages. Saccharin is a common sugar substitute. It imparts a bitter taste to foods prepared at normal cooking temperatures and should be added only after cooking or to foods that will not be cooked.

The diet should be adjusted to the patient's ethnic background. Translating the diet into a different language often is only a communication of a typical middle-class American diet of meat and vegetables. It is not suitable for, say, the Mexican American who consistently eats chile, tacos, and

## LIST 3    FRUIT EXCHANGES

This list shows the kinds and amounts of fruits to use for one Fruit Exchange.

| | | | |
|---|---|---|---|
| Apple | 1 small | Mango | ½ small |
| Apple juice | ⅓ cup | Melon | |
| Applesauce (unsweetened) | ½ cup | Cantaloupe | ¼ small |
| Apricots, fresh | 2 medium | Honeydew | ⅛ medium |
| Apricots, dried | 4 halves | Watermelon | 1 cup |
| Banana | ½ small | Nectarine | 1 small |
| Berries | | Orange | 1 small |
| Blackberries | ½ cup | Orange juice | ½ cup |
| Blueberries | ½ cup | Papaya | ¾ cup |
| Raspberries | ½ cup | Peach | 1 medium |
| Strawberries | ¾ cup | Pear | 1 small |
| Cherries | 10 large | Persimmon, native | 1 medium |
| Cider | ⅓ cup | Pineapple | ½ cup |
| Dates | 2 | Pineapple juice | ⅓ cup |
| Figs, fresh | 1 | Plums | 2 medium |
| Figs, dried | 1 | Prunes | 2 medium |
| Grapefruit | ½ | Prune juice | ¼ cup |
| Grapefruit juice | ½ cup | Raisins | 2 T |
| Grapes | 12 | Tangerine | 1 medium |
| Grape juice | ¼ cup | | |

Cranberries may be used as desired if no sugar is added.

## LIST 4    BREAD EXCHANGES (INCLUDING BREAD, CEREAL, AND STARCHY VEGETABLES)

This list shows the kinds and amounts of breads, cereals, starchy vegetables and prepared foods to use for one Bread Exchange.

### BREAD

| | |
|---|---|
| White (including French and Italian) | 1 slice |
| Whole wheat | 1 slice |
| Rye or pumpernickel | 1 slice |
| Raisin | 1 slice |
| Bagel, small | ½ |
| English muffin, small | ½ |
| Plain roll, bread | 1 |
| Frankfurter roll | ½ |
| Hamburger bun | ½ |
| Dried bread crumbs | 3 T |
| Tortilla, 6 inch | 1 |

### CEREAL

| | |
|---|---|
| Bran flakes | ½ cup |
| Other ready-to-eat unsweetened cereal | ¾ cup |
| Puffed cereal (unfrosted) | 1 cup |
| Cereal (cooked) | ½ cup |
| Grits (cooked) | ½ cup |
| Rice or barley (cooked) | ½ cup |
| Pasta (cooked), spaghetti, noodles, macaroni | ½ cup |
| Popcorn (popped, no fat added) | 3 cups |
| Cornmeal (dry) | 2 T |
| Flour | 2–½ T |
| Wheat germ | ¼ cup |

### CRACKERS

| | |
|---|---|
| Arrowroot | 3 |
| Graham, 2½ inches square | 2 |
| Matzoth, 4 × 6 inches | ½ |
| Oyster | 20 |
| Pretzels, 2⅛ inches long × ⅛ inch diam. | 25 |
| Rye wafers, 2 × 3½ inches | 3 |
| Saltines | 6 |
| Soda, 2½ inches square | 4 |

### DRIED BEANS, PEAS, AND LENTILS

| | |
|---|---|
| Beans, peas, lentils (dried and cooked) | ½ cup |
| Baked beans, no pork (canned) | ¼ cup |

### STARCHY VEGETABLES

| | |
|---|---|
| Corn | ⅓ cup |
| Corn on cob | 1 small |
| Lima beans | ½ cup |
| Parsnips | ⅔ cup |
| Peas, green (canned or frozen) | ½ cup |
| Potato, white | 1 small |
| Potato (mashed) | ½ cup |
| Pumpkin | ¾ cup |
| Winter squash, acorn or butternut | ½ cup |
| Yam or sweet potato | ¼ cup |

**TABLE 20-3**
DIABETIC EXCHANGE LISTS FOR MEAL PLANNING (USED WITH PERMISSION OF AMERICAN DIABETIC ASSOCIATION) (*Continued*)

| PREPARED FOODS | | |
|---|---|---|
| | | |
| Biscuit 2 inches diam. | 1 | |
| (omit 1 Fat Exchange) | | |
| Corn bread, 2 × 2 × 1 inches | 1 | |
| (omit 1 Fat Exchange) | | |
| Corn muffin, 2 inches diam. | 1 | |
| (omit 1 Fat Exchange) | | |
| Crackers, round butter type | 1 | |
| (omit 1 Fat Exchange) | | |

| | | |
|---|---|---|
| Muffin, plain small | 1 | |
| (omit 1 Fat Exchange) | | |
| Potatoes, French Fried, length 2 to 3½ inches | 8 | |
| (omit 1 Fat Exchange) | | |
| Potato or corn chips | 15 | |
| (omit 2 Fat Exchanges) | | |
| Pancake, 5 × ½ inches | 1 | |
| (omit 1 Fat Exchange) | | |
| Waffle, 5 × ½ inches | 1 | |
| (omit 1 Fat Exchange) | | |

### LIST 5 MEAT EXCHANGES (LEAN MEAT)

This list shows the kinds and amounts of lean meat and other protein-rich foods to use for 1 Low-Fat Meat Exchange

| | |
|---|---|
| Beef: Baby beef (very lean), chipped beef, chuck, flank steak, tenderloin, plate ribs, plate skirt steak, round (bottom, top), all cuts rump, spare ribs, tripe | 1 oz |
| Lamb: Leg, rib, sirloin, loin (roast and chips), shank, shoulder | 1 oz |
| Pork: Leg (whole rump, center shank), ham, smoked (center slices) | 1 oz |
| Veal: Leg, loin, rib, shank, shoulder, cutlets | 1 oz |
| Poultry: Meat without skin of chicken, turkey, cornish hen, guinea hen, pheasant | 1 oz |
| Fish: Any fresh or frozen | 1 oz |
| Canned salmon, tuna, mackerel, crab, and lobster | ¼ cup |
| clams, oysters, scallops, shrimp, | 5 or 1 oz |
| sardines, drained | 3 |
| Cheeses containing less than 5% butterfat | 1 oz |
| Cottage cheese, dry and 2% butterfat | ¼ cup |
| Dried beans and peas (omit 1 Bread Exchange) | ½ cup |

### LIST 5 MEAT EXCHANGES (MEDIUM-FAT MEATS)

For each exchange of medium-fat meat omit ½ Fat Exchange.

This list shows the kinds and amounts of medium-fat meat and other protein-rich foods to use for one Medium-Fat Meat Exchange.

| | |
|---|---|
| Beef: Ground (15% fat), corned beef (canned), rib eye, round (ground commercial) | 1 oz |
| Pork: Loin (all cuts tenderloin), shoulder arm (picnic), shoulder blade, Boston butt, Canadian bacon, boiled ham | 1 oz |
| Liver, heart, kidney, and sweetbreads (these are high in cholesterol) | 1 oz |
| Cottage cheese, creamed | ¼ cup |
| Cheese: Mozzarella, ricotta, farmer's cheese, Neufchâtel | 1 oz |
| Parmesan | 3 T |
| Egg (high in cholesterol) | 1 |
| Peanut butter (omit 2 additional Fat Exchanges) | 2 T |

### LIST 5 MEAT EXCHANGES (HIGH-FAT MEAT)

For each exchange of high-fat meat omit 1 Fat Exchange.

This list shows the kinds and amounts of high-fat meat and other protein-rich foods to use for 1 High-Fat Meat Exchange.

| | |
|---|---|
| Beef: Brisket, corned beef (brisket), ground beef (more than 20% fat), hamburger (commercial), chuck (ground commercial), roasts (rib), steaks (club and rib) | 1 oz |
| Lamb: Breast | 1 oz |
| Pork: Spare ribs, loin (back ribs), pork (ground), country style ham, deviled ham | 1 oz |
| Veal: Breast | 1 oz |
| Pountry: Capon, duck (domestic), goose | 1 oz |
| Cheese: Cheddar types | 1 oz |
| Cold cuts | 4½ × ⅛ inch slice |
| Frankfurter | 1 small |

### LIST 6 FAT EXCHANGES

This list shows the kinds and amounts of fat-containing foods to use for 1 Fat Exchange.

| | |
|---|---|
| Margarine, soft, tub or stick* | 1 t |
| Avocado (4 inches in diam.)† | ⅛ |
| Oil, corn, cottonseed, safflower, soy, sunflower | 1 t |
| Oil, olive† | 1 t |
| Oil, peanut† | 1 t |
| Olives† | 5 small |
| Almonds† | 10 whole |
| Pecans† | 2 large whole |
| Peanuts† | |
| Spanish | 20 whole |
| Virginia | 10 whole |

| | |
|---|---|
| Walnuts | 6 small |
| Nuts, other† | 6 small |
| | |
| Margarine, regular stick | 1 t |
| Butter | 1 t |
| Bacon fat | 1 t |
| Bacon, crisp | 1 strip |
| Cream, light | 2 T |
| Cream, sour | 2 T |
| Cream, heavy | 1 T |
| Cream cheese | 1 T |
| French dressing‡ | 1 T |
| Italian dressing‡ | 1 T |
| Lard | 1 t |
| Mayonnaise‡ | 1 t |
| Salad dressing, mayonnaise type‡ | 2 t |
| Salt pork | ¾-inch cube |

* Made with corn, cottonseed, safflower, soy, or sunflower oil only.
† Fat content is primarily mono-unsaturated.
‡ If made with corn, cottonseed, safflower, soy, or sunflower oil, can be used on fat-modified diet.

menudo. Exchange lists should be individualized to the patient's usual foodstuffs.

Allowances can also be made for the person accustomed to drinking alcoholic beverages. A limited amount can be incorporated, but it must be done correctly. Distilled spirits such as Scotch, rye, bourbon, vodka, and gin, while high in calories, contain only trace amounts of carbohydrate. Beer and wines have a higher carbohydrate content. The patient should be advised to use the distilled spirits and to mix the drinks with water. Alcohol may not be permitted for patients with some types of hyperlipidemias.

**O**ral Antidiabetic Agents  When dietary management alone does not keep the blood glucose at a satisfactory level, oral antidiabetic agents are considered. The insulin-independent patient is able to secrete some insulin so that these drugs correct a deficiency. Persons most suitable for this therapy are those who have developed diabetes after 40 years of age, are not overweight, have an insulin requirement of 10 to 20 units/day, and have had the disease less than 5 years.

The oral antidiabetic agents (oral hypoglycemic agents) are the sulfonylureas and the biguanides. These are summarized in Table 20-4. The

**TABLE 20-4**
ORAL ANTIDIABETIC AGENTS

| Generic Name | Trade Name | Common Daily Dose Range, (mg) | Usual Doses per Day | Duration of Action, h | Adverse Effects (All Classes) |
|---|---|---|---|---|---|
| SULFONYLUREAS | | | | | |
| Acetohexamide | Dymelor | 250–1500 | 1–2 | 8–10 | Hypoglycemia GI upset |
| Chlorpropamide | Diabinese | 100–500 | 1 | 30–60 | Skin rashes Bone marrow depression Liver toxicity |
| Tolazamide | Tolinase | 100–750 | 1 | 10–14 | |
| Tolbutamide | Orinase | 500–3000 | 2–3 | 6–12 | Counterindicated in: Hepatic disease Renal disease Chlorpropamide counterindicated in the elderly |
| BIGUANIDES | | | | | |
| Phenformin | DBI | 25–150 | 2 | 4–6 | Lactic acidosis GI upsets Metallic taste |
| Phenformin (timed release) | DBI-TD | 50–150 | 1 | 8–14 | Counterindicated in hepatic disease renal disease |

*sulfonylureas* lower blood glucose by stimulating the release of insulin from the beta cells. Sulfonylureas are effective only if the pancreas retains the capability to secrete some insulin. The only *biguanide* used clinically in the United States is phenformin (DBI, DBI-TD). Phenformin is thought to promote hypoglycemia in three ways: (1) inhibiting glucose absorption from the intestine, (2) increasing peripheral utilization of glucose, and (3) decreasing gluconeogenesis.

The use of oral antidiabetic agents has been a source of controversy since publication of the findings of a study undertaken by the University Group Diabetes Program (UGDP). Twelve clinics located in various geographical regions of the United States participated in an 8½ year study. Tolbutamide (Orinase) and DBI were found not to prolong the lives of patients with onset of diabetes in their adult years as compared with the longevity of persons treated only by diet. Most controversial was the increased mortality from cardiovascular disease among subjects using tolbutamide and phenformin when compared with persons treated with diet alone or with the combination of diet and insulin. In the light of these data, it is likely that the oral agents will be used with caution. However, many patients are well controlled on these drugs. Critics of the study argue that inappropriate methods of case selection, nonindividualization of drug doses, and analysis of data with unsuitable biostatistical techniques decreased the validity of the findings.

**U**rine Testing   Urine tests for glucosuria and ketonuria are indices to the control of the diabetic state. The insulin-independent diabetic person utilizes the tests for glucosuria and ketones as an information source about the stability of the diabetic state. Urine test results can reflect dietary indiscretions. The physician uses the information to harmonize the oral hypoglycemic agent with the diet and activity prescription. If glucose begins to show in the urine consistently, the diabetic state may be worsening. Ketonuria in the insulin-independent patient merits immediate attention.

The insulin-independent diabetic usually needs to check the urine for glucose only. Ketonuria develops only if the patient is severely ill. Testing for glucosuria may be done on a daily or weekly basis or in times of stress. A single voided specimen obtained about two hours after a meal is adequate.

Two types of tests are used to test for glucosuria—the *copper-reducing tests* and the *glucose oxidase enzyme strips.* Clinitest and Benedict's test are examples of the copper-reducing tests; Bene-

dict's test is seldom used today. The copper-reduction tests are not specific for glucose but give quantitative information on the amount of any sugar present. It is important to select a test that does not render an erroneous result. Lactose may be present in the urine during the third trimester of pregnancy and during lactation; a reducing test should not be used for this group of women. Similarly, if the client is known to have an inborn error in metabolism such as pentosuria or fructosuria in which pentose or fructose is continually excreted, a reducing test is inadequate. An advantage of the enzyme tests is that they check specifically for glucose.

Patients should be taught that moisture, direct sunlight, and heat deteriorate the reagents. Outdated or discolored agents must be discarded. Clinitest tablets are a robin's egg blue; a dark speckled or black color suggests loss of potency. Tes-Tape becomes brown with deterioration. The color of enzyme strips does not necessarily indicate potency. Reagents can be checked for activity by performing the test with a glucose solution or a freshly opened bottle of regular cola.

Both the Clinitest and the enzyme tests should be done carefully following proper procedure. A common error with Clinitest is failing to observe the test continuously throughout the reaction period. If the patient's urine contains more than 2 percent glucose, a *pass-through phenomenon* may be missed. The reaction changes rapidly from green to tan to orange, and then returns to a dark green-brown color. If the reaction goes unobserved, only the final result is read, leading to misinterpretation. If the pass-through phenomenon is noted, the client should use two drops of urine and 10 drops of water. A special reference color chart which can be obtained from the manufacturer is needed to interpret the results.

Either false positive or false negative reactions with the glucosuria tests can result from intake of some drugs. Table 20-5 summarizes some drugs that can affect urine test reactions.

### Third-Level Nursing Care

The diabetic patient most frequently seen in the hospital is the *insulin-dependent* client. Such a person often experiences an abrupt onset before the age of 20. Poorly controlled insulin-independent patients can become insulin-dependent over time. An insulin-dependent patient whose blood glucose is difficult to control is considered a *labile* diabetic.

**Nursing assessment** A thorough assessment of the diabetic patient must focus on the disruption in glucose metabolism and the widespread complications that can develop. A detailed health history, thorough physical assessment, and diagnostic work-up are indicated.

**H**ealth History The insulin-dependent patient is most likely to describe the classic symptoms of diabetes mellitus—polyuria, polydipsia, polyphagia, and weight loss. For some, these symptoms develop so rapidly that the patient is first seen in an emergency setting. The patient should be questioned about any feelings of lethargy or drowsiness. Complaints of pruritis are common and result from the dry skin associated with dehydration. If vascular changes are present, patients may experience intermittent claudication (see Chap. 29). Blurred and dimmed vision is also common if ketoacidosis is developing or if chronic changes in the eye are present. Any delays in healing or prolonged infections should be explored. Female patients should be questioned about vaginal itching and discharge. All patients should be asked about indications of urinary tract infections—dysuria, urge incontinence, and pneumaturia.

Changes indicative of any neuropathy should be explored. Patients may complain of diarrhea which is intermittent, unpredictable in its occurrence, and not accompanied by straining or abdominal distress. Periods of constipation may be evident between diarrhetic episodes. Diabetic diarrhea worsens at night. Because the anal sphincter is involved, there may be nocturnal fecal incontinence. The patient is often reluctant to discuss this owing to embarrassment.

Since sexual dysfunction is a manifestation of neuropathy, obtaining a sexual history should be a regular part of the diabetic health assessment. Both diabetic men and women experience disorders. Approximately 50 percent of diabetic men have organic impotence. Neurological complaints of painful legs and impaired sensation in the hands and feet should also be explored. The patient should be asked about the presence of other health problems, and, especially important, a detailed dietary history should be taken (see Chap. 16).

**P**hysical Assessment The diabetic patient should be carefully examined to adequately evaluate the changes that have occurred. Initially the patient should be weighed and the results compared with a previous weight record. Insulin-dependent diabetics often consistently lose weight.

*Oxygenation status* should be assessed by evaluating the adequacy of tissue perfusion. This provides an index to the degree of vascular changes. The blood pressure is often elevated. Peripheral pulses especially should be palpated and evaluated. If arteriosclerosis and atherosclerosis are well established, the pulses are often diminished in the extremities. The pulses should be compared bilaterally, and the strength of the posterior tibialis and dorsalis pedis pulses evaluated for vascular competence. In arterial insufficiency the posterior tibial and dorsalis pedis arteries are ropy and pipestemlike. Feet become pale when elevated, but in a dependent position they show rubor. Normal arteriovenous filling time is 10 seconds; in vascular insufficiency it is 20 to 30 seconds. The longer the filling time, the poorer the prognosis.

The lower extremities should be meticulously examined. The absence of hair on the toes and lower legs, a thin, shiny atrophic skin, and thick toenails suggest vascular insufficiency. The legs should also be examined for *necrobiosis lipoidica diabeticorum* and *shin spots*.

Unless nephropathy is present, *fluid and electrolyte status* will not be significantly altered. If the patient has been drinking fluids, dehydration will not be severe. The skin will be dry and tissue turgor diminished. The eyeballs may feel soft if the dehydration is more severe.

The *inflammatory changes* can be assessed throughout the body. All skin surfaces should be examined for infection. Skin folds or intertriginous areas under the breasts, in the groin, and in the abdominal folds should be inspected for beefy red oozing lesions with small pustules on the periphery. The interdigital spaces of the toes should be

**TABLE 20-5**
DRUGS THAT CAN AFFECT URINE TEST RESULTS

DRUGS THAT CAN AFFECT CLINITEST AND TES-TAPE RESULTS:

Ascorbic acid (vitamin C)
Aspirin
Medicines with high sugar content (cough syrups, antibiotic suspensions, and liquid vitamins)

DRUGS THAT CAN AFFECT CLINITEST RESULTS:

Nalidixic acid (NegGram)
Tetracycline
Chloramphenical
Cephalosporin antibiotics (Keflin, Keflex, and Loridine)
Probenecid (Benemid)

DRUGS THAT CAN AFFECT TES-TAPE RESULTS:

Dipyrone (Narone, Pyrilgin)
Meralluride (Mercuhydrin)
Levodopa (Dopar, Larodopa, Bendopa)
Methyldopa (Aldomet)

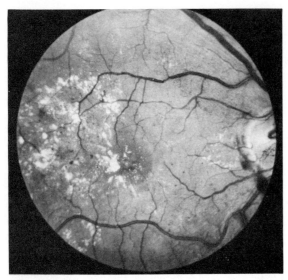

**FIGURE 20-2**
"Hard," discretely outlined exudates found in diabetic retinopathy. *(From M. Ellenberg and H. Rifkin, Diabetes Mellitus; McGraw-Hill, New York, 1970. Used with permission. Photograph courtesy of T. W. Lieberman, M.D.)*

given special attention, and boils or furuncles should be noted. In women, inspection of the perineal area may reveal an extensive vulvovaginitis.

Because of the widespread neuropathies that can accompany diabetes, *perception and coordination* should be carefully evaluated. *Sensation* of the

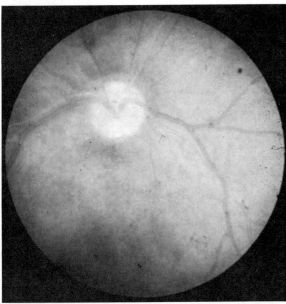

**FIGURE 20-3**
Proliferating new vessels arising from the vasculature of the optic disk. *(Photograph courtesy of T. W. Lieberman, M.D.)*

fingers, hands, and feet should be assessed. Numbness and tingling are often related to the glucose imbalance and, therefore, subside when the blood glucose returns to normal. The *deep tendon reflexes* should be checked. With neuropathy, the Achilles tendon reflex (ankle jerk) is lost first. All skin surfaces should be evaluated for diminished sensation to pain, temperature, touch, and vibration. The feet should be examined for neuropathic changes, and the presence of sores or burns on any extremity that the patient is unaware of should be noted.

Special attention should be given the *eye examination* with diabetic patients. Visual acuity should be tested, and intraocular pressure determined with a tonometer. Movement of the eyelids and eyes should be evaluated. Careful inspection of the *fundus* must be made. If hyperlipemia is present, the retina and its vessels will appear the color of cream of tomato soup rather than the usual dark red. This is called *lipemia retinalis. Microaneurysms* and small hemorrhages appear as pinpoint red dots. *Retinal exudates* that result from absorbed hemorrhages appear as sharply outlined, yellow-white areas (Fig. 20-2). *New-vessel formation* is illustrated in Fig. 20-3 and *fibrous proliferation* in Fig. 20-4. *Hemorrhages* into the liquid vitreous initially form a general haze and then settle in a defined area (Fig. 20-5). Hemorrhages into the solid vitreous clear poorly and after a time appear as white cottony masses (Fig. 20-6). Some of the changes associated with diabetic retinopathy are illustrated in Color Plates 20-3, 20-4, and 20-5.

**D**iagnostic Tests  As with the insulin-independent patient, the various *blood glucose tests* will be elevated in the insulin-dependent diabetic patient. A *lipoprotein typing* should be done to guide in planning dietary restrictions. The insulin-dependent patient often evidences chronic complications, and tests of kidney function, circulation, and cardiac function may be indicated.

**Nursing problems and interventions**  The insulin-dependent diabetic often must cope with difficult and sometimes incapacitating problems. These include not only controlling the blood glucose level, but foot problems, multiple neuropathies, retinopathy, infections, renal problems, and psychological and social adjustments.

**B**lood Glucose Management  Like the insulin-independent patient, management at this level focuses on an activity plan, dietary planning, and

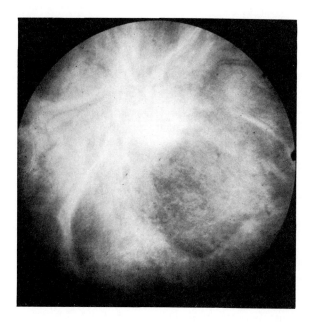 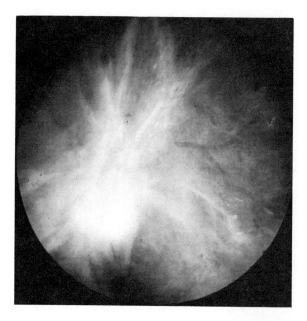

**FIGURE 20-4**
Devascularized fibrous proliferative tissue. Visual acuity is usually reduced at this stage. (*Photographs courtesy of T. W. Lieberman, M.D.*)

urine testing in addition to insulin therapy. The activity and diet plans discussed in Second-Level Nursing Care are applicable to the insulin-dependent patient. Again, regularity in exercise is very important. The insulin-dependent patient should be encouraged to increase food intake prior to any abnormal exertion. Because the insulin requirements will be less, if food intake is not increased, the usual insulin dose will result in hypoglycemia.

The diet should be planned and managed with the type and dose of insulin being taken kept in mind. Since exogenous insulin is absorbed at a fixed rate, meals must often be spaced consistently, not missed, and eaten completely. A bedtime snack should be included when planning meals. For the labile diabetic patient a midmorning, midafternoon, and bedtime snack may also be necessary. It is also helpful to teach patients to carry such foods as peanut butter crackers and raisins with them in case a meal is missed.

*Urine testing* Tests for glucosuria and ketonuria tell the insulin-dependent client how well the diabetes is controlled. The insulin-dependent client needs a regular pattern for urine testing. While the diabetes is being brought under control, testing for glucose and ketones is done four times daily, ordinarily before each meal and prior to the bedtime snack. As the diabetes is controlled, the number of

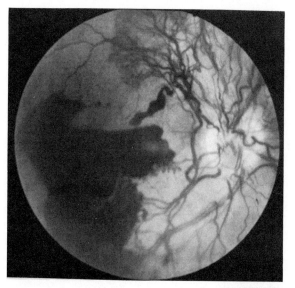

**FIGURE 20-5**
A preretinal (subhyaloid) hemorrhage in a diabetic patient with proliferative retinopathy. The shape of these hemorrhages depends on the form of the detachment of the solid vitreous from the posterior retina. The flat top of these hemorrhages is gravity dependent. (*From M. Ellenberg and H. Rifkin, Diabetes Mellitus, McGraw-Hill, New York, 1970. Used with permission. Photograph courtesy of T. W. Lieberman, M.D.*)

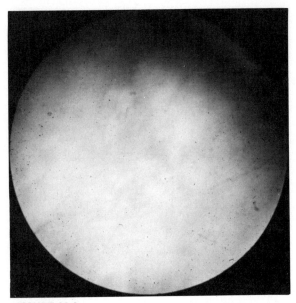

**FIGURE 20-6**
Cottony masses in the vitreous represent old, partially absorbed vitreous hemorrhages. (*Photograph courtesy of T. W. Lieberman, M.D.*)

testing times per day may be decreased. The original pattern should be resumed whenever glucose spillage steadily increases. The criteria used to decide whether urine should be checked for ketones are: (1) a concentration of ¾ percent or more glucose, (2) a 2 percent concentration of glucose more than two times in succession, or (3) illness.

Among the familiar testing agents are the sodium nitroprusside test (Acetest) and Keto-Diastix. Ketone test materials require the same meticulous care as do glucosuria reagents. Protection from

moisture, direct sunlight, and heat prevents deterioration. Freshly voided specimens must be used in testing.

The insulin-dependent client should use a second-voided specimen for the urine tests. The patient should be instructed to empty the bladder. A half hour later the second voiding will yield fresh urine that is more reflective of the blood glucose level. If the patient has an indwelling catheter, the specimen should be collected with a needle and syringe directly from the catheter. This again provides fresh urine for testing.

The patient should be taught the procedures for urine testing, a method for recording results, and the significance of test results. A negative urine test for glucose is not necessarily "good" and a positive test "bad." Continuous negative tests suggest the constant threat of an insulin reaction. Psychologically, a positive test implies a lack of control; however, a trace of glucose in the urine indicates that the patient is in control but is not in danger of having a reaction. Patients should be instructed to contact their physician or nurse practitioner if they begin to spill ketones into their urine.

*Insulin therapy*  Exogenous insulin is needed when insulin production by the islet cells is insufficient. Because insulin is destroyed in the gastrointestinal tract, it is supplied by injection. Insulins are categorized according to their duration of action. The types and characteristics of insulins in use in the United States are presented in Table 20-6.

The type of insulin used will be determined by the patients' specific needs. The time of onset, peak action, and duration must all be considered in light

**TABLE 20-6**
PROPERTIES OF INSULIN PREPARATIONS USED IN THE UNITED STATES

| Type | Preparation | Appearance | Time of Onset, h* | Peak, h* | Duration, h* | When to Anticipate Hypoglycemia (based on insulin dose given before breakfast) |
|------|-------------|------------|-------------------|----------|--------------|-------------------------------------------------------------------------------|
| Rapid-acting | Crystalline zinc (regular) | Clear | 1 | 2–4 | 6 | Before lunch |
| | Semilente | Cloudy | 1 | 6–7 | 8 | Before lunch |
| Intermediate-acting | NPH | Cloudy | 2 | 8–12 | 24 | Late afternoon and during night |
| | Lente | Cloudy | 2 | 8–12 | 24 | Late afternoon and during night |
| Long-acting | Protamine zinc | Cloudy | 7 | 14–20 | 36 | During night and early morning |
| | Ultralente | Cloudy | 7 | 16–24 | 36 | During night and early morning |

* These times are representative but can be expected to vary over a wide range.

of the patient's normal eating and activity patterns and responses to therapy.

The variability in length of action is achieved by combining substances such as zinc crystals or proteins such as protamine and globin with the insulin. These substances modify the insulin and change the solubility of insulin in water, thus delaying absorption. Regular insulin is an unmodified insulin. Crystalline zinc is a more highly purified unmodified form of regular insulin. These are used interchangeably when quick action is needed. They are often used in ketoacidosis, during an acute illness, during surgical procedures, or to stabilize a patient who is out of control. Regular or crystalline insulin is the only type that can be given intravenously.

To stabilize the patient out of control, regular insulin is often given in adjusted doses according to the results of urine tests. The physician will order a "sliding scale" indicating how much regular insulin should be given for the various possible urine results. As the urine tests for glucosuria and ketonuria begin to stabilize, an intermediate-acting insulin will be started with regular insulin supplements. When regular insulin coverage is needed and the blood glucose remains high, the dose of the intermediate insulin is adjusted until the blood glucose stabilizes and regular insulin is not necessary.

The most commonly used insulins for long-term therapy are the intermediate-acting insulins. Their duration allows the patient to develop a 24-hour regime. Most often one injection is sufficient, but two may be used for smoother control.

If a patient responds poorly to the available insulins, one can be tailor-made by mixing different types. The combination of two insulins will give a time-activity curve specifically for the patient's needs. Table 20-7 indicates which insulins can be safely mixed. The procedure for safely mixing insulins is illustrated in Fig. 20-7.

The bottle of insulin that is in current use may be stored at room temperature. If it is kept in the refrigerator, warming it to room temperature before injecting it reduces tissue reaction and the discomforts associated with administering cold solutions. Insulin preparations do not lose their potency for many weeks, or even months, at ordinary room temperature. At higher temperatures (37 to 38°C), they deteriorate. Freezing clumps insulin particles so that they are unevenly dispersed as the dose is withdrawn from the vial. Reserve bottles of insulin should be refrigerated.

Insulin dosages are calibrated in units per cubic centimeters. Recently, concentrations of insulin have been standardized to U-100 (100 units/ml). Patients with diabetes of long-standing may be using older concentrations (40 or 80 units/ml) and should be phased into the use of the U-100 insulin and corresponding syringe.

Insulin syringes are calibrated to units to match the concentration of insulin. A 25- to 27-gauge needle with a length of ⅝ inch is preferred for the injection. The use of a syringe other than one specifically calibrated for insulin is a hazardous practice and encourages dosage errors. Before withdrawing a modified insulin, the vial should be rotated between the palms or inverted gently several times to disperse the particles evenly. Insulin should not be shaken as this results in the formation of bubbles and foam.

It is generally agreed that insulin should be administered deep subcutaneously for optimal absorption. Although it can be given intramuscularly or into the tissue between the layer of fat and muscle, the subcutaneous route has remained the most acceptable. Intravenous administration of regular insulin is reserved for emergency situations.

The injection can be given at a 45 or a 90° angle, depending on the depth of the subcutaneous tissue. For persons with little fatty tissue, injection at 45° may be appropriate, yet for a more corpulent person a 90° position is needed to penetrate to the appropriate subcutaneous depth. Similar judgment should be used in deciding whether the skin should be pinched or stretched.

The sites suitable for insulin injection are shown in Fig. 20-8. The patient should be taught to

**TABLE 20-7**
MIXING INSULINS

| INSULINS THAT CAN BE SAFELY MIXED | | |
|---|---|---|
| Regular (unmodified) | and | Semilente |
| | | NPH |
| | | Lente |
| | | Protamine zinc |
| | | Ultralente |
| Semilente | and | Lente |
| | | Ultralente |
| Lente | and | Ultralente |
| | | Semilente |
| INSULINS THAT CANNOT BE MIXED | | |
| Semilente | and | Protamine zinc |
| | | NPH |
| Lente | and | Protamine zinc |
| | | NPH |
| Ultralente | and | Protamine zinc |
| | | NPH |

devise a pattern for regular and systematic rotation for the insulin injection. This avoids infection, skin deterioration, and delayed absorption. Marking the sites used at each injection on a diagram helps to recall and to plan for the next dose. To prevent retarded absorption and skin complications, a minimum diameter of 3 to 4 cm should be allowed between injection sites, and none of these regions should be injected more than once each month. Patients should be cautioned to avoid a region of approximately 1 cm around the umbilicus because of its vascularity. The waistline should also be avoided because of its increased nerve supply.

The nurse should assess the sites for tissue changes. *Lipodystrophy* refers to changes in subcutaneous fat at the site of injection. Either atrophy or hypertrophy can develop. Although the changes are harmless, they are cosmetically disfiguring. Atrophic changes range from a mild dimpling of the skin to deep pits. Girls and young women are prone to atrophy. Hypertrophy is most frequent in boys and young men. It is mostly seen on the anterior or lateral thigh and gives the appearance of well-developed muscle. Because the masses are rela-

tively avascular and anesthetic, patients often choose them as pain-free injection sites. When lipodystrophy is noted, the nurse should evaluate the patient's injection technique and review the method, sites, and rotation schedule with the patient. The patient should be reminded to administer the insulin at room temperature, as cold solutions predispose to lipodystrophy.

The intermediate-acting and long-acting insulins are administered approximately one-half hour before breakfast. The rapid-acting insulins are given 15 to 30 minutes before a meal. Because their action is coordinated to meals, the nurse should be alert to the time of administration. If diagnostic procedures or tests will delay breakfast, the insulin dose should also be delayed.

When insulin therapy is first initiated, patients often experience blurred vision. This blurring arises from fluctuations in the blood glucose level that causes osmotic changes within the lens and ocular fluids. As the blood glucose stabilizes and ocular equilibrium is restored, vision improves. Patients should be informed that this may happen and that it will subside in 6 to 8 weeks.

**FIGURE 20-7**

Mixing insulins. Sept 1: Inject air into the modified insulin. Step 2: Inject air into the unmodified insulin and withdraw the desired dose. Step 3: Withdraw the dose of the modified insulin. Step 4: Rotate the syringe to mix the insulins. The regular (unmodified) insulin is withdrawn first. If any of the regular insulin accidentally enters the modified insulin, the action of the latter will not be changed significantly.

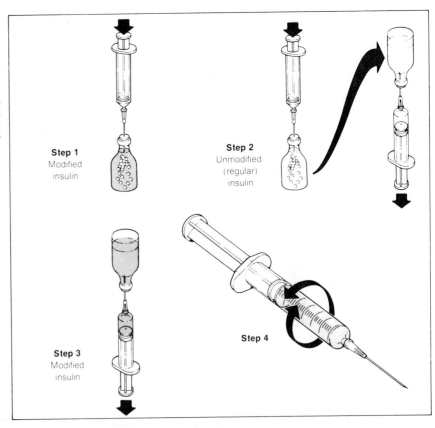

An allergic reaction at the injection site is not unusual when insulin is first administered. Itching, redness, and induration develop at the injection site. This process is self-limiting and subsides spontaneously after 1 to 2 weeks of therapy. Antihistaminic drugs are sometimes given. Intradermal injection or impurities in the alcohol used in skin cleansing can cause these symptoms.

*Hypoglycemia*   Patients taking insulin can develop insulin excess. The excess insulin drives glucose into the cells and *hypoglycemia* results. Because glucose is the primary nutrient used by the brain, cerebral symptoms develop. In most instances hypoglycemia tends to develop rapidly.

A patient's first indications of an insulin reaction are parasympathetic effects of hunger, nausea, and a slowed pulse. Yawning, inability to concentrate or to do simple calculations, lethargy, and disinterest signal that the cerebrum is being deprived of glucose. This stimulates a stress response and epinephrine is released. Patients develop excessive perspiration, nervousness, tremors, and cardiac palpitation. These adrenergic effects make the patient feel "different" or "jumpy." The patient often recognizes what is happening and is able to treat it. If nothing is done, lower brain centers will be affected. The patient will become comatose and obtunded. Repeated, prolonged hypoglycemia can lead to irreversible brain damage.

Insulin reactions develop more slowly with the long- and intermediate-acting insulins so that the premonitory signs may go unheeded. The patient may comment about a feeling of numbness of the hands or around the lips. Associates may notice personality changes and atypical behavior— impaired work performance, inability to study, or mood swings. Staggering, slurring of words, confusion, or behavior ranging from combativeness to uncontrolled weeping occurs and is sometimes misinterpreted as alcoholic intoxication. Whenever a patient appears intoxicated, hypoglycemia should be suspected. As the hypoglycemia deepens, the patient develops double vision, difficulties in coordination, and eventually convulsions and coma.

With the long- and intermediate-acting insulins patients may slip into insulin reactions during the middle of the night. Clues are nightmares, sleep

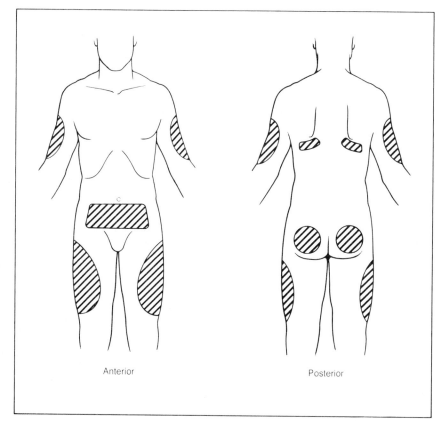

**FIGURE 20-8**
Sites for insulin injection. A different site should be selected for each injection and no spot should be used more often than once each month.

Anterior                    Posterior

walking, and crying out in one's sleep. The nurse must check all patients receiving insulin throughout the night for this impending danger. The patient's skin should be touched for moisture. The *squint challenge reflex* should be tested. This is done by shining a light on the patient's eyes while asleep. If the central nervous system is intact, the sleeping person will compress both eyelids when a light is shone on them. A comatose person shows no response.

To reverse the hypoglycemia, food must be given by mouth or parenterally. If the patient can comprehend and swallow, offer a rapidly absorbing carbohydrate in the form of fruit juice, candy, or carbonated beverage. The amount given should equal 10 to 12 g of quick-absorbing carbohydrate. The following are suggestions: two teaspoons of honey or Karo syrup; five or six Lifesavers; four ounces of orange juice, apple juice, or ginger ale; 10 small gumdrops; or two lumps of sugar. Additional sugar should not be added to fruit juices or beverages since this spikes the blood glucose and impedes reversal of symptoms.

Once there is clinical improvement, supplemental slowly digestible carbohydrates should be eaten. These restore the liver glycogen and prevent recurrence of the hypoglycemia. Milk, cottage cheese, peanut butter, and bread are suitable for this.

If an insulin reaction has advanced to a point where the patient is unresponsive and unable to swallow, the parenteral route must be used. Administering glucagon may reverse the symptoms. It can be given subcutaneously, intramuscularly, or intravenously, and it acts to mobilize the glycogen stores in the liver. Even if there is only minimal glycogen, mobilization of this store can be sufficient to arouse the patient to a point where carbohydrates can be taken orally. Supplemental slow-absorbing carbohydrate must be eaten to replenish the glycogen stores and prevent secondary hypoglycemia.

When the patient does not respond to any of the above measures, glucose should be given intravenously. Concentrations ranging from 10 to 50 percent will reverse the effects of hypoglycemia. The amount needed depends upon the severity of the hypoglycemia. After administration the patient will awaken immediately.

In an emergency, products that are absorbable from the buccal mucosa can be used. Honey or corn syrup can be coated on the buccal surfaces. As this is absorbed, the patient may be aroused enough to take carbohydrate foods. Commercially prepared products include Reactose, Instant Glucose, and Neg-React.

Protection against insulin-induced hypoglycemia requires maintenance of a balance among insulin, food intake, and exercise. Even with the greatest care the patient may occasionally experience an insulin reaction. The patient and family should be well acquainted with the symptoms and the appropriate treatment. Some diabetologists induce an insulin reaction under controlled conditions so that patients know what they will experience.

Patients and their families should be taught what symptoms to expect, the times reactions are most likely to occur, and measures to be taken should they happen. The family must know how to prepare and administer glucagon, and it should be available as an emergency drug at all times. Patients should be encouraged to explore the factors that precipitated a reaction so that future episodes can be prevented. Errors in dosage, missing a meal, excessive exercise, renal failure, excessive alcohol consumption, and medications such as aspirin, propanolol, and sulfonamides can all contribute to an insulin reaction.

Following a hypoglycemic reaction, the patient's blood glucose level may increase. The hypoglycemia activates counterregulation with release of epinephrine, glucocorticoids, and growth hormone. This stimulates gluconeogenesis, and the blood glucose climbs. This is known as the *Symogyi effect.* The cause is too much insulin, but the hyperglycemia may be misinterpreted as a worsening of the diabetic state, and additional insulin is often given. Appropriate therapy is to lower the insulin dose and achieve a stabilized state.

*Diabetic ketoacidosis* Another acute emergency situation that can develop is ketoacidosis. It usually develops slowly, although the time of onset can vary from patient to patient. It develops when insufficient insulin levels result in cellular starvation and hyperglycemia. As hyperglycemia increases, glucose is lost in the urine and acts as an osmotic diuretic pulling water into the urine with it. Large quantities of potassium, sodium, and chloride are lost in this diuresis. Dehydration results and can progress to hypovolemic shock (see Chap. 28).

In response to the cellular starvation, large quantities of fat are mobilized from adipose tissue. Ordinarily the liver metabolizes fatty acids, but with unregulated amounts the liver is unable to proceed with this efficiently. It partially oxidizes them to form acetyl CoA molecules which combine to form the ketoacids, acetoacetic acid and beta-hydroxybutyric acid. These travel to the cells where they can be used as energy. In insulin deficiency, however, muscle cells cannot use ketones for fuel as they do normally. The acids enter the bloodstream and increase the hydrogen ion concentration. The body's buffer system is rapidly exhausted, and acidosis develops. If allowed to continue, severe acidosis, circulatory collapse, renal shutdown, and coma will develop.

In the early stages of ketoacidosis the effects on the patient are indefinite. The patient may feel weak. Glucosuria and ketonuria may be evident. The classic symptoms of diabetes may become noticeable. As sodium becomes depleted, abdominal pain is often present. Hypovolemia may begin to evidence itself.

As ketone bodies build up in the circulation, acidosis becomes evident. The patient's face becomes flushed, and nausea and vomiting often develop. Paresthesias may be noted, vision may become dimmed or blurred, deep tendon reflexes diminished, and the patient progresses from drowsiness to stupor and possibly to coma.

The body tries to compensate the acidosis by blowing off $CO_2$. This results in characteristic deep breathing called *Kussmaul respirations.* Acetone is volatile and is also excreted by the lungs, giving the breath a fruity odor sometimes described as the smell of "new-mown hay."

The patient with suspected ketosis requires continuous medical care and is usually admitted to the intensive care unit. Interventions usually include intravenous fluids, insulin replacement, and electrolyte supplements. A systematic and detailed assessment of the patient will be necessary. Initially, vital signs, urine volume, serum ketones, and serum electrolytes will be monitored closely. Serum glucose and arterial blood gases will also be measured. The patient's level of alertness should be recorded frequently.

The fluid deficit must be corrected first, and this is accomplished with rapid infusions of intravenous iso- or hypotonic saline. Often 1 liter will be given within the first hour. Subsequently 300 to 500 ml is often administered hourly for another 2 to 3 hours. The large fluid volume dilutes the hypertonic extracellular fluid and fosters glucose excretion by the kidneys. In patients with known cardiac or renal impairment, a central venous catheter may be inserted to monitor the volume status.

When the plasma glucose falls to 250 mg/dl, the intravenous fluid should be changed to 5% glucose. This prevents both hypoglycemia and cerebral edema that can accompany the rapid insulin-induced fall in blood glucose. Urine volume, urine glucose, and urine ketones are determined every hour concurrently with the fluid replacement.

Rapid-acting insulin (regular) is used to treat diabetic ketoacidosis. It is given intravenously or intramuscularly in preference to the subcutaneous route since diminished circulation and hypovolemia retard absorption from superficial areas. Currently the optimal method and amount of insulin for ketosis are under investigation. One of several methods may be selected. Insulin may be added to the intravenous fluid; a usual initial amount is 100 units. An objection to adding insulin to the bottle of intravenous fluid is that it binds or absorbs to glass and plastic tubing, hence preventing the full amount from reaching the patient. This binding can be overcome by adding a small amount of albumin to the intravenous fluid.

Another method for administering insulin, and one that is currently advocated, is to deliver it directly into a vein by a slow infusion pump. Amounts ranging from 6 to 8 units/hour can be infused. Hourly blood and urine glucose and ketone measurements serve as guides to the effectiveness of the dose.

The shift of potassium from within the cell to the extracellular compartment that occurs with dehydration and protein catabolism raises the serum potassium to high levels. As the ketosis is corrected and the blood volume is restored, potassium once again shifts intracellularly. Within a short period of time the patient may fluctuate between hyper- and hypokalemic states. Potassium may be added to the intravenous solution after the initial hydration period. It is not supplemented if the patient is anuric or the urine output is low. Nurses should be alert to indications of hypo- or hyperkalemia (see Chap. 12).

With correction of the hypovolemia and progression toward normal metabolism, ketones disappear from the urine and blood, and the acidosis resolves. Blood glucose levels decline. The nurse may notice increased urine output, growing alertness, restored skin turgor, and brightness of the eyes as indices of improvement. Once the patient is alert enough to take solid food, subcutaneous insulin every 6 hours will be started, and high-carbohydrate nutrients given one-half hour after each insulin dose. The patient will be gradually advanced to the usual three-meal pattern and the preillness insulin dose. Reachieving a stable blood glucose level with food, insulin, and activity may require several days.

Identifying the factors that precipitated the ketoacidosis is of prime importance. Ketoacidosis is most often caused by infection. The nurse should inspect all body surfaces for possible infections. The lungs should be carefully auscultated and the abdomen examined for distention or painful areas. Hidden infections such as cholecystitis, pyelonephritis, and appendicitis may persist for some time before becoming noticeable. Influenza or a cold can become a major threat. Because of the increased metabolic rate associated with infections, the body stores of fat and protein are mobilized, and more insulin is needed.

*Hyperglycemic hyperosmolar nonketotic coma* Another comatose condition that may develop in diabetic patients is *hyperglycemic hyperosmolar nonketotic coma* (HHNK). It develops instead of ketosis if the patient produces insulin that is sufficient to prevent ketone bodies from forming, but inadequate to reduce the hyperglycemia. The glucose then accumulates to render the blood hyperosmolar. Analyses of blood parameters are identical to those outlined for diabetic ketoacidosis. The differentiating characteristic is that the ketone bodies are low or absent. The symptoms are similar to ketosis except that coma develops rapidly. Patients do not have the Kussmaul respirations nor the smell of acetone on their breath.

Management and monitoring of the patient are similar to those for the patient in ketosis. The blood volume is restored, and the osmolarity of the blood reduced. Intravenous fluids should be hypotonic, and insulin should be used sparingly.

*Transplantation* An approach to keeping the blood glucose at physiologic levels has been through *pancreatic transplantation.* Pancreatic transplant from a nondiabetic donor to a diabetic recipient has been used experimentally. As with all organ transplants of this type, rejection is a problem (see Chap. 10). More encouraging results have been obtained by *implantation* of clumps of beta cells from the islets of Langerhans. In experimentally induced diabetic rats, the beta cells were injected into the portal vein. The islets lodge in the liver and function by secreting insulin.[8]

Work on development of an *artificial pancreas* or an *artificial beta cell* has been exciting.[9] It is envisioned as a small instrument that would be implanted under the skin and would be responsive to elevations in blood glucose by infusing rapid-acting insulin. A small sensor monitoring the glucose level would feed into a miniaturized computer. This, in turn, would connect with an infusion pump and a reservoir of insulin. Insulin would enter the circulation on the basis of minute-by-minute determinations of blood glucose. A machine has been developed, but it awaits miniaturization.

*Control of diabetes during surgery* When the diabetic patient undergoes surgery, special care is needed to avert serious metabolic complications. The management scheme throughout the operative experience depends largely upon whether insulin is a usual part of the daily therapy. For the insulin-independent diabetic the possibilities range from being permitted to take the oral antidiabetic agent on the morning of surgery to starting an intravenous infusion with 5% glucose and receiving insulin as a replacement for the oral agent. Under most circumstances for the diet-controlled diabetic, insulin is not given, but an intravenous infusion is started to replace the usual oral intake. If the person is controlled with the combination of diet and an oral agent, an intravenous infusion of 5% glucose is started. Whether insulin is given as replacement for the oral agent depends upon the extent of the procedure. The situation is different for the insulin-dependent person. An intravenous infusion of 5% glucose is started, and one-third to one-half of the usual morning insulin dose is given subcutaneously. The reduced insulin dose minimizes the possibility of hypoglycemia during the anesthetic phase.

The basic preoperative preparation of the diabetic patient is identical to that of other patients undergoing surgery. Prior to the surgery the nurse should anticipate that a fasting blood glucose will be drawn. If extensive surgery or prolonged recovery is anticipated, preoperative determinations of blood acetone, carbon dioxide, and blood urea nitrogen are made.

When the patient arrives in the recovery unit, the nurse should observe for and prevent hypoglycemia and ketoacidosis. Insulin, fluids, or electrolyte supplements are prescribed according to the metabolic situation as assessed by blood acetone, carbon dioxide, glucose, and urinary glucose concentrations. Infusions of 5 or 10% glucose are used until oral intake is satisfactorily reestablished. Regular insulin is given subcutaneously during this time to maintain metabolic balance. The insulin dose is managed on a sliding scale based on the results of the glucosuria test. The nurse should anticipate that the urine will be checked for glucose as often as every 4 hours during the early postoperative phase.

Because the diabetic patient is prone to develop vascular and skin complications, astute nursing observation is necessary. Inspection of the wound for evidences of infection, concerted effort to prevent vascular complications such as thrombosis, and utilization of methods to induce voiding and avert catheterization are specific challenges for nursing. As recovery takes place and the stress is reduced, insulin needs are reduced. The nurse should call the physician's attention to the need for the daily adjustments in dosage so that the patient is not subjected to hypoglycemia.

**F**oot Problems  Problems with feet are common in diabetic patients and are a result of neuropathic, vascular, and infectious changes. The insulin-dependent patient with diabetes of long-standing is especially vulnerable. Patients should be impressed with the responsibility of maintaining adequate blood flow to the lower extremities and in preventing trauma to the legs and feet. Patients who smoke should be encouraged to stop as smoking increases the vascular disorders. The following are simple instructions that should be incorporated into the teaching plan for all diabetic patients.

Instructions for care of the feet:

1  Wash your feet every night with a mild face soap and warm water. Check the water temperature with your hand; it is too hot if you must withdraw your hand.

2  Dry your feet without rubbing by using a soft, clean cloth. The spaces between the toes need to be dried carefully. Avoid drawing the towel vigorously between them.

3  Keep your feet warm. During the winter use woolen socks or wool-lined shoes; in summer wear white cotton socks. Change your socks each day.

4  If your feet are cold at night, wear loose-fitting bed socks.

5  Never apply hot water bottles, electric pads, or any kind of mechanical heating device to your legs or feet.

6  Do not wear mended stockings or stockings with seams. Select stockings that allow for toe motion.

7  Wear low-heeled shoes that are made of soft leather with nonrigid shanks. Open-toe or open-heel shoes predispose your feet to damage. When you buy new shoes, wear them ½ hour only the first day and increase the length you wear them by 1 hour each day.

8  Inspect the inside of your shoes before putting them on. If you have numbness of your hands, ask a family member to check for you.

9  Cut your toenails only after you have softened them by soaking them in warm water. Cut them straight across; do not cut down in the corners of the nails. If

you have trouble seeing, ask someone to help you with this.

10  Calluses may be an indication that shoes do not fit well. Rough calluses can be smoothed with pumice stone or an emery board.

11  Wear soft pads over calluses, corns, or bunions; do not cut corns or calluses; do not use commercial preparations to remove corns or calluses.

12  To prevent cracking, lanolin or petrolatum are the best softening agents. These must not be applied between the toes.

13  Do not wear garters or tight clothing that restricts the circulation to your legs and feet.

14  Never use strong antiseptic drugs on your feet, particularly tincture of iodine, lysol, or carbolic acid.

15  Inspect your feet daily for any unusual developments such as blisters, cuts, or scratches.

16  Prevent athlete's foot by wearing a clean pair of socks each day. If you notice excessive moisture, apply a dusting powder lightly on your feet. Seek the advice of your physician.

17  Walking is the best exercise for your feet. If you are unable to walk because of leg problems, move your feet and toes by flexing and extending them several times each day.

18  Consult your physician if you have questions about the care of your feet. Do not follow the advice of well-meaning friends, neighbors, or family.

**I**nfections  Diabetic patients are also prone to infections which can have devastating effects. The skin should be inspected for cutaneous infections. Moist skin folds should be kept as dry as possible. *Candida* is a common offending organism and can be treated with nystatin. Antibiotics are used for frequently occurring boils and furuncles.

The interdigital areas of the feet require inspection for fungal infections. Preventive measures to suggest are drying well between the toes, using a prophylactic dusting powder, and wearing clean stockings each day. Using lamb's wool between the toes helps absorb moisture and keeps the skin surfaces from touching. Fungal infections can be treated with fungicidal powder.

For the female diabetic patient vaginal infections are common. Exploring ways to control these infections is a nursing responsibility. Wearing cotton rather than nylon underclothing and sitting on chairs with caned or wooden seats are practical hints to offer patients. Nystatin is used to treat these infections.

**N**europathies Diabetic patients must often cope with multiple neuropathies. Peripheral neuropathies often result in varying degrees of *paresthesias.* To prevent injury, patients should be taught to compensate for this. Being especially careful when smoking or cooking, measuring the temperature of bath water, avoiding the use of heating pads, keeping an adequate distance from heat sources, and dressing warmly in cold weather are ways of compensating for the decreased sensation.

The visceral neuropathies often cause disturbing problems. If *diarrhea* is a problem, Lomotil, Sonnaton, or tetracycline may be used. The use of tetracycline prevents bacteria from overgrowing and forming "puddles" in an atonic bowel. This neuropathic diarrhea is not infectious.

Neuropathic *bladder paralysis* can also develop. This is often treated with bethanecol chloride which increases bladder contraction. A regular voiding program should be established to prevent urinary tract infections from bladder distention. If conservative management does not restore satisfactory bladder emptying, surgically cutting the internal sphincter relieves the inability of the bladder to propel urine against the sphincter. Incontinence does not develop because the external sphincter remains in control.

If the patient is experiencing *sexual dysfunction,* counseling of the patient and the spouse must be undertaken. This relieves anxieties and eliminates misinterpretation about the problem. As a last resort for the male a silastic implant can be inserted to keep the penis semierect. While this is not obvious when walking, it allows for penetration during intercourse.

**R**etinopathy The most conscientious efforts of both the physician and the patient may not be able to prevent *visual problems.* Many diabetologists stress that there are fewer visual complications if the diabetes is kept well in hand the first 10 years of the disease.

Because of the variety of visual problems that plague the diabetic, assessment of visual acuity and completing a fundoscopic examination every 6 months by the physician or nurse are essential. An ophthalmologist should complete a thorough examination of the retina at least every 2 years.

Today the most beneficial treatment for retinopathy involves application of an intense light source, such as the xenon arc lamp or the argon laser, to specific lesions of the retina. As the melanin of the retina and the hemoglobin of the retinal vessels absorb the light, heat is generated that coagulates the specific points to which it was directed. Both newly forming vessels or lesions within existing vessels can be coagulated. This procedure retards the growth of new vessels.

**R**enal Problems Because of the nephropathy associated with diabetes, renal failure can develop. The care is that for any other patient with uremia: limiting dietary sodium and protein, controlling the blood pressure with antihypertensive agents, hemodialysis, and renal transplantation.

The outlook for diabetic patients with advanced nephropathy has been dismal. Hemodialysis seems less satisfactory than renal transplantation for diabetic patients. Shunts or fistulas are difficult to maintain owing to the vascular changes. Blood glucose levels fluctuate markedly with dialysis, and in the nephrectomized client urine specimens are not available for glucose monitoring.

Even though the number of diabetic patients with renal transplants is small, the results are promising. Not only are the pathologic kidneys replaced, but retinopathy improves and neuropathic symptoms seem less severe to patients. However, health personnel and patients are confronted with managing two complex situations: diabetes mellitus and renal transplantation. It is much too early to draw general conclusions about the benefits to the diabetic population.

**P**sychological Problems The psychological reactions of patients to a diagnosis of diabetes mellitus will depend on the individual's personality structure and conceptions of the disease. In general, reactions vary greatly. Some patients will accept the diagnosis with apparent ease. Others evidence severe reactions requiring long-term therapy.

For the adult an initial reaction may be relief. Often adults fear that the symptoms they are experiencing are indications of "catastrophic" disease such as a malignancy. This is often followed, however, by a reactive depression. Patients will utilize a variety of coping mechanisms to handle the situation. Anxiety is common. This can be increased significantly if the patient is aware of complications that can develop. Some patients become compulsive, adhering to the therapeutic regime in every respect. These patients are often critical of health professionals who do not advocate the strictest control. Other patients may react with denial. Urine may not be tested, the diet not followed, nor the insulin taken properly.

Diabetes can have significant effects on several aspects of the patient's life. Individual reactions will vary not only with personality structure, but with the age and developmental stage of the patient. Adolescents with diabetes may resist any restriction that makes them different from their peers. Resentment and rebellion may develop. The elderly may be unwilling to change lifelong habits that they associate with pleasant memories. The requirements of glucose control can significantly alter the individual's life-style. Some patients are able to adjust to the changes, while others find this extremely difficult.

The nurse should be aware that patients react differently and be tolerant of various coping mechanisms because coping mechanisms protect the patient. At the same time considerate but firm parameters must be set for the uncooperative patient. Individual psychotherapy, group therapy, and family group therapy may be helpful.

**Fourth-Level Nursing Care**

A goal for all diabetic patients is attainment of their customary life-style and a quality of life that allows them to pursue activities enjoyed by nondiabetics. The person with diabetes cannot lead a completely normal life, but by taking steps to control the disorder, a high quality life is possible.

Diabetes is a serious health problem, and its ramifications in management may be overwhelming to some clients. Family members, too, may be unable to cope. Participating in a diabetic group or club and sharing ideas, concerns, and problems may make adjustment easier. Clients should be informed of round-the-clock information services for emotional crises. The Joslin Clinic in Boston maintains this type of service with the purpose of helping diabetics deal with crises. Psychotherapy is recommended for patients and families who are emotionally overwhelmed with the disease.

The client may become more comfortable with the condition through learning about the problem and reading some of the publications that are designed as communication media for and to diabetics. *Forecast,** a bimonthly publication of the American Diabetes Association, relates current information about research, tips in management, and personal experiences of diabetic clients. Booklets

giving facts about diabetes and meal-planning suggestions are also available from this organization. *Diabetes in the News,†* a newspaper-like publication designed for the diabetic population, provides helpful hints about physical management, dietary modifications, and new products.

The nurse should be aware of the economic status of the diabetic client. Minimal equipment for injections includes syringes, needles, a small jar of cotton balls or a roll of cotton, and a bottle of alcohol. Disposable needles and syringes are preferred, but some clients cannot afford these. If the disposable type is used, a proper method for discarding the equipment must be worked out.

The client who uses nondisposable equipment needs instruction on sterilization and storage of the syringe and needle. Setting a strainer into a small saucepan of sufficient depth and covering the equipment with water is a way to boil and handle it without contamination or damage. The client may find it more suitable to soak the needle and syringe in alcohol, but they still must be boiled weekly.

The nurse should also discuss management of daily activities. Clients and families who have difficulty with meal planning may benefit from cookbooks designed for diabetics. These are obtainable from bookstores or from the American Diabetes Association. If weight reduction is a goal, attending Weight Watchers, Inc., may provide incentive. No weight reduction plan should be initiated without the physician's consent. Since susceptibility to hypoglycemia is greater at the end of a workday and occasionally symptoms develop while driving home, sugar supplies should be carried in the car. Insulin can be managed on vacations by preparing an insulin kit using a thermos vacuum or by purchasing a commercially available kit. If clients are sensitive about being observed while injecting insulin, they can seek privacy in a clean restroom or in the car. When driving long distances, diabetics should stop every few hours and snack on crackers to ensure alertness. Getting out of the car and walking around will stimulate peripheral circulation.

The diabetic patient should carry an identification card at all times. The card distributed by the American Diabetes Association is most appropriate for it identifies the client and gives pertinent information about management. The American Diabetes Association also advocates that every diabetic wear a Medic-Alert identification bracelet. Patients

* American Diabetes Association, Inc., 600 Fifth Ave., New York, N.Y. 10020.

† Ames Company, Division of Miles Laboratories, Inc., Elkart, Ind. 46514.

should be instructed to notify their dentists so a proper anesthetic agent can be selected and a prophylactic dental program initiated. Beauticians should also be notified because neuropathy may diminish perception of burns by chemicals or hair dryers.

**Teaching plan** Teaching the diabetic about management is a complex problem. Principles of teaching are presented in Chap. 2. Effective teaching requires sound assessment of the patient's condition, learning abilities and learning modes, adjustment to the illness, and normal life pattern. Teaching should focus on those aspects that are pertinent to the patient as an individual diabetic. The patient may not need to know everything about diabetes and its management. The nurse should differentiate between what is significant for the insulin-dependent and the insulin-independent client.

Instruction about diabetes should begin immediately when the diagnosis is made, and it must continue throughout the patient's lifetime. Teaching sessions in either the hospital or ambulatory care settings should be scheduled. There is no best way to teach the diabetic client. On the basis of the nurses' assessment, methods of teaching and use of teaching materials should correlate with the patient's learning style. A general guideline is to use a variety of methods that will appeal to many senses. Among the available diabetic education materials are videotapes, records, self-instruction booklets, pamphlets, and books. Some hospitals and clinics have computer-based diabetic instruction or a television channel which carries a daily diabetic program. It is important to remember that the diabetic college professor might enjoy the computer-based program but it is unsuitable for the person who has vision problems or neuropathy of the upper extremity and "numb" fingertips.

The nurse may find it necessary to prepare, write, or draw materials to fit the learning abilities of some clients. A variety of booklets about diabetes are available from pharmaceutical companies, but these are not appropriate for all clients. Some may not be able to understand the contents or read them. The words of diabetic care are complex and unfamiliar to clients, requiring that they first learn their meaning. Some diabetic materials are available in foreign languages.* The client who is disadvantaged in reading English may benefit from this material.

* E. R. Squibb and Sons, 909 Third Ave., New York, N.Y.

Equally significant is that individual and group instruction should be planned. Group instruction helps patients realize that others have the same condition, allows for sharing of problems, and encourages learning how others manage their condition; individualized instruction provides an opportunity to work on specific details or aspects unique to that person.

A learning plan must be developed, and the nurse must decide on the outcomes desired for the client. Outcomes must include behaviors in the cognitive, psychomotor, and affective domains. In the *cognitive* domain the patient needs to know the basic elements of the disease; how it is controlled; its effects; the action of insulin; the action of oral antidiabetic agents; information about dietary management; adjustment of food intake; how to plan menus; how to control hypoglycemia and ketoacidosis; information about an exercise plan; and how to handle injuries and infections. Among the *psychomotor* outcomes are performing and reading the urine test for glucosuria and ketonuria accurately, preparing and injecting insulin safely, and carrying out foot care and other aspects of hygiene properly. Within the *affective* domain acceptance of the disease is a desired outcome. The degree of acceptance can be evaluated by the clients' willingness to seek help with questions about complications and to keep a record of insulin taken and the urine tests for glucosuria, among others. Individualized teaching plans should be developed for each patient. In line with the format presented in Chap. 2, a sample plan is presented in Table 20-8.

The individualized instructions for the diabetic should be written out so that they can be referred to when necessary. Dietary details, insulin doses and how to make modifications based on glucosuria tests, and specifics of personal care are among the written materials that should be given each patient. Instructions on how to mix glucagon and what to do in emergencies should be available to the associates of the labile diabetic so that they can initiate the proper care if unusual situations arise.

The teaching plan must include the family or an associate designated by the client. Arrangements must be made with these people to come to the clinic or hospital for instruction. This helps them to learn specific aspects of management, to function in emergency situations, and to support and encourage the client in self-management or to assume the care if necessary.

*Diabetic teaching cannot be done in a short period of time.* Factual information and skills are acquired quickly by some clients, but it is only upon returning home or to work that there is recognition of what actually needs to be known. The most highly developed teaching program cannot include everything that every patient needs to know.

It has been shown that diabetics forget details as they manage their condition and that they need to keep abreast of changes in management. Continuing education programs are increasing in number and in importance. Diabetic clients should be informed of these and referred to them so that they keep their health care practices safe and up-to-date. A referral should be made to a community health nurse, clinical specialist, nurse practitioner, or local clinic for follow-up care and teaching. The patient's understanding of management should be periodically reevaluated.

**Visual impairment** The nurse may be confronted with finding ways to promote independence for the partially sighted or nonsighted diabetic. Sometimes other family members can assist with the urine testing and read the color blocks, administer the insulin, or help with physical care. Some must rely on community health nurses or neighbors. It is appropriate to encourage independence so long as it does not interfere with safety. A variety of self-help devices are available for the diabetic. A clip-on magnifier enlarges the tiny calibrations on the insulin syringe (C-Better Magnifier). A dosage monitor helps to withdraw the proper insulin dose. A needle guide can be used to direct the needle into the rubber stopper of the insulin vial. The publication, *Aids for the Blind,* offers other suggestions

and is available from the American Foundation for the Blind.*

Modifications in methods of administering insulin may be necessary for the visually impaired. They should inject the insulin by placing the needle at the skin surface and pushing it through, rather than thrusting it in a short distance from the skin. They need not aspirate after the needle has penetrated the tissue. The possibility of entering a blood vessel is so remote with subcutaneous injection that aspiration is a step which can be eliminated if the client has difficulty in manipulating the injection.

A 7-day supply of insulin can be withdrawn into separate insulin syringes by a community health nurse or a sighted person and placed in the refrigerator for use by the visually impaired diabetic. The insulin will not deteriorate by this method, but maintenance of sterility is a matter of concern.

The visually impaired can use touch to estimate the amount of glucose in the urine. They should be instructed to place one-fourth teaspoon of baker's yeast in a small test tube and add 12 ml urine. A rubber finger cot should be placed over the tube and the contents shaken vigorously. If sugar is present, fermentation of the sugar by the yeast will release carbon dioxide, and the finger cot will inflate. When performed at room temperature, this test is reported to be sensitive to glucose concentrations as low as 0.25 percent in 20 to 30 minutes. A deflated finger cot indicates no glucose or a

* American Foundation for the Blind, Inc., 15 W. 16 St., New York, N.Y. 10011.

**TABLE 20-8**
SAMPLE TEACHING PLAN FOR DIABETIC PATIENT

| Objectives | Content | Strategies | Evaluation |
|---|---|---|---|
| After hearing and viewing a lecture on television and observing a visual demonstration on proper foot care, the student will: <br><br>1 Recall from memory the proper steps in washing feet. <br><br>2 Know the types of socks and shoes to wear as well as other materials used to protect the feet. <br><br>3 List all the materials, treatments, and commercial preparations to be avoided when caring for feet. <br><br>4 Indicate all the reasons for seeking medical attention for any irritation to the feet or toes. | Should be drawn from Instructions for Care of the Foot discussed under Foot Problems in Third-Level Nursing Care. | May include any combination of the following: <br><br>Demonstration, <br>Videotape on foot care, <br>Group discussion, <br>Family involvement, <br>Slide tape on foot care, <br>Booklet, <br>Programmed instruction unit, <br>Television instruction program, <br>Individualized instruction. | Oral quiz. <br><br>Return demonstration on foot care. <br><br>Check selection of appropriate socks and shoes. <br><br>Pick out from a picture those problems that indicate need for medical attention. <br><br>Have patient explain the need for good foot care and indicate what must be avoided in order to prevent foot problems. |

trace; a mushy feeling suggests a medium amount of glucose, while tautness indicates a large amount of glucose.

**Employment**  Prejudices against the diabetic in finding employment have decreased. Objections to hiring diabetic workers focused on concerns of (1) excessive absenteeism, (2) insulin reactions on the job, (3) fears that injuries or disabilities will result from the diabetic state, and (4) fears of adverse effects on group medical insurance rates. Some studies have shown that absenteeism is no greater in diabetic employees than among nondiabetics; other studies have shown it to be even less.

Some states have "second injury" laws that offer incentives to employers to hire workers with certain disabilities. They offer the employer an insurance advantage. In the case of diabetics this type of law guarantees medical expense beyond a fixed sum if diabetes is a factor in causing an injury or if it delays recovery from the injury.

There are certain types of work that are not suitable for the diabetic. Policies of the United States Civil Service Commission are usable as guidelines. Job classes from which diabetics are excluded are those in which the primary responsibility is climbing to high places, working around power-driven machinery, working in sewers, or wading in water. Diabetics should not be placed in positions where sudden loss of consciousness endangers them or others. They should be counseled to avoid jobs that require rotation of shifts and for which physical demands are irregular.

**Marriage and pregnancy**  A frequent question of young diabetics is whether they should marry. In general, fewer diabetics marry, and the fertility problems are well known. Knowing that offspring may become diabetic and develop the long-term complications can generate guilt feelings. Diabetic wives may fear pregnancy because of the additional strain on the body and possible stillbirth. Gestation in the diabetic female is associated with an increased incidence of toxemia and polyhydramnios, but the majority of these pregnancies can be successfully managed with good obstetrical care. Diabetics should be informed that there is a relationship between clinical or chemical diabetes in the mother and congenital defects in the offspring. The risk is higher than for the nondiabetic mother. A characteristic diabetic embryo problem is the caudal regression syndrome which consists of agenesis of the sacrum and coccyx, hypoplasia of both femurs, and urogenital abnormalities.

## HYPOGLYCEMIA CONDITIONS

Recently hypoglycemia has become a "fad" disease, widely publicized in lay journals. While it has been overdiagnosed, correction of true hypoglycemia is essential to preventing irreparable brain damage. Hypoglycemic episodes can follow meals (postprandial) or fasting.

Hypoglycemia can be associated with *obesity*. In the obese patient hyperglycemia follows the excessive eating and absorption of food. This stimulates the release of large quantities of insulin, and as these levels persist, hypoglycemia develops. Increasing the dietary protein content and lowering the carbohydrate in the diet will diminish the signal to the pancreas to produce large quantities of insulin.

Excessive intake of *alcohol* can also precipitate hypoglycemia. Alcohol in sizeable quantities and without food is quickly metabolized in the liver. The formation of acetate inhibits glucose formation, and the blood glucose drops. Refraining from alcoholic intake will alleviate the problem, but gaining adherence to this is a more complex endeavor (see Chap. 19).

Other *drugs,* too, reduce the blood glucose levels. Salicylates, haloperidol (Haldol), propoxyphene (Darvon), antihistamines, and para-aminobenzoic acid are among the commonly prescribed drugs that can lower the blood glucose level and induce hypoglycemia.

*Hormonal deficiencies* must also be considered when symptoms of hypoglycemia are noted. Hypoglycemia occurs in adrenal cortical insufficiency and hypothyroidism. Symptoms subside with hormonal replacement therapy.

The most definitive *diagnostic test* for hypoglycemia is the glucose tolerance test. The procedure is identical to that used for establishing the diagnosis of diabetes mellitus. However, the test is extended to 4 to 5 hours to follow the blood glucose levels after the stressor effect of the glucose. It must show a drop in plasma glucose to 50 mg/dl or below. Extending the test for a longer period of time allows for distinction between the two types of hypoglycemia. Patients with reactive (postprandial) hypoglycemia will not have a low blood glucose level at the end of 5 hours; patients with fasting hypoglycemia will have a low level both at the beginning of the test and at the end of 4 to 5 hours.

The *tolbutamide* response test may also be used. The expected response is an initial drop in blood glucose but a return to 70 percent or more of its fasting level by the end of 3 hours. When *leucine* is given, a drop in plasma insulin is suggestive of an insulinoma. Similarly, an exaggerated increase in serum insulin levels after giving *glucagon* hints of a pancreatic islet cell tumor.

### Postprandial Hypoglycemia

Postprandial hypoglycemia is most often associated with early diabetes mellitus, a gastroenterostomy, or emotional lability. Spontaneous attacks of low plasma glucose occurring 3 to 5 hours after eating develop in the early phases of development of diabetes mellitus. Gastrectomy or surgical bypass of the pylorus allows ingested glucose to be more rapidly absorbed in the small bowel. The rapid rise in blood glucose provokes a greater-than-normal release of insulin. Glucose is transported across the cell membrane rapidly, the plasma glucose falls to pre-eating levels, but excessive insulin remains in the blood. The hyperinsulinism prompts development of hypoglycemia.

Functional hypoglycemia also develops in healthy young adults with no history of gastric surgery or diabetes mellitus. These persons are usually thin, emotionally unstable, tense, anxious, and compulsive. They comment about gastric hyperacidity, nausea, vomiting, and an irritable colon. Speculated as causes are excess catecholamine production and increased glucose absorption.

The nurse should be alert to patients who describe symptoms arising 2 to 3 hours after eating, usually after lunch. Sweating, jitters, inward trembling, racing pulse, and a headache are often noted. Numb lips and fingers, shaky handwriting, or inability to speak are a part of the clinical picture. Symptoms are not progressive, and subside in 15 to 30 minutes. There is no loss of consciousness or convulsions.

Nursing functions revolve around the dietary therapy. High-protein intake is advocated. If the problem stems from gastroenterostomy, six small high-protein feedings may allay the symptoms. For the obese and suspected diabetic, weight reduction, caloric restriction, and a decreased intake of sugar-containing foods is prescribed. Phenformin may be added to halt the rise in blood glucose and exaggerated insulin response.

The emotionally labile person should avoid caffeine-containing beverages and cigarettes. Anticholinergic drugs have been employed to inhibit vagal action and delay gastric emptying. As the patient's emotional status improves, the hypoglycemia subsides spontaneously.

### Severe Hypoglycemia

Among the more severe causes for hypoglycemia is excess insulin secretion by pancreatic islet cell tumors. About 10 percent of insulinomas are malignant. Hypoglycemic episodes are often more intense with malignant conditions. Information about the episodes should be sought. In tumors of beta cells excess insulin is discharged sporadically, and the episodes may be unpredictable.

The desired therapy is surgical removal of the tumor. Prior to surgery pharmacologic or hormonal management will keep the blood glucose at nondangerous levels. Glucagon or epinephrine may be given to elevate the blood glucose for several hours. Infusions of 5% glucose solution are used to keep the patient symptom-free.

If surgery is successful, the patient will be cured of the hypoglycemia. However, excision of a large portion of the pancreas will produce a diabetic state. The severity of the diabetes will depend upon the extent of the pancreatic resection. Replacement of insulin, as well as pancreatic digestive enzymes, will be required. The patient will need the same instruction and meticulous care as that described for any patient with diabetes mellitus. Pancreatin, a medication prepared from powdered animal pancreas and available in enteric-coated capsules or as granules, is used as pancreatic digestive enzyme replacement. The granules are taken with water or milk or sprinkled on food.

If removal of the tumor cannot be considered, the patient may be a candidate for diazoxide therapy. This thiazide derivative with diuretic properties elevates the blood glucose and decreases plasma insulin levels. It also produces nausea, vomiting, and hypotension. The blood pressure should be monitored, and for ambulatory patients, the final blood pressure check should be made with the patient standing. The drug also increases growth of body hair. Women should be alerted to this often distressing side effect.

Streptozotocin may also be used. It acts to destroy pancreatic islet cells and is given intravenously on a weekly basis. This is an experimental drug, and patients should be informed that its long-term effects are unknown.

## REFERENCES

1  Singal, D. P., and M. A. Blajchman, "Histocompatibility (HL-A) Antigens, Lymphocytotoxic Antibodies and Tissue Antibodies in Patients with Diabetes Mellitus," *Diabetes,* 22(6):429–432, June 1973.

2  Rayfield, E. J., et al., "Virus-induced Pancreatic Disease in Venezuelan Encephalitis Virus," *Diabetes,* 25(7):623–631, July 1976.

3  Unger, Roger, and LdLio Orci, "Hypothesis: The Essential Role of Glucagon in the Pathogenesis of Diabetes Mellitus," *Lancet,* 7897(1):14–16, January 4, 1975.

4  Feldman, Robert, A. Joseph Sender, and A. B. Siegelaub, "Difference in Diabetic and Non-Diabetic Fat Distribution Patterns by Skinfold Measurements," *Diabetes,* 18(7):478–486, July 1969.

5  Mowat, Alastair, and John Baum, "Chemotaxis of Polymorphonuclear Leukocytes from Patients with Diabetes Mellitus," *N Engl J Med,* 284:621–627, March 25, 1971.

6  Rimoin, D., "The Genetics of Diabetes Mellitus," in M. Ellenberg and H. Rifkin (eds.), *Diabetes Mellitus: Theory and Practice,* McGraw-Hill, New York, 1970.

7  Steinberg, B., "Heredity and Diabetes," *Eugenics Q,* 2:26–30, March 1955.

8  Matas, Arthur, David Sutherland, and John Najarian, "Current State of Islet and Pancreas Transplantation in Diabetes," *Diabetes,* 25(9):785, September 1976.

9  Botz, C. K., et al., "Comparison of Peripheral and Portal Routes of Insulin Infusion by a Computer Controlled Insulin Infusion System (Artificial Endocrine Pancreas)," *Diabetes,* 25(8):691–700, August 1976.

## BIBLIOGRAPHY

Assal, Jean-Ph., et al.: "Metabolic Effects of Sodium Bicarbonate in Management of Diabetic Ketoacidosis," *Diabetes,* 23(5):405–411, May 1974.

Bierman, E. L., and R. Nelson: "Carbohydrates, Diabetes, and Blood Lipids," *World Rev Nutr Dietetics,* 22:280–287, 1975.

Brazeau, P., and T. Guillemia: "Somatostatin: Newcomer from the Hypothalamus," *N Engl J Med.,* 290:963–964, April 25, 1974.

Cohen, E., and Leonard Mastbaum: "Employment for Patients with Diabetes," *Minn Med,* 57(3):241–243, March 1974.

Ensinck, John, and Robert Williams: "Disorders Causing Hypoglycemia," in Robert Williams (ed.), *Textbook of Endocrinology,* Saunders, Philadelphia, 1974, pp. 627–659.

Felig, Philip: "Current Concepts, Diabetic Ketoacidosis," *N Engl J Med,* 290:1360–1362, June 13, 1974.

Fletcher, H. Patrick: "The Oral Antidiabetic Drugs: Pro and Con," *Am J Nurs,* 76(4):596–599, April 1976.

Fletcher, Mary, et al.: "Helping Diabetics Adapt to Failing Vision," *Am J Nurs,* 74(1):54–57, January 1974.

Guthrie, Diana, and Richard Guthrie: "Coping with Diabetic Ketoacidosis," *Nursing 73,* 3:17–23, November 1973.

Hayter, Jean: "Fine Points in Diabetic Care," *Nursing 76,* 76(4):594–599, April 1976.

Kjellstrand, Carl, et al.: "Renal Transplantation in Patients with Insulin-Dependent Diabetes," *Lancet,* 2:4–8, July 7, 1973.

Ma, King, Donald Masler, and David Brown: "Hemodialysis in Diabetic Patients with Chronic Renal Failure," *Ann Inter Med,* 83(2):215–217, August 1975.

McMillan, Donald: "Deterioration of the Microcirculation in Diabetes," *Diabetes,* 24(10):944–957, October 1975.

Permutt, M. Alan: "Postprandial Hypoglycemia," *Diabetes,* 25(8):719–733, August 1976.

Schumann, Delores: "Coping with the Complex, Dangerous, Elusive Problems of Those Insulin-Induced Hypoglycemic Reactions," *Nursing 74,* 4:56–60, April 1974.

————: "Tips for Improving Urine Testing Techniques," *Nursing 76,* 6(2):23–27, February 1976.

————: "Assessing the Diabetic," *Nursing 76,* 6(3): 62–67, March 1976.

Semple, R., D. White, and W. Manderson: "Continuous Intravenous Infusion of Small Doses of Insulin in Treatment of Diabetic Ketoacidosis," *Br Med J.,* 2:694–698, June 29, 1974.

Steinke, Jurgen, and George W. Thorn: "Diabetes Mellitus," in Maxwell M. Wintrobe et al. (eds.), *Harrison's Principles of Internal Medicine,* 7th ed., McGraw-Hill, New York, 1974, pp. 532–550.

Williams, Robert, and Daniel Porte, Jr.: "The Pancreas," in Robert Williams (ed.), *Textbook of Endocrinology,* Saunders, Philadelphia, 1974, pp. 502–626.

Witt, Karen: "HHNK (Hyperglycemic Hyperosmolar Nonketotic Coma); A Newly Recognized Syndrome to Watch For," *Nursing 76,* 6(2):66–70, February 1976.

# 21
# HORMONAL DISTURBANCES AND THEIR EFFECTS ON METABOLISM*

Ann Gill Taylor
Ann Ziebol Hamory

The endocrine system is a widespread and highly specialized group of tissues that synthesize and secrete hormones within the body. These hormones function to elicit specialized physiological responses from the human system. Their activity affects target organs and elicits responses that aid the body in interacting with its environment. The activities of the various body systems are, in part, controlled by hormones. As the secretion of a particular hormone increases, so does the corresponding physiological response. Conversely, as hormonal secretion decreases, the physiological response decreases. Hormonal disturbances involve either overproduction or underproduction of a particular hormone. In Chap. 15 the endocrine system is overviewed, and its relationship to metabolism explored in detail. There the thyroid gland and adrenal cortex are shown to play a significant role in the body's metabolic processes. In this chapter the consequences of hypo- and hypersecretion of the thyroid gland and adrenal cortex are explored.

## THYROID MALFUNCTION

Because of the complexity of the thyroid gland's response to disease, understanding the terminology commonly used to describe thyroid function is helpful. *Euthyroid* is indicative of normal functioning of the thyroid gland. *Hypothyroidism* involves a decrease in normal thyroid gland activity, while *hyperthyroidism* is characterized by increased glandular functioning. *Myxedema* is often used synonymously with hypothyroidism but is more appropriately the term applied to a severe degree of long-standing hypothyroidism characterized by skin changes and tissue swelling. The possibility of thyroid disturbance arises when there are symptoms suggestive of hypo- or hyperthyroidism or some physical abnormality of the gland.

### Hypothyroidism

Hypothyroidism is a systemic disorder which results from a deficiency of thyroid hormones. In the adult, hypothyroidism is divided into two types—primary and secondary. *Primary hypothyroidism* involves changes within the gland itself which result in a decreased production of thyroid hormones. In *secondary hypothyroidism* changes in pituitary

* The authors acknowledge the critical review of the manuscript of this section by William T. Cave, Jr., M.D., and Steven L. Pohl, M.D., Department of Internal Medicine, Endocrinology Division, University of Virginia.

function and, therefore, thyroid-stimulating hormone secretion compromise normal thyroid secretion. Primary hypothyroidism accounts for 96 percent of adult hypothyroidism.

**Causes**  The various causes of primary and secondary hypothyroidism are summarized in Table 21-1. Hypothyroidism may develop *spontaneously* with atrophy of the thyroid gland. Extensive studies have disclosed a high incidence of antibodies against thyroid antigens in patients with spontaneous atrophy, suggesting a possible autoimmune reaction.[1] Hypothyroidism may also occur as a result of the autoimmune disease *Hashimoto's thyroiditis* (see Chap. 10). It is probable that hypothyroidism thought to occur from "spontaneous atrophy" of the thyroid gland may be, in general, an expression of the end state of Hashimoto's thyroiditis.

*Iatrogenic* hypothyroidism can be inadvertently caused in the process of treating hyperthyroidism. In fact, the most common cause of hypothyroidism today is radioactive iodine treatment for Graves' disease (hyperthyroidism) where radioiodine therapy results in overdestruction of thyroid tissue. Another important cause of hypothyroidism is surgical removal of the thyroid gland. This often develops even while functioning remnants of the gland remain after surgery. Its occurrence seems to correlate with the presence of antibodies to thyroid antigens. Thus, continuing destruction of the residual tissue by thyroiditis may be the pathogenic mechanism involved.[2] Finally, a variety of drugs, especially antithyroid drugs, if given over a sufficient period of time and in large doses, can impair the function of the thyroid and result in hypothy-

roidism. These drugs deplete the thyroid of its hormone stores.

*Secondary* hypothyroidism may occur because the pituitary fails to secrete sufficient thyroid-stimulating hormone. This can result when the pituitary is destroyed by either compression from a nonsecreting pituitary tumor, necrosis following blood pressure changes associated with postpartum hemorrhage or head injury, surgical removal of the pituitary, or pituitary insufficiency.

**Pathophysiology**  Hypothyroidism is a disease occurring four to seven times as often in females as males. It is found to occur in warm and cold climates equally and may develop at any age in adult life. The incidence has risen with the use of radioactive iodine.[3]

Although there are a variety of causes of hypothyroidism, the effects on the patient resulting from deficiencies of the thyroid hormones are the same. Symptoms may begin at any age and usually occur insidiously over many months to years. The patient, family, and friends are often unaware of the changes. The onset following overtreatment of hyperthyroidism is more abrupt, however, and may occur within several months. The severity of the symptoms will be dependent upon the degree and duration of thyroid hormone deficiency. The changes can be explained almost entirely on the basis of a deficiency of thyroid hormone action in the peripheral tissues.

**C**hanges in Fluid and Electrolyte Dynamics  The effects of the thyroid hormone are dispersed throughout the body. Thus, a deficiency in the hormone causes widespread changes. A decrease in thyroid hormone will alter the fluid and electrolyte dynamics, with total body water and extracellular fluid being increased while plasma volume is decreased. Capillary permeability is also increased causing the accumulation of mucoprotein deposits in tissues. This leads to *fluid retention* and results in thickened, edematous, puffy skin most noticeable in the eyelids, hands, and feet. It is a nonpitting type of edema. There may be sticky secretions on the eyelids, and patients awaken with their lids stuck together.

The fluid retention also causes the tongue to enlarge and the patient's *speech* to be thick and slurred. The speech is deliberate and slow as a result. Swelling of the vocal cords gives the voice a hoarse tone. The patient may experience an overall *weight gain* attributable to the fluid changes as well as the acquisition of fat.

**TABLE 21-1**
CAUSES OF HYPOTHYROIDISM IN THE ADULT

| Type | Cause | Rationale |
|---|---|---|
| Primary | Idiopathic | Possible autoimmune reaction |
| | Hashimoto's thyroiditis | Autoimmune reaction |
| | Iatrogenic | Surgical removal of thyroid gland<br>Destruction of thyroid gland by radioiodine<br>Overuse of antithyroid drugs |
| Secondary | Decrease in thyroid-stimulating hormone | Destructive pituitary tumors<br>Necrosis of pituitary gland (postpartum)<br>Pituitary insufficiency<br>Surgical removal of the pituitary gland |

Hypothyroid patients tend to drink small amounts of water and to have *diminished urinary output.* The decrease in renal function correlates with the decrease in cardiac output. Certain deviations from normal renal function are revealed by laboratory tests. Minimal amounts of protein may be seen in the urine which could be due to the increased capillary permeability typical of hypothyroidism.

Hypothyroidism decreases formation and absorption of bone, yet the serum calcium and phosphorus concentrations usually remain normal. Calcium in the urine is reduced. Recent research studies reveal that an increased secretion of parathyroid hormone occurs in hypothyroidism, apparently as a homeostatic mechanism to keep the serum calcium level normal in spite of the slowed bone metabolism.[4]

**C**hanges in Cellular Growth and Proliferation  A decrease in thyroid hormone will also affect cellular growth and proliferation. This hormone is not only essential for normal growth and development, but also affects both male and female reproductive systems. In the female excessive and irregular *menstrual bleeding* results from endometrial proliferation. This problem persists because of decreases in progesterone secretion. In both sexes *libido* is usually *decreased.* Likewise, *reduced fertility* is also seen in both sexes. Women who do become pregnant often abort.

Associated with hypothyroidism is an overgrowth of the horny layer of the epidermis known as *hyperkeratosis.* This causes the skin to become unusually dry and rough and decreases the activity of the sweat glands. The skin may show fine wrinkling and scaling. Hyperkeratosis also affects the appendages of the skin. The hair becomes dry, coarse, and brittle and often lacks luster; its growth is retarded, and it tends to fall out. The eyebrows are often sparse, especially in the temporal areas. The nails become thin and brittle with longitudinal and transverse grooves. Another change indicating cellular growth and proliferation is increased subcutaneous fat with definite fat pads being formed, especially above the clavicles. In addition, the hands and feet may have a broad appearance because of the thickening of subcutaneous tissue.

**M**etabolic Changes  Hypothyroidism has especially profound effects on metabolism. In fact, perhaps the most common physiological deviation in health status is lowering of the *metabolic rate.* In the gastrointestinal tract there are not only decreases in gastric hydrochloric acid secretion, but generalized *decreases in peristalsis* and *slowed absorption.* A lowered food requirement and decreased peristaltic activity combine to make the patient feel *anorectic* with frequent complaints of *constipation* and *fecal impaction.* The overall decrease in metabolic rate leads to a reduction in *body temperature* and intolerance to cold. Protein synthesis is slowed; this is complicated by the diffusion of albumin through capillary walls into the tissues, leaving less protein available for growth and body healing.

The lowered metabolic rate slows *cholesterol metabolism* and increases the levels of cholesterol in the blood. Another of the metabolic effects of hypothyroidism is a decrease in the *conversion of carotene* to vitamin A in the liver. This leads to increased serum carotene and accounts for the slight yellowish coloring of the skin.

Adrenal steroid metabolism slows to accommodate the reduced needs of the hypothyroid patient. Under stress, however, the plasma cortisol concentration is normal and sufficient to respond to the needs of the patient.

**C**hanges in Oxygenation  The effects of hypothyroidism on oxygenation are also widespread. The generalized decrease in the body's metabolism decreases oxygen consumption by the cells. The body compensates for the lessened demand for oxygen by decreasing *cardiac output* and increasing *peripheral resistance.* The decrease in cardiac output results in a slowing of the heart rate (*bradycardia*), a decrease in *blood pressure,* and a narrowing of the pulse pressure. These combine to slow peripheral circulation time allowing more complete extraction of oxygen. However, in the presence of peripheral vasoconstriction the skin becomes cool and pale and further increases the patient's tendency to cold intolerance.

The body further compensates for the decreased need for oxygen by decreasing the number of *red blood cells.* That is, hypothyroidism causes diminished blood cell formation, probably as a response to the decreased oxygen demand. The resultant normocytic, normochromic anemia may be complicated by other factors. Excessive menstrual bleeding and decreased iron absorption because of lack of hydrochloric acid can superimpose an iron deficiency anemia on the already existing condition. Similarly, diminished intrinsic factor in the stomach can interfere with the normal absorption of vitamin $B_{12}$ necessary for the maturation of red blood cells (see Chap. 23). A relationship between hypothyroidism and pernicious anemia has been reported and is probably related to a vitamin $B_{12}$ deficiency which results from an underlying progressive gastritis brought on by an autoimmune phenomenon.[5,6]

Decreases in circulation throughout the body can create systemic effects. For example, the decrease in *renal blood flow* lessens the glomerular filtration rate and tubular reabsorption. This impairs excretion of the body's water and further complicates the fluid retention and electrolyte balance. The changes in circulation also affect the body's ability to fight infection and heal itself.

As stated earlier, capillary permeability also increases in hypothyroidism. In more severe cases it is probably the cause of *pericardial effusion* which can develop. In addition, *capillary fragility* is increased and may cause the patient to bruise more easily.

**Changes in Perception and Coordination**  Perception and coordination are also affected in the hypothyroid individual. The patient's movements tend to be slow and clumsy with *muscle weakness, stiffness, cramps,* and *transient pain.* These symptoms are thought to be due to mucoprotein edema which causes a separation of the muscle fibers. Slowed muscle contraction and relaxation times compound the muscle weakness and pain. This is especially evident in the relaxation time of the ankle jerk (Achilles tendon), although these findings may be within the normal range.

*Sensory changes* often involve numbness and tingling of the fingers due to compression of the median nerve by mucoprotein deposits. Night blindness occurs due to a deficiency in vitamin A. An adequate supply of vitamin A is necessary to maintain levels of retinene, the pigment required for dark adaptation. As discussed earlier, conversion of carotene to vitamin A is decreased in the hypothyroid individual. Deafness is also a very characteristic and troublesome symptom. This can be due to VIIth-nerve damage from pressure by mucoprotein deposits, conduction problems, or a combination of these.

In addition, perception and coordination are affected by a decrease in cerebral blood flow which often leads to *cerebral hypoxia.* Consequently, there is a general slowing of all intellectual functions. The patient may experience memory defects, lethargy, somnolence, psychological reactions, and, in more severe cases, coma. Table 21-2 summarizes the pathophysiological changes and effects manifested in hypothyroidism.

**First-level nursing care**  It is difficult to prevent hypothyroidism because there is no clear understanding of the causative factor in the majority of cases. Hypothyroidism as a result of surgery to treat overactivity of the gland occurs in approximately 20 percent of the patients and is an unpreventable consequence of the treatment. Radioiodine should certainly be used judiciously with an appreciation for its destructive effects. The nurse's most significant task in preventing hypothyroidism is associated with the use of antithyroid drugs. Individuals taking these drugs should be monitored closely and taught the side effects. A more thorough discussion of this may be found in Hyperthyroidism below.

**Second-level nursing care**  The nurse in the community or outpatient clinic is in a unique position to become involved in case finding, referral, and early treatment of hypothyroidism. The school nurse should consider the possibility of thyroid dysfunction when a child's mental alertness and attention span wane. Accurate assessment of patients with thyroid disease involves a history, physical assessment, and laboratory tests.

**Nursing Assessment**  The *health history* is especially important because patients may be asymptomatic or symptoms may be so vague that they escape detection. In fact, these patients are often identified in the course of seeking health care for unrelated symptoms. Any past history of thyroid disease and/or goiter should be explored. Questions regarding thyroid surgery, radioiodine therapy, antithyroid drugs, or thyroid hormone therapy should be asked if thyroid dysfunction is suspected. The nurse should also be especially cognizant of current complaints being expressed by the patient. The patient often presents with vague complaints of easy fatigability, lethargy, increased need for sleep, muscle weakness, nonspecific muscle pain, hypersensitivity to cold, and inability to concentrate.

During the interview the patient's voice should be evaluated for quickness of speech and vocal tone. The patient should be asked if any changes in voice quality have been noticed. Menstrual histories should be taken, and the patient asked about any changes in appetite or bowel habits. Intellectual functioning should be observed throughout the interview, and the patient should be questioned regarding memory difficulties, attention span, lethargy, and the like. Through a careful survey of the health history the nurse may disclose many mild changes affecting the patient.

Assessment of the adult with hypothyroidism

who has not reached the stage of myxedema may be difficult since the alterations from normal are often not very distinct. However, *physical assessment* often reveals symptoms of which the patient is unaware. To assess changes in cellular proliferation, the skin should be examined. It is often found to be cold, dry, rough, and scaly with brittle nails and hair. The changes in fluid and electrolyte dynamics cause swelling which also may be observed. The eyelids, hands, and feet should especially be noted. Edema may also be assessed by weighing the patient and comparing the results with the previous weight record. The thyroid gland itself should be palpated for enlargement. It may initially proliferate to compensate for the lower levels of thyroid hormones.

The decreased metabolic rate can be partially assessed through taking the patient's temperature which may be lower than normal. The reduced body temperature causes the skin to feel cold and demonstrates the ability of the skin vasculature to perform its major function: heat conservation. Slowness in skin healing can be noted through observation of any cuts and scratches while ascertaining from the patient the time of their occurrence. The yellowish coloring associated with hypercarotemia will not likely be present in mild hypothyroidism. However, it is best observed on the palms and soles of the feet. The abdominal examination may reveal gaseous distention and diminished bowel sounds as a result of the decreased peristaltic activity.

Assessment of the oxygenation status should include evaluation of heart rate and blood pressure, both of which will be lowered. Extremities will feel cool to the touch, and nailbeds may appear pale with fair to poor capillary refill time. Breath sounds may be essentially normal, although the rate and depth may be diminished. However, dyspnea may be observed in some patients as a result of congestive heart failure due to some other cause such as pleural effusion, anemia, obesity, or pulmonary disease. The patient with hypothyroidism often has a generalized pale appearance which is best observed in the nailbeds and mucosa of the eye. During the physical examination the nurse should also be alert to any bruising which could be related to increased capillary fragility.

Perception and coordination should be assessed through muscle strength and reflex testing. Reflex contraction and relaxation times are usually noted to be prolonged because of the slow rate of muscle contraction and relaxation. The strength and tone of the muscles may be normal, or they may be weak and flabby. The patient should also be questioned regarding any weakness and poor coordination. The nurse may assess the patient for inability to make rapid alternating movements. Constant involuntary movements of the eye (nystagmus) and intention tremors may be observed. The patient should be questioned about any night blindness, hearing difficulties, or sensory phenomena such as numbness and tingling in the extremities.

*Diagnostic tests*   There are a large number of diagnostic tests which can be done on an outpatient basis and aid in assessing a patient with possible thyroid dysfunction. Thyroid function tests assist in evaluating the metabolic level of the body which is

**TABLE 21-2**
SUMMARY OF PATHOPHYSIOLOGICAL CHANGES AND CLINICAL EFFECTS IN HYPOTHYROIDISM

| Changes | Effects |
|---|---|
| ALTERED FLUID AND ELECTROLYTE DYNAMICS<br>Increased capillary permeability<br>Mucoprotein deposits in tissues | Fluid retention<br>Enlarged tongue<br>Slurred speech<br>Hoarseness<br>Exophthalmos<br>Edema of eyelids<br>Edema of face<br>Peripheral edema<br>Gain in weight (attributable in part to fluid retention) |
| CHANGES IN CELLULAR GROWTH AND PROLIFERATION<br>Endometrial proliferation<br>Decreased progesterone secretion<br>Hyperkeratosis<br>Increased subcutaneous fat | Menorrhagia<br>Decreased libido and fertility<br>Dry skin<br>Coarse skin<br>Decreased sweating<br>Coarseness of hair<br>Loss of hair<br>Sparse eyebrows<br>Brittle nails |
| DECREASED METABOLIC RATE<br>Decreased HCl production<br>Decreased peristalsis<br>Slowed absorption<br>Decreased vitamin A metabolism | Decreased body temperature<br>Intolerance to cold<br>Anorexia<br>Constipation<br>Yellowish skin coloring |
| DECREASED OXYGEN CONSUMPTION<br>Decreased cardiac output<br>Increased peripheral resistance<br>Increased capillary permeability | Pallor of skin and lips<br>Cold skin<br>Cold intolerance<br>Bruising<br>Bradycardia<br>Decreased blood pressure<br>Decreased RBC production |
| ALTERED PERCEPTION AND COORDINATION<br>Separation of muscle fibers<br>Compression of nerves<br>Conduction problems<br>Cerebral hypoxia | Weakness (generalized)<br>Lethargy<br>Slow movements<br>Slow intellectual functioning<br>  Slow speech<br>  Impaired memory<br>Slow muscle contraction and relaxation<br>Muscle pain<br>Paresthesias<br>Night blindness<br>Deafness |

controlled by the thyroid hormone circulating in the bloodstream and in identifying the cause of the thyroid disease.

The *basal metabolic rate,* which measures the rate of oxygen consumption, is the most direct measure of metabolic activity due to thyroid hormone, but this test has fallen into disuse today because it is influenced by so many clinical variables. Today reliance is placed primarily on measurement of the levels of thyroid hormones in the blood. The most useful test for obtaining an accurate reflection of total circulating hormone is the *serum $T_4$* by competitive binding or radioimmunoassay. This test measures the total level of $T_4$ in the blood. Either method requires only a sample of the patient's blood and is not affected by exogenous iodine. Results are expressed as micrograms of $T_4$/100 ml plasma. The serum $T_4$ is reduced in hypothyroidism. Previously used tests for thyroid hormone measurement such as the *protein-binding iodide* (PBI), *butanol-extractable iodine* (BEI), and *$T_4$ by column* are little used today because of the many sources of contaminating iodides which interfere with these tests.

The *$T_3$ resin uptake test* measures the binding capacity of serum proteins for the thyroid hormones. This information together with the measurement of the total serum $T_4$ allows one to estimate the amount of physiologically active hormone (nonprotein-bound hormone) from a sample of the patient's plasma. Normal values vary with the specific laboratory method used; however, the test results are low in hypothyroidism.

Since most of the serum $T_4$ (99.96 percent) is bound to serum proteins, the small remaining percent of non-protein-bound hormone is the "free" thyroid hormone in the blood which is the component that is physiologically active. This *serum-free thyroxine* may be estimated by measuring the total serum $T_4$ and the hormone-binding capacity of the serum as noted above.

Perhaps the most useful test for diagnosing primary hypothyroidism is the *serum thyroid-stimulating hormone* (serum TSH). It is a very sensitive determinant of the state of the thyroid system. The level of the serum TSH is determined by an assay method using a small sample of the patient's serum. Values differ moderately in various laboratories. However, in the patient with primary hypothyroidism it is invariably elevated about 10 $\mu$U/ml serum. The elevated blood levels of TSH occur whenever the normally functioning pituitary-hypothalamic system senses a deficiency of thyroid hormone in the plasma, as is the case in primary hypothyroidism.

The activity of the thyroid and its production of thyroid hormone can be measured by the *radioactive iodide uptake (RAIU) test.* A tracer dose of [131]I is given, and then through the use of a scintiscanner the amount of [131]I taken up by the thyroid after 24 hours is measured. A profile of the gland reveals both the extent of glandular tissue and areas of increased activity within the gland. In hypothyroidism the uptake of [131]I is decreased. However, there is considerable overlap between hypothyroid and normal patients.

A number of factors can distort the results of this test by inhibiting radioiodine uptake. For example, there has been a general increase of iodide in our diets from bread and numerous other sources.[7] For this reason it is important for the nurse to take a careful history prior to the test. The patient should be asked about recent dietary habits and ingestion of large amounts of iodine-containing foods such as fish and shellfish. The use of iodine-containing drugs such as Quadrinal, saturated solution of potassium iodine (SSKI), Lugol's solution, Combid, and Ornade should be noted. The use of antiseptics containing iodine and recent x-ray studies with contrast media can also distort the findings. The contrast media used to visualize the kidneys and blood vessels is cleared within days with normal renal function, but contrast agents used in visualizing the gallbladder may suppress iodide uptake for 4 months or more. Thus, because of the problems associated with determining the normal range for the test results and the effects of prior exposure to iodide, the radioactive iodide uptake test has relatively little value in assessing hypothyroidism. It is, however, more reliable in patients with hyperthyroidism.

*Scanning procedures* are commonly used, although they often do not provide much diagnostically helpful information. The purpose of the scanning procedure is to evaluate the anatomical features of the thyroid, to recognize areas of increased or decreased hormone synthesis, and to identify any tissue outside the thyroid which is active in accumulating iodide. The scanning technique involves administration of a radioactive isotope that is concentrated by the thyroid such as technetium or [131]I. The [131]I scan is conventionally performed after 24 hours, when the RAIU is also measured. The procedure involves a mechanical device with a detector moving back and forth across the thyroid and recording the intensity of the signals received on a sensitive paper and on a photographic film. Scans are interpreted in conjunction with other laboratory tests.

Another clinically useful indicator of the level of metabolism is reflex relaxation time. This is especially true of the *Achilles tendon reflex time.* It is prolonged in hypothyroidism and shortened in hyperthyroidism. Although some offices and hospitals have elaborate machinery for recording the reflex time, experienced individuals using their practiced eye can gain almost as much useful information as the more elaborate machine provides.

A reliable indicator of thyroid disease is the detection of antibodies by a number of *thyroid autoantibodies tests.* The presence of antibodies directed against thyroid tissue antigens indicates that autoimmunity is present, but it does not reveal the nature of the clinical disease process. The presence of antibodies directed against thyroglobulin or thyroid tissue antigen may be revealed in primary hypothyroidism. However, because of problems of interpretation, lack of standardization of technique, and difficulty in performing some of the tests, the measurement of thyroid autoantibodies has limited clinical value in some laboratories.

Although *serum cholesterol concentration* is not specific to thyroid function, it is known that thyroid function affects the level of lipids in the serum, especially cholesterol. There is a greater rate of excretion of cholesterol in hyperthyroidism and a reduction in hypothyroidism. Thus, the hypothyroid patient will usually have an elevated serum cholesterol.

In summary, it is important to remember that most tests are only an indirect assessment of thyroid gland status and that the ranges of normal are quite wide. The tests should be considered only as indicators of thyroid dysfunction and not as conclusive evidence. A good deal of clinical experience may be necessary to fully correlate them with the actual patient.

**N**ursing Problems and Interventions   Whenever hypothyroidism is suspected, the nurse should refer the patient for appropriate medical care. The patient may be seen on an outpatient basis during the initial evaluation and treatment. At that time assistance can be offered which will help the patient cope with problems.

One of the first problems the patient may experience is *increased sensitivity to cold.* The patient is generally able to cope with this by maintaining the living area at an unduly warm temperature.

However, the nurse should advise the patient to dress adequately, eliminate drafts if possible, and use extra blankets at night. Sometimes patients will first note the problem of *lack of energy or fatigue.* This is especially bothersome to some patients because the demands made upon them in daily life usually remain unchanged even though they find themselves slowing up. It may be helpful for the nurse to reassure the patient that the reason for the fatigue is being explored and in the meantime to evaluate ways of adjusting the patient's daily schedule to include more rest periods.

Probably one of the most important tasks of the nurse at this time is providing reassurance that the problem is being explored in order to alleviate it. This may be especially true in relation to the *menorrhagia* and the *changes in sexual function* the patient may be experiencing. If the patient complains of *anorexia,* it may be helpful to suggest smaller, more frequent meals. The nurse may also recommend drinking hot water, coffee, or tea upon rising, eating foods high in cellulose and fiber content, and drinking six to eight glasses of water a day. If difficulty with bowel movements persists, stool softeners or mild laxatives may be helpful.

*Dry skin* can be an especially bothersome problem, and the nurse should recommend a reduction in the patient's use of soap. The use of lanolin and various skin creams is helpful. Patients should also be warned that excessive pressure on the skin or bony points could cause bruising.

With mild hypothyroidism thyroid replacement therapy is often begun on an outpatient basis. These medications are discussed in detail below.

**Third-level nursing care**   In the hospital setting the nurse is more likely to encounter patients with myxedema, a more severe degree of hypothyroidism. During *nursing assessment,* the *health history* of myxedema patients is similar to that taken in second-level nursing care with the exception that the nurse may uncover a history of lack of health care or a misunderstanding regarding continuation of thyroid replacement therapy during earlier treatment. *Physical assessment* reveals an intensification of all the signs and symptoms associated with hypothyroidism. Figure 21-1 illustrates the typical facies of the myxedematous patient with edema of the face and eyelids especially noticeable. The skin changes, weight gain, slowness, and changes in gastrointestinal, cardiac, and mental functioning will be exaggerated.

*Myxedema coma* represents the end stage of

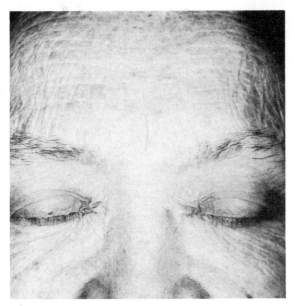

**FIGURE 21-1**
Facial appearance of a myxedematous patient.

failure to correct hypothyroidism for many months. It constitutes a true medical emergency. It is a disease of neglect characterized by progressive stupor ending in a comatose state. The typical patient seen in myxedema coma usually is elderly, lives alone, rarely leaves his or her living quarters, and is severely hypothyroid. These elderly people are generally economically deprived, and presumably they do not seek or cannot obtain adequate health care until they become seriously ill. The precoma or myxedema coma per se is often precipitated by low environmental temperature. Thus, it may be seen more often in winter months.

The patient, when first seen, may appear to be asleep. The body temperature may be too low to be measured with a clinical thermometer. The patient will often hypoventilate which results in carbon dioxide retention. Hypotension, severe hyponatremia, and hypoglycemia all lead to severely disturbed cerebral metabolism, shock, and finally death unless interventions are promptly begun.

**N**ursing Problems and Interventions   The patient hospitalized with myxedema will experience not only the difficulties associated with mild deficiency, but many additional problems. These often present a special challenge to the nurse.

Perhaps one of the first problems the nurse will assess in the myxedematous patient is an *altered ability to perform self-care activities.* Occasionally, a family member may provide evidence on admission of the patient's slowly changing status relative to performing the more routine hygienic and self-care habits. This is compounded by the associated problem of *impaired thought processes* due to the decreased cerebral function. It is essential for the nurse to carry out the nursing care at a pace consistent with the patient's ability to respond. Sufficient time should be provided for the patient to think, speak, and act during nurse-patient interactions.

Encouragement to participate in activities of daily living and other activities requiring decision making and judgment should be started by the nurse as the patient becomes more alert. The nurse in consultation with the occupational therapist should select activities and crafts which will enhance the patient's feeling of adequacy and relieve the boredom of the inactivity associated with hospitalization.

A common sensory problem for some myxedema patients is *paresthesia* and decreased sensation over the thumb and index and middle fingers with weakness of the thumb. This requires the measurement of water temperature and suggests areas for further patient education. If heating pads and hot packs to the hand are indicated for any reason, they should be used cautiously to avoid burning the patient.

In addition to the sensory problem, the patient with myxedema may experience *impaired mobility* associated with muscle weakness, pain, and joint stiffness. The nurse should be alert to the arrangement of furnishings in the patient's hospital environment and provide a traffic pattern that will facilitate ease in movement and lessen the possibility of the patient falling.

Another frequent problem for the patient is *dyspnea on exertion.* This problem along with the *anemia* that is often seen makes it necessary for the nurse to consciously reduce stress on the patient's cardiovascular system. This is especially true during the introduction of thyroxine replacement therapy. The nurse should space all patient activity allowing for periodic rest opportunities. The anemia often requires iron supplements and an iron-rich diet (see Chap. 23).

Because the patient with myxedema experiences the problem of *increased sensitivity to depressants* including barbiturates, tranquilizers, and morphine, the nurse should try to avoid the use of these drugs. If depressants are necessary, reduced dosages should be used, and the nurse should closely monitor the patient, being especially alert to signs of respiratory distress. Likewise, the nurse should be alert to increased sensitivity to other drugs, including digitalis. Administration of the usual dose of digitalis to a hypothyroid patient may cause nausea and cardiac irritability.

*Thyroid replacement therapy* The primary objective in treating inadequate thyroid function is to return the patient to a euthyroid state as rapidly, safely, and inexpensively as possible. The program of therapy varies in relation to the patient's age, severity of the hypothyroid state, and the patient's cardiovascular status. Except in myxedema coma, which is a life-threatening emergency, the replacement therapy is always started slowly. The hormone increases cellular metabolism, thus increasing the need for oxygen. The patient's heart must be given time to adjust to the increased workload. If this is not done arrhythmias such as atrial fibrillation, angina, and, in more severe cases, congestive heart failure can result. Therefore, attempts to restore a normal metabolic rate too rapidly are unnecessary and dangerous. The daily replacement dose is usually achieved over a period of months.

Various preparations of thyroid hormones are currently available. For many years *desiccated thyroid,* a medication prepared from a mixture of pork and beef thyroid, has been used. *Synthetic sodium* L-*thyroxine, sodium* L-*triiodothyronine,* and physiological combinations of these two are being used increasingly today. A summary of drugs used in thy-roid replacement appears in Table 21-3. Generally synthetic sodium L-thyroxine (levothyroxine) is preferable since it is well absorbed from the intestine and slowly penetrates the tissues from the blood.

Monitoring the effect of thyroid hormone replacement is a major responsibility of the nurse. In a patient being treated for typical uncomplicated hypothyroidism, the nurse can expect the patient's metabolic activity to improve within a week. Careful observations and recording should be made of the temperature, pulse, respiration, and blood pressure. Coincidental to the increased metabolic rate, over a period of 2 weeks or so, the nurse should observe an increase in the basal pulse rate, a widening pulse pressure, a rise in the temperature from subnormal to normal range, and an increase in respirations.

Because a diuresis develops after 2 or 3 days of thyroid hormone therapy, the patient's intake and output should be closely monitored. An increase in water intake is usually observed as sweating returns. Similarly, daily weights should be obtained in an effort to follow the patient's weight loss. Initially it will result from water loss and later from loss of fat stores. Associated with the water loss is a change in the patient's appearance. The "puffy" look will disappear and normal expression return. An increase in energy, initiative, and spontaneous activity can be expected. In addition, specific attention should be given to other bodily functions in-

TABLE 21-3

DRUGS USED IN THYROID REPLACEMENT

| | Composition | Average Dose in Treatment of Hypothyroidism* | Comments |
|---|---|---|---|
| Desiccated thyroid | | 120 mg | Made from the thyroid glands of animals slaughtered for food. |
| Thyroglobulin (Proloid) | $T_4$ and $T_3$ in a ratio of 2.5:1 | 120 mg | This compound is the purified extract of pig thyroid. |
| Levothyroxine sodium, U.S.P. (Synthroid, Letter, Levoid) | Synthetic $T_4$ | 0.2 mg | An active principle of the thyroid gland prepared synthetically as the sodium salt. |
| Liothyronine sodium, U.S.P. (Cytomel) | Synthetic $T_3$ | 0.05–0.75 mg | A synthetic form of the natural hormone prepared as the sodium salt. It has a short duration of action which permits quick dosage adjustments. May be used in patients allergic to desiccated thyroid or thyroid extract derived from pork or beef. |
| Liotrix | Synthetic $T_4$ and $T_3$ in a ratio of 4:1 by weight | | Manufacturers differ in the amount that is equivalent to 1 g. |

* In practice, the exact dose must be adjusted for each individual patient on the basis of clinical response.

cluding the appetite and bowel function, both of which will improve.

Because the dosage of thyroid hormone varies from patient to patient, these observations are important in establishing the optimal dosage for each individual. The appearance of untoward effects should be noted immediately, and the hormone stopped until the effects disappear. The patient should be evaluated for the possibility of other medications potentiating the thyroid effects. The nurse should be especially alert for any pain suggestive of angina pectoris or the development of an agitated or psychotic state in the patient.

*Myxedema coma*  Treatment for myxedema coma is generally initiated on health history and clinical assessment of the patient since there is no time to await laboratory tests values. The goals of therapy are (1) to replace thyroid hormones and (2) to detect and manage the secondary complications. Because of the very sluggish circulation and the hypometabolism, intravenous medications are used if possible. However, this often can be difficult because the veins may be collapsed. Thyroid hormone is generally given as a single intravenous dose ranging from 300 to 500 $\mu$g sodium levothyroxine which rapidly replenishes the circulating hormone.

Treatment is then aimed at the decreased respiratory function usually by means of assisted ventilation and controlled administration of oxygen. Because of the likelihood of adrenocorticoid insufficiency, especially as the metabolic rate increases, the nurse can anticipate that hydrocortisone may be given daily. Despite the fact that the patient is hypothermic, external warming should be avoided as it may cause vascular collapse.

Nursing intervention should be directed toward avoiding further heat loss by using ordinary blankets. Other aspects of nursing intervention include turning the patient and prevention of aspiration. The nurse should continue to assess the patient for reasons that may have precipitated the coma. Early diagnosis and treatment of hypothyroidism are the best approach to prevention. Untreated myxedema coma is usually fatal.

**Fourth-level nursing care**  After the initial establishment of a daily thyroid dose, the patient can expect a fairly normal, active life. This is dependent, however, on patients' cooperation in taking thyroid replacement for the rest of their lives. The nurse plays a vital part in establishing and reinforcing the need for this continuity of treatment. This role begins in the hospital with the development and

implementation of a teaching plan and continues in the community with referral and follow-up.

Before beginning the teaching, the nurse should assess the patient's and family's ability to understand the need for the unceasing and consistent treatment. Likewise, an assessment of economic status should be made in relation to purchasing the drugs. The plan itself should focus on the mechanics of taking the drug and the side effects to be aware of with appropriate action if they occur. A schedule for taking the drug should be set up and discussed with the patient. In addition, the patient should be instructed not to take any drugs other than those prescribed by the physician because certain drugs may cause unusual and undesired responses. The patient and family are given a printed list of symptoms including headache, palpitations, and angina pectoris to report immediately to the physician should they occur. These symptoms may be reflective of overdosage and are associated with thyrotoxicosis. Thus, they indicate the need for the drug to be withheld until the symptoms disappear. The teaching plan should emphasize the need for the patient to be seen from time to time to be sure the plan of therapy is appropriate.

### Hyperthyroidism

Hyperthyroidism results from an excess of thyroid hormones. It generally takes the form of toxic diffuse goiter or toxic nodular goiter. *Graves' disease, Basedow's disease,* and *exophthalmic goiter* are terms used synonymously with toxic diffuse goiter. *Thyrotoxicosis* refers to hyperthyroidism but may be reserved to designate an excess of thyroid hormone which does not originate in the thyroid gland. Hyperthyroidism is predominantly a disease of females, affecting women over four times as often as men. It occurs most frequently in the third and fourth decades of life.[8]

Since hyperthyroidism is not a reportable health disruption, data on cultural, social, and economic status and geographic factors specific to those affected are difficult to establish. However, the problem is widespread among the population, occurring in all people. There is some evidence that individuals with long-standing multinodular goiter may be predisposed to developing toxic nodular goiter with hyperthyroidism.

**Pathophysiology**  The most common cause of hyperthyroidism is *Graves' disease,* a problem which is not well understood. Researchers have been unable to confirm a specific etiological factor. However, there is evidence that it is a disease of apparent autoimmune etiology with an associated thyroid-stimulating factor. The exact biochemical nature of the factor is unknown, but in some patients a circulating serum immunoglobulin called long-acting thyroid stimulator (LATS) has been identified. Presumably, LATS causes hyperplasia of the thyroid gland and excessive stimulation of it.

The possible role of *emotional factors* in the emergence of Graves' disease has been suggested, but thus far no conclusive evidence exists. It has been noted that the disease often becomes evident after a severe emotional stress such as actual or threatened separation from a significant person or after emotionally traumatic happenings like an automobile accident. In the female, it tends to become evident during puberty, pregnancy, and the menopause. However, there is no proof that the cyclic factors are anything more than coincidental.

*Toxic multinodular goiter* is the second most common cause of hyperthyroidism. The reason individuals with long-standing thyroid nodules develop hyperthyroidism is perhaps that the nodules have a tendency to become autonomous and, as they increase in size, produce more hormone than the patient needs. The thyroid may be stimulated by factors such as iodide deficiency, dietary goitrogens, defects in hormone synthesis, or a combination of these, resulting in growth of hyperactive nodules. Hyperthyroidism resulting from toxic multinodular goiter usually first appears in the fifth through seventh decades.

A third cause of hyperthyroidism is *toxic adenoma* which is a solitary, autonomously hyperfunctioning nodule which suppresses the remainder of the thyroid gland. These nodules usually occur in patients of younger age and are much less common than the toxic multinodular goiter. Generally, with removal of the nodule, normal levels of thyroid-stimulating hormone return, and normal thyroid function resumes.

**M**etabolic Changes   Like hypothyroidism, the effects of increased thyroid hormone secretion are widespread. The *elevated metabolic rate* is among the most obvious effects. As a result of the increased *catabolism,* protein formation and destruction are both accelerated. Consequently, nitrogen excretion is increased, and a negative nitrogen balance may develop leading to muscular weakness and wasting of muscle mass. Loss of weight may occur from the increased catabolism. However, the appetite is characteristically increased which tends to offset, in many instances, the weight loss.

The hypermetabolic rate increases the need for insulin, causing a change to occur in *carbohydrate metabolism.* There is an acceleration of the rate of glucose absorption from the intestinal tract, and insulin secretion increases in response. The result is an abnormally rapid rise and fall in blood glucose. *Fat metabolism* is accelerated. As fats are oxidized to meet the energy requirements, weight is lost and the serum cholesterol decreases.

In the *gastrointestinal tract* there is an increase in peristaltic activity which leads to loose stools. Patients who had difficulties with constipation may, with the development of hyperthyroidism, have more regular bowel movements.

Hyperthyroidism also increases the activity of other *endocrine glands.* As secretion of the adrenocorticotropic hormone increases, the patient may experience increased pigmentation of the skin. Because of the *heat* produced by the accelerated metabolic reactions, patients are unable to tolerate hot weather. Thus, the individual develops a preference for cold weather and desires less clothing and bed covering.

**C**hanges in Oxygenation   The overall increase in metabolic rate raises oxygen consumption. The *vasomotor system* becomes overactive in an effort to rid the body of the increased heat. Dilatation of the superficial capillaries for the purpose of dissipating the heat causes increased peripheral blood flow and increased cardiac output. In addition, it leads to warm, moist, and red skin, especially typical in the palms of the hands and soles of the feet where the sweat glands are under sympathetic control. Likewise, redness of the elbows is frequently observed. It results from a combination of increased activity, an exposed part, and a hyperirritable vasomotor system. First and foremost of the symptoms resulting from the *increased cardiac output* are palpitation and tachycardia. Extrasystoles are frequently observed, and paroxysmal atrial tachycardia and atrial fibrillation occur in approximately 10 percent of the patients (see Chap. 25).

**C**hanges in Perception and Coordination   The increased metabolic rate and accompanying increased oxygen consumption also result in varied and striking changes in perception and coordination. For example, the *increased blood flow* to the brain and the *increased adrenergic activity* result in hyperactivity, irritability, nervousness, restlessness, insomnia, and hyperexcitability. Likewise, the increased blood flow to the muscles and the increased adrenergic activity tend to speed muscle

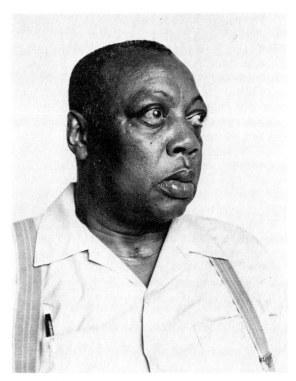

**FIGURE 21-2**
Noninfiltrative ophthalmopathy.

contraction and relaxation. This is made most evi-dent by the shortened Achilles tendon reflex time and the fine muscle tremors observed in the out-stretched hand. In addition, the adrenergic activity presumably causes retraction of the upper eyelid made evident by increased scleral exposure as illus-trated in Fig. 21-2. Although the eyes may appear exophthalmic in these individuals, no protrusion is evident upon measurement. Movements of the lids are jerky and spasmodic, and the individual has a staring, bright-eyed or popeyed look. These eye changes are referred to as *noninfiltrative ophthal-mopathy.*

**C**hanges in Cellular Growth and Proliferation   Cell-ular growth and proliferation are also affected by increased thyroid hormone secretion. In some in-stances, this is perhaps most evident by enlarge-ment of the thyroid gland itself (*goiter*). However, it is quite possible for hyperthyroidism to exist with-out a visible goiter. Changes in the growth of the *skin* and its *appendages* also occur. Although the skin is thinned, other manifestations due to altered growth in tissue are less evident. An example is the nail changes, often called *Plummer's nails,*

wherein the nails tend to leave the nail beds and become soft and flat with wavy margins where they do contact the nail beds. The hair tends to be fine, soft, and straight. Thinning of the hair is common.

Changes in the reproductive system in both males and females are also observed. *Menstruation* is characteristically decreased in volume. However, in severe hyperthyroidism, the menstrual cycle may be either shortened or prolonged with the eventual development of amenorrhea. *Fertility* is decreased, but pregnancy can occur. Increased sexual desire and activity or the opposite may develop in either sex. *Gynecomastia,* enlarged mammary glands, may occasionally occur in the hyperthyroid male for rea-sons not yet fully explained.

**F**luid and Electrolyte Imbalances   Two of the more characteristic features resulting from Graves' dis-ease are associated with changes in the body's fluid dynamics. One of these changes is an ophthalmic phenomenon referred to as *infiltrative ophthal-mopathy,* the cause of which remains obscure. However, altered mucopolysaccharide metabolism is thought to lead to interstitial inflammatory edema of the orbital contents, the lid, and periorbital tis-sues, and to cause protrusion of the eyeball (exoph-thalmos) and paralysis or paresis of the extraocular muscles. This ocular manifestation, illustrated in Fig. 21-3, is distinct from the noninfiltrative ophthal-mopathy referred to earlier that almost all hyper-thyroid patients have as a result of the hyperactivity of the sympathetic nervous system.

A second alteration in fluid dynamics may de-velop in association with infiltrative ophthalmopa-thy in Graves' disease and is referred to as *localized pretibial myxedema.* Pretibial myxedema is the result of deposits of material rich in mucopolysac-charides in the skin of the lower legs and occasion-ally over the phalanges. These deposits cause localized edema. The skin over the pretibial area of the leg becomes firm, thickened, and nonpitting, having the texture of orange peel or pigskin.

**First-level nursing care**   Prevention of the major causative factors in hyperthyroidism is not yet pos-sible since the exact etiology remains unclear. There exist information gaps about the relationship between genetic and emotional influences and the connection between these factors and the auto-immune basis for the problem. However, finding and treating individuals with nontoxic goiters using T₄ replacement can prevent them from developing toxic goiters. In addition, close follow-up of pa-tients receiving thyroid hormone replacement therapy may prevent the patient from overtreatment and thus from becoming hyperthyroid.

**Second-level nursing care**   During the initial onset of hyperthyroidism or with an uncomplicated course of the illness, the patient will be assessed and treated on an outpatient basis. *Nursing assessment* involves a health history, physical evaluation, and diagnostic tests.

**N**ursing Assessment   *History taking* is especially important in assessing the patient with hyperthyroidism since this disease state assumes many forms. Patients may present for health care with a variety of symptom patterns. They may complain of weight loss, weakness, dyspnea, palpitation, increased thirst or appetite, irritability, profuse sweating, sensitivity to heat or increased tolerance to cold, or tremor. Occasionally, prominence of the eyes or diplopia will be cited by the patient as the reason for seeking health care. On the other hand, during the interview it may be revealed that a relative or friend noticed eye changes, goiter, or a nervous phenomenon before the patient was conscious of any departure from his or her usual health status. The patient may be able to produce photographs to demonstrate the changes in appearance. Often the onset of the symptoms will have been so gradual that it will be difficult or impossible to date their beginning. During the interview the nurse should be alert to any emotionally laden life episodes expressed by the individual and explore them in relation to the onset of the hyperthyroidism. Psychic trauma is perhaps the most frequent and important of these. It is worthwhile to identify any relationship between the patient's illness and any prolonged periods of anxiety, sorrow, or fear.

Any past history of thyroid problems and/or goiter in the patient or family should be explored. This is especially true in Graves' disease. The history may reveal that the patient knew of the existence of a goiter for months or years prior to the development of toxicity. Menstrual histories should be taken, and the patient questioned about changes in weight, appetite, and bowel function. Questions should be explored regarding sexual desire and activity. During the interview, discussions should be directed toward identifying any musculoskeletal weakness that might be evidenced by such activities as climbing stairs or rising from a chair.

Throughout the interview the nurse should observe for evidence of hyperkinetic behavior, thought, and speech. The patient should be questioned regarding nervousness, irritability, emo-

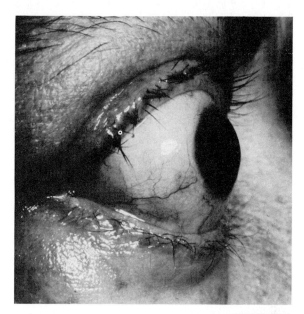

**FIGURE 21-3**
Infiltrative ophthalmopathy.

tional lability, and insomnia or decreased sleep requirement. Except in atypical cases or in those in whom the disease is so mild or early as to be unconvincing, the nurse should be able, through a careful history, to disclose the combination of eye symptoms, goiter, and other characteristic symptoms of hyperthyroidism.

*Physical assessment* of the adult with hyperthyroidism may reveal many changes. The increased metabolic rate and accompanying increased oxygen consumption can be partially assessed through the patient's pulse which will be bounding and generally average over 90 beats per minute. Monitoring the blood pressure will demonstrate a widened pulse pressure. Respirations may be essentially normal, although the rate and depth may increase on exertion. Occasionally, signs of congestive heart failure and paroxysmal tachycardia or atrial fibrillation may be observed.

The abdominal examination will be essentially normal except for the increase in bowel sounds relative to the increased peristaltic activity. Catabolism can be assessed by weighing the patient and comparing the weight with previous weight records, since loss of weight, in spite of increased appetite, is nearly always observed. In elderly patients with significant anorexia, weight loss may be marked.

To assess cellular proliferation and growth, the thyroid gland, the skin, and its appendages should be examined. The thyroid gland itself is generally enlarged, making the neck conspicuous if a palpable goiter is present. Inspection of the integument will reveal velvety soft, warm, moist skin. During the physical examination the patient should be questioned about excessive perspiration. The hyperthyroid individual is often observed to have a more or less continuous erythema of the face and neck. Patchy hyperpigmentation is also frequently seen. The hair will be finer, softer and straighter than normal. Frequently, females may comment that it will not hold a "permanent wave." During the physical examination inspection of the nails, especially of the fourth and fifth fingers, will often reveal separation of the nail from the nail bed. Gynecomastia may be present in the male.

Changes in fluid dynamics may be evidenced by the presence of peripheral edema. Therefore, the periorbital tissue, lower legs and phalanges should be especially observed. The extent of edema of the orbital contents can be sensed by applying gentle digital pressure on the globe. Often it cannot be displaced backward. Likewise, measuring and recording protrusion of the globe beyond the lateral margin of the orbit using an ophthalmometer can be helpful in documenting any progression of exophthalmos.

Perception and coordination should be assessed through muscle strength and reflex testing. Reflex contraction and relaxation times are usually noted to be brisk and quickened. Tremor is usually observed and is attributed to altered neural function. Fine tremors can be evaluated by having patients spread their fingers in the air, palm down, and placing a piece of paper over the fingers to detect tremors. Muscular weakness and atrophy can be assessed by asking the patient, seated in a chair, to hold one leg out straight and in a horizontal position. The thyrotoxic patient may be able to do this for 25 to 30 seconds only, whereas the normal person can maintain such a position over 60 to 120 seconds. Asking patients to rise on their toes or climb steps is also a means to assess muscle weakness which otherwise could be missed.

*Diagnostic tests* The diagnostic tests associated with thyroid function are discussed in detail in Hypothyroidism. Generally, a composite of several *laboratory tests* is used in confirming the diagnosis of hyperthyroidism. Among the tests used are the serum $T_4$, $T_3$ resin uptake, and the $^{131}I$ uptake tests. These tests are characteristically elevated in Graves' disease. Scanning of the thyroid gland may be helpful when the gland is difficult to feel or where nodules are present and require evaluation. The results of those tests in hyperthyroidism as compared with hypothyroidism are summarized in Table 21-4.

**N**ursing Problems and Interventions The initial evaluation and treatment of the hyperthyroid patient are usually carried out on an outpatient basis. During this time nursing intervention can help the individual cope with problems resulting from the hyperfunctioning thyroid gland. The nature of the symptoms and the problems encountered by patients are dependent on the action of the hormones and the personality, constitution, and reaction pattern of the individual. However, one problem almost all hyperthyroid individuals experience is *alterations in emotional stability.* Some are severe enough to cause a change in personality. The increased nervousness, irritability, and occasionally irresponsible behavior can lead to the problem of *altered relationships with others.* Therefore, an important part of the nurse's responsibility involves evaluation of the adjustment of significant others to the patient's illness since the more severe hyperthyroid individual can be a trial for those family members with whom the patient lives. Often the problem involves the marital partner. During the initial and subsequent interviews the nurse should spend sufficient time with both the patient and the family to determine the nature of any stresses they may be experiencing. Frequently, the major emotional problems surface after the patient recognizes the sincere interest expressed by the nurse and physician. At this point the patient may feel comfortable enough to discuss any *alterations in sexual functioning* which may be bothersome. In some instances, the patient may have sufficient insight to realize that the problems of emotional instability, hyperactivity, and nervousness are a result of the thyroid malfunction.

One of the first and very significant problems the hyperthyroid individual may encounter is a change in reaction to external temperature manifested by *heat intolerance.* Physiologically, the body attempts to compensate for this alteration in environmental comfort level by sweating. In addition, the patient is generally able to cope with this through preference for cooler external environmental temperature and the use of less clothing and bed covering.

In other patients *hyperactivity* combined with marked *increase in fatigability* may be an initial problem cited. This disruption is especially bothersome because the hyperthyroid individual's mind is very active, causing *insomnia* in spite of physical exhaustion. It is helpful for the nurse to reassure the patient that progress will be made in alleviating these problems with appropriate therapy. Probably one of the most important tasks of the nurse at this time is to discuss with the patient and family the importance of rest and time away from normal duties. Carrying out daily activities and work will not affect the drug therapy. The patient should be advised, however, that time away from the usual daily regime can make the symptoms more tolerable while awaiting the full effects of the drug therapy. A quiet, nonstressful environment will aid in this process.

Another important aspect of the nurse's role is attention to the nutritional needs of the hyperthyroid individual. This is especially true in relation to the problems of *weight loss* and *irregular bowel function* (frequent stool or diarrhea). A brief diet history may be helpful when discussing with the patient the need to increase the caloric and protein intake until metabolism is restored to normal. Recording the weight on each visit to the clinic can provide an additional parameter in determining nutritional balance. An increase of bulk in the diet may decrease the frequency of stools.

*Drug therapy*    In spite of the progress made in managing the problems manifested by the hyperthyroid patient, therapy does not cure this hormonal disturbance. However, the patient can be maintained in a euthyroid state. Therapeutic methods used in treatment include drugs, radioactive iodine, and surgery. In uncomplicated cases treatment with drugs or radioiodine can be accomplished on an ambulatory basis.

*Antithyroid agents* are the most widely used drugs in the treatment of hyperthyroidism. Propylthioruacil (Propacil) and methimazole (Tapazole), which block the formation of thyroid hormones, are examples of commonly used antithyroid agents. These drugs are administered initially in high dosages, and the daily dose gradually reduced to that which will maintain the patient at a euthyroid level. Since these drugs block the formation of new thyroid hormones without affecting hormone secretion, a remission in the hyperthyroid state does not take place until there has been a major reduction in thyroid hormone stores. This may require 3 or more weeks. Thus, the nurse should instruct the patient that weeks may pass before the symptoms disappear. The patient on antithyroid therapy must also be made aware of the need to take the number of prescribed pills at the proper intervals. Likewise,

the patient should be aware that the goal of the therapy is to maintain a euthyroid state and ultimately to achieve a permanent remission of the hyperthyroidism after the drug therapy is discontinued. However, only about one-third of the patients undergoing long-term antithyroid therapy achieve permanent euthyroidism. The nurse should emphasize to the patient that management of the hyperthyroid state is greatly dependent upon cooperative participation. This usually includes frequent visits to the physician during the first 6 weeks and less often thereafter.

In some patients the use of antithyroid drugs is accompanied by *toxic reactions.* Manifestation of these changes occur in the form of a skin rash, pruritus, and fever. Other toxic reactions include sore throat, joint stiffness, pain, or swelling. The nurse should instruct the patient to be alert to and report any skin lesions, fever, sore throat, malaise, or unusual infections. These warning signs of toxicity should be given to the patient in printed form. Agranulocytosis, although rare, can occur and has the potential for causing serious problems. In the event agranulocytosis develops, the patient may be

**TABLE 21-4**
SUMMARY OF THYROID FUNCTION TESTS
IN HYPO- AND HYPERTHYROIDISM

| Test or Index | Hypothyroidism (primary) | Hyperthyroidism (Graves' disease) |
|---|---|---|
| Basal metabolic rate (BMR)* | Decreased | Increased |
| Serum $T_4$: By competitive binding or radio-immunoassay | Decreased | Increased |
| Protein-binding iodide (PBI)† | Decreased | Increased |
| Butanol-extractable iodine (BEI)† | Decreased | Increased |
| $T_3$-resin uptake test | Decreased | Increased |
| Serum-free thyroxine | Decreased | Increased |
| Thyroid-stimulating hormone (TSH) | Increased | Decreased |
| Radioactive iodine uptake (RAIU) | Decreased | Increased |
| Achilles tendon reflex | Slow | Rapid |
| Serum cholesterol‡ | High | Low |

* BMR is the most direct measure of metabolic activity due to thyroid hormone, but this test has little clinical use today because it is disturbed by many variables.
† PBI and BEI are less reliable tests of thyroid hormone in the presence of interfering sources of iodine and have been replaced by the determination of serum $T_4$.
‡ Serum cholesterol is not a specific test for thyroid function. The normal range of serum cholesterol is very large, and individual values vary considerably.

hospitalized and given adrenal steroids and antibiotics. Special care should be taken by all personnel to ensure against the patient's exposure to infection. As with radioiodine therapy, attention must be given to the lactating woman who might be administered antithyroid drugs. These drugs appear in high concentration in the breast milk, and their use is discouraged in these patients. It is possible for these drugs to be responsible for goiter in the nursing infant as well as the serious side effect of agranulocytosis.

Several other drugs are used in adjunctive therapy and have been proved successful in reducing clinical features of hyperthyroidism. *Reserpine* and *guanethidine,* drugs that deplete tissue catecholamines, reduce nervousness and anxiety, tremor, fatigue, and heat intolerance are examples. The pharmacology of these agents in relation to hyperthyroidism is not completely understood. *Propranolol,* a potent beta-adrenergic blocking agent, is another drug very useful in alleviating many of the symptoms of hyperthyroidism. It controls palpitation, tachycardia, excessive sweating, nervousness, and tremor. Some investigators have used long-term propranolol therapy as the only means of treatment for thyrotoxicosis. While it is an effective adjunct to treatment, it has no effect on the disease process, does not completely reverse the metabolic and cardiac abnormalities, and can precipitate congestive heart failure in patients with heart disease.[9]

*Radioiodine therapy*  Treatment of hyperthyroidism with *radioiodine* is accomplished with relative ease. Likewise, there are a number of advantages for those patients for whom radioactive iodine is considered the treatment of choice. The patient is spared the risks, emotional strain, and trauma of a surgical procedure. The cost is low, hospitalization is seldom required, and patients can continue their customary activities during the course of the treatment.

Since iodine is readily absorbed from the gastrointestinal tract, the procedure, which simply involves drinking a calculated dose of radioiodine mixed in water or some other liquid or taking a capsule filled with a calculated dose of radioiodine, can be easily administered. The thyroid gland then picks up and concentrates the radioactive iodine. Consequently, the cells in the thyroid gland which are responsible for concentrating iodine from the blood and making thyroxine are destroyed. The $^{131}$I which is not taken up by the thyroid is excreted in the urine.

Preparation of the patient for $^{131}$I therapy generally involves ascertaining the patient's thyroid uptake level in an effort to determine the dose of radioactive iodine necessary. In addition, where there is any question of the possibility of thyroid storm (discussed in Third-Level Nursing Care), the patient should be brought under control with antithyroid drugs before the iodine therapy is given.

Once the $^{131}$I has been administered, the patient receiving less than 30 millicuries (mCi) is allowed to leave the clinic. Before leaving the clinic, the patient should be told of the possibility of the thyroid gland becoming very tender immediately after the $^{131}$I therapy. In addition, the patient needs to be well informed about the special precautions necessary after taking the radioactive drug. The patient must be instructed not to eat solid foods for 2 hours following the administration of the drug in an effort to reduce the likelihood of vomiting the isotope. Since the radioactive iodine is excreted by the kidneys, the patient should be instructed to drink fluids frequently and to empty the bladder often during the first 24 hours, flushing the toilet three times after each use. If small children are in the home, close contact should be limited to only needed care, and the patient instructed to sleep alone for two nights.

Occasionally, radioactive iodine will be selected as the treatment of choice for a nursing mother. In such a case, the patient should be instructed to stop breast feeding for approximately one week, returning to the laboratory to have a sample of her milk tested before resuming breast feeding. During this period, the mother should be instructed in manual expression of her milk. The milk should be disposed of in the toilet.

In the event a dose of $^{131}$I larger than 30 mCi is given, the patient is hospitalized. It is preferable for the patient to be placed in a single room as remote as possible from the nurse's station. However, in some instances, a private room may be either impractical or not considered necessary, provided the beds of other patients are at least 6 feet away. Since iodine is excreted not only by the kidney, but also through perspiration, protective plastic or rubber coverings should be used under the pillowcase and mattress coverings. No other special precautions are necessary with regard to bed linens unless the patient vomits, has urinary incontinence, or perspires profusely. In any of these events, the nurse should wear rubber gloves and a protective gown while handling the patient's clothing and bed linens. Contaminated linens should be placed in a waterproof bag or metal container and turned over to the radioisotope personnel as soon as possible.

Patients who are not acutely ill and ambulatory

may use the regular bathroom and toilets on the nursing unit. If a tub bath is taken, the tub should be thoroughly rinsed after use. The toilets should be flushed three times after each use. If the patient is not ambulatory, the nurse giving the bed bath and handling the bedpan and urinals should wear rubber gloves. For the patient who has an indwelling catheter, the urine from the collection bag should be emptied frequently during the first 48 hours. Likewise, during any dressing changes, gloves should be worn, and the discarded dressing should be surveyed by the radioisotope personnel before being thrown into the general waste containers. No special handling of food trays is necessary. In addition, there need be no restrictions on visitors, except for children and pregnant women. Generally, all precautions may be lifted at the end of 48 hours.

**Third-level nursing care**  While ambulatory care is becoming increasingly more feasible, a patient with uncomplicated hyperthyroidism may be admitted to the hospital for diagnostic work and initial treatment. More often, however, the hyperthyroid patient seen in a hospital setting will be a candidate for surgery or experiencing thyroid storm. The *nursing assessment* findings including *diagnostic test* results will be similar to those discussed under Second-Level Nursing Care.

**S**urgical Intervention  The first effective treatment for hyperthyroidism was surgery. Today, however, the use of surgery to correct hyperthyroidism is limited to those patients who do not respond to or are unable or unwilling to undergo treatment with antithyroid drugs or radioiodine. Surgery is also the treatment of choice for patients with unusually large goiters or those experiencing compression of the structures around the thyroid gland.

Surgical intervention includes the removal of the thyroid gland, leaving intact a small functioning remnant of the gland. Although subtotal thyroidectomy is unquestionably effective in relieving hyperthyroidism, the incidences of postoperative hypothyroidism and other surgical complications are considered before selecting the treatment for an individual patient. The incidence of hypothyroidism developing in patients followed for 1 to 16 years has been reported as 28 percent, and the incidence in patients followed for 10 years was 43 percent.[10]

The *preoperative care* for a patient who is to undergo a subtotal thyroidectomy is aimed at restoring the patient to a normal metabolic state in order to prevent thyroid storm and at reducing the vascularity of the thyroid gland in order to prevent hemorrhage.

To achieve the euthyroid state, antithyroid therapy is begun while the patient is at home. These antithyroid drugs deplete the glandular hormone stores. After a normal metabolic state is achieved, the patient is given a course of iodine therapy. The iodine is administered in the form of saturated solution of potassium iodine (SSKI) or Lugol's solution for 7 to 10 days. The iodine prevents release of the thyroid hormone into the circulation and also makes the gland firmer and less vascular. Another adjunct to preoperative preparation is the use of propranolol, a beta-blocking drug, which is very effective in slowing the heart and in controlling the sweating and nervousness.

Generally, no definite date for the surgery can be planned in advance since it may take weeks to months for the physician to bring the patient to a euthyroid state. However, after this initial preoperative care, the patient will be hospitalized and preoperative teaching instituted. The patient should be instructed regarding the usual postoperative matters (turning, coughing, deep breathing, and possible accompanying nausea and headache), and, in addition, should be told to avoid abruptly turning the head or extending the neck. The patient should be shown that the head and neck can be supported with one's hands when getting up. In addition, the patient can be alerted not to be alarmed at the headache which may be experienced. Headache is particularly common, especially since the cervical spine may have been forcibly extended under anesthesia. Likewise, the patient should be prepared for the discomfort that will be experienced upon swallowing. A female patient may be especially concerned about the scar the surgery will leave. Therefore, preoperative teaching should include assurance that the incision is usually a low one, following the lines of the neck, and that the scar resulting will, in time, be no more than a fine hairline. If the patient is bothered by the anticipated appearance of the scar, the nurse may suggest wearing an attractive neck scarf or necklace to cover it.

The *postoperative care* of the patient experiencing thyroid surgery focuses on three major goals. The first is to prevent strain on the suture line and thereby maintain its integrity. This is done by elevating the head of the bed at a 30° angle with the patient's head well supported. As was discussed preoperatively, abruptly turning the head or extending the neck should be avoided. Assistance should also be offered in supporting the head and neck when the patient gets up.

The second goal is to relieve the discomfort associated with tracheal irritation. As soon as the patient is alert enough to drink, fluids are encouraged even though initial discomfort is experienced when swallowing. However, soreness associated with swallowing generally lasts only 1 to 3 days.

The third and most immediate goal in nursing the patient after thyroid surgery is to prevent, detect, and/or relieve complications that may occur. Injury to the recurrent largyngeal nerves that supply the vocal cords is always a concern. The patient's voice should be assessed every 30 to 60 minutes in the first few hours postoperatively with attention given to the quality of the tone and any changes in it. Hoarseness and weakness of the voice are expected and are usually temporary. Today, modern techniques of surgery allow the surgeon to carefully identify and preserve the recurrent laryngeal nerves. As a consequence, injury to these nerves is limited to that which is accidental. The incidence of recurrent nerve paralysis has been reported to be between 0 and 0.6 percent.[11] The paralysis is transient in nature in most instances. However, should both nerves be injured or cut, respiratory obstruction may occur, requiring a tracheostomy.

The patient who has undergone thyroid surgery must also be observed closely in the immediate postoperative period for bleeding. The highly vascular nature of the thyroid gland and surrounding tissue increases the possibility of hemorrhage. Occasionally, when the patient is returned to the nursing unit, as the blood pressure rises postoperatively, and coughing occurs, hemorrhage may develop. The blood, unable to escape, may fill the wound, compressing the trachea and causing difficulty in breathing. Bleeding is best detected by careful observation of the back of the neck and the pillow and by noting complaints of sensations of pressure and fullness in the neck. Because of the danger of obstruction to the airway, a tracheotomy tray should be available at the patient's bedside. If bleeding does occur, the nurse should immediately notify the physician. Generally, the skin clips or sutures will need to be removed and the muscles separated in the midline by inserting a pair of scissors from the tracheotomy tray in the wound and opening the blades to allow the clots to escape. The nurse should monitor the breathing and prepare the patient to return to the operating suite to determine the bleeding point.

A temporary *hypoparathyroidism* is common following thyroid surgery and usually does not require treatment. It is evidenced by a temporary drop in the serum calcium 24 to 48 hours postoperatively and a positive Chvostek's sign. Chvostek's sign, which is normally positive in 10 percent of adults, consists of a twitching of facial muscles, especially noticeable in the upper lip, when a sharp tap is given over the facial nerve located in front of the ear.

Permanent damage to the parathyroids rarely occurs following thyroidectomy if careful identification of the parathyroid glands is made at the time of surgery. This is seen more often following a total thyroidectomy as is the case in cancer of the thyroid gland. Tetany will occasionally develop from the hypocalcemia associated with removal of the parathyroid glands. This is discussed in greater detail in Chap. 12.

**T**hyroid Crisis  Thyroid crisis, or thyroid storm, is an extreme form of hyperthyroidism. It is so severe as to be life-threatening, and it constitutes a medical emergency. Fortunately, it is a syndrome which has become increasingly rare. In the past it occurred frequently in patients who underwent thyroidectomies without being adequately treated preoperatively. Today, it occurs most commonly as a medical problem in uncontrolled hyperthyroid patients. This problem can be evoked by such stressful factors as infections, trauma, or acute cardiovascular disease. The way in which such physiological stresses bring on thyroid crisis is uncertain. There is some speculation that alterations in thyroid hormone binding in the blood, which occurs in some illnesses, may cause an increase in free thyroid hormone concentrations. This would increase even more the already existing hyperthyroid state of the individual.

A patient in thyroid crisis is in a state of severe hypermetabolism. All the problems associated with hyperthyroidism are exaggerated. The onset of thyroid crisis will be accompanied by severe persistent tachycardia, hypertension, and fever. Tremulousness and restlessness are almost always present. Without treatment, the patient will progress to a state of delirium, congestive heart failure, and death.

Of primary concern is the goal to decrease the metabolic rate. This is achieved by inhibiting hormone synthesis and release and decreasing the peripheral effects of thyroid hormone. Large doses of an *antithyroid drug* such as propylthiouracil are administered to prevent synthesis of the thyroid hormone from iodine. *Iodine* administered in the form of SSKI or sodium iodine reduces the release of hormone from the thyroid.

Since thyroid hormone increases the body's

sensitivity to the sympathetic nervous system, a *beta-receptor blocking agent* such as propranolol is given to antagonize the adrenergic aspects of thyroid crisis. Thus, it reduces the systolic blood pressure, decreases heart rate and cardiac output, and lessens cardiac irritability. This leads to improvement in nervousness, fatigue, palpitation, dyspnea, and heat intolerance. Because these drugs are myocardial depressants, they require close monitoring of vital signs by the nurse.

Another adjunct to therapy in hyperthyroid crisis includes the use of *adrenal corticosteroids,* since the rate of metabolism of the patient's endogenous glucocorticoids is greatly increased. Therefore, to prevent the likelihood of an addisonian crisis during the acute emergency, the nurse should anticipate the parenteral administration of hydrocortisone sodium succinate. Addisonian crisis is discussed in detail in the section on adrenocortical malfunction.

During the drug therapy the patient will experience other intensified problems associated with hyperthyroidism. A major problem encountered by all patients in thyroid crisis is *fever.* This is often the "cardinal sign" that heralds the onset of thyroid storm. Monitoring the temperature and reducing the patient's fever are important aspects of the nurse's role. Measures to combat the failure in thermoregulation include administration of aspirin and sponging the patient. The use of hypothermia may also be helpful in reducing the fever.

The problems of *hyperirritability* and *increased excitability,* likewise, need to be considered in planning nursing care. A quiet, nonstimulating environment should be provided. If available, an air-conditioned room away from the mainstream of activity on the nursing unit is preferable. Noise should be controlled outside the patient's room. Screening the patient's visitors and limiting the visiting time helps to eliminate unnecessary stimulation. As the patient's condition improves, nonstimulating activity such as simple puzzles or simple needlework can be made available.

Although there is generally no altered ability of the individual to perform established hygiene activities and self-care habits, the patient who is hyperirritable and readily upset for periods of time should be bathed and assisted with all aspects of care. This may be done despite the patient's ability to carry out this aspect of care alone. Promotion of rest for the patient is essential to a more rapid recovery as it gives the body a chance to store energy sources.

Another major consideration for the individual in thyroid crisis relates to the *emotional problems* experienced. Anticipation of the patient's needs will help to reduce frustration. Answering the patient's call light and administering medications and treatments promptly are examples of nursing intervention which can reduce the patient's frustration level. Likewise, continuity of care can be maintained by assigning the same nurse to care for the patient over a period of time. The nurse who is patient and mild mannered can help create a more relaxing environment and should be considered for the assignment. In addition, recovery can be facilitated by offering support and reassurance.

**Fourth-level nursing care**   With proper care a hyperthyroid patient can be maintained in a relatively euthyroid state indefinitely. Teaching and follow-up of a patient taking antithyroid drugs are discussed in Second-Level Nursing Care. For the patient who underwent radioiodine therapy or surgery, long-term follow-up is of utmost importance.

Care after [131]I therapy is especially important, since the effects of the radioactive iodine on the patient are so variable that even individualized dose calculation does not guarantee what effect the treatment will have. Therefore, close follow-up during the first year after therapy is necessary to determine the patient's thyroid status. Hypothyroidism is the most common sequela. The patient should be made aware that this may be a complication if adequate treatment of hyperthyroidism is to be achieved.

For the patient who has undergone subtotal thyroidectomy, recurrence of hyperthyroidism due to inadequate removal of thyroid tissue may be experienced. As in the case of [131]I therapy, the patient who has been surgically treated can also become hypothyroid. Instructions on the importance of yearly evaluation should be given to the patient in view of the insidious development of hypothyroidism. The signs of hypothyroidism should be reviewed and a printed copy of them given to the patient and/or family for later reference.

### Goiter

Perhaps the most common of all disorders of the thyroid gland is goiter, a general term applied to any enlargement of the thyroid gland. It is most often associated with normal thyroid hormone production. Like most thyroid disease, it is more common in women than men. There are three types of goiter: (1) familial, (2) goitrogenic, and (3) endemic. The pathogenesis of *familial goiter* involves inborn errors in the metabolic apparatus of the thyroid gland which impair the delivery of a normal amount of thyroid hormone into the blood. This inherited block in thyroid hormone synthesis or secretion leads to increased thyroid growth and distortion of its structure. Most nontoxic goiter in the United States is of this type and involves congenital enzymatic defects.

*Goitrogenic goiter* develops occasionally in patients because of goiter-producing substances (goitrogens) either in their diet or from drugs that have been given for other conditions. Goitrogens cause thyroid enlargement in an effort to compensate for inefficient production of thyroid hormone caused by chemically induced partial blockage of hormone synthesis. Iodide is a goitrogen. Likewise, the following foods, when consumed in excessive amounts over long periods of time, can produce goitrogenic goiter: rutabagas, radishes, turnips, spinach, cabbage, soybeans, peas, carrots, peaches, and strawberries. These foods all contain substances which convert progoitrin into goitrin, an active antithyroid.

Perhaps more than in any other health problem, the complexity of the relationship between man and the environment is revealed in the development and prevention of endemic goiter. *Endemic goiter* is generally thought to result from thyroid enlargement in response to a deficiency of iodine. Although genetic and dietary factors may contribute, iodine deficiency remains the central and preventable element in this disorder. At the same time that iodine deficiencies persist in some parts of the population, there is high and excessive iodine intake by others. This excessive iodine intake is partly from the iodate in bread and from other sources not under control of health authorities. In the past the incidence of goiter varied considerably throughout the United States, and definite zones of high frequency where diets were deficient in iodine were identified in the Middle West and Northwest. These differences have diminished sharply in recent years, and goiter is not presently endemic in the United States. However, it remains one of the most important diseases in the world population, and its occurrence seems to closely correlate with the amount of iodine in the soil.

Prevention of endemic goiter is relatively simple and consists of a prophylactic program with iodine that reaches the entire population. The most economical, suitable, and reliable goiter prevention program has been the use of iodized salt. Approximately 50 $\mu$g/day is sufficient, but it is recommended that salt should be iodized to allow for 200 $\mu$g iodine per day. However, one-half of today's table salt is not iodized, and consumption of table salt in general is decreasing because of the widespread use of preprocessed food prepared with noniodized salt both at home and in public eating facilities. An important aspect of the role of the community health nurse in goiter prevention relates to educating the public to the use of iodized salt. The nurse may determine whether the daily salt intake is adequate by taking a brief diet history. Asking to view the type of salt purchased is a simple measure to aid in determining a family's intake. In addition, the nurse may assist in emphasizing the need for stricter controls on all additions of iodine to foods, drugs, and household and industrial chemicals.

## Thyroid Cancer

Malignant tumors of the thyroid are rare. Thyroid cancer accounts for only ½ to 1 percent of all clinical cancer. However, there has been an increased incidence of thyroid cancer in the last 20 years. This may be associated with better recognition of thyroid cancer but could be a result of increased exposure to carcinogenic agents such as drugs and radiation. Thyroid carcinomas are generally of four types: papillary, follicular, medullary, or anaplastic.

The most common variety of thyroid carcinoma is *papillary carcinoma,* which accounts for 50 percent of thyroid cancers. It occurs from the second to seventh decades, with the peak incidence in the third decade. It is slow growing with lymphatic spread. The overall 10-year survival rate is 82 percent. *Follicular carcinoma* causes 15 percent of thyroid cancers. It is most frequent in the sixth and seventh decades and is slightly more frequent in women. *Anaplastic carcinoma* spreads rapidly to adjacent neck structures, with a 75 percent mortality rate in 3 years.

The symptoms of thyroid carcinoma are associated primarily with enlargement of the gland with local compression. The thyroid scan is a valuable tool in evaluating thyroid cancers. Most malignant thyroid tumors will show little or no accumulation of radioiodine following a thyroid scan, whereas benign adenomas frequently show normal or at times increased retention of $^{131}$I. Final diagnosis of thyroid cancer, however, is ultimately dependent upon microscopic examination of the tissue.

Carcinoma of the thyroid, especially if it is localized, is usually treated by surgical thyroidectomy. The extent of the surgical procedure may range from simple removal of the malignant lobe to total thyroidectomy with bilateral radical neck dissection. Thyroid surgery is discussed more fully in Hyperthyroidism. After a thyroidectomy, the patient will often have some functioning thyroid tissue remaining. This is true even for many patients who have had a "total" thyroidectomy and can be detected by a careful scanning procedure. Therapeutic radioiodine used postoperatively can destroy any remaining malignant tissue. After a thyroidectomy, replacement therapy with thyroid hormones is started. Time of initiation of full thyroid hormone replacement varies with the physician's approach to treating thyroid cancer.

## Thyroiditis

Thyroiditis is a general descriptive term indicating an inflammation of the thyroid gland. The term by itself is nonspecific with regard to the pathologic etiology. There are three basic forms: (1) lymphocytic thyroiditis, or autoimmune thyroiditis (Hashimoto's disease), (2) subacute thyroiditis, and (3) acute suppurative thyroiditis. Lymphocytic thyroiditis is an autoimmune disturbance and is discussed in Chap. 10.

**Subacute nonsuppurative thyroiditis** Also known as *de Quervain's thyroiditis,* subacute nonsuppurative thyroiditis is considered a self-limiting inflammation of the thyroid thought to be caused by any of several viral agents. Among the viruses implicated are mumps virus, influenza, ECHO viruses, and adenoviruses. Subacute thyroiditis is uncommon, yet the condition often follows upper respiratory infections. Women are more often affected than men, with the highest incidence occurring in the fourth and fifth decades. The symptoms generally include malaise, fever, and severe pain in the region of the thyroid aggravated by coughing, swallowing, or turning of the head. Some patients complain of symptoms of hyperthyroidism such as nervousness, tremulousness, some weight loss, heat intolerance, and rapid heartbeat. The course of this problem is variable, with an average duration of 2 to 4 months. Although patients may initially present with symptoms simulating hyperthyroidism, a quarter of the time the disease will progress to a transient hypothyroidism. This results when there is depletion of the colloid stored in the thyroid due to the destructive process involved in the pathophysiology and consequently failure of formation of new thyroid hormone. Normal thyroid function resumes as the colloid is repleted in the gland.

Treatment is generally supportive with the use of analgesics such as aspirin and Darvon. In more

extreme cases, corticosteroids are usually recommended to reduce inflammation. In the majority of cases there are no residual effects.

**Acute suppurative thyroiditis** This form of thyroiditis is an uncommon condition that is caused by invasion of the thyroid gland by microorganisms. There are signs of acute inflammation in the gland and surrounding tissue. In addition to severe pain and tenderness in the region of the thyroid, patients may complain of dysphagia, fever, and malaise. Treatment is generally with antibiotics appropriate to the invading organism. Incision and drainage of the gland may be necessary in some cases.

## ADRENOCORTICAL MALFUNCTION

Maintenance of a homeostatic state in health and disease is dependent upon the presence of a normally functioning adrenal cortex. The adrenocortical hormones play a vital role in the interaction between man and the environment. Deficiencies or excesses of these hormones disturb the normal physiologic mechanisms essential for man to cope effectively with stress. The consequences of malfunction of the adrenal cortex will be discussed here.

### Adrenocortical Insufficiency

The incidence of adrenocortical insufficiency is thought to be relatively rare, but accurate statistics are difficult to obtain. It is estimated that primary adrenocortical insufficiency (Addison's disease) occurs in approximately 1 person per 100,000 population, while insufficiency secondary to hypopituitarism is seen in approximately 1 of every 1000 hospitalized patients.[12] However, because the onset of this problem is usually insidious and symptoms do not appear until late in its course, it is probable that many undiagnosed cases exist. Both sexes and all age groups are affected, although the disorder seems to occur more commonly in middle age. No significant differences in incidence have been observed among various socioeconomic, cultural, or racial groups. The etiology of Addison's disease may be influenced by the prevalence of other diseases (e.g., tuberculosis, systemic fungal infections) in different geographic regions.

**Pathophysiology** Adrenocortical insufficiency results from hypofunction of the adrenal cortex with deficiencies of one or more of the adrenocortical hormones. The disorder may be classified as primary or secondary, depending on its etiology. *Primary adrenocortical insufficiency* (Addison's disease) results from disturbances within the gland itself. The most frequent cause is atrophy of the adrenal cortex of idiopathic origin. The possibility of an autoimmune process has been implicated, as a significant number of addisonian patients with idiopathic atrophy have been observed to possess circulating antibodies which bind specifically to adrenal tissue. A good percentage of these patients have associated extraadrenal endocrine disorders, particularly ovarian failure, hypothyroidism, hypoparathyroidism, and diabetes mellitus. A familial tendency toward the development of adrenocortical insufficiency has also been observed.[13]

Adrenocortical tissue can also be destroyed by tuberculosis or fungal invasion, leading to primary dysfunction. Amyloidosis, tumors, adrenal vascular thrombosis and adrenal hemorrhage associated with overwhelming sepsis (Waterhouse-Friderichsen syndrome) or anticoagulant therapy rarely cause adrenocortical hypofunction.

*Secondary adrenocortical insufficiency* results when there is inadequate secretion of ACTH by the anterior pituitary gland. ACTH is necessary to stimulate secretion in the adrenal cortex; without ACTH, an otherwise normal adrenal cortex cannot function. The most common causes of hypopituitarism include pituitary tumors (particularly chromophobe adenomas), postpartum pituitary necrosis (Sheehan's syndrome), and surgical removal of the pituitary gland. Prolonged administration of supraphysiologic doses of corticosteroids causes adrenal insufficiency by suppressing the secretion of ACTH with resultant adrenal atrophy and decreased responsiveness to ACTH. It is the commonest cause of secondary adrenocortical insufficiency. Table 21-5 summarizes the causes of adrenocortical hypofunction.

**Metabolic Changes** The many pathophysiologic changes in adrenocortical insufficiency are attributable to deficiencies of cortisol, aldosterone, and, in females, adrenal androgens. Cortisol deficiency results in altered metabolism of carbohydrates, proteins, and fats. *Gluconeogenesis* does not occur readily during prolonged periods of fasting to maintain normal serum glucose levels, and liver *glycogen stores* may be depleted. The patient develops a tendency toward *hypoglycemia,* particularly in the early morning and 1 to 3 hours after a high-carbohydrate meal. The blood sugar threshold at which symptoms of hypoglycemia are manifested may be decreased, and extreme sensitivity to insulin is common. This problem is more exaggerated in adrenal insufficiency secondary to hypopituitarism because of the concurrent deficiency of growth hormone, which also stimulates gluconeogenesis. When hypoglycemia does occur, the effects are similar to those seen in an insulin reaction—weakness, tremulousness, irritability, sweating, headache, blurred vision, slurred speech, and confusion.

Of great significance is the body's compromised *ability to cope with stress* of any nature. Even minor

**TABLE 21-5**
CAUSES OF ADRENOCORTICAL INSUFFICIENCY

| Type | Pathogenesis | Etiology |
| --- | --- | --- |
| Primary (intrinsic disease) | Adrenocortical atrophy | Idiopathic (questionable autoimmune process) |
| | Destruction of the adrenal cortex | Tuberculosis |
| | | Tumor |
| | | Amyloidosis |
| | | Fungal infection |
| | | Hemorrhage (Waterhouse-Friderichsen syndrome) (anticoagulant therapy) |
| | | Bilateral adrenalectomy |
| Secondary (pituitary-hypothalamic failure) | Hypopituitarism | Pituitary tumors (chromophobe adenomas) |
| | | Postpartum pituitary necrosis (Sheehan's syndrome) |
| | | Infection |
| | | Irradiation |
| | | Hypophysectomy |
| Iatrogenic | Hypothalamic-pituitary-adrenal suppression | Prolonged corticosteroid therapy |

injuries or infections may precipitate severe prostration, progressing to shock and death if adrenocortical reserves are inadequate.

A variety of *gastrointestinal symptoms* may be manifested. Anorexia, nausea, and vomiting occur with increasing frequency as the disease progresses and contribute to weight loss and fluid and electrolyte imbalance. These problems result from disappearance of the hydrochloric acid–secreting cells of the gastric mucosa and decreased gastric and intestinal motility secondary to reduced cortisol levels.

Decreased serum cortisol levels activate the hypothalamic-pituitary-adrenal feedback mechanism to stimulate secretion of ACTH by the pituitary gland. Secretion of a similar hormone, *melanocyte-stimulating hormone (MSH),* is also increased. Both MSH and, to a lesser degree, ACTH have the capacity to stimulate melanin synthesis. Deposition of melanin produces areas of *hyperpigmentation* in the skin and mucous membranes. The degree of pigmentation is dependent upon the duration of the disease and the natural coloring of the patient. Increased pigmentation may precede other symptoms by many years. It is most obvious in those areas exposed to light, pressure, or friction. Initially, the patient may notice a generalized tan over the entire body which later becomes more exaggerated over the exposed portions of the skin. Elbows, knees, skin folds, recent scars, and the areolar and genital areas are particularly prone to hyperpigmentation. The mucous membranes of the mouth, conjunctiva, and vagina also develop dark bluish brown spots. *Vitiligo,* patchy areas of depigmentation surrounded by areas of increased pigmentation, occurs in some patients. Fair-haired individuals may note a darkening of hair color. Generalized darkening of the skin and increased pigmentation in the creases of the palms may be observed in Negroes. Hyperpigmentation is minimal or absent in secondary adrenal insufficiency due to hypopituitarism, as both ACTH and MSH secretion are inadequate.

**F**luid and Electrolyte Imbalances Some of the most striking effects of adrenocortical insufficiency are precipitated by changes in aldosterone secretion. In primary insufficiency aldosterone secretion is often deficient or absent, and disturbances in fluid and electrolyte balance result (see Chap. 12). Because aldosterone secretion is less dependent on ACTH, it is only slightly decreased in hypopituitarism, and fluid and electrolyte changes are usually less pronounced.

Decreased aldosterone production in Addison's disease causes decreased reabsorption of sodium by the renal tubules. This inability to conserve sodium also promotes urinary loss of chloride and water, leading to depletion of extracellular fluid volume, *dehydration,* and *weight loss.* Tissue turgor is decreased, and the mucous membranes are dry. Depletion of extracellular fluid volume and sodium frequently causes muscle cramps.

As *hypovolemia* progresses, renal perfusion is reduced, and the glomerular filtration rate decreases. With severe insufficiency, waste products normally excreted by the kidney accumulate, and the blood urea nitrogen level becomes elevated. *Hyponatremia* also promotes hydrogen ion retention, since these ions are not exchanged as readily for sodium ions in the renal tubules. As a result, there is a tendency toward development of *metabolic acidosis.* Other side effects of hyponatremia are vomiting and diarrhea, which may further aggravate the sodium imbalance.

Potassium excretion is affected by deficient aldosterone levels. While sodium ions are lost, potassium ions are conserved and hyperkalemia develops. If severe, it may precipitate serious cardiac arrhythmias.

Patients with adrenal insufficiency do not excrete free water normally and are prone to *water intoxification.* The exact mechanism for the abnormality is unclear.[14] It may be due in part to the hypovolemia and resultant decrease in renal blood flow and glomerular filtration rate. At the same time, cortisol's effect of antagonizing the antidiuretic hormone (ADH) is decreased. The water-conserving effects of ADH are intensified, and free water is not readily excreted. This effect is less evident in primary insufficiency where the sodium loss associated with decreases in aldosterone causes water loss as well. However, in insufficiency secondary to hypopituitarism, water intoxication is more likely to develop, as aldosterone levels are usually normal and do not counteract the water-conserving effects of ADH.

**C**hanges in Oxygenation Alterations in fluid and electrolyte balance contribute to changes in oxygenation status, as decreased extracellular volume and hypovolemia lead to a *reduced cardiac output.* With time, the heart becomes smaller in response to the decreased workload. Most patients with Addison's disease have a reduction in *blood pressure,* and the *pulse* may be weak. Peripheral vascular tone is diminished when cortisol levels are inadequate, and the normal reflex mechanism of vasoconstriction in response to hypotension is impaired. Symptoms of lightheadedness, dizziness, and syncopal episodes related to *orthostatic hypotension* are experienced. Cardiac arrhythmias may be precipitated by hyperkalemia, further reducing cardiac output. In severe adrenal insufficiency, hypovolemia progresses to circulatory collapse and shock.

**C**hanges in Perception and Coordination   Muscle *weakness* is common in adrenocortical insufficiency. The degree of weakness and fatigability are directly related to the severity and duration of the disease and the patient's previous muscular development. With the insidious onset of adrenocortical insufficiency, fatigue is initially mild. As the disease progresses, weakness becomes more exaggerated, and exhaustion develops with even minimal effort. The symptoms are usually improved by sleep and rest and intensified by disturbances in electrolyte balance.

Mental status of the addisonian patient frequently deteriorates as the disease progresses. Drowsiness, apathy, and inability to concentrate are common characteristics. Restlessness, irritability, negativity, and insomnia may be observed. Emotional disturbances range from mild neurotic symptoms to severe depression.

**C**hanges in Cellular Growth and Proliferation   The decreased levels of androgens alter the secondary sex characteristics. These changes are more prominent in females, as the adrenal cortex is the major source of androgens. Axillary and pubic hair become sparse or absent. Disturbances in menstruation and male potency may occur, but these are usually related to the degree of debility. Changes in secondary sex characteristics and gonadal function are more pronounced when adrenal insufficiency is secondary to hypopituitarism because of the concurrent gonadotropin deficiency, and both sexes may exhibit more severe symptoms of androgen and estrogen deficiency. The pathophysiological changes in primary and secondary adrenocortical insufficiency are summarized in Fig. 21-4.

**First-level nursing care**   Prevention of primary adrenocortical insufficiency is difficult since, in the majority of cases, its etiology is not known. Tuberculosis was once a significant causative factor, but increased case finding and the development of more effective antituberculous chemotherapy have decreased the incidence of tuberculosis with its potential pathological effects on the adrenal cortex.

The nurse can play a significant role in the pre-

vention of adrenocortical insufficiency secondary to the prolonged use of corticosteroid therapy in nonendocrine disease entities. Normally, secretion of the adrenocortical hormones, particularly cortisol, is controlled through a negative feedback mechanism. As the hormone level decreases, the hypothalamus secretes corticotropin-releasing factor (CRF), which stimulates the anterior pituitary to produce ACTH. As adrenocortical hormone levels increase, CRF and, therefore, ACTH secretion are suppressed. Administration of supraphysiologic doses of corticosteroids similarly suppresses the release of CRF, ACTH, and cortisol. With prolonged therapy the secretory ability of the anterior pituitary is reduced, atrophy of the adrenal cortex occurs, and production of their hormones ceases. Consequently, corticosteroid therapy should never be abruptly discontinued. Rather, the dosage should be gradually tapered to allow these glands adequate time to reestablish normal function. If therapy is stopped abruptly, the individual may develop acute adrenal insufficiency (discussed under Third-Level Nursing Care). Complete recovery of the feedback system usually requires several months.

To minimize glandular atrophy, exogenous steroids must be administered judiciously and correctly. Alternate-day steroid administration has been shown to reduce many of the undesirable effects of prolonged corticosteroid therapy in nonendocrine disorders. The total dosage of corticosteroid for 2 days is given as a single dose on the morning of the first day. Administration of the drug in the early morning simulates the normal peak secretion of cortisol. Because the therapeutic effects of steroids persist longer than their metabolic effects, symptoms of the underlying disease process can often be adequately suppressed, while more normal activity of the hypothalamic-pituitary-adrenal feedback system is permitted on the off-medication day. If the corticosteroid therapy is eventually discontinued, the degree of adrenal insufficiency and pituitary suppression is reduced significantly. The patient needs to understand the rationale for the alternate-day regimen and be made aware that some symptoms of the disease process may be evident shortly before the administration of the next steroid dose. The importance of taking the medication as prescribed and not discontinuing its use abruptly should be emphasized. Other aspects of health teaching related to steroid therapy in adrenocortical insufficiency are discussed in Fourth-Level Nursing Care.

**Second-level nursing care**   The onset of Addison's disease is usually insidious. Approximately 90 percent of the adrenal cortex must be destroyed before the problem becomes clinically evident. Even then, adrenocortical reserves may be adequate to meet daily needs under nonstressful conditions. Because of this slow onset the patient may remain undiagnosed for an indeterminate period of time. It should be kept in mind, however, that the patient may experience a rapid onset of symptoms when adrenocortical reserves are suddenly inadequate to cope with an acute stressful situation, such as an infection, injury, or surgical procedure.

**N**ursing Assessment   The *health history* of a patient with adrenocortical insufficiency is often unremarkable, revealing symptomatology that is rather vague and nonspecific. A thorough assessment is necessary to elicit information which will facilitate case finding and early referral for diagnosis.

The patient should be asked about muscular weakness, any decrease in activity tolerance, easy fatigability, or inability to concentrate. Changes in dietary habits related to anorexia, nausea, vomiting,

increased thirst, or an unusual craving for salt, as well as a history of recent significant weight loss, need to be explored. Symptoms of hypoglycemic episodes, such as weakness, sweating, tremulousness, nervousness, and irritability should be noted. Evidence of orthostatic hypotension may be elicited by questioning the patient about symptoms of lightheadedness, dizziness, or syncope related to changes in posture. The patient should be asked if any changes in skin color have been noted, although a negative answer does not rule out the diagnosis of adrenocortical insufficiency. Abnormalities in menstruation should also be assessed.

Knowledge of any history of previous steroid therapy, particularly within the last 6 months to a year, is extremely important when evaluating the patient. Evidence of long periods of convalescence following any illness or surgery should be explored. A history of other medical problems and a thorough family history should be taken to determine the existence of other disease processes, such as tuberculosis or other endocrine disorders, which might

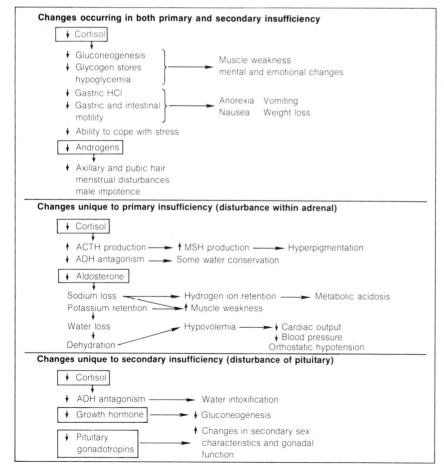

**FIGURE 21-4**
Pathophysiological changes in primary and secondary adrenocortical insufficiency.

indicate a predisposition toward adrenal insufficiency.

Findings upon *physical assessment* vary with the severity and duration of the disease. To evaluate fluid and electrolyte status, tissue turgor and the appearance of the mucous membranes should be noted. In the dehydrated patient tissue turgor is poor with loose skin and dry mucous membranes. The weight should be taken and compared with previous recordings to detect significant losses.

The effect of fluid and electrolyte changes on oxygenation are evaluated by assessment of changes in cardiovascular status. The systolic blood pressure is usually lower when compared with previous recordings. Lying, standing, and sitting blood pressures should be taken and compared, since a decrease indicating orthostatic changes is frequently observed. The pulse should also be evaluated for significant increases in rate associated with episodes of postural hypotension. Heart sounds may be diminished on auscultation and the pulse weakened with the peripheral pulses difficult to palpate. Abnormalities in the rate and rhythm of the apical pulse may be detected if potassium levels are extremely elevated or fluid losses severe.

Patients with adrenocortical insufficiency are characteristically thin. An emaciated or debilitated appearance, if present, is an indication of the extent of the disease. The abdominal examination is usually within normal limits, although the patient may complain of costovertebral pain and tenderness.

Neurologically, the patient is normal, although evaluation of mental status may demonstrate a variety of symptoms ranging from drowsiness and apathy to restlessness and irritability. Symptoms of neurosis or severe depression may be noted.

An assessment of color changes in the skin should be made. Hyperpigmentation will be manifested as a generalized tan that does not fade. This is difficult to detect in dark-skinned individuals and is best observed in the creases of the palms. Areas especially prone to increased coloring, such as elbows, knees, skin folds, belt lines, recent scars, areolae, and genitals, should be inspected. A spotty bluish-brown pigmentation of the mucous membranes, particularly of the mouth, is almost universally present. The recent appearance of dark freckles may also be noted. Assessment of hair distribution often reveals a noticeable decrease in axillary and pubic hair in the female.

*Diagnostic tests* There are several routine blood tests that aid in the evaluation of a patient with suspected adrenocortical insufficiency. Measurement of *serum sodium* and *potassium* levels provide an indication of the adequacy of mineralocorticoid secretion. A serum sodium less than 130 meq/liter and a potassium greater than 5 meq/liter are frequently observed in primary adrenal insufficiency. The *ratio of sodium to potassium* is also calculated, since the serum sodium may be falsely high due to dehydration. The ratio, normally greater than 30:1, approaches 20:1. In adrenal insufficiency secondary to hypopituitarism, hyponatremia may be more severe. The impaired ability to excrete free water in the presence of normal aldosterone levels increases the risk of water intoxication and hyponatremia.

*Fasting blood sugar* levels may be significantly decreased as a result of diminished gluconeogenesis. Mild acidosis due to the retention of hydrogen ions is common, and the *plasma bicarbonate* is decreased. As a result of decreased glomerular filtration rate, the *blood urea nitrogen* is elevated.

With decreased cortisol levels the destruction of *lymphocytes* and *eosinophils* is inhibited. Their release is augmented and levels are increased, while the *total white blood cell count* is decreased. Anemia occurs commonly, although the *hematocrit* may be normal or elevated due to hemoconcentration secondary to aldosterone deficiency and dehydration.

The *nursing problems* associated with adrenocortical insufficiency are generally not managed on an outpatient basis. In the community the nurse's primary role is *case finding* and *referral*. Patients suspected of having the disease should be referred immediately for evaluation and diagnosis. Untreated, the patient is susceptible to life-threatening complications if adrenocortical reserves are inadequate to help body systems cope with stress.

**Third-level nursing care** Because of the precarious nature of untreated adrenocortical insufficiency and the testing methods utilized, more extensive evaluation of the patient is carried out in the hospital under close supervision. During the *nursing assessment,* the health history and physical assessment findings will be similar to those discussed in Second-Level Nursing Care. Evaluation of the patient in the hospital will involve more specific diagnostic studies.

**D**iagnostic Tests Adrenocortical hormone secretion is evaluated by measuring the specific hormone to be evaluated or one of its metabolic byproducts. Determination of *plasma cortisol levels* is usually done with the patient at rest. The primary by-products of cortisol metabolism are *17-hydroxy-corticosteroids* (17-OHCS) and *17-ketogenic steroids* (17-KGS). 17-KGS are 17-OHCS that have been converted in the laboratory to facilitate analysis. The by-products of androgenic hormone metabolism are *17-ketosteroids* (17-KS). In many of the diagnostic studies the urinary levels of these by-products are measured. Valid interpretation of the tests for adrenal function depends on the accuracy and efficiency of urine collections. Creatinine excretion is frequently evaluated at the same time to monitor the completeness of the urine collection.

Patients should be instructed in collection procedures, and the importance of accurate collections emphasized. Stress should be avoided during the collection period to minimize difficulty in interpreting results. Urine volume may influence steroid secretion, and the patient should maintain a fluid intake adequate to ensure a urinary output of 1000 to 1500 ml. However, excessive output should also be avoided. Because some antibiotics, analgesics, and tranquilizers may interfere with the chemical determination of urinary steroids, they should not be administered during collection periods. Glucosuria above trace amounts can produce abnormally low values, and careful regulation of diabetes during testing is important.

The most reliable and specific diagnostic study used to determine the presence of adrenocortical insufficiency is the *8-hour intravenous ACTH test,* which measures levels of adrenocortical hormones secreted in response to the administration of corticotropin. The day before the test a 24-hour urine for 17-OHCS and 17-KS is collected to measure baseline levels. After a blood sample for determination of the baseline plasma cortisol level is drawn, an infusion of 25 to 50 units ACTH in 500 ml isotonic saline solution is begun and administered over a period of exactly 8 hours. The length of the infusion period is critical since the total adrenocortical output changes semilogarithmically with time. Therefore, close observation and regulation of the infusion are crucial. A second 24-hour urine measurement is begun at the time of ACTH administration. After at least 1 hour and at the end of the infusion, a plasma cortisol is drawn. Normally, cortisol levels rise to at least 30 $\mu$g/100 ml, and urinary steroid excretion increases two- to fivefold in response to ACTH. In the patient with primary adrenocortical insufficiency there is little or no rise in plasma cortisol or urinary steroid levels because the adrenal cortex is nonfunctional. A gradual rise in steroid levels will be noted in the patient with insufficiency due to hypopituitarism if the test is repeated over 3 to 5 days. This response is due to the slow recovery

of the adrenal cortex when its secretion has been temporarily suppressed secondary to decreased ACTH. *Eosinophil counts* may be measured before and after the ACTH infusion. A decrease in eosinophils of less than 50 percent at the conclusion of the test is indicative of adrenocortical insufficiency. Table 21-6 summarizes these test results.

Since anaphylactic reactions may occur when nonsynthetic preparations of ACTH are used, the nurse should be alert to the warning signs of impending anaphylaxis. If they occur, the infusion should be discontinued immediately and the physician notified. To prevent this complication, dexamethasone may be administered orally prior to and during the test. The drug does not interfere significantly with the test results.

A more rapid screening test using a synthetic ACTH preparation is the *Cortrosyn* (cosyntropin) *test.* After a sample to determine a baseline plasma cortisol level is drawn, 0.25 mg Cortrosyn is given intramuscularly in 2 ml saline. Thirty minutes later another blood sample for cortisol determination is drawn. Cortisol levels should rise at least 2½-fold in normal subjects, while the patient with adrenocortical insufficiency demonstrates little or no increase. Advantages of this testing method are its rapidity and the rare occurrence of anaphylactic reactions. A similar test may be performed with a natural ACTH preparation.

**N**ursing Problems and Interventions   The patient with adrenocortical insufficiency may present with a variety of problems which require nursing intervention. Potentially, the most serious of these is the *inability to cope with stress.* Hospitalization in itself is often a stressful situation, and the nurse can be instrumental in facilitating the patient's adjustment. The patient should be thoroughly oriented to the

**TABLE 21-6**
TESTS TO EVALUATE
ADRENOCORTICAL INSUFFICIENCY

| Test | Results* | |
|------|---------|----|
| | Primary | Secondary |
| Plasma cortisol | Decreased | Decreased |
| Urinary 17-OHCS | Decreased | Decreased |
| 17-KS | Decreased | Decreased |
| 8-Hour intravenous ACTH stimulation test | Minimal or no increase | Gradual increase over several days |
| Cortrosyn test (IM) | Minimal or no increase | Gradual increase over several days |
| Plasma ACTH (if available) | Increased | Decreased |

* Normal values are not included here as they vary with the laboratory method utilized.

physical environment and hospital routine. Activities related to diagnostic testing and care should be coordinated to ensure that the schedule is realistic in light of the patient's physical limitations. Special attention should be given to the administration of testing materials and collection of specimens to avoid unnecessary repetition or delay in obtaining test results.

Measures to protect the patient from exposure to infection are essential. Contact with any patient or staff member with a respiratory infection should be avoided. Any symptoms of infection, such as a sore throat, rhinorrhea, or increasing temperature, must be reported immediately. Early treatment could be crucial in the prevention of adrenal crisis.

*Generalized weakness and easy fatigability* may compromise the patient's ability to independently perform activities of daily living. Physical limitations should be assessed and assistance provided as necessary to minimize stress. Activities which require exertion or overtire the patient should be avoided. Patient care activities and testing procedures can be scheduled so that several periods of uninterrupted rest are provided throughout the day.

*Dehydration* is a common problem, and close observation of the patient's state of hydration is crucial. A careful record of intake and output and daily weights should be kept. Dietary intake of sodium should be adequate to maintain normal serum levels. To promote optimal hydration, it may be necessary to increase fluid intake, particularly with fluids containing electrolytes—broths, carbonated beverages, and juices. If the patient is experiencing *orthostatic hypotension,* changing from supine to upright positions slowly to prevent syncopal episodes and possible injury should be emphasized.

Small, frequent feedings should be provided throughout the day to alleviate the problem of *hypoglycemia.* Prolonged periods of fasting for testing purposes must be kept to a minimum to prevent hypoglycemic episodes. Early signs and symptoms of hypoglycemia should be treated immediately by administering a quickly absorbed source of glucose, such as juice, nondietetic carbonated beverages, or sugar.

If *nausea* is a problem, an antiemetic may be prescribed. Administration of medication shortly before meals may help to improve the patient's dietary intake. Every effort should be made to provide a pleasant environment during mealtime. If vomiting prevents adequate oral intake, intravenous therapy must be instituted to prevent further fluid and electrolyte losses.

The degree of *mental fatigue* may affect the patient's ability to concentrate for long periods. It is important that the patient understand the relationship between this and the hormonal imbalance. Instructions and explanations should be presented simply and concisely. Repetition may be necessary. In-depth teaching should be delayed until the patient is improved and able to fully participate in the learning process.

*Drug therapy* Adrenocortical insufficiency is treated by oral replacement of *adrenocorticosteroids.* Several natural and synthetic glucocorticoid preparations are available. Varying with the biological potency of the medication used, the dosages prescribed are equivalent to the 20 to 50 mg cortisol normally secreted each day under nonstressful conditions. The exact dosage is determined by the needs of the individual. A schedule which simulates the diurnal rhythm of cortisol release is generally recommended, although a single dose may also be prescribed. For example, 25 mg cortisone may be administered in the morning and 12.5 mg in the early afternoon. If prednisone, a less expensive synthetic preparation is used, the dosage might be 5 mg in the morning and 2.5 mg in the afternoon. If weakness or anorexia persists, the amount of glucocorticoid is increased. Side effects of glucocorticoid therapy in the presence of adrenocortical insufficiency are usually minimal, as dosages represent normal physiologic levels. Under stress, the dosage of glucocorticoid must be increased two to four times to meet increased body demands during that period.

In secondary adrenocortical insufficiency glucocorticoid replacement alone is usually adequate because mineralocorticoid secretion is minimally affected. In primary insufficiency, however, replacement of the *mineralocorticoids* is also necessary. This is accomplished through the use of 9-$\alpha$-fluorohydrocortisone (Florinef). A dose of 0.05 to 0.2 mg taken daily at breakfast is usually sufficient to maintain normal fluid and electrolyte balance. A long-acting preparation of deoxycorticosterone, given intramuscularly every 3 to 4 weeks, may also be used. Side effects of mineralocorticoid therapy include edema, hypertension, and hypokalemia. Reducing the dosage of mineralocorticoid, however, will usually alleviate these problems.

The patient who is addisonian generally cannot tolerate sodium deprivation. *Salt intake* must be adequate (100 to 300 meq daily) and should be increased during periods of increased sweating. If salt tablets are used, they should be given with meals to reduce gastric irritation.

Response to therapy usually begins within 24 hours. Fluid and electrolyte levels move toward normal as evidenced by improving blood pressure and electrolyte values. Physical and mental strength increase, and the patient's general feeling of well-being improves. In many instances, there is a reduction in pigmentation after several weeks.

*Addisonian crisis* A patient with chronic adrenocortical insufficiency may develop an episode of acute insufficiency known as addisonian crisis. This results when adrenocortical hormonal reserves are suddenly inadequate to meet the body's needs. It most frequently occurs after an acute stress with which the patient is not physiologically able to cope, such as an infection, trauma, surgery, or exposure to excessive heat or cold. Addisonian crisis can also occur after adrenal thrombosis or trauma, adrenal hemorrhage associated with overwhelming infection or anticoagulant therapy, surgical removal of the adrenal or pituitary glands, or sudden withdrawal from steroid therapy after prolonged use.

Addisonian crisis, as the term implies, is a medical emergency. The patient experiences many of the symptoms of chronic adrenocortical insufficiency, but to extreme degrees. Dehydration, hypovolemia, and hypotension progress to circulatory collapse and shock. The patient becomes extremely weak, lethargic, confused, restless, and eventually comatose. These symptoms are compounded by hyponatremia and hyperkalemia, as well as metabolic acidosis and hypoglycemia. Gastrointestinal symptoms are intensified with nausea, vomiting, diarrhea, and abdominal pain. Hyperpyrexia frequently occurs to further compromise fluid and electrolyte balance.

Early recognition of impending addisonian crisis is crucial in reducing mortality. The nurse should be alert to early symptoms, particularly in patients who by history or nature of their disease are more prone to develop adrenocortical insufficiency. It should be suspected in anyone who develops unaccountable shock after the administration of anesthesia or a surgical procedure. Treatment should be initiated as soon as the diagnosis of addisonian crisis is suspected. A blood sample can be drawn for later analysis of electrolyte and cortisol levels to aid in confirmation of the diagnosis.

Treatment focuses on alleviating or minimizing the life-threatening problems the patient is experiencing. *Circulatory collapse* is initially the most pressing problem. Hydrocortisone or dexamethasone as a bolus dose and/or added to dextrose in isotonic saline solution are rapidly administered intravenously. Increasing serum cortisol levels begin to restore the body's ability to cope with the stressful event. Saline therapy replaces *water losses* and *depleted sodium levels,* while the dextrose corrects *hypoglycemia.* If the blood pressure does not respond to cortisol and fluid replacement, plasma may be given and vasopressors prescribed with dosages titrated according to blood pressure. The patient will require extremely close monitoring of vital signs, central venous pressure, and intake and output. Urine output and specific gravity should be measured hourly to evaluate renal function and state of hydration. If *hyperkalemia* is severe, the patient should be placed on continuous cardiac monitoring.

*Hyperpyrexia* usually begins to resolve with adequate cortisol therapy. If the temperature remains elevated, sponge baths or hypothermia may be employed to reduce the fever. Antipyretics may also be prescribed.

At this time the patient is *unable to cope with* any additional *stress.* Physical and emotional stresses should be identified and minimized. Strict bed rest is essential. The room should be quiet, with activity around the patient kept to a minimum. Reassurance with brief explanations regarding procedures will help to allay anxiety.

If the crisis was precipitated by an infection, appropriate antibiotic therapy should be instituted. With early and effective medical treatment and skilled nursing care, the crisis will begin to resolve within hours. Glucocorticoid therapy is then tapered to maintenance doses over the next 2 to 3 days.

**Fourth-level nursing care** The prognosis with adrenocortical insufficiency is excellent provided that the patient is able to cooperate with permanent daily replacement therapy of adrenal steroids. Patient teaching is of primary importance, and the nurse is instrumental in accomplishing this. Teaching focuses on three areas—medication, recognition of stressful situations, and safety. Patients should know the names of all medications and be able to discuss the rationale and action of each, including the signs and symptoms of both under- and overdosage. They should be able to recognize both emotional and physical stresses that affect their health state and discuss methods of modifying or avoiding them. It is imperative that the patient know how to adjust the medication dosage according to instructions and recognize when to seek medical assistance. Glucocorticoid dosages are usually increased two- to threefold in acute illness, as this represents the body's normal cortisol output under stress. An adequate supply of medication must be kept on reserve at all times for use during periods of stress. If medication cannot be taken orally, the physician should be notified. As an additional precaution, the patient should have a kit which includes an intramuscular glucocorticoid preparation, needle and syringe and instructions for emergency use, especially when traveling. Both the patient and family should be instructed how to prepare and administer the solution. A Medic-Alert tag should be worn, and an identification card carried listing medications and instructions for emergency treatment. Patients should inform any physician or dentist treating them of their condition.

Financial resources should be explored to determine the patient's ability to purchase medications. If problems arise, social service should be contacted and arrangements made prior to discharge from the hospital.

Following discharge, the patient will require long-term health care follow-up. The importance of continued supervision should be emphasized. Periodically, the patient's understanding of adrenocortical insufficiency and the prescribed medication regimen should be reevaluated by a nurse in the community. Assessment for indications of excessive or inadequate steroid replacement should also be made.

With adequate therapy there is no reason the patient cannot lead a productive life. Resumption of previous activities should be encouraged. The responsibility of assisting the patient with the medical regimen, particularly in emergency situations, may be overwhelming to family members. They should be included in teaching sessions and provided opportunities to discuss their concerns regarding the patient's care. The patient and family working together can help to promote the patient's optimum health and prevent complications.

### Adrenocortical Hyperfunction

*Cushing's syndrome* is a relatively rare disease that results from chronic overproduction of cortisol. It can be found in all geographic locations and does not seem to be influenced by racial, cultural, or socioeconomic factors. Cushing's syndrome has been reported with greatest frequency in females between the ages of 20 and 60.[15]

**Pathophysiology**    There are three major causes of Cushing's syndrome. *Primary Cushing's syndrome* occurs as a result of cortisol-secreting adrenal tumors, the majority of which are benign. With hypersecretion of cortisol by the adrenal

tumor, ACTH production by the pituitary is suppressed through the feedback mechanism. This results in atrophy of the healthy adrenal tissue.

*Secondary Cushing's syndrome* can occur as a result of pituitary hypersecretion of ACTH or ectopic ACTH-secreting tumors. Bilateral hyperplasia and hypersecretion of the adrenal cortices is caused by overproduction of ACTH by the pituitary in 60 to 75 percent of the cases of Cushing's syndrome.[18] The hypothalamic-pituitary-adrenal feedback system apparently fails, and pituitary release of ACTH is relatively unresponsive to elevated cortisol levels. The diurnal fluctuations of both ACTH and cortisol are absent. The exact mechanism behind this phenomenon is unknown. In approximately 10 percent of the cases pituitary tumors are the cause of excess corticotropin production.[16] This condition is referred to as Cushing's *disease.* However, in the majority of cases hypersecretion of ACTH occurs in the presence of a normal-appearing pituitary gland and may be due to excessive stimulation by the hypothalamus.

Elevated ACTH levels may originate from a source other than the pituitary gland. Ectopic secretion of ACTH can occur with several types of tumors, particularly bronchogenic oat-cell carcinoma and, less frequently, malignant thymomas or carcinomas of the prostate, breast, or pancreas. This phenomenon is called the *ectopic ACTH syndrome.*

*Iatrogenically induced Cushing's syndrome* (Cushing's syndrome medicamentosus) results from the prolonged use of glucocorticoid therapy. Supraphysiologic doses of glucocorticoids produce changes similar to those caused by hypersecretion of the adrenal cortex. As use of glucocorticoid therapy in various nonendocrine disease entities increases, this disorder is becoming more prevalent.

**Metabolic Changes**    The pathophysiologic changes of Cushing's syndrome primarily result from the effects of excess cortisol levels on carbohydrate, protein, and fat metabolism. The increased level of cortisol accelerates the rate of gluconeogenesis in the body. To supply the materials needed, proteins and fats are mobilized.

The serum glucose level is elevated, stimulating insulin secretion by the pancreas. Approximately 90 percent of the patients with Cushing's syndrome exhibit some impairment of glucose tolerance. When *hyperglycemia* persists over prolonged periods, the pancreatic beta cells may actually "burn out" with the development of frank diabetes mellitus. This occurs in about 20 percent of the cases.[17] Administration of exogenous corticosteroids may unmask previously undiagnosed latent diabetes.

The persistently elevated serum cortisol and insulin levels also contribute to *abnormalities in fat metabolism* and deposition. Weight gain is common. Although obesity is generalized in about half the patients, fat distribution classically tends to be centripetal in the cushingoid individual. The torso becomes large with comparatively thin extremities and the abdomen pendulous. Fat pads develop in the supraclavicular regions, on the back of the neck, and in the cheeks. This gives the patient the characteristic "buffalo hump" and "moon face" associated with Cushing's syndrome (see Fig. 21-5). The tendency of cortisol to stimulate the appetite may contribute to actual weight gain. Patients with an ectopic ACTH-secreting tumor do not usually exhibit these classic characteristics of the cushingoid individual. As a result of the malignant process, they are generally wasted and debilitated.

The catabolism that results from the protein mobilization occasionally results in a marked decrease in skeletal muscle mass, and the patient's extremities may appear wasted. Lassitude and muscular weakness occurs early and may progress to the point of incapacitation in severe cases.

Loss of protein from the bone and alterations in calcium excretion lead to *osteoporosis.* Backache is a common early symptom. Spontaneous pathologic fractures, particularly compression fractures of the vertebrae, may occur, and a decrease in height and curvature of the thoracic spine may be evident. The increased amounts of calcium mobilized from the bone may be deposited in the kidney, and renal calculi may develop.

Protein loss from collagen fibers weakens tissue structure. The *skin* tends to be very thin and fine, almost paperlike in texture. It is susceptible even to minor trauma and breaks down easily. Wound healing is impaired, permitting infection and ulceration. Pink and purple striae are formed where streaks of capillaries have become visible under the skin or weakened subcutaneous tissues have torn, particularly over the abdomen, thighs, upper arms, and breasts. Capillaries are fragile and rupture with minimal trauma, resulting in numerous ecchymoses. The face and neck develop a ruddy or *hyperemic appearance* due to the transparency of the skin and vasculature.

**F**luid and Electrolyte Imbalances   Changes in fluid and electrolyte dynamics also occur in Cushing's

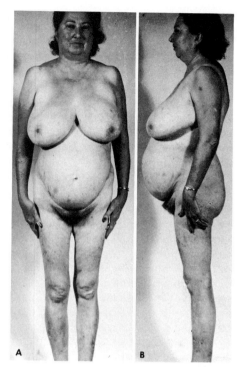

**FIGURE 21-5**

Cushing's disease. (*a*) Note the round face and the increase in preauricular fat pads. Despite the marked obesity and protuberance of the abdomen, the extremities are disproportionately thin. There are a few striae over the lower abdomen. (*b*) A side view of the same patient, again showing the marked protuberance of the abdomen and central fat, with thin extremities. (*From S. I. Schwartz et al.: Principles of Surgery, McGraw-Hill, New York, 1974. With permission of the publisher.*)

syndrome. Although hypersecretion of aldosterone is rare, the mineralocorticoid effects of large quantities of cortisol may become evident. *Sodium* and *water* are retained, while *potassium* is lost. However, edema and hypokalemia occur infrequently and usually only in severe cases.

**C**hanges in Oxygenation   Hypertension is one of the most frequent changes in adrenocortical hypersecretion. Several factors contribute to this phenomenon. The enhanced metabolism of fat increases serum cholesterol levels and accelerates the development of atherosclerosis. Cortisol enhances the responsiveness of blood vessels to norepinephrine in addition to causing mild sodium and fluid retention. Other sequelae of hypertension and the atherosclerotic process are left ventricular hypertrophy, cardiac failure, coronary artery disease, stroke, and nephrosclerosis.

**C**hanges in Inflammation and Immunity Excessive amounts of cortisol alter the body's normal inflammatory and immune responses. The enhanced *anti-inflammatory* properties of cortisol impair the body's ability to fight infection and retard normal healing. T lymphocytes are depressed. The individual's response to trauma or illness is ineffective, and minor localized infections may disseminate and become chronic. The infection is often more severe than the symptomatology indicates, as fever, inflammation, and discomfort may be minimal or absent.

**C**hanges in Cellular Growth and Proliferation When Cushing's syndrome is associated with excessive production of androgenic steroids, as in adrenal carcinoma, changes in cellular growth and proliferation occur. Secondary sex characteristics are altered. Masculinization in females is exhibited by the appearance of dark, coarse facial hair and acne. Thinning of scalp hair is frequently noted. The catabolic effects of cortisol are often counteracted, and muscle size is preserved or increased. The frequency of menstruation is diminished and may progress to amenorrhea. Occasionally, there is enlargement of the clitoris and deepening of the voice. Symptoms of virilism are usually milder in secondary Cushing's syndrome. Changes in males are generally not clinically significant, although gynecomastia, loss of body and facial hair, and reduced sexual potency may occasionally develop.

**E**motional Changes Excessive cortisol secretion also precipitates alterations in the patient's emotional status. *Emotional lability* is common, and the patient often bursts into tears for no apparent reason. Irritability, insomnia, depression, and euphoria are characteristic symptoms which may be noted in varying degrees. With severe disruptions in cortisol secretion, frank schizophrenia or other psychosis may develop.

**First-level nursing care** Currently, prevention of most causes of Cushing's syndrome is virtually impossible. No one can predict with any certainty who will develop adrenal or pituitary dysfunction or a malignancy which will result in hypercortisolism. As in adrenocortical insufficiency, judicious use of corticosteroids in the treatment of nonendocrine disease conditions can prevent or minimize the cushingoid effects produced by chronic therapy. The dosage of exogenous glucocorticoid necessary to cause the development of symptoms varies with individuals. The daily administration of as little as 10 mg prednisone/day may precipitate the onset of cushingoid changes. Dosages of corticosteroids should be adjusted so that the patient is taking the minimal amount necessary to control the disease process. Again, there is evidence to support use of an alternate-day schedule, when feasible, to reduce the incidence of these complications. Additional details regarding steroid therapy and its nursing implications are discussed in the section on adrenocortical insufficiency.

**Second-level nursing care** The onset of Cushing's syndrome is insidious. The presenting symptoms are dependent upon the etiology, severity, and duration of the disease. Many of the classic signs and symptoms of Cushing's syndrome are absent early in the course of the illness. Although diagnosis may be facilitated by the characteristic combination of physical changes, occurrence of similar symptoms in noncushingoid patients complicates case finding and evaluation.

**N**ursing Assessment Significant symptomatology elicited during the *health history* and *physical examination* focuses on the effects of altered metabolism on physical appearance. The patient should be questioned regarding changes in body structure and facial appearance, particularly weight, muscle size and development, and fat deposition. Changes in appearance may have occurred so gradually as to be unnoticed by the patient, family, or close friends; comparing the patient's present appearance with that in old photographs may be helpful. The patient may appear generally obese or an obvious disproportion between the size of the trunk and extremities may be noted. While the trunk is comparatively large and heavy, the extremities are thin and wasted (see Fig. 21-5). However, if excess androgen production is a part of the syndrome, muscle size may be preserved or increased. In the ectopic ACTH syndrome, the individual is frequently thin and emaciated secondary to the malignant process. The weight should be obtained and compared with previous recordings.

A thorough assessment of the integument should be performed. Patients may report that they bruise more easily and that skin breaks down after minimal trauma. Wounds heal slowly or not at all. The skin should be examined for ecchymoses and evidence of poor healing and infection. The presence of pink or purplish striae, particularly over the abdomen, thighs, breasts, and upper arms should be noted. Assessment of facial coloring may reveal patchy hyperemic areas. The presence of dark, coarse facial hair, thin scalp hair, and acne in females may be indicative of excess androgen levels.

Symptoms of osteoporotic changes may be elicited by questioning the patient regarding the incidence of frequent or persistent backache. Changes in body alignment, posture, and height should be noted on physical examination.

Changes in sexual characteristics should also be assessed. In addition to alterations in distribution of hair and in muscle size, the female with Cushing's syndrome should be asked about disturbances in menstruation or voice changes. Examination of the genitalia may reveal enlargement of the clitoris. The cushingoid male may report problems with decreased libido and impotence.

Questioning should be directed toward changes in activity tolerance and behavior patterns. A history of progressive physical weakness may be reported. The patient or family may have noted unusual behavior, such as inappropriate crying, euphoria, irritability, or depression. Changes in sleeping habits should also be elicited, as insomnia may be a problem.

Cardiovascular status should be assessed. The blood pressure is measured and compared with previous recordings. The lower extremities should be examined for evidence of edema, and the patient questioned regarding symptoms of shortness of breath or chest pain.

Changes in bladder patterns, such as polyuria or nocturia, may be reported, possibly indicating glucosuria. The presence of any symptoms of urinary tract infection, such as frequency, burning on urination, cloudy urine, or flank pain should be elicited and urinalysis performed, if indicated.

*Diagnostic tests* Several routine screening procedures may be employed to assist in confirming the diagnosis of Cushing's syndrome and evaluating the need for further testing. The mineralocorticoid effects of excessive cortisol levels may result in elevated *serum sodium levels* and depressed *potassium levels*. A metabolic acidosis may be associated with hypokalemia. Fasting serum glucose levels are elevated in some patients, while glucose tolerance tests are abnormal in the majority of cases. Disturbances in the rate of gluconeogenesis and increased insulin resistance are responsible for these effects. *Glucosuria* may also be present.

Glucocorticoids in high concentrations shrink lymphoid tissue and inhibit the production and release of lymphocytes and eosinophils. *Lymphocytes* are decreased to less than 15 percent and *eosinophils* to less than $50/mm^3$, while the *total white blood cell count* itself is increased.

Various *radiologic studies* may be helpful in establishing the diagnosis or etiology of Cushing's syndrome. These include evaluation of the sella turcica and adrenals by x-ray and angiography. The presence of adrenal or pituitary tumors or other nonendocrine neoplasms may be ascertained, as well as evidence of osteoporosis and pathologic fractures.

More specific diagnostic studies may be performed on an out-patient basis. The *free urinary cortisol,* the biologically active non-protein-bound cortisol which is excreted unaltered in the urine, provides a definitive index of adrenocortical hyperfunction. Its concentrations in a 24-hour collection are increased in patients with Cushing's syndrome.

The low-dose or the standard *dexamethasone suppression test* may be used as a screening procedure. The low-dose test involves the administration of 1.0 mg of the drug at 11 or 12 P.M. and measurement of plasma cortisol levels the following morning. Normally, suppression of cortisol levels occurs. This study is discussed in greater detail in Third-Level Nursing Care.

**N**ursing Problems and Intervention The nurse's primary role in the community is *case finding* and *referral* of patients suspected of having Cushing's syndrome. Early diagnosis and treatment can help to prevent or minimize damage to body systems which would occur if the disease remained uncontrolled for a prolonged period of time. Initially, hospitalization is often necessary for a more extensive diagnostic evaluation and treatment of problems.

**Third-level nursing care** As in adrenocortical insufficiency, the nature of many of the specific diagnostic tests for Cushing's syndrome usually necessitates hospitalization for close supervision. *Nursing assessment* reveals a health history and physical assessment similar to that discussed in Second Level Nursing Care. Because adrenocortical hypersecretion may be due to abnormalities in the hypothalamic-pituitary-adrenal system or a paraendocrine tumor, diagnostic studies must indicate the cause of the cortisol excess before appropriate treatment can be instituted.

**D**iagnostic Tests Many aspects of the diagnostic tests used to evaluate the patient with Cushing's syndrome are discussed in detail in the section on hypofunction of the adrenal cortex. The reader should refer to that section to supplement this discussion. The results of studies to evaluate Cushing's syndrome are summarized in Table 21-7.

Loss of the circadian rhythm of cortisol secretion occurs early in the development of Cushing's syndrome. *Plasma cortisol levels* may be evaluated initially to determine the existence of *diurnal patterns*. Specimens are drawn between 6 and 8 A.M. and 10 and 12 P.M. Normal levels in nonstressed patients range from 10 to 25 $\mu$g/100 ml in the morning and gradually decrease to less than 10 $\mu$g/100 ml in the evening. However, several factors may affect the reliability of this test. Any form of stress may obliterate the normal diurnal variation. The episodic pattern of cortisol secretion can produce misleading results when spot samples are relied upon. Plasma cortisol levels are increased in women on oral contraceptives and many obese individuals, while the diurnal variation may be lost in severely depressed individuals and in some disorders of the central nervous system. Normal values may be transposed in individuals who have worked at night and slept during the day for a long period of time.

In those centers with appropriate laboratory facilities a *plasma ACTH assay* may be drawn to help differentiate the etiology of Cushing's syndrome. Normally, ACTH synthesis is suppressed when cortisol levels are elevated. ACTH is usually undetectable with adrenal tumors. When adrenocortical hyperplasia is secondary to pituitary hypersecretion of ACTH, levels are only slightly elevated or at the upper limits of normal. Levels are significantly elevated when the origin of the disorder is a paraendocrine tumor.

The *dexamethasone suppression test* differentiates adrenal hypersecretion due to pituitary dysfunction from that due to ectopic ACTH syndrome or an adrenal tumor. Dexamethasone is a potent synthetic corticosteroid which suppresses ACTH release but does not significantly interfere with the measurement of steroid levels. Emotional or physical stress can produce a resistance to dexamethasone suppression of ACTH. Exposure to any stressful situation would precipitate a physiologic increase in ACTH and cortisol production and interfere with test results. For this reason, it is particularly important that the nurse identify potential stresses and assist the patient in avoiding them. Sedation may be prescribed, if necessary.

Baseline plasma cortisol and 24-hour urinary 17-OHCS are measured. A dose of 0.5 mg dexamethasone is then given orally every 6 hours for eight doses, and plasma cortisol and 24-hour urine specimens are collected. In the normal individual suppression of plasma cortisol and urinary 17-OHCS is observed at this dosage. However, the patient with Cushing's syndrome is relatively resistant to the suppressive effect of dexamethasone, except when administered in high doses. If suppression does not occur, the dosage of dexamethasone is increased to 2.0 mg every 6 hours for eight doses. Plasma cortisol and urinary 17-OHCS will be partially or totally suppressed if the adrenal gland is under pituitary control. There is no suppression in most cases of adrenal tumors or ectopic ACTH syndrome. Exceptions do occur and complicate determination of the exact etiology of the syndrome.

The *metyrapone (Metopirone) test* differentiates the presence of adrenocortical hyperplasia from adrenal tumor by revealing whether the

**TABLE 21-7**
DIAGNOSTIC STUDIES TO EVALUATE
ADRENOCORTICAL HYPERFUNCTION RESULTS

| Test | Cushing's Disease | Adrenal Tumor | Ectopic ACTH |
|---|---|---|---|
| Plasma cortisol | Normal to increased No diurnal variation | Increased No diurnal variation | Increased No diurnal variation |
| Free urinary cortisol | Increased | Increased | Increased |
| Plasma ACTH | Increased | Not detectable or low | Greatly increased |
| Urinary 17-OHCS | Normal or increased | Usually increased | Increased |
| Dexamethasone suppression test | No suppression on 2 mg Suppression 50% control on 8 mg 1 day (<10 mg 1 day) | No suppression | No suppression |
| 8-Hour intravenous ACTH stimulation test | Hyperresponsive | Usually no response (may be response with adenoma) | Usually no response |
| Metyrapone test | Increased two- to fourfold over baseline | Minimal or no response | Usually no response |

pituitary-adrenal feedback mechanism is intact. Metyrapone blocks cortisol synthesis, thus decreasing cortisol levels. Through the negative feedback mechanism the decrease in cortisol stimulates ACTH secretion. Since cortisol itself cannot be synthesized, large amounts of cortisol precursors are formed which may be measured as urinary 17-OHCS. Interpretation of the test requires that adrenal responsiveness to ACTH first be proven. An *ACTH stimulation test* should be performed prior to the metyrapone test. (See Table 21-7 for results.)

Before the test a baseline 24-hour urine for 17-OHCS is collected. Metyrapone 750 mg is given orally every 4 hours for 24 hours. Owing to its brief half-life, failure to give the drug on time can affect test results. Another 24-hour urine is collected concurrently and on the following day. The level of 17-OHCS will normally rise two- to fourfold. This response is exaggerated in Cushing's disease, while there is no response with adrenal tumors owing to suppression of pituitary ACTH secretion.

Because metyrapone inhibits cortisol synthesis, the nurse should be alert to signs of impending addisonian crisis. These symptoms are discussed in Adrenocortical Insufficiency. Nausea and vertigo, which may result with the rapid absorption of metyrapone from the gastrointestinal tract, are minimized by giving the drug with milk or a small amount of food.

**N**ursing Problems and Interventions   The psychological and emotional changes induced by the excessive levels of cortisol influences the patient's self-image and reactions to the environment. The frequently pronounced and undesirable changes in body image often decrease self-esteem. *Emotional lability* with mood swings and periods of *euphoria, irritability,* or *depression* affect interpersonal relationships. The patient, family, and friends should be aware of the physiologic basis for the altered behavior patterns. Acceptance and reassurance from family members and hospital personnel are important to help the patient to deal with these physical and emotional changes. An opportunity should be given to express feelings, and patients should not be condemned for inappropriate behavior. Realization that the physical and emotional changes may be reversible with treatment may relieve much of the patient's apprehension and concern. The nurse should be supportive not only in the nurse-patient relationship but by working with family members to help them cope with the patient's behavior.

The degree of *weakness* and *muscular wasting* varies with the severity and duration of the disease.

Motor ability and exercise tolerance should be assessed and interventions regarding assistance with activities of daily living planned accordingly. Scheduled periods of rest should be provided. Range of motion exercises can be performed daily to maintain muscle tone. If insomnia prevents the patient from getting adequate sleep at night, appropriate nursing measures can be employed to promote relaxation. If necessary, sedation may be prescribed.

When osteoporotic changes are severe and involve the spine, the patient may have *difficulty maintaining balance.* Assistance with ambulation is especially important to prevent accidental injury. Use of a walker or cane may increase stability. The patient's call bell should be within reach at all times. If the patient is disoriented or receiving sedation at night, side rails and a night light will help to reduce the possibility of injury. A firm mattress can be provided, and a brace may be prescribed for support. The patient should avoid direct bending and be instructed in the use of correct body mechanics.

The immunosuppressive and anti-inflammatory effects of excessive cortisol *impair* the patient's *ability to cope with infection.* Protection from other patients, visitors, and staff with respiratory infections should be provided. Close observation for minor signs of infection, such as a slight increase in temperature, is necessary, as the normal body responses are often depressed. The patient may be prone to urinary tract infections if glucosuria is present. The appearance of the urine should be assessed, and the patient questioned regarding symptoms of frequency, urgency, and burning on urination. Catheterization should be avoided.

The characteristically *paperlike skin* of the cushingoid patient is easily injured. Skin integrity should be assessed for evidence of breakdown. Paper tape rather than adhesive should be used to secure dressings or tubing. If the patient is extremely weak or on bed rest, precautions such as frequent turning, skin care, proper positioning and support, and flotation pads or sheepskins can be employed to prevent loss of skin integrity.

The patient with Cushing's syndrome exhibits a tendency toward *easy bruising* due to capillary fragility. Therefore, direct pressure must be applied over all injection and venipuncture sites to reduce bleeding into the subcutaneous tissues. Precautions should be taken to prevent trauma when the patient is ambulating or being transported.

When *hyperglycemia* and *glucosuria* occur or *diabetes mellitus* has been diagnosed, urine sugars should be checked routinely before meals and at bedtime. While the patient's diet may be sodium- and calorie-restricted, high intake of protein is encouraged to counteract the catabolic effects of excessive cortisol. Small, frequent feedings throughout the day help satisfy the patient's increased appetite.

Blood pressure and weight should be monitored to assess the degree of *hypertension* and *sodium and water retention*. If the patient is on digitalis or diuretic therapy, potassium levels must be assessed at intervals. Serum potassium should be maintained well within normal limits to prevent symptoms of digitalis toxicity. Supplements may be provided in the diet or with pharmaceutical preparations.

*Treatment*   The therapeutic goal in the treatment of Cushing's syndrome is to reduce excessive cortisol production. The specific method of therapy employed is dependent upon the nature and origin of the underlying lesion. It may involve chemotherapy, irradiation, adrenalectomy, or hypophysectomy.

In primary Cushing's syndrome removal of the tumor by *adrenalectomy* is the treatment of choice. If the tumor is not surgically resectable due to widespread metastases or the carcinoma recurs, chemotherapy is utilized. In secondary Cushing's syndrome associated with pituitary hypersecretion and adrenal hyperplasia, the choice of therapy remains controversial. Several approaches have been employed with varying degrees of success. These include *pituitary ablation* by irradiation or cryosurgery, surgical removal of the pituitary (*hypophysectomy*), and *bilateral adrenalectomy.*

When Cushing's syndrome results from an ectopic ACTH-secreting tumor, the prognosis is usually poor. Removal of the tumor will relieve the hypercortisolism; however, these tumors are often malignant and widely metastasized by the time diagnosis is made. Treatment measures are generally palliative and often include the use of adrenal inhibitors.

In mild cases of Cushing's syndrome *external pituitary irradiation* with 4000 to 5000 rads over a period of approximately one month has been effective in reducing cortisol secretion in a small percentage of patients. *Proton beam irradiation* has been somewhat more successful in effecting a remission. Several weeks to months are required before the patient may appreciate the maximal benefit of therapy. *Adrenal inhibitors* may be used in conjunction with irradiation to reduce cortisol levels pending maximal benefit of radiation therapy

or when cortisol levels remain only marginally elevated. Hypersecretion of cortisol frequently recurs, necessitating further therapy by other methods. Hypopituitarism with secondary hypogonadism and hypothyroidism is an occasional side effect.

Local needle implants of *yttrium 90,* a radioactive isotope, and *cryosurgery* are also used to ablate the pituitary gland. Panhypopituitarism occurs frequently. Leakage of cerebrospinal fluid and secondary development of meningitis are additional side effects with these methods.

If pituitary hypersecretion has resulted in advanced cushingoid symptoms or if severe hypertension, severe diabetes, rapidly progressive osteoporosis, or serious psychological problems are present, *bilateral adrenalectomy* is the treatment of choice. *Pituitary irradiation* may also be used in conjunction with adrenalectomy, as it is thought to reduce the later development of pituitary chromophobe adenomas and prevent hyperpigmentation due to elevation of ACTH and MSH (Nelson's syndrome).

*Adrenal surgery*   The technique used for adrenal surgery varies with the type and extent of the lesion and the surgeon's preference. Four different approaches have been advocated: the transabdominal, abdominothoracic, posterior, and posterolateral. Frequently, both adrenal glands are explored simultaneously for evidence of pathology with total removal of one or both glands as indicated. Subtotal adrenalectomy has generally proved unsuccessful, as the adrenal remnant either produces insufficient amounts of adrenocortical hormones or again becomes hyperplastic.

Adequate *preoperative preparation* is important in reducing serious complications during and after surgery. Explanations regarding the surgical procedure and results should be provided and reinforced as necessary. The importance of coughing, turning, and deep breathing should be stressed, and the correct techniques practiced by the patient preoperatively. Adequate dietary intake should be encouraged to improve nutritional status, promote a positive nitrogen balance, and provide supplemental potassium. Blood pressures and weight should be monitored closely for signs of severe hypertension and fluid overload. Urine samples should be evaluated frequently for glucose, and insulin given as indicated.

Supplemental steroid therapy is begun prior to surgery in anticipation that the surgical procedure may precipitate acute adrenal insufficiency. Excessive cortisol levels secreted by the tumor suppress production by the normal adrenal tissue. It may take several months for the suppressed gland to completely recover. Meticulous attention must be given to administering the patient's prescribed replacement regimen before, during, and after surgery. *Postoperatively,* the patient should be monitored closely for signs of hemorrhage or impending addisonian crisis. A relative deficiency of cortisol may exist despite preoperative therapy when compared with excessive presurgical levels. Blood pressure and pulse should be monitored frequently, and urine output checked hourly. Intravenous fluids and vasopressors are administered as indicated.

If the surgical approach involved entry into the pleural cavity, the patient should be observed for symptoms of pneumothorax, such as dyspnea or sudden chest pain. Coughing, deep breathing, and turning should be performed by the patient at least every 2 hours to prevent atelectasis and respiratory infections.

Because of the instability of the vascular system, elastic support hose may be prescribed to prevent venous stasis. Flexion and extension exercises can be performed as tolerated to promote circulation in the lower extremities. Medication for pain is administered as needed to reduce stress and promote rest. Nausea and vomiting with paralytic ileus occur commonly when the abdominal approach is used, and nasogastric suction may be necessary until symptoms diminish.

The major complications of adrenal surgery in the patient with Cushing's syndrome are hemorrhage and wound infection or breakdown which occur as a result of the long-term effects of hypercortisolism. The surgical incision should be observed closely for signs of infection or impaired healing. Strain on the incision can be avoided by providing proper splinting or support when the patient is active. Sterile technique when changing dressings is essential.

Postoperatively, many patients note improvement in physical appearance. A fine desquamation of the skin develops after a few days, and striae begin to heal within a few weeks. While some patients regain normal weight within a few months, others who have always been obese remain so. If hypertension has existed for only a short period before treatment, blood pressure will usually return to normal after 4 to 8 weeks. Patients frequently develop a psychologic dependency on the euphoric effects of hypercortisolism. Emotional problems may be enhanced after the sudden decrease in cortisol levels, with the patient experiencing severe depression, fatigue, and anorexia. Slow withdrawal

by tapering replacement dosages of glucocorticoids over a period of months may be necessary. However, marked improvement in emotional symptoms usually occurs after a few days of maintenance therapy. Symptoms of bone tenderness are usually relieved, although osteoporosis often persists on x-ray. Clinical manifestations of diabetes usually improve markedly after surgery.

*Pituitary surgery Hypophysectomy* may be performed when irradiation of the pituitary is ineffective or there is an enlarged pituitary tumor causing visual field changes (usually bitemporal hemianopsia) or symptoms of increased intracranial pressure. Surgical approaches include the transsphenoidal, transethmoidal, and transcranial. The transsphenoidal microsurgical approach is being used with increasing frequency and success. This route involves entry into the sella turcica via a small incision made under the upper lip.

Preoperative preparation is similar to that discussed under Adrenal Surgery above. The patient should be given an opportunity to express concerns about the procedure, future chemotherapy, and possible sterility. Postoperatively, the patient is observed not only for symptoms of adrenal insufficiency but also for symptoms of increased intracranial pressure. Vital signs, pupillary equality and response, level of consciousness, and motor function should be evaluated frequently. The head of the bed is elevated to facilitate venous return and reduce intracranial pressure and headache.

Urine output and specific gravity are measured hourly to detect excessive output of dilute urine indicating a deficiency of ADH. Pitressin may be ordered if output is excessive. The deficiency is usually temporary (2 to 3 weeks), as the hypothalamus is responsible for the production and secretion of ADH.

After transsphenoidal hypophysectomy the nose is packed with gauze for a few days. The patient should be observed for symptoms from leakage of cerebrospinal fluid, which include a clear nasal drip or constant swallowing. Cerebrospinal fluid can be differentiated from nasal secretions by testing the drainage for glucose with a glucose-sensitive strip. A positive test indicates a cerebrospinal fluid leak. An elevation in temperature associated with headache should be reported, as meningitis is a serious postoperative complication. Antibiotics may be given prophylactically because of the increased risk of infection with the transsphenoidal route. The patient should avoid nose-blowing, coughing vigorously, or initiating a Valsalva maneuver for 48 hours postoperatively to prevent bleeding or accidental dislodgement of any packing in the sella turcica. Cold compresses may be applied to the eyes to reduce the edema and discomfort. Long-term care following hypophysectomy is discussed in Fourth-Level Nursing Care.

*Chemotherapy* Chemotherapy with *dichlorodiphenyldichloroethane (o,p'-DDD)* has been shown to decrease the tumor size and control hypersecretion of cortisol in cases of adrenal carcinoma. The drug has a direct toxic effect on adrenal tissue, inhibiting only cortical synthesis through destruction of the zona fasciculata and zona reticularis. Several weeks or months of therapy may be necessary before cortisol levels decrease to normal. Close monitoring of therapy is necessary to minimize the risk of total loss of cortisol secretory capacity. The drug is given orally in gradually increasing doses until the desired effect is obtained or toxic symptoms develop. Toxic symptoms include nausea and vomiting, vertigo, ataxia, and, less frequently, skin rash, diarrhea, and central nervous system depression with somnolence and lethargy. Side effects persist for extended periods after the drug is discontinued, since it is stored in fatty tissue and released slowly. Because *o,p'-DDD* alters the extraadrenal metabolism of cortisol, plasma levels of 17-OHCS are measured to assess response to therapy. Glucocorticoid therapy may be administered prophylactically as a precaution against development of adrenal insufficiency. Mineralocorticoid replacement is unnecessary, since aldosterone production is unaffected.

Metyrapone and *aminoglutethimide* (Elipten) have been used in conjunction with *o,p'-DDD* therapy to block cortisol synthesis. Dosages must be carefully monitored to prevent development of adrenal insufficiency. Adrenal inhibitors may also be used for several weeks preoperatively to control hypercortisolism, improve the patient's physical status, and decrease the surgical risk.

**Fourth-level nursing care** The prognosis with Cushing's syndrome is significantly improved with appropriate therapy in most cases. Unfortunately, patients are usually dependent on some form of daily hormonal replacement for a period ranging from several months to the remainder of their lives. The choice of therapy and patient response determine the hormones and dosages to be prescribed. Patient education and follow-up are important aspects of care, and the necessity for continued intervention and evaluation of the therapeutic regimen should be emphasized.

If *bilateral adrenalectomy* is performed, care is similar to that of the patient with adrenocortical insufficiency, discussed in detail earlier in this chapter. Mineralocorticoid replacement may not be necessary if the patient was significantly hypertensive before treatment. Adequate salt intake should be encouraged.

Hypersecretion of cortisol by an adrenal tumor results in suppression of pituitary ACTH secretion and atrophy of the opposite adrenal gland. Therefore, with *unilateral adrenalectomy,* glucocorticoid replacement is usually required during the first postoperative year. The steroid is given in the lowest dose possible to permit recovery of the hypothalamic-pituitary-adrenal system. Laboratory studies are conducted at intervals to evaluate the degree of recovery. Patients should be advised that supplementary glucocorticoid therapy may be necessary in times of stress for at least 1 year after removal of the tumor as a precautionary measure against addisonian crisis.

Following loss of the *pituitary gland* either by surgical removal or destruction with irradiation, the pituitary trophic hormones will be deficient. Consequently, their target glands often develop insufficiency. Steroid replacement will be necessary. In addition, patients should be instructed regarding symptoms of hypothyroidism. Development of symptoms usually occurs gradually over a period of several weeks and includes tiredness, lethargy, dry skin, intolerance to cold, and constipation. Replacement therapy with a thyroid preparation is prescribed as indicated. Replacement of antidiuretic hormone may be temporarily necessary. The patient should be taught what symptoms indicate deficiency and how to administer the medication.

Testosterone is frequently prescribed to alleviate the impotence and loss of libido experienced by males. In younger women estrogens may be administered to correct vaginal mucosal atrophy. Fertility can now be restored in some patients, particularly females, with the use of human pituitary gonadotropins.[18] Patients and their spouses should be provided opportunities to discuss their feelings and concerns about sexual and reproductive functioning. Resources for counseling and therapy can be suggested and referrals made to appropriate agencies.

When adrenal tissue has been destroyed by *o,p'-DDD* therapy, the amount of glucocorticoid therapy prescribed will depend on the degree of glandular destruction. Maintenance dosages may be necessary on a daily basis or only when the patient is under stress. The patient should be alerted to the signs and symptoms of hypo- and hypersecretion of cortisol and instructed in the action to take if they occur.

The patient and family need to realize that, depending on the therapy used, several weeks may pass before physical appearance and emotional behavior return to the preillness state. If the syndrome has existed for several years, some sequelae of the disease related to cardiovascular and osteoporotic changes will remain. Although the symptoms of the syndrome may be resolved with therapy, any malignant process is frequently only temporarily affected.

Follow-up care for a patient with Cushing's syndrome is essential. With all forms of treatment the normal mechanisms used by the body to combat stress have been altered. At regular intervals the nurse should reevaluate the effectiveness of treatment. Symptoms of either over- or undertreatment with glucocorticoids and recurrence of the disease should be observed for. The patient and family's understanding of this complicated disease and the treatment regimen should be reinforced periodically. Counseling should be provided to help the patient and family cope with the emotional changes and alterations in body image that occur.

## PITUITARY DYSFUNCTION

The anterior pituitary gland (adenohypophysis) is responsible for the secretion of the growth hormone and several trophic hormones which regulate the function of other endocrine glands in the body. Clinical manifestations of pituitary dysfunction are dependent upon the hormones involved; hypo- or hypersecretion of pituitary hormones precipitates a similar response in the target glands or tissues.

### Hypersecretion of Growth Hormone

Excessive levels of growth hormone (*somatotropin*) generally occur as a result of a hypersecreting pituitary tumor. Prior to the age of puberty and closure of the epiphyses of the long bones, excessive production of somatotropin causes *gigantism.* Growth is enhanced, and individuals may reach heights of 8 to 9 feet. In adults, overproduction of growth hormone causes *acromegaly,* a condition characterized by thickening of bones and hypertrophy of soft tissues. Onset of the disease is insidious, beginning most commonly in the third and

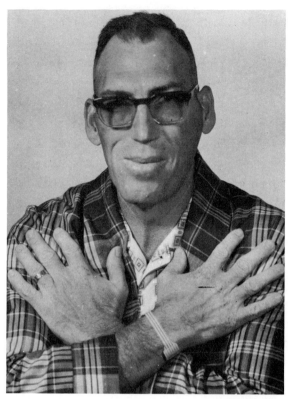

**FIGURE 21-6**
Patient with acromegaly. Note the large, broad hands, stubby thumbs, thick lips, and prominent jaw. The classic full-blown features of acromegaly are seldom seen at the present time, since treatment is instituted at a much earlier stage than formerly. (*From S. I. Schwartz et al.: McGraw-Hill, New York, 1974. With permission of the publisher.*)

fourth decades. It occurs two to three times more frequently in women than men.

Elevated somatotropin levels affect most organs and tissues, and patients may show a variety of symptoms. *Changes in physical appearance* are striking but develop so gradually that they may initially be unnoticed by the patient, family, or friends. Facial features become coarse and heavy. The mandible is enlarged and elongated. Lips and tongue thicken. The nose increases in size. Enlargement of the sinuses causes the forehead to become prominent (Fig. 21-6). The skin thickens and becomes leathery. Pores and skin markings are more noticeable. Sebaceous and sweat glands increase in number and size; excessive sweating and oiliness of the skin are common. Body hair becomes coarse and increases in amount.

The hands and feet widen, and the first symptoms usually noted are increases in show, glove, and

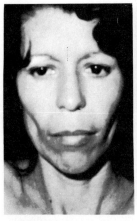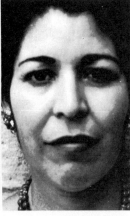

**FIGURE 21-7**
Photographs of a 40-year-old woman when first seen with hypopituitarism (Simmond's disease) and after 6 months' therapy. (*From M. M. Wintrobe et al.: Harrison's Principles of Internal Medicine, McGraw-Hill, New York, 1974. With permission of the publisher.*)

ring sizes. Overgrowth of bone and soft tissues predisposes the individual to degenerative changes in the joints, and arthritis or severe arthralgias occur. Compression of peripheral nerves causes the development of paresthesias. As with the cushingoid individual, adverse changes in body image contribute to the development of emotional problems.

*Enlargement of visceral organs* is common. With an increase in heart size (cardiomegaly), hypertension and congestive failure may develop. The thyroid, parathyroid, and adrenal glands, spleen, kidneys, liver, and pancreas may also be enlarged. Other *endocrine problems* frequently occur in conjunction with excessive growth hormone levels, including diabetes mellitus, impotency, and amenorrhea.

If the pituitary tumor is large and compresses neighboring structures, symptoms of increased intracranial pressure may be noted. Headache is common. Compression of the optic nerve produces changes in visual fields, particularly bitemporal hemianopsia. Visual acuity may also be impaired, progressing to total blindness.

Early diagnosis of acromegaly is difficult because of its insidious onset. Various radiologic studies may be performed to confirm the presence of a pituitary tumor and bony changes. Serum growth hormone levels are drawn to detect any elevation.

Physical changes in acromegaly are irreversible, and therapy is aimed at arresting the disease process. The treatment involves pituitary ablation by irradiation, cryosurgery, or surgical removal of the gland. Hormone replacement therapy and nursing care are similar to those discussed in the section on Cushing's syndrome. Other aspects of nursing care include proper positioning and support of painful joints, frequent hygiene to reduce skin oiliness and body odor, and maintenance of proper nutrition to meet increased body demands.

### Hypopituitarism

*Hypopituitarism* refers to a deficiency of one or more of the hormones secreted by the anterior pituitary gland. *Panhypopituitarism* indicates an absence of all hormones released by the pituitary. The terms *pituitary cachexia* and *Simmond's disease* (originally describing septic infarction of the gland following postdelivery pelvic inflammation) have been used synonymously.

Pituitary insufficiency in the adult is caused by nonfunctioning tumors, surgical removal or irradiation of the gland, postpartum necrosis of the pituitary (Sheehan's syndrome), and, less commonly, granulomatous disease. The lack of pituitary hormones results in a reduction in the hormones released by the target glands. Clinical features of hypogonadism, hypothyroidism, and/or hypoadrenalism may develop, depending on the hormones involved. When hypopituitarism results from intrinsic disease or irradiation, symptoms develop gradually and are usually absent until approximately seventy-five percent of the gland has been destroyed. After hypophysectomy, secondary adrenal insufficiency develops within days and hypothyroidism after a month.

With hypogonadism, which is often the initial imbalance, there is regression of secondary sex characteristics. Facial and body hair decrease and reproductive organs and muscle tissue atrophy. There is loss of libido, impotency, amenorrhea, and infertility. Symptoms of secondary thyroid and adrenal deficiency appear later. (These are discussed in detail in their respective sections.) Hypoglycemia may occur due to a deficiency of growth hormone.

In hypopituitarism there is also a loss of normal skin pigmentation, which becomes pale and waxy in appearance. Fine wrinkles develop around the eyes and mouth, making the patient appear older than normal. When pituitary deficiency is severe, there is extreme weight loss and emaciation with eventual coma and, if untreated, death. Figure 21-7 shows a patient with panhypopituitarism (Simmond's disease).

Because pituitary hormones are destroyed in

the gastrointestinal tract, treatment of hypopituitarism involves replacement of the deficient hormones of the target organs—thyroid, adrenals, and gonads. Only glucocorticoid replacement is usually necessary in pituitary-induced adrenal insufficiency since mineralocorticoid secretion remains adequate. Surgical intervention is indicated if a tumor is causing signs of intracranial pressure or optic nerve damage.

## REFERENCES

1  DeGroot, Leslie J., and J. B. Stanbury, *The Thyroid and Its Diseases,* Wiley, New York, 1975, p. 408.
2  *Ibid.,* 410.
3  *Ibid.,* 411.
4  *Ibid.,* 436.
5  *Ibid.,* 439.
6  Castle, William B., and Ralph O. Wallerstein, "Blood," in S. C. Werner and S. H. Ingbar (eds.), *The Thyroid,* Harper & Row, New York, 1971, pp. 786–789.
7  Pittman, J. A., G. E. Daily, and R. J. Besch, "Changing Normal Values for Thyroidal Radioiodine Uptake," *N Engl J Med,* **280:**1431–1434, June 26, 1969.
8  DeGroot, L. J., and J. B. Stanbury, *op. cit.,* p. 264.
9  Mazzaferri, E. L., et al., "Propranolol as Primary Therapy for Thyrotoxicosis," *Arch Intern Med,* **136:** 50–56, January 1976.
10  Ingbar, S. H., and K. A. Wolber, "The Thyroid Gland," in R. H. Williams (ed.), *Textbook of Endocrinology,* 5th ed., Saunders, Philadelphia, 1974, pp. 95–232.
11  Thomas, C. G., Jr., "Surgery," in *The Thyroid and Its Diseases,* Wiley, New York, 1975, p. 695.
12  Liddle, G. W., "Adrenal Cortex," in P. B. Beeson and W. McDermott (eds.), *Cecil-Loeb Textbook of Medicine,* 14th ed., Saunders, Philadelphia, 1975, pp. 1733–1746.
13  Bondy, P. K., "The Adrenal Cortex," in P. K. Bondy and L. E. Rosenberg (eds.), *Duncan's Diseases of Metabolism,* Saunders, Philadelphia, 1974, pp. 1105–1180.
14  Quintanilla, A. P., C. Delgado-Butron, and J. Zeballos, "Renal Hemodynamics and Water Excretion in Addison's Disease," *Metabolism,* **25:**419–425, April 1976.
15  Liddle, G. W., "The Adrenals," in R. H. Williams (ed.), *Textbook of Endocrinology,* 5th ed., Saunders, Philadelphia, 1974, pp. 233–283.
16  Bondy, P. K., *op. cit.,* p. 1148.
17  Liddle, G. W., *op. cit.,* p. 257.
18  Daughaday, W. H., "The Adenohypophysis," in R. H. Williams (ed.), *Textbook of Endocrinology,* 5th ed., Saunders, Philadelphia, 1974, pp. 31–79.

## BIBLIOGRAPHY

Besser, G. M., and C. R. W. Edwards: "Cushing's syndrome," *Clin Endocrinol Metab,* **1:**451–490, July 1972.

Bledsoe, Turner: "Surgery and the Adrenal Cortex," *Surg Clin North Am,* **54:**449–460, April 1974.

Blount, Mary, and Anna Belle Kinney: "Chronic Steroid Therapy," *Am J Nurs,* **74:**1626–1631, September 1974.

Burke, C. W.: "Cushing's Disease Treatment by Pituitary Implantation of Radioactive Gold or Yttrium Seeds," *Q J Med,* **42:**693–714, October 1973.

Conn, Harold O., and Bennett L. Blitzer: "Nonassociation of Adrenocorticosteroid Therapy and Peptic Ulcer," *N Engl J Med,* **294:**473–479, Feb. 26, 1976.

Egdahl, Richard H.: "Surgery of the Adrenal Gland," *N Engl J Med,* **278:**939–949, April 25, 1968.

Forsham, P. H.: "The Adrenals," in R. H. Williams (ed.), *Textbook of Endocrinology,* 4th ed., Saunders, Philadelphia, 1968, pp. 287–354.

Graber, Alan L., et al.: "Natural History of Pituitary-Adrenal Recovery Following Long-Term Suppression with Corticosteroids," *J Clin Endocrinol Metab,* **25:**11–16, January 1965.

Hamdi, Mary Evans: "Nursing Intervention for Patients Receiving Corticosteriod Therapy," in Kay Corman Kintzel (ed.), *Advanced Concepts in Clinical Nursing,* Lippincott, Philadelphia, 1971, pp. 236–245.

Hawkens, Patty: "Hypophysectomy with Yttrium 90," *Am J Nurs,* **65:**122–125, October 1965.

Hill, C. Stratton, Jr.: "Thyroid Cancer—Iatrogenic and Otherwise," *CA,* **26:**160–164, May/June 1976.

Hume, David M., and Timothy S. Harrison: "Pituitary and Adrenal," in Seymour I. Schwartz (ed.), *Textbook of Surgery,* 2d ed., McGraw-Hill, New York, 1974, pp. 1363–1390.

Illingworth, R. S.: "Abnormal Substances Excreted in Human Milk," *Practitioner,* **171:**533, November 1953.

Irvine, W. J., and E. W. Barnes: "Adrenocortical Insufficiency," *Clin Endocrinol Metab,* **1:**549–594, July 1972.

Knowles, John A.: "Excretion of Drugs in Milk—A Review," *J Pediatr,* **66:**1068–1082, June 1965.

Liddle, Grant W.: "Cushing's Syndrome," in A. B. Eisenstein (ed.), *The Adrenal Cortex,* Little, Brown, Boston, 1967, pp. 523–549.

———: "Pathogenesis of Glucocorticoid Disorders," *Am J Med,* **53:**638–648, November 1972.

Luckman, Joan, and Karen C. Sorenson: *Medical-Surgical Nursing: A Psychophysiologic Approach,* Saunders, Philadelphia, 1974, pp. 1366–1385.

Orth, David N., and Grant W. Liddle: "Results of Treatment in 108 Patients with Cushing's Syndrome," *N Engl J Med,* **285:**243–247, July 29, 1971.

Peake, Robert L.: "New Concepts in Graves' Disease," *Hosp Med,* **11:**74, October 1975.

Powaser, Mary M.: "The Patient with Metabolic Disorders," in Harriet C. Moidel et al. (eds.), *Nursing Care of the Patient with Medical-Surgical Disorders,* McGraw-Hill, New York, 1976, pp. 834–855.

Read, Sharon P.: "Clinical Care in Hypophysectomy," *Nurs Clin North Am,* **9:**647–654, December 1974.

Scott, William H., Jr. and Robert K. Rhamy: "The Pituitary and the Adrenals," in David C. Sabiston, Jr. (ed.), *Davis-Christopher Textbook of Surgery,* 10th edition, Saunders, Philadelphia, 1972, pp. 668–698.

Stowe, Sharon W.: "Hypophysectomy for Diabetic Retinopathy," *Am J Nurs,* **73:**632–637, April 1973.

Temple, T. Eugene, Jr., et al.: "Treatment of Cushing's Disease," *N Engl J Med,* **281:**801–804, Oct. 9, 1969.

The Adrenal Gland (Clinician 1) MEDCOM, New York: 1971 prepared for G. D. Searle, pp. 7–36.

Thorn, George W. (ed.): *Steroid Therapy,* MEDCOM, New York, 1971, pp. 6–42 (prepared for Upjohn Company).

——— and David P. Lauler: "Clinical Therapeutics of Adrenal Disorders," *Am J Med,* **53:**673–684, November 1972.

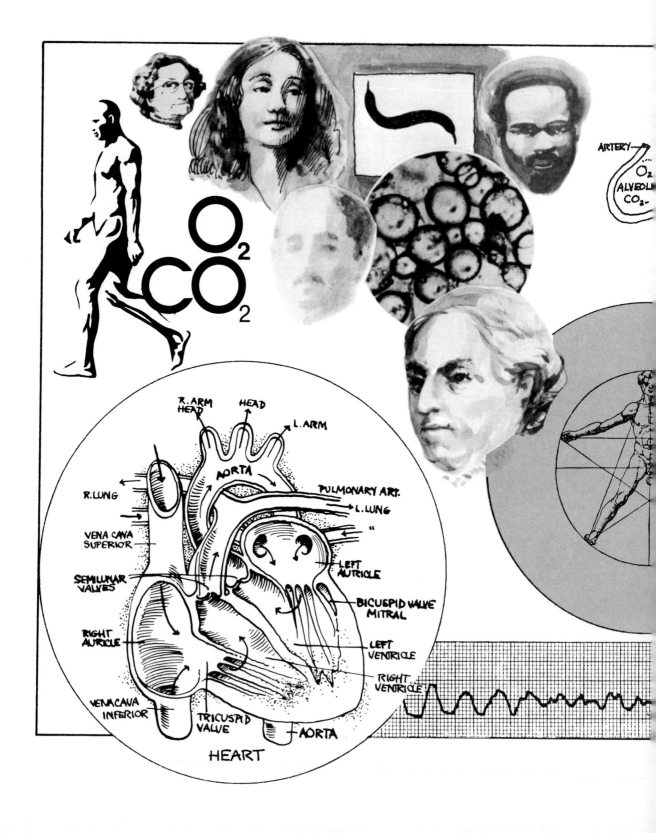

ARTERY
$O_2$
ALVEOLI
$CO_2$

$O_2$
$CO_2$

R. ARM
HEAD

HEAD

L. ARM

AORTA

R. LUNG

PULMONARY ART.

L. LUNG

VENA CAVA
SUPERIOR

"

LEFT
AURICLE

SEMILUNAR
VALVES

BICUSPID VALVE
MITRAL

RIGHT
AURICLE

LEFT
VENTRICLE

RIGHT
VENTRICLE

VENA CAVA
INFERIOR

TRICUSPID
VALVE

AORTA

HEART

# PART 6

## OXYGENATION

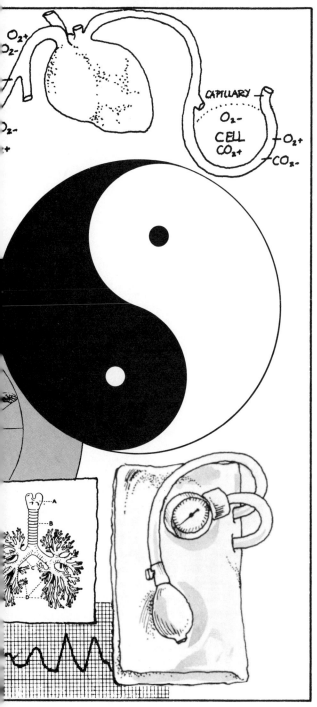

# 22

# THE CONCEPT OF OXYGENATION*

First the auricle contracts and in so doing it sends the content of blood into the ventricle of the heart.

When the ventricle is full the heart raises itself, forthwith tenses all its fibers, contracts the ventricles and gives a beat. By this means it ejects at once into the arteries the blood discharged into it by the auricle, the right ventricle doing so into the lungs through the vessel which is called the artery-like vein but is in fact in both structure and function . . . an artery, the left ventricle doing so into the aorta through the arteries into the whole of the body.[1]

Dorothy A. Jones
Joyce S. Martin

This theory of oxygenation, presented to the world by William Harvey in 1628, revolutionized the concept of circulation and oxygenation and set the stage for growth and progress in the field.

A neonate's introduction into the "human" world consists of the inspiration of oxygen into the body and the abandonment of the fetal oxygen transport system. This process initiates a system of oxygenation which will terminate only at the time of death. The concept of oxygenation then is the dynamic interaction involved in the transportation of oxygen to all body parts and the removal of carbon dioxide. This process includes the oxygen-carrying mechanism, the vessels as the transporting network, the heart as the pump, and the lungs as that component responsible for $O_2$ and $CO_2$ exchange.

## THE RED BLOOD CELL

*Blood* is composed of plasma and cells. Plasma and interstitial fluid make up the components of the extracellular fluid in the body (see Chap. 11). The hematocrit level represents the percentage of blood that is cells; an individual with a hematocrit level of 42 percent has blood which is composed of 42 percent red cells, while the remaining 58 percent is made of plasma.[2] The normal hematocrit level in the female is 42 percent and in the male 45 percent.

The cells of the blood include the erythrocyte (red blood cell), the leukocyte (white blood cell) (see Chap. 7 for a complete discussion), and the thrombocyte (platelet). The production of these elements is called *hemopoiesis,* while the production of red blood cells alone is referred to as *erythropoiesis.* Since the function of the leukocyte has already been discussed, this chapter will focus upon the production and function of the erythrocyte and the thrombocyte.

The production of red blood cells is an essential component of oxygenation. This process is a continuous one, and the underproduction or overproduction of red blood cells can interfere with circulation and contribute to tissue anoxia and changes in oxygen and carbon dioxide exchange.

### Erythrocyte Formation

The red blood cell (corpuscle), or *erythrocyte,* is shaped as a biconcave disk. This shape offers the

---

* The section on Physical Assessment was written by Joyce S. Martin. The section on Electrocardiogram was contributed by Mary B. McFarland.

erythrocyte the capability of passing easily through the veins, arteries, and capillaries throughout the body.

The most important function of the red blood cell (RBC) is to transport hemoglobin (with oxygen and other nutrients) from the lungs to the body tissues and vital organs. In addition, the RBC removes carbon dioxide from the tissues and returns it to the lungs. Finally, the hemoglobin within the RBC can act as an acid base buffer and is responsible for over 70 percent of the entire buffering power of whole blood.[3]

The red blood cell evolves from a hemocytoblast formed in the bone marrow. Figure 22-1 shows evolutionary stages in erythrocyte development. In early fetal development red blood cells are concentrated in the yoke sac. As the fetus grows, the liver takes over RBC development. As birth nears, RBCs are produced in the bone marrow as well as in such components as the liver, spleen, ribs, and long bones.

The basophil erythroblast begins hemoglobin synthesis.[4] As the cell passes through other stages of growth and development, red blood cells are produced. After the cytoplasm normoblast is filled with hemoglobin up to a concentration of 34 percent, the nucleus is absorbed and the reticulocyte or immature red blood cell, is formed.[5] The erythrocyte does not emerge until after 2 to 3 days following the production of the reticulocyte. This is due to the fact that some basophil reticulum is still present in the reticulocyte for a few days.

There are an average of 5,400,000 ($\pm$600,000) RBCs/mm$^3$ in the normal male and 4,600,000 ($\pm$500,000) RBCs/mm$^3$ in the normal female.[6]

**Factors influencing RBC production**   Physical activity affects the number of red blood cells produced. A very active individual can produce RBCs more rapidly than an individual lying in bed. Therefore, the RBC count of an active individual will be above normal limits, whereas the less active individual may have an RBC count below normal limits.

Tissue anoxia stimulates RBC production by a feedback system involving erythropoietin (see Fig. 22-2). Erythropoietin (hemopoietin) is a glucoprotein that is formed in the body in response to anoxia;[7] it is formed in the kidneys during anoxia, as well as in the liver. Erythropoietin acts upon the bone marrow to increase RBC production.

Several other factors influence the production of RBCs. As the individual *ages,* the bone marrow becomes less productive. In adulthood erythropoiesis occurs only in the proximal ends of the femora and humeri, the bones that form the ribs, stenum, skull, vertebrae, hands, and feet.[8] If the amount of atmospheric oxygen inspired decreases, the amount of oxygen transported will also diminish. The body compensates, however, by rapidly increasing the number of RBCs in the circulation.

Vitamin B$_{12}$ is an essential nutrient for cell growth and is vital for RBC production. If vitamin B$_{12}$ is inadequate, RBC production decreases and larger-than-normal erythrocytes (megaloblasts) are formed (see Chap. 23).

*Folic acid* is also necessary for RBC maturation. Both vitamin B$_{12}$ and folic acid are essential to formation of deoxyribonucleic acid (DNA), while vitamin B$_{12}$ is necessary for formation of ribonucleic acid (RNA). Folic acid and vitamin B$_{12}$ have similar functions in terms of RBC growth and maturation

**FIGURE 22-1**
Genesis of RBC formation.

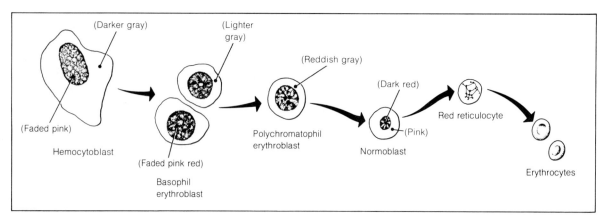

and can often substitute the functions for one another. However, vitamin $B_{12}$ alone is essential for maintaining the integrity of the central nervous system.

**H**emoglobin Formation    Hemoglobin is composed of two parts: *heme,* the iron-containing pigment, and *globin,* a protein made from a combination of 574 amino acids. In the adult hemoglobin there are two alpha chains of 141 amino acids each and two beta chains each containing 146 amino acids. Each chain is linked to one heme group. The heme and amino acid chain join together to form a hemoglobin molecule. Hemoglobin combines easily with oxygen and result in thousands of hemoglobin molecules within the mature erythrocyte. In the adult the average range of hemoglobin is 14 to 16 in the male and 12 to 14 in the female.

*Iron* is an essential component needed for hemoglobin formation. It is absorbed from the small intestines and combines with a beta globulin to form transferrin.[9] Excess iron is stored in the liver where it combines with a protein *apoferritin,* to form *ferritin.*

Iron is lost daily through excreta (feces) and through bleeding. Normally about 0.6 mg iron is lost each day. During menstruation up to 2.1 mg can be lost daily.

## Destruction of RBCs

Erythrocytes enter the circulation and undergo multiple metabolic changes during their 120-day lifespan. As they age they become more fragile and suddenly fragment. The fragments are destroyed by phagocytosis. Iron is released and stored in the bone marrow for new red blood cell production. The hemoglobin diffuses throughout the plasma, and the destroyed cell membrane is removed from the blood by the reticuloendothelial system (which includes the lymph nodes, bone marrow, connective tissue, liver, and spleen). Here the cells are broken down into their component parts (hemoglobin), and bilirubin production occurs.

**Bilirubin formation**    Bilirubin is a waste product formed from hemoglobin. It combines with plasma proteins throughout the body and is removed from the protein by the liver cells (conjugated bilirubin). In the liver it is formed into *bilirubin glucuronide,* secreted into the bile, and excreted from the body. In the presence of disruptions of liver function, excretion of bile may be altered. (See chapter 19 for a more complete discussion.)

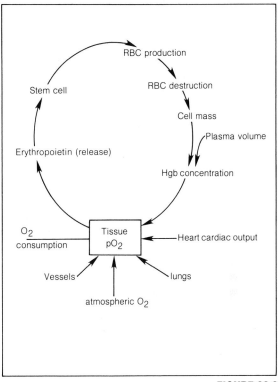

**FIGURE 22-2**

Feedback system for tissue oxygenation. (*Adapted from W. Williams, Hematology, McGraw-Hill, New York, 1972.*)

## BLOOD COAGULATION

The term *hemostasis* means prevention of blood loss.[10] There are three components of the hemostatic mechanism. These are platelets, blood vessels, and coagulation factors.

### Blood vessels

Several theories have been developed to explain the mechanism of blood clotting. Since no one theory is absolute, the following discussion is used to describe a sequence of events.

When trauma occurs to a blood vessel, the integrity of the vessel wall is interrupted and blood escapes from the area. Platelets travel to the area and adhere to the damaged endosurface to form a plug. This plug slows and eventually terminates the bleeding process. The degradation of the platelets causes a reuse of the platelet factor (incomplete thromboplastin) which interacts with other substances to form a *fibrous* clot at the injured site. Within 3 to 6 minutes after the initial injury the injured end of the vessel is filled with a clot. Within an hour the clot begins to retract.[11] See Fig. 22-3.

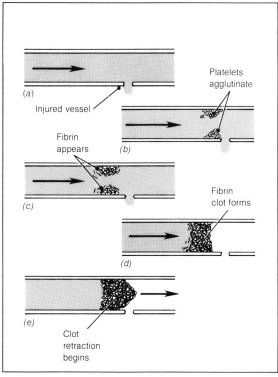

**FIGURE 22-3**
Blood vessel trauma and clot formation. (*Adapted from Arthur Guyton, Textbook of Medical Physiology, Saunders, Philadelphia, 1970.*)

## Platelets

Platelets are composed of a variety of cellular substances with the exclusion of DNA (see Table 22-1). Proteins are the major components of platelets. Approximately 15 percent of the total platelet protein is composed of adenosine triphosphate (ATPase) or thrombosthenin.

**TABLE 22-1**
COMPOSITION OF PLATELETS

|  | % weight, g/100 g |
| --- | --- |
| Water | 77.00 |
| Protein | 11.9–14.8* |
| Lipid | 2.9–4.9 |
| Carbohydrates | 1.94–1.10 |
| Ash | 2.2 |
| RNA | 0.20 |
| Amino acids | 0.59–0.53 |
| Adenine nucleotide | 0.20 |
| Reduced glutathione | 0.02–0.19 |

\* Major constituent of platelets: 15% of total protein is composed of adenosine triphosphatase and thrombosthenin.
SOURCE: William Williams, *Hematology*, McGraw-Hill, New York, 1972, p. 999.

Platelet factor II, also called fibrinogen-activating factor, and platelet factor IV (the antiheparin factor) are called *true* platelet proteins (that is, the ones not absorbed from the plasma).[12]

**Platelet production** Recent research seems to indicate that hormonal factors affect the production of platelets. Estrogen hormones seem to decrease platelet production, and steroids (corticosteriods) have been reported to supress platelet production.[13, 14] The spleen also influences platelet production. The platelets that are produced by the fragmentation of giant multinucleated cells are called *megakaryocytes.* These cells are the precursors of the thrombocytes. Maturation of a megakaryocyte takes about 4 to 5 days in human beings. Approximately 2000 to 7700 platelets are released by each megakaryocyte.[15,16]

Platelet membranes differ from the plasma membranes of other cells. The platelet membrane consists of two thick outer layers and a less dense inner layer. The outer layers are protein in nature, the inner is lipid.

The life-span of a platelet is 8 to 12 days in humans. This is altered in specific health states such as Hodgkin's disease, aortic valve prosthesis, cirrhosis, and carcinoma.

Platelets store metabolic substances, have a role in phagocytosis (see Chap. 8), and play an integral part in blood coagulation.

Thrombocytopenia occurs when the level of circulating platelets drop below 100,000 cells/min$^3$ blood. The time between the development of thrombocytopenia and the stimulation of platelet production is between 3 and 5 days.[17,18,19]

**Platelet destruction** Depletion in platelets can occur as a result of hemorrhage, exchange transfusions, or injection of antiplatelet antibodies.[20,21] The bone marrow's ability to compensate for this is limited.

Little is known of the sites in which human platelets are destroyed or utilized. From research gathered thus far it is thought that most of the activity occurs in the liver and spleen.[22]

### Coagulation Factors

Clotting factors are essential to prevent loss of blood due to a disruption in the coagulation process. There are over 30 different substances which have been found within the body that relate directly to promoting clot formation. These are referred to as *precoagulants.* Other substances inhibit coagulation and are called *anticoagulants.*

In addition there are a series of *clotting factors* (see Table 22-2) which directly influence clotting of blood. When any of these factors are not present in the body (through genetic inheritance or destruction), there is an interruption in blood clotting mechanisms and severe blood loss may result.

Stages of clot formation are depicted in Fig. 22-4. In order for clotting to occur, intrinsic and extrinsic systems must interact (see Fig. 22-5) to facilitate the process. Alteration in any of these factors will disrupt clot formation and result in potential blood loss.

## THE HEART

The heart is a precise, durable, and efficient structure. It is a pulsatile four-chambered pump composed of two atria and two ventricles.[23] Human hearts contract on the average of 72 times per minute, resting approximately 0.4 second between heartbeats. The heart pumps blood into the arterial network and the capillaries through the aorta with each contraction for the purposes of transporting oxygenated blood and nutrients throughout the body and removing cell metabolic wastes via the venous system and pumping blood into the lungs to be oxygenated.

### Cardiac Muscle

The heart is made up of atrial muscle, ventricular muscle, and specialized excitory muscle called syncytium. The muscle structure contains striated muscle and monofibrils and is similar to skeletal muscle throughout the body (refer to Chap. 31). *Syncytium* muscle (see Fig. 22-6) is more unique in that its structure is composed of a series of *intercalated disks* which run throughout the muscle fibers. In addition, they are connected in a series of inter-

**TABLE 22-2**
BLOOD-CLOTTING FACTORS

| Factor | Synonyms | Comments |
|---|---|---|
| I | Fibrinogen | Produced in liver; forms fibrin when acted upon by thrombin. |
| II | Prothrombin | Produced in liver; vitamin K is essential component; forms fibrin when acted upon by thromboplastin |
| III | Thromboplastin | Found in tissue, plasma. Acts upon prothrombin to form thrombin. |
| IV | Calcium | Diet is main source; needed in all stages of clotting. Stimulates enzyme activity. |
| V | Labile factor, AC globulin, proaccelerin | Present in plasma; needed in clotting of blood; stimulates conversion of prothrombin to thrombin. |
| VI | Not assigned | |
| VII | Stable factor, serum prothrombin conversion accelerator, SPCA proconversion | Main source is the liver. Present in normal serum, stimulates prothrombin to form thrombin. |
| VIII | Antihemophilic factor A, antihemophilic globulin (AHG) | Plasma globulin derivation. Used up in clotting; necessary for thromboplastin formation and change of prothrombin to thrombin. |
| IX | Christmas factor, antihemophilic factor B, plasma thromboplastin component | Source: Liver. Influences production of thromboplastin. |
| X | Stuart-Power factor | Found in liver. Vitamin K necessary in normal plasma. Similar to Factor VII. |
| XI | Plasma thromboplastin antecedent/antihemophilic factor | Original site unknown. |
| XII | Hageman factor | Origin and function unknown. |
| XIII | Fibrin stabilizing factor | Origin unknown. Helps maintain clots. Formed in plasma. |

Adapted from Joan Luckman and Karen Sorensen, *Medical Surgical Nursing: A Psychophysiologic Approach*, Saunders, Philadelphia, 1974, p. 792, and R. M. French, *Nurses' Guide To Diagnostic Procedures*, 3d ed., McGraw-Hill, New York, 1971.

connecting fibers which bind the tissue close together. As a result when one cell within the heart musculature becomes excited, the energy potential spreads laterally until the entire muscle is involved. This is referred to as the *all-or-none principle*.[24] When this principle is applied to cardiac muscle, it refers to the excitation of an entire functional system rather than a single skeletal muscle fiber.

Other properties of cardiac muscle include its rhythmicity, irritability (excitability), conductivity, contractability, automaticity, and extensibility.

**Rhythmicity** The heart contracts and relaxes in a rhythmic pattern anywhere from 60 to 100 beats per minute. When the impulses are initiated at the sinoatrial (SA) node, they are transmitted throughout the conduction pathway in a continuous pattern. Within the range listed above, the heart may increase or decrease its rate. The pattern remains continuous and regular in the absence of pathology.

**Irritability** The term *irritability* (excitability) refers to the component of cardiac muscle tissue that con-

tinuously responds to stimuli (all-or-none law). When a cardiac muscle cell is irritated (or stimulated), it responds to that stimulus and irritates other cells until the entire muscle is responding to the initial irritant.

There are several factors that influence cardiac irritability. An adequate oxygen supply, normal neural and hormonal functioning, and a balanced diet are essential to maintaining normal initiation of the muscle tissue. Drug therapy, infection, lack of oxygen, and disruptions in neural and hormonal balance can increase muscle irritability and lead to conduction disturbances.

**Refractoriness** Refractoriness prevents the heart muscle from responding to additional new stimuli while the heart is contracting from another stimulus. Cardiac irritability is most vulnerable during the refractory period because of this factor.

During the *absolute* refractory period the muscle will not respond to new stimuli of any magnitude. During a *relative* refractory period the muscle begins to be ready for response for new stimuli and regains its irritability. (See Electrocardiogram for an additional discussion.)

**FIGURE 22-4**
Stages of clot formation.
(Adapted from G. Scipien et al (eds.),
Comprehensive Pediatric Nursing,
McGraw-Hill, New York, 1975.)

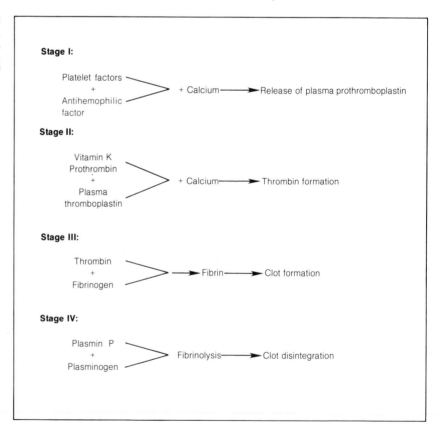

**Conductivity—contractability**  The ability of the heart to effectively transmit impulses through the muscles is influenced by two properties, conductivity and contractability. *Conductivity* refers to the ability of cardiac muscle fibers to transmit electrical impulses throughout the heart in a continuous rhythmic pattern. The conduction pathways begin at the SA node located in the atrium and terminate in the Purkinje fibers in the ventricle wall. *Contractability* refers to the shortening of the cardiac muscle fibers in response to a stimulus. This contraction occurs rhythmically and is followed by a relaxation period which corresponds to the filling and emptying of the cardiac chambers. At rest the heart pumps approximately 2 oz of blood with each beat, 70 barrels in 24 hours, and in a lifetime of 70 years over 18 million barrels of blood are pumped.[25]

**Automaticity**  The automaticity of cardiac muscle is a unique phenomenon. The term refers to the ability of the heart to automatically beat spontaneously and repetitively without external neurohormonal control. This property is sensitive to changes in body fluid and electrolytes and can be disrupted when electrolyte imbalances occur.

**Extensibility**  The ability of heart muscle to expand (stretch) while the chambers fill with blood between muscle contraction is termed *extensibility*. This property of cardiac muscle is governed by the principles of Starling's law which states that the greater the stretch (expansion) of cardiac muscle, the more forceful the contraction of the heart. Overexpansion of the muscle can result in alterations in muscle filling and decrease the forcefulness of contraction.

### The Conduction System

The transmission of impulses throughout the heart is controlled by the autonomic nervous system and influenced by many other factors. Within the heart there is a specialized conduction pathway which accepts the initial innovation and transmits it throughout the conduction system of the heart. This impulse will occur anywhere from 60 to 100 times per minute in the healthy adult. Figure 22-7 shows the conduction system and should be referred to throughout the following discussion.

**Sinoatrial node**  The SA node is a C-shaped disk located at the junction of the superior vena cava and the right atrium. The SA node is under the influence of the autonomic nervous system. Impulses are initiated at the SA node, which is the official

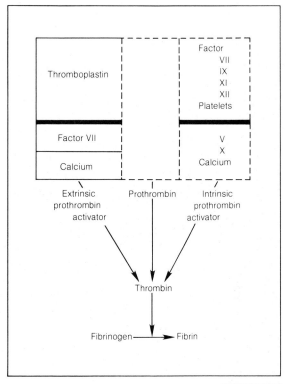

**FIGURE 22-5**
Intrinsic and extrinsic factors needed for blood clotting. (*Adapted from Arthur Guyton, Textbook of Medical Physiology, Saunders, Philadelphia, 1970.*)

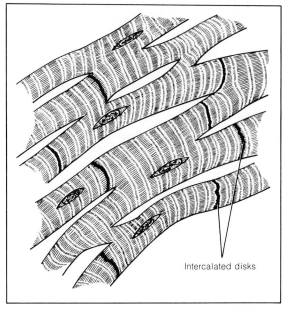

**FIGURE 22-6**
Syncytium tissue found in cardiac muscle.

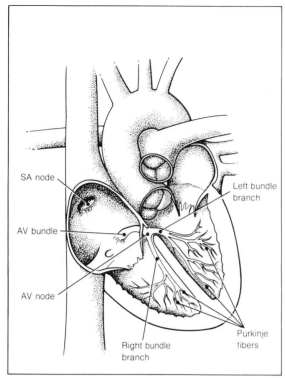

**FIGURE 22-7**
Conduction system.

*pacemaker* of the heart. The heart rate, rhythm, and regularity are controlled by the SA node which stimulates conduction every 60 to 100 times per minute. While other components of the conduction pathway may have the potential to discharge impulses independently, the SA node releases impulses more rapidly and therefore assumes control over the process. Impulses travel from the SA node to the atrioventricular (AV) node in 0.3 to 0.4 second.

**Atrioventricular node**   The AV node is located in the lower interatrial system. The AV node receives impulses from the SA node, delays them slightly before they travel into the AV bundle, or *bundle of His.* The length of time between entry of the impulse to the exit at the bundle is approximately 0.07 to 0.11 second. The AV node discharges impulses rhythmically approximately 4 to 6 beats per minute. If the SA node fails, the AV node will take over and conduct impulses through the ventricle.

**Bundle branches**   The bundle branches contain special cardiac muscle fibers that originate in the AV node. After leaving the bundle of His, the im-

pulses travel into the right and left bundle branch which lie beneath the endocardium to the right and left of the septum. The *right* bundle branch contains a main branch with fibers which originate from the common bundle branch. The *left* bundle branch contains three main branches. The two bundles bring electrical impulses in an anterior apical direction and cover the ventricular endocardium.[26]

**Purkinje fibers**   The Purkinje fibers extend from the AV node through the AV bundle into the ventricles intraventricular septum.[27] They discharge impulses at a rate of 15 to 20 beats per minute. They transmit impulses anywhere from 1.5 to 2.5 meters per second.

Along the course of the bundle branches are many small branches of Purkinje fibers spreading in many directions, transmitting and conducting impulses throughout the muscle.

**F**actors Influencing Conduction   The stimulation of the *sympathetic* nerves (vagal) results in the release of acetylcholine of the vagal endings. This hormone acts upon the SA node and slows down the heart rate. In addition, it acts upon the AV node and decreases its excitability, thereby slowing impulse transmission to the ventricles.

Stimulation of the sympathetic nervous system can also result in an increased heart rate and increased muscle excitability.

*Exercise* will increase heart rate because of the body's demand for increased oxygen and elimination of $CO_2$. Exercise also stimulates body metabolism, which increases oxygen demand, thereby increasing overall heart rate.

*Age* also influences heart rate. In the fetus, the heart rate may range from 120 to 160 beats per minute. As the person grows older, the heart rate may range from 60 to 100 beats per minute. However, in the absence of significant pathology, the elderly have a slower heart rate. *Females* usually have a faster heart rate.

There are three *electrolytes,* namely, sodium, potassium, and calcium, which have a significant effect upon the cardiac membrane potential and transmission of impulses. When the distribution of these substances is altered within the body, disruption in conduction of impulses occurs.

Excess *potassium* causes the heart to dilate and become flaccid. This results in decrease in the membrane potential and results in weaker, less forceful, contractions.

*Excess calcium* results in spastic contraction of the heart muscle. The excess calcium in the body excites cardiac muscle and stimulates contractions. A *decrease in calcium* below normal limits causes an effect similar to that of potassium excess.

*Excess sodium* within the body decreases cardiac function and results in weak contractions and muscle flaccidity. For some unexplained reason the greater the excess of sodium ions, the less effective calcium will be in producing cardiac muscle contractions.

A *decrease in sodium* ion concentration allows the calcium ions to improve cardiac output by strengthening muscle contraction.

The higher the body temperature, the more rapid the heart rate. The lower the body temperature, the slower the heart rate. "The effect of temperature . . . results from increased conductance of the muscle membrane for the different ions, resulting in all states of self-excitation."[28] If the arterial pressure drops below normal limits, the heart will beat faster in order to increase cardiac output and increase blood volume.

In addition, *hormones* such as thyroxine and epinephrine can affect heart rate, causing an increase in rate and potential rhythm change.

### Structures of the heart

The heart is a cone-shaped, hollow muscle located in the midiastinum between the lungs and the thoracic cavity.

The *base* of the heart is directed toward the right side of the body, while the *apex* (the point) is toward the left side of the body, resting on the diaphram. Apical impulses are palpable between the fourth and fifth intercostal spaces (see Fig. 22-8).

The *pericardium* is a thin covering which loosely surrounds the heart. It is composed of tough fibrous membranes which are attached to the great vessels. The *pericardial space* is located between the visceral and parietal layers and contains approximately 5 to 20 ml pericardial fluid. This fluid is clear and thin, lubricating the visceral and pericardial surfaces as the heart contracts. In addition the presence of this fluid decreases friction between the heart surfaces with each heartbeat and facilitates the regularity of each contraction.

**Layers of the heart**   There are three layers which line the heart muscle. These are the epicardium, the myocardium, and the endocardium.

The *epicardium* is the outer layer of the heart and is similar in structure to the visceral pericardium. It covers the cardiac muscle and protects its inner structures.

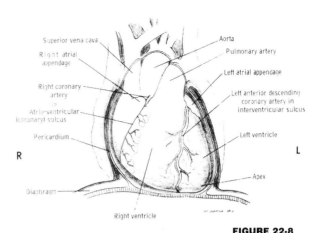

**FIGURE 22-8**
Structure of the heart. Coronary blood supply. (*From J. W. Hurst et al. (eds.), The Heart, 4th ed., McGraw-Hill, New York, 1978. Used with permission of McGraw-Hill Book Company.*)

The *myocardium* is the middle layer of the heart. It is composed of striated muscle interconnected to form muscle bundles. This is the muscle of the heart itself (the pump) which is ultimately responsible for the contraction and relaxation of the heart and the distribution of blood throughout the heart structures and systemic circulation. Multiple autonomic nerve fibers innovate the muscle responses. Coronary blood supply is responsible for oxygenation of this muscle.

The *endocardium* is the innermost layer of the heart composed of endothelial tissue and blood vessels. The endocardium lines the cavity of the heart and covers the valves.

**Chambers of the heart**   The heart is divided into the right and left side. The *right side* of the heart removes deoxygenated blood from the heart and pumps it into the lungs to be oxygenated. The *left side* of the heart receives the oxygenated blood from the lungs and expels it into the circulation through the aorta. Within this division there are four chambers which are responsible for the reception and distribution of blood throughout the body. These chambers are the right atrium, the right ventricle, the left atrium, and the left ventricle (see Fig. 22-9). Each chamber contains specific oxygen percentages and pressures. Fig. 22-10 depicts each reading.

**R**ight Atrium   The right atrium is located behind and to the right of the right ventricle and to the right of the left atrium.[29] Venous blood enters the right atrium through the superior and inferior vena cavae. The deoxygenated blood is stored in the right

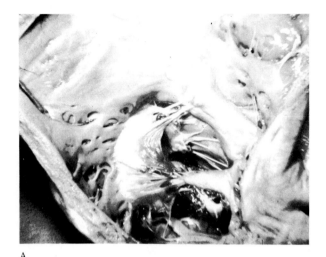

A

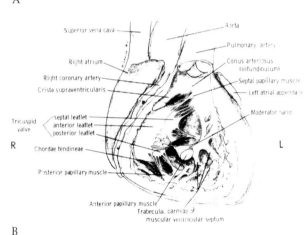

B

**FIGURE 22-9**
Frontal view of the heart. (*From J. W. Hurst et al. (eds.), The Heart, 4th ed., McGraw-Hill, New York, 1978. Used with permission of McGraw-Hill Book Company.*)

atrium during diastole and empties into the left ventricle following diastole. The wall of the right ventricle is thinner than that of the left ventricle owing to decrease in pressure and output (see Fig. 22-11).

**R**ight Ventricle   The right ventricle is a crescent-shaped chamber located beneath the sternum and is the most anterior cardiac chamber, most palpable at the left lower sternal border.[30] The right ventricle receives blood from the right atrium. During ventricular contraction it forces unoxygenated blood into the pulmonary artery and remaining pulmonary circulation.

The interventricular septum forms the middle wall of both the left and right ventricle. However, for purposes of function it belongs to the right ventri-

cle. The right ventricle is smaller in size than the left ventricle owing to a decrease in the wall thickness and decrease in right-sided pressure.

**L**eft Atrium   The *left atrium* is located posterior to other cardiac chambers.[31] Often it is not observed on x-ray. The walls of the left atrium are thicker than those of the right atrium owing to increased pumping effort. Two pulmonary veins enter the left atrium on the posterior side and empty oxygenated blood into the chambers. In addition, the left atrium serves as a conduit during left ventricle filling. When the left atrium contracts, it provides a significant increment of blood into the left ventricle, stretching the ventricle and priming it for ventricular ejection.[32] Special muscle bundles called *trabeculae carneae* line the anterior and inferior wall of the right ventricle and work with other valves and muscles to control and direct the blood flow to the ventricular chamber (see the discussion below).

**L**eft Ventricle   The muscle of the left ventricle is bullet shaped and is two to three times thicker than the wall of the right ventricle (see Fig. 22-11). This is necessary since it is the left ventricle that is responsible for ejecting oxygenated blood into the aorta and systemic circulation. The *septum* is triangular in shape. The upper one-third of the septum is made up of smooth endocardium.[33] The lower two-thirds of the septum are the trabeculae carneae. The ventricular wall that is not in contact with the septum is referred to as the *free wall* of the ventricle (see Fig. 22-12).

**Valves**   Within the chambers of the heart are several structures referred to as *valves.* These include the tricuspid valve, the mitral valve, and the semilunar valves. These valves open and close with diastolic and systolic contractions and influence the amount of blood transmitted (see Fig. 22-13).

**T**ricuspid Valve   The *tricuspid valve* is located between the right atrium and right ventricles. The valve contains three leaflets: *the anterior, the medial* (septal), and *the posterior leaflets.* These leaflets are thin and easily defined. The tricuspid valve is larger than the mitral valve and functions to control blood flow from the right atrium to the right ventricle. Upon closure, valves prevent blood flow from returning (regurgitating) to the right atrium. (Refer to Figs. 22-12 and 22-13.)

**M**itral Valve   The mitral valve (or bicuspid valve) contains two triangular-shaped leaflets, the *anterior*

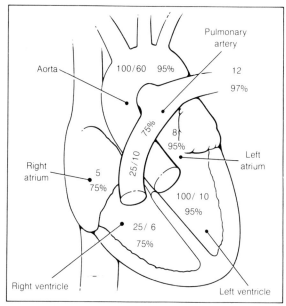

**FIGURE 22-10**
Pressures and oxygen concentrations within heart structures.
(*Adapted from J. Kernicki et al., Cardiovascular Nursing, Putnam, New York, 1970.*)

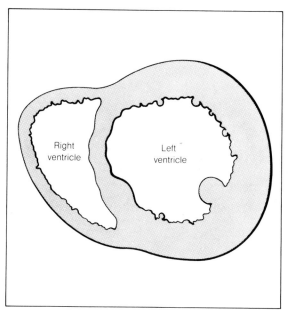

**FIGURE 22-11**
Comparison in the sizes of the right and left ventricles.

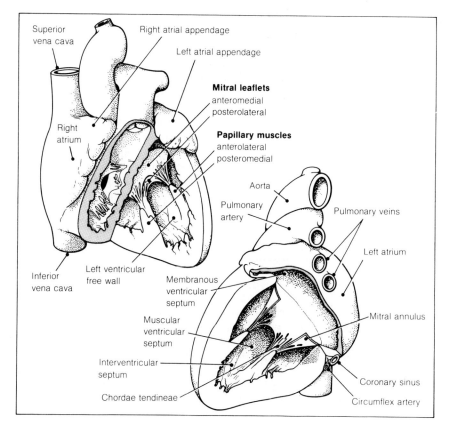

**FIGURE 22-12**
Right ventricle—interventricular septum.

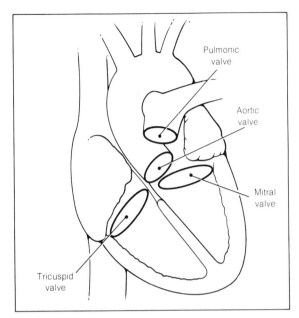

**FIGURE 22-13**
Valve position.

*medial leaflet* which is larger and more mobile, and the *posterolateral leaflet* which is longer and less mobile. These two leaflets contribute significantly to the closure of the mitral valve (refer to Figs. 22-12 and 22-13). Upon ventricular systole both mitral leaflets are propelled upward, connecting the entire left ventricular into an expulsion chamber.[34] When the valve relaxes, leaflets separate and permit blood flow into the ventricle.

**S**emilunar Valves    Both the aortic and pulmonary valves are referred to as the *semilunar* valves (refer to Fig. 22-13). Each valve contains three fibrous cusps (*anterior, right,* and *left*) which are suspended from the root of the pulmonary artery or the aorta. Behind each cusp there is a pouchlike dilatation referred to as the *sinus* of valsalva.

The *pulmonary veins* that bring oxygenated blood from the lungs to the right atrium do not have true valves. However, the muscles from the right arterial wall surround the pulmonary veins, acting like a sphincter.

**Muscular structures**    There are several muscular structures contained within the heart muscle to facilitate contraction and circulation. These include the trabeculae carneae, the papillary muscle, and the chordae tendineae.

The *trabeculae carneae* are muscle bundles that line the inferior wall of the right ventricle (see Fig. 22-14). They are also found in the ventricular walls of the septum. They act to support contraction of the ventricular wall during diastole.

The papillary muscles project from the trabeculae carneae and are located below the valve openings. These muscles receive their blood supply from branches of the right and left coronary arteries (see Fig. 22-14).

There are three papillary muscles in the right ventricle below the tricuspid valve, the *anterior* papillary muscle which is the largest, the *posterior* papillary muscle which is located below the junction of the posterior leaflets, and the *conus* papillary muscle which is the smallest of these three muscles and develops from the wall of the infundibulum.[35] The *left ventricle* contains two papillary muscles located below anterolateral and posteromedial commissures at the mitral valve. Because of their particular structures, the papillary muscles are able to pull the leaflets of the mitral valve and tricuspid veins downward when the ventricles contract. This motion closes the valves, prevents blood from entering the ventricles during contraction, and allows for complete emptying of the ventricles. Disruption in blood supply to the papillary muscle may contribute to disturbances in muscle function.

The *chordae tendineae* are strong fibrous tissue that arise from the tip of each papillary muscle. They can be an integral part of the ventricle, run along the unattached edges of a valve, or be attached to a fibrous band (see Figs. 22-12 and 22-14).

Because of their attachment to the edges of each valve, the valve leaflets are able to balloon upward against each other and eventually distribute the force of ventricular systole. When there is a disturbance or rupture of the papillary muscle or a tearing of the chordae tendineae, the support to the valvular leaflets is diminished. Blood from the ventricles may flow back into the atrium. This process is called *regurgitation*.

## CIRCULATION

Oxygenated blood leaves the left ventricle, travels into the aorta, and is ejected into the arteries and smaller branches (arterioles), traveling throughout the body through a dynamic interactive vascular network. In addition to the arteries, veins, capillaries, and the lymphatic system compose the remaining circulatory structures (see Fig. 22-15). The end result of this process is the return of unoxygenated blood to the right side of the heart by way of the inferior and superior vena cava. Circulation to the myocardium is referred to as *coronary* circulation; when blood circulates through the periphery (extremities), the term *peripheral* circulation is used. Pulmonary circulation occurs when unoxygenated blood is transmitted to the lungs and oxygenated blood is returned to the left atrium. Additional circulation patterns occur throughout specific organs in the body: *portal circulation* (Chap. 15), *renal circulation* (Chap. 31), *cerebral circulation* and *circulation to the skin* (Chap. 8). All forms of circulation consist of a similar exchange of oxygen and carbon dioxide; the reader is referred to the specific chapter for a more complete discussion.

## Arteries

Arteries are the body's distribution system originating from the aorta and its branches. The purpose of the arteries is to carry oxygenated blood and nutrients from the left ventricle to the systemic circulation. The pulmonary artery, however, originates in the right atrium and transports unoxygenated blood, returning from the circulation, to the lungs where it will be oxygenated (see Pulmonary Circulation).

The *aorta* and the pulmonary artery are similar structures in that they both are derived from the division of the embryonic structus arteriosus.[36] The aorta has a thicker wall than the pulmonary artery because of its function in adult life. The aorta is a fibrous pulsating tissue which assists the flow of blood to the arteries or acts as a reservoir for blood during ejection of the ventricles.[37]

*Arteries* transport blood to the systemic circulation and originate in the aorta or its branches. The arteries then branch into smaller arteries and *arterioles,* which form a regulating system and offer the major source of resistance to systemic circulation. The arterial wall is strong and pulsating. It is composed of several layers, namely, the intimal, the elastic membrane, the media, and the adventitia (Fig. 22-16).

## Capillaries

Capillaries are small vessels composed of a single endothelial wall. They hold about 5 percent of the total blood volume. Normally, blood flows through the capillary veins and lungs and supplies oxygen and nutrients. Bloodflow through the capillary bed is sluggish; therefore, stasis may result. The normal capillary pressure in the systemic circulation is between 25 and 35 mmHg, while in the lung the normal capillary pressure is between 7 and 10 mmHg.[38]

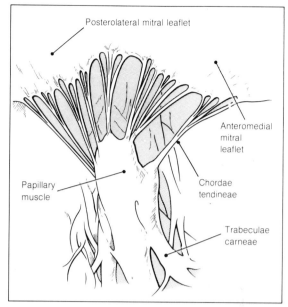

**FIGURE 22-14**
Muscular structures of the heart.

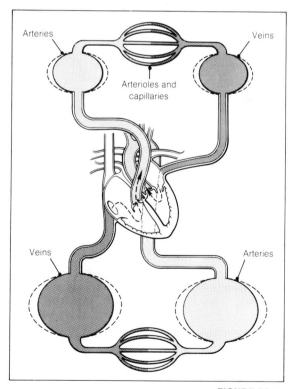

**FIGURE 22-15**
Systemic circulation.

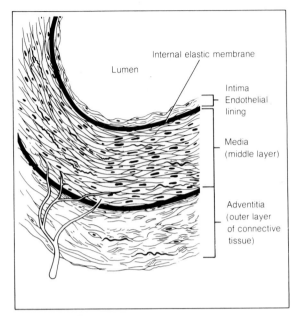

Internal elastic membrane

Lumen

Intima
Endothelial
lining

Media
(middle layer)

Adventitia
(outer layer
of connective
tissue)

**FIGURE 22-16**
Arterial wall lining.

### Veins

Veins are thin-walled contracting and expanding vessels, capable of storing and transporting blood to the heart. Venous blood is drawn from capillaries and collects in smaller veins, then passes to other venous tributaries. It carries oxygenated blood and body wastes from the systemic circulation and returns it to the right atrium by way of the inferior and superior vena cava. Veins tend to be under less pressure than arteries; therefore, some larger veins, especially those in the legs, contain special valves (see Fig. 22-17). These valves help to direct the flow of blood toward the heart, in response to contraction of muscles of the arms and legs as well as to pressure changes in the abdominal and thoracic vessels. In a resting state approximately 50 to 65 percent of the total blood volume is contained in the venous circulation.[39]

### Lymphatic Vessels

Circulation throughout the cardiovascular system is thought to be contained within a closed system. However, some fluid and protein filters from the capillary bed into the interstitial tissue. This fluid must be returned to the heart, usually through the venous system or by way of the lymphatic circulation. There are three major terminal vessels of the lymphatic system. These are the thoracic duct, left brachiocephalic vein, and the junction of the jugular and left subclavian vein.

A considerable amount of blood volume is returned to the heart via the terminal vessel of the lymphatic system, the *thoracic duct*.[40] The myocardial lymphatic vessels bring nutrients to the heart, especially in the presence of ischemia, infection, and structural damage.

**Pulmonary circulation** As unoxygenated venous blood returns from the systemic circulation to the right ventricle, it flows into the pulmonary artery. From here it is transported to the lungs, oxygenated, and returned to the left ventricle by the pulmonary veins.

In addition to the fact that the pulmonary artery carries unoxygenated blood to the lungs, the arterial structure differs in several other ways. The pulmonary artery is thin-walled, and blood passes through the artery at a rate of about one-sixth that of the systemic circulation. The tissue has less medial muscle, and circulation tends to be more passive. Pulmonary blood vessels tend to respond less to neural and hormonal stimulation, thus making them less reactive to vasoconstriction.

Local regional vasoconstriction, produced by alveolar hypoxia, and constriction of local branches in underperfused areas help maintain normal balance between pulmonary circulation and exchange of oxygen and carbon dioxide.

The normal capillary pressure within the lungs is between 7 and 10 mmHg. The interstitial fluid is kept at a minimum by this pressure and normal osmotic pressure. Blood flow to the lungs can increase significantly in the presence of increased need (for example, chronic obstructive pulmonary disease). The pressure gradient between the pulmonary artery and left atrium can change, altering blood flow to the area.

The pulmonary veins return oxygenated blood to the left atrium to be distributed throughout the systemic circulation.

**Coronary blood supply** Supplying blood to the myocardium is the function of the right and left coronary arteries and the coronary veins. The *left coronary artery* (refer to Fig. 22-9) is located in the upper half of the coronary sinus of the aorta. It has three main branches, the left circumflex artery, the anterior descending artery, and the posterior descending artery. The *left circumflex* artery originates near the aorta and the pulmonary artery and travels along the margin of the left ventricle. The *left circumflex* artery supplies most of the left atrium and the lateral and posterior walls of the left ventricle. The *posterior descending artery* is a continuation of the left circumflex artery and sulcus. The *anterior descending* artery has two major branches which cover the wall of the left ventricle and penetrate the interventricular system. Smaller branches distribute to the right ventricle.

The *right coronary artery* (Fig. 22-9) arises from two ostia of the coronary sinus. The smaller ostium gives rise to the conus artery. This artery has the potential of serving as an alternate route for collateral circulation. The right coronary artery divides into two directions; one or more branches descend toward the apex of the heart while the other branch descends to the left ventricle. Several branches emerge to serve the right ventricle.

There are three systems of veins in the heart. These are the *thebesian vein,* the *anterior cardiac vein* from the anterior wall of the right ventricle, and the *coronary sinus* and its tributaries.

The coronary sinus is the primary means of drainage from the left ventricle. Smaller tributary veins from the left ventricle empty into the *great cardiac* vein. These veins all work to transport unoxygenated blood from the myocardium.

The *interventricular* septum is located between the right and left ventricle and receives its blood supply from the anterior and posterior descending arteries. Coronary circulation changes in accordance with cardiac output, the degree of oxygen consumption, diastolic blood pressure, vascular resistance, blood volume, and neurohormonal influences.

*Microcirculation* is that circulation which occurs throughout the capillaries and lymphatics. The rate of circulation through this network is influenced by cardiac output, blood volume, and heart rate. Decrease in blood flow through the microcirculation causes trapping of blood cells and venous stasis.

**Factors regulating circulation** Circulation is influenced by several major systems. The *nervous system* regulates heart rate and influences arteriolar constriction and blood pressure. Reflexes in the vasomotor center of the medulla influence dilatation and constriction of blood vessels and inhibition and acceleration of the heart rate.

In addition, *pressoreceptors* (or baroreceptors), specialized nerve endings located in the superior and inferior venae cavae, are stimulated by changes within the arterial wall (see Arterial Blood Pressure below). Changes in oxygen and increases in carbon dioxide stimulate chemoreceptors, producing an *ischemic response.* This results in vasoconstriction of small blood vessels due to hypoxia.

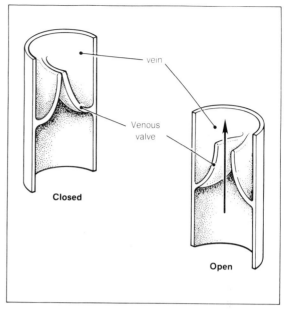

**FIGURE 22-17**
Vein valve structure.

The *peripheral vascular* circulation is influenced by the *hypothalamus* which in turn influences peripheral vasomotor activity. Cerebral centers interact in governing peripheral circulation. *Hormonal influences* affect peripheral vascular dilatation and constriction and affect peripheral resistance. Table 22-3 lists the hormones involved in

**TABLE 22-3**
HORMONES THAT REGULATE PERIPHERAL VASCULAR BLOOD VESSELS

| Hormone | Effect on Peripheral Vascular System |
| --- | --- |
| Histamine | Causes vasodilation of small blood vessels; can also cause vasoconstriction of larger arteries. |
| Epinephrine | Constricts superficial blood vessels. |
| Norepinephrine | Constricts all blood vessels. |
| Angiotensin | Constricts arteries. |
| Bradykinin | Powerful vasodilator, especially of the cutaneous vessels. |
| Acetylcholine | Vasodilator most often noted in face and upper limbs. |
| Serotonin | Released from platelets; causes vasoconstriction of cutaneous arterioles; dilates capillaries. |
| Muscle metabolites | Vasodilator action. |

peripheral resistance and their effects on peripheral arteries and veins.

## CARDIAC OUTPUT

Cardiac output is dependent upon two factors, namely, stroke volume and heart rate.

Stroke volume + heart rate = cardiac output

*Stroke volume* refers to the amount of blood expelled by the heart with each contraction. *Heart rate* refers to the number of contractions (beats) that occur per minute. *Cardiac output* (CO) is the amount of blood expelled by the heart (aorta) each minute. The average cardiac output for adults is approximately 5 liters/minute.

Effective cardiac output is dependent upon many variables including the amount of venous return, extensibility of the cardiac muscle, contractability of the muscle (strength of contraction), heart rate, and blood pressure. In addition, *body size* influences cardiac output, for as body surface increases, cardiac output increases. As individuals *age* and *grow,* the demand for cardiac output changes. However, output declines only slightly above the age of 80. *Standing* causes a drop in cardiac output of as much as 20 percent. *Exercise* and increased *metabolic* needs place a greater demand on output, probably owing to increase in oxygen consumption.

Two major factors regulate cardiac output. These are the overall effectiveness of the blood pumping action of the heart and the way blood is capable of flowing throughout the systemic circulation without undue resistance. Effective *cardiac pumping* is influenced by sympathetic (constricting) stimulation, enlargement (hypertrophy) of the cardiac musculature, decreased arterial blood pressure, and disruption in the parasympathetic (slowing) inhibitors of the heart.

*Extracardiac pressure* also influences cardiac output. Alteration in respiration or changes in thoracic pressure influence cardiac demand.

*Resistance* to *blood* can be altered by the main systemic pressure and sympathetic stimulation and blood volume.

Cardiac output can be increased by such factors as exercise, stress, occlusion of blood vessel, and increased demand. Output is diminished by hypovolemia, venous stasis, and pump failure.

The ability of the heart to adjust to and cope with the body's demands for increased output is referred to as *cardiac reserve.*

## BLOOD PRESSURE

The pressure exerted by the blood against the walls of the arteries, veins, and capillaries is termed *blood pressure*. The blood pressure gradient is that force that allows blood to flow throughout all components of the circulatory system.

*Mean arterial pressure* is the average pressure that exists throughout the pressure pulse cycle. It is the average pressure, that pressure needed to force the blood through the systemic circulation. Arterial blood pressure is regulated according to the following formula:

Blood pressure = cardiac output × total peripheral resistance

*Arterial blood pressure* refers to that pressure exerted by the blood against the arterial walls. *Systolic blood pressure* is the maximum pressure of blood exerted against the wall of an artery when the heart is contracting. The normal range is between 115 and 120 mmHg. *Diastolic blood pressure* refers to the force of blood exerted against the wall of the artery when the heart is at rest. The average range is between 75 and 80 mmHg.

*Pulse pressure* refers to the difference between diastolic and systolic arterial blood pressure. Normally this difference should not exceed 40 mmHg.

### Arterial Blood Pressure

Blood flow within the vessels is laminar. The blood flow that is farthest from the heart usually has the lowest pressure. Pressure tends to be the highest in the arteries, lower in the capillaries, and lowest in the veins. The viscosity of the blood also influences arterial pressure; the greater the viscosity, the higher the arterial pressure. *Autoregulation* refers to the tissues' ability to regulate their own blood flow and adjust blood flow to changes in blood pressure. The *myogenic* theory suggests that this regulation occurs in response to the intrinsic contracting of smooth muscles to stretch.

Approximately 50 percent of total resistance to blood flow is exerted by the arterioles.[41] There are three *major* factors that help regulate arterial blood pressure. These are the autonomic system (including the sympathetic and parasympathetic systems), the kidneys, and hormones (see Table 22-4). Arterial blood pressure is influenced by many other factors. Table 22-5 lists some of them and the rationale for their development.

## Venous Pressure

Blood pressure within the veins is low and in some instances nonexistent. Smaller veins do not appear to pulsate, while some larger ones do. Venous blood returning from the systemic circulation enters the right atrium through the superior and inferior venae cavae. The pressure within the right atrium is sometimes called the *central venous pressure.* Normal right atrial pressure is usually zero. Under certain situations, e.g., pulmonary edema and heart failure, the pressure can rise 15 to 20 mmHg. The lower limits of right atrial pressure are from 4 to 5 mmHg, reflecting pressure in the pericardial and intrapleural spaces. Large veins entering the thorax can be compressed, resulting in impeded blood flow. Valves located within the large veins of the legs offer added resistance to venous blood flow.

## Capillary Pressure

The pressure against capillary walls is approximately 27 mmHg at the arterial end 12 mmHg in the venous fluid. When capillary pressure increases, capillary filtration increases and causes the fluid to shift from the vascular system to the tissue; edema results. When the capillary pressure is below normal, capillary filtration decreases, and fluids are drawn from the tissue into the circulation to increase blood volume and blood pressure.

The walls of the *lymphatic* capillaries have a thinner membrane. For this reason they offer little or no resistance to the flow of fluid or proteins. Lymphatic pressure is influenced by increased interstitial fluid pressure. Elevated capillary pressure decreases osmotic pressure. This results in an accumulation of fluid and protein in the periphery and contributes to the formation of edema.

## OXYGEN AND CARBON DIOXIDE EXCHANGE

Adequate oxygen and carbon dioxide exchange is the essence of oxygenation. The processes of respiration and ventilation allow for the exchange of oxygen and carbon dioxide, a critical component of the life process.

## Ventilation and Respiration

*Ventilation* consists of those processes necessary to move oxygen into the lungs and remove carbon dioxide. *Respiration* is defined as the transportation of oxygen from the atmosphere to the cells of the body and the return of carbon dioxide from the cells to the atmosphere. Several major structures of the respiratory tract facilitate this gaseous exchange.

**TABLE 22-4**
MAJOR FACTORS REGULATING ARTERIAL BLOOD PRESSURE

| | |
|---|---|
| Nervous system | Sympathetic stimulation occurs in response to activity and increase in blood pressure. Pressoreceptors respond to changes in blood pressure (decreases). They are located in the carotid sinus of the pulmonary arteries and aorta. When stimulated inhibit the vasomotor center, dilate blood vessels, and maintain blood pressure. Pressoreceptors respond to increase and decrease in blood pressure and are referred to as the *moderator reflex.* Central nervous system ischemic response refers to the fact that when there is a drop in blood pressure there is a vasoconstrictor response to increase blood pressure. |
| Kidney | The kidney has the potential of maintaining constant pressure in the arteries. It controls blood pressure by retention and regulation of blood volume and sodium level. It responds to antidiuretic hormone and aldosterone production when there is a decrease in blood pressure by retaining sodium and fluids. When there is an increase in blood pressure, the opposite response occurs. A substance, *renin,* is produced which can increase blood pressure by converting a glycoprotein angiotensinogen I to angiotensin II. This substance causes increased aldosterone secretion and vasoconstriction. |
| Hormones | *Vasopressin* leads to arterial vasoconstriction in significant amounts. *Epinephrine* and *norepinephrine* are secreted by the adrenal medulla in response to sympathetic nervous system stimulation and cause vasoconstriction leading to an increase in blood pressure. Aldosterone increases reabsorption of sodium and water volume leading to an increase in blood pressure. |

**TABLE 22-5**
FACTORS INFLUENCING ARTERIAL BLOOD PRESSURE

| Factor | Rationale |
|---|---|
| Cardiac output (CO) | Increased CO leads to increased BP—decreased CO leads to decreased BP. |
| Peripheral resistance | Narrow blood vessels cause increased BP. Dilated blood vessels cause decreased BP. |
| Arterial elasticity | Elastic vessels accommodate changes in blood flow. Rigid vessels lead to increased BP and pulse pressure. |
| Blood volume | Decreased blood volume leads to decreased BP. |
| Blood viscosity | Increased blood viscosity leads to increased BP. Lowered RBC count causes lowered blood viscosity leading to decreased BP. |
| Age | Newborn: BP lowest. Adult: BP highest. |
| Body weight | Increased body weight (above normal limits) leads to increased BP. |

Figure 22-18 shows these structures and can be referred to throughout this discussion.

**Structures involved in respiration** The *upper airway structures* include the nasal cavity and the nasopharnyx (and turbinates), auditory tube, pharynx, epiglottis, and pharyngeal tonsils. The turbinates and septum initially warm the inspired air. The mucous membrane lining of the nasal pharynx secretes a watery mucus which helps to humidify the inspired air. In addition, the epithelial lining of the nasal passage contains cilia which filter the air and trap large particles in the mucus, passing them to the pharynx where they are swallowed or expectorated. Irritation of the nasal passage by a particular stimulus can initiate the sneezing reflex. This occurs when pressure builds up behind the uvula and is released, thus clearing the nasal passage.

As the air passes through the posterior wall of the mouth (oropharynx), it is dependent upon the functioning of the swallowing reflex in order to reach the trachea. The swallowing reflex acts to move ingested food into the esophagus. The larynx

is stimulated simultaneously to act as a valve, blocking the aspiration of food into the lower airway.

The *larynx* contains several cartilages of which the *thyroid* cartilage is the largest. The vocal cords are contained in the thyroid cartilage and are the narrowest point in the airway passage in adults. Beneath the thyroid cartilage lies the cricoid cartilage. The *epiglottis* is connected to the thyroid cartilage and helps to cover the larynx when it closes in response to the swallowing reflex. The larynx is adapted to act as a vibrator for the vocal sounds and is instrumental in producing speech. In addition, the articulation and resonance of speech are influenced by the structures of the nasopharynx.

When chemical or mechanical irritants enter the larynx, trachea, or bronchi, vagal stimulation occurs, and impulses pass from the respiratory structures to the medulla. This sequence of events results in closure of the epiglottis and the vocal cords and the containment of air within the lungs. The intercostal and abdominal muscles contract, and the pressure in the lungs increases. When the vocal cords and epiglottis open, there is a sudden

**FIGURE 22-18**
Structures of the respiratory tree.

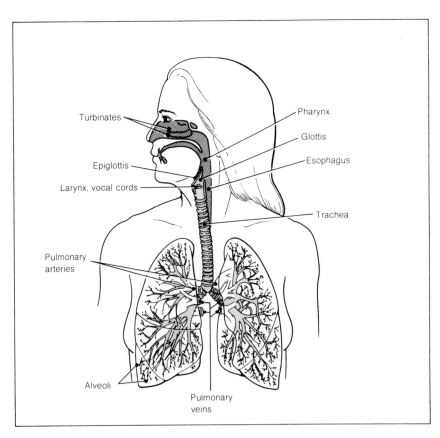

release of air under pressure and the foreign substances are removed from the respiratory tract.

The *trachea,* a cylindrical structure approximately 11 cm long, reaches from the cricoid cartilage to the thorax. The trachea is supported by a
series of C-shaped rings made of cartilage. The
trachea extends downward and branches into the
left and right stems of the bronchi.

There are two *lungs,* a right and a left. They are
served with blood by the pulmonary artery and the
pulmonary vein. The *right* lung is larger than the left
and consists of three lobes, the *upper,* the *middle,*
and the *lower,* whereas the left lung consists of two
lobes, the *upper* and the *lower.* Each lung is contained within a *pleural space* (sometimes called a
*potential space*). The parietal pleural lines the
thoracic cavity. A thin film of liquid lies between the
visceral pleura and the parietal pleura allowing for
smooth movement of the chest wall. The pleural
space is bounded by the diaphragm, the chest wall,
and the mediastinum. The mediastinum is located
between the right and left pleural space.

The *segmental bronchi* further divide the lobes
of the lungs into segments which help to isolate
specific areas. The alveolar surface contains both
liquid and gas. The surface tension results in the
contraction of the surface area. *Surfactant* present
at the liquid surface helps to lower surface tension.
Surfactant increases surface tension during inspiration and reduces the tension during expiration, thus
controlling alveolar constriction and collapse.[42]

The respiratory unit is composed of a respiratory bronchiole, an alveolar duct, atria, and alveolar
sac (see Fig. 22-19). The membranes of these structures are thin and permit gas exchange. The basement membrane is shared by components of the
alveolar membrane, the alveolar epithelium, and
the capillary epithelium.

**Mechanics of respiration**  Respiration is regulated by several components, among them being
muscles, pressure within the thoracic cavity, expansion of the cavity, lung compliance, and airway
resistance.

The diaphragm and the intercostal muscles enhance inspiration and expiration. *Inspiration* involves the contraction of the diaphragm and intercostal muscles and results in the downward expansion of the thoracic cavity and elevation of the rib
cage. *Accessory muscles* can be used in pathological states or after exercise when additional expansion is needed.

*Expiration* is a relatively passive action which
involves the deflation of the lungs, relaxation of

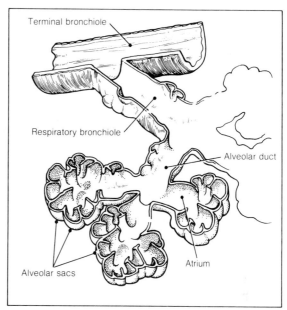

**FIGURE 22-19**
The respiratory unit.

thoracic musculature, and reduction in the size of
the thoracic cavity. The *abdominal muscles* may be
used during coughing.

**Interpleural pressure**  The pressure within the
pleural space is normally negative (below atmospheric pressure). Pleural pressure recorded at rest
is approximately 755 to 760 mmHg. During inspiration it decreased to about 751 to 755 mmHg. Interpleural pressure varies during respiration. During
*inspiration* there is a reduction in interpleural and
intrapulmonic pressure. The air enters the pleural
cavity until the intrapulmonic and atmospheric
pressures equalize. During *expiration* there is an
increase in intrapleural and intrapulmonic pressure, and gases in the pleural cavity are expelled
until intrapulmonic pressures and atmospheric
pressures equalize.

The relationship between pressure change and
volume occurring during respiration is referred to
as *compliance.* Normal compliance for an adult is
about 50 ml/cmH$_2$O when lying at rest. This is altered by inflammation of the lungs (e.g., pneumonia) or pneumothorax. When lung compliance is
lowered, the respiratory effort is increased.

*Airway resistance* refers to the relationship between airflow and pleural pressure. Normally, airway resistance across the tracheobronchial tube is
about 0.5 to 2.5 cmH$_2$O. The highest resistance is
found in the nose and lowest in the bronchioles.

Airway problems, e.g., emphysema, increase airway resistance.

As noted above, the movement of gas volume throughout the lung is termed ventilation. Within the pulmonary tree it is accomplished by the mechanical contraction and expansion of the lungs. With each respiration there is an alteration in the lung volume and capacity which affects pulmonary ventilation (refer to Fig. 22-20).

**Pulmonary volume**  Four different volumes are affected by ventilation. These are tidal volume, inspiratory reserve volume, expiratory reserve volume, and residual volume.

The normal volume of air inspired and expired with each respiration (breath) is called *tidal volume.* The normal amount of tidal volume in the healthy adult male is approximately 500 ml. Tidal volume should be considered in terms of two components: air which fills the bronchial (respiratory) tree is called *dead space;* air entering the alveoli is referred to as *alveoli ventilation. Inspiratory reserve volume* refers to the volume of air that can be inspired above the tidal volume (approximately 3000

ml). *Expiratory reserve volume* is that amount of air that is expired forcefully at the end of normal tidal volume expiration (approximately 1100 ml). *Residual volume* is the amount of air present in the lungs after forceful expiration (approximately 1200 ml).[43,44]

**Lung capacity**  The combination of gas volumes within the lungs is sometimes referred to as *lung capacity.* There are four divisions of lung capacity termed the inspiratory capacity, the functional residual capacity, the vital capacity, and the total lung capacity.

The *inspiratory capacity (tidal volume* plus *inspiratory reserve volume)* is the amount of air an individual can breathe from a resting expiratory level. The *functional residual capacity (expiratory reserve volume* plus *residual volume)* is the amount of air present in the lungs after normal expiration. The *vital capacity (inspiratory reserve* plus *tidal volume,* plus *expiratory reserve volume)* is the maximum amount of air expelled by the lungs after maximum inspiration. (Normal limits equal approximately 4600 ml.) Finally, *total lung* capacity is the

**FIGURE 22-20**
Respiratory excursion.

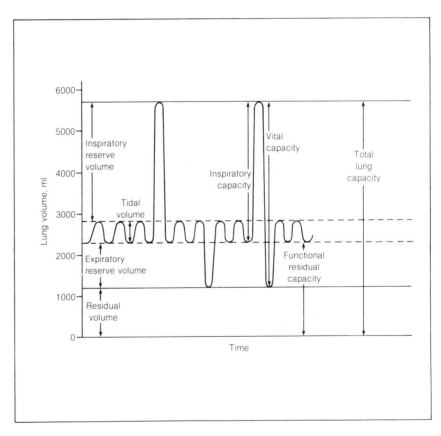

amount of air that is contained in the lungs on maximal inspiration (5800 ml).[45]

Changes anywhere in the pulmonary tracheo-branchial tree can affect both pulmonary volume and pulmonary capacity. Diminished lung volume and lung capacity will affect oxygen and carbon dioxide exchange and seriously affect oxygenation.

**A**lveolar Ventilation   Gases filter through liquid by the process of *diffusion.* This process is influenced by the rate of airflow through water and by the pressure gradient. The respiratory membrane, although containing several layers, allows for easy exchange of gas. *Diffusing capacity* is defined as the volume of gas that diffuses through the membrane each minute for a pressure gradient of 1 mmHg. The diffusing capacity of oxygen for an adult at rest is 21 ml/minute.[46] The diffusing capacity for carbon dioxide is approximately 400 to 450 ml, or about 20 times greater than for oxygen. This difference is due to the rapidity with which carbon dioxide diffuses through the membrane.[47] Figure 22-21 illustrates the diffusion of oxygen and carbon dioxide across the respiratory membrane.

*Perfusion* refers to the amount of blood that supplies the lungs. This is usually attributed to the functioning of the pulmonary artery and the right ventricle. The volume of blood in the pulmonary circulation is approximately 100 ml at any one time.

**Factors regulating O$_2$-CO$_2$ exchange**   The *respiratory center* is located in the medulla oblongata of the brainstem. Multiple neurons are activated to control both inspiration and expiration. The reverse is also true. The respiratory center is stimulated by the concentration of carbon dioxide in the arterial blood. The amount of circulating oxygen is important but less significant.

The *brain chemoreceptors* are located in the anterior medullary chemoreceptor area. They are stimulated primarily by the amount of hydrogen ions and carbon dioxide in the cerebrospinal fluid. When there are excess CO$_2$ and hydrogen ions, these receptors are stimulated and the respiratory rate is increased, thereby blowing off the excess CO$_2$ and restoring the pH balance of the blood. When pulmonary ventilation decreases, a high concentration of carbon dioxide in the blood results in an accumulation of carbonic acid and hydrogen ions. *Respiratory acidosis* results. When pulmonary ventilation increases, the number of hydrogen ions decreases. *Respiratory alkalosis* results.

When O$_2$ levels drop, *peripheral chemoreceptors,* located in the aortic and carotid bodies, are

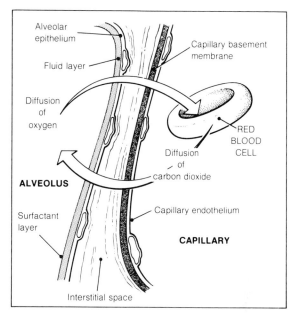

**FIGURE 22-21**
Diffusion of oxygen and carbon dioxide across the respiratory membrane.

stimulated. The respiratory center responds by stimulating the glossopharyngeal, vagus, and phrenic nerve fibers, thereby innervating the diaphragm and increasing alveolar ventilation and oxygen tension.

## THE ELECTROCARDIOGRAM

The electrocardiogram (EKG) is a common test that will be referred to in the succeeding chapters. Therefore it will be discussed in depth here in this concept chapter.

The EKG is a graphic representation of the electrical activity of the heart as detected by leads attached to the body surface. A *lead* is an electrode which picks up and measures electrical currents that occur during a cardiac cycle and are conducted to the body surface.

Standard limb leads (lead I, II, III) are set up by placing one lead on each arm and leg and an exploring lead on the chest (see Fig. 22-22*a*). These are often referred to as *bipolar leads* because they record the difference in electrical potential between two anatomical sites. The augmented *unipolar limb* leads (aVR, aVL, aVF) are placed on either the right arm and left arm or leg. A unipolar lead serves when only a positive lead is used to measure electrical activity in the heart. Chest leads (precordial leads) are also unipolar leads. Figure 22-22*b* shows the sites for placement of chest leads. The recording produced by the electrocardiograph machine (*galvanometer*) represents the currents which occur during the cardiac cycle. The normal EKG pattern is composed of a P wave, a QRS complex, and a T wave (see Fig. 22-23). The P wave represents atrial depoloarization. It indicates the time interval between the origin of the impulse in the SA node and the subsequent spread of the impulse through the atrial musculature. The *P-R interval* represents the time required by the impulse to travel from the SA node through the atria to the AV junction. This interval, from the beginning of the P wave to the beginning of the QRS complex, normally ranges from 0.12 to 0.20 second. The QRS complex represents ventricular deploarization; its normal duration should not normally exceed 0.10 second. There is no manifestation of atrial depolarization in the EKG because it occurs slowly and is buried in the QRS complex. The T wave represents ventricular repolarization. The beginning of the T wave is called the *absolute* refractory period. During this time depolarization

has just occurred, and the cells are unable to accept another stimulus. The middle portion of the T wave is considered the *relative* refractory state, meaning that if a strong-enough stimulus were present, it could cause problems because some cells are polarized while others are still depolarized. The so-called "tail end" of the T wave is very susceptible to the invasion of stimuli and is a source of serious problems for the patient. For example, if a premature or ectopic ventricular beat were to be fired at the tail end of the repolarization process, it could precipitate ventricular fibrillation and even death due to the interruption in conduction.

A U wave on occasion follows the T wave. These waves are observed in the chest leads, and their presence does not always indicate heart disease. They are most often seen in patients with hypokalemia.

A *vectorcardiography* is a test done to record the direction and magnitude of cardiac vectors. An *echocardiography* is a test which uses ultrasound (acoustical waves) to outline the heart structure and motion as well as the great vessels.

**FIGURE 22-22**

(*a*) Standard limb leads. (*b*) Precordial chest leads.

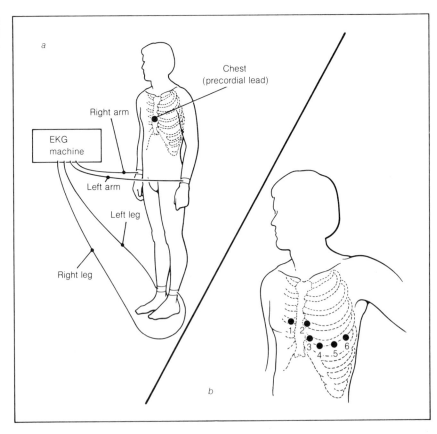

## PHYSICAL ASSESSMENT AND OXYGENATION

Physical assessment of the components of oxygenation will include an evaluation of an individual's circulation, cardiac output, and ventilatory status. This information along with specific laboratory tests and health history will provide essential data when assessing the client's oxygenation status.

The following discussion will focus upon inspection, palpation, percussion, and auscultation of those body systems involved in oxygenation. Each section will review specific assessment techniques in order to help the nurse evaluate specific findings in relation to disruptions in oxygenation.

### Inspection

Physical assessment of oxygenation begins with careful *inspection* of the client. The examiner considers the individual's *general appearance* including physiological and psychosociological developmental stage, body build, posture, skin color, facial expression, orientation, respiratory pattern, pulsa-

tions, edema, and any other aberrations noted while developing rapport and taking the history. The mental status which encompasses the level of consciousness; orientation to time, place, and person; thought content; mood and affect all correlate with the adequate or inadequate supply of oxygen to the brain and should be noted during this part of the examination.

The client's physique may alert the examiner to the presence of possible anomalies related to oxygenation. The posture which a client consistently assumes may require further investigation. If the individual sits in a chair, elevates the shoulders, and leans forward, it is apparent that an attempt is being made to expand the thorax in order to increase the utilization of all available lung space. This posture is typical of adult clients who are experiencing obstructive lung disease.

The client's facial expression may be tense because of exertion on breathing and anxiety. The skin color may also be altered (see Inspection of Skin) and the speech pattern may be disturbed owing to an insufficient intake of air. The client may be able to utter only a few words or phrases at

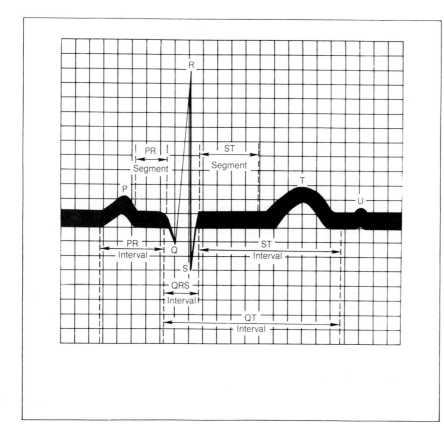

**FIGURE 22-23**
Cardiac cycle, graphically represented by the electrocardiogram.

a time before having to stop and take a breath. When oxygen levels in the body decrease, "the neurologic picture changes from anxiety and restlessness to irritability, to drowsiness, and finally to coma."[48] Should the client appear restless or drowsy, further neurological testing may be needed.

**Skin, mucous membranes, lips, and nailbeds**
The skin, mucous membranes, lips, and nailbeds should be inspected for color, pigmentation, temperature, moisture, and texture. Individuals of certain racial groups who have dark skin or individuals with blood dyscrasias must be assessed carefully (see Chap. 8).

Difficulties with oxygenation may be quickly noted by inspection of the general skin color. Around the mouth the examiner may note either an ashen-blue color or a frank cyanosis. Brightly colored or pale cheeks and lips may also be a significant clue to a dysfunction related to oxygenation and blood formation. To evaluate color, also inspect the mucous membranes under the tongue, roof of the mouth, buccal mucosa, and nailbeds. Diminished oxygenation is suspected if changes in skin color denote cyanosis, if the appearance of cyanosis is sudden in onset, or if the degree of cyanosis increases. Areas of the skin with increased vascularity should also be described.

Normally the *nail base* is firm, and the angle between the nail base and the fingernail is 160°. The examiner may identify the presence of clubbing by inspecting the angle between the skin and nail base. When clubbing is present, the examiner may note that the normal ridges and fingerprints on the touch pads of the fingers are decreased or absent owing to edema. (See Chap. 8 for further discussion.)

**Nose** Inspect the nose for color, drainage, route of air intake, flaring of the nares, and structural deviations. The color and intactness of the mucous membranes, secretions, presence or absence of hair, the size of the air passageways including the inferior and medial turbinates, the presence or absence of polyps, and the structure of the nasal septum should be included in each assessment. The normal color of the nasal mucosa and the turbinates is deep pink. Pale bluish, swollen, or "boggy" turbinates are indicative of an allergy. Polyps of the nasal mucosa are pale, round, and smooth fluid-filled sacs. Polyps are usually found high in the nasal canal (medial turbinate) by using a nasal speculum and light.

Evaluate the nasal septum for deviation and perforation. Use a penlight to occlude one nostril while inspecting the transilluminated septum through the open nostril.

**Sinuses** Transillumination of the sinuses is an additional test used primarily to evaluate a client's progress after an x-ray diagnosis of sinusitis has been made. For this examination the room must be dark. Place the light under the medial aspect of the supraorbital rim for the frontal sinus and above the infraorbital rim for the maxillary sinus.[49] Factors which may decrease the value of this test include under-developed sinus cavities, presence of clear fluid in the sinus cavity giving it a normal appearance, and thick bone and superficial tissues.

**Neck** With the client in a sitting position, inspect the neck for pulsations and distention of the neck veins. Then with the client in a supine position, inspect the neck for venous pulsations. Describe the effects of gradually elevating the head to an upright position. Good light conditions are necessary to accomplish this inspection.

**Trachea** Inspect the trachea for position, deviation from midline, size, shape, and symmetry. Instruct the client to swallow and observe the movement of the trachea. Normally the trachea remains midline with the upward and downward swallowing movement. If clients experience difficulty in swallowing, give them water and observe as they swallow.

**Cough** A cough is produced when there is need to clear the airways; therefore, the presence of a cough is abnormal. When a cough is present, describe the characteristics of the cough, such as whether it is productive or nonproductive of secretions, frequency, incidence in relation to the time of day and changes in position, and sound—hacking, brassy, or barklike. If secretions are expectorated, it is important to note their color, consistency, amount, and odor.

**Respirations** Respirations are carefully inspected to determine whether the route of air intake is oral or nasal. In addition the type of respirations (thoracic or abdominal) is assessed by inspecting the use of accessory muscles such as neck muscle contraction, intercostal or sternal retraction, and abdominal muscle contraction. The rate of respirations per minute, the rhythm of respirations (regular or irregular) and the quality (deep or shallow, quite or labored) are also inspected at this time.

**Thorax** To prepare the client for examination of the chest will require an explanation of the procedure and the patient's cooperation. All clothing must be removed and the female client's chest should be draped. The client is approached from the right side and instructed to turn the head to the left. In addition to the standard landmarks (see Fig. 22-24) of the thorax which are used to describe findings, the examiner may wish to identify and utilize additional landmarks for greater descriptive accuracy. The anterior sternal angle can be identified by finding the bony ridge joining the manubrium to the body of the sternum.[50] The sternal angle is adjacent to the second rib. The interspace immediately below is the second interspace.[51] When identifying ribs or interspaces on the anterior chest wall, start from the sternal angle and second rib, then count downward in an oblique line several centimeters lateral to the sternal edge or costal margin.[52] Posteriorly the inferior angle of the scapula is a helpful landmark, lying approximately at the level of the seventh rib or interspace.[53] The spinous processes may be helpful in describing the location of findings on the posterior chest wall.

Examination of the thorax begins with inspection of its size to determine whether the proportion of the chest is appropriate to body size and whether the rib cage is intact. The shape and contour of the thorax can be determined by observing the client's posture and body alignment. Inspect the anterioposterior diameter by evaluating the right and left lateral views of the chest wall. An extremely convex or concave anterior chest wall indicates alteration of the thorax and lungs. To evaluate the symmetry of the thorax, note the position of the shoulders and the equality of movement of the right and left sides of the chest wall. Any deviation in the body structure of the thorax will compromise the respiratory efforts and therefore alter the oxygen supply. Such bony deviations of the thorax include pigeon chest, scoliosis, and kyphosis. Scars on the chest may suggest a past incidence of oxygen embarrassment. Information about these changes should be elicited from the patient during the health history. Inspect the expansion and synchrony of the thorax. Movement or excursion of the thorax should be equal bilaterally.

**Heart** Inspect the heart by noting the anterior chest for any elevation or prominence which varies from one side to the other (see Fig. 33-24).

Inspect for pulses on the thorax. Describe the location, rate, rhythm, and character of the apical pulse, and point of maximal impulse (PMI), abdominal aorta, and pulsating masses.

**Extremities** Inspection of the extremities is needed in order to evaluate the color of the skin, hair distribution, size, symmetry, and proportion. Observation of the patient's gait, posture, and standing pattern will offer additional data to the nurse.

Examination of the lower extremities for varicose veins is more accurate with the client in a standing position, thereby allowing the veins to fill. The veins should be inspected for size, distortion, and redness.

The skin color and temperature indicate oxygen supply to the periphery. An inadequate oxygen supply or a vascular dysfunction to the extremities may produce clinical findings such as pale, pigmented skin, edema, ulcers, and other trophic changes in the skin.

### Palpation

Palpation is used to provide additional assessment data to the nurse following general inspection. Since palpation and inspection may occur concurrently, much of the data obtained by palpation will increase the overall evaluation of the patient's general health status.

**Nailbeds** The *nailbeds* are normally smooth. The presence of coarse vertical ridges on the nails indicates a possible chronic pulmonary insufficiency. Hyperemia may be suspected when the nails tend "to become periodically flushed and then return to their original color. . . . As the carbon dioxide builds up in the capillaries the arteries dilate, and the blood rushes through the area. When more oxygen has been supplied to the area, the arteries return to their normal size and blood flow becomes normal."[54] The ability of the capillaries to refill is tested by applying enough pressure to blanch the nail bed, releasing the pressure quickly, and noting the rapidity with which the color returns.

Clubbing of the fingers is associated with a severe and chronic decrease in oxygenation. The nails are curved convexly from base to tip and from side to side. The tissue at the base of the nail is spongy and the nail itself is loosely attached; its free edge may be palpable.[55] (Refer to Chap. 8.)

**Nose** The *nose* should be palpated for any anatomical deviations. The patency of each nostril is tested by occluding (with finger pressure) one nostril at a time and instructing the client to close the

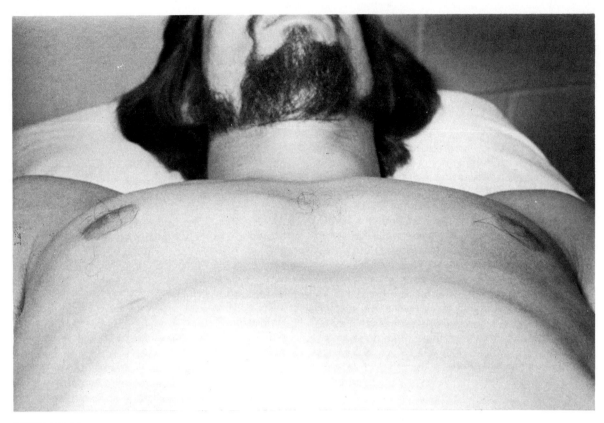

**FIGURE 22-24**
Inspection of the anterior chest for symmetry and elevation. (*Photo by Jeff Collins.*)

mouth and inhale. Examine the interior of the nose by tilting the head back and gently pressing upward on the tip of the nose, using an external source of light for adequate visualization.

In acute sinusitis, redness and edema over the frontal and maxillary sinuses may be observed. In severe sinusitis the eye(s) may nearly close owing to the extreme edema around the orbital region. Palpate the *frontal* sinuses by pressing upward over the superior orbit of the eye and the *maxillary* sinuses by pressing along the ascending processes of the maxillae and the canine fossae. Differences in tenderness can be identified by simultaneous bilateral comparison. The presence of moist secretions in the nose or of a mucopurulent postnasal drip indicates a possible infection of the paranasal sinuses. Pain in the frontal and maxillary sinus regions, edema of the eyelids, and diplopia are symptoms which may be associated with sinusitis.

**N**eck   Palpation of the *neck* includes evaluation of the pulses and a description of the rate, rhythm, amplitude, quality, and vessel wall elasticity. Prior to

evaluating the carotid pulses, instruct the client to turn the head opposite from the side being examined. Palpate only one side at a time in order to avoid the possibility of occluding arterial flow to the brain and to avoid massaging the carotid sinus which decreases the heart rate. While evaluating the pulse areas, include palpation for thrills. (A *thrill* is a high-frequency vibration which may be felt over a vessel, mass, or the cardiac area.) The sensation of a thrill may be likened to the feeling of water running through a hose.

**T**rachea   Palpation of the *trachea* should include assessing its position, along with evaluation of its size, shape, and symmetry. The examiner can place his or her hands on the trachea and ask the patient to swallow. Palpation of the upward movement of the trachea will indicate its proper position.

**T**horax   Findings from inspection may be confirmed or denied and new findings elicited by palpating the *thorax*. The size of the chest wall can be determined by measuring it with a tape measure.

The anteroposterior diameter can be measured by using calipers. Assessment of shape and contour includes palpating the underlying muscle tissue and palpating for masses. If a mass is present, note the location, size, and consistency. Determine the symmetry of the chest wall movement by palpating the anterior and posterior chest walls bilaterally with each respiration. Also evaluate the bone structure as to normal alignment and deviations.

Expansion and synchrony of the thorax are evaluated by measuring the respiratory excursion. The examiner's hands are positioned to grasp the lateral portion of the rib cage with the thumbs placed bilaterally to the tenth thoracic vertebra (see Fig. 22-25). Ask the client to exhale and then to take a deep breath. The character of the movement of thumbs and rib cage should be noted as the client goes from expiratory phase to maximum inspiratory phase (see Fig. 22-26).

The *chest wall* can be palpated to determine the presence or absence of subcutaneous crepitus. If air has escaped and become trapped in the subcutaneous tissues, a crackling sensation will be felt by the examiner. Immediate action must be taken when crepitation is detected, for it progresses quickly, causing rapid obstruction of the airway.[56]

Palpation of the chest wall should focus upon detection of bony prominences and should note the presence of growths or tumors. The thorax can be palpated for rhythmicity of respirations and bilateral uniform chest movement. The examiner can place both hands on the right and left side of the chest wall to assess this movement.

*Tactile fremitus,* sometimes also called *vocal fremitus,* is a palpable vibration produced by the "transmission of the vibration of air resulting from phonation."[57] To palpate for tactile fremitus, ask the client to softly repeat phrases such as "ninety-nine, ninety-nine" or "how now brown cow." Factors influencing the intensity of vocal fremitus include the loudness or frequency of the client's voice, the presence of consolidation in the lung fields, the degree of thickness of subcutaneous tissue, the location of major bronchi in relation to the palpated areas along the chest wall, and the palmar sensitivity of the examiner's hands. Move the hands in a

**FIGURE 22-25**
Starting position to evaluate respiratory excursion. (*Photo by Jeff Collins.*)

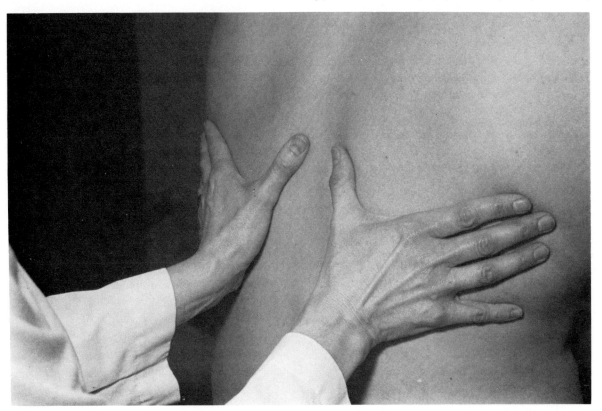

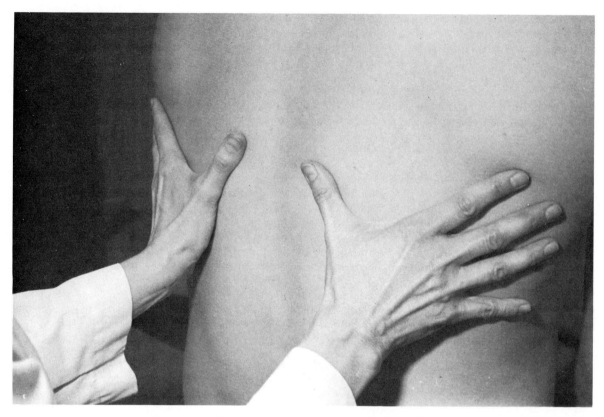

**FIGURE 22-26**
Position of maximum inspiration for evaluating respiratory excursion. (*Photo by Jeff Collins.*)

consistent pattern to evaluate fremitus, by comparing corresponding areas of the thorax. Ask the client to speak at the same audible level during this part of the examination. Note areas of increased or decreased intensity of fremitus and areas absent of fremitus.

Normally, fremitus is most intense "at the base of the neck, both anteriorly and posteriorly, at the first and second interspaces lateral to the sternum, at the right apex, and also between the scapulae."[58] When the density of the lung tissue increases, the vibrations transmitted are intensified. "Increased vocal fremitus therefore occurs in conditions that are associated with consolidation of the lungs."[59] A blockage or obstruction of the upper airway or bronchus will prevent the transmission of the vibration; therefore, fremitus is decreased or absent. "However, air or fluid in the pleural space will diminish the vibrations or make it impossible to feel them."[60]

**E**xtremities   Palpation of the *extremities* is due to evaluate temperature of the skin, hair distribution, size proportion, symmetry, edema, pulses, and dilatation of superficial leg veins. Measurements of the circumference of each leg should be included in the assessment. A tape measure can be placed around the thigh and calf of each leg, and the bilateral measurements compared. A description of the findings should include the rate, rhythm, character, elasticity of the vessel walls, thrills (if present), and the presence or absence of arterial pulses. The brachial, radial, femoral, popliteal, posterior tibialis, and dorsalis pedis pulses should be palpated, and bilateral comparisons for equality should be included (refer to Chap. 29).

The etiology of edema is varied. *Edema* of the feet and ankles (commonly referred to as *dependent* edema) is usually of cardiac origin. *Pitting* edema may be an indication of congestive heart failure. The pit or indentation is produced by a slow, firm, continuous pressure (minimum of 5 seconds) of the thumb over the subcutaneous tissue against the tibia, fibula, medial malleolus, or other bony areas. The pitting may be rated as 1+ through 4+ or the depth of the pit should be estimated and recorded in millimeters.[61] Nonpitting edema may indicate an arterial occlusion of the peripheral vessels. Unilateral edema may indicate obstruction of a major vein.

**H**eart    The *heart* can be palpated by noting the presence of an apical pulsation, rhythm, rate, and character of the impulses, and the presence of thrills. The position of the PMI (Point of Maximum Intensity) should be noted, and the presence of additional pulsating masses detected.

The apical pulse is present over the apex of the heart when the ventricles contract. The PMI is usually seen and palpated on the left side of the chest wall in the fourth or fifth intercostal space near the left midclavicular line. To palpate the PMI, identify the anatomical guidelines on the chest wall for the normally anticipated site, then place the palm or the palmar surface of the fingers over the area and adjacent areas until the maximal impulse is felt (see Fig. 22-27).

### Percussion

Percussion of specific organs such as the thorax, the heart, and the lungs will provide vital data regarding the patient's overall oxygenation potential. It allows the examiner to assess the hollowness or density of a cavity and add the data to the other information collected during the examination.

**T**horax    Percussion of the *thorax* is a method of assessing the amount of air, fluid, or consolidated material in the lungs. The general size of the aerated lungs can also be determined by percussion. A *resonant percussion* sound is normal throughout the thorax except over the heart and liver areas, sternum, and spine.

The percussion of the anterior, posterior, and lateral *chest wall* begins at the top of each shoulder in order to identify the resonant area over the apex of each lung. The client is asked to move the torso to help make the intercostal spaces more apparent. Percussion should occur downward, bilaterally, medially, and laterally in the intercostal spaces. The examiner must avoid percussing over bony structures such as the scapula, clavicle, and ribs (see Fig. 22-28 to 22-30).

Diaphragmatic excursion can be measured bilaterally by percussing the resonant border of the diaphragm at maximum inspiration and maximum expiration. The client is asked to forcefully inhale and hold the breath. By percussing downward, the examiner can mark the point of dullness. The client then forcefully exhales and holds the breath. The

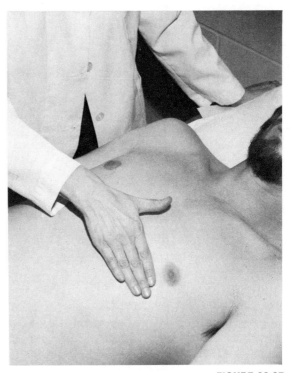

**FIGURE 22-27**
Palpation for PMI. (*Photo by Jeff Collins.*)

examiner identifies and marks the point of dullness once again. The *diaphragmatic excursion* is the distance between the marked areas of dullness. Normally the measured distance is 5 to 6 cm.

The *cardiac borders* can normally be evaluated by percussing the left anterior chest wall to deter-

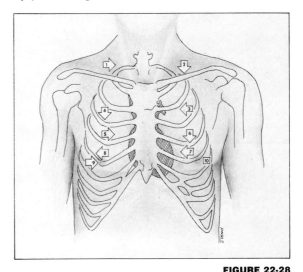

**FIGURE 22-28**
Diagram of areas to percuss and auscultate on the anterior chest wall. (*Drawing by J. Denny.*)

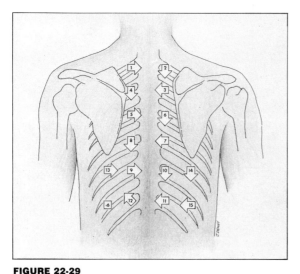

**FIGURE 22-29**
Diagram of areas to percuss and auscultate on the posterior chest wall. (*Drawing by J. Denny.*)

mine the size and position of the heart. Percussion can occur from superior to inferior, lateral to medial, medial to lateral, and inferior to superior. Markings should be placed where dullness is felt or heard in order to outline the borders of the heart.

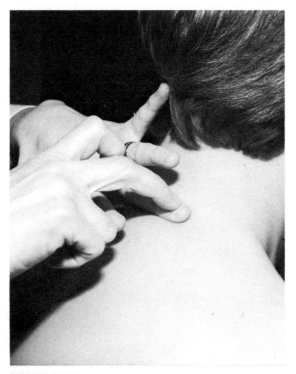

**FIGURE 22-30**
Percussion across top of shoulder. (*Photo by Jeff Collins.*)

The method described offers a rather gross assessment of the heart's size and location, whereas x-ray is the better method of gathering this information.

### Auscultation

Information gathered by inspection, palpation, and percussion can be validated and supplemented by auscultation. In order to perform auscultation effectively, the examiner must have the necessary knowledge of and skill in stethoscope usage, a normal auditory capacity, and a quiet room. Auscultation begins at the superior aspect and proceeds downward with bilateral comparison of each comparable area. Both the bell and the diaphragm of the stethoscope should be used when auscultating the anterior, posterior, and lateral chest walls.

**N**ose   Auscultation of the *nose* is used to further verify the patency of the nasal passages and to assist in determining whether pathological sounds heard in the chest are transmitted from the upper respiratory tract or originate in the lower respiratory tract. To verify patency, occlude (with finger pressure) one nostril at a time, place the diaphragm of the stethoscope under the open nostril, and listen to the air intake. To differentiate the origin of pathological chest sounds, place the diaphragm of the stethoscope under the client's nose. If the sound is the same as the sound heard in the chest, it is probably a transmitted upper respiratory sound. If the sound is not the same as the sound heard in the chest, it is probably originating in the lower respiratory tract and is, therefore, pathological.

**N**eck   Auscultation of the *neck* for bruits is a significant assessment component. A *bruit* is a somewhat harsh, blowing sound heard over a vessel; it may be normal in a child but is usually indicative of vascular pathology in the adult client. In assessing for bruits, include the temporal, carotid, and subclavian arteries.

**Heart sounds**   Auscultation of the *heart* provides additional information about the client's cardiac status. The examiner must understand the anatomy and physiology of the heart's action and the differences in loudness, quality, and pitch which occur in the body at various stages of growth and development. Careful supervision is also necessary to learn and practice the skill.

   The heart should be auscultated in the following order: aortic area (right side of sternum, second interspace), pulmonic area (left side of sternum, second interspace), Erb's point (left side of sternum, third interspace), tricuspid area (left side of sternum, fifth interspace), mitral area (medial to left midclavicular line in fifth interspace) (see Fig. 22-31). Use the bell of the stethoscope to listen to *low-pitched heart sounds* and the diaphragm of the stethoscope to listen to *high-pitched heart sounds.* Note the rate, rhythm, and character of each heart sound. Apical heart rates should be listened to for one full minute. While listening to heart sounds, focus *only* on the heart sounds (one at a time).

Examine the client in both a sitting and a supine position. If the heart sounds are difficult to hear, ask the client to sit up and lean forward. This position brings the heart closer to the chest wall, thereby increasing the hearing potential of the examiner.

The *cardiac cycle* is divided into systole and diastole. During auscultation of the complete cycle the first heart sound heard is $S_1$, which is due to closure of the mitral and tricuspid valves. The second heart sound ($S_2$) results from closure of the aortic and pulmonary valves. A physiological third heart sound ($S_3$) occurs when there is rapid filling of the ventricles, and a physiological fourth heart sound ($S_4$) may occur late in diastole, in conjunction with atrial contraction.

At the apex, the first sound ($S_1$) is louder, longer, and lower pitched than the second sound ($S_2$).[62] The mitral valve closes only a fraction of a second before the tricuspid valve closes, and so a splitting of $S_1$ is normal and common, especially when heard in the tricuspid area. In order to distinguish $S_1$ from $S_2$, gently palpate the carotid artery. The pulse felt is simultaneous with the sound heard ($S_1$).

The second sound ($S_2$) is usually louder than $S_1$ at the base. Closing of the aortic valve is predominantly heard at the apex. The pulmonic valve closure is softer and normally heard along the superior left sternal border. A physiological splitting of $S_2$ may normally occur on inspiration and is best heard over the second interspace to the left of the sternal border. A split $S_2$ may be emphasized by instructing the client to take a deep breath and hold it for a short time.

The physiological third sound ($S_3$) is inconsistent, faint, and low pitched and becomes louder upon expiration. If present, it is best heard at the apex and with the client in a left recumbent position. It usually disappears when the client sits upright. A third heart sound may be normal in young people under age 30, in adults after exercise, and during times of stress.

**M**urmurs  Normally, the interval between heart sounds is silent. When noise is heard between the

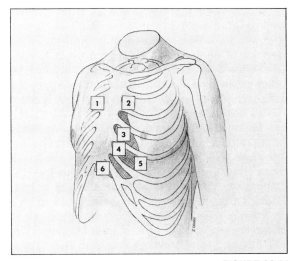

**FIGURE 22-31**
Areas of the heart to auscultate. (*Drawing by J. Denny.*)

heart sounds, it is referred to as a *murmur.* A cardiac murmur is a prolonged series of audible vibrations, characterized by intensity (loudness), frequency (pitch), configuration (shape), quality, duration, direction of radiation, and timing in the cardiac cycle.[63]

It is important to differentiate between murmurs and the normal heart sounds. Generally murmurs tend to be of longer duration and differ in the quality of the sound. When a noise is detected between the first and second heart sound, it is referred to as a *systolic murmur.* If the abnormal sound is produced between the third and fourth heart sounds, it is referred to as a *diastolic murmur.*

Murmurs are caused by a variety of changes that occur within the heart structure. They may be noted when there is constriction in the wall of a blood vessel; when the diameter of a heart valve is narrowed or incompetent (e.g., stenosed), or there is a backflow of blood regurgitation due to defective valves; when there is an increase in the rate or velocity of blood flow (e.g., exercise, pregnancy); or in the presence of an altered or taunt membrane.

The *quality* of a murmur varies with the type and location of the problem. Murmurs may be harsh or rasping (loud), musical or whistle (or high pitched), rumbling (often noted with a mid or late diastolic murmur), or blowing. The *frequency* (pitch) of all murmurs can also vary with the velocity of blood flow. The greater the velocity of the blood flow, the higher the pitch. The lower the overall blood velocity, the softer the pitch.

The *intensity,* or loudness, of a murmur can

range from being barely audible to being audible with the stethoscope removed from direct contact with the skin. For purposes of identification the intensity of murmur has been divided into six *grades* (see Table 22-6). It is essential that a murmur be graded when first noted so that it can be fully evaluated, classified, and reevaluated with subsequent health visits.

Murmurs are transmitted with or in the direction of the bloodstream in which they are produced. They can also be transmitted toward bony structures of the upper extremity, the chest wall, or the posterior or back of the chest. The shape or configuration of the murmur may be referred to as a crescendo, plateau, or decrescendo. A *crescendo* shape is used to describe a murmur that increases in intensity, peeks, and then begins to decrease in intensity. A *plateau* murmur sustains its shape throughout the cycle. A *decrescendo*-shaped murmur decreases in intensity after its point of initial onset.

The *timing* of heart sounds is heard in accordance with the cardiac cycle. These may be divided into three phases and include early, mid, and late systolic or diastolic phases. A *systolic murmur* may begin with or after the first heart sound. A *midsystolic murmur* begins after the first heart sound and ends before the second sound. A *pansystolic murmur* is a sound that is persistent throughout systole.

*Diastolic sounds* that occur early in the diastolic phase are referred to as *protodiastole* murmurs. Diastolic murmurs that appear late in the diastolic phase are referred to as *presystole murmurs.*

Systolic murmurs are the most frequent heart murmurs heard. They are classified as either ejection murmurs or pansystolic murmurs. *Ejection* murmurs are of short duration and begin after the first heart sound and climax during midsystole. They are heard in aortic and pulmonic stenosis and may be noted in the so-called "functional" or "innocent" murmur.

The *pansystolic* (or halo systolic) murmur begins with the first heart sound and continues through part of the second sound. It is associated with tricuspid regurgitation (see Chap. 27) and ventricular septal defects. *Diastolic* murmurs are usually observed in problems related to regurgitant murmurs (semilunar valve insufficiency) and impairment of ventricular filling due valvular constriction or malfunction.

To locate murmurs, the examiner must focus on each phase of the cardiac cycle, listening first to the systolic phase and then to the diastolic phase. Frequently the murmurs are best heard over the cardiac area directly affected. For example, valvular murmurs are best heard directly over the valve that is stenosed or altered in overall functioning. Murmurs that are present with septal defects or congenital anomalies are best heard over the sternal borders, the apex of the heart, or the region of the neck. Additional reference points are discussed in the Assessment section, especially in Chap. 27.

**Breath sounds**  While listening to *respirations,* the examiner should focus (one at a time) on the breath sounds, voice sounds, or any adventitious sounds which may be present. Approach from the client's right side and instruct the client to turn the head to the left and to breathe slowly and deeply with the mouth open, demonstrating if necessary. If the client breathes through the nose, air turbulance may be transmitted to the chest, and extraneous sound may be misinterpreted (see Fig. 22-32).

Additional specifics which may be noted upon auscultation of *breath sounds* include the character of the inspiratory and expiratory phases of respiration, the quality and pitch of the breath sound, and the differentiation between rales and rhonchi.

As the air moves through the trachea and bronchi, a vibration occurs which produces the breath sounds heard on auscultation. Variations in resonance of the breath sounds may occur, depending on the thickness of the chest wall. Careful attention must be given to listening over the intercostal spaces rather than over the ribs and scapulae (see Figs. 22-28 and 22-29).

The breath sounds heard during auscultation may be classified into four categories: vesicular, bronchial, bronchovesicular, and adventitious.

*Vesicular sounds* are described as soft rustling

**TABLE 22-6**
GRADING OF CARDIAC MURMURS

| Grade | Description |
|---|---|
| Grade I | Faint sound barely audible with special effort, e.g., position change. |
| Grade II | Faint sound but recognizable. |
| Grade III | An audible, prominent sound, but not loud. |
| Grade IV | Audible, loud sound. |
| Grade V | Audible and very loud sound. |
| Grade VI | Very audible and extremely loud sound. Can be heard with the stethoscope removed from direct contact with the thoracic area. |

SOURCE: From Willis J. Hurst, *The Heart,* McGraw-Hill, New York, 1974, p. 261.

or swishing sounds. The inspiratory phase is longer and louder than the expiratory phase. Normally, vesicular sounds are heard over all lung tissue except in the upper intrascapular area and beneath the manubrium sterni.

*Bronchial sounds* are louder, harsher, and higher pitched than vesicular sounds. The inspiratory phase is shorter, and the expiratory phase is longer and louder. Bronchial sounds are not normal when heard over lung tissue. The sounds heard when listening over the trachea near the suprasternal notch simulate the pathological bronchial breath sounds.

*Bronchovesicular sounds* are a combination of vesicular (soft, swishing) sounds and bronchial (harsh, louder) sounds. Inspiratory and expiratory phases are nearly equal. The sounds are normal when heard over the manubrium sterni and in the upper intrascapular regions where the large airways bifurcate. Listening to the sounds in these particular areas offers the examiner the opportunity to hear simulated pathological sounds as a base of reference to identify breath sounds.

*Adventitious sounds* are abnormal breath sounds such as rales, rhonchi, wheezes, and friction rub.

*Rales* are fine sounds sometimes described as similar to the rustling of plastic wrap, to the bubbling of a carbonated drink, or to the sound heard when rubbing a few strands of hair together near the ear. Rales are best heard on inspiration. The presence of rales indicates pathology in the bronchioles and alveoli.

*Rhonchi* are coarse, loud sounds which may simulate a snoring sound. They are heard best during expiration. When rhonchi are heard, the client is asked to cough and to clear the nasal passages as the sounds may be transmitted from the upper respiratory tract or may be due to mobile secretions in the bronchus. The diaphragm of the stethoscope is then placed in front of the nares in order to further determine whether the sound originates in the upper respiratory tract or in the lungs. The presence of rhonchi is indicative of pathology in the larger air passages of the lungs.

*Wheezes* are similar to rhonchi but with a squeaky quality best heard on expiration. The sound does not clear with coughing because it is due to constriction of the bronchial tubes.

*Friction rub* is a sound produced by the altered mobility of the pleura and lung tissue during respiration. It is a result of inflammation of the pleura which roughens the surfaces and decreases the lubricant between the surfaces. When a friction rub

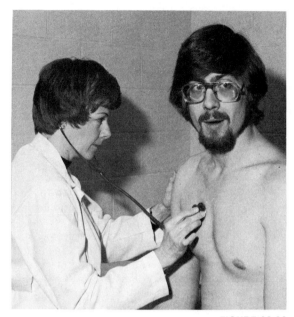

**FIGURE 22-32**
Auscultation of anterior lung fields (client position described).
*(Photo by Jeff Collins.)*

is present, it is most easily heard on the anterior chest wall and at the base of the lung in the lateral axillary region.

The following terms are used to describe the voice sounds heard through auscultation. They include bronchophony, pectorophony, and egophony.

*Bronchophony* describes voice sounds which are exaggerated in clarity and loudness. Normally speech is indistinct except when one listens over the trachea or a large bronchus. Distinct voice sounds are indicative of pulmonary consolidation or compression of lung tissue.[64]

*Pectorophony* is the exaggerated clarity of whispered sounds which are normally indistinct when auscultating lung tissue. When whispered sounds are heard distinctly upon auscultation, it is indicative of small early partial consolidation of the lung tissue.[65]

*Egophony* describes the situation wherein the client says "ee," however the listener hears the sound through the stethoscope as "ay." The change from "ee" to "ay" is abnormal. "Egophony is rarely found except over an area of compressed lung above a pleural effusion."[66]

**Auscultation of blood vessels**  Auscultation for bruits should include both the *femoral* and *renal arteries.* With the client in a supine position, the renal arteries are approximately 10 to 15 cm above the umbilicus and to the right and left of the midline. The femoral arteries can be easily auscultated after locating the pulse in each groin.

Accurate *blood pressure recordings* are significant in assessing the oxygenation status of the client. Consideration must be given to physical factors which influence blood pressure, including height, weight, age, gender, race, and heredity. Technical factors including the size of the cuff (in relation to size of extremity), application of cuff to the extremity, and skill of the examiner in accurate auscultation and recording are also important (see Chap. 28). The normal adult range for systolic pressures is 95 to 140 mmHg; for diastolic pressures it is 60 to 90 mmHg. The difference between systolic and diastolic pressure is *pulse pressure*. The normal adult range for pulse pressures is 40 to 50 mmHg.

Blood pressure recordings between the right and left arms may vary 5 to 15 mmHg. The systolic blood pressure of the lower extremities is normally 10 mmHg higher than that of the upper extremities. When pressures taken while the client is standing and reclining are contrasted, the systolic blood pressure may be found to decrease 15 mmHg and the diastolic pressure increase 3 to 5 mmHg in the standing position.

## REFERENCES

1 William Harvey, *The Circulation of the Blood*, Everyman's Library, New York, 1966, p. 39.
2 Arthur Guyton, *Textbook of Medical Physiology*, Saunders, Philadelphia, 1966, 1970, p. 109.
3 *Ibid.*, p. 111.
4 *Ibid.*, p. 112.
5 *Ibid.*, p. 113.
6 *Ibid.*, p. 112.
7 *Ibid.*, p. 113.
8 Joan Luckman and Karen Sorensen, *Medical Surgical Nursing: A Psychophysiologic Approach*, Saunders, Philadelphia, 1974, p. 751.
9 Guyton, *op. cit.*, p. 117.
10 *Ibid.*, p. 162.
11 *Ibid.*, p. 163.
12 W. J. Williams et al. (eds.), *Hematology*, McGraw-Hill, New York, 1972, p. 1000.
13 A. G. Shaper, "Oestrogens, Progesterone, Platelets," *Lancet*, **2:**569, 1968.
14 P. Cohen and F. H. Gardner, "Thrombocytopenic Effect of Sustained High Dosage Prednisone, Therapy in Thrombocytopenic Purpura," *N Engl J Med*, 265–611, 1961.

15 L. A. Harker, "Kinetics of Thrombosis," *J Clin Invest*, **47:**458, 1968.
16 E. P. Cronkite, "Regulation of Platelet Production in Hemostatic Mechanisms," *Brookhaven Sympos Biol*, **10:**96, 1967.
17 J. R. Krevans et al., "Hemorrhagic Disorder Following Massive Blood Transfusion," *J Am Med Assoc*, **159:**171, 1955.
18 M. G. Davey, *The Survival and Destruction of Human Platelets*, Karger, Basel, 1966, p. 99.
19 N. R. Shulman et al., "Evidence That the Spleen Retains the Youngest and Hemostatically Most Effective Platelets," *Trans Assoc Am Physicians*, **81:**302, 1968.
20 S. Witte, "Megakaryocyten und Thrombocytopoiese bei der Experimentallen Thrombocytopenischen Purpura," *Acta Haematol*, **14:**215, 1955.
21 S. Ebbe et al., "Megakaryocyte Size in Thrombocytopenic and Normal Rats," *Blood*, **32:**383, 1968.
22 Williams, *op. cit.*, p. 1048.
23 Guyton, *op. cit.*, p. 233.
24 Guyton, *op. cit.*, p. 180.
25 Luckman and Sorensen, *op. cit.*, p. 597.
26 J. W. Hurst et al. (eds.), *The Heart*, 3d ed., McGraw-Hill, New York, 1974, p. 57.
27 Guyton, *op. cit.*, p. 184.
28 Guyton, *op. cit.*, p. 189.
29 Hurst, *op. cit.*, p. 23.
30 *Ibid.*, p. 24.
31 *Ibid.*, p. 25.
32 *Ibid.*
33 *Ibid.*, p. 26.
34 *Ibid.*, p. 29.
35 *Ibid.*
36 *Ibid.*, p. 31.
37 *Ibid.*, p. 32.
38 *Ibid.*
39 *Ibid.*
40 *Ibid.*
41 Guyton, *op. cit.*, p. 355.
42 Sharon Spaeth Bushnell, *Respiratory Intensive Care Nursing*, Little, Brown, Boston, 1973, p. 6.
43 *Ibid.*, p. 18.
44 Guyton, *op. cit.*, p. 550.
45 Bushnell, *op. cit.*, pp. 18–19.
46 Guyton, *op. cit.*, p. 571.
47 *Ibid.*, p. 572.
48 Josephine M. Sana and Richard D. Judge (eds.), *Physical Appraisal Methods in Nursing Practice*, Little, Brown, Boston, 1975, p. 135.
49 Richard D. Judge and George D. Zuidema (eds.), *Methods of Clinical Examination: A Physiological Approach*, 3d ed., Little, Brown, Boston, 1974, p. 102.
50 Barbara Bates, *A Guide to Physical Examination*, Lippincott, Philadelphia, 1974, p. 74.

51 *Ibid.,* p. 74.
52 *Ibid.*
53 *Ibid.,* p. 75.
54 Sana and Judge, *op. cit.,* p. 135.
55 Judge and Zuidema, *op. cit.,* pp. 126–127.
56 Sana and Judge, *op. cit.,* p. 155.
57 *Ibid.,* p. 153.
58 *Ibid.*
59 *Ibid.,* pp. 154–155.
60 *Ibid.,* p. 155.
61 Elmer L. Gowin and Richard L. DeGowin, *Bedside Diagnostic Examination,* 2d ed., Macmillan, 1969, p. 324.
62 Judge and Zuidema, *op. cit.,* p. 162.
63 Hurst, *op. cit.,* p. 261.
64 Judge and Zuidema, *op. cit.,* p. 165.
65 *Ibid.,* p. 133.
66 *Ibid.*

## BIBLIOGRAPHY

Andrioli, K., et al.: *Comprehensive Cardiac Care* Mosby, St. Louis, 1968.

Anthony, C. P.: *Textbook of Anatomy and Physiology,* 7th ed., Mosby, St. Louis, 1967.

Barrett, N. R.: "The Pleura," *Thorax,* **25:**515, September 1970.

Baum, G. L.: *Textbook of Pulmonary Diseases,* Little, Brown, Boston, 1973.

Bates, D. B., et al.: *Respiratory Function in Diseases,* 2d ed., Saunders, Philadelphia, 1971.

Beland, I., and J. Passos: *Clinical Nursing, Pathophysiological and Psychosocial Approaches,* 3d ed., Macmillan, New York, 1975.

Betson, C.: "Blood Gases," *Am J Nurs,* **68:**1010, May 1968.

Braunwald, E., J. Ross, Jr., and E. H. Sonnenblick: "Mechanisms of Contraction of the Normal and Failing Heart," *N Engl J Med,* **277:**794, 1967.

Broughton, J.: "Chest Physical Diagnosis for Nurses and Respiratory Therapists," *Heart Lung,* **1:**200–206, March 1972.

Bucholz, P., and C. Gilbert: "Understanding the EKG," *RN,* **35**(2):38, February 1972.

Burch, G., and T. Winsor: *A Primer of Electrocardiography,* Lea & Febiger, Philadelphia, 1966.

Buruner, L., et al.: *Textbook of Medical Surgical Nursing,* 3d ed., Lippincott, Philadelphia, 1975.

Cherniak, R. M., L. Cherniak, and A. Naimark: *Respiration in Health and Disease,* 2d ed., Saunders, Philadelphia, 1972.

Conn, H. F. (ed.): *Current Therapy,* Saunders, Philadelphia, 1974.

Delp, Mahlon H., and Robert T. Manning (eds.): *Major's Physical Diagnosis,* 8th ed., Saunders, 1975.

Early, G.: "The Gaseous Exchange Process: Nursing Implication," in K. C. Kintzel (ed.), *Advanced Concepts in Clinical Nursing,* Lippincott, Philadelphia, 1971.

Egan, D.: *Fundamentals of Respiratory Therapy,* 2d ed., Mosby, St. Louis, 1973.

Erslev, A. J.: "Control of Red Cell Production," *Ann Rev Med,* 315, 1969.

Fraser, R. G., and J. A. Pare: *Structure and Function of the Lung,* Saunders, Philadelphia, 1971.

Friedberg, Charles: *Disease of the Heart,* Saunders, Philadelphia, 1970.

Ganz, W., and H. J. C. Swan: "Measurement of Blood Flow by Thermodilution," *Am J Cardiol,* **29:**241, 1972.

Hedges, J. E., and C. J. Bridges: "Stimulation of the Cough Reflex," *Am J Nurs,* **68:**347, February 1968.

Hobson, Lawrence B.: *Examination of the Patient,* McGraw-Hill, New York, 1975.

Hunsinger, D., et al.: *Respiratory Technology,* Virginia, Reston Publishing Company, Inc., 1973.

Kao, F. F.: *An Introduction to Respiratory Physiology,* American Elsevier, 1973.

Katz, A. M.: "Contractile Proteins of the Heart," *Physiol Rev,* **50:**63, 1970.

Kelman, G. R.: *Applied Cardiovascular Physiology,* Appleton-Century-Crofts, New York, 1971.

Kernicki, J., B. Bullock, and Joan Matthews: *Cardiovascular Nursing,* Putnam, New York, 1970.

Kurihara, M.: "Assessment and Maintenance of Adequate Respiration," *Nurs Clin North Am,* **3:**65, March 1968.

Lagerson, Joanne: "The Bed and the Breath," *Resp Care,* **18:**190–194, March–April, 1973.

Lehmann, Sister Janet: "Auscultation of the Heart Sounds," *Am J Nurs,* **72**(7):1242–1246, July 1972.

Littman, D.: "Stethoscope and Auscultation," *Am J Nurs,* **72:**1238, July 1972.

Longmore, Donald: *The Heart,* World University Library, McGraw-Hill, New York, 1971.

Mahoney, Elizabeth Ann, Laurie Verdisco, and Lillie Shortridge: *How To Collect and Record a Health History,* Lippincott, Philadelphia, 1976.

Marshall, R. J., and J. T. Shepher: "Cardiac Function in Health and Disease," Saunders, Philadelphia, 1968.

Mayer, G., et al.: "Arrhythmias and Cardiac Output," *Am J Nurs,* **72:**9, 1597, September 1972.

Meltzer, L. E., et al.: *Intensive Coronary Care,* The Charles Press, Philadelphia, 1970.

Phillips, R., and M. Feeney: *The Cardiac Rhythms,* Saunders, Philadelphia, 1973.

Programmed Instruction Patient Assessment: "Examination of the Chest and Lungs," *Am J Nurs,* **76:**9, 1453, September 1976.

Randall, W. C. (ed.): *Nervous Control of the Heart,* Williams & Wilkins, Baltimore, 1965.

Riseman, Joseph: P-Q-R-S-T, Macmillan, New York, 1968.

Rushman, Robert: *Cardiovascular Dynamics,* 2d ed. Saunders, Philadelphia, 1967.

Secor, Jane: *Patient Care in Respiratory Problems,* Saunders, Philadelphia, 1969.

Small, Iver, F.: *Introduction to the Clinical History,* 2d ed., Medical Examination Publishing Company, Inc., New York, 1971.

Stein, Emanuel: *The Electrocardiogram,* Saunders, Philadelphia, 1976.

Stroheman, F., Jr.: *Regulation of Red Cell Production in Blood Cells,* Greunwalt and Jamieson (eds.), Lippincott, Philadelphia, 1970.

Thorling, E. B., and A. J. Erslev: "The Tissue Tension of Oxygen and Its Relation to Hematocrit and Erythropoiesis," *Blood,* **31:**332–1968.

Thorn, G., et al. (eds.): *Harrison's Principles of Internal Medicine,* 8th ed., McGraw-Hill, New York, 1977.

Traver, Gayle A.: "Assessment of the Thorax and Lungs," *Am J Nurs,* **73:**3, 466–471, March 1973.

———: "Respiratory Care: Roles of Allied Health Professionals," *Med Clin North Am,* **57:**793–800, 1973.

Vander, A., J. Sherman, and D. Luciano: *Human Physiology, The Mechanisms of Body Function,* 2d ed., McGraw-Hill, New York, 1975.

West, J. B.: *Ventilation/Blood Flow and Gas Exchange,* 2d ed., Davis, Philadelphia, 1971.

Williams, R. A.: *Textbook of Black Related Diseases,* McGraw-Hill, New York, 1975.

# 23

# DISTURBANCES IN THE OXYGEN-CARRYING MECHANISM

Judith M. McFarlane

The interaction of the human body with the internal and external environments can affect the circulation throughout the organism. Oxygen, the essential component of aerobic respiration, is bound to hemoglobin molecules within the red blood cell and transported to every part of the body. When the body's vital organs are deprived of oxygen and nutrients through an increase in erythrocyte destruction, an increase in erythrocyte production, or bleeding and clotting disorders, multiple changes can occur within the individual. This chapter will consider each of these disturbances and the effects they produce on the patient.

## DEFECTS IN ERYTHROCYTE PRODUCTION

Effective erythropoiesis (Chap. 22) requires an adequate intake of specific vitamins, a balanced diet, and adequate absorption of nutrients. Disruptions in erythrocyte production will result in *megaloblastic anemias.* These disorders are characterized by impairment of deoxyribonucleic acid (DNA) synthesis within red blood cells and result in the production of megaloblasts or large abnormal erythrocytes. Anemias caused by these changes are seen in deficiencies of vitamin $B_{12}$ and folic acid, metabolic disorders, and drug-induced megaloblastic anemias.

### Vitamin $B_{12}$ Deficiencies

Normally, vitamin $B_{12}$ is supplied by animal products such as meat and fish. Vitamin $B_{12}$ is stored in liver, where it is released as needed for the maturation of red blood cells. Reserves of vitamin $B_{12}$ may be depleted by a decreased intake of animal products or an increased body need, as in the presence of pregnancy or tumors.

Deficiencies in vitamin $B_{12}$ can impair DNA synthesis within the red blood cells and result in the production of large, abnormally shaped red blood cells, easily destroyed because of their fragile membrane. Vitamin $B_{12}$ is necessary for cell growth and maturation; deficiencies decrease this activity in all body cells.

Several conditions can lead to a deficiency of vitamin $B_{12}$. Because this vitamin is absorbed in the small intestines, the removal of all or a portion of the small intestine can impair its absorption. Bowel strictures necessitating *surgery* (e.g., anastomosis) cause a diversion of gastric contents, bypassing the section of the intestine where vitamin $B_{12}$ is absorbed and resulting in a deficiency of the vitamin.

*Parasites,* such as tapeworm, may also contribute to a vitamin $B_{12}$ deficiency. The parasites lodged in the intestines compete for the vitamin $B_{12}$ that is present and decrease the amount available for absorption. *Sprue* is a malabsorption syndrome which impairs the absorptive membrane of the small intestines. Therefore, food, minerals, water, and vitamins such as vitamin $B_{12}$ cannot be adequately absorbed by the small intestines.

Deficiency in vitamin $B_{12}$ can also occur after a significant *decrease* in the *ingestion of animal products.* However, a deficiency from this cause usually takes many years to develop. The most common cause of vitamin $B_{12}$ deficiency is a *decrease in the production of the intrinsic factor* caused by gastric atrophy or surgical removal of the gastric mucosa. Vitamin $B_{12}$ deficiencies resulting from this change lead to one of the most common megaloblastic anemias called *pernicious anemia.*

**Pernicious anemia** A chronic condition, pernicious anemia is characterized by a deficiency in the production of the so-called intrinsic factor. Absorption of vitamin $B_{12}$ is dependent upon a mucoprotein, or a related substance bound to a mucoprotein, found in the mucus secreted by the stomach. This factor has been called the *intrinsic factor* (IF). When present, it combines with vitamin $B_{12}$, making the vitamin more soluble and absorbable by the body. In the absence of IF the absorption of vitamin $B_{12}$ is poor, altering RBC maturation.

**P**athophysiology When the absorption of vitamin $B_{12}$ is disrupted by the absence of IF, the rate of red blood cell production is slowed, and the shape and structure of the cells are altered. The cell membranes are fragile and easily destroyed. The cells are larger than normal (*macrocytic*), vary in size (*anisocytosis*), and are deformed in shape (*poikilocytosis*).[1]

The growth of all body cells is affected by a vitamin $B_{12}$ deficiency. The cells most affected by this disruption are in the bone marrow and gastrointestinal tract. In the gastrointestinal tract, the gastric mucosa becomes thin, and muscle atrophy occurs. Atrophy of the stomach leads to a decreased hydrochloric acid production and contributes to failure of the gastric fundus to secrete enough IF (thermolabile glucoprotein) to ensure absorption of ingested vitamin $B_{12}$.

*Cause* The cause of pernicious anemia remains obscure. Although a *genetic predisposition* may

exist, the mechanisms of inheritance are unknown. Pernicious anemia does seem to run in families, and the question of heredity must be considered. Approximately 13 percent of the afflicted patients' families have pernicious anemia.[2]

Most current attention focuses upon an *autoimmune* mechanism as a potential causative factor. Serum autoantibodies to gastric parietal cell cytoplasm are found in 90 percent of patients with pernicious anemia. Blocking and binding antibodies to IF can be found in the serum, gastric secretions, and saliva of patients with pernicious anemia. Thyroid antibodies have also been noted in many patients with pernicious anemia. Patients with thyroid disruptions have serum antibodies to gastric and parietal cells.[3] The evidence is not conclusive; however, it does suggest that if antibodies to IF are present, they may inhibit synthesis or release of gastric IF by reacting with parietal gastric cells.[4]

*Iron deficiency* can result in atrophy of the gastric mucosa and lead to decreased production of IF. This usually occurs in the presence of long-term iron deficiency. *Gastric surgery* which includes the removal of the gastric mucosa that releases IF (for example, a total gastrectomy; see Chap. 16) can lead to the development of pernicious anemia, unless replacement of vitamin $B_{12}$ is instituted early.

*Effects on the patient* The primary effects pernicious anemia centers on the reduction in hemoglobin content due to the production of defective red blood cells and subsequent reduction in oxygen-carrying capacity of the erythrocyte. This results in classic anemia with weakness, fatigue, and light-headedness. There is an increased cardiac output to compensate for the reduced circulating oxygen, which can lead to palpitation, dyspnea and orthopnea, and eventually pump failure (see Chap. 24). Disruptions in cardiac rhythm, such as tachycardia and premature beats, can be noted. Hypertrophy and precardial murmurs and angina may result. Decreased hemoglobin supply can lead to tissue anoxia and contributes to fatigue.

Deminished production of mature, well-formed erythrocytes may cause *disruptions* in *growth and development* and degenerative changes in the lateral and dorsal columns of the spinal cord.[5] The earliest *neurological abnormality* noted is the loss of the myelin sheath followed by degeneration of the axon and finally death of the neuron.[6] These changes can be reversed, providing early treatment is initiated. *Peripheral nerve damage* can occur, leading to *disturbances in proprioception* and vibratory senses, ataxia, irritability, and *behavioral changes.* Occasionally, alteration in smell and taste and optic atrophy can occur. Other possible results include *peripheral paresthesia* of the hands and feet, loss of bowel and bladder control, alteration in reflexes, poor memory, depression and/or delirium. In addition, the patient may experience a generalized lack of coordination and an inability to perform fine movements.

Gastric atrophy and decreased production of hydrochloric acid may lead to *achlorhydria* and alter food digestion. Dyspepsia, anorexia, weight loss, a decrease in appetite, constipation, and diarrhea may be noted.

The characteristic "lemon skin" of jaundice is an indication of increased destruction of malformed red blood cells. Unconjugated bilirubin (see Chap. 19) may be seen in blood and in stool and urine, if bilirubin production exceeds the liver's ability to conjugate and excrete this material.

*Glossitis* and *gingivitis* (inflammation of gums) can also occur because of the absence of vitamin $B_{12}$ and disruption of food intake. Nutritional deficits in vitamin $B_{12}$ ingestion along with anorexia can compound the problem.

**F**irst-Level Nursing Care   Pernicious anemia is classically an adult problem, but it has been reported in children.[7,8] Pernicious anemia is uncommon in individuals before the age of 30. It is most often seen in individuals between 50 and 60 years of age. More commonly affected are blue-eyed persons with grey or white hair. These individuals tend to be of Northern European or Scandinavian descent. In the United States the New England and the Great Lakes regions have a higher incidence of the problem because of the population's ancestry. A higher incidence is also noted among individuals with group A blood type. Blacks and Orientals do not seem to have a high incidence of pernicious anemia.

*Population at Risk*   Several groups of individuals are at risk to develop pernicious anemia. Persons who have a total or partial gastrectomy involving the removal of all or part of the gastric mucosa are at risk to develop vitamin $B_{12}$ deficiency and resulting anemia. The absence of the gastric mucosa will also reduce the amount of IF present and impair vitamin $B_{12}$ absorption. In addition persons with a family history of pernicious anemia, or individuals living in the specific areas of the country noted above are also at risk.

Iron deficiency, resulting in atrophy of the gastric mucosa, may cause individuals to become potential candidates for pernicious anemia. In addition, persons with thyroid problems may also be at risk owing to the presence of serum antibodies which react against the gastric mucosa and alter its effect.

*Prevention*   Educating community health personnel to the causes and treatment of vitamin $B_{12}$ deficiency is essential. By alerting members of the health team to early identification of high-risk groups, severe complications of vitamin $B_{12}$ deficiency can be averted. Nutritional counseling is important. Individuals should be taught that vitamin $B_{12}$ is normally supplied in meat, liver, fish, eggs, and milk.

Patients with chronic gastrointestinal problems such as peptic ulcer and diverticulitis should be encouraged to treat the problem early to prevent gastric surgery. If gastric surgery is performed, removal of the gastric mucosa may potentiate development of vitamin $B_{12}$ deficiency owing to the absence of IF. Patients with thyroid problems should have the problem corrected early to avoid changes within the gastric mucosa that might alter vitamin $B_{12}$ absorption. Persons who follow a strict vegetarian diet should be told of the potential effects of such a diet and encouraged to take supplements. If patients have gastric surgery involving the removal of a large portion of the gastric mucosa, they should start vitamin $B_{12}$ supplements immediately. A family history of pernicious anemia should be noted in the health history.

**S**econd-Level Nursing Care   The onset of vitamin $B_{12}$ deficiency may go unnoticed for some time. When the patient seeks medical assistance, it is often because of multiple health problems.

*Nursing assessment*   Patients seeking medical attention frequently give a health history of generalized weakness, fatigue, peripheral numbness, and tingling, along with a sore tongue. In addition there may be a loss of appetite and bowel changes, including diarrhea and constipation. Complaints of indigestion are not uncommon. Irritability and mood swings can also accompany the problem. Palpitations are another common problem, and patients often fear that a cardiac disorder is at the root of the physical and emotional changes.

On *physical assessment* several changes will be observed in a patient with early pernicious anemia. The individual will have a somewhat wasted appearance with a weight loss of 15 to 20 lb. The mouth will appear sore and inflamed, and the tongue will be red. Gingival bleeding may be noted. The skin may or may not be jaundiced. This is usually noted during the acute phase (see Third-

Level Nursing Care). Dyspnea may be present but often only with exertion. Upon heart auscultation, tachycardia may be noted.

Neurological changes may be minimal at this time. However, alterations in balance may be noted when the patients are asked to close their eyes and balance on one foot. They may find it difficult to do so, losing their balance easily. Disruptions in proprioception, smell, and touch may also be noted during tests (see Chap. 31).

As one of the *diagnostic tests* available, a trial test of IM vitamin $B_{12}$ may be administered to the patient suspected of having pernicious anemia. If anemia is present and is due to a vitamin $B_{12}$ deficiency, the physical symptoms will reverse themselves within a few days, and fatigue and weakness will disappear.

Bone marrow examination is crowded with many cells. The degree of hyperplasia and the degree of the immaturity of cells are proportional to the severity of the anemia.[9]

The erythrocyte count will be reduced below 3 million/mm³. Neutrophils may be exceptionally large, and leukocyte abnormalities are not uncommon.[10]

Increased *reticulocytes* will be noted owing to generalized increased red blood cell production. *Platelets* are reduced and altered in appearance. Increased *serum bilirubin* as well as *urinobilogen may* be present as results of increased red blood cell breakdown. Vitamin $B_{12}$ deficiency in anemic patients is classically determined by two methods, the $B_{12}$ serum assay test and the Schilling test. The Schilling test is used to differentiate pernicious anemia from other vitamin $B_{12}$ disorders. The most commonly used form of the test is dependent upon the amount of vitamin $B_{12}$ excreted in the urine following the parenteral administration of a radioactive vitamin $B_{12}$ substance. Individuals who are able to absorb the vitamin $B_{12}$ will show radioactivity in the urine within 48 hours of an oral dose of 2 $\mu$g. If pernicious anemia is present, the patient will excrete only a small amount of vitamin $B_{12}$ (less than 5 percent).[11] When an oral dose of IF is given to these same patients, the amount of radioactivity in the urine is increased. Patients with a malabsorption problem will not be affected by the addition of IF.

*Nursing problems and intervention*  The patient in the community with chronic pernicious anemia must cope with a variety of problems that are a consequence of the vitamin $B_{12}$ deficiency. These include fatigue, weakness, dyspnea, nutritional dys-

pepsia, glossitis, and constipation. Correction of these problems begins with the administration of vitamin $B_{12}$.

*Vitamin $B_{12}$ therapy* usually involves administration of cyanocobalamin two or three times a week intramuscularly, until remission of the symptoms occurs. This remission usually takes 10 days to 2 weeks. However, an initial response to vitamin $B_{12}$ is usually seen within 48 to 72 hours after administration is begun. By the end of the second week, the erythrocyte count is elevated, and symptoms begin to reverse. Dosages are based upon the severity of the anemia and diagnostic studies. Cyanocobalamin 200 $\mu$g IM can be given monthly, or 100 $\mu$g IM every 2 weeks after the initial dosage. Oral doses are also available in doses of 500 to 1000 $\mu$g daily. If it is necessary. IF may have to be supplemented orally. The patient should be observed for any signs of allergic reaction to vitamin $B_{12}$ injection. Some individuals may experience pain on injection, but the incidence of this is rare.

*Diet counseling* will provide added vitamin supplements. Patients should be taught to include in their menus the basics for restoring optimum health. Therefore, fish, milk, and eggs will be important components of this diet. In addition, animal products including meat and liver will help supplement vitamin $B_{12}$ reserves. The patient should eat a well-balanced diet and avoid skipping meals. Nutritious snacks and food supplements should be encouraged between meals.

If the patient has *dyspepsia,* spicy foods should be avoided. These may be irritating to the stomach lining and intensify the problem. Milk and dairy products, good for providing added vitamin $B_{12}$, may also help alleviate dyspepsia. Hydrochloric acid (HCl) diluted in large amounts of water can be taken after meals to enhance food digestion. This drug can be administered as long as the symptoms last and then is terminated as the condition improves. Since HCl can stain the teeth, patients are encouraged to drink the well-diluted medication through a straw. When *constipation* is a problem, patients may have to alter their dietary intake to include larger amounts of fluids. In the absence of dyspepsia, foods high in roughage can be considered.

*Fatigue* and *generalized weakness* are common problems associated with pernicious anemia. As the initial therapy begins, frequent rest periods should be encouraged, especially if the patient is frequently tired. Strenuous activity should be kept at a minimum since this places an added strain on the individual and could increase fatigue. *Dyspnea* is often more noticeable upon exertion and can also increase fatigue. In the early stages of pernicious anemia, the patient should be encouraged to avoid exercise or other activities. Bed rest is often encouraged until the treatment begins to take effect and there is a remission of symptoms. Initially, complete bed rest may be recommended.

*Gum bleeding* and irritation can be painful to the patient and interfere with nutrition. Proper oral hygiene will help relieve the symptoms and offer the patient some comfort. Good dental care and the use of an antiseptic mouth wash or warm saline several times daily should be encouraged.

**T**hird-Level Nursing Care   The patient with severe pernicious anemia usually presents a matrix of acute care problems. Neurological involvement, anemia, infection, and cardiac decompensation may necessitate immediate hospitalization.

*Nursing assessment* Patients with severe untreated pernicious anemia will require a complete nursing assessment during the acute phase of illness. A careful *health history* and physical assessment may reveal many health disruptions requiring both immediate and long-term interventions. Patients with severe pernicious anemia will complain of extreme fatigue and weakness. Further investigation may reveal that the patient has little physical strength to carry on activities of daily living. In addition, patients complain of tinnitus. Some are very sensitive to sound, usually because of auditory nerve damage, and complain that loud noises are very upsetting. Tingling and numbness of one of the extremities may also be discussed. Dyspnea as well as orthopnea are often present. Weight loss will continue. Anginal pain may be a frequent complaint, along with complaints of nausea, vomiting, and diarrhea. Constipation may be a problem for some patients.

The family may also have to become involved in the health history, since mental confusion is often seen in these patients. The family may report changes in the patient's personality and describe paranoia and delusional behavior, along with generalized irritability.

The *physical assessment* of an individual with pernicious anemia will reveal the following changes. Upon general observation, the patient will appear pale and lethargic and manifest signs of varying degrees of weight loss. The patient's skin will have a "lemon" hue, and the sclera will appear slightly jaundiced. The tongue may appear beefy red, and gum bleeding is not uncommon.

Upon palpation, the liver will frequently be enlarged. The spleen may also be palpable. Bowel sounds are usually noted and accelerated if diarrhea is present, or slowed or altered in the presence of altered neurologic change.

The neurological examination will reveal an alteration in the individual's sense of balance and gait caused by the spasticity of the lower extremities. Apragnosia (impaired sense of position) will be apparent as the patient will lose his or her balance easily. Altered sensory proprioception will be seen when the patient's responses to touch, hot, and cold, as well as pain, are evaluated. The patient will exhibit a hyperactive response to mild sounds.

In addition, depending on the degree of neurologic involvement, the reflexes may be hyperactive or flaccid. A positive Babinski and Romberg's sign (see Chap. 31) are often observed. Fine finger movements may be absent. When given a command to complete an activity, the patient may be unable to perform well. Tremors may develop. If severe involvement of the spinal cord is present, there may be loss of bowel and bladder control as with a paralysis of the extremities. Changes in vision may be present, and the eye examination may reveal muscle atrophy and neurological involvement. Diplopia, blurring, or even diminished vision may be reported.

Dyspnea will often be observed resulting from defects in red blood cell production and from decreased oxygen cell capacity. Shortness of breath is often increased when the patient moves or changes position. Auscultation of the arterial blood pressure should be taken in the standing and sitting positions. Postural hypotension is often present. Inspection and palpation of the capillary refill will detect a slowed return of blood to the fingernails, and nail tips appear pale.

Heart auscultation will reveal a sinus tachycardia, and premature ventricular beats may be heard. A precordial murmur (see Chap. 22) may be heard and cardiac enlargement palpated. Signs of congestive heart failure (pump) may be present (see Chap. 24). Basal rales may be heard in auscultating the breath sounds. Palpation of the extremities may reveal pitting edema. These changes may accompany the dyspnea.

In addition to those tests discussed under Second Level Nursing Care *diagnostic tests* often used to evaluate the severely ill patient include bone marrow examination and gastric analysis.

The *bone marrow* aspiration determines the amount of blood-forming tissue in the bone's cellular composition. The sternum or hip illiac crest are the sites most commonly used. The patient should be told that the area will be anesthetized and that a narrow needle will be inserted into the bone in a twisting motion. The needle contains a stylet which is then removed, withdrawing a specimen with it. During the procedure the patient will experience pressure over the area of insertion. Some patients complain of pain at this time. Upon withdrawal of the needle, pressure should be applied over the site until the bleeding stops. An analysis of the aspirated tissue will show a high number of megaloblasts and few normoblasts or normally developing erythrocytes when pernicious anemia is present. Alteration in the production of leukocytes will also be noted.

The *gastric analysis* (discussed in Chap. 16) will show a decrease in the amount of gastric juice secreted. The specimen will be highly acidic with an absence of free hydrochloric acid. These changes will usually persist after the injection of histamine (a gastric juice releaser).

A gastric biopsy is done on occasion to evaluate the gastric mucosa. Changes may be noted in tissue, especially if specific malignant processes are present. A gastric tumor could be a cause of vitamin $B_{12}$ deficiency.

*Nursing problems and interventions* The problems associated with the acute phase of pernicious anemia tend to be more severe than those discussed in Second-Level Nursing Care. Fatigue and generalized weakness are more pronounced. Dyspnea also is present. Impaired gait, sensory disturbances, paralysis, edema, and postural hypotension are additional problems.

Generalized *weakness and fatigue* persist during the acute phase of illness. In addition to the administration of vitamin $B_{12}$ (see Second-Level Nursing Care), iron supplements in the form of ferrous sulfate may be given daily. This drug is usually given after meals, and the patient should be told that it may cause the color of the stool to become a dark green or black. Since iron deficiency can play a part in the development of pernicious anemia, it is seen as a valuable supplement to be administered in conjunction with vitamin $B_{12}$.

Until the acute phase of anemia has subsided, the patient will be kept on complete *bed rest* for a period of time—often several weeks if the fatigue and generalized weakness are pronounced. Care must be taken to prevent problems of immobility including muscle atrophy and venous stasis. Activity should include good range of motion exercises and frequent position change.

As soon as the gastrointestinal problems such as nausea, vomiting, constipation, and diarrhea

subside, a *well-balanced diet* high in iron and vitamin $B_{12}$ should be encouraged. In the presence of pump failure or peripheral edema, a low-sodium diet (see Chap. 24) should be stressed. Mouth care should be given to reduce the discomfort of *glossitis* and oral irritation and may help stimulate an appetite.

If the hemoglobin is less than 5 g/100 ml blood, a blood *transfusion* will be given. If pump failure is present, washed red blood cells are given in a partial exchange. This means that a volume of the patient's anemic blood equal to the volume of cells being administered is removed. Close monitoring during transfusions requires prompt reporting of any change in pulse rate, arterial pressure, chilling, fever, pruritus, swelling, or other unusual signs indicative of a transfusion reaction. If a reaction is suspected, the infusion should be stopped and the physician notified.

*Infections* which occur frequently are due to defects in leukocyte production and lowered resistance in the genitourinary tracts, especially in patients with neurologic involvement. Vigorous antibiotic therapy is needed because persistent infection may impair the therapeutic response to vitamin $B_{12}$.

Patients should be made aware of personal hygiene. They should be taught good hand-washing techniques, especially before and after urination. If neurological involvement impairs bladder function, then frequent pericare may be needed. The nurse should also be encouraged to maintain asepsis as needed.

If catheterization is performed or a permanent catheter inserted, strict asepsis should be maintained. Urine cultures should be taken if infection is suspected (see Chap. 14 for discussion of urinary tract infection).

Patients should also be observed for systemic infections occurring in other body parts. Open wounds, upper respiratory infections, or inflammation at the infusion site may contribute to infection.

*Dyspnea* often continues to be a major problem. Raising the bed slightly will improve cardiac output and ease dyspnea. Oxygen therapy may be used as needed. Activity should be planned to avoid overexertion. As the therapy brings about improvement in erythrocyte production and the patient's strength and general sense of well-being return, increased activity including ambulation will be allowed.

*Alterations in coordination* Frequently in severe pernicious anemia, the patient's gait is unsteady and mechanical devices will be needed to prevent falls. Additional support can be provided by the nurse when the patient is ambulating. *Paralysis* of the extremities may also be present. This may reverse itself upon therapy but will depend upon the amount of brain damage and spinal column changes that have taken place.

Patients who are paralyzed will require special care (see Chap. 32). It is important to assess the degree of paralysis present before allowing the patient to ambulate.

*Apragnosia,* also present in some patients, may complicate walking. Impairment in one's sense of position will alter balance and increase mental confusion. The nurse must assist the patient with all activities, while continually orienting the patient to the location of items within the environment, as well as to direction when walking. Apragnosia can be a very frightening experience for the patient and can heighten anxiety if support is not continual. Avoiding walking in dark areas or at night may lessen this problem.

Neurological changes may lead to alterations in *perceptual disturbances,* including alterations in touch and temperature perception. Therefore, hot or cold treatments should be applied to the skin with caution. Where changes are present, further diagnostic testing is essential before applying heat or cold directly to the patient.

Loud noises and increases in sound and activity can be very stressful to the patient. A quiet environment eliminating disturbing noise and activity should always be provided. Placement of the patient away from a crowded nurses' station may help to alleviate some of the stress. A mild tranquilizer may help relaxation and induce sleep. Family members should be told of this problem, and visiting may be limited.

In the presence of peripheral *edema* and signs of pump failure, diuretics and a digitalis preparation (see Chaps. 24 and 28) will be used. A decrease in sodium intake will also be prescribed. Care must be taken to observe the patient who is using diuretics and digitalis (see Chap. 24) in order to prevent toxic side effects. Undue pressure or tugging on the edematous areas should be avoided. If bed rest is required, a footboard or bed cradle can be used to reduce pressure on the extremities. Range of motion exercises along with elevation of the legs will decrease pooling of blood in the periphery and reduce the chances of emboli formation.

Neurological changes may also include loss of bowel and bladder control. Therefore, a bowel and bladder retraining program may have to be instituted (see Chap. 32 for a complete discussion). This loss of control may cause the patient to become depressed and withdrawn. The nurse should offer a complete discussion of the nature of the problem along with continual support throughout the retraining period.

Severe pernicious anemia may bring many *behavioral problems* due to anoxic destruction of brain tissue. These problems include irritability, mental confusion, disorientation to time and place, and delusional psychosis. These will be changes frightening to the patient and can increase anxiety. A Posey restraint may be needed at night, but in the presence of irritability and extreme restlessness it can increase fear. When possible, discussion of the need for temporary restraints may help decrease problems. Mild sedation may be used in some cases. Often the initiation of treatment will help reduce or eliminate some of these changes. However, until therapeutic levels of a medication can be reached, the nurse will have to be most supportive to patients and continuously orient them to their surroundings. Family members should be told of anticipated behavioral changes and informed as to how they can help the patient through this difficult period.

**F**ourth-Level Nursing Care Patients with pernicious anemia will require life-long therapy of vitamin $B_{12}$ injections. The amount of health teaching will depend upon many factors including the degree of permanent neurological involvement or other generalized limitations. Patients will be either instructed to go to an outpatient health care facility for administration of vitamin $B_{12}$, taught to administer their own injections, or placed on a daily oral dose of the drug. If patients are to administer their own injections, they must be provided with a supply of vitamin $B_{12}$ for parenteral use and taught proper intramuscular injection technique. Equipment needed will include a 2- to 3-ml disposable syringe and 21-23 gauge needles. Practice sessions should be held so that the patient and family members will have the opportunity to practice correct injection techniques. Identification of injection sites (e.g., deltoid muscle, muscle in thigh, and gluteous maximus) should be included in the teaching plan. The patient should be assured that prognosis is excellent when therapy is adequate. The patient should be told of the need for yearly periodic health review and encouraged to participate in periodic health checks.

The incidence of gastric cancer has been reported higher in patients with pernicious anemia, indicating the need for continued follow-up health care.

Patients must be taught the importance of good nutrition and the need for life-long compliance with drug therapy even when symptoms disappear. Neurologic changes may lessen with therapy, but residual changes may remain. The patient may be told that with adequate treatment these changes will not worsen. If the patient fails to take vitamin $B_{12}$, the symptoms discussed earlier will return, and neurological problems may intensify.

## Folic Acid Deficiency

Folic acid is needed for red blood cell formation and maturation. Unlike vitamin $B_{12}$ deficiency, body reserves of folate are normally small, and so dietary deficits quickly result in a clinical deficiency. Folate is supplied to the diet in green leafy vegetables such as asparagus, broccoli, spinach, and lettuce. Liver, kidney, yeast, mushrooms, lemons, bananas, and melons are also good sources. As folate deficiency is seen among people who cook foods for long periods, it is important to obtain information about food preparation as well as dietary intake in the health history. Groups at high risk to develop folate deficiency are the elderly who may be too weak, anorexic, or depressed to buy and prepare food; the chronic alcoholic; the young infant with infection or diarrhea on a cow's milk diet and not receiving vegetables, eggs, or meat; or the premature infant, with small folate reserves. Also at risk are persons with chronic liver disease due to poor diet and impaired liver storage of folate. Dilantin and some oral contraceptives can block synthesis of folic acid in certain individuals. Pregnancy also increases folate demands five to ten times above normal. Routine folic acid supplementation during pregnancy is advocated not only to meet pregnancy requirements but also to prevent severe folate deficiency and complications of spontaneous abortion, bleeding, and abruptio placentae have been recorded. Folate needs also rise sharply in hemolytic anemia (discussed below), acute or chronic overactivity of the bone marrow, and a chronic hemolytic anemia such as sickle-cell disease.

In folate deficiency, neurological changes described under vitamin $B_{12}$ deficiency are not seen because folic acid does not play a part in nervous system function. Low serum and red blood cell folate levels confirm the diagnosis. Folate is usually administered orally in 1-mg tablets with satisfactory results. The sole indication for folic acid therapy is folic acid deficiency.

## Iron-Deficiency Anemia

The most *common chronic organic condition* of mankind which develops slowly is iron-deficiency anemia. Iron is imperative for hemoglobin synthesis. When deficiencies occur, they result in a decreased red blood cell mass, a reduced hemoglobin concentration, and subsequent lower oxygen-carrying capacity of blood. A classic anemia pattern of pallor, fatigue, and irritability, as well as compensatory cardiac changes of tachycardia, and an increase cardiac output will develop.

Fifteen percent of infants and 25 percent of pregnant teen-age girls (in one homogeneous socioeconomic and racial group) were found to be at risk to develop iron-deficiency anemia.[12] Inadequate dietary iron intake is the primary cause of iron deficiency. Milk products are poor sources of iron, and prolonged bottle or milk feedings lead to iron-deficiency anemia unless iron supplementation is provided.

Dietary deficiencies, pregnancy, intestinal parasites, and bleeding from the gastrointestinal tract are other common causes of iron-deficiency anemia. In adult males and postmenopausal women, iron deficiency is commonly caused by chronic bleeding from stomach ulcers, small bowel polyps, ulcers, vascular occlusions, rectal hemorrhoids, ulceration, or carcinoma. As the patient may manifest symptoms of the primary disorder, for example, an anatomic lesion causing bleeding, and not display classic symptoms of anemia, recognition and hematologic evaluation of high-risk groups is especially important.

*Laboratory parameters* for iron-deficiency anemia reveal reduced hemoglobin and hematocrit values, blood smear observations of hypochromic, microcytic erthyrocytes, low plasma iron concentrations, and increased iron-binding capacity. As the iron deficiency increases, the hemoglobin concentration decreases further, and hypochromia appears.

Replacement iron therapy is administered orally, parenterally, or by transfusion. Oral administration is the safest and most economical. Mild gastrointestinal complaints of constipation or loose stools may be reported after oral therapy. Patients should be told that stool color will become dark green. It is important to continue iron therapy for a sufficient length of time to rebuild body stores. Hemoglobin and hematocrit values need serial reevaluation. If a significant increase of iron deficiency is not seen in 3 to 4 weeks, the initial diagnosis may need reappraising. The possibility of a persistent blood loss and/or incorrect dosage intake by the patient needs to be evaluated. If therapy is stopped as soon as the anemia is corrected and iron stores are not replenished, anemia may reoccur.

If intramuscular injections of iron are necessary, a moderate degree of pain and a dark stain at the injection site are possible side effects. To reduce the discoloration and irritating effects of iron deposition in the tissue, a "Z track" injection pattern is used. When the "Z track" method is used, it is important to withdraw the solution with one needle and inject with another, leaving 0.5 ml air in the syringe. With a 2- to 3-in needle, 19- or 20-gauge, the injection is given deep into the upper outer quadrant of the buttock. The use of the arm should be avoided. After aspiration the nurse should check to see that the needle is not in the vein and then inject the solution. The 0.5 ml air previously withdrawn into the syringe is then injected into the site in order to ensure that the iron dextran has been totally removed from the syringe. This process will help to avoid further staining due to leakage from the needle. The area around the injection should not be massaged.[13] The patient should avoid using constricting clothing and should exercise. The injection site should be observed frequently for inflammation and swelling. Anaphylaxis is rare.

Urticaria, fever, myalgia, and headaches have occurred after parenteral administration of iron dextran. It is important that the patient understand the dosage and specific iron therapy prescribed. Health consumers frequently duplicate therapy by supplementing with commercial products such as Geritol or Vitron-C, not realizing their added iron content. Accurate interviewing during the health history is essential in order to obtain these data. Because of a large contingent of iron-deficient individuals, wide use of therapy, and easy accessibility of over-the-counter iron preparations for self-treatment, *acute iron poisoning* has become a potential health problem. This is most often seen in children.

The earliest manifestations of severe iron poisoning include vomiting and diarrhea, usually within an hour of ingestion, followed by hypotension, tachypnea, cyanosis, coma, and death in a few hours. Initial care of suspected iron ingestion is rapid evacuation of the stomach contents. At home, vomiting can be induced by digital stimulation of the pharyngeal gag reflex or with the use of syrup of ipecac. Oral administration of a tepid solution of baking soda serves to induce vomiting, and the bicarbonate ion combines with the iron to retard absorption. Children who survive 3 to 4 days usually recover.

### Hypoplastic Anemia

*Hypoplasia* of the bone marrow refers to failure of the marrow to deliver blood cells into the circulation. The term *aplastic anemia* is frequently used, but it is an inappropriate synonym for hypoplastic anemia because the marrow is never totally aplastic. Total aplasia is incompatible with life. Ionizing radiation and certain chemical agents are known to induce hypoplasia. Chemicals which in sufficient dosage regularly produce marrow hypoplasia are benzene and antineoplastic agents such as 6-mercaptopurine. Other chemicals which occasionally cause hypoplasia are anticonvulsants and antimicrobial drugs such as chloramphenicol and tetracycline. Infectious states may also cause hypoplastic anemia, especially viral hepatitis.

The effects of hypoplastic anemia on the patient include clinical manifestations of pancytopenia (a reduction in erythrocytes, leukocytes, and blood platelets); thrombocytopenia and bleeding problems (discussed below); neutropenia (a decrease in neutrophils), and the increased susceptibility to infection. Problems associated with anemia (e.g., weakness, fatigue) persist. The onset of hypoplastic anemia is usually insidious. The course may be brief or prolonged, with death occurring within a few months. The morbidity of hypoplastic anemia in adults has been reported at 65 to 75 percent, with a median survival of 3 months. The prognosis in children is slightly better, with 50 percent of children surviving, whether treated with supportive medical care alone or with myelostimulatory agents.

The outstanding *complications* of hypoplastic anemia are *infection* and *bleeding*.[14] The incidence of *infection* correlates with neutrophil counts, age, and whether the patient was receiving *corticosteroid* treatments. With early signs of infection, such as fever or local infestation of throat tissue, a urinalysis and blood culture are obtained, and bactericidal broad-spectrum antibiotics are administered. Reverse isolation should be initiated for the patient's protection.

*Bleeding* may result in deep hemorrhage within organs or external skin or retinal hemorrhage. Patients should be taught ways to reduce the risk of hemorrhage. This may be accomplished by the use of electric razors, soft toothbrushes (softened further in warm water), stool softeners to avoid hard bowel movements, and the avoidance of intramuscular injections and venipunctures, if possible.

When injections are needed, the smallest possible gauge needle should be employed. If restraints are necessary, care should be taken to support extremities and avoid trauma. Catheters, drainage appliances, and suction tubes must be handled gingerly to prevent mucosal bleeding. When and if bleeding occurs, the patient should be reassured that it can be controlled. Local pressure should be used on bleeding sites with care not to interfere with clot formation. Bleeding from puncture sites will require a pressure bandage and observation of the site for signs of coagulation. Bleeding from any site provides an excellent opportunity for bacterial growth. Frequent observation and cleansing of the area are imperative. Salt pork packs used to control anterior nasal bleeding and dry tea bags to control gingival bleeding have been reported effective.[15]

The goal of medical management is to remove the suspected causative agent, if one exists. Supportative care with transfusions of packed red blood cells and platelets is used as hematologic values dictate. Transfusions of concentrates of white blood cells, although feasible, are not routinely available in most institutions. Therapeutic agents sometimes used to induce a remission include drugs such as steroids and androgens. Both types of drugs have been successful to a degree in children but not in adults. Splenectomy and bone marrow transplant are additional treatment regimes. Bone marrow transplants are performed at certain specific centers in the United States with a definite laborious protocol and specific care plan.[16] The success rate has been variable but encouraging.

## INCREASED ERYTHROCYTE DESTRUCTION

*Hemolysis* is the premature destruction of red blood cells. It may result from chemical ingestion, radiation, and inherited spherocytosis. Infections such as mononucleosis and drugs such as alpha methyldopa or penicillin type (hapten) affect the morphologic appearance of red blood cells.[17] Spherocytes are the most common morphologic abnormality noted.[18] These cells have a bizarre shape and are easily identified under the microscope. The changes in the red blood cells cause increased cell destruction and will lead to hemoglobinopathies, membrane defects of erythrocytes, and acquired and nonacquired hemolytic anemias.

### Hemoglobinopathies

Hemoglobin consists of two parts: *heme,* a pigment, and *globin,* a protein. The globin is made from 574 amino acids, whose chemical structure and sequence are known. The heme is an iron component. Conditions of abnormal hemoglobins are termed *hemoglobinopathies.* They consist of a group of problems characterized by the abnormal production of hemoglobin. These changes are usually caused by the substitution of a particular amino acid into the normal structural chain. Most of the over 200 known variations do not cause clinical symptoms. However, there are several which result in serious health problems. These include sickle-cell anemia, sickle-C disease, and sickle-cell thalassemia.

**Sickle-cell anemia** A genetically determined hemolytic anemia, sickle-cell anemia (SCA) is characterized by abnormally shaped red blood cells (sickle cells) which interfere with blood circulation and oxygenation to vital organs.

**P**athophysiology Sickle hemoblogin (HbS) differs from normal hemoglobin by one amino acid substituting a valine which occurs where a glutamic acid should be. This substitution results in an abnormal linking reaction between hemoglobin S molecules and the valine chain when oxygen tension is lowered. With deoxygenation there is increased viscosity, causing the valine substitution to deform the normally smooth-surfaced, flexible, disk-shaped erythrocyte (Fig. 23-1) into a rigid, rough-textured, elongated, crescent-shaped sickle cell (Fig. 23-2).

Several factors influence the degree and involvement of sickling. If the red blood cells contain predominately hemoglobin S molecules (as in homozygous sickle-cell anemia or sickle thalassemia), deoxygenation results in a distorted cell shape. However, if the red blood cell contains a significant percentage of another hemoglobin such as A in sickle-cell trait (Hb AS), or fetal (Hb F) in hereditary persistence of fetal hemoglobin, sickling will not occur in vivo. This is owing to the fact that the dilution effect interferes with the sickling phenomenon and the concentration of hemoglobin S within the red blood cell is not great enough to cause aggregation under normal conditions.

Additional forces affecting sickling of hemoglobin S are the *blood oxygen tension* and *blood pH.* When lowered, both precipitate sickling in the presence of hemoglobin S. The type of sickle cell that develops is also crucial. Two types of sickled cells are usually present. One is a *mildly sickled* or oat-shaped cell that can revert to a normal disk shape with exposure to oxygen. The second is a *filamentous form,* which appears to be *irreversibly sickled.* The irreversibly sickled cell precipitates an unhealthy cycle of additional sickling, stasis, further deoxygenation, and more irreversibly sickled cells.

The time required for red blood cells with hemoglobin S to assume varying sickle shapes is dependent on several factors. Some cells change in seconds; others are normal for hours. All have a shortened survival, varying from 15 to 20 days.[19]

Persons with *sickle-cell trait* (SCT) are not anemic, and their hemoglobin and hematocrit values are normal. They are usually asymptomatic and have a normal life-span.[20]

Under certain circumstances persons with sickle-cell trait may exhibit crisis symptoms. Reduction in oxygen level can be caused by unpressurized aircraft, high altitudes, and scuba diving. A person witn SCT could experience intravascular sickling, vasoocclusions, and infarctions from these causes. Gross hematuria may be seen, and gradual and progressive loss of renal concentrating capacity is observed in adults. Close observation of the patient is required along with improved oxygenation.

*Oxygenation* The effects of sickling on the patient are best exemplified in the cardiovascular system. As the deformed sickle cell is unable to achieve passage through the microcirculation, blood flow is obstructed. Local occlusions cause oxygen deprivation to tissue and an accumulation of metabolic acid waste products. This lowers the blood pH and precipitates additional sickling as previously non-sickled cells arrive. Exercise and/or infection amplifies the tissue anoxia, causing more sickling.

Variations exist in the level of tissue oxygenation and acidity. Therefore, certain organs including the liver, spleen, and renal medulla pose more hazards to the circulatory flow of sickle hemoglobin. Organs such as the brain and muscle, where more oxygen is extracted from the blood owing to a high metabolic rate, are also subject to diminished function in the presence of sickle cells. Almost all clinical manifestations, symptoms, and disabilities associatcd with sickle hemoglobinopathies are the direct result of vasoocclusive episodes, with repeated involvement in vital organs capable of causing fatal complications.[21] The difficult passage of sickled red blood cells through the spleen is seen in Fig. 23-3.

The cardiopulmonary system is affected from chronic sickle-cell anemia and infarctions, with cardiomegaly and tachycardia being common problems. Progressive cardiac decompensation is seen in a few adolescents and adults. Progressive

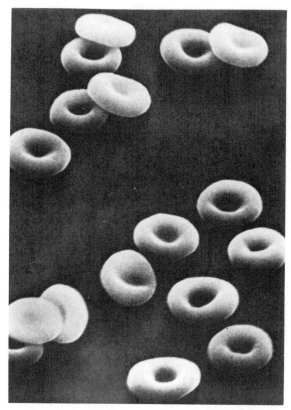

**FIGURE 23-1**

Normal red blood cells from person with hemoblogin AA as seen in scanning electron micrograph (SEM). (*From M. I. Barnhart, R. L. Henry, and J. M. Lusher, Sickle Cell, A Scope Monograph, The Upjohn Company, Kalamazoo, Mich., 1974. Used by permission of the photographer.*)

chronic *congestive heart failure* occurs and may be fatal. *Pulmonary infarctions* are undoubtedly common and may lead to repeated episodes of chest pain, unexplained *dyspnea,* and episodes of pneumonia requiring hospitalization. *Leg ulcerations* are frequent occurrences owing to tissue hypoxia and decreased body temperature. Fifty percent of infants with sickle-cell anemia experience *dactylitis* (hand-foot syndrome). This problem is characterized by ischemic necrosis of the small bones in the hand and/or foot and swelling of soft tissue accompanied by heat and tenderness. Usually several small bones are affected. With each infarction and necrosis, new bone formation develops and healing occurs spontaneously.

*Fluids and electrolytes* In the genitourinary system, the renal medulla is particularly susceptible to damage. Infarctions may occur with subsequent renal papillary necrosis. *Hematuria* and a chronic

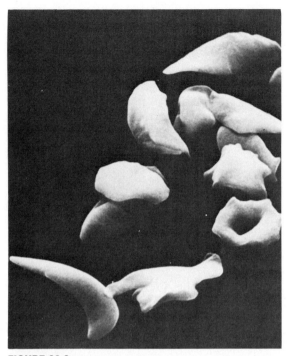

**FIGURE 23-2**
Sickled red blood cells from person with sickle-cell anemia as viewed by SEM. (*From M. I. Barnhart, R. L. Henry, and J. M. Lusher, Sickle Cell, A Scope Monograph, The Upjohn Company, Kalamazoo, Mich., 1974. Used by permission of the photographer.*)

defect in renal concentrating ability are frequently seen. *Pyelonephritis* may be increased if the patient is pregnant. In males, *priapism,* a persistent and painful erection of the penis, may last for hours, days, or even weeks. It is a result of sickling, stasis, and occlusions of venous blood. Prolonged episodes of priapism without surgery may result in impotence.

In addition to the above problems, renal changes leading to nephropathy are not uncommon. *Uremia* and death can be a sequel of these changes.

*Metabolism* The liver, somewhat enlarged and firm, is also congested with sickle cells and shows various degrees of degenerative changes. Enlargement may be more obvious during a crisis. *Jaundice* and *hepatomegaly* are common. Chronic hemolysis predispose the individual to *cholelithiasis.* Gallstones may appear in the second decade of life and are common in the third; they are due to the increased production of urobilinogen. Normal red blood cells can become pooled in the congested area or hyperplastic spleen, where they stagnate,

contributing to the abnormal cell structure.[22] There is a reduction in red blood cell surface area and an inability of cells to filter out of the spleen. This congestion results in *splenomegaly* with ultimate destruction of cells in the spleen. Occasionally patients may be susceptible to developing serum hepatitis following a blood transfusion.

*Inflammatory response* During a sickle-cell crisis an inflammatory response develops. The body temperature can rise to 101 to 104°F, and severe leukocytosis will be present. Patients are often vulnerable to infection because of the anemic state, and the stress of an infection can precipitate a sickle crisis. A sickle-cell aplastic crisis occurs when the bone marrow markedly decreases or ceases production of red blood cells. Excessive red blood cell destruction continues, causing hemoglobin values to drop quickly. These crises may occur in the wake of an infectious illness such as otitis media, tonsillitis, gastroenteritis, or flu-like symptoms.

*Perception and coordination* Changes may be noted in the skeletomuscular system, with *demineralization of the vertebrae* occurring. In late childhood a characteristic laying down of new bone along the cortices of the long bones may be noted. This can result in narrowing of the medullary spaces.[23] Persons with sickle-cell anemia are particularly susceptible to pneumococcal sepsis, pneumococcal meningitis, and salmonella osteomyelitis.[24-27] The majority of pneumococcal infections occur in children less than 3 years of age. Areas of infarction in the usual pulmonary portals of entry for bacteria, as well as splenic defense action impairment, stifle normal bacterial phagocytosis, allowing for bacterial multiplication.

*Retinopathy* is not an uncommon sequela of sickling. The eye vessels may become distorted by the presence of the sickle cells. Temporary or permanent blindness will occur if tissue destruction is severe. Depending on the degree of sickling, cerebral blood vessels often become occluded. This may lead to central nervous system changes including headache, drowsiness, seizure, coma, and paralysis.

*Pain* accompanies crises and can be a spontaneous problem or can occur in response to a stressful event. Emotional problems and temperature change (especially cold), as well as physiologic stress caused by infection, usually induce the pain. It is often severe and radiating, occurring in the extremities, lower back, and joints. The pain will last up to a week and will then begin to subside gradually. *Cerebral hemorrhage* can occur and cause death.

**F**irst-Level Nursing Care   The mutational source of sickle hemoglobin was apparently an original selective advantage in geographic areas where malaria was common. The sickle hemoglobin protects individuals against malaria caused by *Plasmodium falciparum.* Two million Black Americans, or 1 in 10, carry one gene for sickle hemoglobin and have sickle-cell trait. Some Caucasians, particularly those from the Mediterranean and Middle East, as well as parts of India, may have a form of sickle-cell disease. Among Blacks, 1 in every 500 births is a child with sickle-cell anemia. Presently there are 30,000 to 50,000 affected individuals in the United States. Each of these persons has a 50 percent chance of dying before the twentieth birthday.[28]

*Screening*   Individuals may be screened for SCT by a laboratory technique termed *hemoglobin electrophoresis,* which permits separation and identification of different hemoglobins according to their differing electrical properties. This is a highly sophisticated and reliable test for determining the hemoglobin type. New, inexpensive electrophoretic methods using capillary blood samples are dependable and can offer screening possibilities at local community health facilities. Adequate transport of blood samples to a designated, adequately equipped laboratory is essential for reliable results. A Sickledex test is done to quickly determine the presence of sickle cells. Although a positive Sickledex demonstrates sickling, it will not identify the specific sickle hemoglobinopathy nor differentiate between SCT, a totally benign condition, and SCA, a chronic debilitating disease. A complete hemoglobin study is essential to understand the patient's hemoglobin and its implications. The optimum time for hemoglobin testing is debatable. Clear objectives are essential before any screening program is initiated, and ample time should be allowed for pre-education, counseling, and recounseling at a later date to identify and correct misunderstandings. Infant testing is usually not done until after 6 months of age because of the presence of fetal hemoglobin and consequent difficulty in reading capillary samples. Some hospitals will test umbilical cord blood to identify neonates with a sickle hemoglobinopathy.

*Prevention*   The most important aspect of SCT is genetic transmission of the traits to the offspring. Careful nursing assessment of the patient's under-

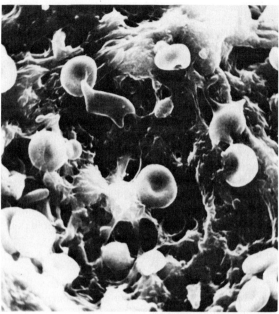

**FIGURE 23-3**
Sickled red blood cells in red pulp of spleen viewed by SEM. Note size of openings in reticular meshwork. Red blood cells must pass through these and others in splenic sinus to return to the venous circuit. (*From M. I. Barnhart, R. L. Henry and J. M. Lusher, Sickle Cell, A Scope Monograph, The Upjohn Company, Kalamazoo, Mich., 1974. Used by permission of the photographer.*)

standing of SCT and its genetic implications is primary to any counseling session. In recent years much information on SCT has been made available to the public through newspaper articles, radio and TV commentaries, and vigorous community screening programs. However, much confusion still exists, and facts have been distorted leading to fear and misunderstanding by many people. The genetics of SCT are simple. If both parents have the trait, each child has a 1:4 (25 percent) chance of having sickle-cell anemia (Fig. 23-4). The chance remains the same with each pregnancy. Many persons with SCA assume that all their children will have SCA. The facts are that if one parent has SCA (Hb SS) and the other parent has normal adult hemoglobin (Hb AA), none of the children will have SCA but all will have SCT; no other possibilities exist. If one parent has SCA and the other has SCT, each offspring has a 1:2 (50 percent) chance of having SCA and an equal chance of having SCT; no other possibilities exist.

*Family planning*   Parents with SCT who have a child with SCA are frequently faced with an agonizing decision on each family addition. Effective contraceptive methods should be offered and explained while decisions are being made. Awareness that one can pass a chronic, life-threatening disease onto an offspring is frightening and guilt producing. Nurses can give support by providing an opportunity for parents to discuss fears and concerns. Meetings of concerned parents are one therapeutic means of offering an exchange of ideas on ways others have coped with the decision. Infant testing of parents known to have SCT should be offered to aid in abating parental anxiety. Lastly, the nurse must present the facts to those concerned, emphasizing that individuals with SCT have normal blood values and should not experience any medical problems from their different hemoglobin except under unusual circumstances. The National Foundation of the March of Dimes provides valuable public information regarding sickle-cell anemia. Local branches can be contacted for help with counseling parents.

People with sickle-cell trait (SCT) should be aware of their condition. They should carry identification stating that they have this trait; appropriate medical personnel (e.g., local medical doctor, public health department) should have documentation of their condition. In case of accident, shock, or need for anesthesia, the attending medical personnel should be aware that the patient has SCT. The need to avoid riding in unpressurized aircraft, scuba diving, and high altitudes should be emphasized. Persons with SCT need counseling and recounseling on the difference between SCT and SCA. Continued emphasis on the fact that SCT will never change to SCA is also important.

**S**econd-Level Nursing Care    Assessment and identification of problems in the nonacute patient with sickle-cell anemia begins with an understanding of the usual hemolytic blood values (Table 23-1). Sickle-cell anemia is characterized by a chronic hemolytic anemia and intermittent "crises" of varying frequency and severity.

*Nursing assessment*    A detailed health history and an accurate physical assessment will help the nurse to distinguish a nonacute from an acute sickle crisis. Since most physicians wish to prevent multiple hospitalizations for the patient, the nonacute phase of a sickle-cell crisis will often be treated on an outpatient basis.

An accurate *health history* can be obtained

**FIGURE 23-4**
Inheritance pattern of sickle-cell anemia. Probability and percentage possibilities for each pregnancy at conception of parental matings of sickle-cell trait (Hb AS).

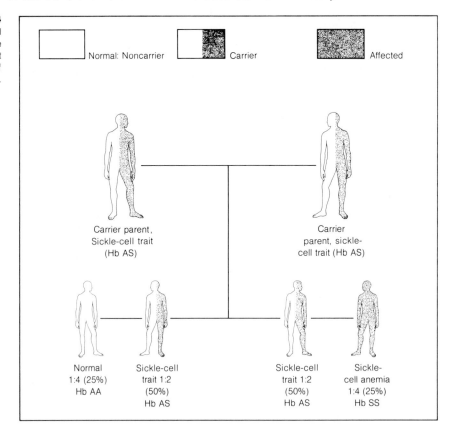

from the patient or family member. The onset of the crisis may be precipitated by stress of any type. Current infections, exposure to cold, dehydration (e.g., fever), stressful exercise, and emotional trauma can all contribute to the crisis state.

Mothers often seek medical attention for the undiagnosed child, giving a 2- to 3-day history of puffy hands, inability to put the child's shoes on, or refusal by the child to walk or use an extremity. The older child and adult describe pain in bones or joints of the extremities, often with swelling and limitation of movement. Abdominal pain is another common complaint. Hematuria may be noted, and, in the presence of fever, dehydration may be present.

*Physical assessment* will reveal an individual who is in much distress, mainly due to pain. If *dactylitis* (see Pathophysiology) is present, there will be noticeable edema of the hands and feet. Joints will be tender to touch, and range of motion will often be limited. During the abdominal examination, distention and tenderness may also be noted. The liver may be enlarged, with organ tenderness noted. The spleen is usually not palpable in adults.

The body temperature may be elevated (101 to 104°F), and there may be slight dyspnea present. Tachycardia may be noted, especially in the presence of a fever. The skin turgor may be poor and mucosa dry in the presence of dehydration. Urinary output may be diminished.

Anxiety may be noted and behavioral changes observed. Investigation of the stress-producing events is critical. If an emotional or occupational stress is identified, it should be carefully explored.

Several *diagnostic tests* can aid in evaluating sickle-cell anemia. *Hemoglobin and hematocrit* levels are done and may remain unchanged or slightly elevated owing to dehydration. A stained *blood smear* is done to reveal the presence of sickle cells. Mean corpuscular volume (MCV) and mean corpuscular hemoglobin (MCH) may be altered.

*Sickle-cell preparation* is a test in which a specimen of blood is collected and then deprived of oxygen. When sickle-cell anemia is present, the red blood cells will sickle. *Hemoglobin electrophoresis* is done to differentiate between SCA and SCT. During the test, blood hemoglobin is separated, and the shapes of the cells are examined. If sickling is present, it can be noted at this time.

**N**ursing Problems and Interventions  In general, the "crisis" phase may last from a few hours to 4 to 6 days, with gradual, spontaneous subsidence of pain. The main problems confronting the patient are pain, dehydration, and fever. Usually these problems can be treated at home, providing the family has received adequate health teaching.

*Pain*  The *pain* of sickle-cell crisis is often severe and stressful to the patient. This problem must be discussed with the patient and families. *Narcotics* are usually avoided as much as possible to prevent addiction. Analgesics most often used are aspirin, empirin, and acetaminophen preparations (i.e., Tempra and Tylenol). The *analgesic* dosage should be effective, yet not so high or frequent that the patient is continuously drowsy or sleeping and unable to consume fluids. Dosage is based on patients' experience. Planned and varied analgesic schedules are helpful. For example, alternating an acetaminophen preparation and aspirin, rather than using the same chemical preparation continuously, may be effective. The patient and/or family should evaluate the response to the medication and assess overall comfort. The patient must be taught that a *heating pad* or hot water bottle is comforting and can be used as needed. The patient should be encouraged to change position frequently. Local application of pressure by rubbing the aching area is an additional measure to provide temporary relief.

*Dehydration*  An important component in treating sickle-cell crises is *fluid administration* to prevent dehydration. This will also prevent further sickling and aid in mobilization of trapped sickled cells. Families or parents should be instructed to offer water, soda, weak tea, juices, milk, popsicles, ice cream, sherbet, or any mixtures of liquids which are appealing to the individual. Solids should be offered but not forced. Liquids are of prime importance. Coaxing a disinterested person to consume liquids is a nursing challenge needing creative persistence. Drinking small amounts of liquid every 30 minutes is more readily accepted than drinking 8 oz every 2 hours. Older children and adults may be enticed with an eggnog or milkshake.

The importance of fluids can not be overemphasized. During routine clinic visits, patients are shown a blood smear of their sickling and

**TABLE 23-1**
USUAL BLOOD VALUES OF PERSONS WITH SICKLE-CELL ANEMIA

| | |
|---|---|
| RBC life-span | 15–20 days |
| Hemoglobin | 5.5–9.5 g/100 ml |
| Hematocrit | 17–29% |
| Reticulocyte count | 5–30% |
| WBC count | 12,000–35,000/mm³ |
| Bilirubin (T) | 1.5–4.0 mg/100 ml |

sickled red blood cells. The etiology of pain crises can be explained in relationship to the blood smear. Patients should be advised that if the pain is severe, or if vomiting and dehydration ensue, a physician or nurse must be consulted as IV hydration may be necessary. Many institutions provide IV fluids in the outpatient area, thus circumventing hospitalization. Four to six hours of IV hydration may have dramatic pain-relieving results.

*Fever* Elevation in body temperature often accompanies sickle-cell crisis. Patients should be taught to take their temperature before administering an analgesic. Oral *temperature* elevations greater than 100°F that persist for 48 hours, or an initial fever of 102°F or higher, warrants a physician's attention.[29] A temperature elevation frequently signals infection, and observation for infection during and following a crisis is imperative. An increase in body temperature contributes to dehydration. Lethargy, sleepiness, or disinterest in play and surroundings indicates a need for fever evaluation. Assessing whether the patient and family possess a thermometer and their knowledge of care, accuracy of reading, and reporting is an important evaluation and teaching responsibility.

*Health promotion Nutritional requirements* with SCA are the same as without it. No special foods or diet will correct hemolytic anemia. Supplemental vitamins without iron are recommended until age 3 and can be continued indefinitely if a nutritional assessment dictates a need. Folic acid may be prescribed if normal dietary intake is lacking, but it does not halt or reverse sickling. Transfusions, with the associated risk of reactions, hepatitis, and hemochromatosis are not indicated except for specific reasons in acute-care episodes. Routine immunizations should be given according to the established schedule for optimal well-child care. If mumps vaccine is not available through community facilities, inoculation from a private physician is advisable. Although many *infections* can not be prevented, good prophylactic care is advised with prompt cleansing and care of cuts, bites, and other prime infection portals, as well as routine dental evaluations and adequate clothing for damp and cold weather. Infected lacerations or a dental abscess may present potentially serious problems to the individual with SCA and should be treated early. No restrictions are placed on the child's or adult's *activities.* Persons with SCA are advised to establish their tolerance level for activities and to rest as needed. Competitive sports, where team goals take precedence over individual tolerance levels, are to be discouraged.

*Chronic, nonacute health problems* are apparent in the teen-ager and adult with SCA. Chronic problems are best explained via major organ involvement. Splenic congestion with subsequent splenomegaly usually persists until 5 to 6 years of age, when repeated infarctions result in fibrosis, scarring, and atrophy. A state of *functional asplenia* exists with bypassing of the reticuloendothelial elements of the spleen, a state contributory to overwhelming infections.

*Prevention of "crisis"* Prophylactic care and health maintenance are crucial in any chronic disease. Monthly or bimonthly hematologic evaluations and teaching sessions are recommended for children. Adults need follow-up assessments every 3 to 6 months. During these evaluations, aspects of daily health care needs should be reviewed.

**T**hird-Level Nursing Care Nursing assessment of persons with sickle-cell anemia having an acute crisis differs radically from child to adult. In children, acute care is usually necessitated by a sudden, unexpected sequence of events, usually precipitated by infection. Symptoms progress rapidly, and if medical attention is not quick and vigorous, the child may die. While adults can also develop sickle-cell crisis, acute care is often necessitated by gradual major organ damage; however, infection and aplastic crises can also occur.

*Health history* An accurate *health history* should be obtained from the patient or family. The patient will often appear lethargic and complain of extreme fatigue and weakness. Headache may also be present. A decrease in visual acuity may be reported. Pain will be a common problem and is usually severe. Often the patient will complain of pain in the abdomen, chest, and muscles. The pain is often so severe that movement of any kind will increase its intensity. Chest pain may also persist because of pulmonary infarction or atypical pneumonia. An elevation in body temperature can be reported for several days.

Discussion of precipitating events often reveals the presence of an acute stressful episode. Anorexia may also be a problem, contributing to fatigue.

*Physical assessment* After a complete history is taken, a physical assessment will be performed. Patients in acute crisis will be pale; in fact, *pallor* is often a signal that an acute crisis is impending. The patient will appear *lethargic,* tired and sleepy, or even in a comatose state. *Jaundice* may be present, but it is often minimal. The patient will be warm to touch. Signs of dehydration including loss of *skin turgor, dryness of the buccal mucosa,* and *decreased urination* may be observed. Upon auscultation of the heart, diastolic and systolic *murmurs* can be heard (Chap. 22), along with sinus arrhythmias. If the sickle-cell crisis involves the heart, signs of *pump failure* including basal rales, cyanosis, dyspnea, and peripheral edema may be noted. Cardiac enlargement may be present (see Chap. 24).

*Urinary output* may be altered and *hematuria* observed. The penis may be enlarged and painful. Central nervous system changes will be indicated by the persistence of *pain.* If destruction of peripheral nerves and spinal tissue is present, hemiplegia, aphasia, paralysis, and seizure activity may be observed. Reflexes and general muscle tone can be altered.

*Changes in vision* may also occur. Examination of the conjunctiva will reveal short comma-shaped segments, often seen separated from the normal vascular network. Temporary or permanent blindness may also be present.

*Diagnostic tests*   There are several diagnostic tests that will be performed during the acute crisis. *Hemoglobin and hemotocrit* levels continue to be below normal. The tests discussed in Second-Level Nursing Care will also be performed. In addition, urine and blood urobilinogen will be tested and are usually elevated during crisis.

Selected tests to assess the effects of the sickling process on major organs will also be done; e.g., the *blood urea* will be elevated with renal obstruction; the electrocardiogram may show sinus arrhythmia and tachycardia; the *bone marrow* may show red blood cell depression; and urinalysis may indicate the presence of hematuria.

**N**ursing Problems and Intervention   The adult in acute crisis usually has several major problems, including anemia, leg ulcerations, dyspnea, and anxiety. Pain and the potential for dehydration discussed under Second-Level Nursing Care still exist.

Hemoglobin levels may fall rapidly during acute sickle-cell crisis, and severe *anemia* may result. Blood transfusions are used to keep hemoglobin levels above 10 g/100 ml. Transfusions are usually given in the form of packed red blood cells. Monitoring of blood transfusions is the responsibility of the nurse. Two to five percent of all transfusions result in an unfavorable reaction. Nursing intervention for a possible transfusion reaction includes stopping the transfusion, obtaining blood samples, and notifying the physician of the changes. The most dangerous type of transfusion reaction is a hemolytic or blood incompatibility reaction. A potentially lethal condition, the hemolytic reaction occurs once in 2500 transfusions with a 20 to 25 percent mortality rate. Most hemolytic as well as other transfusion reactions are due to clerical or technical error or limits of cross-matching procedures in the institution. A *hemolytic reaction* usually occurs within the first 5 to 10 minutes of the transfusion, accompanied by chills, headache and fever, tachycardia, chest pain, dyspnea, nausea, vomiting, facial flushing, apprehension, and backache. (Refer, to Chap. 10 for a complete discussion of transfusion reaction.)

Careful screening of donors is the only preventive means. Other complications can ensue from blood transfusions, but hemolytic, allergic, and pyrogenic reactions are the most common. Once the transfusion is begun, initial observation for 15 minutes followed by a check of vital signs every 15 to 30 minutes is essential for rapid detection of a reaction and intervention.

Because of decreased circulation to peripheral tissue, *leg ulcers* are common. Tissue hypoxia makes healing difficult. The ulcerated area should be cleansed frequently with saline soaks and debrided as needed. A dry sterile dressing should be applied to the area with careful aseptic techniques. Removal of bed clothes from direct contact with the skin can be achieved through the use of a bed cradle. Skin grafts may be needed if the area of ulceration increases and healing does not occur.

*Pain* and *dehydration* still present a problem for the patient. Nursing care as discussed under Second-Level Nursing Care continues to be pertinent in reducing these problems. In addition, IV administration of fluids and electrolytes may be used. Urea therapy has been suggested with the thought that it could potentially "unsickle" the sickle cells by diffusing into the sickle cells that are clogging the microcirculation and unclogging them.[30] Since there are multiple side effects of this therapy, including thrombophlebitis (see Chap. 29), the treatment is still controversial.

Narcotics will be used if necessary for the relief of pain. If other problems related to *paralysis* (see Chap. 32) or *hemiplegia* (see Chap. 34) occur, appropriate nursing care is required.

*Dyspnea* may be present due to infection (pneumonia), cardiac pathology, or even pump failure. Whatever the reason, the administration of oxygen is essential. This can be done through the use of a nasal catheter or oxygen mask. Reduction of activity and adequate rest during the crisis state will reduce oxygen consumption and help relieve the dyspneic state. Care must be taken to prevent *venous stasis* secondary to immobility. When pain subsides, range of motion exercises should be instituted.

Patients who are experiencing an acute sickle-cell crisis may be extremely *anxious.* They are acutely aware of the debilitating effects of this health problem and fear death. Increasing signs of vascular occlusion and central nervous system damage in the form of hemiplegia or blindness may intensify the anxiety already present. Emotional support is critical. Careful discussion of the disease process as well as the overall effects of the sickling process may help decrease fears. Mild tranquilizer may be necessary to reduce the stressed state; when needed, counseling may be suggested.

The sickle cell acute sequestration crisis is rare but very dangerous, occurring predominantly in infants and young children. It is a sudden and massive entrapment of large amounts of sickled red blood cells in the splenic sinusoids. The child is pale, lethargic, and in hypovolemic shock. Death usually occurs if the patient is not treated with oxygen and blood transfusions.[31-33] If the child survives (75 percent mortality has been reported for these crises), a splenectomy is recommended. The young child is usually placed on intramuscular prophylactic prolonged-action Bicillin every 28 days to, it is hoped, reduce the incidence of bacterial infections. These surviving children will need close hematologic monitoring and close parenteral attention to possible infectious states.

**F**ourth-Level Nursing Care   Care of the individual with a chronic life-threatening disease is an ongoing nursing challenge. Patient anxiety can be decreased with implementation of some basic health maintenance principles.[34] A thorough discussion of the disease and reiteration of the physiology and accompanying symptomatology will maximize understanding and foster a trusting relationship among the nurse, patient, and family. Parent and patient education with pamphlets, audiovisual aids, and group discussion is a meaningful, supportive way of evaluating the client's understanding of the illness and instigating needed teaching. Frequently patient education needs are ignored on the assumption that a patient who has had the disease a long time knows everything. The availability of an interested and knowledgeable nurse and/or physician who can consult with family

or patient during crisis states at home will decrease anxiety and frequently circumvent a hospitalization or emergency-room visit. Continuity of care is best achieved with written and verbal correspondence from subspecialty clinic personnel to primary-care nurses and physicians in the community. It is advisable to include other nonmedical community professionals in the total care of the individual. This should include a conference with parent, nurse, and teacher early in the school year. During this conference, exercise needs and abilities of the child with SCA should be discussed. Emphasis should be placed on the fact that SCA does not affect intelligence. The young adult with SCA will need vocational counseling and realistic planning for future employment. Guidance counselors at school and vocational rehabilitation personnel are valuable sources of advice. Employment that requires a great deal of physical energy should be avoided.

Reproduction and sexual function are added concerns that need exploration based on facts. Both males and females with SCA usually have a delay in secondary sexual characteristics. Females have a delay in estrogen stimulation, thus a later onset of menarche. The preadolescent and adolescent girl with SCA may become anxious and/or depressed as peers develop sexually and begin their menses. The nurse should reassure the patient that sexual maturity will occur. The pregnant woman with SCA requires close medical supervision. Complications of increasing anemia, pyelonephritis, congestive heart failure, and toxemia are common. A substantial increase of stillbirths, spontaneous abortions, and neonatal deaths exists.[35] Counseling parents as to the realities of pregnancy and the exact inheritance patterns of SCA is essential. (See First-Level Nursing Care.) Some women with SCA use oral contraceptives, others use an IUD, a diaphragm, or other methods. Coordination between hematologist and gynecologist is important.

The clinical picture of SCA is variable. Some individuals have little symptomatology, others die or become severely disabled as youngsters. Presently, all treatment is symptomatic; no cure or identified agent to attack the basic problem of sickling of the red blood cell exists. Numerous agents have received clinical trials, the most recent being urea[36] and cyanate.[37] None have proved therapeutic. Patients frequently ask about longevity in light of the seriousness of the disease. The most common quoted statistic is that 50 percent of patients die before age 20, most not surviving beyond 40. However, good statistical data are lacking, and these figures may not be absolute. Sickle-cell anemia is a chronic, complex disease calling for accurate transmission of knowledge and ample medical support for each patient.

**Sickle-C disease (hemoglobin SC)** Sickle-C disease is an inherited chronic hemolytic anemia. It results from the inheritance of a hemoglobin S gene from one parent and a hemoglobin C gene from the other parent (Fig. 23-5). Sickle-C disease occurs in an estimated 0.06 to 0.25 percent of the Black population in the United States,[38] 1 in 800 is affected. The onset of symptoms, owing to the presence of both hemoglobin S and hemoglobin C, usually appears later in life than for SCA, with 50 percent of the children having musculoskeletal and/or abdominal pains before age 10.[39] The pain crises are less frequent and less severe than in SCA, with moderate anemia, i.e., hemoglobin averaging 8 to 13 g/100 ml blood.[40] Individuals with sickle-C disease frequently have splenomegaly in adult life. Cardiomegaly and cardiac murmurs are only occasional occurrences, in contrast to the frequent car-

diac changes seen in SCA.[41] Sickle retinopathy is strikingly higher in sickle-C disease with a 60 to 70 percent occurrence as compared with 10 percent in SCA.[42] Clinical symptoms and significant stages of retinopathy are usually observed between 20 and 30 years. The retinopathy is progressive and may lead to retinal detachment and loss of vision. Frequent ophthalmology examinations are crucial for these persons. Women with sickle-C disease often become gravely ill during the third trimester of pregnancy with frequent episodes of bone pain. An increased incidence of abortions, stillbirths, and neonatal deaths is usually seen. Persons with sickle-C disease have an increased incidence of bacterial infections which can precipitate a life-threatening crises. While the crisis and subsequent problems are similar to those in SCA, sickle-C disease usually follows a much more benign course, and the patient can expect greater longevity.

**Sickle-cell–thalassemia disease** An estimated 0.1 percent of American Blacks who have inherited a sickle gene from one parent and a thalassemia gene from the other parent (Fig. 23-6) are

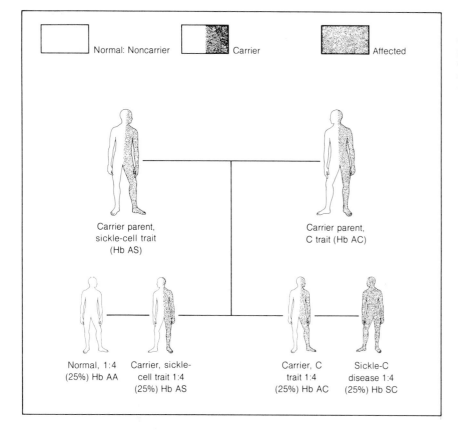

**FIGURE 23-5**
Inheritance pattern of sickle-C disease. Probability and percentage possibilities for each pregnancy at conception of parental matings of sickle-cell trait (Hb AS) and C trait (Hb AC).

affected by sickle-cell–thalassemia disease.[43] As discussed earlier, thalassemia results from a decreased production of a specific hemoglobin chain, thus a decreased amount of hemoglobin. Thalassemias are mild in the heterozygote and more severe in the homozygote. A decreased production of hemoglobin coupled with a sickle hemoglobin results in a variable clinical picture. The patient can have mild to moderate vaso-occlusive crises and mild to moderate splenomegaly. Hemoglobin values range from 6 to 13 g/100 ml. Patient teaching regarding symptomatology, pain crises, infection, and life-threatening episodes is similar to that for sickle-cell anemia.

**Thalassemia** When there is an insufficient amount of polypeptide chains owing to a genetic deficit, thalassemia occurs. The disease without the sickle gene may be termed either thalassemia minor or thalassemia major. In *thalassemia,* the hemoglobin type is normal, but the rate of hemoglobin synthesis is altered. *Thalassemia minor* develops in the heterozygotes in the form of a mild anemia. In *thalassemia major,* the person suffers from severe anemia owing to the impairment of hemoglobin synthesis. Alpha or beta chains can be affected by the impaired synthesis. Beta thalassemia is the most common form and is often referred to as class B thalassemia.[44] Infants with *thalassemia major* are anemic and fail to thrive. Growth retardation continues throughout life. Infections are frequent. Marked pallor, anoxic leg ulcers, anorexia, and retarded mental development are common. Complications occur from the chronic hemolytic process and repeated transfusions. Adults with thalassemia major are especially prone to cardiac hemosiderosis (a pathological accumulation of iron-substance glycoprotein), accompanying arrhythmias such as heart block, and cardiac failure (see Chaps. 24 and 25). Primary treatment includes routine blood transfusions to maintain the hemoglobin at 10 g/100 ml. If hypersplenism exists and is accompanied by increased red blood cell destruction and constant thrombocytopenia, splenectomy may be required. Because of the serious threat of infection following a splenectomy, the patient is placed on prophylactic intramuscular penicillin therapy for at least 2 years.

Thalassemia minor produces few symptoms and may not require any specific treatment. Since

**FIGURE 23-6**

Inheritance pattern of sickle-cell–thalassemia disease. Probability and percentage possibilities for each pregnancy at conception of parental matings of sickle-cell trait (Hb AS) and thalassemia trait (Hb A thalassemia).

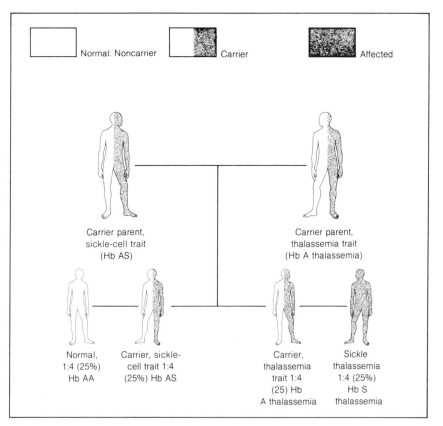

the person with thalassemia minor does carry the genetic trait for the disease, genetic counseling will be necessary.

## Membrane Defects of the Erythrocyte

Defects in the erythrocyte membrane can cause an increased destruction of erythrocytes and result in anemia. *Hereditary spherocytosis* (HS) is a congenital hemolytic anemia which occurs in 1 of 4500 births in the United States.[45] It affects all races and is acquired via autosomal dominant inheritance, thus appearing in both sexes equally. Children of an afflicted parent have a 0.5 degree of probability of inheriting the disease. It is the most common hereditary hemolytic disorder among persons of Northern European descent. Although the exact biochemical defect in HS remains unknown, the erythrocytes are intrinsically abnormal and prematurely destroyed in the spleen.

The filtering mechanism of the spleen requires that erythrocytes be smooth and malleable. The abnormal erythrocytes of HS are spherical in shape and destroyed by passage through the spleen, producing a hemolytic anemia. Frequently, because of their size the spherocytes are trapped in the splenic sinuses, and the spleen becomes enlarged and overworked. Following splenectomy, spherocytes have a life-span equal to that of normal erythrocytes, indicating that they were previously sequestered in the spleen but not elsewhere. Erythrocytes have normal survival times when transfused into persons with HS; therefore, the defect in HS is intrinsic, nontransferable, and causes erythrocyte destruction only in the presence of a spleen.

Clinical features of this problem include anemia, malaise, jaundice (due to the hemolytic process), and gallstones (due to increased levels of bilirubin). Splenomegaly is pronounced, and patients often complain of left upper quadrant pain. Classic laboratory studies reveal anemia, presence of spherocytes, and increased concentration of reticulocytes. Diagnosis is established by presence of an abnormal red blood cell osmotic fragility curve and presence of disease in another family member.

Recommended therapy is a splenectomy after 3 to 4 years of age and before 8 to 10 years of age. In young children prophylactic penicillin is usually given monthly in order to prevent infection. Generally, anemia is usually mild; however, patients can have episodes of bone marrow failure, usually termed *aplastic crises,* which are commonly precipitated by infections. Blood transfusions can be administered during crisis, but a splenectomy is the preferred treatment. Usually, most patients will experience a complete reversal of symptoms after the spleen is removed.

## Metabolic Defects in the Erythrocyte

Metabolic defects in the erythrocyte can also result in anemia. A sex-linked hereditary abnormality, a deficiency in *glucose 6-phosphate dehydrogenase* (G-6-PD) is the most common red blood cell enzyme deficiency causing a hemolytic anemia. This is an X-linked disorder, and the gene determining the structure of the enzyme is transmitted from mother to son. Since males have only one type of enzyme, they have either normal or deficient levels of G-6-PD. Women may be homozygous or heterozygous for the condition, making them normal, carriers of the trait, or deficient. The deficiency occurs most frequently in African and Mediterranean populations, affecting 13 percent of American Negro males and 3 percent of females. An estimated 1.5 percent of American Caucasians are affected.[46] A deficiency in G-6-PD acts upon the erythrocytes by causing them to be more susceptible to hemolysis following ingestion of certain drugs or chemicals (Table 23-2). The exact cause of this hemolysis is not known. Anemia in individuals deficient in G-6-PD is also

**TABLE 23-2**
AGENTS ASSOCIATED WITH HEMOLYSIS IN INDIVIDUALS DEFICIENT IN G-6-PD

| | |
|---|---|
| ANTIMALARIALS | Bromo Seltzer |
| Primaquine | Black Draught and other senna |
| Pamaquine | preparations |
| Plasmoquine | |
| Pentaquine | |
| Quinacrine (Atabrine) | ANALGESICS |
| Quinine | Acetylsalicylic acid |
| | Acetanilid |
| SULFONAMIDES | Acetophenetidin (Phenacetin) |
| Sulfanilamide | Aminopyrine (Pyramidon) |
| Acetylsulfanilamide | Antipyrine |
| Sulfacetamide (Sulamyd) | |
| Sulfamethoxypyridazine | SULFONES |
| (Kynex, Midicel) | Sulfoxone (Diasone) |
| Salicylazosulfapyridine | Thiazolsulfone (Promizole) |
| (Azulfidine) | Diaminidephenyl sulfone (DDS) |
| Sulfisoxable (Gantrisin) | |
| | OTHERS |
| NITROFURANS | Dimercaprol (BAL) |
| Nitrofurantoin (Furadantin) | Methylene blue |
| Furazolidone (Furoxone) | Naphthalene (moth balls) |
| Furaltadone (Altafur) | Aminosalicylic acid |
| Nitrofurazone (Furacin) | Phenylhydrazine |
| | Acetylphenylhydrazine |
| NONPRESCRIPTION ITEMS | Probenecid (Benemid) |
| CONTAINING PHENACETIN, | Vitamin K (water-soluble |
| ACETANILID, OR QUININE | analogues) |
| 666 | Chloramphenicol |
| APC | Quinidine |
| Super Anahist | Trinitrotoluene |
| Anacin | Fava beans and similar |
| Empirin | vegetables |
| Stanback | Para-aminosalicylic acid (PAS) |
| 4-Way Cold Tablets | |

seen during the neonatal period and with infections.[47]

Shortness of breath and fatigue accompany the hemolytic anemia. The rapidity of development and severity of the anemia depend on the amount of chemical as well as the specific drug ingested. Jaundice and dark urine are additional signs of hemolysis. The patient usually experiences 7 to 12 days of acute hemolysis, followed by an increase in reticulocytes and hemoglobin. Heterozygous females will usually have mild anemia or experience no difficulty following exposure to most offensive agents; however, naphthalene and other chemicals listed in Table 23-2 should be avoided.

Screening for G-6-PD can be completed with a direct blood assay test. Once screened and diagnosed, patients should be given information on the disease and provided with a list of drugs and chemicals to avoid. Instructions should be given on how to read drug labels, as many of the offending agents are included in nonprescription medicines. Additional lists should be left with pharmacists, health workers, physicians, and others who may prescribe or monitor drugs for the individual. Each patient should know the importance of not taking any medicine, over-the-counter or otherwise, which is not prescribed by a pharmacist or physician knowledgeable about the individual's G-6-PD deficiency.

### Acquired Hemolytic Anemias

*Acquired hemolytic anemias* (AHA) are caused by the premature destruction of red blood cells. These anemias are induced in extrinsic ways, such as extravascularly in the spleen or liver when hemoglobin is converted to bilirubin, or intravascularly when free hemoglobin is liberated within the blood. Acquired hemolytic anemias are categorized as being immunohemolytic or nonimmune anemias.

**Immunohemolytic anemias**  *Immunohemolytic* states are further classified as being *isoimmune* or *autoimmune*. Isoimmune reactions occur between antigens and antibodies from different sources but within the same species, as in transfusion reactions or erythroblastosis fetalis. In autoimmune reactions the destructive hemolytic agent originates in the person. The hemolytic agent may be a serum protein, for example, an immune globulin protein, functioning like an antibody producing the hemolysis.

At present, two hypotheses are offered to explain abnormal immune reactions. One hypothesis maintains that the abnormality is within the immune system itself. Here the immune mechanism loses its capacity for self-recognition. The second hypothesis suggests that pathogenic changes occur within the red blood cell membrane forming a new antigen which stimulates a normal immune system to respond.

The predispositions that may precipitate an autoimmune hemolytic state are conditions such as chronic lymphocytic leukemia, lymphosarcoma, and reticulum-cell sarcoma. Systemic lupus erythematosus accounts for many symptomatic patients. Autoimmune hemolytic anemia is also associated with rheumatic fever, acute and chronic liver disease, and viral disorders such as infectious mononucleosis. The clinical features are extremely variable with symptoms appearing when a significant degree of anemia has developed. Jaundice may be an initial symptom. Onset and relapses may be precipitated by infection, trauma, pregnancy, surgery, or psychologic stress. The physical findings are extremely variable; some patients have no related physical findings, while others in a hyperacute hemolytic state may show jaundice, pallor, air hunger, and cardiovascular failure.

The Coombs' test is a diagnostic test used to identify antigen-antibody reactions within blood serum, distinguish between types of hemolytic anemias, and identify blood types. There are two forms of this test, the direct and indirect. The *direct Coombs' test* is used to demonstrate the presence of a serum globulin on the red blood cell membrane. Globulins are proteins present in blood serum where antibodies are also associated. The *indirect Coombs' test* is used to detect red blood cell antibodies in the serum. Abnormal warm or cold antibodies active against the patient's red blood cells are also identified in the serum. In autoimmune hemolytic anemias the patient is expected to demonstrate a positive Coombs' test and the presence of an abnormal cold or warm antibody.

Hemolysis is an active process and may have mild to severe effects. The treatment of choice is corticosteroids, usually prednisone, which induces an initial remission after 2 to 4 days of treatment in 80 percent of patients. High dosages of prednisone are given until some evidence of hematocrit stabilization is seen. The dose is then tapered slowly. Patient teaching regarding side effects of prednisone should be incorporated into the plan of care. (Refer to Chap. 21 for a complete discussion of steroids.) Increased appetite and weight gain are consistent side effects of prednisone. The weight gain may produce a feeling of tightness and fullness in the abdomen. The immunosuppressive effects of prednisone predispose patients to increased incidence of infection. The patient should avoid persons with known infections and large crowds, and completely avoid all live virus vaccines (e.g., measles, rubella, mumps, smallpox, and polio). To alleviate peptic and gastric ulcerations, Maalox or a similar antacid is usually recommended. General measures supportive of cardiovascular function are indicated.

Transfusions should be avoided whenever possible as they result in accelerated hemolysis. The duration of autoimmune hemolytic anemia is measured in terms of months to years before recovery or death. The mechanism producing the antibody in these conditions is unknown, and treatment is care of the underlying disorder in the hope of eliminating possible causative agents.

Drug reactions involving antibody reaction with normal red blood cells can cause hemolysis. This *immunohemolytic process* does not involve any known abnormality in the red blood cell. Drugs capable of inducing an immunohemolytic disorder are antibiotics, such as penicillin or streptomycin, or anticonvulsants and sedatives, such as Mesantoin, Dilantin, and Chlorpromazine. Most patients having this type of a drug-induced hemolytic anemia, will have mild or moderate hemolysis. Occasionally thrombocytopenia and bleeding occur. The treatment includes discontinuing the offending drug(s) and educating the patient regarding the drug sensitivity.

#### Acquired nonimmune hemolytic anemia

Mechanisms that can cause nonimmune hemolytic anemia include cardiac valvular prostheses which produce trauma and subsequent hemolysis and physiochemical factors such as exposure to heavy metals, benzene compounds, and inhalation of arsine gas. Arsine arises in the course of many industrial processes (e.g., those involving carbon tetrachloride), and sufficient exposure will cause anemia, jaundice, and hemoglobinuria. Sufficient exposure to lead and copper salts will also produce hemolysis in human beings. Bee stings and spider bites have also been linked with hemolytic anemias and hemoglobinuria.

### INCREASED ERYTHROCYTE PRODUCTION

*Polycythemia* is an increase in the number and volume of circulating red blood cells. This increase in red blood cell production may exceed the normal cell growth by as much as six to ten times. There are three types of polycythemias, namely, polycythemia vera, secondary polycythemia, and relative polycythemia.

#### Polycythemia Vera

A chronic disease of unknown etiology, polycythemia vera is characterized by an increase in the number of circulating erythrocytes and total blood volume. Thrombocytosis, leukocytosis, and splenomegaly are additional problems of the disorder. Formerly addressed as a separate entity, polycythemia vera is now considered one of a group of diseases termed *myeloproliferative disorders* (that is, problems related to overproduction or proliferation of bone marrow).[48]

As the numbers of red blood cells, leukocytes, and thrombocytes increase, a series of changes occur having a serious effect on the patient. These changes include an increase in blood volume, increased blood viscosity, increased hemoglobin production, and severe congestion within vital organs and body tissue. The overall effects on the patient are widespread. Increased blood volume and viscosity cause an increase in arterial blood pressure, dizziness, tinnitus, and a feeling of fullness in the face and head. Increased viscosity also results in thrombus formation, especially within vessels supplying the lower extremities and vital organs. (See Chaps. 26 and 29.) As blood volume increases, cardiac demand will intensify, resulting in overload and pump failure. (See Chap. 24 for a discussion of pump failure.) An increase in the number of erythrocytes accumulating in the liver can lead to portal congestion and result in an enlargement of the liver and spleen.

Hemorrhage may occur owing to defective platelet functioning, defective clot formation, and rupturing of vessels due to congestion, and distention with capillaries, vessels, and arteries. Bleeding can begin in the gastrointestinal tract, as well as in the nose, mouth, and brain. Severe bleeding may accompany minor accidents and surgery.

As hemoglobin synthesis is accelerated, an iron deficiency develops. In addition, painful joint swelling may occur owing to increased cell destruction. This results in an increase in nucleoproteins. Uric acid is a by-product retained by nucleoprotein breakdown and may contribute to the increase in uric acid levels. Gout may also appear as a result of these changes (see Chap. 40).

Since the *cause* of polycythemia vera is unknown, it cannot be prevented. Careful analysis of serum hemoglobin helps to screen patients with polycythemia. Generally, the patient affected is over 60 and is often a male of Jewish extraction. The problem is rare in Blacks.

The onset of this condition is usually insidious, with the problem present for some time before medical personnel are contacted. Patients with polycythemia are often seen in an acute health care setting for observation. Nonacute as well as acute problems secondary to the polycythemia may also be noted.

A family *history* of polycythemia is rarely noted. The patient with polycythemia will complain of dizziness, headache, fullness in the head, and tinnitus. Mild dyspnea may be apparent, and joint pain may be experienced. Gastrointestinal complaints such as nausea, vomiting, and abdominal pain may also be present.

During the *physical assessment,* observation of the patient will reveal an individual with a ruddy complexion (*plethora*) caused by congestion of capillaries in the skin and mucous membrane. This redness is also noted in the conjunctiva and mucous membranes of the mouth. If early heart failure is present, tachycardia and lung congestion may be noted (see Chap. 24). Spontaneous bleeding such as nose bleeds, gingival bleeding, and bruising may be seen.

The spleen and liver may be enlarged. Upon abdominal examination, the liver will be palpable. Joint pain may be present, especially in the big toe, if gout has developed. Swelling may also be noted in the joints. Complaints of pruritus and urticaria are common. This problem may be due to an increased release of histamine into the circulation. Hypertension is also noted as a result of increased blood volume. Thrombophlebitis may be apparent in extremities (see Chap. 29) and can lead to more complicated health problems.

During the *diagnostic testing,* a routine complete blood count will reveal an elevation in the number of red blood cells (8 to 12 million/mm$^3$) and a rise in hemoglobin (8 to 25 g/100 ml). A *granulocytic series* will demonstrate granulocytosis in many cases. An increase in the production of granulocytes is seen in the presence of polycythemia vera. Examination of peripheral blood smear shows abnormally shaped *platelets.* In addition, blood coagulation reveals a disorganized platelet fibrin network. This may be related to a decrease in platelet dendrite formation often observed in the disease. *Fibrinogen* levels are usually normal. *Bone marrow* tests will reveal a proliferation of red blood cells and an active growth of hematopoietic bone marrow.

The *uric acid* levels are increased by the increased production of nucleoprotein, an end product of red blood cell breakdown. *Arterial* oxygen saturation levels are normal. This feature seems to distinguish polycythemia vera from secondary polycythemia. *Alkaline phospatose* levels are increased, and *hyperhistaminemia* is noted in many patients not being treated for polycythemia.

The major *nursing problem* in patients with nonacute polycythemia vera is the *increase in blood volume.* For the nonacute patient with polycythemia vera, the primary goal of treatment will be reducing blood viscosity. This is usually done by means of a *phlebotomy,* a procedure whereby a needle is introduced into a vein and blood is withdrawn. In the patient with polycythemia vera, this procedure is done to reduce the circulating blood volume quickly. Up to 350 to 500 ml blood may be withdrawn every other day until the hematocrit levels are reduced. The patient usually responds well to the treatment. However, the patient should be observed for signs of hypovolemia in case rapid withdrawal of blood leads to hemodynamic changes. It should be noted that removal of blood by means of a phlebotomy can lead to iron deficiency. Replacement therapy may be given as needed.

*Control of cellular proliferation* and shrinking of enlarged organs are managed with chemotherapeutic agents. Radioactive phosphorus and sodium phosphate have been reported to be successful. Education of the patient and close monitoring of the chemotherapeutic regime are essential. Myelosuppressive agents and radiation may also be used to decrease cell proliferation.

*Gastrointestinal symptoms,* including fullness, pain, and dyspepsia, may be present. Through nutritional assessment, meal planning to include small nourishing servings, and attention to environmental and cultural factors the nurse can promote optimal health.

Acute *complications* of polycythemia vera include *vascular effects* of hypervolemia and hyperviscosity resulting in vascular distention, impairment of blood flow, stasis, and tissue hypoxia. *Venous thrombosis* occurs in half of the patients composing a significant cause of morbidity and mortality. Anticoagulants are used with caution because of the increased danger of hemorrhage; however, heparin and vitamin K antagonist have been used safely and successfully in treatment of thrombotic complications. Exercise should be encouraged since the threat of thrombus formation will increase with immobility. Patients on bed rest should engage in frequent passive exercises.

*Fluid and electrolyte* balance must be carefully assessed. Fluids should be encouraged to reduce blood viscosity. In the presence of pump failure, careful measurement of intake and output is required.

Pain due to *joint swelling* can be relieved by the use of analgesics, application of heat, and elevation of the extremity (see Chap. 40). When circulating blood volume decreases and the uric acid levels become lowered, the symptoms may reverse themselves.

Follow-up health care centers on continuity. The patient is often elderly, and the disease may run a course of 10 to 15 years if complications do not intervene. Education of the patient to basic needs of nutrition is essential. Deficiencies in iron, vitamin $B_{12}$, and folic acid frequently result from accelerated erythropoiesis and long-term use of phlebotomy. Therefore replacement of these substances may become necessary.

### Secondary Polycythemia

*Secondary polycythemia* occurs when an external or internal stimuli causes an increase in the body's oxygen demands. When this happens, the bone marrow is forced to increase the number of circulating erythrocytes in an attempt to prevent tissue hypoxia. When the tissue is deprived of sufficient oxygen for a long enough time, secondary polycythemia will develop. These changes often occur when people are in high altitudes above 7000 ft (acute mountain sickness) and in mountain areas. Persons with chronic lung disease or structural defects of the heart may also have this response. Nausea, vomiting, weakness, lethargy, and emotional responses may be noted.

The only significant laboratory findings are essentially the same as for polycythemia vera. Leukocytes and counts are normal, while reticulocytes are increased. Splenomegaly and jaundice are more noticeable. Treatment, if necessary, involves removing the cause. In many instances, secondary polycythemia is a normal physiologic response.

### Relative Polycythemia

*Relative polycythemia* occurs when there is a loss of plasma while the number of red blood cells remains within normal limits. The amount of red blood cells in the circulation becomes greater relative to the amount of existing plasma; in other words, the red blood cell concentration is increased. This problem can be seen in patients with burns or dehydration, or following vigorous diuresis. Relative polycythemia will usually reverse itself when the initial problem is successfully treated and the patient is adequately hydrated.

## BLEEDING DISORDERS

Bleeding disorders are caused by a disruption in platelet coagulation, rupture of fragile, easily damaged blood vessels, alteration or absence of clotting factors, or disruption in fibrinolysis. There are two major classifications of bleeding disorders, purpura and coagulation disorders. The following discussion will focus upon these two problems and related nursing care.

### Purpura

Purpura is the extravasation of small amounts of blood into the tissue and mucous membrane.[49] It is of two types, vascular purpura and purpura caused by a disruption in platelet formation (idiopathic thrombocytopenic purpura and secondary purpura thrombocytopenia).

**Vascular purpura**  This type of purpura is the result of the rupturing of small blood vessels with bleeding into the tissue usually following the application of undue pressure. Vascular purpura may be inherited (familial hemorrhagic telangiectasis), it may occur in response to an allergen (anaphylactoid purpura), or it may be caused by poisons or other toxins as in toxic purpura.[50] Hypertension, inflammation, and poor diet can be contributing causes of this problem. Bleeding can occur in the gastrointestinal tract, kidneys, or joints. The patient will complain of joint pain, fever, hematuria, abdominal pain, and gastrointestinal problems.

**Idiopathic thrombocytopenic purpura**  Purpura due to disruption in platelets is called *idiopathic thrombocytopenic purpura* (ITP). It is caused by the *premature destruction* of red blood cells. The exact cause of the disorder is unknown. However, it may be caused by an immune response following infection or may be drug induced.

**P**athophysiology  ITP is characterized by a low platelet count, short platelet life-span, abundant megakaryocytes in the bone, and an immunologic pathogenesis.[51]

A *congenital immunologic type* of thrombocytopenia includes neonatal low platelets due to immunization of the mother against fetal platelets. This disorder is similar to erythroblastosis fetalis except that fetal platelets, not erythrocytes, provide antigen stimulus. Acquired types of increased platelet destruction include the thrombocytopenias associated with bacterial, viral, or rickettsial infections. Direct interaction between platelet and virus or bacteria may contribute to this lowering of platelet numbers. This may be the result of antigen-antibody complexes which have an affinity for sites on the platelet surface. Antibody-coated platelets, like antibody-coated red blood cells, are selectively sequestered and destroyed in the spleen.

*Acute ITP,* sometimes termed *postinfectious thrombocytopenia,* is predominantly a disease of childhood, typically affecting children 2 to 6 years of age. Characteristically, the abrupt onset of severe thrombocytopenic purpura follows a viral infection. Effects of this problem include petechial hemorrhages, purpura, and frequent bleeding from the gums, gastrointestinal, and urinary tracts.

*Chronic ITP* is primarily a disease of adults. The condition usually occurs in the 20- to 50-year old female where no familial tendency exists, and a history of preceding infection is rarely obtained. These changes result in scattered petechiae or minor bleeding, a bruising tendency, menorrhagia, and recurrent epistaxis present for months. Petechial and purpuric lesions of a noninflammatory nature may occur anywhere but are common on distal upper and lower extremities.

**F**irst-Level Nursing Care  Several groups of individuals are at risk to develop ITP. Neonatal rubella occurring in the newborn can result in platelet counts of 70 to 200/mm³. Prenatal ingestion of a thiazide diuretic has resulted in thrombocytopenic purpura in infants. Decreased platelet production, as in aplastic anemia, alteration in bone marrow infiltration by carcinoma such as acute or chronic leukemia, ionizing radiation and myelosuppressive drugs such as methotrexate, 6-mercaptopurine, or drugs that act specifically on platelet production such as alcohol, estrogens, and thiazide diuretics, can also predispose an individual to thrombocytopenia. Nutritional deficiencies including folic acid deficiency or pernicious anemia may predispose and contribute to the risk of developing ITP. Cyclic thrombocytopenia occurs in normal women, with platelet counts decreasing up to 20 percent during the 2 weeks preceding menstruation. Therefore, accurate interviewing as to the current medications in use, a dietary assessment, and history of infections can help to identify a population at risk.

*Prevention*  Since the etiology of ITP involves an autoimmune response of unknown origin, prevention of acute problems rests with early detection and treatment of infection. Identification of high-risk persons, and follow-up of individuals who complain of easy bruising, petechiae, and bleeding gums, are important for health promotion. All patients should be encouraged to eat a well-balanced diet, especially in the presence of an infectious process. Injections of thiazide diuretics during pregnancy should be avoided. Women of child-bearing age should have rubella titers checked and be properly immunized if necessary. They will thus avoid the potential of developing rubella during pregnancy.

**S**econd-Level Nursing Care  Patients with early ITP seek medical attention because of physical symptoms and bleeding manifestations. A careful health history, including a bleeding history, and physical examination are important components of care at this level.

*Nursing assessment*  Prior to the health history and physical assessment, history of bleeding tendency should be completed. The acquisition of an accurate *bleeding history* is an initial assessment skill vital to helping the nurse identify bleeding and coagulation disorders.

An understanding of possible causes responsible for decreased platelet production or increased platelet destruction is also necessary. Bleeding is termed either spontaneous or traumatic. *Spontaneous,* or purpuric, bleeding is confined to the microcirculation and usually involves the mucous membranes and platelet disfunction. Epistaxis (nosebleed), gingival bleeding, and gastrointestinal hemorrhages are common examples. *Traumatic* bleeding results from injury to arterioles and small arteries, exemplified by hemarthrosis, hematuria, and deep intramuscular bleeding. Coagulation defects, for example, hemophilia, are associated with traumatic bleeding. Determination whether the bleeding is spontaneous or traumatic is an important component of the bleeding history. The nursing assessment must take into consideration other factors commonly responsible for decreased platelet production or increased platelet destruction, as both congenital and acquired factors may cause thrombocytopenia.

Patients with ITP often will offer a *health history*

of a tendency to bruise easily. They may observe a frequency of petechiae (small hemorrhages) or ecchymoses (large areas of hemorrhage) appearing with the slightest degree of skin pressure. Epistaxsis may be common but often goes unmentioned by the patient unless questioned. There is usually no family history of bleeding disorders; in children, a previous history of a viral or bacterial infection may be obtained. Complaints of frequent gum bleeding may also accompany the history.

The physical effects of ITP may vary from patient to patient. Generally, upon *physical assessment,* ecchymatic areas may be noted anywhere on the body including the extremities. Hemorrhagic petechiae may also be noted in the oral mucosa. Generally, these lesions are not inflamed. The liver and spleen are often palpable but not enlarged. Vital signs are usually within normal limits with no marked difference in neurological findings.

*Diagnostic tests* used to establish a diagnosis of ITP include an examination of a *blood smear, platelet count,* and *bone marrow* to demonstrate megakaryocyte production. A normal platelet count ranges from 200,000 to 400,000/mm$^3$. Counts of less than 50,000/mm$^3$ may be associated with hemorrhagic phenomena. Counts less than 10,000/mm$^3$ may be life-threatening.

Bleeding time may be checked to evaluate qualitative platelet disorders. A simple technique, *bleeding time* (BT) is determined by placing a puncture wound 2.5 mm deep on the volar surface of the forearm after a blood pressure cuff has been placed on the arm and the pressure maintained at 40 mmHg. The blood is blotted at half-minute intervals until bleeding ceases.[52] Prolongation of the BT when the platelet count is normal implies a qualitative platelet disorder that is an abnormal platelet function due to congenital or acquired abnormalities.

*Nursing problems and interventions*  Only a small percentage of adults have spontaneous remissions to ITP (less than 10 percent). Many present acute symptoms for which hospitalization will be required. Therefore, identification of problems and related interventions for the adult will be discussed in Third-Level Nursing Care.

Most children with ITP can be managed at home with allowances for their developmental age. Eighty percent of children recover completely and permanently regardless of the treatment.

**T**hird-Level Nursing Care  Adults with acute ITP require hospitalization and a careful assessment of

physical status since less than 10 percent have a spontaneous recovery. The onset of hemorrhages and related changes may be severe. Early detection of changes can help prevent more serious complications.

*Nursing assessment*  In addition to the *health history* discussed in Second-Level Nursing Care, patients in the acute phase of ITP may report the presence of tarry stools and hematuria. Gingival bleeding may increase, as well as the frequency of nosebleeds. If bleeding into an organ has occurred, dyspnea, limited joint movement, and pain in addition to complaints of fatigue and generalized weakness may be added to the history.

The significant addition to the *physical assessment* noted under Second-Level Nursing Care is the increase in bleeding sites. Ecchymotic areas may be larger, deeper, and more painful to touch. There may be an increased distribution of *petechiae* over the body, and an immediate bruising noted upon the slightest application of pressure to an area. If bleeding is continuous, the patient often appears restless and agitated.

In the presence of *hemorrhage,* frank bleeding will be observed on the gums or oral mucosa as well as in the stools. Signs of *hypovolemia* (see Chap. 28) including a decrease in blood pressure and skin temperature may be noted. *Increased intracranial pressure* (see Chap. 32) is rare, but patients should have a complete neurological assessment with frequent checks to assess changes in their current health status. If *anesthesia or weakness* is observed in the extremities and pain is present, bleeding into the nerve may be present. If there is bleeding into the thoracic cavity, *shortness of breath* and changes in respiration will be seen. Signs of *pump failure* (see Chap. 24) may also be noted.

*Diagnostic tests*  In addition to the tests mentioned in Second-Level Nursing Care, a *coagulation time* and *prothrombin time* (see Chap. 29) will be done and the results will be normal. The test of stool with guaiac will be positive in the presence of gastrointestinal bleeding, and hematuria will be noted if there is urinary tract hemorrhage. *Clot* retraction is done to assess the number and function of platelets. The tests attempt to measure the time it takes for contraction (or clot retraction) of an undisturbed clot to occur. (Clot formation usually begins within 2 hours after the sample is placed in the test tube and is completed within 24 hours.)

*Rumpel-Leeds capillary fragility test* (tourniquet test) is used to demonstrate vascular resistance and the function as well as the number of platelets present. The test is accomplished by placing a tourniquet or blood pressure cuff on the patient's arm for approximately five minutes and noting the appearance of petechiae. Usually there will be no petechiae present. However, in the presence of thrombocytopenia petechiae will be noted.

**N**ursing Problems and Interventions  The major problem faced by the patient in the acute phase of ITP is *hemorrhage.* Therefore, the goal of treatment is to control the bleeding.

During early treatment, the patient should be observed for signs of cerebral hemorrhage (see Chap. 34). It is important to reduce the degree of stress in the external environment and help the patient relax. Patients are often kept on complete bed rest to combat generalized fatigue and weakness. Avoiding physical exertion, straining at stool, and coughing is important.

*Platelet transfusions* can be used during the acute phase of bleeding as this will increase the platelet count and may help control hemorrhage. Since the platelet life-span is reduced in the presence of ITP, transfusions are only a temporary intervention. Antibody formation can also occur which will render this treatment ineffective on subsequent occasions.

*Steroid therapy* is usually given to the patient as an initial intervention to control bleeding. The value of adrenocortical steroids lies in their suppression of phagocytic activity of the reticuloendothelial system and splenic sequestration so that the life-span of antibody-coated platelets is prolonged. Generally prednisone is given in divided doses of from 0.5 to 2 mg/kg daily. Patients should be observed for side effects of steroid therapy (see Chap. 21). Frequently, the use of steroids is a temporary intervention, as it can only control rather than cure the problem. If there is no marked improvement after several weeks of treatment, a splenectomy is usually performed.

*Splenectomy*  The most effective intervention for ITP is a *splenectomy.* The removal of the spleen is thought to stop the early destruction of platelets, although the exact mechanism is unknown. Routine preoperative teaching is done, and the administration of steroids is usually a part of the initial preparation. Steroids are administered to raise the platelet count.

Following the surgery the nurse should be alert to signs of restlessness and alterations in vital signs. These changes may indicate hemorrhage

and/or impending shock. Since patients with ITP have an increased bleeding tendency, they need to be carefully observed for hemorrhage. Transfusions postoperatively may help, should bleeding occur. Abdominal distention may be present because of manipulation of the bowel during surgery or fluid retention due to decreased voiding. Catheterization may be needed along with continued assessment of bowel sounds and presence of flatus. Pain may also be present, and analgesia can be provided according to the patient's need.

Preoperative teaching should be directed toward an explanation of the impending procedure and its overall effect on the patient and family. The patient should be told the anticipated outcome of the procedure and its impact on his or her life.

Upon the removal of the spleen, its functions are taken over by the reticuloendothelial organs such as the lymph nodes, the liver, and bone marrow.

Splenectomy is usually performed because of beneficial effects of removing a major site of platelet destruction. Seventy to ninety percent of patients improve after splenectomy, and platelet counts are restored to normal in about two-thirds of patients.[53–57] There is no way to predetermine which patients will respond to splenectomy and which will not. Following splenectomy, steroids may be withdrawn gradually over a period of time from 2 to 4 weeks. Relapses of ITP do occur, some as long as 10 years later. The use of immunosuppressives may be considered if a splenectomy is unsuccessful. However, current research on this intervention is not conclusive.[58]

**F**ourth-Level Nursing Care  Follow-up of persons with ITP by the community health nurse involves serial platelet counts until they return to normal levels. Then routine platelet counts and total health evaluations are done as deemed appropriate. The splenectomized patient should receive prophylactic penicillin orally or intramuscularly. Constant explanation of the importance of routine administration of this medicine is extremely important. The steroid preparation will be discontinued after a course of treatment and should never be continued indefinitely nor withdrawn abruptly.

Patients with ITP must be informed that relapses may occur and educated as to identification of initial symptoms and importance of prompt medical evaluation. They should be taught about the need for repeated activity and a well-balanced diet and encouraged to report any signs of bleeding in the stool, urine, or vomitus. Feelings of fatigue, weight loss, or pallor should be reported immediately.

## Coagulation Disorders

The term blood coagulation is used to denote a sequence of reactions which lead to the formation of a fibrin clot. The complex of factors involved in coagulation are individually identified by the roman numerals I to XIII. These numerals were assigned by the order of their discovery and do not indicate sequential activity. Except for factor IV, which is calcium, all the plasma coagulation factors are proteins.

To explain the cascading sequence of coagulation, three systems will be referred to, the *extravascular* (surrounding tissue), the *vascular* (blood vessels), and the *intravascular* (plasma and platelets) as shown in Fig. 23-7.[59] If any one of these systems fails, bleeding will occur. With trauma, the extravascular system releases tissue thromboplastin (factor III) which converts serum prothrombin (factor II) to thrombin in the presence of calcium (factor IV) and factors V, VII, and X. Thrombin then polymerizes fibrinogen to form fibrin. Simultaneously, the vascular system constricts, and platelets adhere to each other to form a seal, a temporary plug against further bleeding. The intravascular system forms the fibrin clot. The fibrin in this system is formed without the help of tissue thromboplastin, provided that platelet thromboplastin (factor XII) is present. Factors VIII and IX are necessary for conversion of prothrombin to thrombin and the final step of polymerization of fibrinogen (factor I) to fibrin. This added fibrin adheres to the previously formed platelet seal, making a firmer clot. (See Chapter 22.)

**Hemophilia** Hemophilia results from a failure of the intravascular clotting system to release factors VIII and IX, resulting in prolonged bleeding. Hemophilia occurs in 1 of every 10,000 births in the United States. It is an inherited, congenital, hemorrhagic disease transmitted from mother to son by a sex-linked recessive gene. All male offspring of a female carrier have a 50 percent chance of being affected. All female offsprings of a female carrier have a 50 percent chance of being a carrier of the hemophilia gene and a 50 percent chance of being a non-carrier. Identification of a female hemophilia carrier is now possible in greater than 50 percent of cases by immunochemical means. Two principle types of hemophilia exist: hemophilia A, or classic hemophilia, and hemophilia B, or Christmas disease. The

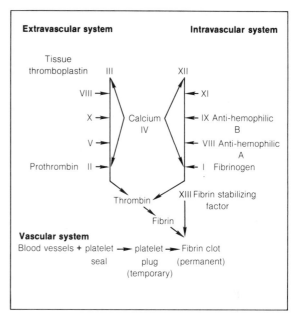

**FIGURE 23-7**
Sequence of coagulation.

symptoms of the two types are similar, but they differ in the specific type of clotting protein that is absent in the blood. (Refer to Table 22-2 for a complete list of the blood-clotting factors.)

Hemophilia A is the most common of all hereditary coagulation disorders and occurs five to six times as frequently as hemophilia B, C, or Von Willebrand's disease. (Von Willebrand's disease is an inherited factor VIII deficiency which also causes defective platelet dysfunction. It is an autosomal dominant trait transmitted to both males and females.) Male children with hemophilia are usually identified soon after birth by excessive bleeding from the severed umbilical cord or following circumcision. Later the parents note that the child bruises very easily; when the child begins to walk, bleeding can occur in the large joints (hemarthrosis), especially of the knees, elbows, ankles, and wrists, causing painful swelling. Hematuria, epistaxis, hematemesis, and melena are also common bleeding experiences.[60] Although this problem is classified as a childhood disease, it is now seen in adults owing to improved treatments in prolonging life.

*Class coagulation tests* are utilized to determine the type of bleeding disorder affecting these patients. These tests include determination of bleeding time, platelet count, prothrombin time, partial thromboplastin time, specific factor assay, and pre- and postinfusion response.

Once hemophilia is diagnosed, therapy is based on replacement of the deficient factor. From 1950 to 1965 fresh frozen plasma was the mainstay of treatment. Owing to the low concentration of the clotting protein in plasma, large volumes were needed to control bleeding. Use of large volumes resulted in an excessive quantity of circulating blood and lead to congestive heart failure. In 1966 cryoprecipitate, a plasma concentrate, began to replace fresh frozen plasma and became the primary mode of treatment. In 1970 high-potency concentrates were made available. Only small volumes of the high-potency concentrates are needed, and the dosage can be administered by syringe. The cost of plasma concentrates is high. It is not unusual for a child with hemophilia to use a quantity of plasma concentrates costing $12,000 a year. With the National Hemophilia Foundation estimating 40,000 males in the United States having moderate to severe forms of hemophilia, this presents an enormous financial problem.[61,62]

Infusions of factors VIII or IX are used for severe spontaneous bleeding episodes or following major trauma. *Prophylactic infusions* of factor VIII are advocated in some situations. For prophylactic care, the concentrate must be given on a fixed schedule, usually two or three times a week. This prophylactic approach is often prescribed for patients who have severe muscle and joint degeneration and require extensive physical therapy. It is also used for a patient in a bleeding cycle where symptomatic concentrate treatment is as frequent as a scheduled prophylactic protocol. In the past, patients were caught in a vicious debilitating cycle. Hemarthrosis necessitated joint immobilization to reduce bleeding and pain. With immobilization, muscle atrophy, fibrosis, and scarring of the joint occurred. Physical therapy to correct atrophy led to recurrence of bleeding. The person eventually became an orthopedic patient with casts and/or braces, which again *increased* muscle atrophy. Prophylactic administration of factor VIII breaks this cycle as the patient can tolerate physical therapy, improve range of motion, and maintain muscle mass. Prophylactic treatment is expensive but must be measured against plasma cost and administration, multiple hospitalization, orthopedic and further subspeciality medical care, loss of education and job potential, and loss of self-independence and esteem.[63]

Special nursing considerations for persons with hemophilia center on parent and patient education regarding identification, treatment of bleeding episodes, and general maintenance for optimum health. Families and patients need careful instruction regarding when to contact health personnel. Indications for hospitalization include severe pain and swelling of muscles or joints, causing limitation of movement or producing sleeplessness; serious or hard blows on the head; swelling in the tissues of the neck and/or floor of the mouth; severe abdominal pain; hematuria; or melena. All deep muscular hematomas should be given careful attention. Superficial bruises and cuts rarely result in serious bleeding.

Local treatment for bleeding close to the surface includes ice bags for vasoconstriction, immobilization to prevent clot dislodgment, and elevation of the area above the heart to decrease blood pressure in the vessels and allow for vasoconstriction. Firm manual pressure or a dressing will usually suffice for a mild cut or abrasion. Topical administration of coagulants such as thrombin may be helpful. Application of these measures for 15 minutes should be successful in stopping bleeding from small wounds. If these measures are not successful, further treatment with infusion of a factor concentrate is necessary. Since pain usually accompanies bleeding episodes, choice of an analgesic is important. As aspirin, Indocin, and Butazolidin are known to affect normal platelet function and prolong bleeding time, they should be avoided.

Joint bleeding is painful and may be dangerous. With initial joint pain, the patient should be instructed to begin rest without delay and immobilize the joint. An elastic bandage or a plaster cast may be applied according to the severity of bleeding. Prompt treatment will reduce trauma and delay onset of chronic orthopathy.

General management of the child or adult with hemophilia requires good oral hygiene and dental prophylactic care. This includes nutritious meals, dental examinations every 6 months, use of a softened toothbrush for mouth hygiene, and rapid attention to any dental discomfort.

School attendance is vital to prepare for an occupation not involving physical labor. Parents are advised to permit children to attend regular classes and interact with peers in activities appropriate for their age and condition.

Acute-care complications do occur, and families must be acquainted with their potential, to foster rapid assessment and appropriate intervention. Complications from bleeding include airway obstruction due to hemorrhage into the neck and pharynx, intestinal obstruction due to bleeding into intestinal walls, nerve compression with paralysis from hemorrhaging into deep tissue, and intracranial bleeding with the patient presenting convulsive seizures due to hemorrhaging into or around the brain. These are frightening thoughts for any family to cope with. Continual support and counseling are needed for both patient and family. The nurse can provide much guidance for the family and help improve the patient's overall health status. If parents have a positive attitude toward the hemophilia, the child usually develops a healthy, productive, self-confident attitude about himself and his health problem. Parents who have children with hemophilia can lend support to parents who are experiencing them for the first time. Nurses involved in parent groups should facilitate the group interaction by furnishing families with factual, up-to-date information on hemophilia. Informing families about the National Hemophilia Foundation and local chapters will facilitate dispersal of accurate information.

An increasing percentage of individuals with hemophilia are receiving their clotting factors at home by self or family administration. Advantages of the home transfusion program include improved school or work attendance, decreased utilization of medical facilities for major complications of hemophilia, and decreased frequency of serious orthopedic problems. Possible dangers of home transfusions include poor long-term care, improper handling of materials resulting in sepsis, wrong dosage, decreased potency, damage to veins, serious transfusion reactions, and overuse or delay or omission of therapy.[64] Families expressing an interest in home therapy need a thorough evaluation by the health team weighing all positive and negative factors. If home care is initiated, close medical and nursing supervision is needed with constant availability of consultation, periodically scheduled follow-up visits, reappraisal of technical skill, and home record review to evaluate therapy.

**Diffuse intravascular coagulation** Unlike the life-long bleeding characteristic of hemophilia, *diffuse intravascular coagulation* (DIC) is an acute bleeding disorder resulting from defibrination that occurs as a complication of a primary underlying pathologic process. Synonyms for DIC include *defibrination syndrome, fibrination syndrome,* and *consumption coagulation.* Differences in terminology arise from the various presentations of this disorder, although all refer to a generalized activation of the hemostatic mechanism beyond that normally confined to areas of local vascular injury.[65]

Diffuse intravascular coagulation is best understood by reviewing two basic processes involved in the clotting system (Fig. 23-7). A definite sequence of events leads to the production of thrombin and, ultimately, clot formation. A second protective chain of events defends the body against generalized clotting that would occur in the absence of unchecked thrombin. *Defibrination* refers to low or absent fibrogen levels. This results when the balance between circulatory clot-promoting substances and the mechanisms for their inactivation and removal is disrupted. Certain illnesses introduce into the general circulation substances which can initiate or accelerate intravascular coagulation or interfere with the body's ability to remove intermediate products of coagulation. For example, in abruptio placentae, cellular material, rich in tissue thromboplastin, enters the maternal circulation and initiates intravascular coagulation.

Defibrination states occur in association with other obstetrical complications such as toxemia and retention of a nonviable fetus. Infections, malignant diseases, heat strokes, massive trauma, burns, hemolytic transfusion reactions, and snake bites can precipitate DIC by introducing into the general circulation substances which can initiate or interfere with the body's ability to remove intermediate products of coagulation. As a result, the circulatory plasma is depleted of clotting factors that are consumed by the clotting process and transformed to serum. Because of the consumption of platelets and clotting factors, a potential for increased bleeding is created. In addition, widespread deposits of fibrin within the arterioles and capillaries cause an increase in clotting with a decrease in blood flow to vital organs, resulting in ischemic tissue damage. Therefore, the patient with DIC has widespread clotting within the microcirculation accompanied by decreased tissue perfusion and at the same time an increase in bleeding.

The onset of DIC with accompanying signs and symptoms tends to be acute. Bleeding may be severe. If the episode is acute, DIC may last hours to several days. Once the precipitating event has ended, fibrinogen can be reconstituted by a normal liver in 24 hours. Under other conditions, symptoms may persist for days or weeks.

Significant nursing problems of severe bleeding from DIC include shock, ischemic renal damage, oliguria or anuria, and iron-deficiency anemia. The mechanisms of shock cascade from oligemia and subsequent fall in cardiac output to decreased circulation to vital tissues, an anaerobic metabolism, acidosis, and eventual cellular injury and death. Interventions for shock include restoration of blood volume, oxygenation, and monitoring of vital signs with special attention to urinary output records.[66] Therapy may include heparin to stop intravascular clotting, although there is a risk of increased hemorrhage. Generally heparin is used unless bleeding is severe. Administration of fibrinogen, platelet concentrates, cryoprecipitate, and fresh plasma will replace depleted hemostatic factors but also supply fresh ingredients for new fibrin to be laid down in the microcirculation. The most important component of treatment is correcting the underlying problem. In some cases the problem may be self-limiting. If complications such as severe hemorrhage, renal failure, or organ damage occur, this problem could be fatal.

## REFERENCES

1   G. W. Thorn et al. (eds.), *Harrison's Principles of Internal Medicine,* 8th ed., McGraw-Hill, New York, 1977, p. 1660.

2   *Ibid.,* p. 1659.

3   W. J. Williams et al. (eds.), *Hematology,* McGraw-Hill, New York, 1972, p. 267.

4   *Ibid.,* p. 267.

5   Thorn, *op. cit.,* p. 1660.

6   *Ibid.,* p. 1660.

7   O. R. McIntyre et al., "Pernicious Anemia in Childhood," *N Engl J Med,* **272:**981–985, May 13, 1965.

8   D. R. Miller et al., "Juvenile Congenital Pernicious Anemia," *N Engl J Med,* **275:**978–983, Nov. 3, 1966.

9   Thorn, *loc. cit.,* p. 1660.

10   *Ibid.,* p. 1660.

11   *Ibid.,* p. 1663.

12   H. Pearson, F. McLean, and R. Brigety, "Anemia Related to age," *JAMA,* **215:** 1982–1984, March 22, 1971.

13   Joan Luckman and K. Sorensen, *Medical-Surgical Nursing—A Psychophysiologic Approach,* Saunders, Philadelphia, 1974, p. 761.

14   P. C. Vincent and G. C. Grunchy, "Complications and Treatment of Acquired Aplastic Anemia," *Br J Hematol,* **13:**977–998, 1967.

15   Vincent, *op. cit.,* pp. 977–978.

16   G. Schwitter and J. Beach, "Bone Marrow Transplantation In Children," *Nurs Clin North Am,* **11:**49–57, March 1976.

17   Thorn, *op. cit.,* p. 1676.

18   *Ibid.,* p. 1675.

19   J. F. Desforges, P. R. McCurdy, and H. A. Pearson, "Sickle Cell Anemia: Improving the Odds for Your Patient," *Patient Care,* **6:**116, Feb. 15, 1972.

20   J. Lin-Fu, "Sickle Cell Anemia: A Medical Review," Department of Health, Education, and Welfare, GPO #0-468-993, 1965, p. 17.

21   *Ibid.,* pp. 5–17.

22   Thorn, *op. cit.,* p. 1674.

23   Williams, *op. cit.,* p. 417.

24   D. R. Powers, "Natural History of Sickle Cell Disease: The First Ten Years," *Semin Hematol,* **12:**276, 1975.

25   E. Barrett-Connor, "Bacterial Infection and Sickle Cell Anemia," *Medicine,* **50:**97–112, 1971.

26   R. Johnson, "Increased Susceptibility to Infection in Sickle Cell Disease," *South Med J,* **67:**1342–1347, November 1974.

27   M. Robinson and R. Watson, "Pneumococcal Meningitis in Sickle Cell Anemia," *N Engl J Med,* **274:**1006–1008, May 5, 1966.

28   H. Abramson, "Introduction," in H. Abramson et al. (eds.), *Sickle Cell Diseases: Diagnosis, Management, Education, and Research,* Mosby, St. Louis, 1973, p. 1.

29   P. Gilman and R. Luddy, *Your Child and Sickle Cell Anemia,* University of Maryland Medical School and Department of Pediatrics, 1972, p. 7.

30   Luckman and Sorensen, *op. cit.,* p. 775.

31   M. Jenkins, R. Scott, and R. Baird, "Studies in Sickle Cell Anemia: Sudden Death During Sickle Cell Crises in Young Children," *Pediatrics,* **16:**30–37, January 1960.

32   R. A. Seeler, "Deaths in Children with Sickle Cell Anemia," *Clin Pediatr,* **11:**634–637, November 1972.

33   ——— and M. F. Schwiaki, "Acute Splenic Sequestration Crises (ASSC) in Young Children with Sickle Cell Anemia," *Clin Pediatr,* **11:**701–704, December 1972.

34   M. Green, "Care of the Child with a Long Term, Life-Threatening Illness: Some Principles of Management," *Pediatrics,* **39:**441–445, March 1967.

35   J. Pritchard et al., "The Effects of Maternal Sickle Hemoglobinopathies and Sickle Cell Trait on Reproductive Performance," *Am J Obstet Gynecol,* **117:** 662–670, November 1973.

36   Y. Frances, "Management of a Comprehensive Care Sickle Cell Clinic," in H. Abramson et al. (eds.), *op. cit.,* pp. 270–271.

37   J. Manning et al., "Cyanate Inhibition of Red Blood Cell Sickling," in H. Abramson et al. (eds.), *ibid.,* pp. 180–182.

38   Lin-Fu, *op. cit.,* pp. 19–20.

39   M. I. Barnhart, R. L. Henry, and J. M. Lusher, *Sickle Cell,* A Scope Monograph, Upjohn Co., Kalamazoo, Mich., 1974, pp. 58–60.

40   A. Tuttle and B. Kock, "Clinical and Hematological Manifestations of Hemoglobin SC Disease in Children," *Pediatrics,* **56:**331–340, March 1960.

41   E. Hook and G. Cooper, "The Clinical Manifestations of Sickle Cell Hemoglobin C Disease and Sickle Cell Anemia," *South Med J,* **51:**610–635, May 1958.

42   M. Barnhart et al., *op. cit.,* p. 62.

43   Lin-Fu, *op. cit.,* p. 19.

44  Thorn, *op. cit.,* pp. 1696–1697.

45  N. E. Morton et al., "Genetics of Spherocytosis," *Am J Hum Genet,* **14:**170, 1962.

46  L. A. Eisenhauer, "Drug-Induced Blood Dyscrasias," *Nurs Clin North Am,* **7:**799, December 1972.

47  C. Mengel, E. Metz, and W. Yancey, "Anemia During Acute Infections: Role of Glucose-6-Phosphate Dehydrogenase," *Arch Intern Med,* **119:**287–290, March 1967.

48  Luckman and Sorensen, *op. cit.,* p. 776.

49  *Ibid.,* p. 793.

50  *Ibid.,* p. 794.

51  M. Baldini, "Idiopathic Thrombocytopenic Purpura," *N Engl J Med,* **274:**1245–1251, June 2, 1966.

52  *Ibid.,* p. 1304, June 9, 1966.

53  R. M. French, *Nurse's Guide To Diagnostic Procedures,* McGraw-Hill, New York, 1971, p. 89.

54  A. Norday and G. Neset, "Splenectomy In Hematologic Diseases," *Acta Med Scand,* **183:**117, 1968.

55  D. Charlesworth and H. B. Torrence, "Splenectomy in Thrombocytopenic Purpura," *Brit J Surg,* **55:**432, 1968.

56  A. F. Carpenter et al., "Treatment of Idiopathic Thrombocytopenic Purpura," *JAMA,* **171:**1911, 1959.

57  Luckman and Sorensen, *op. cit.,* p. 796.

58  Williams et al., *op. cit.,* p. 1055.

59  P. C. Patterson, "Hemophilia: The New Look," *Nurs Clin North Am,* **7:**780, December 1972.

60  C. Burke, "Working with Children with Hemophilia," *Nurs Clin North Am,* **7:**777–785, December 1972.

61  K. Brinkhous, "Changing Prospects for Children with Hemophilia," *Children,* **17:**222–227, November-December 1970.

62  J. Lazerson, "The Prophylactic Approach to Hemophilia A," *Hosp Prac,* 99–109, 1971.

63  C. Kasper, S. Dietrich, and S. Rapaport, "Hemophilia Prophylaxis with Factor VIII Concentrate," *Arch Intern Med,* **125:**1004–1009, June 1970.

64  J. Van Eys et al., *Home Therapy for Hemophilia: A Physicians Manual,* Hemophilia Foundation: Medical and Scientific Advisory Council, June 1974, pp. 3–23.

65  G. Deykin, "The Clinical Challenge of Disseminated Intravascular Coagulation," *N Engl J Med,* **283:**636–644, Dec. 17, 1970.

66  F. A. Simeone, "The Nature and Treatment of Shock," *Am J Nurs,* **66:**1289, 1966.

## BIBLIOGRAPHY

Balarzak, S., and E. Munsey: "Disorders of Iron Metabolism," in *Hematology Principles and Practice,* Year Book, Chicago, 1972, pp. 43–65.

Barrett-Connor, E.: "Bacterial Infection and Sickle Cell Anemia," *Medicine,* **50:**97–108, 1971.

———: "Infection and Sickle-C Disease," *Am J Med Sci,* **262:**163–168, September 1971.

Beck, W. S. (ed.): *Hematology,* M.I.T., Cambridge, Mass., 1973.

Brown, K., et al.: "Prevalence of Anemia Among Preadolescent and Young Adolescent Urban Black Americans," *Pediatrics,* **50:**714–717, October 1972.

Brunner, L. S., et al. (eds.): *Textbook of Medical Surgical Nursing,* Lippincott, Philadelphia, 1970, pp. 302–325.

Butler, E.: "Drug-Induced Hemolytic Anemia," *Pharmacol Rev,* **21:**73, 1969.

Canale, V.: "Beta-Thalassemia: A Clinical Review," *Pediatr Ann,* **3:**6–23, September 1974.

Clement, D.: "Pitfalls in the Diagnosis and Treatment of Iron-Deficiency Anemia in Pediatrics," *Pediatrics,* **34:**117–121, July 1964.

Conn, H. F., and R. B. Conn (eds.): *Current Diagnosis,* Saunders, Philadelphia, 1968, pp. 297–388.

Cooke, R. E., and S. Levin (eds.): *The Biological Basis of Pediatric Practice,* McGraw-Hill, New York, 1968, pp. 421–475.

Dallman, P., and J. Pool: "Treatment of Hemophilia with Factor VIII Concentrates," *N Engl J Med,* **278:**199–202, Jan. 25, 1968.

Dyment, P. F., and E. M. Donowho: "Fatal Pneumococcemia and Sickle Cell Anemia," *South Med J,* **64:**758, June 1971.

Foster, S.: "Sickle Cell Anemia: Closing the Gap between Theory and Therapy," *Am J Nurs,* **71:**1952–1956, October 1971.

Garby, L.: "Iron Deficiency: Definition and Prevalence," *Clin Hematol,* **2:**245–365, June 1973.

Gaston, L.: "The Blood Clotting Factors," *N Engl J Med,* **270:**236–242, Jan. 30, 1964.

Gelpi, A. P., and R. P. Perrine: "Sickle Cell Disease and Trait in White Populations," *JAMA,* **224:**605–608, April 30, 1973.

Jackson, D.: "Sickle Cell Disease: Meeting a Need," *Nurs Clin North Am,* **7:**727–741, December 1972.

Linman, J.: "Physiologic and Pathophysiologic Effects of Anemia," *N Engl J Med,* **279:**812–818, Oct. 10, 1968.

McCormick, W.: "Abnormal Hemoglobins—The Pathology of Sickle Cell Trait," *Am J Med Sci,* **241:**329, 1961.

Murray, R. F.: "Genetic Counseling in Sickle Cell Anemia and Related Hemoglobinopathies," *Urban Health,* **2:**28–35, December 1973.

Nathan, D., and F. Oski (eds.): *Hematology of Infancy and Childhood,* Saunders, Philadelphia, 1974.

Pearson, H.: "Progress in Early Diagnosis of Sickle

Cell Disease," *Children,* **18:**222–226, November-December 1971.

Phillips, J. R.: "Mental Health and SCA: A Psycho-Social Approach," *Urban Health,* **2:**38–41, December 1973.

Pochedly, C.: "Sickle Cell Disease: Recognition and Management," *Am J Nurs,* **71:**1948–1951, October 1971.

Rabiner, S., and M. Telfer: "Home Transfusion for Patients with Hemophilia," *N Engl J Med,* **283:**1011–1015, Nov. 5, 1970.

Sojania, M., and S. Gross: "Hemolytic Anemias and Folic Acid Deficiencies," *Am J Dis Child,* **108:**53–60, July 1964.

Valaes, T., S. Doxiadis, and P. Fessas: "Acute Hemolysis due to Naphthalene Inhalation," *J Pediatr,* **63:**904, 1963.

Vaz, D.: "The Common Anemias: Nursing Approaches," *Nurs Clin North Am,* **7:**711–725, December 1972.

Williams, W. J., et al.: *Hematology,* McGraw-Hill, New York, 1972.

Wintrobe, M.: *Clinical Hematology,* Lea & Febiger, Philadelphia, 1974.

# 24
# DISTURBANCES IN THE BLOOD-PUMPING MECHANISM

Nancy Fairchild Clark

As human beings interact with the environment, the heart (pump) reacts with a highly complex and most dynamic response. Efficient pumping action provides vital organs with needed oxygen and nutrients to carry out their unique functions. Alterations in the efficiency of the pump are usually induced by both intrinsic and extrinsic variables which hamper effective muscle contractility. Changes within the pump itself may be due to congenital abnormalities, valve damage, or coronary artery problems. Other factors that precipitate diminished pumping activity are often external to the pump itself and include such factors as anemia, environmental stressors, vitamin deficiencies, and emotional problems.

When these changes occur, the pump attempts to cope with the disruption by developing mechanisms to handle alterations in muscle contractility. When these mechanisms fail, cardiac output diminishes and pump failure results.

## PUMP FAILURE

*Pump failure* can be defined as the heart's inability to pump blood, oxygen, and nutrients to the body in proportion to its metabolic needs. Pump failure is not a disease; it is a syndrome resulting from a variety of pathophysiological disruptions that place increased demands on the heart. These disruptions usually affect either the contractile functioning of the myocardium or the inflow or outflow of blood from the heart. *Left-sided failure* is due to a weakness in the left ventricle to adequately pump blood returning from the lungs into the arterial circulation. This blood backs up into the lung tissue and leads to pulmonary edema. *Right-sided failure* is due to a weakness of the right ventricle to circulate blood from the superior vena cava and inferior vena cava to the lungs. Venous blood backs up into the systemic circulation and results in peripheral edema. The exact pathophysiologic mechanisms responsible for pump failure are not entirely understood and will vary according to the pathological disruption present.

Pump failure usually begins gradually and, without adequate treatment, continues into the chronic state. The *pump failure syndrome* can be chronic or acute, and often an acute exacerbation of pump failure may be superimposed upon a chronic low-grade but refractory pump failure. The emphasis of this chapter will primarily be focussed on chronic pump failure and its effect on the individual. Acute pump failure can lead to cardiogenic shock and will be discussed in Chap. 28.

### Causes of Pump Failure

As seen in Table 24-1, disruption in cardiac function as well as extracardiac disorders may lead to the development of pump failure. The causes of pump failure are multiple and can be attributed to any disorder which places a continuous stress on the heart's ability to pump and circulate the blood required for normal bodily processes.

Generally, it is important to isolate the underlying as well as the precipitating causes of pump failure. The *primary causes* of pump failure are usually associated cardiac abnormalities produced by congenital or acquired problems. These include coronary artery occlusions, valvular disturbances, and primary vessel disturbances such as hypertension.

Often, disruptions may not become obvious until an acute disturbance occurs elsewhere and precipitates pump failure. These *precipitating causes* include hyper- and hypothyroidism, obesity, anemia, pregnancy, and environmental and emotional stressors. Identification of both the primary and the precipitating cause of pump failure is needed before adequate health care can be planned.

**Primary heart disturbances** As *coronary vessels* become occluded, blood flow to the myocardium decreases. Oxygenation of the cardiac muscle is disrupted, impairing its ability to function prop-

erly. Coronary artery disease most commonly produces vessel narrowing, due to arteriosclerosis. Although arteriosclerosis has several etiologies, atherosclerosis is by far the most common cause of this narrowing. Atherosclerosis is defined and discussed in more depth in Chap. 26.

When angina pectoris or reversible ischemia occurs because of coronary occlusion, the myocardium has a transient reduction of oxygen supply and it is consequently unable to sustain its normal contractile functioning. As the cardiac output drops, pump failure may develop. If the ischemic episode passes quickly, the myocardium will not show any significant damage and it may return to a cardiac output sufficient to meet the body's needs. Thus the pump failure will be alleviated.

In cases where occlusion of the coronary artery is prolonged, the cardiac muscle becomes increasingly hypoxic until death of the myocardium occurs (myocardial infarction). Approximately 65 percent of persons who have sustained a myocardial infarction will show some signs of pump failure. The extent and seriousness of the failure depend on the location and extent of myocardial necrosis. Necrotic muscle does not participate in the contractile process, and when muscle death is located in the left ventricle, a fall in cardiac output may result.

*Valvular defects* cause primary failure by interfering with the heart's ability to move blood from the venous to arterial system (see Chap. 29). In aortic stenosis the aortic valve is narrowed. Consequently, when the left ventricle contracts, the stenotic valve inhibits the blood flow from the left ventricle to the aorta. This elevated resistence to flow across the valve creates an increase in the work of the left ventricle. The strain placed on the ventricle leads to hypertrophy, with some dilatation usually present. Persistence of this state will lead to decompensation of the heart and resultant pump failure.

*Valvular insufficiency* is an additional problem that results from a defective valve not closing completely. This incompetence allows blood to regurgitate through the valve during systole into the antecedent chamber. In mitral insufficiency, for example, blood regurgitates into the left atrium during ventricular systole. This inefficiency in blood flow from one chamber to the next causes a volume overload of both the left ventricle and the left atria. The left ventricle compensates by dilatation with some hypertrophy, but as the disease process worsens, the left ventricle eventually decompensates for reasons previously discussed, and pump failure ensues.

*Electrical disturbances* affecting the rate and/

**TABLE 24-1**
CAUSES OF PUMP FAILURE

1 Primary heart disruptions
    *a* Coronary artery occlusion
    *b* Valvular defects
    *c* Arrhythmias
    *d* Primary muscle disturbances
    *e* Pericarditis and cardiac tamponade
2 Primary vessel disturbances
    *a* Hypertension
    *b* Arteriovenous fistulas
3 Precipitating causes of pump failure
    *a* Hyperthyroidism, hypothyroidism
    *b* Oxygenation disturbances and infection
    *c* Obesity
    *d* Paget's disease
    *e* Volume overload
    *f* Anemia
    *g* Beriberi
    *h* Pulmonary emboli
    *i* Environmental and emotional stress
    *j* Pregnancy

or rhythm of the heart's conduction system can lead to primary pump failure by affecting the amount of blood expelled by the heart. Heart rates over 100 beats/minute as in tachycardia usually cause a shortening of diastole, the time when the ventricles are receiving blood from the atria. When diastole is shortened, the ventricles do not receive sufficient blood from the atria, thus reducing the stroke volume. Although the increased heart rate may compensate for the reduced stroke volume at rates between 100 and 150 beats/minute, at rates over 150 beats/minute the stroke volume becomes so small the cardiac output diminishes. Similarly, output is decreased with the bradyrhythmias where the heart rate falls below 60 beats/minute. A decrease in heart rate may result in an ineffectual contraction and diminish cardiac output. (See Chap. 26 for a discussion of arrhythmias.)

*Primary muscle disturbances* may be divided into two classifications: *cardiomyopathies* and *myocarditis.* Cardiomyopathy indicates a state where the symptoms of pump failure result from primary myocardial dysfunction, secondary to the disorganization in the heart muscle, with loss of its contractile elements. Myocardial dysfunction may result from many causes such as alcohol, genetic predisposition, or neuromuscular disease or may arise from unknown or idiopathic causes. Many of the cardiomyopathies are considered "congestive" and are characterized mainly by heart dilatation with some hypertrophy. Signs of both left and right heart failure are evident, and the failure is said to be *refractory.* Research is currently being conducted to find ways in which congestive cardiomyopathy can be detected before it reaches the advanced stage.

*Myocarditis* is an inflammation of the myocardium usually caused by a virus and frequently associated with acute pericarditis. When this problem is present the heart is unable to contract properly because the inflammatory process interferes with the contractile function of the myocardial cells and eventually may cause cell death. The treatment of myocarditis may be difficult since an inflamed myocardium has the propensity to develop arrhythmias with relatively low doses of digitalis preparations.

Inflammation of the pericardium, or *pericarditis,* can be either acute or chronic and can occur from multiple causes: viral, neoplastic, autoimmune, traumatic, or congenital disorders. However, the cause may be unknown or idiopathic. Pericarditis often leads to an increase in the amount of fluid in the pericardial sac or to a decrease in the sac's elasticity. Both phenomena produce pressure on the heart and interfere with myocardial contraction and alter emptying of the ventricular chambers. Heart failure may then ensue. When large amounts of fluid develop in the paricardial sac, *cardiac tamponade* is said to occur. Should the fluid accumulate rapidly, the tamponade may be fatal. If discovered in time, aspiration of the fluid will relieve the contricting effect on the heart, and the cardiac function will return to normal.

**Primary vessel disturbances** These disturbances include those problems associated with hypertension and arteriovenous (AV) fistulas.

*Hypertension,* the pathologic elevation of arterial blood pressure, causes damage and scarring to the walls of arterial blood vessels with a resultant decrease in the size of their lumina. Atherosclerotic deposits on the vessel intima will also decrease lumen size. The increased resistance of the systemic vasculature associated with hypertension increases the workload of the heart. As a result, the left ventricle hypertrophies and eventually may fail if treatment is not instituted.

*Arteriovenous fistulas* (AV) are abnormal communications between arteries and veins. Blood flow in an artery follows the least resistant pathway, and, therefore, if an AV fistula is present, the blood enters the vein directly, thus bypassing the arterial and capillary network. Nutrients and oxygen from the blood to that tissue are impaired.

The most common type of AV fistula is that created for the purpose of renal dialysis. Others can be congenital, develop from a traumatic injury such as gunshot or stab wounds, or arise after surgery. They also are known to occur secondary to malignancy, arterial aneurysm, and infection.

Since an AV fistula shunts blood away from the normal circulation, the heart must increase its output to maintain a reasonable blood flow through the arterial system. The size of the fistula determines the amount of extra work demanded of the heart. When the fistula is large, the heart can become overburdened as the cardiac output increases above normal. High-output pump failure may result.

**P**recipitating Causes of Pump Failure *Hyperthyroidism* is commonly associated with pump failure (see Chap. 21). With elevated thyroid hormone levels the entire body's metabolic processes can speed up, increasing the demand on the heart to supply the tissues with nutrients. Tachycardia and an increase in cardiac output develop. If hyperthyroidism, particularly in the elderly, is untreated, high-output cardiac failure occurs and contributes to a syndrome known as *thyrotoxicosis.*

*Hypothyroidism* is the condition which results when the thyroid gland is not producing a sufficient amount of thyroid hormone. If it is left untreated, hypothyroidism predisposes the patient to the development of atherosclerosis and coronary artery disease and the disorder eventually leads to pump failure.

Disruptions in oxygenation caused by *emphysema, chronic bronchitis,* or *neuromuscular disorders* may lead to *cor pulmonale.* Cor pulmonale is defined as dilatation and hypertrophy of the right ventricle associated with pulmonary pathophysiology. The reasons that cor pulmonale and ultimately right heart failure develop are multiple, but generally are related to the pulmonary arterial hypertension caused by the lung disorder. The increased pulmonary pressure exerts a constant, heavy work load on the right ventricle analogous to the increased work of the left ventricle caused by systemic hypertension. This extra work load is the cause of right ventricular dilatation and hypertrophy, and it finally leads to a decrease in cardiac output.

*Infections,* particularly those affecting the respiratory tract, which produce tachycardia, hypoxia, and fever, make demands on the heart and may precipitate failure. Elderly individuals as well as those prone to lung problems may have an increased chance of developing pump failure secondary to infection. It is also important to note that elevated pulmonary pressures seen in compensated left ventricular failure and cor pulmonale can predispose an individual to respiratory infection and eventual pump failure.

An individual who is *obese* runs a much higher risk of developing cardiac disturbances. Obesity predisposes an individual to the development of atherosclerosis which can lead to coronary artery disease. In addition, the heart must work harder in order to meet the obese person's increased tissue needs for oxygen and to eliminate the increased waste products of metabolism. Over a period of time when severe obesity is present, pump failure will occur.

*Paget's disease* of the bone (see Chap. 40) is characterized by external and internal bone deformity. It is a chronic, progressive, idiopathic disease with increased vascularity of the involved bone. Many patients have no symptoms; however, if the disease is widespread, the marked increase in the vascularity of the involved bones requires an increase in the blood flow through the skeleton which may contribute to cardiac enlargement and high-output heart failure.

*Volume overload* presents the heart with an increased amount of fluid to pump. The heart enlarges and the rate increases in an attempt to circulate the extra fluid into the vascular system. Eventually the heart becomes overwhelmed and failure occurs. Volume overload can result from many causes, including (1) renal failure accompanied by an increase in sodium and water retention, and (2) excessive or rapidly administered intravenous fluids.

*Anemia* can also lead to pump failure. When erythrocytes are below normal limits or hemoglobin content is low, tissue hypoxia can occur. The heart, in an attempt to provide the tissues with the needed oxygen, increases its rate and force of contraction. In mild cases of anemia an increase in cardiac output may provide adequate oxygen to the tissues. However, if the individual who has anemia takes part in strenuous exercise or activity, the heart will no longer be able to cope with the demand for additional oxygen. Insufficient cardiac oxygenation will decrease cardiac contraction, and symptoms of pump failure will develop.

Beriberi is a deficiency in body thiamine (vitamin $B_1$). It is usually seen in countries where polished rice is the dietary mainstay. A decrease in thiamine interferes with the biochemical reactions necessary for the heart to convert chemical energy to mechanical energy. Tachycardia, as well as hypertrophy, are compensatory mechanisms frequently seen in individuals with beriberi.

In addition to the aforementioned causes of pump failure, other physical, emotional, and environmental stressors can contribute to its development. The frequency of *pulmonary embolism* in individuals with heart disease is well known. Inactivity and venous stasis coupled with a low cardiac output facilitates thrombus formation in the veins of the lower extremities. A dislodged thrombus is called an *embolus* and may travel to the lungs where it causes an elevation in the pulmonary arterial pressure by obstructing the pulmonary artery and by triggering a reflex pulmonary vasoconstriction. This sequence of events places additional strain on the right ventricle, and cardiac output may decrease further.

*Overexertion* by the individual increases the tissues' demand for oxygen. In the compromised heart, this demand may prove excessive, with the signs of failure becoming evident. *Emotional stress* causes activation of the autonomic nervous system with a subsequent increase in circulating catecholamines, creating additional strain on the heart.[1] The amount of physical activity a person with cardiac problems can tolerate without precipitating symptoms of failure is highly individualized and will be discussed in more detail later in the chapter.

*High altitudes* and *excessive environmental humidity* or *temperature* tax the heart and precipitate failure in an already compromised heart. Lack of oxygen in the air (high altitudes) or increased metabolic needs of the tissues produced by high temperature or increased humidity can activate signs of failure, especially in the presence of anemia or cardiac disruptions.

During the sixth or seventh month of *pregnancy,* when the fetus demands extra blood and there is an expanded fluid volume, pump failure may ensue for the first time in a woman with previously compensated rheumatic valvular disease. Although treatment is required, the heart usually returns to its compensated state following delivery. Careful history taking by the nurse may identify the potential causes of failure and make both the nurse and physician increasingly aware of potential pump failure.

### Pathophysiology

Cardiac output is adjusted by the heart according to body needs; for example, in exercise and stress the output is appropriately increased. However, when the heart is under continuous stress, certain *compensatory mechanisms* are put into play to maintain output consistent with body demands. These compensatory mechanisms include *dilatation* and/or *hypertrophy* of the heart and *autonomic nervous system activation.* These responses are the body's way of reacting to and coping with external and internal stressors. All are designed to augment cardiac output at a level that satisfies body requirements and maintains a desired healthy state.

Both hypertrophy and dilatation increase the size of the heart and improve function, thus enhancing stroke volume. The interactive mechanisms of dilatation and hypertrophy are not totally clear, although some researchers feel that chronic dilatation precedes hypertrophy. When these mechanisms are operating and there is an absence of overt failure, the heart is said to be *compensated.* However, when these mechanisms fail and the patient manifests symptoms of failure, the heart is said to have *decompensated.*

**Dilatation**　As pressure within the heart chambers increases, dilatation occurs. *Dilatation* is an enlargement of the chamber(s) of the heart. The left ventricle is the most common chamber in which this process initially occurs. The dilatating process within the cardiac chambers causes the muscle fibers of the heart to stretch, thus increasing their force of contraction. According to Starling's law (see Chap. 22), this dilating process increases stroke volume and cardiac output. Dilatation can maintain adequate pumping activity with no overt signs of pump failure. However, given the same stressors over a prolonged period of time, the additional muscle fibers reduce their contractile tension and eventually fail in their ability to provide adequate cardiac output.

In addition to the above response, it should be noted that within the dilatated myocardium there is a higher wall tension than normal. This increases the energy requirement for contraction and consumes more oxygen. Both of these processes become self-defeating mechanisms for continued circulatory maintenance. The process of dilatation is therefore an attempt by the heart muscle to cope with increasing blood volume. If it fails, the pump begins to decompensate and symptoms of failure appear.

**Hypertrophy**　*Hypertrophy* refers to an increase in the muscle mass and wall thickness of the cardiac chamber under strain; usually the left ventricle is most often affected. Since time is necessary for the heart to produce more muscle tissue, dilatation usually precedes hypertrophy as a response to volume overload. Nevertheless, chamber pressure overloads such as that produced by aortic stenosis or hypertension tend to cause hypertrophy before dilatation. With pressure overloads or long-standing dilatation, there is an increase in cardiac protein synthesis increasing muscle cells (hypertrophy). Initially in hypertrophy, capillary circulation is able to increase in proportion to the new muscle size, thus maintaining oxygenation. The hypertrophied myocardium is usually able to maintain circulation in spite of work loads that are two to three times normal. However, there are upper limits of its adaptive capabilities. As the hypertrophy continues, its additional blood supply does not continue, and the chamber outgrows its supply of oxygen and nutrients, thus producing overt manifestations of heart failure.

**Changes and effects in perception and coordination**　As cardiac output is reduced in proportion to body requirements, the *autonomic nervous system* attempts to augment the amount of blood pumped by the heart. By activation of the sympathetic nervous system, norepinephrine is released in the heart and blood vessels, and epinephrine is released from the adrenal cortex. The release of these catecholamines results in a redistribution of blood flow, an increase in cardiac rate (chronotropic effect), and stronger myocardial contractions (inotropic effect). In most forms of heart failure one will find peripheral vascular vasoconstriction, a decrease in urine output, diaphoresis, and tachycardia, all the result of sympathetic nervous system stimulation.

The sympathetic nervous system when stimulated will affect the sinoatrial (SA) node by speeding the rate of electrical impulse release and increasing the rate the impulse travels through the atrioventricular node. This results in an increased heart rate. Myocardial contractability is also significantly improved by the presence of catecholamines through their ability to increase both the rate and force of contraction. It is important to note that catecholamines, when released, can stimulate production of premature beats.

Stimulation of the autonomic nervous system also provides vital organs of the body, namely the heart and brain, with needed oxygen, through its influence on the redistribution of blood flow. While *vasoconstriction* is occurring in the skin, splanchnic viscera, kidneys, and skeletal muscles, reciprocal dilatation is occurring in the brain and heart. As with the other compensatory mechanisms, the ability of the autonomic nervous system to augment cardiac output eventually fails. Current research indicates that the failure is due to the depletion of norepinephrine stores in the heart secondary to abnormal local synthesis. Although heart failure is characterized by a well-known constellation of symptoms and physical signs, the physiologic and biochemical changes of heart failure prove to be more difficult to characterize or define.

The patients may become extremely anxious during these changes. As the heart rate increases, *tachycardia* will become evident. Anxiety associated with autonomic changes as well as the fears associated with other physical changes of pump failure may intensify the problem. Diaphoresis may also be present.

Skeletomuscular changes are expressed by *fatigue and weakness.* Although fatigue and weakness may have multiple causes, early fatigue of exercising muscles is perhaps the most common symptom of an inadequate cardiac output. Patients will find activities such as walking tiring, and their gait may be unsteady and lack coordination.

*Deviations* from the individual's *normal behavior* may occur as a result of diminished cerebral circulation. Decreased cerebral circulation can lead to mental cloudiness and confusion and diminished attention span.

**Changes and effects in fluids and electrolytes** The mechanisms by which the patient in pump failure *retains sodium and water* are complex and not totally understood. The inadequacy of cardiac output found in the failing heart has its effect on various organs and tissues of the body, particularly the kidneys. A decrease in cardiac output caused by diminished circulation results in a decrease in renal blood flow and a reduction in the glomerular filtration rate. This prevents the normal amount of sodium from being reabsorbed by the renal tubules. With increased amounts of sodium being retained, water is reabsorbed by osmosis. As heart failure becomes more severe, the decreased cardiac output, diminished glomerular filtration rate, and heightened sympathetic activity cause certain cells of the kidney to release renin. Renin interacts with a component of the blood plasma to activate angiotensin. Angiotensin in turn acts directly on the adrenal cortex, stimulating the release of aldosterone. Sodium is further retained by the action of the aldosterone on the distal renal tubules. The liver is primarily responsible for the destruction of aldosterone in the body; however, with a decrease in cardiac output and elevated venous pressures, there is a decline in hepatic blood flow. This results in congestion and impairment of aldosterone destruction. Research indicates that in addition to the reninaldosterone mechanism, there are other hormonal factors involved which at this time are not completely understood.[2] Most individuals experiencing dyspnea have elevated pulmonary capillary and venous pressure and engorged pulmonary vessels with interstitial pulmonary edema. The fluid in the interstitial spaces replaces the volume of air normally found and triggers the Hering-Breuer reflex, causing shallow and rapid respirations.

With elevated pulmonary venous and capillary pressures, fluid is found initially in the interstitial spaces of the lungs and eventually in the alveoli, both of which inhibit gaseous exchange. This fluid serves as an irritant, and the lungs attempt to rid themselves of excess secretions by initiating the *cough* mechanism.

Increased systemic venous pressure and the retention of sodium and water foster the development of edema in the dependent portions of the body. In advanced pump failure *ascites* and *ana-scara* may be present. Ascites is another form of edema localizing itself in the abdomen. Fluid canals collect in the pericardial and pleural cavities. Anasarca is a generalized edema of almost the entire body and is the ultimate form of edema. It is a late sign of right-sided heart failure. Due to the feeling of fullness in advanced edema, *anorexia, nausea,* and *vomiting* may occur. Decreased urinary output is influenced by vasoconstriction and intensifies the problems caused by edema.

**Changes and effects in oxygenation** The exact *biochemical defect* which results in the myocardium becoming weak and unable to contract properly is not entirely understood. Animal studies have shown that the intrinsic contractile state of the myocardium and its individual fibers is greatly depressed when heart failure is present. The three levels at which this depression might take place have been suggested and are discussed below.

*Cardiac muscle contraction* depends on conversion of chemical energy to mechanical energy. Within the units that make up individual muscle fibers (sarcomeres), two protein strands or filaments, actin and myosin, interreact chemically, causing the strands to slide over each other, thereby shortening the length of the muscle fiber (cardiac contraction). Initially, it was felt that the compensatory mechanisms of hypertrophy and/or dilatation caused overstretching of the actin and myosin filaments and possibly their disengagements prevented the substances from fully acting in the chemical process necessary for contraction. This has recently been proved incorrect.[3-5]

The *chemical energy* needed to generate mechanical energy of actin and myosin is supplied normally by the oxidation of free fatty acids and glucose in the mitochondria of the myocardial cells. This oxidation causes the release of ATP containing a high-energy phosphate bond which is broken by the enzyme ATPase in myosin. The cleavage of this bond provides the energy for the actin filaments to slide over the myosin strands causing contraction of the muscle fiber. The amount of ATP consumption is directly dependent upon the amount of tension of physical work produced by the myocardial fiber. When pump failure is present, defects in this energy metabolism may occur, altering the amount of ATP produced and interfering further with muscle contraction.

*Calcium* has long been known to be an important contributor to myocardial contraction, since its presence is necessary for ATP utilization in the contractile process. It is released from areas near the protein strands by the electrical stimuli (depolarization) traveling through the conduction system. This process is called *excitation-contraction coupling,* although the exact mechanism is unknown. Current research in this area indicates that a defect in excitation-contraction coupling contributes to the decompensation of the biochemical machinery within the myocardial cells during heart failure.[6,7]

It has been found that manifestations of pump failure can be related to both low- and high-output failure. *Low-output failure* is the more common occurrence and is characterized by a decrease in cardiac output. This problem is associated with such disruptions as valvular stenosis, myocardial infarction, and hypertension.

*High-output failure* on the other hand, develops when cardiac output is normal or increased but not adequate to meet the metabolic and oxygen demands of the body. This problem is often seen in thyrotoxicosis, anemia, beriberi, and pregnancy. Whether cardiac output is high or low, the amount of blood pumped into circulation is not sufficient, and the oxygen needs of the vital organs cannot be sustained.

As the cardiac output of the failing heart diminishes, the left ventricle develops both a volume and pressure overload. The *volume overload* occurs because the left ventricle is unable to empty its contents completely during systole. The blood that remains in the ventricle during diastole causes an increase in the pressure, or pressure overload. As the *end diastolic pressure* continues to increase, the left atria must work harder to pump blood into the ventricle. Consequently, the left atrial pressure increases, and this increased pressure is transmitted back to the pulmonary veins and the capillaries of the lungs. When the hydrostatic pressure in the capillaries of the lungs exceeds their colloid osmotic pressure, then fluid seeps out of the capillaries into the interstitial spaces of the lungs.[8]

Thus through pulmonary venous hypertension, respiratory symptoms consistent with *left-sided failure* occur. If the increases in pulmonary venous pressure persist and/or increase further, the fluid in the interstitial spaces will spill into the alveoli, bronchi, and bronchioles, reducing lung vital capacity. This results in *pulmonary edema,* which, if untreated, can lead to death.

Left ventricle failure when not properly or adequately treated may lead to right-sided failure, producing symptoms of venous congestion. The most common cause of right-sided pump failure is left-sided pump failure. However, certain conditions such as cor pulmonale and valvular pulmonic stenosis can cause the right side of the heart to fail initially. (See the discussion in Chapter 27.)

As pulmonary vascular pressure increases, it places an added stress upon the right ventricle as it attempts to pump blood against an already congested pulmonary artery and lungs. As a result backup pressure increases in the right atria, superior vena cava, and the venous system. When this occurs, symptoms consistent with venous congestion or *right-sided failure* result. Although right- and left-sided failure may occur separately, the left side, being the major pump and subjected to the most strain, usually fails first.

*Dyspnea on exertion* is one of the first symptoms manifested by an individual with left-sided failure and is usually accompanied by rapid, shallow breathing. It is a subjective feeling of difficult breathing and is dependent upon the individual's age, conditioning, size, etc., and varies widely. The physiologic changes that occur in the lungs lead to a loss in lung compliance elasticity.

In order to move the "stiff" lungs, the respiratory muscles must work harder and thus consume more oxygen. The failing heart is not able to supply the needed oxygen, and respiratory muscles become fatigued, which may also contribute to the sensation of dyspnea.

As dyspnea progresses, *orthopnea* may result.[9] This term is applied to a condition characterized by dyspnea at rest, soon after the individual assumes a supine position. However, assumption of a semi- or high Fowler's position relieves the breathlessness. The upright position reduces the capillary and venous pressures and allows the diaphragm and abdominal organs to drop. The lungs' vital capacity is increased, allowing more space for the exchange of oxygen and carbon dioxide.[10]

*Paroxysmal nocturnal dyspnea* (*PND*), sometimes referred to as cardiac asthma, involves severe decompensation of the left ventricle.[11] The individual is aroused from a recumbent position at night with a feeling of suffocation. Gasping for air and frequently sweating profusely, the person must assume an upright position and often will go to an open window and take deep breaths. The mechanisms responsible for PND include the factors that produce orthopnea and depression of both the respiratory centers and myocardial functions associated with the sleeping state. The presence of PND indicates severe decompensation of the left ventricle which could lead to acute pulmonary edema.

A complication of left-sided failure which constitutes an emergency situation is *acute pulmonary edema.* It is the result of a severe and acute decompensation of the left ventricle. The patient presents with manifestations of acute respiratory distress which must be treated immediately. Tachycardia will be present, and arrhythmias can occur owing to increased heart rate and the presence of catecholamines.

As pulmonary edema is associated with left ventricular failure, right-sided pump failure presents with *venous hypertension* and dependent edema. As pressure in the right side of the heart becomes elevated, it may be reflected in the superior vena cava by *jugular vein distention.* Distended neck veins frequently precede the other prominent manifestations of right ventricular failure, namely, dependent edema and hepatomegaly.

Elevation of pressure in the inferior vena cava causes the *liver* to become *congested, enlarged,* and *pulsating.* Jaundice usually does not occur; when it does, it is a late sign.

*Cyanosis* may or may not be observed in individuals with right-sided pump failure. If observed, it is due to the decreased circulation time, causing reduced hemoglobin to be concentrated in the congested veins.

### First-Level Nursing Care

In the United States today, there are several million individuals who have had or who are presently experiencing some degree of pump failure. The populations primarily affected are both males and females over 55 years old. The underlying problem most responsible for pump failure is heart disease. Approximately 50 to 60 percent of individuals who have cardiovascular pathophysiology develop some manifestations of pump failure. The severity and longevity of these manifestations relate directly to the underlying problem and how this underlying problem is being controlled.

As noted from the previous discussion, the causes of pump failure are multiple and can include any disorder which places a continuous strain on the heart's ability to pump and circulate the blood required for normal bodily processes. If the causative factor of pump failure is identified and adequately controlled, manifestations of pump failure will be minimized or eliminated. Therefore, the best means of controlling pump failure is through early detection and treatment of the predisposing factors.

There are several groups of individuals who are at *risk* to develop pump failure. Patients who sustain a myocardial infarction, individuals with elevated cholesterol, rheumatic heart disease, infections, as well as hypertension, alcoholism, and structural heart defects are all at risk to develop pump failure. In addition, individuals who are obese, anemic, or have a vitamin deficiency can develop symptoms of pump failure. For some women, especially those with previous cardiac health problems, pregnancy may cause an added stress which can lead to cardiac decompensation and failure.

**Prevention** Early detection of hypertension, congenital anomalies, valvular disorders, and arteriosclerosis as well as atherosclerotic disturbances can ensure the patient early treatment and prevention of complications. Individuals likely to develop upper respiratory infections, especially the elderly and those with chronic obstructive lung problems, should be encouraged to obtain an annual vaccination against the influenza virus. In addition they need to be taught early signs of infection and encouraged to contact their nurse or physician if respiratory or other problems develop.

Individuals having predisposing factors to pump failure should be instructed to avoid high altitudes or unpressurized airplanes. Today, commercial airline cabins are pressurized and do not present a problem in this area. The individual should also be cautioned against environmental changes related to increases in temperature or humidity. If the situation does arise, patients should be instructed to use an air conditioner or dehumidifier to correct potentially harmful environmental stressors.

Various preventive measures which help to eliminate venous stasis and resultant thrombosis are beneficial. Patients should be encouraged not to wear constricting socks, hosiery, or garter belts and not to place extra pressure on their legs by crossing them or holding heavy objects in their laps. Exercise programs should be established for each patient in all settings. Research has shown us that putting a healthy individual to bed for a 24-hour period leads to muscle atrophy; therefore, we nurses must be aware of mobilizing the hospitalized patient as soon as possible.

All individuals should be encouraged to engage in a regular exercise program, avoid exhausting activities, eat well-balanced meals, and maintain a body weight within prescribed limits. Prevention of anemia as well as other vitamin deficiencies (thiamine) can also aid in eliminating signs of failure.

Hospitalized patients requiring administration of intravenous fluids should be carefully assessed during the administration proceedings. Stressful situations which increase anxiety and associated cardiac output need to be avoided. When necessary the nurse should clarify potentially stressful events with the patient and seek appropriate counseling.

### Second-Level Nursing Care
Many individuals in the community have health problems which potentially could lead to pump failure. Ideally, to prevent the onset of pump failure, the underlying cause must be properly identified and controlled. When the problem cannot be controlled, manifestations of pump failure will appear.

**Nursing assessment** Identification of the early onset of cardiac failure may allow therapeutic means to be instituted on an outpatient basis. Careful identification of predisposing factors as well as evaluation of presenting problems will aid in planning appropriate interventions.

**H**ealth History Obtaining a thorough *health history* from the individual will aid in determining the extent of pump failure. With a diminished amount of oxygen being delivered to the musculoskeletal system, the individual frequently complains of being more *tired* than usual. A *slumped posture, slower speech* with less animation, an *altered tone of voice,* and changes in facial expression are other changes noted.

Complaints of *restlessness* and *insomnia* are common; in fact, insomnia and restlessness during the night may be an initial indication of dyspnea. The individual may appear slightly more *confused* or *anxious* and complain of *memory lapses* and a *decreased attention span.* Any subtle behavior change appearing in an individual who is a likely candidate to develop cardiac decompensation should be assessed further.

If an individual complains of dyspnea, it is important to find out what activity (or activities) produce(s) dyspnea, when the symptom began, and when was the last time the individual was able to perform the specific physical task without difficulty. Sudden change in one's ability to tolerate routine activities may be an indication of the severity of the failure. When simple activities are accompanied by shortness of breath, *dyspnea* on exertion then becomes the problem.

Dyspnea following a normally routine activity can be a frightening experience for any individual. Unfortunately, this initial phase of left-sided pump failure may go undetected. Careful history taking by the nurse and/or physician is essential since the optimum time to treat patients with beginning left-sided heart failure is when they first experience mild dyspnea.

An increase in *cough* frequency with expectoration may also be an early indication of left ventricular decompensation. The cough of pump failure may initially occur only with effort or emotional stress, while later it may occur at night and interfere with sleep. The nurse should observe the patient and inquire about the persistence of a cough, the frequency, and the precipitating factor(s), and obtain a description of the amount, color, and consistency of expectoration.

*Orthopneic* individuals avoid attacks of breathlessness by sleeping with their head and thorax elevated on several pillows. As the problem becomes progressively worse, individuals may need to sit in a chair at night. The nurse, in obtaining data to substantiate the existence and severity of orthopnea, must carefully question the individual. When asking how many pillows are used for sleep, the patient may respond one, which is considered normal. However, upon further questioning, it may be discovered that the individual folds the one pillow in half in order to raise the head and thorax to diminish the feeling of dypnea and finds it necessary to sleep in front of an open window. Once manifestations of orthopnea appear, moderate to severe pump failure exists and prompt treatment is required.

The development of *paroxysmal nocturnal dyspnea (PND)* may constitute another reason an individual first seeks medical attention, as the breathlessness experienced while in the supine position is a terrifying experience. It may be necessary for the nurse to pursue the frequency of these attacks, identify how they were relieved, and learn whether they were triggered by other factors. PND usually subsides when the patient assumes an upright position but can reoccur several times during the night. The development of a PND attack can be caused by other factors such as coughing, an increase in heart rate associated with nightmares, or digestion of a heavy meal, all of which can further increase the pulmonary venous and capillary pressures.

*Dependent edema,* when mild, is difficult to detect. However, prior to overt swelling, the individual may recall pitting depressions on the feet or legs as a result of extra fluid volume and or constrictive clothing. These changes should be explored with the patient and documented.

**P**hysical Assessment   The effects of early pump failure are often most evident during an examination of the chest and thorax. The sound of *rales* can be heard at the base of the lungs when fluid accumulates in the alveoli.[12] As more alveoli become edematous, these sounds will be heard higher up in the lungs. The crackling of rales signifies early left-sided failure and resembles the sound produced when a lock of hair is rubbed between two fingers. Rales are heard on inspiration and may be auscultated at both bases (bilateral), in one base (unilateral), or heard widely over the entire lung field. Frequently, rales are accompanied by an expiratory wheeze which results from edema of the airways with subsequent narrowing of the lumen. Upon palpation there may be some dullness at the base of the lungs; the extent will depend upon the amount of fluid present.

Early pump failure may also be evidenced by fluid accumulations. This may be a gradual process, and the extremities should be carefully inspected for evidence of edema. Pedal edema may be noted when the feet are dependent for prolonged periods. It is unlikely that fluid accumulation and liver congestion will be noted during the abdominal examination in early pump failure.

In addition to peripheral edema, the extremities may feel cool to touch. The peripheral pulses may be diminished and somewhat difficult to palpate.

The individual with pump failure not only has a faster resting heart rate, but with exercise has an excessive increase in rate and a delayed return to the resting-level pulse. Assessment of this factor is mandatory, especially when the rate becomes so excessive it is self-defeating.

The appearance of a *third heart sound* may herald the onset of left ventricular failure. Upon auscultation of the heart, a triple rhythm produces a sound similar to that of a horse galloping and is therefore called *gallop rhythm.* This rhythm has also been referred to as the "Kentucky rhythm" because it sounds like the audible third sound heard upon rapid repetition of the word *Kentucky.*

**D**iagnostic Tests   Pump failure is primarily diagnosed through the symptoms the individual presents and knowledge of the underlying cause. Although there is no one diagnostic test that will completely confirm the presence of pump failure, certain tests may be done on an ambulatory basis to assist in the diagnosis.

These tests should include a routine *chest x-ray,* which will indicate the presence of fluid in the lungs and cardiac enlargement. In addition, a 12-lead *EKG* should be done; in the presence of failure it will indicate abnormal axis deviation and enlargement of the QRS complex with ventricular hypertrophy. *Vital lung capacity* (discussed in Chap. 30) will be decreased in the presence of failure.

The initial assessment of cardiac output may also include the *circulation time* test. In this arm-to-tongue test, a rapid injection of sodium dehydro-cholate (Decholin sodium) is injected into the peripheral vein in the arm. The time required from the initial injection until the patient experiences a bitter taste in the mouth is measured with a stop-watch. The time normally ranges from 9 to 16 seconds. In pump failure the circulation time is usually prolonged. As with the injection of any substance, the nurse should be aware of a possible allergic response to the drug and be prepared to intervene, should this problem occur. The physician may choose to give a test dose in order to prevent an adverse reaction.

**Nursing problems and interventions**   An individual with early pump failure usually manifests several major problems. These include *dyspnea,* at times associated with exertion, *fatigue, tachycardia, anxiety, orthopnea,* and *mild edema.*

There are three main goals of care which the nurse needs to consider. These are: (1) improvement of tissue and organ oxygenation, (2) reduction of the volume of venous blood returning to the heart, and (3) increase in the strength of myocardial contractability. Early intervention in mild failure and careful patient education can help reduce the incidence of more acute problems.

**A**ctivity   A balance between *physical and mental rest* and *activity* functions to reduce the body's requirement for oxygen and thus improves tissue and organ oxygenation. With improved tissue and organ oxygenation, the kidneys will increase output, the heart rate will decline, decreasing cardiac work load, respiratory muscle functioning will improve, and dyspnea will diminish. In mild congestive failure, rest or a decrease in normal activity may be all that is needed to alleviate the symptoms. The *health history* obtained from the individual assists the nurse in planning appropriate types of activities.

Physical rest is not without complications. Prolonged rest at home can lead to the complications of immobilization. Slowed circulation accompanied by dependent edema makes the individual particularly prone to the formation of thrombi with resultant pulmonary emboli. The family and patient should be taught how to avoid these complications. Therefore, passive range of motion exercises should be taught while the patient is in bed or sitting in a chair. Constricting clothing such as garter belts,

tight stockings or pantsuits, or tight shoes should be avoided. Teaching plans should indicate that any constriction will impede venous return and enhance pedal edema. Use of elastic stockings should be encouraged, thereby reducing the effects of immobility. Frequent *position change* may help to reduce dyspnea.

Mental as well as physical rest is required to reduce the burden of pump failure. If an individual is tense and upset emotionally, the demands of the body are raised due to increased metabolic activity. (Measures associated with energy conservation are discussed under Fourth-Level Nursing Care.)

Anxiety may result from any number of causes: finances, separation from job or family, and fears about death, as well as the physiological changes and resulting difficulty in breathing. The underlying cause of the anxiety needs to be identified by the nurse so that proper supportive measures can be implemented. Involving the family members in the counseling assists in identifying and reducing potential stressors in the home. If the cause of the emotional unrest cannot be identified or dealt with effectively, sedatives or tranquilizers may be needed. Oversedation, however, must be avoided.

**R**estricted Sodium Diet   Individuals with pump failure tend to retain sodium. Although some consumption of sodium is necessary, modification of the dietary intake of sodium is usually mandatory for all patients with pump failure. In mild cases of pump failure, sodium restriction may take the place of diuretic therapy and thus alleviate the potential side effects which accompany the use of diuretic agents.

The amount of sodium an adult consumes on a regular diet is between 3 and 7 g (3000 to 7000 mg) a day. The wide variations in the intake of sodium are attributable to differences in food and the amount of supplementary salt added.

There are three sodium-restricted diets: strict, moderate, and mild. A *strict sodium diet* allows the patient between 250 and 500 mg sodium per day and is generally employed for hospitalized patients or for patients who have not responded adequately to a moderate sodium-restricted diet or to medications. On this diet, absolutely no table salt is used, and all salty foods or products must be avoided. *Moderate sodium restriction* allows a daily intake of 1000 mg sodium and is frequently used as the maintenance diet for the pump failure patient at home. Again, salt should not be used at the table or in the preparation of food. However, the patient is allowed either one-fourth teaspoon of salt a day or a *mea-*

*sured* amount of a food high in sodium. This makes the diet more palatable.

*Mild sodium restriction* is prescribed for individuals in mild failure who require some sodium restriction to alleviate or control sodium retention. The individual is allowed between 2400 and 4500 mg sodium daily, which essentially constitutes a normal diet. Salt may be used lightly in the preparation of foods but is not to be added after cooking.

*Diet teaching* should stress reading the labels of food products to learn the ingredients. This will reduce frustration of a patient on a restricted sodium intake. It is extremely important for the nurse working with a dietitian to assist the patient in learning what brands or food products are high or low in sodium and how much sodium is allowed in the diet. For example, the largest amount of sodium is obtained through the free use of table salt (40 percent sodium by content), preservatives such as sodium benzoate and sodium propinate used by manufacturers in order to maintain freshness and taste of their products, and natural ingredients of the product itself. Anyone on a sodium-restricted diet must be taught how to read labels and what foods are high in sodium. Products that contain the words *salt, sodium* (Na), or *soda* on their label contain sodium and, depending on the degree of the patient's sodium restriction, must be decreased or eliminated. Table 24-2 lists various food products and their sodium content.

Protein foods such as meat, fish, shellfish, cheese, milk, poultry, and eggs tend to be high in sodium. Since protein and vitamins are supplied by

**TABLE 24-2**
EXAMPLES OF FOOD PRODUCTS AND SODIUM CONTENT

| Food Products | Sodium Content, mg, (approximate) |
| --- | --- |
| 1 slice *regular* bread | 200 |
| 1 large olive | 130 |
| 1 oz *processed* cheddar cheese | 420 |
| 1 oz *natural* cheddar cheese | 200 |
| ½ cup sauerkraut | 500 |
| 2 cups *regular* milk | 250 |
| 1 serving cooked cereal with salt added as directed | 500 |
| 1 tsp baking powder | 500 |
| 1 tsp salt | 2300 |
| 1 tsp monosodium glutamate | 750 |
| 1 tsp baking soda | 1000 |

these foods and are essential for body hemeodynamics, they are allowed in *measured* amounts on all the sodium-restricted diets. The strict sodium diet, however, may require that vitamin supplements be ordered. Repeated boiling with intermittent discard of the water will drastically reduce the sodium content in meat, poultry, fish, and shellfish.

Although fruits and vegetables are generally low in sodium, some, such as artichokes, celery, carrots, beets, spinach, kale, mustard greens, sauerkraut, white turnips, and whole hominy, possess a relatively large amount of sodium and should be eliminated from the strict and moderate sodium-restricted diets. They can be used with discretion on the mild sodium diet. The labels of canned vegetables and vegetable juices should be carefully read to be sure they are low in sodium; unfortunately, even if a label states that the product was *prepared* without salt, it does not mean that the product *itself* is low in sodium. Also, if the label states that salt or an ingredient containing sodium has been added, it usually does not indicate the exact amount. The names and quantities of all ingredients *should* be included on all products utilized.

There are other hidden sources of sodium which most people are not aware of. Certain toothpastes are high in sodium; any individual on a sodium-restricted diet, particularly one on a strict low-sodium diet, should avoid their use.

The accumulation of fluid in the dependent areas of the body is usually gradual, and a person can experience a weight gain of as much as 10 lb edematous fluid without it becoming obvious on visual inspection. Patients with signs of mild failure should be taught to weigh themselves daily. Since body weight does not usually fluctuate from day to day, the individual should be instructed to take his or her weight (preferably before breakfast) at the same time every day and with the same amount of clothing. Weight comparisons can then be made and weight gains due to fluid retention can be confirmed before they become physically obvious as dependent edema.

**C**ardiac Glycosides   Digitalis preparations are fundamental drugs employed in the treatment of heart failure, especially when the failure is associated with low cardiac output. They are not, however, as effective in individuals whose heart failure is due to beriberi, AV fistulas, thyrotoxicosis, myocarditis, or certain forms of cardiomyopathies.

Although these drugs were first written about in 1785 by William Withering, the *exact mechanism* of their action is still not completely understood. A digitalis preparation affects the heart in various ways: it *slows* the heart rate (negative chronotropic effect) through its action on the SA node and vagal activity; it slows the impulse conduction through the atrioventricular node (negative dromotropic effect), and it causes reflex dilatation in the peripheral vasculature.

*Drug action* In pump failure the most important action of the cardiac glycosides is to increase the force of myocardial contractability (positive inotropic effect). The drug accomplishes this, it is believed, by allowing more calcium ions to participate in the contractile process. However, digitalis' effect on the normal sodium and potassium exchange and ATPase activity may also play a role on its positive inotropic properties. Increasing the *force* of myocardial contractability increases cardiac output:[13] the left ventricle is able to empty more of its contents. With more complete emptying of the cardiac chambers, the left ventricle and diastolic, arterial, venous, and pulmonary pressures decrease. The heart then is better able to handle the circulating blood volume. As cardiac performance increases, circulation improves, the heart reduces in size, and kidney function improves. As sodium is excreted in larger amounts, there is a reduction of venous pressure and edema improves.

*Types of preparations* There are two categories of dosages for cardiac glycosides (see Table 24-3). These are: (1) the digitalizing or loading doses, and (2) the maintenance dose. The *digitalizing* dose for the patient in pump failure is aimed at administering the drug in divided dosages over a period of hours or days until an "optimum" cardiac effect is reached.[14] This effect is judged by the disappearance of most of the signs of pump failure. Once

this is achieved, the patient is then placed on a daily maintenance dose which is smaller in amount and designed to replace the digitalis lost by excretion while maintaining "optimal" cardiac functioning. The difficulty with all the digitalis preparations is the amount of the drug needed by each patient to reach a desired effect without producing toxic effects. Unfortunately there is a fine line between the therapeutic and toxic doses. This requires that the dosage selection be highly individualized. There is no specific test to determine the correct dosage.[15,16] The fact that digitalis preparations cause cupping or sagging of the ST segment, shortening of the QT segment, and flattening or inversion of the T wave on the 12-lead EKG is not documental proof that either optimum or toxic effects have been reached.

*Nursing responsibility* The nurse must assume a large responsibility in evaluating the effectiveness of the dosage, toxic effects, and predisposing factors to digitalis toxicity and in determining whether to administer or withhold the drug. In order to accomplish these goals, many factors must be evaluated.

The nurse must be aware of the actions and different usages of these cardiac glycosides (see Table 24-3). Deslanoside and ouabain are given either by intravenous (IV), and/or intramuscular (IM) injections and therefore are primarily used in emergency situations where rapid digitalization is required. They are excreted rapidly and their absorption is not reliable, which makes them unsuitable for long-term maintenance use.

*Digoxin,* which can also be administered intravenously for rapid effect, may also be given orally for maintenance dose. This drug is excreted less rapidly than ouabain and deslanoside but more

**TABLE 24-3**
COMMON CARDIAC GLYCOSIDES USED IN PUMP FAILURE

| | Total Digitalizing Dose (usually given in divided dosages over a period of time) | Maintenance Dose (daily) | Onset of Action* | Peak Effect* | Gastro-intestinal Absorption | Means of Elimination |
|---|---|---|---|---|---|---|
| Digoxin | 2.0–3.0 mg po<br>0.75–1.5 mg IV | 0.25–0.75 mg po | 15–30 min | 1–5 hr | 60–85 % | Renal |
| Digitoxin | 1.2–1.6 mg po<br>1.2–1.6 mg IV | 0.05–0.2 mg po | ½–2 hr | 4–12 hr | 90–100 % | Hepatic-renal |
| Deslanoside | 1.2–1.6 mg IV or IM | | 10–30 min | 1–2 hr | Erratic | Renal |
| Ouabain | 0.25–0.5 mg IV | | 5–10 min | ½–2 hr | Erratic | Renal |

* The onset of action and peak effect are based on the initial IV administration of the digitalizing dose.

rapidly than digitoxin. Consequently if digitalis toxicity develops, the toxic manifestations usually are of shorter duration upon discontinuation of drug than with digitoxin. However, if a daily maintenance dose is missed, manifestations of heart failure may be evident.

*Digitoxin* is slowly but almost completely absorbed in the intestinal tract which accounts for the same digitalization and maintenance dose; it is metabolized in the liver and excreted in the kidneys. It is excreted slowly by the kidneys, thus offering the advantage of maintaining a digitalized state for a longer time even though the patient may have skipped a dose. However, if toxicity develops because of its slow excretion and cumulative effects, digitalis toxicity usually lasts much longer than in those patients receiving digoxin.

*Toxicity* The nurse must be aware of the toxic effects produced by the digitalis preparations. In order to detect early signs of digitalis toxicity, the nurse must be aware of, and continually evaluate the presence of, both the extracardiac and cardiac manifestations of toxicity. Early extracardiac symptoms include nausea and vomiting which frequently continue for a day and may be followed by moderate or complete anorexia. Other symptoms of *toxicity* occurring outside the heart include diarrhea, abdominal pain, confusion, drowsiness, and visual disturbances, particularly yellow vision. Elderly patients, who tend to have an increased sensitivity to the drug, usually exhibit vague complaints of general malaise. The nurse should, however, be very suspicious of the possibility of digitalis intoxication and review their health histories accordingly.

Cardiac manifestation in the form of *arrhythmias* are a common indication of digitalis intoxication. Because digitalis is an irritant to the heart muscle itself, it can cause almost any arrhythmia. Frequent premature beats, bigeminy, paroxysmal atrial tachycardia with block, first-degree heart block, or a striking increase or decrease in rate are cause of high concern of digitalis toxicity. (These changes are discussed more fully in Chap. 25.) Although arrhythmias can best be detected through the use of a cardiac monitor or an electrocardiogram, the nurse can often detect rhythm disturbances by taking the apical and radial pulses. It is essential that the nurse check the apical pulse because often beats may be too weak to produce a palpable radial pulse. If the nurse finds that the patient's pulse has suddenly become markedly irregular, the patient may be receiving too much digitalis. Excessive slowing of the pulse (below 60 beats/minute) is also a clinical sign of digitalis overdose. In either case, the nurse should withhold the digitalis preparation and notify the physician immediately. Usually the extracardiac signs of toxicity will disappear after the drug has been stopped. However, if arrhythmias are present, other drug measures may be necessary. Concentrations of cardiac glycosides in the serum can then be determined when digitalis intoxication is suspected.[17]

There are several factors which, when present, will increase the likelihood of digitalis toxicity. Since digitalis preparations are excreted primarily by the kidneys, any problems with renal function may result in a toxic accumulation of digitalis in the body. Although the creatinine clearance test best mimics the kidneys' ability to excrete digitalis, the blood urea nitrogen (BUN) will serve as a rough guide to kidney function. When there is severe renal impairment, digitalis should be given in reduced dosages.

Depletion of potassium sensitizes the myocardium to digitalis and actually enhances its effect. As a result, dosages of digitalis which may in ordinary situations be nontoxic can induce toxicity in the presence of low serum potassium levels (hypokalemia). The increased incidence of arrhythmias in individuals receiving digitalis is frequently related to the widespread use of potassium-depleting diuretics and other factors such as vomiting, diarrhea, and corticosteroid therapy which allow too much potassium to be lost from the body. Patients with pump failure, receiving digitalis and diuretic preparations together, are often given potassium supplements either in the form of a medication or an increase in potassium-rich food. Hypokalemia is discussed more fully in Chap. 12.

Since digitalis appears to act on the heart by increasing the amount of calcium in the contractile process, the administration of IV calcium presents a danger of precipitating digitalis arrhythmias, particularly ventricular arrhythmias. In order to prevent complications from arising in individuals receiving digitalis preparations, the nurse must have a thorough understanding of all aspects of the therapy. Since many patients will be required to take these preparations daily for years, patient teaching is mandatory.

*Patient teaching* The patient as well as the family should possess an understanding of the necessity of digitalis medication, its action, and its adverse effects. Writing the information down and planning with the patient the best time to take the medication are helpful in assuring patient compliance. Caution to the individual, especially the elderly, not to double the dose of the digitalis preparation when a dose is forgotten will decrease the incidence of toxic effects.

When possible, patients and their families should be taught to check their pulse rates so that changes can be detected and toxicity reduced. It is important that this teaching component be discussed and agreed upon with the physician on an individual basis. It may be advisable to avoid the learning experience for some patients as it could be an overwhelming or a threatening issue.

As the teaching plan is developed, patients need to be informed about the action of digitalis as well as its side effects. Patients should be instructed to notify the nurse or physician concerning untoward side effects. They should be instructed to seek medical attention when they experience persistent anorexia, nausea, vomiting, diarrhea; alterations in vision such as seeing rainbows or yellow hazes around bright lights; chest pain; shortness of breath; swelling of the hands or ankles; progressive weight gain, dizziness or fainting; or any change in heart rate or rhythm. A general guideline is that if the pulse falls below 60 beats/minute, the

digitalis preparation should be withheld until notification of the physician. However, in some cases the physician may want the individual to take the medication with a pulse below 60 beats/minute.

Communication between the health team and patient is vital. Follow-up examinations need to be stressed. In this way the effectiveness of the treatment can be more fully evaluated.

**D**iuretic Agents   In the treatment of pump failure diuretic agents are often employed. Their use is usually dependent upon the degree of respiratory problems and/or dependent edema. Diuretics can, however, be considered one of the mainstays in therapy for pump failure.

There are basically five categories of diuretics; they can be administered either singly or in combination to patients in pump failure. These are the thiazides, organomercurials, carbonic anhydrase inhibitors, aldosterone antagonists, and the so-called "potent diuretics." Because of its specific action, method of administration, and rapidity of action, a particular diuretic may be chosen during an acute episode of pulmonary edema.

Table 24-4 lists the specific diuretics and their potential use in pump failure. Chapter 28 offers the

**TABLE 24-4**
DIURETICS USED IN PUMP FAILURE

| Drug Classification | When Used | Dose | Toxicity |
|---|---|---|---|
| Thiazide diuretics | Used in treatment of moderate edema due to pump failure. | 0.5–2 g po daily | Loss of Na, hypokalemia, blurring of vision, dryness of mouth |
| Organomercurials (Mercuhydrin) | Used less frequently, in hospital settings for more rapid diuresis or in combination with other diuretics. | 1–2 ml IM or sq Daily or as ordered | Gastric symptoms, irritating to kidney tubules; can cause mercury sensitivity, dizziness, nausea, rash, ventricular arrhythmias |
| Carbonic anhydrase inhibitors (Diamox) | Limited use in pump failure; relatively ineffective diuretic, can cause systemic acidosis. | 250–375 mg q.d. po | Inefficient diuretics; can cause systemic acidosis, nausea, and vomiting |
| Aldosterone antagonists | Protein-sparing, potassium-sparing diuretic used in mild failure, not a potent diuretic, blocks action of aldosterone. | Up to 3 g daily | Hepatic and renal damage, skin rash, tinnitus, dry mouth, drowsiness |
| "Potent" diuretics Furosemide (Lasix) | Edecrin and Lasix are "potent" diuretics used in acute failure and pulmonary edema. Because of their rapid effect, electrolyte imbalance can be a problem. | Average dose 40–200 mg q.d. or q.o.d. | Disturbances in electrolyte balance, e.g., hypokalemia, leads to weakness, G.I. complaints, muscle weakness, and paralysis, also hyponatremia, gastric disturbances, and diarrhea (see Chap. 12) |
| Ethacrynic acid (Edecrin) | | 25–200 mg po daily | |
| Sodium ethacrynate | — | 0.5–1 mg/kg body weight IV | |

SOURCE: M. Rodman and D. Smith: *Pharmacology and Drug Therapy in Nursing,* Lippincott, Philadelphia, 1968, pp. 299–304.

reader a complete discussion of diuretic interventions and selected usages. Whatever the diuretic of choice, the nurse must closely observe the patient for signs of electrolyte imbalance, especially if the patient is receiving a digitalis preparation. Because of the high rate of proximal tubular sodium removal (hence low distal tubular sodium delivery), maximum potassium excretion may approach ceiling levels. Since the body cannot store excess potassium, extracellular potassium may rise and increase cardiac toxicity.[18]

*Patient teaching* Patients receiving diuretics should evaluate their weight loss on a daily basis. Therefore the patient should be taught to check body weight at the same time each day, wearing the same amount of clothing, and to keep an accurate daily record. The physician should be notified if there is a gain of 2 lb in one day or a slow, persistent weight gain. The patient with dependent edema should know the essentials of good skin care since edematous areas are more easily subject to breakdown.

If the patient is taking diuretics, the toxic effects of the diuretic should be taught (see Table 24-4). If symptoms are experienced, the physician or nurse should be notified. When a potassium supplement is not being used the patient must be encouraged to eat foods high in potassium. The nurse should assist the patient in planning a proper diet so that it includes foods high in potassium such as *juices,* including orange, grapefruit, and pineapple; *fruits* such as oranges, bananas, strawberries, watermelon, and raisins; *vegetables* such as tomatoes, corn, spinach, and lima beans; and *meats* including beef chuck, turkey, and chicken.

The teaching plan should place emphasis on routine follow-up care. A 12-lead EKG and serum electrolyte levels should be checked often. The patient should be cautioned about related problems which may indicate that failure is persisting and should be encouraged to contact the nurse or physician if these changes occur.

### Third-Level Nursing Care

Many individuals with pump failure are able to remain in the community and carry on their activities of daily living with varying degrees of modification. The reasons for hospitalizing an individual with pump failure are diverse. The problems associated with pump failure may have become more severe or advanced and require supervised administration of digitalis and diuretic preparations, as well as other measures to reduce the edema and improve myo-

cardial performance. In addition, individuals currently on the maintenance program of rest, restricted sodium diet, and medications may not be adhering to the plan of care, leading to manifestations of overt pump failure. Also, the underlying cause of the failure may have increased in severity, aggravating the cardiac status. Subsequently hospitalization is required to stabilize and reassess the patient.

**Nursing assessment** When the patient is admitted to the hospital, a careful health history and physical assessment are essential. In the presence of severe failure the nurse may have to rely upon the family or a close friend for an adequate evaluation of the problem.

**H**ealth History  If the failure has progressed and previous treatment has been ineffective, or if precipitating causes have induced the onset of failure, the *health history* will reveal *dyspnea* as a critical problem. This disturbance will often be aggravated by any physical activity. In severe failure the patient may report that even the most routine activity produces shortness of breath. *Decrease in urine output,* and in some instances *oliguria* may be present. In the presence of this problem it is important to identify any medications the patient may have been receiving, including diuretics and digitalis preparations.

Generally, the patient in severe failure is *weak* and exhausted by the respiratory distress. *Ascites* is evident in advanced failure (right side). The patient may complain of severe discomfort when tightening a belt or girdle. Massive ascites can elevate the diaphragm in the supine position, thus aggravating dyspnea and orthopnea. In the presence of *edematous fluid* and congestion of the bowel, the patient may give a history of experiencing *anorexia, nausea,* and *vomiting.* This may also be associated with the use of digitalis preparations. Patients in severe failure may look somewhat *cachexic* due to *malnutrition* of tissue and decreased oxygen.

A decrease in oxygen to the brain may also lead to *cerebral anoxia.* This problem can be manifested by *mental confusion, irritability,* and *reduced attention span.* In the elderly, this problem can become acute, interfering with patient care. Increased *anxiety,* intensified by the inability to breathe, can increase the patient's dyspnea and compound the existing problems.

**P**hysical Assessment  As pump failure becomes more severe, there is an increase in the amount of fluids accumulating in the body. Dependent edema is usually observed in the lower extremities and may be pitting at times.

The extremities should be carefully inspected and palpated to evaluate the degree of edema. The extent of involvement should also be noted. With severe failure, visible moisture may be noted over the edematous area. The edema is said to be "weeping." As failure progresses, a more *generalized edema* is found. In addition, there is a noted *increase in body weight* while the patient may appear malnourished. Ideally, the patient should be weighed and the results compared with a previous weight record.

Elevation of pressure in the inferior vena cava causes the liver to become congested, enlarged, and pulsating. During the abdominal examination percussion and palpation of the liver will reveal hepatomegaly and tenderness. During palpation it is often tender. If right-sided failure is severe, the patient may complain of pain in the right upper quadrant and be reluctant to change positions rapidly. *Ascites* will also be evident during the abdominal examination. Testing for shifting dullness and fluid wave and the puddle examination will help to confirm its presence. *Jaundice* usually does not occur—when it does, it is usually a late sign. (Refer to Chap. 19 for assessment of liver function.)

An increase in pressure on the right side of the heart causes the *jugular veins of the neck to enlarge.* Under normal conditions these veins become flat when the individual assumes an erect position. However, if the veins remain full or distended, perhaps pulsating with each ventricular contraction when the person's head is raised to a 45° angle, right-sided failure can be suspected.

*Cyanosis* may or may not be observed in individuals with heart failure. If observed, it is due to a decrease in circulation causing reduced hemoglobin to be concentrated in the congested veins. The nurse, when assessing for the presence of cyanosis, should do so in bright daylight and observe the color of fingernail beds, mucous membranes and mouth and lips, and earlobes for a bluish color. Tissue perfusion can also be evaluated by observing the *capillary refill time.* A fingernail should be pressed and released. Patients with pump failure will show a slower return of color to the nailbed.

*Cheyne-Stokes respiration* is not consistently found in pump failure, but it may be manifested in some individuals with several heart failures or who have compromised cerebral circulation such as seen in cerebral atherosclerosis. This symptom

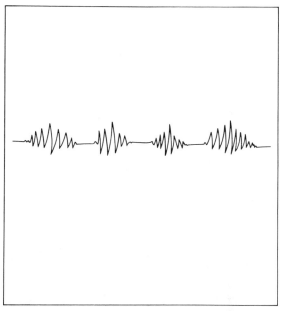

**FIGURE 24-1**
Periodic breathing. The respiratory cycle is characterized by alternating periods of rapid breathing with increased depth becoming increasingly shallow until breathing stops completely.

tends to be seen more frequently in elderly people with left ventricular failure, especially those taking any barbiturate drug. Cheyne-Stokes respiration is characterized by periods of hypoventilation, hyperventilization, and apnea. It is thought to relate to the prolonged circulation time seen with heart failure between the lungs and brain which affects the arterial blood gases function on the respiratory center. There is a fall in arterial $pO_2$ with a subsequent rise in $pCO_2$. The increase in $pCO_2$ (hypercapnia) stimulates hyperventilation in the respiratory center in an attempt to rid the body of excess $CO_2$. Hyperventilation will continue to a peak and then decrease to an apneic state. In assessing the patient, the nurse will notice periods of rapid breathing followed by apnea (so-called "periodic breathing"; see Fig. 24-1).

During the chest auscultation, *fine rales* (crackling) occurring late in inspiration are present. They are often most obvious when the patient is asked to take a deep breath. *Coarse rales* are also audible. These are louder, bubbling sounds produced by air as it passes through fluid. They are heard early in the inspiratory phase of respiration. These sounds tend to originate in the trachea and bronchi.

Upon inspection of the chest, the nurse may observe alternating periods of rapid breathing, followed by slowed respirations and even periods of *apnea.* Palpation of the thoracic wall will reveal alterations in chest expansion depending on the degree of fluid accumulation; rate and depth of respiration, vocal resonance and palpable vibrations heard on the chest wall when the patient speaks will diminish. Asking the patient to repeat words or sounds like "ninety-nine," or "e-e-e" will often indicate diminished clarity of tone. This will depend upon the amount of fluid the vocal vibrations have to pass through before reaching the thoracic wall.

Percussion of lung bases will usually indicate decreased intensity and pitch in the presence of failure. The duration of a sound will be short, and in the presence of excess fluid the base as well as upper lung areas will be dull.

Blood pressure can be altered, especially in the presence of acute failure. Decreased blood pressure will be indicative of shock. Peripheral pulses may be difficult to palpate, and the apical pulse rate will be rapid.

**Diagnostic Tests** In an assessment of the patient's health status, diagnostic tests are performed to confirm specific problems. In the presence of failure, blood electrolytes are altered and circulation time prolonged. When there is decreased kidney function and oliguria, blood urea nitrogen is elevated. Arterial blood gas readings are abnormal due to hypoxemia, increase in pulmonary fluid, increased pulmonary pressure, and limited lung mobility. EKG readings may indicate tachycardia, ventricular hypertrophy, and arrhythmias including the presence of premature ventricular beats.

**Nursing problems and interventions** The major problems confronting the hospitalized patients in severe failure are many. They include dyspnea, fatigue, fluid retention, and tachycardia with decreased oxygenation.

**Dyspnea** Dyspnea continues to be a significant problem for the patient. Oxygen via nose or mask is used to promote physical comfort and alleviate the dyspnea. Mask oxygen may be discouraged with severe dyspnea as it may be occlusive to the patient and compound anxiety. Positioning the patient in a semi- or high Fowler's position will provide expansion of the chest and improve cardiac output and respiratory rate. Overexertion should be avoided and rest encouraged, particularly during the presence of acute symptoms.

**Fatigue** Physical and emotional rest should be maintained and encouraged. Mild tranquilizers may be prescribed in the presence of severe anxiety, although in the presence of mental confusion this is discouraged. When necessary counseling or social service referral may help the patient.

Selected activities can be planned for the patient on a daily basis. Rest periods should be incorporated into the care plan. Physical care can be arranged so as to limit additional stress. Visitors should be restricted so that the patient can have adequate rest. Family teaching concerning this will help gain their cooperation.

While rest is important, the hazards of immobility continue to be a potential problem. Passive range of motion exercises should continue daily. Frequent change of position will also prevent peripheral pooling. Elastic stockings should be used, and constrictive clothing avoided.

**Fluid Retention** Patients in acute failure are usually placed on a low-sodium diet, as discussed in Second-Level Nursing Care. In addition fast-acting diuretics will be used to help remove excess fluid. Patients must be observed carefully for signs of electrolyte imbalance. Frequent checks of blood electrolytes should also be taken. Patients should be weighed daily, at the same time of day whenever possible. The abdominal girth should be measured as well.

For some patients intake of oral fluids may be restricted. Reasons for this intervention must be carefully explained to the patient. Often patients can be taught to record fluid intake and measure output. It is important that the amount of fluid allowed over a 24-hour period be divided according to the patient's need. For example, the patient will usually drink the largest amount of fluids during the day and less at night. Mouth care should be given as needed, and signs of dehydration can be noted early through careful assessment.

As indicated, careful intake and output are critical. In addition, urine specific gravity should be checked to assess the concentration of urine. When intravenous fluids are used, they should be given with caution to prevent volume overload.

**Tachycardia** Digitalis preparations continue to be used to slow the heart rate and improve cardiac contractions. Signs of digitalis toxicity discussed in Second-Level Nursing Care must be observed continuously. When necessary, the drug may have to be terminated.

Blood pressure pulses and respiration should be monitored throughout hospitalization. Significant changes should be reported immediately. Improvement in vital signs may indicate positive response to treatment. When signs of hypovolemia are present, volume expanders may be used (see Chap. 28). When necessary, antiarrhythmic drugs may be given. Careful monitoring of cardiac pulse rate will help detect changes in cardiac rhythm (see Chap. 25).

**P**ulmonary Edema   Pulmonary edema is an emergency situation always requiring immediate treatment in a hospital environment. Acute pulmonary edema may result from severe decompensation of the left ventricle. This occurs most frequently after a massive myocardial infarction but may be seen with any acute exacerbation of the underlying or precipitating causes of failures. Paroxysmal nocturnal dyspnea and Cheyne-Stokes respiration may be the forerunners in its development. Acute pulmonary edema results when the lungs' hydrostatic pressure becomes severely elevated, overriding the capillary colloid osmotic pressure. This causes a large transudation of fluid from the capillaries into the interstitial lung spaces, the alveoli, and bronchioles. Figure 24-2 shows an x-ray of a patient in severe acute pulmonary edema with gross amount of fluids in the pulmonary alveoli. This fluid makes the lung appear opaque on chest x-ray like a solid organ. Figure 24-3 demonstrates changes following successful treatment of acute pulmonary edema. With sudden large increases in the lungs' hydrostatic pressure, alveoli edema and bronchiole congestion will drastically reduce the individual's ability to exchange oxygen and carbon dioxide. The patient may essentially drown in his or her own fluids.

*Nursing assessment*   The *health history* of an individual in acute pulmonary edema is often limited since the severity of the problem usually necessitates prompt intervention. Often a family member will relate specific changes that occurred prior to hospitalization.

During physical assessment clinical manifestations presented include actue respiratory distress due to *hypoxia* and *hypercapnia*. The patient will be extremely *anxious, gasping for air* (marked dyspnea), *coughing and producing pink, frothy sputum,* which is an intraalveolar mixture of fluid, erythrocytes, and air. *Cyanosis* is usually present. The fluid in the lungs produces gurgly, noisy respirations ( *rhonchi*) which frequently are audible without the assistance of a stethoscope. In addition, the individual's heart rate will be rapid and diaphoresis may be profuse due to the activation of the sympathetic nervous system. With *severe shortness of breath,* the individual is struggling for each breath

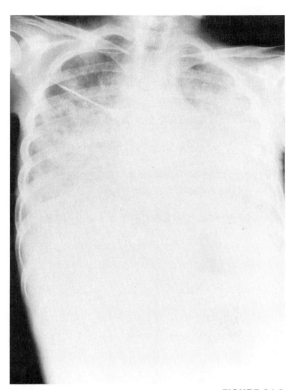

**FIGURE 24-2**
Chest x-ray of patient with acute pulmonary edema.

and *fears death is near.* The severity of the emotional distress further activates the sympathetic nervous system.

**D**iagnostic Tests   Owing to the severity of such a health crisis, a complete diagnostic workup cannot be done; however, a *central venous pressure (cvp)* line may be inserted to assist in the assessment of pump failure. This serves as a guide in determining the circulating blood volume and the rate and amount of fluid the body can tolerate. Since left-sided failures usually occur before right-sided failure and the CVP reflects conditions in the *right* side of the heart, it is not helpful for the early detection of pump failure. *Pulmonary wedge pressure* readings are available for a more accurate assessment of left-sided failure. However this may not be done until the acute phase of pulmonary edema has stabilized. The use of this measurement may be employed when causes of pump failure have not been determined. A complete discussion of CVP and pulmonary wedge pressure can be found in Chap. 28.

*Nursing problems and interventions*   The major problem confronting patients in pulmonary edema

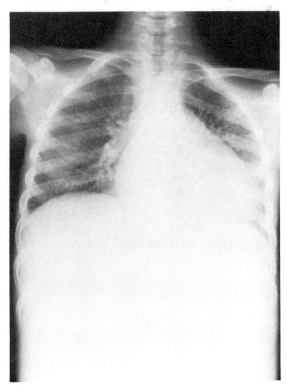

**FIGURE 24-3**
Chest x-ray of same patient following successful treatment of pulmonary edema.

is *dyspnea.* The experience is a most frightening one and tends to increase the patients' *anxiety.* This added stress only serves to complicate the problem. Because of the presence of a large amount of fluid in the lungs, patients feel as if they are drowning in their own secretions. The perception is a most accurate one and requires much support from the nurse in helping to reduce the accompanying anxiety.

Dyspnea is also complicated by the presence of a continuous productive *cough* accompanied by frothy sputum. The experience is an exhausting one for the patient, and complaints of *dizziness, anorexia,* and *weakness* are not uncommon.

Once the nurse has assessed the client's current health status, the individual should be placed in a *high Fowler's position.* This position assists breathing by the gravitational forces which drain the excess fluid from the upper lungs, allowing more alveoli to participate in the needed gas exchange. The treatment of acute pulmonary edema follows the same goals as for less severe pump failure but is intensified and more rapid.

*Oxygen* in high concentrations may initially be used to relieve dyspnea and anxiety. However, before the administration of *high* oxygen concentrations, caution should be exercised to review the health history. If chronic obstructive pulmonary disease is present, high concentrations of oxygen should not be used. The *intermittent positive pressure breathing* (IPPB) machine is also effective in increasing alveolar oxygen concentrations and preventing further capillary exudation of fluid. The increased intrathoracic pressure produced by this machine impedes the venous return from the right side of the heart. *Alcohol* (20 to 50 percent) is sometimes placed in the nebulizer of the IPPB machine along with normal saline or distilled water because of its antifoaming action and its relaxing effects. The patient may find the mask frightening, and careful teaching and support by the nurse may be needed. (Refer to IPPB in Chap. 30.)

An intravenous line is inserted for the *administration of medications.* Aminophylline may be given intravenously or via suppositories to relieve bronchospasm and improve cardiac output. A *urinary catheter* is usually inserted by the nurse so that careful monitoring of intake and output can be made. Hypovolemic or cardiogenic shock may result from acute pulmonary edema or the medications used to treat it, and monitoring of the urinary volume assists in the early detection of these complications. Since arrhythmias may either precipitate or result from acute pulmonary edema, the patient is often placed on a cardiac monitor.

The administration of a *narcotic* by the nurse to reduce the patient's anxiety and restlessness and to help relieve dyspnea is another initial step in the treatment plan. *Morphine sulfate* intravenously is the drug of choice in this instance because it decreases anxiety and slows the patient's rapid respirations and creates some peripheral vasodilatation. This peripheral vasodilatation functions as a medical tourniquet, decreasing the amount of venous blood returning to the heart. However, morphine sulfate has a high incidence of disturbing side effects such as severe depression of respirations, urinary retention, and nausea and vomiting which may prompt some physicians to order meperidine (Demerol) instead. The extreme apprehension of these patients will require much emotional support from the nurse. Both the patient and the family will need careful explanation of all tests and interventions. The patient should never be left alone until the acute phase has subsided.

The reduction of venous return of fluid to the right side of the heart is usually required to reduce the increased lung pressure and pulmonary edema.

The *potent, rapid-acting diuretics* (ethacrynic acid or furosemide) are administered intravenously. These drugs usually cause a profound diuresis within 15 minutes after administration. Intake and output must be carefully calculated to assess the effectiveness of the diuretic and early detection of potential shock. Careful evaluation of fluids and blood electrolytes must continue throughout the acute phase.

The application of *rotating tourniquets* (see Fig. 24-4) also reduces fluid return to the heart by trapping as much as 700 cc blood in the periphery. Tourniquets are generally found in two forms: the blood pressure cuff type utilized[19] by the electric automatic tourniquet machine and the soft rubber tourniquets which requires constant attention by the nurse.

The electric rotating tourniquet machine will automatically inflate and deflate its constricting cuffs at set periods, allowing the nurse more time to attend to other patient needs. Another advantage of the machine is that a more accurate amount of extremity pressure can be applied, which is usually slightly above the individual's own diastolic blood pressure. When rotating tourniquets are used, a certain protocol must be followed by the nurse:

1   Tourniquets must be applied high up on *three* extremities, i.e., near the axilla area of the arms and near the groin area of the legs.

2   The distal pulse must always be palpable since the intent of the tourniquets is to reduce venous return and not obstruct the vital arterial blood flow.

3   The constricting force of the tourniquets on any one extremity must not be applied for more than 45 minutes of occlusion, or ischemia and/or cyanosis of the pressurized limb may result. Consequently the tourniquets should be rotated clockwise every 10 to 15 minutes. While the electric tourniquet machine does this automatically, a diagram showing the location, direction, and times for rotation is necessary when using the soft rubber form to prevent confusion and neglect (see Fig. 24-4).

4   To prevent skin irritation under the tourniquet, a softening adjunct such as a towel may be used. Careful inspection of the area by the nurse is required.

**FIGURE 24-4**
Rotating tourniquets clockwise every 10 to 15 minutes.

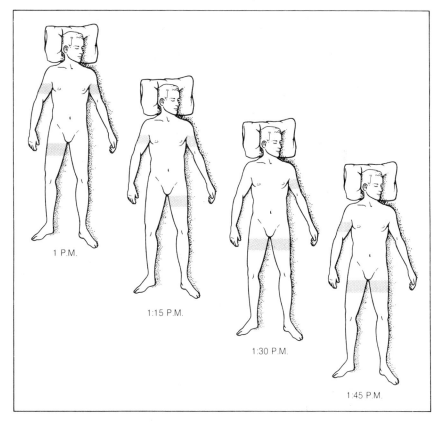

1 P.M.

1:15 P.M.

1:30 P.M.

1:45 P.M.

5 When this therapy is discontinued, the tourniquets must *never* be released all at once. If this is done, the heart is presented with a large volume of blood which could put the individual back into pulmonary edema. Instead, the tourniquets should be removed gradually, one every 15 minutes, allowing the heart time to adjust to the increased venous return.

If the administration of a potent, rapid-acting diuretic and the rotating tourniquets are not sufficient to reduce the venous return, a "wet" phlebotomy may be done. A *phlebotomy, or venesection,* is the actual removal of approximately 500 ml blood from the central circulation. This procedure is contraindicated if severe hypotension is present.

To improve myocardial contractibility or to slow the heart rate, a rapid-acting *digitalis preparation* such as Quabain *may* be administered intravenously. However, with the patient in an upright position the administration of a potent diuretic and a narcotic to depress the overt anxiety generally alleviates the crisis, and digitalis preparations may not be required.

With severe congestion of the bronchioles, *aminophylline,* either intravenously or by suppository, may be used. Aminophylline not only relaxes the bronchioles but also dilatates the coronary arteries and increases the rate of urine formation in the kidneys. Care must be taken by the nurse if this drug is administered intravenously. It must be given slowly for if too rapidly administered, headache, palpitations, dizziness, nausea, and a drop in blood pressure will occur.

Since a patient in acute pulmonary edema has the potential of developing shock, evaluation of vital signs should be processed systematically and continuously. Fluid and electrolyte balance is one parameter which requires continuous reevaluation. The recording of intake and output and the serum electrolyte levels are good indices of fluid and electrolyte balance. Other valuable information of fluid balance can be obtained through the pulmonary wedge pressure and the monitoring of central venous pressure. The monitoring of both vital signs and the heart assists in the evaluation of circulation and oxygenation. Cerebral functioning directly relates to the degree of oxygenation. As oxygenation of the brain falls, behavior changes such as confusion and restlessness are observed.

Once the crisis of acute pulmonary edema has subsided, the individual will usually be placed on a cardiac regimen which may include all or some combination of a digitalis preparation, a diuretic, restricted sodium diet, and rest. Continued nursing assessment of the physical and psychosocial influences must be recorded, and an appropriate plan of care revised to reflect transition from the more acute phase of illness to the rehabilitation process.

**Fourth-Level Nursing Care**
Following an episode of pump failure, the underlying cause and the precipitating factor need to be identified. Whenever possible, the cause for the failure should be corrected immediately and the precipitant removed or controlled as previously discussed; however, some causes of pump failure such as a myocardial infarction and some of the cardiomyopathies may not be able to be adequately controlled or modified. The individual with valvular insufficiency or regurgitation may not be a good candidate for surgery. Consequently, many individuals with the problem of pump failure will be temporarily or permanently placed on some form of the aforementioned therapeutic regimen.

**Patient teaching** Education is essential to help the patients function within their capabilities and to decrease the number of hospitalizations. It has been shown that education of the family or a close friend or colleague will directly influence the patient's acceptance and adaptive capabilities. A team approach is necessary for successful rehabilitation. The nurse, whether working in a hospital, clinic, physician's office, the community, or industry, plays a primary role in coordinating the rehabilitative program and the follow-up assessment and teaching activities. Rehabilitation begins in the hospital and is continued after discharge of the patient. The American Heart Association is most helpful in providing the heart failure patient, as well as the nurse, with information, relevant support services, and teaching materials.

For the rehabilitative program to be successful, the individual must be motivated. A thorough understanding of the current condition, restrictions, and activities to restore and maintain optimal level of functioning are needed. In addition, the patient must be aware of those potential stressors within the environment that can disrupt the healthy state.

Many individuals misinterpret pump failure and often associate it with an actual stoppage of the heart. The nurse should first determine what the patient knows about the condition, then expand teaching to include the normal functioning of the heart, the cause and meaning of pump failure, the symptoms produced, and the treatment employed. Reinforcing and explaining what will be experienced will make it easier for the patient to understand and remember.

The avoidance of physical and mental activities that cause undue fatigue, weakness, dyspnea, and palpitations should be included in the teaching plan. Measures to prevent the recurrence of pump failure and the importance of medical supervision must be stressed.

When a digitalis and/or a diuretic preparation are prescribed, the patient must understand their purpose, untoward effects, and when to notify the physician of complications. A careful teaching plan should be developed to clarify a follow-up health program of diuretics, digitalis preparations, and diet control.

A *sodium-restricted diet* is frequently the most difficult area for patient compliance. Consultation with a dietitian may help the family and the patient cope with diet changes.

A balance between *rest* and *activity* is always included as part of the treatment for pump failure. Bed rest for a few days or weeks is generally required after the failure has been controlled. When bed rest is prolonged, the person is subject to all the complications of immobility. The prevention of these complications should always be included as one of the paramount goals of the nursing care plan.

**Activity** The amount of energy expenditure, whether physical or psychological, must always be correlated with the individual's requirements to lead a meaningful life. It is usually economically and psychologically necessary to keep the patient employed for as long as possible. Many individuals with a mild degree of heart failure may not have to change their activities, others may have to modify them only slightly. Some patients, however, will have to adopt a new daily routine. For example, a homemaker may have to hire domestic help and/or reorganize the housework activities; a business person may have to decrease work hours and have someone else drive him or her to and from the office. In some cases, failure may be so severe that any normal activity results in symptoms, and the individual must be confined to bed to remain symptomless. Consequently, the amount of activity a person can safely engage in is highly individualized, but all individuals must plan for rest periods during the day. Physical rest is easier to accomplish than mental relaxation, and a mild sedative may be required.

Guidelines prescribing activity levels for individuals with heart failure have been developed by the New York Heart Association. These guidelines classify the individual into one of four groups depending upon the way physical activity is tolerated. (See Table 24-5.) Assignment into various classifications is usually made by evaluation of the patient's history and by observation. Scientific information is now available that delineates the approximate amount of energy required to perform various job and recreational activities. The cost to the patient in performing the specific activity is estimated in terms of a unit known as a *metabolic equivalent* (MET).

A MET is based on the amount of oxygen consumed for kilogram of body weight per minute. For example, approximately 3.5 ml oxygen per kilogram of body weight per minute is required for 1 MET. An individual at *rest* expends approximately 1 MET. The approximate number of METs an individual can tolerate without producing signs of pump failure is correlated with the New York Heart Association's classifications. Examples of activities according to their MET expenditures are included in Table 24-6.

Although the physician can usually employ the "commonsense" approach in prescribing activity levels for individuals with heart failure, some individuals need more standardized tests and/or sophisticated methods of tolerance testing before a more accurate, safe activity level can be determined. Standardized tests have been developed which require an individual to perform a specific amount of exercise followed by an evaluation of the response to it. A common example is *Master's two-step exer-*

**TABLE 24-5**
NEW YORK HEART ASSOCIATIONS' FUNCTIONAL CLASSIFICATIONS AND APPROXIMATE METABOLIC COST OF ACTIVITIES FOR A 70-KG PERSON

| Functional Classification | Metabolic Cost, METs |
| --- | --- |
| **CLASS 1**<br>No limitation of physical activity. Ordinary physical activity does not result in symptoms. | 7 |
| **CLASS 2**<br>Slight limitation of physical activity. No symptoms at rest *but* symptoms *may be* produced with ordinary activity. | 5–6 |
| **CLASS 3**<br>More severe limitations. Usually comfortable at rest; symptoms manifested with many less than ordinary physical activities. | 3–4 |
| **CLASS 4**<br>Inability to carry on any physical activity without producing symtpoms, and symptoms may be present at rest. | 1–2 |

*cise test* (discussed in Chap. 26). Sophisticated methods utilizing a treadmill or an ergometer (a device which measures oxygen consumption) may be employed for a more precise appraisal of the person's response to various exercise loads.

Actually assessing an individual in a trial work situation can be most helpful in determining how well a specific activity can be tolerated. Since physical exertion is only one parameter of an individual's ability to perform a certain task comfortably, a trial work period affords an opportunity to observe how other factors such as temperature, humidity, exposure to toxins, coordination and rate of work, and anxiety affect the person's ability to work. Vocational counseling may be necessary if occupational change is required.

Evaluation of the home setting by the nurse is necessary for the patient with activity restrictions. Questions relating to the location of the bedroom and bathroom, the arrangement of the kitchen, the amount of stair climbing demanded, and so forth assists the nurse in helping the individual make

**TABLE 24-6**
APPROXIMATE ENERGY EXPENDITURE IN METS
OF ACTIVITIES FOR A 70-KG PERSON*

| Energy Expenditure, METS | Housework and Industrial Activities | Recreational and Self-Care Activities |
|---|---|---|
| 1–2 | Sewing by hand, knitting, needlework<br>Desk work<br>Typing (electric)<br>Driving an automobile<br>Watch repairing | Bed rest, sitting<br>Eating<br>Conversing<br>Washing hands and face<br>Walking level, slowly 1 mph<br>Playing cards |
| 2–3 | Kneading dough<br>Washing small clothes<br>Peeling potatoes<br>Auto repair<br>Radio, TV repair<br>Machine sewing<br>Custodial work<br>Typing, manual | Dressing and undressing<br>Using bedside commode<br>Walking level, 2 mph<br>Golfing, using electric cart<br>Playing piano<br>Volleyball<br>Horseback riding, slow |
| 3–4 | Scrubbing floors<br>Window cleaning<br>Making beds<br>Laying bricks<br>Machine assembly<br>Plastering | Showering<br>Using bedpan<br>Walking level, 3 mph<br>Badminton<br>Power mower, light pushing<br>Bowling |
| 4–5 | Beating carpets<br>Light carpentry<br>Hanging wallpaper<br>Ploughing by horse | Walking downstairs<br>Walking level, 3½ mph<br>Golf, carrying clubs<br>Rowing<br>Bicycle riding, 8 mph |
| 5–6 | Garden digging<br>Light dirt shoveling<br>Heavy carpentry | Walking level, 4 mph<br>Bicycle riding, 10 mph<br>Ice skating, 9 mph |
| 6–7 | Shoveling snow, 10 min, 10 lb<br>Mowing lawn by hand<br>Cutting down trees | Walking level, 5 mph<br>Walking with braces or crutches<br>Water skiing |
| 7–8 | Ascending stairs with 17-lb load<br>Carrying 80 lb level<br>Heavy digging | Jogging level, 5 mph<br>Bicycle riding, 12 mph<br>Basketball<br>Touch football |
| 8–9 | Shoveling snow, 10 min, 14 lb | Running level, 5½ mph<br>Bicycle riding, 13 mph<br>Fencing<br>Squash, social |
| 10 or more | Shoveling snow, 10 min, 16 lb | Squash or handball, competitive |

* Psychological factors will increase metabolic needs. Also, activities should begin gradually and maximum tolerance worked up to overtime.

modifications in the home. For example, a commode may need to be placed on the first-floor level, the kitchen may need to be rearranged to conserve energy expenditure, or the individual may be required to move to a first-floor apartment to eliminate stair climbing.

Teaching measures to conserve energy allows the patient to participate in more physical activity. Principles of work simplification aid the person to plan a task, to utilize good body mechanics, to use mental and physical relaxation methods, and to pace activities. Table 24-7 identifies some common principles of work simplification.

The prognosis of patients who have developed pump failure is as variable as the causes. Treatment of the primary and precipitating causes, as well as the pump failure itself, has improved through scientific research. Discovery of new methods of surgical and medical intervention, the advent of modern

**TABLE 24-7**
PRINCIPLES OF WORK SIMPLIFICATION

1 An activity well thought out and planned for can be completed more efficiently and with less energy expenditure.
   *a* Select a job to be improved.
   *b* Break the job down in terms of preparation, doing, and cleaning up.
   *c* Question whether the job is necessary, what is the best way of accomplishing it in terms of the time it should be done, equipment necessary, work area, etc.
   *d* Develop a new method of accomplishing the job that saves energy (eliminate unnecessary details, combine and simplify motions, change sequence of performing job).
   *e* Utilize the new method by rearranging necessary equipment, adjusting the work areas including their height to meet your needs.

2 Simplification of tasks is accomplished through correct utilization of muscles and proper body mechanics.
   *a* Keep back straight, bend at hips, avoid twisting.
   *b* For improved balance and weight distribution, keep knees straight forward, bent slightly.
   *c* Carry packages close to body with even distribution, to both sides.
   *d* When rising from a chair, move forward on chair, then lean forward to rise.

3 To avoid undue fatigue, utilize the principles of mental and physical relaxation.
   *a* Physical relaxation:
     (1) Utilize muscles correctly.
     (2) Muscle movement should be smooth and continuous.
     (3) Obtain appropriate equipment for your job.
     (4) Dress in suitable attire for your job, including good supporting shoes.
   *b* Mental relaxation:
     (1) Lie with feet elevated.
     (2) Rest in a dark room with soothing music.
     (3) Take a warm tub bath.

4 To accomplish more with less fatigue, activities should be paced.
   *a* Balance activities with periods of rest.
   *b* Use your own natural speed.
   *c* Do not rush, use a steady pace.

drugs, and the earlier recognition of pump failure allow the individual to live longer.

The nurse, by assuming more responsibility in the areas of prevention, assessment, evaluation, consultation, and education, has contributed greatly to the prolongation of a meaningful life for the individual afflicted with pump failure.

## REFERENCES

1 L. F. Bishop and P. Reichert, "Emotion and Heart Failure," *Psychosomatics,* **12**(6):412–415, November-December 1971.

2 M. E. Nicholls et al., "Aldosterone and Its Regulation during Diuresis in Patients with Gross Congestive Heart Failure," *Clin Sci Mol Med,* **47**(4):301–315, October 1974.

3 M. Rabinowitz and R. Zak, "Biochemical and Cellular Changes in Cardiac Hypertrophy," *Annu Rev Med,* **23:**245, 1972.

4 A. M. Katz, and A. J. Brady, "Mechanical and Biochemical Correlates of Cardiac Contractions," *Mod Concepts Cardiovasc Dis,* **40:**39, 1971.

5 A. M. Katz, "Contractile Proteins of the Heart," *Phys Rev,* **50:**63, 1970.

6 Rabinowitz and Zak, *op. cit.,* p. 258.

7 Katz and Brady, *op. cit.,* p. 39.

8 H. Smulyan, R. Gilbert, and R. H. Eich, "Pulmonary Effects of Heart Failure," *Surg Clin North Am,* **54**(5):1077–1087, October 1974.

9 *Ibid.,* p. 1085.

10 A. Ramirez and W. H. Abelmann, "Cardiac Decompensation," *N Engl J Med,* **290**(9):499–501, Feb. 28, 1974.

11 Smulyan, *op. cit.,* p. 1085.

12 *Ibid.,* p. 1085.

13 K. Cohn, et al., "Variability of Hemodynamic Responses to Acute Digitalization in Chronic Cardiac Failure due to Cardiomyopathy and Coronary Artery Disease," *Am J Cardiol,* **35**(4):461–468, April 1975.

14 R. J. Hoeschen and T. E. Cuddy, "Dose-Response Relation between Therapeutic Levels of Serum Digoxin and Systolic Time Intervals," *Am J Cardiol,* **35**(4):469–472, April 1975.

15 Cohn et al., *op. cit.,* pp. 461–468.

16 Hoeschen, *op. cit.,* pp. 469–472.

17 *Ibid.,* p. 469–472.

18 J. William Hurst, *The Heart,* 3d ed., McGraw-Hill, New York, 1974, pp. 440–441.

19 P. A. Habak, et al., "Effectiveness of Congesting Cuffs ("Rotating Tourniquets") in Patients with Left Heart Failure," *Circulation,* **50**(2):366–371, August 1974.

## BIBLIOGRAPHY

Abramson, F. P.: "What is "Refractory" Cardiac Failure?" (letter), *N Engl J Med,* **292**(1):49–50, Jan. 2, 1975.

Anderson, M. I.: "Development of Outcome Criteria for the Patient with Congestive Heart Failure," *Nurs Clin North Am,* **9**(2):349–358, June 1974.

Braumwald, B.: "Mechanics and Energetics of the Normal and Failing Heart," *Trans Assoc Am Physicians,* **84**:63–94, 1971.

Braumwald, E.: *The Myocardium: Failure and Infarction,* HP Publishing Co., New York, 1975.

Burch, G. E.: "Proper Digitalization," *Postgrad Med,* **55**(4):165–169, April 1974.

Chidsey, C. A., et al.: "Catecholamine Excretion and Cardiac Stores of Norepinephrine in Congestive Heart Failure," *Am J Med,* **39**:442, 1965.

Chrisman, M.: "Dsypnea," *Am J Nurs,* **74**:643–646, April 1974.

Clark, H.: "Nursing Care Study: Left Ventricular Failure with Acute Pulmonary Edema," *Nurs Times,* **71**(27):1040–1042, July 3, 1975.

Clark, N. F.: "Pump Failure," *Nurs Clin North Am,* **7**:3:529–540, September 1972.

Cogen, R.: "Cardiac Catheterization: Preparing the Adult," *Am J Nurs,* **73**:77, January 1973.

Cohn, J. N.: "Indications for Digitalis Therapy. A New Look," *JAMA,* **229**(14):1911–1914, Sept. 30, 1974.

Daly, S., et al.: "Central Veneris Catheterization," *Am J Nurs,* **75**:820–824, May 1975.

DeBerry, P., et al.: "Teaching Cardiac Patients to Manage Medications," *Am J Nurs,* **75**:12:2191–2193, December 1975.

Fleming, J. S.: "Heart Failure and Cardiac Arrhythmias," *Practitioner,* **213** (1276 SPEC NO):448–453, October 1974.

Foster, S. B.: "Pump Failure," *Am J Nurs,* **74**(10):1830–1834, October 1974.

Fournet, K., and O. Carm: "Patient Discharged on Diuretics: Prime Candidates for Individualized Teaching by the Nurse," *Heart Lung,* **3**:1:108–116, March 1974.

Frohlich, E. G.: "Use and Abuse of Diuretics," (editorial), *Am Heart J,* **89**(1):1–3, January 1975.

Habak, P.A., et al.: "Rotating Tourniquets: How Effective in Left Heart Failure?" *RN,* **38**(1):ICUI-2, ICU5, January 1975.

Hanchett, C., and R. Johnson: "Early Signs of Congestive Heart Failure," *Am J Nurs,* **58**:1457–1461, July 1968.

Ingelfinger, L. A., and P. Goldman: "The Serum Digitalis Concentration—Does It Diagnose Digitalis Toxicity?" *N Engl J Med,* **294**:16:867–870, April 15, 1976.

"Intractable Heart Failure" (clinical conference), *NY State J Med,* **75**(8):1235–1246, July 1975.

Jones, P.: "Rotating Tourniquets: The Nurse's Role," *RN,* **38**(1):ICU6, January 1975.

Kannel, W. B., et al.: "Vital Capacity and Congestive Heart Failure. The Framingham Study," *Circulation,* **49**(6):1160–1166, June 1974.

Kimble, M. A., and R. M. Elenbaas: "Congestive Heart Failure," *J Am Pharm Assoc,* **14**(7):362–375, July 1974.

Kleint, S., et al.: "Diuretic Therapy—Current Status," *Am Heart J,* **79**:700–712, May 1970.

Larson, E.: "The Patient with Acute Pulmonary Edema," *Am J Nurs,* **68**:1019–1021, May 1968.

Littman, P.: "Stethoscope and Auscultation," *Am J Nurs,* **72**:1238, July 1972.

Mason, D. T., et al.: "Digitalis—New Facts about an Old Drug," *Am J Cardiol,* **22**:151, August 1968.

Mechner, F.: "Programmed Instruction Patient Assessment: Examination of the Chest and Lungs," *Am J Nurs,* **76**:9:1453–1475, September 1976.

Perez-Stable, E. C., and B. T. Matesson: "Diuretic Drug Therapy of Edema," *Med Clin North Am,* **55**:359–372, March 1971.

Posner, M. D.: "Cardiac failure: tourniquets vs. phlebotomy," (letter), *N Engl J Med,* **290**(26):1485–1486, June 27, 1974.

Powell, A.: "Physical Assessment of the Patient with Cardiac Disease," *Nurs Clin North Am,* **11**(2):251–258, June 1976.

Rasmussen, S., J. Noble, and C. Fisch: "The Pharmacology and Clinical Use of Digitalis," *Cardiovasc Nurs,* **11**(1):23–28, January-February 1975.

Reubi, F. C.: "Combination Diuretic Drug Therapy," *Cardiovasc Clin,* **2**(3):197–210, 1971.

Roberts, W. C., et al.: "Congestive Heart Failure and Angina Pectoris: Opposite Ends of the Spectrum of Symptomatic Ischemic Heart Disease," *Am J Cardio,* **34**(7):870–872, December 1974.

Tikoff, G., and H. Kuida: "Pathophysiology of Heart Failure in Congenital Heart Disease," *Mod Concepts Cardiovasc Dis,* **41**(1):1–6 (editorial), January 1972.

Vaisrub, S.: "Reducing the Work Load of the Failing Heart," (editorial), *JAMA,* **266**(11):1350–1351, Dec. 10, 1973.

Walker, B.: "Nursing Care To Assess and Prevent Common Cardiovascular Problems," *Nurs Clin North Am,* **10**(1):43–48, March 1975.

Walker, W. J.: "Treatment of Heart Failure," *JAMA,* **228**(10):1276–1278, June 3, 1974.

Walther, J. U.: "Ouabain in Heart Failure," (letter), *Br Med J,* **1**(5956), March 1, 1975.

Waxler, R.: "The Patient with Congestive Heart Failure: Teaching Implications," *Nurs Clin North Am,* **11**:2:297–308, June 1976.

Whight, C., et al.: "Diuretics, Cardiac Failure and Potassium Depletion: A Rational Approach," *Med J Aust,* **2**(23):831–833, Dec. 7, 1974.

Winslow, E.: "Digitalis," *Am J Nurs,* **74**:1062–1065, June 1974.

# 25

# CONDUCTION DISTURBANCES AS A CAUSE OF PUMP FAILURE

Mary B. McFarland

The action of the heart as a pump includes both mechanical and electrical components. The mechanical components include the structures of the heart (Chap. 27) and the muscle action of the myocardium (Chap. 26). The electrical components initiate cardiac response and are therefore vitally important to life. As man interacts with the environment, certain physical, emotional and sociocultural factors can influence electrical stimulation and cardiac conduction.

The mechanical or pumping response of the heart is directly influenced by electrical conduction. When changes occur in electrical stimulation, disruptions in cardiac rate, rhythm, and output can result. If conduction disturbances persist, pump failure may develop and death can follow.

Modern techniques of evaluating the electrical conduction of the heart, along with the expanding role of the nurse in assessing, evaluating, and treating patients, make an in-depth understanding of arrhythmias essential. The information in this chapter should be a stimulus to further study of conduction disruptions of the heartbeat.

## PATHOPHYSIOLOGY

Changes in cardiac rhythm due to alterations in conduction are called *arrhythmias.* An arrhythmia is defined as any change in the rate, rhythm, or conduction of impulses that ultimately affects the quality of cardiac output. (*Dysrhythmia* is a term used interchangeably with arrhythmia.[1]) In the normal heart (refer to Chap. 22), electrical conduction is stimulated by the sinoatrial (SA) node at the rate of 60 to 100 beats per minute. These conducted impulses travel throughout the heart muscle, stimulating the pumping and contracting mechanism. Interruptions in this process result in an arrhythmia. Arrhythmias may themselves be life-threatening or may indicate more serious pathophysiology elsewhere in the body. An understanding of the significance, causes, and effects of alterations in cardiac rate and rhythm will lead to improved patient care.

Arrhythmias can occur at any point in the normal conduction pathway (refer to Chap. 22). When arrhythmias occur in the SA node, they are called *sinus arrhythmias.* Increased excitation of the SA node can produce an increase in heart rate, or *sinus tachycardia.* A lack of sinoatrial stimulation can result in a slowing of the heart rate, or *sinus bradycardia.*

Alterations in the atria due to ischemia of the muscle walls can lead to *atrial arrhythmias.* An increase in the atrial rate is referred to as *atrial tachycardia*. When the irritability of the atrial muscle increases, *premature* atrial beats can occur. An increased irritable focus within the atria can lead to *atrial flutter* or *atrial fibrillation*. Both these problems increase the amount of electricity discharged at the beginning of the conduction cycle and can result in pump failure if not corrected.

Arrhythmias occurring at the atrioventricular (AV) node are called *AV junctional arrhythmias.* Two problems can occur at the AV node: first, the AV node may replace the SA node as the cardiac pacemaker (nodal rhythm); second, the AV node can block impulses coming from the SA node. Both *incomplete heart block* (first- and second-degree heart block) and *complete heart block* are examples of the second problem. Again, failure to correct this rhythm will lead to diminished cardiac output and result in pump failure.

Rhythm changes occurring in the ventricles are the most life-threatening. These changes can result from irritability in the ventricle wall leading to ectopic beats, as in *premature ventricular contractions.* Rhythm disturbances can also occur when there is damage in the ventricular branches (*bundle branch block*) and, finally, when ischemia in the ventricle causes repeated and rapid stimulation of an ectopic electrical stimulus, as in *ventricular fibrillation.* Unless ventricular arrhythmias are corrected immediately, they can lead to cardiac standstill and death.

With all arrhythmias, there are alterations in myocardial tissues, automaticity, regularity, and excitability (see Chap. 22). These changes can lead to hemodynamic alterations affecting the force of contraction and overall cardiac output. The following discussion focuses on the changes, causes, and effects in each arrhythmia and their impact on the patient.

### Sinus Arrhythmias

All sinus arrhythmias originate in the sinoatrial node and are conducted along the normal conductive pathways. The variations from normal are observed in either the rate or the rhythm of the heartbeat and are usually due to overactivity of the autonomic nervous system. When the sympathetic nervous system is in control, the heart rate is rapid. When the parasympathetic nervous system (or vagal response) is enforcing its action, the heart rate is slowed down. Major sinus arrhythmias include sinus tachycardia, sinus bradycardia, sinus arrest, and wandering pacemaker.

**Sinus tachycardia** In sinus tachycardia, the automaticity of the sinoatrial node is enhanced and the heart rate is increased to between 100 and 180 beats per minute. Usually normal conduction continues through the system. However, at the higher rates there is a decrease in ventricular filling and the stroke volume begins to diminish. The result is decreased cardiac output and subsequent pump failure. When this occurs in the presence of cardiac pathology, myocardial cellular oxygen tension may develop and irreversible changes may follow (i.e., shock).

The *causes* of sinus tachycardia may include sympathetic stimulants such as pain, exercise, hypoxia, pulmonary embolism (see Chap. 29), hemorrhage (Chap. 28), or hyperthyroidism (Chap. 21). Fever can also cause the heart rate to increase, because a rise in body temperature increases the metabolic rate and intensifies the excitability of the cardiac muscle. Overeating, excessive ingestion of caffeine, and drugs classified as sympathomimetics (e.g., epinephrine and isoproterinol) and parasympatholytics (e.g., atropine) may lead to sinus tachycardia as a result of sympathetic stimulation.

Anxiety, tension, and emotional stress can induce sinus tachycardia due to adrenal stimulation. In addition, anger, rage, or fright increase the heart rate significantly. After the stressful event is removed, the heart rate usually returns to normal. Ischemic changes due to a myocardial infarction can result in edema of the SA node and increase its vulnerability to rhythm disturbances.

The *effects* of these changes on the patient, which are usually minimal, include mild dyspnea and complaints of palpitations. However, the pulse rate is rapid, and the cardiac rhythm and its quality are unaffected. The *EKG* demonstrates a normal rhythm with a rapid rate. If the rate is very rapid, the P and T waves may appear close together (see Fig. 25-1). In the presence of myocardial disease, sinus tachycardia can place an added burden on the heart muscle and can lead to irreversible changes (cardiogenic shock; see Chap. 28) and death.

**Sinus bradycardia** In sinus bradycardia the automaticity of the sinoatrial node is depressed and the heart rate is decreased to below 60 beats per minute. This is due to an increased rate of parasympathetic (vagal) stimulation that can be induced by ischemia of the vagal fibers following myocardial infarction. Vagal stimulation may also occur during the Valsalva maneuver or vomiting. *Carotid sinus syndrome* results from arteriosclerosis in the carotid sinus area and can cause excessive sensitivity of pressor receptors. Consequently, mild pressure on the neck can cause intense vagal stimulation and extreme bradycardia. Sinus bradycardia may also be caused by ischemia of the sinoatrial node, hypothermia, hyperkalemia, depression, or by drugs such as digitalis and propranolol. Older persons with sinus bradycardia tend to have disruptions of the atrioventricular junction or the interventricular conduction system.

Anesthesia and surgery cause alterations in body function that lead to the development of arrhythmias. These arrhythmias often result from tissue hypoxia, anoxia, vagal reflexes, or myocardial irritation, as well as from the anesthetic agent and the type and length of the operation. Sinus bradycardia may increase the response to the anesthetic used during surgery. The presence of coronary artery disease greatly increases the possibility of multiple rhythm changes.

Sinus bradycardia produces no specific symptoms unless the rate becomes very slow. Normally, sinus bradycardia is not dangerous to the patient. It is common in older age groups because of physiologic changes in the conduction system and arteriosclerotic heart disease. The most significant finding is a pulse rate below 60. Highly trained athletes frequently have sinus bradycardia, probably because of a greater stroke volume output, with larger quantities of blood being pumped into the arterial tree with each beat.

The EKG indicates normal conduction with a regular rhythm. The most significant change is a slowed heart rate. If the heart rate becomes significantly slow, syncope (fainting) may occur. In the presence of cardiovascular ischemia, circulation to the vital organs may be decreased and irritable foci stimulated along the conduction pathway.

**Other sinus arrhythmias** In sinus arrhythmia, the impulse originates in the SA node, but the rhythm is irregular. This arrhythmia, considered normal, is seen more often in young adults.

Several cardiac reflexes are involved in this arrhythmia. These include reflexes which slow and speed up the heart rate when baroreceptors are alternately stimulated or there is excitation of the respiratory center. An increase and decrease in the number of impulses sent to the heart by the vagus nerves results.

Although it may be a normal rhythm for many persons, sinus arrhythmia may be indicative of heart pathology. Sinus arrhythmia unrelated to respiration or external forces may prove clinically significant.

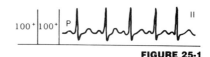

**FIGURE 25-1**

Sinus tachycardia. (*From Harrison's Principles of Internal Medicine, 8th ed., by G. W. Thorn et al. Copyright 1977 by McGraw-Hill, Inc. Used with permission of McGraw-Hill Book Company.*)

Sinus arrest and wandering pacemakers are two additional sinus arrhythmias. In *sinus arrest* a heart beat may be completely missed because of failure of the SA node to discharge a stimulus. Increased vagal stimulation or digitalis toxicosis may be the precipitating cause. An increase in potassium can decrease muscle excitability and slow conduction and can result in a sinus arrest.

A *wandering of the pacemaker* can occur within the sinoatrial node or may move to various locations within the atria and the atrioventricular junction. The *cause* of a wandering pacemaker is usually a slowing of the sinus impulses associated with increased vagal stimulation, organic heart disease affecting the fibers of the sinoatrial node, or parasympathetic drugs which cause slowing of the heart rate. Usually a sinus arrhythmia of this type produces no serious patient effects but requires observation. Changes in the regularity of the P-R interval are noted on the EKG.

### Atrial Arrhythmias

Atrial arrhythmias are a manifestation of abnormal electrical activity which results in stimulation outside the SA node but within the atria. An ectopic focus or a circus movement of impulses within one of the atria results in arrhythmias that range from harmless, with no effect on cardiac function, to severe, with decrease in cardiac output. Premature atrial contractions, paroxysmal atrial tachycardia, atrial flutter, and atrial fibrillation are included in this discussion.

**Premature atrial contractions** Premature atrial contraction (PAC) occurs when an ectopic focus within one of the atria fires prematurely. The impulse then travels in an abnormal fashion throughout the atria. Premature atrial contractions may be a normal phenomenon in some persons but may also be caused by emotional disturbances, fatigue, tobacco, or caffeine. They may also be an early sign of abnormal electrical activity associated with organic heart disease such as congestive heart failure, electrolyte imbalance, or more serious atrial arrhythmias.

Normally, the patient is unaware of this rhythm

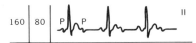

**FIGURE 25-2**
Paroxysmal atrial tachycardia (PAT). (*From Thorn et al., with permission of McGraw-Hill Book Company.*)

change. On auscultation, a heart beat may be heard sooner than usual. In the presence of cardiac pathology, PAC may herald the onset of more serious atrial arrhythmias.

The *EKG* reveals an abnormally shaped P wave followed by a normal QRS complex. The P wave is often difficult to find, but except for its earlier than normal occurrence, the rate and rhythm are normal.

**Paroxysmal atrial tachycardia**  In paroxysmal atrial tachycardia (PAT), there is a rapid rhythmic discharge of impulses originating from an ectopic focus within the atria. This continuous run of premature atrial contractions is followed by a normal ventricular response at a rate of 160 to 250 beats per minute. The onset and termination of the episode may be sudden while the duration of an attack may range from a few minutes to several days.

The most frequent *cause* of PAT is atrial-muscle ischemia. Abnormalities such as rheumatic heart disease or acute myocardial infarction can precipitate PAT, as can psychological factors such as anxiety, stress, or other forms of emotional trauma. A decrease in potassium leads to cardiac irritability and may result in PAT. Smoking and caffeine, along with exercise, often stimulates sympathetic nerve fibers and can result in PAT. Ingestion of large meals and excessive swallowing increases the metabolic rate and elevates the heart rate, precipitating tachycardia.

When tachycardia is prolonged, the period of ventricular filling is shortened, the stroke volume is reduced, and cardiac output falls. Pump failure, hypotension, and additional arrhythmias can result.

Most patients are acutely aware of the increased activity of the heart. They feel the pulsing sensations and become restless and dizzy. Syncope may be present, and light-headedness and anxiety may intensify the problem. The arrhythmia rhythm frequently disappears as quickly as it began.

The EKG (see Fig. 25-2) shows a rapid conduction rate. P waves are difficult to distingush, especially with a rapid rate. They are often buried in the QRS or T waves, so that these waves appear ab-

normal. A normal ventricular response follows each conducted atrial beat.

**Atrial flutter**  Atrial flutter is an infrequent arrhythmia which arises from an ectopic focus within the atrial wall. The origin of this arrhythmia is controversial. One theory holds that a single ectopic focus stimulates atrial depolarization; another, that a circular band of cardiac muscles containing the sinoatrial node gives rise to electrical impulses which create a continuous wave, called a *circus movement*. A third theory suggests that several pacemaking centers exist in the atria.[2]

Whatever the circumstances that precipitate atrial flutter, the stimulated atrium contracts 250 to 400 times per minute. Fortunately, most of these impulses are blocked by the AV node, which protects the ventricle from receiving every impulse from the atrium.

Atrial flutter may be *caused* by stress, trauma, or hypoxia. Drugs such as digitalis, quinidine, and epinephrine may also precipitate atrial flutter. Chronic heart disease, hypertension, arteriosclerosis, rheumatic heart disease, constrictive pericarditis, and cor pulmonale may be additional factors in the development of atrial flutter.

The *effects* of atrial flutter depend on the extent of heart damage. Some patients are completely unaware of the arrhythmia, whereas others may experience palpitations, weakness, dizziness, or fainting.

The pulse rate will be regular as soon as the extent of block becomes established. The EKG pattern of atrial flutter is characteristic and usually easy to identify (see Fig. 25-3). The P waves are replaced by flutter waves (or F waves) which are saw-toothed in configuration and not always followed by QRS complexes, because the refractory period of the atrioventricular junction blocks conduction of some of the impulses originating in the atria. Since the degree of block varies, the ratio of atrial to ventricular beats may be 2:1 to 6:1 or higher. In severe cases all impulses may be conducted. If this occurs, the ventricular rate is so rapid that a low cardiac output results and leads to pump failure. Once a pattern has been established, the rhythm of atrial flutter tends to be regular. The QRS is normally shaped and the pulse rate ranges from 60 to 160 beats per minute, depending on the number of conducted ventricular beats.

**Atrial fibrillation**  Atrial fibrillation occurs when several ectopic foci within the atria discharge 350 to 500 or more times per minute (see Fig. 25-4). As in atrial flutter, the origin of this arrhythmia is controversial. The circus movement in this case is thought to occur in several bands of muscle fibers instead of only one, with multiple rapidly firing ectopic foci replacing effective muscular contractions.

*Atrial fibrillation is the most common atrial arrhythmia* and is most frequently *caused* by chronic lung disease, organic heart disease, and heart failure. It may be associated with rheumatic heart disease, and it is the most common arrhythmia following mitral-valve replacement. Atrial and ventricular septal defects and other congenital defects which cause anoxia or ventricular strain may lead to atrial fibrillation. In rare instances, atrial fibrillation may occur without evidence of heart disease.

Atrial fibrillation may be associated with metabolic disorders such as hyperthyroidism. An increase in thyroid hormone affects the heart by directly impairing the heart muscle, while increasing its sensitivity to catecholamines and cardiac work load. As a result, in oxygen consumption, cardiac output, heart rate, and stroke volume lead to alterations in rhythm. Some of these changes (e.g., the tachycardia) occur as compensatory mechanisms, attempting to meet the oxygen needs of the body. Increased thyroid levels cause a rapid ventricular rate which is difficult to control but disappears spontaneously when the thyroid returns to normal.

The *onset* of atrial fibrillation is often sudden. Patients with atrial fibrillation have a grossly irregular pulse rate, with ventricular rates between 110 and 150 beats per minute. Confusion, syncope, and dizziness may occur if severe hypoxia is present. Pump failure may result. Often pulses heard at the apex of the heart may not be palpable in the periphery (pulse deficit). In the presence of hyperthyroidism the patient may exhibit additional changes, including increased anxiety. Pulmonary emboli can occur in the presence of atrial fibrillation and may be a serious threat (see Chap. 29).

The EKG characteristics of atrial fibrillation (see Fig. 25-5) include abnormalities in the rhythm, P waves, and P-R intervals. The rhythm is grossly irregular, and P waves are replaced by small irregular fibrillation waves (f waves). Because the P waves are absent, the P-R interval is not identifiable. The QRS complexes are normal in shape but irregular in occurrence. The rate varies and the rhythm is irregular. When controlled by medication, the pulse rate may be below 100 beats per minute. In uncon-

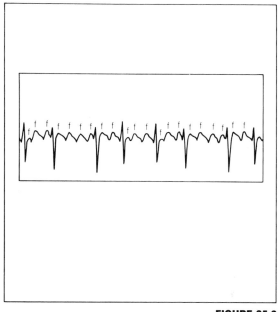

**FIGURE 25-3**
Atrial flutter, with multiple F, or flutter, waves occurring in a variety of ratios (3:1, etc.).

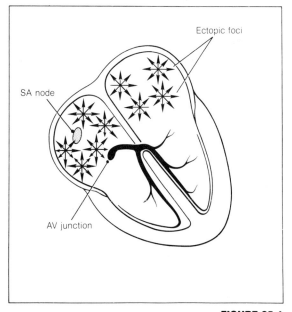

**FIGURE 25-4**
Schematic drawing of atrial fibrillation. Note the multiple direction of each ectopic focus.

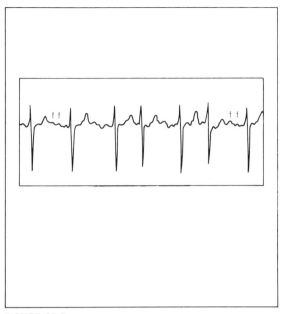

**FIGURE 25-5**
Atrial fibrillation (EKG).

trolled cases the pulse rate will be above 100 beats per minute. If this rapid rate persists, signs of pump failure may become evident.

### Junctional Arrhythmias

In atrioventricular (AV) junctional (nodal) arrhythmias an ectopic focus within the junction takes over the pacing function of the heart. When this occurs, the impulse travels in both directions: forward in an antegrade fashion and upward in a retrograde direction. Arrhythmias may originate in different portions of the AV junction; the terms upper, middle, and lower junctional (nodal) arrhythmias have been used to describe the location of the abnormal rhythms.

*AV junctional rhythms* usually occur when there are abnormalities in the functioning of the sinoatrial node. These may be *caused* by vagal stimulation, injury due to inflammation, medications such as digitalis and atropine, and myocardial infarction. This disruption in impulse formation results in minimal hemodynamic impairment. The signs of AV junctional rhythms are similar to bradycardia, except when the patient has a junctional tachycardia. When junctional arrhythmias are present, the only abnormalities seen on the EKG are changes in the P wave and the P-R interval. The P wave may be inverted before or after the QRS complex or buried within it. The P-R interval varies, depending on the location of the P wave.

### Ventricular Arrhythmias

Ventricular arrhythmias occur when one or more ectopic foci arise within the ventricles. These arrhythmias range from premature ectopic beats to fatal ventricular fibrillation.

**Premature ventricular contractions** Premature ventricular contractions (PVC) occur when one or more ectopic foci stimulate a premature ventricular response (see Fig. 25-6). The irritable foci can develop from ischemia due to a myocardial infarction, from infection (e.g., carditis), or from mechanical damage due to pump failure.

Deviations in concentration of electrolytes, particularly potassium and calcium, are also *causative* factors in the development of PVCs. A decrease in potassium may result in cardiac enlargement and increased cardiac irritability. Hypocalcemia may be associated with ectopic rhythms such as premature beats.

Nicotine can affect the heart by causing an initial slowing due to vagal stimulation followed by stimulation of the cardiac sympathetic ganglia and a concomitant increase in heart rate. Ectopic beats may develop in persons with coronary artery disease.

Coffee, tea, and alcohol can increase the cardiac rate and lead to PVCs. Exercise, or drugs such as digitalis and reserpine, as well as psychogenic factors such as stress, anxiety, and fatigue may result in ectopic beats. In these situations the central nervous system stimulation affects the autonomic nervous system and the endocrine system. The resulting catecholamine secretions of epinephrine and norepinephrine produces electrophysiologic changes in the myocardium which cause arrhythmias. It has also been noted that parasympathetic effects may be present along with sympathetic activity, causing production of acetylcholine and resultant arrhythmias.[3]

Acute and chronic lung disease may lead to right heart stress and eventual right-sided heart failure (cor pulmonale). Arrhythmias resulting from these conditions may be due to anoxia, pulmonary disease, vagal stimulation, coughing, or electrolyte changes. Prolonged right-heart strain and distention of the right atrium and great vessels leads to increased cardiac irritability and stimulation of ectopic pacemakers. PVC may also occur in persons who have no evidence of heart disease.

The hemodynamic *effects* of PVC depend on the frequency of occurrence and site of origin. When PVCs occur frequently, they decrease the efficiency of the heart's pumping action because the heart is forced to contract before ventricular filling is complete. Premature beats that arise in the right ventricle do not adversely affect the systemic hemodynamics as much as those which arise in the left ventricle.

When more than five to six PVCs occur within a minute, it may indicate acute irritability. Three or more PVCs occurring consecutively by definition constitute *ventricular tachycardia.* A PVC, even if infrequent, that falls on the end of a T wave can precipitate ventricular fibrillation.

The patient's physical response to PVCs ranges from unawareness to palpitations, with a feeling of an irregular heart beat, a "lump in the throat," or the heart "skipping a beat." The pulse rate is usually normal.

The EKG (see Fig. 25-7) shows a normal conduction pattern except for the PVC, which has a bizarre-appearing QRS complex that is wide and slurred. In addition, the T wave is in the opposite direction from the QRS complex. The QRS complex is not preceded by a P wave, and the PVC occurs prematurely and is followed by a full *compensatory pause.* When a cardiac cycle has been interrupted by a PVC, this compensatory pause will occur prior to the start of the normal cycle.

**Ventricular tachycardia**   Ventricular tachycardia often occurs in paroxysms and is indicative of severe myocardial irritability. It is considered clinically present when three or more PVCs occur in a row. Paroxysmal ventricular tachycardia is seen infrequently in healthy persons. It is a serious arrhythmia because of its association with severe organic heart disease and the fact that it may develop into ventricular fibrillation. All forms of heart pathology, especially myocardial infarction, can *cause* ventricular tachycardia due to muscle ischemia or conduction damage. Cardiac catheterization may precipitate an episode of ventricular tachycardia, due to mechanical irritation as the catheter travels through the ventricles. When the catheter passes through the heart chambers it may strike the ventricular wall and stimulate ectopic beats.

The appearance of this arrhythmia may be sudden, but often it is precipitated by PVCs. The *effects* of these changes include chest pain, dizziness, fainting, occasional collapse, and cardiogenic shock. The pulse rate is rapid and the blood pressure falls. In ventricular tachycardia the EKG is grossly abnormal, the pattern resembling several PVCs in a row. The ventricular rate is usually be-

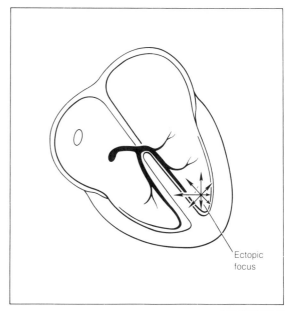

**FIGURE 25-6**
Premature ventricular contraction.

tween 140 and 220 beats per minute, and the rhythm is slightly irregular. The P waves occur independently of the QRS complexes and are buried within the QRS complex, which is wide and slurred. Usually ventricular tachycardia does not last long before it becomes ventricular fibrillation.

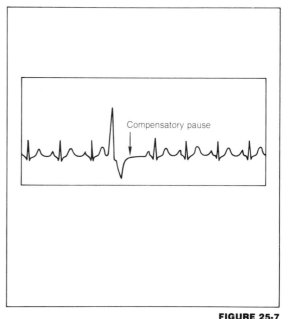

**FIGURE 25-7**
Premature ventricular contraction (EKG).

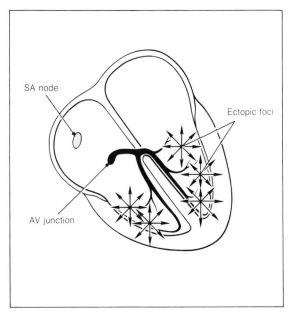

**FIGURE 25-8**
Ventricular fibrillation.

**Ventricular fibrillation** Ventricular fibrillation is the *most serious* of all arrhythmias, because it will result in cardiac standstill and death if not treated. The problem occurs when several ectopic foci within the ventricles are discharged at a very rapid rate (see Fig. 25-8).

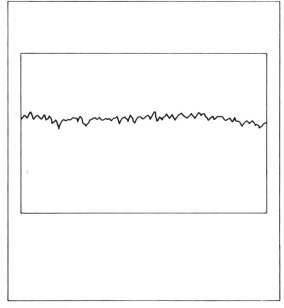

**FIGURE 25-9**
Ventricular fibrillation (EKG).

The *cause* of ventricular fibrillation is usually organic heart disease such as acute myocardial infarction, hypertension, or rheumatic or arteriosclerotic heart disturbances. It may also occur following open-heart surgery. Hypoxia or emotional trauma with increased sympathetic activity may be predisposing factors. Ventricular fibrillation can result when an electric current is received during the last phase of ventricular repolarization. This may occur in a hospital when electric equipment is not grounded properly.

When ventricular fibrillation occurs, pulses and audible heart sounds disappear, the blood pressure is unobtainable, and the patient becomes unresponsive. Circulation ceases, and unless blood flow is restored by cardiopulmonary resuscitation (discussed in Chap. 26) and the arrhythmia interrupted (by defibrillation), death will result within 90 seconds to 5 minutes.

The EKG pattern (see Fig. 25-9) is very irregular, showing a wavy or fibrillation line. There are no identifiable PQRST waves, rate, or rhythm, indicating the absence of effective myocardial contractions.

## Conduction Defects

The term *heart block* refers to a delay in the conduction of impulses within the atrioventricular system, present when the AV junction (node) or the bundle of His does not conduct impulses to the ventricles within the normal time period. (Normally it takes the AV junction 0.12 to 0.20 second to conduct the impulses to the bundle of His.) Defects in this nodal conduction may be partial (incomplete) or complete.

**Bundle branch block** Bundle branch block occurs when the right or left branches of the bundle of His (see Chap. 22) are blocked, causing the impulses to change their path of conduction or pass through the myocardial tissue. In left bundle branch block, either the posterior and anterior fascicles are obstructed or the branch itself is blocked.[4] Right bundle branch block occurs because the entire branch is blocked.

The *cause* of the block is usually myocardial ischemia or digitalis toxicosis. Left bundle branch block tends to be more serious and indicates left-sided heart problems. Bundle branch block is usually not considered an acute problem, but it can lead to complete heart block if it intensifies.

The EKG usually shows a widened QRS complex beyond 0.10 to 0.12 second. In right bundle branch block, there is also an M-shaped notching of the peak of the QRS complex (see Fig. 25-10).

*Hemiblock* is the term used for a partial block in the left branch—a left posterior block (LPB) or a left anterior block (LAB). This change in conduction often goes unnoticed but indicates the onset of more serious conduction blocks.

**Incomplete heart block** Incomplete heart block includes both first- and second-degree block. *First-degree block* occurs when the AV junction conducts all impulses, but at a slower than normal rate (longer than 0.20 second). *Second-degree block* occurs when the AV junction conducts some but not all impulses arising in the atria.

Incomplete heart block may be *caused* by infections, digitalis toxicosis, coronary artery disease, fibrosis of the conduction system, or myocardial infarction. Vagal stimulation can also result in partial heart block. In addition, nodal edema resulting from myocardial ischemia can slow conduction of an impulse.

The *effects* of incomplete heart block vary with the degree of block. Changes may include a slow heart rate with fainting and loss of consciousness. The pulse rate is decreased and blood pressure may be lower than normal.

In *first-degree* heart block the patient experiences no significant changes. The only abnormality seen on the EKG is a prolongation of the P-R interval which may cause a slow pulse rate (see Fig. 25-11). The P, Q, R, S, and T waves are normal in shape, and the heart rate and rhythm are usually slow and regular. If the problem is drug-related, withdrawal of the medication may produce improvement in the pulse rate as well as the conduction pattern.

*Second-degree* heart block occurs as the AV node blocks every second, third, or fourth impulse and conduction to the ventricles. Variant forms include Mobitz I, or the Wenckebach phenomenon, and Mobitz II. In Mobitz I there is a gradual prolonging of the conduction time through the AV node until one beat is blocked and fails to appear (dropped beat). The cycle then repeats itself in a pattern and may lead to a more serious block. Mobitz II is seen on the EKG as a normal flow of P waves followed by a QRS complex. Then, without warning, there is a dropped beat. This phenomenon can repeat itself and be indicative of serious conduction damage. The more frequently the beats are dropped, the slower the pulse rate and the more vulnerable the patient to the development of irritable foci (PVCs).

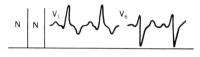

**FIGURE 25-10**

Right bundle branch block (EKG). (*From Thorn et al., with permission of McGraw-Hill Book Company.*)

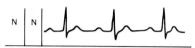

**FIGURE 25-11**

First-degree heart block. (*From Thorn et al., with permission of McGraw-Hill Book Company.*)

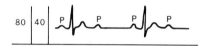

**FIGURE 25-12**

Second-degree heart block. (*From Thorn et al., with permission of McGraw-Hill Book Company.*)

The effect on cardiac output depends on the degree of block present. When there is a high degree of block there is diminished cardiac output and pump failure. The pulse rate is slower than in first-degree heart block. Second-degree heart block is usually a short-lived arrhythmia, often proceeding to complete heart block if not interrupted.

The EKG in second-degree block (see Fig. 25-12) shows a slow and regular ventricular rate. P waves are normal in shape, and several are seen before one is conducted to a QRS complex. While not every P wave is conducted, the QRS is normal in shape.

**Complete heart block** In complete heart block the AV junction blocks all impulses to the ventricles. In time the atria and ventricles dissociate and beat independently, each with its own pacemaker establishing a rate. The ventricular rate is slow, 20 to 40 beats per minute.

Complete heart block may be *caused* by either a congenital defect or an acquired heart problem such as vascular insufficiency, fibrosis of the myocardial tissue, or myocardial infarction. It may also be a result of cardiac surgery, especially if hypoxia occurs.

Stokes-Adams syndrome is a grouping of symptoms characterized by angina, syncope, mental confusion, convulsions, and unconsciousness. It is the most frequent cause of death in untreated complete heart block.

The hemodynamic *effects* of congenital complete heart block differ from those of the acquired

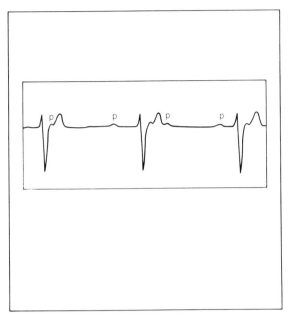

**FIGURE 25-13**
Complete heart block.

type. In congenital heart block there is an increase in stroke volume and diastolic heart volume. During exercise the ventricular rate may increase to 100 beats per minute.[5] In acquired complete heart block there is a prolonged diastolic period of ventricular filling with an increased stroke volume.

Complete heart block is a serious conduction problem which, if not treated immediately, will lead to death. The initial effects of complete heart block include palpitations, dizziness, syncope, dyspnea, mental confusion, and cyanosis.

The characteristics of complete heart block seen on the EKG (see Fig. 25-13) differ from those indicative of partial heart block because the atria and ventricles are disassociated. The atria maintain a normal rate, and P waves are present. The ventricular rate is usually between 20 and 40 beats per minute, and the QRS complexes are abnormally shaped, according to the site of origin. There is no measurable P-R interval, since the atria and ventricles are beating independently. Occasionally P waves are difficult to identify, as they are buried within the QRS complex. Although the atria and ventricles beat independently, a regular rhythm is often noted within each. If complete heart block is not corrected it will lead to death. When complete heart block is precipitated by myocardial infarction, pump failure may ensue. Recovery is often limited in the presence of myocardial damage.

## FIRST-LEVEL NURSING CARE

In order to prevent the occurrence of arrhythmias, it is important for the nurse to identify those persons at risk of developing arrhythmias. Elimination of potential stressors which could precipitate alterations in cardiac rhythm must be carefully considered.

Early treatment of all health problems is essential. Many disruptions in oxygenation will require long-term care and management. Until the underlying problems of coronary artery disease (Chap. 26) and hypertension (Chap. 28) and structural problems resulting from rheumatic heart disease (Chap. 27) are corrected, patients with these conditions are always at risk of developing arrhythmias.

Many drugs used in the treatment of cardiac disturbances can also precipitate arrhythmias. Patients receiving medications such as digitalis preparations, sympathomimetic drugs (e.g., epinephrine and isoproterenol), quinidine, and lidocaine should be observed closely for arrhythmias. These drugs can depress the heart rate (digitalis) or stimulate it (isoproterenol) and lead to the development of tachycardia or ectopic beats or even to death. Health teaching is essential for patients taking these drugs outside the acute-care setting. The nurse should be sure that the patient is familiar with all drugs and encourage them to report all side effects early.

Hormonal problems such as hyperthyroidism and electrolyte imbalances (sodium, calcium, and potassium) should be treated and corrected as soon as possible. Patients taking diuretics, especially with digitalis preparations, should be observed often for electrolyte imbalances.

Overeating, eating large meals quickly, and high ingestion of caffeine and nicotine have been cited as precipitants of rhythm disturbances. Patients, especially those with oxygenation problems, should avoid drinking large amounts of coffee, tea, or cola drinks. In addition, they should avoid smoking. The public at large should be taught a well-balanced diet and be encouraged to avoid large meals or eating too quickly.

It has been noted that some arrhythmias have a familiar tendency. Among these are paroxysmal tachycardia, junctional tachycardia, atrial fibrillation, sinus tachycardia, and multifocal premature contractions. A careful family history should therefore include questions related to the incidence and types of arrhythmias noted in family members.

Anesthetics are also cardiac depressants and

may lead to the development of arrhythmias. Older patients or patients sensitive to the anesthetic being used should be observed for arrhythmias. Emphasis should be placed on the patient's psychological status, since stress and tension are important in the development of arrhythmias. When a person has a high degree of anxiety, tranquilizers, as well as counseling may help reduce the tension. Occupational demands can also cause much stress. If this is severe, a change in position may be required. Sociocultural components of the patient's background should be part of the health assessment and should be evaluated accordingly.

## SECOND-LEVEL NURSING CARE

Few patients are treated initially in the community for an arrhythmia. The discussion of this level of care, therefore, focuses on early identification of an arrhythmia and referral to an appropriate acute-care setting.

### Nursing Assessment

Patients who are having arrhythmias often seek medical attention for other health problems. When changes in cardiac rate and rhythm are noted, a careful health history and physical examination must be performed.

**Health history** In an initial health history, a family history of cardiac problems and arrhythmias, as well as a list of current medications, should be elicited. The patient may complain of palpitations, a "lump in the throat," the feeling of the heart "skipping a beat," dizziness, fainting, fatigue, shortness of breath, and chest pain. "Spells" often described by elderly patients should be investigated, as these could be periods when the patient has experienced a major cardiac arrhythmia.

The health history should be used as a point of reference for the nurse to evaluate other physiologic changes when assessing the presence of cardiac arrhythmias. The psychological status of the patient should be examined, with particular attention to the personality, ways of handling stress, anxiety level, significant stressors such as a death in the family or loss of a job, and any previous causal relation between psychological stress and development of arrhythmia.

**Physical assessment** The physical assessment should include auscultation of the heart (see Chap. 22), with careful evaluation of the regularity of rate,

rhythm, and quality of the heartbeat. Assessment of the first heart sound demonstrates variation in its intensity. Determination of the point of maximum impulse (PMI) and the left border of cardiac dullness will provide information about heart size. Peripheral pulses (discussed in Chap. 29) can be checked and their rate, rhythm, and quality compared to the apical pulse. Pulse deficits should be noted. The blood pressure is an essential part of the cardiovascular assessment. The patient's neurologic status should be evaluated, since some arrhythmias are first identified when manifestations of central nervous system disorders become apparent. Tremors, gait problems, and changes in sensorium should be closely evaluated to determine whether they might be caused by a clinical disorder of the heartbeat.

**Diagnostic tests** The *electrocardiogram* (EKG) is the most effective diagnostic tool for evaluating cardiac muscle conduction. Chapter 22 offers a complete discussion of the EKG and its function in demonstrating cardiac rhythm.

*Echocardiography* provides another diagnostic measurement especially helpful in valvular problems as well as in failure. Here a unidirectional probe is used to pick up inaudible pulses and amplify the sound (or echo), displaying the electrical potential on an oscilloscope. Evaluation of the recordings aids in the diagnosis of special problems which under ordinary circumstances cannot be fully assessed. Other, more sophisticated, testing of electrical cardiac potential would be completed in the hospital setting.

Blood electrolytes are checked to evaluate blood, calcium, and potassium levels. $T_3$ and $T_4$ are checked when thyroid disturbances are suspected. If digitalis toxicosis is suspected, blood levels can be checked to assess the amount of digitalis present in the circulation.

### Nursing Problems and Interventions

Sinus arrhythmias may be treated in the community. Uncomplicated sinus bradycardia and sinus tachycardia are often controlled on an outpatient basis. Paroxysmal tachycardia and occasionally premature ventricular contractions may also be treated in the community, but most arrhythmias are initially treated in the hospital. Until the cause of the problem can be clearly identified, careful patient screening and evaluation should take place in the acute-care setting. For this reason, all nursing problems and interventions related to arrhythmias are discussed under Third-Level Nursing Care.

### THIRD-LEVEL NURSING CARE

Arrhythmias usually imply a serious health problem requiring care in an acute-care setting. While some arrhythmias, such as sinus arrhythmias, may occur in the community, the more severe rhythm changes usually accompany major cardiac problems. This presentation first discusses care of acute arrhythmias in general, then the specific therapies for each arrhythmia.

### Nursing Assessment

An arrhythmia may have varying clinical symptoms. Careful health history and physical assessment are essential to measure the overall effects of these changes.

**Health history** Patients experiencing arrhythmias often have cardiac problems associated with rhythm change. Frequently a myocardial infarction is the precipitating factor; however, anesthesia, medications, hyperthyroidism, valve replacement, and pump failure may contribute to development of arrhythmia. The patient often complains of palpitations, feeling as though the heart is "skipping a beat." On occasion these symptoms are accompanied by generalized weakness, syncope, precordial tightness and pain, confusion, and restlessness. The uncomfortable sensations often make patients anxious and fearful, and emotional stress may intensify the rhythm changes. Vomiting and nausea may accompany arrhythmias, especially in the presence of digitalis toxicosis and myocardial infarction. Decreased attention span and memory loss may also be reported.

The patient should be asked about activities that preceded the rhythm change. Exercise must be evaluated as to amount and type, and fatigue should be considered. Ingestion of a large meal and use of coffee, tea, cola drinks, tobacco, drugs, and alcohol must be assessed and evaluated.

The onset of the more serious arrhythmias is often sudden. Such actions as brushing the teeth or washing the face can simulate a ventricular fibrillation–like pattern on the monitor. All arrhythmias should always be evaluated in the light of physical findings.

Assessment of the patient's type of employment is another important component of this evaluation. Stressors precipitated by occupation may contribute to arrhythmias, especially if other cardiac problems exist. Social obligations should also be incorporated into the assessment and evaluated as a component of the patient's total profile.

**Physical assessment** In addition to the parameters examined in Second-Level Nursing Care, an accurate assessment of the apical rate is of critical importance. Evaluation should be based on the rate, rhythm, and quality of the pulse. Each assessment should last for one full minute or longer. In addition, pauses should be noted, as well as intermittence of pulse beat. The *quality* may not be strong and rebounding, especially in the presence of pump failure. There may also be a *pulse deficit—* i.e., a diminished peripheral pulse (Chap. 24)—in the presence of pump failure. Dyspnea may also accompany pump failure.

When failure occurs, there may be altered heart sounds (see Chap. 24), including a wide splitting of heart sounds with gallop (S₃) sounds.[6]

*Blood pressure* may also be affected by changes in pulse rate. Slowed heart rate will lead to decreased cardiac output, and blood pressure may drop as a result. Urinary output may also diminish.

*Respirations* are usually normal except in the presence of failure. The appearance of basilar rales is an early indication of this problem.

With life-threatening arrhythmias there may be an absence of apical and peripheral pulses, inaudible blood pressure, syncope, cyanosis, low level of consciousness leading to coma, dilated pupils, and anoxia which may lead to respiratory arrest and seizures. Body reflexes also diminish.

**Diagnostic tests** *Electrocardiographic* changes distinguish the sinus, atrial, and ventricular arrhythmias and conduction disturbances. Arrhythmias present alterations in the rate, rhythm, and quality of pulse and show alterations on EKG reading. Regularity of the rhythm is disrupted, and changes are seen in the P, QRS, and T complexes, depending on the location of the conduction disturbance.

Levels of triglyceride and other enzymes, such as the serum transaminases are elevated in the presence of myocardial damage (see Chap. 26).

*Thyroid levels* should be evaluated for hyperthyroidism in the presence of atrial flutter and fibrillation or sinus tachycardia.

### Nursing Problems and Interventions

The major problem is the arrhythmia itself. As a result of this condition the patient usually experiences dyspnea, weakness, syncope, pain, nausea and vomiting, restlessness, and anxiety.

The use of antiarrhythmic drugs (see Table 25-1) is the most common intervention used to control arrhythmias. These drugs can slow or speed up the heart rate, block ectopic foci (irritable foci), enhance conduction through the system, improve the quality of myocardial contraction and increase the force of expulsion, and depress or stimulate cardiac contractility. Specific arrhythmias will require additional interventions, which are discussed below.

**Monitoring** Patients with changes in cardiac rhythm will require monitoring. Monitors are used to obtain a continuous picture of the electrical activity of the heart. In the presence of arrhythmias, monitoring allows the nurse and the physician to view the changes that develop within the conduction system and provide for prompt termination of rhythm disturbances.

The leads or wires attached to the patient's body surface provide the pattern observed on the monitor (*oscilloscope*). There are two recording leads, usually placed on the chest wall, in addition to a third lead called a *ground.* The ground can be placed at any comfortable site not close to the two recording leads (see Fig. 25-14). The purpose of the ground is to limit electrical interference from extraneous current leakage within the environment. It is important that the leads not be placed directly over a muscle, since some muscles such as the pectoral muscles, as well as breast tissue, contain electric potential which could interfere with EKG recording.

Whenever monitoring equipment is to be used, its purpose should be explained to the patient and the various components of the devices (such as the alarm system) discussed. The sites of the electrodes should be cleansed and rubbed with alcohol, to reduce skin resistance and enhance electrical transmission. A paste or jelly may then be applied along with the electrode secured to the skin. A heavy growth of chest hair may interfere with conduction and should therefore be shaved. Electrodes should be changed as needed, depending on the type being utilized.

It should be noted that the cardiac monitor is only one device available to detect changes in the patient's cardiac status. Each patient being monitored should be assessed continuously for changes in vital signs, level of consciousness, color, etc. Support and explanation will be required to help alleviate fears and anxieties about monitoring, and

the nurse can provide this information to the patient and the family members.

**Dyspnea** Dyspnea often accompanies arrhythmias, especially in the presence of diminished cardiac output. It may be an early sign of pump failure, secondary to ischemia or altered circulation. Alterations in $PCO_2$ and $PO_2$ levels due to disruptions in the pumping mechanism can induce it. Pain (angina), activity, and emotional stress can also enhance respiratory difficulties. Restlessness, in the presence of cerebral anoxia, will contribute to shortness of breath, as will exertion.

Administration of nasal oxygen (3 to 6 liters) will increase the amount of circulating oxygen. This will elevate the $O_2$ level in the brain tissue and bring additional oxygen to myocardial tissue. Drugs such as digitalis preparations (see Chap. 24) and diuretics will relieve pump failure and reduce the dyspneic state. An upright position such as sitting in a chair may ease respiratory distress. If pump failure is present, passive exercise and other nonstressful activities should be encouraged.

**Syncope** Dizziness, weakness, and fainting are often associated with a decreased cardiac rate and slowed cerebral circulation. This is observed in sinus bradycardia and Stokes-Adams syndrome (complete heart block). Stimulation of the SA rate and improved conduction through the AV node can be achieved through drugs such as atropine and isoproterenol (see Table 25-1). Mask oxygen will increase the blood $O_2$ level, thereby increasing the supply of nutrients to the tissue. Patients with syncope should be told why the problem exists and should be protected from fall or injury during periods of dizziness.

**Pain** In the presence of a myocardial infarct or coronary artery ischemia (see Chap. 26), pain may become severe. Unrelated cardiac pain can be stressful for the patient and can induce an arrhythmia by stimulating the release of epinephrine which can be irritating to a damaged myocardium. Analgesia (see Chap. 39) and reduction of stress can help alleviate pain, as can an increased oxygen supply to ischemic coronary arteries. Overexertion should be avoided, and frequent position change may increase the patient's overall comfort.

**Anxiety** Stress can lead to arrhythmias because of the potential adrenal stimulation and release of catecholamines. Premature beats occurring in response to stress unrelated to cardiac problems

**TABLE 25-1**
ANTIARRHYTHMIC DRUGS

| Drug | Administration | Pharmacologic Effects | Indications | Contraindications | Toxic Effects |
|---|---|---|---|---|---|
| Lidocaine (Xylocaine) | IV: Bolus, 1–2 mg/kg infused over 30 s; drip; 60–200 mg/h (1–4 mg/min) | Increases threshold for stimulation of ventricles during diastole, depresses automaticity of His-Purkinje fibers | Ventricular arrhythmias, PVCs, ventricular tachycardia, prevention of arrhythmias after countershock | History of hypersensitivity to local anesthetics; severe AS, AV, intraventricular block | Depression of AV conduction, hypotension, dizziness, drowsiness, convulsions, coma |
| Procainamide (Pronestyl) | po 250–500 mg q4h, IM 0.5–1 g q6h, IV 0.2–1 g in diluent given 25–50 mg/min | Depresses myocardial metabolism, reduces atrial excitability, and increases threshold to electrical stimuli; has anticholinergic action | Ventricular arrhythmias, PVC, ventricular tachycardia, supraventricular arrhythmias (generally less effective than quinidine) | Hypotension, complete AV block, bundle branch block, severe cardiovascular damage and shock, allergies | Lupus erythematosis-like syndrome (polyarthritis, pleuritic pain, pericarditis), depression of myocardial contractility, hypotension, rashes, anorexia, nausea and vomiting, transient psychoses |
| Quinidine sulfate | Dosage for conversion to normal sinus rhythm: 0.3 g five times/day to 0.6 g qid po; maintenance dose po 0.3 g qid; IM 0.4 g, IV 0.3–0.8 g for emergency treatment | Depresses myocardial contractility, inhibits generation and maintenance of action potential and vagolytic effect (i.e., reduces vagal tone) | Conversion of atrial flutter and atrial fibrillation to normal sinus rhythm; treatment of atrial, functional, and ventricular premature beats; maintenance of normal sinus rhythm after conversion from atrial flutter and atrial fibrillation | Partial or complete A-V block, bundle branch block, hypotension, hypersensitivity to drug, digitalis intoxication and hyperkalemia; administer with caution in congestive heart failure. | Dizziness, nausea and vomiting, diarrhea, tinnitus, blurred vision, thrombocytopenia, fever, rash, depression of atrial activity, ventricular arrhythmias |
| Propranolol (Inderal) | po 10–30 mg 3–8 times/day; IV 1–5 mg slowly (may be repeated in 2 minutes) | Beta-adrenergic blocking agent resulting in reversal of sympathetic effects present; decreases sinus rate, decreases AV conduction velocity, lengthens AV junctional refractory period, decreases ventricular irritability | Selected cases of sinus tachycardia (due to pheochromocytoma, thyrotoxicosis, or severe anxiety), supraventricular tachycardias associated with Wolff-Parkinson-White syndrome, ventricular arrhythmias not responsive to other antiarrhythmic agents | Slow heart rate, second-degree and complete AV block, cardiogenic shock, congestive heart failure, bronchial asthma | Slow ventricular rate (bradycardia), aggravation or precipitation of congestive heart failure, sudden depression of ventilatory function |
| Diphenylhydantoin sodium (Dilantin) | po 200–400 mg daily for maintenance, IV 3.5–5 mg/kg body weight | Lowers myocardial threshold for stimulation, increases conduction velocity of Purkinje fibers | Digitalis-produced arrhythmias, arrhythmias of obscure origin | Hypotension, severe bradycardia, high degree of AV block, congestive heart failure, hypersensitivity | Hypotension, bradycardia, AV block, prolonged AV conduction, ventricular standstill |
| Atropine | IV 1.8–3 mg; for complete autonomic blockade, 0.04 mg/kg | Increases rate by altering vagal effects on SA node by blocking effects of acetylcholine | Sinus bradycardia (below 50 beats/min) due to increased vagal tone, sinus arrhythmia, SA block, partial AV block due to increased vagal tone, digitalis intoxication | Hypersensitivity to drug, hepatic disease | Difficulty swallowing, disturbed speech, headaches, weak pulse, pupil dilatation, hallucinations, and coma |

are infrequent and are usually not treated. In the presence of cardiac pathology, irritable foci can intensify rhythm change and precipitate serious arrhythmias.

Antiarrhythmic drugs may be given to correct the arrhythmia. In addition, mild tranquilizers, along with emotional counseling, may be used, especially when the patient cannot control the anxiety. Reduction of the use of stimulants such as coffee, tea, cola drinks, and cigarettes may also improve the situation. If hyperthyroidism is present, treatment of this problem will relieve the related rhythm changes. A patient's personality can influence the way stress and anxiety-provoking events are handled. These patterns of stress response should be carefully evaluated and altered when necessary.

**Nausea and vomiting**  Nausea and vomiting can serve as a vagal stimulus and induce a change in heart rhythm. Infection, gastrointestinal problems, and drug toxicosis (digitalis), as well as fluid and electrolyte imbalance and myocardial damage, precipitate rhythm disturbances that in the presence of muscle changes, may lead to sinus bradycardia and ectopic beats. Removal of the stimulus that induces the vomiting, along with antiemetics such as compazine help to correct the problem. Anxiety and stress also potentiate nausea and vomiting and may necessitate a relaxant or mild tranquilizer to ease the distress.

**Specific therapies**  Many of the problems induced by arrhythmias can be alleviated by the interventions mentioned above, but specific therapies for individual arrhythmias are considered separately below.

**S**inus Arrhythmias  In general, sinus arrhythmias respond to interventions such as relief of pain, decreased anxiety, reduction of stress, and correction of a health problem; but in some instances they may lead to more serious problems such as pump failure. In the presence of *carotid sinus syndrome,* the patient should be instructed to avoid constriction about the neck area. Ties or tight collars should be eliminated or closed loosely.

**A**trial Arrhythmias  There are three atrial arrhythmias that require specific treatments: paroxysmal atrial tachycardia, atrial flutter, and atrial fibrillation.

*Paroxysmal atrial tachycardia*  When a patient with paroxysmal atrial tachycardia is hospitalized, the

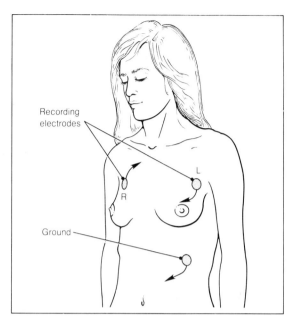

**FIGURE 25-14**
Chest heads.

physician may attempt conversion to a normal sinus rhythm. Often this is done by using some form of *vagal stimulation.* When carotid sinus therapy is planned, the nurse should tell the patient that the physician will press on the carotid area of the neck in an attempt to interrupt the rapid rate and restore the heart to a normal rate. Because of the serious nature of this intervention, the nurse must carefully observe the patient's vital signs as well as other physical changes. The nurse must be ready to institute cardiopulmonary resuscitation should the heart rate slow or the heart stop. Patients should *never* be taught this procedure, as they could accidentally occlude circulation to the brain and cause temporary cerebral anoxia.

Less dangerous forms of vagal stimulation that are used include the Valsalva maneuver, the use of an ice collar around the neck,[7] blowing into a balloon that is difficult to inflate, and pressure on the eyeballs. The *Valsalva maneuver* involves holding the breath and bearing down as if to strain at stool. This increases interthoracic pressure and temporarily slows cardiac intake of blood from outside the chest; when the breath is released, there is a sudden rush of blood into the heart, placing an increased demand on the pump.[8] This activates a vagal response at the SA node, interrupts the tachycardia, and restores a sinus rhythm. Blowing into a balloon that is difficult to inflate is another way to terminate PAT using the above rationale. Eyeball pressure and application of an ice collar to the neck also alter peripheral blood flow and create a vagal response that may interrupt the tachycardia and cause the heart rate to return to normal. Patients may be taught these interventions with physician approval and careful supervision.

*Digitalis* can relieve attacks of PAT by sensitizing the carotid sinus so that carotid sinus pressure will be more effective; it also prolongs the refractory period of atrial muscle, thereby increasing atrioventricular conduction time and slowing the heart rate. *Quinidine* acts to terminate PAT by its ability to increase the refractory period of atrial muscle and decrease the automaticity of ectopic pacemakers. *Procainamide* has an effect similar to that of quinidine and may also be used to treat PAT (see Table 25-1). Patient teaching should focus upon drug therapy and avoiding stimuli which precipitate PAT such as stress, overeating, or fatigue.

When carotid sinus pressure and drug therapy do not correct this arrhythmia, *electric countershock* may be used, particularly when signs of early pump failure are apparent. This procedure, along with appropriate nursing interventions, is discussed under Atrial Fibrillation.

*Atrial pacing* is another mode of therapy used when other treatments have failed. An artificial pacemaker electrode is inserted into the atria and electrical stimulation is delivered to the atrium in an attempt to override the ectopic pacing site within the atria (see discussion under Cardiac Pacing later in the chapter).

*Atrial flutter and atrial fibrillation* Because the atrial rate is the major variant distinguishing atrial flutter from atrial fibrillation, the treatment for these problems is essentially the same. Since atrial fibrillation involves a more rapid heart rate, pump failure is usually a complication.

Digitalis and quinidine are two drugs frequently used in atrial fibrillation, either alone or in conjunction. *Digitalis* is also used to control a rapid ventricular rate. When pump failure is present, digitalis will help improve cardiac output. In both situations, frequent evaluation of the apical pulse is essential. Patients should be told that digitalis therapy is used to control but not cure this abnormality. The patient receiving a digitalis preparation must be observed for toxic side effects, including nausea, vomiting, and visual changes (see Chap. 24).

*Quinidine* may be given to patients in an attempt to convert either atrial flutter or atrial fibrillation to normal sinus rhythm. It eliminates ectopic foci, permitting the SA node to conduct all impulses. Nursing care of patients receiving this drug focuses on the cardiac response, so constant evaluation of the EKG pattern and apical pulse is essential. If conversion to normal sinus rhythm occurs with drug therapy, the time should be noted. Occasionally digitalis and quinidine may be used together to retain the effect of the conversion.

Another mode of treatment for atrial fibrillation is *electrical cardioversion.* In this procedure an electric shock is delivered to the myocardium in order to interrupt or terminate an arrhythmia. An electric current administered through electrodes placed on the chest wall simultaneously depolarizes the electrical conduction system of the heart. It is hoped that the SA node will resume its normal pacing function first and become the pacemaker. This procedure is often performed when there is pump failure or when the patient is not responding to drug therapy. Digitalis may or may not be discontinued before cardioversion is performed. In the presence of digitalis toxicosis, however, it is withdrawn. Antiarrhythmic drugs such as quinidine may be given prior to cardioversion to improve the success of the conversion. Lidocaine can be used if other arrhythmias occur during the procedure. Some physicians give patients with atrial fibrillation anticoagulants to decrease the chance of thrombus release.[9]

The patient is given sedation prior to cardioversion for relaxation and to reduce the stress associated with the procedure. Anesthesia may also be used if necessary. The choice of an anesthetic depends on the clinical status of the patient: diazepam, methohexital, or sodium Pentothol may be used. In most hospitals cardioversion is done either in the patient's hospital room or in the coronary-care unit. A medication such as Valium is given intravenously until adequate sedation is reached. An electric countershock is delivered which will be synchronized with the R wave so that the heart will receive the impulse during ventricular depolarization. This avoids the period of vulnerability at the peak of the T wave when the heart is in a relatively refractory state. More than one shock may have to be given before conversion to normal sinus rhythm is achieved. Usually the current is delivered with 24 to 50 watt-seconds of energy, with increasing strength if the arrhythmia does not convert. In occasional cases of long-standing atrial fibrillation, it may not be possible to convert the arrhythmia to normal sinus rhythm.

Assessment of the patient's level of consciousness and respirations after the procedure is extremely important, since severe respiratory depression may occur after intravenous administration of Valium and other anesthetics. The cardiac status is also closely watched and any changes in rhythm reported promptly. Occasionally a patient's heart rhythm may return to atrial fibrillation after cardioversion.

Teaching is essential for patients receiving this type of therapy. The teaching plan should include a discussion of the procedure itself, why it must be performed, where it is to be done, who will be present, and the type of anesthesia to be used. Some patients may experience a period of confusion following the procedure, and others will report loss of recent memory. Patients should be told that this can happen from the effect of the shock itself and be given support by the nurse to allay fears. Discussion of the experience following the procedure gives the patient an opportunity to ask questions about the cardioversion.

When quinidine therapy is continued following elective cardioversion, patients should be taught the importance of continuing this therapy and reporting any symptoms which may indicate drug toxicosis. If patients were receiving digitalis prior to cardioversion, the nurse should be alert to any signs or symptoms of digitalis toxicosis, since a return to normal sinus rhythm will improve cardiac output and decrease the need for cardiac glycosides. In some instances the use of digitalis preparations may be continued following cardioversion.

**V**entricular Arrhythmias  Ventricular arrhythmias requiring specific therapy include premature ventricular contractions, ventricular tachycardia, and ventricular fibrillation. These are all potentially life-threatening arrhythmias and without prompt treatment can result in death.

*Premature ventricular contractions*  Premature ventricular contractions (PVC) require immediate treatment, especially when they follow a myocardial infarction. If not treated, PVCs can lead to more serious arrhythmias such as ventricular tachycardia. The occurrence of six or more PVCs per minute necessitates the use of antiarrhythmic drugs. The medications most frequently ordered to treat PVCs are lidocaine (Xylocaine), procainamide (Pronestyl), quinidine sulfate, and diphenylhydantoin (Dilantin). They are usually administered intravenously so that their action will be immediate. Accurate recording and reporting of the occurrence of premature ventricular contractions and their treatment is essential. Table 25-1 lists the variety of antiarrhythmic drugs available, indications for use, and intended

as well as toxic effects. A thorough understanding of these drugs is critical if the nurse is to appropriately measure their effect on patients. It should be noted that in the presence of anxiety, a mild tranquilizer may be used to decrease stress and the potential catecholamine effects.

Patients also need to become involved in eliminating controllable stimuli leading to the formation of premature beats. Smoking should be decreased if not eliminated, as the nicotine can stimulate PVCs. Caffeine found in coffee, tea, cola drinks, and cocoa must be evaluated separately and eliminated from the diet if necessary; Sanka or other caffeine-free substitutes may be utilized.

Patients need to be cautioned against eating large meals, which stimulate the development of PVCs. While considering these interventions, both the nurse and the patient need to explore those stress-producing situations which predispose the individual to premature beats. Families also need to be counseled to help reduce stressful events.

When PVCs are noted, the patient should be hooked up to a monitor and observed frequently. Vital signs should be carefully assessed and rhythm strips analyzed. When PVCs increase to more than six per minute, treatment should be started immediately. The patient should be told why the monitor is being used and when it will be discontinued, to avoid unnecessary dependence on the machinery.

*Ventricular tachycardia*  Ventricular tachycardia is considered a *medical emergency.* The mode of treatment used will depend on the type and duration of the tachycardia. If antiarrhythmic medications are ordered, the nurse should administer them at the onset of the arrhythmia. Direct-current electric countershock (see Ventricular Fibrillation) using 100 to 400 volts (or joules) may be needed to correct the arrhythmia. In some instances a blow to the precordium (the anterior surface of the lower part of the thorax) can successfully terminate this arrhythmia; but its possible use should be discussed with the medical staff, since it may also precipitate ventricular fibrillation.

Continuous *reassessment* of the patient's vital signs is essential to effective nursing care. After the arrhythmia is corrected it can easily return, especially if the precipitating cause is not eliminated. Ventricular tachycardia can quickly lead to ventricular fibrillation, which, if not immediately terminated, can cause death.

*Ventricular fibrillation*  Ventricular fibrillation will result in death if not terminated promptly. In the absence of vital signs, resuscitative measures should begin immediately. A lag of time in restoring effective circulation beyond 3 to 4 minutes results in impaired circulation to vital organs. (See Chap. 26 for complete cardiopulmonary resuscitation procedure.) When a patient is successfully resuscitated, the nurse must continue to observe the monitor pattern for signs of ventricular irritability and administer antiarrhythmic drugs as ordered. Patients who have had an episode of ventricular fibrillation must be carefully observed.

*Defibrillation* involves the delivery of asynchronized shock to the chest in an effort to interrupt ventricular fibrillation. The number of volts (or joules) used varies with the physician and the degree of success in converting the arrhythmia. Some arrhythmias are more difficult to convert and require higher voltage, others lower: some ventricular arrhythmias can be corrected with 50 joules, while others require 400.

Often this is an emergency situation with no chance to prepare the patient. The patient may be unconscious. An intravenous catheter is usually inserted, so that additional antiarrhythmic drugs can be rapidly given along with sodium bicarbonate. Two paddles connected to a defibrillator are used to deliver the shock. The paddles are lubricated *well* with a special salt-base paste in order to protect the skin from burning and improve the conduction of the electric current. One paddle is placed over the right sternal border, the other at the apex of the heart. The current delivered may have to be increased and redelivered should the patient not respond.

It is important to turn off all other electrical equipment that may be functioning prior to ventricular defibrillation, in order to reduce electrical hazards. Personnel standing at the bedside should be told to stand back prior to administration of the shock.

Since recurrence of ventricular fibrillation within a 24-hour period is frequent, careful assessment and continued evaluation of the patient is critical. Often signs of hypovolemia occur which affect resuscitative efforts and lead to continuing conduction problems and eventual death.

**C**onduction Defects  The effects of heart block range from mild problems to life-threatening consequences necessitating the use of pacing devices.

*First-degree heart block*  When a patient is found to have first-degree heart block, the nurse should find out whether the patient is taking digitalis, as this altered rhythm may indicate digitalis toxicosis (see Chap. 26). Depending on the physician, the use of this drug may be terminated. In general, first-degree heart block does not require any specific nursing care. If first-degree heart block occurs suddenly in a patient with organic heart disease, it may be a precursor of a more serious conduction defect, and the monitor pattern must be watched closely. The *pulse rate, vital signs, chest pain,* and *mental status* should be carefully evaluated. Accurate check of urinary output is also important. A decrease in output can increase toxic levels of digitalis by preventing its adequate excretion. Diuresis can alter electrolyte balance and potentiate the action of digitalis.

*Second-degree heart block*  When second-degree heart block is present, both treatment and nursing care will depend on the severity of the block and the underlying organic heart problem. The major intervention will be a *slowing* of the pulse rate. Patients receiving antiarrhythmic drugs (see Table 25-1) should be observed for any signs that the heart block is responding to medication. Atropine is given to reduce the block and improve cardiac output. (It should be noted that if atropine is used in the patient with glaucoma, pilocarpine 2% should be instilled into each eye every 6 hours to prevent further eye damage.) A return to normal conduction will be evidenced by increased pulse rate and improved cardiac function.

Patients with more severe forms of second-degree heart block should be observed for the development of syncopal attacks or other signs of impending complete heart block, as well as pump failure and hypotension. Frequently a pacemaker will be inserted to maintain the heart rate within normal limits (see Cardiac Pacing).

*Complete heart block (third-degree block)*  When a patient develops complete heart block, monitoring should be initiated immediately. Although medications are rarely able to convert third-degree (complete) heart block to a normal sinus rhythm, atropine may be given to reduce vagal tone and accelerate the ventricular rate. During this time the nurse should observe the monitor pattern for any changes in the rate. Vital signs need to be continually assessed and developing pump failure monitored. In most instances a *pacemaker* is inserted temporarily (see Cardiac Pacing). Figure 25-15 shows a graphic representation of complete heart block. Note the regularity of the rate and absence of a conducted P wave. Figure 25-16 shows the same rhythm after the insertion of a pacemaker. Note the pacing line shown; it represents the SA node action and initiates a ventricular response.

*Cardiac pacing*   Cardiac pacing is used to initiate the heartbeat by means of electrical stimulation in the absence of proper conduction from a functioning SA-AV node. Two types of pacemaker units may be used by the patient requiring direct electrical stimulation of the myocardium: external pacemakers and internal pacemakers. The *external pacemaker* unit (see Fig. 25-17) is a self-contained battery pack with terminals to which pacing electrodes are attached. The unit may be secured to the patient's arm, where the controls are readily available. If the patient is ambulatory, the external pacemaker (Fig. 25-18) may be worn on a belt around the waist. This unit is used for *temporary pacing.* The *internal pacemaker* unit is a small, self-contained battery pack that is surgically implanted in a subcutaneous pocket under the breast, near the clavicle, or in the abdominal region. It is used for *permanent pacing.* There are several types of internal pacemaker units, including mercury-powered battery cells, lithium-generated cells, and nuclear-powered units.

The pacemaker unit chosen is attached to either an endocardial or an epicardial electrode. *Endocardial electrodes* (Fig. 25-19) used for transvenous pacing are passed into the right side of the heart under fluoroscopy by way of the venous system. When temporary pacing is used, the electrode is inserted through the veins in the antecubital fossa or femoral area. When used for permanent pacing, the subclavian or jugular vein is selected. In both cases, the electrode is advanced until the tip reaches the apex of the right ventricle and is wedged under the trabeculae. In an emergency, an endocardial electrode may be passed into the right or left ventricle by inserting it substernally or through the fourth or fifth intercostal space.

*Epicardial electrodes* are surgically implanted on the ventricular wall through a thoracotomy incision (see Chap. 30). They may be implanted during open-heart surgery when the need for postoperative temporary pacing is anticipated. Epicardial electrodes are used less frequently than endocardial electrodes but may be needed if transvenous pacing is ineffective.

*Patient teaching* for either temporary or permanent pacemaker units should begin as soon as the physician decides on this mode of treatment. The nurse should tell the patient why the pacemaker is needed and how it will be inserted. Patient teaching

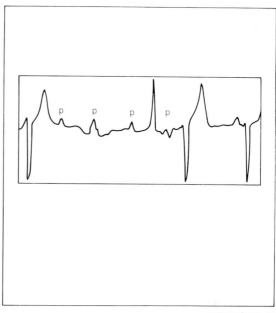

**FIGURE 25-15**
Complete heart block before pacing.

will depend on the amount of time the nurse has to prepare the patient, since insertion of the pacing unit may be an emergency procedure. When time permits, the nurse should give the patient a brief explanation of how the heart functions. A description of how cardiac conduction has been altered by

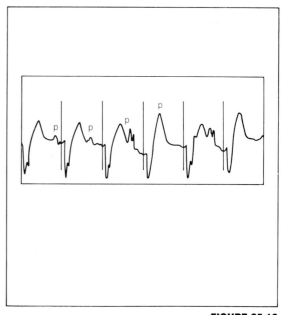

**FIGURE 25-16**
Complete heart block after pacing.

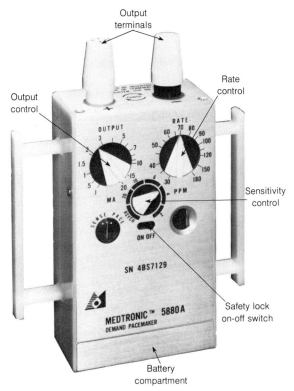

Output terminals

Output control

Rate control

Sensitivity control

Safety lock on-off switch

Battery compartment

**FIGURE 25-17**
External pacemaker unit. (*Courtesy of Medtronic Inc., Minneapolis.*)

a particular conduction defect may also be included. The amount and depth of information included in the teaching plan will depend on the nurse's assessment of the patient's interest and ability to learn. When a temporary pacemaker is to be used, the patient should be told about the room in which the procedure will take place and the fluoroscopic and monitoring equipment. The patient should also be told that there will be nurses and physicians present during the insertion of the pacemaker and that the patient will be awake. If a pacemaker unit is available, it should be shown to the patient. Additional nursing care during the period following pacemaker insertion will depend in part on whether a fixed-rate asynchronous pacemaker or a demand pacemaker has been used.

The *fixed-rate pacemaker* is set to stimulate the ventricles to contract at a preset rate and will continue to do so until the batteries fail, regardless of the metabolic demands of the body. This mode of pacing is not often used, because it suppresses normally conducted beats and precludes a return to normal sinus rhythm. In some instances a fixed-rate pacemaker has been found to compete with a nor-

mal sinus rhythm. This situation can lead to ventricular fibrillation if a pacemaker impulse occurs during the vulnerable period of ventricular repolarization (see Chap. 22).

*Demand pacemakers* are used more often because they stimulate ventricular contraction when beats originating in the sinoatrial node are unable to be conducted through the atrioventricular junction to the ventricles. The pacemaker will fire when the patient's own heart rate falls below a preset level and will continue to pace without interruption until the patient's heart is again able to beat at a rate higher than the preset level.

While caring for a patient with a fixed-rate pacemaker, the nurse should be sure that every QRS complex seen on the cardiac monitor is preceded by a pacemaker artifact. If it is not, the physician should be promptly notified, since this change may indicate either a malfunctioning of the pacemaker unit or failure of the pacing electrode to make constant contact with the ventricular wall. When a demand pacemaker is used, the nurse must evaluate the apical pulse as well as the pattern on the cardiac monitor. Occasionally competition between the patient's own heartbeat and the pacemaker will occur. If a normal sinus beat or a premature ventricular contraction is noted, this should be reported at once and the patient observed closely. Ventricular fibrillation may occur if a pacemaker stimulus occurs during the vulnerable period of the cardiac cycle. The pulse should be maintained at or above the rate at which the demand pacemaker has been set. A pacemaker artifact will not be seen on the cardiac monitor unless the normal heart rate falls below the preset level. If the nurse finds that the patient's pulse has fallen below the preset level, the physician should be notified.

In addition to these signs of pacemaker malfunction, the patient may also complain of weakness, dizziness, and fainting—the same symptoms experienced prior to pacemaker insertion. Since *displacement of the endocardial electrode* is frequent during the first few days following pacemaker insertion, the patient's movement in bed may be moderately restricted during that time. Patients who have an external transvenous pacemaker must be *protected from electrical hazards,* since the pacing electrode which comes out through the skin provides a direct pathway to the heart. Thus any escape of electric current could reach the heart and cause ventricular fibrillation. All equipment in the room should be properly grounded and routinely checked for current leakage. The electrodes attached to the output terminals of the pacemaker unit should be insulated. Frequently a light-colored rubber glove is used for this purpose. The nurse should also watch for any signs of *thrombophlebitis* or infection at the site of entry of the transvenous pacing catheter and report any signs of an *elevated systemic temperature.* Precautionary measures of cleansing the arm daily with an antiseptic soap and applying an antibiotic ointment and sterile dressing to the catheter site are encouraged.

*Prevention of displacement or breakage of the catheter* is another important aspect of nursing care. The patient should be instructed to limit movement of the arm in which the pacing electrode has been placed, and an arm board should be used to immobilize the patient's elbow. When the need for a pacemaker is only temporary, the nurse should assess the patient's emotional state and psychological dependence on the pacemaker so that adequate support can be given during the weaning process. Constant evaluation of the monitor pattern is also important, particularly after the pacemaker is discontinued.

*Permanent pacemakers*  The majority of patients who have a temporary pacemaker will eventually need a permanent one. Nursing care prior to insertion of a permanent pacemaker should include a complete explanation of the reason a permanent pacemaker is needed. A patient anticipating a cure for the heart problem following the insertion of a temporary pacemaker may need much emotional support upon learning that a permanent pacing device is needed. Routine preoperative teaching is also important and should include a description of the type of surgery needed. Most patients will have an internal pacemaker attached to endocardial electrodes. The battery pack will be placed under the breast in women and beneath the clavicle or under the axilla in men. Women should be told that if a slightly larger brassiere is worn the battery pack will not be noticeable. If the nurse has a pacemaker model available, the patient should handle it to feel its size and weight. Patients who will have epicardial electrodes implanted on the myocardial wall should be given the same information preoperatively as is provided for patients who have a thoracotomy (see Chap. 30). In addition, they should be told that the battery pack will probably be placed in the anterior abdominal wall (Fig. 25-19).

The *postoperative nursing care* for these patients is the same as for any postoperative patient. Prevention of infection is important. The nurse should check the temperature every 4 hours initially. Proper asepsis is vital. Careful assessment of

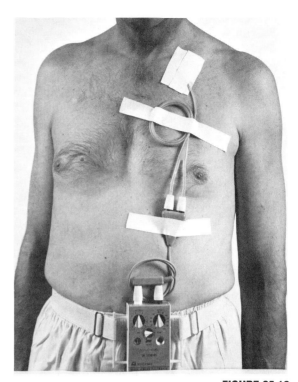

**FIGURE 25-18**
Patient wearing external pacemaker unit. (*Courtesy of Medtronic Inc., Minneapolis.*)

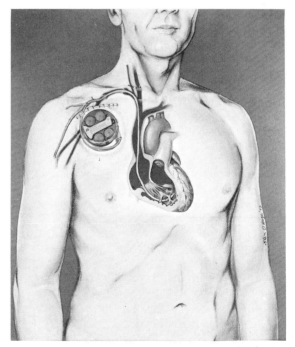

**FIGURE 25-19**
Endocardial pacing. (*Courtesy of Medtronic Inc., Minneapolis.*)

vital signs, along with observation of the functioning pacemaker, is essential. The nurse should also evaluate the patient's attitude toward having a pacemaker, and the emotional reactions discussed openly. If the pacemaker interferes with occupation or employment, a change in jobs and its impact may have to be explored. The patient can be reassured that the pacemaker is safe and that it will allow an increase in activity, although the patient may tire more easily than prior to the onset of the health problem.

With the exception of contact sports, which may damage the pacemaker or dislodge the pacemaker electrode, the patient may resume any *activity*. Such things as swimming, jogging, playing golf and tennis, and sexual activity engaged in prior to surgery can be continued afterward. *Range of motion* of both arms should be promoted, particularly if the patient had a temporary pacemaker with restricted arm movement prior to insertion of the permanent unit. Careful observation of the patient for signs of thrombophlebitis (see Chap. 29) at the site of catheter entry is important. Changes noted should be corrected immediately.

Once the surgical wound is healed, the patient is free to take baths or showers. The teaching plan should indicate that some electrical equipment may affect the functioning of the pacemaker unit. Most pacemakers will malfunction in the presence of microwave ovens. Other types of equipment that may also affect the pacemaker include airport radar, high electrical fields, and large power plant generators. In some instances power lawn mowers and automobile carburetors may also cause pacemaker malfunction. Usually these changes manifest themselves by a change in pulse rate. It the pulse is slowed, the patient may feel dizzy or faint.

Patients should be told the average life span of the pacemaker unit being used and given information about how pacemaker functioning will be evaluated. In some areas patients are taught to take their pulse for one full minute every day and report any irregularities in rate or rhythm. Some physicians believe that this self-evaluation places too much responsibility on the patient and recommend that the patient's pacemaker be evaluated every few months. In order to assess pacemaker effectiveness, a magnet is placed over the pacemaker which is designed to evaluate the state of the batteries. Another method is to place the pacemaker over a radio which is turned on and set at 550 kc. If the pacemaker is functioning properly, it will produce a click before every heartbeat it initiates.

## FOURTH-LEVEL NURSING CARE

Rehabilitation of a patient with an arrhythmia involves identification and elimination of the precipitating cause of the disruption. Frequently correction of the arrhythmia will involve long-term use of such drugs as digitalis and Inderal (see Chap. 26 for a list of potential toxic effects). When other problems such as hyperthyroidism or anxiety are present, additional medication, including mild tranquilizers, may be used. Patients should be taught the necessity of each medication and the importance of compliance. Daily doses must be taken as prescribed in order to eliminate the potential cause of arrhythmias. Families should be taught the importance of the medication and urged to foster compliant behavior.

Elimination of arrhythmia precipitants such as caffeine and nicotine should be stressed. Careful nutritional counseling should also be included and dietary patterns adjusted as needed. Avoiding ingestion of heavy meals should be stressed. Planning meals and developing good eating habits may help reduce the rhythm changes. If obesity is a problem, nutritional counseling and a weight-reduction program will be important components of care.

The patient's life-style and the events which have precipitated previous attacks should also be evaluated. Deep inspiration, hyperventilation, emotional stress, exercise, changes in position, swallowing, and heavy meals have been cited as specific causes.[10] The nurse should attempt to determine whether there is any relation between events such as these and arrhythmias. If such a relation does exist, a plan to alleviate the problems should be developed. The patient can be made aware of those social situations which induce stress. Job-related pressures should be looked at and changed as needed. If the family environment is stressful, the nurse may need to discuss these issues with family members; referral for counseling may be needed.

Activity or lack of it should also be carefully evaluated. In the presence of such conditions as obesity or increased stress, activity may place an added burden on the heart and result in arrhythmia. Patients should be encouraged to engage in activity with moderation. If they find that an activity is too strenuous, they should avoid it.

Patients with organic heart disease who are prone to develop atrial flutter or fibrillation should be advised to seek medical assistance if they experience palpitations or any of the other signs and symptoms associated with these arrhythmias. They should also be taught to keep a record of events preceding the onset of the irregularity to determine specific precipitating factors.

Persons in whom atrial fibrillation occurs spontaneously, should be advised to seek medical care if this rhythm recurs. A patient with a long-standing history of atrial fibrillation should be advised to continue medications as ordered and to keep all heath-care appointments. Patients should be aware of the signs of drug toxicity and report them immediately. The community health nurse who cares for patients with this arrhythmia should be alert for an increase in heart rate, since the cardiac output decreases with rates over 100.

Patients who have had heart surgery, particularly valve replacement, should be assessed for developing signs of atrial flutter or fibrillation. The nurse should also review the patient's record to determine whether either arrhythmia was present prior to surgery.

Although pump failure may be present prior to the development of either atrial flutter or atrial fibrillation, it may also be a sequela of the arrhythmia. Consequently, nursing care must include constant assessment of a patient's respiratory status, which includes evaluation of breath sounds to determine whether specific changes are present. The appearance of bibasilar rales may be an early indication of pulmonary congestion. (See Chap. 24 for a complete discussion of pump failure.)

When recurrent PVCs develop, as a result of organic heart disease, the nurse should teach the patient about arrhythmia and how to identify PVCs when they occur. The patient should be advised to notify a physician if the PVCs suddenly increase in number. Persons with a history of PVCs seen in the community should have an apical pulse checked for several minutes. Increased chest pain should be reported to the physician. The nurse should help the patient to identify events which may precipitate an increase in the frequency of PVCs and to make appropriate modifications in activity.

Patients with varying degrees of heart block should be evaluated accordingly. Usually first-degree block is the only problem seen in the community on a continuing basis. These patients should always be evaluated for signs of digitalis toxicosis.

A heart rate that becomes progressively slower may be a sign that the functioning of the atrioventricular junction is becoming more disrupted. When patients with a history of second-degree heart block are discharged from the hospital, the nurse in the community should check whether the patient is taking the prescribed medication. She should also assess complaints of dizziness or fainting, since patients with second-degree block may develop complete heart block.

Patients in the community with pacemakers require continued follow-up care. Since many persons with pacemakers are elderly, the nurse should be sure that the patient understands what he or she has been told about the pacemaker, how it functions, and what can be done when signs or symptoms of battery failure occur. The nurse should observe the patient taking the radial pulse and check to be sure it is correct. Patients should be able to travel if they desire, as long as health providers are informed prior to departure. If a lengthy trip is planned, patients should be given the names of physicians to contact should the need arise. Questions about sexual activity should be answered and patients assured that sexual activity may be resumed without danger to cardiac function. Sudden failure of the pacemaker requires return to the hospital. In this circumstance the heart rhythm may revert to the prepacemaker level, so the danger of cardiac standstill is minimized. The patient's family should be included in teaching sessions and be reassured that a person with a pacemaker can continue to lead a productive life.

## REFERENCES

1   G. Thorn, R. Adams, E. Braunwald, K. Isselbacher, and R. Petersdorf, *Harrison's Principles of Internal Medicine,* 8th ed., McGraw-Hill, New York, 1977, p. 1187.

2   J. W. Hurst and R. B. Logue, *The Heart,* 3d ed., McGraw-Hill, New York, 1974, p. 525.

3   S. Bellet, *Essentials of Cardiac Arrhythmias,* Saunders, Philadelphia, 1972, p. 109.

4   Hannelore Sweetwood, "Patients with Pacemakers," *Nursing '77,* **7**(3):47, March 1977.

5   Bellet, op. cit., p. 126.

6   Hurst and Logue, op. cit., p. 523.

7   Bellet, op. cit., p. 109.

8   G. Whipple, M. Peterson, V. Haines, E. Learner, and E. McKinnon, *Acute Coronary Care,* Little, Brown, Boston, 1972, p. 129.

9   Ibid., p. 294.

10   Bellet, op. cit., p. 103.

## BIBLIOGRAPHY

### Books

Bergerson, B. S.: *Pharmacology In Nursing,* 13th ed., Mosby, St. Louis, 1976.

Bilitch, M.: *A Manual of Cardiac Arrhythmias,* Little, Brown, Boston, 1971.

Furman, S., and D. Escher: *Principles and Techniques of Cardiac Pacing,* Harper & Row, New York, 1970.

Goldman, M. S.: *Principles of Electrocardiography,* 8th ed., Lange Medical Publications, Los Altos, Calif., 1973.

Kernicki, B. R., and J. Matthews: *Cardiovascular Nursing,* Putnam, New York, 1970.

Marriott, H. S.: *Practical Electrocardiography,* Williams & Wilkins, Baltimore, 1971.

McFarland, M. B.: *Interpreting Cardiac Arrhythmias: A Basic Guide,* Springer, New York, 1975.

Phillips, R., and M. K. Feeney: *The Cardiac Rhythms: A Systematic Approach to Interpretation,* Saunders, Philadelphia, 1973.

Sanderson, R. G.: *The Cardiac Patient,* Saunders, Philadelphia, 1972.

Shamroth, L.: *An Introduction to Electrocardiology,* Blackwell Scientific Publications, Edinburgh, 1971.

Zalis, E. G., and M. H. Conover: *Understanding Electrocardiography,* Mosby, St. Louis, 1972.


### Periodicals

Bain, B.: "Pacemakers and the People who Need Them," *Am J Nurs,* **71:**1582–1585, August 1971.

Barold, S. S.: "Modern Concepts of Cardiac Pacing," *Heart and Lung,* **2:**238–251, March–April, 1973.

Belling, D. I.: "Nursing Care of Patients with Mechanical Cardiac Pacemakers," *Nurs Clin North Am,* **7:**509–515, September 1972.

Butler, H. H.: "How to Read an ECG—Part I," *R.N.* Vol. 36, Jan. 1973, p. 35–45.

Butler, H. H.: "How to Read an ECG—Part II," *RN* **36:**49–61, February 1973.

Butler, H. H.: How to Read an ECG: Part III," *RN,* **36:** 50–59, March 1973.

Cortes, T. S.: "Pacemakers Today," *Nurs '74,* **4:**22–29, February 1974.

Culbert, P., and B. Kos: "Teaching Patients about Pacemakers," *Am J Nurs,* **71:**523–527, March 1971.

Foster, Sue: "Pump Failure," *Am J Nurs,* **74:**1830–1834, October 1974.

Fowler, N. O.: "Sinus Tachycardia: How To Identify Common Causes," *Consultant,* vol. 12, March, 1972.

Gans, J. A.: "Cardiac Drugs Today: Part 4, Antiarrhythmias," *Nurs '73,* **3:**29–34, August 1973.

Hochberg, H. M.: "Effects of Electrical Current on Heart Rhythm," *Am J Nurs,* **71:**1390–1394, July 1971.

Kleiger, R. E., and G. Wolff: "Indications and Contraindications for Cardioversion for Arrhythmias," *Heart and Lung,* **2:**552–560, July–August 1973.

Mayer, G. G., and P. B. Kaelin: "Arrhythmias and Cardiac Output," *Am J Nurs,* **2:**1597–1600, September 1972.

Mond, H., D. Grant, R. McDonald, and S. Graeme: "Telephone Pacemaker Clinic: Transmission of the Pacemaker Artifact and Peripheral Pulse," *Heart and Lung,* **2:**253–259, March–April, 1973.

Meehan, M.: "EKG Primer: A Programmed Instruction Unit," *Am J Nurs,* **71:**2195, November 1971.

Miller, R. R., et al.: "Procainamide: Reappraisal of an Old Antiarrhythmic Drug," *Heart and Lung,* **2:** 277–283, March–April 1973.

Pinneo, R.: "Cardiac Monitoring," *Nurs Clin North Am,* **7:**457–467, September 1972.

Shinn, A. F., D. N. Collins, and Ellen J. Hoops: "Drug Interactions of Common Arrhythmias: CCU Medications," *Am J Nurs,* **74:**1442–1446, August 1974.

Williams, C.: "The CCU Nurse Has a Pacemaker," *Am J Nurs,* **72:**900–902, May 1972.

# 26
# MYOCARDIAL ISCHEMIA

Sue B. Foster

The ability of the pump (myocardium) to meet the many environmental demands placed upon it is dependent on an adequate blood supply. Occlusion of one or more of the coronary blood vessels results in ischemia and infarction of muscle tissue, thereby decreasing myocardial efficiency. The clinical problem that results from these changes is *coronary heart disease,* of which atherosclerotic heart disease, coronary insufficiency, angina pectoris, and myocardial infarction are integral components.

As humans interact with the internal and external environments, variables such as emotional stress, smoking, dietary habits, and inherited predisposition work together to produce changes in cardiac function. This chapter examines coronary heart disease, its causes, the changes it produces, and its effects on the individual.

## CORONARY HEART DISEASE

Coronary heart disease (CHD), also referred to as coronary artery disease (CAD) and ischemic heart disease (IHD), is caused by occlusion of the right or left coronary arteries or both. The occlusion within the arteries creates an imbalance between the oxygen supply available and the overall demands on the heart muscle. This reduction in blood flow to myocardial tissue is called *ischemia.*

In most persons the *underlying* process leading to ischemia and muscle damage involves the formation of fatty plaques in the lining of arterial blood vessels, a process termed *atherogenesis.* Nonatheromatous obstruction of coronary blood vessels can be caused by an embolus, coronary artery spasms, luetic aortitis, or congenital anomalies. The most common cause of reduction in coronary blood flow, however, is *atherosclerosis.*

### Atherosclerotic Heart Disease

Atherosclerotic heart disease (ASHD) is the most common form of CHD. It involves the progressive narrowing of the lumen of coronary blood vessels because of an accumulation of lipids, calcium, fibrous tissue, complex carbohydrates, and blood products in the lining of the arterial wall. These changes can occur in peripheral vessels (see Chap. 29), cerebral blood vessels (see Chap. 34), and coronary blood vessels. Whatever the site of the narrowing, the phases of progressive occlusion are similar.

**Pathophysiology**  The atherosclerotic lesion first observed is fatty streaks or spots which appear as thin lines in the intimal wall. These changes can begin in childhood. Fibrous plaques then develop. These are firm white or grey masses, increasing in size while encroaching on the circumference of the intimal lining. Atheromata or atherosclerotic plaques, characterized by fatty softening, can undergo multiple changes, including ulceration and calcareous deposits. Several major complications can follow atheromata formation, such as luminal narrowing, intramural/intimal hemorrhage, thrombosis, and embolism.[1]

Other theories have been offered for plaque formation, but all theories seem to agree that there is a patchy accumulation of fat, triglycerides, cholesterol, etc., either intracellularly (foam cells) or extracellularly, in the intimal and the inner and medial layers of the arteries. Accumulation of this substance leads to increase in internal thickness and calcification of the vessel. The lumen of the vessel constricts, and changes such as those described above occur.

The degree of narrowing of the arterial lumen is dependent on the size and surface area covered by the plaque formation. This narrowing leads to necrosis, calcification, and vascularization of the plaque. *Intimal hemorrhage* commonly occurs in atheromata. Hemorrhage may cause rupture of the intimal wall and provide a stimulus for thrombus formation. As the atheromatous material leaves the site of rupture and flows into the lumen, it can set the stage for development of an embolism.

When atherosclerotic occlusions occur, under normal conditions collateral circulation develops to meet the heart's nutritional and oxygen demands. Although the actual mechanism of the development of collateral circulation is unknown, the potential for its development seems to exist within each individual. Generally, if collateral circulation is sufficient, there will be no clinical symptoms. It is only when the ischemic myocardium is unable to cope with increased demands that clinical symptoms begin to appear.

The individual may undergo two phases of atherosclerotic changes before the appearance of clinical symptoms: an asymptomatic phase and a symptomatic phase. The *asymptomatic* phase refers to changes due to atherosclerosis that may occur without clinical symptoms; only when an autopsy is performed can changes be noticed. Another group within the asymptomatic classifications are those individuals with pathophysiologic changes due to atherosclerosis who remain symptom-free because of the development of collateral circulation.

The *symptomatic* phase is manifested by the presence of significant clinical symptoms. These include angina (chest pain) and severe occlusion resulting in myocardial infarction. *Angina* is caused by mild ischemia due to temporary or partial occlusion of the coronary artery. *Myocardial infarction* results from a sudden and complete occlusion of one or more coronary arteries or their branches, resulting in irreversible tissue death. Once symptoms occur, the individual clinical course may be one of improvement, stabilization, progressive deterioration, or death. The average mortality rate following entry into the symptomatic phase is 4 percent per year.[2]

**T**heories of Causation  The exact cause of atherogenesis is not known. To date, no single causal factor has been found to entirely explain the process. Many predisposing factors can exist in any individual at a given point in time. These predominant factors and mechanisms may vary and assume importance at different times in a person's life.[3]

Several theories have been formulated to explain atherogenesis. The modern interpretation of the *Virchow-Aschoff lipid infiltration theory* suggests that in response to mechanical or inflammatory trauma to the intimal endothelium, greater than normal amounts of lipids actively enter the endothelium and accumulate in the smooth muscle.[4] The smooth-muscle cells and enzyme systems become ineffective, the lipoproteins are trapped, and damage occurs.[5]

The initial mechanical or inflammatory trauma which sets the stage for the events that follow may be initiated by environmental and physical factors, such as cigarette smoking, emotional stress, automobile driving in congested areas, and elevations of blood pressure. These factors may in turn produce hypoxia, alter membrane permeability, or release catecholamines, kinins, and prostaglandins, which are capable of altering endothelial permeability.[6]

Other theories also help to explain atheromatous complications or the contribution of mechanical factors to atherogenesis. The *thrombogenic theory* attempts to relate atherogenesis to the accumulation of red blood cells, lipids, and platelets in the intima of the arteries. Microthrombi are formed, which become part of the intima. Upon activation, platelets release substances that alter endothelial permeability. A cycle is established in which the thrombus mass extends and the degree of arterial occlusion increases. It is doubtful that thrombogenic theory offers the sole explanation of atherogenesis or that the early development of atherogenesis can be explained by this theory.[7]

The *vascular dynamics theory* emphasizes the importance of mechanical factors in initiating and accelerating atherogenesis. Mechanical factors such as hypertension increase intraluminal pressure, thereby altering endothelial membrane permeability and promoting lipid infiltration, as suggested by the Virchow-Aschoff theory. Atheromatous plaques have a predilection in arteries for areas of bifurcation, tortuosity, and vessel narrowing, as well as areas subject to twisting and bending. In the coronary arteries, plaques are found most commonly in the proximal or epicardial segments of the three main coronary arteries (see Chap. 22).[8]

According to the *capillary hemorrhage theory*, lipids accumulate in phaques as a result of capillary hemorrhage from the vessel lumen or from the vasa vasorum. Obviously, this theory best explains progression, not initiation, of atherogenesis.[9]

The *lipid metabolic theory* suggests that there is a migration of low-density lipoproteins into the arterial wall; these begin to accumulate over time in the internal and medial layers of an artery. Low-density lipoproteins are responsible for transporting cholesterol; thus along with lipoprotein, cholesterol is also being deposited within the vessels.

Additional theories such as the *metabolic theory* suggest that atherosclerotic lesions may be due to the presence of large amounts of lipids because of disruptions in lipid metabolism. The *aging theory*, on the other hand, suggests that atherosclerotic changes occur within everyone's blood vessels to a greater or lesser degree. Occlusive changes occurring in the coronary arteries are therefore an expected part of the aging process. Table 26-1 summarizes the theories of the process of coronary atherogenesis and indicates the section of the artery most often affected.

**C**hanges and Effects of Atherogenesis    Coronary artery disease gradually progresses to acute coronary occlusion and myocardial ischemia. As it does, it can lead to coronary insufficiency, angina, myocardial infarction, and sudden death.

*Angina pectoris*    The process of angina (chest pain) usually reflects widely distributed coronary artery disease. It is a clinical syndrome that results from a disparity between myocardial oxygen demands and the availability of oxygen to the heart. Figure 26-1 depicts the major and minor factors that determine oxygen supply. These factors are highly interactive, and alteration in one group of variables will influence the effectiveness of the other.

Angina represents partial or transient myocardial ischemia. In healthy hearts, 65 to 75 percent of the oxygen in the coronary circulation is extracted by the muscle. Since myocardial oxygen extraction is nearly maximal under normal conditions, increased oxygen demands are met primarily by increasing coronary blood flow. In persons with atherosclerotic coronary arteries, however, the affected coronary vessels are unable to dilate sufficiently in response to metabolic needs.[10] Other factors responsible for compromised coronary blood flow include low blood pressure, low blood volume, arterial vessel spasm, drugs causing vasoconstriction, and aortic stenosis.[11-13] Lowering of the oxygen-carrying capacity of the blood as in anemia and oxyhemoglobin disorders, may also contribute to ischemic states.[14]

The interplay of environmental and psychological factors with these hemodynamic factors may also produce ischemia in persons with heart disease. Anger, fright, exercise, mental tension,

**TABLE 26-1**
SYNTHESIS OF THEORIES OF
CAUSES OF ATHEROGENESIS

| Section of Arterial Wall Affected by Atherogenesis | Mechanisms for Atherogenesis |
|---|---|
| Lumen | Increased hydrostatic pressure<br>Increased entrance of low-density lipoproteins (LDL) and very-low-density lipoproteins (VLDL) into arterial wall<br>Increased platelet adhesiveness and aggregation (clotting)<br>Decreased $O_2$ tension<br>Questionable increase in circulating lipophages |
| Intima | Increased intimal permeability due to hypertension, stasis, mechanical strain, hypoxia, vasoactive substances, injury, or shock<br>Fragmentation or plugging of internal elastic membrane as a result |
| Media | Increased accumulation of lipoproteins intracellularly and extracellularly<br>Increased noxious products from lipoproteins causing damage or cell necrosis<br>Decreased metabolism of smooth muscle cells<br>Altered activity of enzymes associated with metabolism and removal of lipoprotein products<br>Decreased $O_2$ tension<br>Fibrocalcific tissue reaction |
| Adventitia | Decreased lymphatic drainage<br>Decreased vasa vasorum blood supply to outer media and adventitia |

Adapted from G. S. Getz, D. Vesselinovitch, and R. W. Wissler, "A Dynamic Pathology of Atherosclerosis," *Am J Med*, **46**:457, 1969.

sexual intercourse, a heavy meal (*post-prandial angina*), cold weather, smoking, and dreaming (*nocturnal angina*) are examples of extracardiac states that can precipitate increased oxygen consumption or oxygen demand. If the coronary blood vessels are occluded, oxygen supply to the area is decreased. These extracardiac factors create an imbalance between myocardial oxygen supply and demand, and myocardial ischemia, along with anginal pain, results. The cause of the pain is not known. Some research indicates that a chemical irritant such as a polypeptide may be responsible for nerve stimulation. Others attribute pain to the stretching of the coronary blood vessels. This stretching process stimulates the many nerve endings contained within the vessel, and pain results. The afferent fibers of the sympathetic nervous system carry the ischemic pain impulses to the brain. In the brain, the intensity of the pain experienced is subject to a host of modifying factors (see Chap. 39). The pain may be intolerable for some or a minor discomfort for others. Since the pain is often transient, patients with angina often learn to increase their pain tolerance. Partial or temporary myocardial ischemia due to coronary insufficiency may become chronic and more intense with time.

*Myocardial infarction* At some point, ischemic intracellular changes become irreversible, and necrosis results. This change is due to sudden occlusion of a coronary artery followed by cessation of blood flow to a part of the myocardial tissue. The abrupt cutting off of oxygen and nutrients to the myocardium can be disastrous to the entire functioning of the body, and death can quickly follow.

When the entire thickness of cardiac muscle within a segment is involved in the occlusion, the condition is referred to as a *transmural infarction*. Acute coronary artery occlusion is almost always present when this occurs. If, however, the infarction is confined within a restricted segment of myocardium, acute occlusion may not be present. This type of infarction is referred to as a *subendocardial infarction*.[15]

When the oxygen supply to the myocardium is obstructed or limited, a sequence of morphologic and biochemical changes occurs in the ischemic tissue (see Table 26-2). The viability of the affected

**FIGURE 26-1**

Factors determining myocardial oxygen supply and demand.

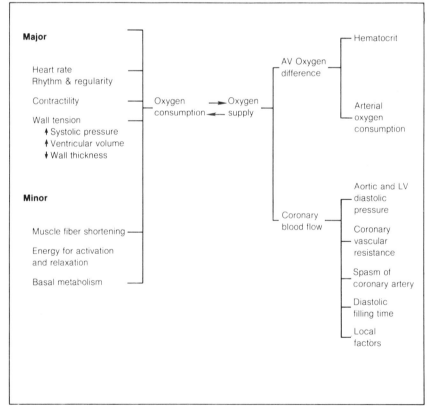

tissue determines the eventual size of the infarcted area of the heart. The location of the area of occlusion is also an important factor in determining damage. The most common sites for infarction are the anterior wall and the posterior wall of the left ventricle. When the anterior wall is involved, there is usually thrombosis in the descending branch of the left coronary artery. When the posterior wall is infarcted, the problem is due to occlusion of the right coronary artery or the circumflex branch of the left coronary artery.[16]

The initial response to coronary occlusion is reflected within the first 10 seconds by cyanosis in the affected area of heart muscle and EKG changes begin to appear. Within minutes of the onset of ischemia, contraction ceases in the injured area. Immediately thereafter, oxygen is no longer available for aerobic glucose metabolism. Anerobic metabolism then occurs, and lactic acid begins to accumulate. Electrolytes such as potassium and creatine are lost from the cell interior, and lysosomes enter the circulation. Enzymes such as creatinine phosphokinase (CPK) are released into the circulating blood, indicating muscle injury. Although metabolically injured, cardiac cells are viable for about 20 minutes under ischemic conditions.[17] If blood flow is reestablished during this time, aerobic metabolism and contractility are restored. The reparative process is then activated to regain cell function, but cell multiplication or regeneration is lacking.[18] Necrotic cells are replaced by nonfunctional connective tissue. Leukocytosis occurs as the inflammatory response is activated. The affected ventricular area becomes fibrotic and stiff (noncompliant). The stiffened wall, an inert area, is unable to pump, and this is reflected by asynergic or uncoordinated wall motion. This can lead to ineffective muscle action, and pump failure can result (see Figure 26-2).

The course after infarction is dynamic. The myocardium beyond the site of occlusion undergoes many changes, including the development of local areas of low pressure and the development of collateral circulation. Some areas of poor perfusion recover as intravascular pressure improves, while others become temporarily or permanently starved as flow ceases altogether.[19]

Systemically, in response to myocardial infarction, catecholamines are released from postsympathetic ganglionic fibers and from the adrenal medulla.[20] Catecholamine-mediated lipolysis and glycogenolysis are responsible for elevated blood levels of free fatty acids and glucose, respectively. Plasma glucose and free fatty acids perfusing the

myocardium can then be used for anaerobic metabolism by the oxygen-poor myocardium.[21] However, this metabolic process supplies only one-fifth as much energy as is supplied under normal conditions of oxidative phosphorylation for contractile events.[22] With continued ATP depletion, anaerobic metabolism eventually ceases.

The five major causes of death following an infarction are congestive heart failure, shock, arrhythmias, rupture, and embolus formation. *Pump failure* (congestive heart failure) occurs because of extensive loss of muscle, papillary muscle involvement leading to mitral insufficiency (see Chap. 27), loss of synchronous muscle contractions (caused by previous scarring of the myocardium), or paradoxic movement of the ventricular wall. Usually left-sided failure is present and can progress to pulmonary edema (see Chap. 24). If the precipitating factors listed above are extensive, or if the complicating pulmonary edema cannot be corrected, *cardiogenic shock* may occur (see Chap. 28 for complete discussion).

*Arrhythmias* are seen in 80 percent of patients with a myocardial infarction. Control of life-threatening arrhythmias has been facilitated by the development of coronary care units. Serious arrhythmias occur more frequently in the presence of pump failure, anterior wall infarctions, and shock. Complete heart block is seen with extensive infarction, and ventricular fibrillation may also be present. *Sudden death* with or without infarction was reported to be the largest single type of death from coronary artery disease[23] and may have ventricular

**TABLE 26-2**
MORPHOLOGIC AND BIOCHEMICAL CHANGES IN RESPONSE TO ACUTE CORONARY OCCLUSION AND MYOCARDIAL ISCHEMIA

| | |
|---|---|
| 5 s: | Cyanosis |
| 30 s: | Swollen mitochondria, hydrogen ion accumulation, lactic acid accumulation, reduced glycogen, potassium loss |
| 1–5 min: | Nonspecific electrocardiographic changes, decline in contractility |
| 20 min: | Mitochondria enlargement, granule formation, loss of matrix density, severe ATP depletion, cessation of glycolysis, lysosomal degradation |
| 1 h: | Myocardial CPK depletion |
| 8–12 h: | Disorganization of myofibrils |
| 12–18 h: | Maximal collateral blood flow to ischemic zone |
| 4–10 days: | Necrotic area clearly identifiable |
| 6–10 days: | Following complete infarction, scar tissue begins to form |
| 10 days–6 wk: | Continued growth of scar tissue replacing necrotic tissue |

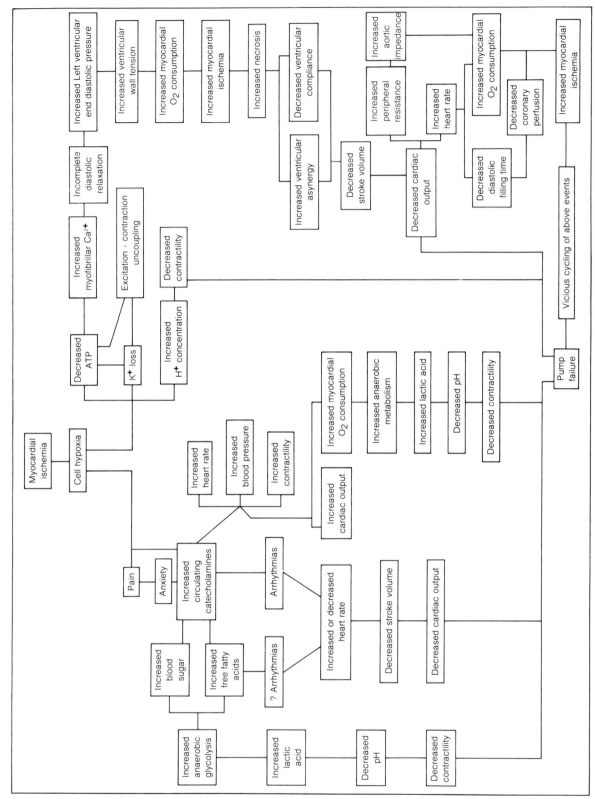

**FIGURE 26-2**
Schematic diagram of sequence of events leading to pump failure as a result of prolonged myocardial ischemia.

fibrillation as its precursor. (For a complete discussion of arrhythmias, refer to Chap. 25.)

*Rupture* of the ventricular wall can occur following an infarction. It is seen more frequently in women than in men. The most common site of rupture is the left ventricle wall. The ventricular septum and papillary muscle may also rupture, but this occurs less frequently. Myocardial rupture can occur as early as 3 to 4 days after infarction.[24]

A *ventricular aneurysm,* caused by a thinning of the cardiac wall, is often associated with rupture. This form of rupture is referred to as a *false aneurysm.* The expression is used to describe a pathogenic sequence of cardiac rupture, confinement of the resulting hematoma, and organization of the periphery of the hematoma.[25]

*Embolus formation* is another cause of mortality following infarction. The main source of emboli tends to be the left ventricular cavity and systemic veins. Generally, larger areas of infarction are more likely to develop thrombosis. Left ventricular mural thrombosis is a potential source of systemic arterial embolism affecting the brain.

*Anterior wall* infarctions usually involve a large mass of myocardium and subject the patient to many complications, such as pump failure and shock. *Lateral wall* infarctions involve a smaller muscle mass but are often associated with arrhythmias and heart block. Patients with *posterior or inferior wall* infarctions are prone to arrhythmias and heart block. Patients with this type of infarction may also experience a difficult recovery period, but because a small muscle mass is involved, the prognosis is good.

A person who sustains a myocardial infarction will experience a variety of physical and psychosocial effects, of which chest pain is the most formidable. This pain ranges from mild, transient pain to the acute and severe pain associated with complete occlusion. Dyspnea, fatigue, generalized weakness, fever, and anxiety can accompany the ischemic attack. Dizziness and syncope due to decreased cerebral circulation and mental confusion, especially in the elderly, may be noted. Alterations in blood pressure, pulse rate, and respirations and signs of pump failure and arrhythmias may appear soon after the infarction has occurred.

**First-level nursing care** The development of atherosclerotic heart disease is thought to be related to an affluent Western life-style, sedentary living habits, and the consumption of rich, fatty foods. Of interest is the fact that over the past decade, a decline in mortality in males 35 to 60 years of age

has been found.[26] Possible explanations include renewed emphasis on physical conditioning, public awareness of the dangers of cigarette smoking and of dietary intake of foods high in cholesterol and saturated fats, and publicity in the mass media on techniques (e.g., transcendental meditation, yoga, relaxation exercises) to combat the stress encountered in daily living.

Annually, over a million persons experience a myocardial infarction and over 600,000 deaths result from coronary atherosclerosis.[27] Two-thirds of these patients die prior to reaching a hospital. In the light of escalating costs and an overburdened health-care delivery system, the future direction of efforts for CHD control logically lies in preventive care. This includes identifying those individuals at high risk and preventing complications in those with existing disease. The mainstay in a program of preventing atherosclerotic sequelae is based upon encouraging adherence to preventive and therapeutic regimens. This necessitates formation of a therapeutic alliance between the nurse and patient based on the premise that atherosclerosis is a lifelong process which can be controlled but not cured.

**A**therogenic Risk Factors Epidemiologic and experimental animal studies have contributed to knowledge of the factors found in persons having or at risk of developing atherosclerotic heart disease. Therefore careful consideration must be given to the results of such research. These results are often based on large-population studies and may not be entirely predictive on an individual basis. Moreover, risk factors operating in one setting may not be as prevalent or as predictive for atherosclerosis in another locality. For example, glucose intolerance is thought to be a major risk factor in certain European countries, but it is considered only a minor risk factor in the United States. Major risk factors, such as hypercholesterolemia and hypertension, elucidated in the Framingham study (see below) are significantly less prevalent in Hawaiian, Japanese, and Puerto Rican studies.[28]

*Risk factors* can be categorized as alterable and unalterable (Table 26-3). Those referred to as *unalterable* include age, sex, and genetic inheritance. It is generally accepted that atherosclerosis is prevalent in middle-aged males and is of similar incidence in men and women past 65 years of age. Why premenopausal women have less atherosclerosis is not known, but speculation focuses on estrogen secretion as a source of this protection. Recent evidence suggests that mortality from atherosclerotic heart disease in young women may be rising.[29] The reasons for this are unclear, but stress, increasing responsibility, and changes in life-style may play an important role.

*Alterable risk factors* can be approached, using the designations of the American Heart Association, as major (probably causal) or minor (suggestive but not markedly significant). Evidence for these risk factors lies in large-scale epidemiologic studies such as the Framingham study,[30] the Tecumseh study,[31] the Evans County Georgia study,[32] and the Western Collaborative Group Study.[33,34]

The *Framingham study* observed a cohort of 5209 men and women over a 20-year period. These individuals were between 30 and 60 years of age and had lived in Framingham, Mass., from 1948 to 1950. This study revealed through biennial physical examinations and concurrent recording of illness or death that serum cholesterol values of 250 mg/100 ml, systolic blood pressure greater than or equal to 160 mmHg, and smoking of one or more packs of cigarettes a day were associated with increased risk of coronary heart disease. Each factor independently increased this risk of CHD, and in combination the risk was four times greater than that for any one factor alone. Furthermore, the younger the subject the greater the likelihood that these factors would predict coronary heart disease. Risk of coronary events was also increased, but not so strongly, in persons with impaired carbohydrate tolerance,

sedentary habits, EKG abnormalities (left ventricular hypertrophy, intraventricular block, nonspecific S-T and T wave abnormality, and atrial fibrillation), and reduced vital capacity.[35] In this study, risk of sudden death was associated with obesity and lack of physical activity.[36] Lately, reduced vital capacity as a risk factor for myocardial infarction and sudden death has been confirmed in a study of the *Kaiser Permanente Medical Care Program.*[37]

*The Evans County Georgia study* is the only black-white epidemiologic study in the United States, and it and the Tecumseh study are the only two total-community epidemiologic studies.[38] The basic economy in Evans County is agricultural, which further differentiates the sample from the samples in other studies. The study, beginning in 1960, observed every adult over 40 years and 50 percent of those between 15 and 39 years for a period of 10 years. For all levels of risk factors, manifestations of coronary heart disease were consistently less frequent in blacks than in whites. None of the risk factors could account for the ethnic differences in prevalence rates. Of the factors studied, the only factor providing a clue was occupation, probably because of differing levels of physical activity. All persons, black or white, engaged in sustained physical activity such as that involved in farming had a low incidence of heart disease, whereas nonfarmers (a predominantly white group) had an extremely high rate of heart disease. However, other factors, not investigated, such as psychosocial processes, may have constituted part of the mechanism mediating these differences.

Many other research studies have been pooled into the National Cooperative Pooling Project, whose follow-up studies over a 10-year period strengthen the correlation between standard risk factors and coronary heart disease.[39]

**P**sychological Risk Factors   Psychosocial and behavioral factors, as mentioned earlier, may partially account for the variability in expression of CHD among different groups. An extensive review of the literature published from 1970 through early 1975 suggests that the psychosocial factors most consistently related to the risk of coronary disease are disturbing emotions such as anxiety and depression, interference with sleep, and the Type A behavior pattern (see Table 26-4).

Furthermore, evidence in recent research studies suggests different psychosocial precursors of angina pectoris and of myocardial infarction.[40–42] For example, anxiety, depression, neuroticism, and

**TABLE 26-3**
RISK FACTORS IN DEVELOPMENT OF ATHEROSCLEROTIC HEART DISEASE

---

Unalterable:
  Age (over 60)
  Sex (predominantly male)
  Genetic predisposition

Alterable (major):
  Hypercholesterolemia
  High blood pressure
  Cigarette smoking
  Hyperlipidemia

Alterable (minor):
  Family history (environmental factors)
  Obesity
  Low level of physical activity
  EKG abnormalities
  Glucose intolerance
  Reduced vital capacity
  Gout
  Psychosocial tensions

Questionable:
  Water hardness
  Coffee-drinking habit
  Lack of dietary fiber
  Lack of ingestion of oil of garlic and onion

interpersonal problems were found prospectively to be precursors of angina and sudden death but not of myocardial infarction. Evidence from retrospective studies links obsessive tendencies and overcontrol of emotions to myocardial infarction. Finally, sleep disturbances and the Type A behavior pattern can be linked to both.

The *Type A behavior pattern* deserves further comment. The Type A behavioral style is described as including some or all of the following personal characteristics: intense striving for achievement, competitiveness, easily provoked impatience, time urgency, abruptness of gesture and speech, overcommitment to vocation or profession, and excess drive and hostility.[43] Support for the association of the coronary-prone Type A behavior pattern with clinical coronary disease is found in several independent retrospective studies and a major prospective study, the Western Collaborative Group Study.[44]

Evidence for the role of psychosocial factors in mediating coronary proneness looks promising. However, before psychosocial risk factors are generally accepted, tightly designed clinical trials are necessary to establish the relation of psychosocial factors to coronary heart disease. In all likelihood the central nervous system plays a major role in converting psychological distress to physiologic responses, but until these data are forthcoming, massive intervention trials are probably not warranted. Appropriate strategies can be negotiated with patients at high coronary risk on an individual basis. The purpose is to lower behavioral susceptibility to coronary heart disease by reducing psychological stress and modifying bothersome symptoms or behavior traits.

**A**ssessment of High-risk Patients   A coronary-risk assessment involves obtaining a patient history and conducting a physical examination. Appropriate laboratory tests can then be ordered to complete the data base.

Areas to be covered in the patient interview are summarized in Table 26-5. The information obtained in a health history contributes to the coronary artery disease profile.

The *family, environmental,* and *psychosocial components, genetic predisposition,* elements of *life-style* such as *dietary habits, exercise,* and *cigarette smoking,* life *stress,* and *Type A behaviors* are all included in the assessment. *Occupational data* should also be obtained in order to gain knowledge about job performance, requirements, work-related stress, and exposure to environmental *pollutants*

and allergens. The latter assume importance in proportion to the amount of exposure to atherogenic and cardioactive pollutants and allergens.[45] For example, chronic exposure to nitrites in an explosives factory is known to be associated with angina pectoris during nonworking hours; withdrawal from the nitrites probably produces reflex coronary artery spasm. Long-term proximity to auto fumes raises carboxyhemoglobin levels, and the ensuing hypoxia may be an intimal endothelial irritant. A

**TABLE 26-4**
CONSISTENCY OF RELATIONSHIP BETWEEN PSYCHOSOCIAL RISK FACTORS AND CORONARY HEART DISEASE

Consistent relationship:
  Anxiety
  Depression
  Sleep interference
  Type A behavior pattern
  Exaggerated blood pressure response to cold-pressor test

Inconsistent relationship:
  Work overload
  Chronic conflict
  Number of life-changing events
  Educational level
  Social mobility
  Migration

**TABLE 26-5**
SCHEDULE FOR DETERMINING CORONARY RISK PROFILE

HISTORY:
  *Family:* History of risk factors; coronary events or sudden death in grandparents, parents or siblings

  *Environmental:* Eating patterns, nature of diet, activities, level of exercise

  *Psychosocial:* History of cigarette smoking, recent deaths in family, Type A behaviors, recent life stresses (positive and negative events), disturbed sleeping, anxiety and depression, amount of alcohol ingestion

  *Occupational:* Place of work, type of work, exposure to pollutants and allergens, level of activity, emotional stress, amount of activity engaged in during work

  *Educational:* Level of education achieved, adult education programs (important for later teaching)

  *Medications:* Medications taken, e.g., antihypertensive or hypolipedemic agents; past experience with medications; estimate of medication adherence

  *Symptoms:* Unusual fatigue, angina, intermittent claudication, dyspnea

  *Additional health problems:* Gout, diabetes, stroke, hypertension, angina, myocardial infarction

  *Attitudes and beliefs:* Cardiovascular illness and health

PHYSICAL ASSESSMENT (see Chap. 2):
Total head-to-toe assessment of physical findings: general physical appearance, cardiovascular findings, pulmonary changes, skin changes, (fluid and electrolyte) kidney function; also congenital anomalies, cardiac changes, including arrhythmias of unknown etiology

final example is the job stress which occurs at peak flight times in air traffic controllers. This stress is thought to predispose individuals to hypertension.

Information about *educational achievement* is primarily useful for developing teaching strategies with patients. Current medications and experience with medications in the past provide information about pill-taking habits. Patients should be queried about coronary events and related health problems such as *gout* and *diabetes.* The risk of developing coronary heart disease increases in the presence of related metabolic problems.

Finally, *attitudes and beliefs about coronary heart disease* should be explored. In doing so, the nurse can correct misconceptions about CHD, discuss risk factors, and realistically weigh beliefs about personal susceptibility to heart disease. At the same time the nurse can reinforce in a positive manner existent risk-reducing behaviors. Intent to mutually develop plans to help the patient eliminate risk-enhancing behaviors may be discussed at this time.

The *physical examination* may contribute clues to hyperlipidemia, which may precede the development of atherosclerosis. *Xanthomata* (collections of lipids) may appear as lumps (yellow masses) over the Achilles tendons and knuckles and along the tendons of the arms. *Xanthelasma* (yellowish lipid-filled cells) may surround the eyes as cream-colored plaques. These are indicative of hyperlipidemia and may be reversed with therapy.[46]

To assess *obesity,* the patient's desirable weight should be estimated by comparing actual weight with a table of mean weights for persons of the same age and sex. The relative weight (actual value divided by the mean group weight) can then be calculated. A skinfold-thickness test using calipers to measure the amount of subcutaneous tissue under the triceps muscle is another reliable index of relative weight.

An accurate estimate of *blood pressure* can usually be obtained by taking an initial measurement with the patient sitting and repeating it a few minutes later with the patient recumbent. If the reading exceeds 140 mmHg systolic pressure or a diastolic pressure of 90 mmHg, measurements should be repeated on two subsequent occasions (see Chap. 28). For persons over the age of 50, readings of 160/95 or over indicate the need for secondary screening. If the patient's average diastolic pressure on three separate occasions exceeds 105 mmHg, drug therapy is usually instituted. The patient with a diastolic pressure between 95 and 105 mmHg is generally evaluated at 3- to 6-month intervals, and drug therapy is individualized.

A major component of the coronary-risk profile is the *blood lipid content.* Coronary risk rises in proportion to the plasma cholesterol concentration. A serum cholesterol of more than 260 mg/100 ml—an arbitrarily chosen value—can be considered "abnormal." Probably less important as a risk factor and certainly more difficult to obtain is the fasting triglyceride. A serum triglyceride value over 150 mg/100 ml is excessive. For those with elevated triglyceride levels, xanthomas, or family histories of premature coronary events, lipoprotein electrophoresis is indicated. Table 26-6 describes the significance as well as the overall classification of the hyperlipoproteinemias.

*Sugar* and *uric acid* levels are also part of the assessment data. A fasting blood sugar of more than 120 mg/100 ml, decreased glucose tolerance, or significant glycosuria are indicative of at least a twofold risk of coronary disease. A uric acid level over 7.5 mg/100 ml contributes further to coronary risk (this change is often noted in patients with gout).

The risk factor of *emotional stress* is difficult to test and most often is judged subjectively. Two tests, the *cold-pressor test* and *stress provocation,* may be used to evaluate cardiovascular reactivity. In the cold-pressor test the forearm is inserted into a container of ice water while the blood pressure is measured. A rise in diastolic pressure during the test is strongly suggestive of subsequent coronary disease.[47]

Another diagnostic tool is the quiz electrocardiogram. A 12-minute tape-recorded quiz designed to provoke psychological stress is administered during electrocardiographic monitoring. Heart-rate and blood-pressure increase and S-T segment depression are the parameters used to determine cardiovascular physiologic and ischemic responses.[48]

Persons who ingest large amounts of *alcohol* are also predisposed to coronary artery disease. Research has shown that ethanol can depress ventricular performance, thereby decreasing myocardial uptake of fatty acids. Excessive alcohol ingestion can increase the uptake of triglycerides, a known cause of myocardial cell injury.[49] Persons with a chronic alcohol problem may also have a thiamine deficiency, which has been associated with systemic vasoconstriction and alterations in cardiac output.

The effects of excessive cigarette smoking on the myocardium cannot be overemphasized. As indicated by the Framingham study and other studies, the vascular constriction caused by smoking results in constriction of coronary as well as

**TABLE 26-6**
CLASSIFICATION OF HYPERLIPOPROTEINEMIAS*

| Type | Mechanism | Cholesterol | Triglycerides | Lipoproteins | Therapy | Clinical Features |
|------|-----------|-------------|---------------|--------------|---------|-------------------|
| I (rare) | Loss of enzymatic step in removal of chylomicrons | Normal or elevated | Elevated | Chylomicrons elevated | Low-fat diet; not drug-responsive | Xanthomas, hepatosplenomegaly, lipemia retinalis, abdominal pain, pancreatitis |
| II† (common) | Excess production or inadequate clearance of low-density lipoproteins (LDL) | Elevated | Normal or slightly elevated | Beta-lipoproteins elevated | Low-fat diet, low cholesterol intake; drugs: cholestyramine D-thyroxine, nicotinic acid | Homozygote: xanthomas, arthritis, premature vascular disease (childhood); heterozygote: tendon and tuberous xanthomas xanthelasma (adult), premature corneal arcus, premature vascular disease |
| III (less common than II and IV) | Block in metabolism of very-low-density lipoproteins (VLDL) causing abnormal intermediate form to circulate in plasma | Elevated | Elevated | Abnormal beta-lipoproteins present | Weight control; low cholesterol intake, carbohydrate restriction, low saturated-fat intake; drugs: clofibrate, D-thyroxine, nicotinic acid | Eruptive and tendon xanthomas (ages 30–40), plantar xanthomas, orange-yellow deposits in palmar and digital creases, xanthelasma, corneal arcus, premature cardiovascular disease (ages 40–50) |
| IV (common) | Excess production or inadequate clearance of VLDL | Normal or elevated | Elevated | Pre-beta-lipoproteins elevated | Weight reduction; restriction of alcohol and carbohydrates; drugs: clofibrate, nicotinic acid | Lipemia retinalis, eruptive xanthomas, hepatosplenomegaly, abdominal pain, premature corneal arcus, premature vascular disease |
| V (uncommon) | VLDL excess combined with poor chylomicron removal | Elevated | Elevated | Chylomicrons and pre-beta-lipoproteins elevated | Restriction of alcohol; weight control; high-protein, low-fat, carbohydrate-restricted diet; control of diabetes; drugs: clofibrate and nicotinic acid | Obesity, abdominal pain, pancreatitis, lipemia retinalis, eruptive xanthomas |

* These may be inherited, acquired, or secondary to other diseases. All types are not atherogenic. Most frequently associated with coronary heart disease is Type IIa.
† Type II may be subdivided into groups IIa and IIb, the latter characterized by pre-beta- and beta-lipoproteins.

peripheral blood vessels. This hazard, along with other risk factors, increases the likelihood of myocardial vascular occlusion.

Persons with a *sedentary job,* such as bus or truck drivers, are also at risk of cardiovascular occlusion. Lack of exercise and circulatory stimulation will result in irreversible changes in peripheral blood vessels and can lead to peripheral pooling. Again, this factor is also complicated by the presence of other risk factors such as high ingestion of fatty foods and excessive cigarette smoking.

**P**revention   When a person at risk to develop CHD is identified, a plan of prevention can be enacted by the nurse to decrease or eliminate potential risk factors. Knowledgeable, well-motivated persons may desire to lower the risk of coronary problems. For many persons, however, the task of risk-factor reduction for an obscure, remotely possible health problem lacks priority over daily habits and needs.[50] Moreover, in the absence of symptoms, few persons are stimulated or able to maintain healthful behaviors. The challenge in assisting people to change attitudes and habits and to maintain healthy cardiovascular behaviors is therefore a demanding and complex one. Before attitudes and habits can be changed, risk factors must be precisely identified and explained to patients. Data collection is the first step in obtaining a coronary-risk profile. Once the level of coronary susceptibility is known and the presence of risk factors is determined, the nurse can plan strategies to meet individual needs.

*Health education*   The most important point to stress in health teaching is that careful adherence to a few simple health habits can prolong life and halt progressive and destructive changes within coronary blood vessels. Helping people recognize their control over heart problems may be the best motivator to compliance.

Health teaching for prevention of coronary heart disease should include dietary control, weight reduction, detection and control of hypertension, elimination of cigarette smoking, reduction of alcohol ingestion, increased planned activity, and reduction of stress. Correction of other medical problems such as anemia and hyperthyroidism, as well as congenital anomalies, is also critical prior to implementing effective health teaching.

*Dietary control* includes decreasing the use of saturated fats and increasing the use of polyunsaturated fats. Reducing ingestion of dietary cholesterol to less than 300 mg/day is advised in limiting atherogenesis. (Refer to Chap. 24 for a listing of the recommended foods.)

Hyperlipidemia can frequently be controlled by diet alone. If dietary measures fail to restore the plasma lipids to normal, lipid-lowering drugs such as clofibrate, cholestyramine, and nicotinic acid can be added (Table 26-6).[51]

*Maintaining optimum weight* for age, sex, and body size is another important factor in preventing coronary occlusion. This may necessitate significantly reducing caloric intake to achieve and maintain weight levels. Limiting the ingestion of pure sugar, which adds only calories to the diet, should be discussed. Parents should be encouraged to limit weight gain in young children, as the number of fat cells deposited in childhood is thought to influence weight control in adulthood. Normally, a low-fat, low-calorie diet, along with a daily exercise schedule, will maintain body weight within normal limits and reduce potential accumulation of fat deposits. Avoiding large meals and overeating, as well as eating in a relaxed environment, will enhance digestion and decrease cardiac work load. Yearly serum cholesterol as well as triglyceride blood tests will help to keep a close check on the atherogenic process.

Recognition and control of *high blood pressure* is another critical factor in eliminating coronary heart disease (see Chap. 28 for complete discussion). Early detection of hypertension through blood pressure screening programs as well as during physical examination can help identify the population at risk. Patients should be encouraged to have their blood pressure checked routinely during the periodic health examination. Should hypertension be noted, careful follow-up should be requested. Extensive health teaching will be required in order to ensure drug compliance and prevent recurrence.

Eliminating *cigarette smoking* is difficult for many patients. Although national recognition has been given to the problem, the cigarette industry is still most successful. Limiting smoking or terminating the habit requires much internal motivation. Even in the presence of serious health problems, many patients will continue to smoke. At times, eliminating smoking altogether is more stress-producing for the patient than the actual effects of smoking. Patients need to be taught the personal risks involved if smoking continues. Referral to groups whose goal is to help people to stop smoking may be useful. Many physicians have supported the use of hypnosis for persons who cannot limit their smoking. If initial attempts to stop smoking fail, the patient should be encouraged to try again, and alternative approaches should be considered.

The ingestion of *alcohol* while smoking increases the risk of coronary artery disease still further. Insidiously, increased ingestion of alcohol may be related to social aspects of a job or professional group. People should be cautioned against the continual and excessive use of alcohol on a daily or even frequent basis and made aware of the risks involved and the potential effects on the cardiovascular system over time.

*Activity* and *planned exercise,* beginning in childhood and continuing through adulthood, should be encouraged for everyone. Adults should engage in some type of daily activity in order to exercise the heart muscle, as well as the body as a whole. Those with sedentary jobs should be encouraged to increase their daily activities as tolerated. Persons who drive trucks or sit for long periods of time should plan breaks in the day when they can walk or exercise in order to stimulate peripheral circulation. Families can plan outdoor activities as a group to satisfy the need for exercise. Recreational activities are also a means of releasing stress and tension and can improve the general sense of well-being.

*Stress* is a constant risk factor in today's highly technological and mobile society. Financial crises, health problems, increased cost of living, social pressures, and occupational stressors all contribute to the development of unhealthy stress responses. Recognition of particularly stressful events within an individual's environment is the first step in removing or modifying those physiological, psychological, or environmental variables that influence the stress response.

*Behavioral strategies*  Because individual attitudes and behavioral patterns are strongly implicated in the causation and chronicity of coronary artery disease, educational strategies for behavioral change must be considered.

Several strategies are available for modifying behavior and increasing self-confidence in dealing with the reduction of coronary risk factors and the maintenance of cardiovascular health (see Table 26-7). Each patient will have different needs, so various combinations of behavioral strategies will be required. In helping patients reduce the risk of cardiovascular problems, awareness of counterproductive behaviors and habits is an important component. The patient should be encouraged to keep diaries, records, or calendars which will facilitate an awareness of the many habitual behaviors performed daily. Individually set realistic goals and methods for achieving these goals can then be determined.[52] With continued follow-up, progress can be monitored and problems mutually con-

fronted by the nurse and the patient. Once a desired goal is achieved, behavior to maintain it, be it cigarette elimination, weight reduction, or physical conditioning, is identified and practiced. Maintenance behavior may require family participation, group sessions, or periodic counseling to ensure continued compliance.[53]

**Second-level nursing care**  In the community setting the nurse will often see patients who have asymptomatic CHD or mild, transient attacks of ischemia (angina). Careful health history and physical assessment are critical, since early atherogenesis may be predominantly asymptomatic.

**N**ursing Assessment  During the health assessment the nurse should ask about angina and other symptoms, as this information serves as a baseline in the event that changes develop in the future.

*Health history*  As indicated under First-level Nursing Care, a careful health history must include the components listed in the coronary-risk profile (refer to Table 26-5). These can be incorporated into the overall health history. A frequent complaint of patients with mild CHD is angina. *Anginal pain* is located in the substernal chest region. The pain may occur with or without radiation to other sites.[54] Most frequently the pain radiates upward to the interscapular region, downward along the medial aspect of the left arm, and then to the hand over the ulnar nerve. The attacks are usually of short duration, lasting less than 3 to 5 minutes. Frequently the onset of pain follows the ingestion of a heavy meal. The pain is often described as a tightness or burning or a gripping or squeezing feeling in the chest, and the problem is often confused with acute indigestion or other gastrointestinal problems.

Angina is characteristically produced by any form of exertion. The patient may describe physical exercise, emotional excitement, sexual intercourse, anger, a heavy meal, or exposure to cold weather as associated with the onset of anginal pain, with relief of pain generally resulting from cessation of the activity.

Patients may describe their attacks as occurring during the night or interrupting sleep. A form of angina called *nocturnal angina* may occur during sleep, particularly in the phase of rapid eye movement (REM) associated with dreaming.[55] Sympathetic activity is probably heightened at this time, and arrhythmias may occur concurrently. If the angina occurs early in sleep, it may be related to anxiety; in late sleep, it may be associated with concomitant depression.

**TABLE 26-7**
ANTIANGINAL PHARMACOLOGIC AGENTS

| Medication | Dosage | Cardiovascular Effects | Side Effects | Patient Counseling |
|---|---|---|---|---|
| Nitroglycerin | 0.15–0.6 mg sublingually (SL) as needed | Decreases arterial pressure, decreases venous tone, reduces ventricular volume, reduces ventricular diastolic pressure, decreases cardiac ejection time, decreases rate of rise of left ventricular pressure | Dizziness, syncope, headaches, flushing | Know drug's purpose and action, know side effects, know how to administer; if side effects occur, take in sitting position; report lack of relief from drug (may be drug loss of potency, or refractory or crescendo angina). In addition to above, for nitroglycerin: Report smallest dose that consistently provides relief; do not take unless chest discomfort is present or anticipated; take early in anginal attack; take 2–3 min prior to strenuous activity; store in tightly stoppered brown bottle without cotton filler; replace supply every 6 months; carry in pill container number of tablets anticipated to be needed when away from home; repeat × 3 if required during an anginal attack; notify practitioner if relief not produced. |
| Long-acting nitrates: Pentaerythrityl tetranitrate (Peritrate) | 10–20 mg 3/day po | | | |
| Erythrityl tetranitrate (Cardilate) | 10–15 mg 3/day SL or chewable | | | |
| Isosorbide dinitrate (Isordil) | 10 mg 3/day–4/day po or SL | | | |
| Nitrol ointment | 2% topically lasts 4 h | | | |
| Amyl nitrate | Inhalation | Decreases arterial pressure, decreases intramyocardial tension, decreases ventricular volume | Dizziness, syncope, headaches, hypotension | Not applicable, since rarely used on ambulatory basis. |
| Propranolol (Inderal) | 10–40 mg 3/day–4/day po (larger doses may be used); peak action: 90 min | Decreases heart rate, decreases myocardial contractility, decreases arterial pressure, decreases rate or rise of left ventricular pressure | Fatigue, headache, diarrhea, nausea, bradycardia, postural hypotension, bronchospasm, sexual problems, depression; contraindicated in heart failure, COPD, bradycardia, asthma, severe valvular disease, diabetes | Know drug's purpose, action, and side effects; do not stop taking without medical supervision, since gradual weaning is recommended; report symptoms of heart failure, severe bradycardia, bronchospasm, and any sexual problems to practitioner; may keep pill calendar or store in prominent place as reminders to take pill; when away from home, carry number of pills needed to maintain regimen. Do not take extra pills to "make up" for doses missed. |

*Angina decubitus* is that form of angina which occurs when the patient is in the recumbent position. The patient usually states that he was awakened from sleep by chest discomfort and shortness of breath. It is thought that angina decubitus may be a form of left ventricular failure. The expansion of intrathoracic blood volume which occurs with recumbency may increase myocardial oxygen requirements.[56] Dreaming has also been associated with this problem. A shift in position may terminate symptoms. Anginal histories should therefore include questions exploring timing of angina at night, presence or absence of dreams, usual sleep positions, quality of sleep (restful or not), and related emotional disturbances.

A less common form of angina, called *variant, or Prinzmetal's, angina,* is manifested as a resting pain unrelated to physical exercise. Its etiology is unknown. Mechanisms contributing to its occurrence include coronary spasm, abnormal oxygen release, carbon monoxide toxicosis, sympathetic hyperfunction, small-vessel disease, and recanalization of thrombi.[57, 58]

In association with the painful discomfort from myocardial ischemia, persons with transient ischemia frequently report *dyspnea.* Since both angina and dyspnea may be described as substernal tightness, the two must be clearly differentiated. The dyspnea is probably produced by an acute decrease in left ventricular compliance. Increased ventricular stiffness leads to an elevation of left atrial and pulmonary pressures. This, in turn, causes early interstitial pulmonary edema and increased lung stiffness. The work of breathing then becomes more difficult.[59,60]

Dyspnea can be classified according to the circumstances of its appearance. *Orthopnea* characterizes dyspnea relieved by sitting. *Paroxysmal nocturnal dyspnea* (PND) is a dyspneic episode occurring at night. *Effort dyspnea* (dyspnea on exertion; DOE) is precipitated by exertion and should be qualified by activity level (e.g., one flight of stairs, one block of walking). *Dyspnea at rest* rarely occurs with uncomplicated angina but may be present with coexistent heart failure.

Complaints of *fatigue* due to cardiac problems should be distinguished from fatigue due to other causes, such as depression. When anginal patients experience fatigue, it may be a forewarning of an impending myocardial infarction. The fatigue may or may not be accompanied by an increase in the severity and number of anginal episodes.[61] Worsening angina is termed *preinfarctional angina, crescendo angina,* or *intermediate coronary syndrome.*

*Anxiety* may accompany these problems. The patient will often describe an uneasy feeling associated with the anginal pain. Since emotions can play an important role in anginal pain, psychological assessment is important.

*Physical assessment* Observation of the patient with CHD usually reveals a person who is overweight and occasionally obese. Xanthelasma (yellowish plaques around the eyelids) and xanthomata (gross yellow masses found in the subcutaneous tissue, often around tendons) may be noted. Usually the skin color is good, and in the absence of pain the facial expression is normal.

Included in the physical assessment is auscultation for the presence of any abnormal heart and lung sounds. Usually rales (see Chap. 24), diastolic heart sounds, murmurs, and arrhythmias (see Chap. 25) are heard when CHD is advanced. A bruit (sound produced by turbulence of blood in the vessels; see Chap. 29) should be listened for over all the major arteries, as coronary atherosclerotic deposition occurs simultaneously with plaque formation in other areas of the body.

During an ischemic attack, a third and fourth heart sound can sometimes be heard. These sounds are best heard when the patient is in a recumbent position (refer to Chap. 22). On occasion, paradoxical splitting of the second sound may be noted. Tachycardia may be present and, in the presence of anxiety, premature beats may be noted.

Heart size may be determined by chest percussion. However, chest percussion for this purpose is becoming outmoded because of the ease and accuracy with which heart size can be measured by chest x-ray. Heart enlargement may occur in asymptomatic persons and may become more obvious over a period of years.

An ophthalmic examination provides the examiner with the only opportunity for observing the living blood vessels and nerves of the body. On inspection of the eyes, arcus senilis, a clouding of the iris, is not uncommonly associated with atherosclerotic changes in the corresponding carotid artery. Using an ophthalmoscope, the fundus of the eye can be examined for atherosclerotic and arteriolar sclerotic (i.e., hypertensive) eye changes.[62]

*Diagnostic tests* Electrocardiographic evidence of significant asymptomatic coronary disease can best be appreciated on the postexercise electrocardiogram (EKG) (see Chap. 22 for complete discussion of the EKG). Ischemic EKG changes provoked by exercise include S-T segment and T wave abnormalities and arrhythmias, particularly premature ventricular ectopic beats.[63]

*Exercise tests* can involve exercising on a bicycle with an ergometer, walking on a variable-speed and -grade treadmill, or walking up and down steps (Master's test). The patient may be stressed to a predetermined heart rate, usually 80 to 85 percent of the predicted maximum heart rate (submaximal testing), or until symptoms such as chest pain and fatigue develop (maximal or near-maximal testing). In the laboratory an emergency cart and defibrillator should be on hand, and personnel licensed to carry out emergency procedures should be present.

Arrhythmias, particularly ventricular ectopic rhythm disturbances, have been observed in studies to significantly increase the risk of sudden cardiac death. Whether or not premature ventricular contractions act independently of other factors (such as left ventricular hypertrophy and severity of coronary disease), their increase of coronary risk remains controversial.

The technology for *24-hour screening for premature ventricular contractions* using Holter-type rhythm recordings is now available. Transient arrhythmias occurring during normal daily activities at home and at work can be detected. Rhythm disturbances such as atrial fibrillation and premature ectopic beats superimposed on other risk factors add to the risk of coronary morbidity.[64-66] *Ambulatory monitoring* shows promise of becoming even more useful once the exact relation of arrhythmias to sudden death and to atherosclerotic events is determined.

The *resting 12-lead EKG* is both practical and useful to obtain. The electrocardiogram is scrutinized for EKG abnormalities such as atrial fibrillation, S-T segment and T wave changes, and left ventricular hypertrophy, all of which increase coronary risk. In fact, evidence of left ventricular hypertrophy is associated in the Framingham study with a mortality comparable to that of persons who survive a symptomatic coronary attack.[67]

Other laboratory tests may be positive during the anginal phase of CHD, revealing elevated blood sugar and uric acid levels, heart enlargement on x-ray, hyperlipidemia, and elevated cholesterol and triglyceride levels.

**N**ursing Problems and Interventions   The primary problem experienced by the patient with transient ischemia (angina) is *chest pain,* often accompanied by anxiety. Risk factors such as cigarette smoking,

hypertension, obesity, and emotional stress may also be present.

*Chest pain*   Relief of chest pain due to transient ischemia includes the use of medications as well as behavioral strategies and exercise training. The main emphasis of antianginal therapy is to help the patient manage angina at home while assuming responsibility for self-care.

*Pharmacologic therapy* for managing stable angina consists of the nitrates and beta-adrenergic blocking agents[68] (Table 26-7). The mainstay of treatment is nitroglycerin taken sublingually. The precise mechanism of the drug's action remains unclear, but nitroglycerin seems to relieve angina by reducing myocardial oxygen consumption rather than by increasing coronary blood flow. Experimental evidence suggests that the use of nitrates may increase regional perfusion of an ischemic area of myocardium while the coronary blood flow remains unaffected. Myocardial oxygen requirements are reduced indirectly by arterial and venous vasodilatation, which decrease ventricular volume and systemic resistance and reduce myocardial workload.

*"Long-acting" nitrates* have been used with varying degrees of success. Their use should be adjunctive to other antianginal therapy, and then only if sublingual nitroglycerin alone is ineffective. Since the absorption of nitrates from the gastrointestinal tract is unpredictable when it is taken orally, the dosage should be carefully titrated to avoid untoward effects and to ensure optimum benefit.[69]

*Topical nitroglycerin ointment,* another antianginal agent, is of particular value in the prophylactic treatment of nocturnal angina.[70] Its vasodilating effect is sustained for longer periods than the "long-acting" nitrates. The ointment is applied directly to the skin substernally and rubbed into the area. Reapplication may be needed after 3 to 6 hours.

It the patient continues to have angina despite trials with nitrates, a drug such as propranolol (Inderal) may be added to nitrate therapy.[71,72] Propranolol (a beta-adrenergic blocker) is frequently effective in reducing the oxygen requirements of the myocardium, especially when the results of other drug therapy have been poor. Side effects of propranolol are transient and include nausea, vomiting, diarrhea, and occasional depression. Unusual tiredness, sexual difficulty, or symptoms of heart failure are additional side effects requiring regular monitoring. Exercise tolerance has been reported to improve significantly with propranolol therapy. Propranolol therapy should never be discontinued abruptly; rather, the dosage should be gradually reduced over a 2-week period in order to avoid severe withdrawal problems such as arrhythmias, angina, and even infarction.[73]

*Behavioral techniques* (refer to Table 26-8) of self-observation and stimulus control may be useful in identifying and managing factors precipitating angina. A pain chart can be kept at home for recording severity and frequency of attacks, associated activities and emotions, and self-management techniques (e.g., rest, stimulus avoidance, cues or reminders to facilitate stress reduction, medications). Patients should be counseled concerning control of emotional tensions and refraining from vigorous activities. Behavioral modeling and rehearsal and role playing may be extremely effective as counseling techniques.

*Exercise training* with medical supervision is another nonpharmacologic method of improving the status of patients with angina. With exercise conditioning, patients can attain pain-free activity levels previously associated with the onset of angina.[74] Walking, jogging, bicycling, and swimming are examples of endurance activities producing cardiopulmonary conditioning. An example of a graduated exercise regimen is to walk 1 mile in 15 to 20 minutes after 4 to 6 weeks of training.

*Anxiety*  Patients with angina are often anxious and fear the chest pain they are experiencing. Careful explanation of angina by the nurse is essential. Mild tranquilizers can be given not only to calm the patient but to help decrease the frequency of anginal attacks. If anxiety persists or intensifies or if there are other long-term emotional problems, the patient may be referred for counseling.

*Obesity*  Patients with angina who are overweight are encouraged to start on a weight-reduction plan immediately. Health teaching should focus on helping the patient plan well-balanced meals, low in cholesterol and saturated fats as well as carbohydrates.

Diet teaching should focus on the ingestion of smaller meals. Patients should eat in a relaxed environment, avoiding a rushed, hurried meal when possible. Weekly records of food intake should be kept by the patient and checked by the nurse. A dietary diary should be kept so that problem foods can be discussed and hunger periods identified. Well-paced activity and exercise programs, as well as a well-balanced diet, will aid in weight reduction.

Patients need much support in order to comply with the dietary regime. The nurse should encourage the patient's achievements and isolate areas that need further improvement. Involving family members in dietary planning and implementation will provide added encouragement for the patient.

*Continued risk factors*  The most important component of nursing intervention continues to be pre-

**TABLE 26-8**
BEHAVIORAL STRATEGIES FOR CARDIOVASCULAR HEALTH

---

For general use in changing eating habits, eliminating cigarettes, increasing exercise levels, stress management, and medication adherence:

1  Self-observation: Discriminating between behaviors, counting, charting, evaluating and goal setting.

2  Social reinforcement: Providing praise and encouragement.

3  Family support: Training spouses and family members in social reinforcement strategies which help maintain changes.

4  Internal reinforcement: Establishing self-regulated incentive systems (e.g., tangible self-reward, self-praise) when goals are achieved and maintained.

5  Guided practice: Demonstrating (e.g., food preparation, reading food labels, trying recommended foods, selecting meals from a restaurant menu).

6  Small group sessions: Using peer influence and support to shape behavior.

7  Role models: Identifying and imitating behavior of persons with desired habits who exert strong social influence over an individual.

8  Integration with routines: Using regular routines as a setting for practicing behaviors (e.g., walking up steps instead of taking the elevator, scheduling short "quiet" times into work routine, substituting healthful snacks for "junk" foods at work or at home).

9  Self-cueing or stimulus control: Choosing "reminders" to serve as cues for behavior, such as placing medication calendar beside mirror, making weekly meal plans and corresponding shopping lists, storing gym shorts or bathing suit in a prominent place.

10  Undesired-behavior extinguishment: Providing self-regulated punishment or unpleasant reinforcement before or following undesired behavior, e.g., verbal statement or nonverbal gestures indicating dissatisfaction with behavior, making self do something disliked, imagining something extremely unpleasant when encountering taboo stimulus.

11  Counterconditioning: Providing noxious or aversive stimuli immediately following undesired behavior.

12  Contingency contracting: Goal setting in which regimen is negotiated, specified, and agreed to by patient in writing (formal contract.)

13  Self-confidence strengthening: Improving patient's ability to manage his problem by role playing, behavioral rehearsal, problem clarification, or cognitive restructuring.

For specific uses:

1  Eating habits: Environmental control (training for improving shopping habits, food storage, and access); self-control in food preferences (making deliberate efforts to develop new food preferences, since tastes and preferences are probably the result of consuming certain foods over a period of time).

2  Stress management: Relaxation training, meditation, yoga, biofeedback, or other activities which promote physical and psychological rest.

---

vention of continued risk factors. Avoiding stressful activities, reducing alcohol and caffeine ingestion, eliminating smoking, and engaging in a program of daily activity are essential. Any complicating medical problems present, such as hypertension, anemia, or hyperthyroidism, should be corrected as soon as possible.

The course of angina is usually prolonged. The frequency of anginal attacks depends on the amount of collateral circulation present and correction of the precipitating cause. When angina is complicated by arrhythmias and heart failure, additional drugs may be used to correct these disturbances and ameliorate angina. *Digitalis* (Chap. 24), *diuretics* (Chap. 28), and antiarrhythmic drugs (Chap. 25) may be beneficial. Emotional disturbances that adversely affect angina may require the judicious use of sedatives, tranquilizers, and antidepressants, but nortriptyline HCl, thioridazine, and amitriptyline should be used with caution, since they raise the heart rate and blood pressure and may aggravate the angina.[75,76]

**E**mergency Intervention in Cardiorespiratory Arrest Patients with transient ischemia (angina) are at risk of developing an acute myocardial infarction. This sudden occlusion of coronary artery supply to a portion of the myocardium may result in cardiorespiratory arrest. Immediate nursing assessment and interventions are imperative and can be life-saving if carried out immediately.

*Cardiorespiratory arrest* (sudden death) is always a danger with myocardial ischemia. It is most frequently caused by ventricular arrhythmias. Cardiorespiratory arrest can also be precipitated in otherwise healthy adults by, for example, trauma, carbon monoxide poisoning, electric shock, suffocation or drowning. Clinical problems occurring in an acute-care facility can also induce arrest—e.g., hypotension, anesthesia, airway obstruction, drug anaphylaxis, and myocardial infarction.

*Nursing assessment* The person with cardiorespiratory arrest presents a striking picture. *Initial* cardiac arrest is manifested by acute pain, with the patient clenching at the chest. This will be followed by faint heartbeat on auscultation, weak or absent peripheral pulses (especially the carotid and femoral), alterations in levels of consciousness, and visual disturbances. The patient may vomit and become diaphoretic. Initial respiratory arrest may be manifested by shortness of breath, gasping dyspnea, or apnea. Respirations are irregular, and cyanosis is observed. The airway may or may not be obstructed. With increasing loss of consciousness, the patient's tongue begins to slip backward, occluding the trachea.

In *well-established* cardiorespiratory arrest, respirations are absent and there is cyanosis (especially about the face, lips, and nail beds), along with loss of consciousness, tremors of the extremities, and on occasion seizures. The skin is cold and clammy to the touch. Pupils appear dilated and unresponsive to light. The corneal reflex may be absent. The heartbeat is absent, and peripheral pulses are lost. Vomiting may persist, and muscle relaxation may cause involuntary bowel and bladder evacuation.

*Nursing intervention* Teaching patients and family members to cope with a myocardial infarction can help minimize cardiac damage and prevent cardiorespiratory arrest. To prevent unnecessary delay, patients should be taught the early signs of a "heart attack," which include prolonged, oppressive pain or unusual discomfort in the center of the chest. The patient with angina should note any change in the frequency, severity, character of the pain (e.g., from a burning sensation to a severe tightness), or failure of the pain to respond to nitroglycerin, as these changes may be indicative of an impending myocardial infarction. Moreover, pain that radiates to the shoulder, arm, neck, or jaw and chest pain accompanied by sweating, nausea, vomiting, and shortness of breath signal danger. Patients and their family members and friends should understand what to do if any of these changes occur. Telephone numbers of the patient's physician, hospital, and ambulance or mobile emergency unit should be displayed above the telephone or in an easily accessible place. The patient and family members should know exactly what to do in an emergency, especially cardiopulmonary resuscitation.

The purpose of *cardiopulmonary resuscitation (CPR)* is to reestablish $CO_2/O_2$ exchange and adequate circulation so that oxygenated blood can be delivered to vital organs. *Resuscitative efforts must begin immediately.* Ventilation must begin within 4 to 6 minutes after the cessation of respirations at most. Failure to institute prompt ventilation will result in cerebral anoxia and brain damage.

The resuscitative procedure should be organized, prompt, and carried out by knowledgeable persons. The following steps should be carried out:

*Summon help.* It is almost impossible for one person to continue resuscitative measures effectively for a long period of time.

*Place patient on a hard, flat surface* (the floor is most effective). If a bed has to be used, place a tray or other hard object under patient's back before beginning.

Strike a *precordial blow* with the fist to the lower third of patient's sternum, taking care to avoid xiphoid process located below sternum.

If necessary, *turn patient's head to one side* and clean out mouth. Remove dentures and vomitus.

*Hyperextend patient's neck* by placing one hand under the neck, the other on the forehead. Then place hand on the patient's mandible and pull jaw forward in order to prevent tongue from obstructing airway (see Fig. 26-3).

*Close off patient's nostrils* and, with the rescuer's mouth covering the patient's mouth, blow into mouth in a rhythmic pattern (see Fig. 26-4) 12 to 15 times/ minute; or if working alone, give four deep initial ventilations.

In the absence of heartbeat, as indicated by nonpalpable pulse, begin *closed heart massage.*

*Place heel of hand on lower third of patient's sternum* (see Figs. 26-5 and 26-6).

*Apply downward vertical force* sufficient to depress sternum 2 to 4 cm at a rate of 60 to 70 times/minute. In children, less pressure is used. In some cases (e.g., with infants) two fingers gently pressing rhythmically on lower sternum 80 to 100 times/minute may suffice.

*Coordinate rhythm* with person giving mouth-to-mouth respiration. Patient should be given approximately one ventilation to every four to five sternal compressions (a 5 to 1 ratio). This pattern should not be disturbed until patient's condition is stabilized or more sophisticated equipment is available.

If working alone, give four, full ventilations quickly. Compress patient's chest approximately 15 times, then give two ventilations, and continue chest compression in this pattern until help arrives.

During resuscitative process, patient should be *assessed to see if resuscitative efforts are successful,* as indicated by return of pulse, improved skin color, pupil contraction, return of corneal reflex, patient movement, and return of unassisted respirations. Continuous reassessment is essential in order to assure rescuer that pumping is effective. Observe the abdomen for gastric distentions, which may suggest improper hyperextension of the neck.

**When resuscitation efforts are successful, the patient can be moved to an acute-care facility for**

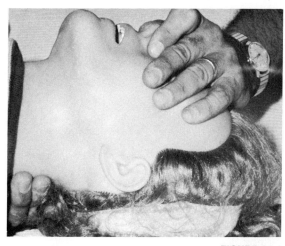

**FIGURE 26-3**
Hyperextension of the neck. (*From The Heart by J. W. Hurst et al. Copyright 1978 by McGraw-Hill, Inc. Used with permission of McGraw-Hill Book Company.*)

more aggressive treatment. Throughout cardiorespiratory resuscitation the family needs continued support. They are fearful of the sudden change in the patient's status and need to be reassured that the acute-care setting will provide optimal care for the patient. If possible, family members should be allowed to accompany the patient to the hospital.

In some situations patients may not respond to resuscitation, either because of delay in beginning the procedure or because of irreversible damage caused by the precipitating events. They may become comatose, have absent or barely palpable pulses, lose corneal reflexes, and have pupillary dilatation. The goal is to move these patients to an acute care setting where intubation can be per-

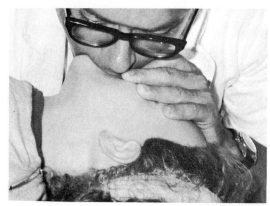

**FIGURE 26-4**
Ventilation. (*From The Heart by J. W. Hurst et al. Copyright 1974 by McGraw-Hill, Inc. Used with permission of McGraw-Hill Book Company.*)

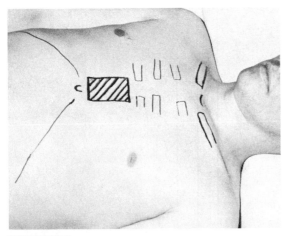

**FIGURE 26-5**
Landmarks for closed heart compression. (*From The Heart by J. W. Hurst et al. Copyright 1978 by McGraw-Hill, Inc. Used with permission of McGraw-Hill Book Company.*)

formed and they can be placed on assisted ventilation (see Chap. 30).

Resuscitation efforts may result in fractured ribs, pneumothorax, trauma of the liver, brain damage, metabolic acidosis, and seizures. These problems complicate the patient's recovery and prolong hospitalization. Nurses in all health care settings should constantly review and practice resuscitative procedures. The public should be encouraged to learn resuscitative techniques so that immediate CPR can be given when a life-threatening crisis occurs.

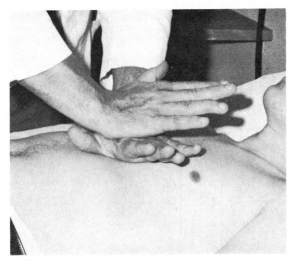

**FIGURE 26-6**
Closed-heart massage. (*From The Heart by J. W. Hurst et al. Copyright 1978 by McGraw-Hill, Inc. Used with permission of McGraw-Hill Book Company.*)

The "cafe coronary syndrome" is asphyxiation due to obstruction of the airway by food lodged in the trachea. Because of the sudden onset and the physical symptoms, this syndrome may be confused with a myocardial infarct. When food occludes the airway, the victim becomes speechless as the obstructed trachea presses against the larynx, causing the victim to choke and clutch the throat. Facial cyanosis will become apparent, and the eyes will bulge. The victim's face shows panic as the threat of death from impaired breathing becomes apparent. Within a few minutes the patient will lose consciousness.

The critical point in rendering care is to determine whether the symptoms are due to a tracheal obstruction or a myocardial infarction. One of the quickest ways to determine this is to ask the person to speak; the person having a heart attack will usually be able to communicate with the rescuer, but someone with food lodged in the trachea will not. In addition, the person who is choking will often clutch at the throat, whereas the person with an infarct will not.

Several methods are available to relieve airway obstruction caused by lodged food. Initially, the mouth should be explored with the fingers and easily accessible objects removed. The victim's head should be tilted back to straighten the airway. The tongue can be held down with a napkin or piece of cloth so that the rescuer can reach inside the mouth with the middle or index finger and remove the obstructing object. This method is most effective with unconscious patients, as they will be more relaxed. In most restaurants today, owners are encouraged to have available at all times a pair of 9-inch plastic tweezers called *choke savers.* The instrument is constructed to slip easily into the oral cavity and grasp the food in its curved tips.

Another method for the successful removal of food lodged in the trachea was devised by D. H. Heimlick and is referred to as the *Heimlick maneuver.* If the patient is standing or sitting when the obstruction occurs (see Fig. 26-7), the rescuer stands behind the victim and envelops the victim in a "bear hug." The rescuer's arms are placed above the umbilicus, and below the xiphoid process. The rescuer then grabs his or her right wrist with the left hand and exerts a sudden strong upward pressure against the abdomen. This should result in compression of the lungs, dislodging the food upward and restoring an open airway. If the patient is lying down (see Fig. 26-8), the procedure is carried out with the rescuer kneeling astride the victim. One hand is placed on top of the other, and the heel of the bottom hand is placed on the victim's abdomen above the umbilicus. A quick upward thrust is exerted against the abdomen and repeated if necessary.

The *Guildner procedure* is another method used to dislodge food from the trachea. In this procedure the rescuer's hands are placed above the xiphoid process and on the sternum. Pressure is exerted in a backward, inward motion to help dislodge the food.

The overall effectiveness of both the Heimlick maneuver and the Guildner procedure are still being studied. Since many people die from choking on pieces of food lodged in the trachea, it is important that both these procedures be studied carefully. Many states are attempting to pass legislation encouraging restaurant owners to require that all personnel know how to treat someone choking on a piece of food and how to institute cardiopulmonary resuscitation.

According to the American Heart Association, choking can be prevented by cutting food into small pieces, chewing food slowly and thoroughly, eliminating laughing while swallowing food, avoiding running with food in the mouth, and decreasing excessive alcohol intake while eating.

**Third-level nursing care** When the ischemia associated with coronary heart disease and coronary artery occlusion progresses to myocardial infarction, hospitalization is required. Patients with severe unrelieved angina may also require intensive nursing care to adequately evaluate current health problems and to prevent serious complications.

**N**ursing Assessment  Patients who sustain a myocardial infarction are acutely ill and susceptible to life-threatening complications. For this reason, an accurate health history and prompt physical assessment with appropriate diagnostic workup are essential.

*Health history*  The health history is probably the most important single factor in determining therapy. The patient or a family member should therefore be interviewed quickly but efficiently concerning changes that occurred prior to hospitalization. The symptom most often described is chest pain.

The *chest pain* of acute myocardial infarction is usually sudden and is more intense and continuous than that of angina pectoris. It is usually not relieved with nitroglycerin and is commonly described as a heavy crushing or squeezing pain. It is often located in the central area of the chest (epi-

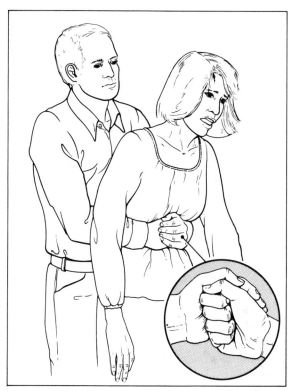

**FIGURE 26-7**
Heimlick maneuver (patient standing).

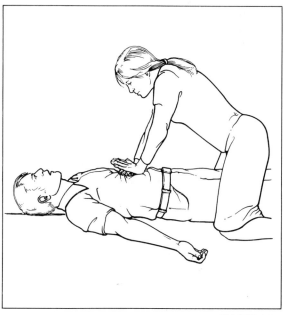

**FIGURE 26-8**
Heimlick maneuver (patient lying down).

gastric area) and may radiate to the jaws, arms, neck, teeth, etc.

Fear of impending death is voiced by many infarct patients. About one-third of the patients experience *premonitory symptoms* such as unaccustomed indigestion, sleep disturbances, excessive fatigue, or changes in their anginal pattern.[77] Patients may experience shortness of breath and anxiety. They are apprehensive about the changes they are experiencing, and often fear of death is a dominating thought. The patient may complain of feeling dizzy and may faint. Complaints of fatigue are not uncommon. Five to fifteen percent of infarct patients may be asymptomatic: the infarction may be discovered fortuitously during routine physical examinations or treatment for other health problems. Lack of symptoms can be a function of denial, cultural norms, differences in pain-sensitivity level, or absence of nerve endings in the ischemic area. The examiner needs to phrase questions about chest pain sensitively in order to obtain an accurate description of recent events and health status prior to the examination.

*Physical examination*   The physical examination of a patient with a myocardial infarction reveals changes that vary in severity according to the extensiveness of the infarction and the presence of complications. On observation, the patient appears pale and in some cases ashen or mildly cyanotic, and the nail beds may also appear cyanotic. The skin will be cool but clammy, and diaphoresis is common. Response to the chest pain continues, and the patient becomes restless and unable to find a comfortable position.

Nausea and vomiting (due to vagal stimulation), often seen with a posterior-wall infarction, can persist, and belching is not uncommon. The apical and radial pulse rate and rhythm will be within normal limits unless an arrhythmia is present. Sinus bradycardia and tachycardia (see Chap. 25) may be noted. Other arrhythmias, including premature ventricular beats, can occur at any point in the postinfarction period. The apical pulse may be difficult to palpate in some patients with anterior-wall infarction, because of changes that occur within the affected ventricle wall as a result of the infarction, and the radial or carotid pulse may have to be used. In the absence of shock (hypovolemia), peripheral pulses should be palpable (see Chap. 29 for sites of peripheral pulse).

The presence of $S_3$ and $S_4$ heart sounds (atrial and ventricular filling) may be auscultated. Intensity of the $S_1$ and $S_2$ heart sounds will be decreased, and a gallop rhythm may be noted. A transient apical systolic murmur may be heard. This is due to mitral regurgitation (see Chap. 27) caused by damage to papillary muscles. A precordial friction rub may be heard in one-third of patients with transmural infarctions usually 2 to 5 days after the infarction has occurred.

A temperature elevation is not uncommon as the inflammatory response is activated. Elevations can range from 100 to 103°F and can persist for a week after the infarction. When a temperature remains elevated (100 to 103°) over a period of days, it is suggestive of extensive cardiac ischemia.

Alterations in blood pressure may be noted, depending on the degree of cardiac damage and the systemic vascular resistance. In the presence of hypovolemia, the blood pressure will be significantly lowered. A systolic pressure below 80 mmHg is indicative of shock (see Chap. 28).

Respirations may be rapid and irregular, especially in the presence of pain. Dyspnea and orthopnea may be noted. In pump failure, basal rales, along with audible sounds of pulmonary edema (see Chap. 24), are often heard. Apprehension and anxiety can accelerate respiratory rate and increase dyspnea.

In the presence of right-sided heart failure, peripheral edema will be observed, especially in the ankles. In the presence of renal hypoxia, usually secondary to pump failure, decreased urinary output (oliguria) may be noted.

There is much fear associated with myocardial infarction. Frequently the patient has been in seemingly good health until the infarction, and the suddenness of the interruption increases apprehension on the part of the patient and the family. This stress is often manifested in a variety of coping behaviors such as denial and depression. Although these behaviors may not initially be manifested, they should be observed and evaluated throughout the recovery period.

*Diagnostic tests*   Several tests are used to support the diagnosis of acute myocardial infarction. These include the measurement of serum enzyme levels, electrocardiography, and coronary arteriography.

The principal *enzymes* which enter the circulation after release from ischemic cardiac cells are serum glutamic oxaloacetic transaminase (SGOT), lactic dehydrogenase (LDH), and creatine phosphokinase (CPK). Generally, the rise in enzyme level is in direct proportion to the size of the infarcted area. The earliest enzyme level to rise after onset of infarction, and the most cardiospecific, is CPK, particularly the MB fraction or CPK isoenzyme.[78,79]

*CPK* is found in heart, skeletal muscle, and

brain. After a myocardial infarction, CPK appears in the blood serum within 6 hours. The level returns to normal in 48 to 72 hours. Serial CPK enzyme levels are measured to detect extension of the infarcted area and reinfarction in other myocardial tissue. Because of the early response of CPK following an infarction, its measurement is most valuable. Normal CPK values range between 0 and 4 units.

The *SGOT* level following cardiac infarction exceeds the normal value of 8 to 40 units within 6 to 8 hours. It usually peaks in 24 to 48 hours and returns to normal in 4 to 8 days. Because other disorders such as hepatic disturbances are associated with elevated SGOT levels, a diagnosis of myocardial infarction should not rely solely on this test. A high SGOT level due to myocardial infarction corresponds to a poor prognosis.[80]

The serum *LDH* measurement is a useful evaluation tool when infarction is diagnosed late. The rise in LDH level is similar to SGOT but persists longer (5 to 7 days). $LDH_5$, an LDH enzyme subgroup contained in heart muscle, has been used to diagnose myocardial infarction when the level of SGOT is normal.[81]

If serum enzyme levels are not immediately or significantly elevated, the *EKG* may contribute significant information about an individual's cardiac status (refer to Chap. 22). The primary changes associated with myocardial infarction are Q waves (0.04 second), S-T segment elevation, and T-wave inversion in the leads overlying the affected cardiac areas. The Q waves signify infarcted tissue, whereas S-T segment elevation and T-wave inversion represent injury and ischemia. *Leukocytosis* (10 to 20 WBC per ml) will appear several days after infarction, and the *sedimentation rate* is elevated in response to the inflammation present. *Blood gases* (arterial) may be altered in the presence of pump failure.

Other noninvasive tests may be helpful in establishing a diagnosis or identifying complications. Vectorcardiography, echocardiography, apex cardiography, and systolic time intervals are gaining wider application (see Chap. 22 for description of these tests). In addition, sophisticated invasive tests such as myocardial perfusion scanning and radarkymography offer new advances in determining infarct size and ventricular wall motion abmormalities.[82] Coronary arteriography is done to identify occlusion sites within the coronary arteries and to determine whether atherosclerotic changes are the cause of the infarction. This test, discussed in Chap. 29, is done prior to coronary surgery to determine the need for a coronary bypass.

**N**ursing Problems and Intervention   Once the diagnosis of an acute myocardial infarction is made, the patient is brought to an intensive care unit, preferably a coronary care unit. Since the concept of coronary care units was first introduced in the early 1960s, care of the patient with a myocardial infarction has significantly improved, as has the prognosis.

The *coronary care unit* (CCU) is usually located in an area of the hospital with easy access to the operating room and contains a multiplicity of resuscitative equipment. The overall purpose of the CCU is to provide continuous, supervised care following a myocardial infarction. Qualified nursing personnel carefully monitor the patient to identify and treat changes in health status without delay.

The immediate problems facing the patient following admission to the CCU are *pain, dyspnea, fatigue,* and *anxiety.* The protocol of the CCU can also be frightening to the patient and family and can intensify fears. When possible, both the family and the patient should be oriented to the procedures of an intensive care unit and told about the equipment they can expect to see being utilized.

*Pain*   Immediate pain is usually treated with morphine sulfate, 1/6 to 1/4 grains. Selection of the route of administration will depend upon the physician, nurse, and patient. Demerol is not often used, because it induces vomiting and a vasovagal response. Careful assessment of vital signs should ensue, since morphine can depress respiration and lower the blood pressure. Frequently the anxiety associated with the presence of chest pain increases emotional as well as physiologic responses to the infarction. Therefore treating pain early will help relieve the additional stress of the situation. Since morphine sulfate often gives the patient an increased sense of well-being, the nurse must continue to emphasize that even though the pain no longer persists, there is significant cardiac damage. For some patients, the absence of pain reinforces denial of the severity of the cardiac problem.

*Dyspnea*   Dyspnea may be relieved by the use of nasal oxygen, 3 to 6 liters. If desired, mask oxygen up to 10 liters can be given. The administration of oxygen will increase the arterial oxygen level, improve the efficiency of vital organs, relieve chest pain, and improve color.

*Positioning* will also help relieve dyspnea. Placing the patient in a semi-Fowler's position lowers the diaphragm, improves lung expansion, and eliminates pooling of blood in pulmonary vessels. This position change will also improve the overall $CO_2/O_2$ exchange and increase the circulating oxygen levels. The use of a footboard, along with proper positioning of pillows, will provide support for the patient in various sitting positions and avoid strain in maintaining any position for long periods. Analgesics and hypnotics can help reduce anxiety and relieve stress, thereby relaxing the patient and easing respiratory effort. Arterial blood gases should be checked to assess the $CO_2/O_2$ exchange level.

If pump failure or pulmonary congestion is severe, diuretics will be used to reduce fluid retention and limit the development of acute right- or left-sided heart failure. Frequently a Foley catheter is inserted on admission to accurately assess the degree of renal perfusion by hourly measurements of urinary output. Nursing measures related to the care of the patient in pump failure are discussed in Chap. 24.

*Fatigue* An acute myocardial infarction produces a dynamic stress on the entire body system. In order for the damaged myocardium to recover, adequate rest must be carefully planned. Generally the patient will be on complete bed rest for an average of 24 hours to 5 days. In some situations patients can begin to move about within a day after the initial attack if there is no pain or serious complications.

Initially, all patient *activity* is limited. Stretching and pulling should be avoided. Complete physical care must be provided by the nurse between planned rest periods. Gradually, as the patient's health begins to improve, simple activities of self-care or feeding may be permitted. For many people, complete relinquishing of self-care activities such as washing the face and hands increases frustrations and emotional tension. In such cases it may be more beneficial to have the patient participate in simple tasks such as shaving or making phone calls in order to relieve the stress. When self-directed activities are permitted, the supplies needed for the activity should be made available and placed within easy reach of the patient. It is important that the need for rest and the purpose of limiting physical as well as emotional stress be discussed with the patient. For the more independent, compulsive personality, these restrictions may be the most difficult limitation to cope with. At times, talking to the patient will help. Often the emotional tension is a manifestation of a deeper unresolved emotional conflict. *Mild sedatives* such as Librium, phenobarbital, or Valium have been used to reduce anxiety and promote rest. Patients receiving these drugs should be observed closely for untoward effects of barbiturates.

*Planned rest periods* without interruption must be incorporated into the nursing care. Visiting hours need to be controlled in order to enforce these rest periods; generally, cooperation can be ensured by discussing the necessity for rest with the family.

*Immobility* Immediately after the infarction, the patient will spend time in bed or in a chair, and the hazards of limited mobility must be carefully considered. *Range of motion exercises* should be used when possible, to help keep muscles in tone and decrease stress when they are put into action once again. Many physicians activate their patients early with limited movements so as to prevent muscle atrophy and reduce threat of embolism.

*Elimination* is another problem for the immobilized patient. Changes in diet, as well as decreased activity and medications, can create elimination problems. The nurse must explain to the patient the effect of straining on elimination. Research has shown that using a bedpan can be most fatiguing for the patient. When possible, a bedside commode should be provided for bowel movements. Colace can be used as a stool softener to prevent straining on elimination. The patient must be told to avoid the Valsalva maneuver (bearing down and straining on defecation) at all times. If a Foley catheter is not being used to drain urine, a bedside urinal can be provided for the male patient. The patient should be able to contact the nurse easily for the use of the commode or bedpan. If diarrhea occurs, the patient will be treated with specific medications such as Kaopectate, or Lomotil. If constipation is a problem, a mild laxative or stool softeners may be used on a daily basis.

Emboli can result from prolonged bed rest, increased viscosity of blood, and immobility. This problem occurs in about 10 to 20 percent of patients. Usually elastic stockings, passive range of motion exercises, and anticoagulant therapy (although controversial) will prevent the formation of emboli. Patients who sustain extensive wall damage due to an infarction or those who demonstrate signs of failure, are initially treated with intravenous heparin. A complete discussion of anticoagulant therapy and related nursing care is found in Chap. 29.

*Gastrointestinal upset* Initially nausea and vomiting may be a problem for some patients following a myocardial infarction. If vomiting is severe, medications such as Compazine may be given to suppress it. As the vomiting and nausea subside, the patient can be given a liquid diet for the first 24 to 48 hours. Smaller amounts of food in the stomach reduce the alimentary diversion of blood for digestion and thus the demand on the myocardium.

After the first 48 hours the patient is put on a soft diet. Each dietary change should be discussed with the patient. At times the sudden disruption in dietary habits can be frustrating. Often this is aggravated by the fact that the person who is a smoker can no longer enjoy this pastime. This limitation, plus food restrictions, can be an added stress. Careful evaluation of usual dietary habits may help to make this transitional period more tolerable for the patient.

Assessment of fluid intake and output is also essential. Patients will be maintained on limited fluids to prevent circulatory overload and pump failure. Fluid intake of between 1500 and 2000 ml may be adequate. Dietary sodium may be restricted to avoid sodium retention. A Foley catheter is often used to measure accurate fluid output. Diaphoresis, vomiting, and diarrhea should be included in the evaluation of fluid output. A reduction in urinary output (e.g., 30 ml/hour) may be indicative of pump failure. A specific gravity above normal limits may be observed in patients who are dehydrated.

*Alteration in vital signs* Continual assessment of vital signs will provide the nurse with valuable data about the patient's progress. The patient may initially experience a temperature elevation, which may persist for several days. Usually, continuing temperature elevation suggests pulmonary infection or severe cardiac pathology. Frequent temperature checks are important. The temperature is usually taken orally, as rectal measurements may act as a vagal stimulus.[83]

Antipyretics (such as Tylenol) may be used to reduce the fever, along with a warm or tepid sponge bath. Fluids should be administered with caution. Aspirin should be avoided if anticoagulant therapy is being used. The patient should be continually assessed for signs of dehydration, and electrolytes should be checked daily.

Initially, following an infarction, the blood pressure should be checked every 1 to 2 hours. Hypotension is frequently noted during the immediate postinfarction period. Any drop in blood pressure should be reported, as it may indicate pump failure or impending shock. A rise in blood pressure is suggestive of hypertension.

Changes in pulse rate may occur at any time during the postinfarction period. An increase in pulse rate may be associated with anxiety and an irregularity in pulse rhythm may denote an arrhythmia, while a slowed pulse rate may be observed in response to medications such as morphine sulfate or digitalis or may indicate impending heart block.

Respiratory rates are initially rapid and at times irregular as a result of pain, dyspnea, and anxiety. Relief of the pain, along with mild sedation, can help restore respiratory regularity and rhythm. Sudden dyspnea or significant slowing in respirations should be carefully assessed as a possible indicator of increased myocardial ischemia, pulmonary embolism, or morphine sulfate toxicosis.

*Psychosocial reactions to a myocardial infarction* Patients who sustain an acute myocardial infarction often go through periods of anxiety, denial, and depression.[84] They may rationalize their cardiac problems or displace and project their anger and fear onto others. For many, a "heart attack" can mean several things. The patient with a myocardial infarction is often male and around middle age or younger. There is fear of potential loss of masculinity, sexual activity, and personal drive and success. In addition, many patients are coping with the fact that they are halfway (more or less) through their life and are adjusting to the middle years. Middle age is often a period when people reflect on the achievements of their lifetime. It is also a time when retirement is approaching and physical evidence of the aging process is apparent. The fact that the patient has sustained a heart attack can be viewed as evidence of "growing old." Denial and depression can become exaggerated, and when this occurs the patient is more difficult to care for.

The cardiac care unit is a most active place even under the best conditions. It is not unusual for the patient's normal biological rhythms such as eating and sleeping habits to be disrupted. Frequently patients experience sensory overload from a variety of sources. Constant monitoring can be distracting and upsetting to the patient. Continual interruption of rest periods by nurses, physicians, and other health providers is irritating. Such disruptions interfere with normal body rhythms and can heighten anxiety.

Patients may become obsessed with the functioning of the equipment, which can also increase their stress levels. Some patients will initially focus their complete attention on the sounds from the monitoring equipment, as if it were a lifeline to their recovery. All the machinery being used should be carefully explained so that the patient will not become frightened by a change in expected sounds.

Patients' anxieties will also be revealed in dreams. EKG readings may be altered during dreaming, and the patient may wake up frightened by the experience. Frequently tachycardia and premature beats are noted at such times.

Anxiety can also be intensified by the seriousness with which the family treats the problem of myocardial infarction. The initial attack may come unexpectedly and without warning. The patient is usually brought to the hospital quickly, connected to a multiplicity of machines, and separated from loved ones. This rapid transition can increase the anxiety of both patient and family members.

Nursing care should focus on reducing potential stressors. Careful orientation to the coronary care unit and the equipment is essential. The patient and family members should be allowed to ask questions about the equipment and its use; explanation will help reduce the patient's initial fears and help with the transition to a postcoronary setting as the patient's overall health begins to improve.

Patients should be allowed time to discuss significant changes that have occurred as a result of the infarction. They should be given time to discuss dreams and fears which increase anxiety. Death should be discussed freely, as it is often at the root of the patient's anxiety. Reassurance and support should be given constantly. When the patient appears anxious, a mild tranquilizer may be used to help reduce tension.

The infarction process should be discussed. The nurse should help the patient begin to identify those factors which may have contributed to the coronary occlusion. The patient, family members, and the nurse should strive to change or modify those risk factors which predisposed the patient to the initial attack. Extensive health teaching may be difficult in the setting of the coronary care unit, but the temporary nature of the stay in the coronary care unit and the need for follow-up nursing care during the rehabilitation phase should be emphasized.

*Cardiac arrhythmias*  Most patients will develop an arrhythmia in conjunction with a myocardial infarction. Arrhythmias can occur at any stage of the infarction process. Frequently patients die at the time of infarction or shortly thereafter because of a life-threatening arrhythmia (e.g., ventricular fibrillation). Arrhythmias such as premature ventricular beats are often precipitated by pain, damage to the conduction pathways as a result of the infarction, or pump failure. Prompt relief of pain, careful assessment of cardiac output, and prevention of pump failure, along with early identification of arrhythmias (see Chap. 25), will help reduce the risk

of a life-threatening crisis. If frequent premature ventricular contractions (more than 3 to 5/minute) develop, they should be treated immediately. Antiarrhythmic drugs (discussed in Chap. 25), analgesia, and nasal oxygen therapy should also be used as the need arises.

Precordial electric shock is used to terminate ventricular arrhythmia and resulting cardiac arrest. *Precordial shock* involves the delivery of a high-voltage electric current either externally (directly on the chest wall) or internally (through the myocardial wall) in order to terminate a life-threatening arrhythmia. The current is delivered to the heart through paddles placed over the chest wall. This results in depolarization of the myocardium, thereby terminating the arrhythmia and restoring the SA node as pacemaker.[85] There are two forms of precordial shock: defibrillation and cardioversion. (Refer to Chap. 25 for a complete discussion of both interventions.)

*Congestive heart failure*  Congestive heart failure (CHF) may develop at any time in the postinfarction period. Its presence is frequently determined by the amount of muscle damage and tissue ischemia. Careful observation for signs of right- and left-sided failure are essential (see Chap. 24). Fluid restriction, low-sodium diet, bed rest, and careful analysis of $PO_2$ and $PCO_2$ levels are important to avert pump failure. Treatment of CHF should begin early so that pulmonary edema and cardiogenic shock can be avoided.

Infarct patients who develop overt or incipient heart failure require careful monitoring of vital signs and serial measurement of blood gases. Taking of vital signs should not be neglected in favor of pressure readings from sophisticated machinery and cardiac-rhythm monitoring. When one stops to consider the sensitivity of heart and respiratory rates to left ventricular function, it becomes apparent that with all the technology available, clinical measures performed at the bedside are still valuable tools for assessment.

Oxygen therapy, diet therapy, and bed rest are important. Diuretics continue to be useful when pump failure is complicated by pulmonary edema. The value of digitalis in acute myocardial infarction is controversial. Experimentally, in the nonfailing heart, digitalis increases infarct size by increasing myocardial oxygen needs, but in failing hearts the inotropic action of digitalis overrides the increase in myocardial oxygen consumption to produce a beneficial effect,[86] hence its use in heart failure is probably justified and efficacious.

*Cardiogenic shock* Persistent pain, extensive loss of myocardial tissue due to infarction, pump failure, and arrhythmias may lead to the development of cardiogenic shock. Shock can be averted by early correction of predisposing problems. (A complete discussion of shock is found in Chap. 28.) Significant decrease in blood pressure, rapid and at times irregular pulse rate, pallor, restlessness, a dulled sensorium, and diminished urinary output may herald the onset of shock.

When shock is present, the objective of care is to reduce the body's oxygen needs by reducing oxygen consumption or by supplementing oxygen delivery. Cardioactive drugs such as isoproternol and norepinephrine may be used. Vasopressors and vasodilators are given to stimulate circulation and increase arterial blood pressure. Volume expanders, such as dextran, are used to increase overall blood volume. An intraaortic balloon may be inserted in an attempt to enhance coronary artery perfusion and hence to salvage ischemic myocardium. Central venous pressure and pulmonary wedge pressures (discussed in Chap. 28) are monitored to assess the patient's response to treatment. The reversal of cardiogenic shock following a myocardial infarction is often difficult because of the amount of damage to the myocardial tissue and the muscle wall.

*Rupture* Rupture of the myocardial wall is rare but can occur 4 to 10 days after infarction. Repeated infarctions lead to necrosis and thinning of the ventricle wall. Massive infarction also increases the area of necrosis and contributes to the problem of rupture. Persistent hypertension, along with physical exertion, can also potentiate ventricular rupture. Patients should be encouraged to rest and to avoid straining at stool. Laxatives may be used as needed. If cardiac tamponade (see Chap. 24) is present from excessive bleeding, pericardial aspiration may be necessary. Ventricular aneurysm due to weakness in the ventricular wall can also occur. An *aneurysmectomy* may be beneficial for patients with significant paradoxical wall motion accompanied by arrhythmias or intractable heart failure.

*Surgical intervention* for coronary occlusion may be considered for patients with severe anginal pain. A nonpharmacologic alternative and recent innovation is *electrical stimulation of the carotid sinus nerves.* The procedure consists of implanting a radio-frequency stimulator in the subcutaneous tissue of the anterior chest. Two bipolar electrodes are then attached to a carotid sinus nerve. Stimulation of the carotid nerve reduces the heart rate, arterial pressure, and myocardial contractility. Surgery with general anesthesia is required. This therapy has so far been confined to patients in whom pharmacologic treatment and exercise have been unsuccessful in controlling angina and for whom coronary bypass graft surgery is not possible.

*Coronary bypass graft surgery* offers an alternative to patients with intractable angina refractory to previous therapeutic efforts.[87] The goal of revascularization surgery is to improve the myocardial oxygen supply. This procedure bypasses one or more obstructed coronary arteries by grafting the saphenous vein graft from the aorta to a coronary vessel distal to the lesion (see Chap. 29 for complete discussion).

A less commonly used procedure involves the use of the internal mammary artery. The artery is directly anastomosed to the coronary artery. Improvement following surgery varies among patients, although there is evidence of increased exercise tolerance and improved ventricular function. Possible loss of graft patency, surgical mortality, and risk of further ventricular function decline after surgery are all problems to be considered prior to choosing this approach. Despite these problems, the surgical modality appears promising. Future data on long-term function of grafts may provide information on the overall clinical effectiveness of the procedures.

**Fourth-level nursing care** Patient *counseling* regarding the physical and emotional adjustment imposed by a myocardial infarction is an integral component of patient care. Following successful physiological and psychological adjustment, the patient should begin to prepare for transfer from the intensive care unit. During the period of *monitor weaning* the patient may verbalize fears. Often the transitional period can be facilitated by the use of battery-operated EKG telemetry, which allows the patient to walk without restriction by electric wires.[88]

**T**ransition Period *Transfer* from the intensive care area has been associated with catecholamine elevation, arrhythmias, heart failure, anxiety, and depression.[89] Prior to the transfer the patient should be counseled about the activities that can safely be performed, the process of myocardial healing, and personnel who will be providing care in the less acute area. Follow-up visits by intensive-nursing personnel during the first few days may help alleviate some of the patient's concerns. Continued monitoring by telemetry, if possible, is recommended.

A *graduated activity* regimen is usually begun. Progress from passive limb exercises to ambulation and stress testing depends on the absence of complications and the patient's tolerance.[90] Changes in respiratory rate and in pulse rate and rhythm, presence of gallop sounds, tachycardia and rales, and level of fatigue should be assessed when activity levels are increased.

Generally, activities permitted in the acute phase, such as lying in bed relaxed, standing still, or sitting in a chair, require an energy expenditure of 1.0 to 1.8 calories/minute. In the semiacute recovery phase, activities can increase to 1.8 to 3.0 calories/minute. Self-care activities, walking (slowly), and sewing can be considered during this period. In the convalescent period, expenditure of up to 3.0 to 4.0 calories/minute will be tolerated, as in showering or walking briskly. It should be noted that physicians will frequently advise patients to bathe rather than shower following an MI.

**H**ealth Teaching   The period following the acute phase of illness may be an appropriate time to begin dealing with the consequences of the myocardial infarction. Patients who sustain an infarction usually go through psychological phases in response to their infarction. These include anxiety, denial, and depression. It is important to assess these psychological states, as they could enhance or distract from the teaching-learning interaction.

*Teaching* should begin early, but information is best retained after the patient has had a chance to adjust to the health crisis. By this time the patient will have passed through crisis phases of shock and disbelief and entered or completed a phase of developing awareness. Anger and depression may be reactions when the reality of the situation is grasped and its consequences set in.[91] Teaching will need to be reemphasized following resolution of emotional conflicts. Research has shown that for some patients, teaching does not become an important component of care until discharge nears, perhaps because the prospect of being in one's own home leaves the patient more ready to respond to teaching. The teaching plan should include a discussion of the nature of the cardiac problem, physical activity, medications, smoking, and psychological factors related to cardiac illness and stress, as well as resumption of daily activity.[92,93]

Throughout the course of illness the patient should receive information about the nature and extent of the cardiac problem. The anatomy and physiology of the heart muscle, risk factors, the patient's particular area of ischemia, and the healing process can be included under this topic.

Almost every patient is discharged from the hospital on some *medication* following a myocardial infarction. *Digitalis* is the most common drug (see Chap. 24). Patients should know the action of digitalis and the potential side effects, and if the physician agrees, should be taught to take their own pulse rate. In addition, the family members as well as the patient should be told the signs of impending heart failure, and the patient should be instructed to see a nurse or physician if these changes are observed.

*Nitroglycerine* is another commonly used drug. The patient should know that tolerance to the drug will not build up over time, so that the same dosage will continue to be effective. A patient who knows that a particular activity may induce pain should be encouraged to take nitroglycerine prophylactically prior to the activity. Since nitroglycerine can change its composition when exposed to light over time, the patient should follow storage directions closely. Some manufacturers may have corrected this problem; the patient should be encouraged to check with the pharmacist about drug decomposition.

*Antiarrhythmic drugs* (see Chap. 25) may be used by some patients following discharge. Specific information regarding each drug should be reviewed with the patient.

*Diuretics* are used with some patients following a myocardial infarction (see Chap. 28). Signs of hypokalemia should be discussed, especially if digitalis is taken in conjunction with a diuretic. Oral potassium can be supplemented by foods such as bananas and orange juice (refer to Chap. 24 for additional foods). The patient should be encouraged to have blood electrolytes checked frequently (every 3 months) so that hypokalemia can be averted.

If *anticoagulants* are used (see Chap. 29), the patient must be taught the need for frequent laboratory blood tests. Usually the physician will decide, with the patient, the frequency of these blood checks. In addition to the effects of anticoagulants, emphasis should be placed on not terminating the medication without specific medical orders, and the patient should be warned to avoid salicylates.

*Mild tranquilizers* can be used to help reduce stress and tension. Moderate use of alcohol may be encouraged, unless the patient is taking such medications as sedatives or tranquilizers.

*Physical activity* is best prescribed in conjunction with exercise testing on a regular basis, but if this is not possible, a graduated program of activity can be safely devised using heart rate and physical status as guides to increasing activity levels.[94]

Frequently metabolic equivalents (or Mets) are used to calibrate specific activities. One Met is equal to the amount of energy required at rest. Activities are assessed according to the amount of oxygen needed per kilogram of body weight. Chapter 24 discusses the functional classification of metabolic equivalents and lists activities with approximate levels of Mets used. Most crafts and hobbies have a low expenditure level and can be engaged in freely, but bicycle riding, gardening, and swimming are considered high-energy activities.

Tachycardia occurring 10 minutes after the termination of exercise indicates lack of coronary reserve. The activity should then be reduced to the next lower level (see Met scale, Chap. 24) at which prolonged tachycardia does not occur. During the recovery period, patients should be given specific advice about the hazards of sustained static exercise such as handgrip or weight-carrying activities.[95] Physical-conditioning programs should not be entered into without a physical examination and professional supervision. It is important to approach all planned activities gradually and with caution. Emphasis should be placed on developing a long-range program of activities which will help the patient regain a preinfarction health state.

Patients should *avoid overexertion* and gradually rebuild their stress tolerance. Frequent rest periods should be encouraged. Normal energy expenditure should be taught through correct body mechanics, work-simplification methods, and correct breathing techniques during activities. Because of the overall improvement in health habits, the patient is often at a higher health level than before the infarction occurred.

*Sexual activity* is frequently neglected in teaching patients and is an area that deserves special attention. Specifically, patients should know that sexual activity can be resumed 4 to 8 weeks after infarction if the hospital course was uncomplicated. The average person who has recovered from an uncomplicated acute myocardial infarction has a maximum capacity of 8 to 9 Mets.[96] This would permit bicycle riding at 12 to 13 mph, jogging at 5 mph, or playing squash. The maximum energy expenditure during coitus is approximately 5 Mets for less than 30 seconds; during pre- and postorgasm periods it is about 3.7 Mets. Thus the energy cost is relatively low. Certain suggestions can be made about sexual intercourse, such as avoiding extremes of temperature, delaying intercourse after

eating or alcohol ingestion, waiting until rested after normal routines, and experimenting with positions of intercourse producing less strain, such as side by side, seated on a low chair with the partner facing on the lap, or lying down with the noncardiac partner on top.[97,98] Onset of chest pain, dyspnea, fatigue, or palpitations after sexual or any physical activity should caution the patient to moderate or cease the activity for a short period before resuming.

*Nutritional counseling* is important. Both the patient and the family members should be involved in discussing dietary limitations. A low-sodium (see Chap. 24), low-calorie, low-cholesterol diet is advisable. Frequently, sociocultural customs and trends will have to be discussed and resolved to obtain dietary compliance.

*Smoking* must be eliminated if at all possible. It is not an easy task. The patient must want to stop smoking and be motivated to do so. Continuing to smoke in the face of serious cardiac pathology is a form of denial. Patients must be given information about the hazards of smoking and impressed with the need to terminate the habit immediately. For some patients, gradual easing away is helpful, such as reducing the number of puffs or the number of cigarettes smoked per day. Hypnosis or the help of organizations devoted to ending the smoking habit may be needed.

To initiate and *maintain desired behaviors*, individual therapy, family counseling, group sessions,[99] or "coronary clubs" are useful. Peer setting of behavioral norms and provision of social support through groups are valuable mechanisms for maintaining behaviors. Ongoing concerns, personal suggestions for overcoming problems, and reinforcement are all part of the group process. The patient should know the psychological changes that can be expected following an infarction. The nurse should encourage complete discussion of these responses. Support and reassurance about personal feelings and behaviors are important concerns for both the family and patient. In addition, value clarification, an innovative approach geared toward setting priorities on required illness adjustments in relation to normal life events, may be an effective educational approach in helping patients who do not use denial to cope with their illness.[100] Effective educational strategies for patients who do use denial are less clear, and hazards may be associated with attempts to overcome denial.[101] Personality accommodation, behavioral modification strategies, and confidence training may be helpful but are as yet unproved.

**C**ompliance Recent research findings suggest that helping the patient to value and to focus on specific measures to restore health may determine the patient's ultimate long-term survival after an acute myocardial infarction.[102] The tactics appropriate to the patient's personal situation should be chosen only after an adequate assessment of strengths and weaknesses. Furthermore, patients can be helped to eliminate or manage their psychophysiologic or stress arousal. Identification of potentially stressful situations may help. Personal coping strategies can be greatly facilitated by actively listening, responding to verbal and nonverbal cues, and providing feedback.[103] Helping the patient learn to live within specific limits is a nursing challenge. Follow-up home visits a few weeks after discharge will be helpful. The patient should be given a phone number where a nurse may be contacted should questions about follow-up care arise. Finally, the patient's family should be taught cardiopulmonary resuscitation, and both the patient and the family should know exactly what to do and whom to call if chest pain recurs.

## REFERENCES

1 J. W. Hurst et al., *The Heart,* McGraw-Hill, New York, 1974, p. 988.

2 G. Thorn, R. Adams, E. Braunwald, K. Isselbacher, and R. Petersdorf, *Harrison's Principles of Internal Medicine,* McGraw-Hill, New York, 1977, p. 1263.

3 W. B. Kannel and T. R. Dawber, "Contributors to Coronary Risk—Implications for Prevention and Public Health: The Framingham Study," *Heart and Lung,* **1:**797–809, November–December 1972.

4 G. A. Gresham, "Early Events in Atherogenesis," *Lancet,* **1:**614–615, March 15, 1975.

5 Hurst et al., op. cit., pp. 992–994.

6 Ibid., pp. 996–997.

7 Ibid., p. 998.

8 Ibid., p. 999.

9 Ibid., pp. 999–1000.

10 E. H. Sonnenblick and C. L. Skelton, "Myocardial Energetics: Basic Principles and Clinical Implications," *N Engl J Med,* **285:**668–675, September 16, 1971.

11 Marie Castellan Clark, "Chest Pain," *Heart and Lung,* **4:**956–962, November–December 1975.

12 T. B. Denzler, E. W. Fuller, and R. S. Eliot, "Angina Pectoris and Myocardial Infarction in the Presence of Patent Coronary Arteries: A Review," *Heart and Lung,* **3:**646–653, July–August 1974.

13 L. S. Dreifus, "Angina Pectoris with Normally Patent Coronary Arteries," *Heart and Lung,* **3:**571–572, July–August 1974.

14 M. A. Nevins, "Oxyhemoglobin Equilibrium in Ischemic Heart Disease," *JAMA,* **229:**804–808, August 12, 1974.

15 Hurst et al., op. cit., p. 1008.

16 J. Luckman and K. Sorensen, *Medical-Surgical Nursing: A Psychophysiologic Approach,* Saunders, Philadelphia, 1974, p. 667.

17 B. E. Sobel, "Biochemical and Morphologic Changes in Infarcting Myocardium," *Hosp Pract,* **7:**59–71, February 1972.

18 R. Zak and M. Rabinowitz, "Metabolism of the Ischemic Heart," *Med Clin North Am,* **57:**93–103, January 1973.

19 M. F. Oliver, "The Metabolic Response to a Heart Attack," *Heart and Lung,* **4:**57–60, January–February 1975.

20 S. D. Fritz, "Energy Metabolism in Shock," *Heart and Lung,* **4:**615–618, July–August 1975.

21 M. F. Oliver, loc. cit.

22 S. D. Fritz, loc. cit.

23 Hurst et al., op. cit., p. 1007.

24 Ibid., p. 1012.

25 Ibid., p. 1015.

26 Ibid., pp. 989–992.

27 "Report of Inter-Society Commission for Heart Disease Resources: Primary Prevention of the Atherosclerotic Diseases," *Circulation,* **42:**A55–A95, December 1970.

28 T. Gordon et al., "Differences in Coronary Heart Disease in Framingham, Honolulu and Puerto Rico," *J Chron Dis,* **27:**329–344, September 1974.

29 M. F. Oliver, "Ischaemic Heart Disease in Young Women," *Br Med J,* **4:**253–259, November 2, 1974.

30 Kannel and Dawber, loc. cit.

31 T. Francis, Jr., and F. H. Epstein, "Survey Methods in General Populations: Studies of a Total Community, Tecumseh, Michigan," *Milbank Mem Fund Quart,* **43:**333–342, 1965.

32 J. C. Cassel, "Summary of Major Findings of the Evans County Cardiovascular Studies," *Arch Intern Med,* **128:**887–889, December 1971.

33 R. H. Rosenman et al., "Coronary Heart Disease in the Western Collaborative Group Study: A Follow-up Experience of 4½ Years," *J Chron Dis,* **23:**173–190, September 1970.

34 R. H. Rosenman et al., "Coronary Heart Disease in the Western Collaborative Group Study: Final Follow-up Experience of 8½ years," *JAMA,* **233:**872–877, August 25, 1975.

35 W. B. Kannel et al., "Electrocardiographic Left Ventricular Hypertrophy and Risk of Coronary Heart

Disease: The Framingham Study," *Ann Intern Med,* **72:**813–822, June 1970.

36 Kannel and Dawber, loc. cit.

37 G. D. Friedman, A. L. Klatsky, and A. B. Siegelaub, "Lung Function and Risk of Myocardial Infarction and Sudden Cardiac Death," *N Engl J Med,* **294:** 1071–1075, May 13, 1976.

38 Cassel, loc. cit.

39 Report of Inter-Society Commission for Heart Disease Resources, loc. cit.

40 J. H. Medalie et al., "Myocardial Infarction over a Five-year Period. I. Prevalence, Incidence and Mortality Experience," *J Chron Dis,* **26:**63–84, February 1973.

41 J. H. Medalie et al., "Angina Pectoris Among 10,000 Men: 5 Year Incidence and Univariate Analysis," *Am J Med,* **55:**583–594, November 1973.

42 A. M. Ostfeld et al., "A Prospective Study of the Relationship between Personality and Coronary Heart Disease, *J Chron Dis,* **17:**265–276, March 1964.

43 C. D. Jenkins, "Recent Evidence Supporting Psychologic and Social Risk Factors for Coronary Disease, Part Ii, *N Engl J Med,* **294:**1033–1038, May 6, 1976.

44 C. D. Jenkins, R. H. Rosenman, and S. J. Zyzanski, "Prediction of Clinical Coronary Heart Disease By a Test for Coronary-prone Behavior Pattern," *N Engl J Med,* **290:**1271–1275, June 6, 1974.

45 Hurst et al., op. cit., p. 992.

46 Ibid., pp. 1038–1042.

47 A. Keys et al., "Mortality and Coronary Heart Disease among Men Studied for 23 Years," *Arch Intern Med,* **128:**201–214, August 1971.

48 Hurst et al., op. cit., pp. 1040–1050.

49 Thorn, et al., op. cit., p. 1298.

50 Howard Leventhal, "Changing Attitudes and Habits To Reduce Risk Factors in Chronic Disease," *Am J Cardiol,* **31:**571–580, May 1973.

51 Hurst et al., op. cit., pp. 1052–1056.

52 A. L. McAlister et al., "Behavioral Science Applied to Cardiovascular Health: Progress and Research Needs in the Modification of Risk-taking Habits in Adult Populations," *Health Educ Mongr,* **4:** 45–74, Spring 1976.

53 L. W. Green et al., "Two Years of Randomized Patient Education Experiments with Urban Poor Hypertensives," Paper presented at First International Congress on Patient Counseling, Amsterdam, Netherlands, April 21, 1976.

54 M. C. Clark, "Chest Pain," *Heart and Lung,* pp. 956–962.

55 J. B. Nowlin et al., "The Association of Nocturnal Angina Pectoris with Dreaming," *Ann Intern Med,* **63:** 1040–1046, December 1965.

56 Thorn et al., op. cit., p. 1264.

57 Denzler et al., loc. cit.

58 Dreifus, loc. cit.

59 E. K. Butler, "Dyspnea in the Patient with Cardiopulmonary Disease," *Heart and Lung,* **4:**599–606, July–August 1975.

60 C. J. Pepine and L. Wiener, "Relationship of Anginal Symptoms to Lung Mechanics during Myocardial Ischemia," *Circulation,* **46:**863–869, November 1972.

61 P. G. F. Nixon and H. J. N. Bethell, "Preinfarction Ill Health," *Am J Cardiol,* **33:**446–449, March 1974.

62 Hurst et al., op. cit., p. 1038.

63 V. E. Friedewald, "Maximal-Stress, Multiple-Lead Exercise Testing: The Significance of ST-Segment Changes in the Detection of Coronary Arterial Occlusive Disease, *Heart and Lung,* **5:**91–96, January–February 1976.

64 D. C. Harrison, "Ambulatory Monitoring: A 1975 Overview," *Heart and Lung,* **4:**537–539, July–August 1975.

65 Kannel and Dawber, loc. cit.

66 J. S. Schroeder and J. W. Fitzgerald, "Indications and Techniques for Ambulatory Electrocardiogram Monitoring," *Heart and Lung,* **4:**540–545, July–August 1975.

67 W. B. Kannel et al., "Electrocardiographic Left Ventricular Hypertrophy and Risk of Coronary Heart Disease," *Ann Intern Med,* pp. 813–822.

68 W. S. Arnow, "Management of Stable Angina," *N Engl J Med,* **289:**516–520, September 6, 1973.

69 F. J. Goicoechea, "Ischemic Heart Disease: Angina Pectoris," *Drug Intelligence and Clinical Pharmacy,* **8:**382–391, June 1974.

70 Ibid.

71 A. S. Nies and D. G. Shand, "Clinical Pharmacology of Propranolol," *Circulation,* **52:**6–15, July 1975.

72 David Shand, "Propranolol," *N Engl J Med,* **293:** 280–285, August 7, 1975.

73 Ibid.

74 E. A. Amsterdam et al., "Management of Angina Pectoris: Therapeutic Methods and Physiologic Mechanisms," *Adv Cardiol,* **11:**175–190, 1974.

75 C. S. Alexander and A. Nino, "Cardiovascular Complications in Young Patients Taking Psychotropic Drugs," *Am Heart J,* **78:**757–769, December 1969.

76 I. H. Raisfeld, "Cardiovascular Complications of Antidepressant Therapy," *Am Heart J,* **83:**129–133, January 1972.

77 E. K. Chung and L. S. Chung, "Chest Pain, I: As a Coronary Symptom," *Drug Ther,* **6:**161–177, February 1976.

78 Robert Roberts and B. E. Sobel, "CPK Isoen-

zymes in Evaluation of Myocardial Ischemic Injury," *Hosp Pract,* **11:**55–62, January 1976.

79 B. E. Sobel, "Biochemical and Morphologic Changes in Infarcting Myocardium," *Hosp Pract,* pp. 59–71.

80 Hurst et al., op. cit., p. 1048.

81 Ibid., pp. 1048–1049.

82 E. Braunwald et al., "Research on the Diagnosis and Treatment of Myocardial Infarction" *Calif Med,* **114:**44–63, May 1971.

83 Patricia Ann Gruber, "Changes in Cardiac Rate Associated with the Use of the Rectal Thermometer in the Patient with Acute Myocardial Infarction," *Heart and Lung,* **3:**288–292, March–April 1974.

84 N. H. Cassem, and T. P. Hacket, "Psychiatric Consultation in a Coronary Care Unit," *Ann Intern Med,* **75:**9–14, 1971.

85 Luckman and Sorensen, op. cit., p. 650.

86 P. R. Maroko and E. Braunwald, "Modification of Myocardial Infarction Size after Coronary Occlusion," *Ann Intern Med,* **79:**720–733, November 1973.

87 T. J. Reeves et al., "Natural History of Angina Pectoris," *Am J Cardiol,* **33:**423–430, March 1974.

88 Estelle Beaumont, "ECG Telemetry," *Nurs '74,* **4:** 27–34, July 1974.

89 W. D. Gentry and T. Haney, "Emotional and Behavioral Response to Acute Myocardial Infarction," *Heart and Lung,* **4:**738–745, September–October 1975.

90 B. L. Johnston, J. D. Cantwell, and G. F. Fletcher, "Eight Steps to Inpatient Cardiac Rehabilitation: The Team Effort—Methodology and Preliminary Results, *Heart and Lung,* **5:**97–111, January–February 1976.

91 Cynthia Scalzi, "Nursing Management of Behavioral Responses Following an Acute Myocardial Infarction," *Heart and Lung,* **2:**62–69, January–February 1973.

92 P. Deberry, L. P. Jefferies, and M. R. Light, "Teaching Cardiac Patients to Manage Medications," *Am J Nurs,* **75:**2191–2193, December 1975.

93 R. H. Rahe, C. Scalzi, and K. Shine, "A Teaching Evaluation Questionnaire for Postmyocardial Infarction Patients," *Heart and Lung,* **4:**759–766, September–October 1975.

94 Millie Lawson, "Progressive Coronary Care," *Heart and Lung,* **1:**240–253, March–April 1972.

95 D. J. Ewing et al., "Weight Carrying after Myocardial Infarction," *Lancet,* **1:**1113–1114, May 17, 1975.

96 A. W. Green, "Sexual Activity and the Postmyocardial Infarction Patient," *Am Heart J,* **89:**246–252, February 1975.

97 G. C. Griffith, "Sexuality and the Cardiac Patient," *Heart and Lung,* **2:**70–73, January–February 1973.

98 Scalzi, loc. cit.

99 Ibid.

100 Bonnie Berger, J. W. Hopp, and V. Raettig, "Values Clarification and the Cardiac Patient," *Health Educ Monogr,* **3:**191–199, Summer 1975.

101 Gentry and Haney, loc. cit.

102 Ibid.

103 T. F. Garrity and R. F. Klein, "Emotional Response and Clinical Severity as Early Determinants of Six-month Mortality after Myocardial Infarction," *Heart and Lung,* **4:**730–737, September–October 1975.

## BIBLIOGRAPHY

Adams, Nancy R.: "Reducing the Perils of Intracardiac Monitoring, *Nurs '76,* **6:**66–74, April 1976.

Allendorf, E. E., and M. H. Keegan: "Teaching Patients about Nitroglycerin," *Am J Nurs,* **75:**1168–1170, July 1975.

Amsterdam, E. A., et al.: "Evaluation and Management of Cardiogenic Shock. Part I. Approach to the Patient," *Heart and Lung,* **1:**402–408, May–June 1972.

Amsterdam, E. A., et al.: "The Use of Diuretics in Acute Myocardial Infarction," *Heart and Lung,* **2:** 434–438, May–June 1973.

Andreoli, Kathleen G., et al.; *Comprehensive Cardiac Care: A Text for Nurses, Physicians, and Other Health Practitioners,* Mosby, St. Louis, 1975.

Berne, R. M., and M. N. Levy: *Cardiovascular Physiology,* Mosby, St. Louis, 1972.

Bloom, B. S., and O. L. Peterson: "End Results, Cost and Productivity of Coronary-care Units," *N Engl J Med,* **288:**72–78, January 11, 1973.

Bolognini, Vicki: "The Swan-Ganz Pulmonary Artery Catheter: Implications for Nursing," *Heart and Lung,* **3:**976–981, November–December 1974.

Bordia, A., et al.: "Effect of the Essential Oils of Garlic and Onion on Alimentary Hyperlipemia," *Atherosclerosis,* **21:**15–19, 1975.

Boston Collaborative Drug Surveillance Program: "Coffee Drinking and Acute Myocardial Infarction," *Lancet,* **2:**1278–1281, December 16, 1972.

Carleton, R. A., and A. D. Johnson: "Coronary Arterial Spasm: A Clinical Entity?", *Mod Concepts Cardiovasc Dis,* **43:**87–91, May 1974.

Castellanos, A., et al.: "Didactic Electrocardiography: General Concepts," *Heart and Lung,* **4:**697–723, September–October 1975.

Coats, Kathryn: "Noninvasive Cardiac Diagnostic Procedures," *Am J Nurs,* **75:**1980–1985, November 1975.

Cooper, T.: "Arteriosclerosis: Policy, Polity and Parity," *Circulation,* **45:**433–440, February 1972.

Corbalan, R., R. Verrier, and B. Lown: "Psychological Stress and Ventricular Arrhythmias during Myocardial Infarction in the Conscious Dog, *Am J Cardiol,* **34:**692–696, November 1974.

Cox, J. L., et al.: "Coronary Collateral Blood Flow in Acute Myocardial Infarction," *J Thorac Cardiovasc Surg,* **69:**117–125, January 1975.

Frank, M. J., and S. Alvarez-Mena: *Cardiovascular Physical Diagnosis,* Year Book, Chicago, 1973.

Forker, A. D., H. Starke, and R. S. Eliot: "Loop Logic: An Introduction to Vectorcardiography," *Geriatrics,* **30:**87–95, June 1975.

Forrester, J. S., K. Chaterjee, and H. J. C. Swan: "Hemodynamic Monitoring in Patients with Acute Myocardial Infarction," *JAMA,* **266:**60–61, October 1, 1973.

Foster, Sue B.: "Pump Failure," *Am J Nurs,* **74:**1830–1834, October 1974.

Fulton, Mary, et al.: "Natural History of Unstable Angina," *Lancet,* **1:**860–868, April 22, 1972.

Gentry, W. D., and R. B. Williams (eds.): *Psychological Aspects of Myocardial Infarction and Coronary Care,* Mosby, St. Louis, 1975.

Glagov, S.: "Mechanical Stresses on Vessels and the Non-Uniform Distribution of Atherosclerosis," *Med Clin North Am,* **57:**63–77, January 1973.

Goldstrom, D. K.: "Cardiac Rest," *Am J Nurs,* **72:**1812–1816, October 1972.

Gorfinkel, H. J., R. Haider, and J. Lindsay: "Diagnosis and Treatment of Hemodynamic Abnormalities after Acute Myocardial Infarction," *Med Ann DC,* **43:**395–400, August 1974.

Griffith, G. C.: "The Life Cycle of Coronary Artery Disease," *Heart and Lung,* **1:**63–67, January–February 1972.

*Heart Facts, 1976,* American Heart Association Publication 50-008B.

Heaton, K. W., and E. W. Pomare: "Effect of Bran on Blood Lipids and Calcium," *Lancet,* **1:**49–50, January 12, 1974.

Houser, Doris: "Ice Water for MI Patients? Why Not?," *Am J Nurs,* **76:**432–434, March 1976.

Hrubec, Z.: "Coffee Drinking and Ischemic Heart Disease," *Lancet,* **1:**548, March 10, 1973.

Hutter, A. M., et al.: "Early Hospital Discharge After Myocardial Infarction," *N Engl J Med,* **288:**1141–1144, May 31, 1973.

Jahre, J. A., et al.: "Medical Approach to the Hypotensive Patient and the Patient in Shock," *Heart and Lung,* **4:**577–587, July–August 1975.

Jenkins, C. D.: "Recent Evidence Supporting Psychologic and Social Risk Factors for Coronary Disease, Part I, *N Engl J Med,* **294:**987–994, April 29, 1976.

Jennings, R. B., and K. A. Reimer: "Salvage of Ischemic Myocardium," *Mod Concepts Cardiovasc Dis,* **43:**125–130, December 1974.

Kasl, S. V.: "Issues in Patient Adherence to Health Care Regimens," *J Hum Stress,* **1:**5–17, 48, September 1975.

Klatsky, A. L., et al.: "Coffee Drinking Prior to Acute Myocardial Infarction," *JAMA,* **226:**540–543, October 29, 1973.

Kones, R. J.: "Oxygen Therapy for Acute Myocardial Infarction: Basis for a Practical Approach," *South Med J,* **67:**1322–1328, November 1974.

Kramer, Barry: "Wiser Way of Living, Not Dramatic 'Cures', Seen as Key to Health," *Wall Street Journal,* March 22, 1976, p. 1.

Lesch, M., and R. Gorlin: "Pharmacological Therapy of Angina Pectoris," *Mod Concepts Cardiovasc Dis,* **42:**5–10, February 1973.

Levy, R. L., J. Morganroth, and B. M. Rifkind: "Treatment of Hyperlipedemia," *N Engl J Med,* **290:**1295–1301, June 6, 1974.

Lichstein, E., and S. G. Seckler: "Evaluation of Acute Chest Pain," *Med Clin North Am,* **57:**1481–1490, November 1973.

Loeb, H. S., et al.: "Assessment of Ventricular Function after Acute Myocardial Infarction by Plasma Volume Expansion," *Circulation,* **47:**720–728, April 1973.

Luchi, R. J., et al.: "Use of Cardioactive Drugs in Acute Myocardial Infarction," *Heart and Lung,* **5:**44–61, January–February 1976.

Martin, S. P., et al.: "Inputs into Coronary Care during 30 Years: A Cost Effectiveness Study," *Ann Intern Med,* **81:**289–293, September 1974.

McFadden, R. B., E. J. Jahnke, and J. H. K. Vogel: "Natural and Unnatural History of Acute Coronary Artery Disease," *Adv Cardiol,* **11:**136–142, 1974.

McIntyre, H. Mildred (ed.): *Heart Disease: New Dimensions of Nursing Care,* Trainex Co., Garden Grove, Calif., 1974.

McNeer, J. F., et al.: "The Course of Acute Myocardial Infarction: Feasibility of Early Discharge of the Uncomplicated Patient," *Circulation,* **51:**410–413, March 1975.

Medical Division, Royal Infirmary, Glasgow: "Early Mobilisation After Uncomplicated Myocardial Infarction," *Lancet,* **2:**346–350, August 18, 1973.

Moskowitz, Lani: "Vasodilator Therapy in Acute Myocardial Infarction," *Heart and Lung,* **4:**939–945, November–December 1975.

*National Heart, Blood Vessel, Lung and Blood Program,* Second Annual Report of the Director of the National Heart and Lung Institute, DHEW Publication (NIH) 75-748, 1975.

Nielsen, M. A.: "Intra-Arterial Monitoring of Blood Pressure," *Am J Nurs,* **74:**48–53, January 1974.

Ramirez, A., and W. H. Abelmann: "Cardiac Decompensation," *N Engl J Med,* **290:**499–501, February 28, 1974.

Rebuck, A. S., J. F. Cade, and E. J. M. Campbell: "Pulmonary Aspects of Myocardial Infarction," *Mod Concepts Cardiovasc Dis,* **42:**17–21, April 1973.

Roberts, C. J., and S. Lloyd: "Association between Mortality from Ischemic Heart-Disease and Rainfall in South Wales and in the County Burroughs of England and Wales," *Lancet,* **1:**1091–1093, May 20, 1972.

Roberts, W. C.: "Coronary Arteries in Fatal Acute Myocardial Infarction," *Circulation,* **45:**215–230, January 1972.

Romhilt, D. W., and N. O. Fowler: "Physical Signs in Acute Myocardial Infarction," *Heart and Lung,* **2:**74–80, January–February 1973.

Rotman, M., et al.: "Pulmonary Arterial Diastolic Pressure in Acute Myocardial Infarction," *Am J Cardiol,* **33:**357–362, March 1974.

Schamroth, L., and J. B. Jaspan: "Variant Angina Pectoris: Atypical Prinzmetal's Angina Pectoris," *Heart and Lung,* **2:**431–433, May–June 1973.

Schiffer, F., et al.: "The Quiz Electrocardiogram: A New Diagnostic and Research Technique for Evaluating the Relation between Emotional Stress and Ischemic Heart Disease, *Am J Cardiol,* **37:**41–47, January 1976.

Segal, B. L., et al.: Echocardiography: Current Concepts and Clinical Application, *Am J Med,* **57:**267–283, August 1974.

Sonnenblick, E. H., and R. Gorlin: "Reversible and Irreversible Depression of Ischemic Myocardium," *N Engl J Med,* **286:**1154–1155, May 25, 1972.

Stitt, F. W., et al.: Clinical and Biochemical Indicators of Cardiovascular Disease among Men Living in Hard and Soft Water Areas, *Lancet,* **1:**122–126, January 20, 1973.

Tuzel, I. H.: "Sodium Nitroprusside: A Review of Its Clinical Effectiveness as A Hypotensive Agent," *J Clin Pharm,* **14:**494–503, October 1974.

Weiss, S. M. (ed.): *Proceedings of the National Heart and Lung Institute Working Conference on Health Behavior,* Basye, Va., May 12–15, 1975, DHEW Publication (NIH) 76-868, 1975.

Weissler, A. M.: "Noninvasive Methods for Assessing Left Ventricular Performance in Man," *Am J Cardiol,* **34:**111–114, July 1974.

Williams, D. O., et al.: "Physical Activity in the Rehabilitation of Patients Following Myocardial Infarction. I. Basis of Early Ambulation," *Heart and Lung,* **5:**317–321, March–April 1976.

Zelis, R., et al.: "The Pulmonary Edema Symptom," *Drug Ther,* **5:**39–51, November 1975.

Zola, I. K.: "Culture and Symptoms: An Analysis of Patients' Presenting Complaints," *Am Socio Rev,* **31:**615–630, October 1966.

# 27
# STRUCTURAL DEFECTS OF THE HEART

Frances J. Storlie

The heart muscle is a remarkably strong organ. Its action is governed by a mechanical pumping system as well as an effective conduction system. The internal structural components of the pumping mechanism operate interdependently and help promote effective oxygenation. Malfunction of any structural component affects the total pumping action of the heart. As human beings interact with the environment, certain external factors (such as dietary habits and inflammatory processes) as well as internal factors (including genetic and chromosomal alterations) can change cardiac structures and disrupt their synergistic functioning. When these changes occur, they produce specific effects on the individual which can significantly alter their health status.

This chapter will focus upon those congenital and acquired structural changes that most frequently occur during human beings' interaction with the environment. Mitral stenosis, a common structural defect observed in adults, will be highlighted as a focal component of this discussion.

Structures within the pumping system can be disrupted by stenosis (narrowing), obstruction, deformity, malposition, damage, or absence. The changes that occur can be attributed to either congenital or acquired causes. When these defects lead to a fall in cardiac output, pump failure results.

## PATHOPHYSIOLOGY OF CONGENITAL HEART DEFECTS

Congenital defects in the structural components of the heart can be divided into three groups on the basis of the physiological changes observed. These groupings are classified as volume overload, obstruction of forward flow, and conditions of desaturation. Each problem is precipitated by specific changes within the heart structure due to a congenital aberration.

### Volume Overload

When a greater than normal amount of blood enters either of the ventricular chambers, volume overload can occur. The work load of that side of the heart increases to meet the extra demand placed upon the muscle owing to the defect. Atrial and ventricular septal defects are two major problems that cause an increase in blood volume in the ventricle receiving the abnormal influx.

*Ventricular septal defects* are among the most common cardiac malformations of congenital origin. The problem is most often observed in com-

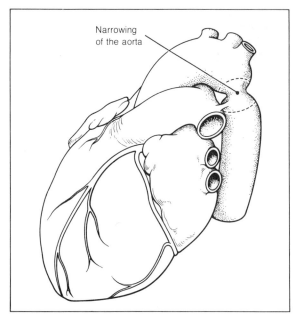

Narrowing
of the aorta

**FIGURE 27-1**
Coarctation of the aorta.

bination with other cardiac anomalies. The main defect occurs in the orifice (opening) of the membranous portion of the ventricular septum. The degree of disruption caused by this opening will depend on size. In a small defect, the opening is slight, and therefore less pressure is exerted on the ventricle. As the opening becomes larger, there is an equalization in ventricular pressure. With progressive enlargement of the orifice there will be an elevation in right ventricular pressure and pulmonary artery pressure. Left-sided failure can also occur. Patients with small defects may experience no physiological effects. However, patients with larger openings may show signs of increasing cardiac insufficiency and pump failure.

An *atrial septal defect* is an opening between the atria that allows blood flow across both sides of the heart in either direction. It is one of the most common congenital defects recognized in female adults. The defect can occur high in the atrial septum near the entry of the superior vena cava or at the fossa ovalis or midseptum (an anatomic patency not to be confused with patent foramen ovale).[1] Other defects can occur adjacent to the atrioventricular valves, which may be either deformed or incompetent. These changes are often seen in patients with Down's syndrome. Again, the magnitude of this problem is dependent upon the size of the opening. In a small opening, there may be an in-

crease in left atrial pressure; however the pressure tends to equalize when the atrial opening becomes larger. These changes result in overloading of the right ventricle and increased pulmonary blood flow (left-to-right shunt). Patients with atrial septal defects are usually symptom-free until the middle adult years.

## Obstruction of Forward Flow

A second class of structural defects includes those caused by obstruction of forward flow of blood from the heart. Coarctation (narrowing) of the aorta or stenosis of the aortic valve will result in stress upon the left ventricle. Pulmonic stenosis and pulmonary hypertension, however, are defects which can create a pressure overload on the right ventricle. With each defect, the forward flow of blood is obstructed, and cardiac efficiency and output are reduced.

*Coarctation of the aorta* is a problem caused by a narrowing of the aorta, usually in the descending portion, distal to or below the origin of the subclavian artery (see Fig. 27-1). The normal lumen of the aorta is often reduced in diameter as much as 1 to 2 mm. The severity of the problem will depend on the amount of additional defects that accompany this problem. Patent ductus and ventricular septal defects are two such defects that may be observed along with coarctation of the aorta. This problem is seen in about 7 to 9 percent of the patients with congenital heart pathology. Males are more commonly affected than females.

The adult or postductal form of aortic coarctation is frequently seen. Generally the patient experiences few symptoms because the left ventricle can pump blood directly through the stricture or through collateral blood vessels which bypass the stricture. Usually surgical intervention corrects the problem, but the greatest complication is hypertension.

*Aortic stenosis* is characterized by the fusion of the three cusps of the aortic valve at the commissures (region of union). The result is a greatly reduced diameter of the outflow tract. According to Sanderson[2] true congenital valvular stenosis occurs when the tissues of the right and left coronary cusps are fused into a single functional cusp, but with an insignificant "shadow commissure" in the center. The orifice is often slitlike and deviated from the center of the tract.

In many cases *congenital pulmonic stenosis* is combined with a ventricular septal defect (VSD) or an atrial septal defect (ASD). Normally the outlet valve between the right ventricle and the pulmonary artery consists of three cusps. When commissures between these cusps become fused, the orifice through which blood must pass on its way to the lungs is reduced, often to only a fraction of its normal size. If, however, the valve is severely stenotic, extremely high pressure must be generated by the right ventricle to move the blood forward. Right ventricular hypertrophy will result from the increased work load (see Fig. 27-2). If VSD or ASD is a component of the pathology, any increase in pressure within the right ventricle will accentuate the right-to-left diversion of unoxygenated blood.

## Conditions of Desaturation

Conditions of desaturation can occur when there is a shunting of oxygenated blood back to the right side of the heart (*left-to-right shunt*), or there is a diversion of blood into the left side of the heart without the blood being oxygenated by the lungs.[3] Defects in which desaturation is marked are the most serious of the congenital heart anomalies and require early correction.

A *right-to-left* shunt is defined as a diversion of unoxygenated blood from the right atrium through an atrial septal defect into the left atrium. Blood from the right ventricle can also flow into the left ventricle through a ventricular-septal defect. This blood mixes with oxygenated blood and is circulated throughout the body. The degree of cyanosis and dyspnea present will depend upon the amount of blood being diverted through the shunt.

*Tetralogy of Fallot* is a structural defect in which there is complex shunting of blood due to multiple structural alterations (see Fig. 27-3). This defect is accompanied by pulmonary stenosis, a ventricular septal defect, right ventricular hypertrophy, and malposition or shifting (dextroposition) of the aorta to the right, thereby overriding the ventricular septum. These changes result in a right-to-left shunting of blood. Pulmonary stenosis causes right ventricular hypertrophy. As blood passes from the right to left side through the ventricular septal opening, pulmonary blood flow is decreased. The size of the right-to-left shunt, the amount of oxygen contained in the shunted blood, and the degree of diminished blood flow through the lungs will be reflected by the amount of cyanosis observed clinically. Surgical correction is usually performed in childhood.

An *atrioventricular septal defect* is a condition in which the right atrium and the left ventricle are in communication with one another. This is due to the formation of a fissure in the septal leaflet. Unoxygenated blood from the right ventricle becomes

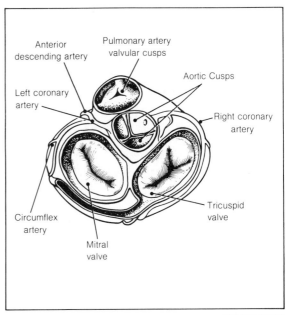

**FIGURE 27-2**
Pulmonic valvular stenosis.

mixed with oxygenated blood of the left ventricle and decreases the level of oxygen content in the circulating blood.

*Patent ductus arteriosis* is another commonly observed structural defect in children. The open channel between the right and left atria, vital during fetal life, fails to close 2 to 3 weeks after birth. This results in a left-to-right shunting of blood from the aorta to the pulmonary artery and then through the lungs and into the left atrium and ventricle.[4] This will result in ventricular hypertrophy (enlargement) if the defect is uncorrected. The severity of the resulting complications will depend upon the size of the opening. The smaller the opening, the fewer residual effects will be noted.

Additional structural changes may be seen; they include such problems as transposition of the great vessels, coronary artery defects, and tricuspid atresia. Table 27-1 gives the frequency of the more common congenital anomalies.

## Causes of Congenital Heart Defects

Congenital cardiovascular structural defects are the result of alterations in embryonic development caused by external environmental factors or genetic aberrations. It is difficult to isolate one specific cause for these defects. Viral infections, drugs, and gene mutations have been cited as three possible

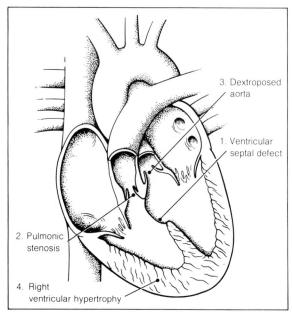

3. Dextroposed aorta

1. Ventricular septal defect

2. Pulmonic stenosis

4. Right ventricular hypertrophy

**FIGURE 27-3**
Tetralogy of Fallot.

factors that interact to produce cardiovascular defects.

*Rubella* (maternal) is cited as a major cause of congenital heart defects. The virus affects the mother early in pregnancy (first trimester) and proceeds to invade fetal tissue, causing structural changes.[5] A rubella syndrome results and may include problems such as motor and somatic retardation, cataracts, and deafness. Patent ductus arteriosus, arterial stenosis, ventricular septal defect, and pulmonic stenosis are the most common results. These changes can occur singly or in combination with one or more problems.

There is some evidence to suggest that the *Coxsackie virus* may also contribute to the forma-

tion of cardiovascular defects. The Coxsackie virus is responsible for a variety of clinical syndromes including aseptic meningitis, myocarditis, and pericarditis. Researchers suggest that the acute phase of illness may be followed by a continuing chronic phase which, if the mother was pregnant, could contribute to cardiovascular defects in the unborn fetus.[6]

*Thalidomide,* if taken by the mother early in pregnancy, has been associated positively with various congenital cardiac defects. In addition, parents who have taken lysergic acid diethylamide (LSD) before conception has occurred have borne children with congenital heart abnormalities. The research suggests that the LSD produces chromosomal alterations which can contribute to congenital heart anomalies.

A *genetic defect,* or malarrangement of certain specific chromosomes, has been identified in some syndromes in which cardiovascular defects are consistently found. Table 27-2 identifies several of these syndromes and the physiological defects associated with them. It is important to note that many of these syndromes may result in a single or multiple cardiovascular defects.

The identification of one isolated cause of a congenital cardiac problem and its direct effect on cardiac structures is difficult. The Inter Society Commission for Heart Disease Resources has indicated that familial clustering of congenital heart disease suggests that an interaction of environmental genetic, or chromosomal factors may be operative in producing these defects.[7]

## PATHOPHYSIOLOGY OF ACQUIRED HEART DEFECTS

Acquired heart disease and related structural defects can be attributed to two specific causes. These are atherosclerotic changes and inflammation of one or more structures of the heart.

*Atherosclerosis* results in cardiac structural changes due to the deposition of fatty plaques that collect in the intimal walls of the arteries and their branches. The coronary arteries are most often affected by these changes, and valvular incompetence can develop as a secondary response to the problem. When this occurs, supporting structures such as the chordae tendineae are affected (see Chap. 22). If this persists, there is calcification of the commissure, and the valve's normal opening and closing can become interrupted.

Inflammation of the myocardium, the endocardium, or the pericardium is the second most

**TABLE 27-1**
FREQUENT CONGENITAL HEART DEFECTS

| Problem | Percentage* |
| --- | --- |
| Ventricular septal defect | 30.5 |
| Atrial septal defect | 9.8 |
| Patent ductus arteriosus | 9.7 |
| Pulmonary stenosis | 6.9 |
| Coarctation of the aorta | 6.8 |
| Aortic stenosis | 6.1 |
| Tetralogy of Fallot | 5.8 |
| Tricuspid atresia | 1.3 |

* 2310 cases equals 100%.
SOURCE: Thorn, George et al., *Harrison's Principles of Internal Medicine,* 8th ed., McGraw-Hill, New York, 1977, Table 241-1, p. 1219.

common cause of acquired structural defects. *Streptococcus viridans* is the organism most responsible for initiating the inflammatory process in the majority of cases.[8] Bacterial infections caused by other organisms can also invade cardiac tissue and will be discussed in the following pages.

## Rheumatic Fever

Rheumatic fever is caused by an invasion of the beta-hemolytic group A streptococcus. These infections are seen most frequently in the early summer and fall. Although the interrelationship exists between the development of rheumatic fever and the onset of cardiac structural defects, the exact process is not clearly understood. Rheumatic fever is classified as a collagen disease and is discussed completely in Chap. 10.

There is evidence to suggest that rheumatic fever may be caused in part by an *antigen-antibody* response. It has been reported that rheumatic subjects form hyperactive antibodies which respond excessively to the stimulus of the streptococcal infection.[9] Other research suggests that the predisposition to rheumatic fever may have an *inherited* basis and is transmitted through a Mendelian recessive trait, while others suggest that the problem "tends to run in families."[10]

*Socioeconomic* and *racial factors* also seem to correlate with the development of rheumatic fever. Poverty, crowded living, poor nutrition, and lack of heat through a cold winter, all seem to contribute to the development and transmission of the streptococcal virus. The northeastern region of the United States appears to be an area of high incidence for many of the reasons listed above.

Whatever the cause, rheumatic fever usually begins with an upper respiratory infection, caused by a streptococcal virus. The individual experiences acute streptococcal tonsillitis, fever, chills, and swollen lymph nodes. After a 2- to 5-week period, the patient appears to recover from the acute infection. Subsequently, the patient becomes ill and begins to experience the effects of rheumatic fever once again (the poststreptococcal hypersensitization theory). During this phase the target organ most often is the heart.

Rheumatic fever can affect any of the three layers of the heart. When *all* three layers are involved, the condition is called *pancarditis.* When *rheumatic myocarditis* occurs, Aschoff's bodies (lesions of interstitial tissue) or nodules can be occasionally found in the myocardial fibers. *Myocarditis* is an inflammation of the myocardium,

usually a temporary problem. However, as the inflammatory process persists, it can affect the myocardial contractibility.

*Rheumatic endocarditis* produces ulcerations of the endocardium along the edges of the leaflets of the valve, where the leaflets are normally opposed in systole. This results in the deposition of tiny, beadlike nodules of fibrin and platelets along these surfaces, leading to fusion of the leaflets at the commissures, fibrosis of the leaflets themselves, and cardiac insufficiency. Calcification may further extend the impairment to normal hemodynamics and valvular incompetence may result.

*Rheumatic pericarditis* does not usually produce any specific lesions in the heart. *Pericarditis* refers to any inflammation of the pericardium. When this occurs, pericardial surfaces loose their lubrication (fluid) owing to the inflammatory response. A pericardial friction rub occurs as the heart moves in a nonlubricated area. Pericardial effusion, or escape of fluid into the pericardial sac, may accompany pericarditis. If the pericardium thickens because of chronic inflammation of the pericardium, movement of the heart may be limited. The stricture will usually be reduced by pericardial aspiration or surgery (pericardiectomy).

In general, the initial attack of rheumatic fever subsides without significant damage to the valve leaflets; however, repeated attacks of fever even-

**TABLE 27-2**
COMMON GENETIC SYNDROMES OR DISEASES AND CONGENITAL HEART DEFECTS

| Syndrome or Disease | Defect |
| --- | --- |
| Ellis–van Creveld syndrome (possibly inherited) | Single atrium, atrioseptal defect |
| Halt-Oram syndrome (possibly inherited) | Atrioseptal defect |
| Marfan's syndrome (connective tissue disorder) | Dilatation of the aorta, and/or pulmonary artery, aortic and mitral insufficiency (aneurysms) |
| Pompe's disease (inborn metabolic error) | Glycogen storage disease of the myocardium |
| Turner's syndrome (XO) (chromosomal) | Coarctation of the aorta, pulmonic stenosis |
| Trisomy 21 (Down's syndrome) (chromosomal) | Coarctation of the aorta, pulmonic stenosis, atrioventricular canal, ventricular and atrioseptal defects (tetralogy of Fallot) |
| Trisomy 18 (E) (chromosomal) | Ventriculoseptal defect, patent ductus arteriosus, pulmonic stenosis |

SOURCE: Thorn, George, et al., *Harrison's Principles of Internal Medicine*, 8th ed., McGraw-Hill, New York, 1977, Table 241-2, p. 1222.

tually lead to valve pathology. Such changes in the valves and supporting structures are the most frequent basis for inefficient blood flow and the problems associated with valvular heart disease. The mitral valve is most frequently involved, the aortic less often, and the tricuspid only rarely. The pulmonary valve is almost never affected. The noncardiac problems observed include joint pain, an elevated temperature, subcutaneous nodules (adhering to tendon sheaths), generalized malaise, weight loss, liver enlargement, abdominal pain, and a migratory rash appearing in the warm body areas.

Damage to one or more of the cardiac layers can be temporary or permanent. If early treatment is instituted, permanent destruction of endocardial tissues and valves can be limited, if not averted. When valve damage occurs, the valves become stenosed (narrowed) or shortened and lead to regurgitation. *Valvular stenosis* results in the need for a greater force to move the blood forward through the atria, ventricles, and aorta. This places an added stress on the pumping mechanism and can lead to decreased cardiac output.

When *regurgitation* occurs, the valve leaflets become shortened and do not close completely after contraction. The blood, therefore, leaks back into the chamber from which the blood has just been removed (ejected). This increases the amount of blood that is to be pumped out into the circulation and places an added strain on the heart.

When the aortic valve is affected, *aortic stenosis* and/or *regurgitation* occurs. When the tricuspid valve is involved, *tricuspid stenosis* and/or *regurgitation* occurs. The most frequently affected valve is the mitral valve, leading to *mitral stenosis* and/or *regurgitation.* A complete discussion of mitral valve disturbances will follow this introductory section.

### Bacterial Endocarditis

An inflammation of the endocardium or inner layer of the heart is termed *endocarditis.* It is characterized by valvular leaflet involvement and is the most common complication of rheumatic fever.

The characteristic lesion of bacterial endocarditis is a friable vegetation composed of bacteria, fibrin, and necrotic tissue.[11] This vegetation attaches to the leaflets of the valves, the endocardium, and the endothelium of blood vessels. Severe structural changes may occur in the course of the infection, and pump failure will result in a few days due to valvular incompetence. Alterations in intracardiac hemodynamics, particularly turbulence in and around the cardiac valves, may be involved in the pathogenesis.

There are two forms of bacterial endocarditis: acute bacterial endocarditis (ABE) and subacute bacterial endocarditis (SBE). ABE is a severe systemic infection caused by *Staphylococcus aureus.* The inflammatory process is accompanied by high-fever cardiac murmurs, splenic enlargement, and increased capillary fragility. An embolic phenomenon may develop due to the dislodging of the fragments formed on the leaflets of the valves during the inflammation. These fragments may be released into the bloodstream and cause circulatory occlusion to the vital organs. ABE can affect normal valves if not treated immediately.

SBE is a less acute inflammatory response caused by *Streptococcus viridans* or on occasion by *Staphlococcus aureus.* The onset of SBE is often insidious and the course prolonged. Weight loss, joint pain, fever, and splenic enlargement may develop as the problem persists.

Individuals with ABE or SBE usually have a history of heart disease or valve injury from an episode of rheumatic fever, syphilis, atherosclerosis, or congenital valve disease. Bacteremia caused by *Streptococcus viridans* often follows an acute infection of the lungs, tonsils, gums, or teeth. Surgery can also offer a portal of entry for bacteria, especially if the patient has existing valvular destruction.

*Staphylococcal bacterial endocarditis* is a bacterial infection that may follow the introduction of a contaminated needle or syringe into the body. *Streptococcal fecalis,* on the other hand, is commonly associated with genitourinary conditions or surgical intervention.

As the calcification and "scarring" of the valves develop, valvular stenosis or insufficiency results. *Insufficiency* denotes an inability of the valve to close adequately due to calcification of the leaflets. Pure or isolated insufficiency is rarely seen. The process that scars and contracts the valve cusps also shortens and fuses the chordae tendineae so that valvular opening as well as closing is impaired. When the area of the cusps is no longer able to close the valve orifice, regurgitation occurs, forcing the blood back into the heart chamber from which it is flowing. The anterior leaflet is almost always normal while the smaller, posterior leaflet may prolapse backward against the left ventricular wall and interfere with blood flow.

Myocardial ejection pressures must be greater than normal to overcome such a physiological handicap, and the myocardial workload likewise increases. There may be a normal cardiac output until the pump begins to fail. Over time (and in some cases this is a period of years) the muscle is stressed beyond its physiological limits, which is to say that it functions on the descending limb of the Frank-Starling curve (see Chap. 22). Hypertrophy compensates to some extent by engaging a larger muscle mass in contraction; however, unless the primary defect is corrected, the end result is pump failure. In addition, rupture of the valve leaflets can occur along with an extension of the infectious process to the aorta, the pericardium, or the chordae tendineae.

## EFFECTS OF CONGENITAL AND ACQUIRED STRUCTURAL HEART DEFECTS

Structural changes and hemodynamic alterations result in similar effects whether they are due to acquired or congenital causes. These alterations can be classified into three main categories: (1) Abnormal variations in intracardiac pressures, (2) reduced oxygen saturation of the arterial blood, and (3) hypertrophy of the cardiac chamber upon which the major pumping load is placed. These changes can result in retardation of physical as well as mental growth, hypertension, cyanosis, dyspnea, periods of anoxia, and syncope. The patient's ability to tolerate stress and activity will decrease depending upon the severity of the defect. Emboli, vessel rupture, aneurysm, and pump failure may result as the problem persists. Timing of the correction of the problem will depend upon the degree that each defect interferes with the individual's activities of daily living.

## MITRAL STENOSIS

Mitral stenosis is an acquired structural defect caused by a progressive thickening of the mitral

**TABLE 27-3**
DISTRIBUTION OF MEAN INTRAVASCULAR PRESSURES
IN THE SYSTEMIC AND PULMONARY CIRCUITS

| Location | Pressure, mmHg |
|---|---|
| Left ventricle | 120/80 |
| Aorta | 120/80 |
| Arterioles | 35 |
| Right ventricle | 25 |
| Pulmonary artery | 13 |
| Pulmonary veins | 7 |
| Left atrium | 7 |

valve cusps and stenosis (narrowing) of the valve orifice. It is one of the most common lesions of the mitral valve.

### Pathophysiology

The mitral valve in normal adults offers little if any impedance to the flow of blood. The valve orifice is 4 to 6 cm wide with no measurable pressure gradient necessary to propel blood from the left atrium to the left ventricle. Table 27-3 shows the normal pressures found within the cardiovascular circuit. If the valve is obstructed owing to stenosis or narrowing, the valvular orifice decreases in size (see Fig. 27-4). When this occurs, blood can flow from the left atrium to the left ventricle only if propelled by an abnormally elevated left atrioventricular pressure gradient. Such a gradient is a hallmark of mitral stenosis.[12]

The amount of force required to move blood past a stenotic mitral valve is directly proportional to the diameter of the mitral orifice. If the opening is no more than a slit, the left atrium must generate greater pressures to force blood into the left ventricular cavity (see Fig. 27-5). A rise in left atrial pressure requires increased contractile work, and,

**FIGURE 27-4**
Mitral stenosis. (*From J. W. Hurst et al. (eds.), The Heart, 4th ed., McGraw-Hill, New York, 1978.*)

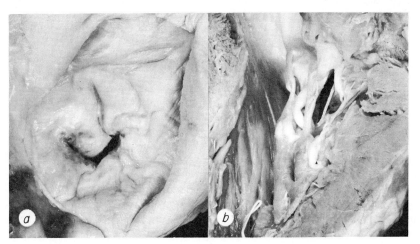

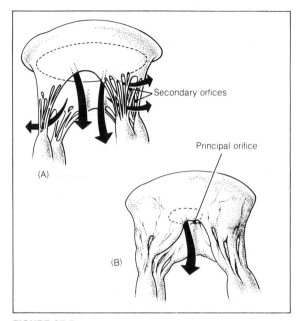

**FIGURE 27-5**
(a) Normal mitral valve. (b) Orifice changes in mitral stenosis.

to a point, such an increase is compensatory. However, over time, the effective point on the Frank-Starling curve (see Chap. 22) is surpassed, and the left atrium hypertrophies to provide additional muscle mass for contraction. Eventually even these contractions are ineffective.

The pathophysiological mechanisms by which the strength of contraction of the myocardial fibers diminishes during hypertrophy are not clearly understood. It is thought that the myocardial cells either cannot utilize the substrates or that the increasingly anaerobic metabolism of the hypertrophied muscle cells leads to ineffective contractions. Whatever the cause, the efficiency of contraction is decreased, and marked strain and hypertrophy of the left atrium result.

Beyond a critical size in the orifice, a point which varies among patients, the cardiac output remains fixed. No increase in left atrial pressure is sufficient to increase the volume of blood that can be forced across the valve. Tachycardia is a reflex mechanism; however, fast heart rates have the disadvantage of shortening the time during which the ventricle can fill (diastolic filling time), and the cardiac output is, again adversely affected. Left atrial pressures may continue to rise or remain stable at an elevated pressure, with the elevation being reflected backward through the pulmonary circuit. Such a backward flow mechanism is physiologi-

cally possible because the pulmonary veins are not protected by valves. Should the hydrostatic pressure within the pulmonary capillaries (that tends to push fluid out) exceed the colloid osmotic pressure (that keeps fluid in the capillaries) of the plasma proteins, pulmonary edema and congestion will follow. An elevated pulmonary vascular resistance is usually seen as a complication of long standing mitral stenosis.

Increased pulmonary capillary pressure requires an increase in the pressure within the pulmonary artery to overcome the pulmonary gradient and maintain an adequate output from the right ventricle. Stress is placed upon the right ventricle, and eventually it, too, enlarges. Since the mass of the right ventricle is less than that of the left, it is even less able to function at high pressures. Right-sided failure culminates in dependent edema, ascites, and congestion of the liver.

A decrease in cardiac output is a natural consequence of mitral stenosis. Persons with moderate stenosis may experience few symptoms; however, if stenosis is severe, or if exercise is greatly increased, dyspnea will result.

**Cause and effects of mitral stenosis** The major *cause* of mitral stenosis is rheumatic fever, although other bacterial inflammatory processes as well as atherosclerosis may also precipitate mitral incompetence. Rheumatic changes affect the valve leaflets. As fibrous tissue accumulates, the valves calcify. The mitral commissures fuse, the chordae tendineae may fuse (mitral regurgitation), and the valve narrows and becomes rigid. Mitral insufficiency results (see Fig. 27-6).

The *effects* of these changes vary with the degree of stenosis and resultant elevation in atrial and pulmonary capillary pressure. In mild stenosis symptoms may be minimal and may include fatigue, dyspnea on exertion, a slight cough, and a vulnerability to infection.

In more severe stenosis, arrhythmias such as atrial fibrillation and flutter and premature atrial contractions (see Chap. 25) may be present. An elevation in pulmonary capillary pressure may result in a cough and dyspnea. Limited activities can produce extreme dyspnea, and inability of the heart to cope with returning blood from the periphery may lead to orthopnea and pulmonary edema. Hemoptysis may be present due to rupture of a pulmonary vein. Chest pain occurs in about 10 percent of the patients with mitral stenosis.[13] Thrombi may also form in the left atria, particularly behind the atrial enlargement. The problem of emboli is intensified in the presence of atrial fibrillation, because the blood tends to clot on the uneven surface of the fibrillating atrial wall. Fatigue will increase with valvular incompetence and increasing pump failure.

### First-Level Nursing Care

The preferred treatment for mitral stenosis is prevention. Identification of the population at risk and implementation of preventive nursing health measures may decrease the incidence of rheumatic fever, infection, and resulting structural cardiac defects. Although the incidence of rheumatic fever has steadily declined over the past 20 years, there are still approximately 100,000 new cases reported yearly in the United States. In 1968, 16,000 deaths from rheumatic fever and rheumatic heart disease were reported. Almost $28,000,000 was paid for physicians' visits and clinic care.[14] Yet, of all the causes of acquired heart disease, rheumatic fever is undoubtedly the most easily prevented.

**Population at risk** Those at risk to develop rheumatic fever are young children exposed to streptococcal infections and persons who are poorly nourished or who live in crowded, poorly heated dwellings. In addition, individuals with a family history of rheumatic fever are at risk as well as those who have previously had rheumatic fever.

Individuals with cardiac problems, as well as elevated cholesterol levels and hyperlipedemia, are at risk to develop mitral stenosis due to atherogenic changes of the valve. Obesity and hypertension are also contributing causes to the atherogenic process (see Chap. 26).

**Prevention** Approximately 85 percent of the cases of rheumatic fever reported are first attacks;

however, the number reported is probably but a fraction of actual cases. Since rheumatic fever is confined largely to school-aged children, the school nurse and family health practitioner bear primary responsibility for identifying the problem in a community. The schoolteacher can also be a valuable contributor if aware of the early symptoms of the disease. Information stressing the association between streptococcal sore throat, rheumatic fever, and heart disease should be made available to parents and persons (such as teachers) whose occupations place them in an advantageous position for case finding.

Children and young persons with pharyngitis should be examined and throat cultures obtained routinely at no cost to the family. If the culture is positive, the child and family are treated with penicillin or (if allergic) another antibiotic for 14 days. If continuous "strep throats" appear in a family, all the family members should have throat cultures as there may be a *carrier* not yet identified.

In some instances, documented streptococcal throat infections occurring in the presence of tonsillitis may necessitate the removal of the tonsils. The number of infections will vary; some physicians believe that three or more streptococcal infections within a year require further investigation and surgical evaluation.

Early diagnosis of a rheumatic infection following streptococcal sore throat is sometimes difficult. Subcutaneous joint nodules usually occur; however, their onset may be as late as 4 weeks after the initial infection. In a small number of cases erythema appears which is extremely transitory in nature. The five minor manifestations are: fever, arthralgia, prolongation of the PR interval of the electrocardiogram, increased erythrocyte sedimentation rate and

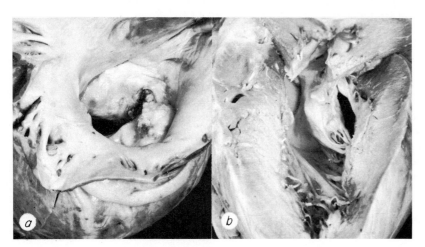

**FIGURE 27-6**
Mitral insufficiency. (*From J. W. Hurst et al. (eds.), The Heart, 4th ed., McGraw-Hill, New York, 1978.*)

white blood cell count, and the presence of C-reactive protein in the blood.[15] Antistreptolysin (ASL) titers may also be done to assess the presence of systemic streptococcal invasion.

Health counseling should be made available to all families with a positive history of congenital or rheumatic heart disease. Familial disorders such as certain of the hyperlipidemias should be followed clinically, for these metabolic disorders are associated with a wide range of heart diseases. Preventive measures aimed at reducing the extent and incidence of atherosclerosis should include a reduction in dietary fat and smoking, increased activity, and a sharp decrease in the amount of daily stress. (See Chap. 26 for a complete discussion.)

Dorsey and Jackson describe persons of ethnic background living in rural or inner-city areas who may exist below the poverty level. For them, "money is spent on food, housing, and other day to day survival needs. Illness and diseases which are manifestations of poverty, often run their course without the benefit of medical attention."[16]

The community health nurse must try to help patients in low socioeconomic areas with selection of essential nutrients while keeping within their budget. They should be told of the need for rest and encouraged to treat all infections promptly. Local hospitals and health clinics should be identified so that the patient will have immediate contact with a health provider. In addition, the school nurse can assist with case finding and instruct teachers and students about prevention of streptococcal infection.

Individuals who have had a streptococcal infection or rheumatic fever must be counseled about adequate nutrition, rest, and prevention of reinfection. Proper dental care followed by prophylactic antibiotics is also essential in preventing further infections. Vaccines for prevention of streptococcal infections are currently in the experimental stages. If perfected, they may hold the answer in preventing repeated streptococcal infections.

**Second-Level Nursing Care**

Problems associated with mild mitral stenosis are similar to those associated with early left-ventricular pump failure (see Chap. 24). A complete health history and physical assessment should help to distinguish some of the more specific changes noted in early mitral stenosis.

**Nursing assessment** Patients seeking health care in the community will usually offer a *health history* of dyspnea, especially upon exertion, and muscular fatigue. These are the most frequent complaints noted by an individual with mitral valve disease. Generally, women below the age of 45 are most often affected by this problem. The greater the degree of pathology (i.e., stenosis and regurgitation), the more marked will be the patient's shortness of breath. Dyspnea may be described in terms of the specific episodes and the activities which trigger them.

Dyspnea may or may not be indicative of pathology. When dyspnea is a relatively recent finding or when an individual complains of tiredness and the inability to participate in activities, these reports should be fully explored. In some cases the patient's initial complaint is one of overwhelming and unusual fatigue, such as, "I just couldn't lift my arm off the table." The reduction in cardiac output that accompanies most cases of mitral stenosis is a contributing factor in this complaint. Emotions also play a part. Anxiety is provoked very quickly if breathing becomes conscious and labored at normal activity levels. It is difficult for the patient experiencing shortness of breath to relax until the pathology is corrected.

Early in mitral valve disease the patient may be successful in balancing the demands made upon the circulatory system through limiting, or even terminating, normal activities and exercise. It must be noted, however, that if the abnormally elevated pulmonary capillary pressures continue over time, the result will be fibrosis and loss of compliance of the alveoli. A concomitant increase in pulmonary vascular resistance will follow so that dyspnea will appear with less and less exertion.

The patient may unconsciously hyperventilate, or be concerned because the pulse rate increases sharply with certain moderate activities. Hyperventilation and tachycardia compensate, to some extent, for the decrease in cardiac output and ineffective gaseous exchange. Since years may pass before the patient requires surgical intervention, it is important to reassess and evaluate physical changes as they occur over time.

Angina at rest is rarely experienced. However, some individuals experience angina as an immediate response to overexertion. A physiological gap thus exists between the effective coronary blood perfusion and the metabolic demands of the myocardial cells. Ischemia results and heart pain is experienced. A detailed assessment should include a history of a sore throat and other infections as well as cardiovascular and related pathologies in the patient and the family members. Careful questioning should ferret out any incidence, diagnosed or not, of streptococcal or other infection.

**P**hysical Assessment  Physical assessment of the patient with mitral stenosis will generally reveal a frail, tired-looking person with pinched and anxious facies. The individual's skin color may be normal since cyanosis is not usually associated with a moderate degree of decompensation. Slight basilar rales may be present, but more often the lung sounds are clear to auscultation.

Percussion of the heart size is of limited usefulness in these patients because in all but the most advanced of cases the heart is of normal size and contour. The apical pulse may be regular, but sinus tachycardia or atrial fibrillation may be present (see Chap. 25).

At the apex of the heart auscultation is often limited to an area 2 to 3 cm in diameter. A marked diastolic murmur is usually present. This is referred to as a *diastolic rumble.* It may be of only grade I or grade II intensity in many patients, but in others the murmur is loud (grades IV to VI), with a palpable purring thrill also present. The murmur may appear only after exercise and when the patient is in a lateral recumbent position. (See Chap. 22 for a discussion of murmurs.) It is important to note that the intensity of the murmur does not necessarily correlate with the severity of mitral disease.

The increased intensity of the first heart sound is brief but sudden and is a distinctive feature in mitral stenosis. An opening snap may also be heard which indicates that the calcified leaflets of the mitral valve are being forced to an immediate wide-open position by the high pressure generated in the left atrium. In pure mitral stenosis, that is, when it occurs without concomitant insufficiency or aortic stenosis, the opening snap is followed by a normal second heart sound. The second heart sound is thought to result from the turbulence of blood and the closing of the pulmonic and aortic valves. A history of shortness of breath, tachycardia upon exertion, and the *classic triad of abnormal heart sounds,* namely, diastolic rumble-murmur at the apex, increased intensity of $S_1$, and an opening snap, complete the assessment of mitral valve disease.

In the presence of atrial fibrillation the blood pressure may be lowered. If early failure is observed, slight peripheral edema may be present.

**D**iagnostic Tests  In many cases of mitral stenosis the *electrocardiogram* (EKG) will be within normal limits. The first observable change is an increase in the P-wave interval. This is an expected finding since the duration of the P interval is a reflection of muscle mass and intracardiac pressures, as well as of the velocity of conduction. Enlargement of a chamber (hypertrophy) or an elevation in cardiac pressure may be noted (ventricular hypertrophy) and the occurrence of atrial fibrillation is not uncommon.

With an increase in pulmonary vascular resistance and subsequent enlargement of the right ventricle, the electrocardiogram usually shows significant deviations from the normal. In this instance, one would expect to observe the classic QRS of right axis deviation. The value of the EKG as a diagnostic tool increases when mitral disease is complicated with other heart disease such as aortic stenosis or left-ventricular hypertrophy.[17]

Detection of even a slight degree of enlargement of the left ventricle is of particular importance in following changes and progression of the disease. A *chest roentgenogram* taken upon the patient's initial visit has value in that the size and silhouette of the left atrium can be visualized. In addition, the initial x-ray can be used as a base with which to compare future films. A lateral film, taken during the administration of barium, will often show the middle portion of the esophagus to be displaced backward so that a slight concavity is formed.

Complete data on blood chemistry will be sought regarding elevation of the serum enzymes, blood sugar, triglycerides, electrolytes, and sedimentation rate, and other determinations may be made. Unless a concomitant inflammatory process is present, one does not expect the serum enzymes or white blood cell count to be elevated. However, patients with long-standing heart disease may show aberrations in hemoglobin and hematocrit, as well as elevations in certain triglyceride levels. If other diseases complicate the process (diabetic or renal), abnormalities of sugar, electrolytes, blood urea nitrogen, and other factors may be present. Elevation of cholesterol and triglyceride levels may be indicative of hyperlipidemia.

**Nursing problems and interventions**  During the early stages of mitral-valve disorders, patients develop several major nursing problems. These include infection, dyspnea, fatigue and malaise, and anxiety. Patients who are fairly well compensated may rarely be ill; therefore, the orientation of nursing care should be directed toward health teaching in the community setting.

**I**nfection  In the early stages of mitral valve disturbances, it is important that the patient not be exposed to bacterial or viral infections. The patient needs to know that particular care should be taken to avoid streptococcal infections when they are present in the household. The school, college, and work settings are more difficult for the patient to control, but personal judgment must be used and care taken to avoid contact with persons who have sore throats or other respiratory problems.

*Antibiotic therapy* may be included in the regimen of the patient with early mitral disease. If so, the nurse will assist the patient in monitoring the effects of the drug and explain the rationale for long-term drug therapy. Although the practice of prescribing antibiotics on a long-term basis for patients is controversial,[18] current indications are that antibiotics can be prescribed for isolated episodes of respiratory infection or sore throats only. Penicillin is the usual agent of choice (unless the patient is allergic to the drug). Other antibiotics, particularly the erthyromycin derivatives, are also effective. The patient on a course of antibiotic therapy requires certain information. Symptoms of toxicity should be carefully reviewed for the allergic response is neither dramatic nor immediate. Patients have been known to take penicillin for an extended period of time before rash, watery eyes, or breathing difficulty has been encountered. On occasion, prolonged use of one antibiotic may lead to ineffectiveness of the drug.

**D**yspnea  The degree of dyspnea will vary with each individual and will depend on the degree of mitral occlusion present. In its mildest form, dyspnea may be experienced only with exertion, exercise, and strenuous activity. The patient should be taught to pace activities and take rest periods as needed to avoid muscle fatigue. Smoking should be discouraged if at all possible, and concerted efforts including the use of hypnosis should be employed if other preventive measures fail. Plans for patient teaching should include the adverse effects of nicotine on the already constricted area of the heart and the need for planned activities.

There is growing support for the development of an exercise plan which is medically supervised and executed gradually. Some research has suggested that the increased activity along with adequate rest, good nutrition, etc., can improve cardiac tolerance and decrease dyspnea, fatigue, and malaise.

**F**atigue  The degree of *fatigue* present will vary with the severity of valvular incompetence. Planning for rest periods throughout the day as well as adequate sleep is essential. Well-paced activities along with planned exercises will increase the patient's physical strength. Well-balanced diets and an adequate nutritional intake will help improve the patient's sense of well being. If the patient is a woman of childbearing age, she should discuss the stress of pregnancy (if any) on the myocardium. Careful assessment and counseling by the physician and nurse may help the patient and her husband decide whether and when children are a possibility.

**S**tress  A general model of stress could be discussed with the patient. In this model stress is conceived as force or load. A given load is suitable to an object; beyond those limits, which in physics are well delineated, strain can result. Strain, when applied to an object over time, results in deformation. When the stress load placed upon a patient with mitral valve problems is increased, it could precipitate exacerbation of the pathologic process. Stress may take many forms, and the patient needs to know this. For example, overtiredness and poor nutrition are physiological stressors that may produce a specific strain on the heart. Psychological stress may take the form of concern for the future, inability to get along with one's peers, or the discomfort of a bad work situation. When the patient and members of the family understand that a relationship does exist between stress and the progression of symptoms, a greater degree of cooperation is usually elicited. With this understanding, anxiety-provoking situations can be more easily reduced, and the working and home environment made less stressful. By providing the patient with adequate information and being supportive and reassuring during this early stage of mitral stenosis, the nurse may prolong the patient's healthy state and reduce the need for immediate surgery.

### Third-Level Nursing Care

When the patient reports a gradual decrease in the amount of exercise that can comfortably be performed and tolerated, the assumption is that the mitral orifice is progressively narrowing or that the left atrium is failing in its capacity to initiate an effective left-ventricular filling pressure. The onset of dyspnea upon exertion (the milder the exertion needed, the more advanced the process) heralds progressive decompensation. The result is a weak and tired patient who becomes increasingly tired with less and less activity. The patient is often hospitalized because of the advanced incompetence of the mitral valve.

**Nursing assessment** Frequently the nurse is able to observe the patient with mitral valve pathology over many months or even years. When the patient is hospitalized with acute manifestations of valvular incompetence, pump failure is often present. A thorough health history and physical assessment will help define the degree of valvular stenosis.

**H**ealth History  Whether the nurse is able to obtain a complete health history will depend upon the patient's clinical status. If severe failure is present, the patient may experience dyspnea, and talking may be an effort. The patient or family member often describes episodes of dyspnea with limited movement. The patient is usually thin; weight loss, accompanied by poor appetite, is not uncommon. Activity is usually limited to the chair or bed rest, as exercise will often be too stressful. The patient is anxious because of the obvious pump failure and dyspnea. In addition, the patient may be frightened of the prospect of surgery. If the patient has been experiencing these changes for any period of time, he or she will appear tired and pale, and complaints of generalized weakness and loss of strength are not uncommon.

Patients with severe dyspnea may be restless, irritable, and confused. They may appear sluggish in their ability to respond and may evidence cerebral anoxia.

**P**hysical Assessment  *Visual inspection* of the patient will disclose a chronically ill, thin, pale individual with anxious (or elfin) facies. Rapid respirations, dyspnea, flaring nostrils, and labored respirations are easily visualized in the acutely ill patient. Inspection of the patient may proceed sporadically for the nurse's responsibility also includes helping the patient into a position which alleviates breathing problems and initiating oxygen therapy. Caution should be used in administering oxygen to the patient whose history is not yet complete in that concentrations of oxygen tolerated well by most persons may depress the respirations of the patient with chronic obstructive lung disease. It is quite safe to begin oxygen therapy at 2 liters/minute until a detailed history is available.

The neck veins must be visually examined for engorgement in the supine and sitting positions. Decreased emptying times are usually noted in these patients if pump failure is a complicating factor. When the patient's chest is bared, inspection may also reveal gross myocardial heaves, as occur with left-ventricular enlargement. Cerebral manifestations can be evaluated as the nurse questions the patient concerning the medical history.

Facial and peripheral cyanosis may be apparent, and dyspnea is often marked. Nail beds may appear blue and skin temperature will vary. If the patient is in acute pump failure, the skin may feel cold and clammy. Skin discolorations and petechiae are not uncommon.

*Palpation* is utilized to evaluate the quality of the patient's pulses. For the patient with mitral or other valvular disorders pulses should be described explicitly as weak, thin, full, bounding, thready, water hammer, or *pulse alternans* (alternating weak and strong beats at regular intervals). The palpable pulses must be compared in rate and rhythm with the apical pulse because a large pulse deficit, and or pulsus alternans, often characterizes pump failure in the early stages.

Carotid pulsations can usually be palpated; however, care must be taken that undue pressure is not placed on the carotid bodies with a subsequent sudden change in heart rate. (See Carotid Sinus Pressure in Chap. 25.) The apical pulse and the point of maximum inspiration can often be observed, rather than palpated, in the patient with a hypertrophied left ventricle. The point of maximum intensity (PMI) which is normally located at the fifth intercostal space at the midclavicular line, may be deviated centrally or laterally in the cardiac patient. Palpation and percussion will indicate whether the contour and size of the left ventricle are within normal limits. When the PMI has been identified, it should be described as being in relation to a specific intercostal space and in numbered centimeters to the right or left of the midclavicular line. The lateral aspect of the hand is often more sensitive than percussion in determining the right ventricular border. A forceful, heaving left-ventricular impulse (PMI) denotes associated disease with left-ventricular hypertrophy. Myocardial heaves and myocardial lifts are usually palpable, particularly in the slender patient, although some practice is required to become skilled in these procedures. Palpation of the liver is possible in right-sided failure. (Refer to Chap. 19 for a discussion of palpation of the liver.) Obviously any tenderness or guarding by the patient indicates that palpation should be discontinued and the findings documented and reported.

Auscultation of heart sounds must be evaluated very carefully in all patients with mitral incompetence. There are usually *three distinctive auscultatory findings in the patient with advanced mitral-valve disease:* a *diastolic murmur* (grade II or III) heard best at the apex of the heart, an *increased intensity of the first heart sound,* and an opening *snap of the first heart sound.* This opening snap is most audible over the apex upon expiration. It can also be heard along the left sternal edge or at the base of the heart. In patients with pure mitral stenosis without concomitant mitral insufficiency, a short murmur may be heard at the apex. Loud, pansystolic murmur (see Chap. 22), however, denotes mitral insufficiency. To differentiate a mitral murmur from that of tricuspid insufficiency, which can also be heard at the apex of the heart, one must determine whether the murmur is accentuated during inspiration as occurs with tricuspid insufficiency. Mitral stenosis is the most common pathological condition which results in an augmented intensity of the first heart sound ($S_1$). The sound, which resembles a snap, may be readily heard at the apex and often results in a sharp apical shock. The opening snap of mitral stenosis depends upon the abrupt cessation of movement by the valve or the valvular ring and may be diminished in intensity as mobility of the valve decreases.

Patients with mitral stenosis may experience atrial fibrillation. If this arrhythmia is present, the pulse will be irregular, and the rate rapid unless controlled by digitalis.

The nurse should observe and evaluate the rate of the patient's respirations and the character of their sounds. Respirations in the acutely ill patient may be greatly increased, depending upon the adequacy of air excursion and the patient's anxiety. An increase in respirations is a physiological compensatory mechanism for inadequate air excursion in the lung. However, fast respirations are often also shallow respirations in which the lower lobes are rarely expanded. Pulmonary edema may be in evidence with the flaring nostrils and use of cervical muscles so characteristic of strained respiratory effort. Sternal retractions may also be noted.

Basilar or generalized rales may indicate that congestion is a problem; however, if the patient has a history of chronic obstructive lung disease (COLD), the rales may not be of recent origin. The more significant rales are those that are generalized and moist, rather than faint, because they suggest acute failure and impending pulmonary edema. These sounds must be compared bilaterally, as well as posteriorly and anteriorly, if meaning is to be gained from their description. The nurse should listen to the lung sounds over each lobe. Chest sounds must be auscultated along the posterior thorax, for when the patient lies supine, the most dependent aspect of the lung will lie inferior and posterior.

Lung sounds may be masked by sounds of digestion, loud, pansystolic murmurs, friction rubs, or sounds emanating from the rubbing of oxygen tubing against bedclothes or from the mechanical activity of an intraaortic balloon. Care and concentration are required to auscultate and note pulmonary sounds accurately.

The patient's body temperature and blood pressure are also measured. The blood pressure is expected to be close to a normal pressure reading or nearly normal, unless pump failure is marked. Then it may be lower than normal. The patient maintains a nearly normal blood pressure with mitral stenosis. However the assumption is that myocardial work load is markedly increased and the myocardial pump is under strain in maintaining an adequate perfusion pressure. Continued assessment will be useful as a baseline for evaluating changes after surgical correction of the mitral structural defect has been completed.

**D**iagnostic Tests  When the patient with acute mitral stenosis is hospitalized, tests are usually done as part of a routine preoperative work-up to assess the degree of stenosis present. Angiography and arteriography are important adjuncts to the diagnosis of any patient with cardiovascular disease. The utilization of these studies, as well as cardiac catheterization, is by no means uniform among physicians. Certain physicians believe the time for diagnostic work-up is early in the course of mitral disease, while other specialists are reluctant to refer patients for extensive studies because of the emotional and financial implications for the family.

Frequently, patients receive information of a general nature early in the course of mitral disease, and, unless the condition worsens suddenly, the patient may have months or years to adjust to the diagnosis. In these cases plans for elective cardiovascular studies can be made well in advance.

An *angiogram* may be carried out on a vein or an artery anywhere in the body. Cardiac angiograms are studies of the heart and great vessels. The test consists of two steps: opacification of the interior of the cardiovascular system by the injection of a radiopaque medium into the bloodstream entering the right heart, and x-rays or fluoroscopic films of the heart chambers and vessels as they fill with blood. The cardiac angiogram will outline the four chambers of the heart, the large veins and arteries, the pulmonary vasculature, and, often, the valve cusps.[19]

*Arteriograms* differ from angiograms in that the

contrast material, which is usually Cardiogreen, Cardiografin, or Pantopaque, is injected directly into the arterial branches of interest. Aortic or coronary arteriograms are those most commonly utilized to provide information about the atherosclerotic process within the lumen of the arteries. (See Chap. 29 for a complete discussion of the procedure, including preparation of the patient and complications.)

*Cardiac catheterization* Cardiac catheterization is a complex procedure used to visualize the specific chambers of the heart as well as valvular structures of the heart. The procedures can be used to study the entire heart or can be confined to the right or left side exclusively. In addition to actual visualization of the heart, cardiac catheterization can give data on the extent and/or progression of structural damage, confirm congenital anomalies, identify the preoperative cardiac status, identify the quantity and quality of cardiac output, provide for assessment of oxygen saturation levels by the withdrawal of samples from the chambers, and allow for additional measurements such as angiocardiography. (This involves injection of a contrast dye, e.g., Ditriokon into the right heart chamber or pulmonary artery to determine the degree of function and/or occlusion.)

The site most often selected for insertion of the catheter is the right or left brachial artery at the anticubital fossa. This area should be shaved and cleansed thoroughly with an antiseptic solution. Preparation of the site by manual cleansing may be a one-time activity, or the patient may be instructed to carry on scrubs for several days prior to the procedure. A local anesthetic, usually 1 or 2% Xylocaine solution, is injected at the cleansed site to lessen the discomfort of the incision for the patient. Subsequently, a cutdown is completed, and when the vessels are adequately visualized a blunt dissection is accomplished to free one end of the vessel for insertion of the catheter.

Because of thromboembolic hazards, the femoral artery is chosen less commonly for retrograde introduction of the polyethylene catheter. In the latter case, a percutaneous needle insertion is done, and a guide wire and catheter are inserted.

Careful *preparation of the patient* for this procedure is essential. Often patients are fearful because of previous catheterization experiences or stories from friends. Therefore, a careful and complete explanation of the procedure is important. Teaching should evaluate the patient's previous knowledge about the procedure, since many pa-

tients with cardiac defects will have multiple catheterizations. The nurse should clarify with the physician those areas that have been stressed with the patient. Support and clarification for family members are of equal importance.

Prior to this discussion the nurse should assess the patient's level of anxiety and readiness to learn. The patient must be willing to focus upon the data being presented if it is to be meaningful. If the patient is apprehensive, the nurse should support an open discussion of these fears.

The anatomy of the heart along with a description of the actual procedure should be carefully explained. Patients should be told that there is little or no pain involved in the procedure. They should be informed that a sense of warmth will be experienced as the dye is injected, as well as an urge to cough. At times fluttering sensations may be felt as the catheter passes into the heart chambers. Reassuring the patient that these are normal responses will help. The biggest problem encountered by patients is the position they are forced to assume during this lengthy procedure. Whether the catheterization is performed in the x-ray department or the cardiac catheterization laboratory, the patient is required to lie flat on a hard surface for up to 6 or more hours. In addition, the arm is usually extended on an armboard for equally as long, and a cutdown with an intravenous solution is present. In addition, an EKG machine will be connected to the patient to detect arrhythmias. This monitoring device can hamper movement and increase patient fatigue.

The room is often darkened, and the patient will be awake during the procedure. If the individual is extremely anxious, a mild tranquilizer can be offered to help reduce stress.

An informed consent will be required for this procedure. It is important that the patient's physician discuss the procedure and potential complications with the patient. The nurse can help reinforce the points discussed and offer support and clarification as needed.

A history of all drug allergies should also be noted. Foods and liquids are often withheld up to 8 or more hours before the procedure. Penicillin (IM) may be given prophylactally to prevent the threat of infection. A relaxant, such as morphine or Nembutal, may be administered.

*Right heart catheterization* provides information about the pressures generated by the right atrium and right ventricle, the adequacy of the tricuspid and pulmonic valves, and the presence of a left-to-right shunt. In addition, mitral stenosis and mitral incompetency can often be identified.

In this procedure, the catheter is introduced into the circulation at the right brachial artery and antecubital space and advanced passively into the right atrium across the tricuspid valve and into the right ventricular chamber. From this position it will be further guided through the pulmonic valve into the pulmonary artery and wedged into one of the smaller arterial branches within the lung. From this position sample pressures are obtained (the pulmonary wedge pressure) which are believed to represent quite accurately pressures within the left atrium. Through the use of a second arterial catheter and a special dye, a curve can be obtained from which cardiac output is readily calculated. However, this latter procedure requires special equipment, such as a thermodilution output computer. Figure 27-7 shows a patient undergoing cardiac output studies with the catheter and equipment in place.

*Catheterization of the left side of the heart* and circulation provides data concerning the function of the left ventricular muscle, pressures in the left ventricle, and the status of the mitral and aortic valves. Left heart catheterization is especially use-

ful for identifying mitral and aortic insufficiency. A catheter can be passed from either the brachial or femoral artery into the left ventricle.

Pressures within the cardiovascular system may be sampled at almost any point within the circulatory pathway. The measurement of left ventricular end diastolic pressure (LVEDP) is of special importance to patients with long-standing cardiac disease. There is usually a concomitant *decrease* in left ventricular compliance if the LVEDP is elevated beyond 20 mmHg. The normal range for left ventricular end diastolic pressure is from 5 to 12 mmHg. Elevated pressures are often seen in a stenosed valve. In many cases a loss of functioning myocardium, or other pathology such as aortic or mitral insufficiency, is also present. To gain more precise information about the contractile properties of the left ventricle, left heart ventriculography is done. This is a procedure by which contrast medium is injected into an area close to the apex of the left ventricle, and measurements of contractility made.

The patient undergoing elective cardiac catheterization is usually mildly sedated, but easily

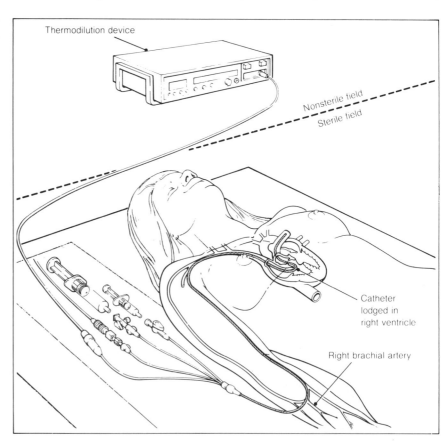

**FIGURE 27-7**
Cardiac catheterization.

Thermodilution device

Nonsterile field

Sterile field

Catheter lodged in right ventricle

Right brachial artery

aroused. The face may be flushed, and often very tense breathing is observed. Many patients exhibit sinus tachycardia, but this rhythm is transient in duration and thought to be a result of anxiety. Premature ventricular contractions can occur and often do as the catheter passes through the tricuspids valve into the right ventricle. While this serves as a useful explanation of premature ventricular contractions during right-sided entry into the heart, other mechanisms appear to be responsible for ectopy during left-sided catheterization.

Several complications can occur during the catheterization. These include: ventricular tachycardia, premature ventricular contractions, and, on occasion, ventricular fibrillation (refer to Chap. 25). Nausea, vomiting, skin irritation, thrombophlebitis at the entry site, and generalized hives may also develop.[20] Major complications include arterial occlusion, pneumothorax (see Chap. 30), and myocardial infarction; even death has been reported, usually due to life-threatening arrhythmias or pump failure.[21,22]

*After cardiac catheterization* the patient should be closely monitored for adverse effects of the procedure. Vital signs should be initially checked every 10 to 15 minutes, then every half hour, and finally every 4 hours for the first 24 hours. Sudden changes in pulse, heart sounds, blood pressure, or body temperature require evaluation as they occur. The cutdown site must be checked frequently for abnormal bleeding, swelling, inflammation, and thrombosis. The skin color, temperature, and peripheral pulses should be carefully evaluated. Warmth of the skin distal to the site of catheter insertion must be assessed for phlebitis. Pulse rate including the quality, rhythm, and regularity should be checked. If being monitored, the patient should be observed for arrhythmias.

Frequently the patient will be exhausted by the catheterization procedure and will need a planned rest period. The patient may wish to describe his or her feelings after the catheterization. The nurse should be supportive and reassuring during this time. Should complications occur, either during the catheterization or immediately thereafter, the patient may be transferred to an intensive-care setting.

*Preoperative diagnostic tests* When the patient is being prepared for surgery, an additional group of laboratory tests is usually performed. Table 27-4 describes each of these tests and their significance in relation to preoperative screening. The nurse shares in the responsibility of reassuring the patient and explaining the rationale for the tests that are

**TABLE 27-4**

DIAGNOSTIC TESTS FOR CARDIAC SURGICAL PATIENTS

| Test | Definition | Purpose |
|---|---|---|
| Antistreptolysin (ASL) titer | Level of ASL titer in blood | Indicates whether infection owes to *Streptococcus* |
| Bleeding time | Time required for puncture wound to stop bleeding | Tests the coagulation process |
| Clotting time (Lee and White) | Rough estimate of coagulation, using venous blood | Tests the coagulation process |
| Blood urea nitrogen | Level of urea nitrogen in blood | Determines whether kidney function has been impaired because of low cardiac output |
| C-reactive protein | Protein precipitation test | Amount of precipitate determines degree of inflammation |
| Differential count | Tabulation of relative number (%) of various types of white blood cells in total count | Assesses active inflammation and autoimmune response |
| Erythrocyte sedimentation rate (ESR) | Rapidity with which blood cells settle out of unclotted blood in 1 hour | Indicates presence of active inflammation |
| Hematocrit | Percent of red-cell mass in whole blood | Assess blood loss |
| Hemoglobin | Percent of iron-containing protein in whole blood | Determines blood iron |
| Nonprotein nitrogen | Ratio of nonprotein nitrogen in blood | Evaluates kidney function |
| Serum electrolyte determination | Levels of Na, Cl, K, and bicarbonate in serum | Compares electrolyte distribution with normal levels |
| Type and crossmatch | Analysis of blood factors | Tests compatability |
| Urine specific gravity | Weight of formed elements in urine | Indicates degree of concentration of urine |
| White blood cell count | Percent of WBCs in whole blood | Gives information about inflammation and infection |

carried out. The patient must feel free to express all concerns and ask questions related to all procedures. The nurse should discuss the rationale for each observation with the family members as well.

**Nursing problems and interventions** Acute mitral stenosis with or without insufficiency can lead to pump failure within hours. Dyspnea, pulmonary and peripheral edema, diaphoresis, fatigue, hypotension, and syncope are a few of the many problems that can occur. The severity of each problem will depend upon the degree of failure that develops. Intervention during pump failure is discussed in full in Chap. 24. The treatment usually includes a combination of diuretics, digitalis, quinine, low-sodium diets, positive pressure oxygen, and/or a phlebotomy. Rest and opiates (e.g., morphine sulfate) are often prescribed.

**S**urgical Intervention  Patients with mitral stenosis will usually progress to the point where surgical intervention is needed to relieve the mitral-valve incompetence. The following discussion will focus upon nursing problems and intervention during the preoperative period, the surgery itself, the immediate postoperative period, and the recovery phase.

*Preoperative care*  Most patients seeking elective open-heart surgery come to the hospital up to a week prior to surgery. The problems encountered by the patient at this time usually include fear and anxiety. The nurse should establish a good rapport with the patient. Since these patients will have a long period of hospitalization, the focus of care should be on continuity. Where possible, a primary nurse should be assigned to plan for the patient's total physical and psychosocial needs. In addition, the patient will need to have concrete information about the surgery. Accurate health teaching is essential. For each patient undergoing open-heart surgery a teaching plan should be individualized.

The main objective of patient teaching is to alleviate apprehension and secure cooperation by dispelling fears of the unknown. If the operation is a lifesaving emergency intervention to be done at the earliest possible moment, teaching will be minimal. If, as in most cases, the patient has been followed through a cardiovascular diagnostic clinic, or if surgery has been planned for many months, teaching should be planned, comprehensive, and detailed. When possible, family members should be included.

At a minimum, the following points should be understood by the patient before surgery is under-

taken: the reason for the surgery, the nature of the procedure (particularly the type of incision), and the length of hospitalization. When possible, the patient should be able to see and touch the prosthetic valve that will be used to replace the defective valve. The patient should be encouraged to get adequate rest and nutrition prior to surgery. When possible, all emotional stressors should be alleviated.

The nurse can discuss with the patient perceptions about the heart, its function, and overall importance to life. Misconceptions about the surgery should be discussed and eliminated by clear, factual data. The patient should be reevaluated on materials taught by some type of posttesting in order to evaluate the degree of comprehension.

Frequently, patients will undergo many tests, including chest x-rays, blood work, cardiograms (to evaluate valvular function), pulmonary function tests (see Chap. 30), and an angiogram. They should know the purpose of each test. In addition, spiritual counseling may be requested and provided as needed.

Many patients fear the postoperative period and are anxious about the intensive-care units. Therefore, it is important for the patient to spend some time with the recovery-room or intensive-care staff. Here the machinery to be used can be viewed. Such items as the monitoring equipment, breathing equipment, and the physical plan of each unit can be more fully described to the patient. By meeting the staff and talking with them, the patient may be reassured by the nurses' skill and overall competence. Practice sessions and a demonstration of breathing techniques, range of motion exercises, and the use of the intermittent positive pressure breathing (IPPB) machine, as well as coughing techniques, will emphasize the patient's role in recovery.

Patients should also be told about some of the physical changes they can expect to experience postoperatively including pain, nausea, discomfort from the endotracheal tube, immobility, chest tubes, and transfusions (either blood and/or IV fluid). Each of these items should be discussed in terms of the reason for their occurrence and what will be done to alleviate the distress. It should be emphasized that if pain is present, medications will be given to reduce it.

The most frightening experiences recalled by the patient following surgery seem to be the psychological changes that occur. These experiences should be discussed with the patient and the family members and the occurrence elaborated upon. The nurse should carefully point out that should these changes occur, the patient should notify the nurse immediately for support. It is also helpful for some patients to discuss the experience with other patients who have been through it. Often small-group teaching and discussion will facilitate this interactive process.

*Immediate preoperative preparation* of the cardiac patient is comparable with preoperative preparation required for any major surgical procedure with several exceptions. An intravenous drip of 5% dextrose in water, or 5% dextrose in 0.2% normal saline, may be started in a peripheral vein. In addition, a *cutdown* for insertion of a polyethylene catheter will be performed by the surgical team. One or more of a variety of potent cardiovascular drugs can be administered through these lines.

Skin preparation may be carried out using a scrub technique with a bacteriostatic soap for several days prior to the procedure. This is also done the evening before and morning of the surgery. For thoracic incisions a wide surface area is cleansed and hair shaved to remove a natural habitat for bacteria. The area of incision may be midline, anterolateral, or posterolateral. It is extremely important that the patient know which type of incision is planned.

Numerous preoperative laboratory tests will be evaluated (see Table 27-4) prior to surgery. Vital signs will be carefully observed, and changes in temperature carefully noted. In some instances prophylactic doses of penicillin may be given preoperatively to decrease the threat of infection. Mild tranquilizers may be used to reduce anxiety, and the support of family and friends is often critical. Drugs such as digoxin and diuretics (see Chaps. 24 and 28) may be discontinued several days before surgery.

Psychological support of the patient and family members continues to be of critical importance. The patient should be allowed to express fears and be reassured as needed. Usually, during this period the patient will be medicated for surgery and vital signs will be evaluated.

*Closed-heart surgery* Mitral stenosis may be treated surgically by either the closed or open technique. When open-heart surgery is performed, extracorporeal circulation, by means of the heart-lung bypass machine, is used. Extracorporeal circulation is almost universally used for children who have either congenital or rheumatic mitral disease. Also, the open technique is necessary in cases in which a valvular prosthesis is needed to replace the

diseased mitral valve. The risk for both the open and closed procedures is about 4 percent.[23]

*Mitral commissurotomy* (closed heart or valvotomy) without heart-lung bypass is performed through a left anterolateral thoracotomy with the patient in the anterolateral position. The chest is entered through the fifth intercostal space, with the entry through the pericardium anterior to the phrenic nerve. A purse-string suture is placed around the left atrial appendage, and the tip of the appendage is incised. The index finger is inserted into the left atrium for the purpose of evaluating the status of the mitral valve and orifice. Loss of blood from the left atrium is prevented by pulling the purse string tightly around the exploring finger. The valve leaflets may be fractured apart with the finger, or, more commonly, a dilator is inserted and its tip guided through the mitral orifice. The dilator is opened maximally to split the commissures. The dilator is withdrawn, the pericardium closed, and the left atrial appendage is oversewn.

Immediate recovery from this procedure is good; however, follow-up studies 5 to 10 years after the initial surgery often indicate restenosis of the valve. Frequently, open-heart surgery with valve replacement must then be performed.

*Open-heart surgery* Open-heart surgery proceeds after a right posterolateral thoracotomy or a midline sternotomy is performed. Cannulations to the heart-lung bypass machine are made from the right atrium and the inferior and superior venae cavae.

In the open-heart method, the left atrium is incised between the intraatrial groove and the right pulmonary veins. The mitral valve can then be visualized. If mitral insufficiency is a complicating condition, sutures are placed in the mitral annulus to shorten the posterior leaflet and thus decrease the diameter of the annulus. Prior to seating the valve prosthesis, the chordae tendineae and papillary muscles may be repaired or excised as needed. The mitral orifice is measured for a prosthetic mitral valve.

The Teflon sewing ring of the prosthesis (Starr-Edwards; see Fig. 27-8) is sutured to the previously prepared mitral annulus with the valve cage projecting downward into the left ventricle. The aorta is cross-clamped during the procedure to prevent aortic regurgitation into the operative field, and is unclamped every few minutes for perfusion of the coronary arteries. At the same time the pump oxygenator performs a suctioning action to clear the operative field of blood. The valve is held incompetent until the heart has filled with blood and all the

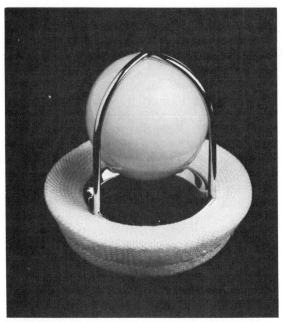

**FIGURE 27-8**
Starr-Edwards silastic prosthetic valve. (*Courtesy of Edwards Laboratories, Division of American Hospital Supply Corporation.*)

air is expelled from the chambers of the heart. The atriotomy is closed and the cardiopulmonary bypass is discontinued.

Generally pacemaking wires are implanted prophylactically during the valvular operation; thus arrhythmias can be treated by intermittent pacing rather than medication. For example, a tachycardia could be depressed by the so-called "override technique" in which the pacemaker is activated at a higher pulse rate, then gradually decreased to allow the myocardium to decrease its rate. Also a slow ventricular rate in third-degree heart block can be treated by pacing the heart from the ventricle at a faster rate. When the operation has been completed and before the incision has been closed, fine copper lead wires are sutured to the surface of the myocardium, one to the atria, and the other to the ventricle. The distal ends of these wires are attached to a pulse generator (external pacemaker). The pacemaker is usually secured to the patient's chest with adhesive tape. (Refer to Chap. 25 for a discussion of pacemakers.)

*Cardiopulmonary bypass*  The purpose of a cardiopulmonary bypass is to (1) divert blood from the heart and lungs during surgery, (2) provide for adequate exchange of oxygen and carbon dioxide,

(3) filter and regulate the temperature of the blood returning to the circulation, and (4) reintroduce oxygenated blood into the patient's arterial blood supply.

The heart-lung machine bypasses blood from the heart through cannulation of the superior and inferior venae cavae (see Fig. 27-9). Instead of flowing into the right atrium, blood enters the cannulas and by gravity flows to a collecting chamber or reservoir which is always placed below the level of the heart. The blood is oxygenated by being run through a special device at modulated pressures, then pumped through a heat exchanger. In the heat exchanger, the blood is lowered in temperature and then filtered before being pumped back into the circulation via one of the large arteries. The iliac, femoral, subclavian, or ascending aorta may be utilized as the receiver channel. A bubble trap is placed between the heat exchanger and the patient entry site to prevent air bubbles from entering the arterial circulation (see Fig. 27-9).

If cannulation is made from the pump into the ascending aorta, the blood flows antegrade (i.e., in a normal manner). When the cannulation is made from other entry sites, the blood may actually flow retrograde. The perfused blood circulates through the various tissue beds of the body and finally back into one of the venae cavae where the process begins anew.

Recent research has shown that *excessive bleeding*[24] and hemolysis[25] occur in a significant number of cases following open-heart surgery. The reasons for these changes in *coagulation* effects are not entirely clear. Several complex mechanisms are thought to lower platelet concentration in these patients and result in postsurgical *anemia*. If anemia is a complication of surgery, the workload of the heart is increased, and pump failure can occur.

*Air embolism* is another complication that can occur from the presence of air in the tubing or poor filtration of air bubbles in the extracorporeal circulation. The air embolus can travel throughout the body and lodge in the lung or other major organ, obstructing blood flow. *Arrhythmias* are a constant threat, and problems such as atrial fibrillation are not uncommon.

*Postperfusion syndrome* produces a myriad of symptoms that occur as a result of extracorporeal circulation. Although the cause is difficult to isolate, manifestations such as hyperthermia, splenomegaly, adenopathy, hepatomegaly, and frequently pharyngitis can occur.

*Postoperative nursing care*  Several immediate problems confront the patient following open-heart surgery. These include alteration in blood pressure, pulse, and respirations, fever, fluid loss, immobility, sensory overload, fear and anxiety, and pain. A patient who has just undergone involved surgery requires complex and intensive nursing care.

Effective pumping action along with adequate circulating volume, proper vascular tone, and tissue perfusion can most effectively be measured through evaluation of the individual's vital signs. Alterations in blood pressure, pulse rate, and respirations will have significant meaning for the patient especially after cardiac surgery.

*Arterial blood pressure changes* must be noted. The patient with a mitral-valve replacement may have a normal blood pressure throughout the postoperative course. Some patients may even tolerate a lowered systolic (80 to 90 mmHg) pressure following surgery. If the pumping capacity is stressed by such things as pain, fear, cardiac tamponade, hemorrhage, or pump failure, the blood pressure level will be unstable. It is essential that a *baseline* blood pressure reading be obtained prior to surgery so that deviations during the postoperative period can be accurately evaluated. Frequent assessments of

the blood pressure readings are essential during the postoperative period.

Information about changes in the arterial blood pressure is also useful when making assumptions about the state of peripheral resistance (diastolic) as well as perfusion of the tissues (systolic). In common with other physical characteristics such as body build, skin color, and weight, there are wide variations between the so-called "normal" pressures. For this reason it is imperative to secure blood pressure measurements preoperatively so that comparisons may be made after surgery.

When signs of hypotension appear (see Chap. 28 for a complete discussion), the cause of the problem must be isolated and appropriate treatment started. Medications (e.g., vasopressors), volume expanders (e.g., dextran, plasma), narcotics to relieve pain, termination of acidosis, and correction of arrhythmias may help reverse the problem.

*Changes in cardiac rhythm* may be noted. Palpation of the radial, carotid, dorsalis pedis, and popliteal arterial pulsations will give important data about the rhythm and quality of the pulses. Several sites should be palpated in order to determine

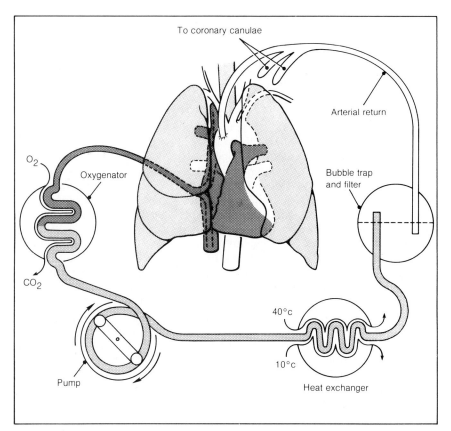

**FIGURE 27-9**
Schematic drawing of heart-lung bypass. (*Adapted from Donald Longmore, The Heart, McGraw-Hill, New York, 1976.*)

whether differences exist. Differences between apical and radial (pulse deficit) should be noted. A pulse deficit is indicative of ineffective cardiac contractions. Irregularities in the pulse rate and rhythm may indicate fibrillation, a common problem associated with mitral valve replacement.

Cross-estimations of tissue perfusion can be made by examining the *capillary filling* time at the fingertips and the earlobes. In addition, inspection and palpation of the veins on the dorsum of the hands or on the feet should provide information about the return of blood to the right side of the heart. Full, dilated veins, when the hand is elevated above the heart (angle of Louis), show that blood is not returning to the right side of the heart adequately.

The warmth and color of the patient's skin must be observed carefully and in several areas of the body. *Cyanosis* should be noted and described by site, exact color, and degree of "coolness." In some patients a generalized loss of pink color is observed, and in others a mottling effect is seen. Cyanosis may result from an increase in peripheral vascular resistance and may be limited to the hands, fingers, feet, cheeks, or earlobes. Or, if cyanosis is of central origin and caused by a gradually failing pump, blueness will be detected in the lips, mucous membranes, tongue, and nailbeds where the small arteries run very close to the surface of the body.

In the presence of pump failure, arrhythmias, fever, dyspnea, or hemorrhage, the pulse rate may vary. The patient's cardiac rhythm will usually be measured via EKG monitoring. This will allow for continuous observation of the apical rate and cardiac conduction.

*Digitalis* therapy is often initiated after surgery to enhance cardiac contractibility and to support a sinus rhythm. If the patient had not been digitalized prior to the surgery, large doses of digitalis preparation (0.75 to 0.87 mg) may be administered intravenously until the desired digitalization level is reached. When this is achieved, smaller daily doses of the desired digitalis preparation (0.125 to 0.25 mg) are administered. Because digitalis can result in a variety of aberrant heart rhythms, any change in the cardiac rhythm or rate should be evaluated, documented, and reported to the physician, depending upon its seriousness. (See Chap. 24 for a complete discussion of digitalis therapy.) It is always hoped that the patient will remain in a normal sinus rhythm postoperatively, but frequently patients revert to atrial fibrillation in spite of the valvular correction. Either quinidine or Pronestyl

hydrochloride may be ordered as an adjunct to the digitalis therapy to decrease the initiation of ectopic foci.

Pulmonary artery wedge pressure readings may also be used to monitor left ventricular function and atrial pressure. Central venous pressure monitoring will offer information about the right side of the heart. (See Chap. 28 for a complete discussion.) When changes in the pump's effectiveness occur, evaluation of the pulse rate will offer early information on impending pump failure.

*Respiration* changes are controlled in several ways. For the first 24 hours after surgery, the patent airway is guaranteed by the use of an endotracheal tube. A positive pressure breathing device may or may not be used postoperatively with this qualification. Patients with long-standing COLD usually require such therapy for several days. A Bennett $MA_1$, Ohio 560, or other breathing equipment may be utilized. (See Chap. 30 for discussion of ventilating machines.) The choice of equipment used will vary with each institution; however, the prophylactic administration of positive pressure breathing treatments is widespread. The concentration of oxygen delivered may vary from 30 to 50 percent or more, while the inspiratory rate, the volume, and sigh volume will depend upon the individual characteristics of each patient. The choice of intubation, ventilator, and treatment varies according to the respiratory and perfusion state of the patient. It should be noted, however, that all patients undergoing cardiac surgery are maintained on some type of oxygen assist if only by mask, nasal cannula, or prongs, for a short period of time following surgery.

The patient with a mitral valve replacement will have arterial blood gases drawn and analyzed immediately upon returning to the cardiac recovery room and periodically thereafter. An arterial puncture is the procedure most often used, although arterial lines for measurement of the blood pressure have the added advantage of being available for arterial blood samples.

For an arterial puncture, a moderate-bore needle and a 10-ml heparinized syringe are used to penetrate a surface artery such as the radial or brachial. Heparin prevents the blood from clotting in the syringe. All air is expelled from the syringe, and the sample is placed on ice for immediate transfer to the laboratory. Approximately 10 ml blood is obtained and analyzed for its dissolved gas distribution. The data obtained include carbon dioxide levels, bases, bicarbonates, and oxygen determinations. The blood pH level, a measure of acidity and alkalinity, will also be ascertained.

The patient whose blood gases remain within normal limits, and in whom respiratory complications are not expected, will be maintained on oyxgen at 2 to 4 liters/minute by nasal prongs or cannula. If the arterial oxygen saturation level decreases below 90 percent, respiratory assistances will be needed. The nurse should observe the retraction of the chest wall or flaring nares which may indicate varying degrees of respiratory distress. Breathlessness as reported by the patient is an early clue to the patient's anxiety. Generalized irritability, especially as a new finding, is also an important sign of reduced oxygenation of the cerebrum. Blood gas tensions should be monitored frequently and ordered at the discretion of the nurse, physician, or inhalation therapist.

Adequate ventilation requires not only evaluation of monitoring devices, but continuous observation of the rate, rhythm, and depth of respiration, patency of the patient's airway, skin color, amount of secretions, and drainage of chest tubes.

A rapid respiratory rate may be observed with anxiety, pain, airway obstruction, anoxia, metabolic acidosis (see Chap. 12), or atelectasis (fluid in the lungs). A decrease in the respiratory rate may suggest poor $O_2/CO_2$ exchange or oversedation. If severe pain, fear of stimulating the cough reflex, or suppression of the respiratory center are present, the patient may be having shallow respiratory exchange.

Shortness of breath (dyspnea) may be noted in association with pump failure or an accumulation of fluids in the lungs. Alterations in respirations with periods of apnea (Cheyne-Stokes pattern) may suggest more severe failure. Assessment of breath sounds may indicate dullness in lobes where there is a density of fluid present or the presence of basal rales especially in pump failure. The presence of wheezing or frothy sputum may suggest pulmonary edema. Palpation of the chest wall may reveal a decrease in resonance upon verbal vibration. Limited bilateral chest movement may also be noted.

Sputum should be observed for thickness, color, and amount. Frequent coughing and deep breathing are essential. Breathing exercises taught during the preoperative period should be utilized often. IPPB with humidity can be used with an aerosol solution to help loosen thick secretions. If needed, clapping and vibration of the posterior chest wall will help loosen thick, lodged secretions (see Chap. 30). Frequent turning will help prevent an accumulation of mucus and secretions in the lungs. If necessary, deep endotracheal suctioning may be needed if secretions can not be removed by

the patient (see Chap. 30). When the patient is coughing, the chest should be splinted with a towel, pillows, or the hands to help reduce pain. The patient can be taught to support the thoracic area during the coughing period.

While chest tubes are being assessed for the amount, color, consistency, and patency of drainage, the lungs should be observed for reexpansion following surgery. As the lungs reexpand, the amount of fluid in the drainage tubes should increase. Approximately 20 to 30 ml fluid can be lost hourly during the immediate postoperative period (24 to 48 hours). Initially the drainage will appear dark red and will become lighter in the days following. Usually the amount of drainage should also decrease with time. Chest tubes should be kept straight at all times. Clots that collect in the tubes can be manually expressed by milking the tubes. Care must be taken to prevent breakage of the drainage bottle or dislodging the tubing. Should the tubes become separated or dislodged, or the bottle break, a Kelly clamp (kept at the patient's bedside) should be placed directly on the tubing, close to the patient's chest wall (see Chap. 30 for a more complete discussion of chest tubes).

If the amount of drainage increases per hour beyond 20 to 30 ml, the nurse should suspect a change in the patient's status (i.e., hemorrhage). These changes may be reflected by alterations in vital signs and cerebral irritability, hypovolemia, dyspnea, alteration in level of consciousness, and hypotension.

Careful cleaning around the chest tubes as well as inspection of the skin site will help alert the nurse to signs of inflammation. Antibiotics may be used prophylactically to avert infection. When drainage is minimal and chest expansion good, a chest x-ray will be taken to assess the lung's total reexpansion.

*Diaphoresis* may be present during the postoperative period; however, unless the skin is cool and damp, there is little clinical significance to this finding other than the presence of a slight fever or a room that is too warm. The temperature should be checked frequently to evaluate the presence of an inflammatory response due to infection, a reaction to the prosthetic device, or a transfusion reaction. Normally the temperature will be elevated 2 to 3 degrees after surgery. The use of antipyretics, a hypothermia blanket, or ice packs may help reduce the temperature.

Therapy with broad-spectrum antibiotics is initiated in the operating room through intravenous infusions and is continued for varying periods of time during the recovery period. In order to prevent postoperative bacterial infection, several *antibiotics* such as penicillin, streptomycin, and kanamycin may be given prophylactically and simultaneously for varying periods of time. The intravenous route is utilized until the patient is able to take foods by mouth.

*Adrenal steroid therapy,* using prednisone, is initiated for the control of fever, edema, and inflammation. Doses may vary but generally range from 2 to 4 mg intravenously every 4 to 6 hours for the first 24 to 48 hours postoperatively. The drug is tapered off gradually over a period of several days to prevent complications from sudden termination. If dehydration is suspected, fluid replacement and evaluation of electrolytes will be required. If atelectasis is suspected, antibiotics, chest x-ray, and more vigorous respiratory therapy will be necessary. Use of careful aseptic technique when changing wound dressings will also help prevent infection.

The importance of maintaining normal *fluid and electrolyte concentrations* in the cardiovascular patient cannot be overemphasized. Myocardial cellular integrity and normal depolarization of the heart are directly affected by aberrations in fluid balance.

Fluid loss is closely monitored in the postoperative course, particularly in patients experiencing vomiting or profuse diaphoresis. Fluid depletion, which occurs infrequently in these patients, is noted by an elevation in the serum sodium concentration and increased serum osmolarity. The loss of electrolytes (isotonic loss) is a frequent finding after major cardiac surgery. Changes in the acid-base balance, hypokalemia, hyperkalemia, and blood electrolytes can occur. Acidosis is associated with an elevated serum potassium, while a sharp decrease in potassium is linked to alkalosis. (A complete discussion of acid-base imbalances is found in Chap. 12.)

*Hypokalemia* is generally anticipated following open-heart surgery and can be prevented by intravenous infusion of potassium. Replacement therapy begins during the surgery and is continued over several days or until the potassium level has been normal for a period of time. The postoperative potassium level should lie between 3.5 and 5.5 meq. However, many surgeons prefer to have the potassium level toward the maximum during the first few hours postoperatively.

Intravenous fluids are administered on a continuous basis during the immediate postoperative period. Accurate and continuous assessment of fluid intake and output is therefore essential. These fluids usually consist of dextrose solutions or Ringer's lactate. When needed, a volume expander such as dextran or plasma is used. Generally, solutions containing sodium are not used as they could increase fluid retention and lead to volume overload. Accurate measurement of urinary renal output will help contribute to the overall evaluation of fluid elimination. Hourly assessment of output may be required during the first 24-hour period after surgery. A urinometer may be used to collect and to measure hourly urinary output. The urine should be observed for color, specific gravity, and clarity. The normal hourly urinary output should range between 40 and 50 ml/hour. When less than 20 to 30 ml is excreted per hour, the patient will be observed for oliguria and dehydration. If the patient is hypovolemic or dehydrated, these problems should be corrected immediately. Mannitol may be used to increase urinary output and blood flow. If anuria and hypovolemia persist, dialysis may be utilized (see Chap. 14). Daily weights enable the nurse to assess fluid loss and retention and should be observed closely.

Following removal of the endotracheal tube, sips of water may be permitted. As the patient's tolerance increases, the diet may progress from clear liquids to soft foods. The patient should be closely observed for abdominal complaints such as pain, nausea, vomiting, or distention. These changes may indicate the presence of a paralytic ileus or stress ulcer. Should any of these problems occur, oral intake should be withheld, and the physician contacted for further evaluation and consultation.

*Hyperkalemia,* while not as commonly observed after surgery as potassium deficiency, has serious effects on the myocardial pump. Adverse effects are probably a function of acidosis when sodium shifts into the cell and potassium is lost to the extracellular fluid. Integrity of the cell membrane is altered in conditions of metabolic acidosis.[26]

Muscular weakness or cramping, abdominal distention, or nausea can be revealed by careful observation and inspection of the patient. In hyperkalemia, the EKG will show the classic pattern of peaked T waves (see Chap. 12), while a prolongation of the QRS interval is observed on occasion.

The treatment for hyperkalemia is a correction of the basic abnormality, namely, a marked increase and retention of the hydrogen ion. In emergency situations, glucose and insulin may be given to correct the acidosis.

Other important *electrolytes* are calcium (a

catalyst for depolarization), sodium, and magnesium. Frequent laboratory analysis is ordered to monitor electrolytes during the immediate postoperative period.

One of the most important aspects of management of the patient at risk of pump failure is *maintenance of adequate blood volume.* An increase in volume will elevate the systemic pressure and overload the left ventricle days following the surgery. Inadequate blood volume causes selective vasoconstriction and poor tissue perfusion and leads to metabolic acidosis. Assessment of blood loss can be accomplished through measurement of the chest tube drainage system, as blood may accumulate within the thoracic or abdominal cavities (silent bleeding). On the first postoperative day chest x-rays may be ordered for as often as every 4 hours and twice daily until the chest tubes are taken out. Blood loss may also be noted in the feces, the urine, or the nasogastric drainage, and may be detected in the hemoglobin and hematocrit readings.

When the amount of blood lost exceeds 10 percent of the total volume, sympathetic tone increases, and blood flow to the splanchnic area, the skin, and limb vessels is sharply curtailed. There will be coldness of the extremities.

When acute blood loss is sensed by sympathetic nerve fibers, and feedback information reaches the adrenal glands, epinephrine and norepinephrine are secreted into the bloodstream. The action of these catecholamines is to increase the heart rate, and possibly to increase the strength of myocardial contraction. Thus tachycardia will be observed. When cardiac output falls, the amount of oxygen delivered to the tissues also falls, and pump failure along with hypovolemia can develop (see Chap. 28).

Blood loss is replaced milliliter for milliliter. Whole blood or packed cells may be used, and in selected cases plasma expanders and plasma fractions are administered to replenish a low circulating volume.

Evaluation of replacement therapy is a nursing measure and includes assessment of the central venous pressure, arterial blood pressure, and pulse rate. Urinary output should be evaluated along with the patient's level of consciousness and responsiveness, skin color, and capillary refill. These parameters indicate the success of replacement therapy. Signs of transfusion reaction (see Chap. 10) should also be noted.

Careful replacement of oral fluids can begin as early as 12 hours after surgery. In the absence of nausea or abdominal distention, the diet can slowly progress from liquids to solids.

Continued assessment of urinary output, electrolytes, hemoglobin, hematocrit, and blood gases is essential to evaluating fluid and electrolyte balance. In addition, accurate recording of intake and output will aid overall nursing assessment.

Patients frequently have *problems of mobility* following surgery due to their attachment to many pieces of equipment as well as to their own physical and psychological exhaustion. However, the dangers of immobility must be counteracted. Although the patient may be weak, activity must begin almost immediately following surgery. When vital signs are stable, the bed can be placed in semi-Fowler's position; frequent turning, every 2 hours, is essential. Passive range of motion exercises to the lower extremities, the use of antiembolic stockings, and elevation of the lower extremities above the head to allow for peripheral drainage are important interventions in preventing venous stasis and phlebitis. (See Chap. 29 for a complete discussion.)

The use of anticoagulent agents in the cardiac surgical patient is controversial. If anticoagulants are ordered, they are titered to the daily prothrombin and proconvertin (P and P) or partial prothrombin times (PPT). The nurse must be aware that the use of anticoagulent agents, their choice, and method of administration are controversial among physicians since the results of research with these drugs vary widely. During the immediate postoperative period there is some danger of surgical hemorrhage, but there is also some risk of thromboembolic complications. The Inter Society Commission for Heart Disease Resources found the need for anticoagulant therapy to be pronounced in patients with recurring atrial fibrillation.[27]

Patients are frequently encouraged to cough and deep breathe to prevent atelectasis. This activity along with frequent turning and respiratory therapy including clapping and vibrating of the chest wall (see Chap. 30) will help reduce the accumulation of fluids in the lungs.

Ambulation should begin the evening of surgery. The patient can begin to dangle and then on the following day can get out of bed into a chair for a short time. The amount of time for this activity will increase daily. As the patient regains strength, walking in the room and in the corridor can be permitted.

Disturbances in sensory stimulation are a frequent postoperative problem. Continuous observation of the patient during this postoperative period necessitates frequent interruption of restful periods. The respiratory therapist, physicians, nurses, and the laboratory and x-ray technicians all must see the patient frequently during the critical post-operative period. Ideally, these stimulation periods should be scheduled around definite rest periods.

Recent literature reports that *sleep deprivation,* and the upset of normal diurnal rhythms, contribute to postoperative psychosis, hallucinations, and confusion in these patients. There are several ways to normalize necessary routine to minimize interruptions in sleep patterns. The lights in the room can be dimmed or turned off during the night so that a routine day-night orientation is not interrupted. If the patient is deprived of the morning (light) and evening (dark) routine for 48 to 72 hours postoperatively, confusion will result. Aberrations and complications are more frequent occurrences in the elderly who rely heavily on daily routine for proper orientation.[28] Assessment of the patient's normal rhythmic patterns can aid in developing a more efficient plan of care. The use of clocks and calendars can help orient the patient to time and the environment, helping to reduce stress.

It is not unusual for the patient to be seen by at least eight members of the staff within the first half hour of the postoperative course. In an uncomplicated postoperative recovery period, the interruptions can be grouped so that more than one activity can be performed with each interruption. Spacing interruptions will also allow for planned rest periods and reduce stressful disruptions in sleep.

Recently much emphasis has been placed upon the sonic, luminous, and physical environment of the patient.[29,30] Research has shown that intensive-care units are very noisy places and further that noise may contribute to the patient's postoperative discomfort. Noise has been implicated in increasing heart rate,[31] as well as increasing the urinary excretion of catecholamines in these persons.[32] While the noise from the machinery cannot be totally eliminated, extraneous noise can be reduced. Discussions about the patient at the bedside should be avoided. The area should be kept as quiet as possible. Visitors should be limited, and when conferences are needed, an area should be assigned specifically for this purpose.

*Alteration in the level of consciousness* is an obvious consequence of long-term deep-plane anesthesia. However, several hours after surgery the patient will begin to respond. A return to consciousness can be complicated by other anesthesia, embolic formation, hemorrhage, hypovolemia, and pump failure. Patients may also have a delayed conscious response depending on the length of time they were attached to bypass oxygenation.

This can contribute to disorientation, hallucinations, and mental confusion.

A neurological assessment including pupil check, limb mobility, sensory perception, and reflexes should be made. Auditory stimulation as well as assessment of the pain response are additional indicators of an intact cerebrum. Extrasensorial stimuli may be perceived as threatening and intensify fear and anxiety. Therefore all nursing activities should be carefully explained to the patient, whether fully conscious or not. Assessment of oxygen saturation levels, oxygen administration, and continuous orientation to time and place will help increase the patient's response during this stressful period.

*Psychological factors* such as the fear of pain, death, or disfigurement can influence the patient's vital signs and affect the postoperative course. The patient is faced with a myriad of uncertainties including the overall success of the surgery and the impact of the surgery on the family and on the person's overall life-style. These fears are intensified by the feelings of disorientation that the patient experiences to time and place. These feelings are understandable, and they are frightening to the patient.

The fear of death, however, is the greatest single cause of apprehension in patients following open-heart surgery. The belief that the heart cannot be separated from the individual[33] seems to precipitate anxiety. The awareness of the nearness of death has been recently described in the literature. Data include detailed accounts given by patients describing individual sensorial experiences while attached to extracorporeal devices. These data offer greater understanding into the postoperative fears and anxieties experienced by patients.

These fears, whether they be precipitated by intense anxiety over a perceived loss or effected by inadequate extracorporeal oxygenation, are threatening to the patient. The nurse, merely by being present, can exert a powerful quieting effect on the patient. Verbal support and reassurance can be most helpful to the patient at this time. Continuous reorienting to time and place as well as careful explanation of all procedures will also be helpful. While coping mechanisms vary greatly among patients, the nurse should be able to help individuals regain control over behavior, feelings, and the environment. This control will be demonstrated by increased verbal communication of fears, control over emotional responses, logical thinking, and a clear perception of the actual situation as well as participation and cooperation in and with self-care.[34] A quiet atmosphere and a comforting and supportive environment will offer the patient the assistance needed to progress through this stressful time.

Frequently psychological problems may become severe and complicate the recovery period. A combination of factors may be responsible for a significant postoperative psychosis including prolonged pump infusion time, personality type, and the atmosphere of the intensive-care unit. Anxiety, tension, and depression may also persist. A variety of psychotropic drugs including diazepam (Valium) are administered routinely. Nursing interventions continue to be directed toward orienting the patient to time and place. If the psychosis is not relieved by these measures, mental health counseling may be needed.

Because of the amount of manipulation of the chest wall and related structures, the patient will often experience much postoperative *pain.* Medication is administered as needed in the postoperative period, and care must be used in dispensing medications so that the respiratory center and vital signs will not be depressed. In most cases morphine sulfate, in small intravenous doses of from 1 to 3 mg, is titered to the extent of the patient's pain. The postoperative patient should be in a state of easy arousal, but not appear restless or grimacing while trying to sleep. Meperidine hydrochloride is also used to alleviate pain during the immediate postoperative period. Both agents have the capacity to alter hemodynamics such as pulse and blood pressure, but to varying extents. In addition, morphine sulfate exerts a depressive effect upon respirations, whereas meperidine generally does not. However, meperidine often produces vomiting in many patients and may not be used with patients recovering from cardiac surgery.

**C**omplications of Mitral Valve Replacement   The complications of mitral valve replacement arise from several sources including disturbances in the blood flow, arrhythmias, respiratory complications, long-standing left ventricular disease, and complications arising from the prosthesis itself.

*Abnormalities of blood flow*   In the majority of cases the patient with a mitral valve correction has had long-standing heart problems. The hematocrit and hemoglobin may be within normal limits; however, there is evidence that mitral stenosis, particularly if accompanied by atrial fibrillation, fractures the circulating red blood cells and causes an *abnormal level of platelets.* According to one large study, thrombus formation on a prosthetic heart valve with subsequent embolization continues to be the most serious of complications after the initial postoperative course. It is thought that the process is related to the adherence of large numbers of platelets and the deposition of fibrosis on the valve.[35]

*Chronic hemolysis* is another recognized complication. In some persons perfusion by the heart-lung machine appears to be the cause of hemodilution, anemia, hemorrhage, or dehydration through processes that are not clearly known. Turbulence of the blood against a rigid mechanical valve has been overcome largely through the use of flexible materials such as Stilastic balls and cloth-covered rings. Other materials, as well as homografts and autografts, are being researched in clinical trials in an effort to find a prosthesis that is totally benign to red blood cells.

*Thrombosis and pulmonary embolization*   The heart is the site of formation of many arterial emboli, called *mural thrombi.* They are often seen in the patient with a severely stenosed preoperative valve and a history of atrial fibrillation. The clot, which theoretically can arise from anywhere within the circulatory system, migrates in the bloodstream to lodge in a femoral, popliteal, common ileac, hepatic, renal, carotid, or pulmonary artery. These clots, arising in the left side of the heart, may occlude the cerebral circulation at some point, and the nurse may observe confusion, irritability, weakness of a side of the body, or other signs of a cerebral vascular accident. Less frequently, the renal, mesenteric, or femoral arteries are involved. A cold, numb extremity is the classic feature if the extremities are involved. Inspection and palpation of the limbs will give the nurse valuable information about peripheral circulation.

Pulmonary embolus after replacement of the mitral valve is generally caused by a thrombus in the veins of the legs, or the pelvis, breaking loose from its primary site and traveling in the bloodstream to the lungs. If the tricuspid or pulmonic valve has also been replaced with a prosthetic valve, the embolus may arise from the suture lines around the valves. A small infarction on the right side of the heart or the septum may also give rise to an embolus.

If the pulmonary embolus occludes a very small artery in the lung, the patient may have few symptoms other than a slight elevation of temperature. However, of the patients who experience a massive occlusion, one-third do not recover. Pulmonary infarction ensues when the lung is deprived of oxygen for more than a very short period of time. Symptoms of pleurisy and pleural effusion are observed in those patients who survive the massive occlusion. Respirations will increase and grow increasingly shallow. The patient may complain of acute pain. Dyspnea is pronounced and diaphoresis is always present. Hemoptysis and fever are usually observed. A complete discussion of the treatment of pulmonary infarction can be found in Chap. 29.

*Myocardial infarction*  In a small number of patients myocardial infarction (MI) occurs shortly after replacement of the mitral valve. When an MI occurs, it is due to ischemia caused by a small, mural thrombus that breaks loose from the area adjacent to the mitral valve and subsequently migrates through the coronary circulation to lodge in one of the smaller branches of the coronary arteries. The seriousness of the episode depends upon the extent of tissue destruction. A complete discussion of myocardial infarction is found in Chap. 26.

*Cardiac tamponade*  Cardiac tamponade is a serious postoperative complication. It occurs when there is bleeding into the pericardial sac resulting in an accumulation of blood around the heart. Consequently the myocardium is compressed and prevented from filling adequately during diastole or emptying properly during systole. Cardiac output is sharply reduced. The patient will demonstrate a low arterial blood pressure, an elevated central venous pressure, narrowed pulse pressure, and pulses that are weak and thready to palpation. The patient becomes extremely anxious as dyspnea increases. Cool, moist skin and varying degrees of cyanosis are also evident. Cardiac tamponade is a medical emergency for the blood must be removed from the pericardial sac and the abnormal flow stopped. Treatment must be immediate if cardiogenic shock and death are to be averted. (See Chap. 24 for additional discussion.)

*Arrhythmias*  Mitral valve correction or replacement is usually followed by a period of atrial fibrillation. This frequently occurs in patients who have no history of atrial arrhythmias preoperatively. It is sometimes caused by alterations in body temperature or a response to the presence of the valve. The exact cause is unknown. According to Brainbridge

the onset of atrial fibrillation can decrease cardiac output as much as 40 percent in the cardiac surgical patient.[36]

If the ventricular response to atrial fibrillation lies within a moderate range (60 to 100 beats/minute) the patient will have few if any symptoms from the arrhythmia. When the ventricular response is very fast (above 100 beats/minute) or extremely slow (50 beats/minute or less), the cardiac output may be decreased, and the symptoms will be those of poor perfusion.

Atrial fibrillation or flutter is usually treated pharmacologically with quinidine sulfate or Pronestyl hydrochloride, and less frequently propranolol. Propranolol is a negative inotropic agent and therefore is rarely given to the patient with left ventricular hypertrophy or pump failure. (A complete discussion of arrhythmias can be found in Chap. 25.)

Careful auscultation of the heart sounds as well as inspection of the EKG is necessary to detect transitional rhythms. It is important to note the appearance of a third or fourth heart sound for all gallop rhythms are associated with either tachycardia or left atrial overload and right-sided overload. Sinus tachycardia, nodal rhythms, ventricular-tachycardia, and heart block may also occur.

*Antiarrhythmic drugs* form another group commonly administered to postoperative cardiac surgical patients. Quinidine, Pronestyl hydrochloride, or lidocaine may be given to depress irritable heart rhythms, particularly those originating in the ventricle.

*Atropine* may be administered intravenously for increasing the heart rate if the rhythm is sinus, but it is far less effective in a slow ventricular rhythm. Isoproterenol hydrochloride (Isuprel) is frequently administered intravenously for slow rhythms initiated by the ventricle.

Of more recent origin is the administration of *dopamine* for a failing pump and *nitroprusside* for elevated arterial blood pressure. Either of these agents is given under very special conditions, as a short-term intravenous infusion and must be monitored continuously. Sympathomimetic agents such as epinephrine and norepinephrine are used less frequently in the cardiac surgical patient, since myocardial work may be increased with their administration.

*Respiratory disruptions*  Both hyper- and hypoventilation can occur during the immediate postoperative period. However, the widespread use of the endotracheal tube for 24 hours postoperatively has either reduced the occurrence of these complications or allowed for early treatment.

It is important to note that normal respiration at the cellular level depends equally upon normal inspiration and expiration, and upon blood flow through the lungs and body tissues. Therefore complications can result from the respiratory aspect or from the perfusion aspect. Deep breathing and coughing exercises are instituted very early after surgery, since respiratory complications due to shallow breathing are the most easily preventable. Effective sedation prevents respiratory complications by allowing the patient to comply with breathing exercises or IPPB treatments. Care must be taken to avoid oversedating the patient and depressing the respiratory center.

The nurse should inspect the anterior chest and thorax frequently for asymmetry, retraction of the sterum, and bulging of the cervical musculature. An increase in respirations or a change in their style is meaningful when plotted over a period of time. *Hyperventilation* generally follows a cerebral thrombosis, pulmonary infarction, pulmonary congestion, or any low-output state.

*Hypoventilation,* a less commonly seen event, occurs in the maximally sedated patient or in the patient with a history of chronic lung disease. Assisted breathing devices, as have been discussed under routine postoperative care, are used to enhance the compliance of the lung and assist in gaseous exchange. Periodic evaluation of blood gas tensions, particularly the $CO_2:O_2$ ratio, will aid in assessing the onset and improvement of this complication.

*Renal disruptions* Renal failure following cardiac surgery usually results from circulatory insufficiency. The amount of urine formed by the kidney depends rather directly upon the flow of blood through the renal artery and its branches. This flow has both a volume and a perfusion pressure. Oliguria and renal failure usually result from low volume (hypovolemia) or poor perfusion states, such as pump failure. Necrosis appears if the renal tissue is deprived of blood for more than a very short period of time.

Low volume is corrected through adequate fluid and blood replacement; however, there are greater difficulties in reversing low-perfusion states such as pump failure. If conservative measures, such as the administration of mannitol, albumin, or fluid loading, fail, azotemia (the accumulation of nitrogenous wastes) may become profound. Renal dialysis has been utilized on a short-term basis for these patients, with some success. (See Chap. 14 for a complete discussion of dialysis.) Obviously, the patient will become most anxious when another mass of machinery is introduced at the bedside. Adequate explanation and assurance must be given to the patient and family. The nurse is in an opportune position to provide this support as the person who has already established rapport with the patient and the family members.

Periodic urinalysis should be done, as well as routine specific gravities. The patient in severe renal failure is critically ill, and the prognosis for final recovery will be guarded.

### Fourth-Level Nursing Care

For cardiac patients, the need for rehabilitation exists in all etiological groups and in mild, moderate, and severe cases. Restrictions may reach across a broad span of activities: work, recreation, diet, and social life. However, a majority of cardiac patients find that reliance upon a cardiac drug and a diet are the only ways in which their lives have changed.

There are three specific goals for rehabilitation of cardiac patients: mobilization, restoration of self-image and family relationships, and education of the patient and family. The responsibilities for these tasks are shared among all disciplines including nursing, medicine, social work, nutrition, and occupational and physical therapy.

**Mobilization** Mobilization has many meanings, from dangling at the bedside, to ambulating in the halls, to returning to full-time work. The hospitalized patient progresses very quickly in activity—from complete bed rest to walking up and down the halls within a week after surgery. Early ambulation has evolved from an increased awareness of the hemodynamic effects of immobilization.

Rehabilitation concerning all phases of life should begin while the patient is still hospitalized, with all members of the team contributing. One cardiac center makes use of a checklist of human needs (such as activity and nutrition) which includes all the services offered by that institution.[37] The patient and the family choose all options in which they wish to participate. One advantage of this system is that the responsibility for defining rehabilitation needs lies with the patient. The assumption is that persons will learn better when they are active participants in defining their own needs.[38]

By the ninth or tenth day the cardiac patient whose recovery has been uncomplicated will be discharged. Discharge planning will have been completed by the hospital, liaison nurses, and the physician. Referrals may be made to agencies such as a visiting nurse service, cardiac rehabilitation program, or social or occupational counseling services.

The great majority of patients who have had correction of their valvular problem will continue a normal productive life. However, cardiac illness of any type, by nature of its chronicity, may give rise to many stresses, long after the primary structural defect has been corrected.

If interpersonal problems between husband and wife, or between parents and children, were present prior to surgery, these same problems are likely to exacerbate. (For example, if marital problems were present, they may begin to surface during this period.) In one large study, for example, wives were *upset* if a shift of roles made them the primary providers for the family.[39] Demoralization was a common finding if the husband wanted to return to work but was physiologically unable, or if he could not be reinstated in his former position. Vocational rehabilitation, a public service provided by most states, may offer some patients valuable guidance in reorganizing a career. Family and/or marital counseling may also be needed.

Large debts contracted prior to the acute illness, prolonged periods of unemployment, or concomitant illness of a second member of the family may place financial stress upon the discharged patient. Fortunately many hospitals utilize social workers and public health nurses who are prepared to assist the patient in resolving such problems.

Regardless of the outcome of the surgery, the return home is characterized by hesitancy and ambiguity. Suddenly the patient is expected to abandon the sick role and return to productive living, with the added burden of a heart prosthesis. It must be emphasized that physiological and psychological events of the recovery process in any serious illness are not well synchronized; psychologic and social function may lag behind the resolution of physical trauma.[40] Furthermore, those afflicted with chronic illness such as rheumatic heart disease cannot help but be influenced by the process. Biorck[41] described patients with valvular lesions as very courageous types who want to fight against their increasing disability and who are ready to accept almost any risk. They want to contribute to the support of their family, or to help in housekeeping, even to the point of overexertion in order to keep their self-respect as useful members of society.

The cardiac patient does not have a one-time

problem, which led to valvular stenosis or insufficiency. Atherosclerosis is a continuous process which will continue to affect the patient. Often by the time the mitral valve has been replaced, other physiologic changes such as hypertrophy or arrhythmias may have occurred. These changes will necessitate continuous dietary control, restrictions in activity, and reduction of physical and emotional stressors as well as planned exercise and gradual resumption of normal activities. Family members will be included in teaching and planning sessions so that the home environment will support the restorative health response.

**Patient education** Nearly all patients are discharged with some explanation of their heart defect and the manner in which it was corrected. However, applying such knowledge about the physiology of the heart to their daily lives is another matter. *Exercise* is one of the specific areas in which guidance is needed. It is difficult for patients to translate knowledge about the oxygen requirements of the heart into meaningful criteria for exercise tolerance. Many postoperative patients will never attain an ideal state of health, especially those whose mitral disease is complicated by diabetes, hypertension, advanced atherosclerosis, or congestive heart failure. These patients may face limitations in work and exercise for the remainder of their lives. Special charts, such as the one shown in Table 27-5, can be utilized by the nurse to explain the energy cost of various occupational duties and activities. If necessary, the patient may be referred to a work classification clinic for a complete analysis of limitations.

The physician may refer the patient to a cardiac rehabilitation clinic where all aspects of cardiodynamics are periodically measured, including cardiac output, left ventricular function, stress and resting electrocardiograms, blood pressure, and weight. The management of the patient will be determined by the results obtained and laboratory evaluations of the patient's cardiac status.

The patient may be *maintained* on medications such as a digitalis derivative or an antiarrhythmic drug such as quinidine sulfate or Pronestyl hydrochloride. Frequently the patient must take a diuretic several times a week to control edema and/or blood pressure (see Chap. 24).

The use of antiarrhythmic agents on a routine basis for cardiac surgical patients is controversial because of the significant side effects and the difficulty of monitoring their effects on a day-by-day basis. When the patient cannot be stabilized in a sinus rhythm and continuously reverts to atrial fibrillation after valvular surgery, digitalis and/or quinidine must be administered to control the fibrillation.[42]

The public health practitioner or the nurse in the adult clinic may be the first to detect abnormalities of heart rhythm in the posthospital patient. A careful history must be recorded for all patients who take anticoagulant or antiarrhythmic medications.

Most cardiac surgical patients are maintained on a low or modified sodium *diet.* Recently attention has turned to the development of diets that are low in sodium and culturally diverse, i.e., for Mexicans, Indian or Black Americans. However, ethnic families and all others of low income meet great difficulty in planning diets with adequate minerals and potassium. In order to simplify menu planning and guarantee compliance, the nurse can teach the patient to recognize and avoid those foods richest in sodium, such as salted meats and fish, potato chips, and milk products. Those patients whom it concerns should be warned of the potassium-depleting effects of digitalis and diuretics when taken together. However, there are some potassium-sparing diuretics on the market, and so the nurse needs to be specific in teaching. Unfortunately, potassium-rich foods are often those that are also high in sodium content. The dietitian is an excellent resource person for patients in whom the several aspects of drug and diet therapy are complex.

The nurse in the primary clinic or physician's office has many opportunities to ferret out diet or drug problems during the health history and physical assessment of patients. A sudden weight gain, elevated blood pressure, arrhythmia, or abnormal electrolytes should alert the nurse to potential problems in diet and drug management. A high level of sodium can be responsible for increases in blood pressure or weight gain, whereas potassium imbalance is often the cause of arrhythmias.

One of the limitations many cardiac patients resent is their inability to eat in restaurants, or as a guest in other homes, owing to their low-sodium diet. The nurse can assist the patient in developing a realistic plan that monitors diet closely at home but allows some flexibility for eating away from home. It is far better that the patient adhere strictly to the diet for 6 days of the week and deviate on the seventh, than to partially maintain the diet all week with a sense of frustration.

If feasible patients should be taught to take their pulse and encouraged to check it daily. They should be taught to report any significant changes in pulse rate and rhythm without delay. Should patients develop a fever, become short of breath, or feel weak or dizzy, they should contact the physician as these changes may indicate valve rejection or impending pump failure.

**Preservation of self-image**   During recuperation at home the patient may become bored and confused about future health problems. Some patients live by unnecessary restrictions either as a result of misinterpreting the physician's advice or in response to an overprotective family.

During discharge planning, the nurse must anticipate such reactions and assure the patient that feelings of role confusion and depression are common during the first few months after cardiac surgery. A mechanism for follow-up care should be established. The patient should be encouraged to contact the nurse when feelings are overwhelming or last more than a short period of time. Teaching may be needed to help the patient cope with fears and focus energies on improvement in health state. Feelings of hostility or depression should be identified and openly discussed before adjustments in life-style can be attained.

Discharge planning must be flexible and reflect the individuality of the patient. The social orientation, cultural background, education, and pattern of family relationships should be taken into account. The patient should be a major participant in any decisions concerning rehabilitation and return to work.

Patients are often concerned about the performance of their normal sexual role. In most cases the individual has been advised to avoid undue ex-

**TABLE 27-5**
ENERGY COST OF VARIOUS COMMON ACTIVITIES

| Activity | Cost, cal |
|---|---|
| Lying in bed (relaxed) | 1.0 |
| Lying on bed (tossing and turning) | 2.0 |
| Sitting in chair | 1.2 |
| Standing still | 1.2 |
| Self-care activities | 2.5 |
| Showering | 4.0 |
| Upright sweeping | 3.0 |
| Sewing | 3.0 |
| Cooking | 3.0 |
| Desk work | 2–3 |
| Bench work | 3–4 |
| Assembly line work | 3–4 |
| Walking (slowly, at 1.5 mph) | 2.0 |
| Walking (moderately, at 2.5 mph) | 4.0 |
| Walking (briskly, at 3.5 mph) | 5.0 |
| Stair climbing | 5.0 |

citement and emotional strain. It has been shown that the physiological cost of conjugal sex is modest, with the maximal heart rate reaching 120 beats/minute for approximately 10 seconds. The equivalent oxygen cost to the heart is that of climbing a short flight of stairs or walking a short distance briskly.[43] The nurse and both partners should discuss the fears associated with sexual activity in light of the patient's cardiac status. The patient needs to be reassured that the average patient can engage in sexual activity with confidence. Should problems occur, the patient must seek medical advice. Literature on cardiac rehabilitation is available from state offices of the American Heart Association.

As nurses become skilled in their physical assessment of hemodynamics, and as their knowledge base continues to grow, their role in the management of cardiac patients will broaden. In colleagueship with physicians, nurses are able to go beyond the physical and add human aspects to their care. The final result is more complete rehabilitation for cardiac patients.

## REFERENCES

1 George Thorn et al., *Harrison's Principles of Internal Medicine,* 8th ed., McGraw-Hill, New York, 1976, p. 1223.
2 R. Sanderson, *The Cardiac Surgical Patient,* Saunders, Philadelphia, 1972.
3 *Ibid.*
4 Jeanette Kernicki, Barbara Bullock, and Joan Matthews, *Cardiovascular Nursing,* Putnam, New York, 1970, p. 225.
5 "Prevention of Congenital Disease," Report of the Inter Society Commission for Heart Disease Resources, American Heart Association, *Circulation,* **XLI:**26, June 1970.
6 M. Lerner, F. Wilson, and R. Milagros, "Enteroviruses and the Heart," *Mod Concepts Cardiovasc Dis,* **XLIV:**2, February 1975.
7 Inter Society Commission for Heart Disease Resources, *op. cit.,* p. 26.
8 Thorn, *op. cit.,* pp. 1222–1226.
9 J. W. Hurst, et al., *The Heart: Arteries and Veins,* McGraw-Hill, New York, 3d ed., 1974, p. 791.
10 Lerner, *op cit.,* p. 249.
11 Harriet Moidel, Elizabeth Giblin, and Bernice Wagner, *Nursing Care of the Patient with Medical-Surgical Disorders,* 2d ed., McGraw-Hill, New York, 1976, p. 511.
12 Thorn, *op. cit.,* p. 1244.
13 Thorn, *op. cit.,* p. 1245.

14 Inter Society Commission for Heart Disease Resources, *op. cit.,* p. A1.
15 A. Johnson, "Rheumatic Fever: A Continuing Threat," *Nursing '74,* **3:**3, 57, March 1974.
16 P. Dorsey, and H. Jackson, "Cultural Health Traditions: The Latino/Chicano Perspective," in N. Branch and P. Paxton (eds.), *Providing Safe Nursing Care for Ethnic People of Color,* Appleton-Century-Crofts, New York, 1976, p. 44.
17 S. Schwartz, (ed.), *Principles of Surgery,* Chap. 18, McGraw-Hill, New York, pp. 642–645.
18 A. Johnson, *op. cit.,* p. 58.
19 G. Robb, *An Atlas of Angiography,* American Registry of Pathology, 1951, p. 12, in G. Wallace (ed.), "Preanesthetic without Narcotics," *JAMA,* **174:**7, 133, 1960.
20 C. Beckman and B. Dooley, "Complications of Left Heart Angiography," *Circulation,* **41:**825–832, May 1970.
21 *Ibid.,* p. 832.
22 H. Machleder, J. Sweeney, and W. Baker, "Pulseless Arm after Trachial Artery Catheterization," *Lancet,* **1:**407–409, Feb. 19, 1972.
23 D. Kahn, R. Strang, and W. Wilson, *Clinical Aspects of Operable Heart Disease,* Chap. 3, Appleton-Century-Crofts, New York, 1968.
24 R. McKenna, et al., "The Hemostatic Mechanism after Open Heart Surgery II," *J Thorac Cardiovasc Surg,* **20:**2, 301–307, August 1975.
25 F. Bachman, et al., "The Hemostatic Mechanism after Open Heart Surgery I." *J Thorac Cardiovasc Surg,* **20:**1, 76–85, July 1975.
26 D. Trunkey, "Review of Current Concepts in Fluid and Electrolyte Management," *Heart Lung,* **4,** 1, January–February, 1975, p. 118.
27 Report of the Inter Society Commission for Heart Disease Resources, *op. cit.,* p. 31.
28 F. Storlie, *Nursing and the Social Conscience,* Chap. 4, Appleton-Century-Crofts, New York, 1970.
29 S. Falk and N. Woods, "Hospital Noise Levels and Potential Health Hazards," *N Engl J Med,* **288:**15, 774–776, Oct. 11, 1973.
30 B. Minckley, "A Study of Noise and Its Relationship to Discomfort in the Recovery Room," *Nurs Res,* **17:**3, 247, May–June, 1968.
31 L. Marshall, "Patient Reaction to Sound in an Intensive Coronary Care Unit," master's thesis, Graduate College Medical Center, University of Illinois, in M. Batey (ed.), *Communicating Nursing Research,* WICHE, Boulder, Col., November 1972, pp. 81–92.
32 A. Wallace, "Catecholamine Metabolism in Patients with Acute Myocardial Infarction," in B. Julian and M. Oliver (eds.), *Acute Myocardial Infarction,* Williams & Wilkins, 1968, pp. 237–242.

33 Much of the material on the previous two pages has been adapted from M. Powers and F. Storlie, *The Cardiac Surgical Patient,* Chap. 6, "The First Critical 48 Hours," New York, Macmillan, 1968.

34 W. Gentry and R. Williams, *Psychological Aspects of Myocardial Infarction and Coronary Care,* Mosby, St. Louis, 1975, p. 66.

35 R. Ahmad et al., "Chronic Hemolysis Following Mitral Valve Replacement," *J Thorac Cardiovasc Surg,* **68:**3, 335, September 1974.

36 M. Brainbridge and P. Ghadiali, *Postoperative Cardiac Care,* Chap. 6, Blackwell Scientific Publications, London, 1965, p. 40.

37 B. Johnston, J. Cantwell, and G. Fletcher, "Eight Steps to Cardiac Rehabilitation: The Team Effort—Methodology and Results," *Heart Lung,* **5:**1, 97–111, January–February 1976.

38 J. Dodge, "Factors Related to Patients' Perceptions of Their Cognitive Needs," *Nurs Res,* **18:**2, 502, 1969.

39 J. Ezra, "Social and Economic Effects upon Families of Patients with Myocardial Infarction," University of Denver Press, 1962.

40 Storlie, *op. cit.,* p. 117.

41 G. Biorck, "Social and Psychological Problems in Patients with Chronic Illness," *Am Heart J,* **58:**3, 414–417, September 1959.

42 A. Moss, "Post-hospital Aspects of Myocardial Infarction," *Primary Cardiol,* **1:**27–29, March 1976.

43 H. Hellerstein and E. Friedman, "Sexual Activity after a Heart Attack," *Primary Cardiol,* **1:**3, 10–13, October 1975.

## BIBLIOGRAPHY

Bradley, R.: "Diagnostic Right Heart Catheterization with Miniature Catheters in Severely Ill Patients," *Lancet,* **2:**941, 1964.

Bruhn, J., and S. Wolf: "Studies Reporting Low Rates of Ischemic Heart Disease: A Critical Review," *Am J Public Health,* **60:**8, 1477–1495, August 1970.

Buggs, H., G. Wetlash, and F. Balguma: "Assessment of Pulmonary Artery End-Diastolic Pressure as an Indirect Measurement of Pulmonary Capillary Mean Pressure—An Index of Left Ventricular Function," *Heart Lung,* **2:**232–237, March–April 1973.

Burton, A.: *Biophysics of the Circulation,* Chap. 15, "The Law of the Heart," Year Book, Chicago, 1968.

Faulkner, S., R. Boerth, and T. Graham: "Direct Myocardial Effects of Precatheterization," *Am Heart J,* **88:**5, 609–614, November 1974.

Folkow, B., and E. Neil: *Circulation,* Oxford, New York, 1971.

Frazee, S., and L. Neil: "New Challenge in Nursing: The Intra-aortic Balloon," *Heart Lung,* **2:**4, 529–531, July–August 1973.

Hirst, A., P. Piyoratn, and I. Gore: "A Comparison of Atherosclerosis of the Aorta and Coronary Arteries in Bangkok and Los Angeles," *Am J Clin Pathol,* **38:**162, 1962.

Keily, W.: "Psychiatric Syndromes in Critically Ill Patients," *JAMA,* **235:**25, 2759, June 21, 1976.

King, G.: in M. Frank and S. Alvarez-Mena, *Cardiovascular Physical Diagnosis,* Chap. 5, Year Book, Chicago, 1973.

Levy, R. (ed.): "Hyperlipoproteinemia," *Curr Probl Cardiol,* **1:**3, 35, June 1976.

McKigney, F.: "The Intensive Care Syndrome," *Conn Med,* **30:**9, 633, September 1966.

Nadas, A., D. Fyler, and A. Castenada: "The Critically Ill Infant with Congenital Heart Disease," *Mod Concepts Cardiovasc Dis,* **XLII:**11, November 1973.

Rosenman, R., and W. Costelli: "Clinical Forum on Risk Factors," *Primary Cardiol,* **1:**4, 26–29, November 1975.

———, et al.: "Coronary Heart Disease in the Western Collaborative Group Study," *JAMA,* **195:**86, 1966.

Storlie, F.: *Patient Teaching in Critical Care,* Appleton-Century-Crofts, New York, 1975.

———, E. Rambousek, and E. Shannon: *Principles of Intensive Nursing Care,* Chap. 2, Appleton-Century-Crofts, New York, 1972.

Udall, J.: "Sedative Interferences with Oral Anticoagulant Therapy," *Practical Cardiol,* **1:**22–24, February 1975.

Voukydio, P., and S. Cohen: "Catheter-Induced Arrhythmias," *Am Heart J,* **88:**5, 588–592, November 1974.

Weissler, A., and C. Gerrard: "Systolic Time Intervals in Cardiac Disease II," *Mod Concepts Cardiovasc,* **XL:**2, 6, 1971.

Winslow, E. H. (ed.): "Teaching and Rehabilitating the Cardiac Patient," *Nurs Clin North Am,* **II:**2, June 1976.

Whyte, H. M.: "Potential Effect on Coronary Heart Disease of Lowering the Blood Cholesterol," *Lancet,* **2:**206, 1975.

# 28

# DISTURBANCES IN BLOOD PRESSURE

Mi Ja Kim

In order to maintain adequate perfusion of the extensive capillary networks in the systemic vascular bed, arterial pressure must be controlled and kept at a specific level. When arterial pressure increases (hypertension) or decreases (hypotension) beyond established parameters, multiple changes occur within the human system. As human beings interact with the environment, chemical substances, stress, obesity, dietary habits, and physiological changes significantly contribute to alter arterial pressure. Because of the dynamic role played by arterial blood pressure, the body is sensitive to changes in blood pressure. When changes do occur, they profoundly affect the oxygenation of the body. A clear comprehension of the interaction of arterial blood pressure and the physiological as well as psychosocial dynamics will aid the nurse when caring for individuals with alterations in blood pressure.

## ARTERIAL BLOOD PRESSURE

Two major factors are involved in the control of arterial blood pressure, namely, cardiac output and total peripheral resistance. *Cardiac output* (see Table 28-1) is determined by heart rate and stroke volume. *Heart rate,* in turn, is influenced by the autonomic nervous system and normally ranges from 60 to 100 beats/minute. *Stroke volume* refers to the amount of blood ejected by the left ventricle during one systolic contraction. It equals the end diastolic volume minus the end systolic volume. *End diastolic volume* (EDV) is the volume of blood left in the ventricle at the end of diastole. It is influenced by the filling pressure, distensibility, and filling time of the ventricles. *End systolic volume* (ESV) is influenced by the vasculature of the aorta, the arterial system, and the strength of myocardial contractibility. *Diastolic blood pressure* refers to minimum blood pressure obtained during ventricular systole. *Systolic blood pressure* refers to maximum pressure obtained during ventricular systole.

Receptors sensing the pressure or volume variations arc located in the aortic arch and the carotid sinuses. Afferent impulses of autonomic reflex arc are transmitted via the glossopharyngeal and vagus nerves to extensive central autonomic connections in the medulla. These synapses connect not only to the sympathetic and parasympathetic nuclei and efferent arcs, but also to the cerebral cortex and hypothalamic nuclei. The hypothalamic nuclei control hormonal secretion via the pituitary gland. Major hormones involved in the regulation of arterial pressure are antidiuretic hormone, adrenocortical hormone (ACTH), renin (from the juxtaglomerular apparatus), angiotensin II (converted from renin), and aldosterone (from the adrenal cortex).[1] Their roles will be described later in this chapter.

*Total peripheral resistance* is controlled by several factors including the radius and length of the vessel and the viscosity of the blood. Among these, the influence of vessel radius is the greatest. For a given level of cardiac output, arterial pressure is largely dependent upon the degree of constriction of the smooth muscle in the walls of the arteriole. Arterial blood pressure is measured by a sphygmomanometer in mmHg.

## HYPERTENSION

Pathophysiological changes involved with cardiac output and arterial resistance can increase peripheral arteriolar resistance and are the primary etiological component of hypertension.

*Hypertension* is present when the arterial blood pressure is 150/90 or higher. Hypertension may be either systolic or diastolic.[2]

*Systolic hypertension* usually occurs in the presence of other pathological processes. This type of hypertension occurs most commonly in elderly patients with decreased elasticity of the aortic wall. Systolic hypertension seen in thyrotoxicosis, severe anemia, fever, and aortic valvular insufficiency is generally a result of an elevated stroke volume.

*Diastolic hypertension,* severe or sustained, is a result of arteriosclerotic changes in the arteries and occlusion of the lumen.

*True systemic hypertension* results in an elevation of both the systolic and diastolic pressures with an increase in the mean arterial pressure. Regardless of the primary cause, the hemodynamic abnormality noted in most patients is an increase in vascular resistance, especially in the smaller arteries and arterioles. In a smaller number of patients, hypertension may result from an increase in cardiac output, hypervolemia, or increased blood viscosity secondary to polycythemia.

### Classification of Hypertension

Hypertension can be classified according to its etiology or severity. These classifications are often referred to as primary and secondary hypertension. *Primary hypertension* accounts for about 85 percent of cases and is of unknown etiology. A diagnosis of primary hypertension is warranted only after re-

**TABLE 28-1**
FACTORS INFLUENCING ARTERIAL PRESSURE

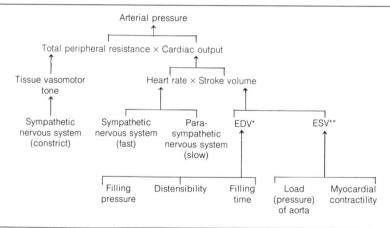

* EDV = End-diastolic volume
** ESV = End-systolic volume

This flow chart indicates those variables that interact to influence arterial pressure. Pressure or volume variations are detected by receptors located in the aortic arch and the carotid sinuses. Afferent impulses of autonomic reflex arc are transmitted via the glossopharyngeal and vagus nerves to central autonomic connections in the medulla. These synapses connect not only to the sympathetic and parasympathetic nuclei and efferent arcs but also to the cerebral cortex and hypothalamic nuclei. The hypothalamic nuclei control hormonal secretion via the pituitary gland.

Modified from C. F. Roth, *Cardiodynamics in Physiology*, Little, Brown, Boston, 1971, p. 71.

peated, and thorough searches for a specific cause have been unsuccessful. Hypertension is transient in the early stages but eventually becomes a permanent health problem.

*Secondary hypertension* refers to hypertension caused by other abnormalities and/or pathophysiologic changes. These include renal problems such as a vascular lesion of renal arteries or the parenchymal lesions of acute and chronic glomerulonephritis. In addition, endocrine pathology including pheochromocytoma, Cushing's syndrome, adrenal insufficiency, and pituitary tumor may be a precipitating factor in the development of secondary hypertension. Toxemia of pregnancy, oral contraception, increased intracranial pressure, and scleroderma may also be included in this category.

A classification according to phases of hypertension is found in Table 28-2. This table offers the nurse another way to view changes in arterial blood pressure and the severity of these changes. This determination aids in deciding future interventions.

**Causes of hypertension**  Because little is known about the causes of primary hypertension, much of the discussion to follow will be related to secondary hypertension. There are several conditions that lead to the development of hypertension. These include structural defects of the heart, renal pathology, stress, and hormonal disturbances.

Dysfunction of the *adrenal gland* is one cause of hypertension. An excessive secretion of epinephrine and norepinephrine by the adrenal medulla results in significant vasoconstriction of blood vessels. *Pheochromocytomas* are tumors which can arise from chromaffin cells and secrete excessive amounts of these hormones. The cells are located in the adrenal medulla, but they may develop along the sympathetic chains (10 percent) where chromaffin cells are found. The incidence of phenochromocytoma among all patients with hypertension is rare, probably less than 0.1 percent.

*Secondary hypertension* usually results from *arteriosclerosis*. This factor is responsible for changes within the large arteries including thickening of the arterial wall, as well as occlusion of the lumen of the smaller arteries and arterioles. These changes lead to an increase in peripheral arteriolar resistance and contribute to an increase in arterial pressure.

When blood pressure is increased in previously normotensive individuals, baroreceptors are activated to decrease sympathetic efferent discharges relaxing vasomotor tone, thereby reducing blood pressure. However, the baroreceptors react to this new blood pressure (which is now hypertension) and "reset" the basal level, causing interference with the compensatory response of sympathetic nervous system used in lowering the pressure in hypertensive states.[3] The time required for these baroreceptor changes has not been established.

Abnormal sympathetic nerve function does account for some increase in peripheral vascular resistance. In addition, reduction of the sympathetic vasomotor tone can reduce blood pressure.

Excessive, unregulated secretion of aldosterone by the adrenal cortex also causes hypertension. *Primary aldosteronism* (or *Conn's syndrome*) is caused by a tumor of the adrenal cortex. It is a relatively rare disorder that is characterized

**TABLE 28-2**
PHASES AND CHARACTERISTICS OF HYPERTENSION

| Phases | Criteria and Characteristics |
|---|---|
| Prehypertensive | Intermittent elevation of blood pressure; systolic pressure below 160 mmHg; diastolic pressure below 90–95 mmHg. Headache, insomnia, irritability, and forgetfulness may be observed. |
| Benign hypertension | |
|   Mild phase | Systolic pressure below 200 mmHg, diastolic pressure between 90 and 114 mmHg. Headache, fatigue, and palpitations may be noted. |
|   Moderate phase | Systolic pressure above 200 mmHg, diastolic pressure between 115 and 129 mmHg. Vascular damage is not apparent at this time. |
|   Severe phase | Systolic pressure up to 250 mmHg or higher, diastolic pressure around 130 mmHg. Abnormal neurologic signs, severe occipital headache, angina may be observed. |
| Malignant hypertension | Sudden sharp elevation in blood pressure: diastolic pressure about 130 mmHg. Retinopathy with hemorrhages, exudate, papilledema, rapidly progressive renal failure with albuminuria, hematuria, increased blood urea nitrogen, and left ventricular failure may be present. Patients die 80 percent in the first year and 100 percent in the second if not treated. Patients should be hospitalized and treated. |
| Acute hypertension | Elevated diastolic pressure (above 140 mmHg). Hypertensive encephalopathy with severe headache, mental confusion, nausea, vomiting, convulsions, coma, papilledema, retinal hemorrhage, and intracranial hemorrhage; acute heart failure with pulmonary edema may be present. |

by diastolic hypertension and hypokalemia. Hypertension is usually mild to moderate in severity, but it may result in left ventricular hypertrophy and narrowing of the retinal arterioles from sustained hypertension.

*Cushing's syndrome* resulting from chronic exposure to excessive secretion of glucocorticoids by the adrenal cortex may also result in hypertension. Systemic arterial hypertension is commonly associated with Cushing's syndrome (see Chap. 21). Possible causes of hypertension are thought to be excess adrenocorticoid production,[4] mineralocorticoid activity of cortisol, and altered vascular responsiveness to pressor agents coupled with increased angiotensin formation.[5]

*Disruptions in the renal blood vessels* are another cause of hypertension. When the diameter of the renal blood vessels is decreased, pathological changes occur which include renal artery stenosis and fibrinoid or necrotizing renal arteritis. These changes tend to cause an increased resistance to blood flow and are frequently seen in malignant hypertension.

*Renal vascular hypertension* and *renal parenchymal hypertension* are the two main subdivisions of renal hypertension. Renal arterial hypertension is caused by stenosis of a main artery or branch and results in decreased renal perfusion. The *stenosis of a main or branch renal artery* causes a decreased renal blood flow and blood pressure to the juxtaglomerular apparatus (JGA) and activates the renin-angiotensin system. Renin is a proteolytic enzyme produced and stored in the granules of the juxtaglomerular cells surrounding the afferent arterioles of the cortical glomeruli.[6]

Two major mechanisms exist in controlling *renin release*. The first mechanism involves a receptor in the afferent glomerular arteriole which is able to respond to either increased or decreased renal vascular resistance raising or lowering blood pressure. The second mechanism consists of receptor cells of the macula densa which respond to changes in sodium concentration in the blood.

Renin acts upon angiotensinogen (a circulating alpha globulin made in the liver) and forms angiotensin I.[7] Angiotensin I passes through the pulmonary circulation and is enzymatically converted to angiotensin II which is a very potent pressor substance causing constriction of arteriolar smooth muscle. In addition to its direct action in increasing blood pressure, angiotensin II acts on the adrenal cortex to cause the release of the sodium-retaining hormone, aldosterone.

The *deficiency of vasodilator compounds* such as the renomedullary prostaglandins (PGs) has been proposed as one of the contributing factors in hypertension. However, the true role of these PGs is not yet fully known. Experimental evidence indicates that PGs decrease blood pressure of patients with essential hypertension by decreasing total peripheral resistance of renal vessels.[8]

*Hypercalcemia* has been shown to have a vasoconstrictive effect which contributes to hypertension. Hypertension is noted in one-third of patients with *hyperparathyroidism*[9] and is usually attributed to renal parenchymal damage owing to nephrolithiasis and nephrocalcinosis. The problem appears to disappear when the hypercalcemia is corrected.

*Oral contraceptives* such as estrogen preparations can precipitate or aggravate hypertension, which usually is reversed when this medication is discontinued. Alternation in the renin-angiotensin system, particularly the abnormal inactivation of angiotensin II, has been considered to be the pathogenesis of this hypertension.[10]

*Hypertensive crisis syndrome* has been related to simultaneous ingestion of drugs that are inhibitors of monoamine oxidase (MAO) (e.g., tranylcypromine and phenelzine) and certain cheeses (such as Cheddar, Camembert, Stilton). It has been postulated that these cheeses might contain a substance (e.g., tyramine) capable of liberating stored catecholamines in the presence of MAO inhibitors which contribute to increased arterial pressures.

Hypertension associated with *coarctation* (narrowing) *of the aorta* may be caused by the mechanical obstruction or constriction of the aorta itself. The process is usually due to structural defects of the heart caused by a congenital constriction of the aorta (see Chap. 27). Blood pressure is elevated in the aorta and its branches proximal to the coarctation, but it is near normal or decreased distally.

*Autoregulation of blood flow* has also been implicated as a cause of hypertension in patients with coarctation of the aorta. The body adjusts to peripheral resistance differently in organs with a normal blood flow, maintaining near normal or slight decreases in pressure in the distal portions of the coarctation. The mechanism of this autoregulation has not yet been determined. Reactive changes seen in this type of hypertension can be observed when a mechanical obstruction is removed by surgery. The vessels below the coarctation are suddenly exposed to a higher pressure than they are used to and at the same time the vessels and organs above the coarctation are exposed to lower pressures than they are used to. The change in pressure stimulates the baroreceptors, and a hypertensive crisis may result. Collateral circulation between the high- and low-pressure aortic segments develops through the intercostal arteries and branches of the subclavian arteries.

The effect of *stressful psychological factors* on the physiological system of the body has been well documented. Psychosomatic disorders are brought about when coping mechanisms of self-correcting adjustments fail to be effective. They involve suppressed or repressed emotions gaining expression through body organs and organ systems. The effect of stress differs according to the structure of the individual's personality, constitution, and previous experience. The nature and degree of the stress are also an influencing factor. There is no unique personality pattern specifically related to patients with hypertension; however, research has shown that these individuals tend to have similar views of life, evaluation of problems and challenges, and manner in which they deal with problems.[11] Anger, severe anxiety, and fear have been known to be related to hypertension via activation of the autonomic nervous system and of the central nervous–pituitary–adrenal system. Paroxysmal tachycardia, vascular spasm, and migraine headaches are other manifestations. The patient with chronic anger tends to have constant hypertension.[12] Hypertension associated with the hypothalamopituitary-activating system is largely related to mineralocorticoid secretion of the adrenal cortex rather than glucocorticoids, even though cortisol plays an essential role in resisting stress.

Tobacco tends to cause vasoconstriction of blood vessels owing to the presence of nicotine. This places smokers at greater risk to develop hypertension than people who do not smoke. This problem can significantly increase hypertension when it occurs in conjunction with other health problems such as cardiac ischemia.

**Pathophysiological changes** As a result of sustained increased arterial blood pressure (hypertension), multiple physiological changes occur throughout the body. Systemic hypertension results in arteriosclerotic changes in large arteries, thickening of the arterial walls, and occlusion of the lumens of small arteries and arterioles. As hypertension continues, widespread pathological changes take place in both the large and small blood vessels and in the vessels of vital organs such as the heart, kidneys, and brain.[13] The large vessels become tortuous, and the lumen narrows.

This results in a decreased blood flow to the heart, brain, and lower extremities.

Damage to the small vessel also occurs with adverse structural changes observed. When the diastolic pressure is severely elevated, it causes damage to the intima of the small vessels; this, in turn, leads to fibrin accumulation in the vessels, local edema, and intravascular clotting. The final result of these changes is a decreased blood supply to the tissue of the heart, brain, and kidneys leading to the functional insufficiency of these organs.

An increase in arterial blood pressure can alter cerebral blood flow and lead to changes in perception and coordination. Circulation through the brain is affected by arterial hypertension. Cerebral infarction (stroke or intracerebral hemorrhage) occurs when systemic hypertension is higher than 170/90.

Hypertensive hemorrhage does not necessarily arise from the large arteries but can occur in any vessel of the brain. The extravasation of fluid which results from rupture of an artery forms a mass which disrupts the tissue. As the bleeding continues, the mass becomes larger (refer to Chap. 34), increasing cerebral tissue hypoxia and contributing to multiple physiological and psychological changes.

Arteriosclerotic or atherosclerotic changes of cerebral blood vessels themselves can cause transient cerebral ischemia. *Cerebral aneurysm* can result from persistent diastolic hypertension. *Hyalinosis* and necrotizing change in the small arteries due to hypertension have also been described as the precursor of hemorrhage, but this cannot be affirmed or denied at the present time.

**Effects of hypertension** Accelerated vascular damage is the major common underlying factor causing changes in the cardiac, renal, and nervous systems. These changes range from an asymptomatic period to clinically observable symptomatic periods. When hypertension does not respond to therapy, it may lead to symptomatic illness and often death.

The earliest symptom of hypertension is occipital headaches, which occur most often in the morning. Dizziness, light-headedness, vertigo, tinnitus, visual changes (including blindness), or syncope may also occur. Cerebral infarcts (strokes) may be manifested as personality changes or memory deficits but larger lesions produce major strokes which account for up to 10 to 15 percent of deaths occurring secondary to hypertension. Damage to brain tissue can increase anxiety and depression and lead to periods of euphoria.

Increased cardiac workload caused by increased arterial pressure may lead to ventricular hypertrophy, and cardiac decompensation may lead to pump failure (see Chap. 24). Frequently patients with hypertension have coronary occlusion, and intermittent anginal pain may be noted. Myocardial infarction and congestive heart failure are the major causes of death due to hypertension.

Patients with hypertension due to the presence of a pheochromocytoma may experience additional effects. Acute onset often brings on a sudden increase in blood pressure, blanching of the skin, and dilation of the pupils. The patient complains of headache, chest pain, palpitation, and profuse diaphoresis. The metabolic effects of excessive circulating catecholamines such as hyperglycemia are usually seen. In most cases, however, the onset of symptoms is slow and less dramatic even though hypertension is sustained. Weakness, tremor, palpitation, and anxiety may also accompany these changes.

The effect of the renal hypertension is an altered glomerular filtration rate and tubular dysfunction. *Protein* and *blood* often leak into the urine as a result of the glomerular lesion. Epistaxis, hemoptysis, and metrorrhagia also occur more frequently in these patients. Renal failure accounts for about 10 percent of the deaths that result from hypertension.

### First-Level Nursing Care

Hypertension is a major public health problem in the United States, producing premature disruptions in health, disability, and death in the adult population. Currently it is estimated that 20 to 25 million Americans have hypertension. The onset is usually between ages 25 and 55.

**Population at risk** Several factors that predispose an individual to developing hypertension are age, sex, obesity, and smoking.

The morbidity and mortality rates of hypertension increase steadily with advancing *age*.[14] The frequency of hypertension is greater for men than for women up to about age 50 years, but at the older ages the reverse is true.[15] Even though the risk of developing hypertension is higher in older women as compared with older men, the probability of developing a stroke is directly related to the systolic blood pressure regardless of sex and age.[16] Most of the available data suggest that elderly women tolerate hypertension better than men of a similar age and that their life expectancy does not decrease appreciably due to hypertension.

If the onset of hypertension occurs during the younger ages, the life expectancy of the individual decreases, and even a modest elevation of blood pressure is associated with a greatly increased risk of death.[17]

At least 50 percent of hypertensive patients in their twenties have primary hypertension. If the problem begins before the age of 30 or after the age of 50, it strongly suggests that the patient may have secondary hypertension.[18] (See Fig. 28-1.)

In every age group, hypertension is more prevalent in *men* than *women,* and the mortality rate of hypertensive disease in men also is higher than women.[19-21] The difference between mortality rates is somewhat less than 3 to 1.[22] However, after menopause the incidence of hypertensive disease due to atherosclerosis in women rapidly approaches that in men,[23] and becomes even higher in older age.

The prevalence of hypertension is twice as high for *blacks* as for *whites.* In addition hypertension is 3.3 times as severe for black men as for white men, and 5.6 times as high for black women as for white women.[24-26] The mortality risk in black patients with hypertension is approximately twice that in white patients with hypertension. Hypertension occurring in blacks under age 50 carries an extremely high risk. Figures 28-1 and 28-2 demonstrate the effect of age, sex, and race on hypertension prevalence and mortality rates and should make more visible the interactive effect these sociocultural variables have on hypertension.

*Elevated* levels of *plasma lipids,* particularly *cholesterol* and *triglycerides,* have been found to be closely related to the development of hypertension. (A complete discussion of cholesterol elevation is found in Chap. 26.)

Even though the relationship between increased risk of coronary artery disease associated with hypertension and high cholesterol levels has been amply demonstrated, the effectiveness of treatment in reducing this risk still remains undecided.

The relationship between *sodium balance* and hypertension has been shown to exist in obese patients and in some patients with renovascular disease. The reasons and mechanisms of this relationship are not clearly understood, but one study reported that reducing dietary salt intake while maintaining the weight in obese patients successfully lowered blood pressure.[27]

The tendency to develop essential hypertension has been long recognized to run in families.[28] Those who have a *family history* of this health prob-

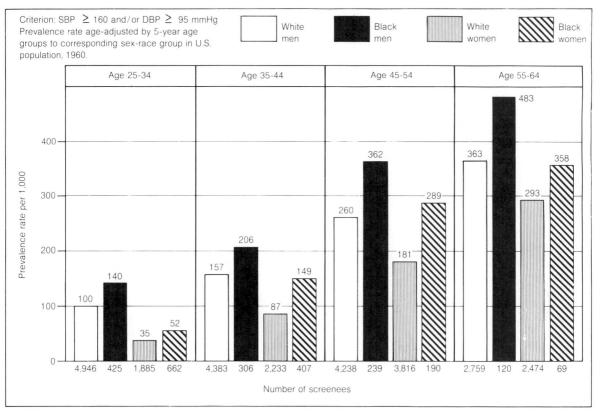

Criterion: SBP ≥ 160 and/or DBP ≥ 95 mmHg
Prevalence rate age-adjusted by 5-year age
groups to corresponding sex-race group in U.S.
population, 1960.

White men | Black men | White women | Black women

**FIGURE 28-1**

Prevalence of high blood pressure by age and sex. (*From J. Stamler, High Blood Pressure in the United States—An Overview of the Problem and the Challenge, Proc. National Conference on High Blood Pressure Education, National Heart and Lung Institute, Department of Health, Education, and Welfare, 1973.*)

lem are more prone to be hypertensive than those who do not. About 75 percent of hypertensive patients have a family history of hypertension. When both parents are involved, the risks are especially great.[29] Observations that were made of identical twins with hypertension suggested the familial clustering is a result of genetic rather than environmental influences.[30] The close similarity of blood pressure levels is seen in monozygotic twins, whereas in dizygotic twins the blood pressure may differ to the same degree as is found in other nontwin siblings.

The presence of positive family history suggests that heredity plays a part in primary rather than secondary hypertension. A history of relatively early death in a parent or sibling from hypertensive complications increases the possibility of progression to a more severe stage from borderline or mild hypertension.[31]

An interrelationship exists between *obesity* and

hypertension. However, the mechanism is not yet understood. The higher the relative weight in youth, the greater the tendency to hypertension in middle age. The greater the gain in weight from young adulthood to middle age, the greater the tendency to hypertension.[32]

Obesity has been identified as one of the factors that lead to atherosclerosis which is one of the well-recognized causes for hypertension. The importance of this factor as compared with hyperlipidemia in the development of hypertension appears to be less. Physical inactivity coupled with obesity seems to have more implication in hypertension than obesity alone.

It is also important to identify any other health problems, *smoking* habits, and whether the patient is using *oral contraceptives* or other medications. Clear identification of baseline data will provide useful information when planning a health education program.

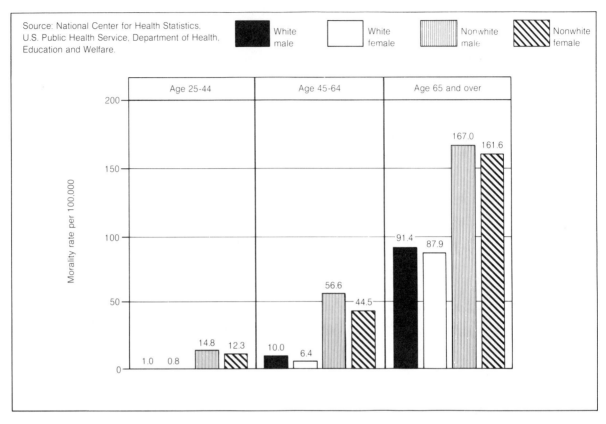

Source: National Center for Health Statistics, U.S. Public Health Service, Department of Health, Education and Welfare.

**FIGURE 28-2**
Hypertensive disease mortality rates.

## Prevention

The majority of these cases of hypertension are usually detected through incidental screening procedures such as insurance examinations, pre-employment examinations, armed forces examinations, blood donor screening, and tests in physicians' offices, emergency rooms, or clinics. This fact points out that a large population of seemingly disease-free subjects may in fact have hypertension. Understanding the predisposing factors to hypertension is essential in order to identify and prevent this health problem.

A careful health inventory should include basic data such as age, sex, and racial background. In an assessment of familial tendency, it is better to use the term *high blood pressure* because lay persons believe that hypertension is synonymous with nervousness and excitability.

Identification of potential stressors including psychosocial background will also provide additional information for the practitioner. Occupational stressors can be isolated and potential life crises clarified so that appropriate changes can be made to diminish stress effect.

**Screening programs** Recently, a number of screening programs have been developed by local and state government agencies. The purpose of these programs is to identify individuals with varying degrees of hypertension, so that early treatment can be started and the risk of developing serious physiological alterations prevented.

Nurses involved in screening programs should be sensitive not only to the previously described predisposing factors but also to the general guidelines for screening procedures.

Guidelines suggested by the Hypertension Study Group of the Intersociety Commission for Heart Disease Resources state that evaluation should be carried out for persons less than 40 years of age who have blood pressure in excess of 140 mmHg systolic and/or 90 mmHg diastolic on at least two of three successive determinations on different days. For patients older than this, the limits are 160 mmHg systolic and/or 95 mmHg diastolic on two of three successive readings. For children less than 15 years of age, limits should be reduced.[33]

Because hypertension has a slow onset and is without specific symptoms at first, a large population of hypertensive subjects are presently undetected and untreated. Community control of hypertension and a centrally organized national screening program have been tried with varying success. Problems related to program success included accuracy of machinery and preparations of the personnel.

A comprehensive approach should be taken with emphasis on a routine blood pressure checkup for *all* patients at *every* visit to the health care system including various subspecialty clinics such as dermatology, ophthalmology, and dentists offices. It is further suggested that all family members and visitors accompanying the patient be checked as well.

The nurse should make every effort to routinely measure the blood pressure and assess the patient's status against any predisposing factors. Because screening programs depend on accurate blood pressure monitoring, it is critical that the nurse be very comfortable with the technique of measuring blood pressure and knowledgeable about its impact upon the human system.

To measure blood pressure, a standard cuff is used except when thigh measurements are needed or the individual is obese. Blood pressure can be measured when the patient is standing, sitting, or lying down. Table 28-3 describes the various positions and related influencing variables on blood pressure.

When the blood pressure cuff is rapidly inflated to pressures greater than systolic pressure, distal arterial flow and venous outflow cease. As the cuff is slowly deflated and pressure is decreased, a series of sounds can be heard through the stethoscope which is applied over the brachial artery in the antecubital fossa. These sounds, called *Korotkov sounds,* are presumably due to vibration of the blood flow against the arterial wall. There are five phases to this sound.

Phase 1     First heard are clear tapping sounds which gradually increase in intensity. Systolic pressure is read as the first regular tapping sound appears during deflation of the cuff.

Phase 2     During further deflation, a softer muffled

sound or murmur replaces the clear tapping tones of Phase 1.

Phase 3     A sharper tone resembling the first phase but less well marked appears.

Phase 4     A sudden change is noted as the tapping sounds of Phase 3 become muffled and have a soft, flowing quality.

Phase 5     All sounds disappear.

Most often, *systolic pressure* is measured at the first regular tapping sound of Phase 1, and *diastolic pressure* is measured at the fifth Korotkov phase (disappearance of sounds). However, both the fourth (muffling sounds) and fifth phases should be recorded if there is more than 5 mmHg difference between the two measurements.

Phase 4 is less variable than phase 5 following exercise and in certain disease states when an increased cardiac output is present (e.g., aortic regurgitation, severe anemia, and thyrotoxicosis). In these conditions and in some individuals, there may be no fifth sound, meaning that the Korotkov sounds can be heard all the way down to zero on the sphygmomanometer.

However, phase 5 (the disappearance of sound) is recommended because this is usually closer to

---

**TABLE 28-3**
FACTORS INFLUENCING BLOOD PRESSURE MEASUREMENT

*Standing position:* Blood pressure measured in the arm when the patient is in a relaxed, standing position is lower than when it is measured with the patient in a supine position.

*Lateral position:* If measurements are made in a lateral position, a lower blood pressure reading may be obtained in both arms. This phenomenon is most apparent in the right arm when the patient is in a left lateral recumbent position.[34]

*Palpatory method:* Blood pressures obtained by this method are as much as 5 mmHg lower than those obtained by the auscultatory method. Blood pressure measured by applying the cuff and palpating the pulses to determine pressure.

*Repeated blood pressure measurement:* Repetition of reading during one session tends to lower blood pressure.

*Heart rate:* Very fast or very slow rates cause a lowered reading.

*Diurnal variation:* During sleep the blood pressure may be as much as 20 mmHg lower than a resting, waking measurement.

*Emotion:* Emotional reactions can result in a rise in blood pressure.

*Environment:* Cold or painful stimulation causes vasoconstriction increase of blood pressure by 10 to 30 mmHg.

*Large meal:* This tends to increase blood pressure because of increased cardiac output to meet metabolic needs.

*Full bladder:* This tends to increase blood pressure because of pressure on abdominal blood vessels.

*Exercise:* Blood pressure increases with exercise because of increased cardiac output.

the true diastolic pressure than is the beginning of phase 4. Recording of phase 5 is more reproducible than phase 4. Considering that some people lack a phase 4, phase 5 is recognized as the correct criterion for measuring diastolic blood pressure.

Blood pressure can be measured on both arms to detect any discrepancy. Consistent differences between the two arms of 10 mmHg or more in systolic or diastolic pressure often signifies an occlusive atherosclerotic plaque in the subclavian artery, usually on the left side. For further evaluation of this type of patient, the blood pressure should be taken in the arm that gives the higher reading.

To establish a baseline blood pressure level, a series of blood pressure readings are necessary on different days. This is because the blood pressure varies considerably over a 24-hour period and is influenced by various factors such as physical, mental, and emotional stress.

**Health education and prevention** Although screening programs help identify individuals with a potential hypertensive health problem, careful health teaching is essential in order to prevent the problem of hypertension. *Nutritional counseling* stressing a well-balanced, low-cholesterol diet is important.

An average meal of natural or aged cheese contains enough tyramine to provide a marked rise in blood pressure and cardiovascular changes. This indicates that when patients are on MAO inhibitors, detailed instruction on food is mandatory. Other foods and beverages implicated in this syndrome are pickled herring, chicken liver, yeast, coffee, broad bean pods, canned figs, and beer. Wine, a favorite cheese companion, is also implicated.

Instructions about the effects of *obesity, smoking, stress,* and *oral contraception* are essential. Reducing diets (see Chap. 16), elimination of smoking (see Chap. 26), and change in method of *contraception* should be encouraged. If physical and psychological *stress* is increased by occupation, social pressure, or family crisis, attempts should be made by the patient and family to resolve these problems.

Counseling related to inherited predispositions and racial tendencies need to be carefully explained so that the patient can be made aware of the potential for hypertension and avoid potential risk factors. General education of the public, especially specific groups such as blacks and those with a positive family history, is needed to increase health awareness. Screening programs should be nation-

wide and must begin with preschool health visits for all children but more importantly with high-risk groups. When needed, family counseling or psychologic therapy may be suggested to help an individual cope with stress as a predisposing factor in hypertension.

### Second-Level Nursing Care

Nurses who are involved in community or public health agencies are likely to come in contact with subjects who are unaware of their early stage of hypertension. These individuals should be thoroughly assessed so that the cause of hypertension can be identified and properly treated.

**N**ursing assessment  Identification of early onset of hypertension and of additional changes that result requires a thorough physical and psychosocial assessment. A detailed health history and physical examination are needed to evaluate the changes that are present. Frequently, early hypertension may be symptom-free. The presence of hypertension may be first noticed during a routine health examination.

**H**ealth History  The health history should focus upon the presence of predisposing factors discussed in Level-One Nursing Care. It should note smoking habits, all health problems, any family predisposition, medications (including oral contraceptive and MAO inhibitors), and dietary habits. The patient will often complain initially of headaches noted upon rising and gradually resolving as the day progresses. Dizziness and fatigue may be reported. Palpitations may be described along with reports of occasional dyspnea noted upon exertion. In early hypertension visual changes are minimal but can include periods of blurring. Patients who offer a history of epistaxsis (nosebleeds) will require a complete investigation of the problem.

Psychological changes including tremors, increased anxiety, and personality changes may be reported. The nurse should assess an individual's coping pattern and response to stress. As noted in First-Level Nursing Care, the patient with chronic anger tends to be predisposed to hypertension.[35]

Assessment of psychosocial variables should also elicit the relationship of the patient with family, friends, and significant others. This investigation should also include interrelationship with co-workers, peers, administrators, and the like. Methods of coping with stressful situations should be identified.

Sociocultural variables, educational background, and related data should be reviewed as appropriate. It is also important to attempt to assess *compliance behavior* early in the course of this health problem. Examining the individual's attitude or understanding of health and health maintenance is helpful. In addition, indications of patients' willingness to help themselves is a positive sign for the practitioner.

**P**hysical Assessment   Auscultation of the blood pressure should be carefully evaluated. Persistent *blood pressure elevations* showing a reading higher than 140 mmHg systolic and/or 90 mmHg diastolic in persons less than 40 years old or 160 mmHg systolic and/or 95 mmHg diastolic in persons older than 40 years of age are indicative of hypertension.

During the eye examination, the appearance of the fundus is an important and reliable index to the severity and prognosis of hypertension. Effects of hypertension on the *retina* can be assessed by ophthalmoscopic examination which permits examination of the progress of vascular effects of hypertension. There is a direct relationship between the severity of ophthalmoscopic grouping and mortality of untreated hypertensive patients. *Vascular changes* such as arteriolar tortuosity, increased light reflex, narrowing, and irregularity of the arteries are indicative of hypertension. The presence of soft exudates and papilledema indicates the vascular damage within the retina, and these are usually found in accelerated or malignant hypertension. Focal spasm, progressive general narrowing of the arterioles, hemorrhage, exudates, and papilledema are associated with increasing severity of hypertension.

Upon physical inspection, the patient's color and overall appearance should be noted. Weighing the patient and assessing overall body weight will provide additional data.

Hypertensive heart disease with concomitant cardiac pathology is common. Changes are best evaluated during auscultation of the heart. The presence of a fourth heart sound ($S_4$, atrial gallop) is one of the earliest physical signs of cardiac involvement, but this is heard only when sinus rhythm is present. Percussion of the heart will help with the evaluation of the heart size (see Chap. 22).

Palpation of the apical impulse gives a good indication of left ventricular hypertrophy and/or dilatation. Normally, in adults the apical impulse is usually located at, or within, the left midclavicular line in the fifth intercostal space. Occasionally, the apical impulse may be located lateral to the midclavicular line. The normal apical impulse is less

than 2 cm in diameter, and in most instances it is considerably smaller. In conditions associated with marked hypertrophy of the left ventricle without dilatation, the apical impulse is characteristically small but forceful and sustained throughout systole, and a powerful atrial impulse (double impulse) may be felt in the left lateral position at the point of maximum apical impulse (PMI). However, in conditions associated with massive dilatation of the left ventricle there is a diffuse apical impulse that has great force and amplitude and is usually displaced significantly, laterally and downwards.

Palpation of peripheral pulses may reveal a delayed or weak femoral pulse as compared with carotid or radial pulses taken simultaneously (refer to Chap. 29). This may suggest the presence of occlusive disease such as coarctation of the aorta. In adults, enlarged and pulsatile collateral vessels may be palpated in the intercostal spaces anteriorly, in the axillae, or posteriorly in the interscapular area.

During the *abdominal examination* palpation of a unilateral mass may be due to an enlarged kidney caused by hydronephrosis or an enlarged adrenal medulla caused by pheochromocytoma. A sharp increase of blood pressure has been observed when the mass was massaged accidentally and is presumably due to pheochromocytoma releasing epinephrine and/or norepinephrine. The nurse may wish to observe the effect of abdominal palpation by assessing the blood pressure following the physical examination and evaluating the results. Upon auscultation an abdominal bruit may suggest hypertension secondary to renal arterial stenosis.

The *neurological examination* may reveal the presence of a positive Babinski, hemiparesis, hyperreflexia, and hemiplegia may indicate pathological changes within the cerebrum.

**D**iagnostic Tests   General diagnostic tests are utilized to evaluate the patient with early hypertension. In the community setting these tests include blood test, electrocardiogram, and chest x-ray. *A fasting blood glucose* (preferably 2 hours postprandial) is done to assess the presence of diabetes mellitus commonly found in hypertensive patients. The *serum cholesterol* and *triglycerides* are measured as they are frequently associated with atherosclerotic changes and hypertension. Serum *calcium levels* are done to evaluate the presence of hypercalcemia which may contribute to increased arterial pressure. Kidney function tests including *serum creatinine* and *blood urea nitrogen* are done to assess renal damage. The *serum potassium* level may help in assessing the possibility of primary aldosteronism in mild or moderate hypertension.

A *urinalysis* is done to further assess kidney involvement in hypertensive problems. Hematuria and proteinuria may be noted in the presence of renal parenchymal disease such as chronic glomerulonephritis. Connective tissue disease or chronic pyelonephritis can be evaluated. If pheochromocytoma is suspected, a *24-hour urine test for steroids* may be done.

*Electrocardiograms* can be used to evaluate cardiac status and assess heart size and electrical as well as structural effectiveness of the heart. EKG changes of left ventricular hypertrophy are often seen in association with hypertension.

*Chest x-rays* can also be performed. They may suggest cardiac enlargement, ventricular hypertrophy, or data to the overall assessment.

**Nursing problems and interventions** Several problems may be present in the individual with mild or early hypertension. These include headache, epistaxis, anxiety, and obesity.

General Therapies Pharmacologic treatment for mild to moderate benign hypertension is varied and dependent upon many factors.

The adverse side effects and potential dangers of drugs should be carefully weighed before treatment is begun. Adverse effects that are common to all types of antihypertensive agents are: (1) Orthostatic and exercise hypotension; (2) delayed or retrograde ejaculation or impotence; and (3) fluid retention.[36] There is little justification for antihypertensive drug therapy in patients at the lower end of the hypertensive spectrum who are over 45 years of age. However, convincing evidence has been reported from a recent study that appropriate drug therapy of hypertension (105 mmHg diastolic) significantly lowered morbidity and prevented cardiovascular complications such as heart failure and stroke.[37] Generally, three classes of drugs are available. These are diuretics, direct vasodilators, and sympathetic inhibitors.

Diuretics are the initial drugs of choice for mild to moderate benign hypertension (diastolic pressure of 100 to 120 mmHg). Oral diuretics (e.g., especially thiazides) given alone often control blood pressure for at least a third of patients with mild hypertension. Most of the antihypertensive effect of thiazide diuretics is attained within 3 to 4 days. The mechanism of decreasing blood pressure by diuretics is probably linked with decreasing plasma and extracellular fluid volume by depletion

of sodium.[38] Since most of the diuretics deplete the potassium store in the body, foods high in potassium should be encouraged (refer to Chap. 12).

Plasma renin activity (PRA) is increased with thiazide therapy and may interfere with the therapeutic effectiveness of the drug and contribute to hypokalemia. Concomitant use of methyldopa with the diuretic has lowered PRA levels, obviating this problem.[39] Common diuretics used for early hypertension are described in Table 28-4.

Patients taking diuretics should be instructed to monitor weights daily in an attempt to observe the effectiveness of the diuretic. In addition to the use of diuretics, mild analgesia, including aspirin and Tylenol, can be given to help relieve the headache.

(A complete discussion of health teaching related to drug therapy can be found under Fourth-Level Nursing Care. Other drugs listed under Third-Level Nursing Care may be used in early hypertension. Refer to Third-Level Nursing Care for a complete discussion.)

**H**eadache One of the most common problems associated with early hypertension is headache. Several factors can aggravate this problem including vasoconstriction due to smoking, stress, and/or a secondary health problem. In addition to reducing smoking and stress and attempting to relieve secondary health problems, antihypertensive drug therapy may be used. The primary goal of antihypertensive drugs is to prolong useful life by preventing cardiovascular complications. Mild analgesia can be used to relieve pain.

**N**osebleeds Often associated with hypertension, nosebleeds (epistaxis) usually occur because of nasal capillary rupture. At times, this problem is a reason an individual seeks medical attention and may serve to make an individual aware of a hypertension problem. The use of an ice pack at the back of the neck or hyperextending the head backward may help relieve the problem. If bleeding is severe, nasal packing may be required. This can be done on an outpatient basis, but often hospitalization may be required (see Third-Level Nursing Care).

**A**nxiety Often present in the individual with hypertension, anxiety manifests itself in the form of tension and/or tremors. This is intensified by the presence of headache, nosebleed, environmental stress, or decreased coping responses. Reassurance and support are needed to help allay problems and fears. The use of tranquilizers may be helpful.

**TABLE 28-4**
ORAL DIURETICS

| Generic Name | Trade Name | Dosage | Action | Side Effects | Remarks |
|---|---|---|---|---|---|
| THIAZIDES<br>Chlorothiazide<br>Chlorthalidone<br>Hydrochlorothiazide<br>Hydroflumethiazide<br>Methylclothiazide<br>Polythiazide<br>Trichlormethiazide | Diuril<br>Hygroton<br>Hydrodiuril<br>Esidrix<br>Enduron<br>Renese<br>Naqua | 50–200 mg<br>50–200 mg<br>50–100 mg<br>50–100 mg<br>2.5–10 mg<br>1–4 mg<br>2–4 mg | Mild diuresis promoted. Causes excretion of calcium, water, sodium, and potassium.<br>Can be taken orally and are effective for long periods of time (6 to 72 h).<br>Have low incidence of side effects. | Hypokalemia, weakness, fatigue, nausea, abdominal pain, hyperglycemia, abdominal distention, diarrhea, rash, hyperuricemia, muscle cramps, and decrease in leukocytes and thrombocytes. | Nurse should check serum electrolyte. Food supplements containing $K^+$ should be encouraged. These drugs should be avoided in patients with azotemia and hepatic failure. Taking alcohol, barbiturate narcotics may result in orthostatic hypotension. |
| POTENT DIURETICS<br>Ethacrynic acid<br>Eurosemide | Edecrin<br>Lasix | 25–200 mg<br>40–200 mg | Rapidly absorbed, patent diuretics. Rapid and continued diuresis. IV diuresis can begin 5 min and reach peak effect 2 to 4 h after administration of Lasix. Endecrin is of shorter duration; water loss with this drug is often more severe. | Tinnitus, hearing loss, diarrhea, vertigo, hypokalemia, hyperglycemia, hyperuricemia, elevated BUN, GI irritation, skin rash, and photosensitivity. | Contraindicated in pregnancy, anuria, hepatic pathology, and profound electrolyte imbalance and water loss. |
| POTASSIUM-SPARING DIURETICS<br>Spironolactone | Aldactone | 100 mg 4 times a day in divided dosage; maximum dosage 400 mg. | Blocks effects of adrenocortical hormone aldosterone resulting in excess excretion of sodium chloride. This drug has been found effective in patients who do not respond well to diuretics. | Usually nontoxic, but hyperkalemia and hyponatremia can occur; skin rash, drowsiness, unsteady gait. | Potassium supplement should not be given unless the patient is also receiving glucocorticoids. |
| Triamterene | Dyrenium | 100 mg twice a day in divided doses; maximum dosage 400 mg. | Blocks aldosterone; not a painful drug, however. | Hyperkalemia, skin rash, blood dyscrasias. | This drug potentiates action of methotrexate and antihypertension drugs. |

The personality of the patient plays an important role in reacting to stressful situations. In addition a logical explanation and teaching of the relationship between stress and hypertension is critical. To the extent that the level of the patient's understanding, education, and willingness permits, the nurse should help the patient to understand hypertension so that the patient can modify life-style and personal behavior accordingly. Rearrangement of activities may be necessary to avoid rushing at the last minute. Individual or group counseling with a nurse or other counselor may be necessary to help the patient (and family) deal more effectively with aggravating interpersonal situations arising in the home, school, or on the job. The nurse should also provide emotional support to the patient and family. It is important to set realistic expectations and easily attainable goals so that progress can be visible.[40]

**O**besity Overweight and elevation of blood cholesterol levels contribute to hypertension. Careful restriction of the intake of fats and a planned activity program can help reduce this contributing risk factor.

Moderate restriction in the intake of cholesterol and saturated fats (i.e., animal fats) is recommended to decrease the hypertensive risk factor and decrease the incidence of arteriosclerotic complications. Restriction in dietary sodium varies according to the individual situation. *Mild dietary sodium restriction,* up to 4 g/day (normal = 2.5 to 7 g/day) may prove to be useful in some cases. Foods with a low sodium content (less than 0.5 g per average serving), medium salt content (0.5 to 1.25 g per average serving), or high salt content (1.25 to 2 g per average serving) all need to be identified for the patient and incorporated into the dietary pattern. (See Chapter 24 for a table listing of all three groupings.) The selection of diet will vary according to the severity of the hypertension and sodium restriction prescribed. Caloric restriction should be urged for the patient who is overweight.

Group therapy focusing on behavior modification has been found to be more successful for long-term reinforcement of a dietary program.[41] A progressive program of *exercise* compatible with the patient's capacity or within the limits of the patient's cardiovascular status is recommended. Limits to physical activity should be carefully determined either by cardiovascular stress testing or by the individual's tolerance level. The patient is encouraged to start with milder forms of exercises (e.g., golf, bowling, and walking) and progress to more strenuous forms (e.g., tennis, handball, and swimming) as desired. Not only is exercise helpful in controlling weight, but, in addition, physical conditioning itself appears to lower arterial pressure.

Extra daily *rest* is not necessary as long as the patient is on antihypertensive therapy. However, regular rest periods or early-to-bed injunctions may serve as constant reminders to some patients that they must reduce stress levels. Mental health in the way of fostering of hobbies and avocations and taking vacations is recommended for hypertensive patients.

**F**ollow-up care Once patients are found to have persistent elevation of blood pressure, they should be fully educated to the necessity of adhering to life-long therapies of diet, drugs, and avoidance of stressful events or circumstances in order to prevent the major cardiovascular and renal complications of hypertension. Securing the *compliance* of the patient requires gradual building of a trusting relationship between the patient and the health team members. Factors that contribute to noncompliance should be carefully assessed. Such things as lack of motivation, especially in the absence of symptoms, cost of health care, family crisis, drugs' side effects, and misconceptions that interventions are only necessary until the blood pressure is normal or symptoms are relieved contribute to this thinking. Care must be taken to evaluate these problems early and seek solutions for each patient. Follow-up of individuals with missed appointments is critical. Careful health education may alleviate some of these problems.

### Third-Level Nursing Care

Patients with severe uncontrolled hypertension, either primary or secondary, are usually hospitalized. In this situation either removal of the secondary cause of hypertension and management of the primary cause is essential.

**Nursing assessment** As the patient's hypertension becomes more severe, the person will complain of a variety of physical and emotional changes. Therefore, the nurse must make a continuous and accurate assessment in order to offer effective care.

**H**ealth History During the health history, the patient with severe hypertension describes many problems similar to those discussed under Second-Level Nursing Care, only with more dramatic and intense physical and psychological responses. The severely hypertensive patient, however, may complain of more serious *headaches* usually confined to the suboccipital or occipital region. Characteristically this problem occurs in the morning as the patient arises, and it wears off as the day progresses. It is a manifestation of hypertensive encephalopathy and is attributed to spasms of cerebral vessels, cerebral edema, multiple small thrombi, or intracerebral hemorrhage. The patient may also experience *shortness of breath,* especially on exertion. Complaints of *anginal pain* may also accompany the patient's history and should be assessed as to time and frequency of onset (refer to Chap. 26 for a complete discussion).

Visual changes including blindness (temporary or permanent), periods of dizziness, syncope, and fatigue may also be present. Increased weight gain may accompany cardiac failure or other health problems, such as Cushing's syndrome. Personality changes may be described as acute, especially if cerebral anoxia is present. The family or patient may describe mood changes that are unassociated with any specific factor. Outbursts of crying are not uncommon.

If a pheochromocytoma exists as a secondary health problem, palpitations, diaphoresis, and postural dizziness may be described.

**P**hysical Assessment   During the physical examination, a variety of systemic changes may be noted. An initial effect is manifested by *left ventricular hypertrophy* which is the physiological compensatory mechanism in response to excessive workload imposed by increased systemic pressure. Furthermore, continuous hypertension causes the ventricular chamber to eventually deteriorate and dilate, leading to heart failure. Signs of both left and right heart failure, including the presence of pulmonary rales, are observable in likewise affected patients (refer to Chap. 24). Physical examination reveals an enlarged heart with a prominent left ventricular impulse. The sound of aortic closure is accentuated, and there may be a faint murmur of aortic insufficiency. Presystolic (atrial) gallop sounds ($S_4$) are frequently heard, and ventricular gallop rhythm ($S_3$) may be present. Tachycardia may also be noted.

Dependent edema may be observed in the ankles, lower extremities, sacrum, buttocks, or posterior thighs. This is usually a result of venous congestion of the kidneys which causes renal vasoconstriction, eventually leading to decreased renal blood flow and filtration. Bruits due to the narrowing of the renal artery may be best heard to the right

or left of the midline and above the umbilicus, or in the flank area.[42] The abdomen should be palpated for the presence of abnormal pulsations that are suggestive of an abdominal aneurysm. The presence of bowel sounds and the normal bowel habits should be evaluated.

During the eye examination, the fundus should be carefully assessed for changes. *Retinal vascular damage* such as scotomas, blurred vision, and even blindness, especially when associated with papilledema or hemorrhage of the macular area, has resulted from the retinal lesions.

The Keith-Wagener (KW) classification of retinal changes in hypertension is useful in identifying and describing the clinical findings. Table 28-5 outlines these classifications and their corresponding retinal changes.

A thorough neurological examination should be done to evaluate the presence of cerebral damage. Range of motion, muscle strength, and gait balance should be checked. Sensory perception should be tested bilaterally. If cerebral damage is present, varying degrees of hemiplegia and hemiparesis may be noted. Calf pain that results from diminished peripheral circulation may be experienced with walking (intermittent claudication; see Chap. 29). Changes in proprioception, and response to smell and taste, may be noted. Additional changes will be present depending on the degree of cerebral vascular anoxia (see Chaps. 32 and 34).

**D**iagnostic Tests   Several additional tests are used to evaluate the physiological changes effected by hypertension. These include the intravenous pyelogram, the renal-vein renin level, the aldosterone level, and urinary catecholamines. The *intravenous pyelogram* (IVP) is a test in which a dye is used to visualize the size, shape, position, and filling of the kidney and the ureters. The radiopaque substance is injected intravenously after which x-ray films are taken at intervals of 2.5, 10, and 15 minutes. When

**TABLE 28-5**
KEITH-WAGENER (KW) CLASSIFICATION OF RETINAL CHANGES IN HYPERTENSION

| | |
|---|---|
| Group 1 | Minimal arteriolar narrowing. |
| Group 2 | More marked narrowing and arteriovenous nicking. |
| Group 3 | Flame-shaped or circular hemorrhages and fluffy cotton-wool exudates. |
| Group 4 | Any of the above plus papilledema, i.e., elevation of the optic disk, obliteration of the physiologic cup, or blurring of the disk margins. By definition, malignant hypertension is always associated with papilledema. |

excretion of the dye is delayed, x-ray films should be taken continually at intervals up to 4 hours or more. If the patient had a lower GI series or barium enema, the barium should be removed before the IVP is done. Care should be taken to evaluate the individual's response to the dye used during an IVP as some patients may experience an allergic response following its administration.

*Preparation of the patient for this test* includes an explanation of the purpose and method of the test. In addition, all food and liquids should be withheld after midnight, prior to the examination day. This will allow the radiopaque substance to become more concentrated when it enters the kidney. A cathartic (e.g., castor oil) is usually given to the patient the night before the test is ordered. This will help to provide a clearer picture of the urinary tract. Following the test, the nurse should be alert to signs of reaction to the dye which may include rash or hives. Fluids should be offered to the patient after the test in order to completely flush out the remaining dye. Care should be taken to assist the patient when getting out of bed since the patient may be weakened by the lack of food.

*A 24-hour test for urinary catecholamine metabolite or vanillylmandelic acid* (VMA) is used to diagnose pheochromocytoma as the cause of hypertension. When pheochromocytoma is associated with paroxysmal hypertension, the most reliable test is to assess the level of epinephrine and norepinephrine in the blood and in the urine. VMA is the catecholamine metabolite excreted in larger amounts when pheochromocytoma is present. High epinephrine levels favor the localization of the tumor within the adrenal gland. If hypertension is intermittent, indicating that the tumor may not be functioning continuously, a provocative test using either histamine or phentolamine (Regitine) IV is performed. This is done immediately before starting a 24-hour collection of urine.

Specific *nursing responsibilities* related to the collection for this 24-hour urine test include an explanation of the purpose and method of urine collection, emphasizing the necessity of having all the urine collected during a 24-hour period. In addition the patient should be instructed and supervised as to the pretest diet, being told to exclude chocolate, coffee, tea, vanilla, and all fruits, especially bananas, for at least 2 days before urine collection begins, as these substances will interfere with the test's results.

The patient should also be instructed not to take any medications for 2 to 3 days prior to testing, as they may alter the findings. Prior to the collection of the specimens, a large-size brown collection bottle should be provided containing hydrochloric acid. The hydrochloric acid acts as a preservative preventing changes in urine composition before testing. When the test begins, the patient should void immediately before the collection begins and then save all urine voided within the next 24-hour period. Immediately before the end of the 24-hour period the patient should void and include that specimen. The patient should be advised to void and save the urine before defecation in order to avoid contamination of the sample.

*Phentolamine (Regitine),* 2.5 to 5 mg IV, is then given rapidly, following the first voiding, preferably into an existing intravenous line during which blood pressure levels have been stabilized. Within 2 to 5 minutes, the blood pressure should show a sustained overall fall of at least 35/25 mmHg in patients with pheochromocytoma.

When Regitine is used in the normotensive patients, histamine is given, 0.01 to 0.25 mg, and mixed with 0.5 ml normal saline. It is drawn into a tuberculin syringe and is given rapidly. Intravenously the needle is left in the vein so that phentolamine can be given in the event blood pressure becomes too high in response to histamine. A blood pressure rise of 60/30 mmHg occurs within 2 minutes when pheochromocytoma is present. Selective *angiography* (see Chaps. 31 and 34) combined with *intravenous urograms* and *tomography* (a photograph of a body part using x-rays) also useful in visualizing adrenal tumors.

The *rapid sequence urogram* is one of the most useful tests to screen for renal arterial stenosis and renovascular hypertension. A dye similar to that used for an IVP is given to the patient. This permits visualization of the renal artery. If renal artery stenosis is present, the urogram may show a delay in appearance of the dye on the affected side, due to a delayed secretion of the dye.

The *renal vein renin level* determination is done to evaluate the renin content in the blood. Serum samples are obtained by catheterization of the renal veins to assess the involvement of renovascular hypertension. This test identifies the degree of renal pathology that can result from hypertension. When there is unilateral renal artery involvement, a higher level of renin is seen in the sample of blood drawn from the stenotic renal arterial lesion. A renal vein ratio greater than 1.5:1 is considered significant. If bilateral renal artery involvement is present, there is no significant difference in renin concentration between the two sides.

An *aldosterone level* is used to diagnose

primary aldosteronism and primary hyperaldosteronism. Urine and plasma aldosterone levels are markedly elevated in primary aldosteronism, above the normal 22 to 23 mg for 24 hour. When this elevation is noted, the patient will have an elevated arterial blood pressure. An increased level of urinary aldosterone is not suppressed by a high sodium intake or the administration of deoxycorticosterone. A low potassium level and an increased sodium level are also found with a diagnosis of primary aldosteronism.

**Nursing problems and interventions**  The aim of all interventions during this level of nursing care is to reduce the blood pressure by identifying and/or eliminating all primary and secondary factors influencing severe hypertension. The initial problem continues to be a sustained elevated arterial blood pressure. Headaches, obesity, epistaxis, and anxiety discussed in Second-Level Nursing Care are present but more severe. In addition, increased fatigue and dyspnea are usually noted.

**E**levated Blood Pressure  In order to establish the range of blood pressure fluctuations during a 24-hour period, the *blood pressure* should be checked on a frequent basis and at the same times each day or more often as the conditions dictate. Blood pressure during sleep may be as much as 20 mmHg lower than a waking measurement. In addition other vital signs including temperature, respiration, and pulse readings should be taken frequently to evaluate the patient's overall status.

**F**atigue  Even though absolute bed *rest* may not be necessary, hospitalized patients with hypertension need to be placed at rest physically as well as mentally in order to conserve energy and avoid unnecessary activation of the sympathetic nervous system. Planned activity should be based upon the individual's general physical health status. In the presence of *dizziness* care should be taken to protect the patient from injury. Often, *relief of emotional and environmental stress* coupled with physical rest improves the clinical conditions of the hypertension. Patients should be properly advised to avoid unnecessary tensions and stress. Family members should be included in this discussion. Reduction of family stress as well as personal anxieties may be achieved through group discussions. When anxiety is high and/or the patient's ability to cope with stress is interfered with, mild tranquilizers may be needed.

**B**ehavioral Changes  *Personality changes* may accompany the use of some antihypertensive drugs or can be associated with cerebral vascular hypoxia. The family as well as the patient should be told of these changes in order to cope with emotional outbursts that may develop. The nurse can support the family through this difficult period by explaining the reasons for the changes noticed. This discussion may help reduce family stress which could be transferred to the patient.

**N**osebleeds  Epistaxis discussed in Second-Level Nursing Care may become severe and require packing. This is an uncomfortable procedure for the patient and can interfere with eating and swallowing if the packing reaches to the back of the pharynx. Frequent mouth care with the planning of a diet that is tolerable can reduce the potential stress of the situation. Mild tranquilizers may also be used to help relax the patient and reduce the discomfort. The nasal packing is usually removed within several days following the initial nosebleed. The patient is observed carefully for any signs of renewed bleeding.

**H**eadaches  These often subside or decrease in intensity as the arterial blood pressure decreases. When necessary a mild analgesic may be ordered. If the headache becomes more severe, it may require the use of a narcotic. It is important to continually assess those other factors which may be contributing to the headache, e.g., stress, and to attempt to reduce those factors. Supportive counseling may be required to assess those factors.

**V**isual Changes  They may subside as hypertension decreases; however, many changes may be permanent. Whether they are is often dependent upon the cause of the hypertension, its duration, and severity. Ophthalmology referrals may be required and the use of eyeglasses suggested. Protection of the patient is critical during this period, especially if the patient is elderly. Family members as well as nursing staff should be reminded to observe safety precautions at all times.

**O**verweight  If *obesity* is a problem, dietary restrictions considered under Second-Level Nursing Care should be enforced. Low-cholesterol, low-fat diets, along with sodium restrictions, will also be suggested. (Refer to Chap. 16 for a more complete discussion.)

*Drug therapy*  One of the main objectives of nursing care related to *hypertension* is reduction of the hypertension. Many categories of drugs are available to achieve this goal. However, each category contains drugs that act upon certain components of the *central nervous system. Vasodilators act on smooth muscles and dilate* peripheral blood vessels. Hydralazine (Table 28-6) and nitroprusside are two examples. Several drugs, e.g., clonidine and methyldopa (see Chap. 37), act upon the *sympathetic nervous system centers* and reduce vasomotor tone.[43] Clonidine, the newest antihypertensive drug, is excluded from Table 28-6 since it is not commonly used. Clonidine, administered intravenously, produces a brief rise in blood pressure in both man and laboratory animals by means of direct stimulation of vascular alpha-adrenergic receptors and not by a release of catecholamines.[44] Following the initial hypertensive response, blood pressure falls as heart rate and cardiac output decreases. This effect is due to a decrease in sympathetic tone that results from a direct action of the drug on the CNS with depression of the vasomotor center.[45]

The oral administration of clonidine produces hypotension without an initial hypertensive response.[46] Effective oral dose is 400 to 3600 mg/day. Additional drugs called *sympathetic inhibitors* (Table 28-7) act on and affect other sites in the nervous system. The *ganglionic blocking agents* (mecamylamine) interfere with parasympathetic as well as sympathetic function and are often used for rapid reduction of blood pressure. Additional drugs such as guanethidine and pargyline (see Table 28-7) act at the *postganglionic nerve endings.* These drugs inhibit the storage of norepinephrine within the vesicles of the adrenergic nerve endings, resulting in a depletion of catecholamine storage.[47]

Phenoxybenzamine (Table 28-7) is an example of an *alpha-adrenergic blocking drug.* Drugs in this group act to block the action of norepinephrine in the bloodstream, at the alpha-adrenergic receptor site. They are usually not as effective in lowering blood pressure as other drugs.

Propranolol (Table 28-7) is an effective *beta-adrenergic blocking agent.* It is a new drug used to treat hypertension. Although the onset of the antihypertensive effect is not immediate, the efficiency of this drug has been confirmed through experiments. The mechanism of its antihypertensive action has not been totally understood; however, the new theory as proposed by Lewis[48] states, "The essential action is to diminish sympathetic nerve output by damping sensory input to the central nervous system from a heart whose capacity to respond to exercise and stress is blunted by beta adreno receptor blockage." A 10-month crossover study of 27 patients with hypertension showed that the re-

sponse of the patient to propranolol was better when the PRA level was higher.[49] This finding supports the concept that the reninangiotensin-aldosterone system may be involved in primary hypertension.

*Diuretics,* discussed in Second-Level Nursing Care, may be used in conjunction with antihypertensive medications. *Sedatives* or *tranquillizers* are sometimes helpful in alleviating the side effects of specific antihypertensive drugs, especially during the initiation of treatment, but sedation itself is neither an integral nor desirable part of modern programs for the treatment of hypertension.

In hypertensive emergencies parenteral administration of such antihypertensive direct vasodilators and sympathetic inhibitors as ganglionic blockers can be given (see Table 28-8). Intravenous administration of either ethacrynic acid (50 to 100 mg) or furosemide (40 to 120 mg) is usually advisable to enhance and prolong the action of the antihypertensive agent and to prevent secondary fluid and sodium retention. This is particularly true in hypertensive crises associated with acute left ventricular failure, eclampsia, and acute or chronic renal disease.

Extensive health teaching is an integral component of antihypertensive drug therapy. A complete teaching guide will be discussed in Fourth-Level Nursing Care.

*Surgery* With the advent of antihypertensive drugs, the use of surgical interventions for an elevated arterial blood pressure has decreased. However, if there is a secondary problem that may contribute to hypertension, surgery is performed. Correction of coarctation of the aorta (see Chap. 27) and repair of a renal stenosis are two such interventions.

If pheochromocytoma is the suspected cause of hypertension, an adrenalectomy, or surgical removal of the adrenal gland, is indicated. Prior to the operation the patient should rest, and emotional tension should be minimized. Dietary stimulants of any kind, including beverages such as coffee or tea, are restricted. In order to keep stress and anxiety at a minimum, sedation may be prescribed. Vital signs are monitored frequently, and antihypertensive drugs are often used.

When surgery is performed, vital signs should be checked every 30 minutes for 24 to 48 hours postoperatively. This is a critical time for the patient as the blood pressure may fall precipitously to hypotensive levels as the blood level of catecholamines drops.

Because the adrenal glands are so highly vas-

**TABLE 28-6**
ORAL VASODILATING DRUGS USED FOR HYPERTENSION

| Generic Name | Trade Name | Dosage | Action | Side Effects | General Remarks |
|---|---|---|---|---|---|
| Hydrolazine (oral administration) | Apresoline | 50 mg divided and given twice daily; maximum dosage 300 mg. | Dilates peripheral blood vessels by decreasing peripheral resistance, increasing cardiac output and renal blood flow. Antihypertensive agent; used with other drug combinations to treat moderate hypertension. | Tachycardia, palpitation, headache, liver damage, nausea, dizziness, sweating, fever, nausea, vomiting, chills. Prolonged use of the drug may result in changes similar to rheumatoid arthritis. | Adverse effects may be minimal when the dose is increased slowly. Tolerance may develop with continued administration. Use with caution in patients with coronary artery disease. Toxic symptoms disappear when drug is terminated. |

**TABLE 28-7**
SYMPATHETIC INHIBITORS USED IN THE MANAGEMENT OF HYPERTENSION

| Generic Name | Trade Name | Dosage | Action | Side Effects | General Remarks |
|---|---|---|---|---|---|
| Reserpine | Serpasil Sandril Reserpoid | 0.1–0.5 mg daily in divided doses two or three times a day | Reduces norepinephrine levels thereby decreasing catecholamines. Stimulation of smooth muscles. | Low toxicity. Predominantly CNS and GI tract effects (drowsiness, sedation, lassitude, nightmares, psychic depression, gastric hyperacidity, abdominal cramps, diarrhea). Incidence of breast cancer associated with long-term therapy. Nasal congestion also occurs. | Should not be given to patients with a history of depressive episodes. Long-term administration was associated with a more than threefold increase in incidence of breast cancer in women. Should not be given to a patient with a history of peptic ulcer. |
| Methyldopa | Aldomet | 0.5–3 g daily; usual dose 500–1000 mg Q.D. | Depletes stores of 5-hydroxy tryptamine, dopamine, norepinephrine in the CNS. Blood pressure by peripheral resistance. | Lassitude, drowsiness, vertigo, lactation. Nightmares and psychic depression less common than with reserpine. Dry mouth, GI upset, postural hypotension, depression, congestion, reduced WBC. | Postural hypotension can develop (less frequent and severe than with guanethidine). Edema with retention of salt and water with weight gain. Contraindicated in liver pathology; and depression. |
| Guanethidine | Ismelin | 10–75 mg; usually only 1 dose daily | Postganglionic blocking agent—inhibits the response of sympathetic adrenergic nerve activation and inhibits indirect-acting sympathomimetic amines (e.g., tyramine or amphetamine) or produces postganglionic sympathetic blockade, depletes tissue stores of norepinephrine. Vascular dilatation occurs. | Severe postural hypotension, diarrhea, weakness, edema, lightheadedness, orthostatic hypotension, impotence, and bradycardia. | Orthostatic hypotension is most prominent shortly after arising from sleep, accentuated with hot weather, alcohol, or exercise. Decreased myocardial competence—congestive heart failure. Therapeutic effect can be antagonized by chlorpromazine. |

**TABLE 28-7**
SYMPATHETIC INHIBITORS USED IN THE MANAGEMENT OF HYPERTENSION (Continued)

| Generic Name | Trade Name | Dosage | Action | Side Effects | General Remarks |
|---|---|---|---|---|---|
| Propranolol | Inderal | 10–40 mg; 30–120 mg daily; available in 10 and 40 mg tab. | β-Adrenergic receptor blocking drug lowers heart rate and lowers myocardial contractility, thereby decreasing cardiac output and plasma renin. | Nausea, vomiting, light-headedness, depression, constipation, diarrhea, fever, aggravation of bronchial asthma, hallucinations. | Watch for signs of pump failure. Avoid in patients with bradycardia or AV blocks. Patients with high or normal plasma renin activities respond better. As effective as methyldopa or hydralazine when added to diuretic treatment. The onset of the therapeutic effect is not immediate. |
| Pentolinium Mecamylamine | Ansolysen Inversine | 40 mg twice daily 5 mg | Ganglionic blockade stabilizes the postsynaptic membranes against the action of ACTH liberated to presynaptic nerve endings. | Orthostatic hypotension, dry mouth, blurred vision constipation, urinary retention, impotence. | Therapeutic use has been diminished considerably with the advent of other drugs. Large IV doses must be given in supine position for effective results. |
| Pargyline | Eutonyl | 10 mg daily | MAO inhibitor acts on the postganglionic nerve terminal; pressor endogenous amines (e.g., dopamine) are accumulated and act as a false neurotransmitter. (Antidepressant). | Postural hypotension, nausea, vomiting, insomnia, nervousness, impotence, urinary retention. | Decrease of blood pressure develops slowly (3 weeks or more). Avoid taking food containing tyramine (certain cheeses, beers, wines, pickled herring, chicken livers) since hypertensive crises and death have been reported. |
| Phenoxybenzamine | Dibenzyline | 20 mg twice a day; maximum dose 80 mg four times a day | α-Adrenergic blockade—a direct action on α-adrenergic receptors only. | Nasal congestion, miosis, orthostatic hypotension, tachycardia, inhibition of ejaculation, GI irritation. | Use cautiously in hypovolemic patient. Exaggerates the depressor effects of narcotics and other agents that act directly to relax smooth muscle. Clinical use has been too limited to find toxicity. |

cular, the patient should be assessed for shock and hemorrhage following surgery. Should shock develop post-operatively, the patient is often treated with vasopressors, intravenous therapy, and frequent monitoring of vital signs (see Hypotension below for a complete discussion of this topic.)

*Complications* The complications associated with severe hypertension are primarily due to the effects of sustained elevation in arterial blood pressure. This results in rapid progression of necrosis of the walls of small arteries and arterioles, with concentric collagenous endothelial thickening leading to diminution or occlusion of the vascular lumen. Prevention of these complications relies on the effectiveness of the therapy. Depending upon the site at which predescribed changes occur, problems such as cerebral vascular accident, renal failure, ischemic heart disease, and hypertensive encephalopathy may be encountered.

Among many causes of *cerebral infarction,* hypertensive intracerebral hemorrhage and ruptured saccular aneurysm most often account for the clinical picture of stroke or cerebrovascular accident. A variety of neurological changers including hemiplegia, aphasia, and changes in the level of consciousness may be present, depending upon the site of the rupture and the brain tissue displaced and compressed (refer to Chap. 34 for a complete discussion of cerebrovascular accidents).

Prolonged and severe hypertension causes renal deterioration and arteriosclerotic lesions which may result in *renal destruction* and eventual *failure.* Massive proteinuria, hematuria, and uremia may develop. Development of these changes may take several days to weeks, and death usually results from uremia. When the therapy for hypertension is not effective, severe vascular damage of the kidneys will necessitate the use of dialysis. (Complete discussion of renal failure is found in Chap. 14.)

Hypertension is one of three major risk factors leading to *ischemic heart disease.* Coronary atherosclerosis coupled with heart failure due to sustained severe hypertension may lead to eventual coronary occlusion, angina, and myocardial infarction. The incidence of ischemic heart disease in men aged 45 to 62 with a blood pressure higher than 160/95 is more than five times that in normotensive men.[50] (See Chap. 26 for a complete discussion of myocardial ischemia.)

*Hypertensive encephalopathy* is caused by spasm of the cerebral blood vessels and cerebral edema. It is associated with extremely severe hypertension (diastolic pressure of 120 mmHg or over). Symptoms including transient paralysis, convulsions, stupor, coma, blindness, and severe headaches can be noted. Treatment with antihypertensive agents may reverse the picture in a day or two. Cardiac decompensation of renal failure becomes apparent when the problem is not controlled; the outcome can be fatal.

**TABLE 28-8**

DRUGS FOR PARENTERAL ADMINISTRATION IN THE TREATMENT OF HYPERTENSIVE EMERGENCIES*

| Drug | IM, mg | Continuous IV, mg | Onset of Action |
| --- | --- | --- | --- |
| DIRECT VASODILATORS | | | |
| Hydralazine (Apresoline) | 10–60 | 50–100 | IM: 30 min<br>IV: 10 min |
| Diazoxide (Hyperstat) | | | 3–5 min |
| Sodium nitroprusside | | 50–150 | Instantaneous |
| SYMPATHETIC INHIBITORS | | | |
| Reserpine (Serpasil) | 1–5 | | 2–3 h |
| GANGLION BLOCKING AGENTS | | | |
| Petolinium (Ansolysen) | 1–25 | 50–150 | IM: 30 min<br>IV: 5–10 min |
| Trimethaphan (Arfonad) | | 1000 | 5–10 min |
| Methyldopa (Aldomet ester) | | | 2–3 h |
| Phentolamine (Regitine) | 5–20 | 100–500 | Instantaneous |
| Furosemide (Lassix) | 40 (repeat 4–8 h prn) | — | 15–20 min |

* When diuretics are given, the smallest dose is given first and infused over 30–60 min. When direct injection is used, the drug is given at a rate of 1 ml/min.
SOURCE: Modified from H. F. Conn (ed.), *Current Therapy,* Saunders, Philadelphia, 1975, p. 220.

### Fourth-Level Nursing Care

The program of rehabilitation for the patient with hypertension and its complications should be carefully tailored to meet the patient's individual needs, personality, habit, life-style, and general health status. The problem of hypertension requires that most patients make some changes in the pattern of their daily lives. Factors which influence hypertension can be altered by change in occupation, response to stress, antihypertensive drug therapy, and other related changes. The progress of rehabilitation depends on the patient's occupation, cultural background, social status, personal motivation, and support from family members.

Following hospitalization the patient usually goes through a variety of emotional reactions to a newly acquired disability. The initial reaction may be *denial* followed by *depression,* and *acceptance.* To make a successful adjustment, the patient must recognize the limitations imposed by the disability and fully cooperate with the rehabilitation program while setting realistic goals for the future. It is important to note that emotional responses can be intensified by antihypertensive drug therapy, and thus mood changes can be more easily accounted for.

Patients having difficulty accepting their disability can become *rebellious.* Others ignore the problem and will not adapt to the prescribed regimen. Often noncompliant behavior is noted after treatment for hypertension is instituted and patients begin to improve. They attribute their improved health to the medication but fail to realize that in order to retain the healthy state they must be faithful to that therapy.

Some patients are anxious about the long-term nature of their problem and fear complications. Careful counseling may be of assistance. Patients who have sustained a cerebrovascular accident will need to spend much time in an extensive rehabilitation program. (See Chap. 34 for a complete discussion of rehabilitation.)

The most important point that hypertensive patients and their families must understand is that hypertension is a chronic condition often without symptoms that cannot be cured but can be controlled by means of continuous antihypertensive drug therapy, weight control through dietary restrictions (such as low-fat, low-cholesterol, low-salt diets), exercise, sufficient rest, and possibly modification of life-style. On occasion, occupational changes may be required if a job is too stressful. Reduction of environmental stress is critical.

The attitudes of family members play an important role in rehabilitation of patients who have suffered a complication of hypertension (e.g., a cardiovascular accident). Undue expression of emotional upset in the presence of the patient may put the patient into further depression. The family should be encouraged and supported to help the patient during the period following hospitalization. The family members should be taught how to perform daily care. As the patient begins self-care, "body image" problems may develop, particularly with patients who have suffered neurological damage (see Chap. 34). This will require the understanding and patience of the family members to help and to remind the patient to give complete self-care. Sexual changes, including impotence and emotional lability, may accompany antihypertensive drugs. Patients and family members should be told that behavioral changes may accompany antihypertensive drug therapy so that both may be prepared for these alterations in mood. Group discussions with family members and patients may allow a time for expression of personal feelings and attitudes regarding this long-term health problem.

**Health teaching** Teaching plans for hypertensive drug therapy should be based on competent knowledge of pharmacology, potential adverse effects, contraindications of drugs, and individual patient needs in order to ensure optimal results. Care must be taken to continuously reinforce the idea that continued therapy is needed to maintain the desired effect of the drug. Two main objectives of health teaching are found in Table 28-9; they encompass information critical to antihypertensive drug therapy. Teaching methods and evaluation should be based upon this knowledge. Implementation of all teaching plans should consider the role of the family members. Therefore, when possible, a family member should always be included in the teaching plan.

Since most patients with hypertension are on long-term antihypertensive drugs, the importance of taking the drug(s) at the right time and regularly can not be emphasized too much. The patient should be explicitly instructed that he or she may not skip the dose or discontinue the drug without the physician's permission. When the patient suffers from other health problems, it is the patient's responsibility to inform the physician about the medicines currently being taken. The patient should also be instructed to take arterial blood pressure readings at home.

In addition to eating *balanced meals,* the patient should be instructed as to the limitation of calorie, cholesterol, and sodium intake as prescribed by the physician. Heavy meals should be avoided since they can put added burden on the vascular system.

## HYPOTENSION

Maintenance of the arterial blood pressure is dependent upon cardiac output, blood volume, and peripheral vasomotor tone. When arterial pressure decreases below normal limits, tissue perfusion becomes impaired and stimulation of pressor receptors (which activate sympathetic outflow and inhibit parasympathetic activity) occurs.[51] Conventionally, the systolic pressure of 90 mmHg, below the subject's normal value, is considered *hypotensive*.

*Hypotension* by itself is not necessarily a pathological finding. Some normal subjects have a blood pressure of 90/60 with no ill effects. The brain can apparently be adequately perfused at systolic pressure as low as 60 mmHg or less even in the upright position. When the blood pressure level is decreased to the state in which blood flow to vital organs (brain, heart, kidneys) is impaired, the condition becomes pathological.

### Shock

Shock is often associated with hypotension; however, the terms are not synonymous. A previously hypertensive patient may develop shock despite an arterial pressure within normal limits. On the other hand, hypotension may be present in the absence of shock.[52] For purposes of this chapter, *shock* will be defined as an abnormal physiological state in which there is widespread, serious reduction of tissue perfusion that, if prolonged, will lead to generalized impairment of cellular function. The following discussion will focus upon causes, changes, and effects related to shock.

**Pathophysiology**  When a decrease in arterial pressure is sufficient to produce a widespread reduction in tissue perfusion, the body attempts to compensate for the physiological changes that ensue. Therefore, the overall purpose of the so-called *compensatory mechanisms* is to utilize the body's readily available energy sources to restore adequate circulation to the vital organs. It is important to remember that although each individual has the ability to compensate for the physiological deficits produced by shock, the overall effect of the compensatory mechanisms will vary from person to person.

A decrease in blood volume, regardless of the

**TABLE 28-9**
TEACHING OBJECTIVES IN ANTIHYPERTENSIVE DRUG THERAPY

1   After health teaching related to hypertensive drug therapy the patient will avoid any activity or movement that will cause orthostatic hypotension. This includes knowledge of the following:

   *a*   Rising from a lying to a sitting and from a sitting to a standing position too fast should be avoided to allow physiological adjustment of the vascular system. Vasoconstriction of the lower extremities which occurs when rising slowly prevents pooling of blood and syncope.

   *b*   Standing still for any length of time should be avoided, especially within 2 hours after taking the drug. Leg vessels are relaxed when standing still, which causes pooling of blood resulting in syncope or weakness. This is more so in the early morning when postural hypotension is often most severe.

   *c*   Leg muscle exercises or recumbency should be encouraged when weakness and dizziness occur. Various muscle activities (e.g., wiggling of toes, flexing calf muscles) promote vasoconstriction, preventing blood from pooling in the lower extremities. A recumbent position with the legs slightly elevated promotes cerebral blood flow and decreases the pooling of blood in the legs.

2   After a presentation on drug therapy the patient will observe the following precautions when taking antihypertensive medications:

   *a*   Prescribed drugs should be taken regularly at the right time continuously even after the problematic symptoms have disappeared.

   *b*   While the use of home remedies, such as vinegar and honey, garlic solution, or other foods, may not be harmful to the patient, the prescribed medicines are still necessary.

   *c*   Take a sedative (if prescribed) as needed without feeling guilty. Even though some patients feel they should be able to relax without medicine, the sedative plays a therapeutic as well as supportive role with other treatment.

   *d*   Be more careful during the 2 hours after taking the medications. The patient should not drive if experiencing blurred vision and should be extra careful when working with or around heavy and dangerous machinery.

   *e*   Heat from hot baths, steam baths, or sun baths should be avoided since this promotes peripheral vasodilatation, causing hypotensive reactions.

   *f*   If impotency occurs, the patient should consult his physician. A decrease in dosage or skipping the dosage may overcome this effect.

   *g*   Abrupt withdrawal of the drug should be avoided in order to prevent hypertensive reactions that occur owing to increased sensitivity to pressor substances.

   *h*   Discontinue the drug if chest pains occur, particularly if there is a history of angina pectoris.

   *i*   The patient should carry an identification card with the name of the drug, dosage, and the times the drug is taken.

   *j*   The patient should sleep with the head elevated or sit up when a headache occurs during the night or early in the morning.

   *k*   Alcohol in moderation has no appreciable effect.

   *l*   Salt intake or ingestion of foods high in sodium content should be modified or decreased.

cause, stimulates both the *nervous and endocrine systems* to respond. The body's energy supplies such as amino acids, fatty acids, glucose, sodium, and water are converted into energy sources and used by the body. The glucocorticoids then mobilize these energy stores. As the body's supply of readily available carbohydrates becomes depleted, fat and protein stores are used. As a result of gluconeogenesis and starvation, protein catabolism and negative nitrogen balance occur.[53]

During the initial stage of the shock the adrenal medulla secretes epinephrine and norepinephrine, which results in peripheral vasoconstriction and an increase in the cardiac heart rate. With an increase in both peripheral resistance and cardiac output, additional blood is available for circulation to the vital organs. Also, the peripheral veins constrict and empty their blood supply into the circulation. This increases venous return and cardiac output.

In an attempt to conserve body fluids, osmoreceptors located in the hypothalamus stimulate the posterior pituitary gland to secrete antidiuretic hormone (ADH). This hormone acts to decrease glomerular filtration and results in added fluid retention. Increased production of mineralocorticoids, such as aldosterone, help to improve blood volume by retaining increased amounts of sodium and water.

As renal vasoconstriction occurs, a renal pressor substance (RPS) is released by the kidneys and empties into the circulation. This substance contributes to the constriction of the arteries. Another substance, angiotensin II, a pressor agent, is released by the ischemic kidneys and has a vasoconstricting effect on smooth muscles.

As compensation for tissue anoxia and hypovolemia caused by shock there is an increased production of red blood cells. These cells are quickly produced and released into the circulation. Many of them are immature and carry less oxygen than the more mature cells. Therefore the overall effect on tissue oxygenation is limited.

Increases in cardiac output and myocardial contractility are stimulated by an increased production of carbon dioxide. This action dilates the coronary arteries and increases myocardial perfusion. In addition, the presence of carbon dioxide stimulates the central nervous system to act upon nonactive tissue, resulting in a shunting of blood to vital areas.[54] When the compensatory mechanisms are no longer functional, an advancement of the shock occurs. This will result in multiple physiological changes.

**Changes That Accompany Advanced Shock** Progressive shock produces multiple systemic changes as a result of decreased cardiac output, hypovolemia, and limited cardiac perfusion. These changes produce alterations in oxygenation, fluid and electrolytes, metabolism, and the body's defense against bacterial invasion.

*Oxygenation* is seriously affected in shock. A decrease in cardiac output is directly influenced by poor myocardial contractility and limited venous return. Initially, the release of epinephrine into the circulation results in an improved heart rate and overall output. Depending upon the cause of shock, and myocardial efficiency, the stress of shock may lead to *cardiac decompensation* and failure. The presence of *pump failure* will intensify the problem of deficient cardiac output.

Along with a deficient cardiac output, there is a decrease in blood volume and a slowing down of blood flow. *Hypovolemia* deprives body cells of oxygen and nutrients needed for cell growth. The *microcirculation* is that part of the arteriolar and venous circulation responsible for transporting oxygen and nutrients to the cells and removing waste products. This circulatory system is widespread throughout the body. Therefore, when the body is deprived of blood from the circulation, many areas are affected and *microcirculatory insufficiency* may result.

The response to shock in the microcirculation is somewhat different than that in the systemic circulation. The systemic circulation attempts to maintain adequate blood volume through peripheral vasoconstriction. The microcirculation responds to shock by vasodilatation in order to secure the necessary nutrients and oxygen for the deprived cells. As this occurs, blood is trapped in the capillary beds, and therefore a limited supply of blood is returned to the systemic circulation.

Decreased pulmonary circulation and tissue perfusion both contribute to significant changes within the *lungs*. Changes such as pulmonary edema and atelectasis as well as capillary thrombi observed in the pulmonary microcirculation may cause additional problems for the patient. When pulmonary failure occurs subsequent to shock, it is called *shock lung*. Changes include pulmonary congestion, decrease in $p_{O_2}$ levels, and loss of pulmonary surfactant (see Chap. 30). This problem can develop after the initial shock has been corrected and may be fatal for the patient. Additional respiratory changes such as *pulmonary edema* may develop as a secondary response to pump failure.

*Respiratory acidosis* and *respiratory alkalosis* can occur owing to a decrease in pulmonary tissue perfusion and a disruption in ventilation.

In addition to changes in peripheral circulation, a decrease in cerebral circulation accompanies shock. *Cerebral hypoxia* will lead to lethargy, alterations in the level of consciousness, restlessness, anxiety, and personality changes. Sluggish circulation and blood hypercoagulability can lead to thrombus formation and cerebral infarction. Disruptions in perception and coordination including aphasia, paralysis, and hemiplegia may result. (See Chap. 34 for a complete discussion.) It is important to note that inadequate filtration of toxic substances by the kidneys as well as an accumulation of metabolic waste products may also contribute to cerebral tissue disruptions.

Inadequate tissue perfusion also affects the body's *metabolism,* resulting in alteration of biochemical substances and accumulation of metabolites. When oxygen is no longer available for cell growth, a substance called adenosine triphosphate (ATP) is produced through the process of *anaerobic metabolism* (or fermentation). While ATP will help provide an additional oxygen supply in an emergency situation, it is an inefficient source on a long-term basis. Anaerobic metabolism also leads to the production of lactic acid in the tissues and can result in metabolic acidosis. (See Chap. 12 for a complete discussion of acidosis/alkalosis.)

Prolonged vasoconstriction in the larger splanchnic blood vessels and inadequate perfusion of the *liver* during various stages of shock can seriously affect the liver's ability to detoxify substances. Alteration in the microcirculation of the portal bed results in blood's being trapped in the small splenic veins, the sinusoids, and the hepatic artery, thereby decreasing hepatic functioning. These changes interfere with liver metabolism and decrease venous return.

The body's defense against *infection* is also altered by shock in several ways. Initially, there is a depression of the body's reticuloendothelial system (RES). This change alters the individual's autoimmune response and disrupts the antibacterial defense mechanism. As a result, the release of bacterial endotoxins is fostered and the integrity of the cells, especially in the microcirculation, is destroyed.

Obstruction of blood flow to the intestines caused by systemic vasoconstriction will result in tissue anoxia of the bowel and in necrosis of bowel tissue. Loss of the integrity of bowel mucosa be-

cause of prolonged shock allows for the transmission of bacteria (such as *Escherichia coli*) into the systemic circulation. The impaired ability of the RES to act as a defense against bacterial invasion may further compound the problem and contribute to a generalized loss of resistance to infection. These changes may result in irreversible shock.

Changes in *fluid and electrolyte* balance occur with shock. Peripheral vasoconstriction caused by the action of norepinephrine results in a shift in fluid from the interstitial tissue to the circulation, thereby increasing blood volume. However, the introduction of increased interstitial fluid in the circulation dilutes the blood and decreases the efficiency of the red blood cells. Depletion of fluid from the interstitial spaces contributes to tissue dehydration. One phenomenon consistently associated with severe hemorrhagic shock is the presumed loss of extracellular fluid into the wall and the lumen of the bowel, resulting in liquid, bloody stools.[55]

Urinary output is diminished (oliguria) in shock to below 40 to 60 ml of urine per hour. This is influenced by a decrease in glomerular filtration and the action of the antidiuretic hormones. As the shock progresses, anuria will result in renal shutdown. This occurs because of a steady decline in blood volume and arterial pressure with resulting decrease in renal perfusion. The afferent and efferent arterioles constrict, and glomerular filtration is reduced. Lack of urination will increase the amount of toxic waste products in the body and seriously affect the function of other body systems (e.g., the brain and liver).

**S**tages of Shock  Shock is a dynamic and interactive process that can occur in various stages. These include the initial stage, the intermediate stage, and the irreversible stage. The rapidity with which shock progresses from the initial onset to a life-threatening stage will depend upon the integrity of the compensatory mechanisms and the cause of shock state.

The *initial stage* of shock occurs when there is a decrease in blood volume by 10 percent of the normal value (500 ml) with diminished cardiac output. This results in inadequate tissue perfusion. The compensatory mechanism is effective, responding with rapid constriction of the arteriolar bed of skin and muscle and increased contractility of the heart by increasing sympathetic discharge of epinephrine and norepinephrine.

In addition, there is a gradual increase in the secretion of antidiuretic hormone, mobilization of

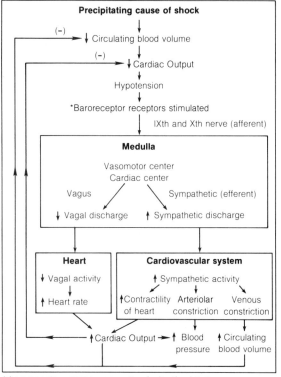

Precipitating cause of shock

(-) ↓ Circulating blood volume

(-) ↓ Cardiac Output

Hypotension

*Baroreceptor receptors stimulated

IXth and Xth nerve (afferent)

**Medulla**

Vasomotor center
Cardiac center

Vagus          Sympathetic (efferent)

↓ Vagal discharge      ↑ Sympathetic discharge

**Heart**
↓ Vagal activity
↑ Heart rate

**Cardiovascular system**
↑ Sympathetic activity
↑Contractility  Arteriolar  Venous
of heart     constriction  constriction

↑Cardiac Output → ↑ Blood  ↑ Circulating
pressure  blood volume

* baroreceptor - sensory nerve terminals stimulated
by changes in arterial pressure.

**FIGURE 28-3**
Initial stage: reversible shock and compensatory mechanism.

energy stores, and secretion of ACTH. As a result cardiac output and blood pressure remain at a normal or slightly reduced level, and the serious effects of shock are averted (see Fig. 28-3).

During the second stage of shock, the *intermediate stage,* the compensatory mechanisms are ineffective, and cardiac output and arterial pressure are low. This is caused by a reduction in blood volume by 15 to 20 percent (a significant reduction). The body attempts to compensate for this loss in volume by creating sympathetic overactivity which leads to intense arteriolar constriction in most vascular beds.

As a result there is splenic ischemia causing a depression of the reticuloendothelial system in the liver and spleen and increased release of endotoxin from the intestine. At the same time the myocardial depressant factor (MDF) is released from the pancreas.

Renal ischemia leads to renin, angiotensin-aldosterone activation which causes excessive arteriolar constriction. As a result, progressive systemic tissue ischemia develops, leading to capillary

endothelial damage and microcirculatory insufficiency. Renal ischemia results and oliguria persists. The overall changes of intermediate shock are diagrammed in Fig. 28-4.

The *irreversible stage* of shock is caused by a decrease in blood volume of more than 25 percent. In this instance compensatory mechanisms are nonfunctioning or no longer effective, and hypotension has reached the critical level to adversely influence the heart and the brain. Advanced changes of splanchnic and renal function are observed.

As the compensatory mechanisms fail, there is rapid deterioration of the microcirculation and surrounding tissue. As a result there is decreased coronary blood flow leading to pump failure, which in turn leads to decreased cardiac output and blood pressure.

In addition to decreased cerebral blood flow there is depressed respiratory neuronal function leading to progressive general hypoxia and damage to capillary endothelium, which results in microcirculation failure and a further decrease in cardiac output and blood pressure. Loss of the central neuronal compensatory mechanism of vasoconstriction results in venous and arteriolar dilatation. This causes peripheral pooling and decreased peripheral resistance, leading to further decrease in cardiac output and arterial pressure.

The overall effects of this shock stage, as noted in Fig. 28-5, are life-threatening owing to decreased cardiac output, arterial pressure, and tissue perfusion.

**T**ypes and Causes of Shock   There are several types or classifications of shock. These include hypovolemic shock, cardiogenic shock, neurogenic shock, and vasogenic shock. Table 28-10 lists the common types of shock and their contributing causes.

*Hypovolemic shock*   A decrease in blood volume (hypovolemia) is a frequent cause of shock. Loss of blood volume diminishes the amount of blood in the circulation and leads to decreased tissue perfusion, decreased venous return, and low cardiac output. This may be affected by the loss of body fluids such as plasma and interstitial fluids.

When *hemorrahagic shock* is present, it is usually due to the loss of whole blood. Acute bleeding following trauma, surgical intervention, bleeding esophageal varices, or rupture of an aneurysm can contribute to the hypovolemic state.

Hemorrhage results in a decreased intravascular volume that causes a decrease in ventricular filling and reduction in stroke volume which, unless compensated for by increased heart rate, will result in a decreased cardiac output and hypotension.

*Cutaneous shock* is most often due to loss of external fluids. The most common cause is burns. *Burn shock* occurs when there is a disruption in body electrolytes and excessive plasma loss. This is attributed to the rapid shift of large amounts of plasma fluid from the vascular compartment into the interstitial area surrounding the burn. A loss of plasma electrolytes and fluid from the body will reduce blood volume and cause the circulating blood to thicken. When this occurs, the general circulation will slow down, thereby diminishing tissue perfusion.

*Gastrointestinal shock* is usually attributed to loss of body fluids and electrolytes (electrolyte shock) in large quantities. Health problems resulting from excessive vomiting and prolonged diarrhea can contribute to this problem (refer to Chap. 17).

*Diabetic shock* is the result of a disruption in the balance of insulin, glucose, water, and electrolytes. Metabolic acidosis and dehydration result, again contributing to a decrease in circulating blood volume (refer to Chap. 20).

*Fractures* of the extremities (i.e., femur, tibia, and fibula) thorax, pelvis, and spine lead to hypotension or shock. This is a result of hemorrhage (both internal and external) and/or loss of extracellular fluid into damaged tissue. Fat emboli may occur as a secondary complication of long-bone fracture and travel to areas such as the lung. (Refer to Chap. 40 for a complete discussion.)

Loss of body fluids can also be observed in *diabetes insipidus.* The *excessive and prolonged use of diuretics* for rapid diuresis and excess loss of body fluids and plasma protein can also create a hypovolemic state. *Ascites* (see Chap. 19) is an additional health problem that can contribute to hypovolemic shock.

**Cardiogenic shock** When the efficiency of the heart as a pump is severely impaired, cardiogenic shock can develop. This can happen when the myocardium has been severely damaged as in a *myocardial infarction,* when the filling of the ventricles is interfered with, as in *pump failure,* or when the heart rate and rhythm are impaired and the efficiency of myocardial contractions is impaired, as with *cardiac arrhythmias.* When the pumping action of the heart is impaired, cardiac output is decreased, lessening the amount of circulating blood volume and impairing oxygenation of the vital

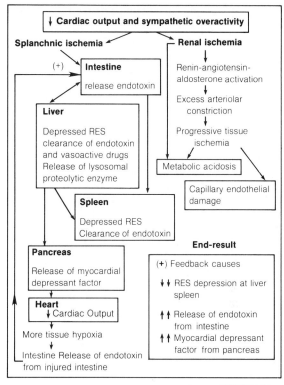

**FIGURE 28-4**

Intermediate stage: involvement of intestine, liver, spleen, pancreas, kidneys and their relationship.

**TABLE 28-10**
COMMON TYPES AND CAUSES OF SHOCK

1  Hypovolemic shock (decrease in blood volume)
   *a*  Hemorrhagic shock
   *b*  Cutaneous shock—burns (external fluid loss)
   *c*  Diabetic shock
   *d*  Gastrointestinal (vomiting and diarrhea) obstruction
   *e*  Diabetes insipidus
   *f*  Excessive use of diuretics
   *g*  Internal sequestration (fractures, hemothorax, ascites)

2  Cardiogenic shock (decreased cardiac output)
   *a*  Myocardial infarction
   *b*  Arrhythmias
   *c*  Pump failure

3  Neurogenic shock
   *a*  Anesthesia (spinal)
   *b*  Barbiturate injection
   *c*  Insulin shock
   *d*  Spinal cord injury

4  Vasogenic shock
   *a*  Toxic shock
   *b*  Anaphylactic shock

SOURCE: From Thorn et al. (eds.), *Harrison's Principles of Internal Medicine,* 8th ed., McGraw-Hill, 1977, p. 186.

organs. Prolonged cardiogenic shock often leads to irreversible shock because of extensive tissue hypoxia and anoxia, as well as extensive myocardial damage.

*Neurogenic shock* In neurogenic shock there is a loss of vascular tone which leads to decreased vasoconstriction and results in systemic vasodilatation. Although blood volume may be within normal limits, it cannot supply capillary beds owing to altered resistance. The loss of the vasoconstricting ability of the medullary vasomotor centers is most probably due to inadequate perfusion of the area.

General *anesthesia* can suppress the body's normal compensatory mechanism to shock if given in large enough doses. *Spinal anesthesia* causes the failure of arterial resistance leading to pooling of blood in dilated vessels. This results in hypotension or shock.

*Insulin shock,* or *hyperinsulinism,* results in a loss of ability of vasomotor nerves to maintain blood vessel tone. This leads to vasodilatation, and hypotension ensues.

*Fracture or dislocations of the spinal cord* re-

sult in squeezing or shearing of the cord, leading to destruction of gray matter and hemorrhage. Immediately after the injury, the patient will develop *spinal shock.* This is followed by a suppression of spinal reflex activity of all spinal segments below the level of the lesion. Paralysis and acute hypotension may accompany the injury. Maximal reflex changes are seen at the level of injury and one or two segments above and below it. As a result of spinal injury, there is a diminished nervous system response and loss of vessel tone. These changes may have systemic effects throughout the body and increase generalized vasodilatation.

Drug *overdose* caused by excessive barbiturates, for example, can depress the central nervous system and contribute to loss of vessel tone. Vasodilatation as well as depression of the vital organs can follow. Hypotension often accompanies these changes with a decrease in tissue perfusion.

*Vasogenic shock* Vasodilatation caused by humoral or toxic substances acting directly on blood vessels can cause vasogenic shock. When this occurs, the peripheral vasculature is dilated, and

**FIGURE 28-5**

Irreversible stage: involvement of heart and brain due to prolonged decrease in cardiac output and arterial pressure with presence of advanced abnormalities on splanchnic system and renal function.

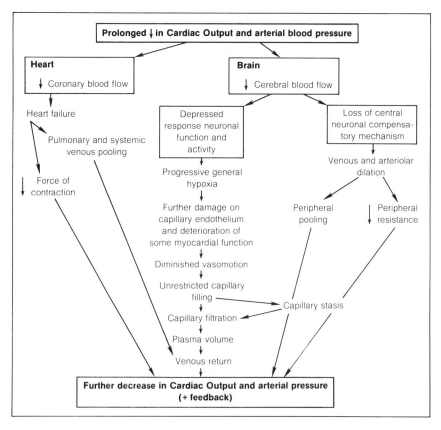

essentially the same phenomena occur as in neurogenic shock.

*Allergic reactions,* such as systemic anaphylaxis, cause hypotension and profound vascular collapse leading to shock and death within minutes unless treatment is instituted immediately. Allergic responses are manifestation of hypersensitivity resulting from the abnormal production of IgE antibodies to otherwise innocuous antigens (allergens) that are in the environment (see Chap. 10 for a complete discussion). Common allergens in humans are various inhalants, insect bites (venom), drugs (i.e., penicillin), and serum (i.e., skin test antigen).[56] Limited experimental data suggested that vascular collapse may be due to the presence of bradykinin, a clinical mediator, which produces vasodilatation and increases vascular permeability.

*Respiratory distress syndrome* associated with anaphylaxis is the result of edema of the hypopharynx and larynx (possibly mediated by histamine) or is due to intractable bronchospasm, possibly mediated by a slow-reacting substance of anaphylaxis (SRS-A). Hypotension may occur secondary to hypoxia induced by respiratory distress. Decrease in ventilation alters oxygen–carbon dioxide exchange and can lead to respiratory arrest and decreased cerebral tissue perfusion.

In *septic shock,* the endotoxin, a lipopolysaccharide, is elaborated from the cell walls of gram-negative bacteria which are released with cellular death or destruction. Examples of these bacteria are *E. coli, Klebsiella Aerobacter-Serratia, Proteus mirabilis,* and *Pseudomonas aeruginosa.* The endotoxin mediates an initial vasodilatation in the peripheral microcirculation. Vasoactive substances such as bradykinin, histamine, SRS-A, and serotonin are released, increasing the permeability of the capillary walls. This allows transudation of plasma constituents into the extracellular tissue fluid. The vasodilatation allows further pooling of blood into the capillary beds and more fluid transudation into tissues, resulting in decrease of venous return, cardiac output, and hypotension.[57]

**E**ffects of Shock on the Patient   Regardless of the primary cause of shock, the general effects of decreased blood volume are similar in each instance. These include a reduction in venous return, a decreased cardiac output, and a decrease in arterial pressure.

Depending on the stage of shock, the patient's symptoms may range from mild hypotension to coma and death. *Tachycardia* due to increased cardiac output and adrenal stimulation will be present. In severe shock the patient's color may be cyanotic. There will be a decrease in urinary output ranging from *oliguria* to *anuria.* Peripheral vasoconstriction will contribute to a *decrease in body temperature* and an *absence of peripheral pulses.* Decreased cerebral tissue perfusion will lead to *anxiety, restlessness,* and *apprehension.* Depending on the cause of shock, *respiration* may be shallow and rapid where the pulse will be weak and thready. A *decrease in arterial blood pressure* will also be noted. *Dehydration* may persist, with alteration in body electrolytes. The patient, if conscious, may complain of thirst. *Nausea* and *vomiting* may be noted depending on the cause of shock. As the stage of shock progresses, the patient's *level of consciousness* may progress from drowsiness and stupor to coma. Signs of *pump failure* may be observed, and *renal failure* will be present. When the changes due to shock become irreversible, death will usually result.

**First-Level Nursing Care**

Hypotension and shock are not diseases but rather are indicators of a health problem, or many problems. Therefore, in order to prevent hypotensive and/or shock states, it is important to identify those persons at risk.

All individuals who experience blood loss by either external or internal causes are at risk to develop shock. Persons who sustain hemorrhage resulting from direct or indirect trauma (e.g., surgery or laceration), gastric bleeding (e.g., gastric ulcers or esophageal varices), and fractures are potential candidates for loss in blood volume. Diabetics, especially uncontrolled diabetics, individuals who use diuretics in large amounts, and patients with diabetes insipidus, may potentially have an increased and rapid loss of body fluids and develop shock from volume depletion. Persons who sustain severe burns may develop shock depending upon the severity of the burn, the extent of internal and external body surface involved, and the amount of fluid loss present.

Patients with chronic health problems such as myocardial ischemia are potential candidates for developing myocardial infarctions. If the cardiac muscle is weakened by the infarct, or if congestive heart failure and/or arrhythmias develop, cardiogenic shock can occur. Excessive use of anesthesia, an anaphalactic reaction to the anesthetic, use of barbiturates (e.g., overdose and in the aged), along with diabetics who receive more insulin than the body can tolerate, can develop a shock state. Trauma to the spinal cord as with spinal cord injury, patients with systemic bacterial infections, as well as persons who are sensitive to noxious sources in the external environment, e.g., drugs (penicillin), insects, poison, or foods such as shellfish, can also be at risk to develop shock.

**Prevention**  In order to prevent hypotension and/or the shock state, care should be taken to correct those states in which hypovolemia can occur. When obvious bleeding occurs, outside the hospital setting, immediate first aid should be instituted to prevent further blood loss. Pressure should be applied directly to the area or above the artery that supplies the injured site. The part affected should be elevated in order to diminish blood flow to the area, and the wound should be covered. If the bleeding sites are extensive, the patient should lie flat with the legs elevated to increase peripheral blood supply to the heart. The patient should be kept warm (covered with a blanket) to prevent chilling. Increases in metabolism can be caused by excessive heat or cold and will result in increased oxygen demand. Both extremes should be avoided.

Following surgery the patient's vital signs should be closely observed for changes which might indicate bleeding. Close observation of the wound site may also indicate internal bleeding. Continued evaluation of drainage (e.g., chest tubes, urinary catheters) will help the nurse evaluate the amount of volume loss, and careful evaluation of blood gases, electrolytes, and a complete blood count will indicate tissue perfusion and fluid balance. Blood pressure should be carefully checked following spinal anesthesia.

Continuous checking of blood sugar levels along with testing of urine can help evaluate the diabetic's response to insulin and indicate control of the diabetic problem. Prevention of atherosclerosis (see Chap. 26) and subsequent myocardial ischemia will decrease the risk of myocardial infarction and the potential for cardiogenic shock. Prompt treatment of arrhythmias and signs of pump failure will help prevent disruptions in heart rate and rhythm and limit the overall disruptions in cardiac output.

Careful identification of individuals with allergic reactions to specific substances will prevent anaphylaxis. Administration of skin tests or utilization of test doses prior to the administration of a drug or potentially noxious stimulus will help identify a potentially allergic reaction and prevent its occurrence. Patients who are sensitive to particular substances in the environment should be made aware of the problem and encouraged to avoid the noxious stimuli. They should be told to report all allergies to health providers and taught administration of intramuscular medications to reverse toxic effect of the causative agent. Special kits containing adrenalin and other preparations are now available for individuals who are specifically sensitive to noxious stimuli in the environment.

Prevention of burns is most important in eliminating the volume loss that may ensue. If a burn does occur, prompt treatment of the victim and early fluid replacement are critical to the prevention of shock (see Chap. 13).

Patients who have been on bed rest for long periods of time should progress gradually from a lying to sitting to standing position to avoid orthostatic hypotension. The patient should be instructed to exercise the legs continually, then gradually sit on the edge of the bed for a few minutes, and then with assistance stand.

### Second-Level Nursing Care

Shock is rarely treated in the community even in its earliest stages. Therefore nursing is directed toward identification of potential shock victims, emergency intervention when possible, and referral to an acute-care setting.

**Case finding and referral**  Individuals who have sustained shock may be bleeding severely either internally or externally. Those who sustain extensive burn injuries, diabetics who develop diabetic coma or insulin reaction, persons who react severely to insect bites, as well as persons with additional injuries due to accidents, such as fractures and spinal cord injury, should be assessed for shock symptoms. Individuals who sustain a myocardial infarction should also be observed for hypotension and cardiac or respiratory arrest. When these individuals are identified as potential shock victims, they should be moved as little as possible. An adequate airway should be established if one is not already present. If needed, cardiopulmonary resuscitation should be started (refer to Chap. 26 for a complete discussion). Changes noted in early shock may include diaphoresis, changes in pupil size, pallor, decreased capillary refill, decreased peripheral pulses, decreased body temperature, respiratory changes, and alterations in level of consciousness.

If bleeding is obvious, attempts should be made to terminate the bleeding by direct application of pressure over the bleeding site and/or the proximal artery or vein as necessary. The affected part should be elevated when possible, and tourniquets should be avoided. A pressure dressing can also be placed over the injury if necessary. When an individual has incurred a burn, the rescuer should be certain the burning process has terminated. When possible the wound should be cleansed, and constricting clothing removed from around the area of the burn (see Chap. 13 for a complete discussion of burn care).

The patient with impending shock should be kept warm to avoid chilling but not hot so as not to interfere with the body's normal compensating response. When spinal injury is *not* present, the legs can be elevated, with the knees kept straight. The head can remain flat or slightly elevated. If neurological damage is suspected (refer to Chaps. 32 and 40), the patient should not be moved.

If possible, a detailed history should be obtained and sent to the hospital with the patient. This should include the nature of the injury and any details that surround the incident, such as the type of fire, a description of an automobile accident, or the nature of an insect bite. A brief assessment including the patient's color, level of consciousness, pulse and respiratory rates, capillary refill index, complaints of thirst as well as indications of nausea and vomiting and skin reaction should accompany the patient's history if possible. If shock is suspected, the patient should be quickly moved to an acute-care setting for more complete treatment.

### Third-Level Nursing Care

Marked hypotension accompanied by signs of shock requires prompt care, and hospitalization. Patients entering the hospital with hypotension must be cared for quickly, and all problems must be assessed immediately. When shock syndrome appears, rapid intervention is needed to prevent the condition from becoming irreversible.

**Nursing assessment**  When the patient is admitted to an acute-care setting, an accurate health history is required. This should be followed by a complete physical assessment in order to evaluate the injuries as well as the stage of shock present.

**H**ealth history  The health history should be obtained from the patient and/or family or friends. Data identified in Second-Level Nursing Care should be incorporated into the history. Identification of past and present health problems as well as current medications being taken should be elicited. Injury (both internal and external), blood loss, myocardial infarction, or exposure to allergens may suggest the precipitating cause for hypotension and/or the shock state. The patient may be restless or irritable and complain of feeling anxious. Depending on the cause, the patient may complain of temperature changes (hot or cold). In some situations, the patient may appear stuporous, confused, or nonresponsive. Weakness and generalized fatigue may also be discussed. Again, depending upon the cause of the shock state, pain, excessive thirst, cutaneous itching, and diaphoresis may be noted.

**P**hysical Assessment  A complete physical examination will reveal a variety of changes depending upon the cause of shock. In the absence of infection there will be a drop in body temperature. The skin may appear cold to touch and clammy. If cardiogenic shock is present, the skin and lips may appear cyanotic. If the cause of shock is infectious, facial rubor (redness) may be observed. In hemorrhagic shock the patient is often pale or ashen. The patient may be shivering owing to peripheral vasoconstriction, and this can lead to exhaustion and fatigue. If the patient has been burned, there may be obvious charring of the skin with a loss of fluid (see Chap. 13 for burn assessment).

When the loss of body fluids is severe, the mucous membranes will be dry and signs of dehydration will appear. Oliguria or anuria may appear before severe hypotention is noted. Signs of metabolic acidosis may also be present. (See Chap. 12 for a complete discussion.)

The apical and radial pulses should be checked, and the pulse deficit noted. The pulse will be rapid at first and often weak. As shock progresses, the pulse rate will become slow. Changes in rhythm may be noted, especially in the presence of severe myocardial ischemia.

Palpation of peripheral pulses is also helpful in assessing shock. Usually in early shock the pulses are weak or inaudible owing to vasoconstriction. In addition, when checking the nail beds, capillary refill time will be slowed in shock. Circulation may also be assessed by evaluating venous collapse in the periphery. This can be observed by applying finger pressure to a peripheral vein and watching whether it collapses. This change is usually noted in shock when little blood is present in the vein because of peripheral vasoconstriction.

Respirations will be rapid and shallow, resulting in an accumulation of carbon dioxide which stimulates the respiration rate. In the presence of pump failure, the patient may experience a cough, and fluid may be heard in the lungs. Auscultation of breath sounds may reveal pulmonary congestion and rales. Dyspnea may also be noted (for additional signs of failure, see Chap. 24). In marked shock Cheyne-Stokes breathing may also be observed.

Hypotension is usually not noted until there is a loss of 15 to 20 percent of blood volume. Some patients do not demonstrate hypotension until there is a 25 percent loss of blood volume.[58] Therefore, evaluation of arterial blood pressure readings in early shock is often unreliable. When changes do occur in blood pressure, a decrease in both systolic and diastolic pressure is heard. Assessment of the distance between these two points (pulse pressure) is often more helpful in assessing hypotension, because the differences reveal overall changes in stroke volume.

There is an instance when hypertension may be observed in the presence of shock. This is referred to as *compensated shock.* It results from vigorous sympathico-adrenal activity which maintains and even elevates the blood pressure.[59]

Alterations in sensorium can range from anxiety and irritability to confusion and stupor. Upon neurological examination increased reflex activity may be noted in early shock, while diminished reflexes may accompany latent stages of shock. As there is decreased cerebral perfusion and brain tissue anoxia, the patient will become stuporous and coma may ensue. Additional systemic neurological changes may be noted.

Nausea and vomiting can be present, and when internal hemorrhage is suspected, the vomitus should be checked for blood. Occult blood may also be present in the stool, which should be checked frequently. Drainage from any orifice should also be evaluated for the amount and consistency. Changes in bowel sounds will vary, depending upon the cause of shock. An absence of all bowel sounds may lead to suspicion of an intestinal obstruction. Assessment of urinary output and concentration will also help to evaluate tissue perfusion. Urinary output of less than 30 ml/hour may indicate a decrease in renal plasma flow and glomerular filtration rate. These changes are usually noted in the early and intermediate stages of shock.

**D**iagnostic Tests Multiple diagnostic tests are used to determine the effects on pump pressure and tissue perfusion. These tests include central venous, pulmonary artery pressure, and intra-arterial pressure monitoring.

The *central venous pressure* (CVP) is measured to assess vascular volume and efficiency of cardiac pumping of the right side of the heart. CVP can be measured by a catheter inserted into the antecubital fossae veins. These veins are frequently used because of ease of puncture, adequate size, and minimal discomfort to the patient. The lateral cephalic vein should be avoided since advancing the catheter through the shoulder region is difficult. An external or internal jugular vein may also be used for catheter insertion, but this procedure may be more uncomfortable for the patient, and it is difficult to control bleeding. However, a low incidence of thrombophlebitis, large-size veins, and high blood flow in these sites make them ideal for long-term indwelling CVP catheters.[60] The subclavian vein may also be used since it provides many of the advantages of the jugular veins. However, potential development of a pneumothorax (5 percent) must be considered when this site is being used, especially if the catheter is dislodged from the site of insertion.[61]

The skin over the *insertion site* should be shaved, if necessary, and an iodine preparation such as providone-iodine complex (Betadine) should be applied and allowed to dry. A solution of 70% alcohol should then be applied. Sterile gloves should be worn, and sterile technique should be maintained throughout the procedure. Prior to insertion the catheter tip is measured. Figure 28-6 demonstrates the position of the catheter in the superior vena cava; the length can be estimated by measuring the horizontal, straight distance between the proposed insertion site and the sternal notch while the packaged or protected catheter is placed along the arm. Note that the arm is extended to make an L-shaped angle to the chest.

The *catheter is inserted* into the vein and threaded through the superior vena cava into the right atrium. The catheter should advance easily without resistance. To prevent air embolism during insertion of the catheter into the jugular or subclavian vein, the nurse may place the patient in Trendelenburg's position. This position also distends the veins for ease of puncture. The patient's head is turned opposite to the side of the insertion site. The insertion site should be infiltrated with a local anesthetic. After the catheter enters the vein and a venous blood return is seen in the syringe, the syringe is removed. The catheter is then advanced and positioned in the midsuperior vena cava (Fig. 28-7). The catheter is sutured in place and taped securely to prevent inadvertent movement from the atria. A *sterile dressing* is applied. The dressing should be changed every 2 or 3 days by the nurse, using aseptic technique to prevent infection.

The *catheter is connected to a manometer* in an IV tubing by way of a three-way stopcock (see Fig. 28-8). An intravenous solution of 5% dextrose and water is usually infused continuously to keep the vein open when a reading is to be taken. The patient should be lying flat in bed in a relaxed position. The zero level of the manometer should be at the level of the right atrium (midauxilliary level). It is advisable to mark the level on the skin so that the subsequent readings can be taken at the same level. If the patient cannot lie in a flat position, the zero level should be adjusted accordingly and marked on the chest wall.

The nurse fills the manometer above the level of the expected pressure by turning the stopcock to connect the IV tubing and manometer, while the flow to the patient by the catheter is stopped. Once the manometer is properly filled, the stopcock is turned to connect manometer and the catheter while the connection to the IV tubing is closed. *The CVP reading* is based upon the equalization of pressures in the central vein versus the effects of gravity on the fluid. As the fluid level of the manometer decreases infusing into the patient, the level is reached at which no further decrease occurs. The fluid level will fluctuate in synchrony with the patient's respirations. The CVP reading is made at this stabilized point. The highest level of fluid in the column represents the central venous pressure. The normal range is between 5 and 8 $mgH_2O$. An elevated CVP reading usually indicates a disruption in cardiac output as seen in pump failure and pulmonary edema. A low or falling CVP reading is indicative of a decrease in circulating blood volume (hypovolemia).

*After the reading* is taken the stopcock should be readjusted to resume the IV infusion. The CVP site should be observed for phlebitis and kept clean. Aseptic technique should be used when changing the dressing.

*Pulmonary artery pressure* (PAP) is a measure of the pressure in the main branch of the pulmonary artery which reflects the function of the left side of heart by measuring the pressure within the pulmonary artery.

PAP can be measured with a venous pressure transducer connected to an oscilloscope to monitor for continuous display. Pressure values are most accurate if the patient is in a supine position and is not on a ventilator. The normal value of a PAP reading should be 25/10 mmHg, mean being 13–15 mmHg.

The *choice of vein* and skin preparation are essentially the same as for CVP measurement. Prior to the insertion of the catheter, the patient is attached to an EKG monitor, so that cardiac rhythm changes can be detected. As the catheter is

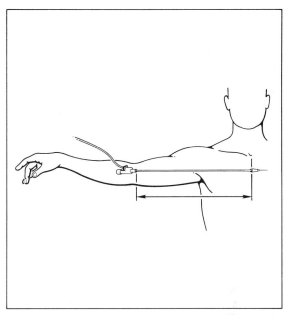

**FIGURE 28-6**

CVP catheter length. Catheter is measured from the place where it will be inserted to the sternal notch. The measurement is an estimate of the length of the catheter required in order to place the catheter tip in the superior vena cava. (*From J. S. Schroeder et al., Techniques in Bedside Hemodynamic Monitoring, Mosby, St. Louis, 1976.*)

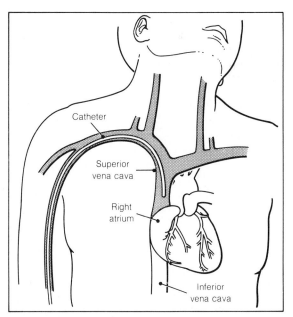

**FIGURE 28-7**

CVP catheter position. The tip of the catheter is in the midsuperior vena cava; the catheter has been advanced from the right basilic vein. (*From J. S. Schroeder et al., Techniques in Bedside Hemodynamic Monitoring, Mosby, St. Louis, 1976.*)

threaded through the atria and ventricles, the catheter tip may hit the ventricular wall and stimulate premature ventricular contractions. The *Swan-Ganz flow-directed, balloon-tipped catheter* is inserted into a selected vein under the guidance of fluoroscopy[62] (see Fig. 28-9). When the balloon enters the vein, it is partially inflated with 0.4 to 0.6 cc air and is propelled into the right atrium by blood flow. An additional 0.2 cc air is injected into the balloon as it propels through the tricuspid valve, right ventricle, pulmonic valve, and into the pulmonary artery. When this occurs there is a slight rise in the diastolic pressure reading. The final position of the catheter can be ascertained by the aid of fluoroscopy. To prevent the formation of a thrombus at the catheter tip, 1 unit heparin per milliliter IV fluid is added. The level of the pressure transducer is to be at midchest height. If the level is higher than midchest level, negative or inappropriately low pressure is recorded. The amplifier (monitor) should be warmed up for at least 30 minutes before the transducer is plugged into it. The "zero" dial on the amplifer is calibrated against the atmospheric pressure by turning the stopcock to room air. If the stopcock is not open to air, buildup of pressure within the transducer gives a false reading.

The PAP should be measured when the balloon is *deflated* and the catheter is properly connected to the amplifier. After the pressure measurement, the nurse keeps the catheter open by slow IV drip. An elevated pressure is usually present with left-sided failure and pulmonary hypertension, associated with pump failure and pulmonary edema.

*Pulmonary artery wedge pressure* (PWP) reflects most accurately the pressure of the left atrium and left ventricle and measures the efficiency of cardiac output. A catheter is guided through the major vein and allowed to flow into the right atrium through the tricuspid valve into the right ventricle and into the pulmonary valve and pulmonary airway. The catheter migrates to a small arterial branch in the lung. A tiny balloon is inflated with normal saline or 0.80 cc air and wedged into an arterial branch where it obstructs the flow of pulmonary artery blood (when inflated) for a few

**FIGURE 28-8**
Procedure for measuring CVP. (a) Manometer and IV tubing in place; (b) stopcock is turned so that the manometer fills with fluid above the level of the expected pressure; (c) stopcock is turned so that the IV is off and the fluid in the manometer flows to the patient; a reading is obtained after the fluid level stabilizes; (d) stopcock is turned to continue the IV flow to the patient. (*From J.S. Schroeder et al., Techniques in Bedside Hemodynamic Monitoring, Mosby, St. Louis, 1976.*)

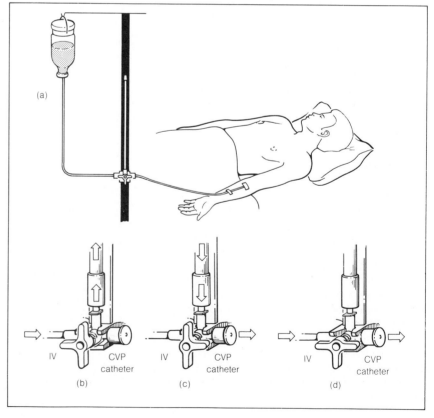

seconds. The pressure is recorded through a transducer and shown on an oscilloscope. The mean pressure ranges between 4 and 12 mmHg.

*Hemoptysis* can occur owing to excessive expansion of the balloon while it is in the wedge position causing rupture of pulmonary capillaries and intrapulmonary hemorrhage. *Rupture* of the pulmonary artery caused by a weakness in the arterial wall can occur as the catheter is placed into the pulmonary artery. *Arrhythmias* are often observed when the catheter passes through the right ventricle. Premature ventricular beats frequently occur when the catheter tip hits the ventricular wall as it passes to the pulmonary artery. This acts as an extra stimulus in the conduction pathway and results in arrhythmias. *Localized* tissue necrosis caused by prolonged inflation of the balloon can also be observed. When the balloon remains inflated, blood flow to the tissue is diminished and tissue hypoxia develops. Sluggish blood flow commonly seen in shock as well as the potential for *thrombus formation* at the catheter site predisposes the patient to the threat of *emboli* and *infarction.* Anticoagulants may be used to prevent this problem.

*Maintaining the patency of the catheter* for continuous recording (for example, of PAP) is essential. To ensure patency, the catheter may need to be irrigated every 15 minutes. A Sorenson Intraflow Device may be used to resolve the problem. This device utilizes a pressure bag IV fluid system and continuously delivers a maximum of 2 to 4 ml IV fluid per hour through the catheter. Periodic quick-high flushes can be performed without stopcock maneuvers. This system works well, if the IV fluid contains 1 unit heparin per milliliter IV fluid, if cardiac output is good, and if there is pulsatile flow at the catheter tip.

The conventional arm-cuff method to measure arterial pressure is not accurate or difficult to obtain in patients with low cardiac output (hypotension) and excessive peripheral vasoconstriction (shock). Blood pressure may be measured by palpation, but this is not a satisfactory method for continuous monitoring. *Intraarterial pressure measurements* provide accurate systolic, diastolic, and mean pressure readings on a continuous basis. This accuracy is vitally important during cardiac surgery and the administration of vasopressor or vasodilator agents. The continuous monitoring enables more frequent measurements in less nursing time. The mean arterial pressure (MAP) can be estimated by the following equation:

$$MAP = \frac{\text{systolic pressure} + (\text{diastolic pressure} \times 2)}{3}$$

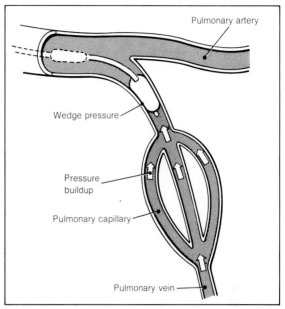

**FIGURE 28-9**
Pulmonary artery pressure. Balloon is deflated during initial positioning of balloon-tipped catheter in the pulmonary artery; catheter is then advanced, and the balloon is reinflated just enough to get a PAP pressure. (*From J. S. Schroeder et al., Techniques in Bedside Hemodynamic Monitoring, Mosby, St. Louis, 1976.*)

Sites commonly used for catheter insertion are the brachial, radial, and femoral arteries. The *brachial artery* can be easily palpated and punctured by a needle. Oozing or bleeding can also be easily controlled, but thrombus formation with an indwelling catheter is the problem. The *radial artery* is easily palpated, but catheter insertion is difficult due to its smaller size. The *femoral artery,* easiest of all to palpate and puncture, is more difficult to use than the other two sites. Control of oozing or active bleeding is much more difficult at this site, causing occult bleeding into abdominal or thigh tissues. The patient's mobility is limited, and the physical care of the patient during the monitoring is also difficult. Since this monitoring device provides accurate and continuous information for the patient in shock, it is usually used during this period. Care should be taken to move the patient carefully and observe for bleeding and oozing from the catheter site.

Additional laboratory tests will include hemoglobin and hematocrit levels (decreased in hypovolemic shock); blood urea nitrogen and creatine levels (increased in the presence of anuria); alteration in $P_{O_2}$ and $P_{CO_2}$ levels (altered in tissue perfusion and hypoxia); elevation or depletion in blood glucose levels (e.g., diabetic coma); elevation in leukocytes (seen with infection), decrease in plasma protein level and disruption in blood electrolytes (especially in hypovolemia). An EKG may also be done to assess cardiac rate and rhythm, and chest x-rays will help evaluate respiratory status.

**Nursing problems and intervention** Many nursing problems can occur with the patient in shock. In general these problems result from a decrease in cardiac output, diminished circulating blood volumes (hypovolemia), and decreased tissue perfusion.

These problems result in hypotension, tachycardia, oliguria, and anuria, disruption in respirations, alterations in level of consciousness, anxiety and irritability, sensory deprivation, changes in body temperature, and immobility.

*Decreased arterial pressure* A decrease in arterial pressure (hypotension) is usually observed in patients in acute shock. This problem may be intensified in the presence of toxic substances, inflammatory processes, myocardial infarction, hemorrhage, or drug intoxication (e.g., anesthesia).

Many opinions are offered on the effectiveness of drug therapy to elevate the arterial blood pressure. The conflict is between using vasoconstrictors or vasodilators to accomplish an increase in arterial pressure. Alpha-adrenergic drugs (such as epinephrine or Aramine) are *vasopressors* used for all types of shock because of their ability to cause peripheral vasoconstriction and elevate the arterial blood pressure. However, routine use of these drugs should be avoided since it is known that an increase in arterial blood pressure may be temporary if the underlying pathology is not identified. The vasoconstricting effect that is achieved may even be detrimental in many instances.

Pharmacologic effects of certain *adrenergic drugs* are given in Table 28-11. The major effect of these drugs is to cause peripheral vasoconstriction thereby depriving the vital organs of needed blood supply. Some research suggests that use of these drugs in the treatment of shock can accentuate the changes that occur with shock such as tissue hypoxia, anxiety, and changes in body temperature.

*Beta-adrenergic blockers* (see Table 28-11) and *ganglionic blockers* which are vasodilators are currently being studied because of their overall systemic effects during shock. These drugs counter the effect of prolonged vasoconstriction. Researchers suggest that if vasodilators are used to treat shock, there will be redistribution of blood to the vital organs and blood collected in the periphery by vasoconstriction can reenter the circulation and increase the total blood volume.

Often drug therapy used to control hypotension involves a combination of several drugs. Drugs which have a mixed alph-beta-adrenergic effect on the patient in shock are often selected (see Table 28-12). Dopamine, which is a mixed alpha- and beta-adrenergic agent, has been used widely due to its favorable effect on renal and splanchnic blood flow. However, its ultimate relative value in the treatment of shock remains to be determined.

Epinephrine is another choice drug because of its great value in the treatment of anaphylaxis, but its use is limited for other forms of shock. The beta-adrenergic stimulating agent isoproterenol may be used as a temporary means to increase heart rate in patients with sinus bradycardia. However, its use is contraindicated in patients with shock following myocardial infarction.

Corticosteroids are used in shock to increase blood flow and decrease blood resistance, thereby augmenting the beneficial effects of vasopressor agents.[63] *Corticosteroids* are particularly beneficial in septic and cardiogenic shock. They can also be used for patients who have allergic reactions. Pharmacological properties of commonly used corticosteriods are given in Table 28-13.

**D**ecreased Cardiac Output Tachycardia is usually present in early shock. It represents the heart's compensatory response to an increase in adrenalin in order to stimulate cardiac output. Inotropic drugs (such as digitalis preparations) are used to slow the heart rate and improve overall cardiac output. Isoproterenol may be used as a temporary means of increasing heart rate, especially in the presence of bradycardia. If tachycardia persists, especially in the presence of myocardial ischemia, pump failure may develop.

In addition, cardiac arrhythmias may develop in the presence of increased catecholamine production and myocardial damage. If *bradycardia* is present, atropine or isoproterenol may be given to stimulate the heart rate. Continuous EKG monitoring is essential to assess changes in cardiac rhythm (see Chap. 22).

*Central venous pressure readings* along with *pulmonary artery wedge pressures* should be checked frequently to monitor the presence of and/or the severity of pump failure (see Chap. 24 for care of the patient with pump failure). If arrhythmias develop, antiarrhythmic drugs may be used (refer Chap. 25). When cardiac output is severely de-

**TABLE 28-11**
ADRENERGIC DRUGS USED IN HYPOTENSION

| Drug | | Vasometer Effect* | | Cardiac Stimulant (inotropic effect)* | Cardiac Output† | Renal and Splanchnic Blood Flow† | Route of Administration and Dosage | General Remarks |
| --- | --- | --- | --- | --- | --- | --- | --- | --- |
| Generic Name | Trade Name | Vaso-constriction | Vaso-dilatation | | | | | |
| ALPHA-ADRENERGIC | | | | | | | | |
| Phenylephrine | Neo-Synephrine | 5 | 0 | 0 | ↓ | ↓ | 0.8 mg IV | Monitor BP, CVP, PAP, PWP, and urine output. Monitor EKG for tachyarrhythmias. Avoid extravasation (may cause tissue necrosis and gangrene). If it occurs, treatment is by infiltrating the tissue with 5–10 mg Regitine (phentolamine). |
| MIXED ALPHA- AND BETA-ADRENERGIC | | | | | | | | |
| Norepinephrine | Levophed | 4 | 0 | 2 | ↓ | ↓ | 8 mg/500 cc 5% D/W continuous IV at 0.25 cc (0.04 mg) to 1.0 cc (0.16 mg)/m | |
| Metaraminol | Aramine | 3 | 2 | 1 | ↓ | ↓ | 5 to 10 mg IM | |
| Epinephrine | Adrenalin | 4 | 2 | 4 | Usually ↑ | ↑ | 500 mg/500 cc 5% D/W continuous IV infusion at 0.25 cc (0.25 mg) to 1.0 cc (1.0 mg)/m | |
| BETA-ADRENERGIC | | | | | | | | |
| Isoproterenol | Isuprel | 0 | 5 | 4 | ↑ | Usually ↓ | 2 mg/500 cc 5% D/W continuous IV infusion at 0.25 cc (0.001 mg) to 1.0 cc (0.004 mg)/m | Monitor continuously for tachyarrhythmias. Defibrillation should be available. Watch for signs of thickening of bronchial secretions. |

* Effects graded on a scale of 0 to 5.
† ↓ = reduced, ↑ = increased.
SOURCE: From Chatton and Krupp, p. 6.

**TABLE 28-12**
ALPHA-ADRENERGIC BLOCKADE USED IN HYPOTENSION

| Drug Generic Name | Trade Name | Action | Route of Administration and Dosage | General Remarks |
|---|---|---|---|---|
| Phenoxybenzamine | Dibenzyline | Improves microcirculation and cardiac output | 1 mg/kg body weight in 100 ml 5% D/W IV drip for 2- to 4-h period | Maintain constant IV flow when drug is given to avoid profound decrease in BP. If BP drops below 70 mmHg, the drug may be stopped and IV fluid increased. BP and CVP should be monitored; keep patient flat. Reflex tachycardia and orthostatic hypotension may persist for 24 h with phenoxybenzamine. |
| Chlorpromazine | Thorazine | | 5 mg IV push with other IV volume expander or IV drip at 0.6 mg/m | |

creased, mechanical circulatory assistance may be utilized.

**Circulatory Assistance** In order to assist the circulation during periods of transient myocardial depression, a method called *counterpulsation* is utilized. The two primary objectives of counterpulsation are to provide temporary mechanical assistance to the patient's circulation until the underlying pathophysiologic condition is corrected and to render optimal conditions for repair of the heart. Two types of devices are available to accomplish the objectives. One of these is the *intraaortic balloon pump,* and the other is the *external noninvasive circulatory assist device.*

The intraaortic balloon pump is used to improve cardiac output and blood pressure during cardiogenic shock. It is a mechanical device made to pump the aortic blood flow back to the aortic notch by inflating the balloon during diastole. This augments coronary artery perfusion, thereby assisting repair or restoration of myocardial function. The balloon is deflated during the systole in order to lower intraaortic pressure (see Fig. 28-10). The basic principles of the intraaortic balloon pump was in-

troduced by Moulopoulos and coworkers in 1962 and was further developed by the Kantrowitz team in 1967. The balloon catheter is inserted into the femoral artery by cut-down method under local anesthesia. The position of the catheter is confirmed by fluoroscope examination; the optimal position is just distal to the left subclavian artery. This position offers two advantages: the balloon is close enough to the aortic valve to optimize diastolic augmentation and yet far enough away that the risk of cerebral embolism is reduced.

When the balloon is positioned properly, the catheter is attached to the gas-pumping apparatus. Helium and carbon dioxide are used for this purpose. Since helium is lighter and has a more rapid delivery time, it facilitates the function of the balloon at fast heart rates and during arrhythmias.

Use of $CO_2$ gas reduces the potential risk of developing gas emboli if the balloon is ruptured. This is due to the high solubility of the $CO_2$ gas in the blood.

One of three types of balloon attached to a gas driving unit is used to achieve essentially the same hemodynamic results. The *single-chambered device* has a single, sausage-shaped balloon. When

**TABLE 28-13**
CORTICOSTEROIDS USED IN HYPOTENSION

| Drug Generic Name | Trade Name | Action | Dosage and Route of Administration | General Remarks |
|---|---|---|---|---|
| Methylprednisolone | Solumedrol | Add to inotropic effect. Decrease peripheral vascular resistance. Stabilization of lysosomes. Prevent MDF formation. Increase urine flow; antiendotoxic, anti-inflammatory; preserve integrity of capillary in the presence of anoxia. | 30 mg/kg body weight IV push | IV push should be given slowly for 5–10 min combined with adequate volume administration. The dose may be repeated in 4 to 6 h. Early administration (as soon as shock is suspected) is recommended. Watch for GI bleeding. Monitor BP, CVP, skin appearance, and $Na^+$ and $K^+$ levels. |
| Dexamethasone | Decadron | | 4.5 mg/kg body weight IV push | |
| Hydrocortisone | Solucortef | | 2 to 10 g IV | |

SOURCE: From Jahre et al.

inflated, the balloon displaces blood volume, both retrograde to the aortic arch and antegrade, to perfuse those areas distal to the balloon. The volume displaced causes more blood flow retrograde to the aortic arch, increasing distolic pressure and coronary perfusion. The *dual-chambered balloon* has a small, round balloon located distally and a large, second balloon more proximal to the aortic root. The smaller chamber is timed to inflate slightly before the large one in order to provide the resistance to the antegrade boost caused by inflation of the second, larger balloon. This results in even greater volume of retrograde flow to perfuse the coronary arteries. The *triple-segmented balloon* is designed to make the middle section of the chamber inflate first and the upper and lower balloons inflate immediately thereafter. This action results in both antegrade and retrograde blood displacement. The balloon size is estimated to be about 85 percent of the diameter of the aorta, since the diameter of the aorta varies with the individual patient and with the mean arterial pressure, and must be estimated accordingly.

The sequence of *inflation and deflation* should be timed exactly for successful therapy. This requires three factors: an EKG, an arterial pressure wave form, and a skilled and knowledgeable nurse. The EKG is used as a sensing mechanism for triggering the gas delivery system. Inflation occurs shortly after the T wave (diastole begins), and deflation occurs at the time of the QRS complex (when systole begins) (Fig. 28-11). Normally EKG precedes the mechanical events of systole and diastole by several fractions of a second. This is why the QRS complex precedes the peak of the arterial systole in the diagram. The dicrotic notch of the arterial wave form is used as the point at which the balloon is inflated. Deflation is timed to occur just before the systolic upstroke of the pressure wave form.

The most frequently encountered *complication* of balloon pumping is vascular insufficiency of the catheterized limb. For this reason, the largest femoral artery with the best pulse should be used for balloon insertion. Heparin may be administered to prevent thrombus formation. The nurse should check carefully and frequently the involved extremities for any changes of color, quality of pulsation, and temperature. Platelet reduction is fre-

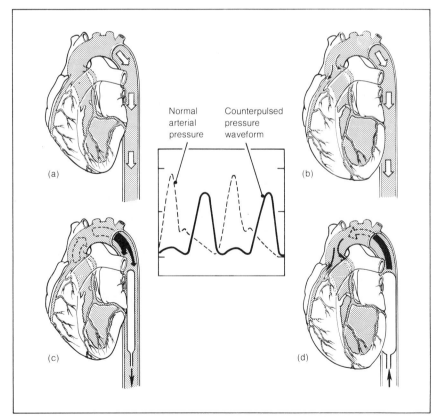

**FIGURE 28-10**

Physiology of counterpulsation. (*a*) Normal systole, characterized by antegrade volume flow and peak intraaortic pressures; (*b*) normal diastole, showing continued antegrade volume flow and adequate intraaortic pressure for coronary perfusion; (*c*) balloon deflation before systole, allowing antegrade volume flow from the aortic arch (systolic unloading); (*d*) counterpulsed diastole, mechanically boosting volume flow retrograde to the aortic arch, heightening diastolic pressure and coronary perfusion. (*From J. S. Schroeder et al., Techniques in Bedside Hemodynamic Monitoring, Mosby, St. Louis, 1976.*)

Normal arterial pressure

Counterpulsed pressure waveform

quently observed in patients with the balloon pump. Injection of heparin may prevent this. Other rarely observed complications are gas embolism due to balloon rupture, aortic damage (aortic wall dissection, intimal laceration, or hematoma), emboli from the balloon and catheter, and hemolysis. Careful technique of balloon insertion, proper size of the catheter, use of $CO_2$ as the inflation gas, and limiting the patient's movement may prevent the aforementioned complications. The nurse should instruct the patient not to flex the legs since this may move the balloon tip up to the aorta, possibly resulting in puncture of the arch.

The *optimal duration* for balloon pumping has not been established. Some investigators believe that pumping should be terminated within 48 hours even though longer assistance is possible. To prevent balloon dependence, however, early termination is recommended.

The systematic weaning process can be achieved by several methods. One method is to alternate the amount of time the patient is on the balloon pump with an equal time off the pump. The other method employs the balloon to pump every other heartbeat, then every third or fourth beat, and

so on, until the patient is finally weaned. This process may take hours to days, depending on the hemodynamic status of the patient.

The *external noninvasive circulatory assist* employs a counterpulsation method externally to the lower extremities (Fig. 28-12). The device consists of two long, rigid support forms that are attached together in a V shape to encase the patient's legs. Inside the rigid casing there are tubelike, inflatable bags that encircle each leg from ankle to thigh. The bags are filled with water at body temperature, and these fill the remaining space inside the rigid support structure completely. Tubes connect the bags to a hydraulic pumping unit which alters the bag pressure synchronously with the cardiac cycle.

Positive pressure (between 150 and 200 mmHg) is applied, by the hydraulic pumping device, (compressing the patient's legs) during *diastole*. This procedure displaces the blood from the arteries and veins in the legs to the heart (it is called *diastolic augmentation*). The procedure will also increase the diastolic pressure, and when this pressure equals or exceeds the systolic pressure, the counterpulsation method is effective.

The pressure is then released just before the

**FIGURE 28-11**

Intraaortic balloon. After initiation of counterpulsation, diastolic pressure is heightened and systolic and end-diastolic pressures are lowered. (*From J. S. Schroeder et al., Techniques in Bedside Hemodynamic Monitoring, Mosby, St. Louis, 1976.*)

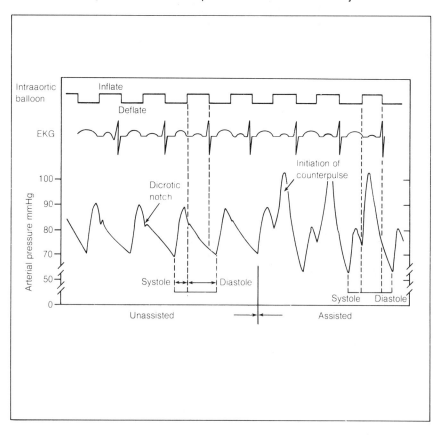

onset of *systole* in order to refill the arteries and veins in the legs (it is called *systolic unloading*). Negative pressure of about −30 mmHg can be applied during systole to facilitate the unloading effect.

Even though it is highly desirable to use this external counterpulsation device because of its noninvasive nature and the ease of initiation of the therapy, *several problems* have been identified. This device has a limited value when used for patients with peripheral vascular disease since it uses intravascular blood reservoirs for its volume displacement. *Discomfort of legs and back,* particularly at higher pumping pressure, may occur. There is also slower inflation and deflation time because of the use of water for pumping compared with the use of gas for pumping, this slower response limits the effectiveness of the device. Patient care and accessibility are limited by the bulk and rigidity of the external device.

Whereas the principles of the two devices are basically the same, the effectiveness of the external counterpulsation device is approximately half that of the intraaortic balloon pump. Table 28-14 lists the factors that would explain the difference.

**H**ypovolemia   Loss of body fluids may accompany shock. Direct loss of fluids will be present in patients who sustain severe burns or hemorrhage. Indirect fluid loss may be precipitated by vasoconstriction which diverts fluid from the circulation and increases peripheral pooling of fluids. In order to increase cardiac output and overall tissue perfusion, body fluids will need to be replaced. Selection of the fluid replacements is based upon the type of fluid that has been lost and the patient's overall health status. Guidelines used to monitor the effectiveness of the therapy are based upon serum hematocrit levels (maintain between 35 and 45 percent of volume), blood electrolytes, pH, and the cardiac and renal status of the patient. Assessment of these variables will define the type of fluids that are being lost and identify what is needed for replacements. The effects of fluid administration should be carefully monitored through PWP and CVP, and the patient assessed for signs of fluid overload or depletion.

*Saline or dextrose solutions* should be given immediately following any evidence of dehydration. IV injection of 500 to 2000 ml sodium chloride (physiologic saline), Ringer's solution, or 5% dextrose in saline should be given rapidly. When this is done, frequent CVP and PWP readings should be taken in order to prevent volume overload and

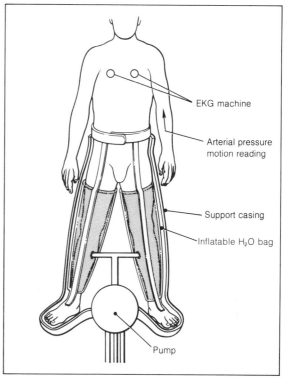

**FIGURE 28-12**
Diagram of external circulatory assist. (*From J. S. Schroeder et al., Techniques in Bedside Hemodynamic Monitoring, Mosby, St. Louis, 1976.*)

resulting congestive heart failure. Crystalloid solutions can also be used. These solutions remain briefly in the bloodstream and cause acute volume expansion and hemodilution. They are used when rapid volume replacement is desired. The need for RBC replacement because of hemodilution however, should be assessed frequently to avoid a lowering in hemoglobin and hematocrit levels.

*Fresh whole blood* is the most effective and longest acting replacement used for treating trauma. Stored old blood is low in diphosphoglyceric acid (2,3-DPG) and coagulation factors, while

**TABLE 28-14**
COMPARISON BETWEEN THE INTRAAORTIC BALLOON PUMP AND EXTERNAL COUNTERPULSATION DEVICE

| Class | Intraaortic Balloon Pump | External Counterpulsation Device |
|---|---|---|
| Diastolic augmentation | Exceeds the systolic pressure | Equals to systolic pressure |
| Systolic unloading | Effective | Less effective |

high in potassium, lactic acid, and hemoglobin saturation. If too much blood is transfused in a short time, it may cause hypothermia. The patient's body temperature should be checked frequently. Packed RBC may be given when the central venous pressure is high and hematocrit levels are low to limit the amount of fluid volume. The nurse should observe for signs of transfusion reaction (see Chap. 10).

*Plasma* is useful particularly for burn patients. It is not routinely used in shock patients owing to the incidence of hepatitis following its use, especially with a pooled commercial plasma.

Dextran and serum albumin are *plasma expenders* which increase the colloid osmotic pressure, thereby controlling the fluid escape from the vasculature. The dextrans have high molecular weights and the necessary viscosity to replace lost blood volume. However, they have not proved as useful as plasma. Dextran should be used cautiously in patients with cardiac disease, renal insufficiency, or marked dehydration in order to avoid pulmonary edema, congestive heart failure, or renal shutdown. If blood samples for typing and cross matching are desired, they should be obtained before the dextran therapy is administered since they can interfere with the overall test results.

When intravenous solutions are being used to replace body fluids, it is essential that the nurse observe for the overall effect of the intervention. Vital signs should be checked frequently and changes noted. In acute shock, vital signs should be taken as often as every 15 minutes. Urinary output should be calculated hourly to evaluate overall volume intake and output. If the amount of output is significantly less than the amount of fluid being infused, the individual may need to be dialyzed. The patient should be observed for signs of cardiac overload and impending failure. Frequent CVP and/or PWP readings should be taken to aid in this evaluation. A complete physical assessment, especially of the chest (heart and lungs) should be performed to evaluate changes in oxygenation. If dehydration is present, the symptoms observed including dryness of the mucous membranes should begin to reverse with fluid replacement. When blood is administered, the patient should be observed for a transfusion reaction. Daily weights are also helpful in determining the amount of fluid being retained.

**D**isturbances in Respiration  Patients in shock will experience rapid and shallow respirations. Dyspnea may be present. Ventilation must be frequently assessed for the patient in shock. Respiratory disturbances are frequently observed in patients with fever, infection and/or metabolic acidosis, coma, pulmonary edema, and cerebral infarction. Arterial blood gases should be checked to prevent metabolic acidosis. A low $p_{CO_2}$ along with a low bicarbonate level indicates that hyperventilation in effective. If, however, the $p_{CO_2}$ rises and the blood pH remains low, ventilatory assistance may be needed (refer to Chap. 30).

The patient's rate and depth of respirations should be carefully observed. In the presence of respiratory failure, the respiratory rate and depth will decrease. Cyanosis may be observed. Respirators (e.g., Bird respirator) may be used, or other forms (e.g., MA-I or Emerson) may be used to assist ventilation. Endotracheal intubation may be needed, depending on the degree of respiratory distress. A tracheostomy may be performed in the presence of laryngeal edema or airway obstruction (see Chap. 30 for care of the patient on respirators and tracheostomies). Continuous respiratory assessment, skin assessment, and evaluation of the patient's level of consciousness will help the nurse determine if the patient is receiving adequate ventilation.

**O**liguria–Anuria  A decrease in urine output usually accompanies shock due to diminished circulation, decreased glomerular filtration, and renal tissue perfusion. Measurement of hourly urine is essential. For this purpose, the patient is usually catheterized immediately following hospitalization. A minimum of 50 cc/hour is indicative of adequate renal perfusion. Urea and mannitol may be given to prevent acute renal tubular damage. Mannitol is a substance filtered in the urine and is neither reabsorbed nor metabolized.[64] It acts as an osmotic diuretic and rids the body of wastes that accumulate in the renal tubes. If anuria is present for a prolonged period of time, or if tubular necrosis is suspected, peritoneal or renal dialysis may become necessary (refer to Chap. 14 for a complete discussion).

**A**lterations in Level of Consciousness  Cerebral anoxia, due to decreased cerebral perfusion, will lead to alterations in the patient's level of consciousness. Initially, the patient will be restless and irritable. Anxiety is common because of fear of the unknown. As the degree of cerebral circulation decreases, or if it increases, as in the presence of toxins (e.g., anesthesia, bacterial invasion), the patient may become more stuporous and lethargic. The sensorium may be clouded and the patient's level of consciousness may lessen.

The nurse must carefully evaluate the patient's response and ease with which the patient can be aroused. Increased confusion and lethargy should be reported. The patient should be asked questions to evaluate the degree of orientation to time and place. Cerebral anoxia, if severe enough, may also lead to seizures and coma. Cerebral infarction (see Chap. 34) and increased intercranial pressures (see Chap. 32) may complicate the shock state and further alter the patient's level of consciousness.

**Immobility** The problems associated with immobility remain a constant threat to the patient, who is often weak and unable to move. Depending on the level of consciousness, there may be difficulty communicating with the individual. In addition, the amount of machinery attached to the patient complicates the problem by limiting activity.

The nurse should provide for adequate rest periods but frequently incorporate passive range of motion exercises into the care plan. When possible the patient should be encouraged to actively participate in movements. Infusion sites should carefully be observed for signs of phlebitis (see Chap. 29), and complaints of chest pain, calf pain, or difficulty breathing should be promptly evaluated for possible emboli formation. Elastic stockings should be used, and in some situations anticoagulants may be administered. (See Chap. 29 for a complete discussion of the patient with venous occlusion due to phlebitis.)

When possible the patient should be turned frequently. Coughing and deep breathing should be encouraged. Lung sounds and body temperature should be assessed frequently to guard against the threat of pneumonia. Adequate skin care is essential in order to prevent decubiti formation. Decreased circulation, lack of tissue perfusion, and immobility will diminish circulation to the tissues. The skin around the pressure points such as the buttocks must be carefully cared for, and frequent turning may help to alleviate direct stress to the tissue.

**Alterations in Body Temperature** When hypovolemia in response to shock first appears, compensatory vasoconstriction will cause the patient's skin to become cold to the touch. Continued use of vasoconstrictors may intensify the problem. If fever is present, the skin may be clammy to touch.

*Antibiotics* are used primarily for septic shock. Specific therapy is instituted according to sensitivity studies. However, in septic shock of uncertain bacterial etiology, a combination of antibiotics is used initially to cover the spectrum of likely organisms until the responsible organism is identified by culture. Even though the major cause for septic shock is gram-negative bacilli, measures to prevent and/or treat gram-positive organisms should also be taken. Combination of gentamicin and oxacillin provides suitable coverage for all common pathogens except *Bacteroides,* enterococcus, and *Hemophilus.* Clindamycin is usually added to the preceding regimen to cover *bacteroides.*

If infection is present, fluids will be administered intravenously and orally when possible. Frequent assessments of level of consciousness, dehydration, and body temperature are essential. Skin care is important when infection is present.

The patient should be kept warm enough to avoid shivering. Care must be taken to increase the body temperature gradually. Extremes in body temperature will increase metabolism and place an added demand upon an already depleted oxygen supply.

**Anxiety** Frequently patients are most anxious during shock because they fear what may happen and they react to the physiological changes occurring in their body (e.g., increase in catecholamine production). These fears are intensified by their physical fatigue, disruption in body rhythms, intense physical care, sensory deprivation, and the amount of machinery that they are attached to. Pain may be a complicating factor, along with the stress of the impending physical changes that may accompany recovery. The patient's greatest fear is often the loss of life. The nurse must be constantly aware of the patient's emotional needs during this critical time. *Analgesics* offer prompt control of severe pain. Usually morphine sulfate, 8 to 18 mg, is given subcutaneously, or 10 to 15 mg IV push is given slowly since the subcutaneous absorption is poor in patients in shock. Morphine should not be given to unconscious patients, to patients with head injuries, or to those with respiratory depression.

When possible, the patient should be given frequent rest periods. Disruptions should be planned so that as much care as possible can be accomplished. During the acute stages of shock it may be difficult to leave the patient for a prolonged period of time since direct observation will be critical. Awareness of the effects of continued interruption on the patient may decrease the amount of direct contact needed.

The patient should be encouraged to discuss all fears freely. The nurse should provide the patient with a complete orientation to all machinery and allow time to answer all questions. The patient's concerns about death should be explored and adequate support given by the nurse.

The family should also be carefully counseled as to the use of machinery and the patient's status. They will require continuous support and reassurance from the nurse. The recovery period may take a long time, and the family members may tire easily. The nurse must be aware of the physical and emotional impact on the family and through counseling offer ways to help them cope with any problems.

### Fourth-Level Nursing Care

Should the patient enter the irreversible phase of shock, death will follow. However, if this does not occur, the patient may recover from shock and begin to recuperate from the precipitating cause. Maintaining this recovery period is often dependent upon the correction of the precipitating cause(s) of shock.

*Prevention* of additional cardiac ischemia and muscle damage, immobilization of fractures, replacement of body fluids, and restoration of fluid and electrolyte balance are essential. In addition, prevention of infection, restoration of adequate respirations and arterial blood pressure, and prevention of drug overdose or introduction of toxins into the body (e.g., insect bites) will all help to decrease the chance of shock reoccurring in the individual.

*Recovery* from serious illnesses such as a myocardial infarction (see Chap. 24), severe burns (see Chap. 13), or massive hemorrhage due to trauma will require prolonged hospitalization and rehabilitation. It is essential that the nurse carefully observe the patient throughout the post-shock phase so that the problems do not reoccur. The patient should be assessed daily for changes in physical and emotional state that may indicate future problems. If the shock was due to an allergic response, the patient should be cautioned against encountering the potential toxin. Health teaching should be directed toward identifying the potential problem, avoiding it whenever possible, recognizing the symptoms, and obtaining treatment early.

*Diabetic teaching* should be directed toward prevention of diabetic coma and insulin shock (see Chap. 20 for a complete discussion). It is important to remember that shock can occur anywhere. The nurse should be able to assess shock quickly, know the contributing causes, and be able to help augment the patient's individual compensatory mechanism.

## IDIOPATHIC ORTHOSTATIC HYPOTENSION

Primary autoimmune insufficiency idiopathic orthostatic hypotension is a rare condition in which there is a degeneration of central and/or peripheral autonomic nervous structures, resulting in severe orthostatic hypotension, syncope, or seizures when the patient arises from recumbency. This syndrome affects men more frequently than women. The obvious neural autonomic involvement is manifested by postural hypotension, loss of sweating, and fixed heart rate; subtle neurologic signs include papillary abnormalities, generalized hyperreflexia, and disturbed bladder regulation. Usually, the sensation and mentality are intact.

In many instances, the disease may represent variants of a syndrome described by Shy and Drager (thus idiopathic orthostatic hypotension is also called *Shy-Drager's syndrome*). Symptoms include dysarthria, rigidity, tremor, ataxia, monotonous speech, diplegia, vertigo, and incontinence, and degenerative changes in the autonomic ganglions, basal ganglions, and cortex. The initial description of the syndrome by Bradbury and Eggleston stressed the triad of postural hypotension, anhidrosis involving most of the body surface, and impotence. Plasma and urinary catecholamines are usually decreased.

No specific treatment is available for most of the neurogenic causes of orthostatic hypotension. Therapy with sympathomimetic drugs (e.g., ephedrine sulfate up to 75 mg daily) may be useful but not effective over prolonged periods. The expansion of extracellular volume by a high salt diet (10 to 20 mg/day) and/or the potent synthetic salt-retaining steroid, 9-flurohydrocortisone (0.1 to 0.5 mg/day) may be helpful. In addition to advising the patient not to rise too rapidly from the sitting or lying position, full-length elastic supportive hose may be tightly applied to reduce orthostatic pooling of blood in the legs. In the most severe cases, pressurized aviator suits may be necessary to permit ambulation.

## REFERENCES

1   C. F. Rothe, *Cardiodynamics in Physiology,* 4th ed., Little, Brown, Boston, 1976, p. 338.
2   George Thorn et al. (eds.), *Harrison's Principles of Internal Medicine,* 8th ed., McGraw-Hill, New York, 1977, p. 1307.
3   J. W. McCubin, J. H. Green, and I. H. Page, "Baroreceptor Function in Chronic Renal Hypertension," *Circ Res.,* **4:**205–210, March 1956.

4   C. M. Plotz, A. I. Knowlton, and C. Ragan, "The Natural History of Cushing's Syndrome," *Am. J. Med.,* **13:**597, 1952.

5   L. Krakoff, G. Nicollis, and B. Amsel, "Pathogenesis of Hypertension in Cushing's Syndrome," *Am J Med,* **58:**216–220, February 1975.

6   G. Thorn, *op. cit.,* p. 525.

7   *Ibid.,* p. 525.

8   J. B. Lee, R. V. Patak, and B. K. Mookejee: "Renal Prostaglandins and the Regulation of Blood Pressure and Sodium and Water Hemostasis," *Am J Med,* **60:** 798–816, May 31, 1976.

9   G. Thorn, *op. cit.,* p. 1309.

10   H. R. Tapia, C. E. Johnson, and C. G. Strong, "Effect of Oral Contraceptive Therapy in Renin-Angiotensin System in Normotension and Hypertension," *Gynecology,* **41:**643–649, May 1973.

11   S. Wolf, et al., *Life Stress and Essential Hypertension,* Williams & Wilkins, Baltimore, 1955, p. 232.

12   F. M. C. Evans, *Psychosocial Nursing: Theory and Practice in Hospital and Community Mental Health,* Macmillan, New York, 1971, pp. 143–213, 194, 198–199.

13   G. Thorn, *op. cit.,* p. 1308.

14   *United States Department of Health, Education, and Welfare: Blood Pressure of Adults by Age and Sex, United States 1960–1962,* National Health Survey, National Center for Health Statistics, Series 11: No. 4, 1964.

15   E. A. Lew, "High Blood Pressure, Other Risk Factors and Longevity: The Insurance Viewpoint," *Am. J. Med,* **55:**281–294, September 1973.

16   W. B. Kannel, "Current Status of the Epidemeology of Brain Infarction Associated with Occlusive Arterial Disease," *Stroke,* **2:**295–318, 1971.

17   E. D. Freis, "Age, Race, Sex and Other Indices of Risk in Hypertension," *Am J Med,* **55:**275–280, 1973.

18   N. O. Fowler, "Essentials of Examining for Hypertension," *Consultant,* p. 74, February 1974.

19   *United States Department of Health, Education and Welfare: loc. cit.*

20   *United States Department of Health, Education, and Welfare: Hypertension and Hypertensive Heart Disease in Adults, United States 1960–1962,* National Health Survey, National Center for Health Statistics, Series 11: Nov. 13, 1966.

21   J. Stamler, *Proceedings of the National Conference on High Blood Pressure Education,* National Heart and Lung Institute, United States Department of Heqlth, Education, and Welfare, Publication (NIH) 73-486, p. 11, 1973.

22   E. D. Fries, "Age, Race, Sex and Other Indices of Rick in Hypertension," *American Journal of Medicine* **55:**275–280, 1973.

23   K. G. Andreolli, et al., *Comprehensive Cardiac Care,* 3d ed., Mosby, St. Louis, 1975, p. 11.

24   *United States Department of Health, Education, and Welfare: Blood Pressure of Adults by Age and Sex, loc. cit.*

25   J. A. Schoenberger, et al., "Current Status of Hypertensive Control in an Industrial Population," *JAMA,* **222:**559, 1972.

26   J. Stamler, *loc. cit.*

27   L. K. Dahl, "Salt and Hypertension," *Am J Clin Nutr,* **25:**231–244, 1972.

28   M. D. Schweitzer, et al., "Genetic Factors in Primary Hypertension and Coronary Disease," *J. Chron Dis,* **15:**1093–1108, 1962.

29   J. Stamler, R. Stamler, and T. N. Pullman, *The Epidemiology of Hypertension,* New York, Grune & Stratton, 1967, p. 105.

30   R. Platt, "Heredity in Hypertension," *Lancet,* **7:**899–904, 1963.

31   E. D. Fries, *loc. cit.*

32   Stamler et al., *loc. cit.*

33   *Hypertension Study Group of the Intersociety Commission for Heart Disease Resources, Circulation,* **44:**A263, 1971 (revised August 1972).

34   M. F. Foley, "Variation in Blood Pressure with Lateral Recumbent Position," *Nurs Res,* **20:**64–69, January–February 1971.

35   F. M. C. Evans, *op. cit.,* 1971, pp. 194–199.

36   A. S. Nies, "Adverse Reactions and Interactions Limiting the Use of Antihypertensive Drugs," *Am J Med,* **58:**495–503, April 1975.

37   Veterans Administration Cooperative Study Group on Antihypertensive Agents: "Effects of Treatment on Morbidity in Hypertension: II. Results in Patients with Diastolic Blood Pressure Averaging 90 through 114 mm/Hg," *JAMA,* **213**(7):1143–1152, August 1970.

38   L. I. Goldberg, "Current Therapy of Hypertension —A Pharmacologic Approach," *Am J Med,* **58:**489–494, April 1975.

39   N. M. Kaplan.: "Antihypertensive Drugs in Combination," *Arch Inter Med,* **135:**660–664, May 1975.

40   J. Gluck, "Hypertension—Caring for the Patient Who Feels Well," *Nursing '74,* **4:**74–76, September 1974.

41   S. B. Penick, "Behavior Modification in the Treatment of Obesity," *Psychosocial Med,* **33:**49, 1971.

42   G. Thorn, *op. cit.,* p. 1310.

43   *Ibid.,* p. 1313.

44   L. B. Page and J. J. Sidd, "Medical Progress: Medical Management of Primary Hypertension" (third of three parts), *N Engl J Med,* **287**(21):1074–1080, November 1972.

45   W. Kobinger, "Pharmacologic Basis of Cardio-vascular Action of Clonidine," in G. Onesti, K. E. Kim, and J. H. Moyer (eds.), *Hypertension: Mechanism and Management,* Grune & Stratton, New York, 1973.

46   G. Onesti, et al.: "Antihypertensive Effects of Clonidine," *Circ Res.,* **28:**suppl. 2, 53–69, 1971.

47   G. Thorn, *op. cit.,* p. 1313.

48   P. Lewis, "The Essential Action of Propranolol in Hypertension," *Am J Med,* **60:**837–852, 1976.

49   B. E. Karlberg, et al., "Controlled Treatment of Primary Hypertension with Propranolol and Spironol-actone," *Am J Cardiol,* **37:**642–649, March 31, 1976.

50   M. M. Wintrobe et al., *Harrison's Principles of Internal Medicine,* 7th ed., McGraw-Hill, New York, 1974, p. 1233.

51   G. Thorn, *op. cit.,* p. 185.

52   *Ibid.,* p. 186.

53   J. Luckman and K. Sorenson, *Medical-Surgical Nursing: A Psychophysiological Approach,* Philadelphia, Saunders, 1975, p. 267.

54   *Ibid.,* p. 268.

55   *Ibid.,* p. 269.

56   N. R. Rose, F. Milgrom, and C. J. Van Oss, *Principles of Immunology,* Macmillan, New York, 1973, pp. 155, 161, 162.

57   M. F. Hayes, R. Posenbaum, and Matsumato, "Diagnosis and Treatment of Hemorrhagic and Septic Shock," *Intern Surg,* **58**(5):299–303, May 1973.

58   K. J. Bordicks, *Patterns of Shock: Implications for Nursing Care,* Macmillan, New York, 1965.

59   J. Luckman and K. Sorensen, *op. cit.,* p. 276.

60   J. M. Daly, B. Ziegler, and S. J. Durdick, "Central Venous Catheterization," *Am J Nurs,* **75:**820–824, May 1975.

61   J. S. Schroeder and E. K. Daily, *Techniques in Bedside Hemodynamic Monitoring,* St. Louis, Mosby, 1976, p. 65.

62   J. S. Schoeder and E. K. Daily, *op. cit.,* p. 81, 1976.

63   J. Luckman and K. Sorensen, *op. cit.,* p. 287.

64   *Ibid.,* p. 267.

## BIBLIOGRAPHY

*1973 Heart Facts,* New York, American Heart Association, 1972.

Beland, I., and J. Passos: *Clinical Nursing,* Macmillan, New York, 1975.

Bergersen, B. S.: *Pharmacology in Nursing,* 13th ed., Mosby, St. Louis, p. 174, 1976.

Chatton, M. J., and M. A. Krupp: *Current Medical Diagnosis and Treatment,* Lange, Los Altos, Calif., 1976, p. 6.

Conte, A., M. Brandzel and S. Whitehead: "Group Work with Hypertensive Patients," *Am J Nurs,* **74:**910–1012, May 1974.

Davies, R., N. N. Payne, and J. D. H. Slater: "Beta Adrenergic Blockade and Diuretic Therapy in Benign Essential Hypertension: A Dynamic Assessment," *Am J Cardiol,* **37:**637–641, March 1976.

Davis, J. O.: "Control of Renin Release," *Hosp Prac,* 55–56, April 1974.

Eipper, D. F., et al.: "Abdominal Bruits in Renovascular Hypertension," *Am J Cardiol,* **37:**48–52, January 1976.

Engel, G. L.: *Psychological Development in Health and Disease,* Saunders, Philadelphia, p. 264, 1962.

Freis, E. D.: *Introduction to the Nature and Management of Hypertension,* Robert J. Brady Company, Bowie, Md., 1974.

Gifford: *The Hypertensive Handbook,* Merck, Sharp and Dohme, Division of Merck and Company, West Point, Pa., pp. 94–95, 1974.

Goodman, L. S., and A. Gilman: *The Pharmacological Basis of Therapeutics,* 5th ed., Macmillan, New York, 1975.

Griffith, E. W., and B. Madero: "Primary Hypertension—Patients' Learning Needs," *Am J Nurs,* **73:**624–627, April 1973.

Hypertensive Detection and Follow-Up Program Cooperative Group: "Hypertensive Detection and Follow-Up Program," *Preventive Med,* **5:**207–215, 1976.

Jahre, J. A., et al.: "Medical Approach to the Hypotensive Patient and the Patient in Shock," *Heart Lung,* **4:**577–587, July–August 1975.

Laragh, J. H.: "Symposium on Hypertension: Part II. Renin Profiling and Drug Therapy, Childhood Hypertension, Prorenin, the Physiology of Renin Secretion." *Am J Cardiol,* **37:**635–691, March 31, 1976.

——— (ed.): "Symposium on Hypertension," *Am J Med,* **60:**733–897, May 31, 1976.

Long, M. L., et al.: "Hypertension," *Am J Nurs,* **76**(5): 765–780, May 1976.

Report from the Boston Collaborative Drug Surveillance Program: "Reserpine and Breast Cancer," *Lancet,* **2:**669–671, Sept. 21, 1974.

Schumer, W.: "Metabolism during Shock and Sepsis," *Heart Lung,* **5:**416–421, May–June 1976.

——— and K. M. Nyhus: "Corticosteroid Effect on Biochemical Parameters of Human Oligemic Shock," *Arch Surg,* **100:**405–408, 1970.

Selye, H.: *The Stress of Life,* McGraw-Hill, New York, p. 11, 1956.

Sodeman, W. A., Jr., and W. A. Sodeman: *Pathologic Physiology,* 5th ed., Saunders, Philadelphia, 1974.

Stamler, J.: *High Blood Pressure in the United States—An Overview of the Problem and the Challenge,* Proc. National Conference on High Blood Pressure Education, National Heart and Lung Institute, Department of Health, Education, and Welfare, no. (NIH) 73-486, p. 11, 1973.

# 29

# BLOOD VESSEL DISRUPTION

Karyn McGaghie Holm

Circulation of blood through the body is essential to oxygenation. Several factors in the human internal and external environment can alter circulation. These include ingestion of a large amount of cholesterol or saturated fats, genetic predisposition, stress, and trauma. When these factors cause an obstruction in the blood vessels, they will interrupt the efficient transportation of oxygen and nutrients to the vital organs.

Vascular disturbances can occur in any blood vessel, be it a vein or an artery. Changes occur slowly, and the onset of pathological disruptions is often insidious. When vessels in the heart are occluded, the result is ischemia to the myocardium, angina, and myocardial infarction (see Chap. 26). When obstruction occurs in cerebral blood vessels, a cerebral infarction results (see Chap. 34). However, when an occlusion occurs in the peripheral arteries or veins, peripheral vascular disease is present. This chapter will focus on those peripheral vascular occlusive diseases that obstruct arterial and venous circulation.

## PERIPHERAL ARTERIOVASCULAR DISEASE

Disruptions in peripheral arterial blood flow are usually caused by arteriosclerosis and atherosclerosis. These changes occur early in life and are compounded by the presence of risk factors such as hypertension, diabetes mellitus, and smoking.

### Pathophysiology

The differentiation between arteriosclerosis and atherosclerosis can be somewhat confusing. Many authors state that *arteriosclerosis* is generalized hardening of the arteries, while *atherosclerosis* involves focal changes on a cellular level. Definitions of atherosclerosis state that it is a pathological process occurring in the intimal layer of large arterial vessels. The arterioatherosclerotic complex becomes clearer when viewed as follows: Atherosclerosis involves changes occurring primarily in the intimal layer of arteries, and arteriosclerosis involves progression of atherosclerosis. As the atherosclerotic process advances, the arteries become nonpliable and the disease process can be termed arteriosclerosis or generalized hardening of the arteries.[1]

For many years the intima was described as the only arterial layer involved in atherosclerosis. Recently medial cell involvement has been consistently demonstrated. The medial cell, it has been

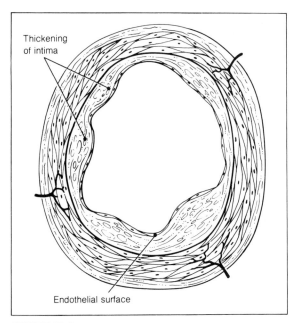

Thickening of intima

Endothelial surface

**FIGURE 29-1**
Endothelial surface. (*From Wiley F. Barker, Peripheral Arterial Disease, Saunders, Philadelphia, 1975.*)

found, is as likely to accumulate lipids and is also prone to injury by lipoproteins.[2]

The initial stage in the progression of atherosclerosis occurs in the first decade of life.[3] During this time fatty streaking is apparent within arterial vessels. This fatty streaking is considered to be a natural phenomenon, but the reason for its occurrence is still unclear. Little advancement of this process is seen in the second decade. In the third decade, if one is predisposed by diet, heredity, or another etiology, plaque formation accelerates with an increase in the deposition of lipids and fibrous protein. Advanced atherosclerosis is seen in the fourth and fifth decades with the presence of true atheromatous plaques. Clinical pathology is seen only in the advanced stages of atherosclerosis, creating numerous problems in prevention and control.

The early stages of atherosclerosis are manifested by small lesions not containing most of the components of the advanced plaque. A pure early lesion contains small amounts of lipid but little collagen, fibrin, elastin, or mucopolysaccharides (see Fig. 29-1). The typical advanced plaque is a complex with a calcified base and a lipid-filled necrotic center encircled by a fibrous cap.[4]

As the blood vessels narrow, blood flow diminishes and tissue ischemia develops. The body develops collateral circulation to the occluded area,

but often this is not adequate. If tissue hypoxia occurs over a long-enough period, tissue necrosis and gangrene will occur (see Fig. 29-2). *Gangrene* is the decomposition and putrefaction of necrotic tissue and cell death. It most often occurs in an area farthest from the heart, e.g., fingers and toes. When bacteria are present in the lesion, the term *gas gangrene* is used. Side effects from the gangrenous process include thrombosis of the small arteries, arterial spasm, and mechanical obstruction.

Atherosclerotic occlusions frequently occur at arterial bifurcations. The reason is the fact that these areas are often subject to trauma from the pulsating bloodstream.[5] The most common sites are the aortic-iliac bifurcation, the femoral artery, and the popliteal artery. Aortic iliac disease is sometimes referred to as the *Leriche syndrome.* This syndrome is characterized by pain in the buttocks and thigh due to claudication of the arteries. When calf pain is experienced, the femoral artery may be obstructed. The problem is seen in males, and physical appearance often includes the presence of thin legs with a lack of gluteal muscle bulk. Impotence may also accompany this syndrome. Pain experienced during this type of arterial occlusion can sometimes be confused with sciatic pain.

**Causes of arterioatherosclerosis** Several theories have evolved to explain the pathogenesis of atherosclerosis. These include the thrombogenic theory, the vascular dynamic theory, the capillary hemorrhage theory, the lipophage migration theory, and the lipid metabolic theory. These theories are discussed fully in Chap. 26.

Psychosocial elements such as stress factors have also been identified in the progression of atherosclerosis. In addition, the normal effects of aging, which lead to a reduction in the elasticity of blood vessels, may contribute to occlusion. Trauma to the artery wall, arterial thrombosis, or arterial rupture can also cause an obstruction in a blood vessel. The presence of *atheromas* (fatty plaques within the arterial system) may result in arteries with decreased diameters. These changes predispose the vessel to further occlusion by causing blood stasis and contribute to thrombus and embolus formation.

**Effects on the patient** *Intermittent claudication* is the earliest effect noted by the patient. Claudication pain is a contraction in the muscles of the leg, brought on by exercise and relieved by rest.[6] Pain may be present in both legs but is more often seen in one. Decreased blood supply to the extremity will cause the limb to be cold, numb, and often cyanotic. When diabetic neuropathy is present, perception of hot and cold may be altered (see Chap. 20).

*Ischemic pain* or pain at rest is often present with arterial occlusion. The cause is not clearly known, but it is suggested that the pain may be triggered by the presence of lactic acid which can accumulate during anaerobic metabolism in ischemia.[7] Bradykinin and histamine released by damaged muscle cells may also stimulate nerve endings and cause a pain experience.[8] Ischemic neuritis can occur, and the patient will experience pain and numbness in the extremities.

With decreased arterial circulation there is *slow healing* and *poor resistance to infection.* Occlusion in circulation prevents leukocytes and antibodies from reaching injured tissue, and healing is slowed. Skin ulcerations can occur and lead to tissue necrosis and gangrene. This may necessitate amputation of a limb. The skin is often dry owing to poor tissue perfusion and has a smooth but taut appearance. Trophic changes, especially around the nailbeds, will usually occur because of tissue malnutrition.

*Arterial edema* can occur in the peripheral extremities owing to structural changes in the arteries. Vasospasm within the arteries can enhance occlusion and cause stasis of blood in the periphery. Decreased blood supply as a result of obstruction of the hypogastric artery and/or terminal artery can lead to impotence. Since atherosclerosis is often seen in the presence of cardiac, renal, cerebral, and metabolic disruptions (e.g., diabetes), additional systemic effects may be noted when arterial changes are present.

## First-Level Nursing Care

Directing nursing efforts toward the prevention of arterioatherosclerosis involves early identification of the population at risk. Recognition of psychosocial influences, familial tendency toward the disease, and the role of nutritional factors in its progression are essential. Because of documentation that initial manifestations and potentials for arterioatherosclerosis appear in early life, nursing care can be directed toward improving the health status of those in the pediatric and young age groups.

*Genetic predisposition* has been indirectly identified by the familial tendency toward atherosclerosis. Our present lack of knowledge concerning genetic predisposition points to a need for fur-

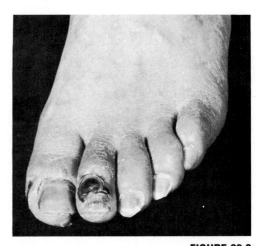

**FIGURE 29-2**
Ischemic gangrenous toe. (*From J. W. Hurst et al. (eds.), The Heart, 4th ed., McGraw-Hill, New York, 1978.*)

ther research in this area, to consider not only genetic factors but other intervening variables such as environment, culture, and nutrition as well.

*Psychosocial elements* involved in the progression of atherosclerosis include age, sex, race, ethnic background, smoking, and obesity. Age and sex are considered secondary-risk factors, while smoking is a primary-risk factor. Atherosclerosis becomes increasingly apparent with advancing age. Males demonstrate a greater incidence of atherosclerosis between the ages of 25 and 64 years. Females, after menopause, demonstrate atherosclerosis at a rate almost equal to males. Researchers have studied effects of race, culture, and structural differences in arteries and have identified interesting relationships. One study found American Blacks to have better-developed intima than Haitian Blacks, while another study, conducted in Israel, discovered that the intima of males with European ancestry contained a richer collagen-tissue fraction than the intima of those with Asian backgrounds. It is interesting to note that the Israelis with European ancestry have a greater incidence of atherosclerosis than those of Asian ancestry.[9] While studies demonstrating racial and cultural differences have been limited, the results must be viewed in combination with the apparent differences in life-styles.

Cigarette smoking continues to be an important risk factor in the development of atherosclerosis. The vasoconstricting influence of nicotine increases the tendency toward vascular disruptions. Many studies have shown that mortality from atherosclerosis (coronary) is higher in younger age groups and that chances of developing atherosclerosis are two to six times greater in cigarette smokers.

Biochemical alterations causing an individual to be prone to atherosclerosis are seen in the obese individual. Another significant finding in the obese population is the elevation of serum lipid protein levels. Elevation of serum lipid proteins is related to arterial lipid deposition. Dietary patterns and their relationship to atherosclerosis provide information that a diet high in calories, saturated fat, cholesterol, and sugar can result in a more rapid progression of plaque formation.[10] Assessment of nutritional patterns is particularly crucial as fat and caloric intake are elements which can be controlled.

**Prevention**    Prevention of arterioatherosclerosis should begin in the prenatal period. Ascertaining the presence of a cultural, racial, or familial predisposition, the presence of risk factors such as cigarette smoking or hypertension, and nutritional patterns of prospective patients provides a beginning focus. Our present knowledge of the multifactorial aspects of this problem indicates that the existence of a single factor does not make one prone to its development, while these factors in combination increase the risk of occurrence. Many of these factors cannot be changed (heredity, sex, culture), but there are many which can be modified or even eliminated (hypertension and cigarette smoking).

The primary consideration in prevention is health education. This important but complex task involves nursing competence in many health care settings. Nurses practicing in offices of obstetricians and pediatricians carry a major responsibility as they have opportunity to educate those potentially at risk. A prospective or new parent can be given verbal and written information pertaining to prevention of arterioatherosclerosis and can also be given opportunity to discuss ways this information can be applied to the home environment. This generalization of health information to the home environment involves behavior modification and is crucial if this disease is to be prevented. There are other health care settings where primary prevention can be employed; waiting rooms in hospitals, the offices of health care practitioners, and waiting areas of clinics are but a few examples.

*Teaching for prevention* of arterioatherosclerosis can occur in all phases of formal education, from elementary school through college. Thus nurses involved in educational settings can provide

a consistent approach to prevention through nutritional counseling, cholesterol screening, blood pressure screening, and weight reduction programs. Shopping areas and other public places such as libraries and recreational centers are additional locations where the public can receive information.

The basic curriculum for prevention of arterioatherosclerosis includes discussion of all factors increasing the risk of this disease process along with specific guidelines pertaining to the modification or elimination of these factors. Every individual should be reminded of the importance of a yearly physical examination, not only to determine general health status, but also to monitor the presence of controllable risk factors. Determining cholesterol levels can aid in reducing the complications of arterial occlusion. The American Heart Association and the National Heart and Lung Institute provide printed and audiovisual material appropriate for public education. Further information regarding these materials can be secured by writing for catalogs or for descriptions of specific publications (Further discussion of the prevention of risk factors is found in Chap. 26.)

Nutritional counseling should focus on (1) total caloric intake, (2) total fat intake, (3) amount of saturated fat consumed, (4) amount of polyunsaturated fat consumed, (5) amount of cholesterol consumed, and (6) carbohydrate intake. Recommendations regarding diet appear in Table 29-1.

Elimination of cigarette smoking and stress is important for prevention. Discussion should focus on the effect of these factors on arterial occlusion. Counseling for stress-related problems may be required. Public groups such as Smokenders may be of some assistance to the patient with a smoking problem. Hypnosis may be effective in some instances.

### Second-Level Nursing Care

In a community setting, professional advice is usually sought because the patient experiences increasing limb pain. Frequently, this pain has begun to interfere with the individual's life-style.[11] Second-level Nursing Care will discuss changes related to *partial arterial occlusion*.

**Nursing assessment**    Critical to the assessment of an individual with suspected disturbances in arterial functioning is an adequate *health history*. This should include a description of current occupation, family history, identification of primary- and secondary-risk factors, analysis of activity, and nutritional intake. Identification of other health problems should be noted at this time.

Limb pain caused by tissue ischemia is the usual reason patients seek professional advice. Arterial vessel disease is usually well advanced before pain is precipitated, but it is not experienced until occlusion produces inadequate tissue perfusion.[12] A thorough analysis of the pain is an important aspect of nursing care. When a nursing history is sought from a patient experiencing limb pain, the following aspects must be included in the history-taking interview. First, the patient should describe the exact location of the pain and when it occurs (at rest or with activity). Next, factors which initiate, exaggerate, minimize, or eliminate the pain such as psychological and cultural responses to pain, should be explored. The effects of external temperature and humidity should also be evaluated.

Males seem to experience claudication more frequently than females, but after menopause females are affected to a greater degree. The patient's age should be elicited as well as a menstrual history. If relief of intermittent claudication is obtained by ceasing the precipitating exercise and resting, or by shifting body weight to the uninvolved extremity, it should be noted.

Pain precipitated by exercise and relieved by rest (intermittent claudication) should be reviewed. Most frequently this type of pain will involve the thigh and limb. The individual will complain of numbness and coldness of the affected limb intensified by external temperature change. Patients may describe being awakened from sleep by the pain as peripheral circulation may be aggravated by position. Male patients may experience difficulty maintaining an erection, and this may contribute to their overall anxiety.

The presence of tension or *stress* can aggravate and intensify arterial occlusion and increase pain perception. Psychosocial assessment is necessary to determine those psychological and cultural variables that may be operating to intensify this problem. The presence of chronic pain can increase anxiety and make the person irritable. Close attention should be paid to the individual's personality, past compliance behavior, and perception of current health problems. These data can be most helpful when developing teaching strategies.

**P**hysical Assessment  General skin color of the affected limb or limbs may be pale or even *cyanotic*. When the limb is raised above the level of the heart,

blanching is noted. The extremity may be *cold* to touch, owing to decrease in peripheral body temperature. *Numbness* may also be present.

*Assessment of gross skin temperature* is also used in diagnosis but is of limited value. In general the temperature of the skin surface of an extremity reflects the balance between the heat lost to the environment and the amount of blood being delivered to the skin. This technique compares bilateral skin surfaces using the dorsal area of the hand or the ventral surface of the fingers. Prior exposure to extremes in temperature as well as increased sympathetic nervous system activity in an anxious patient must be considered. If one or both extremities are cold under a normal environmental temperature, the implication is poor circulation. (A complete discussion and illustration of temperature and assessment of the skin are found in Chap. 8.)

*Peripheral pulses* should be palpated and evaluated bilaterally (see Fig. 29-3). The dorsal pedal pulse as well as the posttibial pulses may be absent or difficult to palpate. The most commonly used sites for peripheral pulse palpation are the temporal, carotid, brachial, radial, femoral, popliteal, dorsalis pedis, and posterior tibialis sites (see Fig. 29-4). Using the first three fingers, the examiner selects the site and places the fingers along the length of the artery, remembering that a normal pulse is usually felt immediately. Pulses are commonly assessed according to the following scale: 4+ refers to a normal pulse, 3+ is slightly weaker, 2+ is weak, 1+ is very weak, and 0 indicates a pulse not palpated. This gradation of pulse strength becomes important when following the course of arterial disease.

As the blood vessel narrows, a characteristic sound called a *bruit* may be heard over the artery. This sound can be auscultated over any location of the artery, by placing the stethoscope directly over the affected artery. A high-pitched sound will be

**TABLE 29-1**
DIETARY RECOMMENDATIONS FOR
FAT AND CALORIC INTAKE

| |
|---|
| Adjust caloric intake to maintain ideal weight |
| Reduce total fat calories by reducing dietary saturated fat (total fat 35%) |
| Reduce dietary cholesterol |
| Avoid excessive salt intake |
| Avoid excessive refined sugar (candy, sweets) |

SOURCE: American Heart Association.

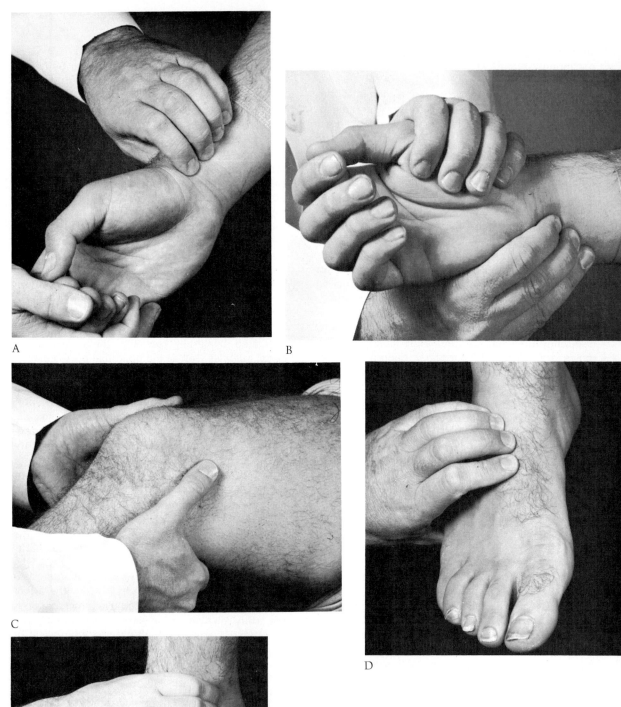

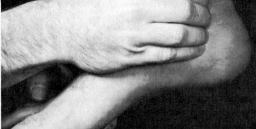

**FIGURE 29-3**
Methods for palpating arteries. (*From J. W. Hurst et al. (eds.), The Heart, 4th ed., McGraw-Hill, New York, 1978.*)

noted during systole as the blood flows through the constricted arterial vessel.

*Joint mobility* may be limited because of decreased joint use and increased pain upon movement. Muscle atrophy may also result. *Leg ulceration* may be noted on the extremities, and local inflammatory response may be noted in the surrounding tissue.

The *skin* is often smooth with a taut appearance. Dryness may also be present. *Trophic changes* or alteration of the skin texture due to decreased blood flow to the tissue frequently occur. As a result there is decreased nutrition to the tissue, and muscle wasting can occur. Hair loss, thickening of the nails, and muscle atrophy can be noted. In addition capillary refill time may be diminished.

**D**iagnostic Tests   *Exercise stress tests* are used to diagnose intermittent claudication. The basic purpose of exercise testing is to detect when the functional capacity of impaired circulation is exceeded. Arteries which are occluded or nonfunctional will be unable to increase blood flow to accommodate an increase in exercise. The patient is timed from the onset of exercise, usually walking, until claudication is experienced. Typically the greater the arterial involvement, the shorter the time required to induce claudication.[13]

*Oscillometry* may also be used to diagnose peripheral arterial occlusion. Oscillometry is a test which locates sites of arterial occlusion not heard through manual palpation of arterial pulses. An *oscillometer* is a manometer connected to a blood pressure cuff. The cuff is usually attached to the calf or thigh and inflated. The oscillometric index, or pressure reading recorded, is the point at which circulation through the deep arterial vessels is halted.[14]

Elevated *serum cholesterol levels* and *serum lipid levels* have been linked to the development of atheromas in certain individuals. The evidence thus far does not demonstrate that all patients with peripheral arterial disease have elevated cholesterol or lipid levels. A *serum cholesterol level* is considered elevated above 220/100 ml, while a triglyceride level above 150/100 ml would also be of concern. When both of these blood levels are elevated, they are suggestive of hyperlipidemia.

**Nursing problems and interventions**   The aim of intervention is to limit the progress of arterial obstruction and identify and minimize those risk factors that can enhance the problem. The major nursing problems presented by the patient with

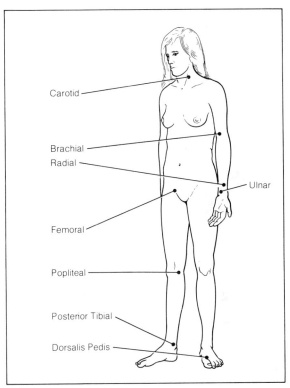

**FIGURE 29-4**
Common sites for palpating arteries.

peripheral arterial occlusion include hyperlipidemia, ischemic pain, anxiety, skin breakdown, and thrombus formation.

**H**yperlipidemia   High lipid levels, obesity, and/or high caloric intake have been identified as major components in arterial occlusion. Nutritional therapy and on occasion antilipemic drugs have been used to reduce blood lipid levels.

The aim of *nutritional therapy* is to retard and/or reverse the development of atherosclerotic lesions. Sporadic reports have alluded to reversal of such lesions in man. While the complete reversal of atherosclerotic lesions may not be possible through diet alone, there is sufficient evidence to warrant the use of a nutritional approach to retarding the atherosclerotic process. Caloric intake should be adjusted to achieve and maintain ideal body weight. Fat should be reduced to become 35 percent of the total caloric intake with less than 10 percent of fat calories from saturated fat (refer to Table 29-1).

*Cholesterol reduction* is another important component of nutritional therapy in both patients with an elevated serum cholesterol and those with normal levels. Three hundred milligrams of cholesterol is suggested for those individuals with normal blood levels, but a more severe cholesterol reduction is appropriate in patients with hypercholesterolemia. (This is discussed in greater detail in Chap. 26.) Reduction of salt intake is generally recommended, especially in those patients with coexisting hypertension.[15]

*Antilipemic agents* are employed to reduce serum lipid concentration by inhibiting gastrointestinal absorption, inhibiting the synthesis of cholesterol, or accelerating of cholesterol breakdown. The use of antilipemic agents is based on the premise that long-term elevations of serum lipids, particularly cholesterol, is basic to the development of atherosclerosis. The choice of a specific antilipemic drug is usually based on the type of hyperlipidemia involved. *Clofibrate (Atromid S)* is used for elevated triglycerides alone or in combination with an elevated cholesterol. *Sodium dextrothyroxine (Choloxin)*, a drug possessing cholesterol-lowering activity, also increases metabolism, which limits its use to patients without heart disease, as increased metabolism can precipitate angina or myocardial infarction. *Sitosterals (Cytellin)* have cholesterol-reducing properties, but their effects are less predictable than other antilipemic agents. *Cholestyramine (Questran)*, an ion-exchange resin, works to promote formation of bile from cholesterol in the liver and is used for type II hyperlipidemia.[16]

To increase blood flow through narrow and obstructed vessels is the rationale behind the use of *vasodilating drugs* which have been employed with limited success in arterial vascular conditions. *Cyclandelate (Cyclospasmol)* directly affects the arterial wall by directly relaxing smooth muscle. *Isoxsuprine hydrochloride (Vasodilan)* produces a slight to moderate increase in blood flow to resting muscle.

**I**schemic Pain   Pain associated with peripheral arterial occlusion is very stressful to the patient. This contributes to contraction of muscles which can lead to vessel spasm, thereby increasing vascular occlusion and intensifying the pain. Analgesia or narcotics can be used if the pain becomes severe.

*Alpha blocking agents* are used to control ischemia by inhibiting the constricting effect of the sympathetic nervous system (circulating catecholamines). Examples of alpha blocking agents are *Regitine* and *Dibenzyline*. Generally, the action of alpha blockers is unpredictable, and side effects are so troublesome that these drugs are not commonly prescribed.

**S**kin Breakdown   Tissue with poor arterial blood flow is poorly oxygenated and nutrient deficient. Maintenance of skin integrity, especially in the lower extremities, is vitally important to prevent injury and infection. Poor arterial flow creates trophic skin changes, causing the skin of the involved body part to be susceptible to lesions and breakdown.

*Fostering skin integrity* is accomplished by the use of mild soaps and lotions to prevent drying of the hands, feet, lips, and arms. Bath water temperature should not be hot; thus the use of a bath thermometer may be warranted to protect lower extremities with poor arterial circulation. Other means to provide protection to susceptible lower limbs include the wearing of well-fitting shoes and slippers when walking indoors. *Exercise* is helpful in promoting circulation. Walking on a flat surface is most effective as it stimulates the development of collateral circulation. Avoidance of unnecessary pressure to an involved extremity, as by constricting clothing or the crossing of the legs for prolonged periods, also enhances circulation. Difficulties in arterial circulation do not respond to extremity elevation unless the venous circulation is also involved. Observing the skin daily for trophic changes such as dryness, cracking, or thickening of the nails is another important measure. Medical assistance is required if corns, callouses, or ingrown toenails are present.

**A**nxiety   Many patients with early signs of arterial occlusion are anxious. Pain intensifies this anxiety as it limits the patient's mobility and can interfere with daily activities. Mild tranquilizers may be ordered if the patient is tense or stressful. Follow-up counseling sessions with the patient and/or family members may be needed to reduce tension. The home environment as well as the occupational setting should be free from stress and calming to the patient.

**T**hrombus Formation   The threat of arterial thrombus formation is often high, especially when edema and severe ischemic pain are present. Activity and exercise are important components of prevention. However, attempts at activity are often thwarted by the presence of ischemic pain.

*Anticoagulant therapy* for arterial obstruction is controversial, but there is increasing evidence available warranting its usefulness. It is known that anticoagulants do not reduce thrombus size but do act to prevent further coagulation of blood. *Heparin* is useful in acute situations as its action is rapid and it must be given parentally. Heparin interferes with the formation of thrombin from prothrombin and also prevents platelets from releasing thromboplastin. The blood test used to control heparin dosage is the Lee-White method for estimating clotting time. Dosage is calculated to arrive at a clotting time of 15 to 20 minutes, well above the normal range of 9 to 12 minutes. Blood to test clotting times should be drawn when heparin activity is least, e.g., just before the next injection. The antidote for heparin is protamine sulfate (see Table 29-2).

*Coumarin derivatives* are oral agents which are prothrombin depressants. It is likely that coumarin competes with vitamin K (see Table 29-2). Vitamin K has an enzymatic action in the clotting process. The onset of coumarin activity occurs in 12 to 36 hours with a cumulative effect of 1 to 2 days. The blood test used to monitor drug dosage is the prothrombin time. The prothrombin time is maintained at a safe level of 35 to 60 seconds or 15 to 30 percent normal. Normal prothrombin time is 12 to 15 seconds. The antidote for coumarin is vitamin K.[17]

*Patient teaching* regarding the use of anticoagulants is critically important. Table 29-3 presents a plan for teaching the patient in the community about anticoagulants.

**Health Teaching** Disturbances in peripheral arterial flow have a propensity to become chronic and to progressively worsen. Thus all aspects of nursing intervention should be explained to patients so they can incorporate these ideas into their daily routines and help reduce arterial occlusion. Nutritional therapy involves a change in life-style necessitating the development of new attitudes about the role of fat in the diet. It may be helpful to form small groups of patients to share experiences and discuss problems, in addition to individualized teaching and consulting. Patients should know the names of the drugs they are taking, as well as the side effects. Characteristics peculiar to each drug should be included. Instructions regarding maintenance of skin integrity should be explained and continually reinforced. All information and suggestions given to patients should be shared with family members to foster understanding in the home environment. Adequate follow-up is required to guarantee patient compliance and to evaluate information regarding skin care, diet, and drugs.

**Third-Level Nursing Care**

Advanced arterial occlusion and the changes that result in tissue hypoxia often require that the patient be hospitalized, sometimes because of the patient's need for more aggressive medical or surgical intervention.

**Nursing Assessment** Many of the changes assessed under Second-Level Nursing Care will persist and intensify. An accurate health history and physical examination will reveal significant health problems requiring immediate and long-term intervention.

**H**ealth History  The patient with advanced peripheral arterial occlusion will complain of pain at rest. This is usually worse at night. The pain wakens the patient, who will often resort to sitting in a chair. Burning, numbness, and tingling may be reported in the lower extremities, e.g., the feet and toes. The patient continues to complain of being cold, even if the environment is warm. Sexual impotence may be reported by male patients. Pain upon exercise occurs rapidly and slowly decreases with frequent rest periods. The patient will often describe a sense of heaviness or fullness in one or both legs. There may be complaints of leg ulcerations that are draining and fail to heal.

**P**hysical Assessment  Skin color in the affected extremity, especially after activity, will demonstrate pallor, particularly in the feet. Changes in skin color can be seen upon elevation of the extremity above the level of the heart. Blanching will also be noted. By having the patient lower the extremities and dangle the legs over the bedside, the nurse can observe the rate of blood return to the feet and toes. Generally, this process should take about 10 seconds. In severe arterial occlusion, this process will slow significantly.

**TABLE 29-2**
ANTICOAGULANTS

| Name | Administration Route | Control Test | Therapeutic Range | Antidote |
|------|----------------------|--------------|-------------------|----------|
| Heparin | Parental | Lee-White clotting time (normal 9–12 min) | 15–20 min | Protamine sulfate |
| Coumarin | Oral | Prothrombin time (normal 12–15 s) | 35–60 s | Vitamin K |

The presence of abnormal amounts of fluid in the extremities creates feelings of heaviness and tiredness. Edema has a tendency toward being self-perpetuating. Typically, pitting or soft-tissue edema is first found in the distal portion of a limb and is generally lessened by recumbency or elevation. Nonpitting edema or lymphedema is firm and less affected by elevation. In the presence of severe arterial impairment, comparison of the affected extremity with the nonaffected extremity will demonstrate the presence of edema, especially in a constant dependent position. This edema may be pitting or nonpitting, depending upon the extent of venous and/or lymph involvement. Arterial edema is due to severe structural changes of the arteries often accompanied by arterial vasospasm.

Decreased blood supply to tissue may limit nourishment to a limb. Assessment of muscle size should be determined by measuring the limbs for symmetry. In Leriche's syndrome there is a loss of bulk in the gluteal muscles due to occlusion of the aortoiliac vessels. Rashes, scars, and ulcerations should also be noted. As discussed under Second-Level Nursing Care, the skin may appear smooth and shiny. Signs of infection should be observed for, especially in the presence of ulceration. Tissue necrosis and gangrene may be noted. If gangrene is present, the area will be hard, dry, and black in appearance.

Skin temperature and appearance undergo changes which generally correspond to the degree of arterial impairment. The skin is cold to touch and cyanotic in appearance with severe disease. Variations in skin temperature can be due to fever, environmental conditions, smoking, or exercise; thus skin temperature is better assessed when the patient is at rest. Skin assessment is similar to palpation of pulses in that comparisons should be made bilaterally. When assessing a limb at rest for temperature change, the nurse should expose both areas to the environment for 10 to 15 minutes. Following this period the areas should be examined bilaterally for gross temperature change (see Second-Level Nursing Care).

Palpation of peripheral pulses gives general information concerning the extent of arterial flow disruption. A decrease in intensity of a peripheral pulse may not only indicate the presence of atherosclerotic plaques but also a thrombus or embolus, as an absent or diminished pulse is the most significant finding of arterial occlusion. As discussed in Second-Level Nursing Care, pulses should be compared bilaterally. Refer to Figs. 29-3 and 29-4.

The presence of a systolic bruit, discussed under Second-Level Nursing Care, still may persist. This is heard most frequently behind the angle of the jaw when there is occlusion of the internal carotid artery.

**TABLE 29-3**
TEACHING-LEARNING PLAN FOR ANTICOAGULATION

| Objective | Content | Teaching Strategy | Evaluation |
|---|---|---|---|
| Following a teaching-learning session an anticoagulant therapy the learner will: | Rationale for anticoagulation | Discuss normal blood flow; how anticoagulants work; name of patient's drug (slide tape and lecture). | Patient describes blood flow and how anticoagulant works |
| 1  Recall from memory normal blood flow. | Laboratory tests | Explain prothrombin time and how results will show changes in response to medication (film). | Patient explains anticoagulants: use and side effects |
| 2  Recall the anticoagulant being used and describe its action. | Medication schedule | Stress importance of adhering to a schedule, not missing a dose (lecture). | Patient lists all factors in therapy, e.g., medication, diet control, use of alcohol activity |
| 3  List all the side effects of anticoagulants. | Other medications | Discuss how other medicines can influence therapy (flow-chart). |  |
| 4  Identify verbally the medication's action and recall specific interventions that accompany use of anticoagulants such as laboratory tests. Understand medication to avoid, diet. | Diet  Signs of overcoagulation | Explain importance of balanced diet, need to avoid foods high in vitamin K (e.g., green leafy vegetables, cabbage, cauliflower). (Demonstration) |  |
| 5  Recall from memory the antidote for specific medication. |  | Tell why unusual or excessive bleeding or change in color of urine or stool should be reported (demonstration) and why alcohol | Weekly reports from the laboratory indicate whether prothrombin time is being affected by |
| 6  Discuss physical needs while taking anticoagulant. | Importance of laboratory evaluation (weekly) and need for compliance | should be avoided. Discuss individual reactions to therapy. | proper ingestion of the anticoagulant |

## Diagnostic Tests

When complete or severe occlusion to an artery is suspected, an angiography is often done. *Angiography* is a technique in which contrast dye is injected into an artery and x-rays are taken to record the course of the dye through the involved arteries. This test is a specific, direct means of ascertaining the location and degree of arterial obstruction whether due to chronic atherosclerosis, acute arterial trauma, thrombus, or aneurysms. Isolated segments of the arterial tree can be studied with angiographic techniques. Angiography can be performed on both arteries of upper and lower extremities as well as cerebral and coronary vessels. This procedure is not without risk; thus patients should receive a full explanation of the test and its risks. Much misinformation exists, making patients very anxious and apprehensive. Patient anxiety could be controlled if explanations are given.

The patient should be told that a dye will be injected intravenously into an artery of choice. (The femoral or brachial artery is commonly used.) During the injection the patient may experience an initial burning sensation around the injection site which will last a few seconds. Since the dye used is calibrated by determining the body weight, the patient's weight will have to be recorded prior to x-ray. Generally, the patient should not eat prior to the x-ray. A mild sedative may be used to relax the patient.

Anaphylactic reaction (see Chap. 28) to the dye may occur. The patient should be told that a skin test will be done prior to the angiography. The nurse should observe the patient for signs of an allergic response (numbness, weakness, nausea, and vomiting).

Venous thrombosis (discussed later in this chapter) can occur due to a leaking of the dye into the vein. A large dose of dye given too rapidly can also act as a thrombus and obstruct a blood vessel. Arrhythmias can sometimes occur, but are rare.

Following the procedure the patient will be put on bed rest; the injection site should be observed for local inflammation or thrombosis formation as well as evidence of hemorrhage. The extremity must be assessed for increased occlusion by noting skin color, pain, numbness, or changes in peripheral pulses. Blood pressure and other vital signs should also be monitored.

**Nursing problems and interventions** The patient with well-established, advanced, or complete occlusion will be faced with many significant prob-lems. These include pain, vasoconstriction, ulceration, tissue necrosis, and anxiety.

**P**ain   Pain continues to be a problem associated with increased arterial occlusion. Increased tissue ischemia and necrosis cause added stimulation to nerve endings and intensify pain. The inflammatory response that results stimulates tissue edema, putting added pressure on free nerve endings. Stronger forms of analgesia should be used to help relieve the pain. Tranquilizers may help reduce the anxiety provoked by the pain experience. Vasodilators can help increase blood supply to the area and reduce the pain.

*Position changes* can also increase blood supply to the lower limbs. By placing the head of the bed on a 6- to 8-inch block, blood flow is forced into the lower limbs by gravity. Frequent position changes will also help prevent venous stasis and stimulate circulation. The patient should be instructed to avoid crossing the legs and feet (at the ankles) in an effort to prevent stasis of fluid.

**V**asoconstriction   With relief of the arterial constriction, circulation to the periphery increases, improving nutrition of tissue and decreasing ischemic pain. In addition to the drugs mentioned in Second-Level Nursing Care, vasoconstriction can be relieved by several additional measures.

Circulation to the extremities can be increased by providing warmth and preventing vasoconstriction. If exposure to the cold is inevitable, patients should be advised to dress warmly. Environmental temperature should be adjusted to provide a consistent temperature range of 70 to 72°F. Direct heat should never be applied to areas possessing poor circulation. Reflex dilatation of arteries of the lower extremities can be accomplished by application of heat to the abdomen. Circulatory status can be maintained or improved by preventing *vasoconstriction*. Smoking, emotional stress, and excessive cold are three situations that precipitate arterial constriction. Patients should be instructed on ways to decrease emotional stress and assisted to eliminate cigarette smoking. *Exercise,* including the *Buerger-Allen exercises,* may be of some value. These exercises involve having the patient lie in bed with the legs elevated above the heart for 2 minutes. When blanching occurs, the legs can be lowered and kept dependent for 3 minutes or until color returns to the extremities and the legs are pink. The patient will lie flat and repeat the activity 4 or 5 times per day. If a patient with peripheral arterial occlusion is receiving antihypertensive medications, care must be taken to maintain adequate arterial pressure.

**U**lceration and Tissue Necrosis   Ulceration of the lower extremity in the presence of peripheral arterial occlusion is a common problem in advanced arterial occlusion. Because of decreased blood supply to the periphery, the slightest skin trauma can become easily infected and necrotic.

*Foot care* is critical, as is generalized care of the legs. Prevention of pressure areas and decubiti is crucial. Use of lotions and skin creams and lamb's wool, as well as exercise and position change, are also essential. Nail care should include warm soaks and cutting as needed. If necessary the patient should be instructed to cut the nails straight across or seek professional help. Patients must be warned against scratching or traumatizing the extremity. Coexisting diabetes mellitus can worsen the problem.

If an ulcerated area occurs and fails to respond to intervention, serious complications can occur. The patient can develop cellulitis (an inflammation of tissue surrounding the injury), ulcerations resulting in tissue breakdown, and necrosis or gangrene. When gangrene does occur, it produces irreversible changes in the main arteries and may lead to amputation of the affected limb.

**A**nxiety   Pain tends to increase the patient's anxiety, and prolonged hospitalization can create an added stress. Healing of the ulceration may be a long process beset by many complications. The potential threat of surgery with the possibility of amputation intensifies the individual's anxiety. Concern for alteration in physical appearance, limited mobility, loss of sexual appeal, and interference with current occupation and potential job advancement must all be considered. The patient needs continuous support from the nurse and family members, and fear of the unknown increases the stress response. The influence of age may also be a factor to be considered when planning alternatives to care. Amputation for a patient 70 years of age, as opposed to a woman of 45 years, has to be dealt with on a very different basis. Therefore careful discussion and clarification of the problem are critical to relieving stress. If an amputation is the intervention of choice, more long-term counseling may be required. Mild tranquilizers and an open discussion of all the issues by the nurse and patient may help to relieve some of the stress.

**S**urgical Intervention   In an effort to control further advancement of arterial occlusion and tissue hypoxia, three surgical interventions can be performed. These are an endarterectomy, femoral popliteal bypass, and amputation.

*Endarterectomy*   An *endarterectomy* is a surgical procedure which increases arterial flow either by removal of the arterial obstruction, usually an atheroma or thrombus, or bypassing the obstructed portion of the artery. In most cases endarterectomy involves both approaches. Patients are evaluated for this procedure following angiography which locates obstruction levels.[18] Preparation of the patient and family for endarterectomy involves adequate explanation of *why* the procedure is necessary and *what* will be done during surgery and a discussion of the patient's anxieties concerning the procedure. *Postoperative nursing intervention* is dependent upon the area of the endarterectomy. Generally a patient is observed for signs of adequate circulation which include the presence of peripheral pulses, changes in skin color and skin temperature, and signs of further occlusion. Patients and families should be taught, prior to discharge, how to assess adequate circulation and to report signs of occlusion.

*Femoral bypass grafting*   *Femoropopliteal bypass grafting* is indicated in the presence of disabling calf pain, rest pain, or impending gangrene. Obstruction of the femoropopliteal area remains a major peripheral vascular problem. Autogenous saphenous vein bypass grafting taken from the patient is often chosen over synthetic grafts because of a decreased incidence of infection and proved long-term patency. The saphenous vein is used most often because it is in close proximity to the femoral artery. Preoperative evaluation is accomplished by angiography.[19] The patient should be told about the procedure and its effects on circulation and should be informed that following surgery, there will be an increase in peripheral blood supply and a decrease in pain and healing of any skin ulcerations. When possible, the type of graft to be used should be viewed by the patient (see Fig. 29-5a). If feasible the family should participate in these discussions.

When an *aortic iliac obstruction* occurs, Dacron polyester fiber grafts are inserted and used to complete the bypass (see Fig. 29-5b). The procedure has added complications in that the patient's body may reject the Dacron materials, inflammatory changes may occur at the site of insertion, and there may be an increase in the incidence of clot formation. Postoperatively, the continued assessment of adequate circulation in the involved limb is imperative. An early postoperative complication of the graft is thrombosis, particularly in the area of anastomosis. The blood pressure and other vital signs should be closely monitored as persistent hypotension increases the likelihood of thrombus formation. Leakage of blood around the anastomosis can lead to hemorrhage. Complaints of pain, tenderness, skin color changes, along with alterations in vital signs and the level of consciousness, may herald the onset of complications.

*Amputation* A severe complication of arterial impairment is observed when nutrition reaching local tissue is inadequate for metabolism at rest. Necrotic and gangrenous tissue associated with marked decrease in arterial flow is often seen. Gangrene produces irreversible changes in main arteries and may eventually require *amputation* of the affected limb.

The decision to amputate a limb requires careful consideration of numerous factors. These include the presence of intractable pain, extension of a gangrenous lesion, the presence of infection, and the possibility of severe impairment of the limb without amputation. Results of diagnostic tests are

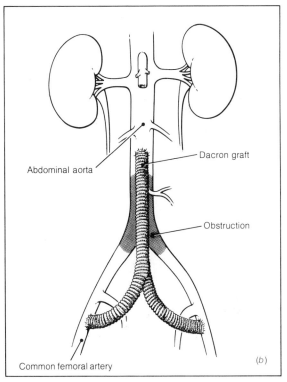

**FIGURE 29-5**

(*a*) Venous autograft. (*Adapted from Sabiston, Davis-Christopher Textbook of Surgery, 10th ed., Saunders, Philadelphia.*) (*b*) Bypass graft.

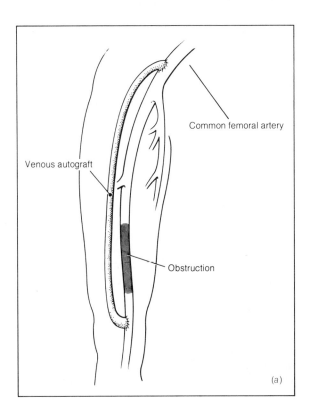

also considered as well as the patient's and physician's attitudes toward the amputation.

*Preoperative preparation* involves both psychological and physical considerations. Maintenance of open, honest communications with the patient and family is the cornerstone of psychological preparation. As the patient is about to lose a body part, both grief and mourning should be anticipated (see Chap. 3). Information should be factual but imparted so as to allow the patient and family to ask questions and ventilate feelings. Individuals may become angry and depressed or refuse to accept the surgery. These behavioral changes will have to be discussed by the patient and nurse and resolved on a day-to-day basis. Teaching preoperatively should also include expectations both pre- and postoperatively and a basic description of the amputation procedure. Physical preparation for a lower extremity prior to amputation involves controlled exercise to strengthen the upper extremities, the trunk, and the abdominal muscles and mobility training to include opportunities to practice transferring, standing, and crutch walking (see

Chap. 40). The patient will require considerable support from the physical therapist and nurse to perform the necessary exercises. Transferring from the bed to a wheelchair or to the commode should be practiced two to three times daily. A patient should also be taught how to modify weight bearing on the affected side.

*Decisions regarding the amputation site* are based upon the amount of circulation in the extremity and the requirements of the prosthesis. Levels of lower-extremity amputation include foot, ankle, above the knee, and below the knee. Below-the-knee amputations are most likely to be successful if the popliteal pulse is adequate. An amputation of the lower extremity due to arterial obstruction is more commonly performed than amputation of the upper extremity.

There are basically two types of surgical amputations: (1) the closed (flap) amputation and (2) the open (guillotine). A *closed amputation* is done by using skin flaps to cover the exposed ends of the amputated bone.[20] The skin is sutured closed and covered with a dressing and an elastic bandage. The primary indication for an *open amputation* is to promote drainage in the presence of infection. In this procedure the skin flaps are not sutured together and the bone ends are left open to drain. The area is covered with a pressure dressing and irrigated several times a day with an antiseptic solution. When the infection has subsided, the stump is surgically closed.

*Below-the-knee amputations* are likely to be most successful if a light plaster cast is used postoperatively. The cast is applied to the entire extremity with a temporary prosthesis incorporated at its distal end. This allows for immobilization of the knee joint and protection from swelling and pain. *Above-the-knee amputations* are most often indicated if tissue involvement is above the ankle level. Levels of upper-extremity amputation include wrist, below the elbow, at the elbow, and above the elbow.

The *postoperative goals* can be summarized as follows: the patient's general health status should be preserved and improved, the stump should be able to utilize the most modern prosthesis, and the untoward psychosocial consequences of the amputation should be decreased. Recent trends in prosthesis fitting of the lower extremities indicate increasing satisfaction with immediate prosthesis fitting to avoid the usual postoperative complications of an amputation. These complications include *phantom limb pain, skin complications, contractures of the joint, hematomas,* and *stump edema.* It should be realized that immediate pros-

thesis fitting creates its own complications due to early ambulation and the presence of a tight-fitting dressing. With early prosthesis fitting it is not possible to assess the wound as the dressing covers it completely. This tight-fitting dressing can become displaced from the stump, resulting in stump edema and wound disruption. Skin breakdown and wound disruption can also result from extensive weight bearing before healing has taken place.

*Stump care* following a closed amputation is an important aspect of postoperative care when prosthesis fitting is delayed. Shrinkage of the stump is facilitated by use of an elastic bandage wrap which also functions to prevent edema (see Fig. 29-6). Fitting of a prosthesis will occur when the stump has achieved maximum shrinkage. *Cleanliness* of the stump is also important. The use of mild soap and water, along with exposure to air and sun, will serve to maintain cleanliness. To allow the stump to accommodate a prosthesis, stump conditioning *exercises,* consisting of pushing the stump against increasingly harder surfaces, should be employed. Massage of the stump will increase blood flow and decrease tenderness and is usually initiated 5 to 7 days postoperatively.

The stump, with or without a prosthesis, is usually *elevated* for approximately 24 hours after surgery to improve venous return and reduce swelling. *Exercise* is particularly important when prosthesis fitting is delayed to retain muscle tone and prevent edema, joint contractions, and muscle atrophy. These exercises can be initiated after the first 24 hours and should include active range of motion to the unaffected limb, exercise to increase the strength of the upper extremities, and stump hyperextension. A patient with an immediate prosthesis is ambulated for increasing lengths of time after the first 24 hours, while a patient without a prosthesis is usually assisted to transfer to a chair on the first postoperative day, with crutch walking initiated as soon as the patient is able to tolerate this progression of activity. Any signs of *hemorrhage,* including an increase in pain, swelling, tenderness, restlessness, and overt blood loss, should be reported. The possibility of gross hemorrhage, although rare, warrants the placement of a tourniquet at the patient's bedside.

*Psychological support* is an important aspect of care. Patients should be encouraged to be as active as possible. Inactivity may increase depression by allowing the patient more time to dwell on the loss, thus focusing all energy on coping. Psychological support consists of not only listening to the patient's fears concerning the future but also providing means to assist coping which can include the opportunity to speak with another amputee who has achieved a state of independence. Changes in body image may result in long-term mourning for the lost limb. Family members need to be helped through this period as it may be lengthy. Emotional counseling as well as occupational planning may be required for some time following the amputation. The way the patient chooses to deal with the loss is often reflective of the way other losses were handled in the past.

### Fourth-Level Nursing Care

*Rehabilitation* of the amputee is directed toward achieving an optimum level of functioning, at an optimum level of independence. It is essential that rehabilitation begin in the preoperative period with initial physical and psychosocial assessments. Successful rehabilitation is dependent not only upon the patient's physical condition and the adequacy of the prosthetic device but also upon the patient's self-perception and acceptance of the physical, social, and psychological implications of the amputation. An organized team approach, incorporating

the skills of the nurse, physician, psychologist, physical therapist, and social worker are necessary to ensure optimum rehabilitation. Exercises, including the Buerger-Allen exercises, should be continued. The patient should use positions which will help reduce and relieve pain. Legs should be elevated when sitting in a chair. Care should be taken to avoid crossing legs or ankles. Rest periods should always follow any activity.

**Health teaching** *Teaching* involves preparing patients for self-care in the home environment. For the patient who has undergone a femoral bypass procedure, it is important to stress that normal activity will be allowed in 1 to 2 months and that flexion of the knee or hip for prolonged periods of time should be avoided. The patient should be encouraged to maintain skin integrity and taught how to provide effective skin care. Alleviation of pressure areas should always be a concern, and care of feet and nails must be included in any care plan. Avoiding constricting clothing and eliminating smoking are critical. The patient should know when adequate circulation is present and should be

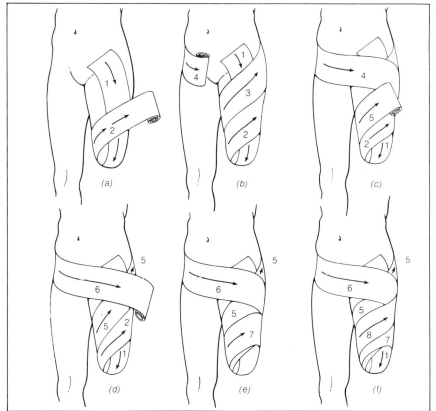

**FIGURE 29-6**
Bandaging an above-the-knee amputation. (*From The University of Washington Department of Prosthetics, Prosthetics-Orthotics.*)

taught to check peripheral pulses. In addition the patient should be helped to recognize alterations in circulation including tingling, numbness, color changes, swelling, and pallor and be encouraged to report these changes immediately.

Educating an amputee for discharge involves stump care, prosthesis care, and instruction for regularly scheduled exercise. Home visits and community referrals, along with occupational counseling, may be important components of continued care. Continuous periodic health reviews will be required to assess overall peripheral arterial status. Dietary counseling may be essential if control of weight is a problem. If pain is present or phantom-limb pain is experienced (see Chap. 39), accurate reporting of the pain is essential.

### Other Peripheral Occlusive Diseases

Several problems other than arterio- and atherosclerotic vessel changes can cause arterial occlusion. These include acute arterial occlusion (embolism, thrombus), aortic aneurysm, Buerger's disease and Raynaud's disease.

**Acute arterial occlusion** This condition is a sudden interruption of arterial blood supply to an extremity due to the presence of a thrombus or embolism. Sudden occlusion of a major artery initially produces a reflex arterial spasm which, if prolonged, creates endothelial damage. The outcome of sudden occlusion is dependent upon the adequacy of collateral circulation. Manifestations of arterial embolism are sequential. There is a loss of distal pulses followed immediately by blanching and cooling of the extremity. In the presence of severe ischemia, pain occurs within 20 minutes. Loss of sensation progresses from the distal to the proximal portion of the limb with loss of motion (most obvious in the upper extremities) in 2 to 3 hours. Muscle necrosis occurs in 6 to 8 hours. Within 48 hours skin breakdown occurs, while gangrene is usually apparent in 72 hours. The majority of arterial emboli (85 percent) arise from the heart, usually owing to mitral and aortic valve stenosis, thrombi, myocardial infarction (Chap. 26), and atrial fibrillation (Chap. 25). Arterial thrombi occur as a secondary response to trauma to artery or vascular disorder. Location of an acute arterial occlusion is usually at arterial bifurcations where an embolus can lodge.

Careful assessment is required for early recognition of acute arterial occlusion. Palpation of peripheral pulses will demonstrate absence of any pulse. Other assessments should include skin temperature to detect coldness and the presence of paresthesia and pain.

The initial therapy is directed toward anticoagulation with heparin to prevent clot formation, either proximal or distal to the location of the embolus. It has been demonstrated that embolectomy can be delayed, if necessary, as long as 3 to 4 days, if the patient has been anticoagulated. Without anticoagulation embolectomy cannot be prolonged for longer than 12 hours. Arterial spasm relief is obtained by use of narcotic analgesics, by wrapping the involved extremity loosely in cotton to conserve body heat, and by maintaining the environmental temperature at approximately 80°F. The ischemic extremity should be placed in a position to promote blood flow by gravity.[21] This necessitates placing the extremity in a slightly dependent position, which can be accomplished by elevating the bed on blocks to direct flow to the ischemic part.

**Aortic aneurysm** An aneurysm is characterized by a weakening of the medial layer of an artery. Atherosclerosis is the most common cause of aneurysms, but infection and trauma can also precipitate their development. Sacculated arteriosclerotic aneurysms (aneurysms involving one area of an artery) most often occur in the abdominal aorta and the popliteal arteries. On rare occasions, a tear may occur in the arterial intima (dissecting), causing blood to make its way between the intimal lining and the arterial muscle layer. This results in the formation of a hematoma in the vessel wall. A complete discussion of aneurysms is found in Chap. 34.

**Buerger's disease** Buerger's disease (thromboangiitis obliterans) is a disease characterized by an inflammation of arteries, as well as veins and nerves of the lower extremities. Structural changes in the vessel wall and thrombosis may result.

The precise mechanism of Buerger's disease is not known, but patients with this condition have been found to possess a high concentration of the heparin-precipitable fraction of fibrinogen in their blood. In addition the disease is associated with arterial (as well as venous) thrombosis and can lead to tissue necrosis and gangrene. Differentiating Buerger's disease from atherosclerosis is done on the basis of the following criteria: the patient is usually male, less than 40 years old, and a heavy cigarette smoker, superficial thrombophlebitis may be present, and arterial involvement of the upper extremities is demonstrated. The presence of all these factors will affirm the diagnosis of Buerger's disease.[22]

This problem may occur suddenly or over time. There may be coldness, numbness, and tingling in the lower extremities. Intermittent claudication may be present, and more persistent peripheral pain noted. Arterial pulses will be decreased or absent. Smoking, cold, and emotional stress intensify the patient's problems.

Assisting a patient to stop smoking is of primary importance, as the incidence of amputation is greater for those individuals who continue to smoke. Relief of the pain associated with Buerger's disease is accomplished by the use of analgesics and by preventing skin breakdown. Ulcerations and gangrene are prevented by maintaining cleanliness and by protecting the extremity from trauma and infection. Vasoconstriction of the involved extremity can be decreased by avoiding exposure to the cold, cessation of smoking, and avoiding constricting garments. Reduction of stress through counseling and isolation of precipitating factors should be evaluated and eliminated when possible. Coexisting diabetes should be detected and controlled, as it could enhance the initial occlusion.

**Raynaud's disease**  Raynaud's disease is a vascular condition in which there are spasmodic contractions of arteries. The upper extremities, particularly the fingers, are most often affected. Occasionally in the lower extremities, the toes are involved. Raynaud's disease is considered a phenomenon which develops in phases. Initially, there is intermittent color change. The *pallor phase* is due to occlusion of affected vessels, which causes the affected digits to appear to have a bluish coloration. A *rubor phase* is a period of excessive *hyperemia* during which the digits appear reddened.

The etiology of this disease is unknown, but there may be a genetic predisposition. Raynaud's phenomenon can be induced by exposure to cold temperatures or by emotional upsets. The presence of *primary Raynaud's disease* is usually precipitated by cold or emotion (see Table 29-4). It is bilateral in origin and gangrene is absent. Normal peripheral pulsations are present, with no other primary disease apparent. The patient usually reports having noted the problem for as long as 2 years.

*Secondary Raynaud's disease* can occur as a result of rheumatoid arthritis, lupus erythematosus, or scleroderma. Generally the presenting symptoms are similar to primary Raynaud's disease, but until the initial cause is removed, problems will persist.

## PERIPHERAL VENOUS OCCLUSIONS

Disturbances in peripheral venous circulation can be precipitated by a variety of causes. These include venous trauma, venous stasis, increased blood viscosity, and inflammation. These changes can lead to occlusion of circulation of blood through the venous system and precipitate the formation of thrombi. This section will discuss in depth the causes, changes, and effects of peripheral venous occlusion due to inflammation of a vein. Terms that will be used to describe peripheral venous occlusion are found in Table 29-5.

### Pathophysiology

*Phlebitis* is a commonly used term which signifies a simple inflammation of a vein. *Thrombophlebitis* refers to the development of venous thrombi accompanied by inflammatory changes in the vessel wall, while *phlebothrombosis* refers to the presence of a thrombus within a vein without accompanying inflammatory changes (see Table 29-5).

The effects of a thrombus within a vein vary depending upon the location, the extent and the depth of involvement, and whether the thrombus is present in a superficial or a deep vein.

**TABLE 29-4**
CRITERIA FOR PRIMARY RAYNAUD'S DISEASE

| | |
|---|---|
| 1 | Precipitated by cold or emotions |
| 2 | Bilateral changes noted |
| 3 | Absence of gangrene |
| 4 | Absence of any primary pathology |
| 5 | Normal pulsations present |
| 6 | Persistence of symptoms for 2 years |

**TABLE 29-5**
TERMS USED IN PERIPHERAL VENOUS OCCLUSION

| Term | Definition |
|---|---|
| Embolism | Movement of solid mass (blood clot) from its origin to a distal point, causing obstruction |
| Embolus | A solid mass (blood clot) carried by the blood |
| Phlebitis | Inflammation of a vein without thrombus |
| Phlebothrombosis | Presence of a venous thrombus without inflammation |
| Thromboembolism | A thrombus which has dislodged from its origin site |
| Thrombophlebitis | Presence of venous thrombi with inflammation |
| Thrombosis | Formation of a solid mass (blood clot) inside a blood vessel |
| Thrombus | A solid mass (blood clot) |

*Superficial thrombophlebitis* usually occurs in superficial veins such as the saphenous vein or in the forearm. Occurrence of this problem in the arm can be precipitated by intravenous injection of caustic material, by the physical trauma of long-term intravenous catheters, or by the irritation of the catheter itself. When the legs are involved, varicose veins often precipitate the thrombophlebitis.

*Deep thrombophlebitis* is the inflammation of deep veins. The severity of the problem varies according to the degree of venous involvement. Usually deeper veins including the femoral, subclavian, and inferior or superior vena cava are involved. At times, the onset of the problem can be insidious, but symptoms usually will manifest themselves as the occlusion progresses.

When the veins of the venous system become defective, the valves contained within the vein become incompetent. As adequate blood flow is maintained toward the pump, the valves are open. This causes a distention of the vein and can render the valves incompetent.

Conditions conducive to thrombus formation include venous stasis, injury to the vessel wall, and hypercoagulability of blood. The pooling of blood or venous stasis is often seen in prolonged bed rest, especially during postoperative and postpartum periods or with the presence of varicosities.

*Varicose veins* are described as dilated and engorged. There is usually hypertrophy of the muscular coat, an increase in fibrous connective tissue, and an increase in the thickness of the intima.[23] As the veins become distended, they lose their elasticity, and their valves become less functional. This results in venous stasis and can lead to atrophy or can render the vein incompetent. Pregnancy, obesity, and occupations requiring limited position change can cause varicosities. Alteration in venous pressure can induce swelling and pain.

**Causes of thrombophlebitis** Rapid blood coagulation accompanied by an increase in thromboplastin is associated with malignancies or blood dyscrasias and can lead to thrombus formation. In most patients, thrombophlebitis is precipitated by a combination of factors. An increase in occurrence is also observed with advancing age, as older persons are more predisposed than younger persons. The role of oral contraceptives in the development of thrombi is still controversial. A federal drug study in the United States (1969), in contrast with earlier British studies, did state that "the pill" may be responsible for only a minimal increase in the occurrence of thromboembolism.

*Venous obstruction* can also be created by use of constricting girdles, crossing legs continuously, and sitting or standing for long periods of time without exercise. They can cause trauma to the vessel walls, venous distention, and stasis and can contribute to varicosities. Chronic edema can also alter venous circulation. In the presence of edema nutrients can be prevented from reaching the tissue. A decrease in oxygen and nutrients can lead to tissue anoxia and ulceration.

*Surgical interventions* involving the pelvic viscera can also increase the incidence of phlebitis. The pelvic area is a highly vascular region, and veins can easily be cut, obstructed during retraction, or occluded by clamps during surgery. Thrombus formation can therefore easily occur. Any roughness or irregularity in the vessel wall tends to attract clotting. A *roughened endothelial surface* as observed in Buerger's disease can lead to thrombus formation.

Platelet changes and alterations in circulating fibrinogen molecules are other possible mechanisms involved in thrombus formation. Events triggering thrombus formation have not yet been specifically defined, but there is widespread agreement that *platelet aggregation* occurs in conjunction with fibrin deposition. The appearance of clotting factors II, V, VIII, X, XI, and XII will be seen, but their precise triggering mechanism is not known. Many questions are still left unanswered, as whether the presence of enough thrombin alters circulating fibrinogen or whether just the half-life of fibrinogen is shortened.

Thrombophlebitis can occur in any of the superficial or deep veins. When the problems are in the deeper veins, they can have more systemic and life-threatening consequences.

**Effects of peripheral venous occlusion** Disruptions in venous pressure, venous engorgement, and edema are observed clinically in the patient with peripheral venous occlusion. An *alteration in venous pressure* is most likely to occur when a large major vein is host to a thrombus. Elevation of venous pressure will be seen distally in the involved limb. Passive congestion of blood flow produces *venous engorgement,* resulting in cyanosis and visible venous distention. *Edema* is initially nonpitting owing to the increase in intravascular volume and capillary venous pressure. The edema evolves from nonpitting to pitting as increased capillary pressures lead to movement of fluid into the tissues.[24] *Pain,* inflammation, and tenderness due to venous distention and compression of nerve endings usually follow. As congestion becomes more severe, *tissue anoxia* is increased and the pain intensifies.

Along with the local inflammation there is a *narrowing of the lumen* of the vein and pooling of blood. This predisposes the individual to thrombus formation. When the thrombus forms, it attaches itself to the intimal wall, decreasing the chance of emboli formation. The threat of the thrombus dislodging and traveling into circulation as an embolus is always present. An *embolus* is defined as any foreign body introduced into the bloodstream; it can be air, fat cells, or a portion of a blood clot. An embolus travels until it reaches a blood vessel too small to pass through. There it lodges, blocking blood flow through the vessel. Only the tail of a fresh thrombus is likely to become detached and give rise to an embolism.[25] Emboli can also travel to the brain, the heart, or the lung (see Fig. 29-7).

When the embolus migrates to the pulmonary area, there is obstruction of the airway and decreased $O_2/CO_2$ exchange. The severity of the occlusion depends upon the area affected. If the major pulmonary branch is occluded, there is a de-

crease in ventilation and lung perfusion. As a result, airways constrict, and there is an increase in dead space in portions of the lung no longer oxygenated. In an attempt to compensate, tachycardia, dyspnea, and hyperpnea occur. There is an increase in vascular resistance, and right-sided pump failure may result. (A discussion of pulmonary embolism can also be found in Chap. 30.) If the embolus travels to the heart, a myocardial infarction can occur (see Chap. 26). If the embolus travels to the brain, cerebral vascular occlusion occurs (see Chap. 34).

### First-Level Nursing Care

Awareness of those situations that predispose an individual to venous thrombus formation is essential if preventive intervention is to be initiated. Patients and individuals susceptible to venous stasis are those who have or will experience periods of immobility and/or prolonged time periods without positional changes. Identification of individuals at risk may be isolated through careful screening. The patient's occupation should be identified, the amount of position changes involved should be noted, and daily exercise habits should be as-

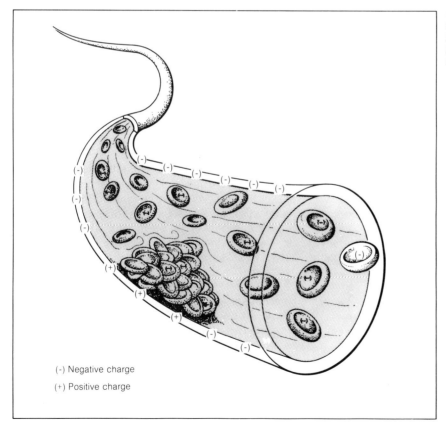

**FIGURE 29-7**
Clot formation. (*From H. Moidel et al., Nursing Care of the Patient With Medical-Surgical Disorders, 2d ed.,* McGraw-Hill, New York, 1976.)

(-) Negative charge

(+) Positive charge

sessed. Patients on prolonged bed rest or immobilized by traction or body cast are also at risk. Surgical patients, especially those having involved vascular or pelvic surgery, are also predisposed to venous stasis. Persons who are obese, wear tight, constricting clothing, or continuously cross their legs, as well as persons who travel a great deal in one position can also be included in a high-risk group. The use of oral contraceptives may also predispose an individual to venous inflammation and clot formation, although this possibility is controversial. In addition, age and sex are important components of the risk assessment. Recognition that thrombus formation may occur more frequently in the elderly owing to arteriosclerotic as well as other physical changes may cause increased focus on this age group.

**Prevention** *Preventive measures taken within the hospital setting* to control the development of phlebothrombosis and thrombophlebitis include early postoperative mobilization, leg exercises for those on bed rest, elevation of the lower extremities to promote venous return, and the use of elastic stockings to compress the superficial vessels directing flow to the deeper veins. Frequent inspection of intravenous sites and changing of intravenous catheters every 24 to 48 hours may help reduce the incidence of superficial thrombophlebitis. Introduction of an intravenous catheter into the lower extremities should be avoided as the veins in the lower limbs are very prone to thrombophlebitis and thromboembolism.

*Antiplatelet agents* may be used, especially if bed rest is prolonged, to decrease the clotting mechanism and reduce the blood viscosity. Dextran, although effective in some situations, can result in hypervolemia and is generally not recommended for primary prevention. The use of low-dose heparin is becoming increasingly popular. Recent literature focuses on its use preoperatively to prevent postoperative embolization. Many trials have indicated that small doses of subcutaneous heparin, 5000 units every 12 hours, used while a patient is immobile, and continued until a patient has fully ambulated, are successful in preventing thromboembolism.

Candidates for thrombus formation are individuals with existent vascular problems creating disruption in blood flow, for example, those with varicose veins or Buerger's disease, individuals receiving intravenous therapy, patients requiring extended periods of immobility such as an elderly person in traction, and individuals experiencing procedures requiring entry into a vein.

An *external pneumatic boot,* although still in the experimental stages, is being used more frequently in prevention. The pneumatic boot is applied as an external legging, does not interfere with blood coagulation, but aids in blood flow. The external boot is connected to an electric pump, which moves air into the legging to compress superficial vessels and aid in venous return.

*Prevention in the community* setting can be best accomplished through health education. Health education within industries where employees engage in limited change of position should encourage increased physical activity, improved circulation of lower limbs, and decreased venous stasis. Individuals working in jobs requiring continuous standing should be encouraged to wear support hose.

Individuals who travel in automobiles or trucks extensively, or people involved in a vacation trip that requires long hours in one position, need to be encouraged to stop frequently and exercise. Getting out of the car or truck every 1 to 2 hours will help stimulate circulation to the periphery.

Avoiding tight, constricting clothing, especially involving the lower extremities, is a critical point in prevention. Women need to be encouraged to avoid tight girdles and occlusive garters. Constriction created by tight clothes can, over time, induce venous incompetence. Individuals having varicose veins need to be encouraged to wear support hose and to be cognizant of the need for frequent position change. They should be aware of the effects of injury to a limb and instructed to increase self-protection against limb trauma.

All persons in any setting, but especially those with oxygenation problems, should be cautioned about the hazards of crossing the legs. Individuals taking oral contraceptives need to be told of the drug's potential effect on thrombus formation and be made aware of the early side effects of such drugs.

### Second-Level Nursing Care

Individuals seen by the community health nurse are usually treated for superficial thrombophlebitis. Patients with deep thrombophlebitis may be first observed in the community, but will be immediately referred to an acute-care setting.

**Nursing assessment** The patient with superficial thrombophlebitis usually offers a *health his-*

*tory* which suggests injury to a superficial vein, chronic vascular problem (such as varicose veins), or the presence of malignancy. Patients will often complain of mild pain and describe an aching tenderness usually localized to a specific area. Activity may or may not increase the pain.

**P**hysical Assessment   Assessment of the extremity involved usually reveals swelling along the course of the involved superficial vein. It tends to be localized in one specific area, and a knot or bump can be felt upon palpation of the vein. Redness is visible and can be observed along the course of the vein. The area involved is hot and tender to the touch. There is no obstruction of peripheral pulses unless other pathology is present. The patient can usually walk without too much discomfort, although there may be a tendency to favor the affected limb. Swelling may be noted around the inflamed area, but skin ulcerations are not apparent.

**D**iagnostic Tests   The tests used in superficial thrombophlebitis are limited. Therefore, a complete discussion of diagnostic tests will take place under Third-Level Nursing Care.

**Nursing problems and intervention**   The major problem incurred by patients with superficial thrombophlebitis is pain due to inflammation of the vein. Secondary to the inflammatory process, the patient may experience swelling and tenderness in the area of inflammation. The prevention of thrombus formation is a third concern for the nurse and patient.

**P**ain   Pain will persist to the degree that the inflammation causes irritation and compression of nerve endings. *Analgesics* are sometimes used to help relieve the pain. If the patient is receiving heparin, aspirin is avoided as it may interfere with platelet aggregation and disrupt the effects of heparin.

Direct application of *heat* to the affected area will also assist in the resolution of the inflammatory process and decrease pain. Two to three days are usually sufficient for the application of compresses. Hot packs are also helpful in providing direct heat to an area and can be purchased from a local pharmacy. Care must be taken to protect the skin from excessive heat. *Bed rest* is usually instituted along with elevation of the involved extremity until tenderness, pain, and swelling subside. It is advised that bed rest not be imployed for longer than 7 to 10

days. During this time, it is critical that the family be taught to utilize passive range of motion exercises to the unaffected limb and other body extremities. Caution should be taken when moving the affected limb so that pain and rubbing of the affected area are avoided. Family members should be taught how to move the limb and avoid massaging the legs.

*Anticoagulants* are rarely used for superficial thrombophlebitis. When used, small doses of heparin can be administered in the physician's office. Refer to Table 29-3 for health teaching related to the use of anticoagulants.

**P**revention of Thrombus Formation   Prevention for a patient with superficial thrombophlebitis should focus upon teaching the signs of thrombus formation. These include pain, tenderness, redness and swelling, and edema. Patients should be instructed not to wear constricting clothing, to avoid maintaining a standing or sitting position for long periods of time, and to establish a plan of daily exercise. Cigarette smoking and obesity should be discouraged and controlled where possible. If taking a long car trip, patients should be taught the need for frequent rest/activity periods. Exercise of the extremity should occur for 5 minutes out of every hour. The patient should be encouraged, when lying down, to elevate the extremity to promote venous circulation. Support hose can be worn, and the patient should be told to avoid trauma to the affected limb.

Follow-up in patients recovering from thrombophlebitis is necessary as residual effects may develop. The *postphlebitic syndrome* is a problem of chronic venous stasis precipitated by thrombophlebitis. As a result of the phlebitis, venous valves become damaged and have difficulty preventing backflow of blood. The presenting manifestations include swelling, skin color changes, pain, ulceration, and the recurrence of thrombosis.

Susceptible patients should be referred to a home health care service, especially those with chronic recurring venous thrombosis. Patients should be advised to notify their physician or primary-care nurse if any signs of thrombophlebitis develop.

**Third-Level Nursing Care**

When a thrombophlebitis of a deep vein occurs and a clot formation is suspected, the patient will usually be hospitalized. Careful assessment and early intervention will help prevent more life-threatening complications.

**Nursing assessment** When patients are seen in the hospital, they will offer a fairly direct *health history*. Pain, severe at times, will again be the major complaint. With deep thrombophlebitis, the description of the pain will vary with the severity of the occlusion. Some patients will describe the pain as a severe cramp, while others have described acute pain. In addition, patients describe a feeling of heaviness in the affected limb. The patient may feel flushed, but the temperature rarely exceeds 101°F. Often the patient will complain of a general malaise, and on occasion nausea and/or vomiting may be present. The health history should also include a list of major health problems which may be related to thrombus formation. The use of oral contraceptives should also be elicited.

**P**hysical Assessment Swelling is the most reliable sign of deep thrombophlebitis. Bilateral measurement of the involved and uninvolved extremity should be done carefully.[26] Since the lower extremities are most often affected by deep thrombophlebitis, they should be measured at the point of largest circumference (the calf) as well as the point of smallest circumference (the ankle). Both limbs should be measured at these two points, and a difference of 5 mm in the measurements is considered significant.

Redness is often not visible in deep thrombophlebitis. However, a reddish, cyanotic color may be present over the area. Generally, the skin will feel warmer on the inflamed, affected side.

Tenderness is usually present over the area of inflammation. It is a less specific sign and should be assessed without excessive pain. Palpation of the calf area should be gentle and should progress proximally from the Achilles tendon. A positive Homans' sign is usually observed when deep thrombophlebitis is present. This sign is usually elicited by asking the patient to bend the knee and dorsiflex the foot. If calf pain is experienced, it may indicate thrombophlebitis, especially in the presence of other clinical evidence.

Additional physical examination may include asymmetrical prominence of the subcutaneous veins and the palpation of the peripheral pulses. (Pulses are usually present.) Vital signs are normal, although the body temperature may be slightly elevated.

**D**iagnostic Tests The *ascending contrast phlebography* is the most complete diagnostic method available at the present time. It is not useful as a screening device because it is time consuming, expensive, and presents a degree of risk to the patient. During conduction of this test, the patient is placed in an upright position with weight shifted to the uninvolved foot. Dye is injected into the dorsal pedal area over a 2- to 4-minute period, filling all deep and superficial veins from the foot to the pelvis. Films are taken under fluoroscopy. This procedure is used infrequently because the need for precise diagnosis has not been deemed a necessity in many situations. Anticoagulants are often used with a degree of success, but if the patient does not improve with anticoagulation, a more precise diagnosis is then attempted.

*The $^{125}I$ fibrinogen injection* is a diagnostic test which is useful as a screening device because its effectiveness is limited to detecting early thrombus formation. The iodine iostope labeled with fibrinogen will locate in the area of a clot along with naturally occurring fibrinogen.

The use of *ultrasound* in detection of venous thrombosis is based upon sound changes that result from the hemodynamic alterations in blood flow created by the presence of a thrombus. Failure to hear normal flow constitutes a positive test. Probes are placed over the femoral, popliteal, or other accessible major vein areas. With the development of collateral channels, the venous flow sounds return, and ultrasound becomes less effective. Thus, its usefulness is limited to the acute period.

**Nursing problems and interventions** During the acute phase the patient will continue to experience pain varying in the degree of severity. There may also be anxiety and decreased peripheral circulation; the danger of embolus formation remains a continuous threat.

**P**ain Pain will continue to be helped by the use of analgesics, heat, and bed rest. In addition, a regimen of anticoagulants and fibrolytic agents may be used.

The patient will continue to be *restricted in activity* and will be placed on bed rest. The affected extremity will be elevated in an attempt to reduce venous congestion or placed in straight alignment to prevent emboli. The affected part should not be massaged or exercised; however, passive exercises to unaffected limbs are important.

*Anticoagulants* used are heparin or coumadin. Heparin interferes with clot formation. The blood test used to control heparin dosage is the Lee-White clotting time, described under Thrombus Formation above.

**A**nxiety  Individuals experiencing thrombophlebitis may be anxious about the potential threat of emboli. Some patients may require a mild tranquilizer such as Valium. Clarification of the experience, treatment, and identification of future problems can help reduce stress. As stress can increase vessel constriction, removing anxiety-provoking events may help reduce the pain as well as the threat of emboli. Counseling regarding anxiety, emotional and environmental stressors, and physical problems may be needed to help reduce the future threats of embolization. Family members should be included in this discussion.

**P**ulmonary Embolism  The major complication of thrombophlebitis is movement of the thrombus from its site of origin to the lungs, causing a *pulmonary embolism.* Assessment of this problem will vary depending upon the location of the occlusion and the amount of lung tissue involved. If the embolus is in the smaller, more terminal branches of the pulmonary arteries, the symptoms will be less severe and can often mimic pleurisy or bronchial pneumonia. If significantly larger, the pulmonary artery is occluded. Severe chest pain and significant disruptions in the hemodynamic state of the individual can result.

*Nursing assessment*  In most situations the onset of a pulmonary embolus is abrupt. Classic manifestations found to occur in approximately 50 percent of patients with a diagnosed pulmonary embolism include: increased intensity of the pulmonic component of the second heart sound, pulmonary rales, increased respiratory rate, increased heart rate, and the presence of a cough and/or hemoptysis.

For most patients with pulmonary embolism the symptoms vary from mild to severe, dependent upon the amount of lung tissue involved. An individual's response to a *mild embolus* may produce only transient dyspnea, mild pleuritic pain or tachycardia, fever, and cough with hemoptysis, while a response to a *major embolus* may result in symptoms which are more persistent. These include gasping, shallow rapid breathing, sharp substernal chest pain, dizziness, hypovolemia, arrhythmias (cardiac), and generalized weakness. *Massive embolism* is least common but, having the highest mortality and morbidity, causes patients to feel a sense of doom and experience air hunger, hypotension, and syncope.[27] Physical examination may reveal increased intensity of the pulmonic component of the second heart sound, pulmonary rales, and a pleuritic friction rub. Signs of pump failure may result (see Chap. 24).

*Lung scanning* is a valuable diagnostic tool for pulmonary emboli as it estimates pulmonary blood flow to the lung regions. With the patient in a supine position, an injection of albumin labeled with $I^{131}$ is given, and scanning of the lungs is conducted. The lung areas with decreased blood flow will have a decreased or nonexistent amount of radioactive material. Lung scanning, although one of the more valuable diagnostic techniques available, is nonspecific, and the results are interpreted as either normal or abnormal. A lung scan is safe and simple to perform and is the preferred procedure for screening patients.

*Pulmonary angiography,* a complex procedure, is the most specific diagnostic aid available for diagnosing pulmonary embolism. Radiopaque dye is injected through a catheter inserted via a brachial vein into the pulmonary artery. Angiography can localize the site of a clot and is a necessary procedure prior to surgery.

*The EKG and chest x-ray* are also frequently nonspecific. For example, EKG changes may be present in less than 25 percent of patients with pulmonary embolism. When EKG changes do occur, the most common are atrial arrhythmias, supraventricular tachycardias, and premature ventricular contractions (see Chap. 25) with evidence of right ventricular hypertrophy in those patients with more severe pulmonary embolism. Although it seems unusual to observe a normal chest film in the presence of an embolus, it does occur in almost half of the documented cases. Chest film abnormalities related to pulmonary embolism include distended pulmonary arteries, elevation of the diaphragm on the embolized side, evidence of pleural effusion, and decreased vascular markings.

Although *laboratory tests* are also nonspecific, they are useful when attempting to negate the presence of an embolism. The *white blood cell count* may be slightly elevated but is most often less than 10,000 cells/mm³ which is within normal range. Elevations of the white blood cell count are more common with coexisting inflammatory pulmonary disease. *Arterial blood gases* can be useful, but only when other cardiopulmonary disease is not present. A normal $P_{O_2}$ is approximately 96 mm; with pulmonary embolism the $P_{O_2}$ would most likely be

80 mm or below.[28] Blood enzymes including SGOT and LDH may be elevated and will help support the diagnosis.

*Nursing problems and intervention* For patients surviving pulmonary embolism (75 percent die within the first few hours) the major nursing problem is the *danger of further embolization.* Bed rest is indicated, and patients should be advised to avoid sudden movements or exertion. Avoiding the occurrence of the Valsalva movement (straining at stool) (see Chap. 25) will decrease the possibility of temporarily increasing intrathoracic pressure which, when released, produces a sudden increase in venous return. This sudden increase in blood flow can dislodge a thrombus.

Patients may also be *dyspneic* and develop *hypoxia.* Oxygen per mask or nasal cannula is indicated, especially if the patient is in distress. Oftentimes patients may become anxious at the thought of a mask, and a careful explanation of the reason for the mask should be given. At times, the use of nasal oxygen, along with elevation of the head of the bed 30° or more, will create increased chest expansion and facilitate breathing.

*Halting of the coagulation process* is another problem requiring intervention. Heparin is the drug of choice for pulmonary embolism. Enough heparin is administered to prolong the clotting time to 25 to 35 minutes. Duration of heparin therapy varies, but estimates are that approximately eight days are required for a thrombus to adhere to the vessel wall or to begin to dissolve. Reduction of the heparin dosage is instituted as the patient begins to ambulate, and oral anticoagulants are commenced.

Other medications which may be useful for an acute pulmonary embolism include narcotic analgesics for the relief of *pain* and fibrinolytic/thrombolytic agents, such as *urokinase and streptokinase* used to dissolve the thrombus. Most of the trial studies have involved streptokinase which has proved to be highly antigenic, precipitating anaphylactic shock and allergic responses in some individuals.[29]

Signs of *shock* are always a threat in severe pulmonary occlusion. The appearance of cold, clammy skin, decreased renal function, and hypotension can indicate massive embolism, requiring the use of vasopressors and/or fluid replacement (see Chap. 28). This is a serious emergency and will require close observation and continuous reassessment of the patient's status.

Provision of *emotional support* is an important nursing intervention. A patient experiencing pain

and difficulty in breathing is frightened. A calm atmosphere must exist. The patient often feels a pervasive sense of doom and thinks death is imminent. Staying with a patient through the crisis period is essential. The nurse should offer support to the patient, and support for the family is also essential. Clarification of all interventions will help the patient relax. Should surgery be needed, the patient will have to be counseled as to the reason.

*Surgical interventions* Generally operative procedures for pulmonary embolism are associated with high mortality and morbidity and therefore are highly questionable. Most often the patient who is a candidate for these procedures is not able to tolerate anesthesia or the impact of major surgery. Surgical treatment for pulmonary embolism is therefore performed with varying degrees of success. Three operative procedures are currently in use. These are a ligation of the inferior vena cava, femoral vein ligation, and pulmonary embolectomy. Angiography is essential prior to surgery in order to detect the exact location of the thrombus.

After a *ligation of the inferior vena cava* the blood from the lower parts of the body returns to the heart through collateral channels. When a caval ligation is performed, the hope is that emboli that develop will be larger than existing collaterals and will become trapped below the site of ligation. At the present time there is insufficient data to justify caval ligation being a procedure of choice. Routine postoperative care for the patient having chest surgery is usually followed (see Chap. 30).

Current knowledge indicates that *ligation of the femoral artery* results in an unacceptable mortality from postoperative embolization. Most patients experience chronic peripheral edema postoperatively. Therefore the procedure is performed selectively.

*Pulmonary embolectomy* involves removal of emboli directly from the pulmonary artery. The mortality rate is very significant, in many reports as high as 82 percent. Many surgeons recommend that this procedure be utilized only for those patients with massive embolism, in shock, for whom no other treatment seems sufficient.[30]

Recently much attention has been directed to the use of *intracaval devices.* The three main types of devices are the *balloon* (Hunter), the *umbrella filter* (Mobin-Uddin), and the *spring covered with Dacron polyester resin* (Pate). These devices either occlude or filter the blood flow. They are inserted through a cutdown into the jugular vein under local anesthesia. General anesthesia is not necessary.

Fluoroscopy or angiography is generally employed to guide insertion into the renal portion of the inferior vena cava. Although little physical preparation of the patient is necessary, emotional support is indicated. The patient and family will require both reassurance and explanation. Hemorrhage, infection, migration of the balloon or filter, and perforation are complications which may occur both during and after the procedure; thus careful assessment of vital signs, level of consciousness, pain, dyspnea, and skin color are necessary to detect their development.

### Fourth-Level Nursing Care

Rehabilitation of the patient with venous disturbances includes much health education. All *teaching* efforts should involve both the family and the patient. The focus of teaching should be directed toward the prevention of future incidences of venous thrombosis. All precautions indicated in First- and Second-Level Nursing Care should be employed, especially in relation to activity, tight constricting clothing, obesity, oral contraception, and occupation. Appropriate changes will be made as each individual situation indicates.

Usually, the patient is discharged from the hospital on oral anticoagulants. Careful instructions regarding the use of *anticoagulants* (see Table 29-3) and the use of antidotes (e.g., vitamin K) should be stressed.

Clear explanation of recurrent *signs of emboli* are necessary. Early treatment and assessment of pain and tenderness in the calf area of the lower extremities should be emphasized.

*Dietary information* should include a list of those foods high in vitamin K which the patient should avoid. Green leaves of plants such as spinach can be used. Kale, cabbage, cauliflower, and pork liver are additional sources. If these foods are normally a part of the patient's diet, substitutions should be suggested. Care should be taken to *avoid stress* on the affected limb and to protect this area from trauma. In some instances when varicose veins are the precipitating cause of thrombophlebitis, removal of the veins may be suggested. This is called *stripping and ligation.*

A patient who has been treated surgically or has had an intracaval device implanted should be instructed as to the signs of complications. Changes suggesting infection would be an important teaching focus for all these procedures. Patients having a femoral ligation or implantation of an intracaval device need to know how to assess the presence or absence of adequate circulation of the lower extremities.

All patients with a history of venous thrombosis, whether treated medically or surgically, should be instructed on *exercises* to combat venous stasis. Generally the values of walking and regular exercise of the extremities are important points to be stressed. Each patient will require specific exercise instruction adapted to his or her particular lifestyle. Consultation with a physical therapist during hospitalization can provide an initial exercise plan. It is extremely important that the nurse, the physician, and the physical therapist work collaboratively to provide the patient with an exercise prescription and opportunity to practice the exercises. Exercise of the lower extremities at least once each hour if prolongation of the sitting position is inevitable due to job constraints or long distance traveling should be recommended. Elevating the lower extremities to promote venous return is another important point which should be discussed with the patient. Avoidance of constricting clothing such as garters or girdles should be stressed. Smoking should be stopped.

The *use of elastic antiembolic stockings* is not advocated by every physician, as these stockings do have a tendency to gather around the knees, producing a constricting effect. If elastic stockings are prescribed, the patient should be instructed to elevate the legs before applying the stocking and to pull them taut above the knee to prevent constriction.

## LYMPHATIC DISTURBANCES

The lymphatic system is a complex network which helps return to the circulation those materials (such as proteins) which cannot be absorbed by the capillaries. Increased formation of lymph as a result of peripheral venous changes can interfere with this process. As a result, the patient may develop enlarged lymph glands and nodes, edema, and inflammation. These changes can interfere with production of immune bodies, antibodies, or lymphocytes. Phagocytosis and hemopoiesis can also be affected.

The causes of an obstruction in lymphatic drainage include an increased venous pressure, venous obstruction causing increased capillary pressure, and alterations in capillary permeability. The following discussion will briefly focus on lymphatic disorders including lymphadenopathy, lymphedema, and inflammatory changes including tularemia, *spirillum minus,* and glandular tuberculosis.

## Lymphadenopathy

Lymphadenopathy is an enlargement of two or more separated chains of lymph nodes. Systemic health problems including inflammation, anemia, and malignancy (Chap. 4) are frequent causes. Infections such as infectious mononucleosis can create lymphadenopathy by stimulation of an antibody response. Many chronic inflammatory responses such as found with syphilis and tuberculosis may also cause node enlargement. Malignancies such as Hodgkin's disease or lymphosarcoma are primary node diseases, while leukemia and metastases from malignancies of other body organs produce secondary lymph node enlargement. Disorders of the hematopoietic system such as sickle-cell anemia can create generalized lymph swelling. This swelling interferes with lymph drainage on return blood flow (see Physical Assessment of Nodes in Chap. 4). Nursing intervention is directed toward treating the underlying cause.

If an infection is present, antibiotics and warm moist packs may be used. If an abscess develops, the area involved may require incision and drainage. Also, if the affected nodes are located in an extremity, elevation of the part may induce a therapeutic response.

## Lymphedema

Lymphedema is swelling of the lymph nodes created primarily by obstruction of the lymph channels. This results in a decreased lymph flow, especially when the limb is in a dependent position. Lymphedema may be observed in an arm following radical mastectomy or in the leg when the problem is associated with varacosities. The swelling is first manifested as soft edema which, if allowed to progress, becomes harder or fixed due to fibrosis. The skin in the later stages becomes folded, thick, coarse, and hard with the descriptive term *elephantiasis* being used.

*Primary lymphedema* is congenital, possibly caused by underdevelopment of the lymph system at birth, such as Milroy's disease which occurs in women during puberty and may be caused by an inherited trait. The process involves edema of a limb which appears gradually; the hand may be initially involved followed by the entire limb. The problem is aggravated by stress and warm weather. Lymphedema is considered *secondary* when it appears in relationship with another condition such as trauma, bursitis, or allergies. Whether primary or secondary, the pathophysiological process results in obstruction of lymph flow and edema. Early detection of lymphedema is essential for adequate treatment. The presence of edema necessitates diuretic therapy and a low-salt diet to attempt to decrease fluid accumulation. Elastic support stockings may be worn to provide a cosmetic effect. The extremity may be elevated to foster lymph drainage. Prevention of infection is critical as an edematous part is very susceptible to breakdown of the skin, providing a pathway for infection-producing organisms. If a patient is resistant to medical therapy, surgery is usually indicated to remove involved tissue.

## Inflammatory Responses in the Lymphatic System

There are several problems that result in inflammation of the lymph system with edema, node enlargement, and obstruction of lymphatic blood flow. These problems include scrub typhus, tularemia, *spirillum minus,* and glandular tuberculosis.

*Scrub typhus* is an acute, febrile condition with gross lymph node enlargement traced to a primary skin ulceration. It is a rickettsial disease, the vector of which is an infected mite that attaches to the skin. The infectious process is treated with tetracycline. The enlarged nodes may benefit from warm compresses, rest, and elevation of the involved part. If the patient lives where mites are prevalent, mite repellent should be used on skin, clothes, and blankets; thorough washing and machine drying of clothing will help destroy this organism.

*Tularemia* is transmitted to humans by insects in contact with infected animals. Ulceration occurs at the primary site of infection. Regional lymph nodes become tender and swollen. The onset is febrile with fever and chills. Control of infection is achieved with streptomycin or tetracycline. Prevention of tularemia can be accomplished in part by instructing patients to thoroughly cook meat, as this can help to destroy the organism if the animal had been infected. Those who work with animal carcasses should be instructed to wear gloves.

*Spirillum minus* is similar to *Moniliformis* as both are initiated by a rat bite. This condition produces lymph node involvement. The sequence of events is as follows: a rat bite occurs, then an edematous lesion forms, and it is followed by regional lymphadenitis accompanied by a febrile response. Care is directed primarily to the control of infection with penicillin or tetracycline. A community-oriented nursing focus includes rodent control, especially in areas where overcrowding is prevalent.

*Glandular tuberculosis* is most often seen in the cervical lymph nodes. It is a blood-borne condition which travels through the lymph channels. The initial manifestation is painless swelling followed by rapid node enlargement and abscess formation. Prevention of tuberculosis, the primary disease, is important. Once glandular tuberculosis is present, focus is directed toward promoting healing with isoniazid therapy and incision and drainage of the abscess if necessary.[31]

## REFERENCES

1   J. W. Hurst (ed.), *The Heart, Arteries and Veins,* McGraw-Hill, New York, 1974, pp. 987–1016.

2   Robert Wissler, "Development of the Atherosclerotic Plaque," in Eugene Brauwald (ed.), *The Myocardium: Failure and Infarction,* HP Publishing Co., New York, 1974, pp. 155–166.

3   Henry N. Neufeld, "Precursors of Coronary Arteriosclerosis in Pediatric and Young Adult Age Groups" *Mod Concepts Cardiovasc Dis,* 93–95, June 1974.

4   Meyer Friedman, "Life History of an Atheromatous Plaque," in Russek and Zohman (eds.), *Coronary Heart Disease,* Lippincott, Philadelphia, 1971, pp. 117–119.

5   S. L. Robbins and M. Angell, *Basic Pathology,* Saunders, Philadelphia, 1976, p. 273.

6   Dorothy Sexton, "The Patient with Peripheral Arterial Occlusive Disease," *Nurs Clin North Am,* **12:** 1, 90, March 1977.

7   *Ibid.,* p. 91.

8   Arthur C. Guyton, *Textbook of Medical Physiology,* Saunders, Philadelphia, 1966, pp. 664–665.

9   Neufeld, *op. cit.,* pp. 93–97.

10   W. E. Stebbens, "Role of Lipid in the Pathogenesis of Arteriosclerosis," *Lancet,* 724–727, March 29, 1975.

11   David I. Abramson, *Vascular Disorders of the Extremities,* Harper & Row, New York, 1974, p. 64.

12   *Ibid.,* pp. 42–48.

13   Wiley F. Baker, *Peripheral Arterial Disease,* Saunders, Philadelphia, 1975, pp. 446–448.

14   *Ibid.,* pp. 105–106.

15   John Mueller, "A Dietary Approach to CAD," *J Am Diet Assoc,* **62:**613–616, June 1973.

16   Allen M. Kratz, "Anti-Lipemic Agents," *Nursing 73,* **3**(9):53–57.

17   Daniel A. Hussar, "Anticoagulants," *Nursing 73,* **3**(4):11–16, April 1973.

18   Anthony M. Imparato, "The Major and Minor Carotid Artery in Arterial Reconstruction," *Curr Conc Cerebrovasc Dis,* **IX:**15–18, July–August 1974.

19   Sylbia Ajemian, "Bypass Grafting for Femoral Artery Occlusion," *Am J Nurs,* **67**(3):565–568, March 1967.

20   Joan Luckman and Karen Creason Sorensen, *Medical-Surgical Nursing: A Psychophysiologic Approach,* Saunders, Philadelphia, 1974, pp. 612–630, pp. 801–848.

21   Barker, *op. cit.*

22   Hurst, *op. cit.,* p. 1628.

23   William Coon, "Operative Therapy of Venous Thromboembolism," *Mod Conc Cardiovasc Dis,* **XLIII:**71–75, February 1974.

24   Hurst, *op. cit.,* p. 1624.

25   *Ibid.,* p. 1625.

26   Hussar, *op. cit.,* pp. 11–16.

27   Luckman, *op. cit.,* pp. 612–630.

28   Dennis A. Bloomfield, "Recognition and Management of Massive Pulmonary Embolism," *Heart Lung,* **3**(2):241–246, March–April 1974.

29   Ruth E. Barstow, "Lymphatic Disorders," in Moidel, Giblin, and Wagner (eds.), *Nursing Care of the Patient with Medical-Surgical Disorders,* McGraw-Hill, New York, pp. 618–623.

30   Coon, *op. cit.,* pp. 71–75.

31   Barstow, *op. cit.,* pp. 618–623.

## BIBLIOGRAPHY

Baron, Howard C.: "Valvular Incompetence and Varicose Veins," *Hosp Med,* 24–39, April 1976.

Bendert, E. P.: "Evidence for a Monoclonal Origin of Human Atherosclerotic Plaques and Some Implications," *Circulation,* 650–652, October 1974.

Blumenthal, Sydney, and Mary Jane Jesse: "Prevention of Atherosclerosis: A Pediatric Problem," in Eugene Braunwald (ed.), *The Myocardium: Failure and Infarction,* HP Publishing Co., New York, pp. 167–176.

Breslau, Roger C.: "Intensive Care Following Peripheral Vascular Surgery," *Am J Nurs,* **76**(1).1670–1676, January 1976.

Cannon, Jack A.: "Peripheral Arterial Disease," in Howard F. Conn (ed.), *Current Therapy,* Saunders, Philadelphia, 1975, pp. 215–223.

Cobey, Jane C., and Janet H. Cobey: "Chronic Leg Ulcers," *Am J Nurs,* **74**(2):258–259, February 1974.

Cowart, Marie, and David W. Newton: "Oral Contraceptives: How Best To Explain Their Effects to Patients," *Nursing 76,* 44–48, June 1976.

Daly, Catherine R., and Elizabeth A. Kelly: "Prevention of Pulmonary Embolism: Intracaval Devices," *Am J Nurs*, **72**(11):2004–2006, November 1972.

DeBakey, Michael E., and George P. Noon: "Aneurysms of the Thoracic Aorta," *Mod Conc Cardiovasc Dis*, **XLIV:**53–58, October 1975.

Elizabeth, Sister Mary: "Occlusion of the Peripheral Arteries," *Am J Nurs* **67**(3):562–564, March 1967.

Fitzmaurice, Joan B., and Arthur A. Sasahara: "Current Concepts of Pulmonary Embolism: Implications for Nursing Practice," *Heart Lung*, **3**(2):209–218, March–April 1974.

Fuller, Magdalene: "Vascular Disorders," in H. Moidel et al. (eds.), *Nursing Care of the Patient with Medical-Surgical Disorders*, McGraw-Hill, New York, 1976, pp. 592–617.

Garrison, Glen E.: "Peripheral Arterial Insufficiency," *Hosp Med*, **2**(3):64–79, March 1975.

Genton, Edward: "Therapeutic Aspects of Pulmonary Embolism," *Heart Lung*, **3**(2):233–235, March–April 1975.

Hass, George M.: "Relations between Human and Experimental Arteriosclerosis," *Mod Conc Cardiovasc Dis*, **XIV**(3):85–90, March 1976.

Hume, Michael: "Examination for Venous Thromboembolism," *Hosp Med*, 56–65, July 1976.

Hussar, Daniel A.: "Antihypertensive Agents," *Nursing 74*, **4**(3):37–42, March 1974.

Keefer, Chester S., and Robert W. Wilkins (eds.): *Medicine, Essentials of Clinical Practice*, Little, Brown, Boston, 1970, pp. 317–350.

Kueler, Lewis H.: "The Transient Ischemic Attack," *Curr Conc Cerebrovasc Dis*, **IX:**23–26, November–December 1974.

Likoff, William et al., "Diseases Accelerating Atherosclerosis," in H. I. Russek and B. L. Zohman (eds.), *Coronary Heart Disease*, Lippincott, Philadelphia, 1971, pp. 147–149.

Moser, Kenneth M.: "Diagnostic Measures in Pulmonary Embolism," *Basics Respiratory Dis*, **3**(3):1–4, January 1975.

Murray, Ruth, and Judith Zentner: "Guidelines for More Effective Health Teaching," *Nursing 76*, **6**(2):44–53, February 1976.

National Heart and Lung Institute: Proceedings of the Conference on Health Behavior, Report on Atherosclerosis, Bethesda, Md., 1975.

Nemer, Paul, and Themic C. Vrachnos: "Surgical Management of Abdominal Aneurysms," *Hosp Med*, **12**(1):46–61, January 1976.

O'Brien, J. R.: "Mechanisms of Venous Thrombosis," *Mod Conc Cardiovasc Dis*, **XLII:**11–16, March 1973.

Olson, Edith: "Hazards of Immobility," *Am J Nurs*, **67**(3):779–797, April 1967.

Porter, John M.: "Massive Deep Thrombophlebitis of the Lower Extremities," in H. F. Conn (ed.), *Current Therapy*, Saunders, Philadelphia, 1975, pp. 224–226.

Purdy, R. T.: "Salvage of the Ischemic Lower Extremity in Patients with Poor Run-Off," *Arch Surg*, 784–786, December 1974.

Rose, Mary Ann: "Home Care after Peripheral Vascular Surgery," *Am J Nurs*, 260–262, February 1974.

Russek, Henry I., and Burton L. Zohman: "The Natural History of Coronary Atherosclerosis," in H. I. Russek and B. L. Zohman (eds.), *Coronary Heart Disease*, Lippincott, Philadelphia, 1971, pp. 167–176.

Sashahara, Arthur, and Vivienne Foster: "Pulmonary Embolism," *Am J Nurs*, 1634–1641, August 1967.

Shapiro, Ruth M.: "Anticoagulant Therapy," *Am J Nurs*, 439–443, March 1974.

Sparks, Collen: "Peripheral Pulses," *Am J Nurs*, 1132–1133, July 1975.

Stamler, Jeremiah: "The Primary Prevention of Coronary Heart Disease," in Eugene Braunwald (ed.), *The Myocardium: Failure and Infarction*, HP Publishing Co., New York, 1974, pp. 219–236.

Strandness, D. Eugene: "Pain in the Extremities," in M. M. Wintrobe (ed.), *Harrison's Principles of Internal Medicine*, McGraw-Hill, New York, 1974, pp. 44–47.

Werko, Lars: "Risk Factors and Coronary Heart Disease—Facts or Fancy," *Am Heart J*, **91**(1):87–98, January 1976.

Wessler, Stanford: "Prevention of Venous Thromboembolism by Low-Dose Heparin," *Mod Conc Cardiovasc Dis*, **XLF:**105–109, June 1976.

Wyper, Mary: "Pulmonary Embolism," *Nursing 75*, **5**(1):31–38, October 1975.

# 30

# DISRUPTIONS IN THE OXYGEN– CARBON DIOXIDE EXCHANGE MECHANISM*

Vickie Edwards
Margaret A. Murphy

Effective exchange of oxygen and carbon dioxide along with the maintenance of blood gas levels is dependent on the integrity and coordination of ventilatory mechanisms. As humans interact with the environment, irritating gases, fumes, and dust can combine with other environmental pollutants (e.g., smoking) and disrupt ventilation. In addition, trauma to the thoracic cavity as well as bacterial invasion of the pulmonary tract can disrupt tissue perfusion and alter the exchange of oxygen and carbon dioxide. This chapter will focus on three major health problems affecting ventilation, namely, chronic obstructive lung disease, traumatic disturbances affecting $O_2$ and $CO_2$ exchange, and pulmonary inflammation.

## MECHANISMS OF RESPIRATION

*Ventilation* is a process which brings oxygen into the lungs. *Respiration* is the actual exchange of oxygen and carbon dioxide through inspiration and expiration of air. Ventilation must be adequate to move air into and out of the lungs, such that sufficient volumes of air reach the alveoli. The process of ventilation requires normal function of muscular and elastic properties of the thorax and lungs, as well as patent airways. In addition, there must be adequate perfusion of the lungs to allow gas exchange to occur between the alveoli and pulmonary capillaries. *Perfusion* of oxygen is dependent on an adequate cardiac output for pulmonary/systemic circulation, the integrity of the pulmonary capillary bed, changes in pressures and resistances within the pulmonary vessel, and gravity.

*Diffusion,* or the actual process of gas exchange, is the movement of gases across semipermeable membranes along pressure gradients. Diffusion occurs in the pulmonary capillary bed as oxygen enters and carbon dioxide leaves the blood and in systemic capillary beds to supply oxygen which is vital for normal cellular function and to remove carbon dioxide. Diffusion is dependent on permeable alveolar capillary membranes, adequate ventilation, and normal circulation with adequate numbers of red blood cells and hemoglobin content.

Finally, there must be adequate *distribution,* or matching of ventilation and perfusion, so that

---

* The section on chronic obstructive pulmonary disease was written by Vickie Edwards; the section on chest trauma was written by Margaret A. Murphy; and the section on inflammation was written by Dorothy A. Jones.

alveoli which are ventilated are perfused and vice versa. The normal lung, in an upright position, has a ventilation/perfusion ratio highest in the apexes, approximately equal in the middle areas, and lowest in the bases of the lungs. (Refer to Chap. 22 for a complete discussion.)

### Disturbances in the Mechanism of Respiration

Any dysfunction in one or more of the above mechanisms will cause impairment of gas exchange and increase the work of breathing. These changes may result in respiratory insufficiency manifested by hypoxemia (decreased oxygen tension in the blood), with or without hypercapnia (increased carbon dioxide tension in the blood). Hypoxemia is primarily caused by ventilation-perfusion abnormalities but may also occur because of right-to-left shunts (perfusion of nonventilated alveoli), hypoventilation, and impaired perfusion. The major physiologic mechanism responsible for hypercapnia is alveolar hypoventilation.[1]

Bronchial-airway obstruction *impairs ventilation* in areas with normal perfusion, resulting in *hypoxemia*. As the disease progresses, or in the presence of superimposed infection, the overall alveolar ventilation is inadequate to cope with carbon dioxide production, and *hypercapnia* develops in conjunction with hypoxemia.

Alveolar destruction affects not only the structural support for airways, but also the pulmonary capillary beds surrounding the alveoli. The individual with "pure" emphysema is generally able to hyperventilate in an attempt to maintain normal blood gases, although more energy is expended for breathing. The alveolar hyperventilation will prevent retention of carbon dioxide but generally does not prevent some degree of hypoxemia, even during early stages of the disease.

*Reduction of the pulmonary capillary bed* reduces the alveolar capillary membrane surface area and diffusing capacity of the lungs. Diffusion time is also reduced as a given volume of blood flows through a reduced pulmonary vascular system with increased velocity. Any diffusion defect will more readily delay movement of oxygen, rather than carbon dioxide, because the latter is twenty times more diffusible.

Pulmonary health problems may be conceptualized as physiologic disturbances which result in hypoxemia with hypercapnia or hypoxemia without hypercapnia. Table 30-1 depicts such a concept but is meant to serve only as a framework for the nurse.

## CHRONIC OBSTRUCTIVE PULMONARY DISEASE

For many years, there has been considerable confusion over the terminology and analysis of a group of chronic pulmonary diseases which include chronic bronchitis, asthma, pulmonary emphysema, and bronchiectasis. Each is a specific entity yet may share certain clinical, pathologic, or physiologic elements. To further complicate the situation, each problem may occur alone or coexist in a given individual. As a result of these difficulties and in order to evaluate prevalence and overall impact of these related pulmonary diseases, the term *chronic obstructive pulmonary disease* (COPD) was coined as a name for diseases characterized by persistent slowing of outflow during forced expiration.[3]

### Causes of COPD

There are several major health problems which can result in COPD. These include asthma, bronchiectasis, chronic bronchitis, pulmonary emphysema, and smoking.

*Asthma* is characterized by an intermittent increase in the responsiveness of the airways to various stimuli. Asthma is manifested by difficult breathing due to widespread narrowing of the airway. During an asthmatic episode airway obstruction occurs as a result of bronchoconstriction, mucosal edema, and hypersecretion of viscus mucus. Asthma has not been clearly documented as a cause of COPD and will not be discussed in this section (see Chap. 10).

*Bronchiectasis* is a disease characterized by permanent dilatation of bronchi and/or bronchioles as a result of inflammation and ulceration. All ages and either sex may be affected, and it frequently occurs in children. There is no single specific cause of bronchiectasis; it generally develops following an airway obstruction, atelectasis, or acute respiratory infection.

When the problem is established, secretions collect in the dilated bronchi, resulting in a chronic productive cough of profuse and purulent sputum. Coughing is particularly stimulated by change of body position which allows drainage of collected pools of secretions into unaffected bronchi. Chronic upper respiratory tract infection, hemoptysis, and breathlessness may also be present.

*Chronic bronchitis* has been defined as a health problem, frequently observed in males. It is characterized by a productive cough for 3 months out of the year for at least 2 consecutive years. When there is no other existing cause which may account for this symptom, chronic bronchitis becomes the given diagnosis. Chronic irritation by inhaled substances, particularly cigarette smoke, is the primary cause of chronic bronchitis. Recurrent respiratory tract infections are common concomitants of chronic bronchitis and are another source of bronchial irritation.

*Pulmonary emphysema* is defined morphologically as a problem characterized by enlargement of the air spaces distal to the terminal nonrespiratory bronchiole, accompanied by destructive changes in the alveolar walls. It is an insidious disease and may be relatively well advanced before symptoms become apparent. The chief manifestation is shortness of breath. The two major types of emphysema are centrilobular and panlobular. *Centrilobular emphysema* (CLE) involves the respiratory bronchiole. This tissue becomes enlarged and destroyed, forming irregular confluent spaces among normal lung tissue. CLE commonly occurs in the upper lobes and is more common in males, being generally associated with chronic bronchitis (necrotizing bronchiolitis). It seldom occurs in nonsmokers.

*Panlobular emphysema* (PLE) is a more uniform enlargement and destruction of the alveoli, with gradual loss of almost all components of the acinus. PLE is diffuse and extensive and involves the lower lungs. It is not generally associated with bronchitis.

The term *bullous emphysema* refers to any dilatation of air spaces in the lung parenchyma greater than 1 cm in diameter. Bullae are common in both CLE and PLE.

*Congenital alpha₁-antitrypsin deficiency* has been associated with PLE since the early 1960s. Alpha₁-antitrypsin is a proteolytic enzyme inhibitor in the blood which protects lung tissue from the digestive activity of leukocytes during in inflammatory process. The individual with a homozygous deficiency generally develops more severe panlobular emphysema, early in the fourth decade, than the individual with heterozygous deficiency. Recent evidence also indicates that the deficiency is more prevalent than previously estimated in patients with emphysema.[4]

*Cigarette smoking* is considered the *most important* cause of COPD. A recent study indicated a linear increase in the prevalence of chronic bronchitis with increased smoking.[5] The inhalation of cigarette smoke inhibits ciliary action, causes bronchoconstriction which increases airways resistance and work of breathing, increases carboxyhemoglobin content, and increases myocardial oxygen consumption by means of increased heart rate and vasoconstriction. The long-term effects of cigarette smoke include most of or all the changes associated with chronic bronchitis along with an elevated closing volume, and squamous-cell neoplasia. Smokers are more susceptible not only to COPD and carcinoma, but also to respiratory infection and decreased ventilatory performance with exertion.[6]

*Air pollution,* while not proved to be a primary cause of COPD, has been shown to aggravate chronic respiratory disease morbidity and increase the mortality rate in individuals with cardiopulmonary conditions.[7] Motor vehicles, combustion of fuel, and industrial processes are common sources of pollution. The four major pollutants are:

**TABLE 30-1**
PHYSIOLOGIC DISTURBANCES LEADING TO RESPIRATORY INSUFFICIENCY

I Hypoxemia with hypercapnia
  A Inadequate ventilation
    1 Inadequate neural/ventilatory drive or muscular power
      a Primary alveolar hypoventilation (Pickwickian syndrome)
      b Drugs—sedatives, narcotics, anesthetic agents
      c High-flow oxygen: Will depress hypoxic drive to breathe in patients with chronic hypercapnia
      d Neuromuscular diseases such as myasthenia gravis, multiple sclerosis, and Guillain-Barré syndrome
      e Head injury with dysfunction of respiratory center
      f Fatigue and pain, particularly after abdominal surgery
    2 Inadequate pulmonary or thoracic mechanisms
      a COPD: Chronic airway obstruction becomes a greater problem if the patient develops congestive heart failure or infection, or is given sedatives or high-flow oxygen
      b Traumatic flail chest
      c Kyphoscoliosis
      d Obesity, abdominal distention
  B Ventilation-perfusion imbalance: Increased physiologic dead space (alveoli are ventilated but not perfused)
    1 Pulmonary emboli
    2 Severe emphysema with a loss of the pulmonary capillary bed
    3 Hemorrhage, hypotension: Gravity and low pulmonary arterial pressure promote redistribution of perfusion to dependent areas of the lung airway from ventilated alveoli[2]

II Hypoxemia without hypercapnia
  A Inadequate oxygen transfer
    1 Inadequate alveolar-capillary membrane: Pulmonary fibrosis
    2 Inadequate pulmonary capillary bed
      a Pulmonary embolism
      b Emphysema
    3 Inadequate hemoglobin
      a Anemia
      b Carbon monoxide poisoning
  B Ventilation-perfusion imbalance: Increased physiologic shunting (perfused alveoli are not ventilated)
    1 Pneumonia, congestive heart failure
    2 Atelectasis: Nonventilation creates right-to-left shunt

*Sulfur oxides.* Produced by industrial fuel consumption, these substances precipitate matter or water and can change sulfur dioxide into sulfuric acid, a particularly irritating corrosive substance.

*Ozone.* This irritating gas is produced from a photochemical reaction of sunlight on vehicular exhausts.

*Carbon monoxide.* This gas is produced chiefly by combustion of fuel in motor vehicles.

*Nitrogen dioxide.* This gas is also produced by fuel combustion and particularly hazardous in areas with high levels of particulate matter.

*Occupational pollutants* are another source of irritants which may aggravate COPD or directly cause lung diseases such as pneumoconiosis and occupational asthma. *Pneumoconiosis* is defined as a reaction to the presence of dust in the lung; among the specific forms are asbestosis, silicosis, and byssinosis. The reactions to three major pulmonary hazards, asbestos, silica, and cotton, have been identified by the US Department of Labor as priority problems for industrial workers. Occupational gases, fumes, and inorganic/organic dust can interact synergistically with other environmental pollution and with cigarette smoking to increase the risk of respiratory distrubances.

The normal *aging process* increases the anteroposterior diameter of the chest and decreases alveolar elasticity, a process which may contribute to emphysema. A recent study indicates a "progressive increase in emphysema with aging" as defined by the presence of alveolar membrane destruction.[8] However, the aging process is not associated with the extensive morphological changes nor the physical disability that are associated with symptomatic pulmonary emphysema.

## Pathophysiology

COPD includes a continuum of pulmonary health problems, ranging from pure obstructive airway disease such as chronic bronchitis to the opposite extreme of air sac disease and the irreversible but not necessarily progressive process of emphysema. Individuals at the extreme ends of the continuum have been given the euphemistic labels of "blue bloater" (chronic bronchitis) and "pink puffer" (emphysema) (see Table 30-2). Most individuals cannot be placed at either end of the continuum and cannot be labeled with either of these terms, since their status is between the extremes.

Chronic bronchitis and emphysema are the most common and most important causes of COPD[9] and coexist most often in symptomatic patients. The basic pathology of COPD involves varying degrees of diffuse inflammatory changes in the bronchial walls, hypertrophy and hyperplasia of mucus-producing glands and globlet cells, and impaired ciliary activity (chronic bronchitis). In addition, the pathology includes loss of alveolar elasticity and structure, hyperinflation of affected alveoli (emphysema), and interference with oxygen and carbon dioxide exchange.

**TABLE 30-2**
CHARACTERISTICS OF CHRONIC BRONCHITIS AND EMPHYSEMA

|  | Chronic Bronchitis (Blue Bloater) | Emphysema (Pink Puffer) |
| --- | --- | --- |
| General appearance | Corpulent, cyanotic | Thin, pink |
| Age, years | 45–65 | 65–75 |
| Cough | Long duration | Short duration |
| Sputum | Copious | Scanty |
| Cardiac enlargement | Yes | No |
| Cor pulmonale with failure | Usually occurs early | May occur late |
| Hyperinflation | Mild to moderate | Severe with increase in total lung capacity |
| Ventilation/perfusion ratio | Marked imbalance | Often minimal imbalance |
| Diffusing capacity | Variable | Low |
| Hypercapnia | Common | Unusual until late |
| Hypoxemia | Usually severe | Mild to moderate |
| Hematocrit | Usually greater than 60 % | Usually less than 65 % |

SOURCE: From G. F. Filley, "Emphysema and Chronic Bronchitis: Clinical Manifestations and Their Psychologic Significance," *Med Clin North Am,* **51**:283, 1967.

Inflammation of the airways with mucosal edema, increased production of mucus, and bronchospasm are major causes of *airway obstruction* in the individual with chronic bronchitis. Chronic inflammatory changes reduce the number and activity of cilia in the tracheobronchial tree so that normal clearing mechanisms are lost, resulting in retention of obstructing mucus. Resistance to airflow is more pronounced during expiration because the airways passively narrow with the deflation and decreasing size of supporting alveolar structures.

Destruction of alveolar walls reduces elastic recoil of the lungs and the structural support system of the membranous airways, thus promoting collapse of small airways during expiration. The airways are further compressed during forced expiration as peribronchial pressures exceed intrabronchial pressure, thereby creating a net force to narrow the airways.

Airway obstruction and premature airway closure, secondary to loss of elastic recoil, results in distal air trapping and *hyperinflation.* As the process of air trapping progresses, lung volume increases. Over a period of time, the chronic increase in total volume of the lungs flattens the diaphragm and forces the ribs upward and outward into a relatively fixed inspiratory position. The anteroposterior diameter of the chest increases characteristically and is commonly described as a ''barrel chest.''

The *work of breathing* is increased to overcome elastic resistance of the thorax and lungs and airway resistance. Normally the work of breathing occurs primarily during the active process of inspiration. Expiration is normally a passive process as the elastic recoil of the thorax and lungs easily overcomes airway resistance to outflow of air. Increased airway resistance, resulting from airway obstruction, early airway closure, and loss of elastic recoil, decreases expiratory airflow. Expiratory time is prolonged, and expiratory flow rates are decreased.

Accessory muscles, the trapezius, pectorals, and sternocleidomastoids, are utilized to assist respiration. Expiration becomes an active, energy-requiring process. Dyspnea and fatigue are intensified as the changes progress and the work of breathing increases.

**Changes and effects of COPD** In addition to the changes already discussed, many other physiological effects can result from chronic obstructive lung disease. These effects occur secondarily to chronic hypoxemia, hypercapnia, or acidosis associated with hypercapnia and can produce multiple changes in the patient.

Interruption in oxygen and carbon dioxide exchange causes *cyanosis.* This is a bluish discoloration of the skin which is observed when arterial oxygen saturation levels are approximately 80 percent. At this point on the oxyhemoglobin dissociation curve (see Fig. 30-1), the oxygen tension is only 50 mmHg. Cyanosis is a late and unreliable phenomenon of hypoxemia. Normal arterial oxygen saturation levels range from 93 to 98%, while arterial oxygen tension levels range from 80 to 100/104. Arterial carbon dioxide tension levels range from 36 to 42 mmHg. (National Tuberculosis and Respiratory Disease Association.)

In an attempt to compensate for the decrease of oxygen level in the circulation, there is an increase in erythrocyte production. The increase in red blood cells can lead to polycythemia (see Chap. 23) and predispose the patient to thrombus formation.

Pulmonary vasoconstriction, secondary to hypoxia and acidosis, may progress to *pulmonary hypertension, cor pulmonale,* and *right ventricular hypertrophy.* Pulmonary hypertension may occur initially in response to an increased blood flow. However in the presence of hypertrophy and dilatation of the right ventricle, the pulmonary hypertension becomes a continuous state. Right-sided heart failure may accompany these changes (see Chap. 24). Cor pulmonale refers to the acute or chronic enlargement of the right ventricle. It is present because of a loss of lung tissue due to COPD, a decrease in the pulmonary vascular bed, increased pulmonary resistance caused by obstruction, and tissue hypoxia resulting in systemic vasoconstriction and elevation of the pulmonary artery pressure (see Chap. 28).

*Arrhythmias* can develop as a result of hypoxia and acidosis. In addition to the stretching of the myocardium and resulting failure, the increased release of circulating catecholamines and stress factors related to dyspnea and medications may cause disturbances in cardiac rhythm. Hypokalemia and digitalis toxicity may occur in the treatment of congestive heart failure and result in other arrhythmias[10] (refer to Chap. 25 for a discussion of cardiac arrhythmias).

*Respiratory acidosis* can occur because of the retention of carbon dioxide accompanied by the metabolic compensation of retention of biocarbonate. *Hyperventilation* may occur in response to increased carbon dioxide levels. As COPD progresses, there may be diminished ventilatory response of the central chemoreceptors to further elevations in carbon dioxide. *Hypoxemia* then becomes the primary drive to breath by stimulating the peripheral chemoreceptors. *Hypotension* may occur as a secondary response to hypoxemia and hypercapnia.

The presence of secretions in the pulmonary tree causes stimulation in the cough reflex. The expulsion of secretions is the body's way of removing airway obstructions to increase oxygen perfusion to lung tissue. Obstruction of alveoli may result in wheezing and spasm of the bronchus.

*Cerebral vasodilatation* also occurs accompanied by cerebral edema, increased spinal fluid pressure, and papilledema. Both hypercapnia and hypoxemia result in cerebral vasodilation and headache. Changes in level of consciousness, syncope, anxiety, unreliability, and generalized sluggishness and drowsiness may result. A reduction of energy for cellular function will result in fatigue and muscle weakness. In addition increased dyspnea will contribute to a decreased exercise capacity, loss of appetite, and loss of body weight. Increased swallowing of air may lead to abdominal distention and discomfort. Disruption in bowel function (e.g., constipation) may also result.

Pulmonary osteoarthropathy, or clubbing of the fingers, may occur or be observed with pulmonary obstruction (e.g., bronchiectasis). Changes in soft tissue and bone structure are thought to result from tissue hypoxia and a subsequent increase in peripheral vascularity. (Clubbing can be observed in Fig. 8-4 in Chap. 8.)

**P**sychosocial Effects  COPD produces many physiological changes which affect psychosocial interaction with others. Sociability is gradually restricted to avoid any emotions or physical activities which may increase respiratory distress, for example, dyspnea. Decreased tolerance for activity forces early retirement, financial burdens, and change in usual family roles. Inability to fill other roles congruent with self-image and dependence on others because of illness compound the feelings of resentment, anger, or anxiety. COPD has been particularly associated with depression, characterized by pessimism and feelings of hopelessness and worthlessness.[11]

**FIGURE 30-1**

Oxyhemoglobin dissociation curves. *(From data of Severinghaus, 1966.)*

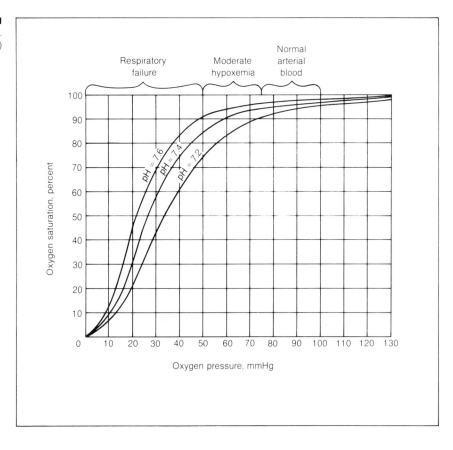

*Psychologic* and *social* factors become more important in the individual with COPD as emotional states can affect carbon dioxide–oxygen exchange. Anxiety and anger may lead to dyspnea, hypoxemia, and hypercapnia secondary to increased work of breathing, increased skeletal muscle activity, and increased cardiac output. Depression and apathy may have the same physiological effect secondary to hypoventilation. The individual with COPD may employ the defense mechanisms of isolation, denial, and repression for comfort and survival.[12] These defense mechanisms also act to inhibit the process of adaptation to chronic illness and responsiveness to treatment, regimen, and health teaching. In summary, it should be emphasized that the processes involved in COPD are dynamic but not necessarily progressive. With adequate pulmonary rehabilitation, the physiological changes associated with chronic airway obstruction may be reversible.

### First-Level Nursing Care

Prevention needs to begin with detection of high-risk individuals before symptoms develop. Major factors upon which to focus assessment and preventive measures include genetic factors, smoking, occupational pollution, and community air pollution.

**Population at risk**  Identification of a population at risk to develop COPD involves careful screening and evaluation of every individual. Those who have a genetic predisposition, such as an alpha$_1$-antitrypsin deficiency, or history of chronic respiratory problems are at risk to develop COPD. Persons with chronic bronchitis or frequent pulmonary infections are included in this grouping. A family history of COPD is also important to determine. Smoking is considered to be a major predisposing factor; statistics seem to indicate that males are more affected by this fact than females. However, in light of recent smoking habits in women, this fact may soon change. The frequency of smoking, number of cigarettes smoked per day, age at which the smoking first began, and number of years the person has smoked should all be noted.

Individuals working with materials such as asbestos or cotton are also at risk to develop COPD. In addition, chemical irritants found in the environment (e.g., air pollution) also can place people living in there in a high-risk category. The incidence of chronic bronchitis, for example, is higher in the northern industrialized cities than in other parts of the country. Therefore it is important to identify the place of residence when attempting to identify populations at risk to develop COPD.

**Screening**  Ventilatory screening tests are used to detect changes in the airways before symptoms develop. Petty encourages ventilatory screening tests, much the same as widespread screening for diabetes and hypertension, utilizing a simple spirometer. He states that if the results are normal it is highly likely the patient is normal. If the results are abnormal, the patient should be rechecked in an established pulmonary function laboratory.[13]

Tests for screening purposes include the following (refer to Table 30-3 for a description of the ventilatory tests):

Timed, forced expiratory volume (FEV) and forced vital capacity (FVC). These tests generally do not show changes in airways smaller than 2 mm in diameter.

Forced midexpiratory flow (FEF). A study by Bates indicated that "very few patients are normal at 30 years of age as judged by the maximal midexpiratory flow rate. Individuals severely affected by emphysema and chronic bronchitis may have abnormal results.

Closing volumes which detect early changes in small airways, a relatively recent test. Closing volume is inversely related to elastic recoil of the lung and will increase with aging and COPD.[15]

As yet, none of the pulmonary function tests have demonstrated that an abnormal test predicts development of obstructive airway disease. Further research will be necessary in order to determine the usefulness of specific tests for early detection of COPD.

**Prevention**  To date, prevention of COPD has been primarily focused on the hazards of cigarette smoking at the expense of other possible causes. Smoking is, in fact, a major cause of COPD, but it is not the only factor to consider in terms of prevention. Particular attention must be given to the vulnerable individual who has a history including one or more etiologic factors or who demonstrates abnormalities on ventilatory screening tests.

High-risk individuals such as those with a family and/or personal history of alpha$_1$-antitypsin deficiency should be counseled to avoid smoking and other forms of air pollution. Counseling should include guidance in selecting occupations which are not associated with pulmonary diseases. Many individuals with documented degrees of alpha$_1$-antitypsin deficiency have lived a normal life when protected against smoking and other irritants.

Counseling against smoking should include objective information emphasizing the immediate adverse health effects of smoking and the combined hazards of smoking with pertinent occupational pollutants. Individuals who smoke should be encouraged to take ventilatory screening tests since the effects of cigarette smoke may not produce significant symptoms. Bates has stated that individuals are likely to reduce, if not eliminate, smoking when confronted with (objective) evidence that damage has occurred.[16] Studies have shown that early structural changes and functional impairment resulting from cigarette smoking are reversible.[17]

Health care agencies and personnel should help to enforce policies banning smoking. Referrals may be made to community agencies such as the American Cancer Society and American Lung Association which offer clinics, helpful hints, and other resources to assist the smoker who wishes to quit. Prospective employees in high-risk occupations should be screened to determine those who might be vulnerable to pulmonary disease. Screening should include a health history, chest x-ray, and pulmonary function tests. Follow-up examinations for pulmonary function should be done routinely, especially for individuals at risk according to their histories. Counseling may be necessary to relocate individuals at risk in certain occupations.

Industrial and governmental agencies have set threshold limits for maximum allowable concentration of occupational pollutants for which no pathological changes can be expected. The 1970 Occupational Safety and Health Act established exposure standards and state assistance for health and safety education and training. The act also established a National Institute for Occupational Safety and Health to initiate, direct, and coordinate research. New materials and processes in industry which might pose a respiratory hazard will be regulated and incorporated with appropriate safety standards.

Other preventive measures include legislative acts to control community air pollution. The 1970 Federal Clean Air Act pertains to standards related to health and adverse effects of pollution. The Environmental Protection Agency sets standards for pollution control according to research findings. This agency recently granted money to the American Lung Association for production of a film entitled "Air Pollution—The Facts."[18] In general, air quality standards in communities are more stringent than in industrial settings.

## Second-Level Nursing Care

Individuals with COPD in the nonacute stage are generally first observed in a community health setting. An individual may not be seeking help because of COPD but because of some other health problem. This person may not even be aware of the disease manifestations of COPD, or their significance. The nurse in the community has a responsibility in the early detection of COPD to prevent irreversible changes, complications, or progression of the disease process.

**Nursing assessment**  In order to prevent irreversible complications of COPD, an accurate health history is essential. In addition, noting early changes during the health history may help prevent additional symptoms.

Health History  The primary symptoms of COPD may be offered as chief complaints or may need to be specifically investigated under review of system.

*Dyspnea* is one of the earliest manifestations of COPD. Dyspnea is a subjective awareness of difficult breathing which may be psychogenic or related to increased work of breathing. Factors which vary the degree of airway obstruction, such as excessive secretions or bronchospasm, will cause fluctuation in the severity of dyspnea. The individual with COPD will usually give a history of progressive exertional dyspnea over a period of time. Severity of dyspnea may be evaluated by determining the minimum level of activity associated with difficulty in breathing. Patients should be asked whether they experience shortness of breath while walking uphill or upstairs, walking on level surfaces; bathing, dressing, or eating; talking; at rest, or lying down.[19]

If the patient complains of a *cough,* the nurse should carefully identify its characteristic features. The character, frequency, time of coughing experience as well as whether the cough is productive should be included in data collection.

The patient should be asked questions to determine the source, consistency, color, and amount of *sputum* expectorated during a 24-hour period. The sputum in chronic bronchitis is usually sticky, mucoid, and grayish in color. The amount gradually increases as pulmonary changes progress. Emphysema is associated with scanty amounts of sputum. Yellow or green sputum indicates infection, a frequent complication of chronic bronchitis. Additional complaints associated with early obstructive lung disease include headaches, impaired motor function, and fatigue.

The patient with COPD might give a past history of allergic disorders which should be investigated. Known allergens, such as drugs or foods, and the allergic manifestations should be recorded. Patterns of respiratory symptoms should be assessed to determine relationship to allergens or irritants. For example, chest tightness, dyspnea, and coughing on Monday mornings has been a characteristic finding in workers exposed to cotton, hemp, and flax.[20]

A complete history should include the following data:

*Previous pulmonary problems:* Such as recurrent respiratory infections, thoracic injury, or surgery should also be recorded under past history.

*Family history of COPD or other respiratory diseases:* May be important in revealing the possibility of hereditary predisposition to asthma, cystic fibrosis, or alpha$_1$-antitrypsin deficiency. History of infectious diseases such as tuberculosis should also be explored.

*Personal and social history:* May be very significant in the etiology and effects of COPD. Areas to be explored include current family roles and relationships, style of living, coping mechanisms, and health resources.

*Smoking habits:* Onset; packs per day times number of smoking years; attempts to quit; if stopped smoking, reasons for quitting.

*Chronological occupational history:* Individual's own description of all jobs and hobbies; nature of industrial work, materials and compounds; duration of hazardous exposures; protective measures in effect; history of respiratory disease in fellow workers.

*Environmental history:* Place of residence and travel; length of time in industrial cities; exposure to industrial exhaust systems; degree of community air pollution.

**P**hysical Assessment   The findings on physical assessment may be minimal during the early stages of COPD. Physical signs become more pronounced in moderate to advanced COPD and are related to airway obstruction, hyperinflation, increased work of breathing, and ventilation-perfusion abnormalities. General appearance of the patient will vary. Often the patient may be of normal weight with good color. As the problem of COPD progresses, weight loss is often noted. The respiratory rate is often increased, and expiratory time will be prolonged. As the disease progresses, the anteroposterior diam-

eter of the chest increases, and accessory muscles of respirations are used. Retraction of the supraclavicular fossae may be apparent in inspiration. Patients may assume a characteristic posture of leaning forward and propping themselves up on outstretched arms. This posture elevates the clavicles and aids in expansion of the chest. Clubbing of the fingers and toes may be associated with advanced cor pulmonale.

Upon palpation of the lateral chest, expansion will be equal but decreased because of hyperinflation. Tactile fremitus (see Chap. 22) decreases as the ratio of air to lung tissue increases.

*Percussion* of the chest in the presence of hyperinflation also results in a hyperresonant percussion noted over the chest wall. The position of the diaphragm will be displaced downward, and diaphragmatic excursion is decreased in more advanced COPD.

Auscultation of breath sounds will be decreased in intensity secondary to decreased airflow, obstructed airways, or destruction of lung tissue. Sonorous rhonchi are produced by secretions in the airways and may clear after productive coughing. Sibilant rhonchi, or wheezes, are high-pitched musical sounds produced by airflow through narrowed airways and are often more pronounced on expiration. They are often heard when airway obstruction occurs owing to bronchospasm, or when mucus secretions are increased.

The patient may be somewhat anxious depending upon the degree of dyspnea present. In the absence of secondary health problems the general health status of the patient is satisfactory.

**D**iagnostic Tests   *Pulmonary function* tests are used to detect early abnormalities in lung function. They are also useful in evaluating the disease process in relation to therapy.

*Spirometry* is used to measure lung volumes, capacities, and flow rates. See Table 30-3 for an outline of ventilatory functions which may be measured by spirometry. Many tests of ventilation require full patient cooperation and will depend on the understanding and effort put forth by the patient.

Indirect methods are used to measure functional residual capacity (FRC) and residual volume (RV). *FRC* is the volume of gas remaining in the lungs at the end of normal expiration. *RV* is the volume of gas remaining in the lungs at the end of maximal expiration. *Total lung capacity* (TLC) can be calculated by adding inspiratory capacity or the maximal volume of gas inspired after a normal exhalation and the FRC. Hyperinflation in COPD causes an increase in RV and, therefore, FRC and total lung capacity. Figure 30-2 shows relationships of lung volumes and capacities.

In the *helium dilution technique,* a known concentration of helium in a known volume of air is rebreathed by the patient in a closed circuit. The final concentration of helium is analyzed, and the FRC can be calculated.

The *nitrogen washout technique* uses an open-circuit method to calculate functional residual capacity. The patient breathes 100 percent oxygen from one source and exhales into a collecting system. The 100 percent oxygen washes all the nitrogen out of the lungs, which is collected and analyzed for nitrogen content.

*Plethysmography* measures thoracic gas volume in an airtight body box system. The air pressure in the lungs and in the plethysmograph are recorded, and the volume of all the gas in the lungs is calculated. This method is more accurate than the indirect methods when areas of the lung contains pockets of air that do not communicate with the outside.[21]

Diffusion abnormalities are determined by *carbon monoxide tests* which require the patient to inhale a low concentration of carbon monoxide. The tests measure the amount of gas which crosses the alveolar-capillary membrane and combines with hemoglobin. The single-breath method can be considered a screening test as it is quick, simple, safe, and does not tire the patient. Diffusion capacity is usually decreased in emphysema as the alveolar surface area and pulmonary capillaries are destroyed.

Distribution of ventilation can be measured by several methods. The *single-breath nitrogen washout test* can be used as a screening test. Nitrogen concentration of exhaled gas is measured after a single breath of oxygen. An abnormal increase in nitrogen concentration toward end inspiration is indicative of uneven distribution. *Multiple-breath nitrogen washout test* will show a prolonged curve in poorly ventilated lungs. Measurement of *closing volume* is a modification of the single-breath nitrogen washout test, with promise for screening large populations. This test analyzes the concentration of gas near the end of inspiration. It is thought to be an early indicator of abnormalities in small airways.

*Chest roentgenogram* is not helpful in the early detection of COPD. Chest films may be read as essentially normal even in moderately advanced COPD. Significant radiologic criteria in advanced emphysema include flattened diaphragm, increased retrosternal space, presence of bullous lesions, and loss of peripheral vascular markings. The chest x-ray is important because it offers baseline data to the health provider which can be used to compare changes that occur over time.

*Fluoroscopy* can serve as an adjunct for a chest film to assess volume changes in the lungs and movement of the diaphragm. Diminished diaphragmatic movement and persistent translucency in the lungs during expiration are characteristic of COPD.

*Arterial blood gases* are used to evaluate the overall adequacy of lung function in maintaining

**TABLE 30-3**
VENTILATORY FUNCTION TEST

| Test | Description | Results in COPD |
|---|---|---|
| Vital capacity (VC) | Maximum volume exhaled following a *maximal* inspiration without forced effort. | May be normal or even high. Is of little value by itself. |
| Forced vital capacity (FVC) | Vital capacity performed with maximal force and rapidity | Decreased due to air trapping. |
| Forced expiration volume in first second (FEV) | Volume exhaled during the first second of FVC. It is often expressed as a percentage of the VC: $$FEV\ 90 = \frac{FEV}{VC} = 100\,\%$$ | Decreased. Degree of reduction correlates with severity of airway obstruction and difficulty in effectively coughing. |
| Forced midexpiration flow | Average rate of flow during middle half of FEV | Decreased. Is an early indication of small-airway obstruction. |
| Maximal voluntary ventilation (MVV) | Volume of air an individual can move with maximal voluntary effort for a given time period | Reduced with evidence of air trapping and increase in FRC during the test. Usually correlates well with complaints of dyspnea. |

SOURCE: From *Chronic Obstructive Pulmonary Disease: A Manual for Physicians,* p. 42.

effective gas exchange. Measurement of arterial carbon dioxide evaluates the adequacy of alveolar ventilation. Increases in the carbon dioxide tension due to hypoventilation in COPD are reflected by a decreased pH (respiratory acidosis). Over a period of time bicarbonate ions will be retained in an attempt to maintain acid-base balance (metabolic compensation). (See Chap. 11.)

Measurement of arterial oxygen tension before and after administration of supplemental oxygen evaluates several mechanisms of lung function. In *hypoventilation* the oxygen will correct the hypoxemia but not the associated hypercapnia. If *impaired diffusion* is present, the hypoxemia may not be apparent at rest but will occur with exercise. Hypoxemia will be corrected with oxygen.

In a *left to right shunt,* hypoxemia will not be corrected by oxygen as shunted blood is never in contact with alveolar air. However, in ventilation-perfusion abnormalities hypoxemia will be corrected by oxygen unless airway is completely obstructed (right to left shunt).[22]

Blood gases may be normal in COPD when the patient is resting. Standard low-intensity *exercise* *testing* can be used in conjunction with multiple blood gas analysis to determine the degree of incapacity. Exercise testing in patients with moderate to severe impairment of lung function will result in hypoxemia. Testing may also be used to evaluate the need for oxygen therapy and in diagnostic problems when complaints of dyspnea do not correlate well with clinical findings.

A *complete blood count* (CBC) may reveal an elevated hemoglobin and hematocrit with secondary polycythemia associated with chronic hypoxia. If the patient has an acute respiratory infection, a neutrophilic leukocytosis may be apparent.

*Alpha₁-antitrypsin* deficiency can be determined by *serum electrophoresis* and will show a flat alpha₁-globulin curve in the presence of a deficiency. A radial immunodiffusion plate impregnated with an antibody to alpha₁-antitrypsin can also be used to detect the alpha₁-antitrypsin deficiency.

*Skin testing* is used to evaluate past and present exposures to allergens. The allergen is pricked into the skin or injected intradermally. Immediate hypersensitivity with development of a wheal may be associated with bronchial asthma. Skin testing is

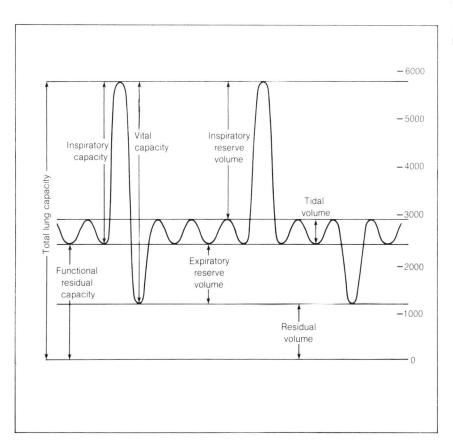

**FIGURE 30-2**
Lung volumes and capacities.

generally of little value in the diagnosis and management of COPD.

**Nursing problems and interventions**  For the patient with early COPD nursing interventions will be related to several major problems. These include cigarette smoking, exposure to hazardous respiratory irritants, dyspnea, airway obstruction, poor nutrition, and the threat of infection.

**S**moking and Chemical Irritants  Once the diagnosis of COPD is established, *avoidance of smoking* becomes an essential part of a treatment program. Many patients are aware of the hazards of smoking and the potential effect on their lives should they continue their smoking habit. At this point patients need factual information and expression of firm belief that further smoking is harmful. Cessation of smoking generally does more than any other treatment toward decreasing airway irritation, sputum production, and cough, while increasing and improving ventilatory function. Continued encouragement and assistance in ways to stop smoking must be given to the patient. A sincere concern and nonjudgmental attitude will be more effective than threats. Family members and significant others should be involved to provide further support for the patient. The patient can be referred to local groups which are working to help individuals stop smoking. In some instances the use of hypnosis has been successful.

Other *respiratory irritants* to be avoided include dry, hot, dusty rooms, smoke-filled rooms, exposure to cold air, strong fumes or toxic gases, and known allergens. Filters in air conditioners and furnaces should be changed frequently to reduce dust and other irritants in the air. Excessive use of alcohol, dehydration, and habitual mouth breathing should be avoided since these are factors which inhibit ciliary activity or produce thicker secretions. When possible the patient should use a humidifier. Patients should be encouraged to live in areas where industrial pollution is low.

*Air pollution* may be a major problem if the patient lives in an industrialized smoggy area or along a busy street. Effective air conditioners may be helpful. During periods of high air pollution, the patient should be encouraged to stay indoors, avoid strenuous activity, and set the air conditioner to recirculate inside air if possible. Any discussion of moving must involve economic, recreational, and psychosocial consequences for the patient and family.

The patient's present occupation should be assessed for respiratory irritants which cause dyspnea, coughing, or wheezing. Patients must utilize appropriate protective devices such as filter masks and protective clothing. Smoking should be strongly discouraged in those job-related diseases linked with or aggravated by smoking. Proper industrial hygiene and monitoring devices should be noted.

Regular periodic examinations are essential and should include assessment of respiratory symptoms and pulmonary function tests. If any changes in respiratory function are detected, the patient should be removed from the source of irritation, even if it necessitates a change in occupation.

**D**yspnea  A change to a more sedentary occupation is sometimes necessary because of *dyspnea on exertion.* This is the major disabling symptom in COPD. When advising a change in occupation, the nurse must be aware of the patient's needs for financial security, as well as higher-level needs of job satisfaction and self-esteem. Occupational changes will have a major impact on patients and their families as occupation provides and determines much of the physical and social environment in which people live, their status within the community, and their patterns for living.[23]

*Bronchodilator* drugs are an important part of the therapy to reduce airway obstruction and dyspnea. Bronchodilators most commonly used can be divided into two groups: catecholamines and methylxanthines, each having different sites of actions.[24]

*Catecholamines* stimulate alpha- and beta-sympathomimetic receptor sites. Stimulation of alpha receptors causes constriction of blood vessels and reduces mucosal edema. Beta$_1$ receptors are primarily located in the heart, and stimulation has an inotropic and chronotropic effect. Stimulation of beta$_2$ receptors relaxes bronchial smooth muscle. Newer drugs are more selective beta$_2$ stimulants and have fewer alpha and beta$_1$ side effects. (See Table 30-4.)

Several methods may be used to administer an inhaled bronchodilator. These include the hand-bulb nebulizer, the pump-driven nebulizer, metered aerosol cartridge, and an intermittent positive pressure unit. The method selected depends on the patient's cooperation and ability to take a deep breath. The patient will need instruction on how to inhale the bronchodilator to maximize its effects and to use the drug as prescribed to avoid overdosage. Metered dosage cartridges are frequently abused through overuse and can cause paradoxical bronchospasm and arrhythmias. Asking the patient to keep a simple record of times and number of inhalations may facilitate assessment of usage. (See Third-Level Nursing Care for teaching components.)

Side effects to be aware of include tachycardia, palpitations, headache, nausea, tremors, restlessness, and insomnia. Patients using drugs with beta₁ effects may need instructions in how to monitor their heart rate. Rinsing the mouth after aerosol treatments will sometimes decrease systemic effects and nausea.

The most important *methylxanthine* is theophylline which is available in many preparations and can be given orally or rectally. Aminophylline is a derivative of theophylline and is one of the most potent antiasthma drugs when given intravenously. Theophylline is generally given orally as absorption is generally better than via rectal administration. It is usually given around the clock at regular intervals to maintain therapeutic levels. Metabolism of the drug varies from patient to patient, and serum levels may fluctuate markedly. Serum theophylline levels may be ordered during the process of establishing an effective dose for a given patient. The nurse must be alert for signs of toxicity such as anorexia, nausea, vomiting, gastritis, and irritability.

**Inadequate Nutrition and Weight Loss**   A nutritious diet is an important defense against lowered resistance and susceptibility to infection. Poor nutrition with subsequent weight loss may be due to dyspnea, nausea, or fatigue, or it may be secondary to medications or difficulty in swallowing. Smaller, more frequent meals will interfere less with abdominal diaphragmatic movements. High-protein, high-caloric drinks and supplemental vitamins can be used to improve nutritional status with minimal expenditure of energy for consumption.

The patient who is overweight should be encouraged to lose weight. Excess weight increases work of breathing and oxygen consumption. Obesity also restricts ventilation and predisposes to hypoventilation.

Patients should be encouraged to maintain an adequate fluid intake as water is the best agent for liquefying sputum. Extremes of hot or cold fluid may cause bronchospasm and should be avoided.

**Rest and Activity**   The patient with early COPD may find that no serious restrictions are placed on activities. The patient should, however, be encouraged to take rest periods as needed and avoid stressful and demanding situations and overexertion. If patients find certain activities taxing, they should be told to reduce the activities or get added assistance as needed. Avoiding overfatigue will help to increase resistance to infection and conserve the energy needed for activities of daily living. Periods of relaxation are critical to reducing stress and excess use of energy.

**Prevention of Infection**   Patients with COPD should avoid exposure to infection. Respiratory infections may contribute to existing pathologic changes and are frequently the precipitating factor in acute exacerbations of respiratory insufficiency. Patients should be encouraged to receive annual influenza immunizations and avoid large gatherings when influenza is prevalent. Patients must be taught to recognize early indications of an infection so that appropriate antibiotic therapy can be started immediately. Ampillicin, erythromycin, or tetracycline is usually ordered for 7 to 10 days. Pa-

**TABLE 30-4**

RELATIVE EFFECTS OF CATECHOLAMINE DRUGS ON ADRENERGIC RECEPTORS*

| Drug | Mode of Administration | | | Alpha | Beta₁ | Beta₂ |
|------|------|------|------|------|------|------|
| Epinephrine | | | SQ† | + + + | + + + + | + + |
| Ephedrine | | Oral | SQ | + | + + + | + + + I |
| Isoproterenol | Aerosol | | | − | + + + + | + + + + + |
| Isoetharine/phenylephrine | Aerosol | | | + | + | + + + |
| Metaproterenol | Aerosol | Oral | | − | + (+) | + + + |
| Terbutalene | | Oral | SQ | − | − | + + + + |
| Salbatamol | Aerosol | | | − | − | + + + + + |

SOURCE: From Irwin Ziment, "The Pharmacology of Airway Dilators," *Resp Ther*, 54, May–June 1974.
* − = No effect
  + = Alpha-beta₁ and/or beta₂ effect on receptor sites. The more +'s, the greater the effect.
† SQ = Subcutaneously

tients should avoid taking tetracycline with milk, milk products, or antacids which may interfere with absorption of the drug. The patient and family members should be taught the dangers of an infection in an individual who already is experiencing difficulty breathing and to avoid contact when infections are present. The patient who begins to show signs of infection should seek medical attention immediately.

**Referrals**  Home visits may be necessary to assess the patient's living environment for potential or existing respiratory irritants and allergens. Follow-up visits may also be necessary to assist the patient in implementing aspects of health care in the home. The family and patient should seek referral to the physician or respiratory clinical specialist in the presence of acute increase in dyspnea, sputum production or fatigue, sudden weight gain, or central nervous system changes such as restlessness, confusion, irritability, or drowsiness.

### Third-Level Nursing Care

The patient with COPD is usually hospitalized because of an acute exacerbation of symptoms which appear, among them being upper respiratory infection, excessive sedation, congestive heart failure, pneumonia, pulmonary embolus, and reaction to heavy environmental pollution. The patient is generally in acute respiratory distress and may even be in acute respiratory failure.

**Nursing assessment**  The patient will not have the energy required for a complete history and physical assessment. Only the information needed for identification of immediate problems should be obtained initially. Further information to complete the data base and plan health care can be obtained from the family or later in the hospitalization period.

**Health History**  The patient with severe COPD or an acute exacerbation generally gives a history of increased dyspnea, wheezing frequency, and severity of coughing (see Second Level Nursing Care). Thicker, yellow, or green sputum and chest tightness are noted. Complaints of generalized weakness are not uncommon. The patient may be anxious and somewhat depressed and unable to speak owing to fatigue.

Other significant manifestations are related to hypoxemia and hypercapnia. Mental acuity, attention span, and judgment are impaired. Family members may note that the patient is drowsy and confused, then restless and irritable. The patient will often complain of headaches and inability to sleep, anorexia, and constipation. As respiratory insufficiency becomes more severe or if the patient is sedated, a gradual loss of consciousness occurs.

**Physical Assessment**  Upon visual inspection the patients will appear thin and generally weak. Their position is slightly bent forward, and they appear exhausted. Their *level of consciousness* must be carefully evaluated as a significant indicator of cerebral hypoxia. The nurse should observe for anxiety, restlessness, and confusion. The patient in severe respiratory failure may be somnolent or comatose. Reaction of pupils to light may be sluggish.

Funduscopic examination may demonstrate changes associated with papilledema (see Chap. 32). In the presence of hypertension, changes in the retina and vascular bed may be observed.

The patients' arterial blood pressure may be initially elevated, then will become hypotensive. Pulsus paradoxus may be present.[25] Capillary refill may be slowed, and cyanosis may be noted in the nail beds. Cardiac monitoring will reveal atrial and/or ventricular tachyarrhythmias in a majority of patients.[26] If cor pulmonale is present, there will be an accentuated precordial thrust of the right ventricle upon palpation of the precordium. In addition there will be an accentuation of the pulmonic sound heard on heart auscultation. Other changes, including jugular venous distention, peripheral dependent edema, diastolic gallop, and hepatomegaly, may accompany right-sided heart failure. Anginal pain may be noted in the presence of coronary artery insufficiency.

Respirations are rapid and shallow. In acute respiratory failure, they will be generally depressed with poor chest expansion. Intercostal retractions and marked use of accessory muscles may be noted. Central cyanosis will be present if hypoxia is severe. Palpation of the chest wall will reveal limited bilateral chest expansion. There may be increased dullness in the lung bases and an increase in pulmonary rales and rhonchi.

The skin may be diaphoretic and clammy. Peripheral extremities may show ankle edema upon palpation. This may be secondary to congestive heart failure. The extremities may be cool to touch and cyanotic because of peripheral vasoconstriction. Asterixis or tremors may be present as a sign of hypercapnia. If dehydration is present, there will be a decrease in skin turgor and dryness of mucous membranes. Clubbing of the toes and fingers may be noted.

Abdominal distention may be noted owing to the accumulation of air in the abdominal cavity. Nausea and vomiting may be present, and epigastric pain may be noted.

**D**iagnostic Tests  *Arterial blood gas* analysis will indicate the severity of the patient's respiratory impairment. Suspected respiratory failure must be confirmed by an oxygen tension of less than 50 mmHg with or without carbon dioxide retention. If the carbon dioxide is greater than 50 mmHg, acute ventilatory failure is considered to be present.

Repeated blood gas analysis will be necessary to evaluate the patient's response to therapy, particularly oxygen administration and correction of acidosis.

*The single-breath xenon test* requires the inhalation of radioactive xenon to determine regional localization of distribution of ventilation. Radiation counters will detect a low level of activity in poorly ventilated areas. A *lung scan* requires intravenous injection of radioactive albumen, $^{133}$Xe, or $^{99m}$Tc to demonstrate distribution of perfusion in the pulmonary vascular system. Consecutive inhalation and injection of radioactive material will demonstrate the relationship between ventilation and perfusion.

*Angiography* of the pulmonary vessels may reveal disruption of the vascular bed secondary to emphysema. This is a very valuable technique in the diagnosis of pulmonary emboli as obstructions in the vessels can be detected. Radiopaque dye is injected into the pulmonary artery through a transvenous catheter in the heart. This procedure is associated with some risk of precipitating right ventricular failure if the patient has severe pulmonary hypertension. A greater risk is the development of cardiac arrhythmias from mechanical irritation by the catheter. The patient must be questioned about allergies to the dye, and cardiovascular status must be carefully monitored during and after the procedure (see Chap. 29).

*Bronchoscopy* allows direct visualization of the airway for diagnostic or therapeutic purposes. The newer fiberoptic bronchoscope is very flexible and can be easily passed through the nose or artificial airways. Direct lung biopsy, bronchial brushings, or bronchial washings may be performed through the bronchoscope. Specimens are obtained for microscopic examination, culture, or cytology. Etiological bases for symptoms such as hemoptysis, hoarseness, or wheezing may also be established. Therapeutic uses include respiration of retained secretions, obstructing mucus plugs, or foreign bodies. For this procedure the patient's naso- and oropharynx are anesthetized topically. After the procedure, nothing should be given by mouth until the gag reflex returns.

A *lung biopsy* is often necessary to establish a diagnosis, especially if neoplastic changes are suspected. A lung biopsy via open thoracotomy (an opening into the chest wall) is the most reliable method of obtaining lung tissue. However it is associated with the risks of chest surgery (see Lung Trauma below). Percutaneous trephining of the lung under fluoroscopic guidance and transbronchial lung biopsy via a bronchoscope are more frequently done and are associated with fewer risks. In pleural effusion of unknown etiology a biopsy of the parietal pleura may establish a diagnosis of malignancy or tuberculosis.

*Sputum* specimens for examination, culture, and sensitivity are essential in the identification and treatment of organisms in a respiratory infection. The best time to collect sputum is in the morning after good oral hygiene to reduce contamination from the oropharynx. The patient should then be instructed to cough from deep within the chest, to obtain a sample of sputum and not saliva. If the specimen is obtained by suctioning, it should be collected directly into a sterile sputum trap to avoid contamination.

*Ultrasound studies* have been useful in diagnosing diseases of the pleura or lung tissue just beneath the pleura. Pleural thickening or effusion, carcinoma, pleural metastasis, or pulmonary emboli may be diagnosed with this technique. There is no special preparation or discomfort for the patient.

*Serum enzymes* may be of diagnostic value. When lung cells are destroyed, the enzymes are released into the blood and can be measured. Elevation of serum lactic dehydrogenase (LDH) without elevation of serum glutamic oxalacetic transaminase (SGOT) may be indicative of pulmonary embolism and infarction. However, atelectasis and pneumonia may have the same laboratory findings. Elevations of LDH may also be found in pleural effusion associated with pleural metastasis as well as myocardial infarction (refer to Chap. 26).

*Serum electrolytes* should be monitored as abnormalities frequently occur in acid-base disturbances or with the use of diuretics. The cause of heart failure can be determined by an *electrocardiagram* (see Chap. 22). Findings of right ventricular hypertrophy will indicate cor pulmonale. Left ventricular hypertrophy will be associated with other diseases such as hypertension. The electrocardiogram may also reveal changes indicative of myocardial infarction. Coronary artery disease is not uncommon in the patient with COPD.

**Nursing problems and interventions** Retention of secretions and hypoxia are major problems for the patient with acute COPD and can become life threatening. Acute exacerbation of COPD is usually associated with increased production of secretions. Retention of bronchial secretions adds to the impairment of ventilation and is a major factor in precipitating respiratory failure. Aggressive nursing care is essential to avoid unnecessary assisted ventilation. Problems affecting the patient include hypoxemia, impaired ventilation, fluid-electrolyte imbalance, inadequate nutrition, anxiety disturbances in rest and sleep patterns, infections, disruptions in activity, and stress. Prevention of future complications is an important consideration.

**H**ypoxemia When associated with tissue hypoxia, hypoxemia due to impaired gas exchange becomes a major concern. Hypoxemia is a deficiency of oxygen in arterial blood. However, even when levels greater than 60 mmHg are present it is still consistent with adequate cellular function. Hypoxia is inadequate tissue oxygenation and is associated with arterial oxygen levels below 50 to 60 mmHg. The most vulnerable organs to hypoxia are the central nervous system and the heart.

Chronic hypoxemia in COPD is due to ventilation-perfusion abnormalities. Acute changes in hypoxemia are generally due to *retention of secretions.* The aim of oxygen therapy is to correct tissue hypoxia until the underlying cause is corrected. In patients with COPD oxygen therapy must be controlled to achieve nearly complete hemoglobin saturation to correct tissue hypoxia without depressing respirations secondary to loss of hypoxemic ventilatory drive. In other words, hypoxemia is improved but not corrected to normal levels.

Understanding the concept of controlled oxygen therapy requires an understanding of the critical level of arterial oxygen tension and the hemoglobin dissociation curve.[27] The critical level of arterial oxygen depends on arterial pH but is generally around 60 mmHg. This is the level at which additional increases in arterial oxygen are associated with only small increases in hemoglobin saturation. This value is determined by the oxyhemoglobin curve which describes the relationship between arterial oxygen tension and hemoglobin saturation (refer to Fig. 30-1).

Below 50 to 60 mmHg, small increases in arterial oxygen are associated with sharp increases in hemoglobin saturation. At 60 mmHg, hemoglobin saturation is close to 90 percent, depending on pH. Administering higher concentrations of oxygen will not significantly increase oxygen content of the blood and may abolish ventilatory drive. The nurse must carefully evaluate and monitor the amount of oxygen being received by the patient. Frequent blood gas analysis and close observation of respiratory rate, rhythm, and depth are essential. Any medication that might lead to respiratory or cough depression must be avoided.

*Oxygen therapy* should not be given intermittently. Withdrawal of oxygen may lead to hypoxemia that is more severe than the initial level.[28] If oxygen is removed, body stores of oxygen are used and the respiratory rate increases, leading to further increases in oxygen consumption. At the same time carbon dioxide production increases. The sequence of events may precipitate respiratory failure.

Oxygen therapy can be delivered by a variety of methods; the choice depends on desired concentration of oxygen and accuracy of control. *Nasal cannulae* are frequently used and can deliver up to 30 to 40 percent oxygen at a flow of 6 to 8 liters per minute. For controlled oxygen therapy flow rates are started at 1 to 2 liters, then adjusted according to blood gas analysis. Cannulae are well tolerated by patients and convenient because they do not need to be removed for eating, expectoration, or oral hygiene. *Nasal catheters* can deliver up to 50 percent oxygen at a flow of 6 to 8 liters but are seldom used because of the need to change them every 8 hours and generalized patient discomfort. The *Venturi mask* (Fig. 30-13) allows delivery of a precise oxygen concentration utilizing the Venturi principle. Four masks are available to provide 24, 28, 35, and 40 percent oxygen concentration when the flow is set as specified on each mask. The major disadvantage is that the mask must be removed for eating, a time when oxygenation may be particularly important. Controlled oxygen therapy is not feasible with other types of face masks. Oxygen concentrations vary from 35 to 60 percent or more and are difficult to regulate. Higher flow rates are generally necessary to prevent accumulation of carbon dioxide in the mask.

**I**mpaired Ventilation A first priority in preventing hypoxia should be maintenance of a patent upper airway. If the patient is semiconscious or unconscious, the tongue may fall against the posterior pharyngeal wall and occlude the upper airway. Other possible causes of large-airway obstruction related to COPD are mucous plugs and severe bronchospasm. Inability to hear or feel movement of air at the nose and mouth indicates complete airway obstruction and requires immediate intervention (see Chap. 26).

Improving ventilation and gas exchange by removal of secretions is best accomplished by vigorous *bronchial hygiene,* which promotes clearing of the airway by use of effective coughing, bronchodilator therapy, inhalation of mist, and chest physiotherapy followed by coughing or suctioning.

*Effective coughing* is the most important first and last step in bronchial hygiene as the most effective method of removing secretions. The patient should be instructed to lean slightly forward and take several slow, deep breaths, inhaling slowly through the nose and exhaling slowly through slightly parted or pursed lips. The patient should then take another deep breath and cough several times during expiration while contracting the abdominal muscles. The patient must be encouraged to cough from deep within the chest and avoid continuous hacking, nonproductive coughing that wastes energy. Dizziness and cough syncope that occurs with marked increases in intrathoracic pressures can be avoided if the patient coughs with an open mouth.[29]

The normal *cough mechanism* may be impaired by extreme fatigue and muscle weakness, central nervous system depression, severely decreased forced expiratory volumes, or intratracheal tubes, which prevent closure of the glottis. If the patient is unable to cough effectively, other steps in bronchial hygiene become necessary.

The *bronchodilators* commonly used and related nursing interventions have been discussed in Second-Level Nursing Care. During acute exacerbation of COPD and particularly respiratory failure, intermittent positive pressure breathing (IPPB) (see Fig. 30-20) devices may be used as a more effective method of administering deep pulmonary aerosol therapy. IPPB also promotes coughing, mobilizes secretions through mechanical bronchodilatation, prevents atelectasis, promotes alveolar ventilation, and can decrease the work of breathing. IPPB may disrupt controlled oxygen therapy if used indiscriminately.

IPPB treatments must not be given using the machine's air entrainment control. Although the control was designed to deliver an oxygen concentration of 40 percent, much higher concentrations are actually delivered. A recent study describes a method of delivering oxygen into the medication nebulizer at the same flow rate that the patient is receiving by cannula under controlled oxygen therapy.[30] The study also indicates the need to evaluate the effects of IPPB by blood gas analysis.

Bronchodilator therapy should be immediately followed by *inhalation of moisture* to liquefy secretions. Two common systems used are the heated, all-purpose nebulizer and the ultrasonic nebulizer. The *ultrasonic nebulizer* can cause fluid overload and may exacerbate congestive heart failure. Mist therapy in conjunction with adequate systemic hydration should make mucolytic agents unnecessary. *Mucolytic agents,* such as acetylcysteine, break up mucus and lower its viscosity. The patient should be observed carefully, and suction equipment should be available as secretions may become profuse and obstruct the airways. Acetylcysteine can also cause bronchospasm and should be given in conjunction with a bronchodilator.

*Chest physiotherapy* is performed after bronchodilatation and mist because the secretions are then easier to move. The purposes of the therapy are to promote removal of secretions with a minimum expenditure of energy and to decrease the need for deep tracheobronchial suctioning.

Chest physiotherapy should begin with frequent *repositioning* from right semiprone to left semiprone positions. These positions promote gravity drainage of peripheral lung segments, enhance ventilator perfusion ratios, and prevent atelectasis.

*Postural drainage* uses gravity to augment impaired mucociliary clearing mechanisms to drain retained secretions. Positioning places segmental bronchi in vertical positions to facilitate drainage into larger airways where they may be removed by coughing or suctioning. Positions may be modified according to the patient's clinical status. Figures 30-3 to 30-6 depict the four most commonly used positions. A sitting position (Fig. 30-7) can also be used to help loosen secretions from the upper lobes. Rotating body movements in various positions can be determined by the respiratory therapist to meet the patient's needs. The frequency and duration of treatment will vary according to the patient's clinical status but generally does not exceed 30 minutes. Postural drainage may be contraindicated in patients with unstable vital signs or extreme obesity, and when dyspnea and fatigue are increased by its use.

*Percussion and vibration* are usually performed during postural drainage to augment the effect of gravity drainage. Percussion is the act of rhythmically striking the chest wall with cupped hands over the area where secretions are retained. If properly

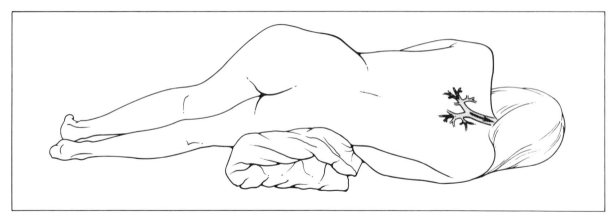

**FIGURE 30-3**
Right lateral decubitus position. (*Adapted from work submitted by Ransom R. Edwards.*)

performed, percussion should not be painful for the patient. It may be contraindicated in hemorrhagic disorders, increased bronchospasm, extreme pain, and pulmonary embolism. After approximately two minutes of percussion, a series of three to five vibrations should be performed. The patient is instructed to take a deep breath. The therapist places both hands over the area just percussed. The hand and arm muscles are tensed and a vibrating pressure is applied to the chest as the patient exhales. Vibrations are also effective for the patient who is given a deep breath with the ventilator or Ambu-Bag. The final step of bronchial hygiene is effective, controlled coughing or suctioning if necessary.

**Increased Ventilation**  If oxygen therapy in conjunction with vigorous bronchial hygiene and removal of secretions is ineffective in maintaining oxygen at or above the critical level, intubation and assisted ventilation may be necessary. Assisted ventilation also provides adequate alveolar ventilation to correct respiratory acidosis. Indication for use includes depressed level of consciousness and inability to cooperate, progressive dyspnea and fatigue, severe hypoxemia (less than 50 mmHg) which is refractory to conservative oxygen therapy, and persistent or worsening alveolar hypoventilation as indicated by increasing carbon dioxide.

*Volume-cycled ventilators* are most commonly used, but *pressure-cycled machines* may also be effective. Ventilation may be assisted when the patient triggers the machine. If the patient has few spontaneous respirations, ventilation can be controlled and delivered automatically by the ventilator.

Mechanical ventilation must be administered by trained personnel and must be continuously monitored. A common hazard is overventilation in

**FIGURE 30-4**
Left lateral decubitus position. (*Adapted from work submitted by Ransom R. Edwards.*)

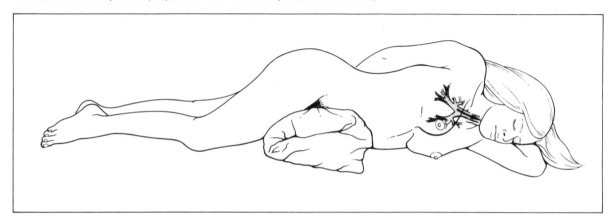

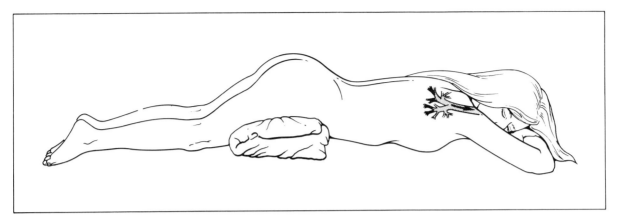

**FIGURE 30-5**
Prone position. (*Adapted from work submitted by Ransom R. Edwards.*)

the patient with chronic hypercapnia which has been compensated by retention of bicarbonate. A severe alkalosis may occur causing convulsions or arrhythmias (see Third-Level Nursing Care under Chest Trauma for nursing care of the patient requiring mechanical ventilation).

*Corticosteroids* may be ordered if airway obstruction is not controlled with catecholamine and methylxanthine bronchodilators, or for patients with rapidly progressing disease; steroids are also useful in patients with allergic bronchial asthma. Short-acting steroids, usually prednisone, should be given in a single daily morning dose every other day to prevent adrenocortical suppression and minimize cushingnoid side effects.

Steroids are never abruptly discontinued but rather gradually reduced in dosage to prevent exacerbation of respiratory symptoms or possible acute adrenocortical insufficiency. Long-term corti-

costeroid therapy is associated with many possible complications and implications for nursing care such as impaired inflammatory and healing responses, peptic ulcers, hyperglycemia, osteoporosis, hypokalemia, hypernatremia, and psychological changes including paranoia and severe depression.

Newer corticosteroids (*aerosol corticosteroids*) such as beclomethasone are administered in aerosol form and have much fewer side effects. These drugs are beneficial in the management of patients with asthma, but further studies are necessary to determine the benefits in patients with COPD.[31]

Anticholinergic drugs can also be effective in patients with acute COPD. A new drug, ipratroprium bromide (Sch 1000), acts like atropine to dilate the bronchi. A recent study compared ipratropium with isoproterenol in patients who were

**FIGURE 30-6**
Supine position. (*Adapted from work submitted by Ransom R. Edwards.*)

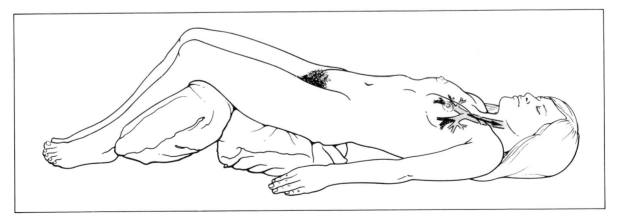

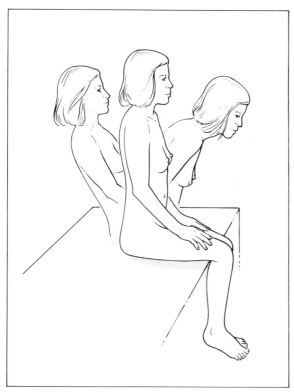

**FIGURE 30-7**
Sitting position. (*Adapted from work submitted by Ransom R. Edwards.*)

responsive to isoproterenol. Ipratropium significantly increased the forced expiratory volume in 1 second and had as rapid an onset but longer duration of action as isoproterenol. Cardiovascular, ocular, and secretion drying effects seemed to be minimal, but further studies are needed.[32]

**Fluid and Electrolyte Imbalances**  A frequent complication of COPD or of medical therapy is fluid and electrolyte imbalances. Sodium retention with fluid overload can occur in congestive heart failure, extreme stress, or steroid therapy. Inadequate fluid intake, fever tachypnea, and mouth breathing may predispose to dehydration. Daily weights and intake and output should be carefully monitored. Palpations of the extremities should be made for pitting edema. Ascultation of breath sounds may detect early changes of congestive heart failure. Dry mucous membranes and thick tenacious mucus are additional indications of underhydration.

Drug therapy which includes steroids and diuretics can cause *hypokalemia,* stress-induced adrenocortical hyperactivity, and metabolic alkalosis;

it can also increase loss of potassium. Hyperkalemia can occur with respiratory acidosis. Manifestations of hypo- and hyperkalemia are generally nonspecific and may be difficult to differentiate. Serum electrolytes should be monitored frequently and correlated with acid-base balance. (See Chap. 12 for a complete discussion of electrolyte imbalances.)

*Acid-base imbalance* is monitored by arterial carbon dioxide and pH. Increased hydrogen ion concentration in respiratory acidosis can be corrected by improving ventilation. Severe hypoxemia may also cause acidosis, secondary to lactic acid production, which may require sodium bicarbonate to correct.

**Anxiety**   The acutely ill patient has two major fears that create anxiety: a fear of the unknown or the biological threats, and fear of biological loss.[33] The patient, preoccupied with loss of respiratory function, is very fearful of suffocating. The individual is often placed in a strange environment and surrounded by unfamiliar equipment and health care professionals. Intensive medical and nursing care compounds the problem of sensory overload. Anxiety must be reduced to decrease oxygen consumption and dyspnea and to promote rest. A supportive, nonthreatening environment and a calm nonjudgmental approach by the nurse are essential. The nurse should explain all equipment and procedures to the patient in understandable terminology. Continuous assessment of overt and covert signs of anxiety must be made daily. The patient and/or family must be assisted in determining the cause of the anxiety. Comfort and reassurance that help is immediately available if needed must be offered frequently. Nursing care, treatments, and visiting hours must be scheduled to provide frequent rest periods. This is essential in order to conserve energy for coping with physiological and psychological stresses. Sedatives must be used with caution to avoid depressing ventilation. The family should be told of the need for frequent rest periods and encouraged to reduce visiting hours during the initial hospitalization period.

The patient and family will also need assistance in coping with the immediate crisis situation and reaction to a chronic illness. The patient's and family's perception of the illness and health care should be assessed and clarification given as indicated. Support systems within the family should be encouraged. Identification of effective coping mechanisms will reduce anxiety and must be encouraged. If, for example, family members use action-oriented coping mechanisms, they may benefit from helping with patient care.

Patients with COPD must make a series of long-term adjustments. They must cope with the loss of physical function, with treatment, and with changes that occur in role identities and interpersonal relationships. This process generally begins when the patient perceives a loss of physical function but is frequently hindered by denial, repression, and isolation. The role of the nurse is not to attempt changing the basic life pattern of the person, but to offer support and guidance as the patient moves toward a way of life that accommodates the illness.[34]

**I**nfections  Existing respiratory *infections* will be vigorously treated with bronchial hygiene and antibiotics. *Allergies* must be checked before any drug is administered to avoid allergic bronchospasm. Careful observations must be made for thrombophlebitis if intravenous antibiotics are given. *Prevention of infection* requires conscientious bronchial hygiene, good handwashing and sterile techniques, protection against exposure to visitors or staff with respiratory infections, maintenance of good personal hygiene, rest, and nutrition by the patient to increase natural defenses. If the patient is on steroid therapy, infections may be more difficult to detect, and white blood cell levels may need to be monitored. A tuberculin skin test is usually done prior to starting steroid therapy, which may activate tuberculosis. Prophylactic tuberculosis chemotherapy may be ordered.

**D**isruptions in Activity  Passive and active exercising of extremities in addition to frequent repositioning is important in reducing the possibility of *thrombus formation.* As soon as possible, the patient must be up in a chair and then ambulating. If the patient is on assisted ventilation, a pressure-cycled ventilator with a portable oxygen tank can be used. Elastic stockings should be worn during hospitalization. Frequently the patient is exhausted by the dyspnea associated with COPD and will resist activity. The nurse will have to identify periods in the day (such as in the morning or following rest periods) when active exercise can begin. Overfatigue must be avoided, and the patient should have planned periods of restricted activity. Good nutrition (see Second-Level Nursing Care) continues to be important and should be encouraged.

**S**urgery  Patients with progressive enlargement of bullae and severe functional impairment may be treated by segmental resection of the lung. If large bullae are compressing normal lung tissue, removal may improve ventilation and gas exchange.

Bronchogenic carcinoma and COPD are both common in male cigarette smokers over the age of 50 and often coexist. A *lobectomy* (removal of a lobe) or *pneumonectomy* (removal of the entire lung) may be necessary. Bronchiectasis may also be treated by any of the above surgical procedures.

Any major surgery and particularly thoracic surgery can be associated with pulmonary complications in the patient with COPD. The patient should be strongly encouraged to stop smoking at least 2 weeks prior to surgery. Admission to the hospital several days prior to surgery will allow time for bronchial hygiene and instruction in coughing. Pulmonary function tests, arterial blood gases, and chest x-ray are usually done at this time. If the surgery is an emergency, bronchoscopy may be done to remove retained secretions. Preoperative medications may be omitted or the dosage decreased.

Postoperatively, nursing management is aimed at preventing retained secretions, atelectasis, pneumonia, hypoventilation, and hypoxia. An adequate airway must be maintained, and oxygen therapy is often necessary. Frequent changes in body position, deep breathing, coughing, bronchial hygiene, and early ambulation are essential. Care should be taken to avoid oversedation and tight abdominal or chest dressings which may restrict ventilation. Frequent assessment of the patient and blood gas analysis are necessary to detect and prevent respiratory failure (see Third-Level Nursing Care under Chest Trauma for a discussion of chest tubes and postoperative nursing care).

**C**omplications  *Acute respiratory failure* occurs when pulmonary insufficiency is severe, resulting in an arterial oxygen reading below 50 mmHg. Acute respiratory failure is defined as the acute inability of the lungs to maintain adequate oxygenation of the blood with or without retention of carbon dioxide. It is a *life-threatening medical emergency.* Most of the problems listed in Table 30-1 can lead to respiratory failure, but COPD is probably the most common cause.

*Management* of the patient in acute respiratory failure, regardless of the cause, has the same emphasis on correcting hypoxia and improving ventilation. Support of circulation, correction of acidosis, and treatment of the underlying cause are problems in addition to those previously discussed. *Artificial airways* with assisted or controlled ventilation may be needed for patients who are unconscious owing to head trauma, neurological illnesses, or drug ingestion; patients with excessive secretions or inability to raise secretions because of chest trauma, chest surgery, or debilitation; and patients with flail chest.

*Cor pulmonale* is a right ventricular disorder resulting from pulmonary hypertension secondary to hypoxia and possibly acidosis. It generally occurs in association with COPD. Cardiac decompensation or congestive heart failure is usually precipitated by acute respiratory failure or chronic progressive pulmonary disease. Treatment is aimed at the underlying problems of bronchospasm, infection, excessive secretions, hypoxemia, hypercapnia, and acidemia. Correcting hypoxemia is a major factor in decreasing pulmonary vasoconstriction and hypertension.

Diuretics and digitalis may be used, requiring careful monitoring of electrolytes, daily weight, fluid intake and output, and digitalis toxicity. There is a greater risk of digitalis toxicity in cor pulmonale because of hypoxemia, hypokalemia, and acidosis. Sodium intake is usually restricted.

It has been shown that daily oxygen therapy for approximately 15 hours significantly reduces secondary polycythemia, pulmonary artery pressure, and episodes of congestive heart failure.[35] See Chap. 27 for a discussion of cor pulmonale and Chap. 24 for a discussion of congestive heart failure.

Dilated air spaces in the visceral pleura, called pulmonary blebs, may rupture spontaneously or secondary to chest trauma. Mechanical ventilation may be a third cause and, if continued, may lead to a *tension pneumothorax* (see Third-level Nursing Care under Chest Trauma for a discussion of pneumothorax).

Steriod therapy also cause gastritis and peptic ulcer disease. Antacids should be given prophylactically, and stools routinely checked for occult blood.

### Fourth-Level Nursing Care

Reliable and valid information regarding the long-term effects of rehabilitation of the patient with COPD is deficient, but most respiratory specialists support the concept of comprehensive health care that covers all aspects of prevention, education, clinical care, and rehabilitation.

The two major objectives of a comprehensive respiratory care program are to control and alleviate as much as possible the symptoms of respiratory impairment and teach the patient how to achieve optimal capacity to carry out activities of daily living, with maximal economy of energy.[36] Components of respiratory rehabilitation include patient and family education, breathing retraining, bronchial hygiene, physical reconditioning, oxygen therapy, vocational counseling, and psychosocial counseling. A multidisciplinary team approach is generally most effective in minimizing the patient's disability within the limits of the disease.

**Patient education** The patient and family need an understanding of the basic anatomy and physiology of the lungs, the disease pathology, and the way COPD affects body function. They should be aware of what is potentially correctable and the purpose of each treatment modality, including medications. Understanding by the patient and family generally increases compliance and problem solving in situations that may arise in the home setting.

Instruction should include the preventive measures discussed in First-Level and Second Level Nursing Care. Prevention of infection and prompt treatment in the event of infection must be stressed. The patient and family should also be aware of signs and symptoms of other complications such as congestive heart failure, peptic ulcer, or acute respiratory failure.

Readiness for learning must be assessed. The patient in the early phases of coping with physiological and psychosocial losses may be using denial and will not be motivated to learn. Teaching should be done in short sessions with frequent reinforcement as patients who are hypoxemic or elderly generally have difficulty concentrating for long periods. Terminology should be concise and geared to the patient's understanding. Simple pamphlets and diagrams may be used to augment individualized instruction. Motor skills, such as use of aerosol devices, should be taught by demonstration and practice sessions. Evaluation of the patient and family's perception is necessary to determine areas for clarification. All teaching plans should be carefully developed according to patient needs.

**Breathing retraining** *Pursed-lip breathing* is the act of inhaling slowly through the nose, followed by a slower exhalation through pursed lips. It is thought to increase intraairway pressure during expiration, preventing excessive airway collapse. It is a more effective pattern of breathing which decreases respiratory rate, increases tidal volume, and improves blood gas tensions.[37] The improvement in blood gases is attributed to slow, deep breathing. Patients may abandon pursed-lip breathing during exercise or respiratory stress and, if so, need encouragement to continue in order to decrease and coordinate respiration. Patients should be encouraged to exhale for approximately twice as long as they inhale to decrease air trapping.

The goal of *abdominal diaphragmatic breathing* is to augment diaphragmatic excursion to decrease the work of breathing and increase alveolar ventilation. As the patient exhales slowly through pursed lips, the abdominal muscles are contracted to help elevate the diaphragm. On inhalation the abdomen should be allowed to protrude. The patient must be encouraged not to use the thoracic cage or accessory neck muscles (see Fig. 30-8*a* and *b*). The breathing pattern should be relaxed, slow, and coordinated. Patients have demonstrated subjective improvement using this technique, although the underlying mechanism is unknown.

**Bronchial hygiene**  The steps of bronchial hygiene have been discussed in Third-Level Nursing Care. These same steps should be individualized and adapted to the home setting. Bronchial hygiene is generally recommended for patients with bron-chiectasis, excessive secretions, or problems with retained secretions.

Patient should be encouraged to use abdominal diaphragmatic pursed-lip breathing when administering aerosols. Long-term use of IPPB to administer aerosols may be beneficial for patients with severe ventilatory insufficiency or excessive secretions. Otherwise, long-term use of IPPB has not been shown to have any greater benefits than the use of a compressed-air device. Bronchial hygiene should be performed each morning and at night before bedtime.[38] If secretions are excessive, patients should perform bronchial hygiene more often. Effective coughing may need to be taught to the patient, in addition to the necessity of examining sputum for changes indicative of infection.

**Physical reconditioning**  When the patient with COPD limits physical activities because of dyspnea, forced inactivity leads to increased functional impairment. Daily graded exercise has been shown to improve exercise tolerance and promote a sense of well-being. Exercise must be individualized according to degree of respiratory impairment and should

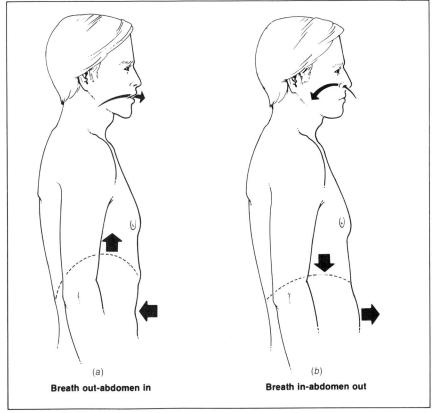

**FIGURE 30-8**
Abdominal diaphragmatic breathing.
(*a*) Breath out, abdomen in.
(*b*) Breath in, abdomen out.

(*a*)

**Breath out-abdomen in**

(*b*)

**Breath in-abdomen out**

be performed daily to be effective. Nutritional counseling may also be needed in order to increase the patient's resistance to infection. Daily well-balanced meals, adequate weight control, and snacks can be encouraged to meet the patient's overall nutritional needs.

*Oxygen therapy* may be necessary while exercising or working to increase exercise tolerance. Long-term oxygen therapy is also used to treat pulmonary hypertension, cor pulmonale, and secondary polycythemia. The patient and family must understand the importance of using oxygen at prescribed flow rates. The risk of higher flow rates must be carefully explained. Oxygen systems for home use have proved to be safe. Since oxygen does support combustion, however, sources of sparks and open flames should be avoided when it is being used. Safety components in the home should be included in follow-up visits.

**Vocational counseling** Vocational counseling should begin early and continue into Fourth-Level Nursing Care. Some patients may be able to return to their previous job on a full-time or part-time basis. Others may need retraining for activities within a limited exercise tolerance. When possible, the patient should be encouraged to select a second career that is less threatening. When functional impairment is severe, emphasis should be placed on self-reliance and minimizing dependence on others, thereby increasing the patient's self-esteem. Patients should be taught ways to simplify their activities and methods of conserving energy. When possible, the patient should be encouraged to select a second career that is less threatening. Physical disability and limitations may require the need for a social worker to help identify other sources of income.

**Psychosocial counseling** Psychosocial history should be evaluated to determine health-related personal adjustments and problems. Perceptions, coping mechanisms, and support systems should be included. Continued assessment regarding adaptation to chronic functional impairment is necessary. When COPD is more severe, patients often use denial, repression, and isolation to protect themselves against emotions that increase respiratory impairment. These defenses may be necessary and should not be destroyed. Emotional support and acceptance should be given. Since compliance may be lacking, rehabilitation should be tailored to minimize need to change life-style.

Goal-setting is often helpful, too, for the anxious patient who needs to regain confidence in the ability to cope with a chronic illness, especially after an exacerbation and acute illness. Successful adaptation to chronic illness involves resolution and identity change wherein the patient works with the consequences of the disease, attempts to set realistic goals, and devises methods to achieve these goals.

The long-term care of the patient should be coordinated by the primary physician and primary nurse. Allied health professionals, such as the physical therapist, social worker, respiratory therapist, and vocational counselor, should be part of the team as indicated. Other resources include the Visiting Nurse Service and various community respiratory rehabilitation programs. A valuable resource for educatonal material is the local branch of the American Lung Association.

## CHEST TRAUMA

Injury to the chest wall resulting from trauma is a common health problem requiring immediate nursing and medical intervention. Trauma to the thoracic cavity results in a disruption in gas exchange, altered diffusion and tissue perfusion, and an interruption in respiratory activity. The following discussion will focus upon those factors that result in chest trauma, their effect on the patient, and related nursing assessment and intervention.

### Pathophysiology

Normally pressure within the pleural cavity is less than atmospheric pressure. That is, intrapleural pressure creates a negative pressure in relation to atmospheric pressure. This factor allows for inspiration of oxygen, expansion of the lungs within the pleural space, and expiration of carbon dioxide into the atmosphere. To maintain adequate negative pressure within the interpleural cavity, the cavity must be closed to the external environment.

Disruption in the integrity of the pleural membrane allows for communication with the outside environment and destroys the negative intrapleural pressure. This causes an immediate compromise in lung expansion and results in collapse of the lung. The movement of air entering from either the parenchyma of the lung or the external atmosphere into the pleural space immobolizes the breathing capacity on the affected side by eliminating the pressure gradient essential for oxygen–carbon dioxide exchange[39] (see Fig. 30-9a and b).

Trauma to the parenchyma of the lung reduces the number of primary respiratory units available to accomplish adequate oxygenation of the blood returned to the lungs from the tissues. Blood will then pass through the alveolar capillary beds without receiving a fresh supply of oxygen (low ventilation/perfusion ratio). This leads to hypoxia and hypercarbia (refer to Table 30-1) when enough units are involved. As air enters the pleural cavity, there is an increase in intrapleural pressure and a decrease in negative pressure.

Collapse of the lung because of communication of a bronchus, bronchiole, or alveolus within the pleural cavity is called a *pneumothorax.* Collapse of a lung due to air collected in the intrapleural space is called a *closed* pneumothorax. When air is able to enter the intrapleural space through an opening in the chest wall, it is called an *open* pneumothorax. Spontaneous pneumothorax occurs when there is spontaneous collapse of a lung, usually caused by the rupture of an emphysematous bleb on the pleural surface. This problem results in a ball-valve action which causes an increase in intrapleural pressure and results in collapse of the lung. As air enters the pleural cavity (inspiration), it is unable to be released (expiration.) The degree of lung collapse is in proportion to the amount of air trapped in the pleural space.

*Hydrothorax* refers to the accumulation of fluid in the pleural cavity. Traumatic laceration of the chest wall is usually accompanied by bleeding. When the blood enters the pleural cavity, it begins to accumulate and results in a *hemothorax.* When the blood is mixed with air, it is called a *hemopneumothorax.*

*Clotted hemothorax* can entrap the lung, causing pleural fibrosis, leading to persistent lung collapse. Infection is common with hemothorax and can lead to suppurative empyema.[40] Empyema is due to pus in the thoracic cavity.

A *chylothorax* occurs when there is an accumulation of chyle in the pleural cavity. This is usually due to rupture of the thoracic duct as it passes through the posterior mediastinum.

### Causes of Chest Trauma

Chest trauma may be caused by either penetrating or nonpenetrating (blunt objects) injuries. *Penetrating* injuries usually result from entry into the chest

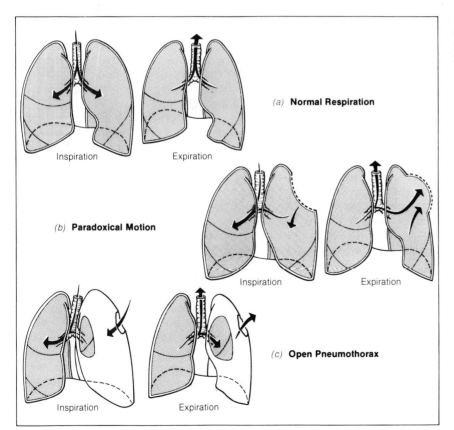

**FIGURE 30-9**
Respiratory phases. (a) Normal respiration. (b) Paradoxical motion. (c) Open pneumothorax.

(a) **Normal Respiration**

Inspiration    Expiration

(b) **Paradoxical Motion**

Inspiration    Expiration

(c) **Open Pneumothorax**

Inspiration    Expiration

wall by a sharp object (e.g., knife) or a high-velocity missile (e.g., bullet). *Nonpenetrating* injuries are caused by forceful contact with a blunt object, electric shock, radiation, immersion, blast injury from an explosion, or alteration in atmospheric pressure.

**Penetrating chest injuries**   Chest injuries may result from any wound causing a hole in the chest and are usually caused by high-velocity missiles or sharp stabbing objects such as bullets, knives, flying shrapnel, or splinters. Damage to the esophagus, trachea, bronchial tree, chest wall, lungs, heart, and/or diaphragm may result in serious and often fatal interference with vital cardiopulmonary functions.

An open sucking chest wound (open pneumothorax) (see Fig. 30-9c) occurs when there is an opening in the chest wall of sufficient size to allow atmospheric air to enter the pleural space with each respiration. If the opening is large enough and does not have a flap of skin to act as a one-way valve, the air will move out of the lung and into the atmosphere through the wound. *Myocardial flutter* may result in sudden cardiac collapse from the alternate flopping motion of the heart and great vessels.

**Nonpenetrating chest injuries**   All structures of the chest can be affected by blunt trauma. Rib fractures, contusion, and bruising of the soft tissues in the lung are the most common injuries. Frequently these fractures are accompanied by rupture of internal organs such as the diaphragm, esophagus, trachea, bronchi, aorta, and the heart.

*Fractures of the ribs and costochondral cartilages* can range from simple injuries with no intrathoracic problems to life-threatening emergencies. Severe complications related to chest injuries are due to a reduction in respiratory excursion and decreased oxygenation and tissue perfusion, and alteration in intrathoracic pressure.

*Electric shock* may act as a blunt trauma by causing powerful tetanic muscular contractions leading to injury of bones or soft tissue including those of the chest. It can also cause paralysis of the respiratory center. *Radiation* accidents or strenuous treatment of carcinoma of the lung can cause burning of lung tissue and result in contusion.

*Drowning* results in asphyxia by inhalation of fluid into the respiratory tract. Following immersion, complicated biochemical and hemodynamic changes occur, and death may ensue from these changes. Causes of drowning relate to shipwrecks,

automobile accidents, water sports or occupations, and intoxication by alcohol or drugs.

*Blast injury* occurs from explosion in air or water and can result in compression of the thorax, rupture of solid viscera, and diffuse hemorrhage with alterations in the capillary bed producing pulmonary edema. Large areas of the lung tissue may consolidate, and inflammation can ensue as often pulmonary contusion.

Disorders due to *alterations in barometric pressure* may cause injury to the lung. Both the nitrogen and the oxygen from the the inspired air become dissolved in the bloodstream and the tissues. These gases become compressed at high barometric pressure such as found below sea level. If ascent to the surface is rapid, the dissolved gases expanded and form bubbles. These bubbles can cause pain and tissue damage, particularly in areas of the body where blood flow is relatively low such as in bone or adipose tissue. This phenomenon, known as the "bends," also has a pulmonary component. (Substernal distress, paroxysmal coughing, and tachypnea are among the chest symptoms.) Use of decompression chambers with simultaneous administration of oxygen can be effective. A type of asphyxia called the "chokes" may occur after decompression. Substernal soreness on deep inspiration is an early symptom. Hemoconcentration and shock may be associated. It is important to realize that bubbles of dissolved gas can expand on rapid ascent from ground level as well as on ascent from below sea level and can require decompression. While deep sea diving and ascent to high altitude are often done under controlled circumstances, in recent years scuba diving has become popular and is often unsupervised. Too-rapid ascent by scuba divers may overexpand the lungs and give rise to air embolism, pneumothorax, and subcutaneous emphysema. Even when diving without scuba gear, a person can incur barotrauma. If divers hold their breath on ascent to the surface, the intrapulmonic pressure tends to increase relative to the hydrostatic pressure. Rupture of blood vessels in the overinflated lungs can occur, and gas may be forced into the lung tissues where it can pass to other parts of the body. On the first inhalation by the diver on reaching the surface, gas may be aspirated into the pulmonary veins and transmitted to the central nervous system, leading to collapse. A similar problem can also occur, of course, to divers using scuba equipment and is not uncommon[41] (see Table 30-5).

Additional causes of chest trauma may be attributed to unrelated health problems. Pathological rib fractures may result from neoplastic processes. Corticosteroid treatment may also result in fractured thoracic vertebrae. Malignant tumors within the thorax can erode or impinge upon any of the soft or bony tissue and result in fracture, pneumothorax, mediastinal emphysema, hemothorax, and rupture of the great vessels.

Head injury can interrupt functioning of the respiratory center and lead to disruptions in respirations. This loss of central control of breathing can lead to ventilatory insufficiency in patients with normal lungs as well as in those who have sustained chest trauma.

Coma can be the result of head injury, accumulations of toxins or alcohol, acidosis, carbon monoxide poisoning, or other metabolic poisons, or it can be secondary to hypocarbia from ventilatory failure. The loss of central control can be determined by observing *levels of consciousness, odors* from the breath of patients, and *reports from companions* or bystanders as to the possibility of ingestion or inhalation. *Medic-alert bracelets* or cards should be noted.

Changes and Effects of Chest Trauma  Trauma to the pleural cavity results in many changes that ultimately affect the individual's health status. Interruption in ventilation can lead to hypoxia, decreased tissue perfusion, and diminished cardiac output (see Chap. 28).

*Fracture of the sternum* can cause myocardial contusion and rupture of the heart and/or aorta. This can be complicated by subsequent aortic aneurysms which may occur years later at the site of aortic rupture. It should be cautioned that these same injuries to the heart and great vessels can occur in the absence of rib fracture when blunt trauma has been sustained.[42]

*Traumatic rupture of the diaphragm* may occur with penetrating or nonpenetrating injuries. The abdominal viscera are forced up against the lung, the diaphragm is ruptured, and surprising amounts of abdominal viscera may enter the thorax. Surgical repair is difficult but often successful.[43] It is necessary to reverse paroxysmal respirations which soon compromise the patient's life.

*Chylothorax* is usually caused by rupture of the thoracic duct with displacement of the lymph into the pleural space. It is rare as a result of trauma. Milky appearance of the fluid aspirated from the pleural space and microscopic demonstration of fat droplets are diagnostic.

Hemorrhage into the mediastinum and pericardium is a particular danger, and the accumulation of as little as 200 cc fluid may be sufficient to cause symptoms of acute *cardiac tamponade*.[44]

Spontaneous pneumothorax results in a shift of the mediastinum and the heart to the opposite side of the chest wall. This causes a sudden decrease in flow in the great veins of the chest and a decrease in cardiac output. The patient will experience unilateral pain and sudden dyspnea. Decrease in oxygen causes the patient to hyperventilate. Dyspnea

**TABLE 30-5**
TOTAL BAROMETRIC PRESSURES AND PARTIAL PRESSURES
OF OXYGEN AT DIFFERENT ALTITUDES

| Feet | Atmospheres | Pounds per Square Inch | Barometric Pressure, mmHg | $P_{O_2}$ |
|---|---|---|---|---|
| ABOVE SEA LEVEL | | | | |
| 50,000 | 0.115 | 1.69 | 87.4 | 18.3 |
| 30,000 | 0.296 | 4.36 | 225.7 | 47.3 |
| 20,000 | 0.460 | 6.70 | 348.8 | 73.1 |
| 10,000 | 0.690 | 10.11 | 522.9 | 109.5 |
| 5000 | 0.835 | 12.23 | 632.3 | 132.5 |
| SEA LEVEL | | | | |
| 0 | 1.000 | 14.70 | 760.0 | 159.0 |
| BELOW SEA LEVEL | | | | |
| −33 | 2.000 | 29.40 | 1520.0 | 318.0 |
| −66 | 3.000 | 44.10 | 2280.0 | 477.0 |
| −99 | 4.000 | 58.80 | 3040.0 | 636.0 |

SOURCE: S. Grenard, G. J. Beck, and G. W. Rich, *Introduction to Respiratory Therapy*, Glenn Educational Medical Services, Inc., Monsey, N.Y., 1970. Used by permission.

may be noted. If pain is present or lung expansion limited, the patient may hypoventilate to avoid pain that accompanies chest trauma.

Trauma can lead to asphyxia due to acute and sustained compression of the thorax or abdomen as occurs when a victim is pinned in a jackknife position or under an automobile or truck. Intrathoracic pressure is elevated, and back pressure on the vena cava and its branches in the head, neck, and shoulders causes a discoloration of the skin varying from reddish brown to black. The eyes bulge with conjunctival congestion and subconjunctival hemorrhage. Extravasation of erythrocytes may occur causing petechia and ecchymosis. Bleeding may occur from the nose, mouth, and ears. Cranial anoxia may cause convulsions or coma, but the syndrome is reversible and recovery may be spontaneous.[45]

Since bullets and missiles penetrating the body do not necessarily follow a straight line, the extent of injury is proportional to the size, type, distance, and velocity of the missile. When missiles rest freely within an artery or vein, the possibility of embolization exists.

A large *chest wall defect* may result from penetrating trauma with massive wounds involving any of or all the ventilatory organs.

*Penetration of the diaphragm* can cause paralysis and subsequent paroxysmal breathing and herniation of the abdominal organs into the thorax. Without the diaphragm, the bellows action of the lungs is not functional, and the pressure gradient necessary to air exchange is lost.

*Hemothorax, cardiac tampanade,* and *esophageal* or *tracheal rupture* may also result from penetrating wounds, depending on the site of entry of the invading object and the anatomic structures penetrated.

*Flail chest* may occur with penetrating or nonpenetrating injuries to the chese[46] (see Fig. 30-10). This phenomenon occurs when a section or sections of the rib cage ride free of the main body of the bony thorax. This happens with multiple fractures of adjacent ribs or the sternum and interferes with the maintenance of the three-dimensional contours of the rib cage. As the chest moves upward and outward on inspiration, that unfixed portion of the chest is sucked in by negative pressure, pre-

**FIGURE 30-10**

Flail chest. Note that upon inspiration there is expansion of the unaffected lung and collapse of the lung on the traumatized side. Upon expiration the unaffected lung is deflated and the affected lung expands with air that travels to the injured side from the uninjured lung.

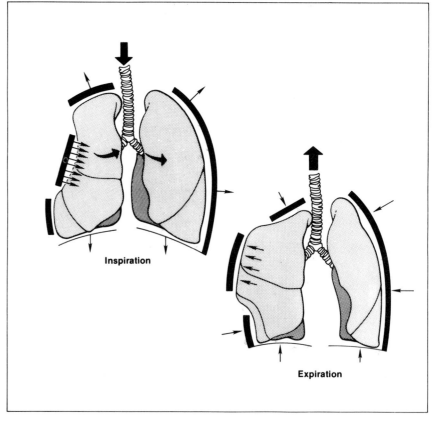

Inspiration

Expiration

venting the expansion of the underlying lung tissue. The unstable portion of the chest wall moves outward on expiration, and the underlying lung tissue does not expire, causing atelectasis, infection, and progressive hypoxemia. This is called *paradoxical breathing* (refer to Fig. 30-9*b*). When one side of the thorax is affected, the opposite hemithorax may in spire part of its air from the injured lung. During expiration, air from the intact lung will be blown back into the injured lung, causing mediastinal shift and a steadily increasing $CO_2$ retention. The harder such patients try to breathe, the more hypoxic they become.[47]

Disruption in fluid and electrolyte balance may also be present. Hypoventilation and decreased chest expansion lead to altered respiration and reduction in alveolar ventilation, decreasing the release of carbon dioxide into the atmosphere. As a result an increased amount of carbon dioxide is retained in the body, and respiratory acidosis results. If the patient begins to hyperventilate, the expiration of $CO_2$ increases, and respiratory alkalosis may develop.

Contusion of the lung tissue (parenchyma and alveoli) results in decreased ventilation and tissue perfusion. Infection may develop (pneumonia), and hemoptysis is often noted. Traumatic "wet lung" syndrome may develop as the tracheobronchial tree is forced to cope with increases in interstitial and intraalveolar fluid. This causes a shunting of venous blood and decreased lung compliance; hypoxia may result.

Acute respiratory distress can occur as the capillary bed of the lung becomes hemorrhagic and edematous. These changes result in hypoxia and hypercapnia (see the discussion COPD), pulmonary edema, and cardiac insufficiency. Death can result if these changes become irreversible.

### First-Level Nursing Care

Prevention of accidents is not a dramatic aspect of nursing care, but it may be the most important. If a nurse can identify a high-risk situation and intervene before the accident occurs, the benefits may be extensive.

Accident causation is a complex subject. Most injuries are caused by a combination of physical circumstances and human motivations. The psychological aspects of human factors are described as absentmindedness, carelessness, or failure to comply with safety regulations, but in truth an accident almost always occurs within a given social context and ecological situation.[48] Factors such as emotional stress, fatigue, and latent unresolved psycho-

logical conflicts may be at play even when the victim has not broken rules or acted hastily. These factors should be incorporated into identifying persons at risk to develop chest injuries.

**Population at risk**  Chest injuries are common in the United States today. Over one-fourth of deaths due to automobile accidents are caused by intrathoracic injury. Therefore individuals who drive at high speeds, or those who fail to wear seat belts, are at risk to develop chest injuries. Divers and individuals who work in areas where there are continuous changes in atmospheric pressures can develop chest injuries because of alterations in intrathoracic pressure.

The effects of crime, especially in large cities, leave the population exposed to injuries incurred by guns, knives, or other weapons. In addition, individuals working with explosives are at high risk of developing crushing chest injuries.

Unsafe living conditions in the home setting may cause individuals to slip in bathtubs or fall down poorly structured stairs. Elderly persons are frequently at risk of tripping on throw rugs or slipping in bathtubs and sustaining fractures.

Persons who have chronic bronchitis, cancer, or an acute upper respiratory infection may develop fractures. Continued expectoration of sputum may traumatize the chest wall and induce rib fractures. Open heart surgery requires that the thoracic cavity be opened and the ribs fractured. This form of chest trauma can lead to complications if the patient is not carefully observed.

**Prevention**  The adverse effects of many of these factors can be alleviated if proper care is taken to ensure that procedures and machines are designed and constructed with regard to the capabilities and limitations of the human beings who are to use them. This interface of people and machines is called the *man-machine system*.[49]

Interest in traffic safety in the last few years has grown because of the awareness of data collected about accidents. Ralph Nader called the country's attention to some unsafe practices in automobile design in his book *Unsafe at Any Speed*.[50] Improved enforcement of safety standards in vehicle design and manufacture has resulted.

Data collection is an important step in identifying the situation which can lead to chest injury. Compilations of epidemiologic data result in information which can point up those faults in the man-machine system which can be rectified. Improvement in safety devices and training can bring about a reduction in the number of accidents. Although the majority of accidental fatalities are in the transportation category, accidents involving the chest are by no means limited to automobile accidents.

Attention to data collection involving all accidents which result in injury to the organs of respiration will help to identify those groups which could benefit from safety training. Factors in occupational accidents have been studied extensively, and large amounts of reliable data have been processed and acted upon to provide improved safety equipment and training to many industries.

The International Statistical Classification of Disease, Injuries, and Causes of Death has been prepared jointly by the World Health Organization and The International Labor Organization (see Table 30-6). It outlines common injuries which can result in chest trauma.

Studying accident reports is a valuable method of assessing populations at risk. This information should be used in the planning of safety training classes. At the primary level the nurse teaches many kinds of safety-oriented classes. Classes on water safety and cardiopulmonary resuscitation are widely attended by the public and offer a fertile field for safety and health teaching.

Many accidents can be avoided by public service programs on television and elsewhere which point up the perils of operating an automobile after alcohol consumption. Young people should be offered regular classes in safety as part of their high school curriculum. Pedestrian, motorcycle, and bicycle safety needs emphasis as well.

Improved gun control laws are essential. Careful instruction on the use of fire arms, reduction of crime, and enforcement of safety rules and regulations regarding the storage of guns may also reduce incidence of injury.

Industrial nurses play a role in the placement and maintenance of emergency equipment and in the surveillance of safety practices on the job. Teaching of safety rules may also help reduce the incidence of trauma.

Regulations for the control of standards for private ambulance services are now a matter of law in many states. Such a service must have personnel trained in the use of emergency equipment available 24 hours a day if a license to operate is to be issued. An enforcement of these laws will contribute to a reduction in the number of casualties which occur because of a lack of emergency equipment and trained personnel at the scene of an accident.

Prevention of hazards in the home as by repair of stairs and use of tub mats and safety bars for the elderly may help in reducing home accidents. The nurse's personal influence as a health professional can be brought to bear to influence legislation at the local and national levels. Mandatory merit reduction of premiums by automobile insurance agencies, the use of seat belt restraints, and driver education courses in high schools have all contributed to highway safety. Legislation at local levels has set standards of safety training for lifeguards and has provided for the presence of employees trained in cardiopulmonary resuscitation and the Heimlick maneuver (refer to Chap. 26).

Health problems such as chronic or acute pulmonary infection and neoplastic processes should be treated early. When an acute cough is present or bone pathology suspected, care should be taken to avoid undue stress on the thoracic cavity. Analgesics and splinting the chest as well as physical therapy may help reduce chest trauma.

### Second-Level Nursing Care

The patient who has sustained a chest injury in the community setting requires immediate attention. The focus of all intervention should be on emergency assessment and intervention along with referral to an acute-care setting.

**Emergency nursing assessment** In assessment of an individual with a chest injury, the simplest and most indicative procedure is a careful count of *respirations* with attention to the quality and depth of excursions. It is helpful to lay the hand lightly upon the chest so that *depth of excursions* may be felt as well as observed visually. This immediately rules out apnea (absence of respirations) and supplies information as to whether the patient has a patent airway. The airway can be occluded by mucus, bone fragments, broken teeth or dentures, blood, and or vomitus.

In evaluating the quality of respirations, the nurse should make note of *tachypnea* (rapid respirations), *bradypnea* (slowed respirations), and *unusual chest movements*. If the patient is exerting great effort to draw breath by using the accessory muscles of respiration or is cyanotic, or if the orthopnic position is sought, this should be noted.

*Assessment of pulse and blood pressure* is second only to the establishment of ventilation. Absence of a pulse or a weak, thready pulse with corresponding low blood pressure reading may indicate hemorrhage, shock, and varying degrees of decreased cardiac output and tissue perfusion. Identification of obvious bleeding sites should be made as soon as possible.

Examination of the chest should be carried out as soon as basic life support has been established. The patient's general appearance, skin color, mental status, and responsiveness should be noted. The quality and intensity of breath sounds over the anterior and posterior chest should be systematically assessed, and adventitious sounds documented according to their location. Abnormality can be pinpointed by reference to the ribs and imaginary vertical lines drawn on the chest[51] (see Fig. 30-11).

**TABLE 30-6**
INTERNATIONAL STATISTICAL CLASSIFICATION OF DISEASE, INJURIES, AND CAUSES OF DEATH

A  Classification according to type of accident.
  1  Falls of persons
  2  Struck by falling objects
  3  Stepping on, striking against, or struck by objects
  4  Caught in or between objects
  5  Overexertion or strenuous movements
  6  Exposure to or contact with extreme temperatures
  7  Exposure to or contact with electric current
  8  Exposure to or contact with harmful substances or radiations.
  9  Other types of accidents

B  Classification according to agency
  1  Machines
    Prime movers
    Transmission machinery
    Metalworking machines
    Wood and assimilated machines
    Agricultural machines
    Mining machinery
    Other machines
  2  Transport and lifting equipment
    Lifting machines
    Rail transport
    Other wheeled transport
    Air transport
    Water transport
    Other means of transport
  3  Other equipment
    Pressure vessels
    Furnaces, ovens, kilns
    Refrigerating plants
    Electrical installations
    Electrical hand tools
    Ladders
    Scaffolding
    Other equipment not elsewhere classified
  4  Materials, substances, and radiations
    Explosives
    Dust, gases, liquids and chemicals
    Flying fragments
    Radiations
    Other materials and substances
  5  Working environment
    Outdoor
    Indoor
    Underground
  6  Other agencies not elsewhere classified

C  Classification according to nature of the injury
  Fractures
  Dislocations
  Sprains and strains
  Concussions and internal injuries
  Amputations and enucleations
  Other wounds
  Superficial injuries
  Contusions and crushings
  Burns
  Acute poisonings
  Effects of weather and exposure
  Asphyxia
  Effects of electric current
  Effects of radiations
  Multiple injuries of different nature
  Other injuries

D  Classification according to bodily location of the injury
  Head
  Neck
  Trunk
  Upper limb
  Lower limb
  Multiple locations
  General injuries
  Unspecified location of injury

SOURCE: World Health Organization and The International Labor Organization.

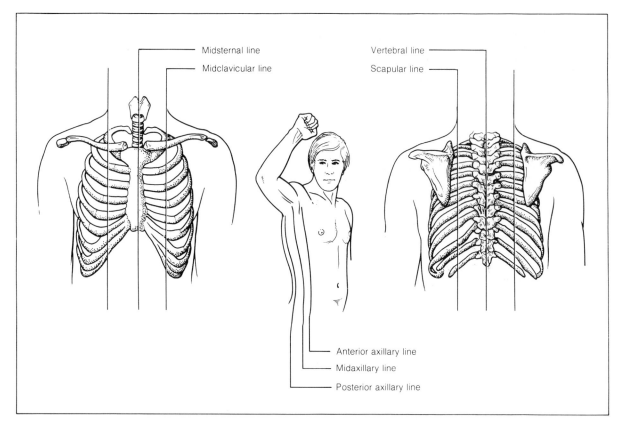

Midsternal line
Midclavicular line
Vertebral line
Scapular line
Anterior axillary line
Midaxillary line
Posterior axillary line

**FIGURE 30-11**
Landmarks of the chest.

*Inspection* includes an evaluation of the three-dimensional configuration of the chest and notes such conditions as kyphoscoliosis and increased anteroposterior diameter (barrel chest). Increased respiratory effort and splinting should also be noted. Obvious bleeding sites should be noted as well as openings in the chest wall.

*Palpation* may reveal areas of tenderness, muscle tone, depth of respiratory excursions, tactile fremitus (transmission of patient's vocal sounds over the chest), and position of the trachea. Percussion of the chest to determine density of the underlying organs is helpful in evaluating fractures, traumatic ruptures, pneumothorax, and equal diaphragmatic excursions. Density will decrease in the presence of a pneumothorax. Peripheral pulses should be assessed for rhythm quality and rate.

It may be impossible to auscultate the chest wall at the accident site. However, the examiner may note some changes in breath sound by placing his or her ear next to the mouth and on the chest wall. (For a full discussion on breath sounds, the reader

is referred to Chap. 22.) Additional changes associated with hypoxia and hypercapnia may develop (refer to Third-Level Nursing Care of COPD).

**Emergency nursing intervention** In the presence of apnea, cardiopulmonary resuscitation should be instituted (see Chap. 26). Measures should be taken to assess the patient's cardiac status as well and to remove any airway obstruction that could potentially interfere with ventilation (see Fig. 30-12).

If hemorrhage is observed or suspected, measures should be taken to terminate the bleeding process. Application of direct pressure may lead to termination and should be accompanied by elevation of the affected area when possible. Emergency interventions related to the patient in shock are found in Chap. 28.

The presence of bloody sputum should be carefully noted as it may herald the onset of the adult respiratory distress syndrome. If this occurs, emergency mechanical ventilation will be needed as soon as possible to offset fatal consequences. *Pain* can help direct the nurse to the site of injury.

Fractured ribs will require no emergency care unless a *flail section* exists owing to multiple fractures of adjacent ribs or sternum (refer to Fig. 30-10). Obvious *paradoxical chest movements* together with cyanosis, dyspnea, tachypnea, and tachycardia require immediate emergency treatment by *immobilization* of the flail section. This is accomplished by turning the patient onto the affected side. External splinting by positioning the patient on the unstable segment or by using compression bandages or sandbags usually results in immediate improvement. If the patient is cyanotic or suffering from labored respirations, application of positive pressure via mechanical ventilation or breathing bag following external immobilization is critical.

If the chest injury is penetrating, the object should not be removed from the wound. This is critical to remember, because removal of the object can result in further damage to the lung and/or surrounding tissue.

The presence of a sucking thoracic wound calls for any form of emergency dressing or continued pressure of the hand over the wound to stop the leakage of air and subsequent *mediastinal flutter* which can develop, causing severely reduced cardiac output and increased venous pressure.

If emergency medical care is available, the nurse may be asked to assist with endotracheal intubation and delivery of positive pressure ventilation via mask and self-inflating breathing bag which may be attached to a portable oxygen supply. Needle pericardiocentesis if a portable EKG defibrillator is available can save lives but is best performed in the operating room.

Emergency tracheostomy is a thing of the past. In the rare instance that an artificial airway is needed immediately, cricothyroidotomy (the insertion of a tube through the small notch between the thyroid and the cricoid cartilage) is preferred since it is simpler to perform. Portable suction units are available in many ambulances for aspiration of secretions. A foot-operated suction unit can supply adequate suction to aid in clearing the airway. (A complete discussion of mechanical ventilators, tracheostomy care, and suctioning will be found under Third-Level Nursing Care.)

Frequently, the patient will be anxious and will fear loss of life. Difficulty in breathing may enforce these fears. Usually the issues surrounding chest trauma may intensify fear. Stress will increase respirations and cause release of catecholamines. The

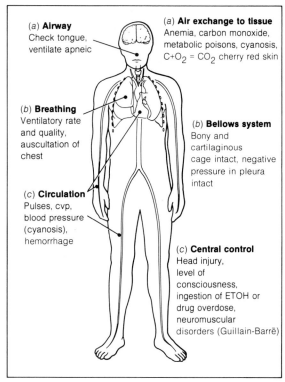

**FIGURE 30-12**
The ABCs of cardiopulmonary resuscitation and oxygenation. The three major steps in cardiopulmonary resuscitation are airway, breathing, and circulation. The components of adequate oxygen supply are air exchange to tissue, bellows system, and central control.

patient should be told what is happening and kept as calm as possible.

Reporting of patient conditions to appropriate health care providers should be done in a clear, concise way with the proper emphasis when judged necessary. If the patient is alert, a statement from the patient regarding the nature of the injury and surrounding events is essential. All information collected at the site of the accident should accompany the patient to the acute-care setting. All patients who have sustained a chest injury will be transferred to an acute-care setting. CB radios, telephone, police, ambulance, or helicopters may be used to summon aid. Care must be taken to incur as little extraneous movement as possible when transferring patients suspected of having chest trauma to an acute-care setting.

### Third-Level Nursing Care

When patients with chest injuries are hospitalized, they will require prompt treatment in order to prevent serious respiratory and systemic complications. They will often be brought to surgery for immediate treatment and/or cared for in an intensive-care setting.

**Nursing assessment** Patients who sustain chest injuries often have a multiplicity of health problems that require continued assessment and evaluation. In order to meet the individual needs of each patient, an accurate health history should be taken and a careful physical assessment performed.

**H**ealth History  Depending upon the degree of injury, the patient may or may not be able to verbally offer information to the nurse. When possible, details surrounding the nature of the chest trauma should be obtained. Identification of the cause of injury will help focus nursing assessment and intervention. The patient will often complain of pain, especially pain which is aggravated by movement. Dyspnea may also be present. A cough may be present and hemoptysis may be noted. The character, consistency, and amount of sputum produced should be assessed. A cough may persist and should also be included in the history. Depending upon the level of consciousness, the patient's sensorium may be dulled and responses sluggish. Coma may develop slowly. (Additional changes as noted in Third-Level Nursing Care of COPD may be present.)

**P**hysical Assessment  Upon inspection, the general appearance of the patient will vary with the degree of the hypoxia and the extent of the injury. The patient's skin and membranes may be cyanotic or pale. Capillary refill time may be diminished. The skin should be observed for openings, scars, or other changes in the chest contour that may indicate injury. Mediastinal shift and deviation of the trachea may be noted.

Palpation of apical pulse may reveal tachycardia, again in response to hypovolemia and/or hypoxia. The peripheral pulses may be weak and thready. Bilateral examination of chest expansion may denote limited movement of the affected pleural cavity. Vocal fremitus (see Chap. 22) will be diminished in the area of the affected lobe, and dullness may be noted in this area.

Hypertension or hypotension may be noted, depending upon the patient's general health state. In the presence of shock, a decrease in arterial pressure will be observed. If air has escaped into the interstitial tissue, it will be felt upon palpation of the

surrounding chest cavity. Crepitus may be noted around the areas of the ribs, indicating fracture.

Upon auscultation of the chest *rales* (a name given to abnormal sounds heard over the lung fields) may be noted. They are usually heard on inspiration and seldom clear with coughing. If pulmonary edema is present, rales may be heard over the entire chest wall.

Ronchi will be heard on expiration and are likely to clear with coughing. They are continuous noises and indicate the presence of secretions in the tracheobronchial tree. High-pitched (musical or sibilant) ronchi are often referred to as *wheezes* and may be present with chest trauma. Vesicular sounds may be heard upon expiration (see Chap. 22). Bronchial sounds (heard over the large airways) over the lung indicate collapse or obstruction of the alveoli if heard over lung fields.[52]

The respiratory rate may vary depending on the type of injury, the presence of shock, and the degree of chest expansion tolerated. Initially, the patient may hyperventilate, and the respiratory rate will be rapid. As chest expansion decreases, the patient's respiratory rate will decrease.

**D**iagnostic Tests  There are many tests that can be performed to assess the patient's respiratory status following chest trauma. A *chest x-ray* will be performed to identify the area and extent of the injury and surrounding tissue destruction. Fractured ribs, atelectasis, and other structural disturbances are also identified at this time. A *complete blood count* (CBC) will be done to assess hemoglobin and hematocrit levels, factors which are especially helpful if hemorrhage is suspected. An EKG will be done to evaluate the patient's cardiac status. Changes in cardiac rhythm may be observed.

A *mediastinoscopy* visualizes the diaphragmatic and mediastinal pleural surfaces. An instrument is introduced via a small incision into the chest wall to allow visualization of pleural surfaces of the mediastinum and diaphragm. If there are disturbances due to the chest injury, they can be quickly observed and treated.

An *open lung biopsy* is performed to observe for changes in the lung tissue. A needle biopsy of lung tissue is most commonly performed to assess lung tissue cells. It is usually preceded by a thoracentesis and pleural biopsy. Serum electrolytes should be checked because they may be altered in the presence of chest trauma. Alterations in acid-base balance may occur.

Assessment of blood gases is critical following

chest injuries. Changes will be noted in the presence of altered oxygen–carbon dioxide exchange.

Additional diagnostic tests that may be performed are discussed under COPD.

**Nursing problems and interventions** A patient with severe chest trauma will encounter several major problems. These include dyspnea, hypoventilation, pain, fluid and electrolyte imbalances, anxiety, and the risk of infection.

**D**yspnea This problem is often intensified by accumulation of secretions in the pleural cavity, decreased oxygenation, and hypoxia. Pain and anxiety may intensify the problem.

The patient's position should be changed frequently so that secretions can be easily dislodged and expelled. The patient can be taught to cough, and the chest can be splinted over the injured site to decrease pain (see Third-Level Nursing Care of COPD). Intermittent deep breathing or "sighing" should be encouraged every 8 to 10 hours to increase chest expansion and expulsion of carbon dioxide.

Frequent uninterrupted rest periods should be provided for the patient. If activity is needed, the patient should avoid exertion. Active and passive range of motion exercises should be done on a planned basis as tolerated by the individual. If the patient is on prolonged bed rest, good skin care will be essential.

*Supplementary oxygen* is needed to ensure adequate tissue oxygenation, especially of the heart and brain, and to eliminate compensatory responses to hypoxia. With hypoxemia there occurs an increase in $CO_2$ content of the blood and an increase in the number of hydrogen ions in the form of carbonic acid. The body is able to compensate by conserving base bicarbonates to maintain the normal 1:20 ratio of acid-base in the body. If oxygen is not supplied, the body will eventually fail to compensate, and the $CO_2$ will act as a poison on the respiratory center causing drowsiness, coma, and death.

If *oxygen* is administered, *humidification* of the gas must be ensured by frequent checking of devices designed to control temperature and humidity. Water levels in reservoirs, temperature gauges, and ventilator water trap bottles should be monitored so that dry gas is not allowed to enter the patient's respiratory system as it will cause encrusting of secretions and make coughing or suctioning traumatic.

*Nasal oxygen* may be administered, between 6 and 8 liters. This flow-rate will deliver 30 to 40 percent oxygen to the patient. Oxygen masks, face tents, rebreathing masks, and Venturi masks can also be used to deliver oxygen (see Mechanical Ventilation).

It is important to remember that in patients with an elevated $CO_2$ level, cerebral receptors which respond to the amount of serum $CO_2$ are nonfunctioning. Instead the respiratory drive is monitored by peripheral receptors which respond only to oxygen levels in the blood. A sudden increase in the concentration of the oxygen inspired by these patients can result in respiratory failure secondary to the loss of hypoxic drive. Assessment of arterial blood gases will help to avoid this problem.

The arterial partial pressure of $O_2$ should be maintained between 70 and 100 mmHg at normal hemoglobin levels for optimum functioning of cells at all levels. Arterial pressure of less than 70 mmHg is not compatible with adequate oxyhemoglobin saturation (see Fig. 30-13).

If the patient with a *flail chest* is cyanotic or suffering from labored respirations even after external immobilization, low-flow oxygen should be administered until mechanical ventilation is available. Three liters/minute by means of a Venturi mask (see Fig. 30-13), connected to a portable oxygen tank, will relieve the hypoxia without danger to the patient since no more than 24 percent oxygen is present in the $FIO_2$. An Ambu-Bag exerts positive pressure and could cause harm if tension pneumothorax exists. Open or closed pneumothorax, hemothorax, or hemipneumothorax occurs in cases of trauma to the chest. Any of these conditions will often require the institution of closed chest drainage tubes and positive pressure assisted ventilation. Positive pressure should not be applied to the patient until chest tubes are inserted to avoid development of tension pneumothorax. A physician may insert a large-bore needle into the pleural space to equalize the pressure of tension pneumothorax until *closed chest drainage* can be instituted.

**S**uctioning When coughing and deep breathing fail to remove secretions from the trachea, suctioning may be required. Secretions may be suctioned from the nasopharynx or the oropharynx, or through tracheostomy or an endotracheal tube (refer to Fig. 30-14). Generally if secretions are thick or the patient is too weak to expel secretions, suctioning will be performed.

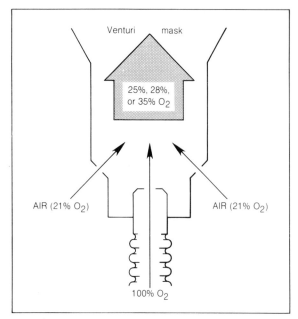

**FIGURE 30-13**
Venturi mask. (*From Emergency Treatment of Acute Respiratory Diseases, Virginia Thoracic Society, 1971. Used with permission.*)

Suctioning is a painless procedure, but it can be potentially frightening to the patient. Careful explanation of the procedure and its overall purpose will help to elicit the needed cooperation from the patient.

Indications for suctioning include noisy respirations, cyanosis due to airway obstruction caused by mucus, increased pulse rate, and tachypnea. Before suctioning, the nurse should be sure the patient is well oxygenated and rested. Increased amounts of oral fluids, humidified air, and chest physical therapy (see Third-Level Nursing Care for COPD) should be performed in order to loosen trapped secretions.

Suctioning should be a totally sterile procedure to avoid infection. A separate sterile catheter should be used for each suctioning period and for each orifice.

A sterile "whistle tip" catheter is selected in the appropriate diameter of the opening; usually a number 14 or 16 inch. The catheter is attached to a low-suction machine. A "I" connector is attached to the catheter so that it can be inserted without suction. It is important to avoid kinking of the catheter since this will cause a pressure buildup in the line and exert harmful levels of pressure on the tracheal membrane when the kink is released. A septic technique with the patient at a 45° angle is

used when inserting the catheter to prevent the entrance of pathogens into the lower airway.

The catheter is moistened with sterile saline and introduced into the nasopharynx. As the catheter approaches the larynx, the patient should be instructed to inhale so that the catheter selectively enters the larynx past a closed glottis. The catheter can then be inserted from 18 to 22 inches in a normal adult. The lower airway can be suctioned without removing the catheter from the larynx. Suction should be applied gently to the catheter for short periods of a few seconds only because oxygen is removed as well as secretions. Oxygen should be administered via the same catheter in place in the larynx between periods of suctioning. Suction periods should be brief, never exceeding 10 to 15 seconds each.[53] Suction should be applied as the catheter is withdrawn to ensure removal of secretions. Oxygen should be reestablished, or nasal oxygen may be administered to the patient throughout the procedure.

There is some controversy as to the efficacy of turning the patient's head to the left and then the right to direct the catheter into the left as well as the right main stem bronchus. Although the procedure is recommended by most authorities, there is much question as to its effectiveness.

Use of a curved catheter is recommended. It must be turned so that the curved portion points toward the left if entrance into the left main stem bronchus is to be successful. The patient should be monitored during the suctioning procedures for cyanosis, respiratory distress, and bradycardia. Prolonged suctioning can lead to hypoxia. If suctioning is done forcefully, it can damage the bronchial tissue and cause ulceration or perforation. In addition excessive suctioning can stimulate the production of an additional secretion and complicate the situation. If the catheter used is too large, it may cause lobar collapse. Continuous suctioning can cause an airway obstruction and lead to sudden death.

When suctioning with a tracheostomy tube the nurse should auscultate the chest wall before and after suctioning. The need for a sterile procedure continues. The suction tip can be inserted 6 to 8 inches into the trachea to remove secretions.

**T**racheostomy  When secretions obstruct the patency of an airway and hypoxia results, a tracheostomy may be performed to create an artificial opening at the level of the second tracheal ring.

A tracheostomy in current medical practice is

almost always an elective procedure. Indications for a tracheostomy are found on Table 30-7.

A *tracheotomy* (the procedure of opening the trachea) is usually performed under sterile technique. The patient lies flat on the back with the neck extended. A pillow can be placed under the shoulder in order to make the location of the trachea more obvious. The skin is then prepared, and a horizontal or vertical incision is made from the circoid cartilage to 2 inches above the sternal notch. Depending upon whether the tracheostomy will be permanent, the opening is then secured to the skin (see Fig. 30-14) and a cannula is then inserted. Postoperatively the nurse should observe the area for signs of infection and hemorrhage. The patient should be monitored for signs of respiratory insufficiency, or pneumothorax. If the cannula is expelled, it should never be forced back into the opening as it could result in undue tissue trauma and asphixiation. A *tracheoesophageal fistula* can develop when there is an erosion of the posterior wall of the trachea. This is often due to weakness in the cell wall. Patients with a tracheostomy should be observed when swallowing food or liquids. If choking ensues after oral intake of food, aspiration may occur and the presence of a fistula should be considered.

*Tracheostomy care*  Prior to tracheostomy care the patient should be rested and adequately oxygenated. Suctioning will be needed in order to remove secretions. Humidified oxygen should be used between suctioning periods along with adequate fluid intake to liquefy secretions. The patient should be allowed frequent rest periods between suctioning periods.

Tracheostomy care is performed at least every 8 hours and involves changing of the dressing and neck tapes which surround the tube and hold it in place. In many settings a sterile kit containing all the materials for cleaning the tracheostomy tube is available. It is important to always tie on clean tapes *before* removing the soiled ones to prevent expulsion of the tracheostomy tube. The tracheostomy wound should be cleaned with a 3% hydrogen peroxide solution and sterile distilled water. Small gauze squares may be cut to fit under the external cannula. If the tracheostomy tube has an inner cannula, it should be removed and soaked in a sterile solution of 3% hydrogen peroxide. By use of aseptic technique the inner cannula should be rinsed in sterile water and replaced. If the patient is receiving oxygen or mechanical ventilation, the

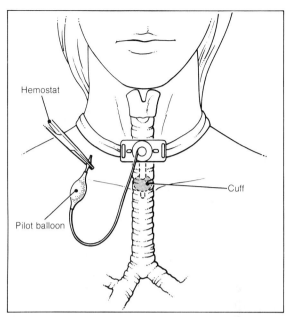

**FIGURE 30-14**
Cuffed tracheostomy.

swivel adaptor should be replaced and the patient reconnected to the ventilator. Should accidental decannulation occur, the nurse should call for help, immediately deflate the cuff, and try to reinsert the cannula gently with the patient's neck hyperextended. An emergency tracheostomy tray should be kept at the bedside with an obturator, an extra disposable tracheostomy tube, and a Kelly clamp to keep the airway patent. If this is unsuccessful, the

**TABLE 30-7**
INDICATIONS FOR A TRACHEOSTOMY

To maintain patent airway

To remove secretions, especially when the patient is unable to do so by coughing independently

In the presence of head and neck burns or suspected laryngeal edema

Following surgical procedures, e.g., radical neck surgery

Following irradiation procedures

Removal of foreign body

Intolerance to endotracheal tube

Neurological disorders involving diaphragm, thoracic cavity, difficulty in swallowing, paralysis

Apnea or unconsciousness

Respiratory failure

Head and neck injury

Ludwig's angina (Chap. 26)

nurse should cover the tracheostomy wound and ventilate with a bag and mask until help comes. Patients who are relying on ventilators to help them breathe must be observed continuously as described under Assessment above. Reports of problems with mechanical ventilation should be made immediately to the physician while artificial ventilation is supplied by a manual resuscitator or by means of mouth-to-mouth resuscitation.

Patients should be *prepared* for the tracheostomy whenever possible. They should be told why this intervention is needed and some of the changes that will occur as a result. They should also be told that they will probably not be able to speak clearly after the tracheostomy. An alternate means of communication should then be established to avoid unnecessary frustration and anxiety.

Initially, fluids will be administered intravenously. However, patients should be told that intake of fluids and solid foods may occur at a later time. Frequently, the patient fears choking and will need to be reassured at that time.

Patients should be told that they will be able to cough up their own secretions. If this is not possible, frequent suctioning will be provided to assist in the process. Support and reassurance are often needed to help patients cope with this physical change in appearance and function.

Use of the tracheostomy is not without *disadvantages* and hazards. A tracheostomy will decrease the cough reflex, diminish an individual's ability to speak, and reduce the humidification of inspired air. In addition, because the inspired air is no longer warmed and filtered, microbes along with dust and other foreign bodies can directly enter the lung. Absence of humidification causes the secretions to become tenacious. Care should also be taken to prevent infections from developing. Careful observation for hemorrhage, aspiration, signs of respiratory failure, and hypoxia is essential.

Complications following tracheostomy often occur because of improper insertion of the cannula, poor selection of site, defective materials, or inadequate cannula size and length.

*Patient teaching* should focus upon instructing the patient and family members how to clean the tracheostomy tube and to deflate the cuffs properly. Prevention of aspiration of food and proper suctioning technique should also be taught. The patient should be encouraged to avoid the use of aeresol powders and lotions as they could irritate the cough reflex. When taking a shower, bath, or washing the hair, care should be taken to prevent water from entering the tube. Covering the opening with a thin face cloth may help to reduce this possibility. Additional irritants such as smoking, dust, and hair should be avoided. The patient should avoid crowds and persons with upper respiratory infections. Shields are available to help filter out chemical irritants, but they are not completely effective.

When the tracheostomy tube is to be removed (extubated), it is done so gradually. The lumen of the tracheostomy tube may be gradually reduced, and the patient's status observed. If this process is well tolerated, the lumen can be completely occluded. A Kistner button is sometimes used for this process.

*Endotracheal intubation* involves insertion of a tube into the trachea via the nose or the mouth. The purpose is to remove secretions and ventilate the patient (see Fig. 30-14). The procedure is rapid and avoids the need for surgical intervention; it is also self-limiting as the tube may be left in place for a short time only (approximately 72 hours to 1 week).

Several complications can occur while an endotracheal tube is in use, often happening when it is inserted too quickly or when the procedure is performed by an inexperienced physician. Problems include infection, damage to the vocal cords, trauma to the nasal and oral mucous membranes, laryngeal edema, pressure ulceration, and tissue necrosis.

Inadequate functioning of the endotracheal tube can lead to displacement of air into the esophagus or bronchus. In addition a malfunctioning endotracheal tube will lead to hypoxia and asphyxiation. Death can ensue unless immediate interventions are performed.

*Cuffed tracheostomy* and endotracheal tubes require special care. In order to stabilize the tube in the trachea, inflation of these cuffs is required (refer to Fig. 30-14). In addition, they prevent aspiration of gastric contents into the trachea, and when attached to mechanical ventilators, they produce controlled positive pressure ventilation.

Continuous inflation of the cuff will result in decreased circulation to the tracheal tissue and lead to ulceration, irritation, and necrosis of the tracheal wall. Tracheoesophageal fistula, tracheostenosis, and tracheitis are not uncommon. Newer cuffs are softer and adapt to the structure of the tracheal rings. Prestretching of the tracheostomy and endotracheal tube cuffs can also make the cuff more pliable.

*Deflating* the cuff is also an important nursing measure done to decrease some of the previously mentioned complications. Before deflating the cuff, the nurse must be certain that all excess secretions have been suctioned or coughed out of the trachea. This will decrease the chance for aspiration of collected secretions. A syringe is then connected to the cuff tube to remove the air. After deflating the cuff, suction the lower airway. Be careful to avoid stimulating the cough reflex as the patient may expel the uncuffed tracheostomy tube easily.

Following this, the patient can be given humidified oxygen for a predetermined period of time. The cuff can then be reinflated. Care must be taken not to overinflate the cuff as it could lead to rupture of the balloon. If the patient is using a respirator, the cuff should be inflated during inspiration. After the cuff is inflated, assess the patient's general status and observe for air leaks.

**H**ypoventilation    Chest trauma may result in a decreased expansion of the chest wall owing to atelectasis, pneumothorax, compression of thoracic organs, and alteration in atmospheric pressure.

Several procedures are performed to remove air and water from the thoracic cavity and restore negative intrathoracic pressure. These include thoracostomy and the use of mechanical ventilation.

*Thoracostomy* is done to remove excess air and water from the pleural cavity and to restore negative intrapleural pressure. A thoracostomy tube is inserted into the chest wall above the area of the second or third rib. A fenestrated tube is used (see Fig. 30-15). A local anesthetic (Xylocaine 1% or 2%) is administered and an incision is then made into the chest wall. A trocar and cannula are inserted into the chest wall, and the cannula is then removed. The tube is clamped, and silk sutures are used to secure the chest tube in place.

If one chest tube is used, it is usually to remove air. If air and fluids are to be removed, a second tube is placed posteriorly through the eighth and ninth intercostal spaces (see Fig. 30-16). Each tube is attached to a closed drainage system.

**C**losed-Chest Drainage    When negative pressure has been lost inside the pleural space owing to pneumothorax, it must be restored by means of closed-chest drainage. The body's ability to reabsorb air and/or fluids from the pleural cavity is limited; therefore, a closed drainage system must be established to remove the collecting fluid and air and to prevent additional air and fluid from entering the pleural cavity.

Careful explanations to patient and family will alleviate some of the anxiety felt by those undergoing such treatment. The nurse's role in caring for

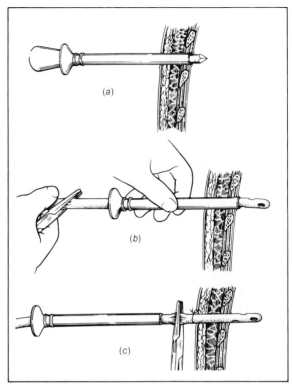

**FIGURE 30-15**

Insertion of chest tubes. (*a*) Trocar and cannula inserted into the pleural space through an incision in the chest wall. (*b*) Chest tube inserted, cannula taken out. (*c*) External portion of the tube is clamped close to the chest wall to prevent entry of air into the chest cavity. The catheter is sutured in place and the tube connected to closed drainage.

patients with *chest tubes,* or *water-seal drainage* as it is also called, is one of ensuring proper functioning and assessing, from the amount and character of the drainage, how successfully the lung is reexpanding. One tube coming from the chest will be located at the second intercostal space anteriorly to allow the escape of air rising in the pleural space. If the presence of serosanguineous fluid is suspected, a tube with a larger diameter is placed posteriorly through the eighth or ninth intercostal space in the midaxillary line. The chest tube leads from the chest via plastic or rubber tubing to a glass container in which the end of the tube is attached to a glass rod submerged in water. An air vent allows the escape of air, which bubbles up through the water. This constitutes the water-seal which prevents air from traveling up the tube to the pleural space in which negative pressure must develop to reexpand the lung.

*One-bottle system*   A simple one-bottle system provides water-seal gravity drainage. The gravity system allows the flow of air or water into the bottle when the pressure in the pleural space is sufficient to displace the water in the glass rod (see Fig. 30-17). The long glass rod is submerged about 2 cm below the water surface; an intrapleural pressure greater than −2 cm in the pleural space will be required to displace it. The reader may demonstrate this concept by taking a drinking straw and blowing air through the straw while it is submerged in a glass of water. More effort is required to blow air through the straw when it is at the bottom of the glass than when it is just slightly under the surface, because a longer column of water must be displaced from the straw. Since the gravity water-seal drainage bottle is covered with a stopper, the short glass rod simply serves to allow the escape of air from the bottle. If this short glass rod becomes occluded, air pressure could build up within the bottle. This increased pressure pushes the water in the bottle up the long glass tube toward the chest, risking back flow of fluid into the chest.

*Two-bottle system*   A two-bottle water seal drainage system involves the addition of a suction source and a suction-control bottle (see Fig. 30-18a). These are added if gravity is not sufficient to clear the air or fluid from the chest. The suction-control bottle allows the entrance of air which bubbles through the column of water in the glass rod, reducing the amount of negative pressure from the suction source. This is sometimes called a *suction-breaking bottle.* When the force of suction exceeds that required to displace the water inside the glass rod from the water level down to the end of the glass rod, air will be drawn into the system to reduce the negative pressure applied to the chest. Failure of the breaker bottle to bubble means that the desired amount of suction has not been reached. The reasons for this should be investigated. Causes may include a leak within the bottle and tube system, an inadequate suction source, and a serious air leak into the pleura from ruptured bronchus or *bronchopleural fistula.*

   The physician may distinguish among them by briefly clamping the chest tube near the chest to determine whether bubbling will resume. Resumption of bubbling indicates an intact drainage system. The problem then is an air leak into the pleura from a physiological source. The tube must not remain clamped as a tension pneumothorax will develop if the air leak into the pleural space has no egress. Air leaks into the pleural space may be

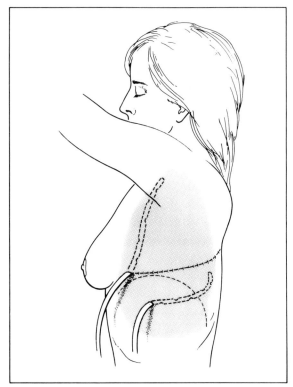

**FIGURE 30-16**
Placement of chest tubes. The upper tube (top) removes air; the lower tube (bottom) removes fluid and blood.

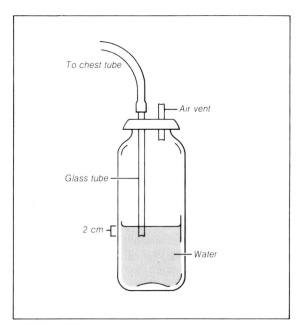

**FIGURE 30-17**
One-bottle drainage system.

localized by careful examination of the chest as discussed in assessment in Second-Level Nursing Care.

A *three-bottle system* involves the addition of a separate collection bottle so that drainage may be measured and inspected as it comes from the chest (see Fig. 30-18b).

*Pleur-evac*  Pleur-evac is a commercially available product incorporating all the features already discussed. It is a single light-weight unit which indicates the amount of air bubbling through the suction chamber from the atmosphere. It calibrates the exact amount of negative pressure in the pleural space and has a patient leak air-flow meter to indicate the amount of air coming from the patient (see Fig. 30-19).

**I**ntermittent Positive Pressure Breathing (IPPB)  In addition to a patent airway, some patients suffering from the effects of hypoventilation will need assistance moving the necessary volume of air in and out of the lungs. Intermittent positive pressure

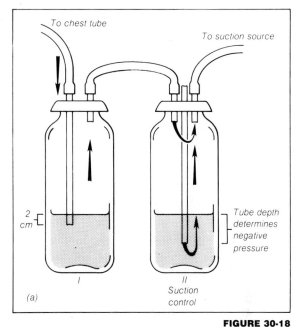

**FIGURE 30-18**

(a) Two-bottle drainage system. (b) Three-bottle drainage system.

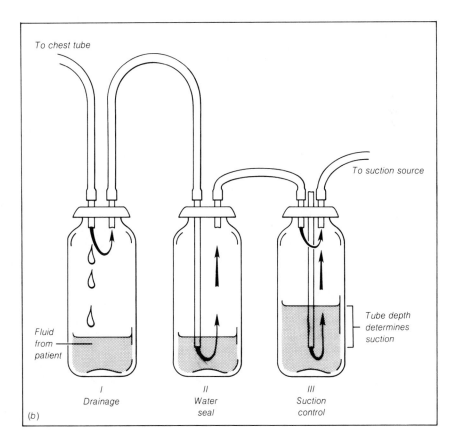

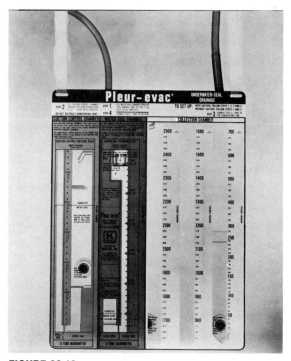

**FIGURE 30-19**
Pleur-evac, a disposable, light-weight closed-chest suction unit.
(*Courtesy of Deknatel, Inc., Queens Village, New York.*)

breathing was developed by US Air Force personnel in 1943 to allow for high-altitude flying. IPPB delivers gas to the lungs during inspiration under higher than atmospheric pressure. When a preset pressure is reached, the machine shuts off and the patient expires normally. IPPB is usually given to augment the patient's own breathing and is not continuous. It refers to treatments that are given to help the patient with his or her own efforts to clear the airways by coughing and to treatments which assist with the expulsion of accumulated secretions.

The patient may be taught to use the IPPB machine during the period of hospitalization. The nurse should instruct the patient as to the best position for achieving adequate chest expansion (usually upright). The lips should be closed tightly around the mouthpiece and the nose pinched off to allow for adequate pulmonary ventilation. The patient should be encouraged to *breathe normally* and relax. If this procedure stimulates coughing, the patient may remove the mouthpiece. Frequently, an aerosol medication may be used to aid in loosening secretions. The frequency of the use of the machine will depend upon the patient's overall health status and the effectiveness of the treatments in raising secretions.

**M**echanical Ventilation  Mechanical ventilators are machines which are capable of delivering air at a positive pressure to the patient. Highly technical machinery is involved in this process, and the nurse must be familiar with not only the principles involved but also the actual machines. The patient's life depends on the nurse's ability to assess the successful functioning of the machines and endotracheal or tracheostomy tubes as well as to be alert to any changes occurring within the patient. Selection of the machine will be based upon the patient's needs.

Hypoventilation can be improved by ventilators which assist or control the respiratory effort. A variety of machines are available to accomplish this, and each patient will be treated according to specific needs. The ventilatory capability of the patient must be considered in conjunction with the capability of any mechanical assistance that is being considered to augment or substitute for the patient's own system. If the nurse thinks of the mechanical ventilator as an extension of the patient's own respiratory system, the importance of checking the vital signs of the machine can be appreciated.

Machine design is of two types. One is the pressure-limited flow-variable type in which the inspiratory cycle ceases when a preset pressure has been reached; the other is the volume-limited pressure-variable type in which the end of inspiration occurs when a certain volume has been delivered. Some ventilators are regulated by a timing device, and others have combined cycling in which flow volume, pressure, and time are set and the preset value that is reached first cycles the inspiratory phase off.

The machine is used to overcome the dangers of respiratory insufficiency. By forcing oxygen into the lungs, it increases the expiration of carbon dioxide. Airflow to the alveoli is well distributed, and the patient's breathing efforts and related energy expenditure are decreased. The machine will improve the effectiveness of coughing and is used to assist with expulsion of accumulating secretions (see Fig. 30-20).

The *pressure-cycled* machine is used when pressure is needed to expand the lungs. The Bird Mark 7 and Bennett PR2 are commonly used pressure-cycled ventilators. Specific controls, e.g., pressure control, sensitivity control, and inspiratory flow rate, are all preset to regulate the rate, volume, and pressure limits of the inspired gas. The *volume-*

*control* machines (e.g., the Bennett MAI, the Emerson, and the Ohio 560) are ventilators which can be preset to control the total inspired oxygen volume received by the patient.

Whatever machinery is chosen, the patient must be prepared carefully for the idea of mechanical ventilation. Frequently, the machinery creates much anxiety for the patient. The nurse needs to prepare the patient for this experience by carefully explaining the machinery and allowing the patient to actively participate. Mechanical ventilators should always be carefully checked for optimal functioning and safety. Power lines should be observed for broken wires, thereby reducing the risk of electrical shock.

The machine may be cycled to inflate the patient's lungs independent of the patient's inspiratory efforts (control), or it can be set so that the patient's inspiratory efforts will trigger the delivering of gas under positive pressure (assist).[54]

*Assisted cycle ventilation* makes use of the patient's own respiratory effort to stimulate the machine. The machine is set to assist the force of the patient's own inspiratory action. When the flow of oxygen ceases, the patient exhales. The machine continues to perform in this manner as long as the patient breathes. When the patient is exhausted by breathing, or when slow, shallow respirations are present, a machine which assists the respiratory effort will allow for increased lung expansion, thereby making maximum use of the patient's own ventilatory capacity.

*Controlled ventilation* also offers continuous oxygen to the patient under positive pressure. The machine sets the respiratory rate and cycles it. Frequently the patient will have an endotracheal tube or tracheostomy. The patient's own respiratory effort can be stimulated if the patient is not relaxed to allow the machine to take over the activity of breathing. This will decrease the effectiveness of the machine and exahust the patient.

When patients become anxious or hyperactive, they must be relaxed. This can be achieved by giving them emotional support and helping them understand the components of the machine. If they continue to fight the machine, their own respirations may be suppressed by medication (e.g., Demerol).

**P**ositive End Expiratory Pressure   It is also possible to apply positive pressure to the lungs during late expiration, a procedure termed *positive end expiratory pressure (PEEP)*. This type of ventilation prevents the patient from exhaling completely and al-

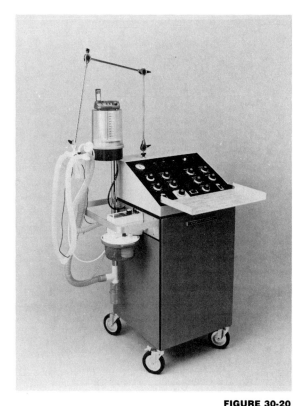

**FIGURE 30-20**
Intermittent positive pressure breathing (IPPB) machine. (*Courtesy of Puritan-Bennett Corp.*)

lows the alveoli at end expiration to retain more oxygen, thereby increasing the functional residual capacity. Partial pressure of oxygen in the arterial blood is determined to a great extent by the amount of alveolar oxygen available to diffuse through the alveolar capillary membrane. Increased perfusion of the capillaries elevates the ventilation/perfusion ratio and supplies more oxygen to the tissues. (It can, however, decrease the action of the cardiovascular pumping mechanism.) Arterial blood pressure, central venous pressure, pulse, body weight, arterial blood gas, fluid intake, and output should be carefully monitored if a patient is on PEEP[55] (see Fig. 30-21). Notice that tidal volume remains the same as long as the upper limit of the capacity of the lung is not exceeded. If PEEP is increased when maximum tidal volume has been reached, significant reduction in the tidal volume can occur.

**C**ontinuous Positive Pressure Ventilation   This type of ventilation assistance involves the application of positive pressure throughout the breathing cycle. Positive pressure applied during expiration offers resistance as the patient expires. The oppos-

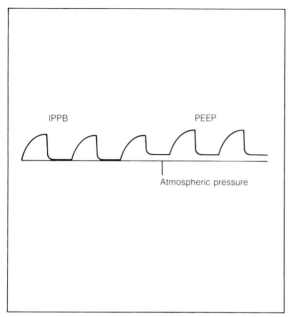

**FIGURE 30-21**
Comparison of wave forms noted with the use of IPPB and PEEP.

ing forces of expiration against a positive pressure cause dilatation of the large and small airways and alveoli, increasing the ventilation/perfusion ratio and achieving increased arterial blood oxygenation with lower inspired oxygen concentrations. Use of the procedure requires the same precautions as discussed under PEEP. Urinary output must be carefully noted on an hourly basis.

Continuous positive pressure breathing or continuous positive airway pressure is the application of the positive pressure during the expiratory cycle in those patients who are not receiving ventilatory assistance.

**P**recautions and Observations  In addition to monitoring the patient's response to ventilation, the nurse should check the machinery frequently to ensure its proper functioning. Parameters will change depending on the type of machine in use, whether it is used for assisted or controlled ventilation, and the sophistication of alarm systems. For each machine in use the nurse should be familiar with safety devices which will regulate volume and pressure or stop flow. The presence of a backup safety limit so that failure of one system activates a second system is also important to note.

*Tidal volume* is the amount of air exhaled with each breath. It is measured by means of an aneroid manometer which can be attached to the expiratory port of the mouthpiece. *Minute ventilation* is the tidal volume multiplied by the number of breaths per minute and should be noted. The *peak pressure* required to deliver the tidal volume is an important indicator of the elasticity of the lung (compliance).[56]

*Temperature* of inspired air as well as *humidity* should be checked hourly. Damage to the trachea from delivery of dry air or gas can cause trauma to the tissues.

*Inspired oxygen concentration* is measured hourly with an oxygen analyzer at a point closest to the patient. This is called the $FIO_2$, and the concentration will be ordered by the physician at a rate to provide adequate oxygenation of tissues without risk of oxygen toxicity.

A sudden increase in *peak pressure* indicates obstruction of the airway via pooling of secretions or a kink in the tubing. A sudden decrease indicates a leak in the system and should be reported immediately to the physician.

In order to determine a preset pressure or volume, the system must be a closed one. A tracheostomy or endotracheal tube will be used to provide continuous delivery of oxygen.

Problems in ventilation should be monitored continuously to avoid unnecessary complications. Vital signs, examination of the chest, inspection of the skin and extremities for cyanosis or clubbing of the fingers and cardiac monitoring for signs of cardiovascular pump failure and arrhythmias are important. The patients level of consciousness and neurological responses are additional important aspects of assessment. In addition, fluid and electrolyte balance and gastric distention should be carefully assessed, and any nausea and vomiting must be noted.

Additional care of the patient on mechanical ventilators should include good oral hygiene, humidification of inhaled oxygen, frequent arterial blood gases check, and monitoring of the tidal volume and pulse pressure gauges.

Patients who are on continuous mechanical ventilation may develop several complications which could be life-threatening. There is an initial danger of *respiratory alkalosis* developing as a result of hyperventilation. The rapid expulsion of $CO_2$ does not give the kidneys sufficient time to release bicarbonate, and alkalosis can result. *Ventricular arrhythmias* (fibrillation) can also result from a rapid reverse in $CO_2$ blood levels.

*Gastric distention* due to increased amounts of air entering the stomach may predispose the individual to a paralytic ileus, vomiting, or gastrointestinal bleeding. Prolonged use of respirators can result in *rupturing of the alveoli* and cause an alveolar block, decreasing oxygen and $CO_2$ exchange. When continuous mechanical ventilation is used, *atelectasis* may develop.

**Ventilator dependency** *Dependence on mechanical ventilation* can be psychological or physiological but is far more often physiological. Old, debilitated patients are most often those who cannot be weaned from the ventilator. The longer a patient is on the ventilator, the more difficult will be the weaning process. Muscles which have been inactive for long periods will be weak and require more adjustment before taking over the work of breathing again.

Many patients equate being alive with being able to breathe. Those whose muscles of respiration have been paralyzed and who have been under controlled ventilation for a long period of time are frequently terrified that they will not be able to breathe off the machine. A technique called *intermittent mandatory ventilation* has been helpful in some cases in weaning patients who might otherwise present long-term problems in ventilator dependency. This technique uses positive pressure breathing during the inspiratory phase but at rates well below those used during the acute stage of illness. The concept is one of slowly transferring control of ventilation to the patient. The ventilator cycles may be set as low as one mandatory breath per minute, two minutes, or three minutes with the rest of the patient's ventilatory needs being met by his or her own efforts.

*Weaning* is usually undertaken when the vital capacity is at least twice the value for tidal volume at rest. Initial trials should be brief, humidified oxygen should be supplied during weaning periods, and a record of the weaning process should be kept. Before a patient is fed with the endotracheal or tracheostomy cuff deflated, the ability to swallow should be tested by giving the patient sterile water containing methylene blue dye to swallow with the cuff deflated. If any blue dye appears upon suctioning the trachea, the swallowing reflex is not intact, and the patient should not be fed with the cuff deflated.

**Fluid and electrolyte imbalance** Depending upon the cause of the chest trauma and the amount of fluid loss, the patient must be carefully observed for electrolyte imbalance (see Chap. 13) and respiratory acidosis.

Adequate fluid replacement is as essential as accurate monitoring of fluid output. If oliguria is present, the patient should be assisted and treated for shock (hypovolemia; see Chap. 28). Frequent checks on serum arterial oxygen gas levels and blood pH levels are essential (see Fig. 30-22). If signs of alkalosis or acidosis are observed, immediate treatment should begin including the correct use of mechanical ventilation and suctioning (see above). Restoration of normal blood pH levels is essential (see Chap. 13).

Fluids should also be encouraged to maintain adequate electrolyte balance and to loosen secretions. A high-protein diet should be encouraged to compensate for negative nitrogen balance. Nourishments should be offered in small, frequent feedings as tolerated by the patient.

**Pain** The body's reaction to pain in the region of the chest always involves two responses. The mechanical response is that of restricting respiratory excursions and immobility. Immobility interferes with the clearing of secretions from the airways. The patient, therefore, has an increased need to cough but resists because of the pain involved in this activity.

*Pain* of even a mild degree will result in some limitation of chest expansion. If splinting occurs it is most serious. Splinting is a severe restriction of motion on the affected side. This produces short, jerky respirations often associated with grunting. Cough and aspiration of secretions are impossible as secretions pool in the chest, leading to *atelectasis* (incomplete chest expansion) and infection. Both objective and subjective signs of pain should be noted by the nurse. Some patients make an effort to be brave and can do themselves real harm by not seeking relief from pain. Physiotherapy will be tolerated and deep breathing and coughing achieved only after pain is relieved.

Pain relief may be accomplished by timely administration of analgesics and in the case of crushing chest injuries by lidocaine injections either locally or as intercostal nerve blocks. Care should be taken to avoid the use of large doses of an analgesic so that CNS depression will not occur. The nurse must coordinate chest physiotherapy, deep breathing and coughing routines, and airway clearance techniques such as suctioning and tracheostomy care with periods of maximum analgesia.[56]

Problems with pain usually arise from fractured ribs or from the kinds of procedures necessary to adequately ventilate the patient. External fixation of flail chest with wires and overhead traction can cause a great deal of pain. Intercostal nerve blocks may be used to help reduce pain and can be repeated in 1 week.

*External immobilization* is rarely used currently except where intubation and mechanical ventilation are not available. It is occasionally used in combination with a ventilator on large-chested patients. Open reduction with internal fixation, external traction, and wiring have all been advocated. Small stab wounds can be made through the skin to allow placement of towel clips through the center of the rib. Overhead traction by the pulley and weight system is used to exert pressure on the flail section. Incorporating elastic in the traction system allows the patient maximum movement and minimum pain (refer to Chap. 40).

Careful observation of the site must be made by the nurse since it can become infected and cause permanent bone loss and chest deformity.

**Anxiety** Patients who sustain a chest injury fear the difficulty they experience in not being able to breathe. They also fear the loss of their life due to their injuries. The amount of pain that is present may create an added stress for the individual and intensify the anxiety.

Not being able to breathe is a most anxiety-producing event. Concentrating upon each inspiration is exhausting. The nurse must recognize this and reassure the patient while supplying information that is needed by the patient or family to reduce their *anxiety.*

There is often a complicated chain of events in accidents, especially those involving motor vehicles. The nurse should be aware of feelings of *guilt* which may be involved in accidents which result in death or injury to another. Many of the seriously injured are teen-agers who are in their formative years and do not have well-developed coping mechanisms. *Fear* of suffocation and impending death are paramount in the patient's mind. Everything that happens to the patient in the hospital should be explained, and reassurance should be offered whenever possible.[57]

Patients involved in disasters such as airplane crashes, bomb blasts, and boating accidents will have need to know about others who were with them at the time of injury. They will also have questions about their role in the event. The patient's ability to respond to therapy can often be hampered by such worries which are not resolved.

**FIGURE 30-22**

Zone of respiratory balance. (*From William E. Neville, Care of the Cardiopulmonary Patient, Year Book, Chicago, 1971. Used by permission.*)

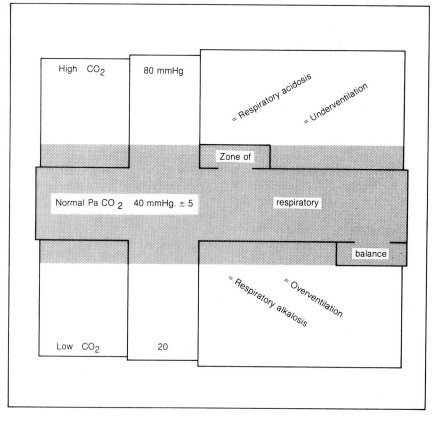

High $CO_2$  80 mmHg  = Respiratory acidosis  = Underventilation

Zone of

Normal Pa $CO_2$  40 mmHg. ± 5  respiratory

balance

= Respiratory alkalosis  = Overventilation

Low $CO_2$  20

Patients should be given an opportunity to verbalize their feelings and freely express their fears and concerns. The nurse should be supportive to the patient at this time.

The level of stress the patient and the family are undergoing can hardly be imagined unless it has been experienced. The atmosphere of intricate machinary with flashing lights, buzzing and beeping monitors, suction pumps, and respirators is one of threat and danger. Nurses dealing with these intensely ill patients must keep in mind the ability of the patients, the families, and themselves to deal with so much stress. Many intensive-care teams are finding it rewarding and helpful to have regular patient care conferences in which they draw upon the expertise of psychiatric specialists. Families are often included in these conferences so that goals for care are mutually arrived at and implications of continued life-support of hopelessly ill patients can be explored and evaluated thoroughly, realistically, and sensitively.

Nurses must be able to draw upon the strength of other team members if they are to be able to help patients deal with injury, dependent status, and fear of death and the unknown.

**Infection** Accident victims are particularly susceptible to infection as they have frequently been injured with grossly contaminated objects which may have penetrated vital organs. Risk of introducing infection in patients with chest trauma is high. Intravenous solutions containing antibodies should be administered on time to maintain blood levels. Fluids should be carefully monitored to avoid overloading the cardiovascular pumping mechanism. Careful intake and output records should be kept. Daily weights and hourly monitoring of urinary output are important determinations in assessing pump failure. Immobility, tracheostomy, improper suctioning, and decreased chest expansion may lead to atelectasis and pneumonia.

The nurse may be asked to assist with thoracentesis, pericardiocentesis, pulmonary lavage, and transtracheal aspiration. *Thoracentesis* involves the placement of a needle into the pleural space through the intercostal spaces in the rib cage and aspirating fluid. *Pericardiocentesis* is needle aspiration of the pericardium when blood has accumulated in the sac and is restricting heart action. This is a life-saving procedure for if the fluid is not removed, cardiac tamponade will occur and death will follow. *Pulmonary lavage* is washing or irrigation of the lung tissue via fiberoptic bronchoscopy. The instrument is passed to the appropriate lung seg-

ment, a balloon is inflated blocking the fluid from the other segments of the lung, and the fluid is instilled and suctioned out through the instrument. *Transtracheal aspiration* is the introduction of a catheter directly into the trachea by way of the cricothyroid membrane. It may be kept in place for 12 to 24 hours under sterile technique. Two milliliter sterile saline may be injected to cause coughing or to dissolve thick secretions.

**Adult resporatory distress syndrome** The most severe complication of serious lung trauma is *adult respiratory distress syndrome* (ARDS). It most frequently occurs after massive trauma, hemorrhage, and shock. The syndrome is known by many other names as noted in Table 30-8. The capillary bed of the lung becomes hemorrhagic and extremely edematous. There is a loss of surfactant, a unique lipoprotein produced in the alveoli which allows them to keep their shape causes complete deflation of the alveoli and massive collapse.[58] Lung compliance is decreased, and oxygenation of the pulmonary capillary beds becomes spotty. Hypoxia is profound. Frothing pulmonary edema is associated with fluid overload and should be carefully avoided in posttraumatic patients. Fluids should be controlled at levels sufficient to produce 500 to 1000 ml urine daily with additions only to replace known losses. Oxygen toxicity is suspected by some to be a cause of ARDS. High-saturation continuous-flow oxygen interferes with the lung's ability to synthesize surfactant. The problem of liberation of other mediators from the lung during hypoxia and anaphylactic shock is currently being studied by pulmonary physiologists.

Treatment in all cases involves the use of a mechanical ventilator to provide adequate oxygen to the tissues. Positive end expiratory pressure is used in which positive pressure is maintained through the expiratory cycle and end expiratory pressure does not return to atmospheric pressure.

**TABLE 30-8**
NAMES USED TO DESCRIBE ADULT RESPIRATORY DISTRESS SYNDROME

| | |
|---|---|
| 1 | Acute respiratory distress syndrome |
| 2 | Acute pulmonary injury syndrome |
| 3 | Shock lung |
| 4 | Traumatic wet lung |
| 5 | Capillary leak syndrome |
| 6 | Adult hyaline membrane disease |
| 7 | Postperfusion lung |
| 8 | Congestive atelectasis |
| 9 | Posttraumatic pulmonary insufficiency |
| 10 | Hemorrhagic shock |

Some have suggested *disseminated intro-vascular coagulation* as having a role in adult respiratory distress syndrome. Shock (refer to Chap. 28) and sepsis must be treated as well as any complicating aspiration pneumonia or fat emboli. Use of corticosteroids and/or heparinization is sometimes helpful in controlling underlying conditions while the lung responds.

The *extracorporeal membrane oxygenator* is the closest thing we have to an artificial lung. It totally filters the blood through a synthetic oxygenator to maintain oxygen levels capable of supporting life. The complications of this therapy are many, but it has been successful in some cases of adult respiratory distress syndrome, especially those involving healthy young people who have been injured in automobile accidents. This treatment must still be considered experimental, but it does offer exciting implications for the future.

**Complications** *Shock* may develop as a complication of chest injury and has been discussed in Chap. 28 and in relations to ARDS in the preceding pages.

*Tracheal stenosis* as a complication of cuff pressure occurs and can be handled by reconstruction of the trachea by surgical intervention. The complication should, of course, be avoided by meticulous care of the artificial airway as previously described. The amount of stress inherent in the care of those injuries to the chest has been alluded to previously. Occasionally, the nurse will see patients who develop gastric stress ulcers under these conditions. Prophylactic antacids are often ordered, particularly if the patient is being treated with steroid preparations.

**Fourth-Level Nursing Care**

*Rehabilitation* of chest-injured patients is aimed toward helping them achieve the optimum level of function that their physical limitations will allow.

Patients who have been immobile and on mechanical ventilators for long periods of time are usually weak and suffer from some degree of muscle wasting. It is important to provide small portions of attractively served high-protein food at frequent intervals throughout the rehabilitation period.

Breathing retraining, with emphasis on breathing through pursed lips and diaphragmatic breathing while gradually increasing activity, helps the patient use lung capacity to its fullest. Attentive pulmonary toilet, dust-free environments, deep breathing, use of aerosol bronchodilators, cough-ing, postural drainage, vibrating, and clapping are of utmost importance.

Long-term continuous *oxygen therapy* may be necessary in some cases. This can be accomplished in the home care setting by means of refillable portable oxygen tanks. These can be carried as the patient ambulates, or they may be wheeled on a cart. Permanent pulmonary problems are rarely the result of accidents since the lungs are basically healthy and surgical reconstruction of crushing injuries is highly successful.

Management of *intractable pain* (see Chap. 39) connected with crushing injuries of the chest can be treated by nerve block or some of the newer methods of pain management evolving from the gate control theory. Chronic pain is a complex malady involving physical, psychological, and social factors. Arthritic pain or causalgia, a searing pain, appearing after sudden systemic shock can cause long-term pain management problems.[59]

Evaluation of *permanent disability* is made on the basis of physical examination. Pulmonary function is tested before and after exercise, and the patient's ability to perform the usual occupation evaluated. Pilots, divers, athletes, people engaged in heavy construction, and others may need job retraining which is provided under social security programs throughout the country.

**Patient teaching** Patients who suffer long-term disability can benefit from knowledge of pulmonary anatomy and physiology, the pathology of their particular disorder, and the rational for the care they are receiving. Knowledge is power, and when the patient is able to understand why care is given and on what basis it is designed, compliance with health care routines will be high. The goal of health teaching should be to make every patient a member of his own health care team[60] and guide him toward that time when he will be the only member of that team. When that occurs, the patient will once again be independent.

The positive aspects of whatever functional ability is left to the patient should be emphasized rather than the deficits by carefully assessing interest, skills, and abilities with the patient. New life-styles can be explored when necessary.

## INFLAMMATORY DISTURBANCES IN O₂-CO₂ EXCHANGE

Several types of inflammatory processes affect the respiratory tract and disrupt ventilation. A complete discussion of the inflammatory process is found in

Chap. 10. One of the most common inflammatory processes which alters $O_2$-$CO_2$ exchange is pneumonia. The following discussion will briefly explore this problem.

## Pneumonia

Pneumonia is an acute inflammatory process which affects the alveolar spaces of the lungs. When this occurs, thick mucous secretions collect in the lungs, and the alveoli fill with exudate. Oxygen–carbon dioxide exchange is disrupted. This results in diminished pulmonary ventilation and diffusion and leads to hypoxia.

Pneumonia can be precipitated by many causes including aspiration of fluid, retention of secretion, anesthesia, upper respiratory infection, inadequate lung expansion, paralysis, immobility, obstructive lung disease, and irritating pollutants.

Perhaps the most common cause of pneumonia is a bacterial infection. Pneumococcal (diplococcal) pneumonia is the most frequent type, being observed in over 80 percent of the patients with pneumonia.[61] Staphyloccal pneumonia is often observed in young children. Frequently, pneumonia occurs as a secondary problem, being superimposed on an upper respiratory illness.

The population at risk to develop pneumonia includes the elderly, smokers, cancer patients on immunosuppressants, immobilized individuals, persons who have had thoracic surgery, persons exposed to noxious gas which has caused paralysis of the diaphragm, and individuals who have COPD. Individuals with congestive heart failure and fibrocystic disease are also at risk. Prevention of pneumonia includes early ambulation following surgery, aggressive chest physiotherapy for any upper respiratory infections, decreased use of narcotics, especially in the elderly, and avoidance of aspiration. In addition frequent position change for immobilized patients and adequate suctioning will prevent complication of pneumonia. Adequate nutrition, early antibiotic treatment of respiratory infections in persons with COPD, and decrease in smoking with also help reduce the incidence of pneumonia.

Pneumococcal pneumonia occurs more often during the winter and early spring. It affects males more than females and has a higher death rate among blacks. It is transmitted via droplets. The bacteria enter the alveoli through the respiratory tract. The inflammation that occurs in the bronchioles drains into the alveoli and is drawn into the respiratory tract. The rusty-color sputum so often observed is due to the escape of red blood cells that pass from the inflamed alveoli into the fluid.[62] Later it will become yellow in color.

Pneumococcal pneumonia usually follows an upper respiratory infection and has a sudden onset. The patient will notice an increase in fever and chills. Early in the course of the problem the patient will have a dry, hacking cough. Chest pain may be present and indicates pleuritic involvement. The patient will often guard and hold the affected side in order to obtain relief from the pain. Dyspnea will be present depending on the amount of lung involvement. Tachypnea and tachycardia will be observed. The patient may be diaphoretic. Upon thoracic auscultation a pleuritic friction rub may be heard. Rales may also be heard. There may be dullness observed upon palpation in one or both lung bases. The abdominal examination should assess for the presence of bowel sounds and abdominal distention. Nausea, vomiting, and diarrhea may be observed.

The patient will usually appear weak and pale and will complain of general aches and pains. A headache is often present. In addition signs of dehydration may be noted about the lips and mouth as well as the buccal membrane.

A *chest x-ray* usually demonstrates consolidation of fluid in the one or more lobes that may be affected. Leukocytosis is usually present with the white blood cell count elevated as high as 20,000 to 35,000/mm$^3$. Sputums are collected, and the infectious agent can often be isolated.

Antipyretics are given to help reduce body temperature. In addition the patient is treated with an *antibiotic.* Crystalline penicillin G is often the drug of choice, although penicillin V can be used for less severe pneumonias.[63] Care should be taken to check for previous allergic responses to this drug. Patients should be kept warm to avoid chills. The environment should be kept as comfortable as possible, and drafts should be prevented.

*Oral hygiene* is important especially if the patient is mouth breathing and expectorating large amounts of sputum. If the lips are cracked or herpes simplex is present, special care should be given to this area.

*Rest* is important and the patient should be encouraged to nap frequently. The environment should be quiet and stress eliminated if possible. If severe dyspnea is present, oxygen may be given. It is important that the patient not be kept immobilized to avoid further lung consolidation. Range of motion exercises and activity as tolerated by the patient may be used.

The patient should be taught to *cough* and to splint the chest in order to expectorate as much mucous as possible. If the cough is dry and pleuritic and pain is present, cough suppresants may be used. *Expectorants* may be used to loosen secretions and aid in expectoration of mucus. *Cool mist humidifiers* as well as increase in oral fluids may also help in the process.

Good *nutrition* and a well-balanced diet will increase resistance to the infectious process. Adequate *intake of fluids* will help loosen secretions and maintain electrolyte balance.

Complications of pneumonia include atelectasis, pulmonary abscess, pulmonary edema, respiratory failure, pleural effusion, and shock. Paralytic ileus, mental confusion, and fluid and electrolyte imbalance may accompany these changes.

Recovery from pneumonia will require long-term convalescence. Treatment of the underlying cause of the problem is essential. The patient will need to follow a well-balanced diet, take frequent rest periods, and avoid overexertion. Avoidance of contacts with individuals who have respiratory infections is critical.

## REFERENCES

1   Robert Rogers and John Juers, "Physiologic Considerations in the Treatment of Acute Respiratory Failure," *Basics RD,* **3:**4, 1–6, March 1975.

2   H. H. Bendixin et al., *Respiratory Care,* Mosby, St. Louis, 1965, p. 19.

3   "Pulmonary Terms and Symbols," A Report of the ACCP-ATS Joint Committee on Pulmonary Nomenclature, *Chest,* **67:**5, 583–593, May 1975.

4   Jack Lieberman, "Alpha-1 Antitrypsin Deficiency," *Med Clin North Am,* **57:**691–706, May 1973.

5   Ira Tager and Frank Speizer, "Risk Estimates for Chronic Bronchitis in Smokers: A Study of Male-Female Differences," *Am Rev Resp Dis,* **113:**619–625, 1976.

6   Stephen Ayres, "Cigarette Smoking and Lung Diseases: An Update," *Basics RD,* **3:**1–6, May 1975.

7   John Goldsmith, "Health Effects of Air Pollution," *Basics RD,* **4:**1–6, November 1975.

8   K. K. Pump, "Emphysema and Its Relation to Age," *Am Rev Resp Dis,* **114:**5–13, 1976.

9   W. M. Thurlbeck, "Chronic Bronchitis and Emphysema," *Med Clin North Am,* **57:**651–668, May 1973.

10   F. Douglas Biggs, et al., "Disturbances of Rhythm in Chronic Lung Disease," *Heart Lung,* **6:**256–261, March–April 1977.

11   D. DeCencio, et al., "Personality Characteristics of Patients with Chronic Obstructive Pulmonary Emphysema," *Arch Phy Med Rehabil,* 471–475, August 1968.

12   Donald Dudley, et al., "Psychosocial Aspects of Care in the Chronic Obstructive Pulmonary Disease Patient," *Heart Lung,* **2:**389–393, May–June, 1973.

13   Thomas Petty, "Test Your Lungs?" (editorial), *Chest,* **70:**450–451, October 1976.

14   D. V. Bates, "The Prevention of Emphysema," *Chest,* **65:**437–441, April 1974.

15   Ronald Knudson and Benjamin Burrows, "Early Detection of Obstructive Lung Disease," *Med Clin North Am,* **57:**681–690, May 1973.

16   Bates, *op. cit.,* p. 440.

17   A. Sonia Buist, et al., "The Effect of Smoking Cessation and Modification on Lung Functions," *Am Rev Resp Dis,* **114:**115–122, 1976.

18   Lucille Fisher, "Air Pollution, the Facts," *Am Lung Assoc Bull,* pp. 6–9, May 1976.

19   Ellen Butler, "Dyspnea in the Patient with Cardiopulmonary Disease," *Heart Lung,* **4:**599–606, July–August 1975.

20   Kaye Kilburn, et al., "Byssinosis Matter from Lint to Lump," *Am J Nurs,* **73:**1952–1956, November 1973.

21   Julius Comroe, et al., *The Lung,* Year Book, Chicago, 1962.

22   Jay Nadel, "Pulmonary Function Testing," *Basics RD,* **1:**4, April 1973.

23   Ruth Murray and Judith Zentner, "Nursing Assessment and Health Promotion through the Life Span," Prentice-Hall, Englewood Cliffs, N.J., 1975, p. 176.

24   Irwin Ziment, "The Pharmacology of Airway Dilators," *Resp Ther,* 51–56, May–June 1974.

25   De Gowin and De Gowin, *Bedside Diagnostic Examination,* Macmillan, New York, 1976, pp. 396–397.

26   H. L. Brammell, "Arrhythmias in Acute Respiratory Failure Associated with Chronic Airway Obstruction," *Heart Lung,* **2:**888–892, November–December 1973.

27   Leonard Hudson, "The Acute Management of the Chronic Airway Obstruction Patient," *Heart Lung,* **3:**93–96 January-February 1974, p. 94.

28   E. J. Campbell, "Oxygen Therapy in Diseases of the Chest," *Brit J Dis Chest,* **58:**149–157, October 1964.

29   JoAnne Lagerson, "Nursing Care of Patients with Chronic Pulmonary Insufficiency," *NCNA,* **9:**165–179, March 1974.

30   Sue Lareau, "The Effect of Positive Pressure Breathing on the Arterial Oxygen Tension in Patients with Chronic Obstructive Pulmonary Disease Receiv-

ing Oxygen Therapy," *Heart Lung,* **5:**449–452, May–June 1976.

31 M. Lentzman and R. Cherniack, "Rehabilitation of Patients with Chronic Obstructive Pulmonary Disease —State of the Art," *Am Rev Resp Dis,* **114:**1145–1165.

32 W. Baigelman and S. Chodash, "Bronchodilator Action of the Anticholinergic Drug, Ipratropium Bromide (Sch 1000) as an Aerosol in Chronic Bronchitis and Asthma," *Chest,* **71:**324–328, March 1977.

33 Sharon Roberts, "Systems Approach in Assessing Behavioral Problems of Arterial Care Patients," *Heart Lung,* **4:**593–598, July–August 1975.

34 Marjorie Crate, "Nursing Functions in Adaptation to Chronic Illness," *Am J Nurs,* **65:**72–76, October 1965.

35 R. Stark, et al., "Daily Requirement of Oxygen to Reserve Pulmonary Hypertension in Patients with Chronic Bronchitis," *Br Med J,* **3:**724–728, Sept. 23, 1972.

36 John E. Hodgkin, et al., "Chronic Obstructive Airway Disease—Current Concepts in Diagnosis and Comprehensive Care," *JAMA,* **232:**1243–1260, June 23, 1975.

37 Robert Mueller, et al., "Ventilation and Arterial Blood Gas Exchange Induced by Pursed Lip Breathing," *J Appl Physiol,* **28:**784–789, June 1970.

38 Ruben Chemack and Edith Svanhill, "Long-Term Use of Intermittent Positive Pressure Breathing (IPPB) in Chronic Obstructive Pulmonary Disease," *Am Rev Resp Dis,* **113:**721–728, 1976.

39 Jimmy Albert Young and Dean Crocker, *Principles and Practice of Respiratory Therapy,* 2d ed., Year Book, Chicago, 1976, p. 149.

40 E. H. Rubin, *Thoracic Diseases,* Saunders, Philadelphia, 1962, p. 891.

41 Paul B. Beeson and Walsh McDermott (eds.), *Cecil-Loeb Textbook of Medicine,* 13th ed., Saunders, Philadelphia, 1971, p. 32.

42 William E. Neville, *Care of the Surgical Cardiopulmonary Patient,* Year Book, Chicago, 1971, p. 253.

43 H. Corwin Hinshaw, *Diseases of the Chest,* 3d ed., Saunders, Philadelphia, 1969, p. 318.

44 Maxwell M. Wintrobe, et al. (eds.), *Harrison's Principles of Internal Medicine,* 6th ed., McGraw-Hill, New York, 1970, p. 1239.

45 Neville, *op. cit.,* p. 253.

46 William Morris (ed.), *The American Heritage Dictionary of the English Language,* Houghton Mifflin, Boston, 1970, p. 498.

47 Sharon Spaeth Bushnell, *Respiratory Intensive Care Nursing,* Little, Brown, Boston, 1973, p. 251.

48 International Labour Office, *Encyclopedia of Occupational Health and Safety,* McGraw-Hill, New York, 1974, p. 21.

49 Ronald M. Pickett and Thomas J. Trigas, *Human Factors in Health Care,* Heath, Lexington, Mass., 1974, p. X.

50 Ralph Nader, *Unsafe at Any Speed.*

51 Francis Mechner, Andrea B. O'Connor, and Barbara Boyce, "Programmed Instruction, Patient Assessment: Examination of the Chest and Lungs," *Am J Nur 76,* 1456, September 1976.

52 Raymond L. H. Murphy Jr., *A Simplified Introduction to Lung Sounds,* Boston Stethophonics, Inc., 1977, p. 20.

53 Irene L. Beland and Joyce Y. Pessos, *Clinical Nursing Pathophysiological and Psychosocial Approaches,* Macmillan, New York, 1975, p. 416.

54 Marvin A. Sackner, "Bronchofiberscopy," in John F. Murphy (ed.), *Lung Disease: State of the Art,* American Lung Association, New York, 1976, p. 276.

55 Peter J. Unguarski, Nina T. Argondizzo, and Patricia K. Boos, "CPR Current Practice Revised," *Am J Nurs,* 236, February 1975.

56 Thomas L. Petty, "Intensive and Rehabilitative Respiratory Care," 2d ed., Lea & Febiger, Philadelphia, 1974, p. 80.

57 Donna C. Aquilera and Janice M. Messie, *Crisis Intervention: Theory and Methodology,* 2d ed., St. Louis, Mosby, 1974, p. 82.

58 Beeson and McDermott, *op. cit.,* p. 881.

59 *Newsweek,* "The New War on Pain," April 25, 1977, p. 48.

60 Petty, *op. cit.,* p. 302.

61 Joan Luckman and Karen Sorenson, *Medical Surgical Nursing: A Psychophysiologic Approach,* Saunders, Philadelphia, 1964, p. 953.

62 *Ibid.,* p. 954.

63 *Ibid.,* p. 957.

## BIBLIOGRAPHY

Abraham, Abraham: "The Management of Patients with Chronic Bronchitis and Cor Pulmonale," *Heart Lung,* **6:**104–108, January–February 1977.

American Red Cross: *Lifesaving Rescue and Water Safety,* Doubleday, New York.

American Thoracic Society: "Chronic Bronchitis, Asthma and Pulmonary Emphysema," *Am Rev Resp Dis,* **85:**762–768, 1962.

Barach, Alvan: *A Treatment Manual for Patients with Pulmonary Emphysema,* Grune & Stratton, New York, 1969.

Barstow, Ruth: "Coping with Emphysema," *Nurs Clin North Am,* **9:**137–145, March 1974.

Bates, Barbara: *A Guide to Physical Examination,* Lippincott, Philadelphia, 1974.

Berzins, G.: "An Occupational Therapy Program for

the Chronic Obstructive Disease Patient," *Am J Occup Ther,* **24:**181–186, April 1970.

Billig, Donald: "Surgery for Bullous Emphysema," *Chest,* **70:**572–573, November 1976.

Block, A. J.: "Low-Flow Oxygen Therapy Treatment of the Ambulant Outpatient," *Am Rev Resp Dis,* **110**(6) Pt. II, 71–83, December 1973.

Blount, M., and A. B. Kinney: "Chronic Steroid Therapy," *Am J Nurs,* **74:**1626–1631, September 1974.

Bouhuys, Arend: *Breathing Physiology, Environment and Lung Disease,* Grune & Stratton, New York, 1974.

Brannin, Patricia: "Oxygen Therapy and Measures of Bronchial Hygiene," *Nurs Clin North Am,* **9:**111–121, March 1974.

Broughton, Joseph: "Chest Physical Diagnosis for Nurses and Respiratory Therapists," *Heart Lung,* **1:**200–206, March–April 1972.

———: "Understanding Blood Gases," Reprint 456, Ohio Medical Products, August 1971.

Bushnell, Sharon S.: *Respiratory Intensive Care Nursing,* Little, Brown, Boston, 1973.

Cardiopulmonary Resuscitation, American National Red Cross, New York, 1974.

Cherniack, Cherniack, and Nainark: *Respiration in Health and Disease,* Saunders, Philadelphia, 1972.

Cherniack, Reuben, et al.: "Home Care of Chronic Respiratory Disease," *JAMA,* **208:**821–824, May 5, 1969.

Chodosh, S.: "Examination of Sputum Cells," *N Engl J Med,* **282:**854–857, April 9, 1970.

Chrisman, Marilyn: "Dyspnea," *Am J Nurs,* **74:**643–646, April 1974.

*Chronic Obstructive Pulmonary Disease: A Manual for Physicians,* 3d ed., American Lung Association, New York, 1972.

*Chronic Obstructive Pulmonary Disease:* National Tuberculosis and Respiratory Disease Association, New York, 1972.

Cochrane, C., et al.: "Early Diagnosis of Airway Obstruction," *Thorax,* **29:**389–393, 1974.

Coe, Nicholas P., and Edwin W. Salzman: "Thrombosis and Intravascular Coagulation," *Surg Clin North Am,* **56:**875–885, August 1976.

Comroe, J. H., Jr., et al.: *The Lung,* 2d ed., Year Book, 1971.

Culbert, P., and B. Kos: "Aging: Considerations for Health Teaching," *Nurs Clin North Am,* **6:**605–613, December 1971.

Douglas, Michael E., and John B. Downs: "Pulmonary Function Following Severe Acute Respiratory Failure and High Levels of Positive End-Expiratory Pressure," *Chest,* **71:**18–23, January 1977.

Ellis, James: "Transbronchial Lung Biopsy: Variations on a Theme" (editorial), *Chest,* **68**(4):485, October 1975.

Fagerbaugh, Shizuko: "Getting Around with Emphysema," *Am J Nurs,* **73:**94–99, January 1973.

Filley, G. F.: "Emphysema and Chronic Bronchitis: Clinical Manifestations and Their Psychologic Significance," *Med Clin North Am,* **51:**283, 1967.

———: *Pulmonary Insufficiency and Respiratory Failure,* Lea & Febiger, Philadelphia, 1968.

Foley, Mary: "Pulmonary Function Testing," *Am J Nurs,* **71:**1134–1139, June 1971.

Foss, Georgia: "Postural Drainage," *Am J Nurs,* **73:**666–669, April 1973.

Fuhs, Margaret, and Alice Stern: "Better Ways to Cope with COPD," *Nursing 76,* **6:**29–38, February 1976.

Garfield, Sidney R.: "The Delivery of Medical Care," *Sci Am,* **222:**14–21, April 1970.

Gracey, Douglas: "Home Oxygen Therapy for the COPD Patient," *Heart Lung,* **4:**792–794, September–October 1975.

Hardy, Harriet, and Joseph Leahy: "Recognition of Occupational Lung Disease," *Clin Notes Resp Dis,* 3–11, Spring 1968.

Herron, Sister Catherine: "Home Care of the Patient with COPD," *Nursing 76,* 81–86, April 1976.

Hirsch, Wlwin F., et al.: "The Lung: Responses to Trauma, Surgery and Sepsis," *Surg Clin North Am,* **56:**909–927, August 1976.

Ishikawa, Sadamy: "The Effects of Air Bubbles and Time Delay on Blood Gas Analysis," *Ann Allergy,* **33:**2, August 1974.

Junod, Alain F.: "Metabolism, Production and Release of Hormones and Mediators in the Lung," in J. F. Murphy (ed.), *Lung Disease: State of the Art,* American Lung Association, New York, 1976, p. 305–320.

Keyes, Jack: "Blood Gases and Blood Gas Transport," *Heart Lung,* **3:**945–954, November–December 1974.

Kimbel, Philip: "Physical Therapy for COPD Therapy," *Clin Notes Resp Dis,* **8:**4, Spring 1970.

——— et al.: "An In-hospital Program for Rehabilitation of Patients with Chronic Obstructive Pulmonary Disease," *Chest,* **60:**65–105 (suppl.), August 1971.

King, E. Garner: "Percutaneous Trephine Lung Biopsy," *Chest,* **70**(2), 212–216, August 1976.

Kinlein, M. Lucille: "Self Care Concept," *Am J Nurs,* **77:**598–601, April 1, 1977.

Kudla, Mary: "The Care of the Patient with Respiratory Insufficiency," *Nurs Clin North Am,* **8:**183–190, March 1973.

Lagerson, J.: "The Cough, Its Effectiveness Depends

on Your Respiratory Care," **18**(4), July–August 1973.

Lentzman, Morley, and Reuben Cherniack: "Rehabilitation of Patients with Chronic Obstructive Pulmonary Disease—State of the Art," *Am Rev Resp Dis,* **114**:1145–1165, 1976.

Luckman, Joan, and Karen Cleason Sorensen: *Medical Surgical Nursing: A Psychophysiologic Approach,* Saunders, Philadelphia, 1974.

Macklem, Peter: "The Pathophysiology of Chronic Bronchitis and Emphysema," *Med Clin North Am,* **57**:669–679, May 1973.

Macklem, P. T., et al.: "Conference Report: Workshop on Screening Programs for Early Diagnosis of Airway Obstruction," *Am Rev Resp Dis,* **109**:567–571, 1974.

Massachusetts General Hospital: *Manual of Nursing Procedures,* Little, Brown, Boston, 1975.

Miller, Wm.: "Rehabilitation of Patients with Chronic Obstructive Lung Disease," *MCNA,* **51**:349–361, March 1967.

Morgan, Wm., and Anthony Seaton: *Occupational Lung Diseases,* Saunders, Philadelphia, 1975.

Mullins, E., and J. Irvine: "Patient and Family Education in Respiratory Care," **19**:273–279, April 1974.

Murphy, Raymond, L. H., Jr., Stephen K. Holford, and William C. Knowler: "Visual Lung Sound Characterization by Time Expanded Wave Form Analysis," *N Engl J Med,* **296**:968–871, April 28, 1977.

Neff, T., and T. Petty: "Mortality in Relationship to Cor Pulmonale Hypoxia and Hypercapnia," *Ann Intern Med,* **72**:621–626, May 1970.

Nett, Louise: "Why Emphysema Patients Are the Way They Are," *Am J Nurs,* **70**:1251–1253, June 1970.

Petty, Thomas: *Intensive and Rehabilitative Respiratory Care,* 2d ed., Lea & Febiger, Philadelphia, 1974.

——: "Pulmonary Rehabilitation," *Basics RD,* **4**:1, 1–6, September 1975.

—— and L. Nett, "Patient Education and Emphysema Care," *Med Times,* **97**:117–130, February 1969.

—— et al.: "A Comprehensive Care Program for Chronic Airway Obstruction," *Ann Chest Med,* **70**:1109–1119, June 1969.

Rau, Joseph, and Mary Rau: "To Breathe or Be Breathed: Understanding IPPB," *Am J Nurs,* **77**:613–

Sagal, P.: *Cardiopulmonary Resuscitation: A Manual for Physicians and Paramedical Instructors,* World Federation of Societies of Anesthesiologists, Norway, 1968.

Schwaid, Madeline: "The Impact of Emphysema," *Am J Nurs,* **70**:1247–1250, June 1970.

Sedlock, Stephanie: "Detection of Chronic Pulmonary Disease," *Am J Nurs,* **72**:1407–1411, August 1972.

Sharp, John T.: "Diaphragmatic Function and Respiratory Failure," *Chest,* **71**:566.

Shaw, James O., and Kenneth M. Moser: "The Current Status of Prostaglandins and the Lungs," **68**:75–80, July 1975.

Simon, Nathan M.: "Psychiatric Consultation with M.I.C.U. Nurses," *Heart Lung,* **6**:497–504, May–June 1977.

Sitzman, Judith: "Nursing Management of the Acutely Ill Respiratory Patient," *Heart Lung,* **1**:207–215, March–April 1972.

Stevens, Paul M.: "Assessment of Acute Respiratory Failure: Cardiac Versus Pulmonary Causes," *Chest,* **67**:1–2, January 1975.

Stringel, Llewellyn W.: "Emergency Treatment of Acute Respiratory Disease," Virginia Thoracic Society, 1971.

Sweetwood, Hannelone: "Bedside Assessment of Respirations," *Nursing 73,* **3**:50–51, September 1973.

——: *Nursing in the Intensive Respiratory Care Unit,* Springer, New York, 1971.

The Health Consequences of Smoking, A Report of the Surgeon General: 1971 U.S. Dept of Health, Education, and Welfare, No. (HSM) 71 7513.

Thurlbeck, Wm: *Chronic Airflow Obstruction in Lung Disease,* Saunders, Philadelphia, 1976.

Tiplitz, Carl: "The Core Pathobiology and Integrated Medical Science of Adult Acute Respiratory Insufficiency," *Surg Clin North Am,* **56**:1091–1129, October 1976.

Travelbee, Joyce: *Interpersonal Aspects of Nursing,* 2d ed., Davis, Philadelphia, 1975.

Traver, Gayle: "Assessment of Thorax and Lungs," *Am J Nurs,* **73**:466–471, March 1973.

——: "Clinical Testing of Lung Function," *Nurs Clin North Am,* **9**:101–110, March 1974.

Trunkey, Donald: "Review of Current Concepts in Fluid and Electrolyte Management," *Heart Lung,* **4**:115–121, January–February 1973.

Wade, Jacqueline: *Respiratory Nursing Care–Physiology and Technique,* Mosby, St. Louis, 1973.

Weed, Lawrence L.: *Medical Records, Medical Education and Patient Care,* Year Book, Chicago, 1970.

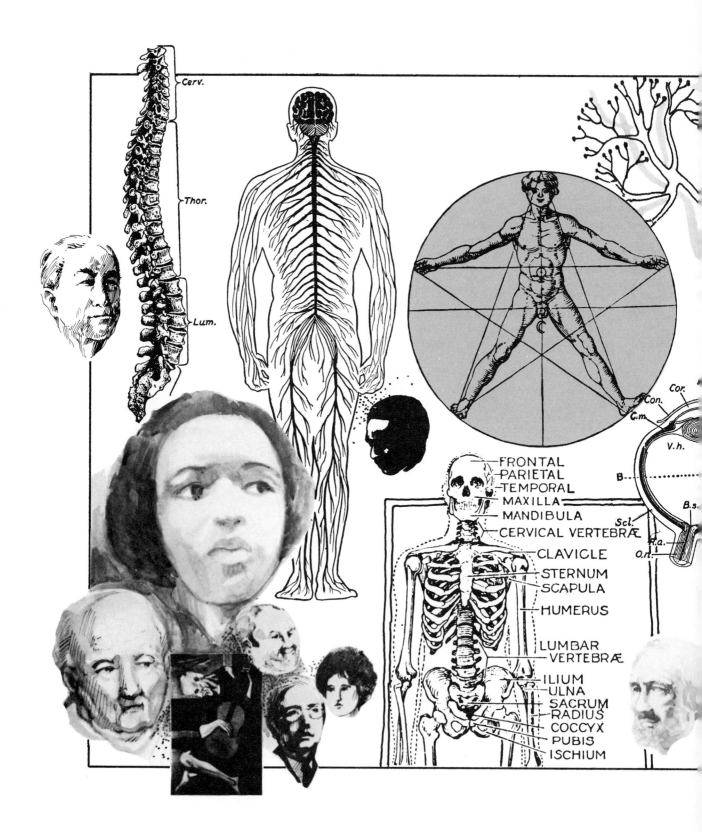

Cerv.

Thor.

Lum.

Cor.
Con.
C.m.
V.h.
B.
B.s.
Scl.
R.a.
o.n.

FRONTAL
PARIETAL
TEMPORAL
MAXILLA
MANDIBULA
CERVICAL VERTEBRÆ
CLAVICLE
STERNUM
SCAPULA
HUMERUS
LUMBAR
VERTEBRÆ
ILIUM
ULNA
SACRUM
RADIUS
COCCYX
PUBIS
ISCHIUM

# PART 7

PERCEPTION AND
COORDINATION

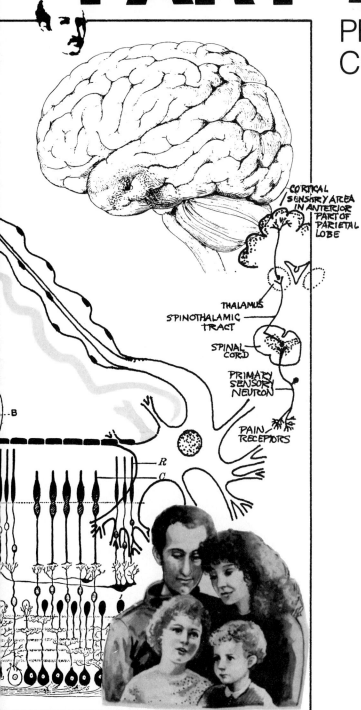

CORTICAL
SENSORY AREA
IN ANTERIOR
PART OF
PARIETAL
LOBE

THALAMUS

SPINOTHALAMIC
TRACT

SPINAL
CORD

PRIMARY
SENSORY
NEURON

PAIN
RECEPTORS

# 31

# THE CONCEPTS OF PERCEPTION AND COORDINATION*

Claire Ford Dunbar
Patricia E. Mahoney

The external and internal environments provide constant stimuli to the human organism. Perception, interpretation, and action upon this input are coordinated by the nervous system, in conjunction with the endocrine system.

## PERCEPTION AND COORDINATION

*Perception* is defined as "recognition in response to sensory stimuli."[1] It is a mental act involving memory and the interpretation of new sensory data in terms of previously encountered information. Disturbances in perception may occur at several levels. There may be a disruption in the reception of sensory data, an interruption in the transmission of the data, or a disturbance in the interpretation of data that is properly received and transmitted.

*Coordination* may be defined as "the combination of nervous impulses in motor centers to ensure cooperation of the appropriate muscles in a reaction."[2] It implies perception of the movement or reaction that is necessary and the subsequent completion of that action via the appropriate bodily activity. Disturbances in coordination may also occur at several levels. Basically, these are at the points of reception, transmission, or interpretation of the incoming stimuli.

Regulation of the activity of striated (*voluntary*) muscles is controlled by the *somatic nervous system.* (The term *somatic* refers to the body wall and limbs.) Data for this system are received by sensory receptors, transmitted by peripheral nerves, and processed in the central nervous system. The heart, nonstriated (*involuntary*) muscles, and glandular cells are controlled by the *autonomic* (visceral) *nervous system.* (The term *visceral* refers to vital organ systems.) The autonomic nervous system is present in both the peripheral and central nervous systems. In this chapter, these systems will be discussed as they pertain to the perception of sensory data and the coordination of actions based upon the reception of those data. The sensory receptors and cranial and spinal nerves (peripheral nervous system) will receive special emphasis because of their unique roles in obtaining sensory information. Following this discussion, functioning of the central and autonomic nervous systems, and the skeletal and muscular systems, as well as physical assessment of perception and coordination, will be presented.

* The section on perception and coordination was written by Claire Ford Dunbar, and the section on physical assessment of perception and coordination was written by Patricia E. Mahoney.

## Sensory Receptors

In the body, *peripheral nerves* relay impulses from the external and internal environments to the central nervous system (brain and spinal cord) via a variety of *peripheral sensory receptors.* The receptors may be classified in several ways. Table 31-1 illustrates the classification of sensory receptors according to their probable functional roles. Most of the body's sensory or afferent receptors may be grouped into five main types:[3]

Mechanoreceptors: Receptors that respond to mechanical stimulation (e.g., pressure) of themselves or adjacent cells; examples are nerve endings in the skin, sound receptors in the cochlea, and baroreceptors in the carotid sinuses and aorta.

**TABLE 31-1**
CLASSIFICATION OF SENSORY RECEPTORS
(PROBABLE FUNCTIONAL ROLES)

I. Receptors of general sensibility
  A. Endings in epidermis
    1. Free nerve endings (tactile, pain, thermal sense)
    2. Terminal disks of Merkel (tactile)
    3. Nerve (peritrichial) ending in hair follicle (tactile)
  B. Endings in connective tissue (skin and connective tissue throughout body)
    1. Free nerve endings (pain, thermal sense)
    2. Encapsulated nerve endings
      *a.* End bulbs of Ruffini [thermal sense, warmth (?), touch-pressure]
      *b.* End bulbs of Krause [thermal sense, cold (?), touch-pressure]
      *c.* Genital corpuscles (thermal sense, touch-pressure)
      *d.* Corpuscles of Meissner (tactile)
      *e.* Corpuscles of Pacini (vibratory sense, touch-pressure)
      *f.* Corpuscles of Golgi-Mazzoni (touch-pressure)
  C. Endings in muscles, tendons, and joints
    1. Neuromuscular spindles (stretch receptors)
    2. Golgi tendon organs, neurotendinous endings (tension receptors)
    3. End bulbs of Ruffini in joint capsule (touch-pressure, position sense)
    4. Corpuscles of Pacini (touch-pressure, vibratory sense)
    5. Free nerve endings (pain, thermal sense)

II. Receptors of special senses
  A. Bipolar neurons of olfactory mucosa (olfaction)
  B. Taste buds (gustatory sense)
  C. Rods and cones in retina (vision)
  D. Hair cells in spiral organ of Corti (audition)
  E. Hair cells in semicircular canals, saccule, and utricle (equilibrium, vestibular sense)

III. Special receptors in viscera
  A. Pressoreceptors in carotid sinus and aortic arch (monitors arterial pressure)
  B. Chemoreceptors in carotid and aortic bodies and in or on surface of medulla (monitors arterial oxygen and carbon dioxide levels)
  C. Chemoreceptors probably located in supraoptic nucleus of hypothalamus (monitors osmolarity of blood)
  D. Free nerve endings in viscera (pain, fullness)
  E. Receptors in lungs (respiratory and cough reflexes)

SOURCE: From C. R. Noback and R. J. Demarest, *The Human Nervous System,* 2d ed., McGraw-Hill, New York, 1975.

Thermoreceptors: Receptors that detect changes in temperature; they are specific for heat or cold.

Nociceptors: Receptors that respond to stimuli such as burning, cutting, crushing, or pressure sufficiently intense to cause tissue damage, whether physical or chemical; examples are free nerve endings for pain detection.

Electromagnetic receptors: These receptors function in light detection and are restricted to the eye (rods, cones).

Chemoreceptors: Receptors that are designed to respond to chemical stimuli such as odors, oxygen and carbon dioxide concentrations, and the osmolality of body fluids.

The *pattern theory of sensation* is currently used to explain the overall role of sensory receptors. This theory contends that groups of specific nerve endings (e.g., free nerve endings or Ruffini's corpuscles) constitute a complex or "spot"; a cold spot, warm spot, pain spot, touch spot, etc., is thus formed. When a specific stimulus activates such a spot, a stream of nerve impulses results, and they are dispersed and transmitted by the innervating fibers to the brain centers. For example, differences in stimulation of a "pain" spot may be interpreted as sensations of pain, itch, or tingle.

The *eye* and *ear* are body structures that house the sensory receptors for sight and hearing. Disturbances in the function of either of these structures may be reflective of a pathologic process in the structure or in the adjacent brain and skull.

**Eye** The sensory receptors (*rods* and *cones*) in the retina of the eye compose approximately 70 percent of the body's receptors.[4] This figure is reflective of the dominant role sight plays in connecting the environment with the organism. Both optical and sensory functions are performed by the eye.

Three coats or *tunics* form the structures of the eye (Fig. 31-1); the *sclera* (a white, fibrous protective covering) and *cornea* (a transparent surface continuous with the conjunctiva) compose the *outer tunic or fibrous coat;* the *choroid* (a vascular, brown membrane that lines the sclera, absorbs light, and prevents reflection within the eyeball), *ciliary body* (controls the convexity of the lens), and *iris* (colored part) compose the second coat or *vascular tunic* (*uveal tract* or *uvea*). The *inner tunic* consists of the *retina.* A biconvex *lens* is situated behind the iris and pupil. It is attached to the ciliary body by *zonular fibers.*

The *anterior chamber* of the eye is located behind the cornea and in front of the lens and iris; the *posterior chamber* is located behind the iris but in front of the lens and ciliary body. A clear, watery substance produced by the ciliary processes and called *aqueous humor* fills both chambers. Between the posterior portion of the lens and the posterior wall of the eyeball is the *vitreous chamber* or body. It is filled with a clear, gelatinous material. Aqueous humor and the vitreous body keep the eyeball firm and distended at an average intraocular pressure of 19 mmHg.[5] The fluid drains into the scleral veins via an opening between the cornea and iris (canal of Schlemm).

The *retina* is the light-sensitive portion of the eye that is located around the posterior wall of the eyeball. Contained in the retina are the rods and the cones which are the sensory receptors for light waves. The *rods* are responsible for vision in the dark and contain a pigment called *rhodopsin* which bleaches in the presence of light. The *cones* function in color vision and contain pigments sensitive to blue, green, and red light waves. Present in the retina are three specialized areas, the *macula,* the *fovea centralis,* and the *blind spot.* The macula appears yellow because of pigment in the neurons of this area. In its center is the funnel-shaped fovea, the area of most acute vision (Fig. 31-1). This spot is composed entirely of cones. The blind spot represents the area at which the optic nerve leaves the eye; it is also referred to as the *optic disk.* This area does not register an image and is located in the upper temporal quadrant of the visual fields (see Physical Assessment of Perception and Coordination). The optic nerve fibers from each eye move toward each other and meet at a point called the *optic chiasma.* Fibers from the inner or nasal half of the retina *cross* to the opposite side in the chiasma. Outer or lateral fibers from the retina remain on the *same* side in the chiasma. Both sets of fibers proceed as optic tracts to the thalamus and then to the visual areas in the occipital lobes.

**F**unctions of the Eye   The *optical functions* may be compared with the action of a camera. Light enters through the iris and its opening, the pupil (Fig.

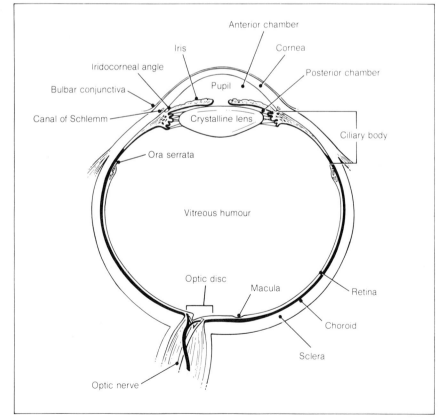

**FIGURE 31-1**
The normal eye. (*Courtesy of the Massachusetts Eye and Ear Infirmary.*)

31-1). Muscles of the iris are capable of constriction and dilation so that the quantity of light entering the eye may be controlled.

Light rays then pass through the lens and vitreous humor and converge to form a two-dimensional image on the retina. In the retina, the *rods* and *cones* assume the *sensory role* of the eye by transmitting input to the optic nerve which conveys it to the brain.

**Ear** The *ear* is a specially designed structure that transmits sounds inward toward its auditory receptors. Anatomically, the ear may be divided into the external ear, the middle ear, and the inner ear.

The *outer* or *external* ear is formed by the auricle and the external auditory meatus. It is funnel-shaped and functions in the collection of sound waves. The inch-long meatus extends inward to the tympanic membrane. Protective hairs and cerumen-producing glands are located near the external opening and serve to keep foreign objects out of the ear. The *tympanic membrane* (eardrum) is formed of thin, fibrous tissue that is sensitive to airborne vibrations (Fig. 31-2). It is cone-shaped and separates the outer and middle parts of the ear.

The *middle ear* is located in the temporal bone and is continuous with the mastoid process. The cavity of the middle ear is bordered by the tympanic membrane and the inner ear (Fig. 31-2). It contains three *ossicles* (*malleus, incus,* and *stapes*) and connects with the nasopharynx via the *auditory (eustachian) tube* (Fig. 31-2). The malleus is attached to the tympanic membrane and the incus, the incus is also connected to the stapes, and the stapes attaches to the inner ear at the *oval window* of the *vestibule* (Fig. 31-2). Equalization of pressure is the function of the eustachian tube. Such a tube is essential because pressure within the middle ear falls as gases within it are absorbed by the circulatory system. Therefore, the act of swallowing permits air to enter or leave the middle ear, equalizing pressure on the outside surface of the tympanic membrane.

The *inner ear* is divided into the vestibule, the cochlea, and the semicircular canals. These structures are located in the temporal bone and compose the *osseous labyrinth.* Within and separated from the osseous labyrinth by a fluid called *perilymph* is a structure called the *membraneous labyrinth* which is filled with a fluid called *endolymph.* The *vestibule* is a chamber located between the semicircular canals and the cochlea and connected to the stapes of the middle ear at the oval window (Fig. 31-2). Beneath the oval window is the *round window.* Within the vestibule are the *utricle* and *saccule* which form the sacs of the membraneous labyrinth.

The *cochlea* is a spiral-shaped structure that is

**FIGURE 31-2**

External ear, middle ear, and inner ear (right ear viewed from the front). (*Reproduced with permission from C. R. Noback and R. J. Demarest, The Human Nervous System, 2d ed., McGraw-Hill, New York, 1975, p. 306.*)

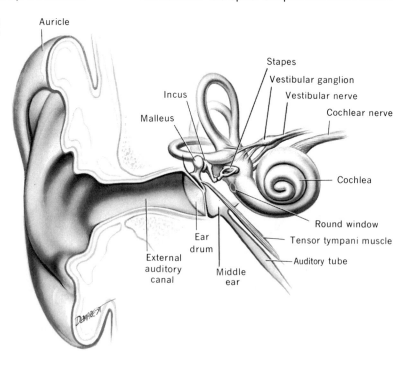

divided into three ducts, the *scala vestibuli,* the *cochlear duct,* and the *scala tympani.* Between the cochlear duct and the scala tympani are located the *basilar membrane* and the *spiral organ of Corti.* At the base of the scala tympani of the cochlea is the membrane of the *round window.*

The *spiral organ of Corti* is significant because it contains the sensory end organs (hair cells) which are the receptors for hearing. These hair cells extend into the endolymph of the cochlear duct. Fibers of the cochlear branch of the VIIIth cranial (vestibulocochlear or acoustic) nerve terminate at the base of each hair cell and connect to the auditory center in the temporal lobe of the cerebrum.

**S**ound Reception and Conduction  Sound waves are collected by the external ear and transmitted to the tympanic membrane. The ossicles receive the sound waves in the form of *vibrations* of the tympanic membrane. They convey them to the inner ear at the oval window. At the oval window, the vibrations are converted into *pressure waves* in the perilymph of the inner ear. The pressure waves travel to the cochlea and are transmitted to the endolymph via the vestibular membrane. The movement of the endolymph stimulates the sensory receptors (hair cells), with the pressure wave ending at the round window. Stimulation of the hair cells results in stimulation of the cochlear nerve endings and conduction of impulses to the cerebrum. There sound is interpreted in terms of the *frequency* (*pitch*) and *amplitude* (*loudness*) of *vibrations.*

**E**quilibrium  The semicircular ducts, the utricle, and the saccule are associated with the *vestibular system* and the maintenance of *equilibrium.* Sensory receptors for the vestibular system are located in the *cristae* (hair cells) of the semicircular ducts, the *macula* of the utricle, and the *macula* of the saccule. These sensory receptors are, in turn, connected to fibers of the vestibular branch of the VIIIth cranial nerve.

The semicircular canals open into the utricle, which is connected to the saccule by a narrow duct. A change of position or rotation of the body causes movement of the endolymph and a deflection of hair cells. This, in turn, sends impulses via the auditory nerve to the cerebellum. There, in conjunction with information received from the eyes and proprioceptive organs in the muscles and tendons, a disturbance in equilibrium is interpreted, and the necessary impulses go out to the body for corrective action.

## Transmission of Sensory Input

The basic cell of nervous tissue is the *neuron* (Fig. 31-3). This microscopic, grayish cell with radiating fibers is found in three forms, according to function. They include the *sensory* or *afferent neurons* which transmit sensory input from the various receptors mentioned earlier; the *motor* or *efferent neurons* which transmit impulses to the muscles; and *association neurons* (*internuncial neurons, interneurons,* or *central neurons*) which connect and convey impulses between sensory and motor neurons.

Each neuron contains receptive fibers known as *dendrites* that receive the impulses and conduct them toward the cell body. There are also fibers called *axons* that conduct the impulse away from the cell body (Fig. 31-3). Axons, which terminate in branches known as *terminal filaments,* are usually surrounded by a *myelin sheath* (discussed below) that is broken at intervals by the *nodes of Ranvier.* These nodes permit the emergence of collateral branches. When the cell bodies of neurons are collected in groups, they appear gray and are referred to as *gray matter.*

Nervous impulses pass from the axon and terminal filaments of one neuron to the dendrites and cell body of the adjacent neuron. This occurs by a process of *synaptic transmission.* Synapses or *synaptic junctions* are the areas of contact between neurons and muscle fibers, or neurons and effector organs. Three types of synapses may be identified, an *interneuronal synapse* (neuron to neuron), a *neuromuscular junction* (neuron to muscle cell), and a *neuroglandular junction* (neuron to glandular cell). Transmission of an impulse at a synapse occurs *chemically* through the release of neurotransmitter substances. Chemical synapses may be *cholinergic* and release the neurotransmitter *acetylcholine* (somatic and parasympathetic nervous systems), or they may be *adrenergic* (sympathetic nervous system) and release *norepinephrine* or *serotonin.*

**Peripheral nervous system**  The cranial and spinal nerves, and their branches, form the *peripheral nervous system.* Peripheral ganglions are groups of cell bodies affiliated with the peripheral nerves.

Peripheral nerves are composed of three basic elements, axons (neurons), neurolemma cells, and connective tissue. The *axons* are the impulse-conducting structures. They are surrounded by

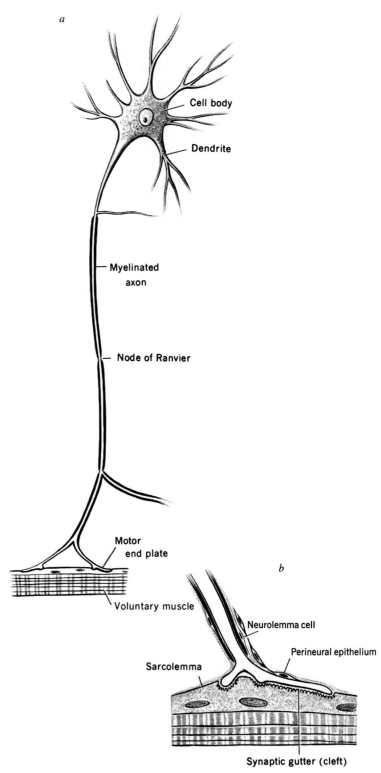

**FIGURE 31-3**
Neuron structure. (a) The neuron, its cell body and processes; (b) a motor end plate. (*Reproduced with permission from C. R. Noback and R. J. Demarest, The Human Nervous System, 2d ed., McGraw-Hill, New York, 1975, p. 47.*)

neurolemma or Schwann cells which may or may not elaborate *myelin.* A fiber that is surrounded with a myelin sheath is described as *myelinated;* one without this sheath is termed *nonmyelinated.* Myelin is a protein and lipid substance that forms a discontinuous layer of insulation around the nerve fiber. *Nodes of Ranvier* are found at discontinuous points along the sheath permitting the branching of nerve fibers and other cellular activities to take place. Impulse conduction on myelinated fibers is more rapid than on nonmyelinated fibers.

The peripheral nerves and ganglions are bound together by several layers of connective tissue and finally by a layer of epithelium. The first layer of connective tissue is the *endoneurium,* which directly surrounds each neurolemma cell. Groups of nerve fibers, known as fascicles, are then surrounded by a layer called the *perineurium.* Groups of fascicles are bound together by the *epineurium.* The entire peripheral nervous system is ensheathed by *perineural epithelium.*

**C**ranial Nerves  There are twelve pairs of *cranial nerves,* which are the peripheral nerves of the brain (Table 31-2 and Fig. 31-4). Assessment of the function of these nerves will be detailed in Physical Assessment of Perception and Coordination below. Each member of the pair of these specialized nerves

**TABLE 31-2**
CRANIAL NERVES

| Number and Name | Type of Nerve | Site of Origin | Site of Termination | Function |
|---|---|---|---|---|
| I. Olfactory | Sensory (afferent) | Sensory receptors in the nasal mucosa | Olfactory bulb in the brain | Smell |
| II. Optic | Sensory (afferent) | Sensory cells in the retina | Occipital lobe of the cerebrum | Vision and associated reflexes |
| III. Oculomotor | Motor (efferent) | Gray matter in the midbrain | Levator palpebrae, superior, medial, and inferior rectus, and inferior oblique muscles | Movement of the eyeball pupillary constriction and accommodation |
| IV. Trochlear | Motor (efferent) | Gray matter in the midbrain | Superior oblique muscles | Movement of the eyeball |
| V. Trigeminal | Sensory (afferent) | Ophthalmic branch: Eye, lacrimal gland, nose, forehead | Sensory: Midpons, below the fourth ventricle | General sensations from the anterior surface of the face, mouth, nose, and tongue |
|  | Sensory (afferent) | Maxillary branch: Teeth and gums of the upper jaw, upper lip, cheek | Motor: Muscles of mastication | Mastication, swallowing; movement of the soft palate, auditory tube, ear ossicles, and tympanic membrane |
|  | Mixed | Mandibular branch: Sensory from teeth and gums of lower jaw, chin, lower lip, tongue. Motor from the midpons | | |
| VI. Abducent | Motor (efferent) | Lower pons beneath fourth ventricle | Lateral rectus muscle | Movement of the eyeball |
| VII. Facial | Motor (efferent) | Lower pons | Muscles of face and forehead; parasympathetic fibers to lacrimal, submandibular, and sublingual glands | Facial expression; lacrimation, salivation, and vasodilatation |
|  | Sensory (afferent) | Anterior two-thirds of tongue, external ear, and facial glands | Geniculate ganglion in temporal bone | Taste; sensation from external ear and glands |
| VIII. Vestibulocochlear | Sensory (afferent) | Cochlear branch: Sensory receptors in cochlea | Temporal lobe of the cerebrum | Hearing |
|  |  | Vestibular branch: Sensory receptors in the semicircular canals and vestibule | Cerebellum | Equilibrium |

**TABLE 31-2**
CRANIAL NERVES (*continued*)

| Number and Name | Type of Nerve | Site of Origin | Site of Termination | Function |
|---|---|---|---|---|
| IX. Glossopharyngeal | Motor (efferent) | Medulla | Muscles of the pharynx, parotid gland via parasympathetic fibers | Swallowing movements, vasodilatation, and salivation |
| | Sensory (afferent) | Tonsils, mucous membrane of the pharynx, external ear and posterior one-third of the tongue, pressoreceptors and chemoreceptors in the carotid body | Medulla | Taste, general sensation to the posterior tongue, tonsils, and upper pharynx; Cardiovascular and respiratory effects from receptors in the carotid sinus and carotid body |
| X. Vagus | Sensory (afferent) | Mucous membrane lining respiratory and digestive tracts | Medulla | Taste and general sensation from larynx, neck, thorax, and abdomen |
| | Motor (efferent) | Medulla | Muscles of pharynx and larynx | Swallowing, movement of pharynx and larynx |
| | | | Parasympathetic fibers to thoracic and abdominal viscera | Inhibitory fibers to the heart; secretion of gastric glands and pancreas; vasodilator fibers to abdominal viscera |
| XI. Accessory | Motor | Cranial portion: Medulla | Pharyngeal and laryngeal muscles | Movement of the soft palate, pharynx, and larynx |
| | | Spinal portion: Upper cervical region of the spinal cord | Sternocleidomastoid and trapezius muscles | Shoulder and head movement |
| XII. Hypoglossal | Motor | Medulla | Muscles of the tongue | Speaking and swallowing, tongue movement |

**FIGURE 31-4**
Basal surface of the brain and roots of the cranial nerves. (*Reproduced with permission from C. R. Noback and R. J. Demarest, The Human Nervous System, 2d ed., McGraw-Hill, New York, 1975, p. 218.*)

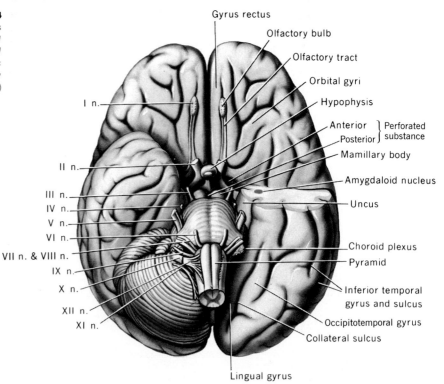

Gyrus rectus
Olfactory bulb
Olfactory tract
Orbital gyri
Hypophysis
Anterior } Perforated
Posterior } substance
Mamillary body
Amygdaloid nucleus
Uncus
Choroid plexus
Pyramid
Inferior temporal gyrus and sulcus
Occipitotemporal gyrus
Collateral sulcus
Lingual gyrus

I n.
II n.
III n.
IV n.
V n.
VI n.
VII n. & VIII n.
IX n.
X n.
XII n.
XI n.

innervates its portion of the right or left half of the body. The origins and basic nature of these nerves are described in Table 32-2.

**S**pinal Nerves   Thirty-one pairs of spinal nerves emerge from the spinal cord through the intervertebral foramena and are distributed throughout segments of the body. There are eight pairs of cervical nerves, twelve pairs of thoracic nerves, five pairs of lumbar nerves, five pairs of sacral nerves, and one pair of coccygeal nerves. These "cord levels" differ from "vertebral levels" because the first pair of cervical nerves arises from the medulla and emerges between the occipital bone and the first cervical vertebra (Fig. 31-5). The first seven cervical nerves are named for the vertebra *below* where the nerve exits (e.g., the fourth cervical nerve leaves via the intervertebral foramen between the third and fourth cervical vertebrae). Beginning with the first thoracic nerve, the name is derived from the vertebra *above* the nerve's exit. This is because the eighth cervical nerve exits between vertebrae C7 and T1. Therefore, the first thoracic nerve exits between the first and second thoracic vertebrae. These differences are important when localizing spinal lesions according to their cord level rather than their vertebral level (see Chap. 32). Also, because the spinal cord is shorter than the vertebral column, the spinal nerves often emerge from the cord at levels above their actual exit from the vertebral column (e.g., all sacral and coccygeal nerves emerge from the cord at vertebrae T12 to L1, as illustrated in Fig. 31-5).

Spinal nerves have a dorsal and ventral root (Fig. 31-6). Sensory (afferent) fibers compose the *dorsal* root which transmits impulses from the various sensory receptors *to* the spinal cord. Dorsal root ganglions (cell bodies) are located within the intervertebral foramen. The skin segments innervated by the dorsal roots are called *dermatomes* (Fig. 31-7).

Motor (efferent) fibers form the *ventral root* which transmits impulses *from* the spinal cord to the muscles and glands of the body. The ventral root cell bodies are found within the gray matter of the spinal cord.

There are several major interwoven networks of the spinal nerves called *plexuses.* It is from these plexuses that the peripheral nerves emerge. The first through fourth spinal nerves form the *cervical plexus* and innervate the back of the head and the neck; the fifth cervical through the first or second thoracic nerves form the *brachial plexus* and innervate the upper extremities; thoracic nerves 3

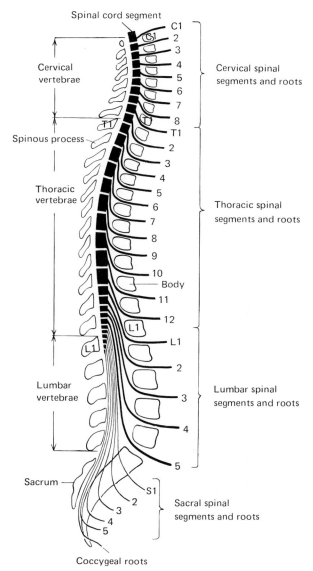

**FIGURE 31-5**
The topographic relations of the spinal cord segments, spinous processes, and bodies of the vertebrae, intervertebral foramina, and spinal nerves. Each spinal cord segment (except upper cervical segments) is located at a higher vertebral level than the spinal nerve emerging through its intervertebral foramen. (*Reproduced with permission from C. R. Noback and R. J. Demarest, The Human Nervous System, 2d ed., McGraw-Hill, New York, 1975, p. 136.*)

through 11 do not form plexuses but innervate directly; the twelfth thoracic *through* the fourth lumbar nerves form the *lumbar plexus* which innervates the lower trunk; the *sacral plexus* is from L4 through S4; and the *coccygeal plexus* composes S4 through the coccygeal nerve. Spinal nerves L4 and S4 contribute branches to both the lumbar and sacral plexuses. The sacral and coccygeal nerves supply the perineum.

Sensory and motor portions of spinal nerves merge as they pass between the vertebrae. This means that all spinal nerves are *mixed* nerves, i.e., contain both sensory and motor fibers.

*Reflex arc*   Simple reflexes such as the knee jerk do not involve brain centers but represent simple nervous circuits in the spinal cord. A sensory receptor, a sensory neuron, an association neuron within the cord, and a motor neuron are the essential elements in reflex arc formation (Fig. 31-6).

The sensory receptor detects the stimuli which are carried to the spinal cord by the sensory neuron. There, association neurons connect the sensory neuron to motor neurons on the same, or opposite, sides of the cord. Impulses are carried to the muscles by the motor neurons.

The *knee jerk* is a common example of the reflex arc circuit. A tap on the patellar tendon causes stretching of the quadriceps femoris muscle. This stretching is a stimulus to the sensory receptors, which transmit it to the sensory neurons. These neurons carry the impulse to the spinal cord, where it is picked up by the association neurons, transmitted to the motor neurons, and carried to the muscle where contraction occurs, causing the leg to jerk forward.

### Central Nervous System

From the peripheral nervous system, information is transmitted to and processed in the spinal cord and brain, which compose the *central nervous system.* The *spinal cord* functions primarily in the reception of impulses from the peripheral nervous system and in their transmission to the brain. It, then, transmits processed impulses from the brain to the muscles via the peripheral nervous system, where a bodily response takes place.

**Spinal cord**   Much of the anatomy of the spinal cord was discussed in connection with the spinal nerves. It is important to note that the cord is surrounded and protected by the *vertebral column* (seven cervical, twelve thoracic, five lumbar, five fused sacral, and the coccygeal vertebrae).

The cylindrically shaped spinal cord extends from the medulla to the level between the first and second lumbar vertebrae (*conus medullaris*). It is surrounded by three meninges, the closely attached *pia mater,* the *arachnoid,* and the *dura mater.* (Meninges are detailed in relation to the brain.) The pia mater continues as the *filum terminale* to the posterior side of the coccyx where it is anchored. The piarachnoid (pia mater and arachnoid) and dura mater fuse with the filum terminale at the level of the second sacral vertebra. The roots of the sacral and coccygeal nerves from the *cauda equina* which extends in a taillike manner below the second lumbar vertebra.

A cross section of the spinal cord (Fig. 31-8) shows that it is arranged as a butterfly-shaped area of gray matter, surrounded by white matter. The *gray matter* is composed of cell bodies and some unmyelinated or lightly myelinated nerve fibers. It is

**FIGURE 31-6**
Cross section of the spinal cord, revealing the essential structures of the reflex arc and a spinal nerve. (*Reproduced with permission from Russell M. DeCoursey, The Human Organism, 4th ed., McGraw-Hill, New York, 1974, p. 202.*)

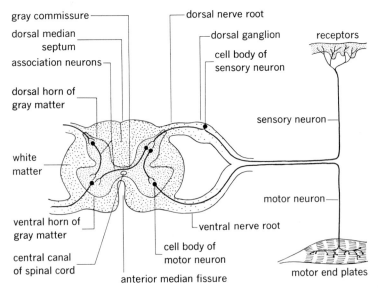

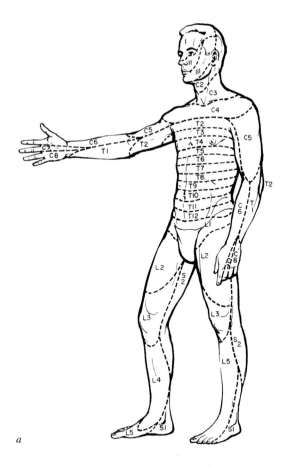

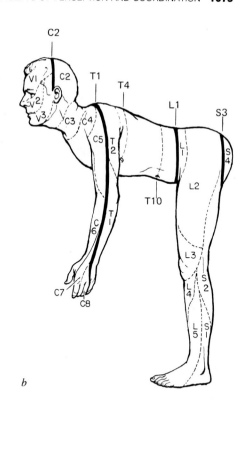

**FIGURE 31-7**

(a) Segmental innervation of the skin (dermatome). Each dorsal (sensory) spinal root innervates one dermatome. The first cervical nerve usually has no cutaneous distribution. The trigeminal nerve supplies most of the general somatic sensory innervation to the anterior aspect of the head (ophthalmic division I, maxillary division II, and mandibular division III). (b) Dermatomes of the skin. The trigeminal nerve is represented by the ophthalmic division, V1; the maxillary division, V2; and the mandibular division, V3. (*Reproduced with permission from C. R. Noback and R. J. Demarest, The Human Nervous System, 2d ed., McGraw-Hill, New York, 1975, pp. 139–140.*)

divided into the posterior horn, the intermediate zone and lateral horn, and the anterior horn. The *white matter* is formed by lightly myelinated and unmyelinated nerve fibers; it does not contain cell bodies. White matter in each half of the spinal cord is divided into three columns, *posterior, lateral,* and *anterior funiculi.* The columns are further divided into *tracts (fasciculi)* which are the sensory and motor pathways of the cord.

Impulses are conducted up the spinal cord via pathways called *ascending tracts.* The major ascending tracts are the *fasciculus gracilis, fasciculus cuneatus, spinocerebellar,* and *spinothalamic* (Table 31-3).

The *descending tracts* conduct impulses from the brain down the spinal cord. The principal descending tracts (Table 31-3) are the *pyramidal* (lateral and ventral corticospinal) and the *extrapyramidal* (rubrospinal and vestibulospinal). These descending motor pathways (from the brain to the spinal cord, as well as from the cerebrum to the brainstem) are formed from neurons referred to as *upper motor neurons.* The upper motor neurons are contained entirely within the central nervous system (brain and spinal cord), in contrast with *lower motor neurons* which begin in the central nervous system but terminate in the muscles.

A significant characteristic of the tracts is the *decussation* or *crossing* of many of the nerve fibers. Many crossed fibers are present in the ascending spinothalamic and anterior spinocerebellar tracts which cross to the opposite side of the cord near

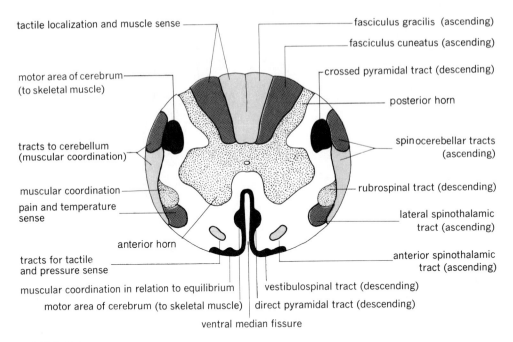

tactile localization and muscle sense

motor area of cerebrum
(to skeletal muscle)

tracts to cerebellum
(muscular coordination)

muscular coordination

pain and temperature
sense

anterior horn

tracts for tactile
and pressure sense

muscular coordination in relation to equilibrium

motor area of cerebrum (to skeletal muscle)

ventral median fissure

fasciculus gracilis (ascending)

fasciculus cuneatus (ascending)

crossed pyramidal tract (descending)

posterior horn

spinocerebellar tracts
(ascending)

rubrospinal tract (descending)

lateral spinothalamic
tract (ascending)

anterior spinothalamic
tract (ascending)

vestibulospinal tract (descending)

direct pyramidal tract (descending)

**FIGURE 31-8**
Diagrammatic cross section of the spinal cord, indicating the general location of some of the principal
nerve tracts. (*Reproduced with permission from R. M. DeCoursey, The Human Organism, 4th ed.,
McGraw-Hill, New York, 1974, p. 235.*)

their point of entrance. The lateral corticospinal
tract crosses over in the lower medulla; the anterior
corticospinal tract decussates in the upper spinal
cord levels; and the rubrospinal tract crosses over
in the midbrain. Fibers of the anterior corticospinal
and vestibulospinal tracts are primarily uncrossed.

Sites of origin and termination, as well as function of the major pathways, are summarized in
Table 31-3. This information is important in understanding the role of the other major component of
the central nervous system, the brain.

**Brain** The human adult brain is a semisolid, pinkish gray organ that weighs approximately three
pounds and functions to control movement, sensation, and thought. It is surrounded by three membranes (meninges): a closely adhering vascular *pia
mater,* a fragile intermediate membrane, the *arachnoid,* and a durable, fibrous outer covering, the
*dura mater.* The dura forms four folds: the *falx
cerebri* which is between the two cerebral lobes;
the *falx cerebelli* located between the cerebellar
hemispheres; the *tentorium cerebelli* which is attached to the falx cerebri, covers the cerebellum,
and is beneath the occipital lobes of the cerebrum;
and the *diaphragm sella* which covers the sella
turcica and part of the pituitary gland.

The brain is usually divided into three areas,
the *forebrain,* the *midbrain* (mesencephalon), and
the *hindbrain.* The forebrain and hindbrain may be
divided even further. The forebrain is composed of
the telencephalon (*cerebral cortex, olfactory bulbs*)
and diencephalon (*pineal body, thalamus, hypothalamus*), while the hindbrain is formed by the
metencephalon (*pons* and *cerebellum*) and myelen-
cephalon (medulla and pyramidal tracts).

The *cerebrum* is formed by the telencephalon,
the diencephalon, and the upper midbrain. The
*brainstem* includes the midbrain and hindbrain except for the cerebellum. The *tentorium cerebelli*
divides the brain in still another way. Those structures above it are referred to as *supratentorial,*
while those beneath it are termed *infratentorial.*

Within the brain is a system of cavities called
*ventricles* (Fig. 31-9) that are filled with cerebrospinal fluid. The brain floats in this fluid, which also
fills the subarachnoid spaces, and is thus protected
from external blows to the head. Four communicating cavities compose the ventricular system which
is continuous with the central canal of the spinal
cord. The largest of these are the two *lateral ventricles* of the cerebral hemispheres. Both lateral
ventricles communicate with the *third ventricle* in
the diencephalon via the *foramen of Monro.* The

third ventricle is in contact with the *fourth ventricle* in the hindbrain via the *aqueduct of Sylvius.* The system is completed as the fourth ventricle is continuous with the central canal of the spinal cord and has openings into the subarachnoid spaces. Each ventricle contains specialized tissue called the *choroid plexuses* which form the cerebrospinal fluid. After circulation around the brain and spinal cord, the fluid is returned to the blood through the arachnoid villi.

**C**erebrum    The cerebrum has four lobes named for the bones overlying them; they are the *frontal, parietal, occipital,* and *temporal* lobes. Each lobe controls specific bodily activities (Fig. 31-9).

The *frontal lobe* is subdivided into the *precentral gyrus (motor cortex), the area in front of the precentral gyrus (premotor area),* and the *prefrontal lobe.* Motor activities are associated with the motor cortex and premotor area. The premotor area also contains *Broca's speech area* which is important in vocalization. Subtle expressions such as anxiety and concern with social attitudes are controlled in the prefrontal lobe.

Receptive areas for the general senses, including touch and pressure, are located in the *parietal lobe.* Vision is controlled by the *occipital lobe,* audition by the *temporal lobe.* Association areas to recognize and comprehend size, shape, weight, texture, and form are also located within the four lobes.

The diencephalon's major structures are the thalamus and hypothalamus. The *thalamus* relays sensory impulses to the cerebral cortex, while the *hypothalamus* is involved in autonomic nervous system activities (body temperature, emotions, endocrine gland function).

**B**rainstem    Structures of the brainstem include the midbrain, the pons, and the medulla. The diencephalon has been discussed as part of the cere-

**TABLE 31-3**
MAJOR TRACTS (PATHWAYS) OF THE SPINAL CORD

| Tract | Spinal Cord Location | Site of Origin | Site of Termination | Function |
|---|---|---|---|---|
| ASCENDING TRACTS Fasciculus gracilis (T7 and below) Fasciculus cuneatus (T6 and above) | Posterior white columns | Spinal ganglions on the same side of the cord | Medulla | Touch, two-point discrimination, position sense, motion, weight perception |
| Spinocerebellar posterior | Lateral white columns | Neuromuscular receptors on the same side of the cord | Cerebellum | Unconscious proprioception (muscle sense) |
| Spinocerebellar anterior | Lateral white columns | Neuromuscular receptors on the same *and* opposite sides of the cord | Cerebellum | Coordination of posture and limb movement |
| Spinothalamic lateral | Lateral white columns | Cell bodies in the posterior horn on the opposite side of the cord | Thalamus | Pain and temperature sensation on the opposite sides of the body |
| Spinothalamic anterior | Anterior white columns | Cell bodies in the posterior horn on the opposite side of the cord | Thalamus | Touch and pressure on the opposite sides of the body |
| DESCENDING TRACTS Pyramidal    Lateral    corticospinal | Lateral white columns | Voluntary motor areas of the cerebral cortex (fibers cross in the medulla) | Anterior gray or anterolateral columns in the spinal cord | Voluntary movement especially of the arms and legs |
| Anterior corticospinal | Anterior or ventral columns | Voluntary motor areas of the cerebral cortex (uncrossed fibers) | Anterior gray or anterolateral columns in the spinal cord | Voluntary movement of the trunk muscles |
| Extrapyramidal    Rubrospinal | Lateral white columns | Red nucleus of the midbrain (fibers cross immediately) | Anterior gray or anterolateral columns in the spinal cord | Muscle tone and coordination; posture |
| Vestibulospinal | Anterior or ventral columns | Vestibular nuclei in the medulla | Anterior gray or anterolateral columns in the spinal cord | Equilibrium and posture |

SOURCE: From R. M. DeCoursey, *The Human Organism,* 4th ed., McGraw-Hill, New York, 1974, pp. 235–237 and C. R. Noback and R. J. Demarest, *The Human Nervous System,* 2d ed., McGraw-Hill, New York, 1975, pp. 149–181.

brum, although it is sometimes classified with the brainstem. The *midbrain* functions largely to relay impulses to the cerebrum from the cerebellum, medulla, and spinal cord. It also contains origins for the IIId and IVth cranial nerves. Fine muscle movement may also be connected with the red nuclei in the midbrain.

The *pons* is a bridge of nerve tracts in the anterior part of the brainstem. It connects the midbrain with the medulla and the rest of the nervous system. At the base of the brainstem is the *medulla oblongata.* It is continuous with the spinal cord and is the site of decussation of the pyramidal tracts. Reflex centers that slow the heart (cardiac inhibitory center), control the respiratory muscles (respiratory center), and constrict the peripheral blood vessels (vasoconstrictor center) are also located here.

*Reticular formation*   Within the white matter of the brainstem is a diffuse mixture of gray matter called the *reticular formation.* It receives fibers from many areas including the cerebral cortex, the hypothalamus, and the ascending sensory tracts. It relays impulses to some cranial nerves and the descending tracts. The role of the reticular formation in sleep and consciousness is perhaps its best known, and least understood, function. It is known that if sensory impulses get through this formation to the cortex, awakening occurs, whereas damage to the reticular area, that prevents the relay of such impulses, produces a loss of consciousness.

**C**erebellum   Below the occipital lobes of the cerebrum are located the two cerebellar hemispheres. They are responsible for the coordination of muscular movements, equilibrium, and muscle tone. Hearing, sight, and tactile sensations are also coordinated in the cerebellum. Each cerebellar hemisphere controls movement coordination for the same side of the body.

### Autonomic Nervous System

The *autonomic nervous system* is concerned with the regulation and coordination of vital visceral activities. It innervates three types of effector cells, involuntary (smooth) muscle cells, cardiac muscle cells, and glandular (secretory) cells. There are two

**FIGURE 31-9**

(a) Ventricles of the brain, lateral view; (b) localized functional areas of the cerebral cortex, medial view; (c) left cerebral hemisphere, lateral view of functional areas. (*Adapted with permission from R. M. DeCoursey, The Human Organism, 4th ed., McGraw-Hill, New York, 1974, p. 218.*)

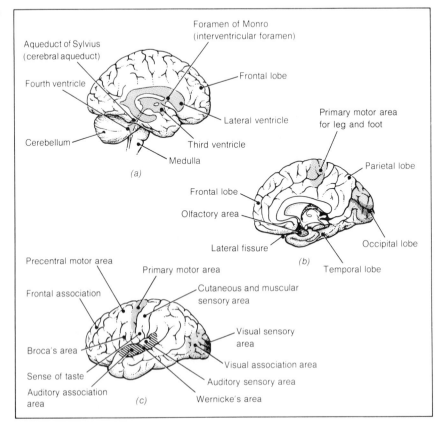

major divisions of the autonomic nervous system, the *sympathetic* (*thoracolumbar*) and the *parasympathetic* (*craniosacral*).

**Sympathetic nervous system** The *sympathetic division* comprises a chain of ganglions and nerves on each side of the spinal cord (Fig. 31-10). This chain extends from the cervical region through the lumbar region. Each ganglion connects, via a communicating branch, to a spinal nerve. *Preganglionic* fibers connect the spinal nerve to the sympathetic ganglion. *Postganglionic* fibers connect the sympathetic ganglion to involuntary muscle tissue or glandular cells. The neurotransmitter *norepinephrine* is released at each junction between a postganglionic (adrenergic) fiber and an effector cell (smooth muscle or gland). Preganglionic fibers are cholinergic.

The sympathetic division is especially active during situations of stress; it is involved in the responses "fight, fright, and flight." This division acts as a total unit producing a widespread, long-lasting response. Major functions of the sympathetic system are summarized in Table 31-4.

**Parasympathetic nervous system** The preganglionic fibers of the *parasympathetic* division exit the brain via the cranial nerves (III, VII, IX, and X) from the brainstem and leave the spinal cord via the second, third, and fourth sacral spinal nerves (Fig. 31-10). Thus, this system is referred to as the *craniosacral division*. Postganglionic fibers are close to the organ they are innervating. The neurotransmitter *acetylcholine* is released at the junction of the postganglionic (cholinergic) fibers and the effector cells. The effects of parasympathetic stimulation are usually brief as acetylcholine is rapidly deactivated by *cholinesterase* at the synapse. Functions of the parasympathetic division are compared with the sympathetic functions in Table 31-4.

**Musculoskeletal System**

Action taken as a result of nervous system stimulation is largely the function of the musculoskeletal system. This system enables the human organism to move and glands and organs to function. It carries out the directions of the nervous and endocrine systems.

**TABLE 31-4**
FUNCTIONS OF THE AUTONOMIC NERVOUS SYSTEM

| Structure | Sympathetic | Parasympathetic |
|---|---|---|
| Eye: Pupil | Dilatation | Contraction |
| Ciliary muscle | Relaxation and distance vision accommodation | Contraction and close-up vision accommodation |
| Glands: nasal, lacrimal, gastric, pancreatic, parotid, submaxillary | Vasoconstriction altering secretion | Increases thin, copious secretions |
| Sweat glands | Profuse sweating | No effect |
| Heart: Muscle | Increased rate and strength of contraction | Slows rate of contraction |
| Coronary arteries | Dilatation | Constriction |
| Lungs: Bronchi | Dilatation | Constriction |
| Blood vessels | Mild constriction | No effect |
| Intestine: Muscle | Decreased peristalsis | Increased peristalsis |
| Sphincter | Increased tone | Decreased tone |
| Liver | Glycogenolysis stimulated | No effect |
| Kidney | Output decreased | No effect |
| Penis | Ejaculation | Erection |
| Blood vessels: Abdominal | Constriction | No effect |
| External genitalia | Constriction | Dilatation |
| Skeletal muscle | Increased strength and glycogenolysis | No effect |
| Mental activity | Accelerated | No effect |
| Blood: Glucose | Increased | No effect |
| Coagulation | Increased | No effect |

SOURCE: From A. C. Guyton, *Textbook of Medical Physiology*, 5th ed., Saunders, Philadelphia, 1976, p. 773 and R. M. DeCoursey, *The Human Organism*, 4th ed., 1974, p. 253.

*a*

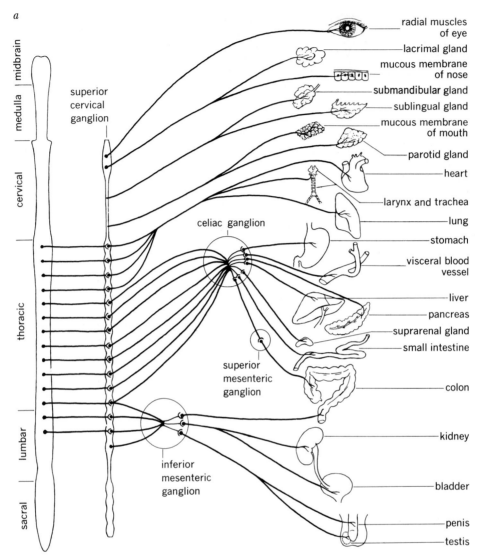

THORACOLUMBAR (SYMPATHETIC) SYSTEM

**FIGURE 31-10**
Autonomic nervous system. (*a*) Thoracolumbar (sympathetic) system; (*b*) craniosacral (parasympathetic) system. (*Reproduced with permission from R. M. DeCoursey, The Human Organism, 4th ed., McGraw-Hill, New York, 1974, pp. 244 and 245.*)

**Muscles** Three types of muscle are found within the human body: skeletal, cardiac, and smooth. Of these, skeletal muscle has a primary role in coordination; therefore, this section will focus upon skeletal muscle, its structure, and function.

*Skeletal* muscles are attached to the skeleton and permit movement (Fig. 31-11). They are *excitable* and capable of *contraction* or *extension*. Arrangement on the skeleton is usually in antagonistic pairs so that one muscle is extended while the other

contracts. After a force that has been applied to a muscle is released, the muscle will return to its normal length because of the characteristic of *elasticity*. The muscles are attached to the bones at points of *insertion* by strong fibrous *tendons*. Each muscle also has a point of *origin*, which is usually more fixed than the point of insertion.

Skeletal or voluntary muscles are composed of many finely striated fibers bound together by a sheath of connective tissue called *fascia*. Each fiber

*b*

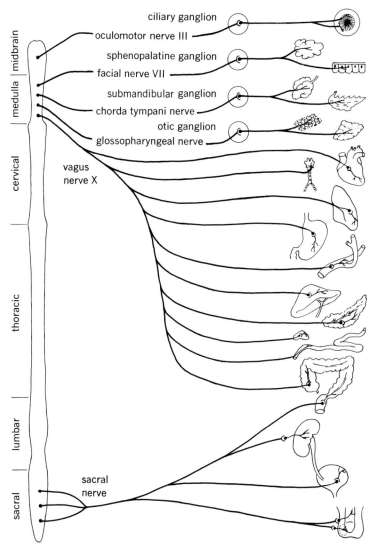

ciliary ganglion
oculomotor nerve III
sphenopalatine ganglion
facial nerve VII
submandibular ganglion
chorda tympani nerve
otic ganglion
glossopharyngeal nerve

midbrain | medulla
cervical
thoracic
lumbar
sacral

vagus
nerve X

sacral
nerve

CRANIOSACRAL (PARASYMPATHETIC) SYSTEM

is surrounded by a plasma membrane, the *sarcolemma.* A semifluid protoplasm, the *sarcoplasm,* lies beneath the sarcolemma. It contains many mitochondria (*sarcosomes*) that function in production of adenosine triphosphate (ATP). Also within the fibers are the *myofibrils.* Myofibrils are the contractile unit of the muscle and are composed of thick filaments called *myosin* and thin filaments called *actin.* The two types of filaments partially interdigitate, causing the myofibrils to have *light*

(isotropic or I) and *dark* (anisotropic or A) bands. In the middle of each I band is a Z line or membrane which divides the myofibril into units called *sarcomeres* (Fig. 31-12). In the middle of the A bands are located the H bands composed only of myosin filaments. The H band is visible only when the muscle is stretched and the A bands are pulled apart. During contraction, the Z bands move closer together as the actin filaments slide inward among the myosin filaments.

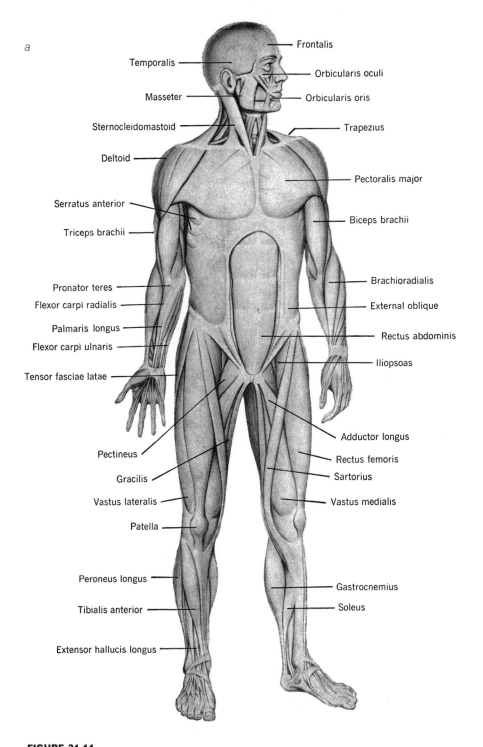

*a*

Frontalis

Temporalis

Orbicularis oculi

Orbicularis oris

Masseter

Sternocleidomastoid

Trapezius

Deltoid

Pectoralis major

Serratus anterior

Biceps brachii

Triceps brachii

Pronator teres

Brachioradialis

Flexor carpi radialis

External oblique

Palmaris longus

Rectus abdominis

Flexor carpi ulnaris

Iliopsoas

Tensor fasciae latae

Adductor longus

Pectineus

Rectus femoris

Gracilis

Sartorius

Vastus lateralis

Vastus medialis

Patella

Peroneus longus

Gastrocnemius

Tibialis anterior

Soleus

Extensor hallucis longus

**FIGURE 31-11**
Major muscles of the body. (*a*) anterior view; (*b*) posterior view. (*Reproduced with permission from R. M. DeCoursey, The Human Organism, 4th ed., McGraw-Hill, New York, 1974.*)

*b*

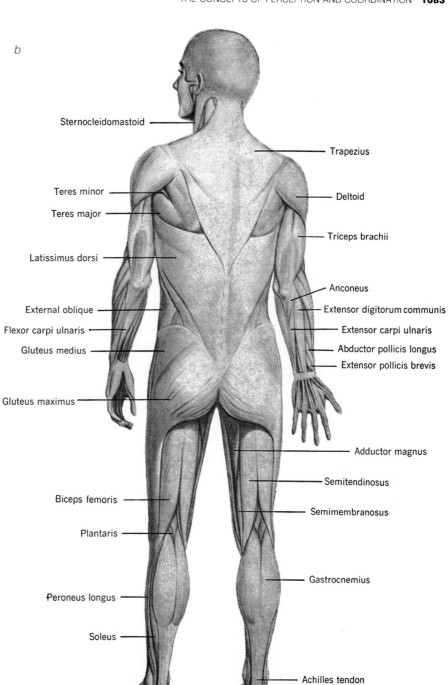

Sternocleidomastoid

Trapezius

Teres minor

Deltoid

Teres major

Triceps brachii

Latissimus dorsi

Anconeus

Extensor digitorum communis

External oblique

Extensor carpi ulnaris

Flexor carpi ulnaris

Abductor pollicis longus

Gluteus medius

Extensor pollicis brevis

Gluteus maximus

Adductor magnus

Semitendinosus

Semimembranosus

Biceps femoris

Plantaris

Peroneus longus

Gastrocnemius

Soleus

Achilles tendon

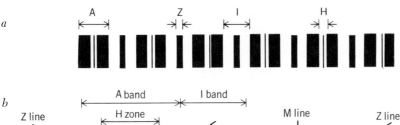

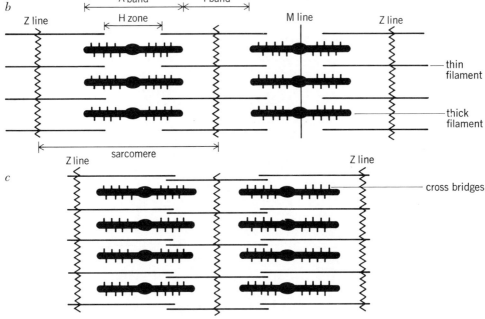

**FIGURE 31-12**

Diagram of muscle zones and filaments. (*a*) A section of striated muscle fiber showing zones and bands; (*b*) resting muscle; (*c*) contracted muscle. In contraction the two sets of filaments slide over each other and the Z lines move closer together. A *sarcomere* is the area between two Z lines. The Z lines pass through I bands. H zones are located in A bands. (*Reproduced with permission from R. M. DeCoursey, The Human Organism, 4th ed., McGraw-Hill, New York, 1974, p. 125.*)

Muscle contraction is initiated by a nerve impulse that reaches the muscle fiber at the myoneural junction. The nerves are located in the middle of the fiber so that the impulse spreads out toward both ends, allowing for more coincident contraction of all sarcomeres. Energy for contraction is supplied by the breakdown of ATP. Oxygen and glucose are also needed for this reaction. During sustained exercise, lactic acid may accumulate in the muscle owing to an inadequate oxygen supply (oxygen debt). After prolonged exercise, an individual will breathe deeply for a period of time in order to replenish the oxygen debt.

Muscle contraction may be isotonic or isometric. *Isotonic* contractions cause a shortening and thickening of the muscle and result in movement. *Isometric* contractions increase muscle tension but do not result in shortening. Such contractions help to maintain body posture.

**Bones** The skeleton or bony framework of the body (Fig. 31-13) is formed from hard connective or osseous tissue. This hardness is created by the presence of inorganic salts, largely calcium phosphate and calcium carbonate.

Bone is constantly being formed by *osteoblasts* and is continually being absorbed by *osteoclasts.* Except in bones that are still growing, bone formation is equal to bone absorption. Bone deposition and strength are proportional to the load or stress the bone must carry; this is because osteoblastic activity is stimulated by continual physical stress.

The parathyroid hormone, thyroid hormone, and vitamin D regulate the blood calcium level and control its deposition in bone. In times of calcium deficiency, the bones may be depleted to maintain the blood level, and vitamin D may promote increased calcium absorption from the intestine.

Bones may be described as long (arms and

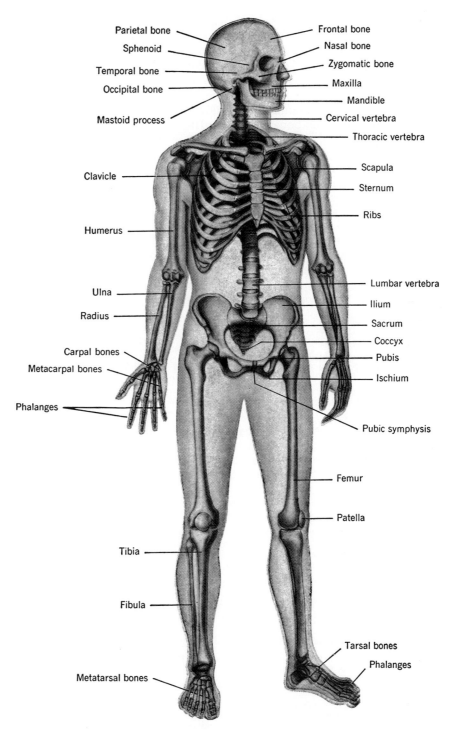

**FIGURE 31-13**

The human skeleton (anterior view). (*Reproduced with permission from R. M. DeCoursey, The Human Organism, 4th ed., McGraw-Hill, New York, 1974.*)

legs), short (wrist and ankle), flat (shoulder blades), or irregular (vertebrae). Only their walls are formed from hard bone. The ends are *cancellous* or spongy bone and contain a central *medullary* canal filled with bone marrow, blood vessels, and fat. The fat gives medullary marrow its yellow color. Red bone marrow, necessary for blood formation, is found in the ends of long bones, flat bones, and ribs. The outside of bone, except at the articulating surfaces, is covered with a tough membrane called *periosteum.* The long bones have a shaft called the *diaphysis* with ends called the *epiphyses.* Bones may have projections or *processes* that provide for muscle or ligament attachment. Examples of such processes are *condyles* and *tubercles.*

The human skeleton (containing 206 bones) has two divisions, the axial and the appendicular portions (Fig. 31-13). The *axial skeleton* is formed from the skull, the hyoid bone, the vertebrae, sternum, and ribs. The *appendicular skeleton* is composed of the bones of the arms, legs, and shoulder and pelvic girdles.

**Joints** Bones join with other bones by means of a variety of joints. These joints may be *immovable* (*fibrous,* or *synarthroses*), *partially movable* (*cartilaginous,* or *amphiarthroses*), or *freely movable* (*synovial,* or *diarthroses*).

The *sutures* binding the cranial bones are an example of immovable joints. These bones interlock and are held together by fibrous connective tissue which later ossifies. Slightly movable joints have a pad of fibrocartilage between the articulating bones. The *intervertebral disks* connecting the vertebrae are an example of this type of joint.

Synovial joints allow movement of the articulating bones. Common synovial joints are described in Table 31-5. A typical joint of this type is pictured in Fig. 31-14. Between movable joints, between tendons, and between muscle and bone are located sacs called *synovial bursae.* These sacs are composed of fibrous connective tissue and are lined with synovial membrane. This membrane secretes a fluid which decreases friction between the moving parts. It also provides nourishment to the joint cartilage.

### Summary

An understanding of nervous, muscular, and skeletal function is vital to the comprehension of how man perceives and coordinates activities within the environment. Pathological conditions can affect the functioning of these three systems and result in an alteration in perception and coordination.

## PHYSICAL ASSESSMENT OF PERCEPTION AND COORDINATION

To adequately assess an individual's perception and coordination, one must understand the neurological examination. It tests the intactness of the individual's ability to relate to the environment. Completing such an evaluation requires that the total person be considered in the interpretation of

**TABLE 31-5**
CLASSIFICATION OF SYNOVIAL JOINTS

| Type | Description | Location (example) |
|---|---|---|
| Ball and socket | One bone contains a socket in which the ball-shaped head of another bone fits | Humerus into the scapula and femur into the acetabulum |
| Condyloid | Modified ball and socket | Between the metacarpals and first phalanges |
| Gliding | Flat, smooth surfaces move along similar plane surfaces | Carpal (wrist) and tarsal (ankle) bones |
| Hinge | Movement is only in one direction or plane; a rounded convex surface fits into a concave surface | Humerus and ulna (elbow joint) |
| Pivot | Rotation of a depression at one bone end with a rounded surface on another bone | The hand: The radius articulates with the capitulum of the humerus |
| Saddle | Movement is from side to side and back and forth; it is a convex-concave joint | Carpal-metacarpal joint of the thumb |

SOURCE: From R. M. DeCoursey, *The Human Organism,* 4th ed., McGraw-Hill, New York, 1974, p. 119.

the results of the various components of the examination. The subjectivity of the patient's response cannot be understated since it serves as the rationale underlying the behavioral and verbal manifestations that are observed by the examiner. The component parts of the neurological examination include *mental status, motor status,* and *sensory status.* The findings in these areas are compared with each other and analyzed as a whole. The patient's ability to understand, cooperate with, and respond to the elements of the testing procedures often require creativity and initiative on the part of the examiner in eliciting patterns of response. Hence, at the time of the examination, the examiner must be aware of the interaction of the patient with the examiner and with the environment. Specifically, the patient's response may vary according to medication administration, fatigue, emotional changes, repetition of the examination, and the physical state of well-being. Therefore, in using the neurological examination as a tool for nursing diagnosis, the nurse must be alert to the subtlety of meaningful observations and the need to repeat and extend some areas of testing when appropriate, in order to obtain a basis for prediction of the patient's course and indicators for nursing action.

For consistency with the format of other sections of the text, the neurological examination will be outlined according to inspection, palpation, percussion, and auscultation. Judgment must be used as to which areas are to be omitted and which areas need to be pursued to a greater extent. For example, a patient with an altered level of consciousness may not be an appropriate subject for detailed examination of mental status, or a patient moving about in bed may demonstrate adequate motor activity so as not to necessitate repetition of that activity during systematic evaluation. Many parts of the testing may be evaluated together. For instance, the patient's ability to comprehend and understand instruction for sensory testing is also indicative of the stability of the mental status. The significance of the findings as related to the functioning of the component parts of the central and peripheral nervous systems will be incorporated throughout Part 7.

### Inspection

The emphasis of the remainder of this chapter will be on inspection of a patient for neurological information. Palpation, percussion, and auscultation all have a large inspection component and will be integrated throughout the neurological examination, whenever appropriate.

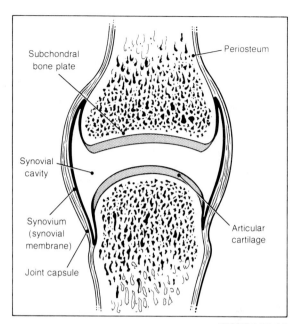

**FIGURE 31-14**
A synovial, or diarthroid joint.

**Mental status**  The assessment of *mental status* should be initiated from the first moment of contact with the patient since the verbal and visual cues which are exhibited will provide information about the emotional and cognitive state. While systematically reviewing the traditional components of an assessment of mental status, the examiner must understand that this process is an ongoing one which depends upon the awareness and perception of the examiner in attaching appropriate significance to the information provided by the patient. Since nursing usually provides for continued contact with the patient, the nurse may best assess the patient parameters of thought process, judgment, etc., without a rigid set of guidelines but should be able to communicate observations according to commonly used categories of reference.

A great deal of information may be obtained through *goal-directed conversation,* but this should be conducted in the appropriate sociocultural context if it is to provide any legitimate meaning. For example, an elaborate English vocabulary would not be appropriate in questioning a patient of limited English-speaking ability, nor would accurate orientation to date and time necessarily be expected of a patient who has spent an extensive period of time in a sensorily altered environment such as an intensive-care unit. Of note, too, is the influence of repetitive cues given by the professional staff in inducing what may be interpreted as a meaningful response. This is often referred to as an *automatic response* and may not be a true indicator of the patient's cognitive ability. For example, when a patient is repeatedly turned to the right in bed and the verbal command "turn to your right" is given, the patient's compliance may not always indicate that he or she is understanding and acting in response to the turning of his or her body. This is especially problematic in the evaluation of an aphasic patient.

Of final note before approaching the specifics of mental status examination is the technique of the examiner. Questions that elicit "yes" or "no" answers from the patient are far less significant, in fact may be meaningless, in a true assessment of orientation or cognition. Instead, the examiner should attempt to encourage answers that contain content, the appropriateness of which can then be determined. There is much to be said for the validity of the nurse's perception in pursuing a specific line of questioning. The patient may provide only the most subtle cues that there is a change in the emotional or cognitive state; the receptivity of the nurse in noting those cues may depend upon the nurse's ability to be a good listener.

The major areas to be assessed in an examination of mental status are: *appearance and behavior, mood and affect, thought processes and perceptions,* and *cognitive functions and sensorium.*

**A**ppearance and Behavior    Information that includes the interviewer's general impression of the total patient, in the initial presentation, is collected. The observations may alert the examiner to an inconsistency between the initial impression and information obtained later in the interview and may signal an emotional and/or organic disorder. The essential components to be noted are:

1    Motor activity and body posture. The presence of tension, agitation, mannerisms, etc., and their relationship to the topics being discussed should be noted.

2    Dress and hygiene. The completeness and appropriateness of dress and grooming are noted according to age, sex, and sociocultural background.

3    Body expression. Visible body and facial expression should be appropriate to subjects discussed. Changes in facial expression should be noted.

4    Speech. The patterns of speech are observed for such elements as quality, quantity, and organization. The ease of articulation is noted, as well as dysphasia,

aphasia, loose association, monosyllabic speech, and scanning speech.

5    General manner and ability to relate to the environment. Observation is made for anger, approachability, uncooperativeness, euphoria, paranoia, etc.

**M**ood and Affect    Observation of mood and affect analyzes any inappropriateness found in an initial assessment of behavior. The examiner should be aware of emotional lability, mood swings, or a lack of appropriate mood change. This may involve specific questioning about an observed emotion such as "Do you think that you feel unusually depressed?" The examiner must remain nondirective and allow the patient to direct the responses rather than to reply in a way that is sensed to be acceptable.

**T**hought Processes and Perceptions    This area of the mental examination may yield information about the patient's interpretation of internal and external stimuli. It indicates the frame of reference from which the individual operates and the subjective nature of the patient's perception of reality. Personality disorders may become evident as the nurse assesses the totality of the patient's response and the organization of thought patterns. The validity of the patient's perceptions must be assessed according to some relative degree of reality, and it is toward this end that the nurse proceeds with the questioning. The specific components to observe are:

1    Organization and appropriateness of thought processes. The composition of the patient's complaints, ability to stay on the subject, and patterns of expression, as well as any consistency of ideation and interpretation of questions, are noted.

2    Thought content. Any tendency toward compulsions, obsessions, indecision, phobias, feelings of unreality, depersonalization, complexes, delusions, or free-floating anxiety should be described.

3    Perceptions. Any illusions or hallucinations, especially any interpretations related to one of the senses, should be noted. These are usually visual or auditory but may involve taste, smell, or touch.

**C**ognitive Functions and Sensorium    This area of testing represents an attempt to evaluate the more objective aspects of the patient's thinking and may often show distortion of an organic nature. Although the objective-subjective aspects of thinking are always intertwined and psychological-organic discrepancies are usually related, it may become apparent that ideation and content are correct but a particular area of function may be limited. Evaluation of this area depends upon the intactness of cerebral function as determined by past experiences, education, interests, memory, self-perception, social background, and culture. Again, it must be emphasized that the questioning should be appropriate for the individual, i.e., attention and concentration should not be evaluated in a highly distracting environment. The specific components of this examination include:

1    Orientation. This is ascertained according to person, place, and time. If the patient shows confusion about time, ask whether it is day or night; if confusion exists about place, ask the patient to describe the place; confused patients will usually retain orientation to person.

2    Attention and concentration. A series of digits are recited randomly and in a nonconsecutive manner; the patient is asked to repeat them. It is wise to begin with two or three digits and extend the numbers. Good technique requires that the numbers be pronounced at a rate of one per second and in a sequence which does not represent a phone number, date, etc. A test with serial 7s is another usual tool. The patient is asked to count backward from 100 by subtracting 7. Normal skill suggests that this can be accomplished in 1½ minutes with about four errors. Other series, with the alphabet, for example, can be used when appropriate.

3    Memory. Both recent and remote memory should be tested. A loss of recent memory may be present with organic brain disease as in progressive senile dementia. The patient can be given several words to remember and asked to repeat them in five or so minutes as an additional test. The patient is evaluated on the basis of accuracy, awareness of accuracy, and tendency to fabricate answers.

4    Fund of information. An oriented and attentive person should be able to answer questions related to current events, word meanings, and significant places and dates. Evaluating the answers will give an idea of the person's level of intelligence.

5    Vocabulary. This area, also, reflects intelligence level. The patient is asked the meanings of some words, and the ability to define them or use them in a sentence is noted. On a very basic level, the general ability to comprehend questions or instructions is described. Cultural background and familiarity with the English language are taken into account in an evaluation of vocabulary.

6    Abstract reasoning. The ability to comprehend both concrete and abstract meanings is noted, as is the relevance of the answer.

7    Similarities. Two objects, for example, an apple and a banana, are mentioned to the patient, and the response is evaluated in terms of concreteness or abstractness.

8    Judgment. This is evaluated by assessing the patient's awareness of his or her present condition and life goals, expectations, and ability to suggest appropriate behavior in specific situations. Again, patients with brain dysfunction, psychological disorders, and retardation may demonstrate poor judgment.

9    Sensory perception and coordination. The patient is asked to copy some common figures ranging from simple to complex. The ability to perform this task is indicative of perceptual, motor, and intellectual skills.

*Consciousness*    Finally, the examination of mental status must include an evaluation of consciousness. Since this is such a fundamental and important concept, it should be dealt with in some detail. Plum and Possner define consciousness as an "awareness of self and environment."[6] They continue to describe the aspects of consciousness as (1) content or the sum of mental functions, and (2) arousal which is the appearance of wakefulness.[7] The two often relate to each other but vary independently in all the normal and altered states associated with consciousness. This is evident, for example, in a patient experiencing delerium tremors after alcohol withdrawal. This person is very arousable yet speech content may be garbled, in contrast to a patient who is somnolent and difficult to arouse but has appropriate speech content. This only emphasizes that a notation of a patient's level of consciousness should include a description of specific responses to stimuli rather than a common term since the interpretation of that term may be subjective and lead to inaccurate assumptions about the patient's state of being. Since the level of consciousness is usually evaluated by behavior, states of psychic withdrawal, sleep, and dreams will constitute altered states of consciousness and serve to increase the difficulty of both evaluation and description. With these considerations in mind, an attempt to define the various levels of consciousness will be made as progressive deterioration occurs, but, again, it is the description which is important and not the selection of a term.

1 Clouding of consciousness. Minimal clouding involves a disturbance in arousal which may include excitability and irritability. The content factor may begin to include audio or visual hallucination. Cognition becomes cloudy and unclear. This progresses to *confusion* which includes a decrease in attention span and deterioration in perception. Disorientation may occur, and arousability decreases.

2 Delerium. A more widespread state than confusion, *delerium* includes fears, disorientation, hallucinations, irritability, and delusions. Delerious patients are more out of touch with their environment, yet are highly arousable.

3 Stupor. The arousal factor decreases in this state, and vigorous and repeated stimuli are necessary to obtain a response.

4 Coma. This is a state of unarousable unresponsiveness. In both stupor and coma, the content of consciousness cannot be determined since the arousal level is so low. Some reflexes may be present.

**Sensory status** Several *general principles* apply to evaluation of the sensory system.

Specific information is required as to the nature, duration, and location of the stimulus and the patient's response.

Extra consideration is given to special complaints such as numbness of a part, tingling, abnormal pain, and temperature.

Generally, if sensation is intact distally, sensation will probably be intact proximally. This understanding conserves time and effort for both the patient and the examiner.

The patient should be alert, cooperative, and calm if accurate responses are to be given. The nurse should be aware of the presence of alcohol, sedation, fatigue, etc.

Evaluation should be bilateral, symmetrical, and extensive enough to provide information about most of the dermatomes. Any abnormality should be mapped to the specific area since the dermatomes overlap.

In testing for sensation, the patient must be prepared to feel something but not to be hurt, with the exception of pain testing. The examiner should modify the examination accordingly.

Technique is crucial to the response. The patient should not be provided with visual or verbal cues. For example, the patient is requested to say when something is felt rather than being asked "Do you feel that?"

The following situations should be avoided:

1 Perseveration: an error of discrimination caused when the examiner increases or decreases the sequence of stimulation without randomization.

2 Summation: an error in sensation in which the patient reports that a stimulus is felt when, in fact, the cumulative effect of the examiner applying many separate stimuli in rapid succession is felt.

3 The application of pressure and pain may be misleading to the patient. To prevent this, the sharp end of a pin is used to test for pain and the blunt end for pressure.

**Smell** To test the sense of smell (IId cranial, or olfactory, nerve), swabs of cotton saturated with strong and familiar odors such as coffee, oil of cloves, or oil of peppermint are obtained. Ammonia and acetic acid should not be used as they test taste and not smell. The patient is asked to close both eyes and occlude one nostril. A swab is held under one nostril and the patient is asked to identify the odor. The procedure is repeated for the other nostril, and each odor is randomly tested. If patients have difficulty in determining the odors, they should be asked whether the difficulty is merely in identifying the odor or in the process of smelling. If the former, the three odors are identified and the test repeated. An abnormality may represent a malfunction anywhere along the sensation transmission from receptor to appreciation of sensation on the cortical level.

**Sight** Intact vision depends upon the ability of the eye (orbit) to *focus* and *accommodate,* the optic nerve (Ist cranial nerve) to receive and transmit the image, and the cerebral cortex to receive and interpret the image. Thus, a deficit in a patient's vision may represent an abnormality in the functioning of any of these components, and separate measures must be taken to test them. The examination of vision involves *a test for visual acuity, a test for visual fields,* and *the ophthalmoscopic examination.*

To begin, the presence of any gross abnormalities is established by asking the patient to read any available printed material. If this presents a difficulty, the patient is asked to determine the correct number of upraised fingers and, finally, to distinguish light from dark. As in any aspect of the visual examination, each eye should be tested separately. The Snellen chart is the usual method of testing for *visual acuity* (Fig. 31-15). This test, it is important to remember, is for actual visual acuity and not for memory. Therefore, the chart should be covered until just before the test, and the patient should be instructed to cover the eye not being examined. In addition, the letters should be read in a reverse or random order when testing the other eye. The procedure is as follows: (1) The patient is seated 20 ft from the chart. (2) When the patient is properly positioned and one eye is covered, the chart is lowered, making sure that it is well illuminated. (3) The patient is instructed to read the top line and then each successive line below it. (4) The number opposite the last line on which the patient was able to read more than half of the numbers correctly is recorded as the denominator of a fraction. The numerator is the distance away from the chart (20 ft). It is important that this distance be constant. (5) The proce-

dure is repeated for the other eye. Interpretation of the results of reading the Snellen chart indicates that the patient could read at 20 ft (numerator) what the normal eye can read at $x$ feet (denominator). Thus, a rating of 20/50 means that the patient sees at 20 ft what the normal eye sees at 50 ft, a visual defect. Acuity decreases as the denominator increases.

While a patient may have excellent visual acuity, an area of peripheral vision may be lacking owing to a lesion in one of the visual pathways (optic nerve, optic radiation, or cortex). The testing of visual fields may be omitted in a routine examination but should be carried out whenever a neurological problem is suspected or should at least be inquired about by the examiner. The test for *visual fields* is performed as follows: (1) The examiner sits approximately 2 ft from the patient. (2) The examiner directly faces the patient and both cover one eye so that the eyes that are opposite each other are open. (3) The patient is instructed to look straight ahead (Fig. 31-16). At an equal distance to

**FIGURE 31-15**
Snellen chart used to test for visual acuity.

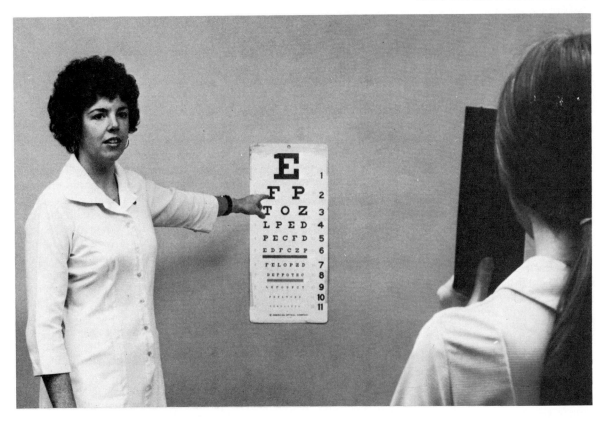

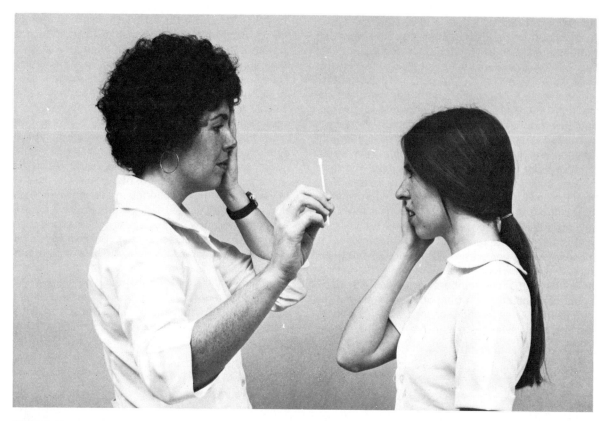

**FIGURE 31-16**
Visual field testing.

both patient and examiner, a test object such as a pencil or cotton-tipped stick should be brought from the periphery to the central vision area, and the patient asked to indicate when it is first seen. (4) When the test object is moved, it is vibrated rather than held still since the eye perceives a moving object more readily. (5) This procedure is repeated at a 45° angle so that the entire circle of vision has been tested. Remember that the patient's temporal (opposite the nose which is called *nasal*) field of vision may be more extensive than the examiner's nasal field, and the examiner may have to initiate the stimulus behind the patient's head. The patient's field of vision should be compared with the examiner's and any deficits recorded, using the angle that is being tested and the eye being tested. (6) The procedure is repeated with the other eye.

Normal visual fields are about a 45° angle for vertical peripheral vision and about an 85° angle for temporal vision as measured in an angle with the straight line of gaze at 0°. Any other variation is significant.

The last test of vision involves the use of the *ophthalmoscope* in examining the interior of the eye (Fig. 31-17). Specifically, the examiner is interested in observing the color, clarity, and size of the optic disk. This is the point at which the optic nerve leaves the retina and proceeds toward the cerebral cortex. These observations include the color and size of the arterioles and veins, the presence of hemorrhages or lesions in the general background of the retina, and the quality of the macula. Also, the ophthalmoscope can yield information about opacities or irregularities of the more anterior structures of the eye.

The use of the ophthalmoscope becomes less formidable with practice. Initially, the examiner should attempt to identify the major normal structures such as the disk, blood vessels, and macula. As one becomes experienced with the normal structures, abnormal findings will become more evident.

A series of numbers called *diopters* are marked on the lens disk of the ophthalmoscope. These units measure the power of a lens to converge or diverge light and are changed according to the need to focus on structures which are closer or farther away, such as the retina of a nearsighted eye or the vitreous humor. If the lens disk is rotated counterclockwise, the minus diopters or red numbers come into focus and allow the examiner to use a longer focus, as in a nearsighted patient whose eyeball is somewhat longer than normal. The reverse or black numbers may be necessary for a farsighted patient and can be focused by rotating the lens disk clockwise.

With the understanding that the use of the appropriate diopter is determined primarily by the examiner's personal requirements for clear visualization of the structures, proceed as follows: (1) The room is darkened and the patient is instructed to stare at a distant object behind the examiner so that the pupils will dilate. (2) Facing the patient and using the right hand and right eye for visualization of the patient's right eye, and the left hand and left eye for the patient's left eye, the examiner places his or her thumb on the patient's eyebrow to provide a fixed point of orientation. (3) The ophthalmo-

scope is braced against the examiner's face, with the examining eye behind its sight hole and the index finger on the lens disk, ready to rotate it if necessary. The light of the ophthalmoscope should shine toward the patient, and the instrument and examiner's head should move as a single unit. Both eyes are kept open while the instrument is in use. (4) The light is directed on the patient's pupil when the examiner is about a foot away from the patient and about 15° lateral to his or her line of vision. This should allow visualization of the "red reflex" which is the orange-red color in the pupil. (5) Movement closer to this red area enables the examiner to look at the retina and to visualize its structures. If the optic disk is not readily visible, a blood vessel should be found and followed centrally until many blood vessels converge. The optic disk should be located at this point. (6) A systematic survey of the entire retina is done next to look for abnormalities. They should be recorded by means of a clockface orientation with the distance from the disk recorded in terms of disk diameters. (7) The macula is visual-

**FIGURE 31-17**
Use of the opthalmoscope to examine the eye.

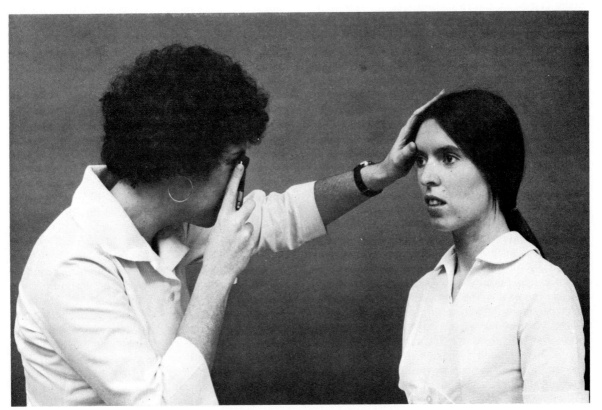

ized by having the patient look directly into the light beam. (8) The examination is repeated for the other eye.

**T**ouch   An evaluation of the sense of touch involves an understanding that the procedure itself must be properly executed, thorough, widespread, and accurately recorded to be of any significance in the determination of a deficit or a change in that deficit. The sensations that are usually tested are pain, temperature, light touch, proprioception, vibration, and discrimination. The examiner must proceed with the awareness that anatomically, the pain, temperature, and light touch sensations are transmitted via the spinothalamic tracts and cross in the cord to the opposite side from which they enter the cord. The sensations of proprioception, vibration, and discrimination, on the other hand, are transmitted via the posterior columns to the level of the medulla where they decussate and proceed to higher centers. The implications of this knowledge not only suggest the location of a disorder but direct the examiner as to how extensive a test to conduct. For example, if pain sensation is intact, there may be no need to routinely test for temperature sensation since they are anatomically similar in their location and transmission; symmetrical lesions may indicate a peripheral rather than a central process; the absence of distal sensation in the presence of proximal sensation may suggest a peripheral nerve lesion. Hence, while seeming to involve a random application of stimuli, the investigator must be aware of the implications of the testing so that important data are not overlooked and applicable nursing measures such as safety and protection may be instituted.

Another key point is the application and notation of the stimulus itself. The nature of the stimulus (pin, cotton, etc.) must be recorded as well as the exact location of the application of the stimulus. The overlapping of dermatomal area demands precision of notation; in addition any spontaneous sensations that the patient reports such as tingling or numbness must be noted.

The test for *pain* sensation is as follows: (1) The patient closes both eyes. (2) A pin is held loosely between the examiner's fingers so that the fingers can slide down the pin during testing. Thus, the patient will respond to the sharpness of the pin rather than to pressure. This is important since deep or heavy touch sensation is transmitted via different tracts than pain sensation. The test for pain sensation does not have to hurt the patient.

(3) The examiner next alternates, in a random manner, between stimulating the patient with the sharp end of the pin and the blunt end of the pin to differentiate between pain and pressure. (4) The patient is asked to report the sensation by stating whether it is "sharp" or "dull." (5) At least 2 seconds are allowed to elapse between stimulus applications to prevent summation. (6) The stimulus is applied in symmetrical distal and proximal areas of the body including the trunk and face. (7) Any areas of discrepancy should be mapped and noted.

*Note:* When a patient's level of consciousness is depressed to the point of semicoma or coma, the only stimulus that evokes a response may be "deep pain." While the goal is to cause a deeply painful stimulus and thus evaluate a response, the examiner is cautioned against injuring the patient. One method of inducing this stimulus is to press down hard on the sternum with the knuckles and to note the reaction. In an arousal response, the patient will move the extremities and/or attempt to withdraw from the stimulus or brush it away. In hemiplegia, there will be no response on the affected side. Subcutaneous bleeding from too frequent and too vigorous stimulation should be avoided. A less harmful way of applying stimulation may be to apply supraorbital pressure over one eye to induce deep pain. Caution should be taken not to apply the pressure to the orbit itself and to be certain that the examiner's fingernails do not leave a mark. The nature of the reaction to deep-pain stimulation should be noted.

To test for *temperature* sensation, proceed as follows: (1) Ask the patient to close both eyes to avoid visual cues. (2) Obtain two test tubes, one filled with cold water and one filled with warm water. Extremes of temperature should be avoided since the objective is to test discrimination ability near threshold, not maximal discrimination. (3) Apply the test tubes randomly to the skin, covering most of the dermatomal areas, and ask the patient to respond by saying "hot" or "cold." Apply the test tubes for a short time only. (4) Record the responses immediately.

To test for *light touch* sensation, proceed as follows: (1) Wrap a wisp of cotton around a stick. (2) Instruct the patient to close both eyes to avoid visual cuing. (3) Apply the touch sensation to the skin, covering most of the dermatomal areas but not visibly depressing the skin surface, since the response might then measure pressure of deep touch sensation. It is important to be aware that sensation is transmitted differently when hair follicles are stimulated, and so skin should be tested, not hair. (4) Ask the patient to respond when the stimulus is felt.

To test for sensation that is transmitted via the posterior columns, the examiner will specifically test for *proprioception, vibration,* and *discrimination sense.* Discrimination sense itself is subdivided into two-point discrimination, stereognosis and extinction phenomenon.

In a test of *position sense,* or *proprioception* (Fig. 31-18), the patient is called upon to sense movement and position of his or her body parts in respect to the rest of the body as well as to the environment. For this test, the examiner should be aware that if sensation is intact distally, it will probably be intact proximally, and so the digits of the four extremities are tested. In addition to the usual precautions against visual cuing, the examiner must also guard against pressure cuing, and so even pressure on the sides of the digit must be maintained. In addition, the patient has a 50 percent chance of responding correctly, particularly if the response is out of expectation rather than true sensation. To reduce this possibility and to aid interpretation, three positions, up, down, and neutral are used. The normal patient should not make any errors. To conduct the test, proceed as follows: (1) Instruct the patient to close both eyes. (2) Support the part to be tested with one hand. With the other hand grasp the digit by its sides and randomly move it in each of the three above positions. Take care to maintain evenness of tone of voice when moving the digits. (3) Ask the patient to report the position of the part. (4) Repeat the examination on all extremities, making sure to test the third and fourth digits since they have less innervation and can give evidence of a more specific lesion.

Another test of proprioception sense is to evaluate the maintenance of the standing position (*Romberg test*). (1) Ask the patient to stand erect with both heels together and both eyes open. Note any swaying or loss of balance. (2) Ask the patient to maintain that position but to close both eyes. Note any abnormal swaying or tendency to fall.

**FIGURE 31-18**
Digital test of proprioception.

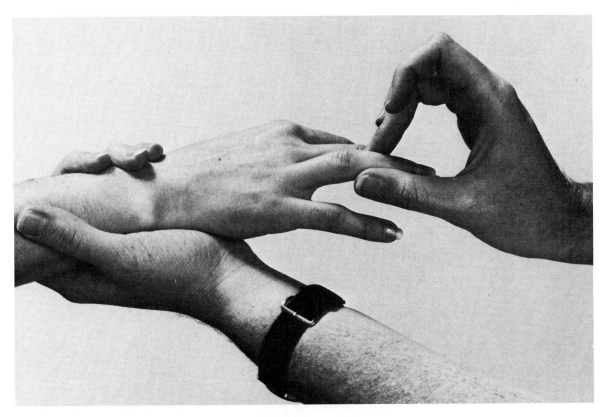

*Note:* The normal patient may sway slightly with the eyes closed, but the patient with impaired proprioception will tend to sway considerably. This person will often use visual cues to maintain a stable position with the eyes open. The patient with cerebellar disease will usually sway with the eyes open *or* closed.

To test for *vibration sensation,* proceed as follows: (1) Ask the patient to close both eyes. (2) Vibrate a tuning fork by knocking it against the palm of the hand. (3) Apply the tuning fork to bony prominences such as finger joints, elbows, knees, ankles, ribs, sternum, and skull. (4) To ensure that the patient is truly responding to vibration and not sound, both ears should be blocked from receiving sound. To prevent additional suggestibility of response by changes in pressure, stimulation should be alternated between a vibrating tuning fork and one that is not. In this case, the fork is struck initially but the vibration is stopped before it is applied to the skin. (5) Ask the patient to report the feeling of a "buzz" and to say when the buzz stops.

Finally, to assess the functioning of the cortex, the *sense of discrimination* is tested by checking the following: (1) Two-point discrimination, or the ability to perceive two points from one when a stimulus is applied to adjacent parts of the skin, (2) stereognosis, the ability to recognize an object by touch, (3) and the extinction phenomenon, or tactile inattention, which is the ability to recognize two stimuli when simultaneously placed on corresponding areas bilaterally.

To test for *two-point discrimination* (Fig. 31-19), proceed as follows: (1) Ask the patient to close both eyes. (2) Hold one pin in each hand and apply them so that the fingers (of the examiner) slide down the pin. (3) Simultaneously, apply the two pins to the same body part, taking care to randomize the distances between the pins. Alternate this procedure with application of both pins to the same spot so that the patient responds to the number of simultaneous stimulations and distance rather than to changes in pressure. (4) Ask the patient to report when one or two pins is/are felt.

Several precautions relate to the above procedure: (1) Visual cuing, pressure cuing, or pain cuing

**FIGURE 31-19**
Test for two-point discrimination.

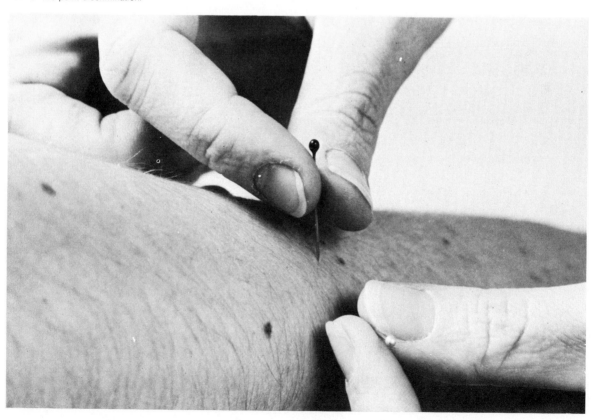

should be avoided by having the patient close both eyes, by always using two pins even if on the same spot, and by allowing the fingers to slide down the pin. (2) Separation of the stimuli in time is avoided by applying the pins simultaneously rather than consecutively. (3) Summation is avoided by allowing several seconds to elapse between each stimulation. (4) Perservation is avoided by randomizing the distances between the pins rather than progressively moving them farther apart or closer together. (5) It should be remembered that there are normal variances in the discrimination thresholds of different parts of the body. Thus, it would be normal for the patient to discern two stimuli at a smaller separation on the fingertips than on the back or chest.

To test for *stereognosis,* proceed as follows: (1) Ask the patient to close both eyes. (2) Place familiar objects, such as a nickel, dime, or quarter, in the patient's hand and ask him or her to identify them. (3) If the person has difficulty with these objects, use simpler ones, such as a comb, a pencil, or a key.

To test for *extinction phenomenon,* proceed as follows: (1) Ask the patient to close both eyes and to report where he or she is touched. The answer should not just state "on the side" but should state which side that is. (2) Brush the back of the patient's hands, feet, cheeks, etc., lightly and simultaneously with the index fingers. The examiner alternates between using one hand and both hands in a random manner.

Some of the cranial nerves are evaluated for their sensory component on the basis of touch. While these would normally be assessed during a comprehensive examination of the head and total cranial nerve function, they will be elaborated upon at this point because of their dependence upon the sensation of touch.

The *Vth cranial nerve,* or *trigeminal nerve,* has both a motor and a sensory component. Its sensory component supplies the sensory innervation of the face, and the distribution of this sensation is consistent with its three main branches: the ophthalmic, maxillary, and mandibular. Thus, sensation of the skin of the face, the oral and nasal mucosa, and the cornea of the eye, as they respond to touch, pain, and temperature, must be tested to obtain information about all three branches.

The procedures already described for testing the sensations of light touch, pain, and temperature sense are repeated in assessing the sensory intactness of the Vth cranial nerve. Using a wisp of cotton, a pin, and warm and cool test tubes, the ex-

aminer evaluates the face, making sure to test over the eyebrow, the cheeks, and the chin. In addition, the *corneal reflex* is tested as follows (Fig. 31-20): (1) Ask the patient to look to one side. (2) With a wisp of cotton, lightly brush the lateral side of the cornea of the opposite eye. This technique is used to avoid a blink reflex caused by entering the field of vision. (3) The patient should blink when stimulated. (4) Any other reactions such as tearing or pain should be noted.

The *IXth (glossopharyngeal)* and *Xth (vagus)* cranial nerves are usually evaluated together, and both have a motor and sensory component. The testing of these nerves is usually considered to be a part of the motor examination with the exception of the taste sensation of the posterior part of the tongue which is sensory and included as a part of the overall evaluation of taste.

In consideration of the sensory modality of touch, the IXth cranial nerve carries the afferent impulses from the pharynx which are involved in testing the gag reflex. It is the Xth cranial nerve which is responsible for the efferent component of this reflex.

To test for the *gag reflex,* proceed as follows: (1) Stimulate the back of the pharynx with a tongue blade or cotton on a stick. (2) The patient should gag or choke if the reflex is intact. (3) In addition, the patient should respond to light stimulation of the posterior pharynx by being able to raise a hand when a tongue blade that is placed against the posterior pharynx is felt.

**T**aste   The sensation of taste is complemented by the senses of smell and vision. This has implications for testing in that care must be taken to avoid visual and olfactory cuing. The cranial nerves involved in sensation include the VIIth (facial) which innervates the taste buds on the anterior two-thirds of the tongue and the IXth (glossopharyngeal) and Xth (vagus) cranial nerves which innervate the taste buds on the posterior one-third of the tongue and tonsillar pillars. The usual test for taste is done as a part of the evaluation of the function of the VIIth cranial nerve since the other nerves can be more definitely evaluated by other procedures. In fact, this is really the only sensory test done for the facial nerve since its other primary function is motor.

To test the *taste* sensation, proceed as follows: (1) Prepare four solutions which are qualitatively different, sweet (sugar), salt, sour (vinegar), and bitter (quinine). (2) The patient may be told what the choices are but care should be taken not to give visual cues and to randomize the order of the stimu-

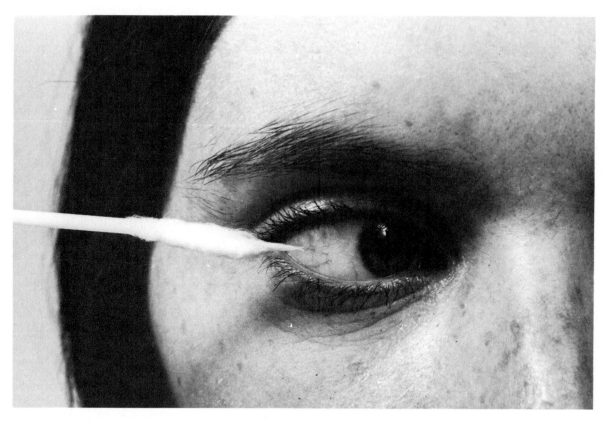

**FIGURE 31-20**
Corneal reflex testing.

lus. (3) Ask the patient to protrude the tongue. (4) Apply a small amount of the stimulus with a cotton applicator to one-half of the tongue laterally. Allow the substance to dissolve in saliva without spreading to the other side of the tongue, and ask the patient to identify the substance. (5) The patient may rinse his or her mouth between applications. (6) Apply the other substances to other areas of the tongue, and record the results.

**H**earing  In evaluating the sense of hearing, the examiner is concerned with a range of the sensation, specifically, the threshold of the sensation. In addition, the conduction of sound is dependent upon the integrity of the VIIIth (acoustic, or vestibulocochlear) cranial nerve which has two components, cochlear and vestibular. It is the cochlear component which is routinely tested. The mechanical conduction of sound depends upon conduction through the external canal, the auditory canal, and the ossicles of the middle ear. This part of conduction is tested by *air conduction,* and any decrease in response is referred to as a *conduction loss.* If the

response is decreased owing to a lesion of the organ of Corti or the acoustic nerve itself, the loss is usually described as neurosensory and is evaluated by testing *bone conduction.*

To begin the examination, one checks the external auditory canal for wax or other obstructions. Then, gross ability to hear can be tested by evaluating the *auditory-palpebral reflex* which involves blinking as a response to a loud sound. Someone stands behind the patient and makes a loud sound by clapping, etc., and the patient should show a blinking or startle response. The results are equivocal, however, since an absence of response does not necessarily signal a hearing loss.

The *watch-tick test* also tells simply whether there is a hearing loss. A watch usually emits a high-frequency sound of low density which is discontinuous and thus is a good standard tool. To conduct the test, proceed as follows: (1) Examine the external auditory canal. (2) Hold the watch on an axis that corresponds with an extension of the auditory canal. (3) Move the watch toward and away from the ear until the point at which the patient can barely hear it is reached. Record this distance. (4) Measure the results against those of another patient in the same test.

If there is hearing loss, the Weber and Rinne tests are performed. The *Rinne* test (Fig. 31-21) involves the following: (1) Place a vibrating tuning fork on the mastoid process and instruct the patient to say when the sound is no longer audible. (2) Transfer the fork quickly, without hitting it again, nearer to the ear canal, and ask the patient if it can still be heard and for how long.

Normally, air conduction is more efficient than bone conduction, and the fork should still be audible when placed in front of the external ear canal. If bone conduction is greater than air conduction, one might infer that the VIIIth nerve is intact but that there is some mechanical impediment in the auditory canal or middle ear.

To conduct the *Weber* test, proceed as follows: (1) Place a vibrating tuning fork at the vertex of the skull. (2) Question the patient as to where the sound is heard. It should be heard equally in both sides. (3) Since this is primarily a test of bone conduction, a mechanical impediment in one ear would make the sound localize to that ear. If there is a lesion of the VIIIth nerve, the sound would localize to the opposite ear.

*Note:* It must be kept in mind that the bone mechanically transmits the vibration to the inner ear and thus stimulates the acoustic nerve. Hence the integrity of the nerve can be tested and a mechanical problem can be defined. Further testing of auditory integrity must be conducted with special equipment.

*Otoscopic examination* of the ear is particularly important to observe the condition of the tympanic membrane. Any bulging, erythema, scarring, discharge, or visible fluid level should be noted. Greater detail on this examination is found in Chap. 38.

**FIGURE 31-21**
The Rinne test of bone conduction.

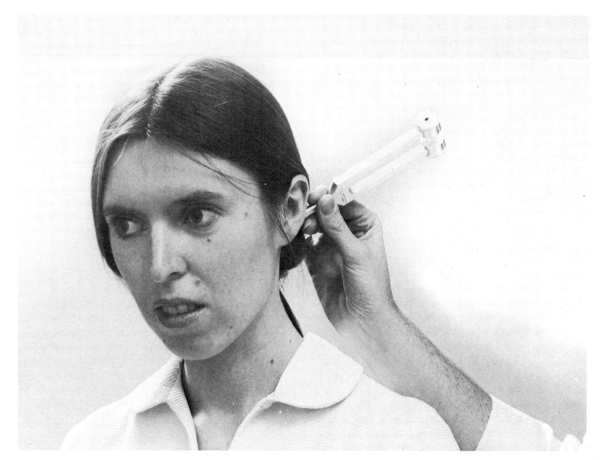

The *vestibular function* of the VIIIth cranial nerve is assessed by nursing history. Inquire whether the patient experiences balance problems, dizziness, vertigo, etc. Further examination may involve caloric testing which is beyond the scope of a routine examination (see Chap. 38).

**S**pinal Reflexes    The spinal reflexes involve both a sensory and motor component and may require the use of a percussive instrument, the reflex hammer. Since their function anatomically involves a sensory modality, they will be discussed as contiguous with the sensory examination. It must be remembered that the response elicited is dependent upon the motor component, and, thus, it is logical to use the reflexes as a bridge to approaching the technique of the motor examination.

The reflexes usually tested are of two kinds: (1) the deep tendon reflexes or muscle stretch reflex, and (2) the superficial reflexes. Essentially the reflexes provide information about the spinal cord segments that innervate the area stimulated. As such, they allow postulation about the location of a lesion and monitoring of the progress of the healing process. They also may serve to differentiate between an upper motor neuron lesion and a lower motor neuron lesion.

*Deep tendon reflexes*    Since the eliciting of a deep tendon reflex (DTR) or a muscle stretch reflex depends upon stimulating receptors deep within the skin, namely, the tendon and thus the muscle spindles, the stimulus must be a sudden and slight stretch of the tendon. This results in a discharge of motor units which causes a muscle contraction and tests the integrity of the reflex arc and the lower motor neurons.

To obtain the most effective response, position the patient so that the muscle to be tested is slightly stretched. The part to be tested is relaxed, and the patient is at rest. The best position is intermediate between full flexion and full extension.

If the response to testing the DTR is insufficient or absent, the examiner should repeat the procedure but first: (1) change the tension on the muscle by moving the position of the limb, or (2) try reinforcement. Reinforcement involves tensing muscles other than those being tested through isometrics which serves to increase reflex activity in the muscles being tested. Examples of reinforcement are asking the patient to lock the fingers of both hands together and trying to pull the hands apart; asking the patient to clench both fists or clench the teeth. If reinforcement is used, it must be noted.

The results of the DTR examination are usually recorded on a "stick figure" by a numerical graduation of 0 to 4 which is interpreted as follows:

0    No response

1    Diminished, below normal

2    Average

3    More brisk than normal

4    Hyperactive; suggestive of upper motor neuron disease

Practice will familiarize the examiner with normal and abnormal results. When the patient is tested, both sides of the body should be symmetrically positioned. Also, the production of any other muscular movements such as clonus (rhythmic oscillations of the limb when the muscle contracts) or fasciculations (the twitching of individual muscle fibers) is significant and should be noted and recorded.

In the actual testing, a reflex hammer is used. The examiner should grasp it so that a rapid blow can be struck. With the wrist loose, the hammer is held loosely between the thumb and index finger so that it swings easily in an arc.

The usual *DTRs* tested are as follows: (1) The biceps reflex (C5, C6). The patient's arm is slightly flexed at the elbow with the palm down. The examiner's thumb is placed on the biceps tendon, and a blow is struck over the thumb. The biceps muscle should contract, and flexion of the forearm at the elbow should occur. (2) The triceps reflex (C7, C8). The patient's arm is flexed at the elbow with the forearm held across the abdomen. The hand of that arm is supported with the palm toward the body, and a blow is struck over the triceps tendon. The triceps muscle should contract, and the arm should extend at the elbow (Fig. 31-22). (3) The brachioradialis reflex (C5, C6). The forearm should rest in the patient's lap. The hand is supported in a semi-prone position, and the tendon over the radius is struck about 1 to 2 inches above the wrist. The result should be flexion and supination of the forearm. (4) The patellar reflex (L2, L3, L4). The patient is usually sitting or lying with his or her knee in a flexed position. The examiner's hand supports the knee, and the patellar tendon (just below the patella) is struck, noting contraction of the quadriceps muscle and extension of the knee. (5) The ankle

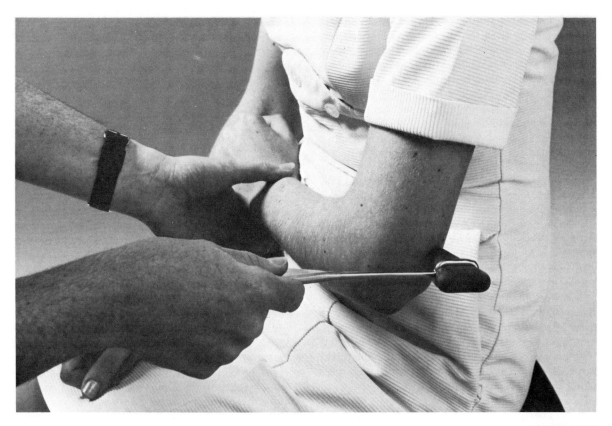

**FIGURE 31-22**
The triceps reflex test.

reflex (S1, S2). With the patient's leg somewhat flexed at the knee and the foot supported with the examiner's hand, the Achilles tendon is struck above the heel. The contraction of the tricepssural muscle and plantar flexion of the foot are noted as well as the speed of relaxation after contraction.

*Superficial reflexes*  The *superficial reflexes* result from stimulation of surface receptors in the skin. Since the reflexes have pathologic responses when there is an interruption in the connections to the upper motor neurons, they are usually indicative of an upper motor neuron lesion. Thus, although the areas tested may innervate a specific dermatomal segment, the eliciting of a pathological response does not as clearly indicate a disorder of that segment as is more often true of the deep reflexes.

As is true for other sensory testing, the nature of the stimulus is significant, and alterations may have to be made in the application of the stimulus to evoke a response. For example, the plantar reflex depends upon the pressure, velocity, and length of the stroke, and this may have to be adjusted to truly assess the patient. Also, the key to a response is its "reproducibility" with some degree of consistency in order to evaluate it as a true response.

In testing for the *plantar reflex* (L4, L5, S1, S2), the patient should be told that pressure on the sole of the foot may be experienced. The patient's position should be supine, the extremities should be symmetrical, and the legs should be extended. A blunt object such as a broken tongue blade, a key, or the end of the handle of the reflex hammer is then placed at the heel and moved along the lateral margin of the foot and lifted before reaching the base of the toes. The object may have to be applied longer by swinging it along the ball of the foot. If no response occurs, the length, pressure, or velocity of the stroke may need to be altered. In the adult, the normal response should be flexion of the toes, while a pathological result would be extension of the toes, otherwise known as the Babinski response, or "upgoing toes."

When tested for the *superficial abdominal* reflexes, the patient should be relaxed. The length of the stimulus and the time of the stimulus may vary in evoking a response. The abdomen of the patient is stroked with a blunt object from the lateral aspect toward the umbilicus on both sides. To test the upper superficial abdominals (T8, T9, T10), the stroke is above the umbilicus. To test for the lower superficial abdominals (T10, T11, T12), the stroke is below the umbilicus. The normal response elicits a contraction of the abdominal muscles with the umbilicus moving toward the side of stimulation. These are present in the normal individual but may not be easily seen in aged, obese, or multiparous patients who have weak abdominal muscles.

The *cremasteric reflex* (L1, L2) may be tested in males; there is no counterpart in females. The skin of the inner aspect of the upper thigh is lightly stroked with a blunt object. Observation is made for elevation of the testicle of that side.

The superficial reflexes serve only to indicate the possibility of a lesion in a specific area. Care must be taken to evaluate the whole patient through careful, complete examination. If there is interference with the efferent sensory supply at a lower level, an abnormal response may occur and necessitate further evaluation.

**Motor status** In assessing the patient's *motor status,* some general principles need to be kept in mind. As in the sensory examination, technique is important, and the motivation and ability of the patient to cooperate have to be evaluated before any conclusions can be drawn. Directions should be simple and clearly stated, especially if the patient is sensorily impaired.

Observations which are relevant to the motor examination persist throughout the entire neurological examination. The examiner should be alert to the patient's movement and coordination ability through all phases.

The patient is tested against himself or herself and an objective "normal." Thus symmetry of body movement is noted, and strength and range of motion can be assessed according to what is normal for a person of similar age, sex, and stature.

In all areas of motor evaluation, strength, fatigability, tone, and coordination are evaluated.

The creative investigator can assess motor strength without specifically putting the patient through the rigors of a formal examination. For example, a great deal of information can be obtained by asking the patient to "chew ice chips," "turn to one side," "pull up in bed," or "transfer from bed to a chair." Observation of flaccidity, ptosis, endurance, etc., provide many cues for necessary follow-up.

Usually, strength noted in distal muscles will indicate that proximal strength and nerve transmission are intact. This does not negate the need to examine both flexors and extensors of a given body area but does indicate a degree of intact function.

The motor examination serves as an indicator of dysfunction. Further investigation is necessary to identify the source of the difficulty, be it a myopathy, neuropathy, or central lesion. A total summation of cues is necessary to begin this process.

**C**ranial Nerves The motor function of the cranial nerves is evaluated specifically for each nerve. Occasionally, several nerves are evaluated together because of their related functions.

*IIId (oculomotor), IVth (trochlear), and VIth (abducens) cranial nerves* The motor components of these three cranial nerves are often concomitantly evaluated since all three innervate the eye and are responsible for eye movement. The third nerve is more extensive in its action as it is responsible for pupillary constriction and dilation and for motor function of the upper eyelid.

In testing eye movements, it must be remembered that all three nerves often act in an interrelated manner, and thus the movements may involve the action of all three nerves. Generally, the IIId cranial nerve moves the eye in four of the six tested directions. If one considers the six directions of gaze (lateral, medial, superior lateral, inferior lateral, superior medial, and inferior medial), which would correspond to four diagonal directions and two horizontal directions, then one can identify the areas of primary innervation of the separate cranial nerves as well as the areas of testing. The IVth (trochlear) nerve is responsible for the downward, inward gaze of each eye, and the VIth (abducens) nerve is responsible for movement laterally. The IIId (oculomotor) nerve is primarily responsible for the other four directions. To test these nerves, proceed as follows: (1) Ask the patient to cover the eye not being tested. (2) Hold an object approximately 12 to 18 inches away from the uncovered eye, and ask the patient to follow it with his or her gaze. (3) Move the object through each of the six directions of gaze (four diagnonal and two horizontal). (4) Note the range of movement of each eye. (5) Test the other eye in a similar fashion, and record the findings. (6) Repeat the procedure with both eyes in unison, and note any abnormality in the conjugation of movement.

The smoothness of movement and any other abnormality including *strabismus* (lack of coordination of movement in which the eyes do not always move in the same direction in a reciprocal manner), *diplopia* (a subjective complaint due to the above in which the patient reports "double vision"), or *nystagmus* (jerky eye movement which usually involves a fast and slow component and is usually named for the fast component) are noted. Any of these three conditions may require further investigation and may be due to either nerve or muscle dysfunction.

The conventional "testing of the pupils" involves these three cranial nerves (IIId, IVth, and VIth), but the emphasis is on the third nerve. *Pupil testing* includes checking size, reaction to light (pupillary constriction), consensuality, and convergence constriction (often known as *accommodation*). Often, normal functioning of the pupil according to size, reaction to light, and accommodation is noted as PERRLA, or pupils equal, round, and reactive to light and accommodation.

In an evaluation of *pupil size,* both eyes are examined together. The size of the pupils is observed as well as their location and relative degree of stability in remaining that size under constant external conditions. Evaluating pupil size in very dark eyes may be difficult, and thus a dim environmental light may be used. The best recording of pupil size is done in terms of actual millimeters, but merely noting equality may be sufficient.

To evaluate the *reactivity to light* (or pupillary constriction), the room is darkened to allow for dilation; a beam of light is aimed directly into the eye being tested, a sluggish or brisk constriction is noted, and the procedure is repeated for the other eye. This is a very significant clinical observation, especially in view of the possibility of increasing intracranial pressure. The examiner should, therefore, establish a baseline and report any change immediately. In addition, the test for *consensual constriction* should be carried out. This involves the simultaneous constriction of the pupil that is not receiving the light source. The anatomical distribution of the optic nerve (IId) with its stimulation of both oculomotor nerves results in this effect.

In testing for *consensual constriction,* the room is darkened and the examiner's hand or a card is placed between the two eyes so that a light source

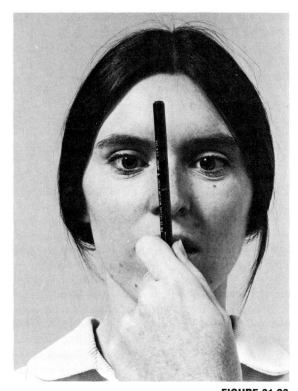

**FIGURE 31-23**
Testing for convergence constriction.

is able to reach only one eye. A light is directed into one eye, and the pupillary reflex is observed in the other eye. The procedure is repeated by shining the light source into the other eye.

The investigator should be aware that three separate reactions are necessary for *convergence constriction* (or *accommodation*). They are pupillary constriction (visible), convergence of the eyes (visible), and bending of the lens (not visible).

To test for *convergence constriction* (Fig. 31-23), the examiner asks the patient to look at an object held 12 to 18 inches in front of the nose. The object is moved closer, and constriction of the pupils and synchronous convergence of the eyes (which should persist until the object is 2 to 3 inches from the nose) are noted.

The oculomotor nerve also controls the *motor function* of the upper eyelid. Any drooping of this lid (ptosis) is therefore due to affectation of this nerve.

*Vth (trigeminal) cranial nerve*  The motor component of the Vth cranial nerve innervates the temporal and masseter muscles which control chewing and jaw movement. Testing these movements is done as follows: (1) The examiner observes for a "sunken" appearance at the temples (atrophy of the muscles). (2) The examiner places his or her hands on each cheek of the patient's face, with the fingers pointing upward; the patient is asked to bite, and the force of muscle contraction on both sides is noted. (3) The patient is asked to move the jaw from side to side against the resistance of the examiner's hands. Symmetry and strength of movement are noted.

*VIIth (facial) cranial nerve*   The seventh cranial nerve innervates the muscles of facial expression including the frontalis, orbicularis oculi, buccinators, and platysma. The patient is inspected for symmetry of movement during both volitional and emotional responses, since their pathways may be different. Testing the motor part of this nerve is done as follows: (1) The patient is asked to raise the eyebrows, frown, show his or her teeth, smile, and puff out the cheeks. (2) The patient is asked to close both eyes against resistance as the examiner attempts to open them. (3) Incomplete closure of the lower lids is noted, if present. (4) Any flattening of the nasolabial fold, putting of the mouth to one side, exaggeration of wrinkles at the side of the eye, and asymmetry of the face are also noted. This is especially important if some motor function of the upper part of the face is retained while that of the lower portion is lost, since it may indicate the area of the lesion. Facial paresis and paralysis may carry significant implications for nursing care, especially in regard to eating (see Chap. 34).

*IXth and Xth (glossopharyngeal and vagus) cranial nerves*   The evaluation of the motor components of the IXth and Xth cranial nerves involves an evaluation of speech, swallowing, and the previously described gag reflex. In assessing *speech,* any hoarseness, problems of phonation (the ability to make sounds via the vocal cord), and/or problems of articulation (the proper formation of sounds) should be determined. In *swallowing* the patient is asked to open the mouth and say "ahh." Observation is made of the position of the palatal arch and the movement of the uvula. Also noted is whether the palate elevates during stimulation of the gag reflex as opposed to voluntary stimulation. If the palate elevates unequally, the direction to which it pulls is significant. Further assessment of swallowing may be made by asking the patient to swallow ice chips which safely takes advantage of temperature and texture in the stimulation.

*XIth (spinal accessory) cranial nerve*   To test the spinal accessory nerve's innervation of the sternocleidomastoid muscles and the trapezius muscles (Fig. 31-24), the examiner places his or her right hand on the patient's left cheek and the left hand on the shoulder for bracing and to force his or her head to midline. The patient is instructed to turn the head to the left and hold it there against resistance. This is repeated for the other side. Contraction of the muscle turns the head to the opposite side and tilts it toward the same side. Both sternocleidomastoid muscles are tested simultaneously by asking the patient to push his or her head forward as the examiner pushes backward on the patient's forehead. The examiner's other hand is used to brace the person's neck. The trapezius muscles are tested by asking the patient to shrug both shoulders while the examiner actively resists the movement.

*XIIth (hypoglossal) cranial nerve*   The XIIth cranial nerve innervates the tongue. To assess its function, proceed as follows: (1) Start by assessing the patient's speech and articulation. (2) Ask the patient to open the mouth, which is observed for atrophy or involuntary movements. (3) Also ask the patient to protrude the tongue, and note any deviation to one side. This will usually indicate a disorder of the nerve on the opposite side. (4) Ask the patient to push the tongue into the cheek, and note the bulge it makes as an indication of strength. Compare both sides.

**Assessment of Intact Musculoskeletal System**   The assessment of the rest of the motor component of the musculoskeletal system can also be carried out in a rather systematic manner. While the maintenance of tone, strength, balance, and coordination is complex physiologically, the examination follows a sensible, organized pattern which looks first at the whole person at rest and in movement and then proceeds to specific muscle groups and follow-up on any specific complaints. Tests for cerebellar function will follow the delineation of the rest of the examination. The formal examination should proceed in a *rostrocaudal* manner by testing the cranial muscles, then the muscles of the neck, shoulder, arm, hand, abdomen, hip, thigh, leg, and foot. The significance of the findings should be evaluated against the total findings, as they may be indicative of local muscle or nerve disorders or dysfunction of the spinal segment innervating that muscle group.

The actual testing is usually done by offering resistance to active movement with the awareness

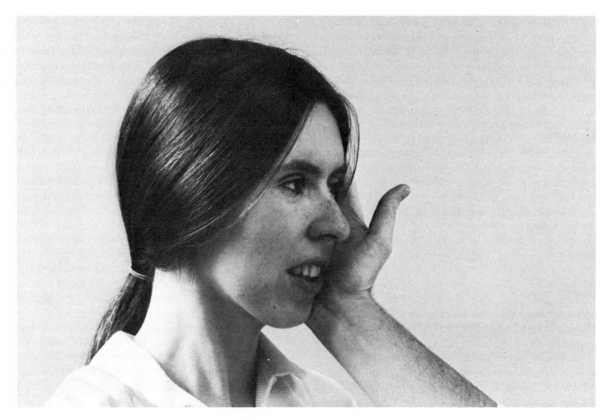

**FIGURE 31-24**
Testing for functioning of the spinal accessory nerve.

that the patient's position of strength is most often achieved when the muscle to be tested is in its shortest position, which usually leads to greater accuracy in testing; i.e., the biceps is usually tested by resisting the patient's flexion of the arm. Very strong muscles, on the other hand, such as the quadriceps, may have to be tested from a position of disadvantage so that evaluation is possible.

The usual method for recording muscle strength is a scale from 0 to 5, with 5 being indicative of normal function. The range is as follows:

0   No contractility

1   Some contractility but no joint motion

2   Complete range of motion without gravity

3   Complete range of motion with gravity

4   Complete range of motion with some resistance

5   Normal function against full resistance

The motor examination begins with the first meeting with the patient. While the patient is in a standing position, the examiner evaluates posture, symmetry, body contour, joint alignment, and any abnormal movements, being alert to atrophy of any muscle groups.

Then the patient should be observed in motion, as in walking across the room. The gait is observed for steadiness, arm swinging, separation of the feet, and elevation of the toes and heels. Balance can be quickly assessed at the same time as gait, by asking the patient to walk in a straight line with one foot in front of the other. Then, the patient should be asked to walk on the toes and on the heels. Finally, a deep knee bend should be accomplished, if feasible.

The motor examination of the musculoskeletal system has two basic components, evaluation of *muscle tone and range of movement* and evaluation of *muscle strength.* The first component involves putting the limbs through their normal range of movement and noting in the process, not only the extent of the *range of motion* but the *tone* of the limb at the same time. The examination progresses systematically in a rostrocaudal fashion beginning with the neck, shoulder, upper arm, lower arm, wrist, fingers, waist, hip, knee, ankle, and toes. Bilateral symmetry is followed to compare one extremity with the other. Flexion, extension, and hyperextension, as well as rotation, abduction, adduction, pronation, supination, inversion, and eversion, should be included where applicable.

In terms of tone, the patient is asked to relax during the above procedure. However, the muscle groups should possess a degree of tension integrity that minimally resists movement. Any deviations from this norm should be noted, such as flaccidity, spasticity, pain, rigidity, or posturing (see Chap. 32).

The second component of the motor examination is the testing for *muscle strength.* This evaluation also proceeds systematically in a rostrocaudal manner, using the body's symmetry to test one extremity against the other.

*Shoulder girdle and upper arm muscles*  *Arm elevation* is tested by asking the patient to hold both arms out to the sides (adduct); the examiner then pushes down on the arms as the patient attempts to resist. To test for arm adduction *downward,* the patient is asked to repeat the position described for testing arm elevation but to resist all efforts to elevate the arms.

*Muscle strength* is evaluated by asking the patient to extend both arms in front and to cross them at the wrists; the degree of strength is noted when the examiner attempts to pull them apart. *Scapular adduction* is tested by having the patient place both hands on the hips and force his or her elbows backwards against the examiner's attempt to push them forward. *Scapular winging* and *serratus anterior weakness* are tested by having the patient lean against a wall with arms outstretched, or by having the patient resist downward force with both arms horizontally outstretched; observation is for protrusion of the tip of the scapula. In testing for "drift" of the lower arms that may be suggestive of hemiparesis, the patient is asked to close both eyes and hold both arms horizontally outstretched with the palms supinated. This position is held for 30 seconds, and the person is observed for pronation of the hands and bending at the elbow. Observation for "drift" may also be made by having the patient close both eyes and vertically extend both arms overhead with the hands pronated. Then, with the patient keeping the arms in the same position, the examiner stands behind the patient and attempts to push the wrists downward. The strength of resistance to this pushing is noted. To test the *triceps*

and *biceps muscles,* the patient is asked to extend both arms horizontally in front with the forearms flexed at the elbow. The examiner attempts first to push each wrist upward and then downward against the patient's resistance.

*Forearm muscles*  To test the functioning of the forearm muscles, the examiner asks the patient to hold both arms with the forearms flexed horizontally and the hands pronated in front of his or her body. The examiner places one hand against the back of the patient's hand and the other hand under each forearm, behind the wrist. The patient is asked to resist attempts to flex the wrist. Weakness may indicate radial nerve disorders. The position of the examiner's hands is then switched to the palmer surface of the patient's hands and the dorsa of the forearm. Again, evaluation is made of efforts to resist dorsiflexion of the wrist.

The muscles of flexion and extension of the fingers are in the forearm. To test these functions, the examiner places his or her middle finger on top of his or her index finger and asks the patient to grip both fingers as tightly as possible. The examiner then attempts to pull the fingers from the patient's grasp.

*Finger muscles*  *Finger flexion* is tested by having the patient make a ring out of his or her fingers by pressing the tip of the thumb against the other fingers. The examiner's thumb is hooked into this ring and attempts are made to break out of it. The patient is next asked to *abduct* his or her fingers and the examiner's fingers are placed against the patient's index and little fingers. The examiner then squeezes his or her fingers together to test the strength of the patient's extensors. Ulnar nerve disorders may cause weakness.

*Abdominal muscles*  The patient is asked to lie in a supine position and is instructed to do a sit-up or to raise both legs or the head. The umbilicus is watched as the abdominal muscles contract. If weakness exists, the umbilicus will move toward the stronger muscles.

*Hip girdle*  For a test of the muscles of the hip girdle, the patient is placed in a supine position and is asked to abduct both legs and to resist all attempts to adduct them. This is repeated with the legs in adduction against attempts to abduct them. The patient is then placed in the prone position and asked to lift one leg at a time off the table to test the hip extensors. Finally, while in a supine position, the patient is asked to lift one leg at a time off the table against resistance to test hip flexors.

*Thigh muscles*  *Flexion* at the knee is tested by instructing the patient to flex each leg at the knee with the foot on a flat surface. The examiner places one hand on the patient's knee and one hand under the ankle. The patient is asked to resist efforts to straighten the leg.

*Extension* is tested similarly by asking the patient to lift each foot 6 to 8 inches off the surface. The examiner places one hand under the knee and the other on the ankle. The patient is instructed to straighten the leg against the resistance.

*Leg muscles*  Plantar flexion is assessed by having the patient walk on his or her toes. The patient should be asked to stand on the toes of one foot at a time. Further evaluation is accomplished by having the patient invert and evert each foot. In a supine position, plantar flexion and dorsiflexion may be tested against the resistance of the examiner's hand.

**G**ait, Balance, and Coordination  The final part of the motor examination involves evaluation of *gait, balance,* and *coordination.* While proper function demands integrity of the entire nervous system, the assessment of these properties introduces several tests which are often significant of cerebellar or basal ganglion function. Smoothness of movement, coordination of movement, or confusion of movement are noteworthy aside from the actual motion of muscle groups. Of course, the patient must be alert and able to comprehend directions, as well as being in a situation where they can be carried out.

*Gait and balance*  In the initial part of the motor examination, the investigator studies the patient's gait while the patient is walking across the room. The description of any abnormality of gait should be objective and comprehensive as to posture, balance, foot placement, specificity of body involvement, and position sense as well as the total pattern of movement.

Some of the more common *gait abnormalities* are these: (1) Spastic hemiparesis. This affects primarily one side of the body. The arm is often flexed and immobile, and the leg is often pulled forward in a semicircle with a toe drag. (2) Scissors gait. The legs tend to cross each other and the steps are short and stiff. (3) Steppage gait. The patient tends to overelevate the foot and then place it with a slap. This is the gait of foot drop. (4) Ataxia. There is a general lack of coordination of movement. The balance is poor; the gait is wide based and staggering, and the swinging of the arms is not coordinated. (5) Parkinsonian gait. This is characterized by akinesia, tremor, and rigidity. The gait is shuffling, the body is still, and the person may demonstrate propulsion or retropulsion in the initiation of the gait.

*Cerebellar function* is tested by observing *whole body coordination* (via the previously described Romberg test) and *arm and hand coordination.* Arm and hand coordination may be evaluated using rapid, rhythmic, alternating movements and the point-to-nose test. Rapid, rhythmic, alternating movements are tested on each hand separately and slowness or awkwardness of movement in these activities is noted. The patient should pat one leg with his or her hand as quickly as possible, pronate and supinate each hand as rapidly as possible, and touch each finger with the thumb as rapidly as possible. In point-to-nose testing, the patient is asked to keep both eyes open and to touch the examiner's index finger and then his or her nose, using the index finger. This is repeated with the eyes closed.

*Leg coordination*  Rapid rhythmic alternating movement is tested by asking the patient to tap the examiner's hand with the ball of his or her foot as quickly as possible. Point-to-point testing is done by asking the patient to place one heel on the other knee and to run it down the shin to the foot; in a normal reaction the heel would not fall off the shin. A final test of leg coordination is to see how quickly and effectively the patient can draw a figure eight with the big toe of each foot.

### Diagnostic Tests

To supplement the physical assessment of a patient, certain diagnostic procedures are frequently used to gain information about a patient's neurological condition. There are several factors which deserve to be considered for patients undergoing many of these neurodiagnostic procedures.

Most of these procedures necessitate the signing of a consent form by the patient, or by a responsible family member if the patient is unable to do so. This, of course, means *informed* consent of the patient and family. While the physician is responsible for explaining the specifics of the procedures, the nurse is responsible for reinforcement of this information, assessment of the patient's learning, and appropriate attention to anxiety.

Specific information about these procedures will vary according to the facility and its policies, such as the place of the procedure (operating room, neuroradiology unit, etc.), the use of equipment, and specific routines for aftercare. These should be investigated by the nurse in the individual setting.

Many of these procedures are used in conjunction with one another, and the nurse will have to convey the total perspective of diagnosis to the patient in order to reinforce the rationale behind these tests. It must be kept in mind that some of the techniques of the procedures, as well as the procedures themselves, will become outdated as technology as a whole advances. This is especially significant in neurodiagnosis since the procedures tend to be invasive, painful, and very anxiety provoking.

**Electroencephalography** The *electroencephalogram (EEG)* involves the use of electrodes to produce a graphic record of the electrical activity of the brain. The test is employed primarily to indicate the focus or foci of seizure activity and to evaluate quantitatively the level of brain function. This is done by interpreting the frequency, amplitude, and characteristics of brain waves.

The usual procedure involves the transportation of the patient to the EEG room where electrodes are applied to the scalp in the prefrontal, frontal, temporal, parietal, and occipital areas. The scalp and hair should be free of hairpins, etc., and an electrode paste is used. The patient is instructed not to move during this procedure as this will create interference and alter the recording. Aside from the cleansing of the electrode paste from the hair, there is no specific aftercare of the patient and no notable side effects.

At times, a sleep EEG is indicated. The purpose is often to demonstrate the presence of temporal lobe epilepsy (Chap. 33). In such cases, a sedative, usually chloral hydrate, is administered 45 minutes prior to taking the EEG, and the procedure is performed as described.

**Echoencephalography** Ultrasound (echoencephalography) is useful diagnostically in that it is a noninvasive way in which to determine if there has been a shift in certain structures of the brain. Ultrasonic impulses are directed through the head where certain structures such as the skull and midline structures reflect the impulses back toward their origin, and these are recorded and projected onto an oscilloscope screen. The time intervals in this process are significant in that they reflect any deviation in the position of the reflecting structures that may be caused by space-occupying lesions, subdural hematomas, etc. There is no specific risk to this procedure and no specific preparation or aftercare.

**Computerized transaxial tomography (EMI scanner)** The computerized transaxial tomography (CTT) scan is a noninvasive x-ray procedure (Fig. 31-25). It makes use of a rotating x-ray beam in conjunction with a computer and an oscilloscope. The machine scans the patient's head 180 times at different angles. Differential absorption by the tissues, in contiguous slices, is calculated by a computer. The information is then displayed in two ways: (1) by a computer printout of numbers corresponding to varying densities of the brain substance, and (2) by an oscilloscopic visualization in shades of gray which also correspond to the density of tissues. This is recorded on Polaroid film. An injection of contrast material can also be used to enhance the detail of the readings.

The CTT scan has been of major significance as a neurological diagnostic tool. It distinguishes normal from abnormal tissue and provides three-dimensional information, whereas traditional scans have provided information in only two dimensions. As such, it has provided direction for further diagnostic tests and eliminated the need in some instances for the more dangerous procedures, for example, pneumoencephalography and arteriography. It is helpful in defining both benign and malignant lesions, like cysts, vascular extremities, tumors, and the presence of blood, CSF, bone calcifications, edema, and air. It also provides information about some areas which are inaccessible to other radiographic studies such as the posterior fossa and the eye and its contents. When used in combination with nuclear medicine scans, the degree of accuracy is improved, and false positives and negatives can be eliminated as with scalp lesions, bone metastases, and tumors.

There are no contraindications to the use of the EMI scanner. When contrast material is used, however, an allergy to the contrast substance may constitute a contraindication.

No specifics of diet or dress are required. The hair should be free of hair spray and bobby pins. The patient lies on a table in front of the scanner, and the head is placed in a rubber cap which projects into a water-filled Lucite acrylic resin cube (Fig. 31-25). The patient is instructed not to move when the machine is in operation but does not have to hold his or her breath. Speech is permitted during the procedure, provided no movement is involved.

The x-ray machine rotates around the patient's head and takes readings at 4- to 6-minute intervals. The entire procedure requires approximately 1 hour. No specific aftercare is involved.

**Brain scan** The *brain scan* was developed prior to the EMI scanner and is often used in conjunction with the EMI scanner, especially when tumors are suspected. Essentially, it takes advantage of the fact that abnormal tissue lesions in the brain often are more vascular and, therefore, accumulate the radioactive isotope more quickly and more freely than normal tissue. The radioactive isotope most commonly used today is technetium-99(m) which has a half-life of 5 to 6 hours and a good energy output.

A test amount of the substance is usually given intravenously before the scan to check for sensitivity. If there is no reaction, the substance is injected; the scan proceeds with the patient in a supine position while the x-ray machine is positioned closely overhead. The procedure takes several minutes, and afterward the patient has no restriction in activity and no specific aftercare.

The brain scan has a high degree of accuracy in the detection of brain tumors, especially the vascular tumors such as meningiomas and gliomas (Chap. 35). Avascular tumors and tumors in the posterior fossa are more difficult to define, in the latter case owing to the muscle mass that is anterior to it. Other irregularities that break the blood-brain barrier or displace normal tissue are also seen, such as clots or infection.

**Arteriogram** Cerebral *arteriography* is a dangerous yet vital procedure in the diagnosis of intracranial pathologies. Essentially, it involves the injection of a radiopaque substance into the cerebral circulation with the simultaneous and subsequent roentgenological examination of selected intracranial and extracranial vessels.

Indications for the use of cerebral arteriography include: (1) Suspicion of an abnormality of the structure of the cerebral blood vessels such as an aneurysm, arteriovenous malformation, spasm, or clot in a vessel. (2) Displacement of the normal cerebral circulation by a space-occupying lesion. (This is informative both diagnostically and in establishing preoperative landmarks.) (3) Identification of certain neoplasms which may either ac-

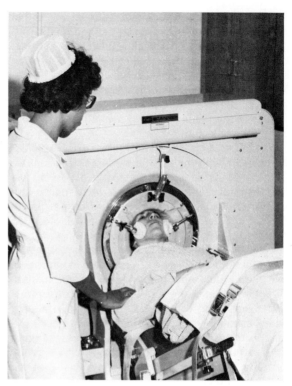

**FIGURE 31-25**
Computerized transaxial tomography.

cumulate or fail to accumulate the dye, depending upon the histology. In this case, arteriography may serve as a "backup" to other diagnostic tests. (4) To check the status of the patient postoperatively, especially after vascular surgery that involved ligation of a vessel or when the patient's condition has changed and bleeding or clot formation is suspected.

The use of cerebral arteriography may be contraindicated when the general condition of the patient indicates that the procedure may be too traumatic, since the procedure itself may induce spasm or thrombosis of the cerebral vessels. Such a contraindication may exist especially in elderly patients who have marked arteriosclerosis or vascular disease. Obviously, the necessity of the procedure in the diagnosis and further treatment of the illness must be weighed against these conditions, on an individual basis, and the patient or responsible family member must be made aware of the risks. The complications which may occur as a result of this procedure include: seizures, petechial hemorrhages of the retina, pupillary irregularities, shock and peripheral collapse, hemiparesis, aphasia, hypertension, respiratory distress, exacerbation of existing neurological signs, and death.

Cerebral arteriography may be of several types: carotid, transfemoral, brachial, or an "arch" (aortic) study, depending upon the location of the lesion. The nursing significance of the above relates primarily to the aftercare at the site of the injection as well as to the predictability of complications owing to the site selected.

In general, a carotid arteriogram involves injection directly into the carotid vessels with visualization of the carotids and the circle of Willis. The transfemoral approach is used to visualize the aortic arch and its branching vessels, as well as the carotid circulation. The vertebral vessels are also explored via a transfemoral approach by way of the subclavian artery. The brachial artery is not one of choice but may be used as an alternate to approaching the aortic arch and subclavian circulation. Direct injection of the vertebral artery is dangerous and painful and therefore not often used except when absolutely necessary since the same information may often be gained via the transfemoral approach. On some occasions, a "retrograde" vertebral arteriogram may be done to visualize the vertebral circulation. This involves injecting the dye directly into the right carotid circulation; the dye is then forced "against the current" into the subclavian artery and vertebral circulation in a retrograde manner.

The preprocedure teaching of the patient (and patient's family) about to undergo cerebral arteriography should specifically include: reinforcement of the serious nature of the procedure without causing undue anxiety; the preprocedure preparation of the patient (nothing taken by mouth after midnight, removal of rings, dentures, etc., premedication); length of time of the procedure; perceptions likely during the procedure such as a warm, flushed feeling, especially in the head, a salty taste in the mouth, and possibly headache; postprocedure care including frequent checking of vital signs and neurological observations, and documentation of the patient's response to and understanding of the above information.

After the arteriogram is completed, the nurse is responsible for assessment of the patient's physical condition. This includes observing for any difficulties and/or complications such as stroke, shock, hematoma, altered level of consciousness, changes in pupil size and reactivity, altered motor strength, and, when applicable, interference with circulation as shown by decreased or absent pedal pulses or radial pulses. Close evaluation for any respiratory compromise caused by edema or hematoma around the trachea should be made. The psychological status is assessed including the presence of anxiety, fear, or relief.

Nursing interventions are specific for the problem. If edema is present around the trachea, an ice collar should be applied. If there is further bleeding, a sandbag is applied, but primarily the site should be checked frequently, keeping the extremity extended and avoiding flexion; bed rest is usually ordered for an appropriate period of time (24 hours). To prevent the hazards of immobility, the patient may turn, provided the injected extremity is extended, and may eat but should remain in bed.

**Cerebrospinal fluid procedures** The other diagnostic procedures which are frequently performed include: lumbar puncture, myelogram, pneumoencephalography, and ventriculogram. These procedures are somewhat associated in that they involve exploration or delineation of the central nervous system's circulatory system (CSF) in order to determine pressure changes, chemical changes, or structural changes. The procedures differ both diagnostically and technically, but all are invasive and involve varying degrees of risk, discomfort, and postprocedure concern to the patient.

Lumbar Puncture   The *lumbar puncture* (LP) is the introduction of a hollow spinal needle into the subarachnoid space of the spinal canal under sterile technique for diagnostic or therapeutic purposes. The needle is usually introduced at the L4 to L5 level so that interception of the cord is minimized, since the cord ends at about L1 to L2.

Diagnostically, an LP is done to: (1) Measure cerebrospinal fluid pressure (opening pressure normally is 60 to 150 mm $H_2O$). (2) Obtain specimens for the appropriate laboratory tests. These usually involve sugar, protein, culture, sensitivity, and cytology. (3) Check for signs of noncommunicating hydrocephalus and pathology such as hemorrhage. (4) Inject air, dye, or drugs into the spinal canal.

Therapeutically, an LP may be done to relieve intracranial pressure, inject therapeutic agents, or administer spinal anesthesia.

A lumbar puncture is contraindicated in the presence of increased intracranial pressure due to an intracranial tumor since herniation of the brain through the foramen magnum may be precipitated. Additionally, an LP would not be performed if another diagnostic procedure which would yield the same specimens were to be carried out in the near future such as myelography or pneumoencephalography.

Complications of the lumbar puncture are

usually relatively minor; however, the patient may experience a great deal of temporary discomfort. The most common complication is spinal headache due, in part, to leakage of spinal fluid around the puncture site and withdrawal of CSF. Additionally, the patient may experience nuchal rigidity due to meningeal irritation, a rise in temperature, local signs of discomfort at the procedure site due to trauma, pain in the back radiating to the leg due to nerve root irritation, and some difficulty in voiding. These should all subside within a few hours.

The lumbar puncture is usually performed with the patient lying in a lateral position, with the head and neck flexed onto the chest, and the knees pulled up into the chest. The back (lumbar area) should be straight and close to the side of the bed. The patient may need assistance in maintaining this position. The physician performs the puncture, using sterile technique after local anesthesia has been injected. It is usually significant to note the "opening pressure" as measured by a manometer. The column of CSF should fluctuate with the respirations. Once the specimens of CSF have been collected, the patient may at times straighten the legs. Often a "closing pressure" will be noted; then the needle is removed, and a sterile dressing is applied to the site.

The preprocedure teaching of the patient should include: an explanation of the purpose of the procedure; perceptions likely during the procedure such as discomfort due to the position; pain from insertion of the spinal needle and possible pain or tingling in the legs, and postprocedure care involving bed rest with the head flat and hydration.

After the lumbar puncture, the nurse should assess the patient's physical status including: movement of the extremities, altered sensation in the extremities, local pain at the injection site, leakage of blood or CSF at the injection site, and the ability to void. It is also important to assess the psychological status predominately evaluating anxiety and headache. Finally, vigilance must continue for the exacerbation of any of these complications, including infection. Headache can be prevented by instructing the patient not to elevate the head, although side-to-side turning is permitted. Hydration is encouraged. The ability to void should be checked to prevent urinary difficulty. Above all, the patient's total response to the procedure should be documented.

**C**isternal Puncture   In principle, this procedure is similar to the lumbar puncture. It is indicated when CSF must be obtained and an LP is contraindicated owing to subarachnoid block, or diagnostically to demonstrate a subarachnoid block. Procedurally, the needle is introduced in the midline below the occipital bone into the cisterna magna. The patient will be in a sitting position.

**M**yelography   The *myelogram* is a diagnostic procedure in which a contrast material is introduced into the spinal subarachnoid space in order to outline the spinal cord, spinal canal, and spinal roots by x-ray examination.

The procedure is indicated when an intraspinal mass causing compression of the spinal cord is suspected or when there is evidence of a root lesion such as a herniated intervertebral disk. The dye will localize the level of compression, outline the mass, and outline compression of the nerve roots. It is important to note that owing to dye permeability, there may be some conditions which are not clearly visualized by myelography. For example, lateral disk disease is, at times, not well defined even though the condition exists. The only contraindication to myelography is intracranial disease where herniation of the brain may result from interference in the dynamics of spinal fluid pressure.

Conceptually, the myelogram is similar to the lumbar puncture, which, in fact, is the procedure involved. The introduction of the dye, however, adds some special considerations to the care of the patient. The dyes used may be either water soluble or oil based, depending upon the clinical indications and the preference of the radiologist. An oil-based substance has the advantage of being relatively nontoxic to the CNS, but its disadvantages include a lack of delineation of detailed structures; an inability to move the dye infratentorially when it has been injected about the tentorium; and the necessity for removal of the substance since it is not reabsorbed. The potential danger of arachnoiditis exists if the substance is not removed. On the other hand, water-based substances may be more toxic to the CNS, and their diffusibility and lack of concentration usually limit their use to the lumbosacral area alone. The choice of a dye may indicate both the preprocedure teaching and the postprocedure care, and the nurse must be aware that as new dyes are found, the indications for use may change. The complications of myelography are similar to those which may occur with a lumbar puncture.

The preprocedure teaching should include the same general points that are important for an LP. Additionally, the nurse should: establish a baseline of neurological vital signs which indicate strength, movement, altered sensation, etc.; instruct the patient as to preprocedure measures (nothing to be taken by mouth from midnight, premedication, and the usual preprocedure routine of the hospital); inform the patient that during the test it is necessary to be tilted into up and down positions on the table so that the dye properly fills the spinal canal, and prepare the patient for the necessity of maintaining a specified postprocedure position either flat in bed or sitting up. The position will be determined by the type of dye used and by the decision as to dye removal.

After the myelogram, the nurse should take the same actions as indicated after a lumbar puncture. In addition, the nurse must pay special attention to: signs of infection or inflammation; dizziness, nausea, or vomiting; any weakness of the extremities, numbness, or inability to void; and positioning of the patient. If the dye has not been removed, the patient should sit up at a 30 to 45° angle so that the dye will not progress rostrally up the spinal canal and cause further complications.

**P**neumoencephalography    The procedure termed *pneumoencephalography* involves the introduction of air into the subarachnoid spaces, ventricles, and cisterns around the brain so that x-ray films may be taken to visualize the ventricular and subarachnoid spaces. It is performed to define any structural abnormality present in the ventricles or subarachnoid spaces. These abnormalities may consist of space-occupying lesions, or they may be unusual structural configurations which can reflect cerebral atrophy, etc. It is used in combination with other diagnostic tests such as the EMI scan to indicate a possible cause of seizures, cerebral atrophy, tumors, or traumatic malformations.

The PEG is contraindicated in the presence of increased intracranial pressure since herniation of the brain may result, particularly if the lumbar approach is used. In such cases, a ventriculogram may be performed instead.

The complications of a PEG involve postprocedure side effects such as an elevated temperature, chills, nausea and vomiting, and headache. The more serious complications might be herniation of the brain as demonstrated by brainstem irregularities or seizures.

The procedure for a PEG essentially follows that for a lumbar puncture which is performed in a sitting position. In this position an opening pressure of 300 to 400 mmH$_2$O is normal. Air is injected, initial films are taken, then some CSF is removed and more air is injected (up to 60 cc). During this procedure the patient is rotated to an upside-down position while strapped in a special chair as x-rays

are taken. Needless to say, it is a most uncomfortable procedure and may indicate general anesthesia in young or confused patients.

The preprocedure teaching of the patient is similar to the preceding procedures (LP and myelogram). Since the procedure is more elaborate and far more uncomfortable for the patient, the teaching should be comprehensive and establish realistic expectations without causing undue anxiety. In addition to the information relative to the lumbar puncture, the preprocedure care of the patient should include: establishment of baseline vital signs and instruction in preprocedure measures (such as taking nothing by mouth after midnight), in the positioning during the procedure, and in the postprocedure complications to expect, including an elevated temperature (within 24 to 48 hours), nausea, chills, and headache. If the patient is suitably informed, and reassured that measures will be taken to ease any discomfort, much of the anxiety may be allayed.

The postprocedure care of the patient will include the care normal to a lumbar puncture. In addition, the patient will be kept flat in bed for a longer period of time, up to 12 hours (air is reabsorbed within 24 to 48 hours); hydration is encouraged to assist the production of CSF; treatment of fever, nausea, vomiting, headache, and chills will be symptomatic. The nurse should also be aware of the possibility of seizures and be vigilant as to their occurrence.

**V**entriculography    A *ventriculogram* is similar to a PEG but involves direct injection of air into the ventricles for x-ray examination of the brain. This is done via burr holes.

The procedure is done for essentially the same reasons that a PEG may be performed. It is chosen instead of a PEG when, because of increased intracranial pressure, herniation might result if CSF is removed from the lumbar area. Since it involves direct injection of air into the ventricles, it does not allow for visualization of the subarachnoid spaces.

It is contraindicated when a less invasive procedure may be performed and when a view of the subarachnoid spaces is necessary. The complications are the same as for a PEG.

The procedure is complicated by the fact that it usually involves taking the patient to the operating room for the placement of burr holes in either the frontal, posterior, parietal, or occipital areas. Approximately 20 to 50 cc air is injected, and a small amount of CSF is removed. The patient is tilted into various positions, and x-rays are taken. The patient may be transported to the x-ray area, or the test may be done in the operating room, depending upon the facility.

The preprocedure care of the patient should include psychological preparation for a serious and anxiety-producing test, establishment of baseline vital signs, and preoperative teaching of the patient. This teaching includes explanation of the procedure, anesthesia, anticipated pain, preparation of the site (shaving of selected areas of the head), and postprocedure care (frequency of vital signs, dressings, position, and bed rest).

After the ventriculogram, the nurse should carefully observe the patient for side effects such as changes in intracranial pressure, headache, nausea and vomiting, diaphoresis, and changes in vital signs. Care relevant to the administration of anesthesia should also be given. Any side effects such as headache, nausea, vomiting should be treated symptomatically. The patient is maintained in the desired position (usually 10 to 15° head elevation) for at least 12 to 15 hours, and the response to the procedure is documented.

## REFERENCES

1   *Blakiston's Gould Medical Dictionary,* 3d ed., McGraw-Hill, New York, 1972, p. 1152.
2   *Ibid.,* p. 358.
3   Arthur C. Guyton, *Textbook of Medical Physiology,* 5th ed., Saunders, Philadelphia, 1976, p. 640.
4   Charles R. Noback and Robert J. Demarest, *The Human Nervous System: Introduction and Review,* 2d ed., McGraw-Hill, New York, 1975, p. 345.
5   Russell M. DeCoursey, *The Human Organism,* 4th ed., McGraw-Hill, New York, 1974, p. 300.
6   Fred Plum and Jerome Posner, *The Diagnosis of Stupor and Coma,* 2d ed., Davis, Philadelphia, 1972, p. 2.
7   *Ibid.,* p. 2.

## BIBLIOGRAPHY

Bates, Barbara: *A Guide to Physical Examination,* Lippincott, Philadelphia, 1974.
DeCoursey, Russell M.: *The Human Organism,* 4th ed., McGraw-Hill, New York, 1974.
DeMyer, William: *Technique of the Neurologic Examination,* McGraw-Hill, New York, 1969.
Guyton, Arthur C.: *Textbook of Medical Physiology,* 5th ed., Saunders, Philadelphia, 1976.
Mechner, Francis, Patricia E. Mahoney, and Lena J. Saffioti: "Patient Assessment: Neurological Examination," Pt. I, *Am J Nurs,* **75:**1511–1536, September 1975.
———, ———, and ———: "Patient Assessment: Neurological Examination," Pt. II, *Am J Nurs,* **75:** 2037–2062, November 1975.
——— and ———: "Patient Assessment: Neurological Examination," Pt. III, *Am J Nurs,* **76:**609–633.
Noback, Charles R., and Robert J. Demarest: *The Human Nervous System: Introduction and Review,* 2d ed., McGraw-Hill, New York, 1975.
Plum, Fred, and Jerome Posner: *The Diagnosis of Stupor and Coma,* 2d ed., Davis, Philadelphia, 1972.
Webb, Kenneth J.: "Early Assessment of Orthopedic Injuries," *Am J Nurs,* **74:**1049–1052.
Wheeler, Patricia: "Care of a Patient with a Cerebellar Tumor," *Am J Nurs,* **77:**263–266.

# 32

# TRAUMATIC DISTURBANCES IN PERCEPTION AND COORDINATION*

Ann E. Hinkhouse
Nell Ann Kirby**

Human beings encounter many hazards in the external environment. All too often these result in trauma to the body. When that trauma causes damage to the head or spinal column, disruptions in neurologic function may result. In the head this frequently results in increased intracranial pressure, and in the spinal cord it may result in sensory or motor disturbances. It is imperative that nurses be able to assess and intervene knowledgeably in the care of patients with these problems.

## HEAD TRAUMA

Craniocerebral trauma from an injury is static. Brain damage that occurs subsequently is a dynamic process that can be controlled or prevented. The hypoxia (insufficient cellular nutrition) and prolonged periods of increased intracranial pressure that may follow trauma can create more brain damage than the initial injury. The nurse's observation of changes in the patient's condition and response to treatment at any level of care can be a significant contribution to a safe recovery.

## Pathophysiology

The skull is a relatively closed structure; therefore, the cranial contents have limitations of expansion. The volume of cerebrospinal fluid (CSF), blood, and brain tissue must remain relatively constant at all times. Cerebrospinal fluid is displaced most easily and blood secondly, while brain tissue is least movable. Changes involving an expansion of any of these can potentially produce signs of *increasing intracranial pressure.* Since neurons do *not* regenerate once they are destroyed, they have the potential of suffering permanent damage from any inflammatory process that causes cerebral edema and a subsequent rise in intracranial pressure.

**Types of trauma** *Traumatic* origins of rising intracranial pressure may be primary or secondary. *Primary trauma* is the direct result of some force applied to the skull resulting in a fracture, hemorrhage, contusion, or concussion. There is no other intervening factor. A *secondary injury* is one in

* The section on head trauma was written by Ann E. Hinkhouse and the section on traumatic impairment of spinal cord function was written by Nell Ann Kirby.

** Ms. Kirby expresses appreciation to Arthur Siebens, M.D., who elucidated many of the principles presented here during two decades of colleagueship in the care of individuals with spinal cord dysfunction.

which some other medical condition causes a person to fall or otherwise to sustain a blow to the head. These conditions include diabetic, cardiac, epileptic, or hysterical problems, and situations following drug and/or alcohol ingestion in which the patient falls, strikes the head, and loses consciousness.

**Fractures, Hemorrhages, and Contusions**  The two primary processes which result from trauma and which produce cerebral congestion and increasing intracranial pressure are *fractures* and *hemorrhages* (Fig. 32-1). The frequency and severity of damage from these two processes can be greater at the base of the skull, which is much less smooth than the vault. Besides the foramen magnum, other irregularities at the base are the sphenoid and ethmoid bones and the sharp edges of the tentorium.

*Fractures*  *Linear* fractures are those in which there is a simple break in the continuity of the bone. *Comminuted* fractures are fragmented interruptions of the skull from multiple linear fractures (Fig.

32-1). In *depressed* fractures comminuted bone fragments penetrate the brain tissue. A *compound* fracture is any of the preceding which also has an opening through the sinuses, eardrums, or scalp.

*Hemorrhages*  An *epidural* hematoma is an accumulation of blood between the outer meningeal layer (the dura) and the skull. It usually results from a laceration of the middle meningeal artery (Fig. 32-1). Epidural hematomas usually follow severe injuries; fractures are often present, and a common location is temporoparietal. Symptoms of increased intracranial pressure develop rapidly owing to the arterial nature of this bleeding.

A *subdural* hematoma is a collection of venous blood between the outer (dura) and middle (arachnoid) meningeal layers (Fig. 32-1). There is little support for the veins crossing this space, and so they can be disrupted easily by trauma. Since a subdural hematoma frequently is associated with an apparently minor injury, assessment should include attention to seemingly trivial injuries. A patient with this problem often reveals slow development of the symptoms of increased intracranial pressure. In

**FIGURE 32-1**
Hemorrhages and fractures.

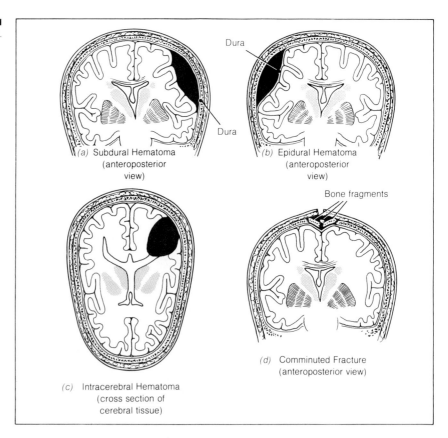

(a) Subdural Hematoma (anteroposterior view)

(b) Epidural Hematoma (anteroposterior view)

(c) Intracerebral Hematoma (cross section of cerebral tissue)

(d) Comminuted Fracture (anteroposterior view)

*acute* cases the blood may spread rapidly and widely since the only limits are the falx cerebri and the tentorium. *Subacute* and *chronic* versions are more common in those with cortical atrophy, such as alcoholics. In subacute or chronic cases the symptoms may be present intermittently;[1] so, unless this variable presence is remembered, the problem may not be accurately assessed.

Sudden compression of the brain tissue on the side opposite the injury (*contrecoup* injury) or penetration of the cerebral tissues by a foreign body can be associated with an *intracerebral* hematoma when deep vessels are torn (Fig. 32-1). Traumatic intracerebral hematomas can follow gunshot or stab wounds. Motor and sensory deficits may be slow (36 to 72 hours) to appear. The way in which the injury was sustained is an important factor to determine. Symptoms of increasing intracranial pressure from this hematoma are as described for the other hematomas.[2]

*Contusions*  Contusions of the brain tissue resemble bruises. There is only slight injury to small vessels with a small amount of bleeding into the surrounding tissues. The resulting effects of increased intracranial pressure are dependent upon the amount of contused brain tissue.

*Concussion*  The condition referred to as *concussion* is essentially a disruption of normal activity among some of the synapses of the neurons. It is a temporary disarrangement of normal nervous activity and by itself is not part of the two processes mentioned previously. Muscular activity and mental clarity usually return within a few minutes after trauma, although there may be residual amnesia for the event.

**Effects of trauma**  These major processes set up an *inflammatory response* that leads to *cerebral edema,* which in turn produces *increasing intracranial pressure.* A displaced fracture immediately reduces the space normally available for the cerebral contents and becomes an irritant to underlying cerebral structures. The reduced space and the inflamed, edematous structures cause a pressure rise. Lacerated veins or arteries permit more of the systemic blood to accumulate within the skull in a fairly short period of time, causing an increased volume of one of the three components (CSF, blood, brain tissue) plus irritation of the surrounding tissues by the extravasated blood, which acts as a foreign body. The extravasated blood increases the osmotic nature of the area in which it is confined.

Thus, more water is drawn to the area, contributing to the space-occupying mass and creating pressure.

Contusions produce some inflammation even with their small amount of blood seepage. Gunshot or stab wounds of the head result in immediate displacement of structures and deposition of a foreign body that diminishes the space usually available for cerebral contents. Unless a concussion is associated with some inflammatory process, it should not cause an increase in intracranial pressure since it does not produce cerebral edema.

**Increased Intracranial Pressure**  Injuries that produce *increased intracranial pressure* can have dramatic effects as the cranial contents have little time to compensate for the increasing pressure after sudden injury. Immediate changes may occur, or if the pressure increases gradually, the effects on the patient may be subtle. Whether the onset is gradual or sudden, the ultimate effects are comparable. The patient's *level of consciousness* is most reflective of changes in this pressure. Progressive lethargy, irritability, indifference to the surroundings, and lack of orientation to time, place, and person may occur. Orientation is lost first to time, then to place, and lastly to person. The foramen magnum, the opening through which the brainstem exits the skull, affords some pressure release. However, as pressure accumulates and before it is released through this opening, *changes in the person's state of wakefulness* will become apparent. This results from pressure on the reticular formation and ranges from drowsiness to coma.

The increasing pressure may also affect the vomiting control center in the medulla. Early after the injury, patients may experience *anorexia, nausea,* and *vomiting.* The vomiting may be projectile, especially in the presence of an epidural hematoma.

More objective measurable symptoms include *changes in motor functions,* such as progressive loss of movement of one or more extremities, loss of hand grip, inability to maintain balance while standing or walking, and paresis. The motor area of the brain, located in the precentral region of the frontal lobe, has descending fibers that form the pyramidal system. They cross in the medulla, and cranial lesions that increase pressure on these fibers above the decussation produce motor deficits on the *opposite* (contralateral) side of the body. *Flaccidity* is possibly the result of destruction of a faciliatory center in the reticular substance between the medulla and the midbrain. Injury to an inhibitory center in the same location results in rigid extension or *decerebrate posturing.*[3] Unless some of the naturally continuous motor activity is allowed, muscle tone is minimal; but unless some of the constant activity is checked, muscle tone becomes too intense. *Decorticate posturing* (rigid flexion) is similar to decerebrate posturing in that there is insufficient inhibition of continuous motor impulses.

Vital functions controlled by the brainstem also become disrupted. Pressure on the respiratory center, located in the medulla, results in *slow, labored respirations.* Slow breathing can lead to carbon dioxide retention with vasodilatation of the cerebral vessels and further aggravation of cerebral circulatory congestion. The extra cerebral blood volume further increases the intracranial pressure. An equally undesirable situation is that in which upper brainstem damage produces rapid respirations and an excessive loss of carbon dioxide. This condition leads to cerebral vasoconstriction and further hypoxia of the neurons. Either process becomes a vicious cycle in which the neurons are deprived of oxygen and basic nutrients. Many factors can cause insufficient ventilation. Some may be unrelated to the head injury but can produce the symptoms of confusion and coma similar to those from neurological deterioration (Fig. 32-2).

Another vital function that is controlled partially by the brainstem is *vasomotor activity.* Pressure on the lower portion of the brainstem can lead to slowing of the pulse. Arterial blood pressure can be affected by pressure in this same area.[4] Initially, after a head injury, the blood pressure is likely to rise and the pulse to decrease. The systolic pressure may show a greater increase as the body attempts to supply more oxygen to the injured neurons. Congestion from cerebral edema increases resistance to vascular flow into the cranium, resulting in a rise in blood pressure. Slowing of the pulse can be a reflex response to these arterial pressure changes. The respiratory and cardiovascular functions of the body are involuntary and are controlled by various processes; increasing intracranial pressure can affect the control exerted on these functions by the brainstem.

After intracranial pressure has had some time to build up, a *positive Babinski's sign* may also be evident. Stroking the bottom of the foot produces a

**FIGURE 32-2**

Results of impaired ventilation after trauma.

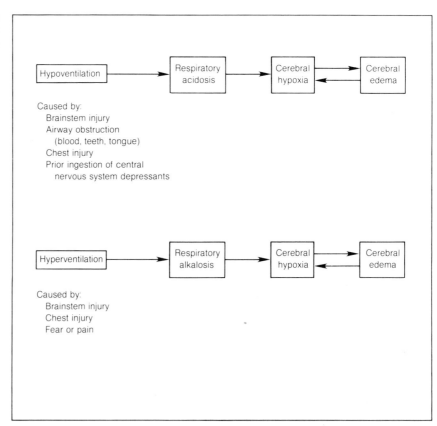

dorsiflexion rather than a plantar flexion of the large toe. This sign is usually evident on the side *contralateral* to the injury owing to compression of the corticospinal or pyramidal tracts before their decussation in the lowest portion of the medulla.

*Papilledema* is another indicator of rising intracranial pressure. Since the optic nerve is sheathed by the meninges, a rise in intracranial pressure involves increasing pressure of the cerebrospinal fluid, which is transmitted to this nerve. The nerve head or optic disk is pushed above the retina, creating a choked disk.[5]

A late visual change is *dilatation* and eventually *fixation of the pupil* from compression of the third cranial or oculomotor nerve. Increasing intracranial pressure that can no longer be accommodated forces part of the temporal lobe around the tentorium and against the brainstem. The oculomotor nerve is compressed at that point, and paresis of normal third-nerve functions occurs. This sign is usually *ipsilateral* (on the same side) to the injury unless there is so much pressure on the brainstem that it is shifted to the opposite side and reverses this sign and motor deficits as well.

The long-term effects of head trauma are dependent upon the severity of the initial injury. Persons who are in a deep coma, with absent reflexes and flaccid extremities, have a very poor prognosis. Those who are in a confused or semicomatose state often have a better prognosis for the resolution of the effects of the trauma.

### First-Level Nursing Care

Avoiding head trauma is a primary focus in preventing increased intracranial pressure. Nurses should be aware of the types of injury patients are susceptible to. They should have knowledge of *medical problems* that may lead to a loss of consciousness and of *environmental hazards* that may precipitate head trauma. In the home, safety varies somewhat with the *age* of the person considered. Children between 6 months and 2 years of age are likely candidates for chronic subdural hematomas of traumatic origin.[6] The accident may result from rolling off a bed and striking the floor, falling off chairs, or falling during early attempts to walk. An apparently minor injury can produce this condition, and child abuse at any age may involve head injuries. Home hazards for the elderly include loose rugs, highly polished or wet floors, and poorly arranged furniture. Disturbances in vision and equilibrium that are common with aging make the elderly susceptible to falls; changes in vascular and bony structures with age make them more vulnerable to head injury from these falls. Falling a considerable distance, as from ladders or roofs, is more common in young and middle-aged adults.

Accidents involving cars, trucks, motorcycles, and bicycles are a major cause of head injuries. Motorcycles and bicycles provide less protection to the rider, who is consequently more prone to sustain a severe head injury. If the driver of any of these vehicles is intoxicated, there may be impairment of reflexes and judgment, creating an additional hazard to the operator and others. The impact to the skull in an accident with a vehicle is potentially great because of the speed with which the head is moving at the time it is stopped. Pedestrians struck by these vehicles are also at risk.

In certain industries some machinery may be hazardous to the skull. Construction work involving the lifting of heavy items by cranes is dangerous to the laborer or bystander who may be unaware of the proximity of the item that is swinging as it is lifted by the crane. Workers with long hair may be at risk in factories if they work around machinery; there is danger of hair being caught in the equipment with a subsequent scalping and possible skull fracture. If floors in factories are wet, there is a risk of falling and striking one's head. Farming can precipitate other kinds of trauma. A farm worker can sustain a head injury when starting a piece of machinery if the upper part of the body is caught in or against it.

At school, children are susceptible to head injuries from falls off playground equipment and from being struck with baseball bats, hockey pucks, or balls. For older students, wrestling and striking the bottom of a swimming pool, when diving, can lead to craniocerebral trauma.

**Prevention of head injuries** Obviously it is desirable to prevent head injuries. Home safety should involve awareness of those physical objects hazardous to the inhabitants and either the correction or elimination of them. Sensitivity to those family situations that are likely to produce child abuse is vital for protection of the child against physical as well as emotional injury. The community health or clinic nurse is frequently the person in contact with high-risk families and should, therefore, assess them carefully.

The matter of safety of vehicles is reflected in nationwide attempts to require motorcyclists to wear helmets. New cars show improved designs of seats and restraints to protect passengers against injuries to the neck region. Children should be safely secured in the seats as well. Establishment of bicycle paths separate from main highways or busy streets indicates a community awareness of the need to protect bicyclists from larger vehicles. As the use of bicycles becomes more popular, this is a need that will probably increase. Prevention of further accidents by someone who operates motor vehicles while intoxicated may involve placement of that person in an educational program that discusses the hazards of such an action. All nurses should teach the public in this regard, within both community and institutional settings.

Industrial safety programs need to emphasize the necessity of wearing hard hats in potentially dangerous areas and keeping long hair covered to avoid entanglement in machinery. The dangerous parts of farm and other industrial equipment should be shielded. The industrial nurse has an infrequently recognized, but critical, role in assessing and preserving employee health.

Prevention of accidents in the school necessitates student awareness of safety regulations and sufficient monitoring by adults to ensure safe performance of activities. The school nurse should assess potential health problems and initiate corrective measures.

Nurses in any patient care situation can teach constantly about reducing hazards within the home environment. Proper use of equipment, such as ladders, should be constantly reinforced.

### Second-Level Nursing Care

The nurse in the community or outpatient situation may be the first person to assess the patient with head trauma. It is imperative that this assessment be thorough and accurate and that subsequent interventions be based upon the potential, as well as the existing, physical condition.

**Nursing assessment**  In the case of severe trauma, symptoms are usually dramatic and progress rapidly. Seemingly trivial injuries, however, may produce only intermittent indications of increasing intracranial pressure and should be thoroughly assessed in the community.

**H**ealth History   Questions should elicit the nature of the injury and when it occurred. The person may notice visual changes such as the presence of *diplopia,* or double vision, and may tilt the head to compensate for this defect. There may also be a sensation of *dizziness* from visual disturbances or from the increasing pressure.[7]

*Anorexia, nausea,* and *vomiting* are other early

symptoms of rising pressure. If the patient is becoming lethargic from rising intracranial pressure, anorexia may occur primarily because of the lethargy.

*Headaches* should be evaluated even in the presence of minor trauma. Duration, consistency, location, and nature of the pain are important factors to determine. A history of headaches prior to the injury needs to be elicited, to compare for any similarities. Any relationship of the pain to visual disturbances may be significant.

**P**hysical Assessment   It is important to look for obvious signs of injury. Lacerations, ecchymoses, and depressed areas on the head may give clues to the location and severity of the injury. *Battle's sign* is a bruise behind the ear indicative of a basal skull fracture. *Otorrhea* and *rhinorrhea* are important clues to identification of basal and frontal fractures, respectively; this drainage of cerebrospinal fluid from the ears or nose may be so slight that only the patient is aware of it, but its presence should be noted.

*Vital signs* should be taken to establish baseline readings. Afterward, they should be monitored closely for any temperature elevation, slowing of the pulse, or widening of the pulse pressure. Respirations may change in rate or increase in difficulty. Systolic blood pressure may increase if there is brainstem involvement, and any elevation should be noted.

The neurological examination is a basic tool in evaluating the patient who has experienced head trauma. Visual, motor, and behavioral assessments are particularly revealing.

The eyes should be observed for *strabismus,* or deviation of one or both eyes. This can occur following compression of the abducens nerve by increased intracranial pressure or by pressure on the oculomotor nerve.[8] At the same time, any *nystagmus,* a jerking movement of the eyes, should be noted. This can result from injuries to the cerebellum or to the brainstem,[9] or from damage to the oculomotor, trochlear, or abducens nerves.[10] Its presence should be described as vertical, horizontal, or both. The ophthalmascopic examination may reveal the presence of *papilledema* if there is pressure on the optic nerve.

If there has been a neck injury along with the head injury, *motor deficits* may also be present; neck injuries should be suspected when craniocerebral trauma exists. However, cranial trauma can also produce weakness or paralysis of parts of the body. The location, amount of weakness, and its progression should be determined by testing motor strength and sensation bilaterally. Frequently, weakness on the side opposite the injury is noted. Reflexes should be tested as well as the Babinski sign. Any absence of reflexes, hyperreflexia, or a positive Babinski's sign should be described.

*Behavioral changes* should be noted as they can be the earliest symptoms of increased intracranial pressure. Progressive *lethargy* or an increasing desire to sleep probably indicates increasing pressure on the reticular activating system (RAS). Even a concussion, which is primarily a physiological disarrangement of cellular activity, may affect the normal function of this system. Other behavioral changes that may be early symptoms are *irritability* and *belligerence.*

Any activity indicative of *seizures* needs attention. This may be a focal disturbance of one part of the body, progressive to several parts, or a generalized grand mal seizure. Besides these signs of electrical disturbances of brain activity, any loss of consciousness after the injury or amnesia for events before and after is a significant symptom. *Amnesia* or *loss of consciousness* for any period of time is usually indicative of a more severe injury.

**D**iagnostic Tests   Early assessment of the head-injured person in the community may involve some diagnostic tests to evaluate the extent of the injury and the need for more acute care. In the presence of a subacute head injury, *visual field* examination may reveal evidence and approximate location of an intracranial lesion. When a person's gaze is fixed in one direction, the space in which objects are visible is called the *field of vision.* To test it, the ability to see targets of different sizes and colors from various distances is plotted on a map of concentric circles. Peripheral vision is determined by moving a white test object along an arc away from the point of fixation until it disappears and then returning it to where it is seen. That point is the edge of the field of vision. Interruption of the optic nerve fiber tracts produces changes in the field of vision. *Homonymous hemianopsia* means a defect in the right or left half of the visual fields of both eyes; this results from interruption of the nerve behind the optic chiasm, where half of the fibers from each eye cross. A lesion at the chiasm produces *bitemporal hemianopsia* or visual loss in the temporal parts of each eye. Visual fields contract with atrophy of the optic nerve that occurs secondarily to papilledema from increased intracranial pressure. This, then, affects visual acuity.[11]

*Roentgenograms* or x-rays of the skull may show conditions causing cerebral congestion. In trauma, fractures or subdural hematomas may be visualized.[12] If the fracture is depressed, it is more likely to cause changes in intracranial pressure as it decreases intracranial space. Recognition of fractures in the bones around the sinuses is important since external openings through the sinuses permit the entrance of bacteria that may lead to infectious processes in the brain.

A very refined radiologic examination that has become available for patient use in the United States in the 1970s is *computerized axial tomography,* or the *EMI scan.* The technique of this procedure is explained in Chap. 31. Computerized tomography is considered to be superior in diagnosing epidural and acute subdural hematomas. Chronic subdural hematomas become diluted with time and are not as easily diagnosed.[13] It is felt that differential diagnosis is also more accurate with the EMI scan because cerebral edema, contusion, and hematoma have distinguishable absorption values.[14] Furthermore, if surgery becomes necessary following trauma to the head, the source of the hematoma or other lesion can be located more specifically.

Another noninvasive technique is *echoencephalography,* which is based on the use of ultrasound. A shift in the midline echo away from its central position is usually indicative of an increased cerebral volume that is causing rising intracranial pressure. The additional detection of a hematoma echo is viewed as even more conclusive evidence of such a process. Echoencephalography is especially useful in diagnosing epidural hematomas because of their usual temporal, parietal, or temporooccipital locations.[15]

*Electroencephalography* (EEG) is a procedure that measures the brain's electrical activity and can be done on an outpatient basis. It is probably most useful following trauma if done serially. Resolution or development of additional pathological waves may indicate posttraumatic abnormalities in cerebral electrical activity arising from some inflammatory process.

One other diagnostic procedure that can be done on an outpatient basis is *brain scanning.* Scanning that is done after trauma can be helpful in identification of subdural hematomas.[16]

A *lumbar puncture* is not recommended in the presence of suspected increased intracranial pressure because of the risk of temporal lobe herniation around the tentorium as some of the pressure is reduced with the removal of cerebrospinal fluid.

**Nursing problems and intervention** Identification of the early subjective and objective problems that follow head trauma varies with the severity of the injury. If the patient has sustained an injury severe enough to have lost consciousness, especially for a prolonged period of time, an immediate *referral* for medical care should be made. Referral should also be immediate if there are obvious depressions in the skull or other major open wounds.

The less obvious and more insidious indications of developing problems are the subjective ones. When the patient *loses consciousness* for only a few seconds or minutes and sustains only *minimal amnesia* for the event, it is difficult to determine whether the need is for immediate attention or only subsequent observation. The patient may appear normal to others and may subjectively notice nothing unusual. This person may be examined as an outpatient and diagnosed as having no neurological deficits; but, when back in the community, this person needs to be observed for *behavioral changes* and other early symptoms listed previously. The person with an apparently minor head injury requires less intense but continuous observation for slowly appearing symptoms. For those who are treated and released from an outpatient service, a relative or friend who will be with the patient should be taught the symptoms which would require the patient to return for further treatment. These symptoms should be written on a form that can be sent home with the patient, and a duplicate should be retained with the person's record at the treatment facility. Also advisable may be telling the relative or friend to awaken the patient every 1 to 2 hours at night for the first night after the injury to determine if there is progression toward a stuporous state. This person should be taught to look for changes in the size of the pupils, especially dilatation. If the patient has sustained a concussion, the sequel is unlikely to be serious since there is primarily a disruption of normal nervous impulse conduction at the synapses that resolves itself with time. Slowly developing *hematomas* eventually produce neurological deficits that an informed person can detect.

**E**mergency Care  If the patient has sustained a severe injury, intervention may involve *emergency care.* Such care includes establishment of a patent airway, assurance of adequate breathing for oxygenation of the cells, and support of an effective rate and volume of circulation. After these basic life functions are maintained, attention can be directed to the monitoring of increasing intracranial pressure. Establishing an initial set of baseline vital signs for subsequent comparison is important. Normal values vary among individuals, and progressive changes in these signs are usually more significant than the values obtained at one isolated time. A *rising blood pressure,* a *widening pulse pressure,* and *bradycardia* may be indicative of increasing intracranial pressure. However, the nurse should not wait for these symptoms to appear before thinking of the possibility of increasing pressure on the cerebral structures. The rapid intravenous administration of 250 to 500 ml 20% mannitol, if available, may be an immediate step to reduce cerebral edema because of its osmotic diuretic action.

If the patient is injured severely enough to necessitate acute care, referral arrangements should be made and potential transport problems anticipated. The *referral* should include a descriptive statement of how the injury occurred. When possible, this information should be obtained from the patient. Otherwise ambulance attendants or other witnesses should be questioned for details unless the patient's condition is deteriorating so rapidly that immediate transfer is mandatory. A copy of the treatments, observations, and assessments performed by those treating the patient initially should be sent. Other treatments specific for that patient may be arranged by verbal discussion between the transfer and the receiving facilities.

The person accompanying the patient should anticipate and be prepared to manage potential *respiratory* and *circulatory problems* during transport. An intravenous site with a solution infusing fast enough just to keep it open should be established, especially if there are other injuries that may lead to hypovolemic shock. An oral airway should be available, and preparations for entubation in transit should be made if the injury is serious enough for that to be a potential need. Respiratory assistance must be available in the form of a bag mask or portable respirator. During transport the attendant must keep a record of vital signs and neurological checks.

**Third-Level Nursing Care**

A patient experiencing increased intracranial pressure as a result of a head injury may be hospitalized soon after the trauma or days to months later, depending on the type of injury. Nursing assessment is a vital part of ongoing evaluation, as well as initial care.

**Nursing assessment** The *health history* should include details of the trauma incurred by the patient. It may be necessary to obtain this information from a witness or family member, depending on the patient's condition.

If the patient is alert, questions should elicit the exact nature and duration of any symptoms, including headaches, changes in sleep patterns, nausea, vomiting, changes in vision, and behavioral or personality alterations. Any pain, bleeding, or nasal drainage or stuffiness should also be noted and described. The patient will often relate a health history similar to that described under Second-Level Nursing Care.

*Physical assessment* requires accurate performance of neurological checks to evaluate changes that may indicate increasing intracranial pressure, as well as evaluation of the factors detailed under Second-Level Nursing Care. In checking the patient's eyes after head trauma, the nurse is primarily concerned with the oculomotor, or third cranial nerve, which controls pupil size and position. Unequal or slow accommodation to light and, especially, a fixed dilated pupil are indicative of increasing intracranial pressure. Reaction of the pupils directly to light should not be confused with *consensual reaction.* A check for consensual reaction evaluates the optic, or second cranial nerve as well as the third. When the examiner places a hand on the patient's nose and shines a light in one eye, the normal reaction is for both eyes to constrict simultaneously since the optic nerve being stimulated carries the impulse to the brain where both oculomotor nerves are stimulated.[17]

*Motor strength* should also be evaluated bilaterally. The patient should be instructed to grasp the nurse's hands and to squeeze them as firmly as possible; strength and equality of firmness should be estimated. The patient's ability to push each foot firmly against the nurse's hand is a comparable indicator of motor strength in the lower extremities. A positive *Babinski's sign* may be present as intracranial pressure increases, and should be tested.

The nurse also needs to see if spontaneous movements in all extremities are equal or if there is an increasing tendency for one or more to be *flaccid. Decerebrate* posture is present when all extremities are in rigid extension, the back is arched, and the toes point inward. *Decorticate* posture describes rigid flexion and abduction of the arms and hands.

Sensation to pain can be checked by gently applying the tip of a pin to various portions of the extremities and trunk in an effort to locate areas of *anesthesia.* The examiner should also determine whether there are areas of *paresthesia,* especially facial.

As mentioned earlier, the serial record of vital signs is more helpful in following the patient's condition than a single apparently abnormal value. With rising intracranial pressure there may be an elevated blood pressure and slower pulse and respiratory rates. A pattern showing a rise in pulse and a decrease in blood pressure early after the injury should cause one to suspect an injury besides craniocerebral trauma. Another vital sign to observe is the patient's temperature. A *temperature elevation* early after injury may indicate damage to the hypothalamus, but temperature elevation from any cause is a problem mostly because fever increases the oxygen and metabolic requirements of the brain.[18]

**D**iagnostic Tests Specific identification of the pathological process occurring in the acute phase may require *angiography.* In the presence of a hematoma, the injection of dye during this diagnostic test shows a local avascular area with displacement of adjacent vessels.[19] Such a procedure can localize the source of the bleeding. A *lumbar puncture* is contraindicated as stated under Second-Level Nursing Care.

**Nursing problems and intervention** The patient who has experienced head trauma with increased intracranial pressure may evidence a variety of nursing problems. Interventions for these problems include repeated neurological assessment, medication, and surgery.

If the hypothalamus is affected, *hyperpyrexia* will be a problem. Sponging the patient with tepid water and using a fan may help to lower the elevated temperature; shivering, however, should not be produced. Another method is to use a hypothermia blanket set at a temperature to keep the patient's body temperature at 38°C (measured rectally) or lower.

If the trauma has caused communication between the brain and nasal or ear passages, the possibility of *infection* becomes a problem. Such an opening may be evidenced by *bleeding, clear drainage,* or a mixture of both from the patient's nose (rhinorrhea) or ears (otorrhea). The clear drainage is likely to be cerebrospinal fluid; a positive reaction for dextrose on a chemical reagent will confirm this. When mixed with blood, this fluid leaves a characteristic ring around the spot of blood when it is placed on white paper. No attempt to obstruct the flow of this drainage should be made. Good hand-washing technique by personnel before working in the vicinity of this drainage is mandatory. Nasal airways and suctioning should be avoided in the presence of rhinorrhea. Prophylactically, antibiotics such as penicillin, cephalothin, and ampicillin are used, especially for open head injuries.

Reducing the patient's *restlessness* is important in keeping peak periods of increased intracranial pressure to a minimum. Restlessness is a part of the patient's behavior and level of consciousness, which are crucial indicators of a changing cerebral status. However, the nurse can control external factors that aggravate irritability. Adequate ventilation and circulation protect the patient against cellular hypoxia, which can cause restlessness; administration of oxygen may be necessary, especially before and after suctioning. Proper drainage of urine controls the discomfort associated with a distended bladder. Judicious use of restraints can decrease the irritation from being completely immobilized and from restricting circulation to the distal parts of the extremities. A quiet environment, simple explanations, and avoidance of a loud tone of voice reduce the amount of distracting sensory input that can aggravate the confusion already experienced by the patient as a result of the primary injury. Unless contraindicated by other injuries, elevation of the head of the bed 30° is also helpful in promoting venous drainage of the cerebral circulatory volume. Eye care with a methylcellulose solution is important for reducing restlessness from eye irritation as well as for preventing *corneal ulcers.*

Although the nurse cannot prevent the patient from *vomiting* or from having *seizures,* it is important to remember that these two events not only may result from but also contribute to rising intracranial pressure. The use of a nasogastric tube may be indicated for prevention of vomiting from gastric distention. Regular administration of anticonvulsant medications for seizure prevention is important. Anticonvulsants may be started prophylactically or after evidence of seizure activity. Diphenlyhydantoin is commonly used in doses of 300 to 400 mg daily. However, it does not achieve therapeutic blood levels for the first 24 to 48 hours after it is initiated. Intravenous administration may be used initially to achieve therapeutic blood levels more quickly and is preferable to the intramuscular route.

Medications and fluid restriction are often used to decrease the *cerebral edema.* Steroids are effective because of their anti-inflammatory action which lessens swelling. Dexamethasone is commonly used in an initial intravenous dose for the adult of up to 10 mg, followed by doses of 4 to 10 mg every 6 hours for several days. It must be tapered slowly rather than suddenly discontinued, and antacids, orally or per nasogastric tube, should be given simultaneously since the patient is already prone to a stress ulcer. Diuretics promote fluid loss and thus reduce cerebral fluid volume. Commonly used ones include mannitol and furosemide. Initially, these are given intravenously, then furosemide may be given intramuscularly (mannitol is given only IV). Narcotics, except for codeine, should never be administered to a patient with a head injury because of potential respiratory depression and changes in sensorium that make it difficult to evaluate the level of consciousness.

To avoid circulatory overload and subsequently increased cerebral volume, fluids may be restricted for several days after the injury. Intravenous therapy is often regulated to 50 to 60 ml/hour for the adult. If there is also some oral intake, the intravenous infusion may be even slower so that the total intake in 24 hours does not exceed 1200 to 1500 ml. A common solution is one with 5% dextrose in water and 0.2% saline. The addition of potassium to an IV solution should be avoided for several days because it is the major intracellular electrolyte and is released to the extracellular spaces in large amounts following cell injury in trauma. If the patient has a nasogastric tube for gastric decompression, the drainage may be replaced per volume with normal saline.

Cerebral edema usually peaks 48 to 72 hours after injury, and this is the time during which fluid restriction seems most crucial. The onset and resolution of this edema can be delayed by 2 days or more if the patient ingested alcohol prior to the trauma. One must also be aware that excessive dehydration from fluid restriction and diuretics during the first 3 or 4 days may reach the point of uremia and coma, which may be mistaken for neurological deterioration. Other factors that can influence fluid and electrolyte balance after craniocerebral trauma include the following: increased aldosterone secretion that causes sodium retention, loss of fluid with excessive dietary protein intake during catabolism, and fever that causes excessive dehydration.[20] The nurse should check for laboratory evaluation of the patient's electrolytes on a daily basis for several days after the injury.

If the nurse notices signs of *shock* in the patient with a head injury, evaluation for the presence of other injuries should be made. Neurogenic shock results from an inhibition of the sympathetic nervous system and produces a sudden vasodilatation of the peripheral vascular system. This is not a particularly common occurrence after craniocerebral trauma. In fact, if the patient has signs of shock such as pallor, cold and moist skin, tachycardia, low blood pressure, and apprehension, it is more likely to be a hypovolemic shock resulting from a thoracic injury, a ruptured spleen, a lacerated liver, a ruptured bladder, or major trauma to an extremity. Nursing action depends on the nature of the other injury. The problem for the patient with shock is the diminished supply of oxygen and glucose available to a brain that is already injured.

The significance of observing for *changes in the level of consciousness* has already been emphasized. This is the one aspect of the patient's care that can, perhaps, be best evaluated by the nurse, who has several hours of continuous patient contact in which to notice subtle changes. The nurse should determine the patient's level of *orientation* to the surroundings by relevant questions. Unless the patient has a clock, questions concerning the actual time of day are unlikely to be answered correctly, but determining the patient's knowledge of the month, year, and ability to distinguish night from day are more significant. If the city and state are not known by the patient, it is important to determine whether there is awareness of being in a hospital as opposed to some other location. Orientation to person involves asking the patient his or her surname, age, and occupation. If the patient cannot respond to verbal stimuli, the nurse should note whether mild or strong pain is required to obtain a response and whether this response is purposeful movement or whether only deep reflexes can be elicited.

In providing nursing care to a patient with a head injury, it is especially crucial in the acute phase to use consistent terminology in documenting the patient's progress. Conflicting terminology can make evaluation of the patient's level of consciousness over a period of time difficult, since that part of the assessment cannot be charted numerically. It may be desirable for the health team to develop specific definitions for such terms as *alert, stuporous, nonresponsive,* and *comatose* and to have personnel use these words only as defined. Or some may prefer to have grades of conditions ranging from alert to complete loss of reflexes and to use these categories in charting the patient's progress. In either situation all personnel must know the definitions thoroughly.

A neurological nursing observation sheet with these terms or grades and their meanings printed on it may be helpful. When such precise definitions are not used, behavior descriptions can be made as explicit as vital signs by writing concise examples in objective terms. For example, instead of saying that the patient is stuporous, it is more meaningful to say that there is response only to a loud tone of voice and only with purposeless movements in bed. Such charting makes it easier for personnel who subsequently care for the patient to evaluate condition changes.

Further *damage to brain tissue* should be avoided. The nurse should be cognizant of activities that are likely to increase intracranial pressure and should not cluster them together. These include suddenly arousing, suctioning, turning, or checking for a fecal impaction. They can be divided so that out of a 3- or 4-hour time period the care needed is distributed slowly and evenly.

**Immobility** If the patient is comatose, several potential problems are associated with immobility. *Pneumonia* is a major respiratory complication due to constant resistance by the bed to chest expansion and to some extent to muscle deterioration from lack of movement. Turning the patient every 2 hours is necessary along with positioning the arms so that they do not further restrict chest expansion. Suctioning and hyperventilating the patient should be done as needed. For a patient with a head injury severe enough to depress the respiratory rate, preventing pneumonia is even more important. If respiratory depression is severe, ventilatory assistance may be necessary.

Muscular activity that would normally facilitate venous return is reduced by immobility so that *venous stasis* and *thrombus formation* become potential problems. Positioning the patient with sharp flexion of the knees or hips inhibits venous return from the lower extremities to the heart. Other factors that may contribute to an increased likelihood of blood coagulation are dehydration and increased serum calcium levels resulting from immobility.[21] Passive exercises by the nurse can help to retain the normal muscle tone needed to allow venous return. Frequent changes of position promote circulatory flow. Sometimes milk products are withheld to decrease dietary intake of calcium. If the patient's fluid intake is restricted, the nurse should be sure that the maximum quantity allowed per day is consumed.

Another potential problem from decreased muscular activity is musculoskeletal deterioration in the form of *osteoporosis* and *contractures*. Contractures (Chap. 40) are especially likely when there is prolonged immobilization of joints. Nursing activities should include maintenance of functional positions of the joints and avoidance of sharp flexion of joints, especially the hips and knees. An additional reason to avoid hip flexion is that it is thought to be a factor in increasing the intracranial pressure. An important nursing activity is getting the patient into an upright position in a supportive chair several times a day to permit some weight bearing by the musculoskeletal system.

*Skin breakdown* is a well-known problem associated with prolonged bed rest. It is generally thought that continuous pressure on one point for 1 hour can initiate skin lesions because of the disruption of circulation to the area. The cells are deprived of their necessary oxygenation and nutrition. Frequent turning and proper positioning can help to prevent this problem. Mechanical devices that may assist this nursing activity include water and alternating air pressure mattresses and flotation pads. If the patient is on a hypothermia blanket to control temperature elevations, these devices cannot be used. Turning then becomes even more crucial, since prolonged coldness against the body may produce burns that precipitate skin lesions.

Adequate urinary drainage can be compromised by immobility. A supine position prevents the force of gravity from helping with urinary drainage from the kidney. *Urinary stagnation* and *calculi* can occur with a risk of fever that is detrimental to the head-injured patient. Unless contraindicated, periodic elevation of the patient into a sitting position can help. Sufficient fluid intake is important as soon as the patient is no longer restricted. Fluids producing an acid ash in the urine are especially helpful because they prevent alkalinity, which promotes the formation of calcium calculi[22] and facilitates bacterial growth. Cranberry juice is one such fluid. Discriminate use of indwelling catheters and scrupulous catheter care need to be included in the patient's treatment.

Decreased activity can lead to *constipation,* especially if the patient is on a fluid restriction. Nursing activities involved in preventing this problem should include observing for small, frequent liquid stools, manual examination for an impaction, accurate records of when the patient has had bowel movements, use of fruit juices, and administration of laxatives, suppositories, and stool softeners as ordered. Straining to have a bowel movement also increases the patient's intracranial pressure and should be avoided.

**Surgical Intervention** Fractures generally do not require surgical intervention unless they are deeply depressed and/or produce fragments that penetrate cerebral tissue. Surgical intervention for the patient with a head injury may be indicated in the presence of an epidural hematoma or focal deficits that localize an expanding lesion, or if the patient's general condition starts to deteriorate rapidly. *Burr holes* may be created to search for the source of the bleeding. Sometimes a *bone flap* must be removed for decompression of the brain. Irrigation of bone fragments and other contaminants is performed as needed. The source of any bleeding is controlled by ligation, and any pulpified brain tissue is removed. If a bullet is present, its location will dictate the chance of removal. The path of a bullet or knife needs to be cleansed and debrided to prevent infection. Postoperatively, the nurse should continue to monitor the patient's neurological signs, observe the dressing for drainage, and not turn the patient on the side from which the bone flap was removed.

The nurse may also be managing an intracranial pressure monitor that gives *continuous* or *intermittent* pressure readings. This device may also be used preoperatively to monitor the status of patients. Monitors measure intracranial pressure via two methods. Insertion of an intraventricular catheter was the earliest type used for pressure determinations. It is still used for measuring pressure and sometimes for removing excessive cerebrospinal fluid. A newer method involves the insertion of a screw that floats in the subarachnoid space (Fig. 32-3). It is inserted through a burr hole in the frontal bone behind the hairline and is connected by high-pressure polyethylene tubing via a transducer to a monitor (oscilloscope) for *continuous* measurement. Intracranial pressure monitoring can be used to detect a rise in pressure early so that medications or surgery can be used to treat the patient before irreversible damage occurs. The intracranial pressure that can be tolerated before additional damage occurs varies from person to person (Fig. 32-4). For this reason, the patient's clinical condition (especially changes in consciousness) must be observed and correlated with the pressure readings.

Continuous measurement gives a good indication of the time when prolonged periods of elevated intracranial pressure occur and sometimes of the cause of this elevation. The use of this method requires scheduled calibrations of the transducer to ensure accurate readings. The equipment should be checked if there is no fluctuation in the readings or if the measurement is constantly at zero. Coughing and straining produce temporary elevations; if after a few minutes the pressure does not decrease and fluctuate with respirations and systemic arterial pressure, the patency of the equipment should be evaluated.

*Intermittent* monitoring can also be done and is a process, similar to measuring central venous pressure, in which a manometer is flushed with heparinized saline solution until there is equalization of the pressure in the manometer with the intracranial pressure; the manometer is joined to the screw on one end and to the bottle of solution on the other.[23]

A major nursing responsibility in caring for a patient with an intracranial pressure monitor is to prevent the development of infection from contamination around the screw or catheter. Placement of the screw requires an opening through the dura, and so there is a risk of meningitis. Cleansing the area around the insertion point with hydrogen peroxide and good handwashing prior to working around it should be practiced. Accidental openings into the system are potential sources of bacteria and should be avoided.

### Fourth-Level Nursing Care

The degree to which a patient recovers from a head injury seems related to the type of injury and to the speed with which neurological deficits resolve. Recovery is slower and not always as complete when loss of consciousness lasts several weeks or months and when paresis, decerebrate posturing, or other abnormal signs persist for prolonged periods of time.

For the patient with minimal response to stimuli, protection against additional increases in intracranial pressure and against the effects of immobility are the important nursing activities to prepare for *rehabilitation.* The assistance of a physical therapist is advisable to direct range of motion exercises and to minimize the risks of foot drop and shortening of tendons through maintenance of muscle tone. Unless the patient is without reflexes or responds only to deep pain, early speech therapy is helpful even though the patient has only incoherent verbalization. Reestablishing the comprehension and expression of words can and should begin early. Besides helping to protect against the dangers of immobility, getting the patient up into a chair several times a day, as soon as it can be tolerated, seems to facilitate a return of environmental awareness.

When the patient does *not* have such severe neurological damage or after recovery from a criti-

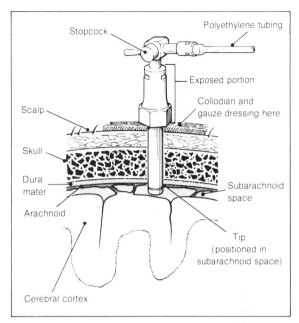

**FIGURE 32-3**

Intracranial pressure screw. (*From Marion Johnson and Judith Quinn, "The Subarachnoid Screw," Am J Nurs, March 1977, p. 449.*)

cal level, rehabilitative efforts can be directed toward regaining the ability to perform activities of daily living. At this point, activities requiring more prolonged attention and finer muscle control may be directed by an occupational therapist. Getting the patient to self-feed again may be the primary goal initially. Relearning previous skills requiring eye-hand coordination might be included. It is important to avoid confronting the patient with more than one or two skills to be regained at one time since frustration develops easily, as fatigue is readily produced by the amount of nervous activity required to perform these activities. At this stage of recovery the patient should be able to reestablish bowel and bladder continence, if that function had been lost, by following a regular schedule for elimination.

Patients with injuries severe enough to produce major neurological deficits frequently show personality changes. Diminished capacity for abstract thought processes may give the person the appearance of being *dull.* Or the patient may be *belligerent* and verbally abusive as consciousness is regained; this can be especially distressing to the family if the patient's behavior and language are usually more refined. Inappropriate laughing and screaming may occur. Sometimes the patient is very depressed. Confusion may even correlate with generalized slowing on the EEG.[24] Undesirable be-

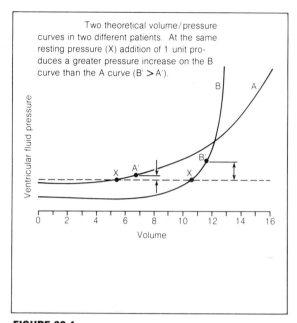

Two theoretical volume/pressure curves in two different patients. At the same resting pressure (X) addition of 1 unit produces a greater pressure increase on the B curve than the A curve (B' > A').

**FIGURE 32-4**

Variations in tolerance to rising intracranial pressure. (*Reprinted with permission from Nursing 76, June 1976. Copyright 1976 by Intermed Communications, Inc., Jenkintown, Pa.*)

havior should not be reinforced by humoring the patient. Repetitious orientation to surroundings and encouragement to assist in self-care are more productive rehabilitative efforts. Relatives and friends need to know that these behavioral changes are part of the recovery process and need to be accepted but not reinforced. These personality changes are not necessarily permanent. The nurse, however, should not attempt to predict how long they may persist.

If the patient sustains an injury involving only cerebral edema that resolves in a short time without deficits, referral to a rehabilitative setting will probably not be needed. Those having more severe injuries may receive initial rehabilitation in the acute care setting of a hospital and then be transferred to a facility specializing in rehabilitation. The availability of such facilities may determine when or if the transfer occurs. After the patient has achieved the goals possible in an institution, there may be a transfer to the home setting with follow-up by community health nurses for extension of care and support of the patient and family. Patients who have sustained severe brainstem injuries or who show little indication of recovery from serious cerebral injuries may be placed in nursing homes for complete physical care.

If the patient is cared for in the home setting

and has minimal ability to do any self-care, support of the family is crucial. Evaluation of the home needs to occur before the patient returns there, not only for the availability of the physical means of care, but also for the assessment of the family's ability to tolerate constant or frequent attention to the patient. A feeling of guilt may be associated with the occurrence of the trauma that can make caring for the patient eventually become a burden; or the family may not be realistic about the physical stress required of them to provide this care. The patient's inability to be left alone for parts of the day or night may not have been recognized by them. Conversely, the family relationships may be so positive that only in that setting will the patient be strongly motivated to continue with a slow process of rehabilitation. Reorientation to daily activities may be best accomplished in a familiar setting. Social service personnel can assist in helping with financial assistance.

For the head-injured patient who has had surgery, postoperative follow-up by the physician may cover several months or a year. If a bone flap had to be removed and could not be replaced owing to severe cerebral edema, months may be required before it is replaced with some substance, often a hard synthetic material. Observation for the late development of a brain abscess may be necessary, especially in the case of penetrating wounds or those in which there was cerebrospinal fluid leakage. Development of chronic subdural hematomas may also occur over this time.

Attention should be directed to the follow-up of the patient who needs medications for control of seizures following trauma (Chap. 33). Not all patients need anticonvulsants. Those needing these medications may be patients whose EEGs normalize and then regain abnormal features or whose EEGs have a persistent abnormality which may change in character.[25] Other candidates are those who sustained deep penetrating wounds, those who are likely to develop abscesses, or those who have had seizures in the acute-care setting. Seizures following trauma in adults may take any form except petit mal. Prophylactic anticonvulsants do not prevent seizures uniformly.[26]

In addition to evaluation of the physiological need for anticonvulsants, the patient's life-style should be considered. If the medications are to be effective, they must be taken consistently every day. The family must understand the need for the medications so that they can encourage the patient to take them.

It may be necessary for the anticonvulsant to be

continued for a year or longer. Many anticonvulsants can precipitate blood dyscrasias, especially in large doses, and so periodic blood counts may be needed during this time. If the medication is diphenylhydantoin, oral hygiene must be emphasized to prevent or to minimize gingival hyperplasia; follow-up should include regular dental checks. If the patient experiences skin rashes or pronounced lethargy on subsequent assessments, decreasing the dose or changing to another medication may be advised.

Counseling and referral of the head-injured patient may involve vocational rehabilitation if there is temporary or permanent inability to perform previous job skills. Recovery of former abilities can be very slow, especially those involving fine muscle control and coordination of several simultaneous activities. It should not be assumed that they can never be regained, however. Several years of persistent rehabilitative efforts may be required along with emotional support when the patient becomes discouraged about the slow progress. In fact, a key element in the nursing care at any level is to avoid predicting the amount of recovery the patient may achieve. Rather, it is better to be objective with the patient and the family about the level of recovery achieved, to recognize the gains and losses experienced, and to make further plans accordingly.

Preventing *reoccurrence* of head injuries is a continuous process for some groups of people. For example, an epileptic has an increased risk of sustaining cerebral trauma with repeated seizure episodes. Contusions of the brain are incurred, and the cerebral tissue becomes more susceptible to subsequent injury.[27] For this person, medications may need readjustment for better control. For one who cannot be kept free of seizures, protection against hazardous jobs, such as in heavy industry, and prevention from operating a motor vehicle may be necessary to avoid severe craniocerebral trauma.

People who have frequent syncope from cardiac arrhythmias (Chap. 25) need to have the basic cardiac problem diagnosed and treated to avoid unexpected loss of consciousness. For arrhythmias particularly difficult to diagnose, a Holter monitor may be useful. This continuous electrocardiogram recorded during several hours of rest and activity may indicate what disorder precedes the loss of consciousness.

Effective counseling of the alcoholic can be an important part of preventing recurrent head injuries sustained during falls resulting from intoxication. Deterioration of the vascular status associated with prolonged use of alcohol makes that person more susceptible to more severe craniocerebral trauma. The alcoholic seems to have a greater risk of intracranial hematoma formation.[28] Even if the existing cerebrovascular damage is irreversible, preventing the extension of it through discontinuation of alcohol usage can be beneficial (Chap. 19).

Rehabilitation can often involve a slow, unpredictable course. Nursing care requires the coordination of diverse health services and the ability to correlate even small improvements with effective nursing approaches.

## TRAUMATIC IMPAIRMENT OF SPINAL CORD FUNCTION

The individual who sustains impairment of the spinal cord is faced with the loss of body functions which produce *a state of physiologic, psychologic, social, and vocational dysequilibrium.* Automatic, familiar, preferred, or even essential patterns of perception and coordination are altered. Bladder emptying, control of defecation, sensory awareness of one's body parts, independence, sexuality, recreational pursuits, and schooling or employment are in all likelihood interrupted.

Just as the patient's functional impairments are complex, so, too, are the *objectives of the comprehensive care* that is required. The aim of care, often called *rehabilitation,* is to help the individual with functional deficits to achieve a state of physiologic, psychologic, social, and vocational equilibrium, compatible with that person's capability and personal desires. While it may be easy to agree to this encompassing objective, the professionals who implement it must have a *commitment* to a philosophy of individual *worth,* individual *right to a meaningful life* (as the *patient* defines it), and individual *potential* for growth, development, and adaptation. In addition, the objective implies a professional *responsibility* for extending help beyond hospital walls into the community and beyond the disabled individual to significant others for as long as help is needed. The multifaceted objective forces nurses to be *interdependent* with many health professionals, each bringing unique knowledge and skills into an integrated service to the individual. The purpose of the following discussion is to provide basic knowledge requisite for providing care and teaching for patients with spinal cord dysfunction.

### Pathophysiology

The primary function of the neurons of the spinal cord is to conduct impulses. When the spinal cord is impaired, there will be abnormalities in the conduction of nervous impulses between the body (peripheral nervous system) and the brain (the central control and coordination centers). From a functional standpoint, the changes in impulses concerned with *motion* and with *sensation* which may occur with spinal cord injury are most significant.

**Motion** Movement of the skeletal muscles can be involuntary or voluntary. A *lower motor neuron* (*LMN*) is a cell body which arises from the *anterior horn* of the gray matter of the spinal cord and its axon which extends out of the cord in the ventral nerve root and becomes a part of a peripheral nerve, terminating in a muscle fiber. The LMN is the essential motor cell concerned with skeletal muscle activity; it must be intact for motion to occur. Reflexes are dependent on the intact LMN. An interruption of the LMN is called a *lower motor neuron lesion.* However, a LMN acting alone can initiate only *involuntary* muscle contractions. Normally, the LMN synapses with and is acted upon by all the descending tracts of the spinal cord (see Chap. 31) as well as by intersegmental reflex neurons. Only through these relationships with higher centers does motion become voluntary and controlled.

*Voluntary* movements of skeletal muscles on the opposite side of the body originate from nerve cell bodies in the *motor cortex* (precentral gyrus) of the cerebrum. The axon of each cell body passes through the internal capsule and brainstem, descends as a part of the pyramidal tracts of the spinal cord, and synapses with the LMN itself or via an internuncial neuron. This cell body plus its axon is called an *upper motor neuron* (*UMN*). Thus, a UMN lies entirely within the central nervous system and extends from the brain to some segmental level within the spinal cord. An interruption of this neuron is termed an *upper motor neuron lesion.* There are nerves from other parts of the brain which descend in different spinal cord tracts and which influence muscle tone and synergy. Together, these nerves with the UMN produce the coordinating, integrating, and mediating effects on the LMN which are essential for purposeful voluntary movement.

The effect of a spinal cord lesion on motor activity is found in both strength and muscle tone. *Paralysis* or *plegia* is a lack of voluntary motion in the affected muscles; weakness is called *paresis.* In the presence of an LMN lesion, there will be *hypotonicity* (flaccidity), indicating that no reflex activity at that spinal cord level is present. For example, in an LMN lesion affecting the quadriceps femoris, there will be no knee jerk when the patellar tendon is tapped. On the other hand, with a UMN lesion, there will be *hypertonicity* (spasticity). Hypertonicity occurs in all muscles innervated distal to the spinal cord lesion in which the reflex arc is intact but uninhibited by higher centers.

In muscles whose LMN is nonfunctional, the muscle fibers will atrophy. If the lesion is that of a UMN, the muscle bulk will be maintained or even hypertrophied through reflex contraction.

If both legs are paralyzed, the patient is termed *paraplegic;* if both legs are weakened, the patient is termed *paraparetic.* If all four extremities are affected, the term is *quadriplegic* or *quadriparetic.* When the arm and leg on one side of the body are affected, the person is said to be *hemiplegic* or *hemiparetic.* The modifying adjective *flaccid* or *spastic* is usually used with the word to denote the type of motor neuron involvement.

**Sensation** There are three types of sensation: superficial, deep, and combined. *Superficial sensation* is concerned with touch, pain, temperature, and two-point discrimination; *deep sensation* with muscle and joint position sense (proprioception), deep muscle pain, and vibration sense. Superficial and deep sensory mechanisms are *combined* in stereognosis (recognition and naming of familiar objects placed in the hand) and in the ability to localize cutaneous stimuli.

Sensation is carried from the receptors in the skin and muscle by a peripheral process to the cell body located in the dorsal root ganglion of the spinal nerve and then into the spinal cord to synapse with cord tracts and intra- and intersegmental neurons. Cutaneous sensation follows the segmental distribution of the spinal nerves. Motor innervation is similar in distribution.

The most severe *sensory changes* are the absence of some or all modalities, expressed as *anesthesia.* A lesser degree of impairment of sensation may be expressed as *paresthesia* (abnormal sensations, numbness, tingling, formication, and prickling), *hyperesthesia,* or *pain.*

**Causes of impairment** Some of the *causes* of spinal cord dysfunction with examples of disease are: (1) anatomic interruptions (accidental or surgical trauma, congenital discontinuity as with myelomeningocele, syringomyelia); (2) anoxic disruptions (arteriovenous malformation, spinal artery thrombosis); (3) pressure-related conditions (spinal stenosis of achondroplasia, extrusion of intervertebral disk, tumor); (4) chemical impairment (tetanus toxin, neurotrophic drugs); (5) degenerative disturbances (spondylosis, multiple sclerosis); (6) inflammatory and infectious diseases, with or without scarring (poliomyelitis, arachnoiditis, transverse myelitis, Guillain-Barré syndrome, syphilis); and (7) autoimmune processes (lupus erythematosus).

Although the pathogenic situations resulting in spinal cord dysfunction are diverse and the nursing care for each common problem area is similar, the emphasis in this chapter will be *trauma* as the inciting cause of impaired spinal cord function. Specific nursing care related to some of the other conditions is discussed in other chapters (Chaps. 33 to 38 and 40).

Approximately 2½ individuals of every 100,000 in the United States annually will sustain traumatic spinal cord injury. Over one-half of these injuries will be a complete spinal cord injury. Automobile accidents, gunshot wounds, and falls will each account for about one-quarter of the injuries.[29]

**T**ypes of Trauma   Trauma to the spine may produce a *vertebral fracture, dislocation* of one vertebra with respect to an adjacent one, or sufficient *ligamentous disruption* to preclude proper alignment of vertebrae if weight bearing (upright posture) is attempted.

Dislocations and fractures occur most frequently at points of junction between relatively fixed and mobile segments of the spinal column. These areas are the lower cervical region, the upper lumbar region which is relatively fixed by the ribs, and the lower lumbar region adjacent to the sacrum. Actual damage to the cord occurs when the vertebrae and attached soft tissue cause *stretching, contusion, anoxia,* or transient *concussive waves* from a bullet or blow on impact. Swelling, hematoma, and circulatory impairment around the site of injury may account for a temporary movement of the lesion upward. The reduction of swelling and absorption of hematoma may improve the neurologic picture over time. Effects of this damage are discussed specifically, according to the level of the lesion, under Second- and Third-Level Nursing Care.

*Herniation* (extrusion) of an intervertebral disk is another potential effect of trauma to the spinal column. It most commonly occurs in the lower lumbar region and, next most frequently, in the lower cervical region (between C5 and C6 or C6 and C7). The disk (nucleus pulposus) may herniate into the vertebral canal or intervertebral foramina. Small, or slowly developing, herniations may produce little or no neurologic deficit. However, *acute* extrusion of a disk caused by severe trauma may result in immediate neurologic deficit as nerve root or spinal cord compression occurs.

### First-Level Nursing Care

In the first level of nursing care the emphasis is on prevention of spinal cord injury. To the extent that such variables as age, behavior, life-style, environment, and other injuries can be identified with a population at risk for spinal cord trauma, the nurse can plan interventions intended to reduce the risks.

**Psychosocial assessment**   *Adolescents* and *young adults* in particular are characteristically challengers. They dispute morals, ethics, and established ways of behaving. Physical limits are also tested. The urge for competition and risk-taking often outweighs judgment. Driven by alternate feelings of omnipotence and self-doubt, the individual strenuously tests personal power in the environment. One may choose to test motor and judgmental skills in sports, through mastery of motor vehicles, and through defying known danger. Most young people learn the reality of their abilities and limitations without serious physical or psychic injury. An unfortunate few suffer the devastating accident of spinal cord trauma resulting in paralysis.

Indiscretion in the ingestion of *pharmacologic agents,* particularly alcohol, is a common finding when the cause of accidents is analyzed. People of *all ages* place themselves and others at risk for central nervous system injury when they allow drugs to adversely influence judgment, coordination, and reaction time.

With an emphasis on leisure time and the rise of a "right to recreation" attitude, our *middle-aged* population is increasingly involved in activities that have a high injury potential such as skiing, diving, racing, sky kiting, and climbing. Often the weekend athlete or vacationer engages in physical pursuits although poorly conditioned and not properly instructed. Physical demands on a body unable to respond can result in dangerous shortcuts, carelessness, weakness, fatigue, and accidents.

**Environmental assessment**   The ways in which one reacts to frustration and threat and the ways in which anger is dissipated have significant implications when coupled with the easy availability of *weapons.* Three decades ago, attack with an ice pick accounted for many spinal cord injuries. Today guns and knives are the instruments of coercion and retaliation, often with devastating results.

We live in an environment in which powerful motorized devices are provided to save human energy and to offer speed. Farm equipment, industrial machines, sports and pleasure devices, and travel vehicles, while a blessing and a necessity in many instances, are also frequent sources of accidental trauma.

*Falls* continue to be the leading cause of accidental injury, and most often they occur in the home. Slippery floors and rugs, rickety ladders, and poorly lighted stairs without handrails are common precursors to accidents. The *aged* population is particularly at risk because of decreased visual acuity and because the osteoporosis of age increases the fragility of bones, including the vertebrae.

**Physiologic assessment** *Strains* to the ligaments and soft tissues of the neck and back are usually self-correcting after a time during which the individual has pain and stiffness. Habitual strain to the lumbosacral area when a person lifts a heavy object from the floor by bending at the waist instead of at the knees, or sudden strain as in cervical whiplash injury, may contribute to extrusion of a portion of the intervertebral disk with impingement on neural tissue.

**Preventive measures** The school nurse has a unique opportunity to observe the motor development of children as well as to note historical data regarding trauma, illnesses, drug ingestion, and behavior in the classroom and on the playground. Over a course of months and years, personality traits appear which can alert one to a child at risk for maladaptive or volatile behavior, excessive daring, and poor judgment. Counseling the child, the parents, and teachers may help. Some objectives might be to direct aggressive behavior into safer channels such as supervised recreation, to structure school experiences to provide success and self-satisfaction in academic and extracurricular settings, and to confront the child with the realities of poor judgment at the time of the incident and suggest alternative behavior. While such interaction with individuals may have to be limited to a few, the nurse can facilitate group education. Topics discussed might include drivers' education, firearm safety, and some precautions in the use of alcohol and other drugs.

The industrial nurse has potential influence over a large adult population. Environmental safety extends from the shop to the home. Body mechanics, general body conditioning, and weight control are appropriate topics to be addressed.

All nurses have numerous teaching opportunities, whether by deliberate design or incidentally, as a model. The particular subjects mentioned here are intended to alert the student to areas in which prevention can forestall some spinal cord injuries.

**Second-Level Nursing Care**

In the second level of nursing care, the focus is on the individual at the time of injury during which dysfunction of the spinal cord becomes apparent. Accurate nursing assessment and appropriate care can minimize further spinal cord damage.

**Nursing assessment** Whenever possible, the patient's perception of body motion and feelings is documented in the *health history*. Some patients who have sustained spinal cord trauma describe the immediate sensation as that of "an electric shock passing through my body," "heaviness in my legs," "a feeling that my head seemed to be floating without a body attached," or "a numbness working its way up my body." The *patient's account of symptoms* should be elicited, if possible, including the presence of pain, its origin and radiation, and conditions which worsen or relieve it. A history of related disease such as spondylosis, arthritis of the spine, osteoporosis, previous injury or surgery of the back, and congenital defects should be noted. From the patient, or an available witness, a complete description of any accidents should be obtained.

**P**hysical Assessment The onset of impairment because of trauma is usually sudden, but may be insidious; some loss of motion and/or sensation of the body is present. The *physical assessment guide* (Table 32-1) can help determine the approximate level of the spinal cord lesion. The most critical immediate determination of motor function in an acutely injured patient is to establish whether the fourth cervical segment is intact since *independent breathing* depends on this segment. If the lesion involves C4 or higher, artificial respiration is required.

If the respiratory status is adequate, the patient's ability to feel and move the extremities should be determined. Each hand and foot should be touched and the patient questioned regarding the sensations. The patient should be asked to squeeze the examiner's fingers with each hand, to move each arm, and to move each leg. If any changes in perception and/or coordination occur, spinal cord injury should be suspected.

Persons seen in community settings who describe the *insidious* onset of symptoms should have a complete neurologic examination. Findings are dependent upon the level of the lesion (Table 32-1). The *neurologic examination* (see Chap. 31) includes an evaluation of motor function and strength in the extremities and trunk, all sensory modalities throughout the body, balance and coordination, sphincter tone, and reflexes.

**D**iagnostic Tests  Most patients will receive comprehensive diagnostic studies at the onset of positive neurologic findings, whether the onset of symptoms be sudden as with trauma, or more gradual as with, for example, spinal stenosis. *Radiographic examination* of the spine at the suspected areas of dysfunction is performed. Movement during the x-rays must be minimal, and a physician should be present. Fractures, dislocations, soft-tissue thickness, bony instability, vertebral deformity, and the location of foreign bodies may be visualized.

**Nursing problems and intervention**  An individual with obvious trauma to the spinal cord, i.e., a *change in sensory and/or motor responses of the limbs,* requires knowledgeable *emergency care.* The person should be *immobilized flat in neutral vertebral alignment* with meticulous care taken to prevent hyperextension, flexion, or lateral rotation of the spine. To accomplish spinal immobilization, an individual in a water accident, for example, can be floated onto an air mattress, a board, or a door and then lifted from the water. A victim of a vehicular accident can be strapped to a board placed behind the trunk and head before being pulled from the wreckage, unless the threat of fire or other danger makes immediate removal imperative. If an injured person must be lifted from the ground, a transport board is placed adjacent to the patient. Then, four people kneel on the board, all on the same side of the patient, so that one pair of hands controls the head, one the shoulders and upper trunk, one the lower back and hips, and one the legs. The patient can then be lifted as a unit onto the board or stretcher. A person with a questionable spinal injury should not be permitted to sit up or try to walk, and nothing should be placed under the patient's head.

Every accident scene needs a *chief.* The most knowledgeable person present should take command of patient handling. Care is more important than haste. If competent rescue squads are available, it is wiser to maintain the patient's respiration, control hemorrhage, prevent panic, and await the arrival of the trained crew and their equipment.

**TABLE 32-1**
ASSESSMENT GUIDE TO DETERMINE APPROXIMATE
LEVEL OF SPINAL CORD LESION

| Cord Level Associated With Motion | Movement To Be Requested of the Patient | Body Part To Be Observed | Cord Level Associated With Sensation in Each Listed Body Part* |
|---|---|---|---|
| S2–S4 | Tighten the muscle around my finger (Finger in anal sphincter) | Perineum | S5 |
| L5, S1, and S2 | Bend and straighten your toes | Toes | L5 |
| L2–L4 | Straighten your leg | Knees | L3 |
| L1–L3 | Bend (flex) your hip | Hips | L2 |
| T5–T12 | Tighten your abdomen | Abdomen<br>Pubis<br>Navel<br>Nipple line | <br>L1<br>T10<br>T4 |
| C8–T1 | Oppose your thumb to each finger tip; make a fist | Thumb,<br>first two digits,<br>little finger | C6<br>C7<br>T1 |
| C6 | Bend your wrist up (only the radial wrist extensor will contract) | Wrist | C6<br>(thumb side of wrist) |
| C5 | Bend your elbow | Elbow | Radial side C6<br>Ulnar side T1 |
| C3, C4, and C5 | Shrug your shoulders; take a deep breath (diaphragms descend causing abdomen to bulge; upper chest does not move) | Shoulder, chest, and abdomen | C4 |

* Light touch, pinprick, position.

"Should neuroinjury exist, one must recognize that only the best facilities will even approach adequacy."[30] When a specialized center is within transportation range, the patient should be taken to it promptly rather than to an inadequate nearby facility.

Patients who give a history of slowly developing sensory or motor impairment should also be referred for further evaluation. Care in transport (e.g., the use of neck braces and immobilization) and in detailing the events of the health history are vitally important here, also.

### Third-Level Nursing Care

Much of the nursing care of the patient with a freshly traumatized spinal cord is similar to the care given during convalescence and perhaps lifelong, should the neurologic deficits persist. Those aspects of care are presented under Fourth-Level Nursing Care. Some nursing care, however, is associated more often with acute illness and is discussed next.

**Nursing assessment** The *health history* of the patient with a spinal cord injury is as described under Second-Level Nursing Care. If the patient is in critical condition, it may be necessary to obtain information from a relative or observer. Subjective symptoms, details of any recent trauma, and the past medical history should be recorded.

**P**hysical Assessment The patient's neurologic findings often change during the first hours and days after injury. The nurse should repeat a *neurologic examination* every few hours initially, and then daily until the patient's status plateaus. Table 32-1 is an assessment guide to approximate the level of lesion. Other significant findings include a change in the patient's sensory acuity, a change in the strength of the motions examined, and the alterations in the symmetry or localization of findings. Sensation should be tested over all body surfaces with a light touch and pin prick. The patient's awareness of pain, position, and temperature should be evoked. Muscle activity should be selectively evaluated and reflexes tested. The sensory level can be mapped with indelible ink on the body with the date and time. The entire examination should be performed in the same way each time so that serial results can be compared.

The Achilles tendon reflexes (ankle jerk) and the quadriceps femoris reflexes (knee jerk) are tested. Initially, *areflexia* is present during a period of spinal shock. The time varies within which reflex activity is reestablished in a person with an upper motor neuron lesion to the lower extremities; hyperactive reflexes and ankle clonus eventually develop. In persons with a lower motor neuron lesion to these muscles, no reflex action is found.

The *vital signs* should be measured. This is especially important in an individual with a high thoracic or cervical cord lesion. In such an individual, the *body temperature* will rise or fall in response to ambient temperature. In a warm room, for example, the temperature may register 39°C (102.2°F), while in a cool room, it might be 36°C (96.8°F). The temperature will also increase in response to infection. The sweat pattern is abnormal because the central control of sweating is lost. Sweating does not occur in response to increased body temperature; thus the cooling mechanism for maintenance of stable temperature is lost. *Diaphoresis* may occur without apparent cause or relation to body temperature. When diaphoresis is present, autonomic causes such as a distended bowel or bladder should be sought. It is important to record the circumstances of the patient when an abnormal temperature is found, i.e., temperature of the environment, amount of body covering, presence and location of sweat or shivering, and the fullness of the bladder or bowel.

*Blood pressure* varies in relation to the dysfunction of the spinal cord. It tends to be lower than normal, particularly in the upright habitus. Blood pools in the lower extremities and viscera because of poor tone of the skeletal muscle and absence of the pumping action which muscle contraction contributes to venous return. Blood pressure can rise suddenly (as high as 260/140) in a patient with a lesion above T6 in response to such sympathetic nervous system stimuli as a distended bladder or rectum. This is evidenced by a severe pulsating headache, bradycardia, red blotches on the trunk and face, diaphoresis, and "goose bumps." This syndrome is called *sympathetic hyperreflexia* (autonomic hyperreflexia). It is caused by an uninhibited sympathetic response of the cord distal to the lesion resulting in vasoconstriction. The normal check and balance of the brainstem and parasympathetic nervous system are ineffective because the spinal lesion prevents the transmission of neural impulses to the sacral portion of the craniosacral division of the autonomic nervous system. It is important to determine and treat the inciting cause promptly.

**D**iagnostic Tests A *myelogram* may be performed to identify the site of spinal canal blockage. In this test, a radiopaque dye (5 to 25 cc) is instilled into the spinal canal through a lumbar or cervical puncture. The dye is denser than spinal fluid and, therefore, will take a gravity-dependent position. Thus, tilting the body up and down will cause the dye to pass up and down the spinal canal, outlining the shape of the canal. A blockage which retards or obstructs the flow of dye can then be visualized. At the end of the test, the dye is allowed to settle in a dependent portion of the canal and as much as possible is withdrawn. Contrast media can be irritating to the lining of the central nervous system and are sometimes implicated in subsequent arachnoiditis. The manipulation of the spine required to permit insertion of the needle and the postinjection positioning on the x-ray table may be contraindicated in an incomplete spinal cord lesion because of the risk of further damage with motion.

*Fluoroscopy of the chest* may be performed to verify the degree of diaphragmatic movement in an individual with a high cervical injury. Fluoroscopy requires that the patient lie on an x-ray table; it cannot be done at the bedside. If C4 is intact, the diaphragms will move down with inspiration one to two rib spaces. If the diaphragms are incompletely innervated, the movements will be paradoxic (i.e., move up into the chest) when the patient inhales rapidly by sniffing.

**Nursing problems and interventions** Four problems provide a focus when caring for a patient during the acute period of spinal cord impairment. They are *vertebral abnormality, joint immobility, impaired respiration,* and *autonomic changes.*

**V**ertebral Abnormality   The normal protective function of the vertebrae is altered, making the spinal cord more vulnerable to tortion and pressure. To prevent further damage, most patients with fractures and/or dislocations of the vertebrae will be placed on a *turning frame* to ensure straight body alignment (Figs. 32-5 and 32-6). Those patients with cervical injuries will usually have traction applied to stretch the neck and allow the vertebrae and bony fragments to become realigned. Traction is applied by insertion of *tongs* into the skull to which a specified weight is attached by a rope over a pulley (Fig. 32-7). The weights should neither touch the floor nor be lifted. The pull on the patient should be constant. Tong sites are cleansed with hydrogen peroxide, and an antibacterial ointment such as Betadine is applied. The hair is clipped in the immediately surrounding area.

An alternative method of cervical traction that

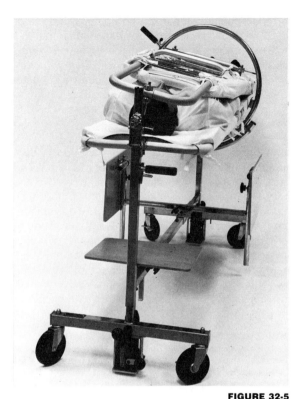

**FIGURE 32-5**
Turning frame on which a patient can be "sandwiched" between an anterior and a posterior frame and then turned from supine to prone or prone to supine by rotation of the joined frames. The uppermost frame is then removed to allow unrestricted access to one entire side of the body. (*Courtesy of the Stryker Corporation, Kalamazoo, Mich.*)

can be used with the patient in a regular bed is called a *halo.* This device consists of a circular band screwed into the skull to which are attached rods which are in turn anchored to a cast or a jacket applied to the trunk. Care should be taken to avoid hitting metal against the rods because the sound will be transmitted through bony conduction to the skull and be distasteful to the patient. The patient in halo traction can be put into the supine, prone, and sitting positions. Supporting pillows or short mattresses are arranged in such a way that there is no pressure against the rods or ring of the halo.

A *laminectomy* (surgical removal of the posterior of a vertebra) to remove bony pressure from the spinal canal or to provide access in order to remove a foreign body or bone fragment may be performed. When the spine is unstable, i.e., anterior or posterior slippage is anticipated with weight bearing, a *posterior fusion,* an *anterior fusion,* or both, using bone grafts or steel rods is done. The bone graft is usually taken from the tibia or iliac crest. It is shaped and then positioned across the unstable area and wired to normal vertebrae above and below the defective vertebra as well as to the defective vertebra itself. Eventually the struts will fuse with the vertebrae to form a solid bony bridge. A cervical collar or a body brace is often applied until the fusion is radiographically solid, and this can take 6 to 24 weeks.

**Joint Immobility** Because motor function is disrupted, normal mobility of the joints is impaired. Each joint of the extremities should be gently moved, either actively or passively, through a normal range of joint motion to a point of resistance about five times, twice a day. Joint limitation should be investigated by a physical therapist and/or the physician. Joints may be limited in motion because of soft-tissue contracture or because of abnormal deposition of calcium in soft tissue. This is called *myositis ossificans*. It is a dreadful complication

since range of motion becomes permanently restricted. The cause of myositis ossificans is not fully understood. However, microscopic hemorrhage into the muscles may trigger the reaction. Vigorous stretching may tear soft tissue. Intramuscular injections to paralyzed muscle may also cause bleeding. Such iatrogenic trauma is thought by some to be the precursor of myositis ossificans. Functional body alignment and mobility may be maintained with the use of splints, sandbags, hand rolls, pillows, and passive exercise.

**Impaired Respiration** If the injury is as high as C4, respiratory function can be disrupted. If respiratory support is required for more than a brief time, a *tracheostomy tube* will be inserted. Since positive pressure ventilation is most commonly used, the tracheostomy tube will have a cuff which is inflated to prevent loss of air from the upper airway while the air under positive pressure is delivered to the

**FIGURE 32-6**

Turning frame with the individual in the prone position. The face is supported at the forehead and chin to allow vision, breathing, and oral functions to continue unhampered. Simulated head traction demonstrates location of pulley, rope, and weights. Traction is not interrupted when the frame is rotated. (*Courtesy of the Stryker Corporation, Kalamazoo, Mich.*)

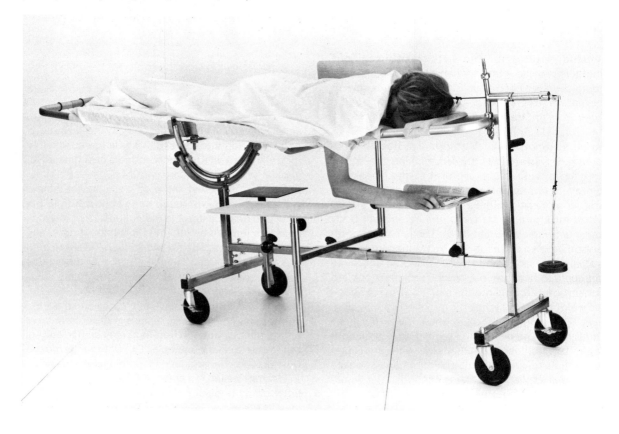

trachea. This technique prevents speech since no air reaches the vocal cords. Every effort should be made to permit the patient to speak. Total body paralysis and loss of sensation are too catastrophic for the able-bodied person to imagine, but it is infinitely worse to be denied, in addition, the expression of one's thoughts and questions. *Speech is possible* if the tube is uncuffed and the patient is taught to control the amount of air leak permitted through the larynx. The patient can watch the bellows or spirometer of the respirator in a mirror to learn to control respiratory volumes. It may be necessary to inflate the cuff during sleep.

To determine the amount of air with which to inflate the cuff of the tube, the nurse should ask the patient to say "ah-h-h" while air is instilled. When vocalization ceases, the cuff is sufficiently full to prevent escape of inspired air. Overinflation of the cuff can cause pressure necrosis and subsequent scarring and stenosis of the trachea. All inflated cuffs should be deflated at least once every 2 hours for a few minutes as a precaution against necrosis of the tracheal lining from prolonged pressure.

When intratracheal suctioning is performed, it should be done in such a way as to prevent hypoxia and vagal irritation. Hypoxia occurs both because respiration is interrupted and because the suction withdraws air (oxygen) present in the trachea and bronchi. Several deep breaths prior to and following suction help compensate for losses during suctioning. Entry of the suction catheter should not exceed 10 seconds. Vagal irritation can be avoided by gentle insertion of the sterile suction catheter and by applying suction only as the tube is withdrawn and rotated to avoid tracheal irritation and trauma.

**A**utonomic System Alterations   Patients may also experience *temperature elevations, diaphoresis,* or the *sympathetic hyperreflexia syndrome.* Generally, a patient will not respond to salicylates as a way to reduce the *fever.* The best way to lower body temperature is to uncover the patient, to apply tepid cloths to the axillae, and to sponge the body, allowing the water to evaporate. When the body temperature is low, it is best increased by covering the patient. Shivering, the body's way of generating heat, may be present only in the normally innervated parts of the body. The physician may prescribe oral propantheline bromide, an anticholinergic agent, to reduce *sweating.* A sympathetic blocking agent may be prescribed for *sympathetic hyperreflexia.* Both excessive hypotension and hypertension should be avoided if this condition exists.

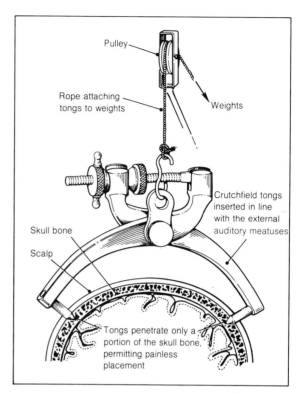

**FIGURE 32-7**
Cervical traction is attached to tongs inserted in the skull.

### Fourth-Level Nursing Care

After lifesaving and reparative measures have been taken for the individual with spinal cord dysfunction, there is a period of time during which body systems stabilize and the physical and psychological tasks of adjustment predominate. The objectives of fourth-level nursing care are to assist the individual to utilize remaining function and to find ways to substitute for lost function in *activities of daily living (ADL),* to teach the patient and significant others to *prevent complications,* and to foster the *psychological integration* of the patient's changed self. Several other health disciplines are required as well as nursing to achieve these objectives. Nursing, however, has major responsibility in reaching some of the objectives and a supportive role in others.

**Activities of daily living**   The patient's *performance of the activities of daily living* is the distillate of many factors. Eight factors are mentioned here. First, the *muscle mass* under volitional control is critical. (Refer to Table 32-2 for the usual functional goals depending on the level of the spinal cord that is intact.) Second, the potential *strength* of normally innervated muscle can be realized only after active exercises counteract the weakening effect of disuse and immobilization. Nursing care should utilize any motion the patient can make. For example, most patients can help turn themselves by hooking an elbow over the siderail and contracting the biceps. Thirdly, patients with paralysis are more functional when *sitting* than when lying. The sooner the patient is able to spend waking hours in a wheelchair, the sooner independence in some tasks will be achieved. Fourth, as with any new skill, *repetition* enhances ability. Allow extra time for tasks since the patient is less efficient and slower in all actions.

Fifth, *spasticity* may be present in muscles below the level of the lesion. Sometimes spasticity is used to complement voluntary action. For example, when a patient is preparing to move from the supine-in-bed position into a wheelchair, a flexor spasm of the knees and hips may be triggered which will make it easier to swing them over the side of the bed. However, spasms may impede performance and force the individual to make all motions more deliberately and slowly.

Sixth, *sequencing* an activity is necessary. Each task is analyzed and its component parts identified so that each component can be mastered before the entire task is attempted.[31] For example, self-feeding while sitting in a chair requires that the individual move his or her arm in the horizontal plane, grasp a utensil, make a scooping or stabbing motion with the utensil, stabilize a dish, keep the food from being pushed over the edge, supinate the forearm, and flex the elbow. Methods of substituting for impaired functions are used when a component of the task cannot be accomplished normally. Positioning the paralyzed arm, using a ballbearing feeder or an overhead suspension arm sling, may help facilitate function. These devices are controlled by shoulder action, and their use is taught by an occupational therapist. When wrist extensors are paralyzed, stabilizing splints to prevent the wrists from dropping into extreme flexion are worn. A universal cuff into which a spoon or fork can be inserted fits over the hand and obviates the need for grasp (Fig. 32-8). The plate guard provides a surface against which to scoop. A dish can be stabilized by a wet washcloth, a suction cup, or a high-friction material placed between the plate and the lapboard or table.

Seventh, *coordination* permits a smooth, predictable, targeted motion. It requires that opposing muscles around a given joint contract and relax harmoniously. For example, lifting the hand from the plate to the mouth depends on movement of the elbow. The elbow is controlled by extensor muscles (triceps) and flexor muscles (biceps). Only when the triceps relax and the biceps contract is the elbow bent to exactly the correct angle to accomplish feeding.

Eighth, *personality* characteristics such as insistence on high standards, the need for immediate reward, distaste for messiness, denial of disability, low level of frustration tolerance, the desire to be independent, sadness, gadget tolerance, reaction to staff expectations, importance to the individual of a given act, and many other attributes influence the performance of the activities of daily living (Table 32-2).

There are two kinds of ADL which deserve special comment: one is the ability to *grasp* with at least one hand and the other is *mobility in space.*

**G**rasp   The radial wrist extensor is innervated by the sixth cervical segment of the cord. The availability of this muscle has immense significance for grasp, and grasp is a fundamental requirement for most activities. To understand the muscle action, sit with one elbow bent and resting on the arm of the chair and let the hand hang limply down. Note that the hand is open. Keep the fingers relaxed but slowly extend the wrist. The thumb and the forefinger will tend to come together in a pinching position. This relationship is called *tenodesis grasp.* Many patients deliberately let their first digits contract into slight flexion in order to improve the thumb-finger contact. Tenodesis grasp, however, is not strong nor is it delicate.

Several different hand splints have been designed utilizing the tenodesis principle. The Siebens-Engel wrist-driven finger flexion hand splint is one of the most versatile (Fig. 32-9). The strength of the wrist extensor is transferred to the thumb and first two digit prehension. An adjustable linkage bar permits the wearer to select a small-pinch opening, say, for a piece of paper, or a large opening, say, for a beer can. Such a splint is readily applied and removed by the patient; its presence does not interfere with wheeling the chair; and it is commonly worn all the time when a person is in a wheelchair.[32] It is possible to connect this type of hand splint by cable to an external power source for the person with a C5 lesion. The total usage is less because the positioning function for the arm and hand are more limited at this higher level.

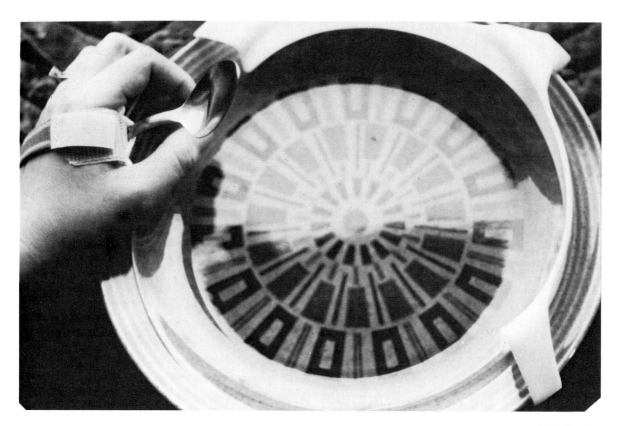

**FIGURE 32-8**
A universal cuff is an elastic band which fits over the forehand. It has a pocket into which a fork, toothbrush, and other objects can be inserted, thus obviating the need to grasp. A plate guard provides a surface against which food can be scooped.

**Mobility in Space** The desire to walk is nearly always expressed by a disabled person. Walking is the most convenient method of getting from one place to another. However, walking also symbolizes a familiar scope of activities, independence, and normalcy. Walking implies that one could "walk out" on the whole catastrophic situation. In discussing walking with a patient, it is best to speak instead of *mobility,* that is, moving from here to there. A wheelchair will provide mobility for the majority of patients with complete lesions through the L2 level.

Because a *wheelchair* is the patient's source of mobility, it is the device in which most waking hours will be spent. It is costly and should be prescribed by a knowledgeable person (usually a physical therapist) according to the needs of the patient. The most common features included in a wheelchair prescription are these: battery power with steering controls activated by chin motion, a mouthstick, head movement, or a puff and suck

device for the individual with a high cervical lesion; projections or knobs on the wheeling rims to enable a person with C5 level to hook the palm of the hand and use biceps contraction to get forward thrust; removable arm rests to facilitate lateral transfer from the wheelchair; removable leg rests to allow the person to get close to other objects such as a car or toilet; heel loops to keep the feet from sliding backward off the foot pedals; extra-long foot plates to support the whole foot and protect the toes; arms with a cutaway front portion (desk arms) to permit the chair to be wheeled under tables and desks; and reliable brakes. Wheelchair cushions are discussed under Skin Care below.

**Prevention of complications** The *prevention of complications* arising from altered body functions is a continuing objective for the patient with spinal cord dysfunction. There are four areas in which nurses carry a significant responsibility for providing the example of appropriate care and for teaching the patient and family how to remain problem-free. The areas are *respiratory care, skin care, bowel management,* and *urinary tract management.*

**R**espiratory Care   When there is a major interruption of neural transmission in the spinal cord, some functional deficits are glaringly apparent: the individual cannot walk, cannot control urination, and cannot sense the changes in the skin and muscle in

**TABLE 32-2**
FUNCTIONAL GOALS AFTER SPINAL CORD INJURY*

| Level at Which Spinal Cord Is Intact | Key Muscle/Function Preserved | Functional Goals |
|---|---|---|
| C3 | Head and neck muscles, trapezius, sternocleidomastoids/Neck control, face and tongue control | Use mouthstick to type, paint<br>Operate microswitches<br>Activate electric wheelchair<br>(will need respiratory assistance) |
| C4 | Diaphragms/Breathing | Breathe without mechanical aids |
| C5 | Deltoids, biceps, supinators/Shoulder control, elbow flexion, forearm supination | Dress upper trunk<br>Feed self using universal cuff<br>Operate wheelchair with projections on wheeling rims and a wrist stabilizing splint (on level surfaces) |
| C6 | Extensor carpi radialis, pronator teres/Wrist extension, forearm pronation, tenodesis grasp | Position hand for grasp<br>Activate wrist-driven finger flexion hand splint for controlled grasp<br>Drive car<br>Transfer to and from wheelchair independently when surfaces are level<br>Compete vocationally for jobs requiring hand skills such as drafting, accounting, computer programming<br>Empty own leg bag of urine<br>Perform most of self-care and simple cooking |
| C7 | Triceps/Push-ups | Perform all transfers easily |
| C8 | Thumb and finger muscles/Normal hand function | Perform all self-care<br>Participate in any activity requiring normal arm and hand function |
| T1–T7 | Intercostal muscles/Chest expansion | Breathe with chest |
| T8–L1 | Abdominal muscles/Deep breath, trunk control | Cough<br>Participate in strenuous sports such as wheelchair basketball, swimming, archery<br>Possibly walk in a limited way with long leg braces and crutches |
| L2 | Sartorius, Iliopsoas/Hip flexion | Walk with long leg braces and Lofstrand crutches with a swing-through or four-point gait |
| L4 | Quadriceps, quadratus femoris, gluteus medius/Pelvic stabilization, leg extension, thigh adduction | Walk with short leg braces and crutches or canes |
| L5–S1 | Soleus, gastrocnemius, tibialis anterior and posterior, gluteus maximus/Ankle dorsiflexion and push-off in gait | Walk without aids |
| S4 | Bladder detrusor, anal sphincters/Voiding, defecation | Empty bladder continently<br>Control bowel evacuation<br>Achieve penile erection and ejaculation |

* The functional goals table assumes the presence of a complete lesion. The levels are spinal cord levels, not vertebral levels. All functions subserved by portions of the central nervous system proximal to the lesion are presumed intact.

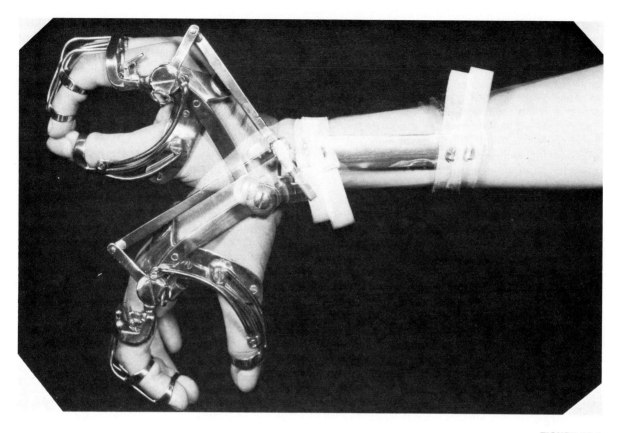

**FIGURE 32-9**
Siebens-Engel tenodesis splint utilizes the power of the radial wrist extensor to provide thumb and two-digit prehension to the paralyzed hand.

certain body parts. Other deficits, such as those affecting breathing, may be more subtle.

The neuromuscular activity in breathing/ respiration has three parts. *Inspiration* is normally accomplished by contraction of the diaphragms, which are innervated by the phrenic nerves from *C3 to C5* and of the intercostal muscles, innervated from *T1 to T8. Expiration* is passive and occurs with relaxation of the diaphragms and intercostal muscles. *Forced expiration,* as in coughing, sneezing, or nose blowing, requires contraction of the abdominal muscles, *T8 to T12,* against a closed glottis to increase the intraabdominal and intrathoracic pressures. Forced expiration is facilitated when a deep breath is taken first, since the elastic recoil of the distended lungs and chest will push air from the chest with greater velocity.

*Assisted respiration* An individual with a complete spinal cord lesion at *C4 or above* will have the use of neither diaphragms nor intercostal muscles to inspire; cough is also impossible since the abdominal muscles are likewise paralyzed. *Inspiratory assistance* may be given by several devices. First, room air or oxygen-enriched air may be forced into the mouth or trachea under *positive pressure.* Second, the individual may utilize a *cuirass,* or *chest shell,* worn over the ventral trunk and connected to a negative pressure source in order to artificially expand the chest and lower the diaphragms. Third, a *rocking bed* alternately tilts the supine patient gently foot-downward, lowering the diaphragms by gravity and causing inspiration, and head-downward, elevating the diaphragms and causing expiration. There are portable and battery-operated positive and negative pressure devices which can be attached to a wheelchair and used in a car. A combination of such devices gives the patient variety and mobility.

In long-term management of the respiration-dependent individual, the emphasis should be on ease and versatility of appropriate assists for inspiration and on the use of the patient's upper airway (nose, mouth, and throat) for humidification and speech. Techniques for assisted forced expiration (cough) are described below.

*Assisted cough* *Both the ability to take a deep breath and the ability to force the air out by contracting the abdominal muscles are prerequisites for effective coughing.* An individual with a lesion between C5 and the midthoracic area will have normally functioning diaphragms to maintain an adequate tidal volume. Although there is no respiratory distress, there will be significant respiratory limitations in forcing the air out and in taking a deep breath. The patient's first inkling that function of the respiratory system is compromised may be that a weak "achoo" is all that can be produced when faced with an insistent desire to sneeze. An attempt at nose blowing results in the discovery that there is no blasting force behind exhalation. Finally, an attempt to cough produces little more than a vocalized sigh. This patient lacks abdominal muscle contraction.

Paralysis of the intercostal muscles precludes the ability to take a breath deep enough to inflate the lungs fully, particularly the upper segments. A deep breath periodically is necessary to distend the alveoli, cleanse the airways, and provide passive range of motion to the otherwise immobile costochondral and costovertebral joints. The simplest way to supplement impaired *deep inspiration,* either as an exercise for the lungs and chest (10 breaths twice a day) or to aid coughing, is to deliver air into the mouth with positive pressure. Several small, uncomplicated respirators are available for home use.* The individual is instructed to lie supine, block the nasopharynx, hold the mouthpiece with closed lips, and allow the stream of air to fill the lungs for a few seconds until the feeling of maximum distensibility is obtained. Assisted breaths are intermingled with normal breaths to prevent hyperventilation. One should observe that the upper chest rises (the anteroposterior diameter increases) during inflation and falls abruptly with expiration. When the chest does not rise, one can conclude that the upper segments of the lungs have not filled or that the rib joints are contractured so that movement is not possible.

In order to substitute for the lack of abdominal muscle contraction required for *forced expiration,* a helper can apply manual pressure over the patient's lower ribs and abdomen at the end of a maximum inspiration to force air out of the lungs and chest. The patient is instructed to take a deep breath (with positive pressure if the intercostal muscles are paralyzed), hold it, and signal the helper by blinking. The helper then pushes once, firmly and quickly, on the lower thorax and abdomen, at the same time instructing the patient to cough. Studies have shown that patients with spinal dysfunction affecting the muscles of inspiration and cough can have a cough which is normal in respect to volume and velocity with these simple techniques.[33] *Assisted cough* should be used as often as the patient has the need to cough and sufficiently often that the patient and the helper maintain their skills.

Pneumonia, atelectasis, and chest cage rigidity on a neuromuscular basis are preventable complications of spinal cord dysfunction if deep breathing and cough assistance are performed. Nursing goals include teaching the patient the reasons for respiratory care and the techniques that should be utilized.

**S**kin Care    Of all the sequelae of paralysis with anesthesia, perhaps the one most universally identified by nurses and most often experienced by individuals with spinal cord dysfunction is decubitus ulcers. These lesions may be insidious in development with destruction of muscle and fat masquerading beneath a callus or a persistently discolored area. They may be forthright with an opening in the integument which exposes viable red tissue or, more often, a sloughing grayish or black mass.

Decubitus ulcers are the most preventable problem of the individual with spinal cord injury. The characteristics which make prevention a realistic goal are that (1) the *high-risk areas* of the body are predictable, (2) the *underlying mechanism of ulcer formation* is known, (3) *signs of incipient ulceration* are identifiable by sight and touch, and (4) *avoidance techniques* can be utilized by everyone.

*High-risk areas*    Any *bony prominence,* particularly in an area with reduced sensation, is at risk for pressure breakdown. All patients who sit for substantial periods of time endanger their ischial areas. Heels are vulnerable from contact with shoes and from friction against bedding. The sacrum bears excessive weight in the supine position, and the trochanters during side-lying. The elbows are particularly susceptible to ulceration in those patients who compensate for trunk instability by leaning on

---

* One is the Thompson Zephyr, made by Thompson Respiration Products, Boulder, Colo.

their lapboards or armrests or who use their arms as levers in shifting body position in bed.

*Origin of decubitus ulcers* Blood flows through capillaries at about 25 mmHg pressure. Constant blood flow provides essential nutrients and oxygen to cells and removes injurious metabolic waste products. Tissues subjected to *external pressure exceeding capillary pressure* (blood flow ceases) undergo metabolic cellular changes within 1 to 2 hours.[34] External pressures as low as 70 mmHg (about the amount of pressure on the heels of a supine individual) applied to tissues for 2 hours produce irreversible changes in cells which ultimately lead to their death.

In addition to ischemia from pressure, tissue can be damaged by shearing forces. *Shearing* occurs when one plane of tissue is pulled in a different direction from adjacent tissue with rupture of small vessels and interference of blood flow. For example, shearing occurs when a supine patient's sweaty buttocks and back stick to the bed sheets. When the head of the bed is elevated, the skin adheres to the sheet, but gravity pulls the internal mass of fat and muscle downward.

Bruises, sheet burns, thermal insults, pustules, and other disruptions of the integument predispose to decubitation, particularly if pressure is placed over them. Maceration from body fluids and irritation from feces compound the incidence of ulcers.

*Signs of an impending decubitus* Visual clues are the most common. Redness which is well demarcated and which does not fade in about 15 minutes after removal of pressure is the earliest sign. Redness which is still present after several hours when it is time for weight bearing on that area again indicates more profound tissue reaction. If pressure is reapplied to such a red area, decubitation is inevitable.

*Tactile clues* can be useful. For example, dark-skinned people cannot determine beginning redness of the skin as readily as is required for decubitus prevention. Waiting until a break in the pigmented skin presents as redness is obviously too late. Careful experimentation with deliberate pressure on the skin to see what shades of difference result is useful for some people. For most, a different technique is needed. A tactile clue is warmth of a specific area of the skin. Detecting changes in skin temperature between weight-bearing areas and adjacent areas can be done grossly with the backs of the fingers (Chap. 8). Circumscribed warmth lasting more than 15 minutes after pressure

is removed is a clue that the tissue is reacting to excessive pressure and circulatory disruption.

Recently a black woman said, "I have some real dry areas but no ulcers." Upon examination, she in fact had a nonsloughing eschar over a far-advanced sacral decubitus and thick callus overlying necrotic heels. The patient's assessment of excessive dryness was understandable because the color was no different from the rest of her skin. Such patients must be taught that dry, hard, or slightly blacker areas should be suspect.

For all patients, a hard or spongy lump, softness under a callus or dried blister, or a depression in the skin from braces or clothing can be tactile clues to a pressure area. Individuals who simply pass a hand over their bony prominences to check for drainage or breaks in the skin, however, are depending on a sign of advanced tissue reaction rather than on an early warning. Sensations, when they can be associated exclusively and predictably with excessive pressure over a body part, are useful reminders to shift weight, a major preventative action.

*Avoidance techniques* Prevention of decubitus ulcers depends largely on the *compensatory behavior* of the susceptible individual. Such behavior, at the very least, *requires that the person value intact skin or fear ulcers and that knowledge of what to do to avoid breakdown is available.*

In one study of 56 experienced patients with spinal cord injuries, the question was asked "Why are decubitus ulcers bad for you?"[35] The increased dependency which results when a person with spinal cord dysfunction is in bed or unable to sit, lowered morale and self-esteem which accompanied job loss, depletion of energy, and strain or worry were most often cited by patients as ways in which ulcers are bad. These were sufficiently powerful threats to the patient's integrity to justify avoidance of ulcers.

A person tends to adopt behavior which protects whatever is most meaningful. *Most meaningful* to patients were mobility, productivity, independence, and freedom from fear of impending catastrophe. Nurses might capitalize on these motivators of patient behavior when they teach the principles upon which compensatory behavior will be based.

While having an accurate respect for the dangers of decubitus ulcers and being highly motivated to prevent them, it is also important that the patient not feel excessively guilty, defeated, or worthless if an ulcer should occur. Such a balanced perspective will foster the patient's compensatory behavior to promote skin intactness but will also permit, should it become necessary, the seeking of help and the taking of proper action to alleviate further skin breakdown.

Once the desire to establish appropriate behavior is present, *knowledge* must be acquired which will enable the individual to choose that behavior. The nurse may impart knowledge either by rehearsal of a list of dos and don'ts (always an incomplete list) or by reasoning. One can hypothesize that the patient who has had only a few directives for behavior, but little understanding of the physiologic process of decubitation, may not know how to compromise safely or to cope with situations not already experienced under professional supervision. On the other hand, the person who has learned to conceptualize and understands the origin of ulcers can apply reasoning to any unique situation in which a decision regarding weight bearing is needed. Six guides to teaching are:

1   Teach patients the *origin of decubitation* through an understanding of the physiologic dynamics of pressure-circulation-cell viability and by applying that knowledge. One might use this example: Ask a patient to press on a nail bed and observe first the blanching, then the hyperemia. This is a graphic demonstration of how small an amount of external pressure is required to interrupt capillary blood flow and of how prompt the tissue response is.

2   Teach patients to *change pressure points:* to lean or push up in the wheelchair every 15 minutes; to sleep prone at night with the feet hanging straight down off the end of the mattress; and to use a cushion in the wheelchair. The search for a practical wheelchair cushion or wheelchair seat which will predictably permit blood flow through stationary weight-bearing areas goes on. In the absence of such a cushion, a 4-inch polyurethane or latex cushion covered with fabric is the cheapest satisfactory kind. Weight shifts are essential no matter what the seating surface. In the wheelchair, the seated individual should have weight on the thighs as well as on the buttocks to distribute the weight more evenly. To accomplish this, lower the footrests so that the knees are below the hips.

3   Teach patients to *inspect* their skin, particularly *bony prominences,* daily prior to weight bearing. Heavy reliance on visual clues can be safe and effective only if the individual can actually see those parts of the body which are most at risk, namely the ischial tuberosities and the sacrum. In order to see these parts, the individual who can grasp can use a long-handled magnifying mirror. One who must rely on a caretaker to hold the mirror can be helped to visualize all body areas by having one mirror held above the area to reflect into another mirror near the face.[36] Tactile inspection, if appropriate, should be performed as regularly as is visual inspection. Teach the patient to remove pressure completely until an incipient area looks and feels normal again.

4   Teach the patient to *think*—to think before plunging into water that may be too hot, before taking risks in body mechanics and falling, before wearing clothes that constrict, before sitting on an already red ischium. Encourage reflection on circumstances that might have precipitated a fresh skin lesion so that repetition of the incident can be avoided.

5   Teach the patient, by example, the *consistent repetitious* nursing care which incorporates the principles of decubitus prevention.

6   Teach the individual that *participation* in health management, whether at home or in an institution, is a patient's right and obligation. The patient must assume responsibility for initiation and supervision of daily care. Family involvement in patient care may be essential, and teaching of involved persons should also be carried out.

Should a decubitus ulcer occur, the principles of care are to remove pressure from the ulcer totally and to keep it clean. Keeping the ulcer clean means debridement of nonviable tissue and promotion of open drainage. Systemic antibiotics are indicated only if cellulitis is present. There are dozens of different topical applications, each favored by some people. For the most part, they are unnecessary, if not harmful. A simple normal saline dressing applied to the open area, allowed to dry, and gently pulled away will cleanse and debride the crater and provide a physiologic medium for growth of granulation tissue. Surgical closure may be a method of choice for some ulcers.

**B**owel Management   Individuals with spinal cord dysfunction affecting the anal sphincters and rectum are commonly found to be either incontinent of stool or impacted before bowel management is introduced. A review of the neurophysiology of the lower gut suggests some interventions to prevent these situations.

*Neurophysiology*   *Innervation* of the bowel is both *intrinsic* and *extrinsic* to its structure. The intrinsic nervous network consists of the myenteric plexus of Auerbach, lying between the circular and longitudinal muscle coats of the bowel, and the submucosal plexus of Meissner. It is unaffected by spinal cord damage; it functions autonomously and is capable of coordinating movements of adjacent segments of the gut necessary for peristaltic progression and delivery of fecal material into the rectum.[37] These intrinsic plexuses extend caudally to encompass the internal anal sphincter, a smooth muscle. However, because they stop at the pectinate line which separates the rectum from the anus, approximately three centimeters of the distal anus is left without intrinsic innervation. Here, under voluntary control, the external sphincter ani, a striated muscle, has extrinsic innervation mainly from branches of the pudendal nerves which originate in the anterior horn cells of sacral cord segments S2 to S4.

The parasympathetic nerves (pelvic nerves) arising from the anterolateral horns of sacral cord segments S2 to S4 are primarily responsible for the coordinated act of defecation. As rectal stretch receptors are activated by bowel contents, the pudendal and pelvic nerves mediate control of both the involuntary intrinsic system and the voluntary external sphincter. Widespread peristalsis and secretions are increased, and the rectum contracts while the sphincters relax. When defecation is delayed voluntarily or by denervation, the rectal musculature adapts itself to continued distention by reduction in stretch stimuli and diminished force of rectal contraction.

The person with spinal cord dysfunction can *expect the fecal mass to be propelled to the rectum by the action of the intrinsic nervous network.* Expulsion from the rectum, however, may be retarded, may be dyssynchronous with sphincter activity, or may occur spontaneously without higher center awareness and voluntary control. When the spinal cord lesion is above S2 (UMN lesion), the anal sphincter will have reflex activity, and bowel emptying by rectal stimulation is possible. If the cord lesion involves S2 to S4 (LMN lesion), a flaccid external sphincter without reflex activity results. The intrinsic network of the sigmoid is also more sluggish in the absence of pelvic nerve innervation. (The vagus nerve controls the intrinsic network down to the splenic flexure and is unaffected by spinal cord dysfunction.) The gastrocolic and orthocolic reflexes are intact; i.e., peristalsis tends to occur after eating and after arising from the supine posture (see Chap. 15).

*Assessment*　Simple tests will determine if the external anal sphincter is flaccid or behaves reflexly. First, the perianal skin is pricked gently. Second, an examining finger is inserted into the rectum. Third, the glans penis or the clitoris is squeezed briskly with the other hand while the finger is in the rectum. If the sacral reflex arc (S2 to S4) is present, the anal sphincter will contract with perianal pinprick, it will tighten around the examining finger, and/or it will contract with stimulation to the glans or clitoris (the bulbocavernosus reflex). If the cord injury includes S2 to S4, the sphincter will remain flaccid during these tests.

*Interventions*　The *goals of bowel management* are to trigger peristalsis and evacuation of the rectum at a predictable time, to achieve prompt, complete defecation, and to avoid inadvertent bowel movements. The approach differs depending on the presence or absence of reflex activity in the sphincters and rectum. Any approach, however, is directed toward the distal gut since the timing of an artificial stimulus introduced to the rectum must be under the patient's control.

The patient with *intact anorectal reflexes* will usually respond to a bisacodyl *suppository* placed above the pectinate line (2 to 3 inches inside the gut) and against the bowel lining and/or to digital stimulation (gentle massage or dilation of the anus).

The patient with a *flaccid sphincter* will usually need to utilize *digital removal* of stool with *straining*. A 2-ounce phosphosoda enema delivered by a 6- to 8-inch tube into the sigmoid colon is an alternative stimulus. The buttocks must be pinched together and the tube left in place (2 to 5 minutes) to prevent premature egress of the solution.

Bowel training for the patient requires a *reasonable time* interval; allow 1 hour from beginning of rectal stimulation to completion of defecation. For the suppository user, up to one-half this time is devoted to suppository melting and neural response. The patient who relies on digital removal generally empties the rectum much faster. A program of bowel training should be on a regular schedule, usually every other day at the same time. Try to build on the patient's previous bowel pattern if there was a regular defecation habit. One should consider orthocolic and postural reflexes as an adjunct to bowel training; i.e., perform bowel care after a meal and put the patient in the upright posture if possible.

It is essential to reach *agreement on a bowel*

*program* which is acceptable from both the patient's and the nurse's points of view. The individual components such as the time required per episode, frequency of care, location (toilet, commode, or pads in the bed), and methods of rectal stimulation should be demonstrated repeatedly to be effective during the rehabilitation period. The aim is for them to become habitual and incorporated into the patient's new self-concept regarding defecation.

Any patient may profit from *stool softeners or bulk formers.* Oral laxatives should be avoided since they increase the unpredictability of bowel movement and thus the incontinence of patients. A diet adequate in roughage and fluid produces a formed consistency of stool.

Thirty-eight patients with spinal cord injury lasting at least 3 years observed themselves and acquired knowledge about the effect of *diet* on their bowels.[38] The specific foods and effects they describe are listed below:

*Laxative: Diarrhea-producing*

| | |
|---|---|
| Applesauce | Licorice |
| Baked beans | Onions |
| Beer, draft | Peanuts (and other nuts) |
| Cabbage | Popcorn |
| Chili | Prunes |
| Corn, whole kernel | Sesame seeds |
| Cranberries | Smoked fish |
| Lasagna | Spicy, rich, gaseous foods |
| Lettuce | Watermelon |

*Helpful for bulk and softening*

Bran flakes

Cheese

Fruits

Graham crackers

Lettuce

Vegetables

Large amounts of food

The consistency of a diarrhea stool or very soft stool will usually result in incontinence. When habituation to a bowel care program has been achieved, rendering an individual accident-free, one should respect this management protocol. The massive catharsis of a "routine preparation" for an intravenous pyelogram, for example, will totally disrupt the predictability of the individual with spinal cord dysfunction. It is wiser to schedule the x-ray within 12 hours after usual defecation and omit administering oral laxatives or other evacuants. Antibiotics, especially ampicillin, cause diarrhea in many patients, and their prescription is appropriately reserved for significant specific infections and then given for as short a course as possible. In the event of brief, spontaneous diarrhea related to food or illness it is suggested that a patient maintain the normal bowel care routine, omitting it only on the day of diarrhea.

Some medications may retard bowel action and should, therefore, be given with caution. Anticholinergic agents, propantheline bromide, for example, are often prescribed to inhibit bladder contractions, but they may decrease bowel peristalsis as well.

A group of patients made the following comments about *teaching methods* that a nurse might use to instruct a paralyzed individual about his or her bowel: "Discuss and explain" were most frequently mentioned, usually with some qualifications: "Don't involve a whole lot of people in it—use a one-to-one approach instead of having two or three bystanders." "Have a male tell the young men; they are a little embarrassed by a woman telling them." "Have group discussions for some who don't like to admit they have to do these things and have problems." Several patients suggested discussion with another experienced paralyzed person. Others wanted a demonstration after which the patient (or caretaker) would perform the care in order to practice and gain experience while in the hospital.

The *goal* for nursing patients with a neurogenic bowel is twofold. One aspect is to establish a *successful program* with the individual and give repetitive opportunity to practice and incorporate the regimen. The second aspect is to give the patient the *bases from which to make judgments* so that bowel management can be modified intelligently to fit changing social and physiologic needs in the future. These bases are an awareness of the anatomy and physiology of the bowel, the deficits and reflex patterns of the patient, the mode of action of the techniques and medications available, and the influence of diet.

**U**rinary Tract Management    The urinary tract comprises an upper portion (kidneys and ureters) and a lower portion (bladder and urethra). Upper-tract function is unimpaired by spinal cord lesions per se; in contrast, the lower tract is often adversely affected. The bladder, a muscular reservoir for urine, commonly fails to contract, or the contractions are of insufficient quality or duration to expel the urine completely. The urethra may fail to open appropriately to permit egress of urine during bladder contraction. In addition, the patient loses volitional control of the bladder both in initiating a stream and in delaying voiding and is, therefore, incontinent.

The upper tracts may become secondarily compromised as a result of lower-tract malfunction. Stasis of bladder urine predisposes to infection; renal function is threatened by ascending infection (pyelonephritis) in which scar tissue replaces glomeruli. Bladder distention when coupled with abnormal intravesical pressure and a constricted urethra creates hydrodynamic changes in the ureters and kidneys (hydroureter, hydronephrosis) in which extrinsic pressure damages renal tissue.

The *primary goal* of urinary care for the individual with a spinal cord lesion is the *preservation of renal function.* Measures designed to treat the lower tract problems are, therefore, oriented toward the upper tracts.

*Neurophysiology* Micturition in the normal, uninhibited state follows this pattern: when the bladder has reached a certain stage of filling (400 to 700 ml), reflex contractions of the detrusor muscle occur; the internal sphincter, the proximal part of the urethra, and the external sphincter relax. As the urine passes along the urethra, the continued *contraction of the detrusor* is assured, together with further *relaxation of the external sphincter.* The voiding reflex is sustained until the *bladder is completely empty.* There is *no backflow of urine* into the ureters or kidneys.

This description of voiding is deceptively simple. The synergistic action of smooth and skeletal muscle and the inhibitory and excitatory influences of somatic, parasympathetic, and sympathetic nerves together with spinal cord, medullary, and cortical centers within the central nervous system are involved. Of particular importance is the spinal cord segment *S2 to S4* from which arise both the *pelvic* and *pudendal nerves.* The sensation of detrusor stretch, the motor action of detrusor contraction, and the relaxation of the smooth muscle of the proximal urethra are mediated through the parasympathetic nerve supply via the *pelvic nerves.* The external sphincter and pelvic floor are skeletal

muscles supplied by the *pudendal nerves.* The role of the sympathetic nerve supply (hypogastric nerves, L1 to L3) is incompletely understood. It is thought that completion of the voiding reflex can be interrupted and voiding postponed by the release of inhibitory impulses from the paracentral lobule of the cerebral cortex; voluntary initiation of voiding also originates in the paracentral lobule.

Cord dysfunctions which occur above S2 to S4 (spinal micturition reflex center) preserve the reflex arc and are, therefore, upper motor neuron lesions to the bladder. This type of bladder is called a *reflex neurogenic* or *upper motor neuron bladder.* There is no voluntary control of voiding. Reflex contraction of the detrusor may be stimulated by a number of visceral and somatic sensory impulses entering the distal cord: bladder distention, leg spasticity, defecation, tapping the abdomen in the suprapubic area, and sensory stimuli to the perineum and inner thighs, for example. Voiding is in short spurts. The residual urine is usually high for three reasons: (1) the detrusor contraction may be weak, (2) the detrusor contraction is unsustained for a time sufficient to empty the bladder, and (3) dyssynergy of the pelvic floor and external sphincter occur such that at the time of bladder contraction the outflow tract is also contracted and resists the flow of urine. In males, surgical intervention to interrupt the external sphincter or to section pudendal nerves may be recommended.

Cord dysfunction which damages the S2 to S4 micturition center or the corresponding nerve roots produces an *autonomous neurogenic bladder,* i.e., a *lower motor neuron bladder* without muscle tone. Voluntary control is absent. The bladder is distensible without contraction. Generally, the outflow resistance is also low. Voiding occurs by overflow with continuous dribbling or by a stream whenever the intraabdominal pressure is increased as in coughing or straining.

Individuals with an incomplete cord lesion have some of the upper motor neuron or lower motor neuron characteristics, depending on the site of dysfunction, but often have frequency, urgency, difficulty starting the stream, a postvoiding residual urine, and some degree of incontinence.

*Assessment Urinalysis* and *urine culture* determine the specific gravity, pH, cell count, and bacterial flora of the urine and drug sensitivities of the infecting organisms. These specimens should be collected midstream after cleaning the urethral meatus or obtained by catheter and sent immediately to the laboratory.

Quantity of *residual urine* is a most significant part of the objective data for the neurogenic bladder. Residual urine is the *amount of urine left in the bladder immediately after a measured void;* it is obtained by catheterization. If the patient is unable to void at all, the amount obtained by catheter is properly termed *bladder volume* rather than residual urine. After the catheter is in place, pressure should be applied suprapubicly to expel all the urine. Pressure should be continued as long as urine flows, then the catheter advanced a few centimeters at a time, with a pause each time for the urine to stop. The record should show the time, the amount, and the circumstances of the voiding, i.e., amounts expelled with spontaneous void, with stimulation, or with straining, and the amount obtained by catheter following the voids.

Several *diagnostic tests* may be utilized to evaluate bladder function. A *cystometrogram* is a record of bladder muscle activity during the introduction of fluid into the bladder. A catheter is inserted which is attached to a manometer to measure the amplitude of intravesical pressure. The presence of reflex contractions of the bladder and the response to voluntary straining are recorded.

*Cystoscopy* is the direct visualization of the urethra and bladder through an instrument inserted into the urethra. Organic obstructions, calculi, bladder inflammation, and the appearance of the urethral orifices are sought.

*Cystourethrography* is the fluoroscopic visualization of the passage, via urethral catheter, of contrast media into the bladder and its expulsion after catheter removal. Of particular interest is the status of vesicoureteral reflux (movement of bladder contents into a ureter), the shape of the bladder and the bladder wall (smooth or trabeculated), and the degree of bladder emptying.

*Intravenous pyelogram* is the radiologic study of the passage of intravenous contrast material from the blood through the kidneys and ureters into the bladder. The outline of the kidney mass, the shape of the renal calyces and the ureters, peristalsis of the ureters, presence of calculi, and the rapidity of dye excretion are noted.

*Intervention* Objectives for the management of the neurogenic bladder are to *evacuate the bladder with minimal residual urine, eliminate infection* of the urine, and provide *continence.* All these are met in such a way as to preserve and protect renal function. The specific techniques of (1) Foley catheterization, (2) intermittent catheterization, (3) catheter freedom, and (4) urinary diversion will be discussed.

During the acute phase of spinal cord dysfunction, most patients have a *Foley catheter* in the bladder. For some persons, this technique is used throughout life. The purpose of the catheter is to provide a conduit for constant drainage of urine from the bladder. Anything that impedes urine flow is to be avoided. An unplanned accumulation of urine in the bladder may cause stretching, tearing, and subsequent scarring of the bladder muscle through overdistention, thus compromising the ultimate recovery of detrusor contractibility. Distention may also cause vesicoureteral reflux of urine into the renal pelvises or may inhibit ureteral peristalsis; damaging pressures occur in the kidneys when urine is not readily propelled into the bladder. A catheter is most often blocked by accumulated sediment which obstructs the eye or the lumen of the tube. In the presence of *dilute urine* and *acid urine,* the catheter will remain patent.

A urine output of approximately three liters per day for an adult ensures adequate dilution (20 ml urine per day per pound of body weight). Usually the patient has to increase fluid intake to achieve this output. Citrus juices produce an alkaline residue in the urine; therefore, such juices should be limited to one serving a day. Daily reporting of the exact output volume with appropriate praise or admonition is a significant factor in helping the patient incorporate the high-output habit.

Normal urine is acidic; when a catheter is present, the urine should remain acidic. In an acid urine, the calcium and phosphates which the immobilized body excretes remain dissolved and are washed out with the urine; in contrast, these minerals precipitate in alkaline urine and may settle in the bladder and catheter, like lime in the bottom of a teakettle. In addition, alkaline urine irritates the bladder and may increase the spasticity of an upper motor neuron bladder. Alkalinity causes the bladder to produce mucus which may clog the catheter. The patient can monitor the *urine pH* (acidity or alkalinity) daily by placing a drop of urine directly from the catheter tip on a strip of pH-sensitive paper in the morning before breakfast or catheter irrigation. Comparison of the color of the damp paper with the standard color scale will determine the pH. A pH above 7 is alkaline, below 7 is acid.

Barring dietary indiscretions, the most frequent cause of alkaline urine is infection. Bladder urine is unavoidably infected in the presence of a catheter. Many infections are compatible with acid urine and are innocuous and, therefore, not treated. However, bladder urine becomes alkaline if it is infected with bacteria which form ammonia from urea, a waste product in urine. These bacteria, the commonest of which are strains of *Proteus,* are called *urea-splitting organisms.* A urea-splitting infection should be *treated with the appropriate antimicrobial* in order to prevent alkalinity of the urine and sedimentation.

The Foley catheter should be *changed before it becomes obstructed* (of course, an obstructed catheter should be changed immediately). Catheters of silicone or other materials have been introduced on the market with claims that they can remain in situ for several weeks or months. The nurse must observe the patient's catheter to determine the time for change. Alkaline or viscous urine and sluggish inflow or outflow of irrigant solutions are warnings of catheter obstruction. When the old catheter is removed, it should be cut across at several places and the lumen examined for sediment. If none is present, the catheter change interval was appropriate; if sediment is present, the catheter should be changed more frequently. A 3-week interval is a guide for changing the catheter, assuming the urine is acid and dilute.

*Trauma* to the urethra is a hazard of catheterization. In the *male,* there are two common sites of trauma—the prostatic urethra and the urethra at the penoscrotal junction. The prostatic urethra can be damaged by forcing a catheter against resistance and creating a false passageway through the soft tissue. It can also be ruptured if the inflation balloon lies within the urethra rather than within the bladder. Trauma to the prostate results in bleeding and may transmit bacteria from the infected urine into the bloodstream causing septicemia, a life-threatening complication. When passing a male catheter, force should not be used if resistance is felt at the bladder neck. A moment should be given for relaxation to occur. If the catheter still does not slip into the bladder, medical assistance should be sought. Once the catheter is in the bladder and urine has begun to flow, the catheter should be inserted another 1½ to 2 inches before the balloon is inflated.

The urethra at the penoscrotal junction is at risk for pressure necrosis because the urethra makes a sharp bend when the penis is in the relaxed position. If the catheter is taped to the thigh with the penis in the flaccid position, there is not sufficient room for erection to occur. If, however, the catheter is taped to the abdomen, the penis will be in such a position that the urethral curves are straightened, and should erection occur, no additional force will be exerted on the catheter and urethra (Fig. 32-10). The course of the urethra along the underside of the penis and scrotum should be

palpated daily, and any induration or lumps which are the first sign of abscess around the traumatized urethra reported.

The *female* is also vulnerable to urethral *trauma.* Inadvertent extrusion of the catheter with the balloon inflated stretches and tears the urethra. Subsequently, there may be leakage of urine around the catheter. To prevent this, the catheter must be taped to the thigh allowing enough slack in the catheter to accommodate all leg positions without pulling on the tube (Fig. 32-11). Should the urethra become stretched and the woman be incontinent despite replacement of the Foley catheter, a small-caliber (No. 16 French) catheter should continue to be used and the soft tissues allowed to constrict to the original size. The use of a larger and larger catheter in an effort to prevent leakage is unwise since this will only further dilate the urethra.

*Irrigation* of an indwelling catheter is a controversial issue. When used, an irrigant should be sterile, innocuous, acid, and *buffered.* The buffered acid will help dissolve precipitates. For this reason, instillation of 30 to 50 ml into the bladder followed by clamping of the catheter for half an hour twice a day is usually recommended. The catheter must be unclamped after the one-half hour period. If hematuria is present, only normal saline should be used to irrigate because many buffering agents have a local anticoagulant effect.

*Periodic decompression* of the bladder with a straight catheter is a practice advocated by some for the initial management of the neurogenic bladder. Others use it as an intermediate step between continuous use of an indwelling catheter and catheter freedom. For some patients, *intermittent catheterization* is a life-long way of emptying the bladder. The advantages cited are the reduced rate of infection as opposed to an indwelling Foley catheter, reduced incidence of urethral trauma, and ease of sexual activity.

The patient should be observed for distention, spontaneous voiding, headache, hypertension, and fever. Distention would indicate overhydration or the need for more frequent decompression. The urinary output is limited to 1200 to 1800 ml in 24 hours. Catheterization is performed at intervals designed to avoid bladder filling in excess of 500 ml. In planning the catheterization schedule, one should note that patients frequently excrete several hundred milliliters of urine within an hour of becoming recumbent after having been in a wheelchair.

In the individual with an upper motor neuron lesion, spontaneous voiding may occur between catheterizations, and it signals the return of function of the detrusor. Attempts to facilitate the micturition reflex arc and cause bladder contraction should be made before each catheterization. Tapping the suprapubic area, brushing the inner thighs, and stroking the abdomen with ice are techniques to try. Should a reflex response occur, repeat the stimulation until no further urine is expelled. Compare the amount voided with the amount of residual urine in order to monitor the progress in bladder efficiency. When residual urine is less than 100 ml, catheterization will probably be stopped, although stimulation to elicit voiding will continue several times a day.

Headache and hypertension are autonomic responses to noxious visceral stimuli in a patient with a cord lesion above T6. In this context, the bladder would be catheterized immediately to reduce the stretch stimulation of the bladder. Fever may indicate the presence of vesicoureteral reflux with pyelonephritis.

When an individual with an upper motor neuron lesion to the bladder develops reflex detrusor contractions sufficient to empty the bladder leaving only a low residual, *catheter freedom* is achieved. Every effort is made to reduce the residual further by repeated stimulation of the voiding reflex; pharmacologic assists such as bethanechol may be given. Since the catheter as a portal for infection is no longer present, sterilization of bladder urine is attempted with the appropriate antimicrobial, and the urinary pH is monitored. A disinfecting agent such as methenamine mandelate or methenamine hippurate is usually given. These compounds are most effective in acid urine.

Since voiding will unpredictably occur with reflex activity of the sacral cord, males will need to wear a urine-collecting device applied to the penis. The device should be reliable, inexpensive, and safe. The simplest type is constructed from a condom fastened to a length of rubber tubing which in turn attaches to a leg bag. To apply it, put a continuous ring of surgical adhesive around the midshaft of the penis. Unroll the condom over the penis and press it down onto the adhesive. Place *elastic* adhesive tape, 1-inch wide, snugly around the flaccid penis over the stuck down part of the condom. The tape should not overlap more than ½ inch.

**FIGURE 32-10**

Taping a Foley catheter (male patient). The objective is to straighten the urethral curve at the penoscrotal area in order to reduce the chance of pressure necrosis within the urethra and to prevent additional force on the catheter and urethra in the event of erection. Positioning the Foley catheter against the thigh would frustrate this objective; therefore, the catheter is anchored on the abdomen instead.

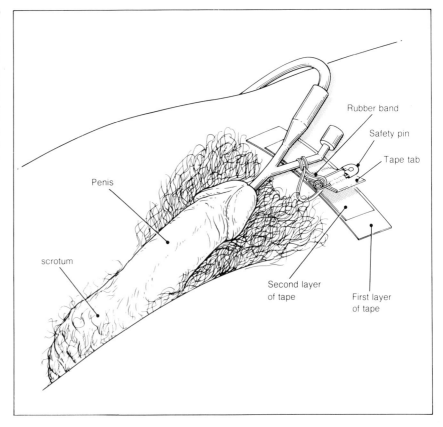

Rubber band

Safety pin

Tape tab

Penis

scrotum

Second layer of tape

First layer of tape

Commercially available devices which attach by rubber bands around the penis or by rubber straps over the crotch and buttocks are dangerous because undue pressure is applied to these insensitive areas.

Females with an upper motor neuron bladder may be able to keep dry by using parasympathetic blocking agents such as l-Hyoscyamine (Cystospaz) to reduce bladder spasticity in combination with emptying the bladder with intermittent catheterization. There is no effective external urinary appliance for women, and most are forced to use a Foley catheter to be dry. It is possible to wear external pads and a waterproof panty to collect the urine. Coating the perineum with petroleum jelly and changing wet pads helps prevent skin breakdown.

Both females and males with lower motor neuron bladders may be catheter-free and continent by expressing the bladder contents at planned intervals. The *Credé maneuver* utilizes external manual pressure with both hands pressing inward and downward over the abdomen starting over the umbilicus and moving down behind the pubis as urine is eliminated. Another technique is

the *Valsalva maneuver* in which the individual takes a deep breath and holds it while contracting the abdominal muscles and straining. The increased intraabdominal pressure forces urine out of the bladder. If neither technique empties the bladder sufficiently, intermittent catheterization can be used. Most patients will wear protective devices or clothing since small voids may occur with the increase of intraabdominal pressure associated with activities such as transferring from bed to chair, crutch walking, and coughing.

A *suprapubic cystostomy* offers an alternative to constant urethral catheterization. Nursing care is the same as with the urethral Foley catheter. Construction of a *substitute bladder* from an isolated loop of ileum into which the ureters are implanted and which empties from a stoma on the abdominal wall is sometimes performed. The selection and application of a collecting device is critical to avoid inadvertent leakage. The loop is not a reservoir but rather a conduit for urine. The peristaltic action of the ileal segment is essential to propel the urine out. If urine fails to exit the loop, reflux will occur into the renal system. The nurse should observe

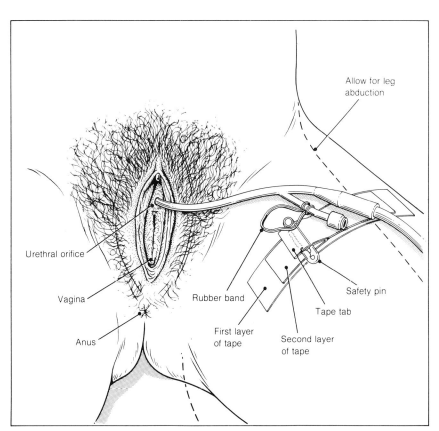

**FIGURE 32-11**

Taping a Foley catheter (female). The objective is to prevent extrusion of the Foley catheter when the balloon is inflated. The catheter is taped to the thigh when the leg is abducted. This allows a sufficient length of catheter to permit leg mobility, transfer activities, etc., without putting stress on the indwelling portion of the catheter.

Allow for leg abduction

Urethral orifice

Vagina

Anus

Rubber band

First layer of tape

Second layer of tape

Tape tab

Safety pin

that the urine spurts from the stoma at frequent intervals (see Chap. 6).

**Fostering psychologic integration** The extensive literature which deals with the psychology of death and dying (Chap. 3) is in large part applicable to the situation in which an individual loses body function. There is grieving for the loss of the familiar "self," for the attributes associated with being physically intact, and for the dreams which are now found to be in jeopardy. There is, however, a major difference between the process of coping with disability and that of coping with death. The disability never ceases, is never finished, can never be put aside and forgotten. The patient with spinal cord dysfunction, the family or significant others, and to some extent the nurses will be faced with the task of adjusting to the fact of extensive disability. One model of psychologic adjustment to loss of body function designates these stages: (1) *denial,* (2) *beginning awareness,* often expressed by anger, (3) *beginning adjustment,* usually marked by anxiety, and (4) *reorganization,* in which learning predominates (modified from Engel).[39]

**D**enial *Denial* of the real situation initially helps the patient to have self-control and to survive the unimaginable psychic and physical shock that the trauma suddenly imposes. Throughout convalescence, the patient may return to denial of the most painful psychologic aspects of the disabled condition despite a gradual mental incorporation of reality. The nurse helps most by giving consistent matter-of-fact care which does not permit the patient to control the quality of care through avoidance or refusal of treatment. It is well to point out the positive aspects of reality. The patient, however, is unable to assume responsibility for personal management which disability requires and will not profit from teaching at this time. As long as problems are denied, lectures about the possibilities of future rehabilitation will go unheard.

The goal in caring for the denying patient is to "establish oneself as a professional person who understands and accepts how the patient feels, but is aware of the fact, and can be depended on to act in accordance with the reality he is not yet able to accept."[40]

**B**eginning Awareness When the realities of the situation are admitted, the patient is faced with the frustrations these realities impose. *Anger* follows. Because of neuromuscular limitations, words may be used to replace physical retaliation. It is often most helpful for the nurse to listen to the patient and give permission for self-expression, without arguing or moralizing in return. The nurse can explore with the patient origins of behavior in order to clarify feelings: "You are swearing a lot today. I wonder why?" "There are many things to be angry about—what bothers *you* the most?" Stay with the patient during verbal outbursts; if you must leave, explain why. The patient must not believe that anger alienates the nurse or that punishment by the withdrawal of a significant person ensues. Angry people need safe outlets for feelings. Talking, games, spectator sports, music, visitors, and involvement in activities outside the hospital room and unit help dissipate anger. The nurse protects the patient from hurting self or staff members.

The goals in caring for the angry patient who is becoming aware of reality are to demonstrate that the patient is worthy and accepted in spite of angry expressions, that help in finding control in safe and appropriate emotional outlets is available, and that the responsibility for care will be assumed by the staff until the patient is ready to accept self-responsibility. The nurse must also find personal outlets for emotions in order to be composed, objective, and understanding when in contact with the angry patient.

**B**eginning Adjustment Patients pose many questions which are unanswerable initially. They wonder about being independent, earning money, having a sexual partnership, being accepted by the general public, and other weighty issues. To the extent that answers are unknown, *anxiety* will increase. Anxiety can deplete the individual's energy resources and distort reality. It can, however, be a motivational stimulus to learning.

There are a number of ways to help the patient conserve energy by reducing anxiety. Through demonstrating ability and willingness to meet needs, the nurse fosters *trust* in hospital caretakers. Setting necessary *limits* indicates that the nurse cares enough for the patient to provide protection. This frees the energy that might otherwise be expended in testing the nurse's concern and in asking for external controls. Most patients do not want the doctor, the nurse, or others to relinquish their *professional roles;* there is less anxiety when staff do not try to become surrogate father, mother, pal, or spouse.

When anxiety distorts reality, the patient becomes frightened. Aberrant behavior, in keeping with the false situation such anxieties have constructed, may appear. Above all, the patient needs to be reassured that such responses are normal and acceptable rather than the result of insanity. The relationship between sensory loss, anxiety, and distorted reality are vividly related by Brian Sternberg, an olympic pole vault candidate, who became quadriplegic in a trampoline accident:

I had no feeling at all below the neck, no proof that I had legs or arms or a torso. I had no sensation of *being* anywhere. Except for the back of my head, I couldn't feel myself touching the air mattress under me. It was as if I were floating around the room. That led to hallucinations—tactile ones. For instance, I could not feel my real arms and legs, but I did have imaginary ones that I could feel and move around. I got so I could 'feel' objects—shapes—in the imaginary hands. At first, I could control it: I could spread the hands apart, think 'basketball,' and be holding one. Then I began to lose control. If I imagined picking up something, I couldn't get rid of it; it stuck to the fingers. Things I didn't invite began appearing in the hands, things you wouldn't want, like razor blades.[41]

The nurse can help the patient put ideas and reality into proper perspective. Honest assessment of improvement, an explanation of benefits from prescribed treatment, and a reiteration of immediate objectives and how to reach them will help build success into the patient's life and replace anxiety with confidence and direction. Some goals in caring for the anxious patient are to conserve the energies needed to cope with the demands of disability, to eliminate perceptual distortions, and to foster the patient's desire to learn.

**R**eorganization   Reorganization is a period of *intense learning*—learning about physical care, about the psychology of oneself, how to cope in an environment that is relatively hostile to disability, how to establish satisfying interpersonal relationships, and about educational, vocational, financial, and health resources. The first of many things the patient has to learn is what has happened to the spinal cord and the functional implications of the lesion. It is important that the painful facts about the self are first realized in a friendly and accepting atmosphere. It is commonly necessary for the staff to provide this atmosphere in the absence of loving parents or relatives who are often infrequent visitors and who may be too distraught by their own grief to support their loved one.

While the patient receives incidental and planned instruction about self-care and about the physiologic reactions of the body to spinal cord dysfunction, the psychologic learning is less structured. The most potent source of psychologic learning about the changed self is found in the attitudes and responses of those closest to the patient. Since nursing staff and other professionals interact with the patient most frequently, it is from them that the patient learns a sense of worthiness and self-esteem. Above all, the patient must learn self-appreciation and self-trust as a reflection of the staff's appreciation and trust.

In the hospital, the entire staff teaches the patient to identify and anticipate difficult situations and to solve problems. *Capabilities have to be tested in actual situations.* Therapeutic leaves of absence with or without a staff member present are part of treatment.

While most patients identify their primary concerns as mobility and independent self-care, *sexual concerns* also arise during all stages of reaction to disability. Patients wonder, for example, whether they will have genital sensation, can engage in intercourse, will be attractive to the opposite sex, and will find their masculinity or femininity threatened. The patient gives cues to sexual concerns in many ways from subtle comments to straightforward questions to overt behavior such as flirtation, use of pornographic material, masturbation, and provocative acts.

Sexual counseling should be a part of the rehabilitative effort, but it is the most sensitive and emotional area for both patients and staff. Staff members should seek guidance from each other and from the most experienced leadership available so that accurate information and perceptive advice are given to the patient. In general, women with spinal cord dysfunction will continue to ovulate and menstruate and can conceive and carry a pregnancy which terminates in vaginal delivery if there is no pelvic dystocia. Men with an upper motor neuron lesion to S2 to S4 will in all likelihood have erection and be able to achieve intromission, but will lack synergism for the complex act of ejaculation. Men with a lesion affecting the lower motor neurons of S2 to S4 will generally not have an erection. The emphasis on intercourse should be expanded to include other forms of sexual expression and experience. The exploration of pleasuring, the satisfaction of giving as well as receiving affection, the psychic comforts of trust and loyalty, and the privilege of sharing another's life are facets of sexuality as available to the person with spinal cord dysfunction as to anyone else.

Reorganization includes planning to *live outside an institution.* Most patients with spinal cord dysfunction can live independently; a few may require a living arrangement which provides for personal assistance during certain times of day. Structural modifications (ramps, larger doorways) and special equipment (grab bars, elevated toilet seat, hand controls on a car) facilitate independence.

Attention to *education, vocation, and recreation* must be given. The United States Division of Vocational Rehabilitation, a federal agency with administrative branches in every state, provides counseling, testing, training, equipment, and financial assistance to clients. Social Security disability benefits may be applicable to a given patient. Referral to both the Division of Vocational Rehabilitation and to local Social Security offices should be made if a patient has a permanent disability.

Patients with spinal cord dysfunction need a base for *medical care* where a *multidisciplinary team* familiar with multisystem impairment can provide regular check-ups and can treat or coordinate treatment should a problem arise. The onset of carelessness, busyness, and a false sense of security ("I've never had a problem") reduce a patient's vigilance. The continuing concern of consistent staff members fosters patient self-care motivation, health, and maturation of judgment.

The realities of one's potentials and limitations are not learned during any specific period of time. This aspect of learning goes on throughout life. Reorganization, then, is never complete, but it can be propelled in a positive direction by informed, sensitive, and caring nurses and other health professionals.

## REFERENCES

1   J. Harold Walton (ed.), *The Pathophysiology of Head Injuries,* CIBA Corporation, Summit, N.J., 1966, p. 91.
2   Frank H. Netter, *The CIBA Collection of Medical Illustrations,* vol. 1, *Nervous System,* CIBA Corporation, Summit, N.J., 1972, p. 110.
3   Joseph G. Chusid, *Correlative Neuroanatomy and Functional Neurology,* Lange, Los Altos, Calif., 1976, p. 32.
4   Arthur C. Guyton, *Structure and Function of the Nervous System,* Saunders, Philadelphia, 1972, p. 213.
5   Arthur J. Gatz, *Manter's Essentials of Clinical Neuroanatomy and Neurophysiology,* Davis, Philadelphia, 1970, p. 126.
6   Netter, *op. cit.,* p. 106.
7   Chusid, *op. cit.,* p. 89.
8   Gatz, *op. cit.,* pp. 58–59.
9   *Ibid.,* p. 77.
10   Francis Mechner, "Patient Assessment: Neurological Examination," *Am J Nurs,* **75:**Pl 11, September 1975.
11   Chusid, *op. cit.,* pp. 87, 269–270.
12   *Ibid.,* p. 246.
13   Juan T. Taveras, "Computerized Axial Tomography—How It Works," *Mod Med,* **43:**49, October 15, 1975.
14   Irving J. Cohen (ed.), "EMI Scan: A Look at Inner Space," *Emergency Med,* **7:**253, January 1975.
15   E. Kazner *et al.* (eds.), *Proceedings in Echo-Encephalography,* Springer-Verlag, New York, 1968, pp. 97, 103.
16   Chusid, *op. cit.,* p. 257.
17   Mechner, *op. cit.,* p. Pl 9.
18   Jeanne H. Quesenbury and Pamela Lembright, "Observations and Care for Patients with Head Injuries," *Nurs Clin North Am,* **4:**244, June 1969.
19   Chusid, *op. cit.,* p. 255.
20   Walton, *op. cit.,* p. 82.
21   Edith V. Olson *et al.,* "The Hazards of Immobility," *Am J Nurs,* **67:**782, April 1967.
22   *Ibid.,* p. 791.
23   Mary S. Tilbury, "The Intracranial Pressure Screw: A New Assessment Tool," *Nurs Clin North Am,* **9:**643, December 1974.
24   Antoine Rémond (ed.), *Handbook of Electroencephalography and Clinical Neurophysiology,* vol. 14 B, Elsevier, Amsterdam, 1972, pp. 20–21.
25   *Ibid.,* p. 76.
26   *Ibid.,* pp. 78, 80.
27   *Ibid.,* pp. 87–88.
28   *Ibid.,* p. 89.
29   Byron Hamilton et al., "Four-Year Outcome: Midwest Regional Spinal Cord Injury Care System," paper presented at National Meetings of the American Congress of Rehabilitation Medicine, San Diego, Calif., November 1976.
30   Daniel Ruge, *Spinal Cord Injuries,* Charles C Thomas, Springfield, Ill., 1969.
31   Jack Ford and Bridget Duckworth, *Physical Management for the Quadriplegic Patient,* Davis, Philadelphia, 1974.
32   William Engel et al., "A Functional Splint for Grasp Driven by Wrist Extension," *Arch Phys Med Rehabil,* **48:**43–52, January 1967.
33   Nell Kirby, Michel Barnerias, and Arthur Siebens, "An Evaluation of Assisted Cough in Quadriparetic Patients," *Arch Phys Med Rehabil,* **47:**705–710, November 1966.
34   Michael Kosiak, "Etiology of Decubitus Ulcers," *Arch Phys Med Rehabil,* **42:**19–29, January 1961.
35   Nell Kirby, Arthur Siebens, and Alice Gifford,

"Teaching Spinal Cord Injured Persons—Exploratory Study," Report of Research Grant #NU-00412, Division of Nursing, Department of Health, Education, and Welfare, 1977.

**36** Connie Becker, Hazel Colletta, and Frances Coover, *Facing Spinal Cord Injury,* Highland View Hospital, Cleveland, 1971.

**37** Frank Netter, *The CIBA Collection of Medical Illustrations,* vol. III, *Digestive System,* Pt. II, *Lower Digestive Tract,* Colorpress, New York, 1962.

**38** Kirby, Siebens and Gifford, *loc. cit.*

**39** George Engel, "Grief and Grieving," *Am J Nurs,* **64:**93–98, September 1964.

**40** Marjorie Crate, "Nursing Functions in Adaptation to Chronic Illness," *Am J Nurs,* **65:**72–76, October 1965.

**41** Brian Sternberg, with John Poppy, "My Search for Faith," *Look,* March 10, 1964.

## BIBLIOGRAPHY

Brobeck, John (ed.): *Best and Taylor's Physiological Basis of Medical Practice,* 9th ed., *Respiration,* William Youmans and Arthur Siebens (eds.), Williams & Wilkins, Baltimore, 1973.

Carini, Esta, and Guy Owens: *Neurological and Neurosurgical Nursing,* Mosby, St. Louis, 1974.

Guttman, Sir Ludwig: *Spinal Cord Injuries,* Blackwell Scientific Publications, Ltd., Oxford, 1973.

Hanlon, Kathryn: "Description and Uses of Intracranial Pressure Monitoring," *Heart Lung,* **5:** 277–282, March–April 1976.

Miller, Marian, and Marvin Sachs: *About Bedsores,* Lippincott, Philadelphia, 1974.

Mitchell, Pamela H., and Nancy Mauss: "Intracranial Pressure: Fact and Fancy," *Nursing 76,* **6:**53–57.

Mooney, Thomas, Theodore Cole, and Richard Chilgren: *Sexual Options for Paraplegics and Quadriplegics,* Little, Brown, Boston, 1975.

Neuman, Ellen, and Mary Price: *Urinary Tract Care,* University of Minnesota Press, Minneapolis, 1976.

Norsworthy, Edith: "Nursing Rehabilitation after Severe Head Trauma," *Am J Nurs,* **74:**1246–1250, July 1974.

Parsons, L. Claire: "Respiratory Changes in Head Injury," *Am J Nurs,* **71:**2187–2191, November 1971.

Pierce, Donald, and Vernon Nickel, *The Total Care of Spinal Cord Injuries,* Little, Brown, Boston, 1977.

Pizzi, Francis J., et al.: "A Protocol for the Management of Head Trauma," *Am Fam Physician,* **10:**163–172.

Ransohoff, Joseph, and Alan Fleischer: "Insult and Injury—Head Injuries," *Emergency Med,* **8:**147–151.

Schwartz, Seymour I., et al.: *Principles of Surgery,* 2d ed., McGraw-Hill, New York, 1974, pp. 1670–1674.

Tindall, George T., and Alan S. Fleischer: "Head Injury," *Hosp Med,* **12:**89–90.

Walton, J. Harold: *The Treatment of Head Injuries,* CIBA Corporation, Summit, N.J., 1967.

Wright, Beatrice: *Physical Disability—A Psychological Approach,* Harper & Row, New York, 1960.

# 33

# SEIZURE DISTURBANCES IN PERCEPTION AND COORDINATION

Gladys Mary Scipien
Margaret Mangan

**A**t birth, the nervous system is immature, and the neonate responds to stimuli from the environment by reflexes. With maturation of this system and subsequent experiences, a human being becomes an individual who has the capability to process, analyze, and interpret data received from a myriad of sources. For example, an internal change such as an increase in one's body temperature, or an external change, be it physical, psychological, or social, precipitates the transmission of electrical impulses to the brain. The afferent impulses are received by the cerebellum which in turn responds by firing efferent impulses to other areas of the nervous system.

The response of a human organism to any sudden, significant change in the internal or external environment is termed *excitability* or *irritability*. While these two ingredients, stimulus and response, are essential, the precise mechanisms involved in the exchanges which subsequently occur are only partially understood. The speed with which the electrophysiological transmission occurs makes its study difficult.

While both the nervous system and the endocrine system have the delicate task of maintaining an incredible balance between bodily activities and responses to the environment, it is the nervous system which makes perception and coordinated movement possible in man. This system, complex and remarkably widespread throughout the body, allows nerve impulses to be transmitted through rich interconnections in thousandths of a second. Obviously complex, it is also governed by order. If an abnormality, imbalance, or disruption occurs anywhere along its communication network, electrical impulses become erratic and unpredictable and result in a seizure.

## SEIZURE DISORDERS

The problem of seizure disorders in the United States is substantial, with approximately 1 million individuals subject to recurrent seizures and about 10 million others who, at some point in their lives, will seek medical advice or be admitted to a hospital because of a seizure.[1] In any discussion of this clinical manifestation it is important to clarify the terms which will be used.

A *convulsion* can best be described as a "sudden, excessive, disorderly discharge of neurons in either a structurally normal or diseased cortex,"[2] "which arises from an instability of the neuronal membrane caused by an excess of excitation, or a deficiency of normal inhibitory mechanisms."[3] The terms *convulsion* and *seizure* are often used synonymously and interchangeably and hence incorrectly. Technically, *convulsion* refers only to those violent, involuntary muscular contractions of voluntary muscles, while the word *seizure* includes clinical manifestations such as disturbances in sensation, alterations in perception and/or coordination, loss of consciousness, convulsive movements, or a combination of any or all of the aforementioned. While these manifestations depend upon the location of the discharge and its spread, it is important for the reader to remember that a seizure, the preferred generic term, is a symptom, not a disease. It is only when seizures become recurrent, or chronic in nature, that the condition is called *epilepsy*. The majority of patients in this category have had seizures since childhood, and in most instances the cause has never been identified; therefore the condition is called *idiopathic epilepsy*.

### Classification of Seizures

The format for categorizing these phenomena can be varied. For example, some clinicians have done so according to: (1) clinical seizure type, (2) electroencephalographic expression, (3) anatomic substrate, (4) etiology, and/or (5) age. Clear-cut distinctions are often difficult because of many variables which can influence classification. As a nurse assesses and intervenes in the presence of a seizure, it is essential that this health care provider understand the clinical components of a seizure.

Five categories have been identified, on the nature of a seizure and its severity. This grouping consists of the most common types in clinical practice and includes (1) generalized (grand mal, major motor), (2) petit-mal (absence), (3) psychomotor, (4) Jacksonian and focal (partial), and (5) miscellaneous. It should be obvious that this listing is not all-inclusive, nor is it meant to be. It does, however, include those seizures which are most significant to a nurse.

### Pathophysiology

Whether an individual has only one seizure in a lifetime, or whether he or she is subject to recurrent episodes, there is no basic difference in the characteristics demonstrated by the seizing patient. Multiple changes occur with the seizure that have distinct effects on the individual involved. The erratic, synchronous discharging neurons are responsible for the initiation of a series of clinical manifestations, and the nurse must know the common types of seizures in order to anticipate the needs of patients.

**Generalized seizures** A generalized seizure (grand mal or major motor) is visually characterized by *prodromal* or *pre-ictal symptoms* which occur hours or days prior to the episode. They may be *paroxysmal,* occurring in the form of "dreamy" states, periods of giddiness, feelings of "strangeness," or palpitations of the heart. *Continuous prodromas* precede a convulsion by a day or two and are accompanied by anorexia, ravenous appetite, headache, euphoria, or depression. These changes in an individual's disposition frequently alert family members to the imminent seizure.

Immediately prior to a grand mal seizure, an *aura* may be experienced by the patient. This can be a motor or sensory symptom such as a flash of light or of color, numbness, tingling, twitching, or a particular taste. Physiologically it is the beginning of the abnormal neuronal discharge. Almost simultaneously with the loss of consciousness the "epileptic cry" occurs and is caused as the thoracic and abdominal muscles force air through the glottis.

An inherent manifestation of a generalized seizure is the tonic-clonic movement. In the *tonic phase,* the extensor muscles of the trunk and extremities are in a rigid, contracted state, while the *clonic* phase consists of rapid, involuntary alternate muscular contractions and relaxations. With the loss of consciousness, a tonic, stiffening spasm of the entire body occurs and usually lasts 10 to 30 seconds as all voluntary muscles are contracted and rigid. Respiratory movement ceases, the face is flushed, and venous engorgement is apparent. As the tonic muscle spasm relaxes, clonic, rhythmic, jerking movements appear and generally last 1 to 5 minutes or longer. As the clonic movements continue, the tonic contractions become stronger and for several minutes these tonic-clonic movements continue until the spasms stop and breathing is restored. During the convulsion, the clonic movements of the chest force saliva and air from the mouth, hence the "foaming at the mouth" associated with grand mal convulsions may be noted. At the onset of unconsciousness, the eyes roll up or to one side, and the pupils dilate and do not react to light. Sphincter control is relaxed so that the patient is incontinent of both urine and feces. After a few minutes, the episode ceases, and the patient regains consciousness for a brief period, usually 15 to 20 minutes. Following this the patient generally falls asleep for several hours.

In periods of wakefulness which follow, there

are complaints of a headache and muscle aches. There may be some mental confusion after such a generalized seizure; however, it lasts only for an hour or two. The period following a generalized tonic-clonic seizure is known as the postictal period and is characterized by the *epileptic coma* during which fatigue, restlessness, and prolonged sleep occur. A serious complication which may develop is *status epilepticus;* it is characterized by one prolonged convulsion or a series of seizures occurring in rapid succession without the patient regaining consciousness.

**Petit mal seizures**   Petit mal (absence) seizures frequently occur in children, and they are seldom seen beyond adolescence. They happen without warning and are characterized by a sudden loss of consciousness. A "blank stare" appears on the child's face; however, this seizure seldom lasts more than 20 seconds. Whatever activity the child is involved in, at the time of the *absence,* is interrupted very briefly. For example, if the child is counting from 1 to 10 at the time of the seizure, a number or two may not be uttered, and counting will resume as if nothing had happened. These seizures are more frequent than grand mal seizures; they can decrease with physical activity and diminish in frequency as the child gets older. Grand mal or psychomotor seizures may occur at any time in a child who demonstrates these petit mal seizures.

**Psychomotor seizures**   These seizures can occur at any age. Prior to their onset patients experience an aura, which takes several forms. These include hearing sounds, seeing objects, or experiencing a feeling of "unreality." There is a sudden change in the individual's level of consciousness, and this type of seizure lasts longer than a petit mal seizure. An important characteristic is the partially coordinated motor activity exhibited by the subject, which takes the form of walking about aimlessly, buttoning or unbuttoning clothes, driving a car, or committing an act of violence. The behavioral changes which occur emphasize the need for a thorough psychiatric assessment. When spoken to, the individual responds irrelevantly and demonstrates lack of contact with reality. A constant smacking of lips or chewing movement may also be noted. There is a partial amnesia regarding the attack. Confusion exists for a short time after the attack, and postictal sleep is common. There seems to be some agreement that a pathological

and/or electrical disturbance of the temporal lobe is involved in this type of disorder.

**Localized motor seizures**   Local, focal, or Jacksonian seizures are tonic and clonic contractions of selected motor groups in a somewhat contained area. *Localized motor seizures* usually occur in those individuals with some form of structural brain disease such as vascular malformations, scars, infections, or brain tumors.[4] A *Jacksonian* seizure has a focal beginning with a progression of the spasm from one area to another but confined to one side of the body. The patient is usually conscious and experiences a twitching which begins within a finger, toe, or angle of the mouth and advances to adjacent areas. For example, a spasm may begin in a finger, then fairly rapidly move to the hand, forearm, arm, trunk, and down to the lower extremity.

**Focal (partial) seizures**   Focal episodes usually involve only a portion of the brain; they most often start in one area of the body, have a limited spread, do not usually become generalized (unless they are severe), and reflect the area of the brain activated by the abnormal neuronal discharge. They are the most transient types of seizures, and the attacks are brief, usually without loss of consciousness. The clinical manifestations exhibited by a patient depend completely on the location of the focus. The variety of disorders in this category extend from one end of the spectrum to the other.

*Sensory seizures* have visual, auditory, olfactory, vertiginous, special sensory, or cutaneous involvement. A patient may complain of seeing bright lights, darkness, or colors or may experience hallucinations about objects' shapes. Strange buzzing sounds or roaring noises can be heard. Peculiar tastes may be experienced, or smells may be projected to an area of the environment. A tingling sensation, numbness, or a "pins and needles" feeling may be described by an individual. Such phenomena are usually confined to one side of the body, without a loss of consciousness or progression of symptoms.

Another type of focal motor disorder is known as *epilepsia partialis continua.* Here, the individual has rhythmic, clonic movements of large groups of muscles in a leg or arm. These seizures may persist for days, weeks, or months.

Yet another type of focal seizure is the *adversive (contraverse) seizure* in which there is an involuntary turning of the head and eyes in one direction, a raising of the upper extremity of the side involved, with a clenching of the fist, and a fixed stare at the raised, flexed arm. The tonic movements are slow in starting and are followed by rapid clonic jerking of the entire portion of one side of the body. At that point the seizure may cease, or it may progress to a generalized, tonic-clonic convulsion.

These examples of focal seizures identify the myriad of manifestations in only three types of the disorder. It should be obvious to the reader that seizure patterns exhibited by the patient subject to focal seizures are many. The causes are unknown in most instances. It behooves the observer to recognize the seizure, identify the anatomical structures involved, and assess the patient's behavior and the course as well as the progression of events. Anticipation of the patient's needs will come only with the knowledge of these basic data.

**Myoclonic seizures** Although the term *myoclonus* refers to several motor disorders which may be localized or diffuse, for purposes of clarification the term *myoclonic seizures* refers to those sudden, involuntary contractions of large groups of muscles as in the trunk or extremities. The seizures may be relatively mild or forceful. Usually, there is no loss of consciousness during the episode and the problem can recur for hours or days.

When the problem occurs in adults, it is usually considered to be benign, unless a progression to major motor seizure activity occurs as in Lafora's disease. On the other hand, massive myoclonic seizures in infants have devastating neurologic consequences.

A myoclonic spasm (infantile spasm, lightning seizures, jackknife seizures) in an infant is forceful and often occurs in a rapid series of successive episodes. These spasms may last only a minute and be as frequent as a few to hundreds each day. When muscles of the trunk, neck, and extremities are involved in a flexor type of seizure, the infant assumes a jackknife position, while in the extensor type of episode, the neck is thrown back, the arms are spread out, and the body assumes the position of a spread eagle. There is rapid neurologic deterioration, and severe mental retardation is the inevitable outcome.

### Causes of Seizures

Seizures can be produced by a number of agents (drugs), systemic metabolic mechanisms, and alterations within the internal environment of the brain. The precise causes of these erratic, abnormal neuronal discharges have yet to be identified; however, much investigative effort is being expended.

Some research into electrocellular function has revealed certain facts.

The normal neuronal cell membrane is selectively permeable; i.e., it is highly permeable to potassium ($K^+$) and poorly permeable to sodium ($Na^+$). There is a high concentration of $K^+$ and a low concentration of $Na^+$ within the cell; the reverse is true extracellularly. The resting membrane potential of a neuron reflects the difference in the charges of ions within the cell as opposed to those outside the cell. It can be altered by several factors including (1) a change in extracellular ion concentration, (2) stimulation, either mechanical (head injury) or chemical (usually by electrical impulses from neighboring cells), and (3) pathophysiological alteration of the membrane itself because of a disease process or genetic malformation.[5]

Diffusion of $Na^+$ and $K^+$ ions across this semipermeable neuronal membrane occurs with stimulation, and the momentary shift of potential is called *action potential.* Following discharge and depolarization of the cell membrane, there is the return of a resting state, with a resumption of previous extracellular/intracellular ion balance. The neuron cannot discharge again until ionic balance is restored.

Since the action potential is greater than the threshold of discharge, it is an effective stimulus to adjacent portions of the cell membrane and its fibers. The spread of this action potential is called *impulse transmission,* and it always moves from the point of initial stimulation. Therefore, it is at the cellular level, with the ionic imbalance and alterations in conditions, that the discharge threshold is affected,[6] initiating the series of events which result in seizure activity. A depletion of $K^+$ and a gain of $Na^+$ in the neuronal cell produce a seizure.

Another possible cause of seizures may occur at the *synapse* when neurotransmitters transfer nerve impulses from one neuron to another. It is the synaptic nerve endings which produce agents essential to impulse conduction. The autonomic ganglions and parasympathetic postganglionic neurons release acetylcholine, while the sympathetic postganglionic fibers produce norepinephrine. The central nervous system is more complex, however, because of its functions which require excitatory and inhibitory systems as well as associated, selective neurotransmitters. One such substance, an amino acid known as *gamma-aminobutyric acid (GABA),* normally has a powerful inhibitory effect on the cortex. Vitamin $B_6$, or pyridoxine, is involved in its metabolism. If there is any *interference with* the synthesis of GABA, a shift of the normal excitatory-inhibitory balance occurs with excitation prevailing and a resultant seizure occurring. Likewise if there is a vitamin $B_6$ deficiency, whether dietary or drug-antagonized, a seizure will occur.[7]

*Alterations in the blood-brain barrier* system may also be involved in the development of a seizure or susceptibility to seizure activity. Normally, this barrier prevents toxic substances from reaching brain tissue. Alterations in the defense, caused by inflammation or trauma, can precipitate a shift in $K^+$ concentration, lowering the convulsive threshold.

The interstitial fluid, which bathes neuronal and glial cells of the brain and maintains a homeodynamic environment for these cells, communicates with the circulating cerebrospinal fluid. With an *insult to the brain* and *damage to the choroid plexus,* for example, the cerebrospinal fluid decreases, thereby impairing this fluid transport system and increasing $K^+$ ion concentration. The hippocampus (grey matter in the floor of the lateral ventricle), susceptible to the change in this $K^+$ ion level, lowers the convulsive threshold, triggering seizure activity.

An *altered oxygen and/or glucose concentration* may also precipitate seizure activity. Both oxygen and glucose cross cerebral capillaries freely and diffuse to all parts of the brain. Since neither is stored, this organ is totally dependent on its vascular supply. Interestingly enough, cerebral circulation has the capacity to identify changes in its metabolic needs and to adjust accordingly.

However, cerebral circulation can be compromised in the presence of certain pathologic conditions such as brain tumors, aneurysms, or atherosclerosis, among other diseased states. In addition, there may be a *hypoglycemia* because of diabetes or altered insulin production, which increases cerebral oxidative metabolism. The energy that is produced results in demonstrable cerebral dysfunction. This deprivation of oxygen or glucose produces a rapid, marked $K^+$ loss and a $Na^+$ accumulation within the cells, depolarizing the membrane and producing those paroxysmal discharges initiating seizure activity.[8]

In the presence of a seizure, it is well known also that oxygen is essential to sustaining that activity and blood flow increases substantially. Yet, hypoxic brain tissue causes seizures in adults and children. What a paradox. Some investigators have suggested that nerve cells become hyperirritable in response to ischemia or the *lack of glucose.* This process is self-limiting, however, for as the metabolic rate increases, there is an exhaustion of substances required for continued stimulation, and an accumulation of inhibitory or depressant substances such as $CO_2$, waste products of metabolism, and amino acids. The latter may well contribute to the cessation of seizure activity.

The above content has dealt with some causes of seizure activity. Some can be anticipated. A blow to the head is responsible for cell destruction and potentiates the occurrence of this phenomenon. An identifiable *infectious process* of the brain also alters one's susceptibility to seizures by cell destruction, fever, inflammation, and possible resultant bacterial toxicity. However, the causes of seizure disorders are oftentimes not known. In *uterine life* a developing brain may be injured by some noxious agent without the injury betraying itself by presenting symptoms prior to a demonstrable seizure. A difficult delivery may be the cause of *birth trauma* in the newborn. In infancy and childhood there are many infections which may be considered trivial and yet may take their toll in years to come. To compound the problem of causation, seizures may occur months or years after a particular cerebral insult has happened. Old scar tissue in the brain, toxicity caused by drugs, and high ammonia levels in patients with liver disease may precipitate seizure activity. Heretofore *undiagnosed neuropathology* also contributes to the incidence of seizures.

There are also several *environmental factors* which must be investigated more fully. Variables such as the presence of flickering lights and altered perceptions of smell and taste have been identified as precipitants of seizure activity, regardless of the age of the individual involved. In addition, the influence of *day and night* as well as the effect of time on a particular individual's body rhythms also must be fully explored in order to identify their roles in relation to seizure activity.

### First-Level Nursing Care

Nurses in all settings must be aware of those factors which may be responsible for precipitating seizure activity in their patients, if efforts to prevent them are to be effective. Abnormally low oxygen levels, head injuries, infections, electrolyte and acid-base imbalance, genetic faults, brain tumors, or other pathologic conditions are some examples of the variables involved.

The seizure activity of most patients with idiopathic epilepsy begins early in childhood and persists into adult life. While seizures can and do occur at a later age, those episodes may be related to the presence of some other pathology.

**Prevention** Preventing predisposing seizure episodes is imperative. If the precipitating factors are known, then efforts should be directed toward decreasing an individual's susceptibility to such abnormal activity. If systemic causes have been identified, then they need to be corrected.

Interference with cerebral oxygenation and the resultant hypoxic state play a vital role in triggering seizure activity. For example, hypoxia has been associated with Adams-Stokes syndrome, pulmonary dysfunction, and transient ischemic attacks. Patients must be treated early, with oxygen administered and blood pressure controlled in order to reduce the likelihood of initiating seizure activity during periods of decreased oxygenation.

Hypoglycemia, which occurs as a result of excessive insulin production, is another systemic cause of seizure activity. It can occur also as a result of a poor dietary intake. Early detection of diabetes, administration of glucose, and improvement of an individual's nutritional status can correct the disequilibrium. Careful teaching of the diabetic patient in relation to nutrition is especially important.

Electrolyte and acid-base imbalance can be responsible for precipitating seizures. Hyponatremia, resulting from diarrhea, infections, fever, a low-sodium diet, tap water enemas, and an increased water consumption are well-defined causes. Electrolyte replacement easily corrects the imbalance. Also, hypernatremia can occur from an increased sodium intake or diarrhea with dehydration. The very careful administration of prescribed hypotonic solutions can correct this faulty mechanism.

Heavy-metal ingestion, such as lead poisoning in children, is another systemic variable. Intramuscular injections of Britial anti-lewisite (BAL) and ethylenediaminetetraacetic acid (EDTA) are most effective in removing this substance from the body.

There are many other systemic deficiencies or defects which enhance seizure activity, among them hepatic or renal insufficiency, endocrine dysfunctions, hyperpyrexia, and alcohol withdrawal. It is essential that they be identified so that the necessary corrective measures may be instituted and seizures can be avoided.

**Second-Level Nursing Care**

When a patient has had a seizure, medical assistance is sought, and at that time it is important to carefully document the events which occurred. This is particularly true if such an attack is the first one for the individual. Remember that not all seizures necessitate hospitalization. Patients can often be seen in ambulatory care or community health settings.

**Nursing assessment** It is important for the nurse to obtain a careful *health history* and details of the seizure. While it would be best to observe an actual attack, such an opportunity is highly unlikely. Although less reliable, eliciting a description of the seizure from a competent witness is most helpful. Probably the least reliable source of information is the patient. This is especially true if a generalized seizure occurred because the person was unconscious and unable to describe what happened. With psychomotor seizures, the same situation prevails; however, in the presence of Jacksonian, or focal, seizures there is no loss of consciousness, and the patient may be able to share the most complete data.

*Descriptions of the prodromal characteristics* and the specifics of an aura, if present, are significant clues which can be obtained from most patients, regardless of the type of seizure experienced. Personal accounts of *incontinence,* a *bitten tongue, bruises, restlessness, confusion,* and *sore muscles* are meaningful.

Although the cause of the seizure is often unknown, it is important for a nurse to question and explore all avenues in an effort to identify that forgotten incident which may be the cause. For children, events surrounding birth should be obtained, i.e., an instrument delivery, cord around the neck, prematurity, or problems associated with establishing respirations. Detailed data including the accomplishment of developmental tasks, childhood diseases, or a seizure with fever are invaluable pieces of information. Such knowledge may not be given unless it is specifically requested. In obtaining *adult histories,* unusual events which occurred prior to the seizure should be pursued, especially those which surround a cerebral insult, such as a fall, an accident, or a severe blow to the head.

Questions which focus on diet, sleep and work habits, alcohol and drug ingestion, or symptoms of an acute illness prior to the seizure should be asked. Parents of a toddler should be questioned about accidental ingestions of harmful substances by their child. If an individual is being treated for a specific health problem, medications which were prescribed should be identified, and the current regimen described. It is also important to learn the time of day the seizure occurred and whether the person was especially tired, performing an unfamiliar task, or in a different environmental setting.

Psychological assessment should also be obtained to isolate behavioral changes.

**P**hysical Assessment   The search for the cause should be as comprehensive as possible. Following the completion of a health history, a complete physical examination should be performed in order to attempt to identify the cause. Special attention should be paid to details of an extensive neurological examination, including gait, muscular strength, symmetry, and visual fields. Positive responses of the Babinski and deep tendon reflexes may indicate diseases affecting the corticospinal tract. Assessing memory, attention span, and cognitive style is informative. This data base and knowledge of any other systemic disorder may lead to more conclusive results. Specific changes may reflect a particular cause of the seizure disorder. For example, the continued presence of certain reflexes may indicate the presence of occlusion or obstruction.

**Diagnostic tests**   By far the most useful tool in diagnosing epilepsy and localizing a specific focus of activity is the *electroencephalogram (EEG)* for it frequently provides the only objective evidence of cerebral dysfunction. This test is used to detect electrical abnormalities and to classify the specific seizure type. In addition to being painless and safe, it can easily be done on an outpatient basis. Since a seizure implies a disorder in the electrical activity of the brain, the value of an EEG is that it records, by electronic amplifying devices, minute electrical impulses which originate in the brain.

In order to perform this test, electrodes are placed on the surface of the scalp over various lobes of the cortex and over the frontal, motor, parietal, occipital, and temporal areas. One electrode is also attached to each ear, which creates an inactive reference area, or an area of the body which does not demonstrate any electrical activity. The electrodes are all connected to wires that lead into the multichannel instrument, and the potentials are recorded on moving paper. The basic normal rhythm varies from the alpha waves, which have electrical oscillations of about 8 to 12 cycles/second and are located in the posterior portion of the brain, to the faster beta waves located anteriorly and which are usually 18 to 30 cycles/second. Each rhythm has its own form, amplitude, and symmetry. *Spikes* and *spike-wave discharges* are often seen in patients with seizure disorders (Fig. 33-1), and they may be either generalized or focal. Localization of a seizure focus is possible when the spike occurs over a specific area of the head as over the temporal lobe

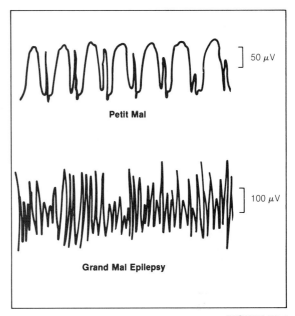

**FIGURE 33-1**
EEG tracings. Changes noted during seizure activity.

in the case of psychomotor seizures. The EEG must be interpreted by a qualified person, and even then a conclusive diagnosis is difficult. Borderline abnormalities can exist in relation to the "normal" population. At the same time, some patients with documented clinical seizures may show no abnormalities.

An EEG is taken with the patient at rest in a quiet environment. Such an environment must exclude those factors which can precipitate a seizure. The EEG may also be done during periods of hyperventilation, sleep deprivation, or during sleep with photic stimulation. Abnormalities which are not present at rest may be manifested by the introduction of these additional stimuli.

On occasion surface electrodes fail to localize foci deep in the brain. Nasopharyngeal leads inserted through the nose and resting against the nasopharynx can record the electrical impulses of the *mesial* portion of the temporal lobe. They may be used in many adolescents and adults with suspected seizure disorders.

Experimental evidence has shown that *depth electrode studies,* done primarily on patients with intractable seizures or on those individuals being considered for neurosurgery, offer more complete and accurate information regarding the existence and localization of epileptic foci. Such a procedure is done in an operating room. Burr holes are made in the skull and electrodes are inserted. The EEG tracings are made and interpreted accordingly.

*Patient education* regarding the EEG is essential if the procedure is to be successful. Clients must know that they will not receive electrical shocks or experience pain. They should also be reassured that this test does not determine their mental status. The sole purpose for such a test is to determine the presence or absence of seizure activity. The entire recording takes from 45 minutes to as long as 2 hours. A nurse should explain the need for a patient to lie still while tracings are being made. Periods of relaxation which are provided between recordings decrease the likelihood of restlessness during the procedure. When informing the patient of episodes of dizziness which occur during the hyperventilation portion of the EEG, the nurse should stress the fact that it is a normal expectation.

Other diagnostic tests can be done; however, the need for them depends on specific clinical findings. In the presence of a generalized seizure it is not unusual to perform: (1) a glucose test which may reveal hypo- or hyperglycemia; (2) a calcium level indicating the presence of hypocalcemia; (3) a blood urea nitrogen test, searching for a renal disturbance; and (4) Na$^+$ and K$^+$ levels for electrolyte imbalance. Skull x-rays are done routinely.

**Emergency nursing care of seizure activity**
When seizures occur initially, the patient is usually found in the community and then, when the condition stabilizes, is transferred to the acute care setting. At this time a complete physical and psychological assessment is done to determine the cause of the seizure activity.

At the beginning of a seizure, with a *loss of consciousness,* there is a potential for *airway obstruction.* A patient's head should be turned to the side, to facilitate drainage of secretions and/or vomitus. Tight, constrictive clothing is loosened to facilitate freedom of movement. Since a patient may bite the tongue during a generalized seizure, placing a soft object (tie, shirt tail) between the teeth may prevent this from occurring. If the teeth are clenched closed, *no efforts should be made* to forcibly open the mouth because the tongue may be pushed back, obstructing the patient's airway. When a seizure has started, one should not attempt to insert a tongue blade or airway because of the danger of injuring the lips, mucosa of the mouth, or teeth. Fingers must *never* be placed into the mouths of seizing patients as injuries can be sustained in the process.

*Documenting all the events* which occurred prior to, during, and after the seizure is a most important nursing action. Disturbances in perception and/or coordination and the presence of an *aura* during the pre-ictal period, an "epileptic cry," and the activity in which the patient was engaged at the time of the seizure, should be noted.

With the beginning of seizure activity, record the loss of consciousness, progression of the convulsion; the type of seizure (generalized, tonic, clonic, focal); anatomic parts affected; changes in the characteristics of the seizure; and the presence of a deviated tongue and unreacting pupils. Incontinence, color, and injuries sustained during the attack are significant notations. Behavioral changes as well as environmental variables should be assessed. While vital signs are monitored, special attention is directed toward assessing the person's respiratory status throughout the seizure. When recording the length of the seizure and the duration of the tonic and clonic phases, make documentation complete. If there are recurring episodes, the frequency and number should be noted.

During the *tonic-clonic activity* of a generalized seizure, the extremities may be injured as they come in contact with hard objects; therefore, all harmful objects need to be removed from the immediate environment. In cribs of infants or toddlers all toys should be removed. If the individual falls to the floor or ground while seizing, his or her head should be protected from injury by a folded blanket or jacket. All efforts are directed toward protecting the patient. No effort should be made to restrain the individual during the seizure.

In the *postictal period* it is important to describe a patient's response to the experience: restlessness; perceptions prior to its onset; complaints of muscle pain; headache; weakness; cramping, and mental status, as well as the sleep pattern which follows are important additions to the individual's health history.

Most seizures are self-limiting; therefore, they should be allowed to run their course. Restraining extremities, forcing the mouth open, or holding the patient back from performing automatic activities are unnecessary interventions and *potentially harmful.* A nurse should remain with seizing patients if possible to protect them from further injury and provide as much privacy as possible. Following the seizure, a patient should be allowed to sleep before resuming normal activities.

Bystanders are often confused about what should or should not be done when a seizure occurs. Nurses are in an ideal position to contribute to the knowledge the public has regarding seizures, thereby making the environment safer for the seizure patient.

### Third-Level Nursing Care

Hospitalization may be required for the individual whose seizures are uncontrolled or have increased for no apparent reason. Regardless of the type of seizure exhibited, observation and documentation by the nurse provide critical data which contribute to diagnosis and subsequent management of the problem.

**Nursing assessment** In addition to collecting data which result from observing a seizure, completing a total health history, and performing a physical assessment, the nurse should pursue the presence of possible precipitants which initiated the seizure. Questions previously described in Second-Level Nursing Care are included and elaborated on at this time.

Alterations in neurological findings may persist and include diminished peripheral reflexes, mental confusion, lack of coordination, muscular twitching, dilated pupils, unsteady gait, and weakened grip. The patient may also demonstrate signs of dehydration (see Chap. 13) or hypoglycemia (see Chap. 21). Complaints of numbness and tingling of body components, facial flushing, and decreased attention span can also be noted. Restlessness may persist and headaches are not uncommon. Frequently, symptoms may be temporary and disappear when the cause is removed.

**Diagnostic tests** The major diagnostic tool continues to be the EEG. Changes as described in Second-Level Nursing Care will be noted as seizure activity continues. In addition, brain scans are performed to detect such things as cellular growth or obstruction. Blood tests discussed under Second-Level Nursing Care will also be performed.

A lumbar puncture also may be performed. An abnormal white cell count may indicate the presence of an infectious process, while an increased pressure reading and an elevated total protein are commonly present in patients with expanding cerebral lesions. After skull x-rays, additional radiologic examinations such as a ventriculogram, arteriography, or pneumoencephalogram may be necessary.

**Nursing problems and interventions** The nursing problems elicited vary and depend on the clinical manifestations exhibited by the patient, as well as the diagnosis. Many of the problems discussed in Second-Level Nursing Care persist; however, if seizure activity is related to a specific pathophysiological alteration, the level of a patient's *anxiety* increases significantly. When other changes associated with disruptions in oxygenation, fluid and electrolytes, metabolism, or perception and coordination occur, additional problems persist.

Certainly, the *safety* of an individual who is experiencing seizure activity is of prime importance. Although all harmful objects in the immediate environment are removed, additional measures such as the padding of side rails or cribs should be taken. Patients whose seizures are poorly controlled may be placed on restricted activity and in very quiet areas of hospital units. Such constraints are implemented to decrease environmental stimuli, agitation, and excitability.

**Medications** Primary treatment for the control of seizures continues to be the effective utilization of anticonvulsant drugs. Nurses are involved in administering these substances as well as documenting the patient's responses to them.

After a diagnosis has been confirmed, one drug is prescribed in order to study its effects on the seizure activity in a patient. Others may be added at a later date. Plasma levels are used to determine an individual's bodily reaction to the anticonvulsant drug. The effectiveness of the specific medication on the seizures, coupled with its plasma level, can necessitate adjustments in the dosage a patient receives. Two or more drugs are sometimes used for their synergistic properties. However, not all seizure disorders can be treated with drugs.

There are several common anticonvulsants which are usually taken by patients prone to seizures. (See Table 33-1.) *Phenytoin,* or *diphenylhydantoin,* is found to be effective against most types of seizures except petit mal (absence) or myoclonus. Although the drug's precise action is not known, it appears to alter the intracellular sodium concentration, making the cell membrane more stable and less readily activated by epileptic dis-

**TABLE 33-1**
COMMONLY USED ANTISEIZURE MEDICATION

| Drug | Therapeutic plasma level, mg/ml | Average adult daily dosage, mg |
|------|---------------------------------|-------------------------------|
| Phenytoin | 10–20 | 300 |
| Phenobarbital | 10–25 | 50–100 |
| Primidone | 5–15 | 500–1500 |
| Carbamazepine | 6–8 | 400–800 |
| Ethosuximide | 40–100 | 300–1200* |

* Usually administered to children with absences; note variations in dosage.

charges.[9] It is usually taken orally. The intramuscular route is rarely used because of unpredictability and slow absorption. Since it has a relatively long serum half-life, phenytoin is taken in a single daily dose, which is most beneficial for the patient who is likely to forget to take a drug several times a day or the individual who prefers not to take a medication while on the job. Although most of the side effects are drug-related, the patient who complains of gastrointestinal upset should be advised to take the drug in two or three divided doses.

Plasma drug levels identify therapeutic and toxic ranges of this medication. In many patients, certain clinical manifestations have been correlated with specific plasma levels, i.e., ataxia in patients whose levels are greater than 300 mg/ml. Some patients' seizures may be controlled at levels below those considered to be therapeutic, while in others, no adverse effects are obvious when toxic plasma levels are being administered. Despite the individual variability, plasma levels are valuable in determining effective doses. The average therapeutic ranges are outlined in Table 33-1. The nurse familiar with this information should utilize it jointly with clinical evidence when requesting a change in the medication order.

One of the oldest anticonvulsants available is *phenobarbital,* which diminishes the excitability of neurons by lowering the postsynaptic potentials or by enhancing presynaptic inhibition.[10] It is effective in controlling generalized, tonic-clonic, and partial seizures. Like phenytoin, phenobarbital can be taken in a single daily dose if tolerated by the adult patient. With children, the daily dose is usually divided. The usual route of administration is oral. While phenobarbital can be given alone for the control of seizures, it also may be used in combination with other drugs, especially phenytoin. During the initial phase of phenobarbital therapy, most patients complain of its sedative effect. This complaint is a very normal expectation which disappears once a tolerance level develops. If the sedation complaint continues, however, a physician needs to be consulted to determine a change in the dosage and/or drug.

*Primidone,* a congerer of phenobarbital, is the third drug of choice in the treatment of generalized, tonic-clonic, and partial seizures. It is not effective in controlling petit mal seizures. Its action is similar to phenobarbital. Since 10 to 15 percent of patients taking this anticonvulsant have side effects, it is important to test a patient's sensitivity with small, initial doses.[11] The side effects of promidone include drowsiness, feelings of intoxication, vertigo, slurred speech, nystagmus, and in some instances loss of libido. It is frequently given with phenytoin. Since a synergistic effect results from this combination, lower dosages are required when both medications are given together.

The last anticonvulsant medication to be considered here is *ethosuximide,* an effective agent in controlling petit mal seizures by increasing the patient's seizure threshold. Toxic reactions include gastrointestinal symptoms, drowsiness, headache, and dizziness. Although these problems are common at the beginning of treatment, they usually disappear with continued use. Should a blood dyscrasia develop, the dose may be lowered or stopped completely, with another anticonvulsant selected for use.

**B**ehavioral Changes   The existence of psychological stressors compounds the problems of a patient who suffers from seizures, and they can usually be identified through a complete health history and assessment. Fear, anxiety, anger, and guilt along with depression are common feelings among patients with continued seizure activity. Patients may verbalize the belief that they are being punished for some wrong of the past, and view these seizures as a reprimand.

It is important for a nurse to assess each problem carefully and encourage the patient to express fears and concerns. Listening, supporting, and accepting are vital to successfully interacting with these individuals. It is crucial to create an atmosphere in which the patient freely discusses alterations in perception and verbalizes the fantasies experienced during a seizure. Careful explanation of the nature of seizures may help reduce the patient stress.

**S**urgery   For those patients whose seizures continue despite extensive attempts to control them with a wide variety of anticonvulsant drugs and/or other regimens, surgical intervention may be considered. Such action certainly applies to those afflicted with brain tumors or abscesses, but surgery can also be performed on some patients with focus seizures which have not responded to vigorous medical management.[12,13]

Criteria for neurosurgery usually include the following: (1) inability to control seizures despite use of various anticonvulsant drugs and maximum dosages; (2) a worsening of epilepsy over a 3 to 5-year period; (3) absence of intellectual impairment or psychiatric disorders; and (4) a focal lesion amenable to surgery without incurring an additional neurologic deficit.[14] A cooperative patient and a hospital equipped for such an undertaking are also imperative. The exact type of surgical intervention varies.

Some children and adults have had *hemispherectomies* for intractable seizures. Other patients have had temporal or frontal *lobectomies* (see Chap. 35). It is important to remember that surgery is done only in a very small percentage of epileptic patients; therefore, its role in the treatment of a seizure disorder is limited.

A recent innovative procedure called *stereotaxy* is another type of surgical intervention which can help control seizure activity. Through use of a probe, nerve fibers or cells are destroyed and epileptogenic foci or cortical tracts involved in spreading the abnormal, erratic discharge, especially those located deep in the brain, are eliminated (see Chap. 39). This approach is considered to be investigative because so few have been done, and as a result an adequate follow-up, essential in its evaluation, has not been possible.

**Status Epilepticus**   Most seizures are self-limiting; however, there is a complication known as *status epilepticus* which occurs on rare occasions in the patient with a seizure disorder. The term refers to a prolonged seizure or one in which there is a rapid, successive series of seizures which does not allow a patient to recover from one episode before the next one begins. It is more commonly found in grand mal seizures, when a patient, especially a child, is unconscious and subjected to repetitive, severe, tonic-clonic convulsive activity for an extended period of time without regaining consciousness. It is a *medical emergency.*

*Airway obstruction* secondary to aspiration is a major nursing problem. The patient should be on one side, and an airway inserted. Any further problems can necessitate a tracheostomy. Suctioning frequently removes the copious secretions being produced.

Intravenous drug therapy is begun immediately, and the drug of choice is diazepam which has a depressive effect on the electrical discharges. Other medications which have been found effective in status epilepticus include nitrazepam, phenobarbital, and phenytoin. The goal of the parenteral therapy is to suppress the recurrent seizure pattern. At times when the drugs being used are ineffective, general anesthesia may be given. The presence of status epilepticus is a serious problem. If these seizures cannot be controlled, death may occur from exhaustion. Although status epilepticus can occur

in patients with seizures originating in the temporal lobe or those with petit mal, they are not as critically emergent as the life-threatening situation which exists in the case of a generalized seizure.

### Fourth-Level Nursing Care

Rehabilitation of the patient diagnosed with epilepsy covers a broad spectrum of activities and involves a variety of health professionals whose primary objective is the restoration of this individual to maximum independence. Effective patient care includes the displacement of myths for specific facts about the disorder, thereby providing support without pity. A majority of patients can be expected and, indeed, encouraged to participate in previous activities. In some instances family counseling is necessary for the spouse and children in order to lessen the frightening genetic fantasies about epilepsy.

It is most important that a patient identify those events or environmental changes which precipitate seizure activity. They must be avoided if possible. Medications being taken and/or protocol should be listed on a card carried in a wallet or on a Medic-Alert bracelet.

Because an epileptic patient is susceptible to uncontrolled seizure activity at any time, any place, adjustments need to be made regarding the uncertainty of these attacks. Open discussions which permit the patient and family to explore and share feelings and attitudes about health are essential in the rehabilitative phase. There must be active involvement by patient and family at all times, but especially immediately after the diagnosis when fear, anger, and hostility are paramount. Parents of children experience guilt, and they require support during this difficult period. Once the individual returns home, an assessment within the context of a familiar environment may identify new problems which need resolution.

Conflicts arise since the patient suffers from a *chronic disease* which has absolutely no cure but usually can be controlled with medication. Such knowledge is not always easy to accept. There are *anxieties* with which patients must deal, in addition to the actual seizures to which they are subjected.

The presence of a *metabolic disturbance* which activates seizure activity may necessitate changes in a patient's nutritional intake. Certainly dietary counseling, which may involve collaboration with a nutritionist, is imperative.

Many individuals experience *abnormal bodily sensations* and/or movements which are frightening and over which they have no control. While such phenomena can influence *changes in an individual's life-style,* convulsive activity also precipitates concerns for safety during these episodes.

For many patients, anxieties related to poorly controlled seizures can be overwhelming. They are fearful about engaging in many activities, including work or travel, because they may have seizures. Adequately educating the patient and family can allay some of these frightening feelings. Knowing their causes and clarifying misconceptions of this health problem lessen apprehensions. In each instance the rationale for treatment should be provided and patient compliance stressed. Because questions may arise or problems develop, mechanisms for contacting appropriate health professionals need to be shared with the patient and family. Assurance that someone is available to help and to listen is a critical component of health care.

**Drug therapy**   The most effective control of seizure activity has been achieved through efficient utilization of anticonvulsant drugs. Patients having more than one type of seizure may receive a combination of drugs. Certain basic information needs to be provided to patients who are being maintained on these medications. It is essential they know that these drugs are safe and effective, and the reason why these anticonvulsants must be taken as prescribed in order to sustain their effectiveness. Successful therapy is dependent upon an individual's seizure threshold and overall compliance with the established regimen. These patients need to be instructed not to skip doses, to be aware of potential side effects, and to report any evidence of toxic symptoms immediately to the nurse or physician. If problems occur, referrals can be made to a physician and alterations in the dosage can quickly relieve the distressing symptom(s). It is essential that the nurse advise patients *not* to stop medications without consultation with a physician.

Long-term administration of phenytoin or diphenylhydantoin may result in gingival hyperplasia, gastrointestinal problems, megaloblastic anemia, hirsutism in young women, as well as nystagmus, ataxia, diplopia, and vertigo.

To minimize the gingival hyperplasia, health teaching should include instruction on meticulous oral hygiene and regular dental care. An increase in any of the aforementioned side effects or an increase in the frequency of seizures should be reported promptly because the dosage may need to be altered or the medication may no longer be effective.

Toxic effects of phenobarbital include: nystag-mus, ataxia, irritability or hyperactivity in children, and confusion in the elderly. The presence of any of these symptoms should be reported to a physician. Newborns whose mothers were treated with phenobarbital during pregnancy have developed hypoprothrombinemia.[15] This condition can be treated with vitamin K.

After three or four seizure-free years the dosages may be decreased and perhaps discontinued providing there are no seizures. Such withdrawal must occur under strict medical supervision. Alcohol is restricted or totally eliminated in all these patients because it is a potential seizure precipitant in addition to being responsible for lowering the effectiveness of anticonvulsants. Alert to specific drugs being taken and knowing their side effects, the nurse must communicate this information to the patient so that there is compliance. Cooperation in taking the medicines prescribed can result in effective control of most seizure disorders.

**Health teaching**   Opportunities for discussion should be made available to the individual and family members, for a better understanding of events involved in seizure activity will give them more confidence in their abilities to deal with these events. Health teaching should include specific information about a seizure as well as its effects on the activities of the person involved, thereby providing those most intimately involved with scientific knowledge, not hearsay, about the process. In the community, those individuals who have extensive contact with large segments of the population (policemen, firemen, teachers, restaurant workers) should receive some type of formalized instruction regarding emergency measures to be instituted when a person experiences a seizure in their presence. Reviewing the medication protocol and identifying measures to be taken in the home to ensure safety also contribute to more effective management of the patient.

The individualized teaching plans that are developed need to deal with physical activity and rest. If seizures are frequent and poorly controlled, activities such as contact sports, horseback riding, and swimming would be dangerous. However, adjustments allowing for such participation may be made for the seizure-free individual or the person who experiences only nocturnal seizures. Participation in some activities can be beneficial. There are clinical results which indicate that activity in the patient experiencing petit mal seizures raises the seizure threshold, thereby decreasing the frequency of these attacks.[16] Although safety factors need to be considered, careful assessment of an individual's particular needs can allow for a thorough activity schedule to be planned.

*Rest and sleep* are to be considered when discussing and planning such activity schedules. It is a known fact that fatigue and overexhaustion precipitate seizures. Therefore, regular and consistent sleep patterns are important. When traveling, efforts need to be made to avoid fatigue, especially when normal body rhythms are disrupted as one travels through different time zones. Well-timed rest periods can diminish the effects of these changes. Those individuals whose work schedules require changes from one shift to another, especially day to night, also risk exposure to stimuli which may initiate a seizure. Such alterations should be thoroughly discussed with the patient.

**Nutrition** Patients often ask if their diet needs to be changed, once they have been diagnosed as having a seizure disorder. There was a period of time when clinical investigations resulted in the utilization of a *ketogenic* diet. This is a specific diet in which an excessive proportion of allotted calories is derived from fats, which are reduced to ketones, and maintain the patient in a state of ketosis and thereby decreasing seizure activity. In the hospital where the diet can be carefully controlled, maintaining ketosis is not difficult, but it is next to impossible in the home. Furthermore, the diet is not palatable and is poorly tolerated. Except for use in selected pediatric patients with myoclonic seizures, the ketogenic diet has for the most part been abandoned. The diet of an epileptic should be wholesome and well-balanced with an abundance of vegetables and fresh fruits. The emphasis is on moderation. Again, avoiding alcohol is important. Since overhydration may precipitate a seizure, women who are premenstrual should be instructed to limit their fluid intake immediately prior to menstruation.

**Public education** It is important for a nurse to look at the patient in a broader social context, in order to understand the bias and prejudice to which an individual with a seizure disorder is subjected. A societal stigma does exist. Employers fear that a seizure will occur on the job and interfere with the individual's job performance or efficiency. Through public education, which nurses coordinate and/or initiate, programs can facilitate a greater understanding of individuals with this disorder. Epilepsy is not synonymous with lower intellectual levels, poor job performance, or psychological problems.

In school systems, nurses can assist the child who is newly diagnosed with seizures to make the necessary reentry into the classroom setting and teach him or her about the limitations on physical activity which may be necessary and can also teach the other children about the nature of seizures. Emphasis needs to be placed on school attendance, an important aspect of a child's growth which needs to be continued, unless contraindicated by a physician. Environmental stressors or problems in those settings can be responsible for lowered drug effectiveness, and they might influence the frequency of seizures or contribute to the toxic effects of the anticonvulsants.

Some aspects of rehabilitation are controlled by law and deserve some discussion. If driving a car was a normal activity prior to the development of a seizure disorder, limitations are placed on continuing to do so. All states require that a person be seizure-free, on or off medications, for a specified period of time, the period varying from state to state. In addition, these individuals must be under the care of a physician. The dangers of driving with this disorder need to be discussed thoroughly with emphasis on peril to the patient as well as the lives of others who might be involved in an accident.

Marriage laws which previously discriminated against the person with epilepsy have been removed in all states. Certainly an individual considering marriage should discuss the disorder with the marriage partner with an honest evaluation of frequency of seizures as well as their control. Medical, psychological, and genetic counseling may be necessary.

Genetic predisposition to epilepsy is controversial at this time. There are some clinical investigators who believe that genetic influences are greatest when epilepsy begins early in childhood and when both parents are epileptics. Genetic liability decreases as the distance between the relationship of individuals involved increases.[17]

Employment is of vital importance in the rehabilitation of a person with epilepsy. Employers should understand that job performance is not affected by a seizure problem. If a nurse knows that the patient is having difficulty finding work, referral to the State Vocational Rehabilitation Agency is appropriate. With offices located in each state capital, information related to vocational training can be obtained. Additional vocational rehabilitation programs are available through the Epilepsy Foundation of America.

The person with a seizure disorder is confronted by a society which regards the individual with fear and hostility because of ignorance. Social stigmas extend to all aspects of that individual's environment. They need to be overcome in order for these individuals to assume their proper positions within our societal structure.

Recent research on the physiology of the nervous system, bioenergetics, and altered stress responses suggests that methods such as transcendental meditation may become successful interventions for patients with seizures. These methods use mind control to help the patients reach levels of relaxation that reduce excitability of brain cells. As science progresses and changes in societal attitudes about epilepsy occur, the future is bright. And in spite of the complex issues which face these patients, they can become active, productive, contributing members of society.

## REFERENCES

1  Raymond D. Adams, "The Convulsive State," in M. M. Wintrobe et al. (eds.), *Harrison's Principles of Internal Medicine,* 7th ed., McGraw-Hill, New York, 1974, p. 131.

2  *Ibid.*

3  Harvey S. Singer and John M. Freeman, "Seizures in Adolescents," *Med Clin North Am,* **59:**6:1461, November 1975.

4  Nicholas A. Vick, "Convulsive Disorders," in *Grinker's Neurology,* 7th ed., Charles C Thomas, Springfield, Ill., 1976, p. 714.

5  Robert B. Aird and Dixon M. Woodbury, *The Management of Epilepsy,* Charles C Thomas, Springfield, Ill., 1974, p. 5.

6  *Ibid.,* p. 12.

7  *Ibid.,* pp. 12–17.

8  *Ibid.,* p. 13.

9  Mervyn J. Eadie and John Tyler, *Anticonvulsant Therapy,* Churchill Livingston, Edinburgh, 1974, p. 73.

10  *Ibid.,* p. 83.

11  Aird and Woodbury, *op. cit.,* p. 257.

12  Francis McNaughton and Theodore Rasmussen, "Criteria for Selection of Patients for Neurosurgical Treatment in Purpura," in K. Perry Dominick and Richard Walter (eds.), *Neurosurgical Management of the Epilepsies,* Raven Press, New York, 1975, p. 38.

13  Raymond D. Adams, "Idiopathic Epilepsy," in M. M. Wintrobe et al. (eds.), *Harrison's Principles of Internal Medicine,* 7th ed., McGraw-Hill, New York, 1974, p. 1867.

14  Aird and Woodbury, *op. cit.,* p. 257.

15  Louis Goodman and Alfred Goodman, *The Pharmacologic Basis of Therapeutics,* Macmillan, New York, 1975, p. 209.

16  W. Gotze, et al., "Physical Exercise on Seizure Threshold," *Dis Nerv System,* **28:**665, 1966.

17  Singer and Freeman, *op. cit.,* p. 1470.

## BIBLIOGRAPHY

Bagley, C.: "Social Prejudice and the Adjustment of People with Epilepsy," *Epilepsia,* **13:**33–45, January 1972.

Boshes, L. D., and H. W. Kienast: "Community Aspects of Epilepsy—A Modern Re-appraisal," *Epilepsia,* **13:**31–32, January 1972.

Brazier, Mary A. B.: *The Electrical Activity of the Nervous System,* Williams & Wilkins, Baltimore, 1968.

Bruya, Margaret Auld, and Rose Norman Bolin: "Epilepsy: A Controllable Disease," *Am J Nurs,* **76:** 388–390, March 1976.

Carini, Esta, and Guy Owens: *Neurological and Neurosurgical Nursing,* Mosby, St. Louis, 1974.

Caveness, W. F., H. H. Merritt, and G. H. Gallup: "A Survey of Public Attitudes toward Epilepsy in 1974 with an Indication of Trends over the Past 25 Years," *Epilepsia,* **15:**523, December 1974.

Cherlow, D. G., and E. A. Serafetinedes: "Speech and Memory Assessment in Psychomotor Epileptics," *Cortex,* **12**(1):21–26, May 1976.

Eadie, Mervyn J.: "The Management of Epilepsy," *Med J Aust,* **2**(2):49–51, July 1975.

Feldman, Robert E.: "Patients with Epilepsy," *Am Fam Physician,* **12**(4):135–140, October 1975.

Gastaut, H.: "Clinical and Electroencephalographical Classification of Epileptic Seizures," *Epilepsia,* **11:**102–113, March 1970.

———: *Dictionary of Epilepsy,* World Health Organization, Geneva, 1973.

——— et al.: "Relative Frequency of Different Types of Epilepsy: A Study Employing the Classification of the International League against Epilepsy," *Epilepsia,* **16**(3):457–461, September 1975.

Gotze, W., et al.: "Physical Exercise on Seizure Threshold: Investigated by Electroencephalographic Telemetry," *Dis Nerv Syst,* **28:**664–666, October 1967.

Guey, J., et al.: "A Study of the Rhythm of Petit Mal Absences in Children in Relation to Prevailing Situations," *Epilepsia,* **10:**441–451, Philadelphia, September 1969.

Guyton, Arthur C.: *Textbook of Medical Physiology,* Saunders, Philadelphia, 1976.

Harris, Phillip and Clifford Mawdsley (eds.): *Epilepsy, Proceedings of Hans Berger Centenary Symposium,* Churchill Livingston, Edinburgh, 1974.

Jasper, Herbert, Arthur Ward, and Alfred Pope: *Basic Mechanisms of the Epilepsies,* Little, Brown, Boston, 1969.

Jennett, Bryan: *Epilepsy after Non-Missile Head Injuries,* Year Book, Chicago, 1975.

Livingston, Samuel: *Comprehensive Management of Epilepsy in Infancy, Childhood and Adolescence,* Charles C Thomas, Springfield, Ill., 1972.

Luessenhop, Alfred, Teodoro Dela Cruz, and Gerald Fenichel: "Surgical Disconnection of the Cerebral Hemispheres for Intractable Seizures," *JAMA,* **213:**1630, September 7, 1970.

Mellor, D. H.: "Precipitating Factors in Epilepsy," *Dev Med Child Neurol,* **12:**800–802, December 1970.

Penfield, Wilder, and Herbert Jasper: *Epilepsy and the Functional Anatomy of the Human Brain,* Little Brown, Boston, 1954.

Richens, Alan: "Sensible Prescribing—Juvenile and Adult Epilepsy," *Practitioner,* **215**(1289):653–659, November 1975.

Shope, Jean T.: "The Clinical Specialist in Epilepsy," *Nurs Clin North Am,* **9**(4):761–772, December 1974.

Strandjord, R. E., and S. I. Johannessen: "One Daily Dose of Diphenylhydantoin for Patients with Epilepsy," *Epilepsia,* **15:**317–327, September 1974.

Taylor, D. C., and B. D. Bower: "Prevention in Epileptic Disorders," *Lancet,* **2**(734):1136–1138, Nov. 20, 1971.

Tharp, Barry: "Epilepsy: Some Comments on Diagnosis and Treatment," *Conn Med,* **40**(2):86–88, February 1976.

Waxman, Stephen, and Norman Geschwind: "The Interictal Behavior Syndrome in Temporal Lobe Epilepsy," *Arch Gen Psychiatry,* **32:**1580–1586, December 1975.

Wilder, B. Joe: *The Clinical Neurophysiology of Epilepsy,* Department of Health, Education, and Welfar, Bethesda, Md., 1968.

Williams, Anne: "Classification and Diagnosis of Epilepsy," *Nurs Clin North Am,* **9**(4):947–959, December 1974.

Wilson, Donald H., et al.: "Disconnection of the Cerebral Hemispheres, An Alternative to Hemispherectomy for the Control of Intractable Seizures," *Neurology,* **25**(12):1149–1153, December 1975.

# 34

# VASCULAR DISTURBANCES IN PERCEPTION AND COORDINATION

Dorothy L. Sexton

It is of critical importance to all human beings that the cerebral vascular system be functional and intact. Brain tissue, which does not store oxygen or glucose, depends on continuous and efficient oxygenation. Without this constant circulation, vital functions involved with perception and coordination may be severely impaired.

Interference with cerebral function caused by obstruction, infarction, or hemorrhage can result in permanent or temporary impairment of the ability to interpret sensation and perceive stimuli. For example, loss of sensory input from a major source (e.g., eye or ear) impairs the ability to perceive and respond to environmental cues. Even the most minor dysfunctions may cause significant changes in a person's ability to engage in simple activities of daily living. An impaired cerebral vascular system therefore carries with it some of the most extensive consequences of any health problem and requires the most skilled nursing care.

## CEREBROVASCULAR INFARCTION

The terms *cerebrovascular infarction* (CVI), *cerebrovascular accident* (CVA), and *stroke* are synonyms used to describe an interruption in oxygen supply to the brain due to the presence of a cerebrovascular lesion. These lesions produce changes in the vessel wall and interfere with cerebral oxygenation. Examples include vessel occlusion by a thrombus or embolus, rupture of the blood vessel (aneurysm), decreased arterial blood supply, atherosclerotic plaque formation, and narrowing of the vessel lumen.[1] A disruption that deprives brain tissue of local oxygen and nutrients can lead to cerebral anoxia.

### Pathophysiology

The absence of oxygen to the brain tissue for more than 5 to 6 minutes leads to irreversible cerebral changes and tissue necrosis. The area of infarction usually appears anemic (pale) and then gradually assumes a muddy appearance. Some areas of infarction may appear congested, while other locales appear to have a scattering of petechial hemorrhage.

In the absence of cerebral oxygenation or in the presence of extravasation of blood into brain tissue, an inflammatory response can occur within the tissue. This contributes to cerebral edema and can cause changes in perception and coordination.

Generalized cerebrovascular interruptions alter fluid and electrolyte balance. When *cerebral edema* is intense, the threat of increased intracranial pressure is present. The edema fluid, which is both extracellular and intracellular, accumulates primarily in the white matter. Tissue edema contributes to the increased intracranial pressure caused by space-occupying lesions. The edematous brain becomes boggy and heavy, and the pressure from the edema compresses the ventricular system.[2]

The neurons and the glia have a narrow and somewhat stereotyped pattern of response to injury. Ischemia of neurons may lead to acute necrosis, which is characterized by contraction of the cell body. Eventually, rupture of the cell membrane and autolysis and phagocytosis of the cell debris occur.[3] After several hours, the necrotic tissue is liquefied and removed by macrophages. A glial and vascular scar replaces the area of infarct.[4]

Changes in the body's ability to excrete urine adequately can be directly influenced by the degree and severity of the cerebrovascular accident and the resultant hypovolemic state that ensues. If the infarction occurs in the hypothalamic area near the fourth ventricle, definite changes occur which interfere not only with temperature regulation but also with ADH (antidiuretic hormone) production. This can also affect urinary output.

Brain tissue metabolism is altered following infarction by the lack of oxygen and glucose. The efficiency of the neurons is affected, since little glucose or oxygen is stored in the neurons. The resulting hypoxia and hypoglycemia increases the irritability of neurons and disrupts nerve transmission. Seizure activity may be one response to these changes. If the temperature-regulating mechanism is dysfunctional, there may be extreme *hypothermia, hyperthermia,* or an unrecognized *poikilothermia* ( a body temperature that varies with that of the environment). Alteration in body temperature affects the basal metabolic rate and increases body metabolism.

**Location of the cerebrovascular infarction and related neurologic deficits** The effects of a CVI are many and vary from person to person, depending on the cerebral blood vessels involved and the amount of brain tissue deprived of oxygen. (Figure 34-1 shows the major cerebral arteries.)

In most cases, a lesion becomes increasingly lethal as it moves caudally from the cerebral cortex (where neurons are dispersed over a fairly large area) toward the medulla oblongata (where nuclei and fibers lie in a relatively compact area). For example, a small infarct in the prefrontal cortex may have no apparent consequence, whereas the same

size lesion in the medulla oblongata may cause instant death.[5]

The territory of any blood vessel (that area directly or indirectly supplied by the cerebral arterial blood source) often determines the psychologic and physiologic effects experienced by the patient. Table 34-1 lists the major cerebral blood vessels usually affected by a CVI, the territory directly involved, other areas indirectly involved, and the effects of these changes on the patient. Table 34-2 lists common terms used to describe CVI problems referred to throughout this chapter.

**Causes and effects of CVI** There are three major causes of stroke (or CVI): thrombus formation, embolization, and hemorrhage. Atherosclerosis, hypertension, spasms, and tumor are additional causes of CVI and are often integral components of the above problems.

A cerebral *thrombus,* or blood clot, occurs most often when a plaque has developed, causing narrowing of the lumen of an artery. Thrombosis is the most frequent cause of CVI. The most common sites for thrombus formation are the internal carotid artery at the carotid sinus, the main bifurcation of the middle cerebral artery, the vertebral and basilar arteries in the region of their junction, and the posterior cerebral artery as it curves upward over the corpus callosum.[13] The middle cerebral artery branches into the internal capsule and supplies the lateral surface of the cerebral hemisphere. The middle nutrient cerebral artery, because of its large blood supply and area, is more prone to infarction than brain tissue in other areas (refer to Fig. 34-1).

Thrombosis may be caused by atherosclerosis or by an inflammation within the vessel itself. When thrombosis occludes an artery, the brain tissue it supplies becomes ischemic. The edema caused by thrombosis may result in more damage than the actual infarction. Usually, as the edema begins to subside, a return of function may be noted.

Cerebral thrombosis presents a more variable picture than embolism or hemorrhage. In approximately 80 percent of cases, minor prodromal (warning) signs precede the more severe attack. *Transient warning disturbances* of the carotid and middle cerebral artery may include mono- or hemiplegia, blindness in one eye, speech disturbances, or mental confusion.

It is common for the stroke or CVI to occur during sleep or after arising. The manifestations of a stroke will vary, depending on the artery occluded. The episode may involve several body parts or one area such as the face or an extremity. If the progression of the CVI is slow and occurs over several hours, other body parts may gradually be affected over time. This may be described as *thrombosis in evolution.*

Most often, *emboli* are dislodged fragments of a thrombus, so the term *thromboembolism* is commonly used. A *cerebral embolus* is usually a fragment which becomes detached from a thrombus within the heart. The most frequent cause of cerebral embolism is chronic atrial fibrillation. The source of the embolus is a "mural" thrombus (along the wall) deposited within the atrial appendage or formed on the damaged endocardium after myocardial infarction. Emboli also originate from the thrombus that occurs in severe mitral stenosis and the vegetation of bacterial endocarditis. Mitral and aortic valve replacement (see Chap. 27), as well as subacute bacterial endocarditis, are also known to disseminate thrombus fragments.

When an embolus travels to the brain, it passes through successively smaller arteries until it becomes lodged in a vessel, obstructing cerebral blood flow. Massive infarction results most commonly from occlusion of the branches of the middle cerebral artery. The middle cerebral artery is a direct continuation of the internal carotid artery and therefore is in direct line for receiving the embolus. As an embolus passes along a cerebral artery, it may produce a temporary neurologic deficit. The deficit clears up quickly as the embolus continues on its passage into a small arterial branch supplying a relatively silent part of the hemisphere.

The onset of a cerebral embolus is rapid and usually without warning. Changes appear within minutes of the infarct. The problem can erupt at any time of the day or night. The degree of subsequent neurologic involvement will depend on the location of the occlusion.

Some patients may experience episodes of recurrent cerebral ischemia associated with transient impairment of cerebral circulation. These *transient cerebral ischemic attacks* (TIA) are reversible episodes of focal neurologic deficit manifested by visual disturbances, weakness and numbness of the arm and other extremities, and aphasia. The attacks may last a few minutes or as long as 12 hours but most commonly from 10 to 30 minutes. It is important to note that the residual deficit does not last for more than 24 hours. TIAs are unrelated to position or activity.

Transient ischemic attacks are associated almost entirely with atherosclerotic thrombosis. Any cerebral artery or cerebellar artery may be involved.

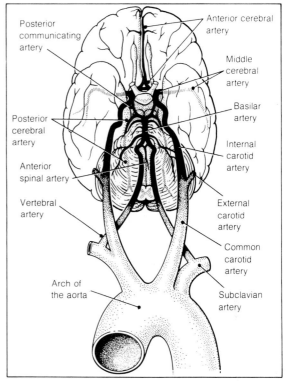

**FIGURE 34-1**

Territories of the major cerebral arteries. (*From Maxwell M. Wintrobe et al. (eds.): Harrison's Principles of Internal Medicine, 7th ed., McGraw-Hill, New York, 1974, p. 1747.*)

At present it is thought that TIAs result from platelet emboli released from sites of atherothrombosis, but evidence to support this viewpoint is lacking. Cerebral vasospasm and transient episodes of systemic arterial hypotension have been considered the basis of the ischemic attacks.[14]

*Hemorrhage* may occur in several sites: outside the dura mater (extradural hemorrhage), beneath the dura mater (subdural hemorrhage), in the subarachnoid space (subarachnoid hemorrhage), or within the brain itself (cerebral or intracerebral hemorrhage).[15] This discussion deals with hemorrhages that occur in brain tissue, or cerebral hemorrhage. A complete discussion of the other hemorrhage sites is found in Chap. 3.

A *cerebral hemorrhage* results from the rupture of a cerebral vessel. When this occurs, there is an extravasation of blood into the parenchyma, the subarachnoid space, or both. The extravasated blood forms an enlarging mass which displaces and compresses brain tissue and disrupts functioning of the areas involved. Pressure can be so severe

**TABLE 34-1**
CEREBRAL ARTERIES COMMONLY AFFECTED BY CEREBROVASCULAR INFARCTION
AND THE RESULTING NEUROLOGIC DEFICITS

| Artery* | Territory | Specific Locations | Effects of Vascular Interference† |
|---|---|---|---|
| Middle cerebral | Middle cerebral | Cortex and white matter of parietal lobe (lateral) | Motor and sensory impairment, paralysis of contralateral face and arm,[6] hemiplegia, interruption of optic-tract fibers with field cut, or homonymous hemianopsia‡ |
| | | Temporal lobe (lateral and superior parts) | Interruption of optic-tract fibers with field cut, or homonymous hemianopsia,‡ diplopia, expressive aphasia, paresis with weakness of leg |
| | | Broca's area (posterior part of inferior frontal gyrus) | Speech disorder, dysphasia, sensory aphasia, expressive aphasia[7] |
| *Anterior cerebral | Medial surface of cerebral hemisphere | Frontal lobe (orbital surface) | Infarction of entire territory: paralysis and profound behavioral changes |
| | | Frontal lobe | Motor and sensory impairment of foot and leg movement,[8] gait disturbance or disruption, urinary incontinence |
| | | Anterior limb of internal capsule | Abulia, whispered speech |
| | | Inferior part of caudate nucleus | Dyspraxia, tactile aphasia |
| *Vertebral | Medulla | Pyramid, medial lemniscus, posterior inferior cerebellar hemisphere | Visual changes, contralateral bilateral paralysis |
| | | Posterior inferior cerebellar artery | Occlusion tolerated |
| | | Posterior medulla | Severe dizziness, nausea, vomiting, ataxia, nystagmus |
| | | Lateral medulla | Coma, contralateral impairment of pain and thermal sense over half the body (sometimes face involved), miosis, ptosis, decreased sweating, dizziness, diplopia, nausea and vomiting, ataxia |
| *Internal carotid | Part of middle cerebral | Frontal lobe | Predominance of unilateral signs but may be asymptomatic |
| | Ipsilateral anterior cerebral | | Contralateral hemiplegia, aphasia (dominant hemisphere) |
| | Anterior choroid artery | | Coma, headache |

that vital centers are compressed and coma and death result.

Cerebral hemorrhage usually has an *abrupt onset* and a fairly rapid evolution. The characteristic pattern is one of gradual and steady progression until the neurologic deficit is established. The time it takes to reach the maximum deficit depends on the rate of bleeding. When the hemorrhage is massive, the patient may survive for several days, until brainstem compression becomes so severe that it affects the functioning of vital centers.[16] It is common for the hemorrhage to occur when a person is up and about daily activities. Frequently the hemorrhage extends to involve the territory of more than one vessel. The sequestered blood displaces brain tissue and gives rise to increased intracranial pressure (see Chap. 32). The extravasate

may also rupture into the ventricles or the subarachnoid space. Once the bleeding has ceased, its recurrence in the near future is rare.

The nature of the vascular lesion that causes cerebral hemorrhage has not been identified. However, rupture of an atherosclerotic cerebral vessel is usually associated with long-standing *hypertension*. There are usually no prodromal symptoms. In most cases the hemorrhage is preceded by physical or emotional exertion which elevates the arterial pressure. Often the onset of hemorrhage is heralded by severe occipital headache, nuchal ridigity, dizziness, fainting, motor or sensory disturbances, and nosebleed.

Neurologic disruptions vary with the size and location of the sequestered blood. The most common sites for hypertensive hemorrhage are the

**TABLE 34-1** (continued)

| Artery* | Territory | Specific Locations | Effects of Vascular Interference† |
|---|---|---|---|
| *Basilar | Pons, upper part of cerebellum, brainstem | Inferior temporal lobe, medial occipital lobe, posterior cerebral arteries | Coma, quadriplegia, bilateral motor and sensory changes, peripheral involvement of cranial nerves III to XII, brainstem involvement leading to compression of vital centers, coma, and death; in lower brain stem: hemiplegia, movement of eyes to side of paralysis, weakness of limbs and spasticity |
| | | Superior cerebellar branch of basilar artery | Dysarthria, ataxia, nausea, vomiting, slurring of speech, loss of pain and temperature sensations contralaterally on face, trunk, and extremities,[9] diplopia, partial deafness, nystagmus |
| | | Inferior cerebellar branch of basilar artery | Deafness, dizziness, nausea and vomiting, ringing in the ear, nystagmus, contralateral loss of pain and temperature sensations |
| Anterior choroid | Posterior limb of internal capsule | Artery and branches | Contralateral hemiplegia, hypesthesia, homonymous hemianopsia‡ |
| *Posterior cerebral | Brainstem, oculomotor nucleus, reticular substance of midbrain | Temporal lobe | Thalamic syndrome characterized by sensory loss (pain, touch proprioception), intention tremor |
| | | Occipital lobe | Hyperpathia, intractable thalamic pain,[10] emotional outbursts |
| | | Ventral tract, spinothalamic tract | Impairment of light touch sensation |
| | | Dorsal and ventral spinocerebellar tract | Impairment of reflex proprioception |
| | | Fasciculus gracilis and fasciculus cuneatus | Impairment of sensations of vibration and passive motion, joint and two-point discrimination[11] |
| | Central reticular formation (diffuse primitive network of fibers and nerve cells from brainstem core | From tegmentum of medulla to pons and midbrain merging into thalamic reticular system | Comatose states[12] |

* See Fig. 34-1 for depiction of major cerebral arteries.
† See Table 34-2 for definitions of various impairments.
‡ See Fig. 34-2 for depiction of visual pathways.

putamen and the adjacent internal capsule, the thalamus, the cerebellar hemisphere, the pons, and components of the central white matter of the frontal lobe.[17] Table 34-1 shows the territories and major cerebral vessels that can be involved. The mortality is especially high in pontine hemorrhage and in those cases in which the extravasate ruptures into a ventricle. Cerebral hemorrhage also carries a high morbidity rate because of the degree of tissue destruction that occurs.

*Thalamic hemorrhage* of even moderate size tends to produce hemiplegia because of extension into the adjacent internal capsule. As would be expected in a thalamic lesion, the sensory deficit is more prominent. When the lesion is on the dominant side, aphasia is present. A lesion on the nondominant side is associated with *apractagnosia,* a perceptual disorder of spatial judgment involving visual and motor elements within the environment. Extension of the hemorrhage into the subthalamic area creates varied occular disturbances.

*Cerebellar hemorrhage* is usually characterized by repeated vomiting, along with inability to stand or walk. Most persons also experience occipital headache and vertigo.[18] Both dysarthria and dysphasia may be present. An ipsilateral facial weakness and a diminished corneal reflex are common. As brainstem compression progresses, the patient passes from *stupor* into a *comatose state.* The eyes may face the lesion, or there may be a forced deviation of the eyes to the opposite side.

The majority of *subarachnoid hemorrhages* are due to rupture of a congenitally weak vessel in the subarachnoid space. The maldevelopment is usually a *saccular aneurysm* (berry aneurysm) that resembles a thin-walled blister protruding from an intracranial vessel (see Fig. 34-2). Saccules, or small sacs, occur in the circle of Willis and its major branches. The most common locations are the internal carotid artery, the posterior cerebral artery, the middle cerebral artery, the anterior communicating artery, and the vertebral basilar system. The saccules usually form at bifurcations and branchings and are considered to be caused by developmental defects in the media and elastica. It is also suggested that arteriosclerotic changes in cerebral arteries may contribute to weakened vessel walls.[19] Because of the local weakness, the intima bulges outward and is covered only by the adventitia. Over time the sac gradually enlarges.

Saccular aneurysms may occur at any age but are rare in childhood. Symptoms are most commonly experienced by the 35- to 65-year age group. Aneurysmal rupture usually occurs while a person is up and about, often engaging in strenuous activity. It is not uncommon for sexual intercourse to precipitate the episode.

In the vast majority of cases the aneurysm is "silent," producing no symptoms until the time of rupture. However, after many years of continued assault, some aneurysms balloon enough to compress brain tissue or cranial nerves. The most common focal symptoms are third or sixth cranial nerve palsies. Infection, brain tumors, blood dyscrasias,

**TABLE 34-2**
NOMENCLATURE OF CHANGES AND EFFECTS ASSOCIATED WITH CEREBRAL VASCULAR INFARCTION

*Dysphasia:* Impairment of ability to speak or to understand language.

*Sensory aphasia (receptive aphasia):* Impaired comprehension of the printed or spoken word.

*Motor aphasia (expressive aphasia):* Disruption of ability to produce speech.

*Acoustic aphasia:* Difficulty in comprehending speech.

*Visual aphasia:* Loss of ability to comprehend visual symbols resulting in difficulty in reading.

*Abulia:* Loss of ability to make decisions.

*Dysarthria:* Difficulty in articulating words, without loss of comprehension.

*Agnosia:* Partial or complete loss of ability (visual, auditory, tactile, or sensory) to recognize familiar objects.

*Alexia:* Loss of ability to recognize or comprehend written or printed words, sometimes referred to as *word blindness.*

*Agraphia:* Loss of ability to write.

*Apraxia:* Loss of ability to perform purposeful movements.

*Amnesic aphasia:* Loss of ability to find the correct word to identify an object, resulting in fragmented speech pattern.

trauma, and rupture of the meningeal vessels are less frequent causes of subarachnoid hemorrhage.

Other causes such as atherosclerosis (see Chap. 26), hypertension (see Chap. 28), brain tumors, and cerebral vessel spasms can contribute to the development of a CVI. *Atheromatous plaques* tend to form at the curve and branching of the artery and can lead to obstruction over time. *Chronic hypertension* will lead to stress on the vessel wall and rupture. *Tumors* of the central nervous system cause disruption in cerebral vasculature by occupying space; that is, neoplasms which are invasive usually destroy the tissues in which they occur and displace the surrounding tissues. In addition to their infiltrative qualities, neoplasms are directly obstructive and tend to compress and distort the vasculature.[20,21] *Spasms* of cerebral vessels and arteries can reduce blood flow to the brain. These spasms are usually of short duration and symptoms are transient.

### First-level Nursing Care

Cerebrovascular infarction is the third most common cause of death in the United States.[22] A CVI (stroke) affects 500,000 Americans annually. It is the most common neurologic disorder seen in adults. In 40 percent of cases the outcome is fatal. More than half the 2.5 million stroke survivors require special care for varying disabilities.[23]

A CVI is usually a disorder of the elderly, but it can occur during the fourth decade or earlier. Population surveys show the following proportions of stroke types: cerebral thrombosis, 62 percent; cerebral hemorrhage, 16 percent; subarachnoid hemorrhage, 12 percent; other cerebrovascular diseases, 10 percent.

**Population at risk** The majority of persons at risk of a stroke have a history of *hypertension* or *atherosclerosis* or both. Epidemiologic studies show that morbidity and mortality increase with an elevation in either the systolic or the diastolic blood pressure. An arterial pressure of 160/90 mmHg or higher in a resting, supine adult is considered to be hypertension. The incidence of hypertension in United States blacks is two or three times higher than that in the general population. Hypertension is thought to be more prevalent among low-income groups generally (see Chap. 28 for a complete discussion). Risk of cerebral infarction is related to elevated cholesterol and triglyceride levels. People who smoke, those with diabetes mellitus or with inherited weakness of vessel walls, and those who have sustained head injury have a high risk of developing a stroke. The use of oral contraceptives has been linked to cerebral vascular disturbances, but the research is controversial.

**Prevention** Many people who are hypertensive remain relatively symptom-free for many years. Therefore it is essential that aggressive screening programs be developed to detect and treat potential cerebral infarct victims (see Chap. 28). Physicians and nurses working in the community are encouraged to take clients' blood pressure at each routine health visit, regardless of the reason for the appointment. If hypertension is suspected, follow-up studies should be done to determine the cause.

Dietary modifications, including low-fat, low-cholesterol, and low-salt diets, are prescribed for patients (see Chap. 26). Patients with hypertension must be carefully checked for drug compliance. Often when the symptoms of hypertension are eliminated, the patient may arbitrarily decide to stop all treatment. Teaching plans, therefore, must stress the importance of following a specific health regimen even in the absence of symptoms. The patient must understand that although hypertension cannot be cured it can be controlled.

Patients who have experienced trauma to skull or brain tissue at an early age may be predisposed to hemorrhage and ruptured cerebral blood vessels as they grow older. It is essential that careful documentation of head injuries in children and young adults be included in the health record or elicited from the client during the health interview. In addition, reports of changes in perception or coordination should be noted and suspected problems clearly described. This will permit early detection and prompt treatment for problems that could become life-threatening.

In elderly patients, oversedation should be avoided, as deep sleep has been noted as a precipitant of cerebral ischemia.[24] Systemic problems such as hypovolemia and anemia should be treated promptly. Rapid diuresis should be avoided. Females using oral contraceptives should beware of the potential side effects of a specific drug. These patients should be encouraged to report severe headaches and seek a follow-up health check immediately. If necessary, oral contraceptives may have to be terminated and another method of birth control substituted.

### Second-level Nursing Care

Patients seen in the community are usually treated for transient vascular changes (TIAs). More than 80 percent of patients who experience transient

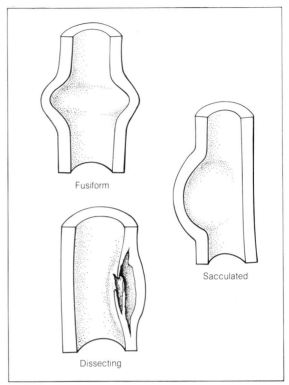

**FIGURE 34-2**
Aneurysms.

ischemic attacks eventually have a major stroke. Medical assistance is often sought by the patient or a family member in relation to milder prodromal symptoms.

**Nursing assessment** Patients with transient cerebrovascular changes may seek medical attention for a variety of physical and emotional changes. A complete assessment must be done to evaluate the extent of the problem and plan appropriate intervention.

**H**ealth History A clear *health history* obtained from the patient or family will reveal a short attack lasting from 10 to 20 minutes to 24 hours. Information obtained from the patient should include any history of hypertension, cerebral trauma, and family predisposition to vascular problems. Physical complaints will be contingent on the vessel involved. If the common or internal carotid artery is involved, the patient may complain of visual disturbances such as tunnel vision and blurring or transient blindness, temporary mental confusion, headache, dizziness, vague auditory complaints, memory lapses or confusion, and weakness of body parts. Patients may describe loss of emotional control and may succumb to crying for no reason. Transient aphasia may also be noted.

During the prodromal period patients may become very frightened. Some become emotional and relate a feeling of impending doom. Increasing loss of body functions and impaired speech along with mental confusion all contribute to increased anxiety.

**Physical Assessment**  Physical changes will vary according to the ischemic area involved. Neurologic changes include weakness of a body part or of one side of the body, and a complete bilateral neurologic examination (see Chap. 31) should be done. Reflex testing may reveal altered or depressed responses. There will be decreased grip response, with weakness noted on the affected side. Hemiplegia may develop to varying degrees, depending on the degree of arterial occlusion.

Muscle rigidity may be noted when the limb is put through range-of-motion exercises. The gait may be slightly unsteady, with staggering movements or dragging of the affected side. When asked to perform rapid rhythmic exercises, the patient may perform them in slow, nonrhythmic movement. Touch testing may reveal diminished perception of stimuli on the affected side. In addition, altered responses to pinprick and to heat and cold may be noted on the affected side.

During the eye examination, accommodation should be tested along with retinal artery pressure. Examination of vessels may reveal specific changes related to hypertension (see Chap. 28). Pupil changes may include unequal responses to light. The eyes may appear glazed, and slight ptosis may be seen on the affected side. Transient speech impairment may be noted, along with visual disturbances.

**Diagnostic Tests**  *Thermography* is done to record infrared radiations emanating from the body's surface, to record temperature, or to identify local thermal changes. Thermography detects hot and cold areas on surfaces such as the face and measures body temperature. When the blood supply to an artery is decreased, its temperature may also be diminished. *Phonoangiography* is a technique which magnifies the sounds made by blood flowing through an artery (e.g., the carotid). Any obstruction in blood flow is detected in monitoring devices set to pick up changes.

**Nursing problems and interventions**  Patients with mild CVI have several problems which require attention. These include hypertension, headaches, stress, dizziness and weakness, visual changes, speech impairments, and thromboembolism.

**Hypertension**  Hypertension may continue to be a problem following CVI, and care must be taken to avoid abrupt reduction in arterial pressure. Antihypertensive drugs should be used with caution, and careful patient education is essential (see Chap. 28).

Blood pressure levels should be checked at frequent intervals to assess drug compliance. Other family members can be screened by the community health nurse to detect hypertension early. Counseling should be directed toward identifying stressful situations and helping the patient reduce anxiety.

Nutritional counseling should focus on decreasing intake of salt, cholesterol, and fat (Chaps. 24 and 26). If the patient is obese, a low-calorie diet should be instituted for weight reduction. Smoking should be discouraged and the patient told of the vasoconstrictive effects of nicotine and its potential effect on arterial blood pressure.

**Headaches**  Headaches frequently accompany hypertension and can be aggravated by stress. Patients often experience the headaches early in the morning, and they appear to lessen as the day progresses. Mild analgesia may be used along with application of cold packs to the affected area. In addition, a quiet environment should be maintained at home to reduce potentially noxious environmental stimuli.

**Stress**  Stressful situations should be carefully assessed in order to identify potentially anxiety-provoking events and eliminate them if possible. Occupational counseling may be needed. If the patient is anxious, a mild tranquilizer may be prescribed. The patient should be given support and help to cope with mood changes and emotional lability. Family counseling may be required to assist family members to cope with this patient crisis. The patient should be given an opportunity to discuss personal fear of loss of bodily functions. The nurse can reassure the patient by explaining the physiologic changes that are occurring and the reason for them.

**Dizziness and Weakness**  *Dizziness* may be present in some forms of cerebral arterial occlusion. This will depend on the artery involved and the amount of obstruction present. Patients and family members should be told about this potential threat, and patients should be encouraged to make some changes in their life-style accordingly. For example, driving should be eliminated, and patients in potentially dangerous occupations, such as working with heavy machinery, should be encouraged to seek less threatening occupations.

Frequently the patient may experience a generalized physical *weakness* of one side of the body, a limb, a hand, or a foot. This may affect ability to walk and result in an unsteady gait. Elderly patients should be especially careful if they are prone to these attacks and not go out without an escort if possible.

**V**isual Changes and Speech Impairments   *Visual changes* may accompany a TIA but are usually temporary. Patients often find blurred vision or blindness, no matter how intermittent, a frightening experience. The patient should be encouraged to have a complete eye examination. If headaches accompanied by visual changes persist, even after the use of medication, immediate medical attention should be sought. Patients should be sure that they have adequate lighting. If eyeglasses are needed, they should be worn, but patients should be told that the use of glasses will not increase vision. Generally visual disturbances are temporary and the side effects will pass.

In addition to visual changes, *transient speech impairments* may also occur. These disruptions can range from slurring of speech to aphasia. The patient and family members should be told that these changes may accompany each attack, so that the problem can be anticipated. Family members should also be taught about speech impairments, as patients may say things that do not seem logical and experience temporary mental confusion (even amnesia). Reassurance and support given by the nurse will help prepare the patient and family for speech and perceptual changes that may occur at a future time.

**T**hromboembolism   Thromboemoblism is a continuous threat to the patient, since thrombus formation accounts for the majority of CVIs. Anticoagulants may be used to help prevent further attacks or massive strokes due to thromboembolism. Transient changes may be eliminated, especially if precipitating problems are due to thrombi or emboli. A full discussion on the use of anti-coagulant therapy is found under Third-level Nursing Care, below.

**E**mergency Intervention   If an ischemic attack becomes severe, emergency intervention may be necessary. Acute cerebral ischemic episodes are often accompanied by headache, dizziness, flushed face, loss of consciousness, paralysis, mental confusion, loss of vision, and difficulty in speaking or swallowing. Immediate nursing responses should include establishment of a patent airway and assessment of the paralysis and respiratory complications, aphasia, and disruptions in swallowing. In the period immediately following the infarction, it is important to loosen or remove constricting clothing such as collars and ties. The conscious patient should be encouraged to gently cough up secretions to maintain an open airway. If the patient is confused, slight elevation of the head may help decrease cerebral edema. In the presence of cardiac and respiratory arrest, cardiopulmonary resuscitation will be necessary (see Chap. 26). Turning the unconscious patient to the affected side will facilitate drainage of secretions and prevent aspiration. A ballooning of the cheeks on exhalation can indicate respiratory problems. Again, it is essential that the airway remain unobstructed. Changes in level of consciousness, cardiac status, and vital signs are important parameters to monitor. Keeping the patient warm will help sustain body temperature. When the condition stabilizes, the patient can be transported to an acute-care setting.

### Third-level Nursing Care

In the time span immediately following the cerebrovascular infarction, nursing care is directed toward maintaining the patient's vital functions. The degree of neurologic deficit may be greater early in the illness because of cerebral edema and resultant swelling (increased intracranial pressure). Neurologic deficits are often most severe 3 to 4 days after the infarct; as cerebral edema and congestion subside, function begins to improve.

**Nursing assessment**   After the patient's physical condition has stabilized, careful assessment will be needed to evaluate the extent of injury. If the patient is unconscious, the health history may need to be obtained from family or friends.

**H**ealth History   A detailed health history and an in-depth assessment of the patient must be obtained. Conversation with the patient will usually reveal the presence of prodromal symptoms prior to the CVI. The patient or family members may describe altered levels of consciousness ranging from mental confusion to stupor to varying degrees of unconsciousness. The patient may be anxious and, depending on the area of the brain affected, unable to speak. Loss of speech accompanied by visual changes intensifies the patient's fear and stress and can increase anxiety. Depression over changes in body image and loss of body movement and sensation may be observed. The family may describe frequent mood swings prior to the onset of the CVI and emotional outbursts are common.

The past medical history is often significant. Major health problems as well as significant health disruptions in other family members are important to the data-collection process. The onset of prodromal symptoms such as speech changes, weakness, and visual changes should be indicated. The approximate frequency of symptoms and the time span between the onset of the initial symptoms and the current symptoms should also be noted. In addition, the nurse should seek a description of the changes that occurred in the patient prior to hospitalization. If the patient is unconscious, stuporous, or comatose, this information can be elicited from family members.

**Physical Assessment** A complete neurologic assessment (see Chap. 31) will be necessary to evaluate physical changes. Assessment of the cranial nerves is essential. Changes affecting the third cranial nerve will cause the eyelid on the affected side to remain partially open. Ptosis may be observed. When this occurs, the presence or absence of the *corneal reflex* should be ascertained. These conditions are often contingent on the level of consciousness and cerebral oxygenation. Absence of the corneal reflex is indicative of severe cerebral anoxia and nerve damage. *Field cut* (homonymous hemianopsia (see Fig. 34-3) may also be present. Patients who have a right-sided paralysis may have decreased vision in the right visual fields of both eyes (see Chap. 31 for assessment of visual fields). Conjugate deviation (the eyes focusing in the direction of the lesion) may be noted. *Pupil reactions* will be altered, depending on the level of consciousness and the increase in intracranial cerebral pressure.

**FIGURE 34-3**

The visual pathways. A, loss of vision in the right field; B, loss of vision in the temporal half of the right and left fields; C, loss of vision in the nasal field of the right eye and the temporal field of the left eye (homonymous hemianopia). (*From Esta Carini and Guy Owens: Neurological and Neurosurgical Nursing, 6th ed., Mosby, St. Louis, 1974, p. 28.*)

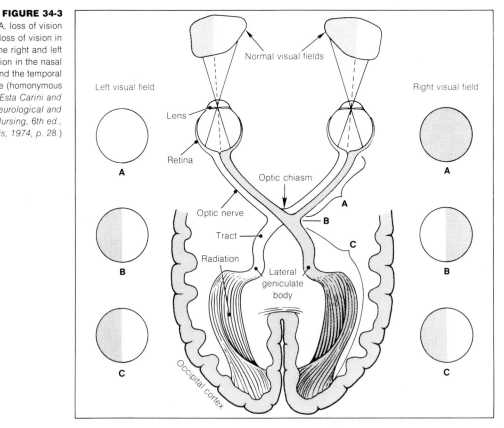

*Facial weakness* may be present on the affected side below the level of the eye. The weakness is demonstrated by facial asymmetry and drooping of the mouth. There is also ballooning out of the cheek during exhalation.

When hemiplegia is present, the affected extremity muscles are flaccid and the leg is everted. Muscle tone is often poor. Gait may be uncoordinated, especially in the presence of paralysis. A *positive Babinski response* may be present because of sensory and nerve damage. (Refer to Chapter 31 for a discussion of this reflex.) Other body reflexes may also be altered or absent. The extremities should be evaluated, using several parameters such as pain and response to touch and to heat and cold, to assess the extent of impairment. Findings should be compared bilaterally. Motor responses can be evaluated by having the patient move the extremities and perform bilateral handgrips. It is not uncommon to detect one-sided weakness.

If stroke is due to hemorrhage, additional changes may occur. As the blood spreads through the subarachnoid space, there will be pain in the lower back and legs. Within a few hours, *nuchal rigidity* and *Kernig's sign* will become evident. Additional symptoms such as aphasia, hemiparesis, field cut, and third-nerve palsy may occur, but this will depend on the location of the aneurysm. Immediate loss of consciousness following a CVI usually carries with it a poor prognosis.[25]

*Seizure activity* may be seen in the presence of hemorrhage. Signs of increased intracranial pressure may also be noted (see Chap. 32). Hypovolemia may eventually lead to shock. Assessment of vital signs reveals altered blood pressure, pulse rate, and respiration, depending on the area of the brain involved and the presence of cerebral edema and shock. Most patients have an elevated blood pressure along with an elevated pulse and respiratory rate in the period following a stroke. Temperature readings are usually 100 to 102°F.

The degree of orientation to time, place, person, and situation should be assessed. It is essential to ascertain the patient's control of language and speech, as well as auditory and perceptual capabilities, for these will influence planning and management of care. Aphasia may be present if the infarction is on the dominant side. Deficits in knowledge, memory, retention of information, and ability to calculate and perform simple activities may be noted (Table 34-2). Difficulty in coordinating activities and making appropriate discriminations may be apparent. The nurse can test for these changes by giving the patient simple math problems, ask-

ing the patient to recall three well-known facts presented a few minutes previously, or asking the patient to arrange colored pieces of string in small groups, each group representing one color. (Chap. 31 discusses these and other sensorimotor checks.) Depending on the degree and location of sensorimotor impairment, disruptions in ability to complete and coordinate these tasks will be observed.

Vomiting may be present. Abdominal examination may reveal distention, altered bowel sounds (which may reflect disruption in sensorimotor stimulation to the bowel), and loss of bowel and bladder muscle control. *Skin color* may also be changed. The face may be flushed initially, and cyanosis may follow.

**D**iagnostic Tests  Physical findings may be augmented by specific diagnostic tests in order to confirm the diagnosis and identify the factors altering cerebrovascular function.

A *lumbar puncture* is performed to determine whether the cerebrospinal fluid is clear or bloody and to obtain a pressure reading. This should be avoided in the presence of increased intracranial pressure. *Angiography* is usually done to demonstrate the site of occlusion, to determine whether surgery can be done, and to assess the presence of narrowed extracranial vessels (see Chap. 29 for a complete discussion of this test). A *brain scan* or *echogram* may be performed to demonstrate the site and size of a blood clot. In some cases an *electroencephalogram* (EEG) will be used to further determine the site of the occlusion. EEG readings reflect the changes through alteration in waves that are observed over the damaged area (refer to Chap. 31 for full discussion). An *EKG* may also be done to check for atrial fibrillation, ventricular hypertrophy, and other changes. *Skull x-rays* may be taken to reveal the location of a specific lesion.

**Nursing problems and interventions**  The major problems confronting the patient at this level include ventilation difficulties, changes in vital signs, hyperthermia, increased intracranial pressure, corneal abrasions, mood swings, immobility, nutritional problems, disruptions in elimination, and aphasia.

Goals of care for patients with cerebrovascular disorders (CVIs) include establishing and maintaining a patent airway, effective communication, and adequate cerebral blood flow and preventing skin breakdown and muscle and joint dysfunction. Rehabilitation should begin as early as possible.

**V**entilation Difficulties   Patients may experience respiratory difficulties as a result of an inability to change position, breathe deeply, or initiate the cough reflex. The patient should be placed in a lateral (unaffected side) or semiprone position with the bed flat. The prone or semiprone position is often avoided because of danger of increasing intracranial pressure, but it promotes gravitation of the tongue forward and facilitates drainage of secretions. Suctioning may be necessary to ensure a clear airway. If the patient is unable to remove the secretions, an endotracheal tube or a tracheostomy may be necessary. A room humidifier or nebulizer is often useful to prevent thickening of secretions. When appropriate, it is important to have the patient begin deep breathing and coughing to avoid the threat of pulmonary infection.

**C**hanges in Vital Signs   The *blood pressure, pulse,* and *respiratory rate* are monitored to ensure an adequate oxygen exchange. Patients who have had an elevated blood pressure for many years continue to need a higher blood pressure for perfusion. In the early phase of a CVI the blood pressure will remain elevated. Antihypertensive medications can be administered to *gradually* decrease the arterial pressure. Blood pressure should be monitored at frequent intervals to guard against a precipitous drop. Frequent monitoring of the vital signs also provides an evaluation of cardiac status. In some patients, the stroke may be the sequel to a myocardial infarction or atrial fibrillation, and the threat of pump failure must be carefully assessed. In addition, arrhythmias may be noted, especially in the presence of brainstem compression.

**H**yperthermia   The patient's temperature (rectal) should be checked frequently, as the body temperature will readily rise in the face of dysfunction of the thermoregulatory center. Patients with a more serious cerebrovascular problem—e.g., brainstem involvement—have an elevated temperature several days before death. Antipyretic preparations are not effective, and increase in fluids is discouraged, especially if increased intracranial pressure is suspected.

The patient can be placed on an electrically controlled cooling blanket. A rectal temperature probe is used to monitor the temperature. Vital signs are taken and a neurologic check made on a scheduled basis and compared with base-line measurements.

**I**ncreased Intracranial Pressure   After a cerebral hemorrhage the extravasate is space-occupying and therefore causes an *increase in intracranial* pressure. Brain tissue edema then adds to the increase in pressure. *Convulsions* are frequently associated with cerebral hemorrhage. In such cases, the patient is given anticonvulsant medication as needed to control attacks. A quiet, darkened environment will help reduce stimuli to the brain. The side rails can be padded to prevent injury. Suction equipment should be at the bedside and ready for use (see Chap. 33).

Careful attention should be paid to the patient's *level of consciousness.* Pupils should be checked frequently for size, equality, and reaction to light. In addition, the orientation to time, place, and environment should be continually evaluated. (A complete discussion of the levels of consciousness is found in Chaps. 32 and 35.) Frequent mouth care will be needed in the presence of coma.

Assessing cerebral functioning will give the nurse a more accurate indication of the severity of the infarction and the degree of damage present. Increased confusion, decreased perception of spatial surroundings, poor memory, inability to think logically, and hypoactivity offer significant cues about the patient's level of consciousness. The nurse should protect the patient from injury, remove objects from the environment that could be potentially harmful, and offer reassurance and support in a calm manner. Family members should also be supported during this period and encouraged to visit the patient frequently, so that they too can help orient the patient to the surroundings.

**C**orneal Abrasion   *Third-nerve palsy, absent corneal reflex,* and facial pain may be present. Patients with trigeminal nerve damage will be unable to close one eyelid. Diminished or absent corneal reflexes require that the eye be protected from corneal abrasion. The eyes should be cleansed daily and artificial tears instilled every 3 to 4 hours. Patients with third-nerve palsy usually experience diplopia and feel more comfortable with an eyepatch. Many patients experience photophobia and need a darkened, quiet environment.

**M**ood Swing   Patients who have had a stroke are subject to mood swings. They may be withdrawn and isolate themselves from others, especially if there are speech problems. They may cry or laugh inappropriately and may exhibit sexually inappropriate behavior. Regression to childhood states, with increased dependency, may also be noted. They are easily frustrated, and failure to achieve specific goals may excite wild, uncontrollable rage ending in loss of consciousness.

The nurse must treat the patient as normally as possible. Successes should be praised and inappropriate behavior pointed out when it seems reasonable to do so. These patients are often confused and frustrated and need support and patience to help them through a very difficult time. If depression ensues, the patient may require formal counseling in order to encourage a more optimistic outlook. Family members must be told of expected changes and be supported in their efforts to help the patient. Mild tranquilizers may be given. Restful environment is encouraged to decrease sensory stimulation and promote a relaxed state. These interventions will also help reduce restlessness and agitation.

For some patients, especially the aged, cerebral infarction can increase the cerebral anoxia that may already be present because of arteriosclerotic changes. Patients may become aggressive, hyperactive, extremely talkative, and delirious (especially at night) and may have difficulty sleeping. The nurse should remember that it is often difficult if not impossible for them to control their behavior. These changes, compounded by memory loss and perceptual difficulties, aggravate the problem. Patients must be protected from injury to themselves and others. Side rails should be in place and mild sedation used as needed. The use of restraints should be a last resort, as they tend to intensify behavioral problems. Patients will require much supervision, especially when eating food or drinking fluids. Often the presence of another person in the room helps decrease the patient's fears and relieves anxiety; a family member may be helpful in this regard. The patient should be kept in a quiet, nonstimulating environment. Soft lighting may be of help. The nurse must maintain a calm, nonthreatening manner with the patient, giving support and reassurance whenever possible.

**P**roblems of Immobility The amount of time a patient will have to spend on complete bed rest will depend on the physician's decision, the type of stroke, the degree of physical limitation, and whether or not cerebral hemorrhage is anticipated. Some patients will remain on bed rest for a few weeks, while others will be immobilized for months. Proper positioning is essential for all patients in order to maintain good body alignment, relieve pressure on bony prominences, and prevent contractures. Abrupt changes in position should be avoided, as they may place added stress on the system. When moving a patient with a stroke, assistance should be obtained in order to avoid undue strain for both patient and nurse. The patient may be maintained in a recumbent position and turned every 2 hours. It is recommended, however, that the patient lie on the affected side for only 20 minutes at a time, because of the increased vulnerability of the paralyzed area to skin breakdown due to decreased peripheral circulation and impaired cutaneous sensitivity.

The skin should be kept clean and free from perspiration and urine. Frequent skin care will help promote circulation and keep the skin dry. Cornstarch can be used to reduce both moisture and the friction incurred during repositioning. When the patient is in a lateral position, a pillow is often placed between the thighs to reduce skin contact and prevent subluxation of the hip joint.

A footboard covered with one layer of sheet or bath blanket should be adjusted to maintain the patient's feet at a 90° angle. The footboard will also help prevent foot drop, keep bedclothes from coming in direct contact with the skin, and provide a sense of pressure to the feet that will stimulate the antigravity muscles. The heels can also be protected with sheepskin. On occasion, a padded posterior splint is used to prevent plantar flexion.

After a stroke, the stronger adductor muscles favor the formation of *contractures*. There is a tendency for the fingers to form a fist and the arm to be drawn to the chest. Contractures can also distort the legs. A trochanter roll (or sandbag) may be placed along the affected leg from the hip to the knee to prevent outward rotation of the joints. Good alignment maintains the bones and muscles in positions of functional advantage. A pillow is used to maintain abduction and elevation of the affected arm, and a hand roll is used to maintain the hand in the position of function. Paralysis of the extremity muscles may cause cessation of the muscle pumping action and thereby affect venous and lymph return flow. Elevation of the extremity will reduce edema.

*Passive exercises* should be started as soon as possible in order to prevent disuse atrophy and loss of muscle strength and to maintain the normal range of joint motion. It is important to support the areas above and below the joint being moved and to avoid grasping the muscle at its belly.

Before beginning *ambulation* the patient needs

time to adjust to the upright position and to practice balancing. Getting out of bed should be progressive, occurring in steps. First the patient should utilize a tilt board for position change, progress to dangling the legs over the side of the bed, then stand for a short period with assistance, and finally begin walking, increasing the distance over time. At each of these steps the patient should be observed for changes in overall health status. When the patient is in the upright position, the affected arm should be supported in a sling (see Fig. 34-4). It is important that pressure be applied over the shoulder to prevent subluxation of the joint. The sling makes it easier for the patient to maintain balance when standing or ambulating. The affected arm should be removed from the sling at frequent intervals for range-of-motion exercises.

**N**utritional Problems  Patients with cerebral infarction may have a disruption in swallowing and an alteration of the gag reflex. Because of this, their nutritional needs are of concern. Fluids are admin-

istered intravenously for the first few days. Tube feedings (discussed in Chap. 16) are also used until the swallowing and gag reflexes return. If high-protein feedings are used, adequate amounts of water must be given to prevent the osmotic diuretic action of a heavy load of solute. Care must be taken to avoid rapid infusion of fluids, especially if increased intracranial pressure is suspected.

Since there is always a risk of aspiration when feeding a patient who has disruptions in swallowing, the nurse should carefully assess the return of the swallowing function before beginning oral feedings. The patient who is ready to take foods by mouth should be turned to the unaffected side. Then small amounts of soft food can be offered (some patients are able to manage soft foods sooner than liquids). Table 34-3 offers guidelines for feeding the dysphagic patient.

Because food tends to accumulate on the affected side, it is important that the patient have mouth care immediately after eating. If toothbrush and toothpaste are not available, *mouth care* can be

**FIGURE 34-4**
Use of the sling. (*From U.S. Department of HEW, Chronic Disease Program, Public Health Service: Strike Back at Stroke, p. 33.*)

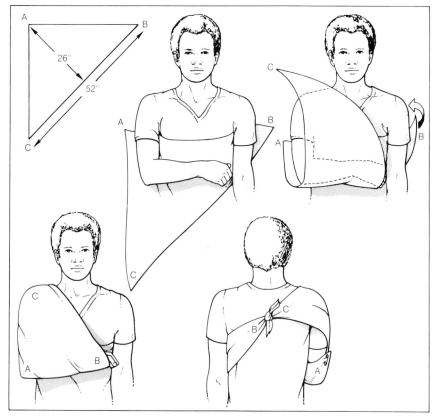

given with glyoxide or an absorbent solution. The lips should then be lubricated to prevent cracking and cold sores.

**D**isruptions in Elimination   Bowel and bladder dysfunction may accompany the cerebral infarction, but the effects may be temporary. Urinary incontinence is a common problem and may necessitate the use of a urinary catheter, although there is some controversy over the use of urinary catheters, since they can lead to bladder infections. Depending on the physician's decision and the age of the patient, catheterization may be used only in those patients who are unconscious or in a coma.

In an attempt to limit urinary incontinence, the patient should be placed on a bedpan or offered a urinal every 2 hours over a 24-hour period. Bladder retraining (discussed in Chapter 32) involves the regulation of fluid intake as well as the emptying of the bladder at planned intervals. Fluid intake should be decreased in the evening to prevent incontinence during the night.

Constipation and fecal impaction are more frequently observed after a CVI than bowel incontinence. Constipation can be prevented by adequate intake of fluids and the use of stool softeners or mild cathartics. Bisacodyl (Dulcolax) suppositories may also be used as needed. The patient should be instructed to avoid straining during the bowel movement, as this could increase systemic arterial pressure and lead to rupture of a cerebral vessel.[26]

**A**phasia   One of the biggest problems confronting both nurse and patient following a stroke is *communication difficulty.* Speech problems can take a long time to improve. The greatest change usually occurs during the first 6 months. Unless aphasic stroke patients begin to recover during the first few weeks, they will probably not regain normal use of language.[27]

The patient experiencing aphasia may have either a sensory (receptive) aphasia or a motor (expressive) aphasia. Most often patients will have both sensory and motor components affected. Both forms of aphasia are frightening to the patient and will increase anxiety.

*Speech therapy* is frequently ordered early in the stroke period and may continue after hospitalization. However, it is helpful if the patient has some control over breathing and lip and tongue movements before therapy begins. It is not uncommon for the patient to become frustrated or angry over these incapacities and to shout obscenities or profanity at family members and care givers. The family needs to know that this is a form of *automatic speech* and therefore, understandably, the patient's early expression. The nurse will need to be supportive and encouraging to the patient during therapy sessions and attempt to follow through with activities practiced during therapy.

Patients with sensory aphasia can follow simple verbal commands and gestures. They should be spoken to slowly, with directions repeated as needed. Patients with motor aphasia may not attempt sounds but will use gestures. The nurse must be patient in attempting to understand the patient's message and beginning to anticipate the meaning of certain gestures. Patients should be asked questions that will require only simple answers, so that they will not become frustrated by the experience.

Families must be taught to continue the speech rehabilitation begun in the hospital. They need to be encouraged to work with the speech therapist and the nurse in order to carry on effective communication at home. Family members should be taught to speak softly and slowly to the patient and to use simple words and phrases. The use of gestures may

---

**TABLE 34-3**
GUIDELINES FOR FEEDING A DYSPHAGIC PATIENT

SUGGESTIONS CONCERNING FOODS
Milk and milk products stimulate thick saliva that is difficult to swallow. They should be avoided.

Foods with some texture stimulate swallowing. Use toast instead of plain bread, boiled or baked potato instead of mashed potato.

Avoid difficult-to-swallow foods such as plums, prunes, hamburger patties; consistency of the food depends on tolerance of the patient.

SUGGESTIONS FOR FEEDING THE PATIENT
Help the patient sit upright ½ h before and after feeding.

If the patient is hemiplegic, place food in the unaffected side of the mouth.

Instruct the patient to move the food around with the tongue.

In the initial stages, small amounts of food should be fed, with a gradual increase as the patient's ability to swallow increases.

Have the patient feel the laryngeal area during the act of swallowing. This demonstrates that he or she can swallow; often patients are afraid they cannot.

Keep the environment quiet while the patient is eating.

Give liquids through a straw if the patient can suck.

Keep a daily chart of the amount and consistency of liquids and solid food the patient takes.

Prepared by John E. Buckley, M.A., CCC, Sp-A, Director of Speech and Audiology, Overlook Hospital, Summit, N.J. and Clinical Instructor, College of Medicine, State University of New York, Downstate Medical Center and Connie L. Addicks, M.A., CCC, Senior Speech Pathologist, Overlook Hospital, Summit, N.J.

also be helpful, as some patients will continue to communicate in this way after discharge. Since patients who sustain a cerebral infarction are often middle-aged or older, they should not be spoken to as if they were children. Correcting them for incorrect or inappropriate speech should be done supportively. The process of speech rehabilitation is a slow one, and progress is often accompanied by much frustration. All evidence of progress should be recognized and praised.

**A**gnosia   Left-sided hemiplegics may be prone to altered spatial perceptions. Their speech may be comprehensive, but they lack awareness of the positioning of body parts and will say they can participate in activities that they cannot handle. Slow verbal communication may help.

Patients with *agnosia* have an inability to comprehend the import of sensations such as touch and hearing. Patients with visual problems should be encouraged to use glasses. Hearing aids may be used, especially if auditory problems existed prior to the stroke. Again, simple instructions and slow activity help patients feel more in control; decreased frustration and anxiety gives them time to organize their thoughts. The nurse should make the patient more aware of the affected side of the body by placing objects and food on the opposite side and helping the patient with self-care to the ignored side. Forcing the patient to turn the head to the affected direction will encourage awareness of the ignored environment. The nurse should be continually observant of patients' movements and protect them from injury by harmful objects.

**T**hromboembolism   Thromboembolism is a constant threat after a cerebral infarct. The use of anticoagulants is controversial, and they are used only when the cerebral infarction is due to a thrombus or embolus. When anticoagulants are administered, heparin is usually given initially, followed by Coumadin (refer to Chap. 29 for complete discussion of anticoagulants). A Coumadin *anticoagulant protocol* requires a large initial dose in order to achieve a rapid therapeutic effect. The initial dose is usually given in divided doses over a period of 2 days. A maintenance dose is then determined on an individual basis. Prothrombin times are determined daily early in the therapeutic period in order to make necessary dose adjustments.

It is usual for patients who are on anticoagulant therapy to have other medications prescribed, so drug reactions are to be expected. Careful instructions must be given to patients regarding the effects of such medications as salicylates and Seconal on prothrombin activity. The nurse needs to be alert for signs of bruising and bleeding. Persantine (25 to 50 mg twice or three times a day) and aspirin may also be used in combination for their anticoagulation effect, but the results are controversial.

*Fibrinolysins* may be used to help dissolve thrombi and emboli; urokinase, which is extracted from human urine, is one fibrolysin now being evaluated[28] (refer to Chap. 29 for complete discussion).

**S**urgical Intervention   The purpose of surgical intervention in cerebral infarction is to restore adequate circulation to the brain. This is accomplished most frequently by removal of a clot or thrombus from a carotid or other cerebral artery or reconstruction of a damaged artery. An *endarterectomy* is performed when an obstructive lesion is present within the extracranial vessels (common carotid or vertebral arteries). The method involves bypassing the occluded cerebral arteries. A new blood supply is created by using scalp arteries, in microsurgical procedures, as bypasses from the carotid or vertebral vessels to cerebral arteries (Fig. 34-5).

When surgery is prescribed, nursing interventions used for patients having brain surgery are followed (see Chap. 35), with attention paid to patency of the airway, stability of the vital signs, positioning of the neck to prevent kinking of the vessels, observation for bleeding and edema, and prevention of hematoma.

In cerebral hemorrhage due to aneurysm, the patient who is to have surgery usually receives an intravenous *hyperosmolar solution* (urea, mannitol) in order to reduce the volume of fluid in brain tissue. *Hypothermia* also reduces cerebral edema and lowers the rate of cerebral metabolism. This makes it somewhat safer to temporarily occlude the cerebral vessel supplying the aneurysm. Aneurysms that have a long neck are occluded with a silver clip, while those with a broad base are wrapped with muscle or fascia or coated with a plastic material. Other aneurysms are trapped with clips. Surgery may also involve the evacuation of a blood clot. Certain aneurysms of the internal carotid artery are treated with progressive occlusion of the carotid vessel with a Selverstone or Poppen clamp. Within the last decade surgery has been performed more frequently because of the high mortality associated with conservative treatment and the incidence of recurrent hemorrhage. Following surgery, vital and neurologic signs are monitored at frequent intervals to detect indications of brainstem compression and herniation caused by rupture. Hyperosmolar preparations are again administered intravenously to reduce cerebral edema.

## Fourth-level Nursing Care

The recovery period which follows a cerebrovascular infarction is often long, involving extensive rehabilitation. About half the victims who survive a stroke have little or no disability. Out of every 1000 persons who survive a stroke for one month, 100 emerge unimpaired, 400 have residual disability, 400 more require specialized care, and 100 need to be institutionalized.[29] If patients do not completely recover by the fourth week following the cerebral infarct, it may take up to 6 or 7 months of rehabilitation before they can begin to function independently.[30] As the recovery period begins, the patient soon becomes conscious of the physical changes that have occurred. These limitations may be frightening to those who view the changes as a temporary or permanent loss of independence. The impact of impaired bodily functions may be profound and result in withdrawal or depression. For older patients the problem is compounded as they see themselves as no longer being in control of their lives and fear becoming a burden on the family. Loss of speech and disruption of thought processes can increase the frustration.

The patient must be helped to deal with these changes, for they are real and must be faced constructively if rehabilitation efforts are to be successful. Continued affection and support are needed from family members, and the patient must be treated as an individual with personal rights despite difficulty in expressing feelings.

The general goals of care should revolve around maintaining the present level of function, promoting effective communication, improving coordination, preventing bone contractures, restoring impaired bodily functions, and improving the overall quality of life by helping the patient regain optimal health status.

**Health teaching** Teaching of the family members as well as the patient continues to be an integral part of the rehabilitative process. For the patient who is able to return home, many limitations are yet to be overcome. The nurse and the patient should begin to plan for discharge as soon as the health status stabilizes. All teaching plans should be modified according to the patient's level of responsiveness and ability to learn. Allowing patients to participate in teaching activities may offer them

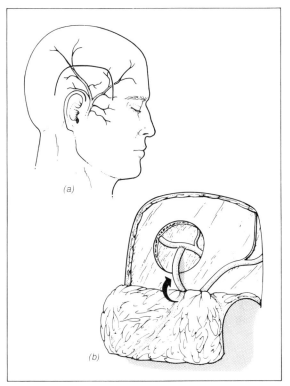

**FIGURE 34-5**
Cerebral artery bypass. (*From Martin S. Bander (ed.): MGH News,* **35,** *Massachusetts General Hospital, Boston, June–August 1976, p. 3. Used with permission.*)

some control over the environmental constraints they are facing.

Range-of-motion joint exercises should be performed at least three times a day as tolerated. The patient and family should be taught to begin exercising the unaffected side first. This will give the nurse an opportunity to observe the actual range of joint motion. The patient can be taught to massage the affected hand and arm with the unaffected hand and should also learn to rest the affected arm and hand on a flat surface and extend the fingers and wrist rhythmically. A small ball or piece of cotton can be placed in the patient's hand to squeeze, which will strengthen the hand muscles. Exercising the unaffected side may result in some transfer of energy to the affected side and increase the action potential of the affected muscles.

Before the patient begins to ambulate, sturdy, supportive shoes that will improve balance and gait are required. A certain degree of spasticity in the lower extremities helps with ambulation. When the patient gets out of bed, the nurse should support the unaffected side, since that is the side used for balance. It is important to have the patient ambulate for 5 to 10 minutes every 2 hours, because reeducation is enhanced by repetition. Each small success should be greeted with encouragement.

The occupational therapist and physical therapist can suggest an increasing scope of activities according to the patient's muscle tone and degree of progress and can advise concerning splints, walkers, wheelchairs, and other support devices (see Chap. 40). In most hospitals and long-term care facilities it is the occupational therapist who teaches the patient to bathe and dress. The therapist can provide the patient with self-help devices for eating. Being able to dress in one's own clothes increases one's self-esteem. The patient using a bedside commode or the toilet seems to have fewer problems with elimination. At night, male patients may be more comfortable wearing a condom drainage catheter to decrease the chance of incontinence.

Speech therapy will continue to be an important component of rehabilitation. Establishing effective communication between the patient and the family members often remains a major problem, but through encouragement and patience the patient can be helped to overcome this problem.

Before discharge, the nurse, working with the family, needs to assess immediate resources and identify the need for supplemental assistance in the community. A home visit is advantageous, and the inclusion of a homemaker in discharge planning may be an asset in helping the patient and family cope. The patient and family must participate in planning if the plan is to succeed. Personal and individual goals must become part of the plan so that an optimal health state can be restored.

Family members need support in their effort to help patients with retraining. It is important that family members not be impatient, or patients will feel themselves a burden. Both patient and family members need to have a realistic idea of the patient's level of ability so that the family will not expect more than is reasonable. On the other hand, the patient will need encouragement to continue with activities and to remain as self-sufficient as possible.

The need for intimacy and love continues all through life. Sex and sexuality continue to provide psychologic and physiologic outlets. Sexual activity may cease because of the impaired physical functions and sensorimotor disturbances resulting from the cerebral infarction. Both the disabled person and the partner may need information or counseling.

As the residual effects of the cerebrovascular disturbance begin to diminish and perception and coordination return, the patient's primary health problem—be it hypertension, heart disease, or diabetes mellitus—must not be overlooked. Careful health assessment and planned counseling are essential. Encouragement and support to continue such measures as medications, diet restrictions, and abstinence from smoking are critical. The patient and family should have a schedule for the taking of medication. It is important that the patient keep appointments to have health status checked. Careful management of the patient's primary health problem may prevent another stroke.

## REFERENCES

1  Maxwell M. Wintrobe et al. (eds.), *Harrison's Principles of Internal Medicine,* 7th ed., McGraw-Hill, New York, 1974, p. 1832.
2  Stanley L. Robbins and Marcia Angell, *Basic Pathology,* 2d ed., Saunders, Philadelphia, 1976, p. 642.
3  Ibid., pp. 639–640.
4  A. Vick Nicholas, *Grinker's Neurology,* 7th ed., Charles C Thomas, Springfield, Ill., 1976, pp. 650–652.
5  Robbins and Angell, loc. cit. p. 641.
6  Wintrobe et al., op. cit., p. 1836.
7  Robbins and Angell, op. cit., p. 227.
8  Wintrobe et al., op. cit., pp. 1837–1838.
9  Nicholas, loc. cit., pp. 650–652.
10  Wintrobe et al., op. cit., p. 1774.
11  Joseph G. Chusid, *Correlative Neuroanatomy and Functional Neurology,* 15th ed., Lange, Los Altos, Calif., 1973, pp. 34–35.
12  Robbins and Angell, op. cit., p 649.
13  Ibid., p. 641.
14  Wintrobe et al., op. cit., pp. 1849–1850.
15  J. Luckman and K. Sorensen, *Medical-Surgical Nursing: A Pathophysiologic Approach,* Saunders, Philadelphia, 1974, p. 437.
16  Wintrobe et al., op. cit., p. 1856.
17  Ibid., p. 1856.
18  Ibid., p. 1856.
19  Ibid., p. 1774.
20  Ibid., p. 1790.
21  Nicholas, op. cit., pp. 393–394.
22  John H. Dingle, "The Ills of Man," *Sci Am,* **229:** 74–84, September 1973, p. 82.
23  Martin Bander, *MCH News,* **35:**1, June–August 1976.
24  Wintrobe et al., p. 184.
25  Ibid., p. 1775.

26  John R. Brobeck (ed.), *Best and Taylor's Physiological Basis of Medical Practice,* 9th ed., Williams & Wilkins, Baltimore, 1973, pp. 6–38.

27  Joan Richl and Jacqueline Chambers, "Better Salvage for the Stroke Victim," *Nurs '76,* **6**(7):29, July 1976.

28  Frederick Meyers, Ernest Jawetz, and Alan Goldfien, *Review of Medical Pharmacology,* 4th ed., Lange, Los Altos, Calif., 1974, p. 174.

29  Richl and Chambers, op. cit., p. 29

30  Ibid., p. 30.

## BIBLIOGRAPHY

Bannister, Roger: *Brain's Clinical Neurology,* 4th ed., Oxford University Press, New York, 1973.

Blount, Mary, and Anna Belle Kinney: "Neurologic and Neurosurgical Nursing," *Nurs Clin North Am,* **9**:4, December 1974.

Bouvette, Jeanne Marie: "Preoperative and Postoperative Care of Patients with Cerebral Aneurysms," *Nurs Clin North Am,* **9**:655–666, December 1974.

Bruya, Margaret Auld, and Rose Homan Bolin: "Epilepsy: A Controllable Disease," *Am J Nurs,* **76**(3): 388–397, March 1976.

Brunner, Lillian Sholtis, and Doris Smith Suddarth: *Textbook of Medical-Surgical Nursing,* 3d ed., Lippincott, Philadelphia, 1975.

Burnside, Irene Mortenson: "Listen to the Aged," *Am J Nurs,* **75**:1800–1803, October 1975.

——— (ed.), *Nursing and the Aged,* McGraw-Hill, New York, 1976.

Crouch, James E.: *Functional Human Anatomy,* 2d ed., Lea & Febiger, Philadelphia, 1972.

Granger, Carl V., et al.: "Measurement of Outcomes of Care for Stroke Patients," *Stroke,* **6**:34–41, January–February 1975.

Guyton, Arthur C.: *Textbook of Medical Physiology,* 5th ed., Saunders, Philadelphia, 1973.

Hinkhouse, Ann: "Craniocerebral Trauma," *Am J Nurs,* **73**(10):1719–1722, October 1973.

Hutchinson, E. C. and E. J. Acheson: *Strokes: Natural History, Pathology and Surgical Treatment,* Saunders, Philadelphia, 1975.

Keller, Margaret R., and B. Lionel Truscott: "Transient Ischemic Attacks," *Am J Nurs,* **73**:1331, August 1973.

Kurtzke, John F.: *Epidemiology of Cerebrovascular Disease,* Springer-Verlag, Heidelberg, 1969, p. 49.

Kuo, Peter T.: "Hyperlipidemia and Coronary Artery Disease," *Med Clin North Am,* **14**:351–362, March 1974.

Langley, L. L., Ira R. Telford, and John B. Christensen: *Dynamic Anatomy and Physiology,* 4th ed., McGraw-Hill, New York, 1974.

McCartney, Virginia C.: "Rehabilitation and Dignity and the Stroke Patient," *Nurs Clin North Am,* **9**: 693–701, December 1974.

Marshall, Carter L., and David Pearson: *Dynamics of Health and Disease,* Appleton-Century-Crofts, New York, 1972.

Mitchell, Helen S., et al.: *Nutrition in Health and Disease,* 6th ed., Lippincott, Philadelphia, 1976.

Mitchell, Pamela H., and Nancy Mauss: "Intracranial Pressure: Fact and Fancy," *Nurs '76,* **6**(6):53–57, June 1976.

Moidel, Harriet Coston, Elizabeth C. Giblin, and Bernice M. Wagner: *Nursing Care of the Patient with Medical-Surgical Disorders,* 2d ed., McGraw-Hill, New York, 1976.

Norsworthy, Edith: "Nursing Rehabilitation after Severe Head Trauma," *Am J Nurs,* **74**(7):1246–1250, July 1974.

Patton, Harry D., et al.: *Introduction to Basic Neurology,* Saunders, Philadelphia, 1976, p. 378.

Plum, Fred, and Jerome B. Posner: *The Diagnosis of Stupor and Coma,* 2d ed., Davis, Philadelphia, 1972.

Rudy, Ellen: "Early Omens of Cerebral Disaster," *Nurs '77,* **7**(2):58–62, February 1977.

Whisnant, Jack P.: "Epidemiology of Stroke: Emphasis on Transient Cerebral Ischemic Attacks and Hypertension," *Stroke,* **5**:68–70, January–February 1974, p. 68.

# 35
# NEOPLASTIC DISTURBANCES IN PERCEPTION AND COORDINATION

Ann Hall Harvey*

It ought to be generally known that the source of our pleasure, merriment, laughter, and amusement, as of our grief, pain, anxiety, and tears, is none other than the brain. It is specially the organ which enables us to think, see, and hear, and to distinguish the ugly and the beautiful, the bad and the good, pleasant and unpleasant. Sometimes we judge according to the perceptions of expediency. It is the brain, too, which is the seat of madness and delirium, of the fears and frights which assail us, often by night, but sometimes even by day; it is there where lies the cause of insomnia and sleep-walking, of thoughts that will not come, forgotten duties, and eccentricities. All such things result from an unhealthy condition of the brain.

Hippocrates

These words of Hippocrates describe vividly the role the nervous system plays in enabling human beings to interact with both the internal and external environments. Neoplastic disruptions in nervous system integrity can profoundly disturb this interaction. Neoplastic lesions of the central nervous system may be *primary* benign or malignant tumors of the brain and spinal cord or *metastatic* lesions affecting the brain and/or spinal cord from systemic cancer. This chapter will discuss the effects of such lesions and the nursing care of patients who possess them.

## BRAIN TUMORS

The embryological development of the human nervous system is a combination of processes of multiplication and differentiation of cells of the neural tube and neural crest. The epithelial cells of the neural tube produce and differentiate into nerve cells (neurons) and neuroglial cells. In the early phases, medulloblasts give rise to neuroblasts and spongioblasts. The neuroblasts mature to become neurons; the spongioblasts are prototypes of astrocytes and oligodendrocytes (neuroglial tissue). The neural crest gives rise to neuroblasts which become spinal ganglion cells and sympathetic ganglion cells (Fig. 35-1).[1,2]

### Pathophysiology

The cells of brain tumors have certain characteristics of embryonic or parent cells. Subsequently, the different types of tumors derive their names from mature glial cells, as an astrocytoma or oligodentrocytoma, or from primitive cells of the embryonic brain, for example, medulloblastoma and spongioblastoma.[3]

Tumors may be located either within or outside brain parenchyma, i.e., intraaxial or extraaxial in location. *Primary brain tumors,* benign or malignant, originate in:

1 The brain's supportive (glial) tissue

2 Coverings of the brain (meninges)

3 Glands and adjacent structures within the brain

4 Cranial nerves

5 Blood vessels within the brain

* The author wishes to express appreciation to Mrs. Louise Schudoma Hall.

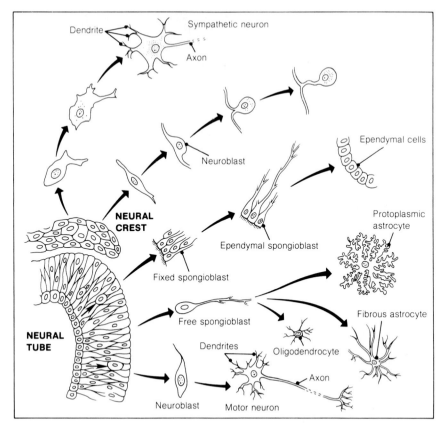

**FIGURE 35-1**

Embryological development of the nervous system. (*After H. Tuckmann-Duplessis et al., Illustrated Human Embryology, vol. III, Nervous System and Endocrine Glands, Springer-Verlag, New York, 1974, p. 10.*)

**Classification** Table 35-1 classifies primary brain tumors as to their type and location. Brain dysfunction is generally greatest in rapidly growing, infiltrative intraaxial tumors, e.g., glioblastoma, owing to marked infiltration, compression, and

**TABLE 35-1**
PRIMARY TUMORS OF THE BRAIN

| Type of Tumor | Usual Site |
| --- | --- |
| Gliomas: | |
| Glioblastoma (multiforme) | Cerebral hemisphere |
| Astrocytoma, cerebral | Cerebral hemisphere |
| Astrocytoma, cerebellar | Cerebellar hemisphere |
| Medulloblastoma | Cerebellar vermis |
| Ependymoma | Ventricles |
| Spongioblastoma | Brainstem |
| Oligodendroma | Frontal and temporal lobes |
| Meningioma | Supratentorial |
| Pituitary adenoma | Hypophyseal fossa |
| Acoustic neurinoma | Cerebellopontine angle |
| Craniopharyngioma | Suprasellar |
| Hemangioblastoma | Cerebellar |

SOURCE: From A. E. Walker, "Diseases of the Nervous System," in P. Beeson and W. McDermott (eds.), *Cecil-Loeb Textbook of Medicine*, 11th ed., Saunders, Philadelphia, 1963, p. 1678.

necrosis of brain tissue. An extraaxial tumor, e.g., meningioma, may slowly compress the brain tissue, reaching a great size with few clinical manifestations.[4]

Secondary tumors affecting the brain are those which invade the intracranial cavity through metastasis from a primary malignant site elsewhere in the body. Melanoma has a greater than 75 percent chance of metastasizing to the brain, while lung, breast, kidney, thyroid, head, and neck tumors metastasize to the brain in 25 to 50 percent of patients.[5]

Figure 35-2 illustrates the anatomical relationship of the different types of brain tumors. Most tumors in adults are located supratentorially.[6]

Brain tumor cells may not be homogeneous and may change their characteristics over time. The greater the degree of *anaplasia* (a loss of differentiation of cells and of their orientation to one another), the greater the degree of malignancy histologically.[7] On the basis of histological examination, brain tumors have been graded from a benign grade I type with a favorable prognosis to the malignant grade IV type with limited survival time.[8] The "clinical" malignancy of intracerebral tumors, i.e., the final outcome of an expanding lesion, is determined by the grade of "histological" malignancy *plus* the following factors:

1   Growth and enlargement configuration

2   Movement with herniation

3   Action upon cerebrospinal fluid pathways

4   Action on arteries

5   Action on vital centers[9]

**Effects on the patient**   The clinical manifestations of brain tumors are diverse and vary greatly according to the type and location. The onset of signs and symptoms may be insidious or acute.

Because an expanding lesion is contained in a rigid skull, its presence is manifested before a lesion of the same size elsewhere in the body. A metastatic lesion to the brain may be the first sign of systemic cancer.

Intracranial tumors give rise to *focal (localized) dysfunction* in the brain and to *increased intracranial pressure. Focal* manifestations occur because (1) brain tissue is compressed or infiltrated by tumor and (2) blood supply to localized tissue is compromised, resulting in (3) necrosis and cerebral edema.[10] *Focal* disturbances in function include: focal seizures, aphasia, hemiparesis, ataxia, disturbances of visual acuity, visual field defects, and cranial nerve involvement. Table 35-2 elaborates the types of clinical manifestations in relation to the location of the tumor. *Generalized* manifestations may also be encountered including signs and symptoms of increased intracranial pressure (headache, vomiting, papilledema, bradycardia, and alterations in mentation leading to coma) or generalized convulsions.

*Supratentorial* masses are more likely to present focal neurological signs. *Infratentorial,* midline masses, usually present signs and symptoms of increased intracranial pressure.[11]

## Theories of Causation

Numerous hypotheses have been formulated in an attempt to define the basic mechanism of cancer and its relationship to the nervous system. Naturally occurring and experimentally induced nervous system tumors are being studied in relation to the following theories in oncology: (1) The somatic mutation theory of cancer and the additive mutagenic action of radiation and alkylating carcinogens;

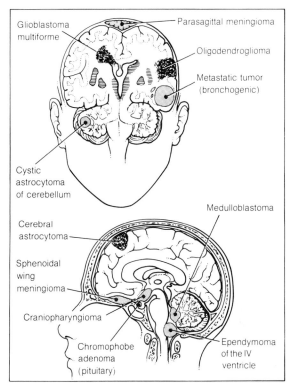

**FIGURE 35-2**
The anatomical relationship of the different types of brain tumors. (*After Helena Kryk et al., "Grand Rounds on Brain Tumors," Can Nurse, September 1975, p. 43.*)

(2) the viral theory of cancer and the production of tumors by oncogenic viruses; (3) disturbances of immunological mechanisms concerned with tumor surveillance involving the central nervous system; and (4) the operation of epigenetic mechanisms in neoplastic systems, the applicability of these mechanisms to embryonal tumors of the central nervous system, and the development of suitable neural neoplastic models for the study of altered patterns of gene expression.[12]

The nature of the vasculature of tumors remains one of the most intriguing mysteries in the field of oncology. Vessel components represent a significant part of tumor bulk as is well illustrated in the glioblastoma multiforme, one of the most vascular of all neoplasms. The electron microscope has facilitated investigations of the tumor-vascular relationship. New information has been obtained through studies of angiogenesis, endothelial proliferation, the permeability properties of tumor vessels, and the morphology of central nervous system capillaries.[13]

### First-Level Nursing Care

Brain tumors have their peak incidence in adults in the fifth and sixth decades in life.[14] Table 35-3 illustrates the incidence of primary and secondary brain tumors. Gliomas compose about 50 percent of all brain tumors, followed in frequency by meningiomas and metastatic tumors.

While there has been much study, no conclusion has been reached about the causation of nervous system tumors. Neither environmental, cultural, nor endogenous racial characteristics appear to have influenced their frequency and distribution.

Inheritance, however, is known to be a causal factor in the development of certain tumors of the nervous system. Tumors (blastomatoses) which have a genetic or familial expression are von Recklinghausen's neurofibromatosis, Bourneville's tuberous sclerosis, von Hipple–Lindau syndrome, and Sturge-Weber syndrome.[15]

Other than genetic counseling, *preventive intervention* for brain tumors is not possible. What is realistic, however, is the early detection and diagnosis of neoplastic disease outside the central nervous system in an effort to prevent metastasis to the brain. For example, yearly gynecological examinations for women should be encouraged since metastatic brain tumors develop from primary lesions of the breast; in addition, all females should be instructed in self-examination of the breast. Yearly physical examination including chest x-ray is also recommended since cord and brain tumors develop from metastatic lesions of the lungs.

### Second-Level Nursing Care

Early detection of tumors of the brain is vital to effective intervention. Frequently, nurses in community settings are the first professionals to see and assess patients with symptoms that reflect the presence of these neoplasms. Even subtle changes in perception and coordination can be indicative of major lesions.

Important early symptoms of intracranial neoplasms that may be revealed during the *health history* include: headache, progressive paralysis, focal or generalized convulsions which have their onset in adult life, failing vision, and mental and personality changes. *Headache* may result from anxiety and depression and is often the first symptom of a brain tumor.[16] Headache associated with a brain tumor is often deep, aching, and dull in nature. It is usually intermittent and of a moderate intensity; i.e., it may diminish in intensity with acetylsalicylic acid or cold compresses applied to the scalp. If there is a variation in intensity during the 24-hour period, it is usually more intense in the early morning.[17] Wolff has described the mechanism of the brain-tumor headache in the following manner:

**TABLE 35-2**
INTRACRANIAL NEOPLASMS

| Location | Usual Clinical Manifestations |
|---|---|
| Cerebrum | Generalized convulsion<br>Increased intracranial pressure |
| Frontal lobe | Changes in personality, behavior<br>Defects in mentation<br>Hemiparesis<br>Aphasia (dominant hemisphere)<br>Focal motor seizures |
| Parietal lobe | Hemisensory impairment<br>Inferior quadrantic hemianopsia<br>Focal sensory seizures |
| Temporal lobe | Defects in memory<br>Nominal aphasia (dominant hemisphere)<br>Superior quadrantic hemianopsia<br>Psychomotor seizures, aura gustatory, déjà vu, and other visual images |
| Occipital lobe | Homonymous hemianopsia<br>Seizures, aura flashes of light |
| Cerebellum | Increased intracranial pressure<br>Ataxia, nystagmus, dysmetria<br>Unsteady gait |
| Brainstem | Hemiparesis<br>Nystagmus<br>Facial paresis<br>Vomiting |
| Pituitary (in relation to sella turcica) | |
|    Intrasellar | Endocrine<br>  Hyperpituitarism |
|    Intra- and extrasellar | Endocrine<br>  Hyperpituitarism<br>  Hypopituitarism<br><br>Optic nerve<br>  Optic atrophy<br>  Decreased visual acuity<br><br>Optic chiasm<br>  Peripheral visual field defects, especially bitemporal hemianopsia<br><br>Hypothalamus<br>  Somnolence, diabetes insipidus<br>  Adiposity<br>  Sexual dystrophy |
| Cranial nerves | Dizziness, vertigo<br>Neurogenic hearing deficit<br>Depressed vestibular response<br>Pain and sensory deficits in trigeminal distribution<br>Depressed corneal reflex<br>Peripheral facial palsy<br>Cerebellar ataxia |

SOURCE: From Guy McKhann, "Mass Lesions," in A. McGehee Harvey et al. (eds.), *The Principles and Practices of Medicine,* 19th ed., Appleton-Century-Crofts, New York, 1976, pp. 1553–1554.

Brain-tumor headache is produced by traction upon and displacement of intracranial pain-sensitive structures, chiefly the large arteries, veins and venous sinuses, and certain cranial nerves. There are two types of traction, which operate singly or in combination: local traction by the tumors upon adjacent structures; and distant traction by extensive displacement of the brain, either directly by the tumor, or indirectly by ventricular obstruction (internal hydrocephalus). Brain tumor may in addition press directly upon cranial nerves.[18]

Data should be collected on the frequency, intensity, and duration of the headache, as well as those measures that have brought the patient relief.

*Seizures* may be the first and only signs the patient with a brain tumor experiences. In patients with seizures developing in adulthood, the possibility of a mass lesion is great. Focal seizures occur as the initial manifestation in 30 to 50 percent of patients.[19] They may be motor, sensory, or both (see Chap. 33). The focal abnormal, excessive neuronal discharges may spread to adjacent tissue, thus causing generalized convulsions.[20] The nature, duration, and frequency of these seizures should be described.

*Mental and personality changes* are manifested differently in patients owing to the time over which the lesion develops, the nature of the lesion (i.e., infiltrative, destructive, or pressure effect), and its location.[21] Much of the information in this area may have to be obtained from a knowledgeable family member. Disorders of mental functioning occur in 60 to 90 percent of patients in which the cerebral tumors involve the frontal lobes.[22] (Tumors of the frontal lobes may be associated with *personality changes, alterations in motor activity,* and *impairment of cognitive functions.*)[23]

Two types of *personality changes* occurring with frontal-lobe lesions have been described: (1) *Apathy* and *indifference* ("pseudodepressed") and (2) *puerility* and *euphoria* ("pseudopsychopathic").[24] Combinations of the two types are more common than the pure form. In the first type the patient appears to have lost all initiative. Responses are usually automatic. The patient does not initiate activities of daily living but follows directions. There is an indifference or lack of concern about the present or future. Slowness and apathy overshadow a near-normal intellect. These changes appear to result from destructive pathology affecting the prefrontal convexity, subcortical centers (basal ganglions and thalamus), and their connections.[25,26]

The second type, or pseudopsychopathic be-

havior, is characterized by the lack of adult tact and restraints. The behavior may be described as coarse, facetious, hyperkinetic, or promiscuous. Such patients often lack social graces and may commit antisocial acts. Erotic behavior, sexual exhibitionism, or lewd remarks may occur. Outbursts of anger or irritability are common and may be the first behavioral change noted. These behaviors are thought to follow injury to the orbital frontal lobe or pathways transversing this region.[27,28]

Personality changes can occur following the onset of temporal-lobe seizures resulting from tumors. The manifestations have been described as follows: "While sexual arousal and response tend to be reduced, there is often a profound deepening of emotional responses. This deepening includes penting up and episodic discharge of anger and rage on the one hand, and intensification of ethical-religious feelings on the other."[29]

*Alterations in motor activity* are also characterized by lack of initiative and spontaneity. There is a general diminution of motor activity. The patient no longer voluntarily gets out of bed in the morning, bathes or feeds self, dresses, urinates or defecates in the toilet. These latter activities may be carried out at any time or place.[30]

**Physical assessment** A complete *neurological examination* should be performed whenever brain

**TABLE 35-3**
INCIDENCE OF TYPES OF BRAIN TUMORS

| Type | Percent* |
|---|---|
| Glioma | 43 |
|    Glioblastoma multiforme | 23 |
|    Astrocytoma | 13 |
|    Ependymoma | 1.8 |
|    Oligodendroglioma | 1.6 |
|    Mixed and other | 1.9 |
|    Medulloblastoma | 1.5 |
| Meningioma | 16 |
| Pituitary adenoma | 8.2 |
| Neurilemoma | 5.7 |
| Craniopharyngioma | 2.8 |
| Sarcoma | 2.5 |
| Hemangioblastoma | 2.7 |
| Pineal tumor | 1.1 |
| Metastatic | 13.0 |
| Other | 6.0 |

* Number of brain tumors studied = 17,580.
SOURCE: From Michael Walker, "Brain and Peripheral Nervous System Tumors," in James F. Holland and Emil Frei III (eds.), *Cancer Medicine,* Lea & Febiger, Philadelphia, 1973, p. 1388.

neoplasms are suspected. Findings are often helpful in identifying alterations in normal function that may aid in localizing the lesion. (Refer to Chap. 31 for a review of the components of the neurological examination.)

Sensory testing should be performed, bilaterally, on all skin surfaces. Impaired sensation to pain, temperature, or light touch may precede deficits in vibration and position sense. Sensory loss may progress to complete anesthesia at a distinct dermatome level.

Assessment of motor function focuses upon changes in reflexes, strength, and coordination. The equality of each of these muscle functions is important to note.

*Confrontation testing* for visual fields utilizes readily available test objects such as pencils, straws, or fingers (see Chap. 31). The basic principle is to bring the test object from an area outside the patient's visual field toward the patient's visual field as in Fig. 35-3. Close observation of the patient's eyes is required in order to ensure that there

has been steady fixation. Often, the first sign that the patient has seen the test object is a movement of the eyes toward the object. In some patients, attention or vision is so poor that the examiner must ask them to state when they see movement of a finger or hand held in each specific field. It may also be necessary to ask the patient to give a total for the number of fingers held in front of him or her (Fig. 35-4). A risk in some of these double simultaneous techniques is that frontal or parietal lesions, which do not affect visual pathways, may suppress the field opposite the side of the lesion in the same way that double simultaneous touch or pressure testing may be suppressed in such patients. Visual-field defects suspected by confrontation should be confirmed by more refined testing.

Fundoscopic examination may reveal the presence of a swollen optic disk and retinal vein fullness. These changes are indicative of papilledema, which is often an early manifestation of brain tumor.

Other visual findings that should be described and noted include nystagmus, impaired ocular

**FIGURE 35-3**

Confrontation method of visual field testing: (*a*) testing the lower right temporal field, (*b*) testing the upper left nasal field.

*a*

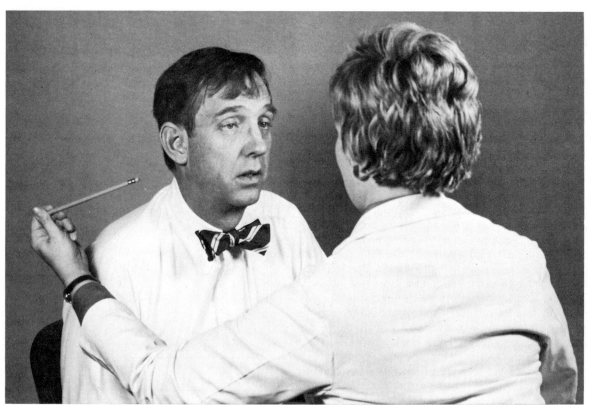

movement, and exophthalmos. Examination should determine whether these findings are unilateral or bilateral.

Evaluation of cranial nerve function should also be completed (see Chap. 31), and abnormalities noted. These include ptosis, facial palsies, and alterations in taste or smell.

*Impairment of cognitive functions* consists of deficits and changes in remembering, perceiving, and thinking (see Chap. 31). Deficits of abstraction, reasoning, and concept formation are considered sensitive indicators of cerebral dysfunction. The most common changes are progressive impairment of abstraction, recent memory and judgment, and a shortened attention span.[31,32] A test of *cortical function* may be undertaken, especially when there have been personality changes and/or changes in mental functioning and abilities (see Chap. 31). In preparing the patient for this test, the nurse should explain that it is not a pass/fail test, but that the patient should try to do his or her best. If the patient wears glasses or a hearing aid, these should be available

for use. The patient may be upset following the tests as this experience may have made evident or reinforced the loss in cognitive functioning and abilities. For example, consider what it means to a successful banker who can no longer do simple subtraction in a checkbook!

**D**iagnostic Tests   The patient may undergo a number of diagnostic tests on an outpatient basis, particularly if there is no evidence of increasing intracranial pressure. Generally, the simpler, noninvasive procedures are performed first.

Preparation of the patient and family includes providing information about the diagnostic procedures. Questions frequently asked about the procedures include the following:

1   What is the test? What is it called?

2   Why is the test being done?

3   Where is the test done?

4   What do I need to do to get ready?

*b*

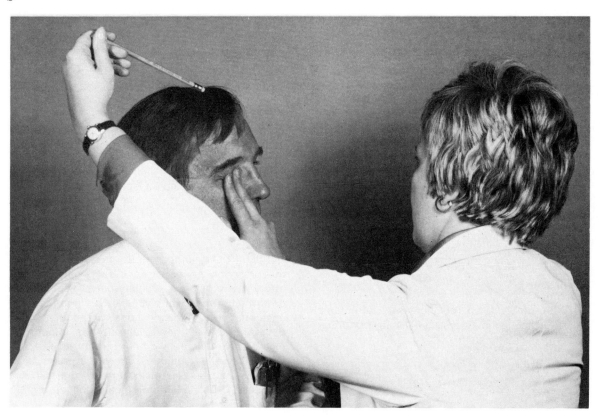

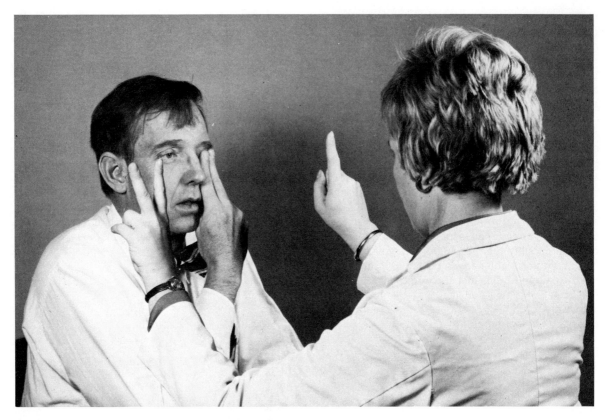

**FIGURE 35-4**
The patient is asked to count the total number of fingers in the double simultaneous technique.

5   What happens during the test?

6   How long will it take?

7   Who does the test?

8   How will it affect me afterward?

9   Who will tell me the results of the test?

10   Does it hurt?

The nurse would obtain this information according to the procedures in the institution or agency of employment. Some institutions provide test information in the form of a pamphlet. Such a tool may be used in combination with nurse-patient interaction.

With no evidence of increased intracranial pressure, the diagnostic tests are usually performed in the following sequence:[33]

1   Neurologic examination

2   Skull roentgenograms

3   Echoencephalography

4   Brain scan

5   Electroencephalogram

6   Lumbar puncture (may be deferred if a pneumoencephalogram is planned later or may follow an angiogram)

7   Computer-assisted tomography

8   Angiography

9   Pneumoencephalography

*Skull roentgenograms* are taken to determine the presence of increased intracranial pressure, atrophy or erosion of cranial bones, displacement of normal intracranial calcifications, and the presence of abnormal calcifications.[34] In addition to the usual anteroposterior and lateral views, tomograms may be taken of specific bony structures. Preparation of the patient includes removing hairpins, hearing aids, and glasses at the time of the test, and requesting the patient to remain still during the actual procedure.

*Echoencephalography* utilizes sound at an ultrasonic wavelength to detect a shift of midline structures in the cranium. This procedure can be carried out quickly and simply as a screening measure with information readily available. The procedure requires no specific physical preparation of the patient, although a thorough explanation should be offered.

*Brain scanning* employs the use of the radioisotope technetium-99m to determine areas of abnormal uptake in brain tissue. It is highly accurate in detecting supratentorial neoplasms, particularly gliomas, meningiomas, and metastatic lesions.[35] The patient is given a small amount of liquid perchlorate which blocks the radioisotope's affinity for the thyroid and salivary glands. Two types of scans are available, i.e., flow (dynamic) and static. Following the intravenous injection of the radioisotope, the scanner records immediately and every 2 seconds for 40 seconds. This phase is the flow or dynamic scan. Approximately two hours later the static views are taken. These comprise four to five different views. Where a brain tumor is suspected, both types of scans are obtained. The patient needs to lie still during the actual scanning, and following the test may resume the pretest level of activity. Figure 35-5 illustrates metastatic melanoma on three views during brain scanning and also by computer-assisted tomography.

*Electroencephalography* (EEG) is utilized to determine focal slowing of brain wave activity or seizure activity. It has localizing value, particularly in superficial lesions of the cerebral hemispheres. More deeply situated mass lesions tend to produce a generalized disturbance of electrical activity.[36] Several small electrodes are attached to the patient's scalp to record the electrical activity of the brain. If the patient is to have a sleep recording of electrical activity, he or she should be kept awake all night. At the time of the actual test, a hypnotic, usually liquid chloral hydrate, is given. Following the procedure it is necessary to shampoo the patient's hair to remove the paste used to secure the electrodes. If a hypnotic has been administered to the patient, it is safer not to allow the patient to drive home.

If there is known increased intracranial pressure, a *lumbar puncture* would not be undertaken as lumbar puncture may cause tentorial herniation. An arteriogram would provide information about potential shifts in intracranial contents.

*Computer-assisted tomography* is considered a major advancement in diagnostic procedures undertaken to detect brain lesions. (See Chap. 31.)

The cranium is scanned in successive layers by a narrow beam of x-rays. The transmission of the x-ray photons across a particular layer can be measured and, by means of a computer, used to construct a picture of the internal structure of the brain, i.e., ventricles, white matter, gray matter.

Lesions are seen as alterations of normal density and are interpreted in light of the pathological changes which are known to occur. Tissue density is artificially enhanced by the intravenous injection of substances containing large atoms.[37] One such substance, an organic iodine composed of diatrizoate meglumine and diatrizoate sodium, has been found to be ideal, and the tissue density of a variety of tumors is enhanced by this means. Figure 35-6 illustrates primary and metastatic neoplastic lesions shown by computer-assisted tomography. Figure 35-5 illustrates a cerebral tumor as demonstrated by both brain scanning and computer-assisted tomography.

Preparation of the patient includes removal of hairpins, glasses, and wigs at the time of the procedure. The procedure usually takes 30 to 60 minutes. Because of the danger of anaphylactic shock, patients allergic to iodine should notify the physician before the injection. The patient is positioned on a table as illustrated in Fig. 31-25. The cheek supports stabilize the head. It is necessary to remain absolutely still during the scanning. Since the patient is in a supine position, if there is an altered level of consciousness or any difficulty with secretions and/or airway obstruction, it is necessary to observe how the patient is handling the secretions and to suction if necessary.

*Visual-field testing* determines the limit of peripheral vision, the space within which an object can be seen while the eye remains fixed on some one point.[38] Supratentorial tumors such as pituitary adenoma, meningioma, craniopharyngioma, or glioma interfere with the visual pathways and thus frequently produce visual-field changes.[39] Figure 35-7 illustrates the course of the visual fibers from the retina to the occipital cortex, the lesions in the pathway, and the resultant visual-field defects.

The three standard methods of testing the visual fields are: the confrontation or hand method, the perimeter, and the campimeter or tangent screen. By confrontation, gross defects in the field of vision may be detected (see Physical Assessment above). To detect more specific defects, the perimeter can be used for testing the peripheral field, and the campimeter or tangent screen for intermediate and central areas. These latter two tests are performed by ophthalmologists, neurologists,

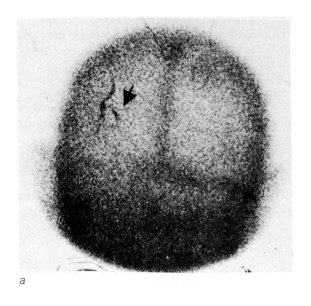

*a*

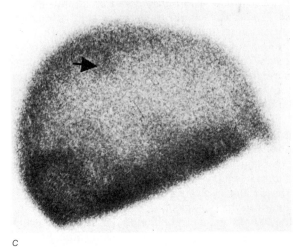

*c*

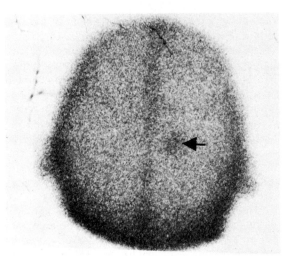

*b*

**FIGURE 35-5**

(*a, b, c*) Brain scan of a patient with metastatic melanoma.
(*d*) Computer-assisted tomography demonstrates the patient's
cerebral lesion.

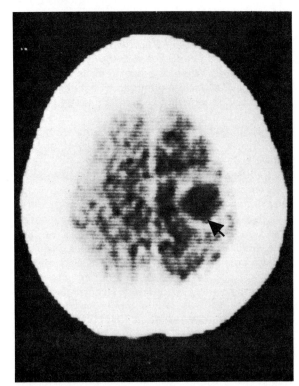

*d*

neurosurgeons, and specially trained technicians.
Perimetry and tangent screen testing requires the
full cooperation of an alert patient. Patients with
brain tumors, head injuries, cerebrovascular accidents manifesting altered levels of consciousness,
aphasia, fatigue, and shortened attention spans
may be unable to cooperate, and the simpler confrontation method may have to be utilized.

**Nursing problems and interventions** Persons
with neoplasms of the brain are referred directly to
a medical facility for further diagnosis and/or intervention. During the initial diagnostic work-up, common nursing problems are the *anxiety* and *uncertainty* that both the patient and the family must
face. During this period it is helpful for the nurse to
allow time to establish a relationship with the pa-

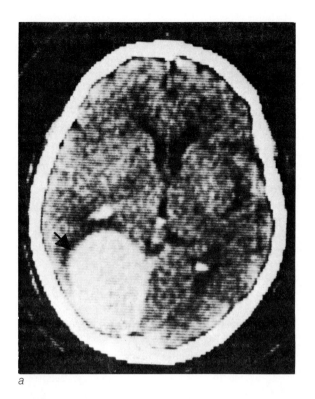

*a*

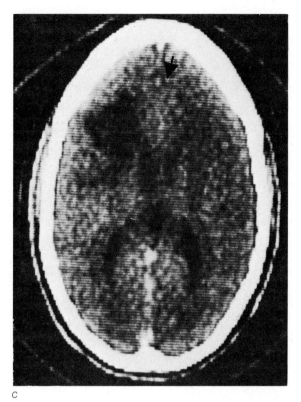

*c*

**FIGURE 35-6**
Computer-assisted tomography. All three patients received contrast media. These demonstrate (*a*) a meningioma, (*b*) a metastatic adenocarcinoma, (*c*) an infiltrating tumor.

*b*

tient and family. The acute onset and progressive manifestations of a brain tumor often do not allow the patient to adapt to a progressive loss of function. It is important for the patient to tell the story of the illness, which may be the most important event in his or her life, and indeed it is, if there is a CNS tumor.

The diagnostic period may be experienced by the patient and family as one of "waiting, and wondering, and worrying." There is waiting to have the scheduled diagnostic tests and waiting for the information revealed by the tests. While waiting, the patient and family are wondering what the tests will reveal. The patient and family worry about what the diagnosis will mean in terms of life, the quality of life, and death.

Approaches the nurse may use with the physician to assist the patient and family during the diagnostic period include: (1) Providing the opportunity for the patient and family to express their perceptions of the events and the meaning of what is happening. (2) Planning the scheduling of tests with subsequent appointments to discuss the results

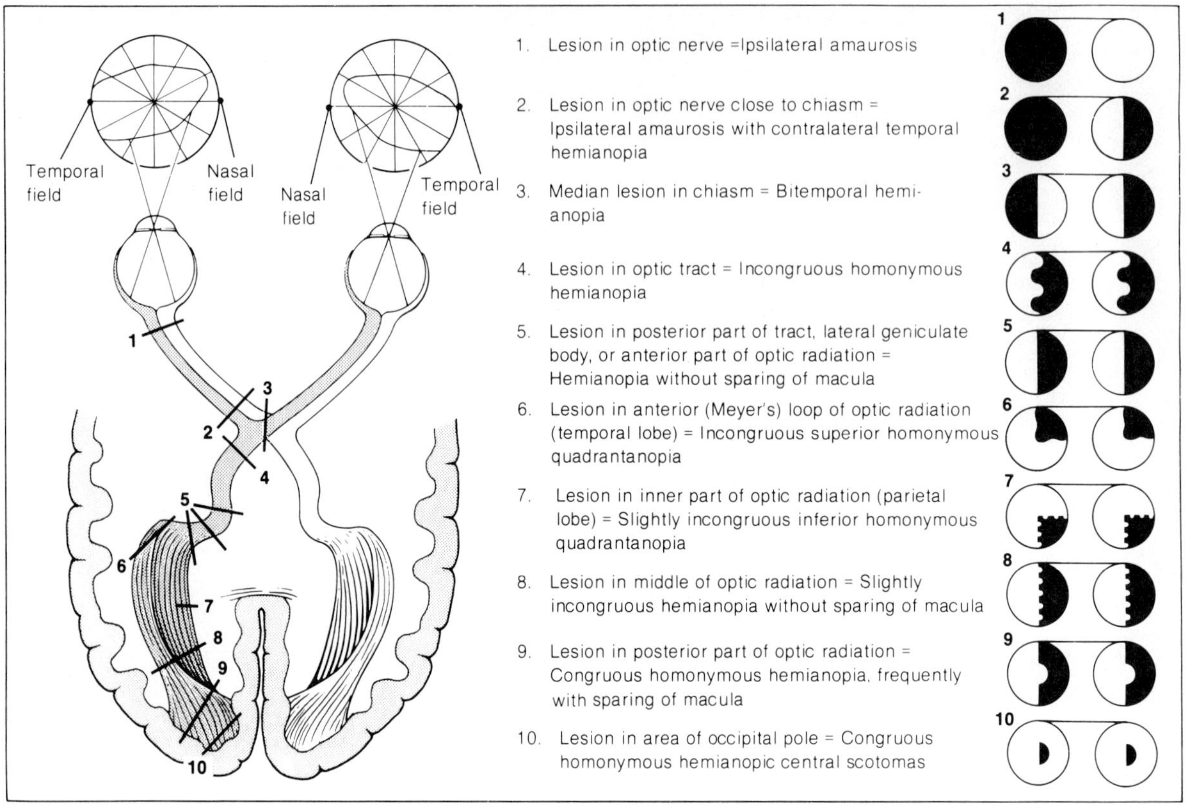

1. Lesion in optic nerve =Ipsilateral amaurosis

2. Lesion in optic nerve close to chiasm = Ipsilateral amaurosis with contralateral temporal hemianopia

3. Median lesion in chiasm = Bitemporal hemianopia

4. Lesion in optic tract = Incongruous homonymous hemianopia

5. Lesion in posterior part of tract, lateral geniculate body, or anterior part of optic radiation = Hemianopia without sparing of macula

6. Lesion in anterior (Meyer's) loop of optic radiation (temporal lobe) = Incongruous superior homonymous quadrantanopia

7. Lesion in inner part of optic radiation (parietal lobe) = Slightly incongruous inferior homonymous quadrantanopia

8. Lesion in middle of optic radiation = Slightly incongruous hemianopia without sparing of macula

9. Lesion in posterior part of optic radiation = Congruous homonymous hemianopia, frequently with sparing of macula

10. Lesion in area of occipital pole = Congruous homonymous hemianopic central scotomas

**FIGURE 35-7**
Diagram of the visual fibers from the retina to the occipital cortex, lesions in the various parts of the pathway (1–10), and the resultant visual-field defects for the lesions. (*After Alfred Huber, Eye Signs and Symptoms in Brain Tumors, Mosby, St. Louis, 1976, p. 87, and Russell N. DeJong, The Neurologic Examination, Harper & Row, New York, 1970, p. 120.*)

with the patient and family. (3) Scheduling tests with consideration of the patient's physical and emotional ability to undergo the tests. A patient may not be able to tolerate closely scheduled tests. (4) Providing a means for the patient and family to communicate with the nurse and physician between tests and appointments to provide information and support, and in case of emergencies.

Patients found to have metastatic lesions to the brain will undergo additional diagnostic tests to determine the primary site if it has not been identified. This is necessary to determine the medical therapeutic approach.

Patients who have inoperable tumors must cope with many problems that are best cared for in the home situation. Frequently, *ptosis* or drooping of the upper eyelid occurs as a result of direct pressure or interference with the pathways of the portion of the IIId cranial nerve supplying the levator muscle. Since the eyelid is weak and not blinking

normally, the goals of nursing intervention include preventing drying and ulceration of the exposed cornea and assisting the patient to compensate for visual changes.

The degree of ptosis should be observed and measured, and the cornea inspected. The patient should be taught to use artificial tears such as methyl cellulose and to close and tape the eyelid at night. The patient and family should be advised to place objects within the patient's view as the patient may have to hyperextend the neck in order to see with the unaffected eye. Arrangements may need to be made with the patient to wear or change to eye glasses if contact lenses are normally worn. Finally, the use of "lid crutches" on eye glasses may be advisable, if ptosis is prolonged or not correctable.

*Visual-field defects,* particularly homonymous hemianopsic defects, either are not noticed at all, or are not disturbing in 25 percent of the patients manifesting them. The patient may not be aware of the defect, but may be aware of its consequences such as colliding with persons or objects.[40] Nursing interventions should be designed to increase the patient's awareness and safety, and to assist the patient to compensate for the defect.

It is important to discuss with the patient any experiences of everyday life which might be affected by the defect and ways to prevent them. For example, a motorist may hit the wall of the garage, or a cyclist may overlook a pedestrian on one side of the street. The nurse and physician should discuss with the patient the safety of driving.

The placement of the patient with homonymous hemianopsia in a room should be considered. Placement should be such that the patient can use the unaffected visual field to see people as they enter the room. The family should be taught to approach the patient on the side of the unaffected visual field and to place objects within the field of vision on that side.

*Headache* is usually intermittent in most patients with brain tumors. Goals of nursing intervention are to ascertain changes in the pattern of the headache and to alleviate the discomfort of the headache.

The intensity of the headache may be diminished by the use of acetylsalicylic acid and/or cold compresses to the scalp. If the headache is intense and/or continuous, the physician may prescribe other or additional analgesics for use at home. Tests or activities should be scheduled during periods of relief from discomfort, if possible.

*Mental and personality changes* may range from very subtle memory problems to more overt outbursts of anger. Generally, objectives of intervention include providing for the patient's safety and well-being and assisting the family in dealing with their feelings and management of the patient.

When the patient is experiencing problems of recent memory and judgment, a family member or other responsible adult will need to know when and where diagnostic tests are scheduled; when medications are to be taken; and when and where medical referral or follow-up appointments are scheduled. The patient may wish to write down information as a memory aid. The nurse may also reorient the patient to time and suggest ways in which the family may reorient the patient daily; i.e., a calendar may be placed in the patient's room, and other reminders of the season such as spring flowers or autumn leaves may be brought in from time to time.

When slowness and apathy are apparent, more time may need to be allowed for activities. Structure and directions in the activities of daily living may have to be provided by the spouse or family.

When outbursts of anger or rage are manifested, it is helpful for the spouse or family to express their feelings and ability to handle the situation. On occasion it may be necessary to hospitalize the patient for more immediate diagnostic studies if behavioral management is difficult or threatening.

When the patient manifests erotic behavior, sexual exhibitionism, lewd remarks, or lack of social graces, the family may express embarrassment and concern. It is helpful for the nurse to explain to the spouse and family that this is a change in the patient's usual behavior that must be managed in an understanding, kind, and respectful way.

Patients may be *referred* for medical and nursing care by family practitioners, internists, or ophthalmologists, as well as from psychiatric settings, the emergency room, and various clinics. When patients are referred from one facility to another, it is important that the nursing data be sent with the medical history, physical examination data, and test results. Initial data provide the baseline against which the nurse may evaluate subsequent changes in the patient. In addition, the patient's ability to provide the data again may change markedly.

### Third-Level Nursing Care

Hospitalization takes place when the patient's physical status changes, when there are new or progressive neurologic deficits, or when further and more invasive diagnostic tests are needed. Frequently, the hospitalization is for the behavioral management and safety of the patient.

The *health history* of patients with progressive neurological neoplasms is similar to that described in Second-Level Nursing Care. However, the severity of symptoms may be increased. Previous motor weakness may have advanced to paralysis; beginning sensory impairment may have become a complete absence of sensation; and symptoms specific to the tumor location (speech difficulties, impaired sphincter control) may now be apparent in severe form (aphasia, incontinence). Pain may be a prominent symptom as the tumor mass enlarges and impinges on sensory nerve endings.

During the *physical assessment* it is most important to collect baseline data about the patient upon admission to the hospital unit. These data serve as the basis for future evaluation of the patient and for the planning of interventions. A complete neurological examination should be done. It will initially focus on signs of *increased intracranial pressure* and *focal neurologic signs* and *symptoms*.

The components of the neurological examination are discussed in Chap. 31. Table 35-2 provides a description of the usual clinical manifestations of patients with intracranial neoplasms on the basis of location of the lesions. Tables 35-4 to 35-6 describe other abnormal findings that may be apparent during the neurological assessment.

**D**iagnostic Tests The patient may have undergone, on an outpatient basis, some of the tests outlined in Second-Level Nursing Care. The more invasive tests which might be scheduled in the hospital are the arteriogram (cerebral angiogram) and the pneumoencephalogram.

An *angiogram* of the cerebral vessels is per-

**TABLE 35-4**
GUIDELINES FOR NEUROLOGICAL STATUS ASSESSMENT

| Parameter | Data Collection* |
|---|---|
| 1. Level of consciousness<br> a. Does the patient respond to verbal stimulation?<br><br> b. Is the patient oriented to person, place, and time?<br><br> c. Is the patient able to speak? Is the conversation coherent and appropriate?<br> d. If not able to speak, can the patient nod "yes" or "no" correctly?<br> e. Can the patient follow directions?<br> f. Is recent and/or remote memory affected? | a. Does patient open both eyes and look in direction of stimuli?<br> b. Ask the patient his or her name, location, and the month, day, and year.<br> c. Ask the patient a question that would not have an automatic or memorized response.<br> d. Ask the patient a "yes" or "no" question to which you know the correct response.<br> e. Request that the patient perform a particular activity.<br> f. Ask the patient a question relative to a recent and a remote event (e.g., recent, last 4 hours; remote, when a child). |
| 2. Pupillary response<br> a. Do the pupils react to light at the same rate?<br><br><br><br> b. Are the pupils equal in size?<br><br> c. What is the size of the pupils? | a. Ask the patient to look at a distant object, or darken the room. With the patient's eyes closed, bring the flashlight from the side, open one eyelid, and observe whether the pupil reacts briskly or sluggishly to light. Repeat and compare with other eye.<br> b. Shine the light into both eyes simultaneously and compare the size of the pupils as they dilate and constrict together.<br> c. Determine the size of each pupil.<br><br> Pupil Size, mm:<br> • • • ● ● ● ● ●<br> 2  3  4  5  6  7  8  9 |
| 3. Vital signs<br> a. Is the blood pressure elevated? Is there a widening pulse pressure? Is there a pattern developing rapidly or slowly?<br> b. What is the pulse rate? Is the pulse rate regular?<br> c. What is the respiratory rate? Is it regular? What is the respiratory pattern?<br> d. Is the temperature elevated? | a. Take the blood pressure and compare with the patient's baseline pressure and the previous reading. Look at the trend over the previous hours.<br> b. Take the pulse for a full minute. Look at the rate for the previous hours.<br> c. Count the respirations for a full minute. Observe the pattern (rate and depth). Look at the trend over the previous hours.<br> d. Take a rectal temperature. Look at the trend from the previous readings. |
| 4. Movement and strength<br> a. Does the patient move spontaneously?<br> b. Does the patient move an extremity to verbal stimulation?<br> c. Does the patient move an extremity to tactile stimulation?<br> d. Does the patient move only to painful stimulation?<br> e. Is the strength of the upper extremities equal?<br><br><br><br><br><br> f. Is the strength of the lower extremities equal? | a. Observe for movement of the extremities and overall posture.<br> d. Ask the patient to move each extremity.<br> c. Touch and apply pressure to the patient's upper extremity.<br> d. Press your thumbnail into patient's nailbed.<br> e. Ask the patient to extend both arms in front to shoulder level. Observe for inability to elevate arm(s), for drift downward of one arm, and/or dropping of the extremity. Ask the patient to squeeze your index and middle fingers. Compare both sides at the same time.<br> f. Ask the patient to elevate each leg. Compare sides. Ask the patient to push against your hands with his or her feet at the same time. Compare sides. |

* These data are recorded on various forms in different hospitals, i.e., progress notes, flow charts, neurological check lists.

**TABLE 35-5**
SIGNS OF INCREASING INTRACRANIAL PRESSURE

| Parameter | Data | Explanation |
|---|---|---|
| Pupils | Dilation of pupil(s) with loss of light reflex (on side of compression) | The downward displacement of the cerebral hemisphere with herniation of the temporal lobe causes compression of the oculomotor nerve (IIId cranial nerve). |
| Blood pressure | Increasing systolic pressure, widening pulse pressure | So-called Cushing reaction, a special CNS ischemic response, whereby CSF pressure rises to equal arterial pressure, with the arterial supply to brain compressed, causing ischemia of vasomotor center which stimulates a rise in arterial pressure. Arterial pressure rises higher than CSF pressure to resume flow to the brain to relieve ischemia.[41] |
| Pulse | Decreasing pulse rate, with an initial bounding pulse | Ischemia or pressure on the medulla causes vagus dysfunction. |
| Respiration | The rate and depth may vary. A pattern or blend may be identified: | Specific patterns of respiratory function are manifested at different levels of brain dysfunction: |
|  | Cheyne-Stokes pattern | Supratentorial dysfunction |
|  | Central hyperventilation pattern | Midbrain level dysfunction |
|  | Apneustic pattern (sustained contraction of the inspiratory muscles) | Pontine level dysfunction |
|  | Anoxic pattern | Medullary level dysfunction[42] |

formed to determine changes in the normal configuration of the blood vessels. (See Chap. 31 also.) A space-occupying lesion may cause a shift in the vessels. There is also an increased vasculature in some types of brain tumors. The angiography is helpful to the neurosurgeon in delineating the approach to surgical intervention. The procedure employs the injection of radiopaque dye into the carotid, brachial, or femoral artery. X-rays are taken to demonstrate the vasculature.

Following the procedure, pressure and a dressing are placed over the injection site and the patient should remain in bed. If the injection site was the brachial artery, the patient should keep the arm in an extended position; the site should be checked for bleeding, the pulse distal to the injection site (radial pulse) checked for presence and quality, and the hand examined for color and temperature. The injected extremity is compared with the other extremity. If the femoral artery was used for injection, the leg should be kept still and straight and not flexed at the hip. In this instance, the pedal pulse is palpated. Should bleeding occur at the site, a pressure dressing and ice packs are applied, and the physician notified. In the absence of a previously palpable pulse, the physician should be notified immediately. In patients with peripheral vascular disease in the lower extremities, the pedal pulses should be assessed prior to the test to obtain a baseline by which to compare.

The patient's blood pressure, pulse, and respirations should be monitored, and the reaction and

**TABLE 35-6**
CONSCIOUSNESS AND ALTERATIONS

| 1 | Consciousness: | An individual's awareness and responsiveness to self, environment, and the impressions made by the senses. The patient is oriented as to person, place, time. He or she is alert and responds to stimuli; recent and remote memory are intact. |
|---|---|---|
| 2 | Lethargy: | Drowsiness with continued or prolonged sleep. The patient can be aroused or awakened by stimuli, responds appropriately, and may fall back to sleep when the stimuli are removed. |
| 3 | Confusion: | State of reduced wakefulness or awareness manifested by defects in memory, attention span, loss of appreciation for and perception of the environment, defects in the spheres of orientation, particularly time. Impaired capacity to think clearly, to perceive, respond to, and remember current stimuli. |
| 4 | Delirium: | Characterized by disorientation, fear, motor and sensory irritability, misperception of sensory stimuli, often visual hallucinations. |
| 5 | Stupor: | An unresponsiveness from which the individual can be aroused only by vigorous and repeated stimuli. Responses are slow and inadequate. In profound stupor the patient responds only to painful stimulation. Corneal and pupillary reflexes are present. |
| 6 | Coma: | Complete unresponsiveness to the environment and to painful stimulation. Corneal sensation and reflexes are absent. No voluntary movement. Pupils do not react; they are either dilated or constricted.[43,44] |

equality of the pupils evaluated. Muscle strength and movement of the extremities should be assessed. Vital signs and neurological parameters should be monitored every 15 minutes for 1 hour, every 30 minutes for 2 hours, every hour for 4 hours, and every 4 hours for the remaining 24 hours. These data are compared with the preprocedure data to determine any new or abnormal developing trends, which should be reported to the physician. Hydration of the patient should be maintained as the dye has a diuretic effect.

A *pneumoencephalogram* (detailed in Chap. 31) is performed to visualize the ventricles of the brain. Changes in the size, shape, and position of the ventricles as well as the subarachnoid pathways provide valuable information in the diagnosis of cerebral neoplasms. Tumors may displace the ventricles and cause obstruction to the flow of cerebrospinal fluid.

Air is injected into the subarachnoid space through a lumbar puncture after cerebrospinal fluid is removed. X-rays are taken as the air circulates to the ventricles, the subarachnoid channels, and cisterns. Following a satisfactory series of x-rays, the spinal needle is removed. A small, sterile dressing is placed over the injection site. The patient should lie flat for 24 hours but can change from prone to supine position, or move from side to side. Lying flat prevents the air from remaining in the upper part of the ventricles and facilitates its reabsorption. Providing additional fluid intake aids the production and replacement of cerebrospinal fluid. Patients are less likely to experience headache while lying flat and still. Analgesics may be indicated. The patient's neurologic status and vital signs are monitored in order to detect and prevent possible postprocedure complications.

*Lumbar puncture* is undertaken judiciously. With evidence of increased intracranial pressure, the lumbar puncture may be deferred until after an angiogram is performed. The angiogram would reveal the potential for shifts of intracranial contents. The shift of intracranial contents can cause herniation of the uncus of the temporal lobe or cerebellar tonsils with compression of the brainstem and its vital centers.

**Nursing problems and interventions**  Patients with neoplasms of the brain may experience one or a combination of nursing problems that must be addressed. One of the most serious of these is seizure activity. Patients with brain tumors can manifest *focal motor* and/or *sensory seizures* or a *generalized convulsion*. Adults experiencing their first generalized convulsion should be taken to an emergency room and admitted to the hospital for diagnostic tests. The seizure activity may be the initial and only sign of a brain tumor, or it can be followed by other signs such as difficulty in speaking, dysarthria, or frank aphasia. Nursing care must include providing a safe environment, assisting in the control of the seizures, and helping the patient to deal with any feelings about the experience.

Important information about the seizure pattern should be obtained from the family or from those persons who have observed the patient's seizure. Subsequently, the patient should be observed for seizures. Documentation of the seizure activity should include: the part of the body involved, the type of movements, any progression of the movements, the duration of the seizure, loss of consciousness, incontinence of urine or stool, and the direction of the eyes during the seizure. At the time of a generalized convulsion, the nurse should position the patient to prevent trauma and ensure a patent airway. After a seizure has begun, it is difficult to insert a tongue blade while the patient is experiencing tonic-clonic movements. If the patient has experienced a generalized convulsion with tonic-clonic movements, the bedsides should be up and padded to prevent bruising and further trauma. If the generalized convulsions are not controlled, the patient should be accompanied to diagnostic tests or when out of bed. Phenytoin sodium (Dilantin) is effective to control generalized convulsions and is administered intravenously in these instances; later when the patient can safely handle oral medications, Dilantin may be given orally. Diazepam may also be administered intravenously for the control of generalized seizure activity. An opportunity should be provided for the patient and family to express their perceptions and feelings about the seizure(s) the patient has experienced.

*Motor weakness and paralysis* result when tumor and edema infiltrate tissue and cause pressure on the neurons of the frontal motor cortex and/or the descending voluntary motor tracts (the pyramidal tracts) of the spinal cord. *Paresis* refers to diminished strength in an extremity; *paralysis* is the complete inability to move an extremity. *Mono-* refers to one extremity, while *hemi-* refers to half the body, or the upper and lower extremities on the same side. Thus, the terms *monoparesis* and *hemiplegia* describe changes in motor function. The goals of nursing care for a patient with motor weakness are to provide for safety when the patient moves and ambulates, to maintain the functional level of the extremity(ies), and to prevent trauma and complications to the affected side.

The strength and range of movement in the affected extremity should be evaluated and compared with those of the unaffected extremity. Range of motion exercises should be provided to the affected extremity twice a day. If the level of consciousness is altered and movement is impaired, it will be important to turn the patient every 2 hours. Inspection of the skin should be made and skin care given with each turning of the patient. The patient and the affected extremity(ies) should be positioned to prevent the complications of dependent edema, contractures, joint dislocation and discomfort, and stretched muscles. Refer to Chap. 34 for a description of correct positioning of the patient. Intramuscular injections and intravenous fluids should *not* be administered in a paretic or paralyzed extremity if at all possible. Medications would not be absorbed as readily in a muscle with decreased movement. There may also be sensory changes in a paralyzed extremity, and the patient may not be able to identify discomfort associated with the complications of intravenous therapy. The nurse should consult with or request a referral to the physical therapist for further planning, intervention, and evaluation of the care of the patient.

*Fever* may occur because of the pathological process and/or the inability of the patient to maintain adequate hydration. Neurologically, a patient cannot maintain an adequate oral fluid intake if there is an altered level of consciousness, disorientation, or dysphagia. Fever can be a sign of pulmonary congestion and thrombophlebitis associated with bed rest and immobility. Hyperthermia may result from hypothalamic involvement, particularly destruction of the anterior portion of the hypothalamus. Also, tumors of the third ventricle often cause hyperthermia.[45]

It is important to identify the factor(s) responsible for the fever. Temperature (rectal), pulse, and respirations should be carefully monitored, and the pattern evaluated. Fluid intake can be maintained through intravenous administration or orally if the patient is able. If there is evidence of cerebral edema, the fluid intake must be monitored closely and restricted. Antipyretic medications may be ordered to reduce the temperature if the cause of the fever is determined; otherwise the cause could be obscured by reduction of temperature. Salicylates are used to act upon the heat-regulating center of the hypothalamus. They increase the elimination of heat by dilating the peripheral blood vessels with heat loss through radiation and the evaporation of perspiration.[46] Other interventions that may be used to reduce the patient's fever include alcohol sponges, minimal use of bed linens, and a hypothermia machine and blanket. The patient's perspiration should be removed by bathing as appropriate; moist gowns and linen should be replaced.

*Mental and personality changes* occur frequently in patients with intracranial neoplasms. A prominent manifestation is confusion consisting of impairment of the patient's awareness accompanied by defects in attention span and memory, and a loss of normal appreciation for and perception of the environment. The chief symptoms may be in the field of orientation: the person may be unaware of time, place, or the identity of self or others. The capacity to think clearly and with rapidity, to perceive, to respond to, and to remember current stimuli is impaired.[47]

In an assessment of the patient's mental and personality changes, the guidelines in Table 35-7 are helpful in differentiating organic from functional confusion. In addition, the family can provide information about specific behavioral changes they have observed and managed. The nurse can elicit from the family those approaches that have been effective in managing the patient and assist the family to deal with their feelings about the manifestations.

The placement of the patient on the hospital unit should permit continuous observation. The family's presence and assistance may facilitate the admission examinations and procedures. The physical environment should be kept simple, uncluttered, and stable. The number of staff the patient must relate to should be kept to a minimum to lessen disorientation and facilitate continuity of care. Reorientation of the patient and memory aids should be used as appropriate. Directions should be simple and given at the time it is necessary for the patient to perform an activity. For a patient who wanders, a chair with a tray table attached may be used instead of restraints. The patient can then be situated in an area where he or she can be observed by staff.

The patient with a brain tumor can manifest *changes in language function,* particularly aphasia. Refer to Chap. 34 for the nursing assessment and interventions.

*Sensory changes* may also be apparent. These include altered sensation to heat and cold, pain, and pressure. Patient and family teaching should be initiated to protect the patient from injury because of these altered sensations. This includes testing bath water to avoid burns, frequent turning to avoid decubiti, and visual checking of sensorily impaired areas for cuts, bruises, or abrasions.

*Surgical intervention, radiation therapy,* and *chemotherapy,* singly or in combination, are the current modes of therapy. The location and suspected type of intracranial lesion are rationale for the selection of the treatment modality. (If the cerebral lesions are metastatic from a primary site elsewhere in the body, the therapeutic approach to the cerebral metastasis is considered in light of the treatment approach to the primary lesion.)

**S**urgical Intervention   A *craniotomy,* or temporary opening into the cranial cavity through a bone flap, is performed to remove cerebral neoplastic lesions (as well as aneurysms, hematomas, and abscesses) and to confirm the diagnosis. A *transphenoidal* surgical approach may be utilized in tumors of the pituitary, particularly where there is an intrasellar tumor. The approaches vary, but modern techniques utilize a binocular dissecting microscope and televised radiofluoroscopic control.[48] A burr hole (a small circular opening) is made into the skull in order to remove a subdural hematoma or to biopsy the cerebral tissue to establish a diagnosis.

Informed consent via an operative permit is secured by the neurosurgeon. If the patient's mental status will not enable him or her to make a decision, the next of kin must be contacted. Patients and families should be allowed time and provided information in terms they can understand in order to make the decision regarding surgery. In emergencies, the decision may need to be made immediately. Patients react in different ways; some will need and want to take care of personal matters before having major surgery; others will want to proceed as soon as possible.

*Providing information* is an important aspect of care and should be done on the basis of the patient's and family's readiness and need. In addition to the procedure to be followed by the neurosurgeon, the patient and family frequently ask about the time of surgery, how long it will last, where the family can wait, where the patient will be cared for after surgery, and when the patient may have visitors. This information can be related and reinforced by the nurse.

While there are various approaches to pre-

**TABLE 35-7**
GUIDELINES FOR DIFFERENTIATING ORGANIC
FROM FUNCTIONAL CONFUSION

| Factor | Organic Confusion | Functional Confusion |
|---|---|---|
| Memory impairment | Recent more impaired than remote | No consistent difference between recent and remote |
| Disorientation: | | |
|     Time | Within own lifetime or reasonably near future | May not be related to patient's lifetime |
|     Place | Familiar place or one where patient might easily be | Bizarre or unfamiliar places |
|     Person | Sense of identity usually preserved | Sense of identity diminished |
| | Misidentification of others as familiar | Misidentification of others based on delusional system |
| Hallucinations | Visual, vivid. Animals and insects common | Auditory more frequent Bizarre and symbolic |
| Illusions | Common | Not prominent |
| Delusions | Concerns everyday occurrences and people | Bizarre and symbolic |
| Confused | Spotty confusion; clear intervals mixed with confused episodes | More consistent |
| | Worse at night | No tendency to become worse at night |

SOURCE: Copyright September 1972, the American Journal of Nursing Company. Reproduced with permission from *Amer J Nurs,* **72**(9):1632.

operative teaching, an important point is that the patient and family be provided the information they request. It is very important that the messages the patient and family receive be accurate and consistent. Information that is frequently provided includes descriptions of: (1) the procedures and care the patient can expect: blow bottles, oxygen therapy, suctioning, intravenous therapy, monitoring devices, possible arterial lines, frequent neurological status evaluation, vital signs (rectal temperature probe), cranial dressing and drains, pain medication, Foley catheter; and (2) the patient's and the unit's physical aspects: head dressing, possible periorbital edema and ecchymosis, and the equipment in the unit. The *emotional* status of the patient needs to be assessed, and opportunities provided for the expression of any feelings. The nurse should be cognizant of and ascertain the patient's and family's need for *spiritual* support. The family may contact its own clergy, or the nurse may call the hospital's chaplaincy services if the patient and family wish.

The patient may be receiving anticonvulsant medications and analgesics for headache. Steroids may be ordered preoperatively in order to reduce cerebral edema. Immediate preoperative medications include injections of atropine sulfate and a hypnotic or relaxant.

The patient's blood is typed and cross matched. Intravenous therapy will be started before surgery. If the patient has evidence of cerebral edema, fluids will be monitored and restricted.

The patient's scalp may be prepared the night before surgery on the unit, or after the patient has been anesthetized in the operating room area. Long hair is braided and cut close to the scalp. The head is scrubbed with an antibacterial agent and wrapped with a sterile towel for the night. The final shaving is done carefully with a straight razor at the time of surgery. Elastic support stockings or elastic bandages may be applied to support venous circulation in the lower extremities while the patient is immobilized on the operating room table.

Bathing the evening before surgery and a back rub may help the patient relax and sleep. A hypnotic may be administered if the patient wishes. The patient whose condition requires frequent evaluation of neurologic status and vital signs *must be awakened.*

Vital signs and neurological parameters should be evaluated prior to medicating the patient. Table 35-4 serves as a guideline for data collection of specific parameters to be assessed. Further interpretation may be guided by Table 35-5, which describes the signs and symptoms of increasing intracranial pressure, and Table 35-6, which describes alterations in consciousness.

Since a patient may initially be admitted to a neurological or medical nursing unit, transferred to an intensive-care unit after surgery, and then transferred to a neurosurgical or surgical nursing unit, providing *continuity of care* is essential. Even if the patient is admitted to a neurosurgical nursing unit and returns to the same unit from the intensive-care unit after surgery, the following interventions should be implemented to provide a means of communication, support, and individualized nursing care. The nurse preparing the patient for surgery should accompany the patient to surgery and interact with the family during surgery to provide support. It is helpful for the nurse to accompany the family into the intensive-care unit for the first visit to the patient following surgery. The intensive-care unit may be a new and frightening environment for the family. The nurse(s) who will care for the patient postoperatively should interact with the patient and family preoperatively to observe the baseline status of the patient and the family's reaction, and to carry out necessary teaching.

In the immediate *postoperative period,* nursing care is directed toward (1) the early detection of increasing intracranial pressure due to hemorrhage and cerebral edema, and (2) the stabilization and maintenance of physiological parameters. Observation of the patient is critical. The parameters to be observed and assessed are the level of consciousness, pupillary signs, movement and strength of the extremities and the vital signs. Refer to Tables 35-4 to 35-6 for guides to the collection and interpretation of data. Changes in these parameters should be reported immediately to the neurosurgeon.

*Intracranial pressure* can be controlled by reduction of the cerebral edema that can result from surgery. Cerebral edema increases the volume in the cranial cavity, thus increasing the intracranial pressure. In order to reduce cerebral edema and prevent arterial and venous congestion in the brain, steroid therapy, positioning of the patient, adequate ventilation, and fluid restriction are significant interventions. The synthetic glucocorticoid steroid, dexamethasone, is often administered postoperatively to reduce cerebral edema, and the dosage is gradually tapered. An antacid is usually administered (when the patient can safely handle oral medications) to prevent gastric irritation from the steroid therapy. Mannitol, an osmotic diuretic, may be administered as a continuous drip or a bolus to reduce cerebral edema and prevent increasing intracranial pressure. Its diuretic effect may be rapid, and so it is necessary to measure the output hourly. Fluids may be limited to 1500 ml the first 24 hours or 70 ml/hour. Electrolytes are maintained and/or replaced on the basis of a daily assessment. A Foley catheter is usually inserted preoperatively and facilitates output measurement. The specific gravity of the urine should be monitored also.

The patient with a supratentorial lesion and surgical approach is positioned in a semi-Fowler's position to facilitate venous circulation from the brain and thereby prevent an increase in the circulating volume of blood. The patient's head and body position should maintain a patent airway and adequate ventilation.

Immediately after surgery, the endotracheal tube is kept in place to provide for ventilation. Inadequate ventilation causes a rise in carbon dioxide in the blood, and the amount of oxygen in the cerebral blood is diminished. In an attempt to increase the oxygen, there is vasodilatation of the cerebral blood vessels and hypertension. With vasodilatation there is an increase in the circulating blood volume in the brain. Therefore, inadequate ventilation is hazardous, causing cerebral anoxia, particularly when increased intracranial pressure exists. Blood gases should be assessed daily. In order to maintain respiratory function, the patient may receive oxygen and be assisted with a respirator. If the patient's ventilation does not require a respirator, deep breathing should be encouraged, and the patient turned every 2 hours in order to prevent pulmonary congestion, infection, and inadequate ventilation.

If the patient's gag reflex is present and the patient is alert and able to swallow, oral fluids may be initiated. The patient's diet may be progressed to include food.

After removal of a pituitary tumor, the patient may manifest diabetes insipidus postoperatively. Management would include strict monitoring of fluid intake and output, specific gravity, fluid replacement, and the administration of vasopressin tannate. (See Chap. 6 for care of the patient having a hypophysectomy.)

*Cardiac functioning* may be assessed through monitoring and observation. Tachycardia may be a sign of shock or cardiac failure, with decreased cardiac output leading to inadequate cerebral perfusion. Blood pressure changes, particularly a widening pulse pressure, may indicate increasing intracranial pressure.

*Musculoskeletal complications* may be prevented by positioning the patient in proper body alignment. Range of motion exercises twice a day to all extremities prevent the development of contractures in weak or paralyzed extremities. The patient's skin should be observed daily, skin care given, and the patient turned every 2 hours to prevent the development of decubitus ulcers.

*Infection* at the operative site is a possible complication. The wound should be observed for signs of infection when the dressing is changed. Temperature elevations should be assessed. A dry, sterile dressing must be kept intact initially; after the dressing is removed, a stockinette cap may be used.

*Hyperthermia* may occur following intracranial surgery. This may be due to hypothalamic dysfunction; however, the possibility of infection should be investigated. Sites to be considered include: the urinary tract, especially if the patient has a Foley catheter inserted; the lungs and bronchial tree, particularly if the patient is immobilized and not handling secretions; and the operative site, which has the potential for meningeal irritation and infection. In addition to specific drug management of any infection, antipyretics, fluids, alcohol sponges, and a hypothermia blanket may be used to reduce the patient's temperature. Insertion of a rectal thermometer probe provides for continuous and accurate determination of temperature.

The operative site is observed for bleeding and the amount of drainage. A drain may have been inserted at surgery to facilitate removal of excessive drainage. The drain usually remains for 48 to 72 hours postoperatively. The drainage system should be observed for patency and maintained carefully to preserve sterility. The degree of periorbital edema and ecchymoses should be noted frequently.

Patients who have experienced surgery for an *infratentorial lesion* should remain flat in bed with the head stabilized (with a restrictive dressing) to prevent flexion onto the chest. The ability to swallow and the gag reflex must be present before oral intake is begun. The patient must be observed carefully for respiratory difficulty.

**R**adiation Therapy  The patient with a brain tumor may have radiation therapy following surgical intervention; this may be on an outpatient basis. In other instances, the patient receiving whole-brain irradiation for metastatic lesions may be hospitalized for the duration of therapy. The hospitalized patient would be observed for signs of increasing intracranial pressure secondary to cerebral edema caused by the radiation. The patient would receive steroids prior to and during treatment to reduce cerebral edema around the tumor.[49]

Patients and their families will have varying

degrees of understanding of the illness and proposed treatment. It is helpful to ascertain their understanding and perceptions. During the initial visit for radiation treatment the patient will receive a physical examination. These data together with any previous data are interpreted in order to make a decision to treat the patient, a decision which is made with the patient and the family.

The next phase of treatment is to define the specific area of the brain to be treated and the dosage calculated for the individual patient. A simulator machine is used to outline the tumor and determine its volume. This information is computerized to select the treatment plan.

In order to restrict radiation only to the specific area being radiated, a focus block is made and attached to the cobalt machine above the patient. It may also be necessary to make a molded lightweight plaster cast to hold the head still and pinpoint the focus of the radiation.

If the patient has undergone intracranial surgery, the sutures should have been removed, the wound healed, and no signs of local infection should be present before radiation therapy is begun. The actual time for a single treatment from the cobalt machine is approximately two minutes.

*Alopecia,* or loss of hair, is manifested after the initiation of radiation therapy to the brain. A deficiency of hair can occur after only one or two treatments. The patient's self-image is affected by the change in physical appearance. The patient frequently feels more comfortable wearing a cap. Women usually prefer attractive scarves or wigs.

*Skin reaction* from treatment may be described as a radiodermatitis or radioepithelitis due to loss of the epidermal or epithelial layers of the skin.[50] Care of the skin includes the following interventions:

1   The calculated markings on the skin delineating the port of the irradiation should not be removed.

2   The skin may be washed gently with a mild soap and water and patted dry.

3   Lotions, oils, and creams should not be applied.

4   Should the reaction become more acute, characterized by weeping of the skin, the therapist may postpone the next treatment.

5   The radiation therapist may prescribe a lotion for application to the site.

6   The skin should always be protected from exposure to direct sunlight by a hat or scarf.

*Fatigue* is experienced by many patients receiving radiation therapy. The nurse may plan with the patient and family to schedule the appointment at a time of day when the patient feels less fatigue or following a rest period. It may be helpful to have a family member or friend accompany the patient for therapy. The patient may be able to select those activities that are most meaningful and use energy resources accordingly. The patient's daily schedule should reflect periods of rest alternating with periods of activity.

An adequate *nutritional* intake is necessary and can be assessed with the patient and family. The ability of the patient or spouse to prepare meals should be assessed, and a referral can be made to agencies for assistance, such as the Meals On Wheels Program, if necessary. The patient's weight should be monitored weekly during treatment. *Dehydration* may occur, and the patient's status should be assessed. Fluid intake should be maintained and encouraged.

Patients receiving radiation treatment may experience a depression of platelets (thrombocytopenia) and white blood cells (leukopenia). Blood is drawn on a weekly basis to monitor these parameters. The patient should report and be observed for easy bruising, gums that bleed, the appearance of petechiae, and any other signs of bleeding, such as hematuria or tarry stools. The use of a soft toothbrush and electric razor reduces the initiation of bleeding. If the white blood cell count is depressed, the patient should avoid crowds and persons with infections, and should report any signs of infection.

**Chemotherapy**   Over the past 20 years several antineoplastic agents have been administered to patients via various routes. Chemotherapy has been used in combination with surgery and radiation therapy. Drugs with certain pharmacological properties cross the blood-brain barrier to concentrate within brain tumors. Two drugs, BCNU and methyl-CCNU (nitrosureas), are being used together and in combination with radiation therapy. These therapies are being studied in patients with malignant gliomas.[51]

BCNU and methyl-CCNU are administered intravenously. The patient may feel a burning sensation at the infusion site. Following administration of these drugs, nausea and vomiting are experienced. Antiemetic medications may alleviate these symptoms.

Other possible side effects are leukopenia, thrombocytopenia, and erythrocytopenia. In addition to the interventions for leukopenia and thrombocytopenia described under Radiation Therapy, interventions for erythrocytopenia include the administration of packed red blood cells, planned periods of rest, and a diet high in protein, iron, and vitamin C.[52] If chemotherapy is used in conjunction with radiation therapy, the reactions may occur sooner and be more severe.[53]

**E**motional Response to Brain Tumor  The emotional responses occurring with a brain tumor vary from patient to patient. These manifestations are similar to those occurring with other catastrophic losses suffered by the individual. Determinants of the response seem related to the patient's premorbid personality and to the rapidity of brain destruction. The premorbid personality is perhaps the best clue, and therefore it is essential to have specific information regarding the patient's preexisting personality.

With a rapidly growing tumor, the patient's psychological defenses often cannot be constructed and perfected fast enough to accommodate for the brain tumor. The patient's response is frequently one of psychologic decompensation and depression that is reflective of the ever-increasing limitations of advancing age.[54]

### Fourth-Level Nursing Care

The process of assisting the patient to become as self-dependent as possible begins in the hospital and continues after discharge. It is of utmost importance that the nurse plan with the patient and family for continuity of care. If the patient is discharged home, referral to community agencies such as the Visiting Nurse Association and the Meals On Wheels Program may be appropriate after evaluation of the patient and family need. Other patients may be referred to a rehabilitation facility where the focus of care will include nursing, physical therapy, speech therapy, occupational therapy, and vocational evaluation as indicated (see Chaps. 32 and 34). Still other patients' conditions will progressively deteriorate, and the nurse will be assisting the patient and family to deal with death (see Chap. 3).

The patient will be returning to an out-patient clinic for further treatment, observation, and evaluation. The nurse will need to assess the patient's physical condition and emotional status, as well as interact with the family to determine their ability to manage the situation and deal with their own feelings. The nurse will evaluate the patient for changes in relation to baseline data.

The status of some patients will change and require hospitalization and a second surgical pro-

cedure for reoccurrence of tumor. Communication of data to provide for continuity of care is essential between nurses in different settings.

As needs are identified, various health team members can share in assisting the patient and family to handle their feelings and other problems, including financial and social. The clergy, social worker, and psychiatrist are team members available to assist in counseling the patient and family.

## SPINAL CORD TUMORS

Spinal cord neoplasms include any new growth within the vertebral canal. Based upon their anatomic relation to the dura mater, tumors affecting the spinal cord are classified as follows:

*Extradural tumors* arise in the vertebral column or in the extradural space; they compose 30 to 35 percent of all primary spinal cord tumors. Neurofibroma, meningioma, and hemangioma are the most frequent types. Metastatic carcinomas to the spine have preference for the extradural space.

*Intradural extramedullary tumors* lie between the dura mater and the spinal cord; they compose a little over 50 percent of primary cord tumors. The most common extramedullary spinal tumors are schwannomas, sarcomas, and meningiomas.

*Intramedullary tumors* arise within the spinal cord itself; they compose 10 to 15 percent of the primary spinal cord tumors. Ependymomas and gliomas are the most frequent histologic types.[55-57]

Most *spinal cord* tumors are primary lesions, while metastatic lesions to the cord are from primary growths in the breast, lung, thyroid, kidney, prostate, and gastrointestinal tract. Approximately 50 percent of cord tumors occur in the thoracic region, 30 percent in the cervical region, and 20 percent in the lumbar region.[58]

### Effects on the Patient

The manifestations of spinal cord tumors occur mainly as a result of their mechanical effects: (1) Irritation and compression of spinal nerve roots, (2) compression and displacement of the spinal cord, and (3) obstruction of the vascular supply. The mechanical alterations result in symptoms of progressive *cord compression,* with focal neurologic signs related to the size, position, and level of the neoplasm. (Review the spinal motor and sensory pathways in Chap. 31.) There is variation in the manifestations of motor and sensory disturbances due to the location of the tumor in relation to the involved pathways in the cord, i.e., whether the tumor is located ventrally, laterally, or dorsally to the cord.

Patients experience three stages in the development of spinal tumors. The *first* stage is a unilateral *radicular* syndrome that is characterized by nerve root pain due to irritation of the spinal nerve roots. The pain is usually intermittent, aggravated by movement, coughing, straining, and sneezing.

During the *second* stage, early cord compression occurs resulting in early *Brown-Séquard* syndrome. There is relative hyperreflexia in the legs compared with hyporeflexia in the arms, early disturbances of posterior column sensory function (vibration sense, pattern recognition), or unilateral disturbances of pain and temperature. The *third* stage is manifested by complete *cord compression* or bilateral paralysis.[59]

General symptoms of spinal neoplasms that may be revealed during the *health history* include pain, sensory impairments, motor impairment, and sphincter disturbances. *Pain* in the back is frequent and may be present for a long time. The pain is a result of nerve root or periosteal irritation or compression. It may be absent at times, severe and constant, or exaggerated by coughing, activity, or straining.

*Sensory impairment* may progress rapidly within several hours or days if the compression is from a malignant tumor or hemorrhage within a benign tumor. Usually the patient describes slowly progressing coldness, numbness, and/or tingling in one extremity. There may be a narrow band of hyperesthesia at the level of the lesion.

*Motor weakness* may be present, keeping pace with the sensory disturbances. Slowly there is increasing weakness, clumsiness, and spasticity. The manifestations may spread homolaterally or contralaterally.

*Sphincter disturbances* initially may be manifested by urgency and difficulty in initiating urination, progressing to retention and overflow incontinence. Difficulty in rectal sphincter control usually is manifested as a late sign.[60]

In the presence of spinal cord tumors, a *lumbar puncture* may reveal increased protein in the cerebrospinal fluid. There is often a partial or complete blockage to the flow of cerebrospinal fluid due to a lesion within the vertebral canal. The diagnosis and localization of spinal cord tumors can be confirmed by lumbar puncture, roentgen studies, and myelography.[61] For spinal cord lesions, a *laminectomy* (the removal of the dorsal arches of the vertebral column to expose the spinal cord) is performed, and the tumor is removed. Radiation therapy and chemotherapy may also be utilized when appropriate.

## REFERENCES

1   H. Tuchmann-Duplessis et al., *Nervous System and Endocrine Glands,* trans. by Lucille S. Hurley, *Illustrated Human Embryology,* Vol. III, Springer-Verlag, New York, p. 2.

2   Helena Kryk et al., "Grand Rounds on Brain Tumors," *Can Nurse,* **71:**42, September 1975.

3   *Ibid.*

4   Robert A. Fishman, *Textbook of Medicine,* in Paul B. Beeson and Walsh McDermott (eds.), 14th ed., Saunders, Philadelphia, 1975, p. 735.

5   Michael Walker, *Cancer Medicine,* in James F. Holland and Emil Frei III (eds.), Lea & Febiger, Philadelphia, 1973, p. 1398.

6   *Ibid.,* p. 1386.

7   Kryk et al., *op. cit.,* p. 42.

8   K. J. Zulch and H. D. Mennel, *Tumours of the Brain and Skull,* in P. J. Vinken and G. W. Bruyn (eds.), *Handbook of Clinical Neurology,* Vol. 16, Pt. I, American Elsevier, New York, 1974, p. 6.

9   *Ibid.,* p. 9.

10   Fishman, *op. cit.,* p. 734.

11   Guy McKhann, *The Principles and Practices of Medicine,* in A. McGehee Harvey et al. (eds.), Appleton-Century-Crofts, New York, 1976, p. 1554.

12   L. J. Rubinstein, *Advances in Neurology,* in R. A. Thompson and J. R. Green (eds.), Raven Press, New York, 1976, p. 19.

13   John D. Waggener and John L. Beggs, *Advances in Neurology,* in R. A. Thompson and J. R. Green (eds.), Raven Press, New York, 1976, p. 27–32.

14   Fishman, *op. cit.,* p. 734.

15   Zulch and Mennel, *op. cit.,* pp. 30–33.

16   Jonathan H. Pincus and Gary J. Tucker, *Behavioral Neurology,* Oxford University Press, New York, 1974, p. 187.

17   Harold G. Wolff, *Signs and Symptoms,* in Cyril M. MacBryde and Robert S. Blacklow (eds.), 5th ed., revised by Helen Goodell et al., Lippincott, Philadelphia, 1970, p. 66.

18   *Ibid.*

19   Zulch and Mennel, *op. cit.,* p. 59.

20   Pincus and Tucker, *op. cit.,* p. 13.

21   Donald Mulder and Wendell M. Swenson, *Tumours of the Brain and Skull,* in P. J. Vinken and G. W. Bruyn (eds.), *Handbook of Clinical Neurology,* Vol. 16, Pt. I, American Elsevier, New York, 1974, p. 728.

22   Henry Hecaen and Martin Albert, *Psychiatric Aspects of Neurologic Disease,* in D. Frank Benson

and Dietrich Blumer (eds.), *Seminars in Psychiatry,* Grune & Stratton, New York, 1975, p. 140.

23 *Ibid.,* p. 138.

24 Dietrich Blumer and D. Frank Benson, *Psychiatric Aspects of Neurologic Disease,* in D. Frank Benson and Dietrich Blumer (eds.), *Seminars In Psychiatry,* Grune & Stratton, New York, 1975, p. 157.

25 *Ibid.*

26 Hecaen and Albert, *op. cit.,* pp. 138–139.

27 *Ibid.*

28 Blumer and Benson, *op. cit.,* p. 158.

29 Blumer and Benson, *op. cit.,* p. 165.

30 Hecaen and Albert, *op. cit.,* p. 139.

31 Zbigniew J. Lipowski, *Psychiatric Aspects of Neurologic Disease,* in D. Frank Benson and Dietrich Blumer (eds.), *Seminars in Psychiatry,* Grune & Stratton, New York, 1975, pp. 14–15.

32 Fishman, *op. cit.,* p. 736.

33 McKhann, *op. cit.,* p. 1558.

34 *Ibid.,* p. 1556.

35 *Ibid.*

36 *Ibid.,* p. 1556.

37 James Ambrose, "Computerized Transverse Axial Scanning (tomography): Part 2. Clinical Application," *Br J Radiol,* **46:**1023, December 1973.

38 Russell N. DeJong, *The Neurologic Examination,* 3d ed., Harper & Row, Hoeber Medical Division, New York, 1970, p. 129.

39 Alfred Huber, *Eye Signs and Symptoms in Brain Tumors,* 3d ed., Mosby, St. Louis, 1976, p. 191.

40 *Ibid.,* p. 4.

41 Arthur C. Guyton, *Textbook of Medical Physiology,* 5th ed., Saunders, Philadelphia, 1976, p. 272.

42 Fred Plum and Jerome B. Posner, *The Diagnosis of Stupor and Coma,* Contemporary Neurology Series, Vol. 10, 2d ed., Davis, Philadelphia, 1972, p. 26.

43 DeJong, *op. cit.,* p. 949–950.

44 Plum and Posner, *op. cit.,* pp. 2–5.

45 DeJong, *op. cit.,* p. 734.

46 Betty S. Bergersen, *Pharmacology in Nursing,* 13th ed., Mosby, St. Louis, 1976, p. 233.

47 DeJong, *op. cit.,* p. 950.

48 David A. Ontjes and Robert L. Ney, "Pituitary Tumors," *CA,* **26:** 6, 346, November/December 1976.

49 Jerome B. Posner, "Diagnosis and Treatment of Metastases to the Brain," Addendum: Nessa Coyle: "Nursing Implications," *Nurs Digest,* December 1975, p. 62.

50 Carolyn Elliott, "Radiation Therapy: How You Can Help," *Nursing 76,* September 1976, p. 38.

51 Michael D. Walker, "New Approaches to Chemotherapy of CNS Tumors," lecture at Turner Auditorium, Johns Hopkins Medical Institutions, February 28, 1977.

52 Janet Barber et al., *Adult and Child Care,* 2d ed., Mosby, St. Louis, 1977, p. 182.

53 Elliott, *op. cit.,* p. 41.

54 Mulder and Swenson, *op. cit.,* pp. 735–736.

55 Fishman, *op. cit.,* p. 776.

56 Frank H. Netter, *Nervous System,* The Ciba Collection of Medical Illustrations, Vol. 1, Ciba Pharmaceutical Company, Division of Ciba-Geigy Corporation, 1972, p. 129.

57 John R. Green et al., *Advances in Neurology,* R. A. Thompson and J. R. Green (eds.), Raven Press, New York, 1976, p. 53.

58 Netter, *op. cit.,* p. 128.

59 Hans Schliack and Dirk Stille, *Tumors of the Spine and Spinal Cord,* in P. J. Vinken and G. W. Bruyn (eds.), *Handbook of Clinical Neurology,* Vol. 19, Pt. 1, American Elsevier, New York, 1974, pp. 24–25.

60 Netter, *op. cit.,* pp. 128–129.

61 DeJong, *op. cit.,* p. 800.

## BIBLIOGRAPHY

Buehler, Janice A.: "What Contributes To Hope in the Cancer Patient?" *Am J Nurs,* **75:**8, 1353–1356, August 1975.

Burrell, Zeb L., and Lenette Burrell: *Critical Care,* Mosby, St. Louis, 1977.

Carini, Esta, and Guy Owens: *Neurological and Neurosurgical Nursing,* 6th ed., Mosby, St. Louis, 1974.

Guyton, Arthur: *Textbook of Medical Physiology,* 5th ed., Saunders, Philadelphia, 1976, p. 272.

Jimm, Louise R.: "Nursing Assessment of Patients for Increased Intracranial Pressure," *J Neurosurg Nurs,* **6:**1:27–37, July 1974.

Mazzola, Rosanne, and George B. Jacobs: "Helping the Patient and the Family Deal with a Crisis Situation," *J Neurosurg Nurs,* **6:**2, 85–88, December 1974.

Morris, Magdalena, and Martha Rhodes: "Guidelines for the Care of Confused Patients," *Am J Nurs,* **72:**9, 1630–1633, September 1972.

Nelson, Gail: "Current Approaches in the Treatment of Malignant Gliomas of the Brain," *J Neurosurg Nurs,* **6:**2, 109–116, December 1974.

Nikas, Diana L., and Rose Konkoly: "Nursing Responsibilities in Arterial and Intracranial Pressure Monitoring," *J Neurosurg Nurs,* **7:**2, 116–122, December 1975.

Pohutsky, Lorraine C., and Karen R. Pohutsky: "Computerized Axial Tomography of the Brain: A New Diagnostic Tool," *Am J Nurs,* **75:**8, 1341–1342, August 1975.

# 36

# INFLAMMATORY DISTURBANCES IN PERCEPTION AND COORDINATION

Rita Kraut

Infectious agents from the external and internal environments may invade the human organism and set up inflammatory reactions throughout the body. Inflammatory processes in the central nervous system are potentially devastating as they affect the brain on all levels. The *cerebral cortex* may be affected; the result, depending on the area, may be changes in the level of consciousness or in higher integral functions, weakness, or paralysis. *Cerebellar* damage due to an inflammatory disease may result in an ataxic gait or a disturbance of proprioception. *Cranial nerve* destruction due to an inflammatory process in the brain stem can result in severe facial, ophthalmological, ear, nose, throat, and respiratory disturbances.

The rapidity of the onset of inflammatory diseases adds to their overwhelming effect. A person can be alert and oriented one minute and stuporous the next. The subtleties of caring for a neurologically ill patient require the astute observational skills of a highly qualified clinician.

Inflammation of the central nervous system is diverse, and its effects are vast. In this chapter some of the most common and most devastating of the group of inflammatory processes will be discussed; these include viral encephalitis, meningitis, brain abscess, rabies, poliomyelitis, and Guillain-Barré disease.

## ENCEPHALITIS

*Encephalitis* is an inflammation of the brain. Usually it is caused by a viral (especially arboviruses and herpes simplex virus) or bacterial invasion. However, protozoa, rickettsia, and worms can also manifest themselves in the inflammatory process. Bacterial encephalitis may be classified under meningitis; for this reason, only viral encephalitis will be discussed in this portion of the chapter.

*Viral encephalitis* is seen when there is transmission of a neurotropic virus (one with a special affinity for damaging nervous tissue) from an intermediate host, such as a horse (equine encephalitis), to man. Encephalitis can be of many types, and the viruses responsible for it are constantly changing. It can occur in epidemic form as a result of viral transmission from an animal to a human, or it can result from a systemic viral infection such as measles, mumps, or chicken pox. The epidemic forms are the most common causes of the disease.

*Epidemic viral encephalitis* usually occurs regionally in limited epidemic form during the summer months. Viruses are named for the region of the world affected. The most severe and destructive type is eastern equine encephalitis, found in the eastern portion of the United States and in Canada, Cuba, and Brazil. Its less severe western counterpart is western equine encephalitis. Probably the most common form of encephalitis is St. Louis encephalitis which is found in the midwestern United States. All these are examples of mosquito-borne viruses. Russian spring-summer encephalitis, found throughout Russia and Central Europe, is an example of a tick-borne disease process.

### Pathophysiology

The *pathophysiology* of viral encephalitis shows perivascular cellular infiltration and proliferation of the glia. A widespread involvement of the nerve cell exhibits changes in, or complete obliteration of, the nucleus. There may be necrosis of the cell wall with deposits of fibrin seen in the area. The vessels may be affected owing to the invasion of neutrophils and leukocytes into the vessel wall. Thrombosis may occur with resultant small infarcts. The white matter (area of myelinated nerve cell fibers) may or may not be affected. Usually the destruction is limited to the cortex, basal ganglions, and brainstem. Destruction of the cerebellum and spinal cord occurs infrequently. The degree of damage done by the viral infiltration depends on the type and the severity of the virus.

Because of the variation in the type of the virus and its severity, the *effects* upon patients are also within a wide range. These effects may be entirely subclinical or may include fever, chills, vomiting, and drowsiness. The drowsiness may progress to coma within a few days. Signs of meningeal irritation may also occur, including head and neck stiffness (Fig. 36-1), altered level of consciousness, and seizures.

The *prognosis* for a person with encephalitis is also dependent upon the causative virus and the severity of the disease. The death rate in any given epidemic has been from 10 to 35 percent.[1] In some epidemics the death rate has been as high as 65 percent. The usual course of the disease is from 2 to 3 weeks, although symptoms begin to subside within 7 to 10 days; the temperature falls to normal and there is a general decrease of other symptoms. At times the encephalitis process may linger in a subclinical form for 1 to 2 months.

### First-Level Nursing Care

Viral encephalitis is seen when there is a transmission of a neurotropic virus from an intermediate host, such as a horse, to man. The mode of transmission is usually via a tick or mosquito (arboviruses). For example, in equine encephalitis birds initially harbor the virus and act as the reservoir. The mosquito vector transmits the virus from the bird to a horse, where it causes a subacute en-

**FIGURE 36-1**

Opisthotonus position: Extreme arching of the back with retraction of the head noted in patients suffering from meningeal irritation.

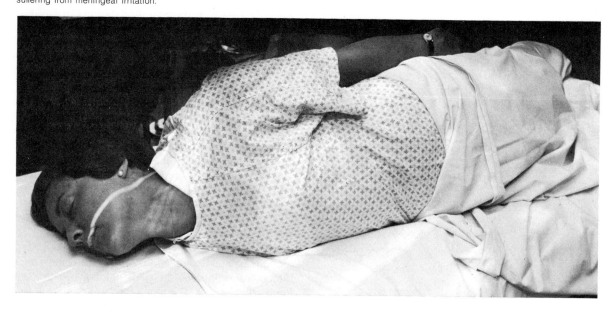

cephalomyelitis (infection of the brain and spinal cord). Then the mosquito transmits the virus from the horse to a previously healthy person.

*Prevention* of encephalitis starts at the level of environmental control. New Jersey, one of the most frequent sites of encephalitis epidemics, contains vast areas of marshland which are infected by mosquitoes. Proper maintenance of marshlands and spraying to prevent mosquito and tick infestation can decrease the incidence of epidemics markedly. Also, proper inoculation of horses and other animals will retard any viral process and prevent its transmission to human beings. Education of the public concerning the importance of avoiding mosquito- and tick-infested areas as well as the value of screening windows and doors is vital. The nurse in the community setting can be very valuable in transmitting this information and ensuring that all measures are taken to prevent the occurrence of this disease.

### Second-Level Nursing Care
Because early symptoms of encephalitis may be subtle, the initial assessment must be particularly attuned to vague findings. The nurse in the community should be aware of these findings when seeing susceptible patients.

**Nursing assessment**  A complete *health history* is of the utmost importance. Questions should be asked concerning the events of the days prior to seeking medical help; the time in question should cover at least the preceding 3 weeks, as the incubation period for encephalitis varies from 5 to 15 days. Has the individual been in contact with farm animals in the last few days? Does the person remember being bitten by a mosquito? Was the individual near swampland or tick-infested bush areas?

The patient may complain of lethargy and generalized malaise. The disease process may also be characterized by a headache that increases in intensity.

*Physical assessment* may reveal the presence of a high fever and nuchal rigidity. Signs of focal damage to the brain such as seizures (Chap. 33), cranial nerve destruction, and hemiplegia are often seen, as are the signs of increased intracranial pressure (Chap. 32). A check should be made from head to toe for insects or imbedded ticks. *Diagnostic tests* are usually performed after hospitalization.

**Nursing problems and intervention**  The problems at this early stage are the presence of a *high*

*fever* and the *history of possible or direct viral contact.* Intervention is careful nursing assessment followed by immediate *referral* to a physician or local hospital for complete evaluation.

### Third-Level Nursing Care
Patients may be admitted to acute-care facilities with symptoms ranging from fever and headache to deep coma. Nurses should be aware of this wide variation when doing the nursing assessment.

**Nursing assessment**  The *health history* for the patient with encephalitis includes those items mentioned under Second-Level Nursing Care. This information may have to be obtained from a family member or knowledgeable acquaintance, if the person is comatose.

Neurological status should be established on *physical assessment* and used as a baseline thereafter. This includes the individual's level of consciousness, orientation, and higher integral functioning. The quality of the patient's speech and ability to articulate should also be evaluated. Blood pressure, pulse, pupil reaction, and the quality of respirations should be assessed and any changes noted. The presence of any motor or sensory changes, weakness, or paralysis should be ascertained by checking the movement of the extremities. The patient should be observed for signs of cranial nerve involvement such as nystagmus, strabismus, diplopia, dysarthria, and ptosis. Any signs of intracranial pressure and/or meningeal irritation should be noted.

**Diagnostic Tests**  A *lumbar puncture* is usually performed to rule out any bacterial invasion. In the presence of an encephalitic process there may be an elevation of cerebrospinal fluid pressure due to cerebral edema. The spinal fluid should appear clear in color, as cloudiness would indicate bacterial invasion. The protein level may be slightly elevated, and the glucose content should be normal.

*Complement-fixation* and *virus neutralization* tests are done to help identify the virus. The results of these tests are of more value in data collecting and classification than for immediate treatment of the illness, because the results cannot be made available immediately. Usually the results are obtained after the acute phase of the disease has passed.

Also of interest is *serological testing* for arthropod-borne viruses. Although human infection may be extremely widespread, as guided by serological testing, only a few of the infected individuals may show clinical evidence of encephalitis.

**Nursing problems and intervention** Treatment of encephalitis is symptomatic. Antipyretic agents are given for the *fever,* along with mechanical means of lowering body temperature. Analgesics are ordered as *headaches* associated with encephalitis become severe. Anticonvulsants are given in the presence of *seizure* disorders (Chap. 33). *Cerebral edema* may be treated with steroids and osmotic diuretics. Because of these problems, ongoing neurologic assessment by the nurse is essential. It is recommended that these observations be made and documented at least every hour.

**R**espiratory Impairment  In severe cases, where *respiratory impairment* is present, a tracheostomy and mechanical ventilation may be necessary (Fig. 36-2). As in any debilitating condition, good pulmonary toilet is essential. An emphasis should be placed on percussing, coughing, and stimulating the patient to deep breathe frequently. In the presence of cranial nerve involvement all measures should be taken to prevent aspiration. The gag reflex should be evaluated frequently, and the patient should always be fed in high Fowler's position.

**I**ncreased Reaction to Sensory Stimuli  Patients with encephalitis, as with many other neurological diseases, react very poorly to increased sensory stimuli. During the acute phase, it is recommended that the patient be kept as quiet as possible and outside stimuli be kept to a minimum. Changes in sleep-wake patterns usually occur; these patients tend to sleep during the day and remain awake at night. All efforts should be made to repattern the patient toward more normal behavior by keeping the person awake during the day and promoting sleep and rest at night.

**I**mmobility  If the inflammatory process is so severe that the patient is comatose, routine care for the immobilized patient should be given (Chaps. 32

**FIGURE 36-2**
Patient with acute bacterial meningitis resulting in complete quadriplegia and respiratory depression necessitating mechanical ventilation.

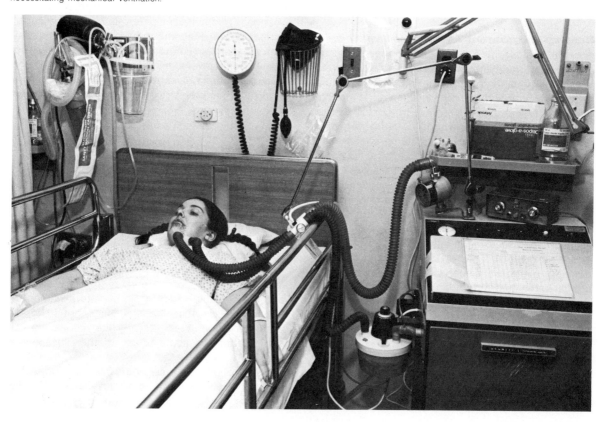

and 40). The patient must be turned every 2 hours. Flotation pads or an air mattress should be placed on the patient's bed to prevent skin breakdown. Range of motion to all extremities should be done every 4 hours to prevent contractures; physical and occupational therapy should be instituted immediately, and corrective devices such as splints and Stryker boots obtained as necessary.

### Fourth-Level Nursing Care

The *residual effects* of encephalitis may be many. The patient may be left with headaches, fatigability, and irritability that can last for any length of time. Mental disturbances, alteration of personality, paresis of limbs, mental retardation, seizure disorders, and Parkinsonism can also occur. The appearance of these neurological sequellae may be transient or permanent.

In terms of the psychological aspects of patient care, the nurse's responsibilities are numerous. The nurse can help the patient deal with the overwhelming frustrations of a devastating disease and help the patient and family understand the disease process. As a coordinator and initiator, the nurse must identify the need for physical and vocational rehabilitation and psychiatric consultation. The nurse can assist these people to return to an optimum state of health, taking into consideration their deficits.

## MENINGITIS

*Meningitis* is an inflammation or infection of the piarachnoid membrane that covers the brain and spinal cord. The disease process may be due to a bacterial or viral invasion of the meninges or to chemical irritation. In all instances the symptoms are similar. The following discussion is specific for bacterial meningitis.

### Pathophysiology

*Bacterial meningitis* is an acute, subacute, or chronic inflammatory process leading to the formation of purulent matter. The causative organism may be meningococcus, staphylococcus, streptococcus, pneumococcus, *Myobacterium tuberculosis,* or *Escherichia coli.* The bacterial invasion stimulates a meningeal hyperemia with infiltration by polymorphonuclear leukocytes (PMN) into the spinal fluid. The PMNs break up, and histiocytes, plasma cells, and fibrin appear. This process is accompanied by an acute vasculitis, thrombosis, and local infarction. The infection and vasculitis can cause areas of local edema and local necrosis

of the brain and ventricular system. The necrosis and resultant stenosis of the ventricles may lead to a hydrocephalus which is characteristic of meningitis. The prognosis is based on the severity and progression of these symptoms. Pneumococcal meningitis has a 30 percent mortality rate, and staphylococcus meningitis an almost 60 percent mortality rate.[2]

The clinical *effects* of meningitis upon the patient include a severe headache, high fever, seizures, and alterations in consciousness (such as delirium and coma). A crucial sign of meningeal inflammation is stiffness of the neck (*nuchal rigidity*). In this situation, the neck resists passive movement, and the head may be retracted with extreme arching of the back (opisthotonus position), as illustrated in Fig. 36-1. Specific clinical effects vary with the causative organism. Of note is the purpuric rash and echymoses that are characteristic of meningococcal meningitis.

### First-Level Nursing Care

Purulent (bacterial) meningitis is usually the result of a septicemia. However, it can be found following a middle ear, mastoid, or sinus infection. Meningitis can also result from a skull fracture or penetrating wound of the skull or spinal cord. There can be iatrogenic causes resulting from spinal taps or intrathecal injections.

As a primary infection, meningitis is most common in infancy through young adulthood. It is very rare in persons over 25 years of age. It usually occurs in epidemics in the winter and early spring. The infection is spread by carriers who constantly have the bacteria in their nasopharynx and who contaminate others via droplet infection. The mode of transmission explains why meningitis epidemics are seen in densely populated or overcrowded areas, such as schools or military camps.

*Preventive measures* can greatly decrease the prevalence of all types of meningitis. Nursing intervention in educating the public to the transmission (via droplets) of meningitis is paramount. Emphasis should be placed on respiratory care. Instruction in utilizing handkerchiefs and disposable tissues to prevent droplet spread should be given to people of all ages. Proper nutritional instruction should be given to people of all ages because the disease process is less likely to affect a well-nourished individual.

Since meningitis also occurs as a secondary infection, preventive measures should be taken in the presence of upper respiratory, sinus, dental, or ear infections, and following neurosurgical procedures or head trauma; prophylactic antibiotic therapy is usually recommended. The nurse's observational skills are invaluable in caring for these people since early signs of meningitis can be identified and communicated to the physician for prompt intervention.

Adolescents with acne should be instructed never to pick or squeeze pimples on their face especially in the nose, lip, and forehead area. This is a highly vascular area with all vessels leading to the brain.

### Second-Level Nursing Care

The nurse in the community may be the first person to see a patient presenting the classic symptoms of meningitis. It is, therefore, important that this initial assessment be a detailed and thorough one.

**Nursing assessment** The *health history* should determine the presence of any current or recent infections, particularly of the upper respiratory or genitourinary tracts. The exact symptoms, their course, and treatment for the infection should be described. The patient will often be experiencing chills, severe headache, vomiting, photophobia, and/or fever.

Upon *physical assessment,* the infectious process may be reflected by changes in the vital signs. An increased pulse and respiratory rate often accompany the elevated temperature. Acute delirium and seizures are seen in the most severe cases and should be described if present. The patient usually experiences reflex contractions of the posterior neck muscles due to meningeal irritation in the posterior fossa and the upper portion of the spinal cord. The head can be moved from side to side, but there is a resistance to passive neck flexion. In severe cases, papilledema may be evident due to increased intercranial pressure. Fifth, seventh, and eighth cranial nerve involvement may also be evident (refer to Chap. 31). The skin should be checked for the presence of any bruises or rashes, and their appearance and location noted.

Key factors in making a diagnosis of meningitis outside the hospital situation are positive Brudzinski's and Kernig's signs. Brudzinski's sign is tested by raising the patient's head quickly while keeping the chest flat. Flexion of both thighs, at the hips, along with flexion at the ankles and knees, is indicative of meningeal irritation. Kernig's sign is the key finding and can be elicited by passively flexing the hip to a right angle and then trying to extend the knee. Spasm of the hamstring muscle will result be-

cause the leg movement produces a pulling on the cauda equina and inflamed meninges. *Diagnostic tests* are usually performed after hospitalization.

**Nursing problems and intervention** Patients with a *high fever* and signs of *nuchal rigidity* should be *referred* to a physician or hospital for diagnosis. Action should be taken quickly to prevent a further increase in the severity of the symptoms.

### Third-Level Nursing Care

Nursing assessment of the patient who is acutely ill with meningitis is critical in preventing complications and permanent deficits. Interventions are similar to those for encephalitis.

**Nursing assessment** The patient's *health history* will reveal findings as described in Second-Level Nursing Care. Relatives and friends may need to be questioned if the patient is confused or unresponsive.

A baseline *physical assessment* of the patient should be done initially. The neurologic examination should describe any changes in the level of consciousness, which may range from alertness to coma. Any seizure activity or evidence of intracranial pressure should be noted, and the presence and degree of any neck and back rigidity (Fig. 36-1) and/or confusion should be described. Vital signs may vary; the temperature reading is particularly important because of the frequent presence of a high fever.

**D**iagnostic Tests A *lumbar puncture* should be performed immediately. In the presence of meningitis, the cerebrospinal fluid (CSF) will be cloudy to milky white in appearance. This is due to the abnormal white blood cell count which may number as high as 50,000/mm³. The CSF pressure and protein levels are usually elevated, while the sugar concentration is decreased.

Blood cultures are obtained to assist in identifying the causative organism. Chest and skull x-rays may also be taken to detect areas of inflammation or abscess.

**Nursing problems and intervention** Once the presence of meningitis is confirmed, intervention focuses on the problem of the *infection* itself. The organism causing the meningitis must be quickly identified and antibiotic therapy instituted. Any delay could result in death or permanent deficits. The drugs of choice in treating meningitis are penicillin G and sulfonamides. Anticonvulsant medication is also given at this time because of the possibility of *seizure activity.*

Since *increased intracranial pressure* is one of the most common sequellae, osmotic diuretics such as mannitol may be given. It should be noted that the effect of mannitol is not permanent. In severe cases where there is stenosis of the ventricles, a ventricular catheter may be inserted to facilitate drainage of cerebrospinal fluid from the ventricles.

If a ventricular catheter has been inserted to relieve *intracranial pressure,* the nurse should be sure that the catheter is secured properly and that the drainage bottle is also secured at the level prescribed by the physician. The nurse should observe the catheter for patency by checking the fluctuation of the cerebrospinal fluid in the drainage tubing. Care must be taken to ensure sterility at the insertion site. The dressing should be removed by the physician and the site thoroughly cleansed.

Neurological observations should be monitored every hour. At this time symptoms such as *nuchal rigidity, headache, photophobia, irritability,* and *malaise* can be evaluated. Symptomatic relief in the form of muscle relaxants, analgesics, and environmental control may be ordered for the patient.

Close attention should be paid to the respiratory status and *prevention* of *pneumonia.* If there is cranial nerve involvement rendering the patient unable to expectorate secretions, frequent suctioning should be done and respiratory assistance maintained (Figs. 36-2 and 36-3).

Accurate recordings of the patient's intake and output are necessary to ensure *fluid and electrolyte balance.* A Foley catheter may be inserted if the patient is subject to either urinary retention or urinary incontinence. Employing this measure is generally considered a last resort because the catheter is an additional source of infection.

A bowel regime should be instituted if *constipa-*

**FIGURE 36-3**
Patient being ventilated with Ambu-bag while tracheostomy cuff is deflated to prevent tracheal necrosis.

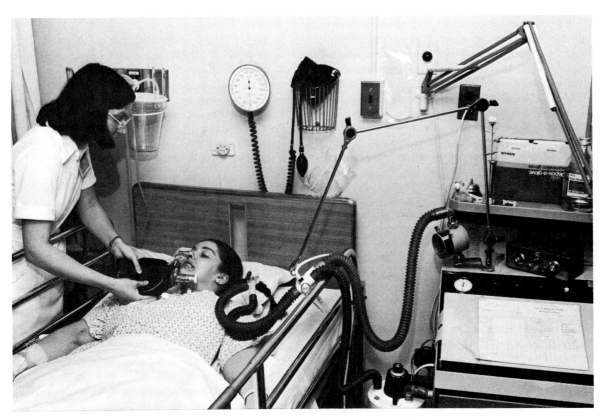

*tion* becomes a problem; this may include giving the patient a suppository every morning and placing him or her on the bedpan an hour later. Stool softeners and laxatives, as well as dietary and fluid adjustments, may also help.

If the patient is lethargic and *unable to move independently,* turning must be done every 2 hours, taking care to maintain proper body alignment. If the nutritional status is poor and the patient is prone to decubitus formation, a sheep skin or flotation pad may be utilized.

In the presence of *paresis* or *plegia,* physical and occupational therapies are instituted (Fig. 36-2). Active or passive range of motion should be done to the affected extremity at least every 4 hours. For lower extremity weakness Stryker boots or high-top sneakers are useful in preventing foot drop.

The patient's *environment* should be similar to that established for patients suffering from encephalitis. That is, a room with minimal stimuli should be provided, and all stressful situations should be avoided. The patient will usually be placed in isolation for a period of time as prescribed by the individual institution. Frequently, the patient is isolated on bed rest until the cultures of the nasal secretions are negative.

If there is a *decrease in the level of consciousness* or if there is an element of confusion, attempts should be made to keep the patient in touch with reality. Realities should be reinforced; misconceptions or misinterpretations should be corrected. There may be great anxiety on the part of the family because it is well known that meningitis is a very severe illness and that even with the most sophisticated medical and nursing care there is a rather high mortality rate. The family needs maximal support from the nurse during this time.

If the patient is in complete control of mental faculties and is aware of the potential seriousness of the condition, many questions may be asked concerning the course of the illness. Clear, concise explanations regarding all aspects of meningitis, as well as the nursing and medical management, are important at this time. The patient must be allowed to express any feelings about the infection and what it means in terms of a future life-style.

### Fourth-Level Nursing Care

Complications of meningitis may be prevented by prompt treatment. Less than 7 percent of patients develop any permanent neurological deficits.[3] Since a form of encephalitis almost always accompanies severe meningitis, many patients are left with symp-

toms of encephalitis. They may have intermittent headache, irritability, dizziness, and decreased memory. These symptoms are usually not permanent. Visual impairment due to opticochiasmatic arachnoiditis can develop. A spastic weakness of the legs due to spinal arachnoiditis may occur. Other complications of meningitis may be acute arthritis, optic neuritis, hearing loss, and endocarditis.

Whatever the deficit present, the nurse and the health team should plan toward returning the patient to optimum health. *Discharge planning* must be initiated early in the illness with the patient, family, and hospital personnel playing equally active roles. If long-term rehabilitation is necessary, a rehabilitation facility or home care should be considered. If the patient is returning immediately to the home, the community nursing service should be contacted to evaluate the home situation. Provisions should be made for patient follow-up either by a private physician or in a clinic. In the presence of emotional disability, or if the patient is having difficulty adjusting, psychiatric consultation should be initiated while the patient is still in a hospital situation and continued on an outpatient basis. If the disease process is devastating to the whole family, family therapy should be initiated.

### BRAIN ABSCESS

The collection of an exudate commonly known as an *abscess* is usually the result of a local or systemic infection. An abscess can occur in any area of the nervous system. It can be extradural, subdural, intradural, or intraspinal. Many of the clinical manifestations are similar to those of meningitis, and in many cases differentiating between the two conditions is difficult.

The most common and most severe abscess is the *intradural* or *cerebral abscess* which occurs predominantly in the white matter. Initially the infectious process starts as a subacute encephalitis. The infection runs rampant, and it may involve the whole surface of the brain causing a diffuse softening, or it may liquefy and become encapsulated. The encapsulated abscess is much less severe as it may become calcified, leaving only a glial scar. In severe cases the abscess may rupture into the ventricles. Cerebral abscesses do not rupture into the surface of the brain. With the rupture there is a blockage of the venous sinus and resultant increased intracranial pressure.

The brain abscess may be the result of a primary infection such as otitis media, mastoiditis, sinusitis, or bronchitis. It can also be seen following septicemia, bacterial endocarditis, pelvic suppuration, and congenital heart disease. Infected emboli reaching the brain via the spinal epidural venous plexus can also cause the disorder. Brain abscess can also result from piercing wounds of the scalp which destroy the bone and dura and reach the brain tissue. This infective process can occur at all ages. However, several studies have found their appearance more common in the 1 to 20- and 50 to 70-year age groups.

As in meningitis, the incidence of disease can be lowered with good *preventive care.* Nurses should help educate the public to the need for proper treatment of sinus, dental, and ear infections. Early treatment should be stressed in the presence of these infections, or other inflammatory processes that could have very serious consequences. In this stage, the process can be retarded by the administration of prophylactic antibiotics.

The nurse in the community often sees a patient with a preexisting infection complaining of the recent onset of a severe headache in the area of the lesion. This may be accompanied by focal epileptic seizures, motor and sensory impairment, a decrease in the level of consciousness and irritability. Many of these patients do not have an elevation of temperature, initially. For this reason, in the beginning stages, it is very difficult to differentiate this infectious process from an expanding intracranial lesion.

The first symptoms may diminish and the patient appear to have recovered. If left untreated, the headaches will become more severe, and signs of *increased intracranial pressure* will be evident. The patient will exhibit a marked deterioration in the level of consciousness, confusion, papilledema, increased blood pressure (especially diastolic blood pressure), decreased pulse, and ataxic respiration.

Many of the focal signs that are seen are dependent on the area of the brain affected. In the presence of a *cerebellar* abscess (Fig. 36-4), there may be transient vertigo, ataxia, nystagmus, and loss or decrease in proprioception. Care should be taken to ensure patient safety at this time. A *temporal lobe* abscess produces a paresis of the face and arm without damage to the leg. There may also be damage to the visual fields. If the abscess is present in the *dominant hemisphere,* dysphasia occurs. An abscess of the *frontal lobe* will eventually affect the motor pathways and cause hemiparesis of the contralateral leg, face, and arm. *Subdural* abscess may produce complete aphasia, hemiplegia, and hemianesthesia.

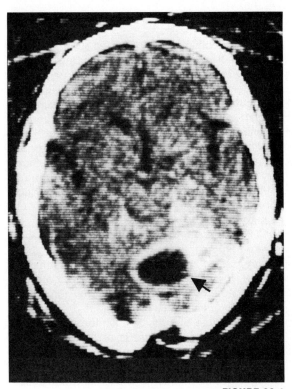

**FIGURE 36-4**
CTT scan revealing a recurrent cerebellar abscess.

A diagnosis of a brain abscess can be made if the patient has a preexisting infection of the face, ear, or nasal sinus and then shows signs of an expanding mass lesion. An *arteriogram* or a *CTT scan* (see Chap. 31) should be performed. *Lumbar puncture* may be done only with great care because there is a danger of precipitating early herniation of the brainstem. It should be performed only when emergency care can easily be instituted. The nurse should be aware of this possibility. The lumbar puncture will reveal an elevated cerebrospinal fluid pressure and an elevated cell count. If the abscess is encapsulated, there will be fewer cells and more lymphocytes. The glucose and chloride levels will be normal unless a meningitis process is present.

Antibiotic therapy is the primary treatment, ideally instituted as soon as the diagnosis is confirmed. The usual treatment is penicillin G, 20 million units daily, chloramphenicol, 50 to 100 mg/kg body weight, and gentamycin, 5 to 6 mg/kg body weight. The dosages may be altered depending on the patient's renal status or associated diseases. All these medications are given intravenously for a period of 4 to 6 weeks. Steroids are given to reduce *cerebral edema,* and prophylactic anticonvulsants are also administered.

The use of an osmotic diuretic such as mannitol may be necessary. A bolus of 50 grams mannitol, intravenously will be effective immediately but is only a temporary measure and lasts only 2 hours. A ventricular catheter can be inserted to ensure ventricular drainage and to decrease intracranial pressure.

In the presence of a quickly expanding cerebral abscess, surgical decompression may be necessary. At this time, the abscess is aspirated and an antibiotic is instilled into the cavity. This is a temporary measure until the encapsulated abscess can be surgically removed.

The remainder of the interventions are directed toward treating the symptoms and preventing complications. The abscess may be so diffuse that the level of consciousness is altered and coma may result. Astute observational skills and quick intervention are of the highest importance. Vital signs in the acute stage should be monitored every half hour, and any changes in the level of consciousness and response to painful stimuli should be carefully noted. If the abscess is severe, careful observation for signs of decortication and decerebration should be made (refer to Chap. 32).

If the respiratory center in the medulla is affected, a tracheostomy and mechanical ventilation may be necessary. As with meningitis and encephalitis, respiratory care is of great importance, and all preventive measures must be taken. If the patient is so severely compromised that mechanical ventilation is necessary, special respiratory care is required, as outlined in Poliomyelitis below.

Proper body positioning and prevention of contractures are of the highest importance in preventing the effects of *immobility.* Physical and occupational therapy should be instituted quickly and corrective devices used.

Accurate assessment of intake and output is extremely important because these patients may develop diabetes insipidis if the abscess disturbs the area around the pituitary gland and prevents the release of antidiuretic hormone stimulatory factors. Any increase in the volume of urine and decrease in its specific gravity should be reported immediately.

Probably the biggest factor in rehabilitative care is the emotional support of the patient and family. Since long-term antibiotic therapy is necessary, a family unit can be disrupted for more than 6 weeks. Even with treatment the outcome is uncertain. Frequent consulting of both the patient and the family is necessary. Diversional therapy is help-

ful during the chronic phase of the illness, taking into consideration the background of the patient and the individual's interests at the present time. Provision should be made early in the hospitalization for an extended-care facility. All community agencies should be utilized if the situation warrants it.

Frequent CTT scans will be done as the patient is recovering and after the patient leaves the hospital situation. They are to ensure that there is no reaccumulation of the abscess. Arrangements should be made for future follow-up examinations before the patient leaves the hospital.

## RABIES

*Rabies,* or *hydrophobia lysia,* is an acute viral disease of the central nervous system which is almost always fatal. The virus is present in the saliva of a rabid animal and can be transmitted to human beings by the bite of the animal.

The disease is characterized by a widespread perivascular infiltration of the brain and spinal cord with lymphocytes, PMNs, and plasma cells. There are diffuse and degenerative changes in the neurons. Inclusion bodies are found in the neurons of the cortex, cerebellum, and spinal ganglions. There is extreme excitability to all peripheral stimuli. Laryngeal and pharyngeal spasms develop and progress to generalized paralysis and death.

The rabid animal is usually a dog; however, cats, bats, wolves, foxes, goats, deer, cows, poultry, and squirrels may also be infected by the virus. The incidence of rabies is largely dependent upon the ability of health departments to control rabid animals through mass innoculation of all domestic pets. It is virtually impossible to innoculate all wild life that may be harboring the disease. Countries such as the United States which have good disease prevention programs have a very low incidence of rabies. However, rabies is still quite prevalent in Southeastern Europe and Asia where programs are not as sophisticated.

The nurse in school or community settings can be invaluable in educating the public (especially children) to be very careful of strange or wild animals. Films may be shown by the nurse to emphasize the severity of the disease and the actions necessary to prevent it.

When a person is bitten, the animal should be confined and observed for a period of 10 days. If during this period the animal begins to exhibit bizarre behavior, it should be destroyed. Its brain should then be examined for rabies virus infiltration. One should remember that not all contact with a rabid animal causes the disease. In fact, only 5 to 10 percent of people bitten by a domesticated animal develop the disease.[4] The percentage is higher in those individuals bitten by a rabid wild animal with about 40 percent of these people becoming afflicted with rabies. One factor determining the incidence of the disease is the proximity of the bite to the head. A bite on the face will most likely manifest the disease, while a bite on the leg may not. The severity of the wound is another factor. Perhaps the most important factor is the amount of saliva coming in contact with the wound. There is a low incidence of rabies in people who have been bitten through clothing because the clothing may clean the infected saliva from the animal's teeth.

If it is documented that the animal is rabid, an *antirabies serum* obtained from horses should be given. A dose is injected locally into the wound. Then, an intramuscular injection of the serum in a dosage of 1000 units/40 lb body weight is given. This should be followed by daily injections over a period of 14 to 21 days of duck embryo vaccine. The vaccine is not without side effects. It can cause a postvaccination encephalitis. The nurse should look for signs of this. Effectiveness of the vaccine will not be known for quite some time because the incubation period varies. The usual incubation period is from 30 to 70 days; however, the disease process has been known to occur anywhere from 20 days to 1 year following exposure.

The earliest symptoms are *pain* and numbness in the area of the wound. These are accompanied by *headache, apathy, drowsiness, anorexia, apprehension,* and *increased irritability.* A period of *excitability* begins after 24 to 72 hours during which any external stimuli may produce twitching or generalized convulsions. There is profuse *salivation* and *spasmodic contractions of the pharynx and larynx* which are usually precipitated by an unsuccessful attempt to swallow. This inability to swallow even water is the source of the name *hydrophobia.* Body temperature at this time may rise to as high as 105 to 107°F. The final stage of the disease is characterized by *generalized paralysis* and *coma.*

From the earliest symptoms of the disease, the patient should be isolated and respiratory precautions employed. These precautions should be maintained throughout the course of the illness. Medical and nursing care involve recognition and treatment of symptoms and prevention of complications. Because the respiratory system is affected in the acute state of the disease, a tracheostomy may be necessary, and the patient may be placed on mechanical ventilation. Routine respiratory and coma care as previously mentioned should be instituted. Passive range of motion should be done with emphasis on preventing contractures. Utilization of intravenous therapy, including prophylactic administration of antibiotics, will probably be necessary.

The disease is almost always fatal. The family requires much help in dealing with the probably imminent death of a once healthy person.

## POLIOMYELITIS

*Poliomyelitis (polio)* is an acute viral disease of the central nervous system, caused by one of three polio viruses, and characterized by destruction of the anterior horn cells of the spinal cord and motor cell destruction of the brainstem. The disease can be manifested in three different areas: *spinal cord poliomyelitis* involves the anterior horn cells; *bulbus poliomyelitis* involves one or all cranial nerves and can occur with spinal poliomyelitis; *encephalitis cerebropoliomyelitis* involves the cerebrum and is difficult to distinguish from other encephalitic processes.

Invasion of the nervous system comes late in the disease. Initially, the virus enters the lymph system via the pharynx and the ileum. It spreads to the cervical and mesenteric lymph nodes and then infiltrates the circulatory system. The virus reaches the nervous system in one of two ways, direct from the bloodstream or by a peripheral sympathetic or sensory ganglion in the gastrointestinal tract or other tissue.

The polio virus has a predilection for the gray matter of the spinal cord, brainstem, and cortex. The large motor cells are mostly affected; however, the inflammatory response also affects the white matter. The viral infiltration of the cell causes a chromatolysis and then a necrosis of the cell. The cell is then phagocytized by polymorphonuclear leukocytes. Accompanying this is an inflammatory reaction in the nearby meninges and in the perivascular spaces. Most of this involvement is seen in the motor area of the cortex. Following the destruction of these cells is a degeneration of the peripheral nerves. There is a *flaccid paralysis* of the muscles innervated by the affected neurons.

Acute poliomyelitis may occur anywhere in the world; however, it is more widely seen in temperate climates. The disease process may occur at any time but is most common in the summer and fall months. The majority of cases of polio are seen in children below the age of 10 years. This age group usually accounts for 80 to 90 percent of those afflicted.[5] Recently there has been an increase in the disease in young adults, with a higher incidence among males than females.

Until 1956, the incidence of polio was extremely high, with about 38,000 cases a year.[6] Usually, it resulted in death or complete paralysis. In 1955 Dr. Jonas Salk discovered a vaccine of formulinized polio virus to immunize people against the disease. Mass innoculation was done with a resultant decrease in the prevalence and severity of the manifestations. In fact, the year after its discovery, the incidence of polio had decreased by 50 percent.[7]

A further decrease in the incidence of poliomyelitis was seen after the discovery of the oral Sabin vaccine in 1961. The Sabin vaccine is a live attenuated polio virus which, after administration, produces an antibody response. This response is initiated by the virus in the gastrointestinal tract. The Sabin vaccine's administration is begun after an infant is 6 weeks old and is followed by two more doses during the first year of life. It is recommended that a fourth dose be given before the child enters school.

The nurse plays a very important role in educating the public concerning the importance of immunization against polio. Mandatory immunization of all children entering school will also decrease its incidence. The physician and nurse should be attuned to the early symptoms of polio because the disease is most communicable in its earliest stage. The infected individual should be isolated for a period of 2 weeks or until the acute phase is over. Stool and respiratory precautions must be instituted because the disease is transmitted via feces and pharyngeal secretions. Children should be cautioned to stay away from large crowds during the summer months. Swimming facilities should be closed if cases of polio are seen. Since one portal of entry for the polio virus may be the tonsils, tonsilectomies are not advisable during the summer months.

The incubation period for poliomyelitis is 5 to 12 days. The nurse in the school or community setting should be well versed with the earliest symptoms of the disease; they are *fatigue, fever, generalized malaise, headache,* and *gastrointestinal* or *upper respiratory problems.* At this point it is very difficult to differentiate polio from other acute infectious disease processes. The second phase of the disease is characterized by an *increased intensity of the headache* and *generalized muscle pain,* especially in the neck and back. In some cases, the second phase of the disease directly follows the first. In other cases there is a disappearance of symptoms and a state of recovery before the second phase begins. *Drowsiness* and *increased irritability* are seen at this time. *Paralysis* may occur after the second to fifteenth days of the disease.

In the hospital, certain laboratory tests may be done to establish a diagnosis. Lumbar puncture reveals a high cerebrospinal fluid pressure, usually 150 to 200 mmH$_2$O. The cell count will also be elevated. The sugar content will be normal. The protein level may be normal or slightly elevated. The presence of polio virus in either the stool, throat secretions, cerebrospinal fluid, or blood gives a positive diagnosis. The prior sequence of events will also be helpful in making a diagnosis, as will the development of the characteristic flaccid paralysis (that is, if this is the paralytic form of the disease).

*Neurologic examination* of the patient may reveal *flaccid paralysis* with *absent deep tendon reflexes.* The affected extremities are cool and cyanotic. Paralysis of the intercostal muscles and the diaphragm can cause *respiratory failure.* Respiratory problems can also be produced by spread of the disease to the medulla. When cranial nerves are affected, transient *nystagmus* can be seen, as can vocal cord paralysis. *Papilledema* is commonly present in conjunction with acute respiratory problems.

Medical care of an acutely ill polio victim is symptomatic, with emphasis on preventing further disease. Strict bed rest is maintained because it has been found helpful in preventing or limiting paralysis. If *respiratory paralysis* is present, a tracheostomy may be performed and the patient placed on mechanical ventilation. Meticulous respiratory care must be given to these patients. Suctioning should be done as necessary and the head turned from side to side, thus facilitating emptying of both mainstem bronchi. Pulmonary therapy should be done to prevent pneumonia. Placing the patient in postural drainage positions and turning frequently in the positions will facilitate drainage of both lungs. If the patient is on a respirator requiring an inflated tracheostomy tube, care should be taken to deflate the cuff every hour to prevent tracheal necrosis. It is important to remember to suction the patient orally before deflating the cuff. If this is not done, all mucus accumulated above the cuff will fall into the trachea, causing aspiration pneumonia.

If the patient has bulbar signs and is unable to take fluids, intravenous therapy should be initiated. If the bulbar paralysis is long-standing, a nasogastric or gastrostomy feeding tube is indicated. In the presence of urinary retention a Foley catheter should be inserted. Prophylactic antibiotics may be given if there is any respiratory or cranial nerve involvement as a treatment for possible aspiration pneumonia.

The most important factor in the treatment of a person with poliomyelitis is the *nursing intervention.* The nurse's observational skills are important. Vital signs should be monitored frequently, with close attention paid to the quality and rate of the patient's respirations. In the early stages of hospitalization, the vital capacity should be measured every 4 hours. Any decrease in the forcefulness of respiration must be reported immediately. The degree of weakness or paralysis, level of consciousness, and mental status are monitored frequently and documented.

If there is *7th cranial nerve involvement* and subsequent inability of the patient to close the eyes, methylcellulose eye drops should be instilled, and the use of clear protective shields employed (Fig. 36-5). Proper body alignment is important, with splints and pillows utilized to maintain positions of function. Stryker boots or high-top sneakers may

be necessary to prevent foot drop. Passive range of motion should be started early to prevent contractures. Active range of motion can be started as soon as the slightest return of function is noted. Meticulous skin care should be given with emphasis on prevention of decubiti. As defecation may be a problem, bowel training may become necessary.

Usually the patient suffering from poliomyelitis is alert and oriented and is completely cognizant of the disease. The manifestations of illness in this once healthy individual may be devastating, for this is an individual whose every movement is dependent on another person. The simplest action such as scratching the nose has become a dependent function. It is both *frightening* and *frustrating* for the patient. The patient lies paralyzed and probably unable to communicate. The nurse can help by teaching the individual to click the teeth when something is needed. An alphabet board such as the one used for aphasic patients may be useful.

At this time it is very difficult for the patient to express feelings because the methods of communication are primitive. The nurse should consider the

**FIGURE 36-5**
Protective eye shield being placed on a Guillain-Barré patient with 7th cranial nerve damage.

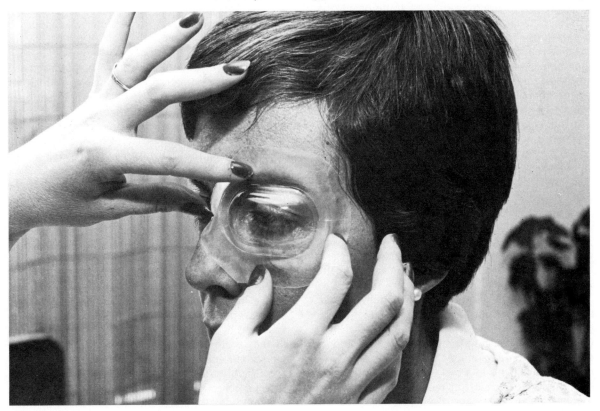

patient's emotional and physical needs before acting and realize that the patient's psychological well-being is greatly dependent upon the nurse. If the nurse can instill confidence, the patient will be made more comfortable.

The prognosis for polio patients is varied. There is a low incidence of mortality, and it is usually associated with respiratory failure. Return of function of affected muscles depends on the severity of the motor cell damage. About 2 percent of those affected are permanently paralyzed.[8] Usually cellular recovery is seen within 2 to 3 months. However, improvement is seen in some patients in 2 to 3 years. Since return of function is possible, physical therapy and occupational therapy should be initiated in the hospital situation and continued. Plans for an extended-care rehabilitation facility should be made as soon as the patient is medically stable. Vocational rehabilitation should be instituted if the disease process causes the patient to be unable to perform at the premorbid level of function.

## GUILLAIN-BARRÉ DISEASE

*Guillain-Barré disease,* or syndrome, or *infectious polyneuropathy* affects the peripheral and cranial nerves and is characterized by an acute onset of a rapidly spreading, ascending polyneuropathy. While the etiology of Guillain-Barré disease is unknown, there are many theories of causation. Some researchers felt that it was the result of a virus. As yet, no one has been able to isolate a virus in the blood, cerebrospinal fluid, brain, or spinal cord of those affected by the disease. Another factor negating the viral theory is that the pathological findings are very different from those of any other viral disease of the nervous system.

In recent years it has been hypothesized that Guillain-Barré disease may be an auto-immune disease. It was found that the injection of extracts of peripheral nerves into animals would precipitate the disease.

Guillain-Barré disease is characterized by changes in the motor cells of the spinal cord and medulla. Segmental demyelination is found in the ventral and dorsal nerve roots.

Guillain-Barré disease is seen equally in men and women. It is most common in adolescents and young adults; however, it can occur at any time. Cases of the disease have been reported in infants and in geriatric persons. At the present, there are no preventive measures that the nurse or physician can employ. Education of the public is limited to recognizing the signs and symptoms.

In approximately two-thirds of the reported cases of Guillain-Barré disease, a mild upper respiratory infection or gastritis precedes the disease by days or weeks.[9] The infective process is seen and then subsides within a few days. About 10 to 21 days following the nonspecific illness, a *polyneuropathy* develops. *Weakness* progressing to paralysis in its most severe form begins in the lower extremities. This weakness is almost always bilateral, though sometimes it is asymmetrical. The motor paralysis has a tendency to ascend the body, involving the trunk and upper limbs. In the majority of cases the disease process keeps ascending and involves the cranial nerves. The ascending process usually takes between 24 and 72 hours. Maximum weakness and paralysis are usually seen within a few days. However, the full impact of the disease may not be seen for several weeks. As this is a progressive disease, characterized by an acute onset of weakness and paralysis, the affected individual should be immediately hospitalized. The person can be closely observed and tests can be done to rule out other disease processes.

The patient with a *flaccid paralysis* will have loss of the deep tendon reflexes. There will also be a loss of sensory proprioception with resultant *ataxia.* The patient may experience *paresthesias.* There may or may not be peripheral sensory impairment. Muscle tenderness or sensitivity of the nerves to pressure is frequently seen with cranial nerve involvement, facial paralysis, bulbar palsy, and weakness of extraoccular muscles (Fig. 36-5). Papilledema is frequently present but may be due to respiratory embarrassment. Motor weakness in the trunk muscles is usually quite severe, and in 25 percent of patients the muscles of respiration are affected. Respiratory involvement is usually seen about 12 days after the onset of the disease. This may be so severe that it necessitates placing the individual on mechanical ventilation. Sphincter control is lost in the most severe cases. Orthostatic hypotension is commonly seen, due to autonomic insufficiency. It is of note that patients suffering from Guillain-Barré disease are usually hypertensive, with pressures of about 160/70 to 200/100. This finding is frequently accompanied by a tachycardia and a low-grade fever. Inappropriate secretion of antidiuretic hormone (ADH) frequently occurs with resultant hyponatremia. There may be disturbances in the levels of consciousness if the disease has caused an encephalitic process.

Since there is no specific diagnostic test, the diagnosis rests entirely upon the presence of the typical clinical picture and the exclusion of other diseases characterized by widespread paralysis of acute onset. Lumbar punctures reveal an elevated cerebrospinal fluid with an absence of cells. There is an increased protein concentration and a change in the colloid concentration.

The treatment of Guillain-Barré disease is mainly supportive and similar to that used in treating polio. Therapy is limited; steroids have been employed, but their effectiveness is questionable.

The nursing care of the Guillain-Barré patient involves all the skills necessary to care for a polio patient. The nurse should remember that every action is significant; it is the nursing care more than the medical care that determines the outcome of the illness. Recovery from the syndrome is usually complete over a period of weeks to months. Residual deficits are uncommon and mild when they do occur.

## REFERENCES

1   Elliot, Frank, *Clinical Neurology*, Saunders, Philadelphia, 1973, p. 295.
2   Merritt, H. Houston, *A Textbook of Neurology*, Lea & Febiger, Philadelphia, 1973, p. 7.
3   Elliot, *op. cit.*, p. 295.
5   *Ibid.*, p. 299.
5   Merritt, *op. cit.*, p. 56.
6   *Ibid.*, p. 226.
7   *Ibid.*, p. 56.
8   Elliot, *op. cit.*, p. 292.
9   Merritt, *op. cit.*, p. 641.

## BIBLIOGRAPHY

### Meningitis

Dodge, P. R., and M. N. Swartz: "Bacterial Meningitis —A Review of Selected Aspects," *N Engl J Med*, 272, 725, 779, 842, 898, 954, and 1003, 1965.

Kremer, M.: "Meningitis after Spinal Anesthesia," *Br Med J*, **2:**4418, 1945.

McKendrick, C. D.: "The Treatment of Pyrogenic Meningitis," *J Neurol Neurosurg Psychiatry*, **31:**528, 1968.

Meade, R. H.: "Treatment of Meningitis," *JAMA*, **185:** 1023, 1963.

Sahs, A. L., and R. J. Joynt: "Meningitis," in A. B. Baker (ed.), *Clinical Neurology*, Hoeber-Harper, New York, 1962, pp. 717–773.

Sanford, J. P., and J. A. Barnett: "Bacterial Meningitis," in Howard F. Conn (ed.), *Current Therapy*, Saunders, Philadelphia, 1971, pp. 27–32.

Smith, H. V., R. M. Norman, and H. Urich: "The Late Sequelae of Penumococcal Meningitis," *J Neurol Neurosurg Psychiatry*, **20:**250, 1957.

### Rabies

Hildreth, E. A.: "Prevention of Rabies," *Ann Intern Med*, **58:**883, 1963.

Kaplan, M. M.: "Epidemiology of Rabies," *Nature*, **221:**421, 1969.

Pawan, J. L.: "Paralysis as Manifestation of Human Rabies," *Ann Trop Med*, **33:**21, 1937.

### Brain Abscess

Brewer, Nelson S., et al.: "Brain Abscess: A Review of Recent Experience," *Ann Intern Med*, **82:**571, 576, 1975.

Carey, M. E., S. W. Chou, and L. A. French: "Long-Term Neurological Residue in Patients Surviving Brain Abscess with Surgery," *J Neurosurg*, **34:** 652–656, 1971.

Sampson, P. S., and K. H. Clark: "Current Review of Brain Abscess," *Am J Med*, **54:**201–210, 1973.

Sperl, M. P., Jr., S. C. MacCarty, and W. E. Wellman: "Observations on Current Therapy of Abscesses of the Brain," *Arch Neurol*, **81:**439–441, 1959.

### Encephalitis

Adams, R. D., and L. Weinstein: "Clinical and Pathological Aspects of Encephalitis," *N Engl J Med*, **239:**865, 1948.

Canady, Marg E.: "Helping the Family Cope," *Am J Nurs*, **72:**94–96, January 1972.

Feenster, R. F.: "Eastern Equine Encephalitis," *Neurology*, **8:**882, 1958.

Fields, W. S., and R. L. Blattner: "Viral Encephalitis," Charles C Thomas, Springfield, Ill., 1958.

Gajdusek, D. C.: "Slow Virus Infections of the Nervous System," *N Engl J Med*, **276:**392–400, 1967.

Scott, McNair, and Wargler: "Penns. Treatment of Encephalitis," *Hosp Med*, **6:**88–97, February 1950.

Seabury, Corinne A.: "Nurse's Observation on Post-Encephalitic Patients," *Nurs Outlook*, **14:**28–29, October 1966.

Zimmerman: *Infections of the Nervous System*, vol. 44, *Res Publ Assoc Res Nerv Ment Dis*, Williams & Wilkins, Baltimore, 1961.

### Polio

Horstmann, D. M., et al.: "Epidemiology of Poliomyelitis and Allied Diseases," *Yale J Biol Med*, 36, 5, 1963.

Medical Research Council Committee: "Comparative Trial of British and American Oral Polio Myelitis Vaccines," *Br Med J*, **2:**142–145, 1962.

Plum, F.: "Poliomyelitis," in *Clinical Neurology,* vol. 3, Harper & Row, New York, 1962.

Salk, Jonas E.: "Present Status of Problems against Poliomyelitis," *Am J Public Health,* **45:**285–297, 1955.

Zaceh, R., et al.: "Mass Oral Sabin Poliomyelitis Vaccination," *Br Med J,* **1:**1091–1098, 1962.

## Guillain-Barré Disease

Rocklin, Ross, et al.: "The Guillain-Barré Syndrome and Multiple Sclerosis," *N Engl J Med,* **284:**803–208, 1971.

Thomas, P. K., et al.: "Recurrent and Chronic Relapsing Guillain-Barré Polyneuritis," *Brain,* **92:**589, 1969.

Tweed, G., et al.: "Guillain-Barré Syndrome," *Am. J. Nurs,* 2222–2226, 1964.

## General

Buescher, E. L., M. P. Arnstein, and L. C. Olson: "Central Nervous System Infections of Viral Etiology: The Changing Pattern," *Res Publ Assoc Res Nerv Ment Dis,* **44:**147, 1968.

Carini, Esta, and Gay Owens: *Neurological and Neurosurgical Nursing,* Mosby, St. Louis, 1974.

Elliot, F.: *Clinical Neurology,* Saunders, Philadelphia, 1971.

Goodman, L., and A. Gilman: *The Pharmacological Basis of Therapeutics,* Macmillan, London, 1969.

Greg, Michael: "Communicable Disease Trends in the United States," *Am J Nurs,* **68:**88–93, 1968.

Jawetz, Ernest: "Axioms on Infections in Adults," *Hosp Med,* **5:**49–59, September 1969.

Merritt, H. Houston: *A Textbook of Neurology,* Lea & Febiger, Philadelphia, 1973.

Morrison, Shirley, and Carolyn Arnolo: "Patients with Common Communicable Diseases," *Nurs Clin North Am,* **5:**143–155, March 1970.

Plum, Fred, and Jerome B. Posner: *Diagnosis of Stupor and Coma,* Davis, Philadelphia, 1972.

Top, Franklin, and Paul F. Wehele: *Communicable and Infectious Disease Diagnosis Prevention, Treatment,* 7th ed., Mosby, St. Louis, 1972.

# 37

# DEGENERATIVE DISTURBANCES IN PERCEPTION AND COORDINATION

Joan Gallagher

The nervous system is a highly complex structure that functions to allow the individual to interact with the environment. Information from both the internal and external environments is received, sorted out, processed, and integrated into a total body response. Chronic degenerative disturbances of the nervous system irreversibly disrupt this intricately balanced system of perception and coordination. The individual's interaction with the environment is interfered with in several ways. Sight, smell, taste, hearing, and touch are often affected, diminishing perception. Coordination is hampered, making movement difficult or impossible and disrupting communication. Because the psyche is part of the nervous system, personality and behavioral changes are often evident.

The chronic, degenerative, neurological disorders exhibit some common characteristics. Their onset tends to be gradual, developing insidiously. Their course generally progresses at varying rates to irreparable damage and disability. Although symptoms are often asymetrical at the onset, as the degeneration is well established, the effects are usually symmetrical.

These degenerative disturbances affect nearly 1 million individuals in our society. At present, their etiology is not well understood. Neither preventive nor curative measures are available, but symptomatic treatment is increasingly effective in prolonging life and minimizing disability. The role of the nurse in early case finding, referral, and treatment is vital.

A discussion of all the degenerative neurological disturbances is not within the scope of this chapter. The more common disruptions will be explored as being representative of degenerative disturbances in perception and coordination. Multiple sclerosis is one of the most common neurological disturbances and represents the demyelinating diseases. Parkinson's disease is a well-known syndrome that includes abnormalities of posture and involuntary movements. These will be explored in detail. Also examined will be Huntington's chorea, a hereditary syndrome that involves progressive dementia with neurological problems, and amyotrophic lateral sclerosis, a syndrome characterized by slowly developing muscle weakness and wasting.

## MULTIPLE SCLEROSIS

*Multiple sclerosis* (disseminated sclerosis) affects primarily the white matter of the brain and spinal cord. The white matter consists chiefly of bundles of myelinated axons which arise from neurons located throughout the nervous system. In the central nervous system, *myelin,* a lipoprotein membrane, is formed when oligodendrocytes, rich in cytoplasm, become wrapped many times around an axon in a spiraling arrangement. Layers of lipid and protein from the oligodendrocyte cell membrane fuse, and tracts of white, glistening, myelinated axons are formed. These tracts compose the bulk of the white matter. Myelin acts as an insulator for the conduction of impulses. Because of this insulation, myelinated fibers have a much higher conduction velocity and a longer activity period before fatigue than do unmyelinated fibers.

**Pathophysiology**

In multiple sclerosis there are irregular patches of demyelination, varying in size and scattered throughout the central nervous system. Some are barely visible, while others are extensive lesions. The effects on patients vary according to the areas affected. In the early stages, myelin loss causes slowing of conduction and intermittent conduction blocks without destruction of axons.

Early lesions appear as shrunken semitranslucent bluish areas. Destruction of nerve fibers appears later or with fulminating forms of the disturbance and is accompanied by gliosis, a proliferation of neuroglial tissue as a replacement process. The scars that form from gliosis appear as hardened (sclerotic), raised, white areas known as *plaque.* Plaques have a tendency to extend into neighboring structures and may invade adjacent grey matter. If the axis cylinder (axon) remains intact, symptoms may remit, but if both myelin and axis cylinder are destroyed, functional impairment becomes permanent. Although symptoms arise from demyelination, there is no consensus as to whether the primary alteration in multiple sclerosis is in the myelin sheath itself, involves destruction of oligodendrocytes responsible for myelin maintenance, or results from altered vascular tissue.

**Causes** The cause of multiple sclerosis is unknown. Understanding of the pathogenesis of this disease is being pursued in three areas—environmental, viral, and immunological. *Epidemiological investigations* seek to find the key to multiple sclerosis in its particular prevalence in countries within the temperate zones. These studies focus on discovering some exogenous or endogenous factor(s) present in the environment giving rise to the

disease. Further epidemiological impetus is derived from migration patterns from high-risk to low-risk countries. The age at migration influences the individual's susceptibility, suggesting the disease may be acquired in childhood.[1-3]

In *virology,* researchers seek to isolate a virus or virion with a long latency period which is capable of damaging central nervous tissue myelin. Because multiple sclerosis patients have been found to have higher antibodies to measles, much viral work has concentrated on measles viruses.[4,5] Viruses have been isolated recently from multiple sclerosis tissue,[6,7] but at present casual links can not be assumed.

*Genetic immunology,* the third area, seeks to discover an intrinsic defect in the immune system of people who develop multiple sclerosis. Autoimmunity is suspected because over half of the individuals with multiple sclerosis have been found to have human-lymphocyte antigen on their lymphocytes. These and other histocompatibility-linked markers are being found to be much more prevalent in multiple sclerosis than in the general population.[8-10] Further, cerebrospinal fluid findings of increased immunoglobulins manufactured within the central nervous system are reported in a significant number of multiple sclerosis patients and are not generally seen in other inflammatory reactions in the central nervous system.[11] The growing body of evidence supports the belief that immunological disorders are a significant component of the disease process. Other theories suggest metabolic disturbances, allergic reactions, and nutritional deficiencies as possible causes.

**Effects on patients** The effects of multiple sclerosis vary widely from person to person and episode to episode depending on the site of the lesion, the depth of myelin loss, and the extent of sclerotic plaque formation. The course of the disease, characterized by remissions and exacerbations, is unpredictable and may involve only minor changes or may be fulminating and rapidly progress to total disability. Both affected individuals and health professionals are forced to deal with uncertainty regarding the effects of multiple sclerosis in a given situation.

The onset of symptoms is often associated with a *precipitating factor.* Emotional stress, injury, infection, fatigue, and pregnancy are among the events that may herald the onset of symptoms or an exacerbation of the process.

*Retrobulbar neuritis* (inflammation of the optic nerve) is often the initial symptom. It occurs because the optic nerves and chiasma are vulnerable in demyelinating diseases. It can be unilateral or bilateral and is characterized by a central scotoma. The center of the field of vision is often blurred or misty and may be accompanied by pain in the eye on movement. About a third of the patients recover complete vision, another third experience partial remission, and the remaining third do not improve.

In more than a third of the cases the onset includes *perceptual changes.* Paresthesias occur more frequently in distal portions of a limb (e.g., fingers and toes) as compared with proximal areas. The numbness is due to plaque in posterior columns of the spinal cord and usually spreads horizontally. The lesions are frequently bilateral, causing symmetrical paresthesias. The patient may experience a feeling of constriction or enlargement of a limb. Spinothalamic tract interruption gives rise to thermal dysesthesias (warm, burning, damp, or cold sensations) in a part of the body. The presence of pain, especially backache, is not uncommon. Other perceptual changes can cause complete loss of awareness of passive motion resulting in motor clumsiness or gait uncertainty. Early sensory symptoms are often associated with lesions in the cervical cord and may be reflected in an "electric" tingling feeling referred down the back when the neck is flexed (*Lhermitte's sign*).

*Pyramidal* involvement can range from increased paresthesia to complete paralysis. Weakness in a limb or one side is a frequent early problem. As involvement progresses, muscle tone increases, resulting in spasticity with extensor and flexor spasms and exaggerated deep tendon reflexes.

*Brainstem* involvement may cause nystagmus (irregular oscillation of the eyeballs) and diplopia (double vision). Brainstem lesions can also cause paresis of other cranial nerves, headache, drowsiness, involuntary outbursts of laughing or crying, and vertigo. Vertigo is usually associated with nystagmus and is experienced as the apparent movement of objects in the environment. The dizziness is decreased by closing the eyes or by lying down. Facial anesthesia or palsy, loss of taste, vertigo, and trigeminal neuralgia are less common manifestations. In advanced stages, difficulty in chewing or swallowing can occur.

When plaques involve the *cerebellum, Charcot's classic triad* of symptoms, intention tremor, scanning speech, and nystagmus, are usually present. Rhythmic movements of *intention tremor* vary from slight hesitation or decreased precision during voluntary movement to an involuntary move-

ment which is so severe that eating, dressing, and drinking activities are impossible. *Ataxic speech* ranges from a slow drawling quality with pauses after each syllable, giving the scanning effect, to explosive utterances difficult to comprehend. *Nystagmus* may be horizontal, an upward jerk type, or seen only in the abducting eye. Other cerebellar manifestations include vertigo accompanied by giddiness and Romberg's sign (unsteadiness when standing with eyes closed). Gait unsteadiness is also attributable to cerebellar involvement, although paresthesias, vertigo, and impairment of postural sense in the lower limbs can contribute to it.

Depending on the severity of the lesion, genitourinary changes may cause frequency and urgency, retention, impairment of normal subjective sensations of the bladder and urethra, or total incontinence. Loss of nervous integrity in the urinary system may also be associated with losses in related structures. Impotence is common among male patients, and bowel problems ranging from constipation to fecal incontinence may occur. Bladder problems and fecal incontinence increase the risk of infective complications of the urinary tract, especially for female patients.

In a small percentage of multiple sclerosis patients epilepsy occurs. Seizures may be local or generalized and may recur or remit spontaneously.

Plaque on the floor of the fourth ventricle may produce vertigo with giddiness, while vestibular vertigo is more often associated with nausea and vomiting. Periventricular plaques often involve the limbic-reticular system, giving rise to altered patterns of communication and mood disturbances. Euphoria, not seen in other neurologic degenerative conditions, may be seen in multiple sclerosis, although depression is more common. Mood swings are common manifestations of limbic involvement; however, intellectual impairment is not seen until late in the course of the disease. Inappropriate behavioral response should not be considered reflective of intellectual status.

The course of the multiple sclerotic changes and their widespread effects are highly variable. The effects on the patient may occur singly or in combination. The majority of patients experience exacerbations followed by remissions. This pattern usually persists for over 20 years. After 25 years one-third of patients with multiple sclerosis are still actively working. Even more are ambulatory.

As the changes progress, each exacerbation will leave some residual impairment. Remissions become less frequent and shorter, and disability increases. In the final state the patient is often bed-ridden and incontinent and suffers from painful flexor spasms.

### First-Level Nursing Care

As long as the cause of multiple sclerosis remains obscure, prevention is not possible. It is helpful, however, for nurses to be aware of patients at risk to its development. Multiple sclerosis has a remarkable, unexplained, world distribution. In both hemispheres the incidence (excluding Japan) is several times higher in the temperate zones than in the tropics or subtropics. Persons migrating after age 15 from temperate to tropic climates carry the higher risk of developing multiple sclerosis with them. Once diagnosed, climate changes do not affect the course of the disease.

In America, multiple sclerosis is the most common disease of the nervous system, affecting an estimated 250,000 individuals.[12] Because it is not a reportable disease, this figure is probably too conservative. The disease attacks adults between the ages of 20 and 40 and affects slightly more women than men. An increased prevalence is seen among relatives, but from the available data no definite genetic pattern emerges.

The onset of multiple sclerosis is often triggered by a recent period of hyperactivity, overfatigue, emotional trauma, infection, physical stress, or trauma. Because the cause remains obscure, prevention is not yet available. Theoretically the nurse, by promoting high-level wellness within communities in high-risk areas, might indirectly reduce the incidence of multiple sclerosis by avoiding precipitating events. Although the impact would be impossible to prove, as an interim measure it would seem worthwhile.

### Second-Level Nursing Care

In second-level care the nurse in the community is in a strategic position to observe early, subtle changes suggestive of multiple sclerosis, facilitate early diagnosis, and promote early rehabilitation programs.

**Nursing assessment** Early case finding is dependent upon thorough and accurate nursing assessment. Because the initial stages of multiple sclerosis are often not remarkable, patients may be seen with other problems. A vigilant nurse can maximize the data base with careful and accurate assessments.

**Health History** History taking is a critical part of the nursing assessment of the individual with multiple sclerosis. The nurse should seek to determine the detailed health history, with special reference to any precipitating physical or emotional events, overfatigue, or hyperactivity. Similarly, existing or recent past infections of the tonsils, sinuses, middle ear, respiratory or urinary system, dental problems, or allergic conditions should be actively elicited. Early in the disease the patient will often experience vague, nonspecific symptoms. Fatigue, irritability, poor memory, and weight loss are common complaints. The patient should be asked about any sensations being experienced. Motor weakness is common, and the patient often feels as if one leg is dragging. The patient should be asked if falling has become a problem. Any changes in vision should be explored. Questions about urinary frequency and urgency should be asked.

During the health history, the interview should focus on the individual's unique perceptions and feelings about the changes she or he is experiencing. The person frequently reports uncommon moods or mood changes. The mood of the patient at interview should be described by behaviors exhibited rather than inferential statements. Because emotional lability is a symptom of the disease, gathering more than baseline data at the initial interview may be impossible. With further interaction and evaluation, the nurse can more effectively identify whether psychological problems exist which warrant intervention or referral.

Information should also be gathered about the individual's education, work situation, and personal, religious, and social affiliations. This not only serves to focus on the worth, strengths, and potential of the patient but also provides background data for planning a meaningful holistic rehabilitation program best suited for that particular individual.

**Physical Assessment** For a patient with early multiple sclerosis, physical assessment must include a complete neurological examination. Depending on the areas involved, findings can vary greatly from patient to patient. Some more common early findings will be discussed here. A thorough discussion of neurological findings can be found in Third-Level Nursing Care.

Early in multiple sclerosis, physical assessment usually reveals visual and perceptual changes and difficulties in coordination. A complete eye examination should be done. Visual fields should be outlined. If retrobulbar neuritis is present, decreased central vision in one or both eyes may be evident. Examination of eye grounds may show pallor of the temporal half of the disk due to myelin loss. Evidence of inflammation or elevation of the optic nerve may be seen. Sluggish pupil reaction may be present in the acute stage but returns to normal as neuritis subsides.

Sensory function should be tested with cotton, pin point, vibration, and recognition of objects by touch. Sensory losses usually involve a decreased appreciation of vibration sensation and sensory stimulation. Areas of paresthesia vary with the location of lesions. They can affect one limb, one side, or bilateral areas. Often paresthesia of one hand is an early finding.

Muscle strength should be evaluated as weakness is an early symptom. Hand grasps, resistance, and maintaining extremities against gravity often reveal unilateral weakness of one or more limbs. Bilateral weakness can also occur.

Symptoms of paresthesias and weakness may be accompanied by exaggeration of some reflexes with depression of others in the limb. Reflexes should be carefully evaluated for hyperactivity or depression. Findings may include (1) depression or absence of abdominal reflexes, (2) hyperactive deep tendon reflexes, and (3) extensor plantar (positive Babinski) response. These abnormalities may disappear spontaneously after a few weeks or months owing to the functional reversibility of the early lesions.

Lack of coordination is not remarkable early in multiple sclerosis. Subtle difficulties, however, may be elicited by having patients touch the nurse's finger and then their own nose, do rapid alternating movements, or perform simple tasks. Intention tremors may be noted at this time.

**D**iagnostic Tests   In the initial phase of multiple sclerosis where no major functional impairments exist, the physician may choose to treat the focal symptoms and arrange for reevaluation if symptoms persist or recur. A diagnosis of multiple sclerosis is not made until the presence of two or more separate central nervous system (CNS) lesions has been documented. Often, however, the patient will be admitted to the hospital for a complete neurological work-up in order to rule out infections or neoplastic processes. These diagnostic tests are discussed in Third-Level Nursing Care.

**Nursing problems and interventions**  Early problems, including *lack of coordination, clumsi-*

*ness, decreased touch sensations, weakness, visual disturbances, extreme fatigability, emotional changes,* and *bladder dysfunction,* occurring singularly or in combination, are usually disruptive enough for the individual to seek treatment. Interference with competent functioning, caused by the symptoms, generates anxiety for the individual and family members. Because multiple sclerosis targets young adults, career goals, marriage, and parenting choices as well as athletic and social activities all may be disrupted.

Even before diagnosis is confirmed, these changes undermine the individual's self-image, independence, and sense of body integrity. The degree of threat experienced depends upon the physical losses themselves, the symbolic meaning these capacities have for the individual, and the response of significant others to changes in the patient. This reaction is further influenced by cultural and religious factors as well as the emotional lability symptomatic of multiple sclerosis itself. Intervention is directed toward relief of symptoms to minimize residual losses and prevent exacerbations and secondary complications.

*Motor symptoms* such as lack of coordination, clumsiness, and weakness need to be evaluated by a physical therapist, and an appropriate regime of therapeutic exercises instituted. If motor problems exist, exercises are geared toward improving muscle strength, coordination, and gait stability. The family can be taught passive exercises for use during acute episodes. Active resistive exercises should be instituted as symptoms abate. The patient and family should be taught that rest between activities and exercises is imperative. Overexertion produced by excessive activity is counterproductive; it serves only to increase the patient's sense of frustration by decreasing rather than building up functional reserve. A balance between rest and independent functional activity must be maintained.

*Sensory losses* create a need for safety measures to be instituted by both the patient and the family. Diminished vision and touch sensation increase the risk of accidents caused by hot liquids, falls, and unfelt bruises. Temperatures of foods, hot beverages, and water for bathing may all need to be adjusted downward to prevent burns without compromising functional independence. Walkways should be free of scatter rugs, electrical and phone cords, and extraneous objects. Use of shoes with good support and nonskid soles provides for safer ambulation. Various rails and supportive devices may be helpful, and social service should be consulted to explore avenues for obtaining necessary equipment.

The patient should be taught to closely inspect body areas with decreased sensation for injury on a daily basis. Any injuries should be treated, and the patient encouraged to identify the cause so that future injury can be prevented.

*Blurred vision* is a common early problem because of the retrobulbar neuritis. It usually involves a portion of the visual field. The patient should be taught to turn the head in order to bring a particular object into the unaffected visual field. If diplopia is present, alternate patching of one eye for a period, then the other, will alleviate this symptom. The person needs to be instructed, however, that depth perception will be impaired by patching.

Emotional care is essential throughout all interactions. The individual's *grieving* is a normal response, both for him or her and family members. Occasionally, a patient may actually be relieved to find an organic cause of symptoms rather than feeling it is "all in my head." The nurse must support the individual through the denial phase of grieving without reinforcing the denial. As the patient moves into the stage of developing awareness of the loss, teaching becomes a major area of need. Multiple sclerosis is not generally a well-known disease; therefore, the attitude and information gleaned from health professionals at this time will significantly influence the patient's concept of this disease. Realistic support should be provided. Ninety percent of the patients with multiple sclerosis have a course of remissions and exacerbations; in the other 10 percent the pathology is steadily progressive. It is usually not possible to accurately predict the tempo or severity at onset.

In general, symptoms occurring abruptly have a better prognosis than insidious changes. Sensory and cranial nerve symptoms remit more frequently than motor symptoms. Groups of symptoms do not remit as readily as isolated symptoms of any type. Full remission is more likely to occur with attacks earlier in life than later ones, except when early symptoms are of cerebellar (rare) origin.

**P**reventing Exacerbations   It must be stressed that the patient can have an impact on the ultimate course of the disease through adherence to treatment programs and maintenance of productive and healthful living. The patient and family members need to be stimulated to function independently at their maximum capabilities. Continued involvement in activities, interests, and socialization by the individual needs to be stressed to maintain a meaningful existence. Residual functional capacities should

be utilized and strengthened through proper exercise, adequate rest, sound nutrition, effective communication, and general well-being. The importance of exercise and rest has already been discussed.

*Nutrition* for the individual with multiple sclerosis involves eating a well-balanced diet that is low in fat, especially cholesterol. Dietary extremes and indiscretions should be avoided. If the patient is overweight, a reduction diet is initiated to reduce the burden fat places on muscles and circulation. The diet should be planned around the cultural and financial position of the family. Evaluation of the home setting by the nurse must address the financial capabilities of the family and available support through social services.

*Effective communication* is essential to maintain the integrity of the family on a long-term basis. Emotional tensions and stresses can trigger exacerbations, but this fact cannot deny the needs of other family members to come to grips with the impact of multiple sclerosis on them. The community health nurse can help individuals in the family to cope with emotional lability as a part of the symptomatology without stifling their own needs to verbalize feelings. It is not the total avoidance of all feelings, but a balanced give and take which provides the desired environment of emotional stability and security.

General well-being involves the *avoidance of injury and infection* and prompt treatment should they occur. Parenting activities are often concerns for individuals with multiple sclerosis. While pregnancy is not contraindicated, most physicians advise 2 years free of relapses before pregnancy. Over time the individual will no doubt identify other situations or events which tend to exaggerate symptoms. Once identified, these factors should be avoided if possible. Assistance in coping with multiple sclerosis is available through local chapters of the National Multiple Sclerosis Society. Patients and families can find support, as well as coping strategies, through membership in the society.

### Third-Level Nursing Care

As lesions progress, exacerbations and subsequent remissions tend to produce evidence of increased neurological dysfunction. As disability increases, hospitalization is often necessary. Most often patients with more widespread involvement require acute care during an exacerbation or acute illness.

**Nursing assessment**   The patient with widespread multiple sclerosis or the patient experiencing an acute exacerbation will often evidence many effects of the pathophysiological changes. The *health history* will be similar to that discussed under Second-Level Nursing Care, but at this stage of the illness the patient often reports more widespread paresthesias and varying amounts of muscle weakness, spasticity and/or paralysis. The patient may complain of blurred and double vision, and incoordination may be common. During the history speech difficulties should be evaluated. The patient should be questioned about changes in bladder, bowel, and sexual functioning.

**P**hysical Assessment   A complete neurological examination should be performed on any patient with multiple sclerosis. This includes evaluation of motor function, sensory perception, cranial nerves, reflex testing, and gait. Besides the findings described in Second-Level Nursing Care, the patient with widespread multiple sclerosis may evidence more diverse changes.

The function of cranial nerves should be investigated. The complete eye examination should include range of ocular movements. Nystagmus often occurs horizontally. The patient may also be unable to adduct one or both eyes on lateral gaze. The presence of retrobulbar neuritis may also be found. Facial anesthesia may be tested with a pin and wisp of cotton. Facial symmetry should be observed when the patient speaks. The patient should be asked to extend the tongue, and its placement, strength, and coordination noted. In advanced stages, the gag reflex may be diminished or absent. The patient's ability to swallow and move the jaw may also be compromised. Tests of smell should be performed. While ocular dysfunction frequently occurs, involvement of other cranial nerves is a less frequent phenomenon.

The tests of motor, sensory, and reflex function described in Second-Level Nursing Care usually reveal more extensive involvement. Paresthesias and muscular spasticity may be more widespread, and paralysis may be present. The patient should be evaluated when walking. Ataxia (muscle incoordination) of gait is often noted.

**D**iagnostic Tests   There are no diagnostic tests that can specifically identify multiple sclerosis. Several, however, may be employed to rule out other problems and gather evidence to support the diagnosis.

A complete blood count and serum studies including electrolytes, electrophoresis of all protein and phospholipid fractions, antibody titers, enzyme levels, and serology are usually done. In multiple sclerosis, serum alterations may include a slightly lowered *albumin level* in the presence of slightly elevated *alpha globulin* and *gamma globulin.* There may also be an elevated *measles antibody titer,* although none of these findings is specific to multiple sclerosis. Plasma lipids are usually normal.

Skull x-rays, electroencephalograms (EEG), cerebral angiography, pneumoencephalograms, echo studies, brain scans, and myelograms may all be done to rule out tumors, herniated intervertebral disks, aneurysms, and other disorders whose symptoms may mimic multiple sclerosis. In each of these tests, the nurse's role includes reassurance and appropriate explanations before the individual undergoes a procedure and close observation and monitoring afterward. Findings in multiple sclerosis are usually within normal limits in all these studies except the *electroencephalogram.* Nonspecific changes in the EEG are relatively common in multiple sclerosis patients, and serial recordings may be of value.

Examination of the *cerebrospinal fluid (CSF)* is of considerable value in the diagnosis of multiple sclerosis. Nursing care involves preparing the patient for a lumbar puncture and maintaining safe positioning during and after the procedure. Cell count and total protein are normal or near normal, but mononuclear cells may be elevated early in the disease. Once neurosyphilis has been ruled out by a negative Wassermann test, a *positive Lange colloidal gold curve,* common to both disorders, points toward a diagnosis of multiple sclerosis. McAlpine points out that a positive paretic Lange curve is likely in 80 percent of cases but that faulty laboratory techniques result in false negatives.[13] Another significant finding strongly supportive of the diagnosis of multiple sclerosis is an *elevated CSF gamma globulin fraction* (over 13 percent) in the presence of normal or near-normal total protein content in Wassermann-negative individuals.

*Immunoelectrophoretic assays* are currently used to detect a variety of immunoglobulins and lymphocytes derived from various body tissue found in cerebrospinal fluid. Of the various measures, an elevation of oligoclonal immunoglobulin G (IgG) is of greatest usefulness, at present, in establishing the diagnosis of multiple sclerosis. Of the phospholipids, cephalin fractions are elevated relative to the total in CSF. All these results support the diagnosis of multiple sclerosis.

To evaluate optic nerve function, the *critical flicker fusion test,* performed by intermittent light flashes, determines the individual's ability to appreciate the intervals between stimuli. Appreciation is abnormally low in multiple sclerosis, resulting in the perception of a steady light.

Recent ophthalmic findings offer considerable promise in the early diagnosis of multiple sclerosis. Examination of the eye grounds may reveal subtle defects. Using an *ophthalmoscope with red-free lighting,* Frisén and Hoyt[14] found funduscopic evidence of focal and diffuse axonal attrition (loss) in a significant number of multiple sclerosis cases even without visual symptoms. Additionally, they observed retinal striae which explained small scotomata (blind spots) that could be documented by *retinal photography.* Sixty-eight percent of multiple sclerosis patients demonstrated similar abnormalities.[15]

In the *visual-evoked response (VER) test,* response to stimuli measured on a graph by means of electrodes has shown delayed responses in a very high percentage of multiple sclerosis patients.[16,17] In both studies, patients with an otherwise normal objective ophthalmic examination demonstrated evidence of optic pathway involvement. Although conduction delays are not specific to multiple sclerosis, this test can be a valuable early diagnostic tool along with other clinical data. Since at least two separate lesions are needed to confirm the diagnosis of multiple sclerosis, the test provides objective evidence of local lesions.

**Nursing problems and interventions** Nursing intervention must take place in the context of total patient management. Again it is critical for the nurse to understand that each patient's course will vary widely and the pattern of progression to complete disability occurs over a period of many years, if at all. The entire health team is mobilized to respond to those areas of needs presented by a particular individual.

The initial nursing problem is the *exacerbation* itself. In general, *complete rest* is indicated for 2 or 3 weeks during an acute exacerbation. Treatment measures are symptomatic and focus on minimizing residual losses, preventing complications, and maintaining independence within the functional limits of the individual. Repeated relapses generally require hospitalization, and residual damage tends to be more pronounced and lasting.

While no medication cures multiple sclerosis, *corticotropin* and *adrenal steroids* are usually prescribed in fairly high doses for 2 to 3 weeks during acute episodes. These anti-inflammatory agents do provide symptomatic relief, but nursing measures must be initiated to detect drug complications such as gastrointestinal bleeding and superimposed infections. Since signs and symptoms of respiratory and urinary infections may be suppressed, the nurse must closely observe the integrity of these systems. Steroids should be gradually reduced as the acute stage of illness passes and never abruptly withdrawn to prevent an adrenal crisis (see Chap. 21).

During an exacerbation, the patient is often bedridden. Nursing problems associated with preventing the *hazards of immobility* should be dealt with. It is decubitus ulcer formation, respiratory and urinary infections, and other complications of immobility that often cause death rather than multiple sclerosis itself. Prevention of these complications falls squarely in the nursing sector of total patient management. The patient should be kept in good alignment and repositioned at least every 2 hours. Periodic use of prone positioning is very helpful in preventing flexion contractures, foot drop, decubiti, and hypostatic pneumonia. Application of a footboard and elastic stockings helps to prevent muscular and vascular complications. Deep breathing and coughing exercises prevent respiratory infections. Promoting high fluid intake serves the dual purposes of liquefying respiratory secretions and preventing urinary complications of infection and renal calculi.

Daily bathing activities afford an opportunity for the nurse to inspect the patient thoroughly for signs of skin breakdown. Extremes of water temperature should be avoided to prevent burns and aggravation of symptoms. Complete passive range of joint motion should be incorporated into bathing activities. Gentle massage with emollient lotion to the back, heels, buttocks, elbows, and other pressure areas will increase the patient's comfort and general sense of well-being as well as provide circulatory stimulation. Supplementary measures such as air or water mattresses, silicone pads, sheepskin, heel and elbow protectors, and bed cradles should all be considered to further reduce pressure on bony prominences or areas of motor or sensory loss.

For *muscle spasticity,* diazepam (Valium) is often prescribed and affords some relief of symptoms. Dantrolene sodium (Dantrium), a peripheral-acting skeletal muscle relaxant, has also been effective in some cases. Another pharmacological approach to the relief of spasticity involves the use of baclofen (Lioresal), a synthetic derivative of the neuroinhibitory chemical transmitter, gamma-aminobutyric acid (GABA), to reduce muscle spasticity. Current studies indicate it is of value in selected cases.[18-20] At present, no drug is completely effective in relieving spasticity. The nurse must observe closely, with the patient, the therapeutic response to drugs as well as dose-limiting side effects. Medication for spasticity is utilized in treatment along with a program of physical therapy.

After evaluation of musculoskeletal status, the physical therapist will prescribe a routine of exercises and if necessary assistive devices. Use of traction and splinting appliances may also be prescribed to prevent contractures in patients with severely spastic muscles. The nurse should be familiar with the use of these aids and inspect splinted and braced areas for signs of injury on a daily basis. The patient and family should also be taught the use of these devices.

As the acute phase subsides, emphasis should be shifted to restoration of self-care in activities of daily living such as bathing, dressing, toileting, transferring, continence, and feeding. Activities must always be balanced with periods of rest. Independence should be maximized by using the remaining strength to compensate for disabilities. This strength can be augmented by coordination and muscle-strengthening exercises. Assistive devices such as rails in hallways and bathrooms and hoists over the bed and tub should be explored to facilitate this goal.

The patient should be taught safety measures to compensate for *motor losses* and *decreased sensations.* Transfer activities and safe ambulation or wheelchair activities should be included in teaching as necessary, with attention to the status of the individual's visual acuity.

In advanced stages of the disease permanent disability and *contractures* may warrant various orthopedic surgical procedures for the release of contractures, relief of pain, and increase in mobility. Nursing care would vary according to the individual patient's needs and the procedure performed.

*Intention tremor* may be helped by using weighted eating utensils and other assistive devices, but in extreme cases stereotaxic surgery may be performed to relieve symptoms of tremor. Unfortunately, since tremor may recur and permanent damage to speech often results from this surgery, it is rarely indicated.

*Genitourinary problems* are common in the course of multiple sclerosis. Problems of frequency and urgency may progress to urge incontinence or complete *urinary incontinence.* Nursing measures to prevent incontinence such as offering the bedpan frequently or providing for the use of a bedside commode may prevent accidents. The incontinent patient should have protective padding and bedding changed as necessary as well as local care to prevent skin breakdown. Care should be given in a manner that minimizes any embarrassment for the patient. Incontinence in the male may be treated by use of a condom catheter but a similar apparatus is not available for females. Because the risk of ascending urinary tract infection and subsequent pyelonephritis and renal failure is high, long-term use of an indwelling catheter is dangerous. Periodic evaluation and attempts to restore continence conservatively are always employed first, but ultimately surgical procedures to divert the urine such as the creation of an ileal conduit may be necessary, especially in the female. Despite the seemingly radical nature of surgical intervention, most patients achieve more independent control in managing the abdominal appliance than with other methods. It can actually improve functional independence and reduce some of the social isolation imposed by the stigma of incontinence.

Some patients experience *urinary retention* rather than frequency if lesions cause decreased sensory awareness of bladder distention or a loss of reflex response of the bladder to distention. Measures to relieve this situation without catheterization include encouraging high fluid intake, providing privacy, normal positioning, running water or pouring water over the area, or gentle manual pressure over the lower abdomen or suprapubic area. If these are ineffective, drugs to promote voiding such as bethanecol chloride (Urecholine) may be prescribed. Catheterization is avoided, if at all possible, but the risk of infection on the one hand must be weighed against the risks of ischemia and subsequent atrophy of detrusor muscle fibers caused by prolonged bladder distention. If catheterized, special hygiene measures, encouraging fluids, and irrigation with saline and antimicrobial solutions may all be employed to prevent secondary infection. If medical management for urinary retention is not effective, surgical bladder neck resection may be helpful in improving the patient's bladder emptying without chronic catheterization.

Problems of *impotence* should be discussed with both sexual partners to explore alternate means of achieving satisfying sexual expressions and to reduce feelings of inadequacy. Sexual capacity may return as the multiple sclerosis symptoms remit or may be permanently lost. Sexual partners need to discuss this openly and in light of their plans for a family. This is often a difficult problem to accept, and alternatives such as artificial insemination should be explored.

The problem of *constipation* can be dealt with by a combination of diet, medication, and exercises.

Foods high in bulk and roughage and a high fluid intake, together with stool softeners or gentle laxatives, are employed along with muscle contraction exercises to promote regularity. Bowel training programs encourage bowel movements in the morning after breakfast when the gastrocolic reflex may assist bowel evacuation. The problem of constipation should not be allowed to progress to fecal impaction. By making sure that the patient does not go more than 3 days without a bowel movement, and by observing the size and consistency of stool, the nurse can effectively prevent this complication. When mobility is limited, use of a bedside commode or portable toilet of the type used by campers can be helpful in bowel and bladder management at home since most have a flush mechanism not available in a bedside commode.

*Speech problems* are common and create frustration for both the patient and those involved in giving care. It is important to teach all personnel to allow the patient time to communicate. Referral for speech therapy may be needed, and the nurse can provide support, reinforcement, and praise as the patient practices the prescribed therapy. Vocal exercises can be done utilizing a tape recorder for feedback and reinforcement without sacrificing privacy. Impatience regarding speech difficulties can be communicated to the individual through both verbal and nonverbal indicators. It is better to tell the person of any time restrictions, rather than to give a body message that could easily be interpreted as rejection. The emotional impact of symptoms on the individual can be compounded by the intellectual awareness of other's responses to them. The nurse is in a strategic position to influence those in the environment to deal with the patient as an adult with dignity and personal significance.

In the late stages of multiple sclerosis, bulbar involvement may result in *chewing and swallowing difficulties.* Since the risk of aspiration pneumonia at this time is great, the nurse must attend to the patient's safe positioning and assist at mealtimes. Alternative routes for providing nourishment such as a feeding tube may have to be considered.

**E**xperimental Treatment  On the hypothesis that multiple sclerosis is an immunological disorder, selected cases of rapidly progressive forms of multiple sclerosis are being treated with immunosuppressive agents such as cyclophosphomide[21] and azathioprine (Imuran). Antilymphocyte globulin (ALG) derived from animal serums has also been used for its action against human white blood cells involved in antibody production.[22,23] Trials have also involved use of ALG and azathioprine in various combinations with thoracic duct drainage of lymphocytes and steroid therapy.[24,25,26] This treatment is complex, costly, and dangerous, needing close, prolonged, medical supervision to prevent complications. Although some positive results have been reported, more controlled experimental trials are necessary. At present it should not be used as a general treatment measure but may hold some future promise.

**Fourth-Level Nursing Care**
Rehabilitation begins at the time of diagnosis when the affected person and family are supported through the grieving process. Grieving is usually triggered by the chronic nature of this illness, interrupted developmental tasks, and perceptions of present and future losses. The patient and family need available resources mobilized and accurate information during this early period. Studies have shown that the survival rate in multiple sclerosis approaches 80 percent of the life expectancy of the general population.[27] Relapses tend to occur 0.66 times per year throughout the course of the disease,[28] averaging less than once a year. Although progressive forms of the disease are seen, for most individuals symptoms remit for significant periods of time during the disease.

**Rehabilitation**  Before discharge, the patient's residual capabilities must be thoroughly evaluated for a meaningful rehabilitation program. In the early stages, goals and teaching outlined in Second-Level Nursing Care are initiated. The community health nurse should assess the patient returning to the home environment. During this evaluation, attention should be focused on the physical environment, emotional tone of the household, and social or economic factors that may impinge on the total rehabilitation. Minor physical changes which may help the individual maintain functional independence should be explored with family members. The local chapters of the National Multiple Sclerosis Society can provide additional information for helpful modifications and assistive devices that are available.

Health teaching should focus on the positive aspects of the patient's status. Continued gainful employment is usually possible and should be strongly encouraged. If a female patient has young children to care for, human assistance such as homemaker or baby-sitting services may need to be discussed to provide for adequate periods of rest during the day. The children's nap time formerly utilized for household chores may provide the patient with a rest period during the day.

Disruptions of normal patterns should be kept to a minimum. Continued involvement in outside interests and social activities should be encouraged within the individual's level of tolerance. Maintenance of social networks provides a sense of interrelatedness, personal validity, and significance for all family members. The nurse can assist the family in coming to terms with the fear of embarrassing symptoms that tend to promote social withdrawal. Public education is especially important in minimizing society's withdrawal from the patient. Employers need to be aware of the strengths and potentials of multiple sclerosis patients. While an occupational change is sometimes required, the patient can often remain gainfully employed for years.

In some cases, when the patient has prolonged difficulty in adjusting to multiple sclerosis, psychiatric counseling may be necessary. Family counseling may also be considered to restore or promote healthy family dynamics. Problems may have preceded the illness or may result from disequilibrium caused by illness. In either case, family counseling often reduces tensions that can trigger exacerbations.

Financial difficulties, resulting from loss of work or other factors, can obstruct rehabilitation efforts. Referral to social services may provide much-needed funds for household appliances, assistive devices, and other financial obligations. If residual losses mandate a change in employment, occupational therapy and vocational retraining possibilities need to be actively explored and appropriate referrals made.

During this early period, when disabilities are minimal, support and community services are most needed and least often provided. Because the individual and his or her family can get by, they are too often left to their own devices. This results in unnecessary loss of the individual's functional potential. The nurse needs to be familiar with the wide variety of services available in order to facilitate referral to the appropriate agencies for these aspects of total care.

**Follow-up care** Since the nature of multiple sclerosis is progressive, follow-up care and periodic reevaluation of the patient's total health status are essential. Both the family and care givers need to realize from the onset that exacerbations characterize the disease process itself and do not reflect a failure of the rehabilitation program.

In order to be feasible, goals must be readjusted to meet the changing patient needs and family situation. With progression of the disease the individual must be helped to cope with limitations and to prevent complications. At each of these critical transition points in the disease continuum, for example, when an ambulant patient shifts to wheelchair status or when an individual's activities become restricted to the house, nursing assessment and intervention are essential to operationalize the judgment made by the physician. Because these shifts may disrupt family equilibrium, the nurse must be actively involved with the family to support and facilitate these transitions. Intervention must again include potential initiation or reactivation of referrals for social services, psychiatric or family counseling, and other community services as needed.

Throughout the rehabilitation process the community health nurse should intervene with the patient, family, and environment to provide comprehensive care. Nursing action can be instrumental in achieving the ultimate objective of the individual participating actively in decision making and functioning independently within the limits imposed by multiple sclerosis.

## PARKINSON'S DISEASE

The debilitating condition known as Parkinson's disease affects about 1 percent of the population over 50. The onset is usually seen in the fifth and sixth decades of life, though it may occur earlier. It is slightly more prevalent in men and knows no race or class boundaries. Geographical patterns do not seem to exist. It begins insidiously and progressively worsens over a period of 15 to 20 years until incapacitation is reached. Within this framework, each individual's course may vary widely.

### Pathophysiology

Parkinson's disease is a syndrome involving the basal ganglions, particularly the substantia nigra and the striatum. The striatum consists of the caudate nucleus and putamen. The basal ganglions function in motor control. A number of anatomical pathways have recently been discovered within them.[29] These pathways, which influence the motor cortex, are composed of excitatory and inhibitory feedback loops which depend upon different synaptic chemical transmitters. A vital balance exists between the inhibitory pathways mediated by dopamine and neighboring excitatory pathways mediated, at least in part, by acetylcholine.

In Parkinson's disease there is degeneration of the melanin-containing nerve cells whose cell bodies lie in the compact part of the substantia nigra and whose axonal terminals lie in the corpus striatum. This causes some areas to be released from higher control (positive signs) and causes deficits in other areas due to damage of specific nuclei or tracts (negative signs). The degeneration includes depigmentation of the substantia nigra and cell loss, resulting in major alterations in the metabolism of the catecholamine, dopamine, in the basal ganglions. The dopamine depletion seen in Parkinson's disease is marked in the caudate nucleus and even more severe in the putamen. As a result of dopamine depletion, the striatum appears to be released from inhibitory modulation. Thus, the balance between the activity of acetylcholine and dopamine in the striatum is tipped in the direction of relative cholinergic dominance. On autopsy, patients are also found to have eosinophilic granular inclusions (Lewy bodies) in the remaining neurons.

In addition to the depigmentation and cell loss previously described, over half of the individuals with Parkinson's disease studied at autopsy demonstrate atrophy and cell loss in the cerebral cortex. This is probably an authentic part of the disease process and may account for increased dementia seen in advanced stages of the disease.

**Causes** *Primary Parkinsonism* (Parkinson's disease, paralysis agitans, idiopathic Parkinsonism) is the major form of the disease described so accurately by James Parkinson in 1817. The cause of this progressive neuronal degeneration is unknown. Neither viral nor genetic causes seem likely. Idiopathic Parkinsonism serves as a prototype for all other forms and will be the focus of subsequent discussion.

*Postencephalitic Parkinsonism* is the classic sequela of encephalitis lethargica (von Economo's disease) which swept the world between 1917 and 1926. Those who survived the acute phase often developed slowly progressive signs and symptoms resembling Parkinson's disease. Postmortem findings in postencephalitic Parkinsonism reveal neuronal depletion in the substantia nigra and dopamine depletion in striatum. Generally, the clinical picture is less severe than in primary Parkinsonism. Pathologic changes develop in the oculomotor nuclei and the reticular substance of the midbrain, producing ocular palsies and oculogyric crises (spasms of the eye muscles which often freeze in a fixed upward gaze) typical of the postencephalitic

form of the disease. Because the last case of encephalitis lethargica was reported in the 1940s, the incidence of postencephalitic Parkinsonism should be rare by 1990.

Other syndromes which resemble Parkinsonism can be produced by *drugs,* especially the phenothiazines; *toxins,* such as, carbon monoxide and manganese poisoning; and *other pathologies* which may involve similar symptoms. Conditions which fall into this pseudo-Parkinsonism category include Wilson's disease, Shy-Drager syndrome, olivopontocerebellar atrophy, progressive supranuclear palsy, familial tremor, hyperparathyroidism, hypo- and hyperthyroidism, Huntington's chorea, and others. Arteriosclerotic Parkinsonism once served as a distinct category of the disturbance, but has been generally dismissed.

**Effects on patients** Parkinsonism affects patients with classic symptoms of tremor, rigidity, and bradykinesia (extreme slowness of movement). Rigidity and tremor represent release from higher cortical control, while bradykinesia and impaired reflexes reflect cell loss. Parkinson's disease is characterized by rhythmic tremors that decrease during purposeful activity and complete relaxation, by rigidity that is manifested in body posture, movements, and facial expression, and by diminished spontaneous and associated movements. Intellectual deterioration is uncommon and usually seen only in the late stages of the disease.

Five stages of Parkinsonism have been established on the basis of the level of disability. In *stage I* there is *unilateral involvement with little or no functional impairment.* Tremor is commonly the first symptom noticed. It is a slow (three to seven cycles per second) resting tremor, which decreases with voluntary movement. In stress situations it increases, but it disappears with sleep. Changes in posture and locomotion include a slight tilt toward the nontremor side, slight abduction at the shoulder, and elbow flexion with decreased walking arm-swing. There is a reduction in arm and facial gestures, as well as the amplitude and inflections of speech. If the involved side is the dominant one, handwriting changes show small writing with a shaky quality and poorly formed loops.

In *stage II* manifestations become more pronounced with *bilateral involvement without impairment of balance* which occurs within 1 or 2 years. Posture is stooped forward at the waist with the spinal column, hips, knees, and ankles slightly flexed. Rigidity is also bilateral, but range of joint motion is usually intact. Feet assume a slight varus (turned inward) position which results in "hammer-toe-like" effects that make wearing shoes and walking uncomfortable. Generalized slowness (brady-kinesia) of all movements develops. This slowness is readily apparent to others while the individual experiences it as fatigue and weakness. Arm swing, facial expression, hand gestures, and spontaneous blinking are also diminished. The individual appears immobile. Walking begins with hesitation (start-hesitation) and is slow and shuffling, and turning requires deliberate effort. Functional capacity is relatively uncompromised, but the effort involved on the part of the individual is considerable.

The onset of *stage III* is heralded by negative signs of pronounced *gait disturbances* that indicate increased alterations in postural and righting reflexes (see Fig. 37-1). Problems include festination gait, a propulsion in which steps become shorter and faster as the individual walks forward. Retropulsion occurs in the same way when the individual is backing up. Walking does not always trigger propulsion. Usually the pace is even slower and more hesitating than before, and may be punctuated by episodes in which the individual's feet seem to freeze to the floor. There is also increasing poverty of motor activities, which results in losses in functional activities such as buttoning, typing, and zipping. The patient needs occasional assistance with the activities of daily living.

Manifestations of *autonomic nervous system dysfunction* also are present. Central sympathetic dysfunction causes the *ocular disturbances* of *miosis* (contraction of the pupil), *enophthalmus* (recession of eyeball in socket), and *ptosis* (partial closure of eyelid) on the more affected side.

Profuse *perspiration* may occur regardless of season, because of disordered temperature regulations, and may result in fever and dehydration. *Seborrhea,* probably caused by dysfunction of the hypothalamus, often results in skin eruptions.

**FIGURE 37-1**
Typical postural changes in Parkinson's disease.

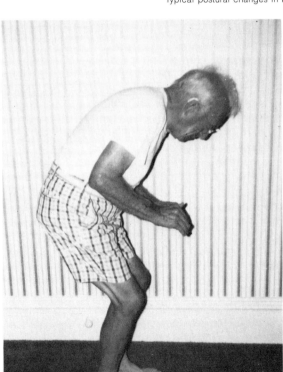

Scoliosis toward unaffected side

Trunk flexed

Posture rigid

Knees flexed

Neck flexed

Facial expression blank

Elbows flexed

Ankles flexed

Feet in varus position

*Drooling* results not from excessive salivation but because of decreased automatic swallowing. Muscular incoordination during swallowing caused by delayed relaxation of the inferior constrictor muscle of the pharnyx results in *dysphagia* which often is severe enough to cause weight loss and dehydration. Because of bradykinesia, the risk of aspiration pneumonia is high.

Generalized slowing of the gastrointestinal system is also found in patients with Parkinson's disease and, combined with poor diet and reduced activity, results in *chronic constipation.* Diarrhea may be present and detectable as liquid stool seeps past impacted stool.

Neurogenic *bladder dysfunction* causes urinary hesitation and frequency and in males can be further aggravated by benign prostatic hypertrophy common in this age group.

Parkinsonian individuals are also occasionally bothered by *thermal paresthesia,* distressing episodes described as burning sensations in a part of or over the entire body. These usually subside after a year or two. Neither the cause of this phenomenon nor treatment measures are known. *Arthralgia* (joint aches) and *myalgia* (muscle aches) are also common and may be caused by immobility and rigidity.

In *stage IV* there is significant disability caused by *increased rigidity, bradykinesia, and akinesia* (inability to initiate voluntary movement). The person can not live alone and needs assistance with many activities of daily living. Turning, rising, and standing activities are performed with great difficulty. Festination gait is present and falls are common. Tremor does not become more severe and may often diminish; nevertheless, finger dexterity is markedly impaired. Assistance may be required for eating and dressing.

*Stage V* involves *complete invalidism;* the patient is confined to bed or chair. Little if any voluntary motor function remains, and the patient, akinetic, contracted, and rigid, lies immobile in bed.

### First-Level Nursing Care

Because the cause of primary Parkinsonism is unknown, its prevention is not yet possible. Nursing care should focus on drugs and toxins that can produce Parkinsonian symptoms. In industrial settings, carbon monoxide or manganese poisoning poses potential health hazards. Safety programs should be instituted and exposure minimized.

Drug-induced pseudo-Parkinsonism is also preventable. Major phenothiazides such as chlorpromazine (Thorazine) and promazine (Sparine),

can cause adverse effects which mimic primary Parkinsonism. Symptoms may also include oculogyric crises and dystonic movements. Iatrogenic Parkinsonism is seen predominantly in psychiatric hospitals and long-term care facilities, but with the trend toward community mental health care it may be seen in any community health setting. Because symptoms are potentially reversible by discontinuing the drug or reducing the dosage, patients taking these drugs should be considered at risk and carefully assessed on a regular basis.

### Second-Level Nursing Care

The onset of Parkinsonism is insidious and often impacts upon the individual's life in a variety of subtle ways. The initial stages seldom require hospitalization and present a unique challenge for the community health nurse.

**Nursing assessment** Because Parkinsonism develops slowly, patients may be unaware of the significance of the changes. Often patients are seen in a clinic or doctor's office for other problems. Whenever Parkinsonism is suspected, a complete health assessment should be done.

**H**ealth History An accurate *health history* will help to identify the onset of symptoms. Some of the early complaints of patients include insomnia, clumsiness, weakness, and vague aches and pains that have persisted for a year or so. Because the patient may not be aware of some of the changes, input from a family member may be useful. During the history, additional observations should be made regarding the individual's posture, facial expressions, coordination, and general demeanor to complete the primary data base. When assessing patients, the nurse must consider the age-related changes that may be occurring.

If the pathology is more advanced, the patient may relate difficulties in walking and performing some of the activities of daily living. Patients should be asked about perspiration, skin problems, difficulty in swallowing, bowel habits, bladder function, sexual difficulties, and any abnormal sensations.

**P**hysical Assessment *Physical assessment* of the patient with Parkinsonism should include a complete neurological examination. When motor function is tested, rigidity will be noted during both flexion and extension (plastic rigidity) regardless of speed. Early in its development the rigidity will be mild, and tremors may appear asymmetrically.

Often the first finding is a slight tremor of the hand or leg. In the hand it appears as pill-rolling movements. Often the patient is able to control the tremor by resting the hand on a table. When tremor is superimposed on rigidity, the alternating resistance-release felt by the examiner is called "cog-wheel rigidity." Facial expressions should be evaluated for decreases in facial mobility. As the condition progresses, the face assumes a characteristic immobile, masklike staring appearance.

Evaluation of muscle strength will reveal weakness in affected extremities. The patient should be asked to perform spontaneous movements and complex tasks. Often the patient will be unable to do two activities at once, such as standing up and blowing his or her nose. During this activity slowness will be noted, and the patient may not be able to spontaneously react to postural changes.

The patient should be observed walking and the gait evaluated. Initially, one leg may be stiff and drag. The arm on the affected side will be flexed at the elbow and abducted at the shoulder. Later, a characteristic shuffling gait will be noted. The patient will take little steps with increasing rapidity (propulsive gait). When this occurs while the patient is walking backward, it is called *retropulsion.*

Reflexes should be tested. The tendon and plantar deep tendon reflexes will be normal. The *palmomental reflex* will be abnormal and is demonstrated by stroking the affected palm near the thumb. In Parkinson's disease, and a number of other central nervous system disorders including amyotrophic lateral sclerosis, the stroking will cause wrinkling of the chin on the stimulated side. The *glabellar reflex* is hyperactive in Parkinson's disease. This is elicited by repeated taps (about one per second) over the smooth prominence on the frontal bone above the root of the nose. The Parkinson's individual will continue to blink or even be unable to open his or her eyes, while normal adults become refractory to blinking after a few taps. These findings point to early Parkinsonism. As the disease progresses, reflex blinking may be lost.

Sensory perception should also be evaluated. Perception usually remains normal in Parkinsonism. The eye should be examined for recession and ptosis. The pupils often contract abnormally.

**D**iagnostic Tests   There are few tests that are diagnostic of Parkinson's disease. Diagnosis is usually made on clinical findings. However, the levels of urine dopamine and cerebrospinal fluid homovanillic acid (HVA is the end product of dopamine metabolism) are depressed in Parkinson's disease.

**Nursing problems and interventions**   The primary problems Parkinsonian patients must deal with are *rigidity, tremors,* and *hypokinesia.* Drug therapy has proved to be effective in controlling these problems in some patients. At present, *levodopa* (L-dopa) is the drug of choice for the treatment of Parkinsonism. It is the immediate precursor of dopamine. Unlike dopamine, it readily passes through the blood-brain barrier where it is rapidly taken up by remaining neurons in the dopaminergic nigrostriatal system. Inside the neurons, it is converted to dopamine, stored, and then transported to axon terminals where it is released as a neurotransmitter.

The most important principle which must be reinforced in family and patient teaching is that treatment must begin with small doses which are gradually increased until a satisfactory response is achieved. Improvement occurs in 1 to 2 months and is seen as decreased bradykinesia with renewed sparkling in the eyes and improved facial animation. Decreased rigidity follows with improvements in walking, posture, and balance. Drooling, dysphagia, and dysarthria also improve. Tremor responds less consistently and in some cases may worsen. Full therapeutic benefits may take 6 months to achieve. Patients and family will need support and encouragement during this phase of treatment.

*Side effects* most commonly encountered include anorexia, nausea, and vomiting. Orthostatic hypotension and cardiac arrhythmias occur, but less frequently than gastrointestinal symptoms. All these side effects are caused by conversion of L-dopa to dopamine outside the brain, where it is widely distributed. Symptomatic relief of nausea can be afforded by taking the drug with meals or milk. Orthostatic hypotension may not produce symptoms of fainting and dizziness, but the newly mobile patient should be cautioned to change positions slowly. Elastic stockings may also be of benefit. Cardiac effects of L-dopa in elderly patients have been found to be relatively harmless.[30] Narrow-angle glaucoma is a contraindication of L-dopa. The patient should be aware that levodopa may change the color of his or her urine to red or brown.

Recently *extracerebral decarboxylase inhibitors,* which reduce conversion of L-dopa to dopamine outside the brain, have been used in combination with L-dopa therapy. Alpha-methyldopa hydrazine[31-33] (Mk 486, carbidopa), used in the United States, and benzerazide (RO 4-4602),[34] used in other countries, have been beneficial in reducing the peripheral actions of levodopa, thus reducing the side effects as well as L-dopa dosage requirements. Combination therapy with L-dopa and peripheral decarboxylase inhibitors is fast becoming the preferred method of symptomatic management for Parkinson's disease.

*Long-range side effects* of levodopa begin to emerge after about two years (earlier with a combination of L-dopa and a decarboxylase inhibitor) and affect 15 to 40 percent of patients treated. The triad of effects known as *akinesia paradoxica* include: (1) subtle changes in cortical function manifested by decreased attention span, poor recent memory, and behavioral changes, (2) persistence of involuntary adventitious (sporadic) movements, and (3) start-hesitation which is accompanied by festination and frequent episodes of freezing in place. Akinesia paradoxica is associated with an "on-off" phenomenon. Attacks occur erratically, are only sometimes associated with dosage times, and are felt to be due to a variety of factors. The "on" period is associated with abnormal involuntary movements, the "off" period with intense akinesia. This is severely incapacitating, and the fear of attacks often keeps the patient housebound.

*Other drugs* used as primary therapy in the pre-levodopa era included cholinergic blocking agents and antihistamines and to a lesser extent cerebral stimulants, tranquilizers, and muscle relaxants. The *anticholinergic agents* are employed now as adjuncts to levodopa therapy. They should be used cautiously with patients who have glaucoma, and they cause atropine-like side effects such as mouth dryness, blurred vision, dry flushed skin, dizziness, tachycardia, urinary retention, and constipation. Other combinations of anti-Parkinson drugs under study include amatadine (Symmetrel), bromocriptine, and propranolol.

The patient should be cautioned against the use of medications other than those prescribed. The excess use of laxatives taken for constipation may cause severe fluid and electrolyte imbalances. Vitamins with high pyridoxine (vitamin $B_6$) content will reverse the therapeutic effects of levadopa. When levadopa is given with peripheral decarboxylase inhibitors, the negative effects of vitamin $B_6$ are not seen. Knowledge of all medications the patient is taking as well as their side effects will give the nurse a solid data base for the analysis of problems the patient may present.

A regimen of physical therapy often helps to relieve some of the *muscle weakness* as well as the rigidity. The patient may come in for regular physical therapy sessions. The family can often be taught the exercises, and a community health nurse can reinforce and supervise the program.

Useful exercises should be taught to the patient and family. Rigidity and its resultant arthralgias and myalgia are helped by application of heat before active and assistive range of motion exercises. Performance often improves when the objective is to accomplish an activity rather than an anatomic motion. Thus, having the patient march to music may be more effective than asking the person to lift his or her feet higher, and at the same time facilitate both high-step gait and renewed arm swing. Working exercise into the patient's daily activities is ideal.

*Postural problems* and *loss of facial muscle strength* can be countered by having the patient make a conscious effort to compensate by standing erect and performing face, eye, and lip exercises in front of a mirror. To increase stability, attention should be given to a high-step gait and wide base (feet 10 to 12 inches apart) when walking and turning. In "freezing" episodes, dorsiflexing the feet will often "unfreeze" them for walking.

*Speech deficits* are treated by having the patient speak loudly with intentionally exaggerated pronunciation. Performance of deep breathing exercises by counting as high as possible during inhalation and again during exhalation improves speech control. These speech exercises may be embarrassing for the patient. The family should be encouraged to provide the patient with complete privacy and let the individual use a tape recorder for feedback regarding his or her progress. Speech classes for groups of Parkinson patients may be beneficial.

**S**afety Parkinsonism is seen primarily among the elderly. Its primary effect is to alter balance, coordination, and locomotion. Treatment side effects add dizziness, blurred vision, and orthostatic hypotension to the problems. All these combine to make the patient a prime candidate for falls. The patient's home should be evaluated for hazards. Good lighting, elevated toilet seats, guard rails in the bathroom, unobstructed hallways, electrical cords kept out of the way, nonslippery floors, and avoidance of throw rugs in areas where the patient walks, as well as properly fitting shoes with rubber soles, all help to reduce the risk of falling. Family members should be encouraged to assist as necessary without taking over for the patient. If changes are necessary in the home environment, social service should be contacted so that financial assistance can be explored.

Safety needs to be considered during mealtimes when tremor on the dominant side might cause burns from spilling hot liquids or when swallowing difficulties are present. Cups with lids are available for hot liquids, and the family should be taught to have someone present when the patient is eating.

**N**utrition  *Proper nutrition* is often a problem for the person with Parkinson's disease because of the disease itself, age factors, and side effects of medication. The edentulous individual or one with poorly fitting dentures may be unable to chew a variety of foods. Difficulty in swallowing may result in decreased intake of fluids as well as solids. Drugs used to treat the condition often cause anorexia, nausea, and vomiting which further jeopardize adequate dietary intake. The individual often turns to soft foods, which are low in bulk and vitamins, but easier to eat without embarrassment.

The lack of bulk and decreased fluid intake add to the tendency to become constipated. *Constipation* causes feelings of lethargy and anorexia, and the individual often responds by taking harsh laxatives or enemas which further deplete fluids and electrolytes. This depletion of electrolytes, especially potassium, causes more muscle weakness and lethargy, and the cycle begins again.

Clearly, dietary counseling is an important aspect of nursing care. Meal planning should provide sufficient calories, fluid, vitamins, and bulk. Foods high in residue and natural laxative properties like bran should be encouraged along with a high fluid intake. These measures along with stool softeners, or gentle laxatives, and exercise promote a more regular bowel pattern. Relief of constipation often has a beneficial effect on the patient's appetite.

Some physicians recommend a reduction in protein intake with L-dopa therapy.[35] Moderate use of alcohol is not harmful and may reduce anxiety, improve appetite, and, at bedtime, promote sleep. If the individual is obese, a reduction diet is indicated to increase mobility potential.

Mouth care before meals will lubricate the mouth for eating and may reduce the metallic taste often associated with L-dopa therapy. After meals, mouth care removes food particles which lead to odor formation and dental caries. Drooling and dexterity problems should be managed with special utensils that are available. The use of a bib is demeaning to some patients.

Meals should be coordinated to meet the patient's food preferences without sacrificing adequate nutrition, rushing the meal, or serving foods cold. It must be remembered that eating patterns have developed over time and it may take time, patience, and family education to correct them.

**A**utonomic Problems  Other problems may be encountered with which the patient and family need assistance. *Reduced frequency of blinking* can cause corneal irritation. Eye drops may have to be obtained from the physician. The patient or family should be taught the proper technique for instilling the drops.

Profuse *perspiration* and *seborrhea* call for fastidious hygienic measures. At home the person may sit on a chair in the shower to ensure cleanliness without falls. Use of a gentle emollient on dry skin may be beneficial. Oily spots should be washed frequently with soap and water and rinsed and dried well.

*Insomnia* is also a frequent problem. The use of Benadryl at bedtime and avoidance of daytime naps may help. Walking, range of motion exercises, and other daytime activities may also encourage more normal sleep patterns.

*Bladder problems* or urinary retention, hesitation, and frequency may result in occasional accidents. As with occasional fecal oozing around an impaction, measures must be taken to accurately assess the situation. This embarrassing loss of control may reflect the patient's inability to reach the bathroom quickly enough.

**E**motional Adjustment  The individual with Parkinson's disease has a chronic progressive degenerative neurological disorder. Smooth coordination and integration of body movements, generally taken for granted, are lost. This loss causes severe alterations in self-esteem, independence, social interactions, work capacity, and all aspects of the individual's emotional life. The grieving process accompanies this irreversible change in body image. If sexual difficulties are present, self-image may be further damaged. Frequently, the patient is overwhelmed and needs support in the work of grieving. Humiliation from symptoms like drooling and the reactions of others to them may cause the individual to withdraw to ease the anguish. The family should be encouraged to actively offer support and explore with the patient the impact of the physical changes.

In order to communicate effectively, the nurse must validate perceptions with the individual. It is important to remember that the hypokinesia, masked facies, and monotone voice are part of the physical symptomatology of Parkinson's disease. These reductions in the individual's capacity to interact with the environment could easily be perceived by the family members, and health professionals, as a reaction to the disease rather than a manifestation of the disease itself. The nurse, sensitive to these difficulties, should provide privacy and ample time for patient and family interviews. The perception of the situation by those involved should be explored. Past successful coping strategies should be discussed to provide perspective on the current situation. Additional supports should be sought from family and community resources. Only then can the nurse set realistic goals to meet the individual's needs for security, self-esteem, independence, affiliation, and interdependence in the context of each patient's unique situation.

**Sociocultural Adjustment** The person with Parkinson's disease, like any other person, participates as a member of a family, community, and society. The individual's interaction patterns need to be assessed by the nurse. Sexual patterns should be part of the nursing assessment. Often sexual activity has been curtailed because of the disturbance. If the individual is not uncomfortable with the change, she or he should not be made to feel inadequate. If the patient feels this is a problem, the nurse can plan care with appropriate resource persons so that mutually satisfying sexual expressions for the individuals involved can be identified.

Other social exchanges such as phone conversations, check writing, and personal correspondence are hampered by the vocal problems and handwriting changes seen in Parkinsonism. The patient's social isolation is often increased.

Often there are significant role alterations within a family constellation as a result of Parkinsonism. If the husband is affected, the wife may have become the breadwinner or may have resumed ego-fulfilling mothering activities that actually encourage the affected individual's dependence. These altered patterns must be assessed relative to the overall family dynamics before a determination can be made regarding their acceptability. Again, perception of the situation by significant others must be evaluated. Cultural and religious factors must also be explored as a framework for planning nursing interventions appropriate for the individual and family. The time interval in which role changes took place must be considered. If new patterns are deeply integrated into the family's life-style, changes will also take time.

A study by Eleanor Singer[36] on the social costs of Parkinson's disease demonstrated that affected individuals are far less likely to work, and if working, lose time to illness far more than the general population. Further, affected persons did less housework, had fewer close friends, and spent more time in idleness than the general population. These findings were more marked among younger patients. She described the net results as "premature social aging." Although the study might underrepresent rural areas in its sample, the findings suggest that both the social and economic impacts of the disease are considerable. In planning at this level, referral to social services for assistance is essential for comprehensive care.

### Third-Level Nursing Care

Despite a good response to therapy, the underlying disease process continues, and patients progress to later stages. During the last stages the patient becomes severely incapacitated and requires complete nursing care at home or in an extended-care facility. The patient is often hospitalized for problems associated with the condition. Falls frequently result in hip fractures. Urinary retention and other neurogenic bladder problems, particularly in the elderly male with prostatic enlargement, often lead to serious urinary tract infections. Rigidity of the muscles of respiration and proneness to aspiration frequently cause respiratory infections such as pneumonia.

During *nursing assessment* the findings will be similar to but more severe than those discussed under Second-Level Nursing Care. The patient will be found to be extremely debilitated and unable to move. Evaluation of range of motion will reveal contractures. The patient often remains rigid, confined to a chair or bed. Communication may be difficult. Muscle strength, range of motion, rigidity, reflexes, and autonomic functions will be greatly impaired. If urinary retention is a problem, the prostate should be palpated.

**Nursing problems and interventions** The patient with advanced Parkinsonism is severely incapacitated and susceptible to all the *hazards of immobility*. Comprehensive nursing care must be planned with this in mind. At the same time nursing care should focus on the *sweating* and *foul body odor*. The latter may result from levodopa therapy. *Adequate nutrition* and *fluid intake* must also be incorporated into the patient's care.

Safety measures outlined previously should be employed in the hospital situation. With L-dopa therapy, increased periods of wakefulness are seen and may be accompanied by confusion. Judicious use of restraints may be necessary for the individual's protection; however, routine employment of restraints is not a substitute for good nursing care.

The increased survival with Parkinson's disease has been accompanied by recognition of *behavioral changes* and *intellectual impairments.* These are considered part of the primary condition but are often aggravated by medications and the unfamiliar surroundings of the hospital. Explanations and orientation to the environment may need to be repeated frequently. The reassurance and patience of the nurse can often help the patient compensate for the many sensory deficits impeding comprehension of the hospital situation. By reducing anxiety the nurse can help restore the patient's sense of control during hospitalization.

**P**arkinsonian Crisis   The patient may be hospitalized for life-threatening Parkinsonian crisis. This is an acute episode of severe loss of symptomatic control with tremor dyskinesia, rigidity, tachycardia, diaphoresis, and hyperpnea. This is usually triggered by acute anxiety or sudden withdrawal of medications. The patient comes to the hospital in an acutely anxious state and needs immediate cardiac and respiratory support measures.

Environmental support in a quiet room with soft lighting and the reassuring presence of the nurse or a significant other combined with immediate medication including phenobarbital or amylbarbital and anti-Parkinson's drugs usually control this episode. Other nursing measures for physical and emotional care and rehabilitation covered earlier in the chapter should also be employed.

**S**urgical Intervention   Rarely, stereotaxic procedures, such as a thalamotomy, are indicated as a mode of treatment. A thalamotomy involves the surgical destruction of a discrete part of the lateroventral thalamus to improve the movement disturbance. In carefully selected individuals with severe unilateral tremor unresponsive to medication and with no mental impairment, major gait problems, or speech impairment, unilateral thalamotomy may provide benefits in reducing tremor and improving fine finger and head movements.

Stereotaxic surgery generally involves placing the patient's head in a metal frame which immobilizes it. The attached needle holder can then guide the insertion of a needle to exact locations in the brain. Cannulas can be similarly inserted and liquid nitrogen used to freeze and thus destroy the area. Ultrasound vibration can produce similar results.

The pre- and postoperative care is similar to that of any patient undergoing neurosurgery (see Chap. 35). If surgical treatment is performed, the nurse needs to be aware that on the first night after surgery the patient is often confused, has difficulty concentrating, and has a tendency to lean to the thalamotomized side. Without adequate safety measures, dangerous early postoperative falls can result.

Long-term studies have shown sustained improvement in tremor and rigidity in unilateral procedures; bilateral procedures showed less sustained benefit.[37,38] Neither procedure necessarily resulted in functional improvement in performing activities of daily living. Patients who have had past stereotaxic surgery, however, still may derive considerable benefits from treatment with levodopa.

### Fourth-Level Nursing Care

The focus of fourth-level nursing care is long-term rehabilitation. Since Parkinson's disease is a chronic progressive disorder, maximizing the individual's functional independence is the most important goal. This means assessing strengths as well as weaknesses. Constant treatment adjustments and teaching needs warrant input by the nurse to promote independence.

Patients should be encouraged to assess their own losses and those anticipated in the future. Coping strategies can then be identified. Continued social interaction and work activities should be maintained. It should be made clear to all concerned with the patient's welfare that facial expression is not necessarily reflective of the patient's mental state.

In order to cope effectively with the disease, patient-teaching needs to be initiated in the areas of diet, medication, exercises, and safety.

*Diet teaching* includes dietary considerations covered in Second-Level Nursing Care. The dietitian should provide the content for dietary management. The nurse can actively utilize data collected to incorporate dietary planning into the patterns, preferences, and cultural trends of the individual. Involvement of family members should accent what the person can and should eat rather than focus on a list of "don'ts."

*Medication teaching* interfaces with diet teaching because of the side effects of anorexia, nausea, and vomiting. The patient needs to know that taking levodopa with food reduces the incidence of vomiting and that the vomiting side effect wanes in a few months. Interim measures may include antiemetic medications for relief.

Levodopa dosage is begun slowly and titrated to meet the individual's unique dosage requirements. This involves increments of the drug until symptomatic relief occurs or adventitious involuntary movements occur. The drug may be given frequently, and measures such as keeping each day's portion of levodopa separate may eliminate the risk of overdose by the elderly patient. Involuntary movements can be the result of accidental overdose or represent a long-term side effect indicating a need for reduction of dosage. The patient should be taught that less medication rather than more will reduce these involuntary movements.

Postural hypotension and cardiac arrhythmias occur less frequently. Elastic stockings and slow changes in position can reduce risk of falls in the former situation; arrhythmias may create the need for cardiac medications and should be watched for during follow-up care.

*Exercise teaching* should be reinforced by the nurse, and therapeutic exercise plans taught. The patient and family need to understand how to perform prescribed exercises as well as the need for faithful execution of them. Activities of daily living such as eating, dressing, washing, and elimination need to be incorporated into these assessments, and appropriate assistance provided.

*Safety teaching* involves environmental factors discussed previously. If able to ambulate, the patient should be encouraged to continue social contacts outside the home. Friends can offer a great benefit by providing assistance in getting in and out of cars and buildings safely. Since stress aggravates the risk of accidents, an environment of emotional warmth and safety maximizes independence for a considerable period of time.

*Other resources* that are available to the nurse for the patient and family include other members of the health team in addition to the dietitian, social worker, and physical therapist. Audiovisual materials may also be of assistance in teaching activities of daily living. If the individual is severely depressed, referral for psychological counseling or psychiatric evaluation may be necessary.

Severely disrupted family dynamics which may have preceded illness or have evolved secondary to Parkinson's disease may require *family counseling*. *Occupational* and *vocational support services* available in the community can also help in any role adjustments the patient must make. *Community services* such as a homemaker and visiting nurse are critical for the individual who lacks available family members. The single or widowed patient is in particular need of community-based follow-up care to compensate for the lack of family support. Information and coping strategies are also available to the

nurse as well as the patient through the *Parkinson's Disease Foundation*. All resources available should be explored and integrated into the total plan of care. The nurse's perception of patient problems and coordination of health team activities can significantly improve the patient's quality of life as the search for the causes and cure of Parkinson's disease continues.

## HUNTINGTON'S CHOREA

*Chronic progressive chorea,* or *Huntington's chorea,* is often characterized by initial features similar to Parkinsonism. Onset in early to middle adult life with choreiform movements (muscular twitching) accompanied by mental deterioration differentiates it from Parkinsonism. This severe neurological disorder, marked by degeneration and selective microneuron atrophy, pursues a downhill course with death occurring 12 to 15 years after onset. Rapid, jerky movements gradually develop, beginning in the face and arms. The movements are purposeless and become progressively more violent, involving the entire body. Huntington's chorea is inherited in an autosomal dominant fashion with complete penetrance. It is probable that a gene-determined metabolic error underlies pathologic changes and resultant symptoms.

Attempts to discover the biochemical basis for Huntington's chorea have shown that gamma-aminobutric acid (GABA) levels are lowered, but drugs to raise the level of this inhibitory neurotransmitter have not yet been successful.[39] However, drugs that reduce dopamine levels or block dopamine receptors have been reported to reduce the chorieform movements of Huntington's chorea. Reserpine, which interferes with catecholamine storage in neurons, is sometimes beneficial in treating choreic symptoms. Thus, the role of neurotransmitters such as dopamine and GABA in Huntington's chorea seems to hold promise and is being actively investigated.

Genetic aspects of the disease are known. Children of a person with Huntington's chorea have a 50 percent chance of developing the disease. In fact, a large number of the cases in America have been traced back to two brothers who immigrated to Long Island, New York, from England. Since onset does not occur until middle years, genetic counseling for individuals potentially having Huntington's chorea is advisable.

At present, treatment of the disease is symptomatic, and the rehabilitation potential grim. Nursing care can provide comfort to the patient and education and support to offspring of individuals with Huntington's chorea who must deal with the uncertainty of their own status.

## AMYOTROPHIC LATERAL SCLEROSIS

Amyotrophic lateral sclerosis (ALS) (motor neuron disease) is a steadily progressive degenerative process involving the corticobulbar, spinal, and lower motor neurons. It leads, by encroachment, to a mixture of spastic and atrophic changes in cranial and spinal musculature. Damage to the myelin sheath, occurring secondary to damage in the lateral columns, may resemble multiple sclerosis in middle-aged patients who show slowly progressive paraplegia associated with muscle wasting. Intact abdominal reflexes, sphincter control, and normal CSF findings plus later age at onset point to the diagnosis of ALS.

This condition affects an estimated 8000 to 10,000 Americans between 40 and 70 years and twice as many males as females.[40] A recent study indicated exposure to heavy metals, increased dietary calcium intake, and involvement in athletics among ALS individuals to be significantly higher than the general population.[41] It is theorized that environmental factors might trigger motor neuron exhaustion in genetically predisposed individuals. The exact cause of ALS is still unknown.

First symptoms may be reflective of either spinal or bulbar involvement. In the former, symptoms include muscular weakness, atrophy, and fasciculations (irregular spasmatic twitching in small muscle groups) in the distal portions of one or more extremity. Bulbar involvement make chewing, swallowing, and speech difficult. Damage above the brainstem may cause sudden outbursts of laughter or tears though cognitive function is intact. Usually either spastic or atrophic changes occur first. As the disease advances, a mixture of spastic and atrophic paralysis with twitching and muscle wasting develops. ALS progresses steadily, but the rate of progression varies widely, depending on the area involved and whether atrophic or spastic changes predominate. Death usually occurs within 1½ years of atrophic bulbar involvement with dysphagia, aspiration pneumonia, and respiratory failure. Death may occur without bulbar damage if spinal involvement causes paralysis of the diaphragm and other respiratory musculature.

The treatment is symptomatic. Respiratory support early in the illness can be beneficial. Nursing care should encourage the individual to maintain good general health and nutrition, avoid infection, and be active within the limits of disability. The prognosis is guarded. Symptomatic care, similar to care of the individual with multiple sclerosis, involves much physical and emotional support. Local chapters of the National Multiple Sclerosis Society provide patient services to sufferers of ALS and can offer a much-needed support group for patients and their families.

## REFERENCES

1  J. D. Millar and R. S. Allison, *Multiple Sclerosis: A Disease Acquired in Childhood,* Charles C Thomas, Springfield, Ill., 1971.
2  M. Alter, U. Leibowitz, and J. Speer, "Risk of Multiple Sclerosis Related to Age at Immigration to Israel," *Arch Neurol,* **15:**234, 1966.
3  Milton Alter and Wojciech Cendrowski, "Multiple Sclerosis and Childhood Infections," *Neurology* (Minneap), **26:**201–204, March 1976.
4  J. A. Brody, et al., "Measles Antibody Titers of Multiple Sclerosis Patients and Their Siblings," *Neurology (Minneap),* **22:**492–499, May 1972.
5  E. Norrby, et al., "Comparison of Antibodies against Different Viruses in the Cerebrospinal Fluid and Serum Samples from Patients with Multiple Sclerosis," *Infections Immunology,* **10:**688–694, October 1974.
6  H. J. Bauer, et al., "Early Sterile Autopsy in Etiological Studies on Multiple Sclerosis," *J Neurol,* **208**(3):159–174, March 1975.
7  R. Carp, G. Merz, and P. Licursi, "A Non-cytopathic Infectious Agent Associated with Multiple Sclerosis," *Neurology (Minneap),* **25**(5):492–493, May, 1975.
8  Milton Alter, et al.: "Genetic Association of Multiple Sclerosis and HL-A Determinants," *Neurology (Minneap),* **26:**31–36, January 1976.
9  L. W. Myers, et al., "HLA and the Immune Responses to Measles in Multiple Sclerosis," *Neurology (Minneap),* **26:**54–55, June 1976.
10  C. Brautbar, M. Alter, and E. Kahana, "HLA Antigens in Multiple Sclerosis," *Neurology (Minneap),* **26:**50–53, June 1976.
11  H. W. Delank, "Clinical and Diagnostic Importance of the Examination of Cerebrospinal Fluid in Multiple Sclerosis," *Acta Neurochir (Wien),* **31**(3–4): 291, 1975.
12  "Multiple Sclerosis and Amyotrophic Lateral Sclerosis," *Stat Bull Metropol Life Ins Co,* New York, **56:**2–5, March 1975.
13  Douglas McAlpine, Charles Lumsden, and E. D. Acheson, *Multiple Sclerosis: A Reappraisal,* E. & S. Livingstone, London, 1965.

14 L. Frisén and W. F. Hoyt, "Insidious Atrophy of Retinal Nerve Fibers in Multiple Sclerosis. Funduscopic Identification in Patients with and without Visual Complaints," *Arch Ophthamol,* **92**(2):91–97, August 1974.

15 Mand Feinsod and W. Hoyt, "Subclinical Optic Neuropathy in Multiple Sclerosis," *J Neurol Neurosurg Psychiatry,* **38**:1109–1114, November 1975.

16 *Loc. cit.*

17 P. Asselman, D. Chadwick, and D. C. Marsden, "Visual Evoked Responses in the Diagnosis and Management of Patients Suspected of Multiple Sclerosis," *Brain,* **98**(2):261–282, June 1975.

18 A. From and A. Heltberg, "A Double Blind Trial with Baclofen (Lioresal) and Diazepam in Spasticity due to Multiple Sclerosis," *Acta Neurol Scand,* **51**(2):158–166, February 1975.

19 J. V. Basmajian, "Lioresal (Balclofen) Treatment of Spasticity in Multiple Sclerosis," *Am J Phys Med,* **54**(4):175–177, August 1975.

20 D. W. Hedley, J. A. Mardon, and M. E. Esper, "Evaluation of Baclofen (Lioresal) for Spasticity in Multiple Sclerosis," *Postgrad Med J,* **51**:615–618, September 1975.

21 D. A. Drachman, et al., "Cyclophosphamide in Exacerbations of Multiple Sclerosis. Therapeutic Trial and Strategy for Pilot Drug Studies," *J Neurol Neurosurg Psychiatry,* **38**(6):592–597, June 1975.

22 D. J. MacFahyen, et al., "Failure of Antilymphocytic Globulin Therapy in Chronic Progressive Multiple Sclerosis," *Neurology (Minneap),* **23**:592–598, June 1973.

23 T. P. Seland, et al., "Evaluation of Antithymocyte Globulin in Acute Relapses of Multiple Sclerosis," *Neurology,* **24**(1):34–40, January 1974.

24 W. Brendel, J. Ring, and J. Seifret, "Immunosuppressive Treatment of Multiple Sclerosis with ALG and/or Thoracic Duct Drainage," *Neurology (Minneap),* **25**(5):490, May 1975.

25 E. M. Lance, et al., "Intensive Immunosuppression in Multiple Sclerosis," *Neurology (Minneap),* **25**(5):491, May 1975.

26 E. M. Lance, et al., "Intensive Immunosuppression in Patients with Disseminated Sclerosis," *Clin Exp Immunol,* **2**(1):1–12, July 1975.

27 J. F. Kurtzke, et al., "Studies on the Natural History of Multiple Sclerosis: V. Long-Term Survival in Young Men," *Arch Neurol,* **22**:215–225, September 1970.

28 F. Lhermitte, et al., "The Frequency of Relapse in Multiple Sclerosis: A Study Based on 245 Cases," *Z Neurol,* **205**(1):47–59, 29 Aug. 1973.

29 K. Fuxe, T. Hokfelt, and U. Ungerstedt, "Morpho-logical and Functional Aspects of Central Monoamine Neurons," *Int Rev Neurol,* **13**:93–126, 1970.

30 J. Wener, et al., "Cardiovascular Effects of Levodopa in Aged Versus Young Patients with Parkinson's Disease," *J Am Geriatr So,* **24**(4):185–188, April 1976.

31 P. Papavasiliou, et al., "Levodopa in Parkinsonism: Potentiation of Central Effects with a Peripheral Inhibitor," *N Engl J Med,* **285**(1):8–13, Jan 6, 1972.

32 G. G. Celesia, and W. M. Wanamaker, "L-dopa Carbidopa: Combined Therapy for the Treatment of Parkinson's Disease," *Dis Nerv Syst,* **37**(3):123–125, March 1976.

33 H. L. Klawans and S. P. Ringel, "L-dopa, B₆ and a-Methyldopa Hydrazine," *Confin Neurlo,* **35**(3):186–192, 1973.

34 Andre Barbeau and Madeleine Roy, "Six Year Results of Treatment with Levodopa plus Benzerazide in Parkinson's Disease," *Neurology (Minneap),* **26**(5):399–404, May 1976.

35 R. Langan and G. Cotzias, "Do's and Don'ts for the Patient on Levodopa Therapy," *Am J Nurs,* **76**:917–918, June 1976.

36 Eleanor Singer, "Social Costs of Parkinson's Disease," *J Chron Dis,* **26**:243–254, April 1973.

37 M. Hoehn and M. Yahr, "Evaluation of the Long Term Results of Surgical Therapy," in F. J. Gellingham and I. M. Donaldson (eds.), *Third Symposium on Parkinson's Disease,* E. and S. Livingstone, London, 1969, pp. 274–280.

38 J. M. Van Buren, et al., "A Qualitative and Quantitative Evaluation of Parkinsonisms Three to Six Years Following Thalamotomy," *Confin Neurol,* **35**(4):202–235, 1973.

39 Ira Shouldson, R. Kartzinel, and T. Chase, "Huntington's Disease: Treatment with Dipropylacetic Acid (DPA) and Gamma-Aminobutyric-Acid (GABA)," *Neurology,* **26**:61–63, January 1976.

40 "Multiple Sclerosis and Amyotrophic Lateral Sclerosis," *Stat Bull Metropol Life Ins Co,* **56**:3–5, March 1975.

41 M. Felmus, B. Patten, and L. Swanke, "Antecedent Events in Amyotrophic Lateral Sclerosis," *Neurology,* **26**:167–172, February 1976.

## BIBLIOGRAPHY

### General

Chusid, Joseph: *Correlative Neuroanatomy and Functional Neurology,* 14th ed., Lange, Los Altos, Cal., 1970.

Dom, R., M. Malfroid, and F. Baro: "Neuropathy of Huntington's Chorea," *Neurology (Minneap),* **26**:64–68, January 1976.

Jameson, R. M.: "Management of the Bladder in Non-Traumatic Paraplegia," *Paraplegia,* **12**(2):92–97, August 1974.

MacRae, Isabel, and Gloria Henderson: "Sexuality and Irreversible Health Limitations," *Nurs Clin North Am,* **10**(3):587–597, September 1975.

Strauss, Anselm: *Chronic Illness and the Quality of Life,* Mosby, St. Louis, 1975.

Yeaworth, Rosalie, and Joyce Friedeman: "Sexuality in Later Life," *Nurs Clin North Am,* **10**(3):565–574, September 1975.

## Multiple Sclerosis

Alter, M., M. Yamoor, and M. Harshe: "Multiple Sclerosis and Nutrition," *Arch Neurol,* **31**(4):267–272, October 1974.

Bradley, W. E., J. L. Logothetes, and G. W. Timm: "Cystometric and Sphincter Abnormalities in Multiple Sclerosis," *Neurology (Minneap),* **23**(10): 1131–1139, October 1973.

Braham, Sara, et al.: "Evaluation of the Social Needs of Non-Hospitalized Chronically Ill Persons," *J Chron Dis,* **28**:401–419, August 1975.

Delmotte, P., and C. Ketelaer: "Biochemical Findings in Multiple Sclerosis: Detailed Study of the Plasma Lipid Fractions of 484 Multiple Sclerosis Patients Compared with 152 Other Neurological Diseases," *J Neurol,* **207**(1):27–43, 1974.

Dillon, Ann: "Nursing Care of the Patient with Multiple Sclerosis," *Nurs Clin North Am,* **8**:653–665, December 1973.

Gelenberg, A. J., and D. C. Poskanzer: "The Effect of Dantrolene Sodium on Spasticity in Multiple Sclerosis," *Neurology (Minneap),* **23**(12):1313–1315, December 1973.

Horne, M. L.: "Treatment of Spasticity of Multiple Sclerosis with Dantroline," *JAMA,* **235**(3):251, Jan. 19, 1976.

Jontz, Donna Lynn: "Prescription for Living with M.S.," *Am J Nurs,* **73**:817–818, May 1973.

Ladd, H., C. Oist, and B. Jansson: "The Effect of Dantrolene on Spasticity in Multiple Sclerosis," *Acta Neurol Scan,* **50**(4):397–408, 1974.

Laitinen, L., A. Ansalo, and A. Hannimen: "Combination of Thalamotomy and Longitudinal Myelotomy in the Treatment of Multiple Sclerosis," *Acta Neurochir (Wien) (Suppl),* **21**:89–91, 1974.

Makay, R. P., and A. Hirano: "Forms of Benign Multiple Sclerosis: Report of Two Clinically Silent Cases Discovered at Autopsy," *Arch Neurol,* **17**: 388–600, December 1967 (reviewed and reprinted by National Multiple Sclerosis Society, February 1971).

McAlpine, Douglas, Charles Lumsden, and E. D. Acheson: *Multiple Sclerosis: A Reappraisal,* E. & S. Livingstone, London, 1965.

Miller, Henry: "Trauma and Multiple Sclerosis," National Multiple Sclerosis Society, New York (reprinted from *Lancet,* April 18, 1964, pp. 848–850) reviewed and reprinted, June 1970.

Olsson, J., H. Link, and R. Muller: "Immunoglobin Abnormalities in Multiple Sclerosis: Relation to Clinical Parameters: Disability, Duration and Onset," *J Neurol Sci,* **27**(2):233–245, February 1976.

Rose, A. S.: "Multiple Sclerosis: A Clinical and Theoretical Review," *J Neurosurg,* **41**(3):279–284, September 1974.

———, et al.: "Criteria for the Clinical Diagnosis of Multiple Sclerosis," *Neurology (Minneap),* **26:** 20–22, June 1976.

Sabin, A. B.: "Multiple Sclerosis— A Critique and Prospective," *Adv Neurol,* **6:**133–140, 1974.

Tolosa, E. S., R. W. Soll, and R. B. Leowenson: "Treatment of Spasticity in Multiple Sclerosis with Dantrolene," *JAMA,* **233**(10):1046, Sept. 8, 1975.

Weinstein, Edwin: "Behavioral Aspects of Multiple Sclerosis," *Mod Treat,* **7:**961–968, September 1970.

Further information and materials may be obtained from:

National Multiple Sclerosis Society
205 E. 42d St.
New York, N. Y. 10017

## Parkinson's Disease

Ansari, K. A., and A. Johnson: "Olfactory Function in Patients with Parkinson's Disease," *J Chron Dis,* **28**(9):493–497, October 1975.

Barbeau, Andre: "Long Term Side Effects of Levodopa," *Lancet,* **1:**395, February 20, 1971.

Bartholini, G., K. G. Lloyd, and H. Stadler: "Dopaminergic Regulation of Cholinergic Neurons in the Striatum: Relation to Parkinsonism," in Fletcher McDowell and Andre Barbeau (eds.), *Adv Neurol,* Raven Press Publishers, New York, 1974.

Bergonzi, P., et al.: "Clinical Pharmacology as an Approach to the Study of Biochemical Sleep Mechanisms: The Action of L-dopa," *Confin Neurol,* **36** (1):5–22, 1974.

Ehringer, H., and O. Hornykiewicz: "Distribution of Noradrenaline and Dopamine in the Human Brain and the Presence of Disease Affecting the Extrapyramidal System," in John Marks (ed.), *The Treatment of Parkinsonism with L-dopa,* American Elsevier, New York, 1974, pp. 47–55.

Erb, Elizabeth: "Improving Speech in Parkinson's Disease," *Am J Nurs,* **73**(11):1910–1911, November 1973.

Haber, Martha: "Parkinson's Disease: Challenge to the Health Professions," *Nurs Clin North Am,* **4**:263–273, June 1969.

Hoehn, Margaret, and Melvin Yahr: "Parkinsonism: Onset, Progression and Mortality," *Neurology (Minneap),* **17**(5):427–442, 1967.

Husby, J., and A. G. Korsgaard: "Proceedings: Late Results of Thalamotomy in Parkinsonism with and without the Influence of Levodopa," *Acta Neurochir,* **31**(3–4):260, 1975.

Kartzinel, Ronald, and Donald Calne: "Studies with Bromocriptine. Pt. I: On-Off Phenomena," *Neurology (Minneap),* **26**(6):508–510, June 1976.

———, Ira Showlson, and Donald Calne: "Studies with Bromocriptine, Pt. II: Double-blind Comparison with Levodopa in Idiopathic Parkinsonism," *Neurology (Minneap),* **26**(6):511–513, June 1976.

Lloyd, K. G., L. Davidson, and O. Hornykiewicz: "The Neurochemistry of Parkinson's Disease: Effect of L-dopa Therapy," *J Pharmacol Exp Therap,* **195**(3):453–464, December 1975.

Marsden, C. D., and J. D. Parkes: "On-Off: Effects in Patients with Parkinson's Disease on Chronic Levodopa Therapy," *Lancet,* **1**(7954):292–296, Feb. 7, 1976.

Murdock, M. I., et al.: "Effects of Levodopa on the Bladder Outlet," *J Urol,* **113**(6):803–805, June 1975.

Nittner, K.: "Review of Parkinsonian Patients Treated Surgically and by L-dopa," *Confin Neurol,* **36**(4–6):360–361, 1974.

Parkinson, James: "An Essay on the Shaking Palsy," (1817), reprinted in *Arch Neurol Psychiatry,* **7:**681–700, June 1922.

Robinson, Marilyn: "Levodopa and Parkinsonism," *Am J Nurs,* **74**(4):656–661, April 1974.

Shapiro, D. Y., et al.: "An Assessment of Cognitive Functions in Post Thalamotomy Parkinson Patients," *Confin Neurol,* **35**(3):144–166, 1973.

Singer, Eleanor: "The Effects of Treatment with Levodopa on Parkinson Patients' Social Functioning and Outlook on Life," *J Chron Dis,* **27**:581–594, December 1974.

Sweet, Richard, et al.: "Mental Symptoms in Parkinson's Disease during Chronic Treatment with Levodopa," *Neurology (Minneap),* **26**(4):305–310, April 1976.

Further information and materials may be obtained from:

The Parkinson's Disease Foundation
William Black
Medical Research Building
640 W. 168th St.
New York, N.Y. 10032

# 38
## DISTURBANCES IN VISUAL AND AUDITORY PERCEPTION*

Irene C. Cullin
Nancy L. Holland

**P**erception of and interaction with one's environment are largely dependent upon one's sensory receptors being intact and functioning. The eye and ear are particularly vital for this communication and interaction. Disturbances in visual and auditory perception may impair functioning and eventually result in a complete absence of sight or hearing. Such disruptions have important implications for nursing care and are detailed in this chapter.

## DISTURBANCES IN VISUAL PERCEPTION

The ability to see enables one to observe and interact with the environment. Disturbances in visual perception are sources of great anxiety and fear. For most of the population, the loss of the sense of vision is prominent in the hierarchy of their fears. In this section some of the more common conditions that may cause deprivation of the visual sense will be presented, and the nurse's role in assessment, prevention, and rehabilitation will be discussed. (To aid in a review of the anatomy of the eye, consult Fig. 31-1, a cross section of the normal eye.)

### Increased Intraocular Pressure—Glaucoma
*Glaucoma* is a condition caused by an elevation in pressure within the eye due to the retention of aqueous fluid. Aqueous fluid is produced by the ciliary body and flows from the posterior chamber through the pupillary space into the anterior chamber. From the anterior chamber the aqueous fluid passes through the iridocorneal angle into the trabecular meshwork and Schlemm's canal and then via the aqueous veins into the venous circulation. This process of production and distribution of aqueous fluid is a continual one and is responsible for maintaining the normal intraocular pressure. Any disturbance in the outflow process may cause a buildup of fluid and an elevation in the intraocular pressure. The eye usually maintains an intraocular pressure ranging from 13 to 22 mmHg.

Glaucoma may be classified as either primary or secondary. In *primary glaucoma* there is no relation to other ocular diseases, while *secondary glaucoma* results from a preexisting condition involving the eye (uveitis, tumor, cataracts, etc.). Primary glaucoma is further divided into *open angle* and *closed angle* and may be *adult* or *congenital*. Any

* The section on disturbances in visual perception was written by Irene C. Cullin, and the section on disturbances in auditory perception was written by Nancy L. Holland.

type of glaucoma may eventually result in a condition known as *absolute glaucoma.*

**Open-angle glaucoma** This type of glaucoma is also referred to as *chronic simple glaucoma* and occurs more frequently than narrow- (closed-) angle glaucoma. There exists a hereditary predisposition for this condition, and it is usually bilateral. In *open-angle glaucoma,* as its name indicates, there is no obstruction to the aqueous outflow at the angle. The obstruction to flow exists somewhere in the trabeculum, Schlemm's canal, or the aqueous veins and may be due to degenerative changes.

The patient has very few complaints of intense symptomatology. Symptoms such as aching and discomfort around the eyes, disturbed adaptation to darkness, blurring of peripheral vision, and halos around lights (uncommon) may be experienced. Unfortunately, the usual onset of this condition is slow, silent, and painless, and damage to the visual field, degeneration of the optic disk, and atrophy of the optic nerve have already occurred before the condition is diagnosed. Without treatment, open-angle glaucoma will result in blindness.

**Closed-angle glaucoma** With *narrow-* or *closed-angle glaucoma,* the patient presents very vivid and observable symptomatology. The onset is of an acute nature. The patient complains of pain, severe headache, nausea and vomiting, colored halos around lights, and blurred vision. The eye is severely injected (redness of the conjunctiva of the eye). Upon measurement with the tonometer, the intraocular pressure will be extremely high, usually from 80 to 100 mmHg. This elevation in pressure is caused by the narrowing or closing of the angle of the anterior chamber due to blockage of the angle by the root of the iris.

Factors which may precipitate an attack of angle-closure glaucoma include: hyperopia (far-sightedness) in which the eye tends to have a shallow anterior chamber, increased thickness of the iris due to pupillary dilatation, and an increase in lens size which might push the iris forward and obstruct the fluid outflow.

An attack of acute-angle closure glaucoma may subside without treatment. However, medical and surgical intervention are usually required to lower the pressure and prevent serious ocular damage. The end result of uncontrolled angle-closure glaucoma will be *absolute glaucoma.* The eye becomes stony hard, sightless, and quite painful; enucleation (removal of the eye) is usually required.

**First-level nursing care** Glaucoma is listed as one of the leading causes of blindness in adults in the United States. It is also classified as being a cause of "preventable" blindness. This means that with proper screening and education of the general population, much of the blindness caused by glaucoma can be prevented.

**P**revention Glaucoma occurs most often in adults over the age of 40. Therefore, it is imperative that measurement of the intraocular pressure of this segment of the population be conducted at least once a year. Many communities now sponsor glaucoma screening programs to promote early case finding and, it is hoped, prevent the occurrence of blindness.

To measure intraocular pressure, the most common tool initially utilized is the hand-held *Schiotz tonometer* (Fig. 38-1). The procedure is quite easy, and it is painless for the patient. The cornea is anesthetized by use of a topical anesthetic medication (e.g., proparacaine HCl); the footplate of the tonometer is placed on the cornea, and the pressure is measured in millimeters of mercury. In the public screening programs, patients are usually referred for further testing if their intraocular pressure measures above 20 mmHg.

**Second-level nursing care** Because the onset of glaucoma may be insidious, it is important that nurses be aware of even subtle symptoms and be prepared to make detailed nursing assessments. Patients with glaucoma may initially be diagnosed on an out-patient basis as a result of a routine eye or physical examination.

**N**ursing Assessment The patient's *health history* may reveal only aching and discomfort with some blurring of peripheral vision, or it may show an acute onset of severe eye pain, headache, blurred vision, nausea, and vomiting. The duration of the symptoms should be noted as well as any precipitating factors in their onset. Patients should be asked about any other preexisting eye diseases or conditions as well as any family history of glaucoma, cataracts, etc.

*Physical assessment* may reveal little by direct observation. With closed-angle glaucoma there may be severe redness around the eye and a widely dilated, nonreacting pupil. Examination by ophthalmoscope may show "cupping" and atrophy of the optic disk.

The most critical *diagnostic* instrument in the

detection of glaucoma is the *tonometer.* The procedure for using the tonometer to measure intraocular pressure is described under First-Level Nursing Care. Pressure readings usually are considered elevated if they are above 20 mmHg. The patient is then referred for further diagnostic testing.

**N**ursing Problems and Intervention  The major nursing problems in caring for a patient with glaucoma, in the early stages, are the *visual loss* or *disturbances* already present and the *potential visual damage* that may occur if the condition is untreated (see the Absence of Visual Perception section).

Whenever the nurse suspects glaucoma or a visual problem, the initial intervention should be referral to an eye clinic or ophthalmologist for further evaluation and diagnosis. Following this medical evaluation, the patient may be placed on a regimen of medication that will require patient and family teaching by the nurse.

Medications vary with the type of glaucoma. *Chronic open-angle glaucoma* is treated with topical miotic agents, carbonic anhydrase inhibitors, and topical epinephrine as prescribed by the physi-

cian. *Miotic agents,* the most common of which is pilocarpine, act by constricting the pupil, thus widening the outflow channels, and providing for an increase in the outflow of the aqueous fluid. The anticholinesterase agents are utilized for a more potent miotic effect. The most commonly used are phospholine iodide and eserine. Diamox, a *carbonic anhydrase inhibitor,* is utilized at times to decrease aqueous production, as is epinephrine. *Epinephrine* is also effective in decreasing production of aqueous fluid and facilitating its outflow from the eye.

It is imperative that the patient with the diagnosis of chronic open-angle glaucoma adhere scrupulously to the medical regime that has been formulated. The nurse responsible for instruction on the administration of eye drops and follow-through care must impress on the patient and the family the necessity of compliance with the regime and the consequences of noncompliance (ocular nerve damage and blindness). (See Table 38-1 and Fig. 38-2).

Because of the insidious and often painless progression of this type of glaucoma, the patient does not usually experience any adverse reaction

**FIGURE 38-1**
Nurse using Schiotz tonometer to measure the patient's intraocular tension. (*Courtesy of the Massachusetts Eye and Ear Infirmary.*)

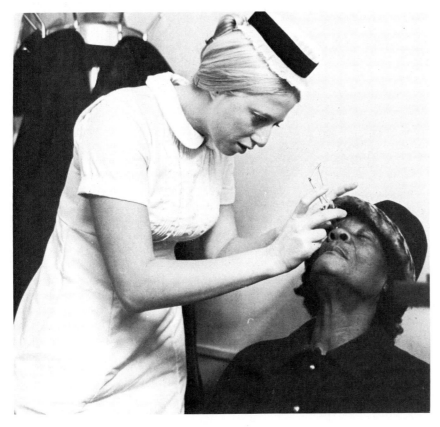

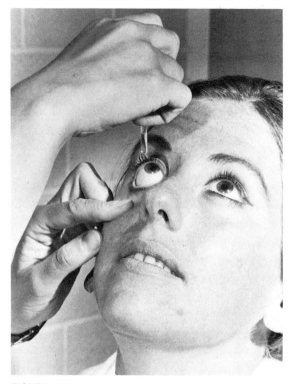

**FIGURE 38-2**
Nurse administering eye drops to patient. (*Courtesy of the Massachusetts Eye and Ear Infirmary.*)

**TABLE 38-1**
GUIDE FOR INSTILLATION OF EYE DROPS AND OINTMENTS

1   Wash hands thoroughly.

2   Inspect the eye in good light and clean it if necessary.

3   If cleansing is necessary close the eyelids and gently wipe the lid with a moist cotton ball, going from the inner canthus to the outer canthus of the eye.

4   Check the label on the bottle of medication.

5   Be sure to identify the correct eye to receive the medication.

6   Check the dropper for any cracks and the clarity of the solution before administering.

7   Gently pull down the lower lid of the eye and instill the drop of medication into the conjunctival sac. Do not touch the dropper to the eye or skin surface.

8   If the patient is to self-administer the eye drops, it may be helpful to steady the hand, holding the dropper by placing it in a "saluting" position on the forehead before instilling the medication.

9   Always have the patient or family member give a return demonstration of the technique.

10. If the patient's vision is poor, establish a labeling code for the bottle of medication to avoid errors.

from noncompliance with the medical regime. In fact, more discomfort is often experienced when taking the medication than when not. Because of the pupillary constriction caused by the miotics, normal accommodation to light is impeded. Good visual perception at night and in dark places is quite difficult, making night driving hazardous. The ability to read for long periods of time is also decreased by the decrease in near-vision accommodation. These restrictions may cause a person to avoid compliance with the prescribed medication regime because of the overriding priorities of daily activities.

Drug distribution via a time-release system is a recent advance. Patients can be provided with a medication device (Ocusert), inserted under the lids, that requires changing only once a week. This system has been of help to those patients who are unable to comply with their medical regime.

When the patient is experiencing an attack of *acute-angle closure glaucoma,* medical intervention must be instituted as quickly as possible in order to decrease the greatly elevated pressure within the eye. Miotic drops are usually administered every 15 minutes. In addition, Diamox and hyperosmotic agents [glycerol (oral), mannitol (IV)] are given to help relieve the pressure. If the pressure is not reduced appreciably through these medical means, the patient is hospitalized and surgical intervention is instituted.

In assessing the needs of the patient experiencing an acute-angle closure attack, the nurse must be aware of many immediate physical needs. The excruciating pain must be abated as well as the attacks of nausea and vomiting. Prompt administration of both pain and antiemetic medications is essential. The patient may also experience increased anxiety and fear for the possible damage or loss of visual perception. The situation is an emergency. However, it is essential that all treatments and medications are properly and clearly explained to the patient as well as the family.

**Third-level nursing care**   Glaucoma that is unresponsive or insufficiently responsive to medication is treated surgically. The hospitalized glaucoma patient requires the same detailed *nursing assessment* that is provided the outpatient. The *health history, physical assessment,* and *diagnostic* evaluation are as described under Second-Level Nursing Care. Now, however, symptoms may become more persistent or acute. *Gonioscopy* may be performed to examine the angle of the anterior chamber. This procedure is done in a darkened room and involves placement of a special contact glass on the cornea. Magnification of the cornea occurs, and under bright illumination the anterior chamber is visualized.

**N**ursing Problems and Interventions  The major nursing problems are *visual losses* and *complications* of surgical intervention. The type of surgery is determined by the type of glaucoma.

If the medical therapy is not totally effective in controlling the elevated intraocular pressure for the patient with *chronic simple glaucoma,* surgical intervention is used. The procedures employed to aid in reduction of the elevated pressure are termed *filtering procedures.* In these procedures, an opening is created in the sclera, therefore bypassing the trabecular meshwork and providing an alternate route for diffusion of aqueous fluid to the subconjunctival space. *Iridencleisis* (scleral opening is maintained by a wick of iris) and *corneal scleral trephination* (removal of a small piece of sclera) are among the procedures that may be performed. The surgical procedure of choice for *acute closed-angle glaucoma* is a *peripheral iridectomy* which provides an outflow channel for the aqueous fluid by removing a piece of iris tissue. This is often recommended even though medical therapy has been successful in controlling the attack. The procedure may be performed bilaterally as a prophylactic means of avoiding future problems.

The period of hospitalization is approximately 1 to 3 days after surgical intervention. After a filtering procedure or peripheral iridectomy has been performed, the affected eye is usually covered with a single eye pad, and the patient is allowed moderate activity with emphasis placed on avoidance of any type of straining, as this causes the intraocular pressure to rise.

**Fourth-level nursing care**  A large part of the treatment of glaucoma, especially the chronic type, is dependent on effective patient and family education. The nurse has a major responsibility in ensuring that a proper understanding of the medical regimes and the eventual consequences of noncompliance are properly understood by both patient and family. The family must also be made aware of the hereditary factor involved with glaucoma; provisions should be made for screening tests for family members. The patient is instructed to continue avoiding those activities which lead to an elevation of intraocular pressure. The proper method of administering eye drops should be reviewed, and return demonstrations given. The importance of maintaining medical follow-up to monitor intraocular pressure should be stressed. The use of group meetings is sometimes an effective means of maintaining an on-going contact with the affected population. A group meeting provides the support that is often needed by the person who has chronic glaucoma. The sharing of ideas and approaches to the medical regime is a feature of these meetings, as well as the presence of medical resource persons to handle any medical problems that are being encountered.

## Disturbances in Visual Clarity—Cataract

A *cataract* is technically defined as an opacity of the crystalline lens of the eye. The crystalline lens is anatomically located behind the iris and in front of the vitreous body. It is normally transparent and is a refractive medium for light rays entering the eye. It is suspended behind the iris by ligaments known as the zonules of Zinn, which arise from the ciliary body and insert in the equator of the lens.

There are several classifications of cataracts. Among these are congenital (present at birth), traumatic (injury to eye), toxic (adverse effect of drugs or steroids), metabolic (diabetes), and senile (aging process). The latter is the one most commonly encountered. The main function of the lens is to focus the light rays on the retina. With the aging process, the lens grows less elastic and the power of accommodation decreases. The aging process also produces various degrees of lens opacification which, depending on the location, will cause a decrease in visual acuity. If the opacity is centrally located and goes untreated, useful vision will be lost. This is particularly destructive since cataracts are usually bilateral, although the opacity may progress at differing rates for each eye.

Because senile cataracts most commonly occur among senior citizens, this group is the target area for public education and screening programs. Case finding should be conducted in community settings as well as in nursing and convalescent homes.

The nurse should therefore ask pertinent questions regarding the visual capacity of all geriatric patients and what types of activities are being avoided because of decreased vision. If there appears to be a significant loss, a referral for ophthalmic evaluation should be made.

**Nursing assessment**  During the health history, the main symptom described by the person affected with an opacity of the lens is dimming or blurring of vision; objects may appear hazy. Usually a cataract is not visible to the casual observer's eye until it has become very dense or "mature." However, after pupil dilation, by use of an ophthalmoscope or slit lamp (bimicroscope), a lens opacity can be identified even in its early stages of development. The slit lamp permits examination of the anterior portion of the eye, by use of high magnification and a finely focused slit of brilliant light.

As previously mentioned, the extent to which a lens opacity affects vision is dependent upon the density and position of the cataract. If the opacity is located peripherally rather than centrally, the effect on visual acuity will not be great.

After a cataract has been identified, the degree of effect on the patient's vision is assessed. Surgical intervention is undertaken only when the lens opacity is interfering with the performance of the daily activities of the patient. Since all individuals have different life-styles and responsibilities, the level at which a cataract poses a problem to daily activities varies greatly.

**Surgical intervention** The surgical approach to the treatment of a cataract lies in the removal of the lens. The procedure of choice for patients with a senile cataract is the *intracapsular cataract extraction.* In this procedure, an incision is made at the limbus (the corneal-scleral junction), and the lens is removed intact. An instrument called the cryoprobe, which produces an "ice-ball" tip, is most often the tool of choice for removal of the lens. When the cryoprobe is introduced into the incision, the lens adheres to the tip, and when it is withdrawn, the lens accompanies it.

Prior to the removal of the lens, an enzyme alpha-chymotrypsin may be instilled into the anterior chamber. The purpose of this procedure is to achieve lysis of the zonular fibers (enzymatic zonulolysis) that hold the lens is place.

If the patient is under 30 years of age, the procedure of choice for treatment of a cataract (usually congenital or traumatic) is an *extracapsular cataract extraction.* In this procedure, the anterior portion of the lens capsule is ruptured through a limbal incision, and the lens nucleus and cortex are removed. The posterior capsule is left in place.

The use of *phacoemulsification* for cataract removal has increased in recent years. In this procedure a probe, which vibrates at 40,000 cycles/second, is introduced into the eye through a small limbal incision. This probe emulsifies and aspirates the lens contents, leaving the posterior capsule in place.

*Postoperatively,* the patient who has had cataract surgery will have the operative eye covered with an eye pad and a protective shield. Topical eye medications to dilate the pupil (mydriatics) and reduce inflammation (steroids) may be prescribed. The activity recommended for the patient is one of moderation. Emphasis is placed on the avoidance of straining activities such as stooping, coughing, sneezing, and vigorous brushing of hair and teeth. Such moderation is encouraged in order to prevent an increase in intraocular pressure. The nurse should arrange the patient's environment to facilitate compliance with the activity regulations. For example, the bedside stand should be placed on the unoperated side, within easy access, so that the patient will be able to see and not have to strain or stretch to reach anything. Also, the use of step-in slippers and shoes to avoid bending and stooping should be recommended.

In addition to elevated intraocular pressure, other possible complications following cataract surgery are hyphema (hemorrhage in the anterior chamber) and wound leak, which might cause a flat anterior chamber. The nurse should caution the patient against forceful squeezing of the eyelids. Also, the nurse should avoid exerting unnecessary pressure while administering eye drops and applying eye pads. Moderation in physical activity and a protective environment must be continually stressed.

Patients will usually remain in the hospital for 3 to 5 days after cataract surgery. The stay is frequently shorter (1 to 2 days) for patients who have had phacoemulsification because the wound is small (usually one suture) and the chance of immediate postoperative complications is less.

Upon discharge, patients should be advised to wear a protective eye shield while sleeping, for at least 1 month. This precaution will help avoid accidental eye injury.

A patient who has had the crystalline lens removed is termed *aphakic* (without a lens). As previously noted, the lens is a refractive medium of the eye. Therefore, some replacement must be made if a high level of visual acuity is desired.

If visual acuity is corrected with spectacle lenses, good central vision may be obtained, but the image will be magnified about 30 percent. The peripheral vision will be greatly reduced and objects will appear distorted if viewed other than through the center of the cataract lens. Also, if the patient is binocular, diplopia will result if a cataract spectacle lens is used, owing to the difference in image size between the two eyes. The spectacle lens of the unoperated eye must be blurred out to avoid double vision.

If the patient is given spectacle cataract lenses

on either a temporary or permanent basis, the nurse should provide adequate education regarding the changes in sensory perception that will occur. Full explanations regarding the distortion and magnification powers of the lenses should be provided. The patient is advised to turn the head when viewing something in the periphery, instead of merely shifting the gaze, as adequate perception is available only through the central portion of the lens. The patient should be instructed in the proper method of putting on the spectacle lenses. That is, the lenses and frames are held by the tips of the temple pieces and guided into place. This method helps to avoid accidental "poking" of the eye. Also, the patient should be told that with these lenses objects may appear larger and closer than they really are, and precautions should always be observed in daily activities until adequate adjustment has been made.

The utilization of a corneal contact lens after cataract surgery provides a tolerable increase in image size, normal peripheral vision, and no significant distortion. If the patient is able to handle its management, the contact lens is more desirable, especially for the monoaphakic patient.

A third alternative for correcting vision after lens removal is the *intraocular lens implant.* This is a relatively new technique that is increasing in use. After cataract extraction, a small plastic lens implant is placed behind the iris and sutured in place. With the use of the lens implant, normal central and peripheral vision can be anticipated. Following the lens implant procedure, the patient will be placed on miotic (pupil constrictor) drops. This regime will be used on a regular basis in order to prevent lens dislocation. It is of extreme importance that mydriatic drops never be placed in an eye that has an intraocular lens implant because of the danger of dislocating the lens.

All patients after cataract surgery, no matter what method of lens replacement is chosen, should be encouraged to adhere to a regimen of moderate activity. The importance of follow-up appointments and adherence to prescribed medical regime should also be stressed. Good patient and family education can help prevent the occurrence of postoperative complications. If the patient is elderly and lives alone, a social service or visiting nurse referral might be of assistance to help evaluate the patient's home resources and ability for self-care.

### Disturbances in Perception of the Image—Retinal Detachment

*Retinal detachment* is a separation between the pigmented epithelial layer (choroid) and the neural or sensory layer (retina) of the eye. (The retina is that part of the eye which receives visual images and transfers them to the optic nerve, which then carries them to the brain for interpretation.) When a tear or hole is present in the retina, vitreous or choroidal fluid exudate accumulates in the subretinal space, causing a retinal separation. The separation may also occur when vitreous leakage has occurred or fibrous bands are present causing vitreous traction on the retina, pulling it away from the pigment epithelium. Situations resulting in retinal detachment include orbital injuries, cataract removal, or myopia (because of the differences in the rate of stretching between the myopic eye's retina and sclera). Retinal separation occurs most frequently in males over the age of 45. Prevention of the condition is not yet possible.

The person experiencing a retinal detachment will usually describe a sensation of seeing "floaters," or spots in front of the eye. "Light flash" sensations are usually present, and definite areas of the visual field will appear blacked out. The patient will usually state that he or she feels as if a curtain or film is being drawn over the eyes. Sudden visual loss usually does not occur if the macula (central portion of the retina and point of most acute central vision) is still attached.

Ophthalmoscopy with the indirect ophthalmoscope (see Fig. 38-3) is essential in order to determine the location of the separation. Because the retinal problem is usually bilateral, it is essential to do a thorough ophthalmoscopic examination on the unaffected eye to determine the presence of any retinal tears, holes, or other degenerative process.

**Surgical intervention** Surgical repair is the treatment prescribed for retinal detachments. Prior to surgery a drawing of the retina is made in which the areas of the attached retina, detached retina, blood vessels, and other anatomical structures are included. This drawing is used as a reference during the surgical procedure. In order to carefully examine the retina and to complete the drawing, the pupil must be kept dilated. Therefore, the patient will be receiving mydriatic eye drops prior to surgical intervention. Bed rest with both eyes covered is usually prescribed prior to surgery to ensure rest for the affected eye. The aim of surgical treatment is reattachment of the retina. This may be achieved by several approaches. The goal of all the techniques described is to induce scar formation to facilitate the sealing of the retinal hole, to promote reattachment of the two retinal surfaces, and to

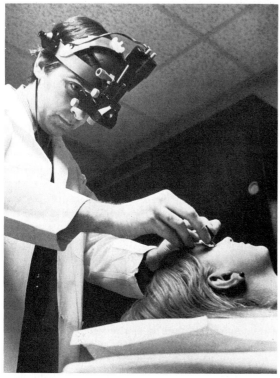

**FIGURE 38-3**
Ophthalmologist examining a patient's eye with an indirect
ophthalmoscope and a hand-held magnifying lens. (*Courtesy of the
Massachusetts Eye and Ear Infirmary.*)

drain subretinal fluid, when present, to further promote reattachment.

In cases in which a retinal tear or hole is present
and a detachment has not yet occurred, *retinopexy*
techniques (photocoagulation or cryosurgery) may
be employed to seal the tear or hole before a detachment occurs. Both procedures produce localized thermal inflammatory responses which result
in scar formation and adhesions that bind the retina
and choroid and seal retinal tears.

*Photocoagulation* is the use of high-intensity
light focused through the eye's refractive media to
a tiny spot in the retina, and *cryosurgery* is the application of a supercooled (cryo-) probe to the scleral
(outer) layer of the eye. Photocoagulation, for which
the *laser* (*l*ight *a*mplification *s*timulated by *e*mission
or *r*adiation) is chiefly utilized, is the treatment of
choice for tears or holes occurring in the posterior
portion of the eye. The *cryoprobe* is utilized for anterior retinal breaks. This choice is made because
of the curvature of the eyeball and the presence of
the pigmented iris. Light cannot be focused efficiently on the front portion of the retina. Therefore,

the cryoprobe is applied to that section of the anterior segment of the retina where the tear is located.

Photocoagulation and cryosurgery are usually
employed as preventive techniques. This means that
when a retinal hole or tear is diagnosed and a retinal
detachment has not yet occurred, these techniques
can seal the break and, one hopes, prevent the progression of detachment. Neither of the above techniques requires an incision into eye tissue.

If a retinal detachment has occurred, a more extensive surgical approach is necessary. The operation of choice for repairing a retinal detachment is
termed a *scleral buckle.* In this procedure the area
of retinal break is identified, and either the cryoprobe or the electrodiathermy probe (high-frequency electrical current) is applied to the sclera,
irritating the choroidal layer and inducing a chorio-
retinal scar formation. The subretinal fluid is
drained so that the retina can settle against the
choroid. A silicone implant is then placed over the
scarred area to indent the eye and bring it in contact
with the detached retina. This internal ''buckle''
creates a high and permanent ridge in the eye which
facilitates sealing of the retinal breaks and minimizes the traction exerted on the retina. At times
the silicone implant is placed under an encircling
silicone band which acts as a belt and permanently
maintains the indentation on the eye (see Fig. 38-4).

The procedures of photocoagulation and cryosurgery for treatment of retinal holes are usually
done in an ambulatory-service minor-surgery area,
under local anesthesia, and hospitalization is not
required. For repair of retinal detachments, the patient is admitted to the hospital. Bed rest with both
eyes covered and head positioning according to
location of the detachment are usually ordered by
the physician. The scleral-buckle procedure is done
under general anesthesia. Postoperatively, the affected eye is covered with a pressure bandage the
day of surgery. A single eye pad is used after the
pressure dressing is removed. The specific head
positioning is ordered by the physician. Usually, the
physician's postoperative orders will also include
mydriatic eye drops to keep the pupil dilated for
facility in ophthalmoscopic examination of the
retina; anti-infective and steroid eye drops are also
usually prescribed. The patient is encouraged, when
allowed, to be ambulatory in order to promote good
circulation and avoid thrombus formation. Leg
exercises are encouraged while bed rest is being
maintained. As with other intraocular surgery,
straining and coughing should be avoided and
medications administered to prevent these occurrences. Emotional support is also a very important

part of the nursing approach to the patient after retinal surgery. The nurse should be aware of the anticipated prognosis for each patient and assist the person in accepting the prognosis. If the prognosis is poor, false hope should not be inspired, but a supportive approach which provides realistic goals for the patient should be employed. Diversional therapy must be provided while the patient is on bed rest or has both eyes covered. Talking books (records supplied by the Library of Congress), a radio, or a family member or volunteer to read to the patient are some of the possibilities to help promote relaxation and prevent restlessness.

The average length of the hospital stay after retinal surgery is approximately 7 days. After discharge, the patient must be encouraged to keep follow-up appointments with the physician. A moderate amount of activity is usually recommended, and the patient is urged to avoid activities that elevate intraocular pressure (e.g., heavy lifting, straining, coughing). Visual acuity will be determined, and if necessary a new prescription for corrective lenses will be given to the patient. The patient is also instructed to report any signs of sudden loss of vision, central or peripheral.

In health teaching, the nurse should counsel those in the patient population prone to retinal detachment (e.g., myopic patients). It is important for them to be aware that if they experience such symptoms as showers of black spots or continuous flickering or shadows in front of one eye, they should consult an ophthalmologist immediately. This type of preventive action might help prevent a small retinal hole from becoming a major retinal detachment.

### Errors in Refraction

*Refraction* is the ability of the eye to focus light rays on the retina. As light rays enter the eye, they pass through the refractive media of the eye. These *refractive media* consist of the cornea, the aqueous fluid, the crystalline lens, and the vitreous body. A visual image occurs only if the light rays are able to pass through the media to a focal point on the retina. If the eye is optically normal (*emmetropic*), parallel rays of light 6 m or more from the eye should come to a focus on the retina. If there are some anatomical abnormalities in the eye structure, refractive errors will occur. *Myopia* (nearsightedness) results when the light rays are focused at a point in front of the retina, and *hyperopia* (farsightedness) occurs when the rays of light are focused at a point behind the retina. *Astigmatism*, which results from defects in the curvature of the

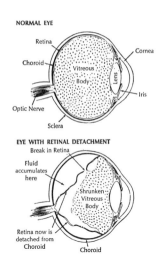

NORMAL EYE

EYE WITH RETINAL DETACHMENT

EYE WITH SCLERAL BUCKLE

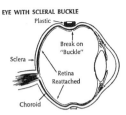

**FIGURE 38-4**

Illustration of normal eye; eye with a detached retina; eye with scleral buckle. (*Courtesy of the Massachusetts Eye and Ear Infirmary.*)

cornea, prevents a sharp image focus by diffusing the light rays on the retina. When objects are nearer than 6 m to the normal eye, the rays of light are no longer parallel and will not come to a sharp focus on the retina unless the crystalline lens becomes more convex (thicker) and "accommodates" for near vision. This process of accommodation is accomplished by the contraction of the ciliary muscle which relaxes the lens capsule, thus making it more convex. This ability of the eye to accommodate for near vision decreases with age as the lens loses its elasticity and can no longer accommodate. This condition usually appears after age 45 and is termed *presbyopia*. (Consult Table 38-2 for further descriptions of these refractive errors.)

### Inflammatory Disturbances of the Eye

Major inflammatory conditions of the eye will be described briefly. They include blepharitis, conjunctivitis, uveitis, sympathetic ophthalmia, trachoma, keratitis, and corneal ulcers.

**Blepharitis** *Blepharitis* is a common chronic bilateral inflammation of the lid margins. The two main types are termed *staphylococcal* and *seborrheic*. They are usually seen in combination, and the patient will often present a history of a seborrheic condition of the scalp. Itching and burning of the eyelids are frequently the initial symptoms. The lid margins will be scaly and red with possible ulcerations. Treatment of this condition is directed toward maintaining cleanliness of the area. Crusts should be removed from the lids; warm saline soaks are recommended prior to crust removal. Application of antibiotic and sulfonamide ointments to the lid margins after crust removal is usually advised. If a seborrheic scalp condition is present, this must be treated if the blepharitis is to be controlled.

**Hordeolum** The term *hordeolum* is applied to a staphylococcal infection of the glands of the eyelid. When the infection affects the Meibomian glands, it is called an *internal* hordeolum. When the infection is located in the glands of Zeis and Moll, it is called an *external* hordeolum, more commonly known as a *sty.* Pain and localized redness and swelling are the primary symptoms. Application of moist warm compresses at least 3 to 4 times a day is the recommended treatment. Antibiotic ophthalmic ointment is frequently used in addition to the compress application.

**Chalazion** A *chalazion* is defined as an inflammation of a Meibomian gland. It is a sterile cyst of unknown etiology which presents as a local inflammation of either the upper or lower lid with external symptoms similar to that of a hordeolum. When the inflammation subsides, a painless lump remains in the lid. If this lump presses against the eye, astigmatism may occur. Surgical excision is recommended if the chalazion is large enough to cause distortion of vision or for cosmetic appearance.

**Conjunctivitis** Inflammation of the conjunctiva (mucous membrane that lines the eyelid, palpebrae,

and anterior or bulbar portion of the eye), or conjunctivitis, is one of the more common inflammatory conditions affecting the eye. It may be caused by a variety of sources including bacterial or viral organisms, allergens, and physical or chemical irritants. The symptoms include redness of the conjunctiva accompanied by tearing, itching, and a watery discharge. A purulent drainage is present when the causative organism is the gonococcus. In treatment of conjunctivitis, precautions should be taken to prevent its communication to other individuals. Good hygiene is essential, especially among immediate family members. Individual towels and washcloths should be used by the affected person. Treatment usually consists of anti-infective ophthalmic ointments as well as warm water or saline irrigants to remove drainage from the eye. With prompt treatment the inflammation usually subsides within 1 to 3 days. Untreated, resolution usually takes place within 10 days. However, if gonococcal conjunctivitis goes untreated, it can lead to corneal perforation and endophthalmitis (generalized infection of the eye).

**Uveitis** The *uveal tract* is the term applied to the pigmented or vascular parts of the eye, that is, the iris, the ciliary body, and the choroid. An inflammation of one or all of these parts is termed *uveitis.* It usually occurs unilaterally and affects young and middle-aged persons. Anterior uveitis, inflammation of the iris (iritis) or of the iris and ciliary body (iridocyclitis), is the most common occurrence. *Posterior uveitis* refers to the inflammation of the choroid (chordiditis) and, as the retina is often secondarily affected, inflammation of the choroid and the retina (chorioretinitis). If the entire uveal tract is involved, the condition is termed *panuveitis.*

Uveitis is further classified as granulomatous or nongranulomatous. *Nongranulomatous uveitis* oc-

**TABLE 38-2**
ERRORS OF REFRACTION

| Error | Description | Symptoms | Corrective lens |
|---|---|---|---|
| Myopia (nearsightedness) | Parallel rays of light focus in *front* of the retina | Blurred distant vision Squinting | Concave (minus) lens |
| Hyperopia (farsightedness) | Parallel rays of light focus *behind* the retina | Headache Burning sensation of the eye Pulling sensation in the eye | Convex (plus) lens |
| Astigmatism | Light rays are not refracted equally in all meridians owing to irregular curvature of cornea | Squinting Tilting head to one side | Cylinder lens |
| Presbyopia | Decrease in accommodative power of the crystalline lens due to aging process | Inability to see comfortably at close range, "arm's length" reading | "Reading glasses" convex lens (for near vision), bifocal lenses for near and distant vision |

curs principally in the anterior portion of the tract and is thought to be a sensitivity reaction. *Granulomatous uveitis,* which generally occurs in the posterior segment, is thought to be related to an organism already present in the body tissues (e.g., *Mycobacterium tuberculosis*).

In nongranulomatous uveitis the onset is acute and is accompanied by pain, injection, photophobia, and blurring of vision. The pupil is constricted, and fine white deposits can be seen on the cornea when the slit lamp is used for examination. In granulomatous uveitis, the onset is insidious, pain is minimal, photophobia is not as severe, and the vision gradually becomes blurred. The pupil is often constricted, and yellowish white patches can be seen on the choroid and retina when the ophthalmoscope is used for examination. In establishing an etiologic diagnosis, skin tests for tuberculosis, histoplasmosis, and toxoplasmosis may be done.

Treatment is directed at the symptomatology. In anterior uveitis of a nongranulomatous source, warm compresses are applied three to four times daily. Mydriatic eye drops (atropine) are prescribed to keep the iris at rest and prevent formation of synechiae (adhesion), which would impede aqueous flow. Dark glasses are recommended for photophobia, and systemic analgesics for the pain. Topical steroid drops may be utilized for their anti-inflammatory and antiallergenic effects. With treatment, an attack of nongranulomatous uveitis will usually last a few days to weeks; recurrence is common.

In cases of granulomatous uveitis, atropine is given as well as anti-infective medication directed at the causative organism; if not effective, systemic steroid therapy is usually initiated. Granulomatous uveitis will usually last months to years with episodes of remissions and exacerbations. These attacks are often accompanied by permanent damage to the eye and resultant visual loss. Cataracts and retinal detachments are frequent complications of this chronic form of uveitis.

**Sympathetic ophthalmia** *Sympathetic ophthalmia* is a bilateral granulomatous uveitis of rare occurrence. It appears after a penetrating injury to the eye in the area of the ciliary body, in a time period that can span from 10 days to several years after injury. The etiology is unknown, and occurrence is rare after intraocular surgery for cataract or glaucoma. Inflammation occurs first in the injured eye and then will appear in the other (sympathizing) eye. The patient complains of photophobia, injection, and blurred vision. Treatment, if sympathetic

ophthalmia is present, consists of local and systemic corticosteroids.

If a severe penetrating injury has occurred in one eye and there is a good possibility for the occurrence of a sympathetic reaction, enucleation of the injured eye may be recommended within 10 days of the injury in order to save the "good" eye. This is, of course, a vary radical approach, and the patient will be confronted with a grave decision. The patient should be given much support as well as the opportunity to thoroughly understand the problem which is being anticipated, before the final decision has to be made. If sympathetic ophthalmia occurs and remains untreated, the condition will slowly progress to bilateral blindness.

**Trachoma** A viral infection affecting the lids and conjunctiva of the eye, trachoma leads to corneal ulceration and blindness. It is the leading cause of blindness, affecting more than 15 percent of the world's population. It is most common in areas with low socioeconomic conditions where bathing facilities are inadequate. Areas of high incidence are found in China and India. In the United States, the disease is well controlled with some incidence of occurrence in the mountains of West Virginia, Tennessee, and Kentucky and among the American Indian population.

The initial symptoms are mild itching and irritation. Follicles form on the palpebral conjunctiva and intensify the symptoms, causing blurring of vision and intense discomfort. As the disease progresses, the upper portion of the cornea is invaded with the development of a network of blood vessels (pannus). Corneal ulceration will follow and eventually leads to scarring and blindness.

Treatment consists of a 3- to 5-week course of oral antibiotics, usually tetracycline. The prognosis is excellent with prompt treatment. Without treatment permanent corneal damage will occur.

Good health education is necessary for prevention of communication of the disease. The World Health Organization has been very active in educating the population of endemic areas and has been successful in reducing occurrences of trachoma in these areas.

**Keratitis** Inflammation of the cornea, *keratitis,* is usually caused by an infective organism. The patient frequently complains of photophobia, tearing, blurred vision, and pain due to the inflammation of multiple pain fibers in the cornea. Ciliary injection and cloudiness of the involved area are noted on examination. Cultures should be taken to determine the causative organism before therapy is instituted. Topical steroids are the usual treatment except in cases of herpes simplex (dendritic keratitis) when, owing to the viral source of the disease, steroids are contraindicated. Idoxuridine (IDU, Stoxil) is the drug of choice for treatment of acute cases of herpes simplex.

**Corneal ulcers** A number of conditions including perforating injuries of the eye, bacterial, fungal, or viral infections, exposure, and allergic reactions can cause corneal ulcers. If untreated or uncontrolled, corneal ulceration can lead to scarring and perforation of the cornea with blindness as the end result.

Symptoms of corneal ulcer include pain, injection, photophobia, and tearing. Simple corneal ulcers are usually treated with topical and systemic antimicrobial and steroid agents (except where contraindicated, as in herpes simplex). Mydriatics are frequently administered, analgesics are used for relief of the pain, and dark glasses are worn to relieve the photophobia. If the ulcer progresses, perforation and scarring will occur leading to a marked decrease in vision. Ten percent of all blindness is due to corneal ulceration.

If scarring does cause blindness, surgical intervention may be attempted. A *keratoplasty* procedure, more commonly known as *corneal transplant,* may be performed. Keratoplasty is performed in cases of corneal opacities, congenital conditions such as keratoconus (cone-shaped cornea), or for chemical burns of the cornea. The procedure consists of removing the damaged corneal tissue of the patient and replacing it with an exactly measured "button" of corneal tissue from a donor eye. The donor corneal tissue is usually obtained from a regional eye tissue bank. After the surgical procedure the patient is placed on high doses of topical steroids to prevent graft rejection.

## Neoplastic Disturbances in Visual Perception

Highly malignant neoplasms may occur within the eye. These include retinoblastoma and malignant melanoma.

**Retinoblastoma** A rare, highly malignant, congenital tumor of the retina, *retinoblastoma* occurs in approximately 1 out of 20,000 births. The condition may arise from a gene mutation or may be inherited. Genetic counseling is quite important because persons who have had retinoblastoma have a 50 per-

cent chance of producing a child affected by the condition.

Retinoblastoma usually occurs unilaterally, but bilateral occurrence may appear in 25 to 30 percent of affected patients. Retinoblastomas occur in early childhood, most by the age of 3 years. They usually arise in the posterior retina, and the growth and dissemination of the tumor unfortunately becomes well advanced before visible symptomatology is present. Usually, a white pupil in the child's eye will bring parents to seek ophthalmic examination. The earlier the diagnosis, the better the chance for survival. In incidences of known familial tendency, where children are routinely examined, an earlier diagnosis can be established.

The treatment of choice is that of immediate enucleation of the affected eye with irradiation of the remaining eye. The patient is followed closely for an occurrence of the neoplasm in the remaining eye. Retinoblastoma obviously produces a tragic family situation. The parents need much support and guidance during and after their child's hospitalization.

**Enucleation** In addition to neoplastic conditions, *enucleation* may be used as the primary treatment for acute traumatic injury, impending sympathetic ophthalmia, and absolute glaucoma. Regardless of the reason for enucleation, the initial impact of an altered body image is much the same for most patients.

The surgical removal of the eye is followed by the insertion of an implant in the fascia of the eye (Tenon's capsule). The rectus muscles are attached to the implant to provide motility for the ocular prosthesis. The ocular prosthesis is usually not fitted until the edema from the surgical trauma has subsided. Immediately after surgery, the patient will have a pressure dressing applied to prevent hemorrhage and hematoma formation. The nurse should also be aware of other possible complications of enucleation such as acute infection and meningitis.

The patient who has had an enucleation will experience the various stages of the process of adjusting to an altered body image. The nurse must allow the patient time to grieve for the lost part and support and encourage the patient toward acceptance and rehabilitation.

When the patient is physically and emotionally ready, the ocular prosthesis can be fitted. The prosthesis is most commonly made from a synthetic plastic, and the color is matched to the patient's remaining eye. The plastic prosthesis is natural looking and nonbreakable. The patient should be instructed in the proper care of the eye socket and the prosthesis. The socket should be irrigated with normal saline, and the plastic prosthesis, when removed, should be cleansed with soap and water. Alcohol should never be used in cleansing as it will cause discoloration and cracking of the plastic. If the prosthesis is made of glass, it is subject to breakage and must be handled very carefully. The nurse should stress the importance of good ocular hygiene with the patient. The patient should be encouraged to wear safety glasses to protect the remaining eye and to seek prompt medical attention at the first signs of irritation or following an eye injury.

**Malignant melanoma**  The most common intraocular tumor is *malignant melanoma*. It usually occurs in persons over age 50, is unilateral and seen only in the uveal tract, and is found predominately in persons of the Caucasian race. The most common site of occurrence in the uveal tract is in the choroid. Melanomas of the choroid give rise to a solid retinal detachment. The sudden or gradual loss of vision caused by the detachment will prompt the patient to seek medical attention. Melanoma in the iris may cause a change in color and possibly a distortion of the pupil. These manifestations prompt the patient to seek medical attention. Diagnosis can be made by ophthalmoscopy and transillumination (a bright light is passed across the sclera; if a solid mass is present, light will not be transmitted), radioisotopes, and ultrasonography (Fig. 38-5).

The treatment of choice for most malignant melanomas of the eye is enucleation. If evidence of extraocular extension is present, an *exenteration* (removal of the eye and surrounding tissues) may be indicated. In cases where the tumor is confined to a small area of the iris, an iridectomy will be performed. Prognosis is dependent on the site of occurrence, iris tumors being the most favorable.

### Traumatic Interference with Visual Perception

Injuries to the eye, no matter how minor they appear, can cause severe damage to eye tissue and

**FIGURE 38-5**

Ophthalmologist utilizing ultrasonography diagnostic testing. (*Courtesy of the Massachusetts Eye and Ear Infirmary.*)

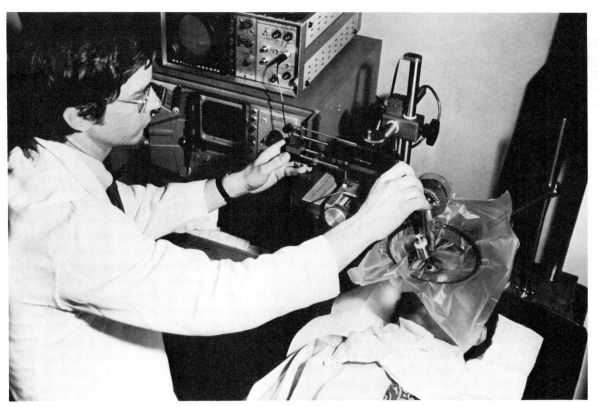

may lead to total loss of vision or loss of the eye itself. Protection and preservation of sight are among the primary goals of public health education. Legislative efforts have been utilized as a means of protecting the public from serious eye injury (e.g., mandatory use of safety lenses). The nurse should be aware of the common eye injuries and the priorities for treatment of ocular emergencies.

**Foreign bodies**  The most frequently encountered cause of eye trauma is foreign bodies. Superficial foreign bodies such as specks of dust or cinders can usually be easily removed with a cotton-tipped applicator by the nurse. If, upon inspection of the eye, the nurse discovers the particle to be on the cornea rather than the conjunctiva, an ophthalmologist should be consulted because of the potential damage that could be done to the epithelial surface of the cornea. If the foreign particle is on the conjunctival surface, it most commonly lodges under the upper lid. Removal of it requires everting the lid first.

If the foreign body has become deeply embedded in the cornea, it must be removed by an ophthalmologist, with the aid of magnifying lenses and special instruments. If the foreign body contains iron and has been in the tissue for any length of time, it may leave a rust residue on the cornea which has to be removed. A special burr drill called the "rust ring remover" is used for this procedure. After removal of a foreign body, antibiotic ointment is placed in the eye, and this treatment is continued for approximately 3 days. An eye pad may be applied to protect the affected area until it heals.

If the foreign body (e.g., a stick) has penetrated the eye and is still in place, the nurse should never attempt to remove the penetrating object. The patient should be seen immediately by an ophthalmologist. An eye pad should never be applied; however, a protective shield that does not press on the penetrating foreign body may be used.

Intraocular foreign bodies must be treated by an ophthalmologist. X-ray examinations are conducted to locate the foreign body and to determine the extent of the penetration. The surgical approach will depend upon the location of the foreign body. If the foreign body is of a metal base, a special surgical magnet may be used to facilitate removal. After removal of the intraocular foreign body, the patient is usually placed on antibiotic and steroid therapy to prevent infection and control inflammation.

**Contusions**  A *contusion* of the eye and surrounding tissue is usually caused by a blow to the eye from a blunt object. The typical results of a contusion injury are subconjunctival hemorrhage and eccymosis of the eye lids (black eye). Treatment of the lid eccymosis generally consists of application of cold compresses for the first 24 hours followed by the application of warm compresses to aid in the absorption of the blood. Although the contusion may initially seem to be superficial, the patient should be urged to have a follow-up examination. Some conditions that could occur following a contusion include traumatic cataract, vitreous hemorrhage, retinal detachment, and optic nerve injury.

**Corneal abrasions**  Abrasions to the corneal epithelium are usually heralded by the sudden onset of severe eye discomfort. Before examination can begin, a topical anesthetic must be administered to control the pain. Fluorescein staining of the eye will assist in the location of the abrasion. Treatment usually consists of the instillation of a topical cycloplegic to make the eye more comfortable and an antibiotic drop or ointment to prevent infection. A pressure patch is often applied for the first 24 hours and a systemic pain reliever prescribed. Anesthetic drops should never be routinely used as they will retard the healing of the corneal epithelium, cause pain, and potentially lead to an addiction to medication for pain relief.

**Chemical burns**  When any chemical enters the eye, the immediate treatment is that of quick and constant irrigation of the eye with tap water, normal saline, or any available nonirritating liquid. All areas of the eye surface and lids should be flushed with the fluid. This treatment should continue for 15 to 20 minutes. Chemicals, especially those of an alkaline base (lye), are extremely toxic to the eye. The irrigation should be done immediately. Time should not be taken to transport the patient to an emergency facility before the irrigation is started. When the patient arrives at an emergency facility the pH will be tested, and further irrigations administered if necessary. A topical anesthetic will be administered for relief of pain and a cycloplegic instilled to minimize iris adhesions. Systemic pain medication will also be of some aid to patient comfort. Severe alkalai burns can lead to deep corneal scarring, cataracts, and glaucoma.

### Absence of Visual Perception
Many conditions affecting the eye can eventually lead to total loss of vision. These conditions include congenital abnormalities, trauma, tumors, untreated cataracts, glaucoma, infections, and retinal detachment.

## Congenital and neonatal visual disruptions

*Congenital* conditions (especially cataracts) that occur are frequently caused by the *rubella virus* or the *spirochete of syphilis* present in the mother during pregnancy. Preventable disturbances in the neonatal period include ophthalmia neonatorum and retrolental fibroplasia.

*Ophthalmia neonatorum* is an infectious condition of the conjunctiva that is contracted as the infant passes through the birth canal. It is most frequently caused by the gonococcus but may also be of staphylococcal, streptococcal, or other bacterial or viral origin.

*Retrolental fibroplasia* is now a rare condition that occurred primarily in premature infants requiring oxygen therapy after birth. It was caused by high concentrations of oxygen administered over prolonged periods of time. The condition is characterized by the growth of new blood vessels in the periphery of the retina and eventual retinal detachment. A retrolental membrane forms from the proliferating connective tissue, obscuring the fundus. Eye growth may also be terminated, resulting in microphthalmus. Reactions to high concentrations of oxygen are individual and may include some, all, or none of the above effects.

**Trauma** Serious head injuries, direct eye trauma, and thermal or chemical burns are the most frequent causes of traumatic blindness. *Head injuries* may result in damage to the sensory receiving areas in the occipital lobe, pressure on all or part of the optic nerve, or fractures of the skull or orbit that cause a penetrating eye wound.

*Direct eye trauma* includes lacerations and intraocular penetration by foreign bodies. Either condition may destroy eye structures and result in blindness. Another serious complication of such injuries is sympathetic ophthalmia (discussed earlier).

**Tumors** Either of the previously discussed tumors eventually results in blindness of one or both eyes. The blindness may be a direct effect of the tumor or of the therapy (enucleation) used to treat it.

**Untreated primary conditions** Primary disruptive conditions of the eye (glaucoma, cataracts, retinal detachment, and infection) may also result in permanent blindness if left untreated. The blindness may be slow and progressive (cataracts) or rapid and complete (acute closed-angle glaucoma).

**Effects on the individual** Whatever the precipitating factor, the result is the same, loss of visual perception—*blindness*—a severe blow to self-perception and a dramatic change in the affected individual's approach to daily living. Sight enables an individual to perceive the external environment and to react to it. Without sight, much of one's surroundings become or remain unknown.

Communication with others is still possible verbally, but not visually. Both written and nonverbal communication pathways are closed to the sightless person. This means that interpersonal relationships may be altered and new acquaintances or experiences are greatly curtailed.

Physically, the blind person is not able to select clothing on the basis of color or apply make-up without direction. Bruises and other skin conditions (rashes, blemishes, stains) are no longer visible but must be detected in another manner. This means additional dependency on others until adjustments in life-style can be made.

**First-level nursing care** Identifying the potential sources and instituting action to prevent the onset of blindness are important nursing responsibilities. Chronic conditions such as diabetes, kidney disease, and hypertension are all potential precursors of blindness. These conditions are in addition to the ones mentioned in the previous section (congenital, trauma, tumor, etc.). Industrial settings with all their hazards create a very large population at risk of eye injury. The preschool age group has the potential for blindness when amblyopia (absent or poor vision) goes undiagnosed. Children of all ages are at risk for traumatic injury when exploring or handling dangerous objects or playing with small or pointed projectiles.

**P**revention *Public education* is the greatest single preventive action that can be taken to curb the incidence of blindness. Programs for glaucoma, diabetes, and hypertension screening are very active in many urban and suburban communities. Persons with these conditions who demonstrate eye symptoms should be urged to consult a physician or ophthalmologist.

Safety programs should exist in all industrial settings to prevent tragic ocular injuries. These programs must establish basic safety standards such as wearing safety goggles, where appropriate, and using shatterproof glass. Basic emergency care for eye injuries should be part of the working knowledge of every industrial, community, clinic, and emergency room nurse.

Through the efforts of local and national organizations, preschool vision screening programs are quite active. These programs are designed to detect the presence of strabismus and prevent disuse blindness (amblyopia) in the crossed eye. Elementary school programs should exist to identify visual disturbances in the school-age child. Frequently, the school nurse is responsible for initiating and carrying out these programs.

Toy safety has recently gained widespread attention. Nurses should promote the establishment of standards for toy safety. This includes the removal of dangerous toys such as BB guns, fireworks, sharp arrows, and playthings with springs or sharp detachable parts.

Ophthalmia neonatorum is prevented by installing silver nitrate solution into the eyes of all newborns. While this procedure is required by law in most areas, it is important for the nurse to be aware of the rationale for this treatment and its necessity, particularly in situations of home delivery.

Blood tests of pregnant women can detect the presence of syphilis or rubella. These tests are invaluable in preventing congenital problems in the infant. Syphilitic mothers can receive treatment, thus protecting the fetus. Some states require that rubella titers be taken prior to the issuance of a marriage license. Women without antibodies for rubella can then be inoculated prior to pregnancy. Nurses can be instrumental in educating the public in both of these areas.

Retrolental fibroplasia is almost nonexistent since knowledge of its cause became known. However, nurses in premature and newborn nurseries should be continually aware of the concentrations of oxygen the infants are receiving to prevent accidental changes in the amounts administered.

Many causes of blindness are preventable. Nurses should urge all persons with eye symptoms to seek immediate evaluation and care.

**Second-level nursing care**   Nurses in a variety of community and outpatient situations may be the first health professionals to evaluate persons with eye disorders that may lead to blindness. It is, therefore, imperative that the initial assessment be thorough and descriptive.

**N**ursing Assessment   The *health history* of patients with ocular problems often includes *visual disturbances, conjunctival discharge,* and/or *pain* or *discomfort.* The visual disturbances may take the form of halos around lights, floating spots before the eyes, blurred vision, diplopia, or loss of peripheral vision. The exact nature, duration, and frequency of these symptoms should be noted.

*Physical assessment* may reveal no observable symptoms, or it may show signs of inflammation,

trauma, or discoloration. The ophthalmoscopic examination may show retinal or optic disk abnormalities. Aged persons may be unaware of or unwilling to admit to visual losses. Often the nurse can observe signs of the deficit such as squinting, difficulty in walking, or lack of recognition of common objects.

*Visual testing* is performed to determine the degree of visual loss. A person is considered *legally blind* when visual acuity is tested at 20/200 or less in the better eye with corrective lenses, or when the visual field subtends an angle no greater than 20°. Complete *absence of vision* is determined by the inability of the person to perceive any visual stimuli.

**N**ursing Problems and Intervention   The basic problem of the sightless individual is *loss of the visual sense* with its accompanying alteration in body image. Persons with severe loss of vision should be referred to an ophthalmologist or medical facility for further evaluation. If this loss has been progressive and inevitable, in spite of medical attention, the person will need assistance in adjusting to the handicap. This may involve referral to social service agencies for financial assistance and to specialty organizations for the blind for seeing-eye dogs or braille-reading information. Adjustment to blindness depends on many factors: age, ability to react to stress situations, significance of the lost part, interpersonal relationships and support systems, and society's attitude toward the disability. Additional information regarding rehabilitation of the blind individual is found under Fourth-Level Nursing Care.

**Third-level nursing care**   Sightless individuals who are hospitalized may be newly blind or may be in the hospital for another medical problem. Much of their care is similar, although the newly blind individual faces additional adjustment problems requiring sensitivity and support.

**N**ursing Assessment   In assessing the needs of the hospitalized patient who is blind, the nurse should first determine the degree of adjustment to the visual loss and the particular approach utilized by the person to the sensory deprivation. To do this, it is necessary to determine the *nature* and *history* of the temporary or permanent blindness.

Some patients, because of a specific surgical procedure or traumatic ocular injury, may be required to have both eyes covered and may thereby be temporarily deprived of their visual sense. Other persons may have experienced an acute, traumatic experience which resulted in a permanent loss of vision. Still others may have been without their visual sense for some time and may be hospitalized for either a related or unrelated condition. In all these situations, there are certain problems that are common. (Physical assessment and tests of visual acuity, where appropriate, are as described in Second-Level Nursing Care.)

**N**ursing Problems and Interventions The primary problem for most blind patients is *identification of personnel.* Whenever a nurse enters the presence of the blind patient, prompt and proper identification of self and the purpose for being there will be of great assistance to the patient. It is important to remember not to physically touch the patient before verbalizing one's presence. The importance of a thorough orientation of the blind patient to the physical environment should be emphasized; once the environment has been arranged and the patient made aware of the arrangement, it must not be altered in any way without informing the patient. This will protect the patient from accidental injury.

It is also important to remember that a blind patient is *unable to see the components of routines and treatments.* Verbal communication is of the utmost importance. Thorough, descriptive explanations should be given. The patient should also be informed when the procedure is complete and personnel are leaving.

*Boredom* may be a problem for the sightless patient. Diversional activities should be provided. Radios, "talking books," and volunteer readers for the patient can be helpful.

In assisting the blind patient in *ambulation,* the nurse should walk slightly ahead and let the patient grasp the back of the nurse's arm. This provides a more secure feeling for the patient. Doors, steps, furniture, curbs, etc., should be pointed out before they are encountered.

In setting up a meal tray, several techniques may be used. One is to use the face of a clock to explain the location of the food (e.g., meat at 12 o'clock, peas at 3 o'clock); another technique is to guide the patient's hand to the various locations of the food on the tray. The patient should be allowed as much independence as possible in all activities. The encouragement of independence in the protected hospital environment is a small beginning step toward achieving it in daily life back in the community.

**Fourth-level nursing care** In assisting in the *rehabilitation process* of the blind adult, the nurse

has many resources to which to refer the patient. Both state and federal governments provide resources for the blind. For example, state and federal departments of vocational rehabilitation, and the Library of Congress, supply talking books. Private national organizations such as the American Foundation of the Blind and the National Society for the Prevention of Blindness are active in their aid to the sightless. Mobility training, an important part of the rehabilitation program, is provided by agencies such as The Seeing Eye, Inc. The nurse who becomes involved with a newly blinded person should utilize the resources known, refer the patient to these resources, and provide adequate follow-up so that the patient may achieve maximum rehabilitation.

Education is possible for both children and adults, largely because of instruction in the use of braille and talking books. Tape recorders take the place of notebooks, enabling many persons to attend colleges and other institutions of higher education. Often family members or friends will serve as "readers," so that the student may benefit from resources not available in other ways.

Occupational opportunities for sightless adults have been expanded in recent years. Referrals to social workers, occupational therapists, and guidance professionals may assist blind persons in maximizing their possibilities.

Grooming, feeding, and self-care activities may be the priorities for a newly blinded individual. These persons need much verbal assistance from family and professionals until they are able to feel secure with these activities.

Touch, listening, and "spatial perception" are senses that can be refined and developed to a greater extent by the blind individual. Greater sensitivity by means of touch permits identification of objects by size, shape, and texture instead of sight. Increased auditory acuity enables the person to identify differences in the pitch of sounds that indicate thickness, depth, or distance. This is particularly helpful to the person who uses the tapping of a cane to guide the path while walking. "Spatial perception" utilizes the echo of sounds to interpret the presence of solid objects in the environment.

In addition to the cane, mobility may be achieved if the sightless person is able to use a seeing-eye dog. These dogs are trained with the blind person and become an inseparable part of all activities. Patients should be made aware of the nearest facilities that provide such training. These dogs should not be touched or given direction by anyone other than their blind owners.

Family members should be included in all aspects of patient counseling. Arranging and maintaining a convenient home environment as well as encouraging independence are two major areas of focus. Family members should be urged to speak and act normally with the patient and to provide assistance only when necessary. Safety is important to prevent discouraging accidents. Open doors, hot stoves or irons, and cluttered stairs all provide unseen hazards. Fear is easily created and much more slowly dissipated. It is therefore better to encourage prevention.

## DISTURBANCES IN AUDITORY PERCEPTION

This section deals with the variety of pathologic conditions which may lead to the impairment of auditory perception. Inflammatory disturbances affecting the external and middle ear are discussed first, followed by the conditions which result in conductive hearing loss. Trauma to the tympanic membrane, mastoiditis, and Ménière's syndrome are examined separately. Finally, deafness, or the total absence of auditory perception, is explored.

### Inflammatory Disturbances in Auditory Perception

Infections and inflammatory disturbances of the external and middle ear occur with considerable frequency. These disturbances are referred to as *external otitis* and *otitis media.*

**External otitis**  Infections of the external ear, that area from the auricle to the eardrum, are termed *acute external otitis* and are most frequently the result of bacterial or fungal invasion. Bacterial infections are most common, with *Staphylococcus aureus* and *Pseudomonas* being frequent contaminants. Fungal infection, or *otomycosis,* is found everywhere but is more prevalent in the warmer climates. Acute external otitis occurs more frequently during the summer months and is often associated with swimming in contaminated water.

A variety of factors may predispose one to the invasion of infecting organisms. Such factors include: poor hygiene; boil or furuncle formation on the external ear; dermatologic conditions such as eczema, psoriasis, and impetigo; and minor injury or abrasion of the auricle or external auditory canal, frequently as a result of attempts to clean or scratch the ear.

The major effect of acute external otitis is *pain* due to diffuse inflammation of the epithelium of the external ear canal and, frequently, the auricle. An aural discharge may be present. Edema and discharge may result in a partial, temporary hearing loss and a plugged sensation in the affected ear (see Fig. 38-6a).

If the infection is allowed to spread unchecked, generalized symptoms of fever and malaise may develop. Postauricular and upper cervical lymphadenopathy may be visually apparent and are quite painful. Manipulation of the auricle or tragus greatly increases the person's pain. In contrast, similar manipulation does not increase pain in cases of otitis media. Acute external otitis usually resolves itself even without treatment, as the body's natural defense system mobilizes to fight the invading organism. Aural drainage helps to debride the external auditory canal of dead and contaminated skin cells. Swelling gradually subsides until healing is complete. However, prompt medical attention is recommended to decrease discomfort and dysfunction and to promote rapid healing.

*Chronic external otitis* is often associated with disorders of the skin, such as seborrheic dermatitis or psoriasis. The external ear is inflamed, but usually there is no infection. The underlying dermatologic disorder often causes dry and scaling skin, itching, and an alteration in the production of cerumen, or earwax. This condition may last for years, resulting in a permanent thickening of the epithelium of the external ear and canal (see Fig. 38-6b).

*Itching* is the characteristic symptom of *chronic* external otitis. Pain is uncommon. Dry, scaling skin may be limited to the external auditory canal or may be visible around the meatus and auricle. The ear may drain but is more often dry. The individual often aggravates this condition by scratching the itchy ear.

**Otitis media**  The middle ear includes the area from the tympanic membrane to the oval window. *Acute otitis media* frequently occurs after upper respiratory infection or childhood illnesses, such as measles and scarlet fever. Infection is caused by a variety of bacteria, most commonly pneumococci and streptococci, which are frequently introduced into the middle ear by way of the eustachian tube. Invasion through the lymphatic system or bloodstream is less common. Infection via the eustachian tube is usually the result of poor nose-blowing practices, such as forceful blowing, which pushes contaminated secretions into the middle ear. During swimming or diving, contaminated water may enter the nose and can also lead to infection.

The "earache" of acute otitis media is especially common during infancy and childhood, in part, it is believed, because the eustachian tube is shorter and straighter than in the adult. In addition, adenoid tissue in the nasopharynx, also common in children but rare in adults, is believed to obstruct the eustachian tube orifice. During respiratory infection, this tissue becomes inflamed and edematous, further increasing the obstruction.

Pain is the major effect of acute otitis media. Pressure builds in the middle ear cavity as purulent material collects and is trapped there. The *tympanic membrane,* or eardrum, bulges and may spontaneously rupture if the pressure becomes too great. Purulent aural drainage is apparent following rupture, but pressure and pain are immediately relieved. Hearing is significantly impaired, although the individual is usually in such discomfort that complaints about hearing loss are infrequent. Malaise and fever up to 40 or 41.1°C (104 to 106°F) are common. Healing will usually occur naturally over time, but prompt medical attention can help relieve pain and prevent residual hearing impairment, which may result if healing is incomplete.

Acute otitis media which does not resolve completely may result in *chronic suppurative otitis media* lasting months to a lifetime. In such cases the eardrum is perforated, allowing a continuous drainage of purulent material which erodes the tympanic membrane and middle-ear bones over the course of months or years. Chronic mastoiditis (described later in this chapter) is virtually always present in cases of chronic otitis media, as the air cells of the mastoid process are contiguous to the middle ear, and infection spreads easily.

Multiple bacteria are usually responsible for chronic otitis media. *Pseudomonas, Proteus, Staphylococcus,* and *Streptococcus* are common pathogens. Frequently these organisms are drug resistant, and *Proteus* and *Pseudomonas* may be particularly difficult to treat.

Some individuals with chronic otitis media develop *cholesteatoma* (Fig. 38-7). In this condition skin from the external auditory canal grows through the perforated eardrum into the middle ear and mastoid air cells. As dead skin cells slough off, they form a soft white ball, the cholesteatoma. Trapped in the middle ear and mastoid, the enlarging ball erodes the surrounding bone, leading to such complications as vertigo, hearing loss, facial paralysis, and meningitis. Cholesteatoma must be surgically removed. Pain is not a symptom of chronic otitis media, and its presence may indicate the existence of an epidural abscess.

*Serous otitis media* may result from a variety of factors, but frequently the cause is unknown. Air pressure changes associated with airplane travel may cause a temporary serous otitis media when the air pressure within the middle ear is not equalized with the atmospheric pressure. Frequently inflamed adenoid tissue is at fault. Swollen tissue occludes the eustachian tube orifice and cuts off the airflow which normally equalizes the pressure in the middle ear. The eardrum becomes retracted as a partial vacuum is formed, and a sterile serous fluid is drawn into the middle-ear cavity. This serous transudate, usually amber in color but occasionally blood tinged, is usually visible through the thin, transparent eardrum. Frequently air is trapped in

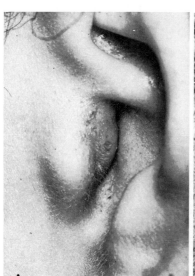
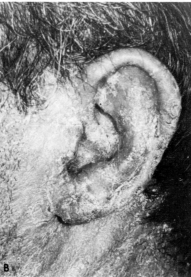

**A** **B**

**FIGURE 38-6**

(a) Acute external otitis with furuncle. Note the swelling of the external auditory canal. (*From Havener, William H., William H. Saunders, Carol Fair Keith, and Ardra W. Prescott: Nursing Care in Eye, Ear, Nose, and Throat Disorders, 3d ed., Mosby, St. Louis, 1974.*) (*b*) Chronic external otitis associated with seborrheic dermatitis. (*From DeWeese, David D. and William H. Saunders: Textbook of Otolaryngology, 4th ed., Mosby, St. Louis, 1973.*)

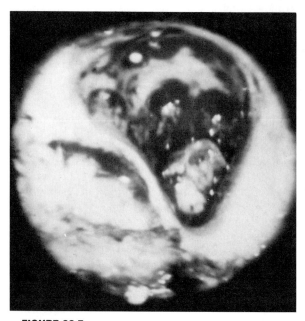

**FIGURE 38-7**
Cholesteatoma with mastoidectomy. The external auditory canal is visible at upper left. Mastoidectomy has been performed (the pear-shaped area at center right), and the white-ball cholesteatoma is visible at the top of the pear. (*Courtesy of Kenneth H. Brookler, M.D.*)

the middle ear, and an air-fluid level is visible across the tympanic membrane. Hearing is impaired, and the individual complains of a plugged sensation or fluid in the ear. Usually this condition resolves itself as the fluid is reabsorbed, but occasionally serous otitis media may persist with no apparent cause and despite all treatment.

**First-level nursing care** Anyone can develop external otitis. The risk of infection increases during the warmer months when water sports are popular and when the increased temperature and humidity encourage the rapid growth of bacterial and fungal organisms. Individuals having poor personal hygiene habits, or those with a poor understanding of safe ear-cleaning techniques, run a higher risk of infection, as do individuals having dermatologic conditions affecting the external ear.

The incidence of acute otitis media is markedly higher in children than in adults. This is partially due to anatomic differences in the eustachian tube and adenoid tissue of children (described in otitis media above). Since acute otitis media and serous otitis media frequently follow upper respiratory infection, tonsillitis, and the childhood diseases, children or adults with these ailments are at higher risk than the general population.

**Prevention** *Health education* directed toward the prevention of disease is the major focus of First-Level Nursing care. The external ear should be thoroughly, but gently, washed daily during regular bathing. Cotton-tipped swabs, which are so widely used to clean and dry the external ear and auditory canal, are a frequent cause of injury when used improperly. These swabs should be used with extreme care. Rubbing or pressing against the canal wall with the swab should be avoided, and the swab should *never* be pushed or forced deep into the auditory canal for any reason. Children and adults should be instructed in the dangers of placing foreign objects in the ear. Frequently this may be done to relieve itching in the external auditory canal, but gently wiggling the auricle in a circular motion often relieves this symptom without risking injury to the ear. Children may need frequent reminders not to stick objects in their ears. An explanation appropriate to the child's level of understanding should be given.

The prompt treatment of upper respiratory infection, colds, and tonsillitis is important in preventing middle-ear infections and its complications, and individuals should be encouraged to seek medical attention during the early stages of illness. Instruction should be given in safe nose-blowing techniques. The nose should always be blown gently with both nostrils open to avoid forcing contaminated secretions through the eustachian tube into the middle ear. Water entering the nose during water sports activities should be allowed to drain out naturally. The nose should never be blown forcefully. Special instructions in nose blowing-techniques should be given to individuals seeking treatment for colds and upper respiratory infection to help prevent the development of otitis media.

Public education can be accomplished in a variety of settings including homes, schools, health facilities, and community organizations. Films, pamphlets, and other media can be useful teaching aides. Health teaching, early disease detection, and prompt treatment are emphasized.

**Second-level nursing care** Individuals with inflammatory conditions of the ear are most frequently identified and treated on an outpatient basis. Nursing assessment is vital to the detection of affected persons.

**Nursing Assessment** A complete *health history* may supply information important to the diagnosis and treatment of the individual's condition. The nurse should elicit information about the person's general state of health, including the presence of any acute illness (particularly upper respiratory infections), chronic disease, or injury which might predispose that individual to ear infection. Any medication currently being used should be noted, as well as any history of drug allergy, especially to antibiotic preparations. It is useful to know whether the individual's tonsils and adenoids have been surgically removed. Persons should be questioned about recent activities in the water, such as swimming and diving, and information about the nature and cleanliness of the body of water involved should be elicited. The patient may be in mild to acute discomfort. Generally this includes ear pain, malaise, and fever.

*Physical assessment*   Included in physical assessment of the affected ear is a visual examination of the auricle and surrounding tissue. In cases of external otitis, the auricle may be edematous and reddened. The presence of scaling, crusting, or fissures may indicate an underlying skin disorder. If discharge is visible, the color, consistency, and quantity should be noted. The auricle may be gently manipulated to determine the presence of malformations, boils, cysts, or other lesions. It is important to note whether this manipulation causes the patient additional pain, a characteristic sign of acute external otitis. Inspection and palpation for regional lymphadenopathy should be carried out. Vital signs may reveal the presence of an elevated body temperature, and the duration and degree of elevation should be noted.

An *otoscope* is used to visualize the external auditory canal and eardrum. In the adult, the canal is straightened prior to insertion of the otoscope speculum to afford better visualization. This is accomplished by gently pulling the auricle up and back. In children, the auricle is pulled slightly down and back.

In acute external otitis it may be impossible to insert the otoscope speculum because of severe pain and swelling. When the otoscope can be used, the speculum is inserted with great care to prevent additional trauma to the inflamed tissue or to lesions which may be present in the ear canal. The external auditory canal is examined for signs of injury, inflammation, infection, lesions, discharge or bleeding, and cerumen (earwax).

If the external canal is relatively clean or can be debrided, the tympanic membrane should be visible, and its condition and color noted. In external otitis the eardrum may be normal or slightly inflamed. In acute otitis media it is always inflamed; frequently it is bulging and may appear whitish in color owing to the accumulation of pus in the middle ear. In contrast the eardrum is characteristically retracted in serous otitis media owing to the partial vacuum which has been created in the middle ear; an amber or blood-tinged fluid may be visible through the relatively thin, transparent tympanic membrane; frequently air bubbles, or an air-fluid level, can be seen (see Fig. 38-8).

*Diagnostic tests*   In cases of acute or chronic otitis media, aural discharge may be *cultured* to identify the invading organisms, which are then tested for their *sensitivity* to various antibiotic drugs. Such testing is particularly important when the patient is allergic to penicillin, the drug of choice for acute otitis media, or does not respond to the drug prescribed. Culture and sensitivity tests are especially useful in treating chronic otitis media which is caused by multiple organisms, some of which may be drug resistant. Two to three days are required before the results of these tests are received, but the individual is usually started on a broad-spectrum antibiotic medication immediately to avoid a delay in treatment.

**N**ursing Problems and Interventions   Because hospitalization is rarely required even in acute cases, nursing interventions focus on helping the individual and family plan and carry out care at home. The major nursing problem is the presence of *inflammation* due to the infectious process. Systemic antibiotic medications are given orally when fever, malaise, and lymphadenopathy indicate infection is generalized. Bed rest is advised, and the nurse should emphasize the importance of a high fluid intake during this period to prevent dehydration. Analgesics such as acetylsalicylic acid or codeine are given for pain. Nasal vasodilators may be used to help open clogged eustachian tubes in otitis media.

The application of wet or dry heat to the affected ear is soothing and produces hyperemia, which is physiologically beneficial. The nurse should instruct the individual in the safe application of a heating pad, hot-water bottle, or wet compress to avoid burning the hypersensitive, inflamed tissue. These materials need not be sterile. The ear should be protected with a piece of cloth or gauze padding before a heating pad or hot water bottle is applied to it.

Whenever possible the auditory canal is cleansed to remove discharge and debris. Medicated eardrops or Burrow's solution may be instilled

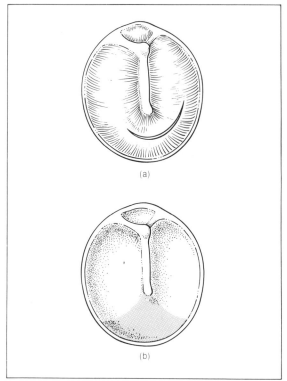

**FIGURE 38-8**
(a) Bulging eardrum in acute otitis media. Note the myringotomy incision in the posterior inferior section of the membrane.
(b) Retracted eardrum common in serous otitis media. A fluid level is visible through the lower section of the membrane.

to treat *local* infection and inflammation. Burrow's solution is often used for its soothing effect; in addition, it encourages the sloughing off of dead skin cells which harbor microorganisms. Antibiotic eardrops are frequently used, and corticosteroid preparations may be applied locally to treat inflammation. To instill eardrops at home, the individual should be instructed to tilt the head sideways until the affected ear is facing upward. The auditory canal is then gently straightened, and the solution instilled by medicine dropper into the auditory meatus. The clean dropper should never touch the affected ear, which is considered contaminated. Gentle pressure on the tragus (triangular cartilage covering the external meatus) helps propel the fluid into the canal. A loose cotton earplug saturated with the same solution can be inserted into the canal to prevent the drops from running out when the head is straightened.

In severe acute external otitis the ear canal may not be patent. A cotton ear wick, saturated with an antibiotic solution, may be inserted into the auditory canal down to the eardrum. The patient should be instructed to return to the office or clinic in 1 or 2 days, at which time the wick is removed and the ear is debrided. Treatment with medicated eardrops may then be instituted. All solutions instilled into the ear should be at room temperature to avoid precipitating a *caloric reaction* (mild vertigo and nausea) in the patient.

In some cases of acute otitis media the eardrum may spontaneously rupture if pressure in the middle ear becomes too great as a result of the *accumulation of pus.* Pain and pressure are dramatically relieved as the purulent material begins to drain. *Myringotomy,* or surgical incision of the tympanic membrane, may be performed when the eardrum is bulging to prevent spontaneous rupture, relieve pain, and allow drainage of the purulent material. This procedure is performed in the physician's office or clinic. Usually no anesthetic is used, as most topical preparations are not effective on the eardrum. The patient is in a prone position with the affected ear uppermost. Children must be restrained, and a mummy restraint is advised for infants. A curved incision is made in the postero-inferior section of the tympanic membrane away from the delicate middle-ear bones (see Fig. 38-8). Sterile cotton in the ear canal absorbs drainage and bleeding. The patient or family should be instructed in the changing and disposal of this contaminated cotton. The patient is advised to keep the ear dry during bathing until the infection is completely resolved. The myringotomy incision may heal within 24 hours, although the procedure may need to be repeated to maintain drainage until antibiotic drugs control the infection.

It is commonly believed that a hole in the eardrum results in impaired or lost hearing. This is not true, and, in fact, myringotomy actually helps to preserve hearing by releasing the pus which can necrose the bones of the middle ear. The incision usually heals completely, and complications are rare. Occasionally a small perforation may remain unhealed, but this does not noticeably affect hearing. However, a careless incision may injure or dislodge one of the middle ear bones, causing marked hearing loss. Both of these conditions can be corrected surgically by the use of tympanoplasty procedures (discussed below).

In cases of serous otitis media a smaller incision may be made in the eardrum, and a small plastic tube inserted to allow for equalization of air pressure in the middle ear. This is most frequently done when the eustachian tube is blocked by inflamed adenoid tissue. The ear must be kept dry as long as the tube provides an open route for infection into the middle ear. When the condition has resolved, usually after several weeks to several months, the tube is removed. Frequently the tube extrudes spontaneously from the eardrum, which then heals rapidly. Adenoidectomy is frequently advised for children having repeated attacks of serous otitis media.

The individual with chronic external otitis usually has no systemic signs or symptoms. Treatment consists of applying soothing salves, such as petroleum jelly containing phenol and salicylic acid, and antibiotic ointments to the external ear and canal to control itching, dryness, and infection. The individual can be taught to make a thin cotton-tipped applicator (commercial swabs are too thick) by covering the end of a blunt toothpick with cotton. The applicator is covered with ointment and inserted carefully into the auditory canal. A gentle twisting motion helps to coat the canal wall and eardrum with salve. The patient may be instructed in the safe application of a wet compress if the ear is draining, but this is discontinued once the ear is dry.

**Third-level nursing care**   Individuals with a long history of acute or chronic otitis media may be left with large perforations of the eardrum and necrotic middle-ear bones. This results in a conductive hearing loss, as the normal route by which sound waves are conducted to the inner ear is interrupted. The individual frequently complains of a marked impairment of hearing. Hospitalization is required for surgical reconstruction of the tympanic membrane and middle-ear ossicles.

**N**ursing Assessment   A complete *health history* and *physical assessment* are completed as previously described in Second-Level Nursing Care. Perforation of the eardrum will be apparent during the otoscopic examination, and the middle-ear bones may be visible if the perforation is large. *Diagnostic tests* are used to confirm and measure the extent of hearing loss. The *audiometric* and *tuning fork tests* used in diagnosis are discussed later in this chapter.

**N**ursing Problems and Interventions   When a *conductive hearing loss* is confirmed in the presence of a normal inner ear, hearing may be improved by *surgical intervention*. As long as the hearing mechanism housed in the inner ear is normal, reconstruction of the middle ear conduction pathway should be attempted.

Before surgery is performed, the ear should be free of infection. The nurse should instruct the individual in how to carry out the prescribed treatment plan at home prior to hospitalization. Once the infection is controlled, the patient enters the hospital to undergo one of a series of operations jointly called *tympanoplasty.*

*Myringoplasty,* or type-I tympanoplasty, is performed to close a residual perforation of the eardrum. A layer of skin from the ear canal, or a section of fascia from the temporal muscle, is grafted across the perforated eardrum. Gelfoam moistened with normal saline or antibiotic eardrops is used to pack the ear and hold the graft in place. When a fascia graft is used, it eventually is covered over by epithelium from the external auditory canal on the outside and by mucous membrane from the middle ear on the inside. Frequently hearing is improved, and the risk of infection is greatly decreased, since the middle ear cavity is protected by an intact eardrum.

*Ossiculoplasty,* or type-II to type-V tympanoplasty, involves the replacement of diseased or missing middle ear bones with plastic or metal prostheses to reconstruct the normal conduction pathway of the ear.

Patients undergoing tympanoplasty procedures are usually hospitalized for 3 to 4 days. Packing in the external ear canal is left undisturbed, but the outer dressing may be reinforced if drainage is extensive. The patient is cautioned to avoid sneezing or nose blowing, as this increases air pressure in the eustachian tube and middle ear and could dislodge the new graft. Mild dizziness and nausea may be experienced for a few days due to stimulation of the labyrinth during surgery. Appropriate safety precautions, including supervised walking and the use of siderails, should be taken to prevent patient injury during this time. The patient is advised to change position slowly to help avoid dizziness. Antimotion and sedative drugs often help relieve nausea and vertigo. The individual is cautioned to keep the ear dry during bathing until healing is complete.

**Fourth-level nursing care**   Prevention of repeated external and middle ear infection is the primary goal of rehabilitation. The importance of good aural hygiene is stressed as well as the dangers of injury to the ear from foreign objects and the improper use of cotton-tipped swabs. The individual is encouraged to seek prompt medical attention for colds and upper respiratory infection. Instruction is given in safe nose-blowing techniques. Any recurrence of ear infection should be treated rapidly to prevent chronic infection and hearing loss.

Recovery is usually complete from ear infection. Individuals undergoing tympanoplasty are followed periodically after discharge from the hospital until the ear is completely healed. The individual can then resume a normal, active life, including air travel and water sports activities. Usually hearing in the affected ear is serviceable as a result of the surgical repair. Depending on the individual results, audiometric testing may be recommended to accurately measure the extent of residual hearing loss. In some cases a hearing aid may be prescribed.

### Conductive Disturbances in Auditory Perception

Hearing occurs, in part, through the conduction of sound waves to the organ of hearing in the inner ear. Sound impulses travel through the external auditory canal and strike the tympanic membrane, causing it to vibrate. The malleus, incus, and stapes of the middle ear each vibrate in turn as the sound impulse is conducted to the inner ear (see Chap. 31). Any condition which interferes with the normal conduction of sound waves to the inner ear results in a conductive hearing loss. The conduction pathway may be interrupted by a foreign body or impacted cerumen in the external auditory canal; by a scarred, thickened, or perforated eardrum resulting from injury or infection; by diseased, injured, or missing middle-ear bones; or by congenital atresia (absence) of the auditory canal. The extent of hearing impairment is related to the extent of damage present. If the inner ear is normal, sound perception is not distorted but is lessened in intensity. Any intervention which helps to restore the conduction pathway helps to restore hearing. Two frequent causes of conductive hearing loss are discussed in this section.

**Cerumen**   Commonly termed earwax, cerumen is usually present in the external auditory canal of all individuals. In normal amounts cerumen helps to protect the ear canal from injury and prevents excessive dryness and itching. Occasionally, the wax may collect and become hard and impacted. Discomfort and hearing impairment may result. This condition is easily rectified by removal of the cerumen plug.

**Otosclerosis**   By far the most common cause of conductive hearing loss is *otosclerosis*. In this gradually progressive condition there is an abnormal proliferation of bone tissue around the foot-

plate of the stapes in the middle ear. Eventually the stapes becomes immobilized in the oval window and is unable to vibrate in response to sound waves. Hearing is markedly impaired at this point, although it may be 10 to 20 years before the disease progresses to this extent. Even when the stapes is totally immobilized, the individual is not deaf, for some hearing occurs by means of bone conduction. *Tinnitus*, a ringing in the ears, and a gradually progressive hearing loss are the major effects of otosclerosis. The exact cause of this condition is unknown, but it is not a result of ear infection. Usually otosclerosis is bilateral, but the ears are not affected equally.

**First-level nursing care**   Although the cause of otosclerosis remains obscure, it is known to run in families and to be considerably more common in females than in males. Negroes rarely develop this condition. Hearing impairment characteristically begins in the late teens or early twenties, although it may be so slight as to be unnoticed by the individual for several years. The degree of hearing loss becomes more pronounced over the next 20-odd years, and this, or the annoying tinnitus, may cause the individual to seek treatment.

**Prevention**   There is no known method of preventing otosclerosis. However, individuals having a family history of this condition should be aware that they are at increased risk. These individuals are advised to seek professional care promptly if tinnitus or hearing loss is noted. Since these symptoms are associated with disorders other than otosclerosis, the importance of prompt medical intervention should be stressed. Some individuals may delay treatment believing that they have the "family deafness," for which there is no treatment. This is incorrect, and prompt case finding can assist in planning proper care.

Anyone may develop a plug of impacted cerumen anytime. *Health education* should stress the importance of having a professional person remove the wax. Some individuals may try to dig the wax out using paper clips, hairpins, or commercial swabs. The danger in placing such objects in the ear is discussed below. The use of proprietary products for removing wax should be discouraged, as they cause inflammation in some individuals.

**Second-level nursing care**   The identification and treatment of individuals having a conductive hearing loss, due to otosclerosis or impaced cerumen, usually occurs in an ambulatory-care setting.

Nursing assessment plays a major role in the detection of these individuals.

**N**ursing Assessment   A complete *health history* is taken as previously described. (See Inflammatory Disturbances in Second-Level Nursing Care.) The individual should be questioned about other family members who may have otosclerosis or a "hearing problem." The presence of tinnitus, and a history of a gradually progressive hearing loss, are of major diagnostic significance if otosclerosis is suspected.

A visual and otoscopic examination is made of the external ear and auditory canal. This *physical assessment* is normal in cases of otosclerosis, unless an additional condition, such as infection, exists concurrently. Impacted cerumen is readily visible during otoscopic examination, and further testing is unnecessary.

*Diagnostic tests*   If the health history and physical examination are suggestive of otosclerosis, additional diagnostic testing may be advised. *Audiometric testing* provides a comprehensive examination of the individual's ability to hear sounds and discriminate speech or words. An electrical device, the *audiometer,* produces pure tone sounds as well as selected words. The individual usually is seated in a specially prepared soundproof room, while the examiner is seated outside at the control console (see Fig. 38-9). In some systems the sounds are delivered through a loudspeaker, but more frequently the individual being tested is fitted with a set of earphones. A series of pure tone sound frequencies is delivered at varying levels of intensity, and the individual is requested to respond in some designated manner whenever a sound is heard. The lowest intensity at which a pure tone sound can be heard is the individual's *hearing threshold.* The *decibel system* is a logarithmic scale used to measure the intensity of sound (see Table 38-3). In a person with normal hearing, speech is comfortably loud in intensities ranging from 40 decibels (dB) to 65 dB. Sound frequency is measured in Hertz (Hz); this unit refers to the number of oscillations per second of a sound wave. Persons with normal hearing may hear frequencies from 20 to 20,000 Hz, although hearing is more sensitive at 500 to 4000 Hz. The decibel system is used to describe the extent of hearing loss. Normal speech may range in intensity from 40 to 65 dB, and in frequency from 500 to 2000 Hz. A bilateral hearing loss of 40 dB or more in the speech frequencies is incapacitating to the individual. Deafness is defined as a bilateral hearing loss of 85 to 90 dB or more in the speech frequencies.

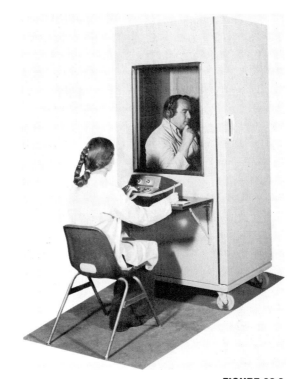

**FIGURE 38-9**
Audiometric testing being conducted in a soundproof room.
(*Courtesy of the Industrial Acoustics Company, New York.*)

Audiometric testing measures any loss in the ability to hear pure tone sounds and indicates which frequencies are most affected. In addition *audiologists* (hearing specialists) can determine the type of hearing loss, conductive or sensorineural (Fig. 38-10). Test signals are administered to each ear separately and reach the inner ear by means of air conduction. A special appliance, the *bone oscillator,* is placed on the mastoid process behind the ear and measures the sound transmitted by bone conduction. This provides a measure of inner-ear function by bypassing the external and middle ear. A comparison of hearing efficiency by bone and air conduction is of particular importance in confirming a diagnosis of otosclerosis. The individual with otosclerosis hears as well or better by bone conduction as by air conduction, whereas the reverse is true of individuals having normal hearing.

*Speech audiometry* measures the individual's ability to hear and understand words. A list of words is read to the individual to determine the lowest intensity at which the person can correctly hear 50 percent of the words. This *speech reception threshold* usually approximates the air conduction hearing threshold. *Speech discrimination* is tested by requesting the individual to repeat a series of common words presented at an intensity level well above the hearing threshold. Individuals with normal hearing have no difficulty with this test. Individuals who do have difficulty understanding the words usually have a nerve-type hearing loss involving the inner ear.

The *Rinne test* also compares hearing efficiency by bone and air conduction. This simple test requires only a tuning fork and may be used as an initial screening device. To test hearing by air conduction, the activated tuning fork is placed near, but not touching, the patient's ear. The length of time the person hears the sound is recorded. Both ears are tested individually in this manner. Next, the handle of the activated tuning fork is placed on the mastoid process behind the ear. Again the length of time the person hears the sound is noted. The individual with normal auditory perception hears the sound by air conduction about twice as long as the sound by bone conduction. The individual with a conductive hearing loss hears the sound by bone conduction longer than by air conduction. How

**TABLE 38-3**
FREQUENTLY HEARD SOUNDS AND THEIR DECIBEL INTENSITIES

| Sound | Decibels |
| --- | --- |
| Air raid siren (painful to ear) | 140 |
| Jet engine | 130 |
| Rock band | |
| Loud shout (1 ft away) | 120 |
| Thunder | |
| Motorcycle | 110 |
| Aircraft engine (propeller) | |
| Power mower (discomfort for pure tones) | 100 |
| Electric food blender | 90 |
| Train | |
| Pneumatic jackhammer | 80 |
| Heavy traffic (outside) | 70 |
| Average conversation | 60 |
| Vacuum cleaner | 50 |
| Automobile | 40 |
| A quiet room | 30 |
| Soft whisper | 20 |
| Breathing | 10 |
| Hearing threshold | 0 |

much longer depends upon the severity of the disorder.

The *Weber test* uses a slightly different technique to test hearing by bone and air conduction. The activated tuning fork is placed either on the forehead at the midline of the skull or on the upper incisor teeth. Normally the sound is heard equally well in both ears. If there is conductive hearing loss (due to disease of the external or middle ear), the individual hears the sound better in the poorer ear by means of bone conduction. If there is sensorineural or nerve-type hearing loss, the individual hears the sound louder in the better ear.

**N**ursing Problems and Interventions When impacted cerumen causes discomfort and interferes with normal hearing, it is usually removed by irrigating the affected ear with an ear syringe and tap water at body temperature (to avoid caloric reaction). The nurse may instruct a member of the family in the proper irrigation technique to be repeated at home in chronic cases.

The ear syringe is first filled with warm water. The individual is seated, and the head is tilted slightly forward toward the affected ear. This allows drainage of the irrigating solution from the ear into a basin which the patient holds just below the ear. The auricle is pulled gently up and back to straighten the auditory canal, and the irrigating solution is injected toward the *upper* wall of the auditory canal (see Fig. 38-11). Injecting the fluid directly into the auditory canal may only force the wax plug deeper into the canal. After irrigation, the canal is carefully dried with cotton and forceps. Occasionally a few drops of warm mineral oil may be instilled in the ear for several days prior to irrigation to soften an especially hard wax plug. In difficult cases the physician or a specially trained nurse may need to remove the wax with a special cerumen spoon and aural speculum.

There is no medical treatment for otosclerosis. Nursing interventions at this stage focus on educating the patient to the nature and course of this problem. The individual should understand that many years of serviceable hearing may remain, but that when hearing is no longer adequate, a widely accepted surgical procedure offers hope for restoration of useful hearing in up to 95 percent of patients.[1] Some individuals may be referred for aural rehabilitation (discussed below) to help maintain and maximize effective communication. If hearing becomes so impaired as to require the use of a hearing aid, surgical intervention should be considered. Periodic medical and audiometric evaluations are required in order to plan appropriate intervention.

**Third-level nursing care**  When the individual's hearing becomes so impaired that normal daily functioning is affected, surgical intervention is indicated. This occurs when the person's hearing loss reaches 40 dB or more in the normal speech frequencies (500 to 2000 Hz).

**N**ursing Assessment  A *health history* and *physical assessment* are completed and usually yield results similar to that described under Second-Level Nursing Care. *Audiometric testing* confirms an incapacitating conductive hearing loss. This is virtually diagnostic of otosclerosis in the presence of a healthy eardrum and a history of gradual and progressive hearing loss.

**N**ursing Problems and Interventions  *Hearing loss* due to otosclerosis is the major nursing problem at this level. Intervention is surgical, and requires hospitalization. A variety of techniques have been developed to reconstruct or modify the air conduction pathway. *Fenestration,* or the "window" operation, was widely used for many years but is rarely performed today since more effective techniques have been developed. This procedure bypasses the middle ear and immobilized the stapes completely. A mastoidectomy is performed (as described below), and a hole or window is created in the horizontal semicircular canal of the inner ear. A skin graft is used to cover this new opening. Adequate hearing is restored as sound, unable to reach the inner ear through the blocked oval window, reaches the inner ear through the newly created window. Normal hearing is not restored, however, and the necessity of performing a mastoidectomy makes fenestration less than desirable.

*Stapes mobilization* has been widely performed with good results. This procedure involves breaking the stapes loose from its fixed position in the oval window. The technique was highly popular because of its simplicity. However, it was found that in as many as 50 percent of the cases, the stapes again became immobilized as the otosclerotic process continued.

*Stapedectomy,* or removal of the diseased stapes, is currently the procedure of choice. An incision is made freeing half the eardrum from its attachment to the wall of the auditory canal, and the membrane is folded back upon itself to provide an opening into the middle ear. A large operating microscope is used to provide magnification of the tiny bones and ensure adequate lighting. The osseous proliferation holding the stapes footplate in the oval window is severed, and the bone is removed. In order to restore the normal sound con-

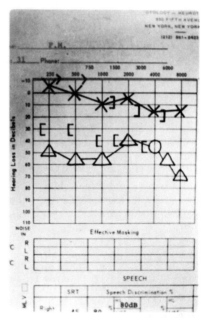

**FIGURE 38-10**

Audiogram of right ear affected with Ménière's disease. Hearing is normal in the left ear (*x*). A moderate hearing loss is noted in the right ear (Δ). The lower frequencies are most affected. (*Courtesy of Kenneth H. Brookler, M.D.*)

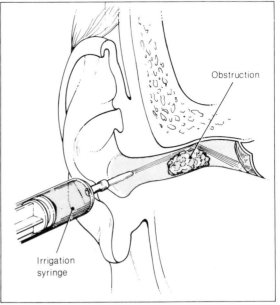

**FIGURE 38-11**

Irrigation of the external auditory canal. Note that the solution is directed toward the upper wall of the canal.

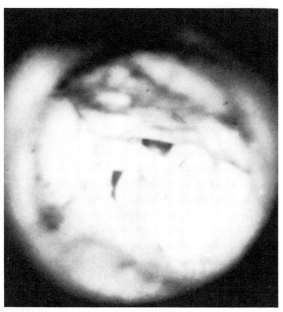

**FIGURE 38-12**
Stapedectomy. The stapes has been removed, and white Gelfoam is visible over the oval window. A stainless steel stapes prosthesis has been crimped around the long process of the incus. At top the tympanic membrane has been reflected to allow access to the middle ear. (*Courtesy of Kenneth H. Brookler, M.D.*)

duction pathway, the oval window must be sealed and rejoined to the incus. A variety of methods are used to accomplish this. A piece of vein or fascia may be used to seal the oval window, and a plastic or wire prosthesis attached to the incus replaces the stapes and completes the conduction pathway. Gelfoam or a piece of earlobe fat may also be used to seal the oval window. If Gelfoam is used, it eventually is reabsorbed and replaced by mucous membrane (see Fig. 38-12). Hearing is restored as soon as the prosthesis is in place and improves once the eardrum is repaired. However, the patient is cautioned that hearing will decrease as blood coagulates in the middle ear and auditory canal following surgery. It may be 1 to 2 weeks before hearing again improves.

*Postoperative care* Following surgery the patient is kept flat for up to 24 hours. Head movement should be avoided, and some surgeons request that a particular head position be maintained to *avoid dislodging the new prosthesis.* Blowing the nose and sneezing are prohibited during the first week to protect the eardrum from air pressure changes which could dislodge it. If sneezing cannot be avoided, the patient is instructed to open the mouth

widely (to help equalize air pressure in the middle ear), and to sneeze as gently as possible.

*Pain* may last several hours after surgery but can be relieved by administration of a narcotic analgesic. The semicircular canals and vagal nerve are often stimulated, and occasionally injured, during surgery. The physician is notified immediately of any complaints of vertigo, nausea, or vomiting. Usually anti–motion sickness drugs are effective in relieving discomfort. Antibiotics are given prophylactically for infection. Side rails and other safety precautions must be used while the patient is experiencing a *disturbance in equilibrium.* The patient is assisted in walking for 2 days following surgery and should be advised to change position slowly and to move the head and upper trunk in unison to avoid vertigo.

*Complications* include injury to the facial nerve or inner ear, infection, and meningitis. Facial weakness or paralysis, or disturbances in taste, may indicate that injury to the facial nerve has occurred. Complaints of stiff neck and generalized headache may be signs of meningitis. All such symptoms are reported to the physician immediately.

Usually the patient is discharged from the hospital 3 to 4 days following surgery. The patient should be given the following instructions: avoid people with colds or upper respiratory infections; avoid taking showers or wetting the head for 10 days; and avoid sudden, rapid movement (elevators) and high altitudes (airplane travel) for at least 1 month.

**Fourth-level nursing care** Once healing is complete, hearing is markedly improved or restored to normal in 90 to 95 percent of the persons having stapedectomy. In a few cases hearing may be worse following surgery. Since results are unpredictable, stapedectomy is performed on only one ear at a time, usually the most affected ear first. Even if surgery is unsuccessful, the patient will never be deaf, as hearing by bone conduction is unimpaired.

The individual is advised to protect whatever hearing remains. The ears should be protected from injury and infection through proper hygienic practices. The individual is encouraged to seek prompt medical attention for upper respiratory and ear infections to avoid further damage to the middle ear and conduction pathway.

For individuals whose hearing is improved, rehabilitation is usually not required. In less successful cases the person may be referred for aural rehabilitation, and a hearing aid may improve hearing to a serviceable level.

## Trauma to the Tympanic Membrane

*Trauma to the tympanic membrane,* or eardrum, may result in perforation, causing pain, impaired hearing, and increased risk of infection to the middle ear. Perforation frequently results from injury due to accidents, foreign bodies in the external auditory canal, extreme changes in external air pressure, or infection.

A *severe blow to the ear or head,* or a skull fracture, may cause injury to the tympanic membrane. This should be remembered in cases of head trauma (see Chap. 32), where the immediate concern may be for the head wound, and injury to the internal ear may be initially overlooked.

The placing of *foreign objects* into the ear is an extremely common phenomenon, especially with children. Any small object, such as paper wads, pencil erasers, or food, may be pushed into the external auditory canal. Such objects can usually be easily removed by irrigation of the canal. However, if the object in the ear is food, especially dried vegetables such as peas or beans, irrigation should not be attempted, as it causes the food to swell in the ear canal and makes removal more difficult. Foreign objects in the external auditory canal rarely pass the isthmus of the ear where the canal is narrowest. Removal of objects past the isthmus should be attempted only by a physician and may require an operative procedure to widen the ear canal.

*Insects* in the ear may be painful, loud, and frightening, but rarely cause injury to the tympanic membrane. The insect may be coaxed out of the ear by holding a flashlight up to the meatus of the external canal. Or the insect may be killed by instilling a few drops of oil or water into the ear. Irrigation will then flush out the dead intruder.

Although foreign bodies in the external canal may cause pain and irritation, perforation of the tympanic membrane rarely results. Perforation is more common, however, when longer, pointed objects are placed in the ear for cleaning or scratching purposes. Pencils, pens, paper clips, matchsticks, hairpins, and the cotton-tipped swab are frequent sources of injury.

Perforation of the eardrum may also be caused by a sudden and rapid *change in air pressure,* as that resulting from a nearby explosion. Brief exposure to high-intensity noise (160 dB) may rupture the eardrum and force the stapes through the oval window. Trauma may also be caused by too rapid a descent during airplane travel, but perforation of the eardrum is rare. More frequently ecchymosis of the tympanic membrane results.

Infection of the middle ear, *otitis media,* is the most frequent cause of spontaneous rupture of the tympanic membrane. Usually the pain is alleviated in such cases because the fluid previously trapped in the middle ear is then free to drain, thus relieving the pressure.

Trauma to the tympanic membrane may cause pain, irritation, edema, bleeding, and impaired hearing. As was noted earlier, contrary to common belief, a perforated eardrum does not result in deafness. Hearing impairment is usually slight to moderate and will improve when the eardrum heals. When healing is incomplete or scar tissue develops, the hearing loss may be permanent.

Interventions are symptomatic; analgesics are given for pain; the ear canal is kept clean; and medicated ear drops may be used to treat infection. Prevention of injury is the best treatment. Children and adults should be instructed in the dangers of placing any foreign object in the ear. Prompt treatment of ear infections decreases the risk of spontaneous rupture of the tympanic membrane. When a myringotomy is performed to release pus from the middle ear in otitis media, the clean incision heals rapidly with little risk of complications.

## Mastoiditis

Prior to the advent of antibiotics, *mastoiditis,* or inflammation of the mastoid process, was a frequent complication of otitis media. The mastoid process is a direct extension of the middle ear, thus providing an easy route for the spread of infection into the mastoid air cells. Although the incidence of mastoiditis has decreased with antibiotic therapy, cases are not infrequent.

Signs and symptoms of acute otitis media are nearly always present in patients with mastoiditis. Usually the eardrum is bulging, and frequently it has ruptured (see Fig. 38-13). Pressing firmly on the mastoid process produces discomfort. Postauricular swelling may be mistaken as a sign of mastoiditis but is most often associated with the lymphadenopathy of acute external otitis. Postauricular swelling due to mastoiditis is a result of abscess formation where purulent material has seeped through the temporal bone. This advanced condition is uncommon. X-ray examination of the temporal bone in this situation shows a hazy appearance in the mastoid area where the air cells are filled with pus. Infection may spread to the labyrinth, causing *labyrinthitis.* Frequently the labyrinth is destroyed by this infection, and permanent hearing loss results.

Treatment for acute mastoiditis consists of high-dosage antibiotic therapy. Myringotomy may

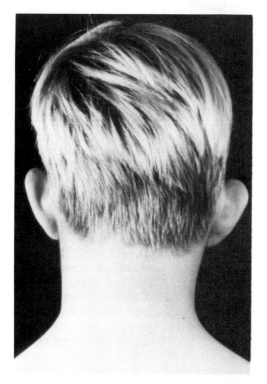

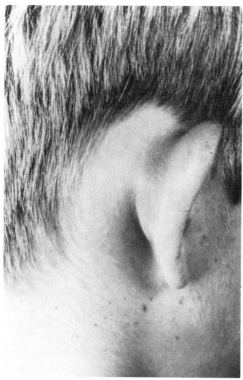

**FIGURE 38-13**

(a) Acute mastoiditis of the right ear. Note the way the right ear protrudes from the head. (b) The auricle is displaced owing to postauricular swelling. The area was noticeably reddened.

be indicated to relieve pressure in the middle ear. Complications of mastoiditis may be severe and include facial paralysis, abscess of the brain and epidural space, and meningitis. Incomplete healing may lead to the development of chronic otitis media and chronic mastoiditis.

Simple or radical mastoidectomy may be performed in cases which do not respond to conventional treatment. In *simple mastoidectomy,* an incision is made behind the auricle, and all the diseased bone and purulent material are removed. The mastoid process remains as an empty hull. Since the mastoid is not involved in auditory perception, hearing should return to normal once the infection has cleared. Simple mastoidectomy is usually reserved for cases of acute mastoiditis in which complications have developed. After simple mastoidectomy, a head dressing may be worn for several days. The physician usually changes the first dressing, but the nurse may reinforce the dressing if it becomes saturated with drainage. Sutures are removed within 5 to 6 days, and eventually granular scar tissue fills the mastoid process.

*Radical mastoidectomy* may be performed in cases of chronic mastoiditis in which the removal of infected material alone is deemed ineffective. It may also be performed to remove cholesteatoma associated with chronic otitis media and mastoiditis. This procedure consists of a simple mastoidectomy plus removal of the eardrum, incus, and malleus. The posterior wall of the internal auditory canal is also removed, and the middle ear and empty mastoid process become one large cavity. The epithelium of the external auditory canal grows into this cavity during healing. The stapes and facial nerve remain intact. This procedure obviously results in hearing loss. However, this is not usually of major concern because hearing has already been greatly impaired as a result of chronic inflammation.

Following radical mastoidectomy, the newly formed cavity is usually packed with gauze permeated with an antibiotic ointment. The packing is removed after 4 to 5 days. This may cause some discomfort, and an analgesic may be given ahead of time. A slight amount of bleeding is anticipated. Gauze padding is positioned behind the auricle to prevent it from becoming depressed, which is painful. Additional gauze is placed over the auricle, and a head dressing is applied. Postoperative pain is managed with a narcotic analgesic, such as meperidine hydrochloride. Vertigo, resulting from inner-ear stimulation, may be a distressing symptom but usually passes within a few days. Anti-nauseant and anti–motion sickness medications may offer some relief. Appropriate safety precautions should be instituted to prevent falls or injury while the patient is experiencing vertigo.

Complications of radical mastoidectomy are serious. Total hearing loss may occur if the stapes is accidentally dislodged from the oval window during surgery. Accidental injury to the facial nerve may result in facial paralysis. The nurse should be alert for signs of this paralysis which include an inability to close the eye or wrinkle the forehead on the affected side. If asked to smile, the mouth is pulled toward the unaffected side.

After discharge from the hospital the patient should be followed until the ear cavity is dry and healed, approximately 6 to 8 weeks. Once or twice yearly the cavity should be observed and cleaned to prevent infection of the new epithelial lining. A hearing aid may improve hearing to a functional level.

### Ménière's Syndrome

A disease of the inner ear, Ménière's syndrome is characterized by tinnitus, vertigo, and unilateral hearing loss. Although the exact cause is unknown, it is thought that autonomic nervous system dysfunction results in episodic vasoconstriction of the inner-ear vessels. This causes the cochlear mucous membrane to become edematous. The resulting increased fluid pressure in the vestibular labyrinth is believed to account for the symptoms of Ménière's disease.

True vertigo is a prominent symptom, and it is essential to differentiate between dizziness and true vertigo. During an attack of *true vertigo,* the individual is disoriented in space. The environment may seem to be whirling around the person, or there may be feelings of spinning in space. Often the individual is unable to maintain equilibrium. There may be staggering or falling, and the person should lie down immediately when an attack begins. In contrast, otolaryngologists consider *dizziness* to be a less severe feeling of unsteadiness or motion than true vertigo.

Characteristically, the onset of vertigo is sudden and unexpected. Attacks are intermittent over a period of days to years. Vertigo crisis frequently lasts several hours to a day, in contrast to dizziness which lasts only seconds to minutes and which is frequently associated with cerebral arteriosclerosis or postural hypotension. At the other extreme, dizziness that lasts several weeks should alert one to the possibility of intracranial disease. Between attacks of vertigo equilibrium is normal, although a few individuals may experience transient dizziness. Tinnitus and hearing loss continue between attacks.

Sensorineural hearing loss in Ménière's disease is generally unilateral, although slight impairment may be noticed in the opposite ear. Impaired hearing is the first symptom to develop in Ménière's disease although its progress is slow and gradual, and the individual may not become aware of it for quite some time.

Characteristically the degree of hearing impairment may fluctuate from day to day. Over a period of years, however, hearing loss becomes increasingly severe, although deafness is rare. Usually functional hearing remains in the less affected ear. Vertigo may not develop until months or years after the onset of hearing loss. Tinnitus is usually constant in the affected ear.

The diagnosis of Ménière's disease is made on the basis of symptoms, audiometric (hearing) testing, and labyrinthine function, as measured by caloric tests. Some degree of hearing loss is always present in Ménière's disease. If *audiometric testing* demonstrates intact hearing in the presence of tinnitus and vertigo, central nervous system disorders should be considered.

The *caloric test* is used to assess vestibular labyrinthine function. The individual may be seated or lying down for this procedure, which involves the rapid irrigation of the external auditory canal with either warm or cold water. This irrigation starts a current flow through the endolymphatic fluid of the labyrinth which stimulates the vestibular end organ, causing the individual to become dizzy. Some individuals experience true vertigo, nausea, and occasionally vomiting. More recently *bithermal caloric testing* has been used to evaluate labyrinthine function (see Fig. 38-14). The ear is irrigated alternately with water 7°C above and 7°C below normal body temperature (30 and 44°C). The individual's reaction is similar to that produced by the caloric test, but the bithermal technique provides more specific information about labyrinth functioning.

*Nystagmus,* a rhythmic oscillation of the eyes, is produced by both tests and is measured by *electronystagmography* (ENG). In this test, electrodes placed around the eyes monitor the electrical changes which occur as the eyes move. These changes are permanently recorded in a manner similar to that used in an electroencephalogram (see Fig. 38-14). In a normal reaction, rapid eye movement is toward the ear not being douched, and the individual experiences the sensation of falling toward the irrigated ear. When labyrinth functioning is impaired or absent, this normal reaction is impaired or absent. Helpful information may be obtained by comparing one ear with the other. This test is neither precise nor diagnostic, as people with normal vestibular function experience a variety of reactions. When used in conjunction with other data, however, caloric testing may help to confirm the diagnosis of Ménière's syndrome.

Unfortunately, no uniformly successful medical treatment has been found for Ménière's disease. Treatment is aimed at preventing attacks, which are acutely distressing to the individual as well as being disruptive to usual life routines. A *salt-free diet* is frequently recommended, and *diuretics* may be added to control edema of the labyrinth. *Vasodilators* help reduce vasoconstriction and vasospasm. Smoking is usually prohibited. Various medical regimes are tried and changed until the individual patient experiences relief. During an acute attack atropine, a vasodilator, 1/100 gr, may be administered intravenously or intramuscularly to inhibit the autonomic nervous system.

In severe cases in which symptoms are unmanageable and hearing loss is severe, surgical intervention may be recommended. The most common procedure is *labyrinthectomy,* or destruction of the membranous labyrinth, thus removing the organs of the inner ear believed to account for the symptoms of Ménière's syndrome. Vertigo is relieved but permanent deafness results. This surgery is not performed if hearing is still functional, or if Ménière's disease is bilateral. The application of ultrasound and cryogenic therapy directly to the horizontal semicircular canal has recently been tried with individuals having serviceable hearing. These interventions relieve vertigo without causing deafness. However, medical and surgical treatment of Ménière's disease remains varied and highly individualized.

Postoperatively, the patient may experience vertigo, nausea, and vomiting for several days. Intake and output are recorded. Antibiotics are used to prevent inner ear infection. Antiemetic drugs may need to be given intramuscularly if vomiting is a symptom. The patient should be assisted in walking while equilibrium is impaired. Transient dizziness may persist for several weeks following surgery, and the patient should be instructed to move and change position slowly and carefully.

Nursing care focuses on *safety, symptom management,* and *supportive care.* During an attack, the individual is safer and more comfortable lying down. All necessary safety precautions should be taken to prevent falls and injury during an episode of vertigo. The individual is often extremely uncomfortable and may become withdrawn, irritable, and anorexic. Antiemetic drugs may offer some relief of nausea and vomiting. Fluid intake should be monitored, especially when vomiting is a problem. It is important to educate the patient, the family, and the employer about Ménière's disease. Attacks occur suddenly and without warning. The individual experiences considerable subjective distress, but outwardly usually appears physically healthy to others who do not understand Ménière's disease.

### Absence of Auditory Perception

Hearing loss is divided into two basic types, conductive and sensorineural. Conditions affecting the

**FIGURE 38-14**
Bithermal caloric test and electronystagmography (ENG). Electrodes are placed around the closed eyes to measure eye movements as the ear is douched alternately with warm and cold water. (*Courtesy of Kenneth H. Brookler, M.D.*)

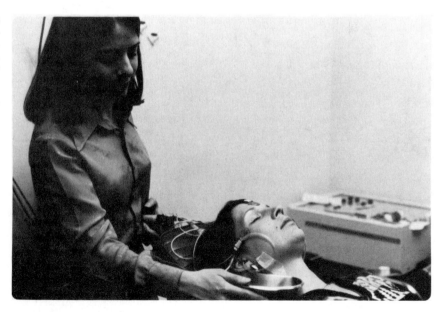

external or middle ear, such as trauma, infection, or otosclerosis, may result in *conductive hearing loss,* as described earlier in this chapter. Individuals with this type of hearing loss rarely become deaf, however, since hearing by means of bone conduction is unimpaired. Even in cases in which medical or surgical intervention is unsuccessful, hearing can usually be improved by using a hearing aid because these individuals have a normal inner ear.

When the sensitive nerve tissue of the inner ear (the organ of hearing and balance) or its neural pathways are damaged, *sensorineural,* or nerve type, hearing loss occurs. The end organ of hearing, the *organ of Corti,* is lined with fine hair cells which can be damaged by mechanical trauma, anoxia, or toxic medications. If these hair cells are destroyed, hearing cannot occur. Once injured, nerve tissue cannot regenerate, and the resulting hearing loss or deafness is permanent.

In practical terms, *deafness,* or the absence of auditory perception, is defined as a bilateral hearing loss of 85 to 90 dB or more in the speech frequencies (500 to 2000 Hz). This section deals with the causes of sensorineural deafness and the needs of the deaf individual in the hospital and community. With proper rehabilitation and the understanding of others, the deaf individual is completely capable of living a full, useful, and happy life.

**Congenital deafness**  Trauma, toxicity, or infection during pregnancy or delivery may cause congenital deafness. Rubella, or German measles, contacted by the expectant mother during the first trimester of pregnancy, can damage the cochlea of the fetus. The child may be born with a profound hearing loss or deafness. The use of quinine, streptomycin, or other drugs toxic to the ear during pregnancy may result in the birth of a deaf child. Prolonged fetal anoxia during delivery can destroy the fine hair cells of the organ of Corti, causing deafness.

**Trauma and infection**  Any *traumatic injury* to the inner ear or VIIIth cranial nerve may result in permanent hearing loss. The most frequent causes of injury are skull fracture, cerebral thrombosis or hemorrhage, and explosive blasts. The inner ear is also susceptible to damage from certain *infections.* Meningitis frequently causes damage to the VIIIth cranial nerve. Scarlet fever can injure the cochlea, and mumps, the most frequent cause of unilateral deafness in children, often attacks the inner ear. Labyrinthitis, a complication of otitis media and

mastoiditis, can destroy the inner ear causing deafness.

**Drug toxicity**  Many frequently used drugs are *ototoxic;* that is, they are toxic to the hearing mechanism of the inner ear. Drugs which damage the cochlea include streptomycin, kanamycin, neomycin, gentamicin, dihydrostreptomycin, and nitrogen mustard. These drugs may cause damage even in small amounts, and deafness may not result until after the drug has been discontinued. Occasionally tinnitus or dizziness appears as an early warning sign, but this is not true in all cases. These drugs should not be given by injection if another equally effective drug can be used. The salicylate drugs, including quinine, quinidine, and aspirin, are also ototoxic in large doses, although they do not usually produce the profound hearing loss associated with the antibiotic drugs mentioned. Tinnitus is usually an early indication of salicylate ototoxicity.

**Noise**  Exposure to loud *noise,* above 85 to 90 dB, for periods of months to years may cause degeneration of the organ of Corti and result in significant hearing loss and deafness. Exposure to industrial noise is the most frequent cause of occupational hearing loss. Initially only certain frequencies (around 4000 Hz) are affected, but as damage continues, hearing at all frequencies is impaired. The higher frequencies are most affected.

The frequent use of firearms by military personnel and sportsmen may also damage the delicate inner ear and cause sensorineural hearing loss. Frequently tinnitus, transient hearing loss, and a feeling of fullness in the ears are early symptoms and indicate that protective measures should be instituted to prevent further damage. Recently much attention has been given to the effects of loud music, especially rock music, on hearing. An intensity of 110 dB at a distance of 30 ft from a music loudspeaker is not uncommon and may produce a significant temporary hearing loss. Many professionals fear that permanent sensorineural hearing loss may result in individuals exposed repeatedly to such high-intensity music.

**Presbycusis**  Hearing loss which occurs as a result of the aging process is called *presbycusis.* It is thought to be caused by degenerative changes and atrophy of the cochlear ganglion cells. Characteristically there is a gradual loss of hearing bilaterally. The high tones are affected first, followed by the middle and lower tones as the degeneration progresses. Eventually deafness results.

**Acoustic neuroma** *Acoustic neuroma,* a tumor of the VIIIth cranial nerve, is a relatively rare cause of hearing loss. Tinnitus is often the first symptom of acoustic neuroma, and a loss of hearing may not be noted for months or years. The tumor must be surgically removed, and the degree of hearing impairment depends upon the extent of VIIIth nerve damage. Squamous-cell carcinomas affecting the ear are rare, but the tumor (in advanced stage), or the treatment (radical surgery and irradiation), may result in profound hearing loss or deafness.

**Effects on the patient** To understand the effects of deafness on the individual, it is necessary to understand the importance of sound in daily life. Sound envelops us and orients us to the environment. Even when we are involved in conversation or activity, background sounds, such as the sound of traffic, of falling rain, or of someone approaching from the rear, serve to alert and connect us to our surroundings. The deaf individual is isolated from conversational interaction with friends and family, as well as from the environmental sounds which are so important to sensory orientation. Sound also provides human beings with enjoyment in the form of music, the sounds of nature, and speech. Words provide us not only with a means to pleasant conversation, but also with a means of conveying thought, information, experience, and feeling tone.

The deaf individual is isolated from the normal interactions and environmental cues involving sound. The individual's feelings of self-confidence, self-worth, and general well-being are jeopardized. Depending upon individual personality characteristics, the deaf person may respond with depression, withdrawal, hostility, and suspicion. In addition, the deaf individual is not highly visible in today's society. The blind person is quickly recognized by a cane or dog, but the deaf individual appears normal to those unaware of this handicap. When spoken to, the deaf person may fail to respond or may respond inappropriately. Frequently the deaf are considered slow or retarded, odd or unfriendly. This cycle of withdrawal, rejection, and isolation may be difficult to break.

The individual with *correctable deafness* often faces as many problems in adjusting to this disability as the person with *noncorrectable deafness.* Much depends upon the individual's own personality structure, although the type and degree of hearing loss and the age at which it occurred are important factors influencing the person's reaction. The important factor to stress is that help is available for individuals with correctable and noncorrectable deafness.

**First-level nursing care** The National Center for Health Statistics estimates that in the United States more than 13 million people have some degree of auditory impairment, with 335,000 persons being classified as deaf.[2] Individuals of all ages and races and both sexes may be born or become deaf. Certain predisposing factors do place some individuals at higher risk, however. Any pregnant woman who contracts rubella, a viral infection, or uses ototoxic drugs during early pregnancy may deliver a deaf child. Premature, anoxic, or jaundiced infants are at higher risk of becoming deaf than full-term, healthy infants. The incidence of deafness increases in children who contract mumps or scarlet fever. Individuals of any age using ototoxic medications may suffer cochlear or nerve damage. Also at high risk are individuals exposed to high-intensity noise over an extended period of time. Persons in this category include factory and industrial workers, individuals using firearms, and those having prolonged exposure to loud music or jet engine noise.

As the elderly population in the United States and in other countries increases, the incidence of presbycusis, a disease of aging, increases. Many individuals over 65 years of age already have some degree of conductive hearing loss, and their hearing problems are intensified by the degenerative changes associated with presbycusis. Progressive hearing loss should always be considered and evaluated when dealing with the elderly, many of whom are already isolated and rejected in our society.

**Prevention** *Public education* focuses on preventing the factors which increase the risk of deafness. The importance of prenatal care cannot be overemphasized, and pregnant women should be encouraged to seek immediate medical attention if they are exposed to or contract measles, mumps, or viral infection. Immunization programs should be encouraged so that all children, especially young girls, are vaccinated for rubella. The childhood diseases can be dangerous, and children contracting these illnesses should receive prompt medical attention.

Health professionals need to be aware of the medications which can be ototoxic, including the new preparations which are constantly being developed. Individuals taking such drugs should be questioned about symptoms of tinnitus, hearing loss, and dizziness. Frequently people attribute these symptoms to the disease for which the drug is being taken and, therefore, do not notify health personnel about these signs. An effort should be made to avoid using these drugs if another medication can be safely substituted.

Recently the public has become increasingly concerned with environmental issues. The health hazards of noise require further discussion and investigation. People whose jobs involve exposure to high-intensity noise should be aware of the potential risks. Special rubber or plastic earplugs and protective ear muffs are worn by many people in high-noise industries. Their use should be strongly encouraged. Audiometric testing is advised periodically to detect early hearing loss. In such cases the individual should be transferred to an area of less noise. Individuals experiencing tinnitus or temporary hearing loss following an exposure to loud noise (music, gunfire, machinery) may be particularly susceptible to hearing injury. They should be advised to avoid exposure to high-intensity noise or to use protective devices in the future.

**Second-level nursing care** The individual with a profound hearing loss or deafness usually seeks medical attention. This person can no longer hear the telephone or doorbell, the car horn, or ambulance siren. These individuals are cut off from all the cues necessary to their daily social functioning and safety. Usually it is this *subjective symptom*—hearing loss—which brings the individual to the health professional. The parents of a congenitally deaf child frequently notice that the infant does not respond to sound or has not begun to talk, and they seek professional help. This is not always the case, however, and nursing assessment may be an essential factor in the detection of these individuals.

**N**ursing Assessment   Often when hearing loss has been gradually progressive, the individual may be unwilling to recognize or admit to the loss, or may actually be unaware of the magnitude of the problem. Many times the elderly believe their hearing loss is due to mental deterioration and are afraid to seek medical help. In many cases family, friends, employers, and health professionals are the first people to recognize the *observable* signs of deafness and encourage the individual to seek help. Frequently the individual speaks too loudly or responds inappropriately during conversation. The person may lean forward or turn one ear toward the speaker in an effort to hear and may ask for frequent clarification or repetition of words or phrases. Some individuals develop headache, neck and back pain, or other somatic complaints as they constantly strain to hear. Unusual, prolonged, or inappropriate withdrawal, irritability, or anger may also be indications of deafness. As the individual strains to understand,

tension, anxiety, and frustration build, and the person may react with hostility, suspicion, and withdrawal. Poor performance at work or school, or the failure of an infant to babble and learn speech, may be the first noticeable effect of deafness.

The individual with observable signs or subjective symptoms of hearing loss should be encouraged to seek prompt medical evaluation. *Audiometric tests* (see Conductive Disturbances above) provide a detailed survey of the individual's hearing capacity and help to determine appropriate interventions.

**N**ursing Problems and Interventions   The major problem for the deaf individual is *impaired communication.* The needs of the deaf person depend upon the type of hearing loss, the age at onset, and the effect these have on speech and language development. Generally the deaf are separated into two categories, each having different problems and needs.

The *congenitally deaf* person, usually identified in early childhood, is at a distinct disadvantage because the development of speech is dependent upon the ability to hear. The psychological and mental development of these children is severely hampered. Visual and sensory perception are impaired, as are emotional and social maturation. The abilities to speak, read, and write are massively impaired, and the congenitally deaf child rarely develops linguistically beyond the age of 11 years. It is imperative that these children be identified and referred for special education as early as possible. Since speech is best learned between ages 2 and 5, the child should be involved in special education as early as the first birthday. Referrals are made to agencies and schools for the deaf in the area in which the family lives.

Persons who were born with normal hearing which later became nonfunctional because of illness or injury are termed *adventitiously deaf.* These individuals should be referred for rehabilitation to conserve and maximize their ability to communicate.

*Aural rehabilitation*   The term *aural rehabilitation* is used to describe a multifaceted approach to the habilitation and rehabilitation of the deaf. The goal is to restore and maintain effective oral communication. Aural rehabilitation is not reserved solely for the deaf, however, as the hard of hearing individual may also benefit from such a program. For the hard of hearing or adventitiously deaf person, the emphasis is on *rehabilitation* and focuses on the restoration, augmentation, and maintenance of oral skills the individual already possesses. For the congenitally deaf child, the focus is on *habilitation,* for the child has no speech or language skills from which to build. A program of aural rehabilitation usually incorporates the use of hearing aids, speech reading and training, and auditory training.

*Hearing aids* are electronic devices which amplify sound. These instruments are composed of a microphone, which receives and converts sound into electrical impulses; an amplifier, which increases the strength of electrical impulses; and a receiver, which converts the impulses back into sound of greater intensity. Since hearing aids amplify sound, they are most helpful to individuals with conductive hearing loss and a normal inner ear. When the inner ear is damaged and speech discrimination is distorted, hearing aids are less beneficial. All sounds, not just speech, are magnified by hearing aids, and the user may find amplified background noise both annoying and distracting.

A variety of hearing aid devices are available, including units which fit into or behind the ear, eyeglass models, and somewhat larger torso or pocket models (see Fig. 38-15). Proper audiometric testing by a competent professional is necessary to determine whether the individual can benefit from the use of a hearing aid, and if so, which type should be used for best results. Hearing aids represent a major financial investment because they range in price from $85 to $350 per unit. In some cases bilateral hearing aids may be recommended, doubling the expense. The individual purchasing a hearing aid should be encouraged to shop carefully and to select a reliable manufacturer and reputable dealer who will guarantee and service the merchandise.

*Speech reading,* commonly called lipreading, is a broad term which describes the use of visual cues in oral communication. Lip movements and facial expressions, body movements and gestures, and the immediate physical environment all provide visible clues which the deaf person can use to supplement hearing. The deaf individual is taught the importance and usefulness of observing these cues and becomes skillful in using visual cues to communicate.

*Speech training* is an important aspect of aural rehabilitation because individuals with inner ear damage can no longer hear their own speech. Often deaf persons speak in a loud or monotonous voice because they can no longer monitor their own voices. Speech training helps conserve normal speech or correct problems involving the loudness, clarity, rate, and inflection of speech.

For the hard of hearing, *auditory training* develops good listening skills to help maximize residual hearing. This is particularly valuable when the discrimination of speech sounds is impaired. The individual is made aware of common errors in sound discrimination and learns to compensate by using alternate speech clues and critical listening techniques.

**Third-level nursing care**   Deaf persons who require hospitalization, no matter what the reason, face special problems. From the moment of admis-

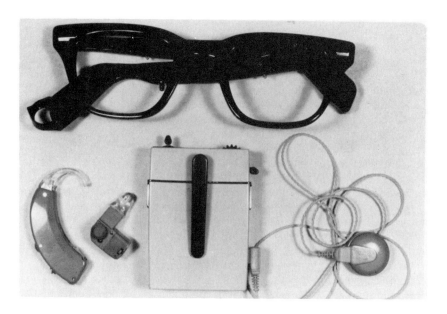

**FIGURE 38-15**
Frequently used hearing aid devices, including eyeglass, postauricular, in-the-ear, and torso models. (*Courtesy of Kenneth H. Brookler, M.D.*)

sion they may be subjected to an endless series of questions, examinations, and procedures, and some hospital personnel may act as if these patients are mute as well as deaf. They may fail to explain procedures and rules to deaf patients because of a lack of understanding, sensitivity, or patience. Deaf persons are usually very apprehensive during hospitalization because their communication disorder isolates them from normal interactions. In addition, the deaf patient who is acutely ill or in pain, or who receives sedation or anesthetics, may be virtually unable to communicate in any way and is truly isolated and alone.

**N**ursing Assessment  When the deaf person enters the hospital, the nurse should assess the extent of the communication disorder and the capabilities of the individual. The nurse should ascertain the degree of hearing and speech impairment as well as the patient's ability to understand. Eliciting information about the patient's capabilities includes discovering whether the person uses a hearing aid and has it in the hospital; whether the patient uses lipreading, speech reading, or sign language; and whether a family member or friend is available to act as translator. Additional factors which may influence the deaf person's ability to communicate include: degree of illness, level of anxiety, and the medications and procedures (such as surgery) which are part of the patient's treatment. This information is essential and should be recorded on the patient's chart and nursing care plan.

**N**ursing Problems and Interventions  The major nursing problems involve *communication difficulties* and *anxiety* which are especially demonstrated by the deaf patient isolated in strange surroundings. Establishing communication is a major step in providing a caring, supportive environment for the deaf patient. Nursing interventions focus on establishing practical methods of communication with the deaf person.

The patient with a hearing aid should be encouraged to use it while in the hospital. It is often a good idea to have the family bring in extra batteries, and the nurse should be sure that the appliance is clean and functioning. At night the patient's hearing aid and eyeglasses, if used, should be kept within easy reach. A small light should be left on in the patient's room at night since the deaf patient relies on sight to communicate.

The deaf patient should be clearly identified so that hospital personnel are immediately aware of the person's handicap. Labels indicating the pa-

tient's deafness should be placed on the outside and inside of the chart to alert staff when the patient is off the unit for tests. Labels should also be placed on the intercommunication switch at the nursing station as well as the patient's door and bed.

It is preferable to have the same nursing staff on each shift care for the deaf patient. This is reassuring to the patient and helps the nurse develop familiarity with the patient's communication methods. Often it is helpful for the nurse to learn a few basic sign language symbols (as for *pain* and *bathroom*) if the patient uses this method of communication. In some cases it may be necessary to have an interpreter assist the patient and staff. The interpreter may be a professional or a competent family member. Hospital policies about visiting and rooming-in may need to be waived when an interpreter is required. This is especially important for the deaf patient in the intensive-care unit or recovery room. An interpreter should be available following surgery, when the use of anesthetics, sedatives, and narcotic analgesics may inhibit the patient's ability to communicate.

In dealings with the deaf patient it is important to remember some simple rules (Table 38-4). The deaf person relies on sight to communicate, and so it is essential to always face the patient when speaking. The use of simple words and short phrases aids lipreading, and supplemental pictures and diagrams are helpful in explaining tests and procedures. A pencil and pad of paper should be kept within reach of the patient. Important, complex, or detailed questions or explanations should always

**TABLE 38-4**
HELPFUL RULES TO REMEMBER WHEN COMMUNICATING
WITH DEAF INDIVIDUALS

Alert the patient to your presence.

Do not approach the patient from behind.

Always face the patient.

Provide good light free from shadows and glare.

Do not stand with your back to the window—glare blocks the patient's vision.

Speak simply, clearly, and naturally.

Do not shout, grimace, or distort mouth movements.

Do not cover the mouth, smoke, or chew gum.

Do not turn or walk away while talking to the patient.

Keep paper and pencil handy.

Write out important words.

Make writing large and dark.

Repeat and rephrase speech to ensure understanding.

Keep conversation short to minimize strain.

be written out for the patient to read to ensure complete understanding. The deaf person has already lost the use of one sensory modality. Darkening the room at night or restricting movement with intravenous tubes and assorted catheters further deprives the patient of sensory stimulation. The nurse should make a special effort to touch deaf patients, not only as a means of reassurance, but also to provide sensory input.

These considerations apply to any deaf individual hospitalized for any reason. The condition which brings the individual into the hospital, whether it is *related* or *unrelated* to the deafness, is also a nursing problem. Nursing interventions are based on the particular condition and the patient's needs. In reality the patient's medical or surgical condition cannot be considered apart from the patient's deafness. They are interrelated and cannot be separated when considering holistic man.

**Fourth-level nursing care** Deaf persons should receive periodic medical and audiology follow-up to maintain a healthy ear and conserve residual hearing. Hearing aid devices should be checked at intervals to ensure maximum effectiveness, and the deaf may benefit from occasional aural rehabilitation "refresher" courses. Many organizations for the deaf sponsor clubs and groups for deaf persons to keep them informed of medical progress, new equipment, and legislation affecting the deaf. In addition these groups provide an opportunity for socialization and recreation.

Deaf persons may need to make many changes in their daily functioning affecting *home, work,* and *school.* The safety of the individual is always of prime concern. In some cases, deaf persons may be unable to continue working at their present jobs, if hearing is essential to their safety or performance. Often counseling may help individuals and employers realize that only minor work adjustments need to be made in order for deaf persons to continue optimal performance at their present jobs. In some cases, however, vocational training or additional education may be required if the individual must learn a new skill or occupation. Indeed, deaf persons need not be cut off from pursuing educational goals. Many special schools provide educational opportunities for the deaf at all levels, from preschool through university study. In addition, many public and private schools and universities provide special programs and support for deaf students.

Many electronic devices are commercially avail-

able to assist deaf persons in the home. Wake-up devices which are connected to alarm clocks or timers wake the deaf individual by vibration or flashing light without disturbing family members. These devices range in price from $12 to $150. Special signaling appliances are available which can be attached to the telephone, doorbell, and baby's crib. When the bell rings or the baby cries, the sound activates a light or vibrator to alert the deaf individual. These devices can cost $100 or more, depending on the number of units desired. Telephone amplifiers, available from the telephone company, are helpful for the hearing-impaired individual who can hear amplified sound, but are not effective for deaf persons. Radio and television amplifiers are also available.

Frequently deaf persons and family members may benefit from short-term professional counseling as they learn to accept deafness and adjust their lives. Frequently local associations for the deaf offer such counseling services. National organizations offering information and assistance to the deaf include:

The American Hearing Society
Washington, D.C.

The Alexander Graham Bell Association for the Deaf, Inc.
Washington, D.C.

The John Tracy Clinic
Los Angeles, California

The National Association for the Deaf
Washington, D.C.

## REFERENCES

1   David D. DeWeese and William H. Saunders, *Textbook of Otolaryngology,* Mosby, St. Louis, 1973.
2   *Hearing Rehabilitation Quarterly,* New York, New York League for the Hard of Hearing, Summer 1976.

## BIBLIOGRAPHY

### Disturbances in Visual Perception

Ammon, L.: "Surviving Enucleation," *Am J Nurs,* 1817–1821, October 1972.
Branson, H. K.: "The Blind Mother," *Am J Nurs,* 414–416, March 1975.
Brown, M. S., and M. Alexander: "Physical Examina-

tion: Pt 5, The Eye," *Nursing 73,* 41–46, December 1973.

Carroll, T.: *Blindness,* Little, Brown, Boston, 1961.

Dupont, J.: "What To Do for Common Eye Emergencies," *Nursing 76,* 17–19, May 1976.

Fernsebner, W.: "Early Diagnosis of Acute Angle Closure Glaucoma," *Am J Nurs,* 1154–1155, July 1975.

Freeman, H.: "Recent Advances in Retinal Detachment and Vitreous Surgery," *AORN J,* 896–906, November 1973.

Fulton, M., et al.: "Helping Diabetics Adapt To Failing Vision," *Am J Nurs,* 54–57, January 1974.

Havener, W., et al.: *Nursing Care in Eye, Ear, Nose and Throat Disorders,* 3d ed., Mosby, St. Louis, 1974.

Hiles, D.: "Strabismus," *Am J Nurs,* 1082–1089, June 1974.

Kelman, C.: "Phaco-Emulsification and Aspiration," *Am J Ophthalmol,* 764–768, May 1973.

Nackazel, D., and J. Smith: "Retinal Detachment," *Am J Nurs,* 1530–1535, September 1973.

Neu, C.: "Coping with Newly Diagnosed Blindness," *Am J Nurs,* 2161–2163, December 1976.

Ohno, M.: "The Eye-Patched Patient," *Am J Nurs,* 271–274, February 1971.

Patient Assessment: Examination of the Eye, Pt. I, Programmed Instruction, *Am J Nurs,* P.I. 24, November 1974.

Patient Assessment: Examination of the Eye, Pt. II, Programmed Instruction, *Am J Nurs,* P.I. 1–24, January 1975.

Paton, D., and M. Goldberg: *Injuries to the Eye, the Lids, and the Orbit,* Saunders, Philadelphia, 1968.

Pilgrim, M., and B. Sigler: "Phaco-Emulsification of Cataracts," *Am J Nurs,* 976–977, June 1975.

Scheie, H., and D. Albert: *Adler's Textbook of Ophthalmology,* 8th ed., Saunders, Philadelphia, 1969.

Schein, H., and B. Scott: *The Ophthalmic Assistant,* 2d ed., Mosby, St. Louis, 1971.

Schulz, J., and M. Williams: "Encouragement Breeds Independence in the Blind Diabetic," *Nursing 76,* 19–20, December 1976.

Schuman, D.: "Assessing the Diabetic," *Nursing 76,* 62–67, March 1976.

Vaughan, D., and T. Asbury: *General Ophthalmology,* 7th ed., Lange, Los Altos, Calif., 1974.

Weinstock, F.: "Tonometry Screening," *Am J Nurs,* 656–657, April 1973.

Wesseling, E. (ed.): "Patients with Sensory Defects," *Nurs Clin North Am,* 453–538, September 1970.

Zucnick, M.: "Care of an Artificial Eye," *Am J Nurs,* 414–416, March 1975.

## BIBLIOGRAPHY

### Disturbances in Auditory Perception

"A Symposium on the Surgery of Deafness," *Nurs Mirror,* **140:**45–55, Feb. 6, 1975.

Chodil, Judith, and Barbara Williams: "The Concept of Sensory Deprivation," *Nurs Clin North Am,* **5:**507–515, September 1970.

Coleman, B. H.: "Chronic Mucous Otitis," *Nurs Times,* **69:**336–338, March 15, 1973.

———: "Deafness," *Nurs Times,* **70:**1661–1663, Oct. 24, 1974.

Conover, Mary, and Joyce Cober: "Understanding and Caring for the Hearing Impaired," *Nurs Clin North Am,* **5:**497–506, September 1970.

Cooke, E. T. M.: "Chronic Supperative Otitis Media," *Nurs Times,* **70:**1846–1847, November 28, 1974.

Cullin, Irene C.: "Techniques for Teaching Patients with Sensory Defects," *Nurs Clin North Am,* **5:**527–528, September 1970.

Delaney, Ramona E.: "Stapedectomy," *Am J Nurs,* **69:**2406–2409, November 1969.

Denhem, Doreen: "Endolymphatic Shunt for the Treatment of Ménière's Disease," *Nurs Times,* **68:**1287–1288, Oct. 12, 1972.

Gibb, Alan G.: "Syringing the Ear," *Nurs Times,* **66:**1264–1266, Oct. 1, 1970.

Goldsmith, John R., and Erland Jonssen: "Health Effects of Community Noise," *Am J Public Health,* **63:**782–793, September 1973.

Golub, Sharon: "Noise, the Underrated Health Hazard," *RN,* **32:**40–45, May 1969.

"How to Buy a Hearing Aid: What Consumers Should Know," Pt. 1, *Consumer Rep,* **41:**346–352, June 1976.

"How to Buy a Hearing Aid: What Professionals Should Know," Pt. 2, *Consumer Rep,* **41:**352–355, June 1976.

Johnston, Dorothy F., and Gail H. Hood: *Total Patient Care: Foundations and Practice,* Mosby, St. Louis, 1976.

Kravitz, H.: "The Cotton-Tipped Swab: A Major Cause of Ear Injury and Hearing Loss," *J NY State School Teachers Assoc,* **6:**33–38, June 1975.

Larsen, George: "Removing Cerumen with a Water Pik," *Am J Nurs,* **76:**264–265, February 1976.

Linnell, Craig, Sister Victorine Long, and Janet Proehl: "The Hearing Impaired Infant: Diagnosis and Treatment," *J Clin North Am,* **5:**507–515, September 1970.

Mechner, E.: "Examination of the Ear," *Am J Nurs,* **75:**P.I. 1–24, March 1975.

Meyers, David, et al.: "Otologic Diagnosis and the

Treatment of Deafness," *Clin Symp,* **22**(2):35–69, 1970.

Moore, Mary V.: "Diagnosis: Deafness," *Am J Nurs,* **69**:279–300, February 1969.

Mulrooney, Jean: "Deaf Patient Care: A Special Concern to Me," *RN,* **39**:69–70, June 1976.

Nilo, Ernest R.: "Needs of the Hearing Impaired," *Am J Nurs,* **69**:115–116, January 1969.

Sabatino, Lois: "Do's and Don'ts of Deaf-Patient Care," *RN,* **39**:64–68, June 1976.

Shafer, Kathleen N., et al.: *Medical-Surgical Nursing,* Mosby, St. Louis, 1975.

"What If Your Patient Is Also Deaf?" *RN,* **39**:59–63, June 1976.

Wright, Joan: "Deaf but not Mute," *Am J Nurs,* **76**: 795–799, May 1976.

Yates, J. T.: "Rehabilitation of Hearing Impaired Adults," *J Rehabil,* **39**:20–22, January–February 1973.

# 39
## PAIN PERCEPTION

Lynne A. Oland

Pain is one of the most explicit examples we have of the complex interrelationships of mind and body. Its perception and expression reflect physical and psychosocial characteristics of the individual affected by the peculiar configuration of the environment at that time. The nature of the stimulus, its transmission through the nervous system, and the various physiologic responses to that stimulus may be diminished, modified, or enhanced by the individual's interpretation of the stimulus. Interpretation of painful stimuli is dependent upon interaction of a number of variables including the level of preexisting and concurrent stress within the individual. No one factor alone is responsible for the existence of pain, as it is well known that neither tissue injury nor an intact nervous system is a prerequisite for pain.[1]

## PAIN

*Pain* may best be described as a perceptual experience derived from a multineuronal, multilevel interaction generated by a perceived stimulus that arises from either the internal or the external environment. It is evidence of a stimulus which threatens to disrupt the integrity of the human system. Pain is experienced by the individual as an unpleasant sensation or sense of hurt referred to the body.[2] Pain can become a stressor evoking a series of psychophysiologic reactions which can further damage the total system. Schweitzer recognized the potential power of pain when he described it as "being a more terrible lord of mankind than even death himself."[3]

Pain is a totally personal experience that can never be fully shared or communicated with others except in the abstract. We can fully know only our own pain, yet as nurses we must become sensitized to the experience, to its meanings, and to the variety of human responses to it. Pain is the primary reason for seeking entry into the health care system whether or not physical illness is present.[4] By exploring the phenomenon of pain and personal responses to it, nurses can skillfully implement the nursing process to aid people in pain. The term *pain experience* will be used throughout the chapter. It includes an individual's integration of noxious stimuli or potentially noxious stimuli with the physical, psychosocial, and environmental variables that affect pain perception. The function of pain and specific responses to painful stimuli are also components of the pain experience and will differ from person to person.

### Functions of Pain

The primitive and evolutionary function of pain is to signal imminent or actual damage to the body. Superficial structures of the body are richly supplied with receptors enabling precise and rapid perception of damage at the outermost physical boundaries. In contrast, less innervated viscera are relatively insensitive to pain. This arrangement reflects the reduced probability of damage to the internal body compartments prior to damage of external structures. As a *warning mechanism,* however, pain is not fully efficient. This can be illustrated when assessing cancer pain. Because of diminished innervation of the viscera, pain may not be experienced despite the presence of a corrosive and metastasizing process. It may be only during more advanced stages of tissue destruction that pain may become a problem.

Pain has a role in the *developmental process.* Numerous instances of minor painful experiences contribute to the child's development of a body image, especially with respect to recognition of boundaries. Children quickly learn how to avoid objects or situations which will produce pain. They recognize the effect pain can have on relationships with others. Early in life the infant begins to identify crying as a way to summon mother, who will offer comfort with much affection. As children grow, they become aware that inflicting or threatening pain can be a way to punish or control others. These and other experiences with pain influence future patterns of pain perception and related behavior.

Pain can also assume meaning as *punishment* or as a way of purging *guilt.* For others, bearing intense pain becomes a ritualistic proof of *strength* and *adulthood.* Pain may be evoked to prove a person's essential reality to himself. It may provide an acceptable structure for a life that would otherwise be intolerable since those sick and in pain are excused from most social responsibility. Occasionally, pain is reported where no pain exists, in a conscious attempt to obtain some desired *gain.* Finally, some use pain as a means of *gratifying* a need such as the need for love and attention which would be inaccessible to them as well persons.

Appreciation of the complex nature of pain grows with the realization that most responses to the presence of pain are learned behavior. Therefore any useful theory of pain must explain these affective and cognitive influences on pain perception.

### Theories of Pain Perception

Originally, it was thought that pain was a primary sense modality. Pain was present when specific pain receptors were stimulated to a predetermined critical or threshold level. Impulses transmitted along pain pathways traveled from the bare nerve endings via the spinothalamic tract to the thalamus where pain was perceived as hurting. From the thalamus, the impulse pattern was projected to the cortex where it was interpreted along spatiotemporal and qualitative dimensions.

The inherent assumption of this construction of pain is that interpretation of a stimulus as painful is a function of the receptors. The *specificity theory* of pain, which supported this concept, was greatly weakened when these receptors were found to respond to cold and pressure stimuli as well as "pain" stimuli. Further, the theory inadequately explained the phenomenon of central pain or why pain pathways could be transsected without diminishing pain.

The most recent, though still controversial, explanation of pain has been developed by Melzack and Wall.[5] The proposed *gate control theory* directly addresses the mind-body interrelationships of pain.

This theory suggests that pain entering from the periphery can be moderated before evoking pain perception. The four main components of the theory include the spinal gate, the central control system, the central biasing system, and the action system. As these components interact, an individual's perception of pain may be augmented or reduced. (Refer to Fig. 39-1 throughout the following discussion.)

The *spinal gating mechanism* (Fig. 39-1a) is made up of large and small fibers, substantia gelatinosa (SG) cells, and transmission, or T, cells. Painful impulses from the periphery travel to the central nervous system through T cells in the spinal cord. Peripheral afferents that enter the dorsal horn of the spinal cord consist of large- and small-diameter fibers. Both pass SG cells in the dorsal horn. These cells act to facilitate or inhibit the passage of the afferent impulse to the T cells. The SG is a functional unit of small cells that extend the length of the spinal cord. As *large fiber impulses* pass the SG, they facilitate SG activity, and entry of impulses into the T cells is inhibited (closed gate). Transmission from the T cells is then diminished or suppressed. Conversely, *small-fiber impulses* inhibit SG activity and, therefore, increase T cell transmission (open gate). The balance of activity between large and small fibers is the primary determinant of T cell transmission with further modification depending on information from the central biasing and central control systems.

The *central control system* (see Fig. 39-1b) is activated by afferents from the dorsal horn which transmit information about the *noxious stimulus* to the thalamus. From the thalamus, information is relayed to the cortical and limbic structures which reside in the central control system (see Fig. 39-1*b*). The system may be hypothetically subdivided into three interrelated components on the basis of function. The *motivational-affective* component involves thalamic, cortical, and limbic structures and determines the discomforting or unpleasant aspect of pain. The *cognitive component* is primarily a cortical function. In its analysis of the significance of noxious stimuli, it integrates information from the peripheral and central structures. Cognitive functions also include formation and initiation of conscious and unconscious response strategies. The *sensory-discriminative component* is also cortically based and determines spatiotemporal and other characteristics of pain sensation.

The interaction of these three subunits of the central control system determines the presence, characteristics, and significance of pain as well as the response to the noxious stimulus or situation.

The T cells relay information to the central control system about the kind, intensity, and location of the stimulus and extent of damage. The motivational-affective subsystem may analyze the information and determine the damage to be painful. The sensory-discriminative subsystem establishes precisely what site is affected and to what degree. The cognitive subsystem uses this information and incoming data from the periphery to determine the nature of the pain, whether and how much pain should be tolerated, what expression of pain is appropriate, and what action, if any, should be taken to protect the person from further pain and/or reduce the pain that exists. Efferent fibers then relay impulses either (1) through the corticospinal tract to the spinal gate area (modifying gate activity) or (2) to the reticular formation, or (3) to the action system to initiate an appropriate response. Under this theory, transmission from the central control system or the biasing system to the spinal gate may be responsible for pain whose origin is primarily psychic.

**FIGURE 39-1**

Components and functional aspects of the gate control theory. (*Adapted from Melzack, R., and P. Wall: "Pain Mechanisms: A New Theory," Science,* **150**:*975, November 1965 and from Bennett, M.: "The Pathophysiology of Pain," Curr Probl Surg, February 1973, p. 11.*)

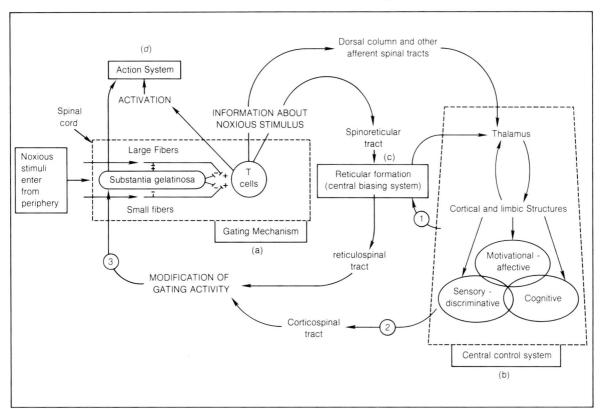

The *central biasing system* (Fig. 39-1c) is a function of the brainstem reticular formation which maintains an appropriate level of sensory input to the rest of the brain. It exerts an *inhibitory effect* on imput from the periphery in direct proportion to the amount of input it receives. As input rises, inhibition increases. However, its action may affect and be affected by information transmitted from the central control system while the efferents modify activity of the spinal gate.

The *action system* (Fig. 39-1d) is a complex sequence of *behavior responses* following the perception of pain including reflex activities, slower physiologic responses such as sympathetic activation, behavioral expression of pain, and initiation of a variety of coping or aversive strategies. At present, gate control theory remains controversial with some conflicting evidence still unexplained. In light of pain response, however, it does offer a comprehensive and integrated approach to describing the psychophysical and environmental responses to pain.

## Sources of Pain Stimuli and Pathophysiologic Changes

Stimuli which are interpreted as painful can be generated by a variety of sources that originate in either the internal or external environment of the human system. These sources may be of a physiologic or psychic nature and can be influenced by a multiplicity of variables that effect pain perception. A summary of these sources is found in Fig. 39-2.

**Physical sources** From the external environment, noxious stimuli applied directly to the body create a pain sensation which originates from a damaged or irritated nerve ending as well as the body's secondary response to the damage. For example, application of direct *heat* or *cold* to the skin causes tissue destruction. This destruction occurs in proportion to the intensity of the stimulus and the length of time the stimulus was in contact with an area. Immediate nerve damage can result along with an inflammatory response precipitated by the body's reaction to this noxious stimuli.

**FIGURE 39-2**
Interaction of variables affecting pain perception, tolerance, and expression.

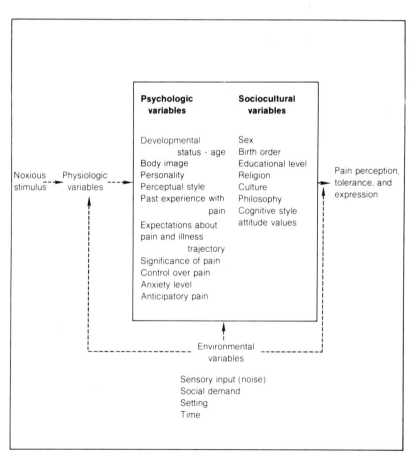

Physical *trauma* occurring through cutting, puncture, or force to the body can result in immediate damage to nerve endings and stimulate an *inflammatory response.* The presence of hemorrhage and fluids in an area can produce pressure on nerve endings, diminish blood supply, and increase the noxious stimuli within a traumatized area. In severe trauma, the sudden disappearance of intense pain may reflect severe nerve damage, indicating injury to pain receptors or pathways which are no longer capable of transmitting information to the brain.

From the internal environment, pain may be derived from *organic disorders,* from normal life processes such as childbirth, or from a central source. Pathologic processes may be associated with pain through direct nerve involvement at the peripheral or central level, pressure or chemical irritation of a nerve, distention of viscera which stretches nerves, or from inhibition of the central biasing system by a disorder of the reticular formation. Such a disorder would permit transmission of stimulus from the periphery without diminution of intensity or frequency.

Diminished blood flow to a specific area, due to muscle spasm, cellular proliferation, or obstruction, can result in *ischemia.* Pain associated with this process is difficult to analyze, but it is thought to result from a buildup in lactic acid caused by an increase in anaerobic metabolism. The presence of this acid in the absence of oxygen creates an irritating effect on nerve endings and causes pain.

*Distention* within vessels or ducts caused by the presence of calculi can cause stretching of the vessel and compression of nerve endings. Pain associated with this experience is often described as excruciating.

*Alteration* in *body fluids* can precipitate a pain experience. For example, when cerebral spinal fluid is removed from the body during a lumbar puncture, the patient may complain of a headache. This may be attributed to position but can also remain a source of pain until the fluid balance has been restored. Fluid accumulation within body tissue can also induce pain if the tissue is *distended* and nerve endings *stretched* or *compressed* owing to the fluid excess. Overdistention can lead to collapse of blood vessels and result in tissue ischemia.

Pain associated with *spastic muscles* may occur as *cramps.* Cramping has a characteristic pattern that increases to severe intensity and then subsides. The process occurs rhythmically every few minutes and is observed in such conditions as menstruation, constipation, or even in labor.

*Perforation* of abdominal organs can lead to release of chemical irritants such as gastric juices, and precipitate pain. Because chemical irritation usually involves a wide surface area, many pain fibers may be stimulated, and the pain experienced is a most severe one.

*Direct irritation* of nerve endings resulting from presence of other chemical substances such as the release of histamine or globulin into tissues can produce pain. Conversely, the *degeneration* and *atrophy* of nerve endings often associated with aging diminish one's response to noxious stimuli.

**Psychologic sources** There are a number of potential psychologic sources of pain. Overall system *tension* may be the source of, or contribute to, increased intensity of pain. Multiple, frequent, or unsuccessfully handled *stressful situations* can create excessive levels of system tension and deplete reserve capacities of the system. When a painful stimulus is then applied, the individual's *tolerance* may be decreased or the pain may be perceived as more intense.

Pain can also be understood as an emotional response to or an attempt to *cope* with a threat to the individual's functioning. The threat may be in the form of unconscious conflicts, especially when strong emotions are present, or the pain may be an identification with the symptoms of a person significant to the individual. There may be evidence of a *hysterical personality,* such that under conditions of stress, tension is manifested as pain. Tension which presents as *chronic depression* is frequently associated with numerous complaints of low-grade pain. Pain may develop in response to a real, threatened, or fantasied *loss* which the individual feels incapable of handling.

In all these situations, unacceptable levels of tension have generated or intensified a perception of pain though no physical source adequate to explain the intensity of pain can be identified. The pain becomes a coping strategy for that individual though perhaps a largely unsuccessful one. The patient with this kind of pain is said to be experiencing *psychogenic pain,* which is defined as pain originating from or strongly affected by a psychologic component. Despite the source, the pain is no less real or less disturbing to the patient than organic pain.

In general, to categorize pain as organic or psychogenic is to artificially dichotomize it. Pure pain of either sort is probably nonexistent. Characteristically with psychogenic pain, the pattern as described by the patient cannot be directly correlated with an anatomic pattern or a physiologic process. The expected pattern is either absent or extensively altered, and there is little or no evidence of organic disease. There appears to be a disparity between the intensity of the pain described and the general appearance of the patient. The patient often presents as a person who is highly sensitive to pain but yet tolerates painful procedures. There is usually a history of multiple medical and surgical treatments for pain, none of which fully relieved the pain. The pain does not usually disturb sleep unless insomnia is present as an associated problem. It tends to occur at precise intervals or at irregular times for no discernible reason. It is usually unrelieved by analgesics or other conventional measures of pain relief. Further investigation may reveal a history of highly stressful situations, especially ones where conflict or loss is involved. In addition, there may be treatment-related disorders that are present such as drug addiction. Pain may disappear with resolution of conflict.

*Phantom pain* may be a type of psychogenic pain though researchers have yet to precisely identify the pain source. After an amputation, the individual usually reports a sensation of the amputated limb which becomes painful in about one-third of all amputees at some time. Phantom pain has four major properties: (1) It endures long after the tissues of the stump are well healed, (2) it may be triggered by stimulation of sites in healthy areas of the body, (3) it tends to develop in patients who have had chronic limb pain prior to amputation, and (4) it may sometimes be abolished for varying intervals by changing the level of sensory input to the stump or appropriate cord level.[6] Since phantom pain often persists after destruction of neural pathways, many researchers feel that a substantial psychologic component is an integral component.

One other kind of pain originates in the internal environment. This is *psychic pain* which is an expression of overwhelming *sorrow* and *grief*. It is not referred to the body except as generalized tension and aching.

**Environmental sources** Other sources of noxious stimuli may exist within the environment. Much attention has recently been paid to the influence of *noise* and high-frequency sound on the human system. Depending on the pain being experienced, these stimuli serve to intensify the amount of sensory input into one's perceptual range. *Drafts* and *wind* have also been noted as stimuli that increase pain intensity.

## Physiological Variables Affecting Pain Perception

There are a number of factors which affect the reception or transmission of noxious stimuli as a sensation. *Integrity of the nervous system* is generally a requirement, though it in itself is not totally responsible for the experience of pain. Pain may be present in the absence of an intact system of receptors or pathways. The point at which an individual first experiences pain is referred to as *pain perception.*

Because attention is a prerequisite, pain perception may be diminished by any factor which directly affects consciousness such as analgesics, anesthesia, or cerebral disturbances such as trauma or hypoxia. Pain perception is increased in the presence of fatigue, anger, boredom, and loneliness.

Experimentally, the *threshold level\** of intensity for pain perception is approximately the same for all individuals over time, though there is a slight variation among body parts. Thus the central control system and environmental factors are very influential in creating the differences in pain experiences. Sex and race differences in threshold level have been cited in the literature but seem to relate to sociocultural variations in tolerance rather than differences in pain threshold.

The presence of one source of painful stimuli raises the threshold to pain from other sources. Pain emanating from several sources does not summate but is as intense as the most intense of the stimuli. For these two reasons, pain relief from a neurosurgical procedure or from a chemical block may seem a failure to the patient whose attention is now drawn to other painful foci.

A reduction in the level or kind of sensory input, be it decreased, monotonous, or nonsensical, is associated with perception of greater pain. With inadequate input from the external environment, the individual focuses on the internal self as a source of stimulation so that peripheral input from the physical body is more readily transmitted and perceived as painful.

There is some evidence that individuals of age extremes are less sensitive to pain. This is purportedly due to an immature nervous system in the young child and to deterioration of the nervous system in the aged person. Both situations are still under investigation.

---

\* *Threshold* is defined as the point of stimulus intensity at which the majority of trained subjects report the stimulus as painful. Threshold point is a function of the physiological capacity of the nervous system.

Pain tolerance* varies among individuals. However, a diagnosis of inability to perceive pain is often misconstrued as total lack of pain perception. The problem is a physiologic one in which the degree of perception varies among the rare individuals unable to feel pain. Though there may be some affective component involved, it is generally felt that either the threshold to noxious stimuli at the receptor level is abnormally high or that there is excessive inhibition centrally. *Absence of pain* perception does not always preclude ability to perceive other stimuli such as temperature or pressure. Physiologically, the problem may be genetic or acquired through traumatic, chemical, or surgical transection which leaves a localized part or region insensitive to pain. Having lost the signal of pain, these persons are highly vulnerable to injury.

**Physiological response to painful stimuli**  An individual's physiological response to pain is triggered by a certain pattern of impulses from the T cells. It is mediated by the sympathetic nervous system and follows the usual pattern of sympatho-adrenal arousal. Blood pressure, heart rate, and respiratory rate rise, with respirations often being irregular. Pupils dilate, and sweating and muscle tension increase. Peripheral vasoconstriction and shunting of blood supply ensure continued function of the vital centers and simultaneously produce pallor. Gastrointestinal motility slows. Activity levels vary with the character of the pain so that the patient is sometimes motionless and at other times extremely restless. If the pain persists, autonomic activity diminishes but remains at greater than normal levels. Unrelieved intense pain of long duration may end in exhaustion of energy reservoirs, with shock and possibly death ensuing.

Pain of visceral origin, especially if severe, may produce a mixed autonomic response, with nausea and vomiting typically present. Blood pressure and heart rate may decrease. In addition, psychic responses accompanying this experience include increased anxiety, heightened awareness to the noxious stimuli, facial grimaces, restlessness, excitability, and irritability.

---

* The term *pain tolerance* as used in laboratory research means the point of stimulus intensity at which the subject requests cessation of the stimulus, because of inability to bear greater pain at the site. Clinically, the term encompasses a broader meaning, referring to the amount of pain a person can withstand without the need for analgesia and without significant depletion of energy for handling pain. *Pain expression* is the individual's peculiar behavioral manifestation of pain including verbal, nonverbal, emotional, and physical responses.

Two major types or patterns of physiologic pain which an individual may encounter are peripheral pain and neurogenic pain. *Peripheral pain* is pain which originates in a structure outside the central nervous system. Superficial pain, deep somatic or visceral pain, referred pain, and radiating pain are some examples.

*Superficial pain* is of cutaneous origin, usually due to trauma which causes strong stimulation of a large number of small-diameter fibers. It is well localized (the patient can point to it) and may have a bright, pricking quality or be dull and burning. Both types are usually of short duration. *Deep somatic or visceral pain* originates in the deeper structures of the body which are poorly localized (less innervation of the viscera). It is often associated with, or manifested solely by, referred pain and tends to have an aching quality. This pain usually depresses most behavioral responses, with inactivity and protective body positioning being common. Nausea and vomiting frequently are present.

*Referred pain* can most often be experienced at a focus of the body separate and removed from the organ where the noxious stimulus is occurring. For example, disruptions in the gallbladder may produce referred pain in an area between the shoulders. This is probably due to a convergence of nerves from the diseased viscera and a skin site at a single cord level. The brain then falsely interprets the message as derived from the more highly innervated skin area. Another factor that may be involved in this pain perception is the lack of experience people have in differentiating visceral pain sites.

*Radiating pain* is a sensation that pain is extending from the initial site to another point. This can be possibly due to recruitment of neurons in adjacent cord segments.

*Neurogenic pain* refers to input modified by a pathophysiologic condition of peripheral afferents or the central nervous system such as dysfunction or trauma. Central pain, neuritis, neuralgia, and causalgia are types of neurogenic pain.

*Central pain* is a form of pain where no peripheral cause can be identified. It is associated with lesions in the central nervous system that directly affect pain pathways, with thalamic lesions probably most common. The pain is characteristically constant though varying in intensity and may be intensified by anxiety, emotional stress, or a variety of ordinarily minor stimuli. It is hypothesized to be caused by a reduction in inhibitory influences within the central nervous system or at the gate level.

*Neuritis* pain occurs in the distribution of one or more nerves. It is often found symmetrically and frequently has a burning quality. *Neuralgia* is pain that arises along the distribution of a single nerve as in trigeminal neuralgia. It is often an intense, burning pain associated with stimulation of trigger points which set off paroxysms of pain.

*Causalgia* is a burning, severe pain due to injury of a large peripheral nerve or plexus. It occurs as a complication of injury in 2 to 5 percent of patients with large nerve damage and is associated with progressive trophic skin changes. The skin is usually hyperesthetic. Pain is exacerbated by emotional, auditory, or visual stimuli, or sometimes any movement of the affected limb. It usually subsides in 4 to 5 months. The pain is thought to result from small-fiber dominance with distortion of sensory input due to destruction of large fibers which normally close the gate.

### Psychological Variables Affecting Pain

Each situation in which pain occurs has its own peculiar characteristic to which the individual's response is partially based on psychological status at that time. Through the developmental process, certain learnings specific to pain are stored as memories to resurface in the cognitive or affective analysis of a painful stimulus. Pain habits or ways of expressing and using pain are learned behaviors. Thus, the nurse must consider how age and developmental status affect beliefs about pain and as affecting the availability of strategies for coping with pain.

**A**ge   The aged person often appears more tolerant of pain. This tolerance is explained by nervous system deterioration, differences in perceptual style, attachment of less importance to pain, and as a result of a greater repertoire of successful coping strategies. Nevertheless, many aged people who are chronically ill and living in constant fear of frequent pain seem more sensitive to pain in a manner consistent with the low tolerance for stress. These reactions are similar to responses found in individuals whose resources have been depleted by chronic illness. Age, per se, does not automatically confer greater ability to cope with pain, though there may be a rough correlation between age and pain tolerance.

**B**ody Image   Body image may be a determinant of pain tolerance. One component of body image is a sense of boundary or perimeter of the physical self. This boundary may be perceived as rather fluid and undefined or as precise and firmly established. In one study, people who were highly cognizant of a definite body perimeter tended to be more tolerant of stress and reported a stimulus as painful at higher levels than did those who had low boundary scores. Low scorers tended to perceive themselves as more vulnerable and would be expected to be less tolerant of pain.[7]

Pain may at times distort body image. The painful part may seem abnormally shaped or weighted. Its use may be limited. That part may seem to be the only part of the body with significance such that it assumes a perceptual dominance with respect to the rest of the body. Because of the damage that produced the pain, the injured part may acquire continued dominance in the unconscious body configuration.

In a situation where the body part involved is highly significant, such as the heart or the genitalia, pain perception may seem more intense. It cannot be assumed that specific body parts are equally significant across cultures, nor that the rules for expressing pain in these areas, especially in private parts, are similar. Many patients are reticent to talk about pain in the anal or genital area, though they are quite comfortable in describing pain elsewhere. Regardless of the components involved, distortion of body image can be a part of pain perception.

**P**ersonality   Character structure or personality affects an individual's usual manner of coping with life stresses including pain. Neurotic and introverted persons tend to be more highly sensitive to pain. With greater attention directed toward the self and bodily processes, even minor bodily pain may be exaggerated. Greater sensitivity need not, however, connote more overt expression of pain. Personality structure may also predispose a person to the development of pain patterns such as psychogenic or chronic pain syndromes.

The manner in which a person processes stimuli is defined as perceptual style and may be described as reducing, augmenting, or moderating.[8] *Reducers* tend to decrease or screen out information and thus do not perceive as much of the noxious stimulus. They tend to be more tolerant of pain, while *augmenters* tend to highlight incoming data in a way that increases the intensity or magnitude of the stress to the perceiver. Augmenters are usually less tolerant of pain. *Moderators* neither diminish nor enhance the data. It is not known whether the difference originates at the sensory receptor level, in the central biasing system, or at the cortical level as a learned behavioral style. However, practical information about an individual's style can be obtained through history, general observation, and use of the Libman test. In this test the thumb is pressed firmly on the mastoid bone which normally causes no pain, then is slipped forward to press on the styloid process. Reducers report mild pain or nothing and show little outward expression of pain. Augmenters, in contrast, may grimace or cry out and report the action as very painful.[9] Though a gross estimate only, the information can be helpful in anticipating responses to pain, determining pain tolerance, and planning coping strategies with the patient.

**P**revious Pain Experience   Past experience with pain is a potent determinant of pain tolerance and expression. One cannot simply disassociate the present experience from expectations about pain that represent an accumulation of thoughts and feelings from the past. For example, a person whose parents paid little attention to minor childhood injuries is likely to tolerate pain fairly well without much overt expression. Where parents displayed love and attention only when the child was injured, pain may become a means of gaining attention.

Few individuals escape multiple encounters with pain of some degree. In each interaction, there is an attempt to subdue or escape the pain, if possible. As the number and/or intensity of exposures to pain increase, each person finds ways of handling the pain that are usually successful and usually approved in his sociocultural group. The person learns to estimate individual capacity to withstand pain. Past experience, then, in part determines the extent and type of coping strategies available. Inability to handle previous pain experiences can make present pain more threatening and influence pain tolerance and perception.

**P**ain Trajectory   The patient's expectations of the pain pattern to be confronted is a function of past experiences and perception of the current *pain trajectory*. Pain trajectory is a construct described by Strauss et al.[10] and is defined as the expected or standard course of an illness or painful experience. Postoperative pain, for example, is expected to be most intense on the first day after surgery, then decrease gradually in a pattern that is usual for the kind of surgery undertaken. Pain that develops slowly following an expected pattern is better tolerated, though the patient may perceive it as more severe. Patients who find that their pain arrives or becomes more intense at unexpected times with no

forewarning are found to be less tolerant of that pain. It is not infrequent that patients' beliefs about the pain trajectory are based upon inadequate or false information. Without accurate information, anxiety rises in response to the unknown dimensions of pain. Inappropriate coping strategies may be tried, leading to lack of control over pain, decreased tolerance, and further fear and anxiety.

**A**nticipatory Pain   Expectation about pain is also influenced by the context of the *anticipatory period* that precedes a known painful experience. Assuming there has been adequate preparation of the patient about the expected pain, a patient has time to mobilize defenses. A short time period is generally inadequate to complete the task, while much time may arouse anxiety and permit development of many fantasies about the pain. Either situation lessens tolerance of pain.

Patients who have recently or chronically experienced pain deserve special consideration since their expectations about pain are likely to be strongly influenced by recent associations or memories of pain. Further, since pain as a *stressor* tends to precipitate the use of large amounts of energy in the process of coping, reserve energy will be unavailable and tolerance to new pain diminished. The net result is a more threatening, exhausting bout with pain. Most people do not adapt to pain and do not become more tolerant of it. Rather, they become psychologically and physically depleted, and tolerance drops.

**P**ain Control   Keeping pain within the bounds of the individual's capacity for coping in an acceptable manner is termed pain control. Therefore, control is dependent upon the availability of coping strategies either from the individual's own repertoire or developed in consultation with the nurse. Knowledge that certain measures have previously worked tends to increase pain tolerance, since the individual feels there are sufficient forces within reach to subdue the pain or at least make it bearable. Active participation in preparing strategies for dealing with pain also increases tolerance.

**A**nxiety   Any condition which decreases an individual's ability to exert control over pain likewise diminished tolerance of pain and increases anxiety. Unexpected pain, fatigue, decreased mobility, lack of information, isolation, absence of family, or a physical disorder are all conditions that may convert bearable pain to more severe and frightening pain. All these situations decrease either the ability to use or develop adequate pain strategies. Lack of control may breed alarming fantasies about the meaning of the pain. The individual may hypothesize that the pain must be a signal indicating serious illness or even death. Anger, fear, and anxiety as well as depression often become dominant behaviors.

Anxiety is a significant factor in nearly all pain experiences. At one extreme, anxiety may be the underlying reason for the pain, which is simply an outward expression of the anxiety. Patients with constantly high levels of anxiety may be more vulnerable to pain and tolerate it poorly.[11] Lack of control or a sense of powerlessness and an unclear notion of the significance of the pain are major anxiety producers. Fear of the unknown can be a significant factor in pain.

Being in pain is a lonely experience that can never be fully understood or shared with another. This loneliness often becomes a source of anxiety. Patients with chronic pain have been observed to undergo both mental and physical deterioration that in turn can become an additional agent of anxiety.[12] Because anxiety is a major cause of low tolerance for pain, its reduction becomes a focal point for nursing intervention.

### Sociocultural Variables Affecting Pain Perception

Along with physiological and psychological variables affecting pain, sociocultural influences must not be ignored. One's cognitive style, attitudes and values, sex, birth order and culture, all influence the way one perceives a pain experience.

**Cognitive style** Data on educational level and cognitive ability provide a rough appraisal of an individual's ability to obtain and process information about painful experiences. Persons with higher intelligence levels and with higher achievement levels in the educational system tend to be more tolerant of pain. This seems to relate to the ability to develop a more varied repertoire of coping behaviors. Though an individual may have little education, intellect and experience may permit development of a wide range of coping mechanisms. Others with considerable education may fail to connect what seems to be obviously related information. For most people, pain is not a familiar experience. They cannot be expected to make associations about pain and thus develop ways to cope that seem simplistic to health professionals. Evaluation of an individual's intellectual competence and

educational background will help to determine an appropriate approach to pain relief.

**Culture** Each person in pain has a religious, cultural, and philosophical foundation which powerfully affects attitudes, values, and beliefs about the meaning of health, illness, pain, and pain relief. Pain may have a negative connotation when it is viewed as destructive or dangerous, or it may have positive value as a character-building experience or as a means of gaining status. For some, pain is a form of God-given punishment or perhaps the unexplained will of God. For others, pain may simply be a destructive force without meaning, or merely a physical response to a noxious stimulus.

Culture becomes a major determinant of the norms of pain behavior. Cultural expectations provide a relatively detailed set of instructions concerning the appropriate level of tolerance for pain, ways of expressing pain, and where, when, and from whom in the health care system to seek help.

Zborowski's classic transcultural study of pain has provided a description of the differences in attitude, belief, and expression as they are found in several groups.[13] In a review of his work, the relative ethnic purity of his groups must be noted.

Zborowski described the behavior of the old American, Italian, Jewish, and Irish groups. Two of these groups are compared here with the intention of directing the nurse in analyzing the contribution of culture to the behavior of patients in pain. In the study the old American group consists of white people, generally born in the United States, of Protestant affiliation, and with no particular identification with any nationality. Members of this group are usually nonexpressive of pain and describe it in very concise, objective terms. They tend to minimize moderate pain but will withdraw to be alone in more severe pain. This group sees pain as unnecessary and expects curative treatment. However, they delay seeking treatment in preference to waiting to see if the pain will subside by itself. Old Americans are future-oriented and show much concern over possible implications of pain as a prognosticator of future health.

The Italian group, in contrast, is more expressive of pain in their utilization of crying, complaining, and gesturing. Family and friends stay in close contact because their presence serves as a distraction and as a support. This group is considered to have low tolerance for pain, and its members seek relief quickly. They focus concern on the pain sensation rather than on the reason for the pain. Pain is seen as decreasing energy and enjoyment of life and thus is often accompanied by depression.

Recognition of different cultural responses to painful experiences is not enough to forestall the common mistake of unwittingly communicating that one approach to pain is more acceptable than another. Appreciating patients' behavior in the context of their cultural heritage rather than in comparison with another culture is more likely to produce a therapeutic effect. Nonacceptance of patients' cultural behavior increases anxiety and reduces patients' ability to control their pain. Therefore pain tolerance decreases proportionately.

**Attitude and values**  Although most people develop a general philosophical orientation toward pain as having positive or negative value, they attribute individual meaning to each painful experience. This meaning is derived from factors such as reasons for the pain, motivation for enduring it, body part involved, and prognosis. Pain may be well tolerated if the experience is valued positively. A painful procedure is somehow less painful or better endured if it affects a cure. In Beecher's classic study of seriously wounded soldiers, many of the men reported no pain at all while civilians with lesser surgical procedures reported intense pain.[14] Beecher attributed the soldiers' lack of pain to their recognition that the wounds would release them from the more threatening front line duty. The civilians, on the other hand, saw their previously secure lives affected by a serious illness. One author has questioned this interpretation and explained the lack of pain as due to inhibition of transmission by the central nervous system in response to overwhelming sensory input.[15] Nevertheless, there is ample evidence that the meaning a person attaches to pain may dramatically change pain tolerance, as well as alter the manner in which it is expressed.

**Sex**  The female of most cultures is generally allowed greater emotional expression of pain. Crying, for example, has been treated as acceptable for girls though a boy would be labeled as a sissy for the same behavior. However, the influence of the women's movement may alter this behavioral pattern in future generations. The question of whether women are more tolerant of pain than men is unresolved.

**Birth order**  Finally, birth order may be related to pain tolerance. In one study firstborn were found to be less tolerant of pain. A tentative hypothesis considered the possibility that parental lack of experience created an atmosphere of emotional overconcern with minor painful incidents.[16]

### Environmental Variables Affecting Pain Perception

The last major variables affecting pain perception are the environmental influences of setting and time. The location in which pain occurs and the time of day seem to be points to consider carefully in pain assessment.

Pain knows no constraints in where it appears or where it is best treated. Patients with orthopedic problems, for example, may experience severe pain amenable only to treatment in a hospital setting. Other patients whose pain is equally intense may prefer to remain at home. Nevertheless, the setting does affect the way pain is tolerated and expressed. Strauss et al. find that pain work, encompassing the diversity of tasks involved in handling pain, "will vary in accordance with the kind of illness experienced by the patients and the organizational features of the particular ward."[17] To illustrate, the primary pain tasks facing patients and staff on an oncology unit may be the endurance or minimization of pain. The milieu is conducive to greater freedom in openly expressing pain. In contrast, staff on a general surgery unit tend to view pain as an unavoidable concomitant of treatment, as a problem to be minimized but not to interfere with necessary work such as ambulation, breathing exercises, or dressing changes. "Excessive" expression of pain is likely to be perceived as a disturbance that interrupts the recuperative process. Clearly the setting is associated with definite expectations of acceptable pain behavior.

Time produces the rhythmic changes of day and night which can affect one's perception of a painful stimuli. During *darkness,* there is an absence of activity, limited distractions, and possibly loneliness. An individual is vulnerable to personal fears, and as a result focuses upon perceived pain continuously. This may be intensified in the presence of insomnia, anxiety, or fatigue resulting in heightened pain perception.

In the *daylight,* people in pain tend to feel somewhat improved. This may be influenced by increased activity, added distractions, the brightness in a room, and the increase in control an individual has over the pain. However, for some individuals, heightened mental and physical activity can become stressful. In addition, people who are used to working during the day may have altered responses to pain during the day. These factors must be considered when dealing with the pain experience.

### Effects of Pain

The physiologic response to pain is far less variable than its behavioral expression but depends to some extent on the nature of pain. To be simplistic, pain occurs as either acute or chronic. *Acute pain* of low to moderate intensity or from a superficial focus elicits physiologic responses that function to protect and maintain adequate bodily integrity in the presence of a painful stimulus. In a sense, acute pain operates as a negative stimulus that persists until the pain is abolished or the damage resolved. Acute pain is usually a temporary, though sometimes intense, phenomenon.

Acute psychic pain can also occur with no less intense an effect. Physical responses accompanying acute pain connote an active fight/flight mechanism induced by the presence of pain. In persons with severe heart disease, increased intracranial pressure, or other similar pathologies, this can have potentially dangerous consequences.

*Chronic pain* does not evoke the same defensive physiologic response. Instead, physical evidence of pain is more often a reflection of the individual's psychological response to the pain, usually with a large overlay of anxiety. One almost inevitable result of chronic pain is physical exhaustion due to the presence of the unrelenting stressor of pain.

Nonverbal pain behavior appears in a pattern quite specific to the individual. Despite the person-specificity of the response, certain manifestations appear frequently enough to serve as valid indications of pain if judged within the context of other data.

Chronic pain is usually accompanied by a disagreeable feeling and by a desire to run away. A sense of fear or depression may pervade. Anxiety is almost universally present when pain becomes more than a minor or fleeting sensation. Irritability is common and may be associated with restlessness. Most patients find themselves focusing on their pain and thus restricting their awareness of, or interaction with, environmental stimuli. Many patients appear preoccupied with pain, especially if the significance of the pain is unclear, or if their coping strategies do not include distraction or some means of disassociating themselves from the pain.

In anticipation of pain, cognitive appraisal of the expected threat is followed by mobilization of defenses such as denial, rationalization, or planning various coping strategies. Later, during a painful period, the nurse will often see evidence of the chosen strategies such as attempts to distract oneself or use of localized activity, often in the form of repetitious small-muscle movements.

## FIRST-LEVEL NURSING CARE

For most of us pain is usually an unexpected experience. However, there are many situations where forewarning of pain is possible. Scheduled therapies, diagnostic tests, surgical procedures, and childbirth are but a few examples. Having knowledge about a potential pain experience can prevent added physical and emotional damage from occurring.

A period of forewarning can be anxiety-provoking. The unknown nature of the expected pain, the often unexpressed fear of not being able to control or relieve the pain, and the basic threat of pain to body integrity may elicit intense anxiety that reduces the effectiveness of coping strategies and decreases tolerance for pain. Alternatively, the anticipatory period can become a supportive time of preparation to increase the patient's ability to handle pain and to provide more data to the nurse to use in determining measures of pain relief or minimization. All individuals must be evaluated accordingly.

### Prevention

The first consideration is when to inform the patient that pain may be expected. In some cases there is no option, such as in an emergency situation when surgery is needed. Preparing the patient should begin immediately. When this decision can be made or influenced by the nurse, it should be determined on the basis of the patient's condition, the reason for the pain, the degree of anxiety present, the proximity of the painful situation, and, lastly, the probability of distraction while discussing the situation with the patient. No one time can be designated as most appropriate for all patients. Patients who are anxious tend to overestimate the threatening nature of the expected pain and doubt their ability to cope with it. Minimizing the time of anticipation usually minimizes further intensification of their anxiety.

Patients anticipating pain generally have several needs which are interrelated but distinct. They need to verbalize their fears and expectations, decrease their anxiety, mobilize their internal resources, determine what pain work will be necessary, and consider what strategies will be most successful for controlling the pain. At this time, moderate anxiety is conducive to the mobilization process and to learning.

*Verbalization* may seem a relatively unimportant and time-consuming process among all those listed. It is probably one of the patient's most important tasks, though sometimes a difficult one for both nurse and patient. It requires a nurse in whom the patient has trust and one who can free the patient to discuss issues freely despite possible embarrassment or imprecision in voicing ideas. Sometimes the nurse will need to point out the evidence of mental discomfort or apprehension such as restlessness, or some other slight changes from the patient's normal behavior. At other times, a direct question about concerns over discomfort or pain is sufficient. Talking about pain and its meaning may reveal misinformation and fantasy as well as place fear and anxiety in perspective. Verbalization is a powerful reducer of anxiety.

*Anxiety* varies directly with the vagueness of a situation and indirectly with the amount of control a person has over that situation. Control may be increased and ambiguity decreased by supplying the patient with specific information about the pain to be experienced and about measures to manage it. Determine first what the expected pain trajectory will be and compare this with the patient's expectations. Many patients expect pain where none might occur. In several studies, researchers found that not all surgical patients have pain and that up to half of the patients needed no analgesics. On the other hand, patients are sometimes unaware of the potential for pain in a study or procedure for which they are scheduled.

Thus, a major nursing responsibility for patients expecting pain is discussion of expected pain both during and after the pain-producing situation. Adequate description of the expected pain includes the location, quality, and intensity of pain expected, purpose of the pain, and the duration of the pain. The nurse should stress the probability of pain rather than the inevitability of it, since the patient may, in fact, not experience pain. Description of the pain should be precise in most instances, since patients are best able to control pain that they are expecting. Though intensity of pain may be modified by a host of factors, some indication of range should be given. The patient should be made aware of situations which may heighten pain, such as coughing postoperatively, and be shown ways to modify its impact.

A description of the expected pain is inadequate if not coupled with an exploration of what to do about it. Patients need to know what they will be expected to do during the pain experience and what kind of pain work will be needed.

If use of an analgesic is contraindicated because the pain produced serves a diagnostic function or because the analgesic would prevent the full participation of the patient, the patient must be so informed. In other situations, as when the patient elects to use various methods to prepare for childbirth, the patient may be allowed to forego use of all pharmacologic agents. Identifying coping strategies that can minimize pain and increase comfort will reduce anxiety and increase pain tolerance. Physical exercise, sometimes in physical therapy, may be useful in maximizing pain tolerance and hastening tissue repair because the increased blood supply that results permits earlier movement and adequate support of injured parts. Adequate sleep is also vital to reduce the fatigue that may decrease tolerance for the upcoming pain.

Past experience with pain to determine the nature of those experiences and estimate the success of the coping strategies used should be explored. If new strategies are to be introduced, the nurse must consider the amount of time needed for practice. Some methods, including relaxation or breathing techniques and certain forms of distraction, require familiarity. Many patients are unaware of pain relief measures beyond analgesics. Many more, especially preoperative patients, feel that there is nothing they personally will be able to do about their pain. Simple explanations of ways of turning, positioning, conscious muscle relaxation, splinting, and the like provide the patient with means to control the pain.

*Group discussion* may offer another option to the patient by permitting verbalization and may offer individuals additional ideas about ways to handle pain. Distraction from thinking about the anticipated pain may interrupt a pattern of increasing anxiety. Patients who require time to plan for demands to be made on them should be encouraged to do so.

If possible, the family (or significant friends) should be included in the discussion of potential painful situations, as they can have the same misapprehensions and anxieties about pain as the patient. Discussions may offer valuable suggestions and explore successful pain strategies.

## SECOND-LEVEL NURSING CARE

*Transitional pain* may be defined as sensation ranging from discomfort to mild pain which is just perceptible to the patient, or which is not significantly interfering with daily activities. There may be minor or intermittent periods of pain experienced from organic disorders, or there may be anxiety, and therefore slightly noxious stimuli may be interpreted as painful. A number of painful experiences are produced by variables within the immediate situation that either increase or decrease pain tolerance or increase perceived intensity of pain.

## Nursing Assessment of Pain Experience

In order to help reduce an individual's pain perception, it is essential that a careful assessment be made before interventions are instituted. Since pain is the body's way of alerting us to the fact that a serious health problem may be present, it is critical that the current health status be evaulated and problems identified.

The first and ongoing step in caring for patients in pain is a thorough assessment of the pain as reported or manifested by the patient. The *history* should reflect a full description of the characteristics of the pain and a representation of the evolving portion of the pain trajectory. The patient's response to the pain is then documented, and the variables affecting the response determined. Influencing variables are the most difficult to ascertain but may be determined through observation, skillful interviewing, and careful analysis of all the variables. Assessment of pain is often more accurate if done on a scale which indicates magnitude. The patient should be asked to select the number from 0 to 5 (0 representing no pain, 5 being severe pain) which most accurately describes the intensity of the pain being experienced (see Fig. 39-3). By charting the patient's responses on a graph over time, the nurse can better assess the pain experience, analyze the precipitating causes, and evaluate the effect of interventions.

An accurate profile of the patient in pain includes thorough analysis of all the following areas:

*Location of pain.* Where is it? Can it be localized? Does it radiate? If so, identify point of origin and pattern of radiation. Is it limited to one portion of the body? Does it follow a particular nerve distribution?

*Intensity.* How is the pain described? Patients can discriminate five levels of intensity: mild, discomforting, distressing, intense (horrible), and excruciating (unbearable). How well does the estimation of intensity correlate with nonverbal and physiologic manifestations of pain? What factors are present that affect level of consciousness? Is anxiety present? Does the

patient feel he or she can control the pain? Does estimate of perceptual style, especially if verbal statement of intensity, correlate well with other clinical indicators (Libman test, described in Personality above)? Does pain interfere with sleep, eating, work, or other daily activities?

*Temporal pattern.* Time of onset? Associated events such as relationship to season, activity, weather? Trigger zones? Is the pattern of pain cyclical or rhythmic in appearance, duration, intensity, or disappearance? Is the pain paroxysmal, steady, or intermittent? How long does it last? Is there any relationship to level of stress?

*Description of the quality of the pain.* The quality of pain, being so subjective, is hard to explain to another person. Patients frequently use analogies such as "cutting like a sharp knife." Note that the patient's ability to describe the pain is partially a reflection of verbal and intellectual capacity, as well as an indication of knowledge about the painful part or area. The description is also influenced by nearly all the variables described earlier. Consider the possibility that the patient is really experiencing discomfort from a sensation to which he or she is unaccustomed and thus has no reference for it except pain.

*Nonverbal and physiologic expressions of pain.* See Effects of Pain above.

*Past experience.* What was the nature of past experiences (include duration, intensity, frequency, recency, and coping strategies)? Be particularly alert for history of emotional stress, loss, or depression.

*Variables.* Evaluate psychological, sociocultural, environmental, and physiological variables as they affect the pain experience or expectations about pain. Of course, not all the information which is summarized in Fig. 39-2 need be obtained in the first instance of pain. In some cases, the patient's immediate need is pain relief. Any attempt to explore the variables influencing the pain beyond very basic information would only prolong the experience and increase distress.

Manifestations of pain at this level may be subtle. There may be a sympathetic response, but probably a modified one with slight variances in vital signs or slightly increased muscle tension. The response may be short-lived, especially if the pain appears only intermittently, or in short bursts. If the discomfort or pain is more or less continuous but mild, minor deviations from normal behavior may be noticed. The direction or character of the deviation depends on personality, past experience with pain, sociocultural norms, and perceived significances of the pain. For example, the individual may converse less or pay less attention to work or favorite activities. Ability to concentrate on complex matters may decrease, and attention is drawn to minor aches or disabilities. The person may be restless or, conversely, abnormally quiet. There is an appearance of tension and usually some degree of irritability. Patients may describe the pain as flickering, pricking, tingling or itchy, dull, nagging, or annoying. The pain is not a dominant factor in their lives, but is causing some concern, especially if the significance of the pain is unknown. Left alone, the stimulus is likely to be interpreted as painful rather than uncomfortable.

After determining the nature of the pain, the nurse and patient should evaluate the adequacy of the patient's coping habits. At this level of pain, no further assistance may be needed. If there is need for nursing, it is based upon the following broad objectives: (1) To eliminate the source of pain, (2) to decrease anxiety, (3) to provide general comfort, (4) to reduce pain or alter perception of the stimulus as painful, (5) and to increase tolerance for pain.

### Nursing Problems and Interventions

Caring for patients with transitional pain proceeds from, and includes, techniques used for patients anticipating pain. Patients need information that will aid them in increasing pain tolerance and clarifying the significance of the pain. *Anxiety,* due to lack of knowledge about the meaning of the pain, often acts as a psychological stimulus to increase the patient's pain experience.

As noted earlier, patients are often unaware of ways to reduce pain other than medication. Admittedly, the administration of drugs, especially narcotics, is an easy way to relieve pain and is frequently the mode of treatment expected by the patient. It is not always a particularly thoughtful or safe way of handling mild pain. The potential risks of analgesics are often greater than the benefits.

**Clarification of pain experience** Nurses should not assume that patients will make what seem to be simple associations between pain and factors which cause or aggravate it. When teaching about controlling pain, it is essential to assess what the patient knows about that pain. It may also be useful to help the patient differentiate between *pain* and *discomfort.* Often minor aches and discomforts are reinterpreted as pain. Recall, too, that the criteria for reporting pain differ greatly among various

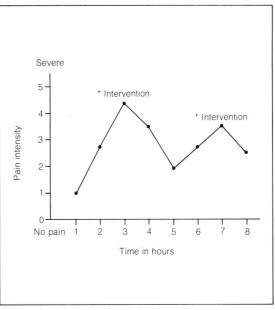

**FIGURE 39-3**
Analysis of pain intensity and related responses to interventions.

sociocultural groups. McBride found that intervention was more appropriate and analgesics frequently unneeded when the nurse took time to explore what the patients meant by pain and to evaluate the parameters of the pain.[18] Often, merely a position change or a brief conversation to clarify a concern will transform pain into discomfort or perhaps alleviate the pain entirely.

**Distraction** Another mode of altering a patient's perception of pain is *distraction.* This method is used by many patients (often unknowingly) and is most successful when pain is of slight or moderate intensity. Distraction is a technique whereby attention is redirected away from the pain to another stimulus. One of the basic axioms of pain perception states that attention to pain must be present for pain to be perceived. Therefore, if one directs attention away from pain, less pain is perceived. Except for periodically determining the nature of the patient's pain, it is best to minimize discussion of it with the patient in mild pain since the talking or thinking about it will merely attract an individual's conscious attention to it.

The efficacy of distraction declines if a single distractor is used for an extended period. Distraction is less useful if the task requires little concentration, is inappropriate to the person, or does not require active involvement. Use of the technique by the nurse may be sufficient to demonstrate its utility to the patient. The nurse can teach the patient to use the techniques consciously and will not need to be present constantly. Where distraction will be used during a known painful period, the nurse should plan appropriate distractors with the patient. Reading, television, a variety of crafts, music, drawing or sketching, talking, mental arithmetic, or planning something with lists or diagrams, and possibly a visit from a friend may all be effective for various patients. As the duration of painful period increases, an array of nonfatiguing, variable activities should be selected. The patient who is at home may have a greater variety of distractors available, but too often patients at home sit in front of a television all day or lie in their rooms where they find themselves bored and brooding about their pain. All efforts should be made to increase their activity level if there is no contraindication to doing so.

**Family teaching**  When the patient with mild pain is staying in the home setting, the nurse may need to discuss reinforcement of wellness behavior with the family. Complaints of pain or other expressions of pain should be responded to objectively, without sympathy or great attention. Family members should be openly responsive to the patient's use of effective strategies for coping with pain and increasing participation in various family or social activities. Through support and consultation, the family can work with the patient and help the individual during this pain experience. It is vitally important that family members be taught to recognize significant changes in the patient's pain experience that require medical attention.

**Activity**  Another important variable to consider is the amount of true rest the patient is obtaining. Pain that interrupts sleep is particularly fatiguing. Virtually no coping strategy will be successful if the patient has insufficient energy to invest in its use. At times mild sedation may be needed to relieve anxiety and allow the patient adequate rest. Relaxation techniques, including conscious muscle relaxation, autosuggestion, meditation, massage, and breathing exercises as used in LaMaze childbirth, may be used to induce rest and relieve energy-usurping muscle tension.

**Touch**  Gate control theory suggests other strategies for reducing pain. One considers raising the sensory input level with music or visual displays to increase the inhibitory influence of the central biasing system, and thus decrease recognition of noxious stimuli. Melzack and Wall state that large-fiber input closes the gate to transmission by small-diameter fibers. Large-fiber stimulation by vibrating or rubbing the skin may be used to diminish perception of pain for periods of minutes to about an hour.[19] Because large fibers adapt, the stimulus must be periodically repeated. This is a simple maneuver that the patient or family members can use to reduce slight to moderate pain. (*Note:* Do *not* rub or massage a painful calf since this movement could dislodge a thrombus.) Last, any measure which maximizes the effect of the central control system can modify the pain experience.

One cannot negate the effect of *touch* on the body. Much research today suggests that this activity can provide both physiological as well as psychological comfort to patients in pain. Individuals caring for a patient at home should be encouraged to touch the patient as a sign of caring as well as an offering of comfort.

## THIRD-LEVEL NURSING CARE

Patients experiencing acute pain are usually hospitalized as a result of a physically traumatic experience, sudden illness, anticipated emergency surgery, or a prolonged pain that is unrelieved by previous measures. A patient may also be hospitalized because pain has interfered with self-care or the pain itself no longer responds to coping measures used in the past.

The person in *acute pain* is experiencing moderate to severe pain, but generally pain of short duration. It differs from transitional pain in both degree and level of awareness. Pain is definitely present, sometimes to the point of frightening and exhausting the patient. It can destroy reason and create a strain on the human system so severe that it can lead to extreme fatigue and even shock.

### Nursing Assessment

Acute pain requires a thorough analysis of the experiences with particular attention paid to variables arising in the context of the situation. These variables may be acting singly or in combination to increase the intensity of pain or decrease the patient's tolerance. The nurse should gather data as previously described in order to formulate a profile of the patient in pain. (See Table 39-1 and accompanying text.) The *health history* is often based on limited verbal input from the patient, physiologic and nonverbal expressions of pain, analysis of variables about which data are available, and knowledge of the etiology and expected pain trajectory. It should be emphasized here that acute pain is acute because of an interplay of intense physiologic stimuli and psychologic variables producing the perception that the pain is severe. Acute pain is not a strictly organic phenomenon.

*Physical assessment* reveals a strong autonomic response with significant changes in vital signs, peripheral vasoconstriction, sweating, nausea, and vomiting. Increased muscle tension is present, sometimes to the point of producing board-like rigidity over the painful part. Extreme restlessness or, conversely, absolute stillness with the body in a protective position may signify acute pain.

Pain becomes a point of central attention. It interferes with sleep, work, and eating. Patients often feel close to loss of control and may become very disturbed if they cannot maintain expression of pain within their own acceptable limits. Frequently, the manner of pain expression may be less upsetting to them during the time of pain than it is on recollection of their behavior. There may be fear, possibly anger, when pain threatens to become overwhelming.

For many patients, the physiologic responses may be the only direct indication of pain, though some behavioral change is rarely absent. Often, the patient will call the nurse with some minor request, and the nurse, while straightening a pillow or checking some equipment, will find the bed soaked through with sweat. The patient may or may not admit to severe pain but clearly requires relief. Overt

**TABLE 39-1**
PROFILE OF THE PATIENT IN PAIN

Location of pain (locate on body drawing, indicating all radiation) _____

Intensity [estimate 1 (mild) to 5 (excruciating)] _____
Temporal pattern _____

_____ Associated or aggravating factors _____
Description of quality of pain _____

Nonverbal behavior _____
Physiologic signs of pain _____
_____ Vital signs _____
General profile of patient (cognitive ability, developmental level, level of anxiety, recent stress level) _____

Age _____ Sex _____ Dominant cultural group _____
Religious affiliation _____ Educational level _____
Perceptual style (Libman test, general observation) _____

Past experience with pain (include coping strategies) _____

Expectations about pain experience _____

_____ Particular concerns _____
Significance of pain (include patient's idea about cause) _____

If pain present chronically: Effect on life-style, personal relationships, activity level, etc. _____

_____ Treatment, current medication _____

Family responses to patient and to patient's behavior _____

Environmental factors _____

Medical diagnosis _____

Other comments:

Nursing diagnosis:

expressions of pain are not necessarily accurate indicators of the presence or intensity of pain.

Other patients are highly expressive of pain with crying, grimacing, moaning, and occasionally screaming. Nurses must be sensitive to their own possibly aversive reaction to this form of pain behavior, as they evaluate the reason for it. The nurse should review personal attitudes toward pain in order to improve the delivery of health care.

**Diagnostic tests** If a painful procedure is planned for a patient already in severe pain, a minimum but precise explanation is needed. Expectations of patient performance during a procedure will be required. The patient should know about measures available to reduce the pain during the procedure. The nurse should expect to have to repeat instructions and possibly have to repeatedly draw the patient's attention away from the pain. Finally, it is important to tell the patient when the procedure is over. Depending on the precipitating source of pain, various diagnostic procedures may be suggested in order to identify the pain source.

### Nursing Problems and Interventions

The primary nursing problem at this level is the *pain* itself. It can be intensified by in the presence of *physiologic problems, anxiety, stress, increased movement,* and *ineffective coping modalities.*

Until the source of pain is identified, the problem of pain can take on proportions of a medical emergency. Increased fatigue to the point of exhaustion depletes the patient of energies and can result in unsuccessful coping. Quick movement through procedures and diagnostic tests places an added stress on the individual and can aggravate the pain experience. Fear of the pain as well as the identification of the potential cause of the problem can be anxiety provoking for the patient.

Interventions may be extremely painful and serve to intensify the pain experience. Debridement of extensive burn tissue, for example, while therapeutic may only intensify anxiety, increase stress, and decrease coping mechanisms.

In all situations the nurse must be supportive and offer encouragement to the patient. Throughout each encounter, the nurse acts as an observer of the pain pattern, assisting the patient in relieving or minimizing the pain or helping the individual endure or express it.

Nurses and other health professionals often act on the assumption that all pain is bad and the goal of all pain work is relief. Such a limited conceptualization could produce dangerous and even fatal re-

sults. For example, a nurse who administers an analgesic to a patient with a headache caused by a head injury places the patient in danger by masking potential changes in the patient's level of consciousness. The type of pain work needed depends upon such factors as the initiating problem, the effect of the pain, the goals of the patient, the objectives of the health organization, and other variables specific to the patient.

Basic to the care itself is informing the patient in acute pain about the pain source and the expected pain trajectory. Patients are not passive receivers of information. Despite their pain they need to share in decisions about their care, to the extent that their energy permits.

Within the constraints of diagnosis, treatment, and patient health status, nurses utilize a variety of strategies to help patients cope with acute pain. Techniques used at the second level of care may still be useful either alone, or as an adjunct to the strategies introduced currently. Anxiety reduction retains major importance along with support and clarification. One measure, *distraction,* will probably be less useful in the presence of severe pain unless coupled with other pain-relieving strategies. As before, the family is a part of the total experience and needs continued support.

**Comfort** Physical comfort measures enhance the effectiveness of other strategies since they are generally relaxing and promote rest. In the process of providing comfort, the nurse's interest and skill are communicated to the patient while at the same time allowing the nurse to continue evaluation of the patient's status. Several nursing researchers have found this kind of interaction with patients often reduced or eliminated the need for analgesics.

The nurse may manipulate the environment of the patient's physical or mental condition to create a state conducive to *rest.* Adequate rest is an essential part of handling pain. Relaxation techniques, anxiety reduction measures, alteration of sensory input, massage to relieve general tension, discussion, repositioning, bathing, or simply being present, are some of the strategies that are frequently effective. Patients also need some time when their pain is minimized in order to recover energy losses. Organized care with well-timed use of analgesics can maximize rest time.

*Position changes* for the patient in severe pain may be an agonizing experience. The pain caused may increase the patient's reluctance to move even if he or she realizes that muscle fatigue and tension directly follow prolonged maintenance of one position. Patients often find that moving themselves can be less pain-provoking than being moved. They can accomplish this movement with greater ease by turning the body as a unit, creating less tension on painful parts. Injured parts should be evenly and fully supported, avoiding pressure or tension. Tubes and other attached equipment should be well taped (except where contraindicated) and positioned to allow the patient maximum freedom of movement. Patients should be helped in maintaining a position of anatomic alignment using supportive equipment as needed.

*Heat and cold* are often used to treat the source of pain or reduce perception of pain. Heat reduces swelling and inflammation, thereby removing noxious stimuli. It also decreases muscle spasm. Cold applications provide local anesthesia and reduce the rate of swelling associated with tissue injury or inflammation.

Any care which protects the patient from other sources of pain or discomfort will enhance pain tolerance. Though the pain derived from several sources do not summate, the presence of additional stressors increases overall tension. A distended bladder, a decubitus ulcer, an awkward movement, or coughing postoperatively without splinting are frequent events that cause additional discomfort. Care must be taken to reduce these added painful stimuli through patient teaching when attempting to reduce pain and increase overall tolerance.

**Analgesia** The nurse may find that the nursing strategies discussed above in addition to the patient's own methods of coping are not effective in accomplishing the necessary pain work. Analgesics may then be needed. An *analgesic* is a substance which alleviates or abolishes pain without causing loss of consciousness. Analgesics act at different sites, some peripherally, some on central pain pathways, and some on structures associated with the motivational-affective component of the central control system. They are almost always needed in the presence of deep pain, but at times they are totally ineffective, such as in some cases of central pain and phantom limb pain.

When a choice of analgesics is made, the minimum-strength drug that is effective is the drug of choice. The age of the patient (the aged tend to report more pain relief from standard doses of analgesics), size (larger patients may need larger doses), recency of anesthesia, likely duration of the pain, and the characteristics of the individual's pain experience also determine the drug of choice. Pain should not be allowed to become too severe before

the drug is administered since many drugs are less effective in the presence of intense pain. Medication should consistently be given as needed according to the patient, rather than when the nurse feels the patient has exhibited sufficient strength. As pain decreases over time, the nurse should gradually wean the patient off the drug instead of abruptly stopping it. *Weaning* involves the use of less potent drugs and substitution of various coping strategies for the drug. Quite frequently, a sedative or other synergistic drug is given with a narcotic to potentiate the action of the analgesic. The most appropriate medication scheduling should be planned with the patient. An effective strategy is to give the drug one-half hour before ambulating or seeing visitors. The nurse has full responsibility for maintaining safety in administering and monitoring the effect of the drug. When narcotics are used over a period of time, it is important to observe for signs of drug dependency, although addiction is unlikely to occur when narcotics are given on a short-term basis. A patient requesting medication every 3 to 4 hours 1 week postoperatively may require a more complete investigation of the pain experience.

The *placebo effect* is a phenomenon. It is caused by the influence of a person's positive belief in the efficacy of a treatment on the actual effectiveness of the treatment. If, because of the nurse's suggestion that this measure or drug *will* relieve the pain, the patient believes that it will help, it very likely will. There is controversy over the fact that use of placebos invades an individual's rights. Some suggest that if a placebo is utilized, the patient should be involved in the strategy planning and discuss the intervention as a possible alternate coping strategy. Others disagree, feeling that the use of placebos is in the patient's best interest.

Two other points about drugs and acute pain are relevant. First, treatment of acute pain frequently includes use of a variety of drugs chosen specifically to combat the problem causing the pain. These include antibiotics, anti-inflammatory agents, immunosuppressants, muscle relaxants, and tranquilizers. Second, analgesic orders should state the minimum interval between doses. If the chosen drug cannot be changed or supplemented, the nurse and patient need to determine what other strategies to use while awaiting the next dose.

In caring for patients in acute pain, as at the other levels, the nurse protects the patient from depletion of all resources in unsuccessful attempts at *coping*. Reducing stress allows the nurse to facilitate an individual's own coping strategies, which can be supplemented as needed. Assuming that acute pain finally subsides, the nurse and patient should review the pain experience together and integrate the various aspects of the period of pain into the total life experience. Determining which strategies were successful will help the patient feel more in control of future pain experiences.

**Surgery** The patient who experiences chronic pain may become a candidate for a neurosurgical procedure (see Table 39-2). Pre- and postoperative care is similar to the care of any neurosurgical patient (see Chap. 35). A complete discussion of additional interventions for chronic pain is found under Fourth-Level Nursing Care.

## FOURTH-LEVEL NURSING CARE

On a long-term basis, care of the patient in chronic or intractable pain incorporates all the nursing knowledge, skill, and art as discussed earlier. Chronic and intractable pain are not synonymous forms of pain, although they may and usually do coexist. *Chronic pain* is pain of longer duration, usually greater than 6 months. *Intractable* pain, on the other hand, is pain that is highly resistant to intervention, especially the more conventional forms of treatment.

In both situations there is no cessation in efforts to eliminate the pain, diminish its effect on the patient, or prevent pain from other sources. Variables affecting pain tolerance or perception become the major focus of nursing intervention. The goal of care is to increase an individual's ability to endure pain which medical science cannot alleviate.

## Profile of the Patient with Chronic Pain

The term *chronic pain* does not imply any particular degree of pain. The sufferer may experience mild to intense pain. The important factor is chronicity, which does not evoke the defensive responses found in acute pain. Several groups fall in the category of patients with chronic pain, that is, pain which lasts more than 6 months. These include: (1) individuals with pain that is primarily psychogenic and whose pain is a persisting adaptive mode, (2) patients with a terminal illness that is associated with pain, and (3) patients whose pain is primarily organic in origin and is not controlled by conventional measures.

LeShan and several others have described the patient who is suffering with chronic pain. The patient often has multiple pain complaints including:

(1) an altered behavioral pattern such as depression; (2) a preoccupation with pain; (3) a history of many procedures and treatments including surgery; (4) fatigue; (5) and a focus only on day-to-day living. Few can tolerate looking ahead to a future full of the same pain that is creating such misery in the present.[20]

There is no time limit or meaning to the pain, although some explain it as God's will. Thus, sufferers turn to themselves and their pain. The withdrawal from other people deprives them of energy and support to cope with pain. Pain becomes less tolerable and exhausting. As the pain grows stronger, without meaning, there is no hope, and without hope there is no reason to live. Severe depression may follow. Suicide may be the last gesture of control over pain. The process does not occur in a month, or even a year. Some individuals find help in religion, others in their family and friends; others in the health care system. Some find no help, yet use their life savings seeking it.

*Chronic pain* whatever its origin is a continuing and unrelenting stressor. It produces either gradual exhaustion or response that very often ends in addiction and depression. Occasionally, chronic pain is a mode of coping that has become vital to the continued functioning of the individual. It may be the "least guilt-engendering and the least disruptive means of relieving deeply situated, unresolved conflict."[21] It is sustained as a set of pain behaviors that are reinforced by gratification of the patient's internal need. Usually, an original pain-producing organic problem can be identified, but though it may still exist, no clear physiologic pattern is apparent. Use of pain in this fashion is an unconscious mechanism. The pain, however, is real and is legitimate.

**Nursing assessment** Because of the myriad of problems that may contribute to, or cause, chronic pain, virtually all members of the health team become involved in planning health care. Determination of the extent of the problem is essential. Nursing contributes data to this analysis and becomes a part of the team that determines the treatment program.

A full description of the pain is obtained as described earlier, including a detailed history and assessment of the pain and related interventions. A review of the profile of patient in chronic pain will reveal the initial cause of the pain, duration, the physical as well as psychological significance of the pain experience, personality pattern, fatigue, personal goals, and interaction with others.

The health team begins to assess the effect of the pain on the individual's life by determining the patient's activity level, by noting changes in social and family relationships and in vocational functioning, and by analyzing the responses of the family to the patient's pain behavior. They seek to determine factors which increase the patient's pain or disability such as patterns of stress, or relationships which reinforce pain behavior. As the collection of pertinent data increases, a determination can be made as to how greatly the pain experience interferes with the patient's performing activities of daily living. The decision about treatment is made at least in part with the patient and family and is dependent on the following factors: etiology and characteristics of the pain, patient's need for pain, age, physical and mental status, life expectancy, obligation to family and community, and available treatment measures and their iatrogenic effects.

**Interventions Used with Chronic Pain**

Table 39-2 lists in detail all the many interventions that can be utilized to relieve chronic pain. Analysis of the particular pain experience unique to the individual and the influence multiple variables have on pain tolerance must precede selection of an intervention.

The patient needs to be informed by the nurse and other health team members about each intervention available while discussing the anticipated effects on pain experience. Since many of the techniques listed in Table 39-2 have been used in various combinations, careful assessment of the individual's particular pain is needed before selecting a program.

After being informed of those resources available in relieving pain, the patient should be invited to participate with the health care team in deciding how pain will be handled. In some areas of the country pain clinics are available where representatives of the major health professions integrate their skills and plan programs for reduction in pain or increased tolerance to the pain experience. By incorporating the patient in the decision-making process, it is hoped that the suggested program will be more closely adhered to. In some settings the patient contracts as to when, where, and how the pain experience will be changed so that pain will no longer dominate the person's life.

For some individuals the objective of a pain program will be to increase pain tolerance, or simply reduce its perception. For others, it may be necessary to reduce negative pain behavior such as drug dependency or the use of pain for secondary gain.

Rehabilitation of the patient with chronic pain may also need to include gradual social reintegration since many patients with chronic pain may have isolated themselves. *Support* of the patient and family is critical. Often this support will be needed during the decision-making process when attempts to alter the pain experience are first discussed.

The patient will need to be encouraged to express fears and concerns about outcome and be prepared for the pain work that will be required. During this time the underlying stressors precipitating maladaptive behavior can be identified and the patient and family guided toward developing more positive coping behavior toward the pain experience.

*Group discussion* and *counseling* still retain much value as a means of working through the significance of chronic pain. Cognitive processes are used to develop methods of coping with pain by enhancing the influence of the central control system. The nurse and the patient need to plan a variety of coping strategies as an adjunct to medical treatments. Of particular import are nursing efforts to interrupt the progression of pain anxiety and increased pain which can become a self-sustaining cyclical pattern. Strategies aimed at increased pain control and anxiety reduction are most effective.

*Operant conditioning* is the treatment of pain based on the idea that learned responses to pain may be positively reinforced so that the pain behavior is either out of proportion to the noxious stimulus or persists in the absence of one. Expression of pain and withdrawal from a productive role are enhanced when wellness behavior is not reinforced or when illness behavior is. A patient, for example, is told to exercise until tolerance. This is done; pain is experienced, and the individual stops for a rest. If rest is seen positively, the patient will show pain more in order to be allowed to rest. The purpose of operant conditioning is reversal of this pattern by first identifying positive reinforcers of pain behavior and then, as an alternate, reinforcing wellness behavior. Currently, operant conditioning is most frequently used to break patterns of drug addiction in patients with chronic pain. Medication is given in liquid form at fixed time intervals rather than on the contingency of pain. Gradually, dosage is decreased in both amount and frequency until the patient is receiving only a placebo.

As discussed earlier, many health professionals object to both the behavior modification philosophy and the use of placebos. There are ethical issues

**TABLE 39-2**
TECHNIQUES USED IN THE TREATMENT OF CHRONIC PAIN

| Technique | Mechanism of Action | Limitations |
|---|---|---|
| Acupuncture | Hypotheses: (1) Produces psychological control over pain perception. (2) Local intense stimulation of large fibers by needles rotated rapidly at specific body sites closes the gate so that noxious stimuli are not transmitted to the brain. | Use of technique not widely accepted by physicians. Repeated treatments often needed. |
| Analgesics | Act at various sites, peripherally and centrally. Some alter reaction to pain, others interrupt transmission pathways. | Side effects common, some lethal. With narcotics, long-term use often results in addiction, possibly with overdosage. Not as effective if they are the only intervention. |
| Biofeedback | Increases an individual's control over pain through reduction of anxiety by developing the ability to control physiologic function, such as producing alpha waves in the brain. (Alpha waves are associated with relaxation.) Distracts person by forcing concentration on inner state and feedback signal. | Poor results to date with maintaining control beyond end of program, which itself requires a high degree of motivation. Has been unable to work with pain directly. Most successful in youth. |
| Electrical stimulation | Hypothesis: (1) Electrical stimulus alters electrical potential of nerve to prevent full depolarization and repolarization. (2) Increased sensory input yields increased inhibition by biasing system. (3) Stimulation of large fibers closes the spinal gate, preventing transmission of intense stimuli to the cortex. | Not tolerated by some patients due to tingling sensation produced. Patients may become habituated and require increased stimulus intensity with greater possibility of skin burn. Inconsistent duration of pain relief. Rarely exceeds 1 week. Can be used continuously. Minimal cost for use. Low success in emotionally unstable patients. |
| (a) Stimulation Trans- or Percutaneous | Uses electrodes positioned over painful area or nerve pathway which provide stimulation for 15 to 20 minutes. | Provides partial or total relief for only about half of those treated. May produce skin irritation or burns. |
| (b) Peripheral Nerve Implant or Dorsal Column Stimulator | Uses electrode attached directly to a major sensory nerve and wired to radio receiver in subcutaneous tissue, or electrode is attached over dorsal column at level determined by pain. Transmitter worn externally so that patient may initiate stimulus as needed. | Requires surgery, a laminectomy in the case of the dorsal column stimulator. Patient must be taught use of the equipment. |
| Group counseling | Encourages sharing of fear and concern, which helps to decrease anxiety. Provides group support, social demand. Use of cognitive system to develop and share strategies. | Group dysfunction. Lack of group availability. |
| Hypnosis | Decreases tension by decreasing anxiety. Increases central control system influence. Acts as a distractor. Promotes relaxation. Produces its effect through suggestion. | Usually insufficient alone. Requires careful screening and extensive training of patients. |
| Neurosurgery | Interrupts transmission of information about stimuli at either the peripheral or central level. In the absence of such stimuli, pain is not usually perceived. | Psychological contribution to pain experience is uncontrolled and may be sufficient to permit persistent pain despite nerve transection. |
| (a) Chemical nerve blocks | May be done to check efficacy of block before surgical transection. Neurolytic agent (alcohol or phenol) destroys nerve fibers, although they can regenerate. Anesthetic blocks transmission temporarily. Both therefore affect physiological capacity to transmit information about painful stimuli to the brain. | Sometimes difficult to find exact pathway to interrupt. May produce uncomfortable numbness and paresthesias. Temporary complications may be urine retention, paresis, headache (1 to 2 days usually). |

**TABLE 39-2**

TECHNIQUES USED IN THE TREATMENT OF CHRONIC PAIN (Continued)

| Technique | Mechanism of Action | Limitations |
|---|---|---|
| (b) Neurectomy | Destroys pain transmission paths by excising the offending nerve. | Does not always alleviate pain. |
| (c) Rhizotomy | Interrupts nerve transmission at anterior nerve root to decrease painful muscle spasm or at posterior nerve root to interrupt sensory function. Root is transected between ganglion and cord. | Requires a laminectomy. Produces loss of all sensation. Sensation may gradually return with pain or severe paresthesias. If bilateral, can sometimes yield postural hypotension. Poor results with nonmalignancy. |
| (d) Sympathectomy | Interferes with transmission by sympathetic afferent nerve pathways. Used primarily for causalgias, phantom pain, pain due to vascular disorders. | May produce some autonomic dysfunction. |
| (e) Cordotomy | Interrupts ascending cord tracts by surgical transection or by diathermy or radiothermy coagulation. Obliterates pain and temperature sensation below level of interruption without affecting other sensations or motor function. May be done via laminectomy or percutaneously. | Sensation may gradually return with pain and paresthesias. Complications of leg weakness and urine retention may last a few weeks, though sometimes may persist. Sexual function may be impaired in the male. Used most effectively for leg and trunk pain due to malignancy. |
| (f) Thalamotomy | Interrupts perception of pain as hurting through stereotaxic procedures such as thermocoagulation. Interrupts transmission of impulses through the thalamus. | Experimental procedure. Used for central pain syndromes or for intractable pain, but is generally reserved for the terminally ill since there may be some alteration in personality. |
| (g) Lobotomy | Modifies motivational-affective component of pain perception through destruction of tissues in frontal lobe. Division of thalamofrontal radiation. | Used as a last resort in patients with intractable pain due to malignancy. Causes alteration in personality. |
| (h) Gyrectomy | Resection of specific cortical areas (gyri) involved in the sensory-discriminative component of pain perception. | Used primarily for treatment of phantom limb pain. |
| Operant conditioning | Decreases negative pain behavior by consistently rewarding positive coping behavior and increased wellness behavior. Negative behavior not reinforced, therefore gradually extinguished. Most often used to break dependence on medication. | Usually requires hospitalization. Informed consent and other ethical considerations remain issues. |
| Physical medicine | Uses various measures (heat, cold, supportive devices, etc.) to remove the source of the pain or to provide general comfort. Examples: Traction to reduce muscle spasm associated with herniated disk, vessel dilation to reduce inflammation and increase oxygenation. | Useful for pain whose source can be readily localized. May be used as an adjunct to other treatments. |
| Psychotherapy | Intensive programs focusing on determination of the underlying cause of maladaptive behavior and on guiding the patient in finding and using more successful modes of coping. | Requires a long treatment period, motivation on part of the patient. May be too threatening to the patient to be of benefit, or even to be acceptable as a form of treatment. |
| Relaxation techniques (e.g., breathing exercises, muscle relaxation, meditation) | Reduce perception of pain by distraction, decrease in fatigue, dissociation of self from pain sensation. | Advanced techniques require practice. Often used as adjunct to other treatments. |
| X-ray therapy | Destroy pain-producing malignancy. | Multiple side effects of irradiation. |

and must be discussed. Possible detrimental effects on the patient/professional relationship must be considered along with the use of the effect of deception and the potential damage it could do to a patient's already weak self-concept. Issues concerning patient involvement in decisions as well as informed consent must be considered. Nurses must determine their role and actively participate in decisions justifying its use for a patient. Surgical intervention is usually made after other sources of treatment prove ineffective (see Table 39-2).

When permanent anesthesia to a body part is produced, through surgery as opposed to genetic inheritance of pain absence, careful instructions about safety precautions will be needed. Patients experiencing pain absence need to be taught self-care activities to compensate for loss of sensation. They will need to establish a daily routine for checking injuries, avoiding activities which would predispose them to unrecognized injury, and avoiding extremes in temperature. Body parts such as the hands, face, and feet should be protected if the potential for injury is high.

While surgical intervention is not the only solution to relief of acute pain, it may be one option available to the patient at this time. Nursing interventions as suggested earlier may need continually to be incorporated into the plan of care should surgical relief be unsuccessful.

## SUMMARY

The final step in caring for patients with all levels of pain is evaluation of the effectiveness of the care given, based on the objectives set in the planning stage. Depending upon the kind of pain work initiated by the nurse and patient, the nurse should determine whether the patient's ability to tolerate pain has increased through effective use of a greater range of coping strategies, whether the patient is better able to control the pain, and whether fewer negative pain behaviors are present. The absence of physiologic signs of pain indicates that acute or transitional pain has been reduced or alleviated. Anxiety level should decline. With successful coping strategies or reduction in pain, the patient's activity level and degree of social and environmental interaction will increase with a concomitant decrease in disruption of family life. Finally, the nurse seeks evidence that the patient has integrated the pain experience into his or her total life pattern.

This analysis reflects only broad areas for evaluation. The nurse should plan more specific objectives for individual patients and conduct an ongoing evaluation of progress made toward those objectives.

Care of the patient in pain is one of the most challenging aspects of nursing. This discussion has provided only a structure for analyzing pain and planning care. It has shown that nursing care may be initiated when a person cannot avoid, reduce, or tolerate pain through the use of the individual's own repertoire; when pain reduces the person's ability to care for herself or himself; or when pain persists and threatens system exhaustion. The nurse's specific actions are geared entirely to the needs of the individual patient precisely because of the highly individualistic nature of pain. The nurse can be a powerful ally against pain.

## REFERENCES

1   C. MacBryde and R. Blacklow, *Signs and Symptoms: Applied Pathologic Physiology and Clinical Interpretation,* 5th ed., Lippincott, Philadelphia, 1970, pp. 44–61.

2   G. Engel, "Psychogenic Pain and the Pain Prone Patient," *Am J Med,* **26:**901, June 1959.

3   W. Wehrmacher, "Introduction to Pain Symposium," *Med Dig,* **42:**20, January 1975.

4   S. Silverman, *Psychological Aspects of Physical Symptoms,* Meredith Press, New York, 1968.

5   R. Melzack and P. Wall: "Pain Mechanisms: A New Theory," *Science,* **150:**971–979, November 1965.

6   R. Melzack, "Phantom Limb Pain: Implications for Treatment of Pathologic Pain," *Anesthesiology,* **35:** 409–419, October 1971.

7   D. Nichols and B. Tursky, "Body Image, Anxiety, and Tolerance for Experimental Pain," *Psychosom Med,* **29:**103–110, 1967.

8   A. Petrie, W. Collins, and P. Solomon, "The Tolerance for Pain and for Sensory Deprivation," *Am J Psychol,* **73:**80, 1960.

9   E. Libman, "Observations on Individual Sensitiveness to Pain," *JAMA,* **102:**335, 1934.

10   A. Strauss, S. Fagerhaugh, and B. Glaser, "Pain: An Organizational-Work-Interactional Perspective," *Nurs Outlook,* **22:**560–566, September, 1974.

11   R. Sternbach, *Pain, A Psychophysiological Analysis,* Academic, New York, 1968, p. 151.

12   R. Black, "The Chronic Pain Syndrome," *Surg Clin North Am,* **55:**999–1011, August 1975.

13   M. Zborowski, *People in Pain,* Jossey-Bass, San Francisco, Calif., 1969.

14   H. Beecher, "Relationship of Significance of Wound to Pain Experienced," *JAMA,* **161:**1609–1612, 1956.

15  A. Fisher, "A Correlative Study of Pain and Its Alternatives," *Headache*, **12:**105–119, October 1972.

16  D. Vernon, "Modeling and Birth Order in Responses to Painful Stimuli," *J Pers Soc Psychol*, **29:** 794–799, June 1974.

17  Strauss, Fagerhaugh, and Glaser, *op. cit.*

18  M. McBride, "Nursing Approach, Pain and Relief: An Exploratory Experiment," *Nurs Res*, **16:**337–341, Fall 1967.

19  Melzack, Wall, *op. cit.*

20  L. LeShan, "The World of the Patient in Severe Pain of Long Duration," *J Chron Dis*, **17:**119–126, 1964.

21  A. Fisher, "A Correlative Study of Pain and Its Alternatives," *Headache*, **12:**105–119, October 1972.

## BIBLIOGRAPHY

Baer, E., et al.: "Inferences of Physical Pain and Psychological Distress in Relation to Verbal and Non-Verbal Patient Communication," *Nurs Res*, **19:** 388–392, October/November, 1970.

Beland, I., and J. Passos: *Clinical Nursing: Pathophysiological and Psychosocial Approaches*, 3d ed., Macmillan, New York, 1975, pp. 270–281.

Belville, J., et al.: "Influence of Age on Pain Relief from Analgesics," *JAMA*, **217:**1835–1841, September 1971.

Bennett, M.: "The Pathophysiology of Pain," *Curr Probl Surg*, 6–15, February 1973.

Bobey, M., and P. Davidson: "Psychological Factors Affecting Pain Tolerance," *J Psychosom Res*, **14:** 371–376, December 1970.

Bonica, J.: "Fundamental Considerations of Chronic Pain Therapy," *Postgrad Med*, **53:**81–85, May 1973.

Botton, J.: "Neurosurgical Procedures for the Management of Intractable Pain," *Clinical Orthop*, **73:** 101–108, November/December 1970.

Carini, E., and G. Owens: *Neurological and Neurosurgical Nursing*, 6th ed., Mosby, St. Louis, 1974.

Casey, K.: "The Neurophysiologic Basis of Pain," *Postgrad Med*, **53:**58–63, May 1973.

Copp, L. A.: "The Spectrum of Suffering," *Am J Nurs*, **74:**491–495, March 1974.

Craig, K., and H. Neidermayer: "Autonomic Correlates of Pain Thresholds Influenced by Social Modeling," *J Pers Soc Psychol*, **29:**246–252, February 1974.

Crowley, D.: *Pain and Its Alleviation, Am Surg,* University of California Press, Los Angeles, 1962.

Dodson, H., and H. Bennett: "Relief of Postoperative Pain," **20:**405–409, April 1954.

Drakontides, A.: "Drugs to Treat Pain," *Am J Nurs*, **74:** 508–513, March 1974.

Engel, G.: "Psychogenic Pain and the Pain-Prone Patient," *Am J Med*, **26:**899–918, 1959.

Fordyce, W.: "An Operant Conditioning Method for Managing Chronic Pain," *Postgrad Med*, **53:** 123–128, May, 1973.

Gildea, J.: "The Relief of Postoperative Pain," *Med Clin North Am*, **52:**81–89, January 1968.

Guyton, A.: *Textbook of Medical Physiology*, 5th ed., Saunders, Philadelphia, 1976.

Hackett, T.: "Pain and Prejudice," *Med Times*, **99:** 130–141, February 1971.

Hardy, J., H. Wolff, and H. Goodell: *Pain Sensations and Reactions*, Hafner, New York, 1967, pp. 262–391.

Jannetta, P.: "Introduction to the Neurosurgical Approach to the Relief of Pain," *Curr Prob Surg*, 3–6, February 1973.

Kane, F., et al.: "A Case of Congenital Indifference to Pain," *Dis Nerv Syst*, **29:**409–412, June 1968.

Kanfer, F., and D. Goldfoot: "Self-Control and Tolerance of Noxious Stimulation," *Psychol Rep*, **18:** 79–85, 1966.

———— and M. Seidner: "Self-Control: Factors Enhancing Tolerance of Noxious Stimulation," *Psychol Rep*, **25:**381–389, March 1973.

Keats, A.: "Postoperative Pain: Research and Treatment," *J Chron Dis*, **4:**72–83, July 1956.

Kolb, L.: "Symbolic Significance of the Complaint of Pain," *Clin Neurosurg*, **8:**248–257, 1962.

Luckman, J., and K. Sorensen: *Medical Surgical Nursing: A Psychophysiologic Approach*, Saunders, Philadelphia, 1974, pp. 545–582.

McBride, M.: "Scientific Bases for Therapeutic Nursing Practice—Evaluation of Nursing Action," *ANA Clinical Sessions*, Appleton-Century-Crofts, New York, 1966, pp. 75–82.

MacBryde, C., and R. Blacklow (eds.): *Signs and Symptoms: Applied Pathologic Physiology and Clinical Interpretation*, 5th ed., Lippincott, Philadelphia, 1970.

McCaffery, M.: *Nursing Management of the Patient with Pain*, Lippincott, Philadelphia, 1972.

Maroon, J., and P. Jannetta: "Pain Following Peripheral Nerve Injuries," *Curr Prob Surg*, 20–32, February 1973.

Mastrovito, R.: "Psychogenic Pain," *Am J Nurs*, **74:** 514–519, March 1974.

Melzack, R., and W. Torgerson: "On the Language of Pain," *Anesthesiology*, **34:**50–59, June 1971.

Merskey, H.: "Pain, Learning and Memory," *J Psychosom Res*, **19:**319–324, 1975.

———— and F. Spear: *Pain: Psychological and Psy-*

*chiatric Aspects,* Baillière, London, 1967, p. 89.

Moss, F., and B. Meyer: "The Effects of Nursing Interaction upon Pain Relief in Patients," *Nurs Res,* **15:**303–306, Fall 1966.

"Pain," Pt. I, "Basic Concepts and Assessment," *Am J Nurs,* **66:**1085–1108, May 1966.

"Pain," Pt. II, "Rationale for Intervention," *Am J Nurs,* **66:**1345–1368, June 1966.

Roberts, A.: "Biofeedback Techniques," *Minn Med,* **57:**167–171, March 1974.

Selker, R., and P. Jannetta: "Central Pain and Central Therapy of Pain," *Curr Prob Surg,* 59–64, February 1973.

Siegele, D.: "The Gate Control Theory," *Am J Nurs,* **74:**498–502, March 1974.

Smith, M.: "Nursing Knowledge and Activity in Relation to the Period of Anticipation of Pain in the Adult," *Solving Difficult Problems in Nursing Care,* American Nurses Association, Monograph #20, 1962.

Soulairac, A., J. Cahn, and J. Charpentier (eds.): *Pain,* Proceedings of the International Symposium on Pain, April 11–13, 1967, Academic, New York, 1968.

Sternbach, R.: *Pain, A Psychophysiological Analysis,* Academic, New York, 1968.

——— and G. Timmerman: "Factors of Human Chronic Pain: An Analysis of Personality and Pain Reaction Variables," *Science,* **184:**806–808, May 1974.

Swerdlow, M.: "Relieving Pain in the Terminally Ill," *Geriatrics,* **28:**100–103, July 1973.

Thomason, R., and S. Kim: Transcutaneous Stimulators in Pain Control, *Med Dig,* **42:**33–34, January 1975.

Voris, H.: "Treatment of Chronic or Intractable Pain by Neurosurgical Measures," *Med Dig,* **42:**35–42, January 1975.

Wolff, H., and S. Wolf: *Pain,* 2d ed., Charles C Thomas, Springfield, Ill., 1958, pp. 13–24, 89.

Wurster, R.: "Mechanisms of Pain and Pain Reflexes," *Med Dig,* **42:**23–30, January 1975.

# 40
# SKELETAL-MUSCULAR DISTURBANCES IN PERCEPTION AND COORDINATION

Elaine Sztyndor Clancy

An intact skeletal-muscular system provides protection for internal organs, gives shape and form to the body, and provides an individual with coordination and balance. As a person begins to interact with stimuli in the external environment, interruptions in the continuity of the bone structure can occur. Such events as trauma, altered auto-immune responses, and infections can produce significant alterations in the structure and function of bones and muscles.

One's perceptions of the surrounding environment are often influenced by the ability to move from place to place selectively and independently. Individuals who sustain skeletal-muscular disturbances are often suddenly faced with an acute health problem complicated by alterations in body image, pain, deformity, and temporary or permanent dependence. With the threat of coordination altered and perception disrupted, the individual will require assistance from health care deliverers in order to continue to carry out activities of daily living in a meaningful way.

## SKELETAL-MUSCULAR TRAUMA

*Trauma* to muscles and bones results when there is an immediate insult to the skeletal-muscular structure. The changes that follow vary in degree of severity depending upon the nature of the trauma, the location of the injury, the age and developmental stage of the individual, and the extent to which injury to a muscle and/or bone disrupts the integrity and functioning of other bodily components.

### Fracture

Perhaps the most frequent health problem associated with skeletal-muscular functioning is the fracture. A *fracture* is an interruption and/or disruption in the normal continuity of a bone due to the exertion of excessive force or stress. Fractures can occur in any bone of the body and can result in altered function of other body components.

Normally a bone has a degree of internal resistance to absorb a force from the external environment. However, when the bone's "elastic limit" (i.e., that point of stress absorption beyond which a bone will break) is reached, a fracture results. *Force* can be defined as a push or pull in any direction. It can be direct or shearing.

The direct forces can be *tensile,* causing the bone to pull apart, or *compressive,* resulting in bones being pushed together. Shearing forces, on the other hand, are those forces which are applied perpendicularly to the long axis of the bone. These forces produce *torsion* or a "twist" in the bone, resulting in a fracture away from the point where the initial force was applied.

**Types of fractures**  The *type* of fracture that an individual sustains will vary with the direction of the force applied. In addition, internal forces of muscle pull on the bone also influence the type of fracture the individual may incur. A bone under stress is pulled toward the strongest muscle into which a particular bone inserts. Frequently the muscle pull can cause overriding of bone fragments.

Several classifications have been developed to aid in describing the appearance of a particular fracture after the bone has been disrupted. Table 40-1 contains a listing of some of the more common fractures along with a definition of the type of bone

**TABLE 40-1**
COMMON FRACTURES

| | |
|---|---|
| Avulsion: | Bone fragment is torn away with muscle damage, e.g., with sprained ankle |
| Capillary: | Hairline fracture, very thin |
| Closed: | No trauma to skin integrity |
| Comminuted: | Bone is broken into many fragments |
| Complete (transverse): | Bone is broken across, with disruption of both sides of the periosteum |
| Complex: | Closed, with soft tissue damage |
| Complicated: | Fracture with injury to adjacent organ, e.g., fractured rib with punctured lung |
| Compound: | Wound communicates from the bone to the surface owing to trauma to both the soft tissue and the bone, or the bone tears through the soft tissue as it fractures |
| Compression: | One bony surface is forced against an adjacent one, as in the vertebrae |
| Displaced: | With dislocations |
| Epiphyseal and epicondylar: | At the respective locations |
| Greenstick: | Incomplete, only one side of the periosteum is disturbed. |
| Impacted: | One part of the fractured bone has been driven into another part |
| Linear: | Occurs parallel to the bone |
| Oblique: | Fractures occurring at a 45° angle to the bone shaft |
| Pathological (also Spontaneous): | Occurs in the presence of a problem or tumor in the bone |
| Simple: | Clean break in the bone; skin not disrupted |
| Spiral: | Results from twisting force; fracture twists around the bone |
| Trophic: | Due to weakening of the bone from metabolic imbalance |
| Undisplaced: | No dislocation of the bony structures |

changes that result. Figure 40-1 contains a composite drawing of some of the most common fractures.

**Pathophysiology**  When a bone is fractured, there is bleeding at the site of injury due to blood vessel rupture and trauma to surrounding tissue. A *local inflammatory response* occurs as a result of the injury, and fluid accumulates. This can cause stretching of tissue, compression on nerve endings, and pain. Ecchymosis is usually present due to trauma to tissue. Muscle spasm may result from involuntary muscle contractions and is often seen in the presence of an overriding bone.

Muscle enzymes are released into the circulation when injury occurs. Metabolites increase in number and are carried to the injured site by circulatory diversion to the area. Oxygen and nutrients are rushed to the area of insult within 24 hours to begin the healing process.

*Healing* occurs in four stages. These are hematoma formation, cellular growth, callus formation, and ossification or bone union.[1] Following the initial bleeding at the site of injury, a *hematoma,* or clot, forms at the break and surrounds the fractured bone. This clot is not reabsorbed but becomes part of the bone itself as healing progresses. The hematoma contains white blood cells and fibrin.

One day after the injury, *cellular growth* begins with capillaries developing into the clot and fibroblasts (spindle-shaped cells) multiplying. Several days later dead tissue and debris resulting from the fracture are removed by phagocytosis. (See Chap. 8 for a discussion of healing in general.)

The formation of soft tissue callus, or *provisional callus,* results from fibroblastic multiplication. In about three weeks, the osteoblast cells of the bone form an osteoid matrix.[2] In this matrix, the callus is developed from the deposition of calcium salts. The callus contains new blood vessel growth. In the adult, this process takes 2 to 3 months, with a characteristic overproduction of callus. Stress or weight bearing is necessary for normal osteoblastic activity. Stress on the callus tissue causes it to resemble parent bone. This process is called *modeling.* The excess callus is then absorbed. With the joining together of new and old bone, *ossification,* or bone union, is completed, and the healing process terminated.

The length of the healing period is usually dependent upon many variables. These include the person's current health status, age, type of fracture, location of injury, and whether bone union is stopped or delayed by other health problems.

Generally, in uncomplicated fractures, healing will occur more rapidly in children (4 to 6 weeks) as opposed to adults, who take much more time (2 to 4 months and longer). If circulation to an area is interrupted by the fracture or obstruction of an artery or vein, healing is further delayed. If the injury occurs in a weight-bearing bone, it takes longer to heal than in a bone absorbing less body stress. In addition, smaller bones tend to heal more rapidly, while long bones can take more time and predispose the individual to more complications. *Contaminated,* complete fractures also can take longer to heal because of the danger of infection. Bones that fracture, injuring other body structures, may also experience prolonged healing times, as well as bones improperly immobilized at the time of injury. Age also influences healing time.

**C**auses of Fracture   Individuals are always subject to traumatic injury of muscles and bones due to excess force. Fractures may result from an automobile accident, a sudden fall, or any movement which would apply a sudden unnatural force to bone or surrounding tissue.

*Fatigue* decreases an individual's resistance to trauma. Normally muscles apply force to a bone and keep it in alignment. Tired, overworked muscles provide diminished support to the bone, and overfatigued muscles can cause an uneven pull on the underlying bone. This force applied to the bone is often compounded by outside stressors. Frequently, skiiers will sustain a fracture on the "last run" of the day. Generally, this occurs because the individual has become overtired by the activity of the day, and during a fall the muscles are less supportive to the bone and cannot absorb the force being exerted. As a result, the bone may fracture.

Bone *neoplasms* affect cellular structure by the formation of lesions that can result in fracture. The cellular proliferation of malignant cells replaces normal tissue and causes the bone to weaken to the point that a very slight force may overstress it, causing it to fracture. This type of fracture is sometimes referred to as a *pathological* fracture.

*Metabolic* disorders such as poor mineral absorption and hormonal changes can *decrease bone calcification* and result in unstable, weak bone tissue. These changes lead to such health problems as Paget's disease and osteoporosis.

*Bed rest* or *disuse* of muscles and bones will similarly result in weakened, atrophic muscle and fragile bones. Osteoporosis may also contribute to fracture formation, owing to demineralization of the bone matrix. Tissue at rest requires decreased oxy-

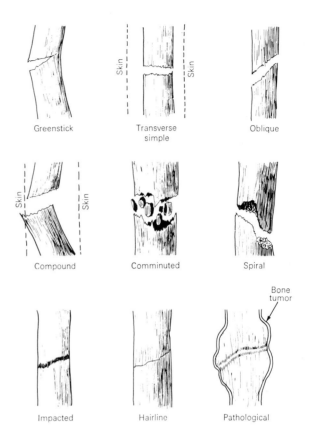

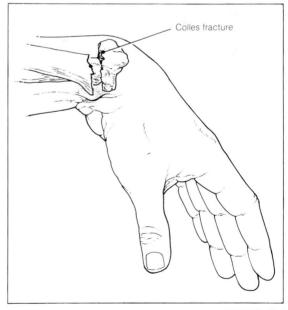

**FIGURE 40-1**

Common fractures. (*Adapted from Moidel et al., Nursing Care of the Patient with Medical-Surgical Disorders, 2d ed., McGraw-Hill, New York, 1976.*)

gen and diminished circulatory demands. The result is little tissue proliferation and decreased stress resistance. Lack of adequate exercise can produce similar problems.

There is some thinking that one's personality can affect one's predisposition to fractures. The so-called *high-risk* individual or the person readily willing to take a dare is often in danger because of personal activities and social encounters. Driving at high speeds or diving into shallow water can lead to serious fracture and related health problems.

**E**ffects of a Fracture   An individual who sustains a fracture will usually experience a variety of effects. *Pain* is generally the most persistent and is usually present immediately following the injury. It is intensified in the presence of *ecchymosis* and swelling at the fracture site which compresses nerve endings and increases tenderness and pain perception. In some injuries to the spine the absence of pain due to trauma to the spinal cord can be most significant.

Normal range of joint motion is limited if not completely eliminated, and a so-called "false motion" is present. The latter term refers to inappropriate movement at a joint. When lower extremities are involved, there is interruption in *gait* and *balance,* and activity decreases.

Fracture of ribs can interfere with normal respiration and inhibit adequate *oxygenation,* particularly, if ribs perforate the lungs. *Bleeding* into any organ or body cavity can occur secondarily to a fracture. The pelvis is a particularly vascular area, and fracturing of bones in this area can lead to bleeding into the pelvis or bladder. Rupture of the uterus along with trauma to the spleen, bladder, or intestines can also occur. When blood loss is significant, signs of shock may appear.

*Metabolic* needs rapidly increase following a fracture as calcification of bone tissue depends on an adequate supply of nutrients to the area. When blood vessels are severed, or their circulation occluded by the fracture itself, oxygen and nutrients are prevented from reaching an area, and tissue necrosis can occur.

In the presence of a skull fracture there may be bleeding into the tissue and an increase in intracranial pressure (see Chap. 32). Alterations in the level of consciousness, mental confusion, changes in vital signs or parasthesia, may occur following injury and increased pressure. Injury to the spine can damage the spinal cord producing *paralysis, numbness, tingling,* and *loss of sensation* throughout the body. These changes can be temporary or permanent, depending upon the level of injury. (See Chapter 32 for a discussion of spinal cord injury.)

The effects of a fracture on the patient are both psychological and physical. Not to be overlooked in fracture causation and effect is the activity in which the patient was involved when the trauma was incurred.

**First-level nursing care**   In any health setting, a nurse should be mindful of fracture prevention. This requires assessment and identification of problems that can lead to fractures. Foremost should be an understanding of the causes of fractures and recognition of their application to clients. Individuals who exercise to the point of fatigue, persons weak and debilitated, those with poor eyesight, or those of poor nutritional status, the elderly with metabolic changes causing a decrease in bone density, or individuals with a neoplastic disorder are people predisposed to fractures.

**P**revention   By being attuned to these problems, the nurse can have much input into care planning and health teaching for each patient. *Safety* is the key point in prevention of accidents and bone trauma. Teaching about the use of good body mechanics to prevent unnatural stress to the skeletal-muscular system is an important component of prevention. Environmental factors including the appropriate use of side rails, proper bed position, locking of wheelchairs when the patient is being transferred, using stretcher straps, and cleaning spills to prevent slippery floors are all important components of safety especially appropriate in hospital settings.

The nurse can also do much teaching regarding the *home environment.* Concern for the age and life-style of the patient and other family members along with knowledge of the patient's home environment are important to facilitate this point. The nurse must encourage use of handrails in bathrooms and on steps, removal of loose rugs underfoot, and improvement of lighting which would cause people to trip or bump into unseen objects. This is especially important when caring for the elderly in the home. Advice can also be given against moving or lifting heavy, awkward articles and standing on an unstable surface, like an unstable stepladder. Prompt removal of ice from pavements and steps is critical. Further, if there are young children in the family, gates at stairways should be used to prevent falling accidents. In the car, seatbelts have been proved effective in decreasing injury during a crash. Special car seats should be recommended for all infants. When packing the car, loose items should be placed in the trunk. In the event of a sudden stop, these objects can become dangerous flying missiles if left inside the passenger compartment.

Careful planning to prevent fractures in patients with identified neoplastic processes is essential, especially when metastatic changes are present. Safety in transferring these patients about is critical.

All individuals should engage in activities which will help strengthen their muscles and help resist external force that could predispose fracture formation. Exercise programs should be planned for hospitalized patients, the elderly, or individuals with long-term illnesses.

Teaching plans should also be directed toward prevention of traffic accidents. Support of reduced speed limits along with reduction in the use of alcohol while driving (see Chap. 19) may help reduce injury.

**Second-level nursing care** Fractures most often occur in the community, and immediate care of the patient is critically important before transferring the patient to an acute-care setting. Therefore, emergency care will be discussed initially. Since many patients are cared for on an outpatient basis, health history, nursing assessment, and identification of problems and nursing intervention will also be discussed.

Nursing Assessment Where possible, a detailed *health history* should focus on the events leading up to the injury, including a description of the injury itself, the setting in which it occurred, and identification of any major health problems. The patient will complain of acute pain and may be extremely anxious. Depending on the severity of these symptoms, the patient may be crying and hysterical. When pain is acute or the fracture severe, fainting, dizziness, and generalized weakness may be present. Immediately following an injury, the individual may be dazed by the experience, but anxiety may intensify with the realization of the accident.

*Physical assessment* Physical assessment should focus on the fracture itself and systemic injury which can affect the survival of the patient. Measurement of blood pressure and pulse rate are important parameters when assessing shock. Bleeding sites should be noted, and peripheral pulses as well as skin temperature checked. The respiratory

rate should be determined, and bilateral chest movements assessed. The airway should be checked for obstruction and made patent. The patient's body warmth and skin color should be ascertained. Level of consciousness, pupillary response, peripheral, sensory, and motor response, and vocalizations should also be determined.

When a bone is fractured, there is an interruption in the normal contour and function of the bone structure. The *cardinal signs of a fracture* are pain or tenderness over the involved area, loss of function to the extremity, and deformity. Pain is present and often difficult to fully assess since bone pain tends to be more diffuse than pain from other causes (see Chap. 39 for discussion of pain). When local swelling and/or hemorrhage are present, the pain may be more intense.

*Muscle spasm* caused by a reflex action of the nerve when stimulated, as with tension or compression of the periosteum in a fracture, will also increase pain.[3]

*Overriding,* as a result of muscle spasms, will cause a deformed-looking extremity. There may also be an open wound or bruising in the area. *Angulation* refers to the placement of a limb in an unnatural position due to fracture and may be seen in the fractured limbs.

*False motion* may also be noted. When determining the presence of a fracture, one should be alert for vascular and nerve impairment to the extremity. Periodic checks should be made to determine the presence or absence of peripheral pulses. Determination of skin color and temperature will help to assess circulation and sensation in the extremities.

*Crepitation,* or the grating sound heard upon movement of broken bones, may be present. In addition, redness, ecchymosis, and swelling may also be observed.

Whenever a fracture is suspected, there should be concern for spinal injury. Even if there is an absence of symptoms, the nurse must be highly suspicious of spinal trauma in any accident where there might have been direct injury to the head, neck, or back. There may be no pain if the patient does not move, but movement to determine the presence of cord damage should be avoided. Tenderness may be observed on palpation of the vertebral area. Deformity may or may not be present. The nurse must be highly suspicious of a neck fracture if the patient does have a facial or scalp wound. A laceration or hematoma on the trunk may be a cue to a thoracic or lumbar injury.

**E**mergency Nursing Care   When a fracture is suspected, top priority goes to immediate lifesaving measures such as extricating an individual from an entangled automobile, using cardiopulmonary resuscitation (see Chap. 26), preventing hemorrhage (see Chap. 28), and assessing vital signs. Massive shock is treated prior to caring for a fractured extremity. In the presence of possible cervical spine injury, care is taken not to cause added trauma to the spinal cord by hyperextending the neck to clear an obstructed airway. The patient should be kept on a flat plane and transported only on a firm, flat surface. In the presence of massive hemorrhage, an attempt should be made to apply pressure in such a way as not to cause greater soft tissue damage at fractured bone ends. Elevation of the extremity will help reduce swelling as well as bleeding.

Often *pain* may be severe. If there are no contraindications (e.g., central nervous system involvement), analgesia may be used to relieve pain and thus decrease muscle spasm. When a fracture is suspected and pain is not present, spinal cord injury should be considered.

If the skin has been broken, it should be cared for as a contaminated wound containing potentially pathogenic substances. Where possible the skin around the break should be cleansed and the open area covered with a sterile dressing. When the patient arrives at an acute-care center, additional wound debridement will be required to prevent infection. Tetanus antitoxin 0.5 cc may be given if the patient had not had a dose in the past 5 years. The fractured site should also be observed for edema. Rings and watches must be removed early so that they will not obstruct circulation if swelling does occur. Again, elevation of the extremity may help reduce this problem.

A fracture is always treated as a true one until it can be positively diagnosed by x-ray. An attempt to realign the extremity without x-ray control could result in even greater soft tissue injury and can cause further periosteal trauma.

Muscle is normally held in slight tension by bone. A fractured bone, however, lends less support to the muscle, allowing for abnormal contraction of the muscle. Splinting will provide support to the muscle and minimize muscle spasm.

*Splinting*   The method whereby an external support made of wood, plastic, plaster, etc., is applied around a fractured site to immobilize the broken bone ends and restrict movement is termed *splinting.*

Splinting a fracture will (1) help reduce additional damage, (2) reduce pain, (3) decrease muscle spasm, (4) limit movement, and (5) stimulate healing. It is an initial step taken by the nurse prior to moving the patient to a health care facility. If the limb is malaligned, it should be splinted as well as possible in the position in which it was found. Attempts to put the injured bone into proper alignment may result in added trauma.

Prior to applying splints, the nurse should make the patient aware of the reason for splinting and should be mindful of any complaints or discomfort caused by the splints, especially paresthesias and increasing pain. Splints should not be constricting but well padded to avoid untoward pressure to the area.

When applying splints, it is important to maintain normal body alignment as much as possible. A single bone is not an entity unto itself, but is affected by muscle groups above and below the area of injury. Therefore, splints should be applied above and below the area of injury. While the splint is applied, a slight use of traction should be employed.

*Air splints,* clear plastic inflatable splints, come in a variety of sizes and shapes and can be used with injuries of the extremities. They provide good support and are easy to apply. Since they are made of plastic, contact with sharp objects must be avoided to prevent puncturing. Air splints cannot always offer adequate immobilization to all fractures. When splinting a fracture of an upper extremity, the upper arm should be splinted to the chest wall for greater stability (see Fig. 40-2).

Materials such as air splints and rigid boards are usually found in an emergency unit or with an ambulance or rescue service. However, if these are not available, such things as pillows, rolled blankets, pieces of wood, or newspapers can be secured with rags to the limb to limit movement.

After an area has been splinted, the *extremity can be elevated* to promote venous return and help prevent edema. Care should be taken so as not to strain the joints by poor positioning.

**D**iagnostic Tests   Upon the arrival to an emergency room or health station, an x-ray will be taken of the affected area and read immediately. X-rays should offer both anterior and lateral views of the injured site as well as functional positions when possible.

**N**ursing Problems and Interventions as an Outpatient   Following the immediate emergency care, the patient will be treated in an emergency room, clinic, or rescue area, then released to home care with follow-up visits. When there is injury, the patient can be referred to an acute health care setting for more extensive treatment.

Generally the patient will still be in *pain* and be *anxious*. If an analgesic has not been administered, it is usually given upon arrival at the health facility. There will still be *edema* and local swelling of the affected part, but if splinted, the affected part may be elevated. If the bone has not yet been aligned, deformity may be present which can enhance both pain and anxiety.

*Reduction of the fracture*  Immediate intervention of a fracture consists of setting the bone and immobilizing it. A procedure called *closed reduction* is done to place the bone in proper alignment. Closed reduction is the manual reduction of a fracture without the use of surgical intervention. It involves maneuvering the injured bone back into correct alignment so that healing can begin. After reduction, a great number of fractures are immobilized by cast application. *Casting* is the application of temporary external support to immobilize the bone and enhance healing. This intervention is advantageous for both the hospitalized patient and the outpatient. Casting affords the injured area protection and firm support. Pain and swelling are alleviated because further trauma to the periosteum and soft tissue has been eliminated. During application of the cast, some traction can be applied to the extremity in order to achieve optimal alignment. *Manual traction* involves exerting a pull by the hands distally to the injured site, in order to achieve healing of the bone. This stress created by traction enhances healing and good modeling.

There is a choice of cast material to be used (see Table 40-2). Because of its easy availability, plaster is still the more common choice. In addition to the cast material, stockinette, felt padding for the bony prominences, and, occasionally, splints are needed prior to cast application. Stockinette is ap-

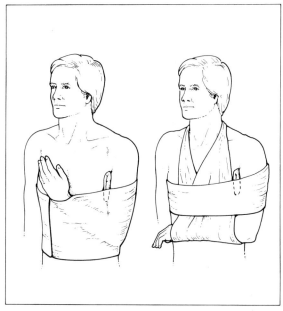

**FIGURE 40-2**
Splinting of upper extremity. (*Drawing by Julie Rotta.*)

plied to the area with care to avoid wrinkles, as this could later be a source of pressure for decubiti formation. Whenever the limb is supported during cast application, the palms should be used instead of the fingers to avoid uncomfortable pressure points for the patient. If a plaster cast is being applied, continued use of the palms of the hand is essential to prevent denting the plaster.

Prior to *cast application,* it is most important to prepare the patient for the procedure to help ensure better cooperation throughout. In order to minimize anxiety and discomfort, the nurse should foresee the patient's need for pain medication prior to cast application. As the cast is applied, the patient

**TABLE 40-2**
TYPES OF CAST MATERIAL

| Material | Advantages | Disadvantages |
|---|---|---|
| Plaster of paris | No special equipment needed<br>Inexpensive<br>Odorless | Heavy<br>Requires long drying time<br>Not porous<br>Easily breaks<br>Softens when wet |
| Light cast | Lightweight<br>Will not soften in water<br>Porous: allows for airflow into cast<br>Sturdy: does not crack | Requires special heat lamp to cure<br>More expensive<br>Unpleasant odor after application, may be irritating to patient |

should know that there will be a feeling of warmth for 10 to 30 minutes as the cast sets. Complaints of intense burning may require removing the cast and checking the skin. A patient with extremely sensitive skin may indeed be burned during a cast application, for a plaster cast will take 24 to 48 hours to dry. The patient should know that there can be no weight bearing until the cast is dry. After the initial warmth, a cool, damp feeling can be expected until the cast is dry. After a cast is applied, the patient often has a great deal of mobility. In the case of a leg cast, assisted ambulation may be feasible. A sling can provide support to the arm as the patient carries out daily activities. (See Chap. 34 for a discussion of sling application.)

Trauma caused by the fracture as well as manipulation of the injured area during reduction will result in *edema.* Elevation of the extremity above the level of the heart will help promote venous return. In some instances casting is delayed one or more days to allow the edema to resolve.

If swelling persists, the chance of *vascular insult* increases. With the extremity contained within a confined space, the tissue will be able to expand only to clearly defined limits. As a result, pressure is created and circulation to the area is compromised.

Edema will cause pressure on the edges of the cast which the nurse can observe. Checks of circulation, including skin color and temperature, and of peripheral pulses of the exposed distal extremity should be carried out hourly for the first 24 hours. If changes in circulation are noted at any time, the patient should be instructed to contact the physician or nurse immediately.

Signs of increasing *pain* due to the presence of edema and compression of nerve endings, as well as the muscle spasm, must be carefully evaluated. Analgesics should be taken as prescribed to help minimize the discomfort. Again, elevation of the affected part will stimulate venous return, eliminate congestion, and reduce pressure on nerve endings. An increase in pain intensity should be evaluated by the physician or nurse. Complaints of increased pain, particularly that pain which is removed from the site of injury or not relieved by analgesia, should be assessed.

If *neurovascular embarrassment* is evident, the physician should be notified immediately. Changes that will be noted include numbness (paresthesia) and tingling loss of sensation. These symptoms should be monitored every 15 minutes and the findings recorded. Increased elevation of the extremity may help promote venous return and limit pressure

on nerve endings. If the problem is not relieved by these interventions, the cast may have to be removed or *bivalved.* Bivalving a cast involves splitting it to allow for improved circulation by reducing compression.

The nurse will need to deal with the patient's discomfort within the confines of a *drying cast.* The cast should be exposed to air to hasten drying. The patient should not cover the cast with heavy blankets. These may keep the patient warm, but will hold in the dampness and prolong the drying time. Exposed areas, like toes, can be covered with a small towel for warmth. A heat lamp can be used to hasten drying of the cast, provided it is not left on one area too long, since plaster will conduct heat if exposed long enough. If the patient can feel heat under the cast, it may mean burning of tissue has occurred.

A dry cast is firm, white, shiny, and odorless. Soft spots or cracks can weaken the cast and should be noted early. The cast edges should be padded to prevent skin abrasion. When edema subsides, the cast should be checked for careful fit. Looking down into the cast with a flashlight to check for skin changes will help detect early signs of infection or tissue breakdown.

*Skin breakdown* Steps should be taken to maintain the integrity of the skin. Skin under a cast becomes very friable. The nurse should check for maceration under the cast edges and foul odors. The use of sticky, slow-drying lotions which can be irritating should be avoided.

Itching is a particular problem of patients with casts. The tendency is to find anything which will fit inside a cast and use it as a scratcher. This can cause a break in the skin, which is then a prime target for infection within the warm, dark environment. Careful explanations of the dangers of this are warranted. Children, especially, must be cautioned against dropping small toys or objects down the cast for safe-keeping. Parents should be taught to check the cast periodically for such items. For the problem of itching, some physicians lay a gauze strip along the extremity before the cast is applied, leaving both ends exposed for use as a scratcher. Also, cool air from a hair dryer can be directed down the cast to alleviate itching.[4]

The stockinette which is placed on the limb prior to casting has a tendency to stretch and wrinkle. It should periodically be pulled taut and the fresh edge taped over the ends of the cast. If the stockinette is not covering the edge of the cast well, the edges should be *petaled,* that is, covered with tape, to prevent loose, crumbly pieces of plaster from falling into the cast.

It is essential to maintain adequate circulation and function in the casted extremity. This can be achieved by engaging the patient in passive exercises such as periodic movement of fingers and toes. Avoiding constriction and reducing edema by elevation of the casted extremity will all contribute to improved circulation.

*Patient teaching*  As care is delivered to the patient, the nurse has a valuable opportunity to teach the steps of cast care. *Teaching plan* should include use of lay terms as much as possible. Assess the patient's knowledge and give a full, clear explanation of what is to be done and why.

As the patient is readied for discharge, explicit written instructions will help to remind both the patient and family what to do for cast care and patient comfort. The patient and family members should be allowed time to read the instructions and ask questions prior to discharge. Teaching plans should stress specific safety factors to be followed in the home. The patient and family should know whom to contact if they have questions at home.

*Teaching content* should also include instructions related to checking for edema, vascular insult, pain, and neurovascular collapse and the presence of "hot spots," localized warm areas over a particular portion of the cast. These are important compo-

nents of a teaching plan, and the patient and family should participate in the teaching-learning activity.

*Maintaining muscle tone*  In order to facilitate recovery and prevent deformity, every attempt should be made to maintain the use of muscle groups not directly casted. A patient wearing a sling should perform range of motion exercises when possible. Toe and finger flexion and extension will also be helpful. The quadriceps muscle of the leg will atrophy within 5 to 7 days of disuse, leaving the patient with weak weight-bearing muscles.[5] Therefore, isometric exercises should be done within the confines of a cast to prevent this.

*Assisted ambulation* is often provided almost immediately after cast application. Crutches and canes are two forms of assistance provided to the individual with a lower limb fracture.

*Crutch walking* is the most common type of assisted ambulation. Occasionally it is the nurse's responsibility to fit the patient's crutches. Proper fit is important to prevent poor posture, instability, and axillary pressure. There are several methods which can be used to fit crutches. The patient must wear the shoes (or shoe) to be used when walking in order to get an accurate fit. (See Table 40-3 for further information.) Crutches must be the correct length, and a space must be present between the top of the axilla and the crutch top.

As the patient ambulates, the posture of crutch-

**TABLE 40-3**
MEASURING FOR CRUTCHES

| Method | Patient Position | Length* | Hand Grasp |
|---|---|---|---|
| Standing | Against wall Feet slightly apart at a comfortable distance from the wall | 1  Place a 2-inch mark on the outside shoe at toe<br><br>2  Measure 6 inches forward and mark again.<br><br>3  Measure the distance from 2 inches below axilla to the second mark. This is the desired length. | 1  Check quality of hand muscle grip<br>2  Elbow flexion at 30°<br>3  Fists clenched<br>4  Wrists slightly hyperextended<br>5  Distance from 2 inches below axilla<br>6  The patient should be able to extend the elbow without the top of the crutch touching the axilla |
| Bed method | Lying on firm mattress Feet against foot board (supine position) | 1  Mark from bottom of heel to 6 inches to the side (laterally).<br><br>2  Mark the distance from 2 inches below axilla to mark<br><br>3  Measure from axilla to 6 inches lateral to the foot | Same |
| Easy method | Any position Used most frequently if the patient cannot stand. | Subtract 16 inches from patient's total height. | Same |

* It is important to be sure the cruches are not too long. The standing crutch should reach the length of the patient from a 2 inch space below the axilla to the floor.

walking should provide a normal progression to good posture for later ambulation without crutches. The patient should stand erect with the pelvis over the feet, the head should be straight, weight should be on the hands, and the shoulders should be back. Flexion of the knee and hip, eversion of the foot, and outward rotation of the hip should be avoided. Cautioning the patient against walking on the ball of the foot with the heel off the floor is essential. Slouching, eyes on the floor, chin on the chest, shoulders and back rounded are all *undesirable.* These postures will cause the patient to tire more easily and to develop poor posture. Further, pressure on the axilla at the point where the radial nerve passes can result in radial nerve palsy.

The patient should be taught to keep the crutches 4 to 6 inches in front and slightly to the side of either foot. Weight should be on the palms of the hands, with the wrists extended and the elbows flexed. The top bar should be pressed against the chest 2 inches below the axilla to provide stability.

Depending on the needs of the patient, one of four types of gaits is used for assisted support. The four are the swing through, the two point, the three point, and the four point. The *swing-through gait* allows for the concurrent forward movement of both crutches. The feet swing through the crutches with the feet usually placed ahead of the crutches. This gait can be used when weight bearing on a lower extremity should be avoided.

The *two-point gait* involves the concurrent advancement of the left foot and right crutch, then the right foot and the left crutch. It can be used to support body weight when excess pressure on either extremity needs to be reduced.

The *three-point gait* is used when weight must be kept off the affected limb. The patient places the weight on the unaffected leg, places both crutches forward and swings through the crutches, using the hands for the weight transfer.

The *four-point gait* allows for partial weight bearing on both legs. It is the safest, most stable gait. The patient will proceed left crutch and right leg, then right crutch and left leg. It is used when equalized assisted weight bearing is required.

When using steps, the patient can be taught to hold the rail on the unaffected side and keep both crutches under the arm on the affected side. Going up the stairs, the pattern should foster the stronger leg and then the weaker leg and the crutches. (Handrails provide more support). The nurse can be most helpful by standing behind the patient. Going down the stairs, the weaker leg and the crutches should go first as the patient holds the handrail, and then the stronger leg follows. The nurse should stand in front of the patient to protect against falling forward.

*Patient teaching* should include emphasis on safety. For stability, crutch ends should be covered with rubber tips and checked weekly. Hand grasps may be padded to prevent blisters. Pads should be firmly in place so they do not slip as the patient ambulates. The top bars should not be padded as this can increase the temptation to lean on them.

Prior to discharge, the home should be assessed for safety. This can be done by the family with the guidance of the nurse. Loose rugs should be removed and highly waxed floors avoided. Care should be taken to arrange furniture so that it will not obstruct the patient's path. Using stairs with handrails is critical.

It is also important to tell patients to avoid large crowds since being in a crowd could precipitate a fall. When patients begin to use crutches, the nurse should be prepared to offer support if the patient begins to fall. The patient should be taught how to fall if alone. If falling is imminent, the crutches should be thrown to the site if possible, and the patient should relax the body and fall limp.

When getting up from a chair or in and out of a car, the patient should be taught to put both crutches together and place them directly in front of the body and move to the end of the chair or seat, then place the unaffected extremity firmly on the floor and the hands on the crutch hand grasps. As the patient begins to rise, he or she should place the weight on the crutches and supportive limb.

A *cane* provides a natural progression from crutches to independent ambulation, or it may be all the patient initially needs for stability. It is used to widen the base of support and improve balance. This will decrease weight bearing on an involved hip or knee. For proper use, a cane should be held in the hand opposite the affected extremity. In this way, the body is supported partially on the affected area and partially on the cane as the unaffected limb moves forward. The cane and the affected limb can then be moved together as the patient is supported on the stronger leg. To correctly fit a cane, measure the distance from the hand with slight flexion of the elbow, to the floor.

*Emotional problems* After the immediate injury a patient may have many negative feelings, not only about the present state, but also about whatever precipitated the accident. There may be feelings of anger, as in the case of an accident caused by another. If the accident occurred while the patient was angry, there may be continued feelings of resentment toward the person or thing which initiated the anger. If this involves a loved one, the patient and significant others may need help in working through these feelings to ensure the patient's physical and emotional recovery. Furthermore, a patient may carry over feelings of fear at the thought of repeating the behavior which caused the injury, e.g., driving a car. Anxiety often appears after the initial shock of the incident is over and the reconstructive process begins.

The nurse must be supportive to the patient and provide an opportunity to discuss the impact the fracture will have on an individual's life-style and occupation. Counseling may be needed to help the person deal with personal loss and guilt. The family should be encouraged to offer the patient needed assistance when possible. If loss of work because of the injury becomes a problem, a social worker may need to be incorporated into the planning.

**Third-level nursing care** Many fractures are not reducible by a closed method. For fractures which are comminuted or in which there is interposition of the muscle between the bone fragments traction and/or surgical intervention may be required. Muscle spasms may also prevent a smooth, closed reduction because the pull which is exerted on the bone may be sufficient to cause overriding of the fragments. If closed reduction is not feasible, the patient will be hospitalized for more extensive treatment.

**N**ursing Assessment Generally, patients who are hospitalized for fractures offer a health history of extensive injury secondary to the fracture, a contaminated injury, or a fracture that is not reducible by manual manipulation. As discussed in Second-Level Nursing Care, there will be *severe pain,* and the patient will complain of tightening over the muscle mass similar to the effect obtained when isometric exercises are performed.

During assessment of the examination, the extremity may appear badly deformed or misshapen. If the fracture is compound, tissue fragments may be noted between the bone and a break in the skin. Pulse should be palpated distal to the injury. If the pulse is absent, vital signs should be evaluated for evidence of shock. Swelling and tenderness along with changes assessed under Second-Level Nursing Care may persist or even worsen.

**D**iagnostic Tests The x-ray continues to be the most effective measure to assess the fracture. When other systemic problems such as malignancy, vitamin deficiency, or metabolic disorders are sus-

pected, other tests may be performed. These may include a calcium and phosphorus level which can be altered in the *presence* of parathyroid problems as well as degenerative bone pathology. Blood enzymes are elevated in the presence of muscle damage and offer some indications of extent of trauma. Lumbar puncture can be done if cerebral fracture is suspected; however, it may be cautioned against in the presence of increased intracranial pressure.

**N**ursing Problems and Interventions Patients hospitalized for a bone fracture will experience problems similar to those discussed under Second-Level Nursing Care but often more severe. *Immobility,* with its problems, often becomes a focus of care. The patient is often in severe *pain* and may experience a variety of *emotional reactions* to hospitalization and the actual trauma. The fracture itself must be reduced. To accomplish this, *traction* or an *open reduction* is often employed.

*Open reduction* Open reduction of a fracture is sometimes the treatment of choice for optimal healing. It is a surgical procedure used when closed reduction is not feasible by external means, when there is displacement of fragments, or when tissue or hemorrhagic matter is lodged between the bone ends. Contaminated wounds requiring debridement and possible irrigation are also treated surgically. If it is decided that closed reduction would cause sufficient immobility to predispose a patient to complications of bed rest, open reduction may be selected.

The timing of an open reduction may vary. For an open fracture, surgery is usually performed immediately to reduce the high risk of infection. A closed fracture, however, can be treated later. In the presence of systemic injury, problems such as hemorrhage and respiratory and cardiac arrest must be stabilized before surgery. Although it is desirable to perform the surgery 24 to 48 hours following the fracture, it can be done as late as 1 to 2 weeks after the initial trauma. During the delay, the blood supply around the fracture increases and the fracture hematoma begins to organize.[6] There is, however, at this point the problem of increased edema at the site.[7]

Prior to surgery, scrupulous preparation of the skin is necessary to prevent cutaneous contamination of the surgical wound. Preoperative preparation of the patient may be limited owing to the emergency nature of the presenting problems. When possible, the patient should receive a clear presentation of the intended surgical procedure, emotional support, and postoperative expectations. The procedure itself may involve the application of vari-

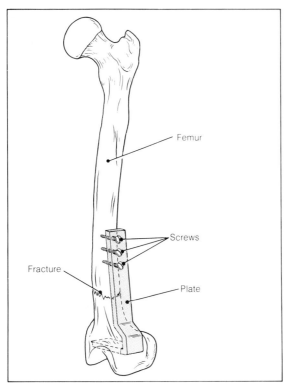

**FIGURE 40-3**
Fractured femur. (*Drawing by Julie Rotta.*)

ous screws, pins, plates, or intramedullary nails needed to maintain bone alignment. It must be remembered that when a hole is made in bone, bone strength is decreased by 50 percent until the bone heals itself.[8] However, physicians can apply stress to an area with a compression plate to promote union while eliminating undesirable forces like side-to-side motion or angulation and thus promote healing.[9] (See Fig. 40-3).

Sometimes, owing to the extent of damage suffered during a fracture, a less than ideal reduction is obtained. In this case, surgical repair is done for maximum function. For example, a hand would be allowed to stay in extension versus flexion, and fingers in flexion versus extension to allow for grasping. *Ankylosis,* or bony growth, causing joint stiffness may be allowed in a functional position.

*Postoperatively,* a patient may be allowed out of bed after 24 hours with no weight bearing on the extremity. In bed, there will be increased mobility, with the ability to sit and turn from side to side. If a distal limb is involved, it should be elevated to promote venous return. Circulation should be monitored for signs of vascular compromise. The surgical wound should be observed for bleeding. Dress-

ing changes should be carried through with strict aseptic technique and the wound closely observed for signs of infection, pain, erythema, odor, or drainage with an odor.

Open reduction is not without risks. Soft tissue healing time is usually longer owing to the creation of a surgical incision. The possibility of infection is ever-present. Postoperatively, scar tissue (adhesions) may limit joint motion. The patient will be subjected to a surgical procedure, usually with the use of general anesthesia. The risks of anesthesia must also be considered.

Occasionally, a patient who has undergone either a closed or an open reduction will have either a malunion or nonunion of the fracture. There will be complaints of pain and instability at the fracture site. A *malunion* is characterized by slow healing of the bone with poor callus formation. In *nonunion,* the bone ends simply do not heal. These conditons are usually a result of a poor reduction of the fracture, ineffective immobilization (too short, not stable), impaired circulation to the area, or poor general condition of the patient. Intervention includes surgical debridement of the necrotic bone ends and internal fixation. A pin or plate may be used to hasten healing and give support.

*Immobility* A problem that must be dealt with for many orthopedic inpatients is that of *immobility.* Fractures that cannot be immediately reduced may require surgery and bed rest to allow for some healing before activity can be allowed. Long-term bed rest with traction is often used to treat an otherwise irreducible fracture. This restricts a patient's mobility.

Injury to blood vessels and bleeding at the site of the fracture with subsequent clot formation predispose the immobilized patient with a fracture to thrombophlebitis and emboli formation (see Chap. 29 for a complete discussion). In addition swelling and altered circulation to the extremity can be intensified by limited movements and lack of exercise. The nurse should observe the patient for changes that might suggest *thrombus formation* including pain, redness, tenderness, and swelling in a localized area. Passive exercises and position change along with reduction of the fracture may help reduce the problem.

Immobilized patients are also prone to the well-known complications of urinary stasis, pulmonary embolus, and decubiti. The nurse should consider the problems of muscle atrophy, contractures, and osteoporosis. *Renal calculi* can develop as a result of disuse osteoporosis. High-calcium diet should be discouraged for bone healing, and the benefits of a high-protein diet should be stressed. Constipation is a problem which can be alleviated by a high-roughage diet, stool softeners, and laxatives.

*Skin breakdown* and the formation of decubitus ulcers are not uncommon problems for the immobilized patient. Careful skin assessment must be done every few hours to observe the skin for areas of breakdown. Pressure areas should be massaged gently to stimulate circulation to the area. Circulating electric beds may be used to reduce pressure on specific areas. Frequent position changes as often as every half to full hour are also helpful. Sheepskin can be used to help reduce skin abrasion, and keeping sheets wrinkle-free will reduce the pressure to affected body parts.

*Muscle atrophy*    If there is *decreased innervation to a muscle mass,* it will atrophy. Furthermore, any patient on *bed rest* will suffer atrophy of the muscles. *Disuse* of the muscle results in decreased circulation to the muscle mass, causing it to decrease in size. Atrophic muscle commonly occurs in the antigravity groups, specifically the quadriceps, the guteals, and the gastrocnemius. Intervention is aimed at breaking the cycle of diminishing muscle mass and increasing the patient's exercise tolerance. Whenever care is delivered to the patient, time should be taken to do active and passive range of motion exercises to areas the patient cannot mobilize. *Isometric exercises* are also important in maintaining and increasing muscular function. Family members, too, can be incorporated into this portion of the plan of care.

*Contractures*    Muscle disuse with decreased muscle tone results in decreased contractility of muscles. Muscles are then held in shortened or lenghened position. Connective tissue deposits form and settle in the joints. These increase with disuse and immobilize the joint. If not corrected within as little as 2 weeks, the limb will have limited function or be useless. Portions of the body most commonly affected by contractures are the hip, the shoulder, the knee, the hand, and the foot.

In the *hip,* the joint may become contracted in the positions of flexion, adduction (convergence), and external rotation. This is often seen in the patient who remains in bed, with knees flexed, outward rotation of the legs, and no abduction of the thighs. This is sometimes referred to as the "sick bed" position.

*Frozen shoulder* means that there is no abduction or outward rotation at the shoulder. Here the pectoral muscles are involved. The patient who sits with the shoulders slumped forward and elbows in flexion, possibly with the hands folded flat across the chest, is a good candidate to develop contractures of the shoulder.

*Drop foot* can occur not only from perineal nerve damage, but also from shortening of the Achilles tendon. The problem can be precipitated by poor support to the foot, or by weighing down the weakened muscles of the feet with heavy covers. Furthermore, patients who are kept in a prone position for extended periods of time, with poor positioning of the feet, will develop this problem. The dorsum of the foot is stretched, and the plantum of the foot and the heel cord shorten.

The nurse must take definite steps to prevent contracture formation. A frequent change of position with attention to the future function of the limbs and an awareness of good body mechanics will prevent contracture formation. When sitting, the patient should be erect with weight on the ischia and thighs and the back straight. A hard, straight-backed chair may help facilitate this. The spine should be supported. The patient should slide the hips back as far as possible to promote this position. Pillows should not be placed behind the back. The head also should not be flexed forward with pillows. The arms should be supported so they do not hang limply and "pull" on the shoulders. Fingers should be held in flexion rather than extension. A rubber ball, putty, or any soft, correctly sized object placed in the patient's hand will promote grasping. Feet can be supported with a footboard, pillows, or a covered box. A *trochanter roll* will help to avoid external rotation of the thigh. This can be made from a rolled blanket and should be placed at the lateral aspect of the thigh and calf. Pillows should be placed between the knees to achieve abduction of the thighs. Encouraging the patient to lie prone periodically will force the joints to be in extension rather than flexion for a time. The patient should be turned from side to side periodically to allow for a change in the position of all the extremities.

The patient should be assessed to determine what *motor function* is present and exercises that will capitalize on these abilities should be encouraged. The patient should understand the rationale for these activities. Passive exercises should be given to those areas the patient cannot move. The patient should be taught to perform a passive range of motion to the involved extremity whenever possible. It is also important to encourage ankle rotation, *quad setting* (isometrics of the quadriceps), and knee flexion. Placing items that the patient would use during the course of the day within reach but at different angles can encourage exercise and increase varying motion. A firm mattress or bedboard helps promote good posture and discourages sagging and stretching of joints while the patient is in bed.

*Activity* It is important to help the patient maintain muscle function so that rehabilitation postimmobilization will not be complicated by a debilitated skeletal-muscular condition. Use of a *trapeze* on the bed (see Figs. 40-2 and 40-3) encourages arm exercises, provides greater mobility, and allows the patient to take a more active part in the care. The patient should do as much self-care as possible, for the benefit of self-esteem as well as for the benefits gained by the active exercise. This will often require an innovative approach on the part of the nurse to set up bedside surroundings in such a way that the patient can eat or bathe without assistance, or reach for necessary items. Do not overlook the value of isometrics and range of motion exercises to keep the patient at an optimal functional level.

The *emotional* effects of immobility on a patient's personality must be carefully considered. The elderly patient with limited sensory stimulation may become disoriented. The child with little tactile demonstration of affection may become withdrawn. A patient with nothing to look forward to except day after day of immobility may become depressed, tearful, withdrawn, and perhaps uncooperative about the plan of care. Awareness of pain may be increased by anxiety and the absence of diversionary activity. Frustration over present decreased abilities and concern over job loss may also be

problems. The attitude of significant others is important. How do family and friends view the present situation? Do they make light of the fact that "it's only a broken leg and no one ever died of a broken leg"? Are they supportive of the patient, or do they resent the hospitalization? Arrangements may need to be made for counseling of the patient and family. It is important to note that the patient's irritability may be the only means available for coping with the situation at this point.

Nursing care can often be effectively directed toward short-term goal setting with the patient in order to further long-term convalescence. In this way, the patient will better be able to assess progress and feel a sense of accomplishment.

*Traction* To help reduce a fracture, traction is often used. This is a mechanical means of applying a pulling force to an area to overcome muscle spasm so that the fracture can be reduced. It may also reduce the patient's pain, and maintain alignment of the bone and allow for more joint and muscle exercising. Traction can be used in nonfracture patients to correct or prevent deformity such as contracture formation.

There are many ways in which traction can be applied (see Table 40-4), but the basic principles apply to all applications. Each time traction or a pulling force is applied, a pull must be exerted in the opposite direction so that the desired force is being applied where it is needed. This opposite pull is termed *countertraction.* It may be obtained by elevating the foot or head of the bed, or by applying shock blocks to the appropriate end of the bed. This allows the pull of gravity to counter the force of traction. Sometimes, the weight of the patient's

**TABLE 40-4**
TYPES OF TRACTION

| Type | Where Force Is Applied | Major Characteristic | Examples |
|---|---|---|---|
| Manual | Directly to skin by hand, indirectly to bone | Static | Used in cast application |
| Skin | Directly to skin by mechanical means, indirectly to bone | Static | Buck's extension Head halter Pelvic traction |
| Skeletal | Directly to bone | Dynamic | Kirschner wire Steinmann pin Crutchfield tongs |
| Skeletal/Skin | Uses skin or skeletal traction Creates a forward and upward pull of the leg by applying direct force to one part of the bone and indirect force to another | Static and/or dynamic | Russell's traction |

body will be sufficient to provide effective counter-traction.

Traction in which the pull is exerted directly against the body weight is referred to as *straight* or *static* traction. In this case, a change in the patient's position will cause a change in the direction of the traction pull. Thus, care must be taken to have the patient maintain a stable position constantly. (See Fig. 40-4.)

Balanced traction is traction in which the limb is suspended in a splint held in place by weights, pulleys, or ropes that are balanced. Here the head or foot of the bed is often adjusted to allow for countertraction. Balanced traction is a *dynamic* traction. Movement of the patient is allowed, so that the patient can indeed turn and sit up without disturbing the line of pull. In the case of a leg in balanced traction (Fig. 40-5), if the angle of flexion at the hip is maintained during movement, there is no disturbance of the line of pull. Slack in the ropes created by movement will be taken up by the pulley system. Ropes and pulleys should be movable and unobstructed in order to be most effective.

Nursing care for the patient in traction is complex and requires much time and patience. After the amount of force required and the desirable direction of force have been estimated, frequent x-rays of the limb are used to guide the physician in adjusting the weight and pull to the varying patient needs. As muscle fatigues and spasms decrease, less traction may be needed.

Except for use in the relief of contractures, the *pull* must be kept constant to be effective. In the case of traction applied to correct the alignment of overriding bone, the absence of the force might allow the bone to resume its overriding position.

In planning care for the patient in traction, be mindful of the need of the patient and family to understand what the traction is for, what may and may not be done, and the rationale for these limitations. Without careful explanations, traction can be a frightening experience to the patient; the effectiveness of the traction may be limited if instructions are not carefully followed.

The nurse will need to check frequently to ensure that the traction is in functional alignment.

**FIGURE 40-4**
Pelvic traction (an example of skin traction). (*Drawing adapted from Julie Rotta.*)

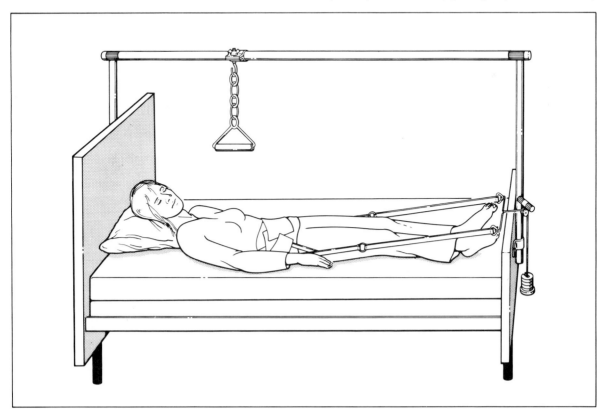

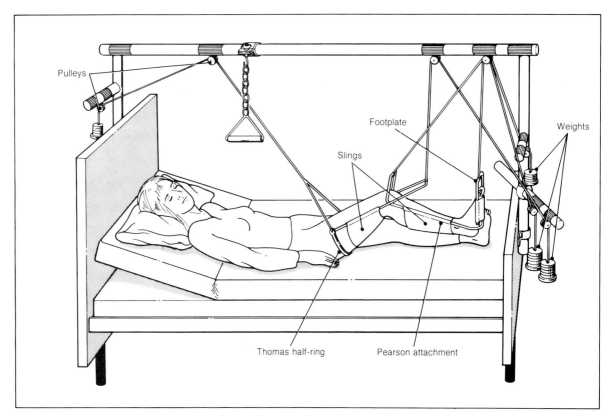

**FIGURE 40-5**
Balanced suspension traction. (*Drawing adapted from Julie Rotta.*)

Ropes should be correctly centered on pulleys to allow for free pull, and weights of the correct size should be hanging freely. Remember that any friction along the system will decrease the amount of traction.

If a patient's leg is suspended in a *Pearson attachment* (see Fig. 40-5), it should be horizontal to the bed. There should be sufficient countertraction to keep the patient from being pulled toward the traction. *Good alignment* is necessary to facilitate the effectiveness of the traction being used.

The affected limb is usually held in a neutral position or in slight internal rotation. As the patient moves from side to side in bed, the limb may be in *abduction* or *adduction*. Check to see that the patient stays in the center of the bed. Slings should also be positioned properly and with no pressure on the foot from the footplate or spreader bar. If a *Thomas splint* is used, additional care is required. A Thomas splint is a balanced traction used with a Pearson attachment. The splint is placed on the affected area beginning at the groin and extending

beyond the foot. These splints also include rings which are placed over the thigh (see Fig. 40-5). These rings are used for temporary immobility or to aid in the management of fractures needing long-term immobilization.

If a patient has a *Thomas ring* (see Fig. 40-5), be sure it is not pressing against the groin. To avoid having to move the patient excessively, a special fracture bedpan and a female urinal can be used. The technique of making the bed from top to bottom is often easier than the conventional side-to-side approach.

Since the person in traction is constantly subjected to friction and pressure, special efforts should be made to maintain the skin's integrity. Susceptible areas should be checked every 8 hours. Areas of potential pressure should be padded. These include areas where the peroneal nerve runs close to the surface of the lateral aspect of the calf, just below the knee, and the sensitive Achilles tendon area. The heel should be kept free from pressure at all times. Bony prominences like the malleoli, elbows, sacrum, and ischea should be observed for signs of redness or irritation. Sheepskin pads and massage can be used to prevent this. Slings should be free of irritating wrinkles, and elastic bandages should be checked frequently. When necessary, they should be reapplied. When traction tapes are used, they may be covered with a bandage to hold them in place. The tape helps to hold the traction in place. The skin should be checked for an allergic response. In addition, tapes should be applied in a lengthwise position to avoid constricting circulation.

*Skeletal traction* can be achieved through the use of wires (Krichner wires) or pins (Steinmann pins), or through the use of metal tongs (Crutchfield tongs) (see Chap. 32). Pins are inserted by drilling into the bone and placing the pin through the bone. With the pin in a perpendicular position, traction is applied.

*Pin sites* should be observed for any redness, swelling, or edema which would indicate possible infection. Erosion of skin and bone around the pin site (*tunneling*) is also a major concern. Pin sites should be observed every 8 hours while pin care is done. The sites should be cleansed to remove crusts and an antibiotic ointment or solution applied to prevent infection. In the event of tunneling, the pin may be removed.

Minimal exercise, positioning, and trauma can all predispose a patient to decreased venous return with resulting vascular compromise. Edema may result due to pooling of fluids in the periphery. Circulation checks should be done every hour for the first 24 hours after the patient is in traction, and every 4 hours thereafter to assess the patient's circulatory status.

**Pain**  The patient with a muscular-skeletal injury will be in pain. *Analgesia for comfort* is often required. Wise use of analgesia will aid the patient by decreasing muscle spasms and will allow for more comfortable rest. Relief of pain will also allow for greater exercise tolerances, including pulmonary exercises and range of motion. The type and amount of medication the patient requires will depend on the extent of the injury and the pain threshold. Other influencing factors will be the patient's past history of medications, current medications, and the present physical status (especially cardiopulmonary and neurological).

Assessing the cause of the *pain* prior to administering medication can help in planning care. Bone pain is generally diffuse, and the patient's complaints may be rather vague. If the pain is caused by

muscle spasms, they can be alleviated by antispasmodics, too. Poor body alignment, causing undue stress on the joints, or constricting wraps can cause added problems and should be corrected to allow time for the patient to appreciate the effects prior to administering medication. Determining other physical causes for the patient's pain is an important component of care. Apprehension, anxiety, and depression should be treated as such and not handled by merely medicating the patient. Since care of skeletal-muscular problems can continue for a long time, it is important not to create a dependence on pain medication when other means will effectively solve the problem at hand.

Occasionally, *complications* will arise from a fracture, causing the nurse concern with even greater threats to the patient's health and requiring skilled intervention. These problems include hemorrhage, paralysis, infection, and fat embolus.

**Hemorrhage**  The tearing of major arteries of the periosteum and bone or excess soft tissue damage can cause a patient to hemorrhage. The nurse should carefully observe the patient for the classic symptoms of hypovolemia (see Chap. 28). Excess bloody drainage may be noted, or, if the bleeding is internal, the presence of a growing hematoma may be observed. The patient may also complain of pain due to the pressure of the hematoma on surrounding soft tissue and nerves.

Pressure to the area will help stop massive hemorrhage. Ice packs may also be used. Any gradually increasing hematoma can be slowed by elevation of the extremity to improve venous return. Fluid replacement and surgical intervention may be required to prevent shock.

**Ischemic paralysis**  Untreated hemorrhage can lead to ischemic paralysis. Also known as *compartment syndrome, ischemic paralysis* is a progressive vascular compromise resulting in necrosis of muscles and nerves if untreated. It usually occurs in muscle groups surrounded by tough fascia which does not expand. Susceptible areas are the anterior, posterior, and lateral compartments of the leg and the flexor muscle groups of the arm. In the arm, the result is often referred to as *Volkmann's ischemic contracture,* which is generally related to a supracondylar fracture of the elbow.

Although fractures commonly cause an ischemic syndrome, anything which will cause trauma or edema to the susceptible areas can potentially lead to ischemia. Other causes may be crushing injuries, anticoagulation, and burns. All these will cause tissue to swell, resulting in venous and arterial compression with ensuing arterial occlusion and muscle ischemia. Since the muscle ischemia leads to further edema, the cycle is then self-perpetuating. It is also thought that ischemia triggers a histamine release, which causes capillary dilatation and "transudation of plasma" into the muscle tissue with resultant swelling.[10] The veins are occluded initially, but arterial blood continues to flow into the compartment until the backflow pressure is great enough to cause it to stop.[11] Uncorrected, this situation could result in permanent damage within 6 hours and complete muscle death with fibrosis within 24 to 48 hours.

The nurse is in an advantageous position to thoroughly assess patients for muscle ischemia. Early detection can prevent irreversible damage. The parameters that are most helpful are referred to as "the five Ps." They are pain, pulselessness, pallor, paresthesias, and paralysis. They should be evaluated periodically to give an ongoing picture of the patient's status.

The *pain* of a fracture is generally relieved by splinting and analgesia. Pain which is not relieved by appropriate intervention or pain which increases without apparent cause is highly suspicious of the presence of an ischemic muscle. Pain is often one of the first indications of ischemia. Pain on passive motion is also an indication of circulatory compromise. Ischemic muscle is resistant to stretching. If the patient cannot move the extremity distal to the wound without pain, ischemia may be present.

As compression progresses, *paralysis* of the extremity occurs. This paralysis should be distinguished from motor nerve dysfunction in which there is no pain on passive motion and no edema over the affected area.

*Pulselessness* distal to the injured area indicates vascular compromise in an advanced stage. For this reason this sign is not used as a sole indicator for quick action.

*Paresthesias* may include numbness, burning, or tingling in the distal portion of the involved extremity (especially fingers and toes) or the complete absence of sensation there.

*Pallor* is the most significant color change. The distal extremity is also significant when neurovascular status is determined. Diminished capillary refill after blanching an area is evidence of arterial impairment. Cyanosis, on the other hand, indicates venous impairment. Checking the *temperature* of the extremity may also reveal changes. If the affected extremity is cooler to touch than the unaffected opposite extremity, the cause may be decreased circulation.

*Nursing interventions* are aimed at prevention and can help reduce the incidence of vascular compromise. An injured extremity should be elevated above the level of the heart in order to maximize venous return. The nurse should continue to avoid placing excess strain on the joints and maintain good body alignment. Ice to an injured area will minimize edema. Monitor the "five Ps" every 15 minutes for the first hour after trauma or manipulation, then every hour for the next 24 hours, and every 4 hours thereafter.

In the event ischemia is suspected, the extremity should be further elevated if possible. Constricting wraps around the limb should be removed. The nurse should continue to monitor the signs every 15 minutes. If no relief is obtained within 30 minutes, the physician can elect to perform a *fasciotomy.* This procedure is a surgical decompression of the area achieved by dividing the fascia, in order to allow for maximal soft tissue expansion.

*Infection*  A patient with an open wound is susceptible to infection by gas bacillus. The offending organism is an anaerobe, generally *Clostridium Verfringens* type A. It is usually found in a puncture wound with a small closed surface or in wounds with much necrotic tissue.

The nurse will often observe the inception of the problem as a local infection with the characteristic erythema, heat, and tenderness. There may or may not be an elevation of body temperature at this point. The infection spreads rapidly, especially to surrounding muscle groups. Here a gaseous infiltrate can be seen appearing as bubbles under the skin.

Prevention is more desirable than attempts to cure since the infection is fatal in approximately 87 percent of the cases.[12] The measures employed include good debridement of an open wound and excellent aseptic technique in the care of wounds. Prophylactic use of antibiotics may be considered, and the patient can be given polyvalent antitoxin to help ward off development of the infection.[13]

Should the patient develop gas bacillus infection, sometimes referred to as *gas gangrene,* the physician will probably elect to do surgical debridement and irrigation of the wound. The patient should be placed under strict isolation to avoid infection of others on the unit. Antibiotics, usually penicillin,[14] will be given. Beneficial effects have been achieved by placing patients in hyperbaric chambers in which the anaerobes are exposed to high-density oxygen.

*Fat embolus*  A curious syndrome may develop in the patient who has had a fracture or surgery to the long bones or the sternum. The syndrome is caused by the presence of fat emboli, and it is often difficult to diagnose since symptoms may mimic those of several other conditions or may be very vague.

The exact cause of the development of fat emboli is not known, but a few theories have been proposed. The *traumatic theory* suggests that fat globules from the bone marrow, or those released from the soft tissue during trauma, enter the venous system and travel to the brain, lungs, heart, kidneys, and skin, causing the resultant symptoms.[15] The *metabolic theory* proposes that "trauma alters the natural physiochemical emulsion of fats in the bloodstream,"[16] thus causing the formation of droplets.

Symptoms are usually seen in young adults and usually occur 12 to 72 hours after trauma or surgery, although they have been observed as long as 3 weeks later. Fat emboli are the major cause of death from fractures, causing 20 percent of all fatalities associated with a fracture.[17]

Assessment of problems varies with the location of the embolus. *Brain involvement* will cause an alcoholic "delirium tremors" type reaction, with memory loss, restlessness, and confusion. There may possibly be headaches, hemiparesis, or coma. If there is involvement of the *hypothalamus,* there may also be an elevated temperature. These symptoms are significant in that they are often dismissed as alcohol withdrawal, and thus the patient may not receive the proper care. Changes in level of consciousness, cyanosis, dyspnea, and the presence of petechiae especially on the chest and shoulders can help differentiate between the two disorders in order to treat the correct one.

If fat droplets travel to the heart and lungs, there will be cardiopulmonary consequences. Significant are the apparent dyspnea and tachypnea. Tests of blood gases will reveal hypoxia. At first, the patient will be pale and subsequently become cyanotic. A chest x-ray may reveal areas of consolidation within the lungs. Symptoms of hypovolemia or shock may be present. There will be hypotension and tachycardia which may also be the result of a decreased hemoglobin and hematocrit levels. (See Chap. 29 for a discussion of embolus.)

Visible changes may also occur in the *skin.*

These include petechiae on the anterior chest, neck, conjunctiva, the axillae, deltoids, buccal membrane, and hard palate. The patches do not blanch with pressure, but may fade very rapidly (within hours) or within a few days.[18]

Intervention is aimed at supporting the patient through the crisis. Generally, if the patient survives through the first 48 hours, recovery will be remarkable.[19] The patient is kept on bed rest to avoid release of even more fat droplets into the bloodstream and to put less stress on the already overtaxed body systems. To counteract the hypoxia, oxygen is administered. IPPB, deep breathing, coughing, and suctioning may well improve the respiratory status (see Chap. 30). The patient may be intubated if oxygenation is not satisfactory. Steroids are used to alleviate the inflammation in the lungs caused by irritation from the breakdown of fat in the lungs, with resultant hemorrhage and edema.[20]

In order to improve blood flow and decrease blood lipids and platelet adhesiveness, so that platelet aggregation is discouraged, heparin is given.[21] Along these same lines, dextran 40 may be given to improve blood flow. Whole blood or packed red blood cells are given to increase the oxygen-carrying capacity of the blood.

*Prevention* of fat emboli should include attention to immobilization of long-bone fractures to prevent the release of fat droplets into the bloodstream. Further, fractured extremities should not be massaged or moved quickly. The nurse will be presented with the special challenge of dealing with any patient who is susceptible to fat emboli and who is confused or agitated for any reason. Ingenuity will be required to keep the patient as immobile as possible. As the patient prepares to ambulate, gradual, slow ambulation will minimize the likelihood of fat release into the bloodstream. Above all immediate recognition of symptoms in order to allow for their prompt treatment will enhance the patient's chances for recovery.

**Fourth-level nursing care**  As care is planned for the patient with a fracture, the ultimate goal should be *rehabilitation.* To implement this, patient teaching is critical. Steps should be taken to prevent deformity and to maintain muscle function. Muscle groups that will be especially important can be further strengthened. For example, a patient who has progressed to crutch walking will require efficient muscles in the upper extremities, and so strengthening exercises may be prescribed to achieve this effect.

In patients with lower extremity involvement, rehabilitation is aimed at weight bearing and ambulation. There are degrees of weight bearing: *no weight bearing* (NWB) means that the patient supports weight on the upper extremities and the unaffected leg; *partial weight bearing* (PWB) indicates a variable amount of weight tolerance, often listed as a percentage of the total, from toe touching to allowing as much weight as the patient can comfortably tolerate; *full weight bearing* (FWB) is the ultimate goal and is generally achieved gradually.

**W**eight Bearing Readiness to progress to weight bearing is determined by the patient's general condition and by the amount of stability in the limb. All the patient's capabilities should be capitalized. Ideally, the patient will be well motivated. To ensure patient cooperation each time a new goal is attempted, the procedure should be carefully explained and demonstrated. A time for return demonstration should be provided.

If the patient has not been allowed to sit up in bed, this maneuver should be taught before progressing to the next activity. It can be facilitated by use of a *tilt table* specially designed to gradually increase the patient's tolerance to the standing position. As this procedure is used, the nurse should be alert for the signs of *orthostatic hypotension.* These changes would include dizziness, a faint feeling, nausea, hypotension, tachycardia, and pallor. By lowering the angle at which the patient has been elevated, these signs can be relieved.

Once the patient is able to tolerate elevation of the head, the next step is *dangling,* that is, having the patient sit over the side of the bed. To achieve this, the bed should be level before the patient sits up; that is, the head should not be elevated nor the knee gatched. The proper use of the overhead trapeze will assist the patient in moving to the edge of the bed (Fig. 40-5). For comfort and safety, allow the patient to place both feet on the floor. This will help increase the feeling of security and will prevent excess pressure on the popliteal space which could result in paresthesias of the feet. Support to the back may be necessary for weaker patients or those with poor posture. Pillows at the back will also give a reassuring feeling of security. The nurse should remain with the patient the first time dangling is done. The patient should begin by dangling for 10 to 20 minutes, then gradually increase this time. Allow the patient to dangle at least twice prior to getting into a chair. This will increase confidence about the ability to progress to the next step.

**T**ransfer to Chair When preparing to get the patient out of bed to a chair, be sure to choose one that is not too low and with good, straight back support. When getting into the chair, the patient should be allowed time to bear weight and pivot on the unaffected leg. Even if the affected leg is to be elevated, it can be dangled momentarily during this procedure. The nurse should help support the patient in *transfer.* In the chair, have the patient maintain good posture. A pillow should rarely be needed under the buttocks or behind the back, but a sheepskin pad will help soften a firm support. Once settled, be sure to place appropriate items within the patient's reach, including a call bell, and diversionary objects, such as books, cards, needlework, or toys. Check the patient frequently to be sure sitting in the chair is being well tolerated.

If the affected extremity is to be elevated, care should be taken to properly support it so it will not fall and so that there is no pressure on the popliteal space or the heel. Do not leave the patient sitting for extended periods. Check every 15 minutes to one-half hour to observe the patient's tolerance. The use of a flotation pad in the chair can help alleviate pressure areas. Also, instruct the patient to periodically raise the buttocks off the chair by using the arms to lift. After the patient is back in bed, check the ischia and sacrum for redness and, if possible, allow the patient to lie on one side for awhile.

After sitting is mastered, ambulation will be initiated. Depending on the patient's abilities, this can take many directions. Prior to commencing this, the nurse should caution patients that they might tire quite easily. Since most people feel stronger in bed, this information may come as a surprise and cause them to be discouraged about their progress. Of course, adequate preparation in terms of exercise can minimize this problem.

**A**ssisted Ambulation *Parallel bars* may be used as the first assistive device in teaching progressive ambulation because they provide maximal stability and will not slip away from the patient. A person can begin any type of weight bearing in this situation. Weight is balanced between the bars and the unaffected leg, with attention to maintenance of an erect posture and use of the quadriceps, abdominal, and gluteal muscles to achieve this posture. Breathing should be slow and even. Shoes with good support should always be worn for any ambulation.

After a person masters ambulation on the parallel bars, walking with a *walker* may be the next step. A walker provides good support because the weight is distributed over four points with good balance. It is often used instead of or prior to crutch walking and has a great value for elderly, debilitated, or unstable persons. Gaits used in walker walking are similar to those used in crutch walking. Crutches and canes may also be used. (Refer to the discussion in Second-Level Nursing Care.)

**E**motional Support  Assessment of both psychological and physical problems must be continuously observed, and family counseling and referrals made. In some cases, as in a spinal cord injury, patients are sent to rehabilitation centers, where there are interdisciplinary health care teams to meet all the patient's needs. Frequently, these regional centers force families to separate and foster emotional distress.

Much of the nurse's time must be spent supporting patients and their families. When possible, early identification of psychological problems will lead to prompt intervention and will facilitate rehabilitation.

It is important to recognize that patients who sustain a fracture, and more especially a complicated fracture, may face a long rehabilitation period. *Depression, anger,* and *frustration* may complicate recovery periods. When the injury is compounded by deformity, paralysis, or loss of others in an accident, a period of grieving may ensue. The nurse must be aware of this and allow the patient an opportunity to ventilate freely.

**C**ast Removal  The length of time required for a bone to heal varies with each individual and depends upon such matters as the type of fracture, the extent of injury, and whether complications were present. An *electric cast cutter* (similar to a saw) is used for cast removal. This machine contains circular blades which are applied directly to the cast. The blades spin as the cutter is moved back and forth over the cast. This motion creates a vibration which separates the plaster. The procedure is somewhat noisy and usually frightening to the patient, who needs to be reassured that the blade will not injure the skin. The patient should be told that after the cast cutter reaches a certain depth, a scissors or separating device will be used to complete the cast removal.

*When the cast is removed,* it is important to remember that the involved muscles and bone are only newly healed and weak from disuse. The affected limb should be supported, and sudden change of its position should be avoided. The ex-

tremity may swell due to venous stasis. Elastic wraps and intermittent exercise will push blood through the extremity and strengthen muscles. The skin will be delicate and should be treated gently. Lotion to soften the scale can be applied and the area washed with soap and water. The skin should not be scrubbed to avoid abrasion. The patient may experience some discomfort as the joint begins to engage in movement. Canes, crutches, and slings may be used to provide additional support during this period of recovery.

**P**hysical Therapy  Following removal of the cast, patients will often receive therapy to help with restoration of limb function and mobility. Therapy is often begun as soon as the condition is stabilized and short- and long-term rehabilitation goals can be determined.

The discipline of *physical therapy* can be useful to the patient with many skeletal-muscular disturbances. The physical therapist can assess the person's abilities and plan a program to maintain and develop muscle function. Furthermore, a therapist can help foresee and solve problems that might occur after discharge, especially involving activities of daily living.

Physical therapy treatment is aimed at restoring and maintaining muscle tone and flexibility. Methods employed to achieve these goals include application of heat, massage, and active and passive exercise.

The nurse needs to understand the regime the therapist prescribes for the patient. There should be communication about the patient's abilities, needs, and tolerance. Involvement of the family in the teaching plan will help ensure correct follow-through with activities begun during hospitalization.

**P**revention of Recurrent Fractures  Patient teaching should focus on helping the patient prevent the reoccurrence of the fracture. Included in the plan should be specific information about safety and avoidance of fatigue. The patient should be encouraged to wear proper shoes. If previous illness or activities caused the accident, pertinent information about these health problems should be included. The patient should be encouraged to interject feelings and concerns about how another accident can be avoided. It may be necessary to discuss specific posthospitalization concerns such as activity, return to work, and use of public transportation. Involving a supportive family member in these conversations will help to give the patient the feeling that someone at home will have an appreciation of any difficulties that might arise.

During discharge teaching, the patient's comprehension of the rationale for follow-up care should be evaluated. Reviewing the date, time, and place of the next appointment and determining convenient times for the patient should be considered. Appointments help ensure patient compliance. Written instructions should include return appointment dates and phone numbers of persons to call if there is a question. Danger signs such as increased pain, numbness, tingling, or increase in temperature should also be discussed. A community-based nurse should follow the patient and send the agency specifics about each individual's needs, abilities, problems, and plans. If the patient is receiving medications such as antibiotics, the drugs action, use, and potential side effects should be discussed.

### Strain

Skeletal muscle stress does not always cause bone to fracture. However, trauma can cause changes in the soft tissue surrounding the bone. A *strain* is an incomplete tear of a ligament.[22] It also may involve increased muscle use and stretching of a tendon. Strains often occur from fatigue or during a sports injury, particularly those resulting in a sudden twisting motion of the ankle. The person will complain of acute pain and swelling to the area. With all such injuries, definitive diagnosis by x-ray is necessary to rule out a fracture.

When caring for the patient with a strain, it is important to avoid further trauma to the area as this can delay healing. Immediate and direct application of ice for the first 24 hours will help to decrease hematoma and edema formation. Following this, heat may be used. Weigh bearing is allowed as tolerated. When at rest, the extremity should be elevated to minimize edema. Acute pain will decrease as the swelling subsides. Tenderness will be present. This should be done until all swelling subsides. Splinting the area with tape or an elastic bandage is sometimes, although not always, employed. Healing will occur within 3 to 6 weeks. Activity and exercise must not be in excess. Should swelling at the injured site appear, the activity should be terminated.

### Sprain

When accidents similar to those which result in a strain cause a complete tear of a ligament, the problem is termed a *sprain.* The synovial membrane, as well as the capsule, can be torn and result in bleeding into the joint. Sprains can occur secondary to dislocations.

Symptoms of a sprain are similar in character but more acute than those of a strain. It is important to remember that an avulsion fracture can occur during a sprain. Therefore, an x-ray is important.

Use of ice and elevation are the same as with a strain. Weight bearing is allowed as tolerated. Casting is sometimes employed with a severe sprain. The use of crutches or a cane may be needed if weight bearing cannot be tolerated.

If healing of the sprain is not complete or if the joint is injured repeatedly, it will be unstable and the chances of injury increase. Healing will occur in 3 to 6 weeks. In order to allow for healing, the ends of the ligaments are approximated by holding the foot, if that is the member affected, in neutral position and applying an elastic bandage. It will be important to teach the patient how to reapply the bandage every 8 hours to prevent skin breakdown from pressure of the bandage. The patient can be shown the degree of tension that should be used when applying an elastic bandage and can be taught dressing so as to assess comfort and secure the bandage without tightness. Care should be taken to cover the affected joint totally in order to give adequate support to the limb. Instructions should be given regarding the presence of excess edema and impaired circulation. The patient should be taught to check for the presence of peripheral pulses, body warmth, and skin color. These changes may occur when the elastic bandage is applied improperly or too tightly. Removal of the bandage, elevation of the limb, and reapplication of the bandage may help relieve the distress. Mild analgesia may be needed to help reduce the swelling and pain.

Where possible, family members should be included in teaching about application of elastic bandages, as they can help with these areas that are difficult to self-wrap.

When the sprain has healed, exercise and activity can be performed in moderation. If sprain occurs in the ligaments of the cervical spine, such as a "whiplash injury," a clinical collar will be applied to the neck to immobilize the part and promote comfort.

Prevention of sprains includes avoidance of shoes with extremely high heels or clogs and taping of susceptible joints for support prior to participation in athletic endeavors. These precautions are particularly important for those who have already suffered one sprain of a particular area.

## Dislocation

A *dislocation* is a separation or displacement of the articular surfaces of a joint, often referred to as a *disarticulation.* It is usually caused by stress greater than that which would cause a strain or a sprain. There may be an underlying pathology which would enhance the likelihood of its occurrence, such as arthritis or a congenital weakness.

When a dislocation occurs, all ligaments at the joint are disrupted. The disruption will cause degeneration of the cartilage due to lack of synovial nourishment to the subchondral bone. If the dislocation is not corrected quickly, or if it occurs repeatedly, the patient will have a painful joint with limited motion. Thus, it is important to reduce the dislocation as soon as possible.

Assessment of the patient with a dislocation will reveal a painful joint with limited motion. There is usually shortening of the extremity and muscle spasms. X-rays will help affirm the diagnosis and guide the reduction. Emergency intervention is aimed at prevention of further trauma by splinting the joint and applying ice to minimize edema.

Manual traction is used to reduce the dislocation. This is done under anesthesia in order to minimize pain and muscle spasm. If closed reduction cannot be achieved because of excess soft tissue damage and edema or because of excessive muscle spasm, open reduction will be performed. After reduction, the joint is immobilized and supported to foster healing. Ice is then applied. Ongoing assessment should include checking for nerve damage and vascular compromise. Instructions should be given to the patient and family concerning these changes. Consideration should be given for the painful muscle spasms the patient is likely to be experiencing, and analgesia or antispasmodics can be prescribed.

Prevention of dislocations is much the same as that for sprains. It is worth noting that even with rapid reduction of the injury, some degree of traumatic arthritis is likely to occur.

A *subluxation* is an incomplete dislocation of a joint. The treatment is the same as that for a dislocation. The important point to remember is that adequate healing is important to prevent a weakened joint which can later be more easily displaced.

## INFLAMMATORY SKELETAL-MUSCULAR DISTURBANCES

Inflammatory changes in the skeletal muscular system can also alter coordination. Some of these more common disturbances will be discussed briefly. Much of the nursing care described under Skeletal-Muscular Trauma is applicable to patients with inflammatory skeletal-muscular disturbances.

## Osteomyelitis

*Osteomyelitis* is an infection of the bone and surrounding soft tissue. It can develop when patient susceptibility is increased by a debilitated condition, decreased resistance to a pathogen, or poor integrity of tissue as a result of inadequate circulation or multiple breaks in the skin. It can also be precipitated by the presence of highly resistant pathogens. It is a secondary infection; that is, it follows an infection elsewhere in the body, such as the skin, upper respiratory tract, or the genitourinary system, and results in bacteremia. This original infection may subside prior to the onset of osteomyelitis.

*Acute infectious osteomyelitis* usually occurs in children and affects the metaphysis of the long bones. It is an inflammatory process which results in edema, local hemorrhage, and abscess formation. Pressure from the inflammatory process forces its way into the bone marrow, causing vascular insufficiency which results in pain and destroyed bone.[23] The osteoblasts, in an attempt to reform bone, isolate *sequestra* (dead fragments), forming *involucra.* These involucra are relatively impervious to antibiotics, and thus the disease may remain in the chronic state for long periods of time.[24]

*Acute localized osteomyelitis* differs from acute infectious osteomyelitis in that it usually results from a direct invasion of pathogens following a compound fracture. The problem, however, follows a similar process.

*Subacute osteomyelitis* is a sequela of the acute process and is generally due to poor response from antibiotics. At this stage, subperiosteal abscesses occasionally rupture, causing soft-tissue abscesses. Furthermore, progressive bone damage may continue to occur.[25]

Another sequela of the acute process is *chronic osteomyelitis.* Here, the patient is without systemic symptoms but may have an involucrum or several involucra. There may be a draining sinus, cellulitis, or an abscess. Intermittent exacerbations may be precipitated by trauma or decreased patient resistance.[26]

Nursing assessment of the patient with acute osteomyelitis reveals a history of previous infection, usually *Staphylococcus aureus,*[27] or a recent compound fracture. The onset is often acute with complaints of severe pain, redness, and swelling at the affected site. In addition there is limited motion and tenderness. Systemic symptoms of the acute infection will include an elevated temperature, tachycardia, chills, and malaise. X-rays of the limb show areas of necrotic bone. A biopsy or culture may be done to confirm the diagnosis.

Nursing care focuses on fighting the inflammatory process locally and systemically. The patient is placed on *bed rest. Adequate fluids,* including blood products, will be administered to combat hypovolemia. *Antipyretics* will be used. A *high-protein diet* should be encouraged. *Antibiotic* coverage will be given for an extended period of time to counter the infection and decrease the likelihood of chronicity. The extremity should be elevated to promote venous return. Warm, moist packs will alleviate local erythema.

Deformity must be prevented. The tendency is to hold the limb in the position of comfort to limit stress on the bone. This is usually accomplished by maintaining nearby joints in flexion, thus promoting the formation of flexion contractures. *Good body alignment* and frequent change of positions need to be encouraged. Because the bone is weakened, there is danger of pathological fracture, and care should be taken in moving the extremity. It may be desirable to splint the area to protect it. As the period of bed rest increases, the nurse should be alert for the complications of bed rest.

When dealing with chronic osteomyelitis, the focus is on the local aspects of treatment. It must be remembered that the infected area is surrounded by avascular periosteum and scar tissue, thus requiring antibiotics to reach the area largely by diffusion, not circulation. *Surgical treatment* may be indicated and consists of incision and drainage of the area followed by long-term irrigation. Prior to surgery, the patient is given coverage with antibiotics to prevent systemic infection. Postoperatively, care will include responsibility for maintenance of strict aseptic technique and monitoring the irrigation.

Occasionally, *amputation* may be necessary for the treatment of osteomyelitis. It is indicated if the patient's life is at risk from the infection or if the infection is so extensive that antibiotics are not successful in treating it. *Amputation* is also the treatment of choice if a proposed bone resection would be so extensive that it would be disabling and the patient would have better function with a prosthesis. (For further discussion of the care of the amputee, see Chap. 29.)

*Psychological support* of the patient with osteomyelitis must never be overlooked. Nurses must remember that it is a frightening, extremely painful process for the patient. Frequently, the person is combatting a problem that could end in amputation. Treatment is sure to be long-term, and the patient is likely to become discouraged and depressed. The nurse's support and concern will help the patient through this difficult time.

After treatment of osteomyelitis, the patient may be in a state of *residual osteomyelitis.* The bone is dense and perhaps larger than normal, with a poor vascular supply. There may be adhesions of the skin to bone. Soft tissue areas may be scarred and susceptible to necrosis from even slight injury. Treatment is directed at the prevention and correction of deformities.[28]

## Acute Infectious Arthritis

*Acute infectious arthritis* is a monarticular form of arthritis caused by various organisms and transmitted via the bloodstream. These organisms cause inflammation of the synovial membrane that surrounds the tissue, with the presence of a purulent effusion noted. This leads to necrosis of the area followed by a spread to the cartilage, resulting in a painful joint and possible ankylosis.

When assessing the patient with this problem, one would find a painful, warm, edematous joint. There also may be symptoms of a systemic infection.

Conservative intervention is usually indicated. *Joint aspiration* may be performed to decrease the pressure within the joint capsule, to remove and culture purulent matter, or to locally instill antibiotics.

The joint should be *immobilized* to prevent damage to it. Traction may be employed to separate the joint surfaces and thus lessen the pressure on the cartilage.[29] This will also relieve *muscle spasms* caused by the periosteal irritation. *Pain relief* can be provided with medication and the local application of heat. Supportive measures should be taken against the systemic infection. As the process progresses to the subacute stage, gradual increase of mobility and passive range of motion exercises can be instituted. If the joint is likely to ankylose, it should be allowed to do so in the position that will be most functional later.

Surgical intervention may be indicated for persistent infectious arthritis. Immediate steps would include incision and drainage of the affected area. Later, joint repair may need to be undertaken.

## Bursitis

Bursae are sacs lined with synovial membranes. Their function is to protect bony prominences from friction caused by skin, tendon, or muscle which rubs over the area. They may or may not communicate with the joint.

*Bursitis* is an inflammation of the bursa caused by acute or chronic trauma, acute or chronic pyogenic infections, or other inflammatory processes like gout, syphilis, tuberculosis, or rheumatoid arthritis. It can occur any place where bursae normally occur. Common sites are in the shoulder, *subdeltoid bursitis,* the patella, *prepatellar bursitis* ("housemaids' knee"), or elbow *epitrochlear bursitis* ("tennis elbow"). There may also be *adventitious bursae,* or those that lack a true synovial lining,[30] which develop an area of swelling due to repeated trauma. *Bunions* are a prime example of these.

Nursing assessment would reveal pain, swelling, and marked tenderness in the area. These disruptions often cause the patient *limited motion at the joint.*

Intervention should be aimed at resolving the primary cause and at treating the symptoms. Local trauma should be avoided, particularly postural or occupational irritants. *Rest, moist heat, elevation,* and *splinting* should be provided to the joint. Inflammatory responses should be treated accordingly. *Aspiration* of fluid from the joint, often with the instillation of an anti-inflammatory agent such as hydrocortisone, will usually produce relief. Surgical intervention may include incision and drainage of the area, excision of the bursa, or excision of the underlying bony prominence.[31]

## DEGENERATIVE SKELETAL-MUSCULAR DISTURBANCES

Skeletal-muscular disturbances can be related to seemingly mechanical changes known as *degenerative processes of the bone.* Again, much of the nursing care discussed in Skeletal-Muscular trauma applies to degenerative conditions. Therefore, some of the more common degenerative problems associated with bone structures will be highlighted.

### Osteoarthritis

Osteoarthritis is a deteriorating process of joint capsules and underlying bone. It can be caused by aging, chronic stress, trauma, infection, or a congenital anomaly. Primarily the lower extremities are involved because of their weight-bearing load.

Two processes are classified as osteoarthritis. The first is *polyarticular degenerative arthritis,* which is of unknown etiology. This form rarely occurs before the age of 35. Because of its polyarticular nature and uncertain course, treatment is difficult.[32] *Monarticular arthritis* is the true degenerative process, confined to the joint where stress is involved. Traumatic arthritis can be classified as this type.

*Traumatic arthritis* is a degenerative form of joint inflammation caused by fractures, dislocations, or other trauma. The clinical symptoms may manifest themselves months or years after the precipitating injury and occur as a result of decreased blood to an area.

Nursing assessment should include a review of the health history to ascertain any underlying causes of the problem. Clinical symptoms would include pain on motion and weight bearing. Pain is often absent at rest. Joint stiffness, grating of the joint with motion, fluid accumulation at the joint, and the need for moderate limitation of motion are common. The presence of *Heberden's nodes* in the distal finger joints may also be noted. These are usually found in women and are of unknown cause.[33]

Intervention includes provision of rest to the joint, pain relief with aspirin and other anti-inflammatory agents such as steroids, and measures to promote comfort such as application of heat and range of motion exercises. Activities of daily living which have caused stress on any joint involved may need to be altered or eliminated. Improvement of posture may be considered in this realm. Occupational therapy can assist the patient with activities and as a result help improve joint motion, although any joint in the body may be affected by treatment. This is successful because the process is self-limiting, generally confined to a single joint.

The care which may be most meaningful to the patient is the emotional support given by the nurse. There is likely to be a feeling of grief over the loss or limitation of function. Adjustment to new ways of doing things may not always fit into the life-style the patient perceives to be essential. Allowing time for the patient to verbalize and work through these feelings and reassuring the patient that the problem does not travel to other joints, as does rheumatoid arthritis, may be helpful.

Surgical intervention most commonly employed is *arthroplasty* (the making of an artificial joint). It is used ". . . to restore motion to a joint and function to the muscles, ligaments and soft tissue structures that control it."[34] This is achieved through use of prosthetic devices, e.g., a cup for the acetabular head. An arthroplasty is indicated to relieve stiffness of ankylosed joints but is more likely to be successful if the joint is ankylosed in a favorable position. It can also be beneficial after trauma because it will relieve the pain in an irregular joint and increase motion blocked by communication of articular surfaces. (Refer to Chap. 10 for a more complete discussion.)

Postoperatively, the joint is immobilized for 10 to 14 days to allow soft-tissue healing. Then, exercises are begun, starting with passive range of motion and gradually increasing to active exercise. Physical therapy is utilized. The therapist can assess the patient prior to surgery to gather baseline data of the patient's ability. As the exercise regime progresses, the patient should be observed for excess pain, tenderness, and swelling. Activity should not be forced to this point, and, if it occurs, provision should be made for rest.

**Total joint replacement**  In the past few years, the concept of total joint replacement has become quite commonplace. The goal of this therapy is the relief of pain. It is also used to restore function and stability of a joint and can be performed on the hip, knee, elbow, and ankle.

Indications for total joint replacement include treatment of osteoarthritis, repair of a traumatized joint in which there is not another feasible alternative, treatment of rheumatoid arthritis, and revision of a previously inserted, painful arthroplasty. Total joint surgery is always done on an elective basis, at a time when the patient is in optimal health. (Refer to Chap. 10 for additional information.)

**Total hip replacement**  *Preparation* of the person for total hip surgery includes routine diagnostic tests to ascertain that the patient is in good general health. Likely candidates for total hip replacement may be elderly with problems of poor nutritional status and anemia. These conditions should be corrected prior to surgery, if possible. Surgical scrubs and prophylactic antibiotics may be used to reduce the likelihood of introducing infection into the surgical area. *Preoperative* teaching should include information about the surgical procedure with specific directions about breathing, range of motion exercises, and the use of the trapeze to increase mobility while on bed rest.

The patient should also be well aware that the surgery is not without risks. Since the risk of bone infection is so great, a "green room," or *laminar airflow room,* is often used during surgery. This is a room in which airflow is controlled in such a way that "dirty air" flows away from the operative area

and clean air is filtered into the sterile field to decrease airborne pathogens.

Candidates for this type of surgery must face long-term disability. The problems this presents to daily accomplishment of routines and establishment of expectations must be considered. The nurse must be prepared to give support when the added stress of surgery and hospitalization is at hand. It is important to help the person set realistic and not grandiose expectations for the postoperative period.

The *surgical procedure* involves replacing the normal ball-and-socket joint of the hip with manmade materials. Briefly, the head of the femur is removed and a metal head, usually of *Vitallium,* a cobalt alloy with high resistance to corrosion, is inserted. The existing acetabulum is reamed out and replaced with a plastic cup. By using two different substances, the greater friction of metal on metal is avoided. These prostheses are cemented into place with *methyl methacrolate,* a quick-setting cement which is relatively free of undesirable side effects. (Refer to Chap. 10.)

In the immediate *postoperative period,* the leg is immobilized in Buck's traction in abduction and slight external rotation to allow for some soft-tissue healing to take place. Care should be taken not to dislocate the joint by placing the leg in internal rotation or adduction. A pillow is kept between the knees and lower thighs for this purpose. A pillow placed under the calf will keep the heel off the bed to prevent ulceration and will put less strain on the operative site. Care must be taken to avoid flexion contractures of the hip by removing the pillow periodically for short intervals.

*Dressing checks* for wound drainage should include checking under the thigh, since gravity causes any excess drainage to collect there. A closed, vacuum drainage system, with or without suction, may be used to prevent formation of a hematoma. Routine circulation checks will also determine the presence of excess hemorrhage or edema into the tissue.

Antibiotic coverage may be given, particularly for the person who has had previous hip surgery or who has suffered an open wound to the area or infectious arthritis.

Encouraging the patient to use the trapeze on the bed will aid in sitting and moving in bed. To allow for elevation of the buttocks off the bed, the patient should be encouraged to use both arms to pull up on the trapeze while pushing up to raise the buttocks with the unaffected foot. This technique can be used for getting on and off the bedpan and during bed making. Top-to-bottom bed making seems to be the most reasonable way to accomplish this task. Use of the fracture bedpan will help prevent stress on the hip and the need for much lifting.

Turning should be allowed only in the presence of a nurse who can maintain external rotation and abduction of the leg. Support for the leg can be provided with pillows.

Within approximately 7 to 14 days traction can be discontinued and the patient will progress to dangling, chair sitting, and then ambulation with a walker. As a patient sits in a chair, the nurse should discourage use of chairs that are so low as to cause excess flexion of the hip and possible dislocation.

If the patient is not able to tolerate the prosthesis, it will be removed, leaving the patient with an unstable, nonarticulating joint. This is because the head of the femur is removed in surgery. Infection and intolerance of cement are two such complications.

Durability of the prosthesis is also a concern. The friction caused by the rubbing of two synthetic surfaces against each other will cause them to wear. The rate of wear varies with the individual and the demands put on the prosthesis. As a rule of thumb, a prosthesis is expected to last about 15 years. Thus, if a total hip replacement is inserted in a young person (age 20 to 40 years), there may be need for revision at a later date. Furthermore, stresses on the prosthesis may cause the cement to crack, causing the joint to be unstable and requiring revision.

## NEOPLASMS OF THE BONE

Both benign and malignant neoplasms can affect the skeletal-muscular system. These usually involve the bone and include multiple myeloma, osteogenic, sarcoma, and giant cell tumor. (A complete discussion of the neoplastic process can be found in Chap. 5.) Much of the nursing care discussed under Skeletal-Muscular trauma will be applicable throughout this discussion.

### Multiple Myeloma

Multiple myeloma is a malignant process associated with protein synthesis and is typified by diffuse, pocked areas of bone, particularly along the midline of the body (ribs, pelvis, skull, and vertebrae).

It is the most frequent tumor arising in bone. It affects men two to three times more often than women, usually during or after the fifth decade.[35] This is significant to the patient because it is often a time of maximal occupational achievement. There may be a family to support. The individual may also be undergoing other stress at this time of life, e.g., the family moving away from home, which make the demands placed by the pathological changes seem even greater.

Nursing intervention can play an important role in prolonging the life expectancy of a patient with multiple myeloma. Because symptoms may be insidious, there is often extensive progress of the pathology prior to diagnosis. Therefore it is important to initiate treatment as soon as possible after the disease is defined. If not treated, 52 percent of the patients may die within 3 months of the diagnosis, and 90 percent will expire within 2 years, with the median fatality rate being 17 months.[36] Life span for the treated patient is from 26 months to greater than 5 years.[37] Death is usually a result of complications and not the primary malignant process.

When the patient is first seen in the community, symptoms may be quite nonspecific. They may include a history of *weight loss* and progressive *weakness.* There may be a general debility, immobility, and *severe anemia. Neurological symptoms* may occur from pressure of an extradural tumor.[38] The patient may complain of *low back pain,* and there may be evidence of a *pathological fracture* of the ribs or vertebrae.

A variety of tests may be used to diagnose multiple myeloma. X-ray evaluation will give evidence of the punched-out bone areas. A *Bence-Jones protein* level may be determined from the urine. The Bence-Jones protein is found only in patients with multiple myeloma. Serum and protein electrophoresis may also be used to detect this. A biopsy and bone marrow aspiration may also be helpful in defining the disease.

Nursing *interventions* for this problem are manifold. Throughout the treatments, it is important to explain all procedures to the patient. This must be done with an empathetic ear to permit the patient to *ventilate fears* and *frustrations* of coping with the disease process. The person may have to adjust a work *regime* to accommodate periodic visits to the hospital for treatment, which will be required for the rest of the patients life. Pain will enhance the patient's frustrations and may lead to unwillingness to cooperate with *exercise* regimes. As much as possible, the patient should participate in the plan of care. This will help the patient retain a feeling of control in the situation.

*Radiotherapy* may be recommended to relieve local pain and attack an isolated lesion. (Refer to Chap. 5 for a complete discussion of the care of the patient receiving radiotherapy.)

*Chemotherapy* is the most important long-term treatment in the care of the myeloma patient. A variety of drug combinations may be used. The nurse should understand the effects and side effects of the chemotherapeutic drugs in use and explain these to the patient. The nurse must then support the patient in dealing with these side effects and be alert for symptoms of toxicity. (Refer to Chap. 5 for a complete discussion of chemotherapy.) Significant in chemotherapy is the use of *steroids,* especially prednisone, in combination with other drugs. The nurse should be alert for the usual problems of steroid therapy (see Chap. 10), especially its ability to decrease resistance to infection and to mask infection. In light of the patient's already debilitated condition, infection can prove to be fatal and must be quickly recognized and treated.

Other interventions are aimed at specific problems caused as the neoplastic process progresses. *Surgical decompression of the cord* may be necessary if neurological symptoms appear owing to a lesion of a vertebra. *Transfusions* may be used to combat anemia. Analgesia should be provided for relief of pain. Care should be taken to avoid pathological fractures, incorporating splinting and braces for support.

*Careful ambulation* is desirable to prevent further physical and psychological debilitation caused by bed rest. *Mobilization* will specifically reduce the likelihood of pneumonia which could be particularly life-threatening. It will also decrease the rapid loss of calcium from bone which will cause it to be even weaker. The patient may be reluctant to ambulate because of the feeling of weakness and fear of pain. Patience and a caring attitude, together with a concrete plan of action including analgesia, braces, and provision of rest periods, will help alleviate the patient's concerns. Furthermore, activity is an excellent morale booster because the person spends less time exhibiting "sick" behavior. However, the nurse should watch for unwarranted euphoria when there is remission of symptoms. This may lead to cessation of treatment by the patient who thinks that cure has been achieved. Family involvement is crucial, since much of the early interventions do not require hospitalization.

## Osteogenic Sarcoma

Osteogenic sarcoma is a primary malignant tumor which usually involves the metaphysis of long bone, particularly the femur but also the proximal tibia, proximal humerus, and the ilium. It occurs more often in males and usually in the second decade.[39] Current statistics place the 5-year survival rate at 15 to 20 percent after "prompt surgical removal of the tumor";[40] thus prognosis is poor.

Initially the patient is likely to seek help for relief of intermittent *pain* and *tenderness* of the involved area. These symptoms usually occur at night. Other complaints may include *tiredness,* a *limp,* and the presence of *swelling without previous trauma* or *infection.* The presence of a pathological fracture is rare.[41] These may be metastasis, most often to the lungs but also to the lymph nodes and other bony sites. There may also be multifocal primary sites.[42] Diagnosis is made from biopsy, the presence of an elevated alkaline phosphatase, and evidence of lung metastasis on a chest x-ray.

Physical treatment includes *amputation* or *disarticulation* of an extremity or extensive radical local excision of other areas. *Palliative radiotherapy* may also be employed.

*Emotional intervention* is necessary to help the patient deal with this health problem. The individual involved is usually a teen-ager or young adult who may have an immature coping process. This person will have to deal with *disfigurement* at a time when the normal person is trying to develop body image and role identification. The prospect of a radically *shortened life-span* must be dealt with at a time when most are planning future life goals. The nurse will have to help this patient work through ways of coping with these psychosocial problems. Counseling will also involve the family who will most likely be experiencing grief of their own at a potential loss of a loved one. Since their grieving may occur at a time when the patient most needs their support, the nurse may have to be supportive and provide counseling to both groups. Peers are important to the patient at this time of life. However, these individuals may easily identify with the patient and may need help dealing with their own feelings of altered body image and mortality.

## Giant-Cell Tumor

A *giant-cell tumor* is a nonmalignant neoplasm thought to be caused by misplacement of growing cells or a pathological disturbance.[43] It occurs slightly more frequently in women who are 20 to 40 years old.[44] Approximately 10 percent of these non-malignant tumors are thought to undergo malignant changes, and so prompt treatment is always indicated.[45] The tumor generally arises in the epiphysis, although it is seen in both the epiphysis and metaphysis. It occurs after the closure of the epiphyseal plate and most often involves the distal femur, proximal tibia, and distal radius.

The patient will usually present a history of *pain,* occasionally with *limitation of joint motion* and *localized weakness.* One might see *muscle atrophy* and *effusion at the joint.* A tender mass may be palpated.

One of the first steps of intervention is to *reassure* the patient that this is a nonmalignant process. However, the potential risks for development of a malignancy should not be dismissed. Surgical intervention is usually indicated. Prior to surgery, hyperparathyroidism will be ruled out, since this will present similar clinical symptoms.[46] The treatment of choice is *total excision of the tumor* and surrounding bone as necessary, with bone grafting as indicated. Surgical intervention does not necessarily mean cure, however, because the rate of reoccurrence is about 50 percent.[47]

### Metastases to the Bone

The most common tumor found in bone usually metastasizes from a primary site in the breast, prostate, intestine, or lung. The neoplastic growth is usually found in those bones which are rich in red marrow, like the spine, pelvis, and ribs. It occurs at any age, although frequency increases with age, as does the frequency of malignancies in general.

Indications of metastasis may include *pain* and *swelling* over the affected area, with a *history of malignancy elsehwere* in the body. A *pathological fracture* may be the first indication of the metastatic process.

Nursing intervention should be aimed, first, at the primary malignancy. Secondly, *chemotherapy* may be used to treat the diffuse malignancy. *Palliative radiotherapy* may be indicated. In the case of a pathological fracture, repair is done after excision of the neoplasm in that area. Certainly, provision should be made for pain relief.

Throughout all, the patient will need *support* to face this new crisis—the development of metastasis. Discouragement may be overwhelming. Encouragement to maintain the treatment regime may be needed.

## METABOLIC SKELETAL-MUSCULAR DISTURBANCE

Bone metabolism requires that there be sufficient uptake, absorption, and proper use of calcium, phosphorus, and vitamin D. Disruption at any point in this process can result in a disturbance of the skeletal-muscular system.

True vitamin deficiencies are rarely seen in the United States, but they do exist. When they occur, they are often due to sociocultural influences which preclude use of foods that contain the necessary nutrients. Another cause is inadequate health teaching which needs correcting. *Rickets,* a disease of children, is the most common vitamin D deficiency.

### Osteomalacia

*Osteomalacia* is the adult form of vitamin D deficiency. It can be caused by insufficient dietary intake of insufficient exposure to sunlight necessary for vitamin D metabolism. These causes are rare today because of health teaching, but should not be overlooked in an era of "junk foods" and air conditioning. Poor absorption of vitamin D in the intestine or inability of the kidney to produce vitamin D in the presence of renal tubular damage constitute other causes of this problem. The result is insufficient calcification of bone, leading to softening of the bone and the formation of deformities.

Prior to treatment, the cause must be determined in order to take steps to alleviate the problem. These steps may include health teaching or appropriate measures to treat the medical problem. Finally, surgical procedures may be necessary to correct bony deformities.

### Gout

*Gout* or *gouty arthritis* is caused by the abnormal metabolism of uric acid causing an elevated blood level and crystallate deposits in the joints, known as *tophi.* It also results in an inflammatory process with effusion into the synovial membrane. Ninety-five percent of the cases of gout occur in men between the ages of 20 and 60.[48] There is also a hereditary predisposition for gout.

The onset is usually abrupt, with the acute attack lasting about 3 to 10 days, characterized by severe, constant pain. The affected joint, most often the great toe, becomes erythematous. Other joints may also be affected, and tophi may be observed in them. The course of this problem varies from a few attacks occurring throughout the lifetime to the existence of a progressive disease which, if left untreated, becomes crippling.

The goals of intervention are to cure the existing attack, prevent future attacks, and provide rest and support for the joint during the acute phase. In the home and the community, teaching to those who have complained of attacks of gout should include encouragement to seek medical advice even though the initial attack has subsided. In this way, further attacks and greater joint damage can be avoided.

Use of specific medications has been helpful in achieving these goals. *Colchicine* is a drug which relieves the pain of gout. Its mode of action is uncertain, and it does not eliminate the tophi. *Probenecid* has been used to prevent further attacks of gout because it increases the excretion of uric acid from the kidney. However, it does not help to alleviate acute attacks. *Allopurinol* is also useful because it reduces the production of uric acid by the body. The latter two drugs must be taken daily for a beneficial effect. Thus, one must stress the importance of continuing to take daily doses even in the absence of symptoms.

Many have heard the old wives' tale that much indulgence in rich food and alcohol will precipitate an attack of gout. In fact, the patient should be instructed to avoid foods with a high purine content, like liver, kidneys, sweetbreads, anchovies, and meat gravies.

*Surgical care* of the patient with gout may be indicated to improve function of a painful, deranged joint. It can also be done to excise tophi in order to prevent ulceration, to improve appearance, and to make the wearing of shoes and gloves possible. Incision and drainage may be indicated to treat a secondary infection of the tophi. Surgery is always done after the acute phase has subsided.

### Osteoporosis

*Osteoporosis* is a general term used for any condition in which the rate of bone resorption is greater than the rate of bone formation. Bone mass is lost due to decreased absorption of protein and minerals. There can be increased resorption with normal formation or normal resorption with a decreased rate of formation. Osteoporosis is the most common reabsorption bone disorder.[49]

Its causes are many. Disuse will lead to an increased rate of bone resorption, as in the patient on bed rest who has no weight bearing and a lack of stress on the bone. Studies have shown that lack of gravity, such as that the astronauts experience, will also cause osteoporosis.[50] Postmenopausal women can develop osteoporosis, which is thought to be due to a change in hormone levels. A diet deficient in vitamins or calcium may also result in osteoporotic changes. This problem is often seen in the elderly where physiological bone changes alter bone density.

Nursing assessment reveals complaints of back pain in the weight-bearing bones. Because bones are brittle, fractures are not uncommon (see Table 40-1). "As many as 70% of patients having hip fracture are diagnosed as having osteoporosis."[51] Diagnosis is made by x-ray which shows thin, porous, but otherwise normal bone (*radiolucent* bone).

Intervention will depend on the cause of the problem. In postmenopausal women, *estrogens* and *androgens* are useful to decrease or arrest the rate of bone resorption. *Exercise* is also useful to decrease resorption of bone. *Support* to the back with a firm mattress, a corset, and good body mechanics will prevent injury and alleviate back pain. For specific *relief of pain,* analgesics and *muscle relaxants* may be used. Adequate *intake of protein,* vitamin D, and calcium will ensure the presence of the raw materials necessary for bone formation.

### Paget's Disease

*Paget's disease,* also known as *osteitis deformans,* is a condition in which there is inappropriate bone resorption, fibrotic changes in the bone, and remodeling with structurally uneven, highly vascular bone. It usually occurs after the fourth decade. The cause is unknown, but there is thought to be a genetic predisposition, with the ultimate problem being one of calcitonin deficiency.[52] *Calcitonin* is a hormone secreted by cells in the thyroid, thymus, and parathyroid. An elevated serum calcium will cause release of the hormone, thus reducing the rate of bone resorption. Its effect is counterbalanced by parathyroid hormone.

Commercially prepared injections of calcitonin offer clinical relief of the symptoms of Paget's disease, including a lower serum alkaline phosphatase, less bone pain, and more normal bone formation. Definitive management with calcitonin has not been established for patients yet, but if it is decided that the person with Paget's disease is to receive daily doses of the drug, the technique for administering an injection will have to be taught.

Measures should be taken to avoid trauma to the delicate bone, including bracing and good body mechanics to prevent stress. Because of the high vascularity of the bone, these patients are poor surgical risks, and long periods of immobilization may be required for bone healing after trauma. The nurse should be supportive and allow the person to vent feelings of frustration. Offering diversionary activities may help to pass the time more quickly.

## AUTOIMMUNE DISTURBANCES AND SKELETAL-MUSCULAR DISRUPTIONS

An extensive discussion of autoimmune responses can be found in Chap. 10. However, several problems will be highlighted here, to indicate their unique effect on coordination. These include juvenile rheumatoid arthritis and ankylosing spondylitis. Much of the nursing care discussed under Skeletal-Muscular Trauma will be appropriate to the care of the patients mentioned in this section.

### Rheumatoid Arthritis

Rheumatoid arthritis is a systemic, inflammatory process which has specific implication to the skeletal-muscular system. Although its cause is not definitely known, it is thought to be an autoimmune response based on the presence of an antigen-antibody complex in the synovial fluid.[53] (See Chap. 10 for a complete discussion of rheumatoid arthritis.)

### Juvenile Rheumatoid Arthritis

*Juvenile rheumatoid arthritis* (Still's disease) occurs before the age of 16. Peak occurrence times are from the ages of 2 to 5 and 9 to 12 years.[54] Assessment of early problems will reveal an *elevated temperature,* an *enlarged liver* and *spleen,* a *rash, pleuritis,* and *pericarditis.* There may be involvement of one to many joints causing *limited movement.* There is generally some cervical involvement, particularly at C2 and C3. If the disease is untreated, the results will be abnormal growth and development.

Treatment consists of the use of *aspirin* and *steroids* to combat the inflammatory process. Inflamed joints are splinted to prevent further trauma to them. The problem often subsides spontaneously. In 70 percent of the cases, there is no joint disturbance later,[55] although some adults will experience acute exacerbation of the disease.

### Ankylosing Spondylitis

*Ankylosing spondylitis* (Marie-Strümpell's disease) involves the sacroiliac joints, the spine, and the pelvis. It is characterized by chronic synovitis which causes ankylosis of the joints. Ninety percent of its sufferers are men, usually between the ages of 16 and 30.[56] There is questionably a hereditary predisposition.

The patient will complain of progressive early morning *stiffness of the low back* and persistent *low back pain* without the presence of neurological symptoms. There may be mild fatigue and weight loss. Palpation over the area will reveal tenderness and straightening of the normal lumbar lordosis. Forward bending may cause spasm of the paravertebral muscles. In the late stages of the disease, there is costovertebral ankylosis.

Intervention cannot stop the progression of the disease but will alleviate its symptoms and help the patient to maintain functional ability. *Relief of pain* can be achieved with aspirin, indomethacin, and phenylbutazone.[57] *Rest* will combat the feeling of fatigue and prevent trauma to the affected area. A *firm mattress* should be used, and the patient should be encouraged to sleep on the back or in the prone position to prevent flexion deformities that result from lying on the side. If there is cervical involvement, a pillow should not be used. Those *activities* which produce pain should be avoided.

*Physical therapy* plays an important role in maintaining good positioning of the vertebrae, strengthening of the paraspinous muscles, and maintaining or increasing breathing capacity in light of the progressive ankylosis of the costovertebral joints. Heat, range of motion, muscle strengthening, and breathing exercises are prescribed. A back brace may be necessary to slow advancing postural deformity which cannot be decreased by exercise. It will also help alleviate otherwise unrelieved muscle spasm.[58]

*Arthroplasties* may be indicated, particularly for hip involvement. Attention must be given to postoperative exercise to maintain range of motion.

## REFERENCES

1   Joan Luckman and Karen Sorenson, *Medical-Surgical Nursing: A Psychophysiologic Approach,* Saunders, Philadelphia, 1974, p. 1206.
2   *Ibid.,* pp. 1206–1207.
3   Carroll B. Larson and Marjorie Gould, *Orthopedic Nursing,* 8th ed., Mosby, St. Louis, 1974, p. 218.
4   Pat Weinhamer and Diana Blazevich, "Guidelines for Cast Care," *ONA J,* **2:**138, June 1975.
5   Jane Farrell, "Preparing a Patient for a Cast Life," *ONA J,* **1:**71, October 1974.
6   A. H. Crenshaw, (ed.), *Campbell's Operative Orthopedics,* 5th ed., Mosby, St. Louis, 1971, p. 479.
7   *Ibid.,* p. 479.

8 F. James Funk, Jr., Lecture, Second Annual Congress of Orthopedic Nurses' Association, May 12, 1975.
9 Crenshaw, *op. cit.*, p. 478.
10 Gerald L. Glancy, "Compartment Syndromes," *ONA J*, **2:**149, June 1975.
11 Arlene Andahl, "Compartment Sundrome," *ONA Newsletter*, **3:**4, February 1974.
12 Crenshaw, *op. cit.*, p. 494.
13 *Ibid.*, p. 494.
14 *Ibid.*
15 Linda Spickler, "Fat Embolism," *ONA J*, **2:**146, June 1975.
16 Dorothy J. Del Bueno, "Recognizing Fat Embolism in Patients," *RN*, **36:**48, January 1973.
17 Spickler, *op. cit.*, p. 146.
18 Del Bueno, *op. cit.*, p. 51.
19 Spickler, *op. cit.*, p. 146.
20 *Ibid.*, p. 146.
21 *Ibid.*
22 Larson and Gould, *op. cit.*, p. 214.
23 Crenshaw, *op. cit.*, p. 1298.
24 Anne M. Wiebe, *Orthopedics in Nursing*, Saunders, Philadelphia, 1961, p. 177.
25 Crenshaw, *op. cit.*, p. 1309.
26 *Ibid.*, pp. 1309–1310.
27 Crenshaw, *op. cit.*, p. 1316.
28 Wiebe, *op. cit.*, p. 177.
29 *Ibid.*, p. 963.
30 *Ibid.*, p. 1507.
31 *Ibid.*
32 *Ibid.*, p. 1004.
33 *Primer on the Rheumatic Diseases*, The Arthritis Foundation, New York, 1973, p. 81.
34 Crenshaw, *op. cit.*, p. 1235.
35 *Ibid.*, p. 1397.
36 Linda Rickel, "Emotional Support for the Multiple Myeloma Patient," *Nursing 76*, **6:**78, April 1976.
37 *Ibid.*, p. 76.
38 Crenshaw, *op. cit.*, p. 1398.
39 *Ibid.*, p. 1379.
40 *Ibid.*, p. 1380.
41 *Ibid.*, p. 1379.
42 *Ibid.*
43 Larson and Gould, *op. cit.*, p. 298.
44 Wiebe, *op. cit.*, p. 167.
45 Crenshaw, *op. cit.*, p. 1357.
46 *Ibid.*, p. 1352.
47 *Ibid.*, p. 1357.
48 Larson and Gould, *op. cit.*, p. 294.
49 Joseph R. DiPalma, "Recent Developments in Bone-Disease Treatment," *RN*, **36:**63, January 1973.
50 Larson and Gould, *op. cit.*, p. 334.
51 *Ibid.*, p. 333.
52 DiPalma, *op. cit.*, p. 68.
53 Pamela Webb Driscoll, "Rheumatoid Arthritis: Understanding It More Fully," *Nursing 75*, **5:**27, December 1975.
54 *Primer on the Rheumatic Diseases*, *op. cit.*, p. 36.
55 *Ibid.*, p. 37.
56 *Ibid.*, p. 67.
57 *Ibid.*, p. 69.
58 *Ibid.*

## BIBLIOGRAPHY

Aultmeier, W. A.: "The Significance of Infection in Trauma, *AORN J*, **15:**92, March 1972.
Bame, K.: "Halo Traction," *Am J Nurs*, **69:**1933, September 1969.
Bray, A. P., and J. R. Thomas: "Severe Fat Embolism Syndrome Following Multiple Fractures," *Nurs Times*, **65:**109, Jan. 23, 1969.
Bruner, L. S., et al.: *Textbook of Medical-Surgical Nursing*, 2d ed., Lippincott, Philadelphia, 1975.
Evarts, C. M. (ed.): "Symposium on Interposition and Implant Arthroplasty," *Orthop Clin North Am*, **4:**233, April 1973.
"Hygiene and the Full Body Cast," *Am J Ortho*, **9:**141, July 1967.
Larson, C. B., and M. Gould: *Orthopedic Nursing*, 7th ed., Mosby, St. Louis, 1970.
May, C. M.: "Wheelchair Patient for a Day," *Am J Nurs*, **73:**650, April 1973.
Powell, M.: *Orthopaedic Nursing*, 6th ed., E. and S. Livingstone, London, 1968.
Ranalls, J.: "Crutches and Walkers," *Nursing 72*, **2:**21, December 1972.
Salter, R. B.: *Textbook of Disorders and Injuries of the Muscularskeletal System*, Williams & Wilkins, Baltimore, 1970.
Shands, A. R., and R. B. Raney: *Handbook of Orthopaedic Surgery*, 7th ed., Mosby, St. Louis, 1967.
Shaefer, K. N., et al.: *Medical Surgical Nursing*, 5th ed., Mosby, St. Louis, 1975.
Wagner, M. M.: "Assessment of Patients with Multiple Injuries," *Am J Nurs*, **72:**1882, October 1972.

# INDEX

# INDEX

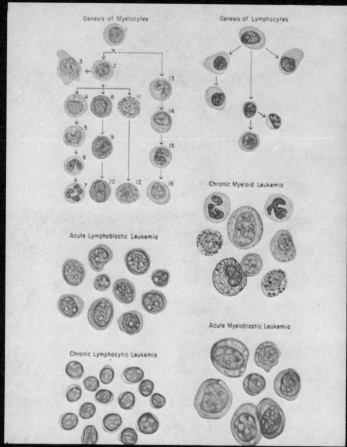

**7-1**

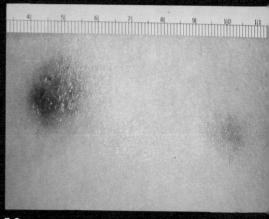

**7-2**

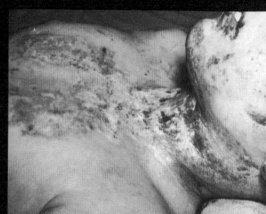

**13-1**

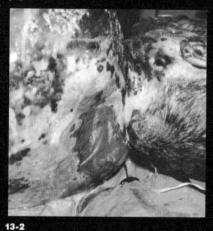

**13-2**

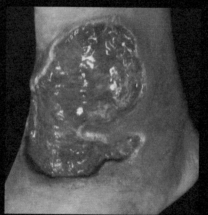

**18-1**

**18-2**

**7-1**  Genesis of white blood cells and the blood picture in different types of leukemia. The different cells of the myelogenous series are (1) *myeloblast*, (2) *promyelocyte*, (3) *megakaryocyte*, (4) *neutrophil myelocyte*, (5) *young neutrophil metamyelocyte*, (6) *"band" neutrophil metamyelocyte*, (7) *polymorphonuclear neutrophil*, (8) *eosinophil myelocyte*, (9) *eosinophil metamyelocyte*, (10) *polymorphonuclear eosinophil*, (11) *basophil myelocyte*, (12) *polymorphonuclear basophil*, (13–16) *stages of monocyte formation*. (Redrawn in part from Piney: A Clinical Atlas of Blood Diseases, McGraw-Hill, New York, 1977.)

**7-2**  Ecthyma gangrenosum, the characteristic skin lesion of *Pseudomonas* septicemia.

**13-1**  Partial-thickness burn injury.

**13-2**  Full-thickness burn injury.

**18-1**  Pyoderma gangrenosum in a patient with ulcerative colitis.*

**18-2**  Ileostomy stoma and abdominal incision. (Courtesy of Cheryl Van Horn.)